Textbook of Medical Physiology

To
the teachers and residents in physiology for their endeavour to dissipate and acquire knowledge.
My parents and teachers for their blessings
my children, Aruj, Bhawna and Arushi,
for their patience and tolerance shown
to loss of many precious moments and
finally to my husband, Dr AK Khurana,
for his understanding, encouragement
and invaluable guidance

Textbook of Medical Physiology

Second Edition

Indu Khurana MD
Senior Professor
Department of Physiology
Postgraduate Institute of Medical Sciences
Rohtak, India

Arushi Khurana MD
Chief Medical Resident
University of Connecticut
School of Medicine
Hartford, Connecticut, USA

ELSEVIER

ELSEVIER

Reed Elsevier India Pvt. Ltd.
Registered Office: 818, 8th Floor, Indraprakash Building, 21, Barakhamba Road, New Delhi 110001
Corporate Office: 14th Floor, Building No. 10B, DLF Cyber City, Phase II, Gurgaon-122002, Haryana, India

Textbook of Medical Physiology, 2e, Khurana

ISBN: 978-81-312-4253-7
e-Book ISBN: 978-81-312-4254-4

Notice

Knowledge and best practice in this field are constantly changing. As new research and experience broaden our understanding, changes in research methods, professional practices, or medical treatment may become necessary.

Practitioners and researchers must always rely on their own experience and knowledge in evaluating and using any information, methods, compounds, or experiments described herein. In using such information or methods they should be mindful of their own safety and the safety of others, including parties for whom they have a professional responsibility.

With respect to any drug or pharmaceutical products identified, readers are advised to check the most current information provided (i) on procedures featured or (ii) by the manufacturer of each product to be administered, to verify the recommended dose or formula, the method and duration of administration, and contraindications. It is the responsibility of practitioners, relying on their own experience and knowledge of their patients, to make diagnoses, to determine dosages and the best treatment for each individual patient, and to take all appropriate safety precautions.

To the fullest extent of the law, neither the Publisher nor the authors, contributors, or editors, assume any liability for any injury and/or damage to persons or property as a matter of product liability, negligence or otherwise, or from any use or operation of any methods, products, instructions, or ideas contained in the material herein.

Although all advertising material is expected to conform to ethical (medical) standards, inclusion in this publication does not constitute a guarantee or endorsement of the quality or value of such product or of the claims made of it by its manufacturer.

Please consult full prescribing information before issuing prescription for any product mentioned in this publication.

Content Strategist: Dr. Renu Rawat
Sr Project Manager—Education Solutions: Shabina Nasim
Content Development Specialist: Shravan Kumar
Project Manager: Nayagi Athmanathan
Cover Designer: Milind Majgaonkar

Typeset by GW India

Printed and bound in India at EIH Limited – Unit Printing Press, IMT Manesar, Gurgaon (Haryana).

Preface

First edition of this book, published in 2006, was primarily aimed for the needs of undergraduate students. Undoubtedly, the text in some parts was a bit detailed, and this very fact was duly mentioned in the preface. However, it was never anticipated that it will become the book of choice for postgraduates in physiology. The undergraduate students also appreciated the text, but always demanded its reduced version. Such a feedback inspired the author to bring out another volume entitled "Medical Physiology for Undergraduate Students" in 2012. In view of the fast changing concepts in physiology and to cater to the needs of postgraduates, the second edition of "Textbook of Medical Physiology" has been thoroughly revised and updated. However, even undergraduates will find it as a useful resource for in-depth understanding of the subject and also for preparing for various postgraduate entrance tests.

SALIENT FEATURES OF THE SECOND EDITION

- Thoroughly revised and updated second edition retains its well accepted unique style of organization of the text in three parts and twelve sections.
- Presentation of the text with various levels of headings, subheadings, boldface and italics has been maintained to help the students easily understand, retain and reproduce.
- Text has been updated incorporating the recent advances in each section including more aspects of molecular physiology.
- Applied physiology has been updated with recent concepts on pathophysiology, and recent advances in the basic investigations and therapeutic principles.
- The book has been transformed into a fully four colored text enhancing lucidity and understanding of the figures and text.
- To further upgrade the book, many new figures, tables and flowcharts have been added.

Second edition of the book has been possible as a result of active criticism, suggestions and generous help of many teachers and students. Surely I owe sincere thanks to them all. Having Arushi Khurana, MD, from the Department of Internal Medicine, University of Connecticut, USA as a co-author has been very useful in updating the text, especially the applied and molecular aspects. I bow with reverence to my teachers: Prof B K Maini, Prof R K Marya, Prof P I Singh and Prof K K Mahajan for grooming me for this task. I wish to express by indebtedness to my husband, Sr. Prof A K Khurana, my son Dr Aruj K Khurana and daughter-in-law Dr Bhawna Piplani Khurana, who have not only helped me during each and every step but also have contributed the updated chapter on 'Sense of Vision'. Sr Prof Sushma Sood, HOD, Physiology has always encouraged and helped me by her academic discussions with a friendly approach. I am thankful to all the faculty members and residents of my department for their co-operation. Of incalculable help to me in updating this edition have been Dr Itika Singh and Dr Harminder. Dr Itika Singh has also contributed as co-author of the chapter on 'Physiology of Body Temperature Regulation'. I am also thankful to Dr Rakesh Gupta, who is just my younger brother and now elevated as Director of PGIMS, Rohtak, Prof Sarla Hooda, a sisterly friend and Registrar UHS and Prof V K Jain, Pro Vice Chancellor UHS, Rohtak. It is my special pleasure to thank Prof O P Kalra, Vice Chancellor, Pt. B D Sharma, UHS, Rohtak for infusing academic atmosphere. The encouragement received from the friends and stalwarts in Physiology especially, Prof Rashmi Mathur, AIIMS, New Delhi, Prof Asha Gandhi, Lady Hardinge Medical College, New Delhi, Prof Rashmi Babbar & Prof A K Jain, Maulana Azad Medical College, New Delhi, Dr Latika Mohan, Dean AIIMS, Rishikesh, Prof K D Singh, Principal GMC, Patiala, Prof Raj Kapoor, HOD, VMMC, New Delhi, Prof D K Aggarwal, JLN Medical College, AMU, Aligarh, Prof Nilima Shankar & Prof Neelam Vaney, UCMS, New Delhi, Dr Nandini Kapoor, HOD, GMC, Chandigarh, needs special mention.

Lastly, it is my special pleasure to acknowledge with gratitude the most assured co-operation and skill of the staff of Elsevier, India especially Ms Shabina Nasim, Mr Shravan.

Dr Saurabh, Dr Ashima and Mr Majumdar deserve a special mention in this Preface for their artistic touch, which I feel provided a considerable beauty to this book.

Sincere efforts have been made to verify the correctness of the text, however in spite of best efforts some inaccuracies, ambiguities and typographical mistakes likely to be noticed by the readers. Therefore, feedback and suggestions from the teachers and students are invited for improving future edition. Feedbacks received shall be highly appreciated and duly acknowledged.

Indu Khurana

Contents

Part I

General Physiology

Section 1

Section 1

General Physiology

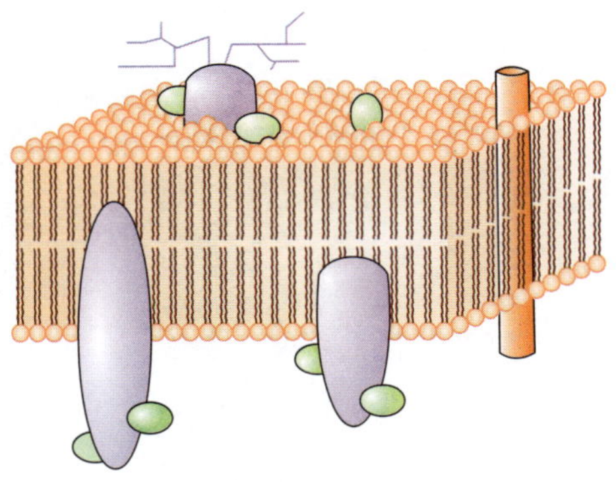

Physiology, in simple terms, refers to the study of normal functioning of the living structures. The *human physiology* is concerned with the way the various systems of the human body function, and the way each contributes to the functions of the body as a whole. In other words, the human physiology is concerned with specific characteristics and mechanisms of the human body that make it a living being, and the mechanisms which help in adaptation and homeostasis, which are the two fundamental features of life.

The *general physiology* envisages the general concepts and principles that are basic to the functions of all the systems. As we know, the fundamental unit of human body is a cell;, therefore, this section includes a short review of fundamental aspect of the cell physiology. Before studying the general biophysiological processes and the cell physiology, it will be worthwhile to have a brief knowledge about the functional organization, composition and internal environment of the human body.

Chapter 1.1

Functional Organization, Composition and Internal Environment of Human Body

FUNCTIONAL ORGANIZATION OF THE HUMAN BODY
- Skin and its appendages
- Skeletal system
- Muscle system
- Nervous system
- Cardiovascular system
- Respiratory system
- Digestive system
- Excretory system
- Reproductive system
- Endocrine system
- Blood and immune system

BODY COMPOSITION
- Total body water
- Body electrolytes

INTERNAL ENVIRONMENT AND HOMEOSTASIS
- Internal environment
- Homeostasis
- Role of different systems
- Modes of action of homeostasis control systems

FUNCTIONAL ORGANIZATION OF THE HUMAN BODY

The human body is actually a social order of about 100 trillion cells organized into different functional structures, some of which are called organs, some organs combinedly form a system. For convenience of description, the human body can be considered to be functionally organized into various systems.

1. Skin and its Appendages

Skin is the outermost covering of the human body. Its appendages include hairs, nails, sebaceous glands and sweat glands. In addition to providing mechanical protection to the underlying tissues, the skin performs following important functions:

- It acts as a physical barrier against entry of microorganisms and other substances.
- It prevents loss of water from the body.
- It is a very important sensory organ, containing receptors for touch and related sensations.
- It plays an important role in regulating body temperature.

2. Skeletal System

The basic framework of the body is provided by a large number of bones that collectively form the *skeleton*. At joints, the bones are united to each other by fibrous bands called *ligaments*. In addition to the bones and joints, the skeletal system also includes the *cartilages* present in the body.

3. Muscle System

Overlying and usually attached to the bones are various muscles. Muscles are composed of many elongated cells called *muscle fibres* which are able to contract and relax. Three distinct types of muscles can be identified, and they are skeletal muscles, smooth muscles and cardiac muscles.

4. Nervous System

The nervous system is made up, predominantly, of tissue that has the special property of being able to conduct impulses rapidly from one part of the body to another. The specialized cells that constitute the functional units of the nervous system are called *neurons*. The nervous system may be divided into: (i) the *central nervous system,* made up of brain and spinal cord, and (ii) the *peripheral nervous system*, consisting of the peripheral nerves and the ganglia associated with them. The nerves supplying the body wall and limbs are often called *cerebrospinal nerves*. The nerves supplying the viscera, along with the parts of the brain and spinal cord related to them, constitute the *autonomic nervous system.* The autonomic nervous system is subdivided into two major parts: the *sympathetic* and the *parasympathetic* nervous system.

5. Cardiovascular System

The cardiovascular system consists of the *heart* and the *blood vessels.* The blood vessels that take blood from the heart to various tissues are called *arteries*. The smallest arteries are called *arterioles.* Arterioles open into a network of *capillaries* that perfuse the tissues. Exchange of various substances between the blood and the tissues take place through the walls of capillaries. In some situations, capillaries are replaced by slightly different vessels called *sinusoids.* Blood from capillaries (or from sinusoids) is collected by small *venules* which join to form *veins.* The veins return blood to the heart.

6. Respiratory System

The respiratory system consists of the lungs and the passages through which air reaches them. The passages are nasal cavities, the pharynx, the trachea, the bronchi and their intrapulmonary continuations.

7. Digestive System

The digestive or the so-called alimentary system includes all those structures that are concerned with eating, and with the digestion and absorption of food. The system consists of an alimentary canal which starts at the mouth and ends at the anus. The alimentary canal includes the oral cavity, pharynx, oesophagus, stomach, small intestine and large intestine. Other structures included in the digestive system are the liver, the gall bladder and the pancreas.

8. Excretory System

Excretion is the removal of waste products of metabolism from the body. *Egestion* (or defaecation) is the removal of undigested food from the gut and is not regarded as excretion because the material taken into the gut through the mouth is not made by the body itself. The organs forming the excretory system are the kidney, the ureters, the bladder and the urethra.

9. Reproductive System

Reproduction is the production of a new generation of individuals of the same species. It involves the transmission of genetic material from one generation to the next. The *male reproductive organs* are the testis, the epididymis, the ductus deferens, and the seminal vesicles (which are paired), and the prostate, the male urethra and the penis (which are unpaired). *The female reproductive organs* are the right and left ovaries and uterine tubes, the uterus, the vagina, the external genitalia and the mammary glands.

10. Endocrine System

Endocrine tissue is made up essentially of cells that produce secretions which are poured directly into blood. The secretions of the endocrine cells are called *hormones.* Some organs are entirely endocrine in function. They are referred to as *endocrine glands* (or *ductless glands*). Those traditionally included under this heading are the hypophysis cerebral (pituitary gland), the pineal gland, the thyroid gland, the parathyroid glands, and the suprarenal (adrenal) glands. Groups of endocrine cells may be present in the organs that have other functions. These include the *islets of Langerhans of* pancreas, the interstitial cells of the testis, the follicles and corpora lutea of the ovaries. Hormones are also produced by some cells in the kidney, the thymus and the placenta. Some workers describe the liver as being partly an endocrine gland.

11. Blood and Immune System

Blood is regarded as a modified connective tissue because the cellular elements in it are separated by a considerable amount of 'intercellular substance' and because some of the cells in it have close affinities to cells in general connective tissue.

Circulating blood normally contains three main types of cells which perform their respective physiologic functions: (i) the red cells (*erythrocytes*) are largely concerned with oxygen transport, (ii) the white cells (*leucocytes*) play various roles in the body defence against infection and tissue injury, and (iii) platelets (*thrombocytes*) which are primarily involved in maintaining integrity of blood vessels and in preventing blood loss. Detailed physiology of each organ system is considered in the relevant chapters.

BODY COMPOSITION

The normal body in an average adult male is composed of *water* (60%), *minerals* (7%), *protein* and related substances (18%), and *fat* (15%). The water, denoted by the term total body water (TBW), and the electrolytes need special emphasis.

Total Body Water

Water is the principal and essential constituent of the human body. The total body water is about 10% less in a normal young adult female (average 50%) than that in average adult male (60%) due to relatively greater amount of adipose tissue in the females. In both sexes, the value tends to decrease with age (Table 1.1-1).

TABLE 1.1-1 Total Body Water (% of Body Weight in Relation to Age and Sex)

Age (years)	Percent (%) of TBW	
	Male	*Female*
10–18	59	57
18–40	61	51
40–60	55	47
Above 60	52	46

The Body Fluid Compartments

The total body water is distributed into two main compartments of the body fluids separated from each other by membranes freely permeable to water (Fig. 1.1-1, Table 1.1-2):

1. Intracellular Fluid Compartment

The intracellular fluid (ICF) compartment comprises about 40% of the body weight, the bulk of which is contained in the muscles.

2. Extracellular Fluid Compartment

The extracellular fluid (ECF) compartment constitutes about 20% of the body weight. The ECF compartment comprises following:

i. Plasma It is the fluid portion of the blood (*intravascular fluid)* and comprises about 5% of the body weight (i.e. 25% of the ECF). On an average out of 5 L of total blood volume, 3.5 L is plasma.

ii. Interstitial fluid including lymph It constitutes the major portion (about 3/4) of the ECF. The composition of interstitial fluid is the same as that of plasma except it has little protein. Thus, interstitial fluid is an ultrafiltrate of plasma.

iii. Transcellular fluid It is the fluid contained in the secretions of the secretary cells and cavities of the body, e.g. saliva, sweat, cerebrospinal fluid (CSF), intraocular fluids (aqueous humour and vitreous humour), pericardial fluid, bile, present between the layers (pleura, peritoneum and synovial membrane), lacrimal fluid and luminal fluids of the gut, thyroid and cochlea.

Transcellular fluid volume is relatively small, about 1.5% of the body weight, i.e. 15 ml/kg body weight (about 1 L in a person of 70 kg).

iv. Mesenchymal tissue fluid The mesenchymal tissues such as dense connective tissue, cartilage and bones contain about 6% of the body water.

The interstitial fluid, transcellular fluid and mesenchymal tissue fluid combine to form 75% of ECF.

The normal distribution of total body water in the fluid compartments is kept constant by two opposing sets of forces: osmotic and hydrostatic pressure.

Measurement of Body Fluid Volumes

Theoretically, it is possible to measure the volume of each fluid component by injecting a substance (indicator) that will stay in only one compartment (provided the

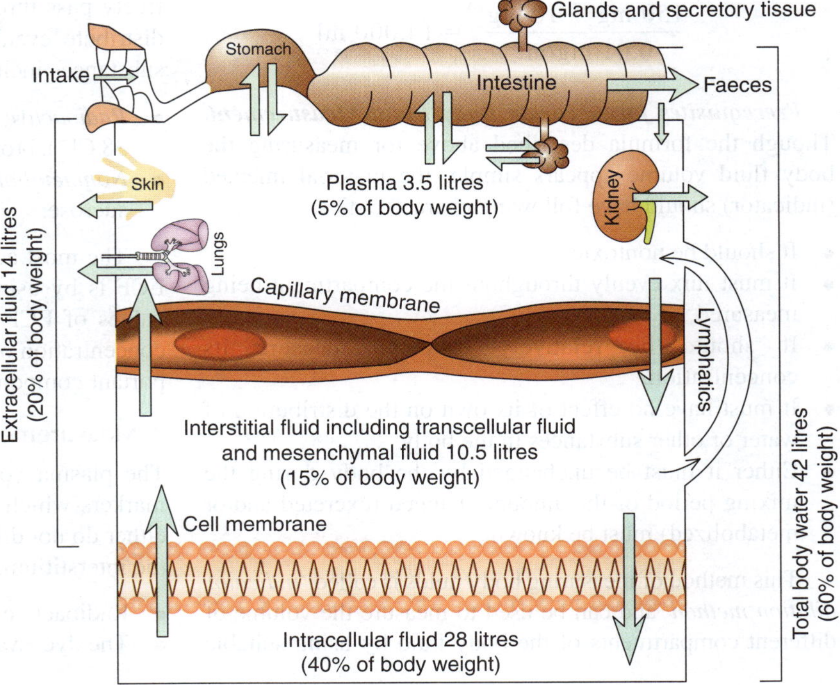

FIGURE 1.1-1 Distribution of total body water in different compartments. Arrows indicate fluid movement.

TABLE 1.1-2 Distribution of Total Body Water in a Normal 70 kg Person

		Percent (%)	
Compartment	*Volume (L)*	*Body weight*	*Body water*
Total body water (TBW)	42	60	100
• Intracellular fluid (ICF)	28	40	67
• Extracellular fluid (ECF)	14	20	33
• Plasma (25% of ECF)	3.5	05	08
• Interstitial fluid, transcellular fluid and mesenchymal tissue fluid (75% of ECF)	10.5	15	25

concentration of the substance in the body fluid and the amount removed by excretion and metabolism can be accurately measured) as:

$$V = \frac{A_1 - A_2}{C} \text{ where:}$$

V = Volume of fluid compartment,
A_1 = Amount of indicator injected in the fluid,
A_2 = Amount of indicator removed by excretion and metabolism and
C = Concentration of the indicator in the fluid.

For example, if 150 mg of sucrose (A_1) is injected into a 70 kg man, 10 mg sucrose (A_2) has been excreted or metabolized and the concentration of plasma sucrose (C) measured is 0.01 mg/ml; then the volume distribution of sucrose is:

$$\frac{150 \text{ mg} - 10 \text{ mg}}{0.01 \text{ mg/ml}} = 14{,}000 \text{ ml}$$

Prerequisites for Accurate Body Fluid Measurement. Though the formula described above for measuring the body fluid volume appears simple, the material injected (indicator) should have following characteristics:

- It should be nontoxic.
- It must mix evenly throughout the compartment being measured.
- It should be relatively easy to measure its concentration.
- It must have no effect of its own on the distribution of water or other substances in the body.
- Either it must be unchanged by the body during the mixing period or the amount changed (excreted and/or metabolized) must be known.

This method of measuring body fluids is called *'indicator dilution method'* and can be used to measure the volume of different compartments of the body fluid by using suitable indicators/markers which will get distributed in that particular compartment as follows:

1. Measurement of Total Body Water (TBW) Volume

The volume of TBW can be measured by injecting a marker which will be evenly distributed in all the compartments of body fluid. Such markers include:

- Deuterium oxide (D_2O),
- Tritium oxide and
- Aminopyrine.

The volume of the TBW can be calculated from the values of the concentration of the marker in the plasma.

2. Measurement of Extracellular Fluid (ECF) Volume

The volume of ECF can be measured by injecting those marker substances which cannot enter the cells but can freely pass through the capillary membrane, and thus can distribute evenly in all the compartments of ECF. Such substances include:

- *Radioactive substances* like sodium, chloride (36 Cl^- and 38 Cl^-), bromide (82 Br^-), sulphate and thiosulphate; and
- *Nonmetabolizable saccharides* like inulin, mannitol and sucrose.

The most accurate method of measuring the volume of ECF is by using *inulin* (polysaccharide, MW 5200). The values of ECF volume are calculated from the values of concentration of *inulin* in the plasma since it makes an important component of the ECF.

3. Measurement of Plasma Volume

The plasma volume can be measured by injecting those markers which bind strongly with the plasma protein and either do not diffuse or diffuse only in small quantities into the interstitium. These substances are:

- Radioactive iodine—^{131}I and
- The dye Evan's blue—T-1824.

The plasma volume can also be calculated from the values of the RBCs which can be measured using radioactive isotopes of chromium (^{51}Cr).

4. Measurement of Intracellular Fluid (ICF) Volume

The volume of ICF cannot be measured directly, since there is no substance which can be confined exclusively to this compartment after intravenous injection. Therefore, values of ICF volume are calculated from the values of TBW and ECF as:

$$\text{ICF volume} = \text{TBW volume} - \text{ECF volume}$$

5. Measurement of Interstitial Fluid Volume

Like ICF volume, the volume of interstitial fluid also cannot be measured directly for the same reasons. Its values can be roughly calculated from the values of ECF volume and plasma volume as:

$$\text{Interstitial fluid volume} = \text{ECF volume} - \text{plasma volume.}$$

The ECF volume/intracellular fluid volume ratio is larger in infants and children as compared to adults, but absolute volume of ECF in children is smaller than in adults. Therefore, dehydration develops rapidly, more frequently and severely in children than in adults.

Body Electrolytes

The electrolytes constitute about 7% of the total body weight and they perform many major functions in the body. The distribution of electrolytes in various compartments differs markedly. Table 1.1-3 shows the distribution of electrolytes in two major compartments of body fluid: the extracellular fluid (ECF) and the intracellular fluid (ICF).

TABLE 1.1-3 Distribution of Ions in the ECF and ICF (Values Are in mEq/L of H_2O)

Ion	Extracellular fluid	Intracellular fluid
Cations		
Na^+	142	14
K^+	5.5	150
Ca^{2+}	5	<1
Mg^{2+}	3	58
Anions		
Cl^-	103	4
HCO_3^-	28	10
PO_4^{3-}	4	75
Proteins	1 g/dL	5 g/dL

From Table 1.1-3, it may be noted that in the ICF the main cations are K^+ and Mg^{2+}, and the main anions are PO_4^{3-} and proteins. It has low concentration of Na^+ and Cl^-. While in ECF, the predominant cation is Na^+ and the principal anions are Cl^- and HCO_3^-. Besides these, a small proportion of nondiffusible proteins and some diffusible nutrients and metabolites such as glucose and urea are also present in ECF. These differences are of great importance for the survival of tissues.

The essential difference between the two main subdivisions of ECF is the higher protein content in plasma than in the interstitial fluid which plays important role in maintaining fluid balance.

It is Important to Note that:

- Essentially all of the body K^+ is in the exchangeable pool.
- Only 65–70% of the body Na^+ is exchangeable.
- Almost all of the body Ca^{2+} and Mg^{2+} are nonexchangeable.
- Only the exchangeable solutes are osmotically active.

Functions of Electrolytes

1. Electrolytes are the main solutes in the body fluids for maintenance of acid–base balance.
2. Electrolytes maintain the proper osmolality and volume of body fluids.
3. The concentration of certain electrolytes determines their specific physiologic functions, e.g. the effect of calcium ions on neuromuscular excitability.

INTERNAL ENVIRONMENT AND HOMEOSTASIS

Internal Environment

Claude Bernarde (1949), the great French physiologist, introduced the term *internal environment* of the body or the *milieu interieur* for the extracellular fluid (ECF) of the body. He said so since all the body cells essentially depend upon the ECF for maintenance of cellular life. Cells are capable of living, growing and performing their special functions so long as the proper concentration of oxygen, glucose, different ions, amino acids, fatty substances and other constituents are available in the internal environment.

The composition of extracellular fluid vis-a-vis intracellular fluid has been discussed in the just preceding pages.

Homeostasis

Homeostasis, a term introduced by WB Cannon, refers to the mechanism by which the constancy of the internal environment is maintained and ensured. For this purpose, living membranes with varying permeabilities such as vascular endothelium and cell membrane play important roles in the exchange of fluids, electrolytes, nutrients and metabolites across the compartments of body fluids.

The factors involved in the maintenance of internal environment can be summarized as:

- Maintenance of pH of ECF (acid–base balance),
- Regulation of temperature,
- Maintenance of water and electrolyte balance,
- Supply of nutrients, oxygen, enzymes and hormones and
- Removal of metabolic and other waste products.

Role of Different Systems of the Body in Homeostasis

Almost all the systems of the human body play vital roles in the maintenance of the internal environment. The details of the role played by each system are described in the relevant chapters. The outlines of the contributions to different mechanisms of homeostasis made by different functional systems of the body are summarized.

1. Transport of Extracellular Fluid The circulatory system plays the most vital role in the transport of extracellular fluid (ECF) in the body. In this way, the ECF everywhere in the body, both the plasma and interstitial fluid, is continually being mixed, thereby maintaining almost complete homogeneity throughout the body.

2. Supply of Oxygen and Nutrients to ECF The nutrients and oxygen are must to provide energy for various cell activities for the growth of the tissue. The respiratory system, digestive system, circulatory system and the musculoskeletal system play major roles in the supply of adequate amount of oxygen and nutrients. Hormones play an essential role in the metabolism of nutrients and other substances necessary for the cells.

3. Removal of Metabolic End Products and Waste Kidneys and other excretory organs are involved in the excretion of end products of metabolism and other waste products. Respiratory system plays a role in the removal of carbon dioxide from the body.

4. Water and Electrolyte Balance in the body is maintained by a combined effort of kidneys, skin, lungs, salivary secretion and digestive system.

5. The pH of Blood and Acid–Base Balance are maintained by the respiratory system, kidneys, blood and the various buffer systems in the body.

6. The Temperature of the Body is maintained affirmably by a combined effort of the skin, cardiovascular system, respiratory system, digestive system, excretory system, skeletal muscle system and the nervous system.

7. Regulation of Body Functions is very important for homeostasis. The nervous system and the hormonal system of regulation play key roles. The autonomic nervous system regulates all the vegetative functions of the body essential for homeostasis.

8. Reproduction Reproduction is not considered a homeostatic function. However, it does help to maintain static conditions by generating new beings to take the place of those that are dying. This perhaps sounds like a permissive usage of the term homeostasis, but it does illustrate that, essentially all body structures are so organized that they help to maintain the automaticity and continuity of life.

Mode of Action of Homeostatic Control System

The homeostasis is a complex phenomenon. The above-mentioned examples of homeostatic control mechanisms are only a few of the many hundreds to thousands in the body, all of which have certain characteristics in common. The mode of operation of all the systems, which are involved in the homeostasis, is through 'feedback' mechanism, and the adaptive control system. Feedback mechanism is of two types: the negative feedback mechanism and the positive feedback mechanism.

Negative Feedback Mechanism

Most control systems of the body act by negative feedback. That is, in general if the activity of a particular system is increased or decreased, a control system initiates a negative feedback, which consists of a series of changes that return the activity toward normal.

The degree of effectiveness with which a control system maintains constant conditions is determined by the gain of the negative feedback.

Examples of a feedback mechanism

1. When the blood pressure suddenly rises or lowers, it initiates a series of reactions that try to bring the blood pressure to normal levels.
2. When thyroxine secretion is in excess, it inhibits the secretion of thyroid stimulating hormone (TSH) from pituitary so that, thyroxine is not secreted from the thyroid gland.

Positive Feedback Mechanism

Positive feedback is better known as a vicious circle. Usually, it is harmful and in some instances even death can occur due to positive feedback. For example, as shown in Fig. 1.1-2, when a person has suddenly bled 2 L of blood, a vicious circle of progressively weakening of the heart is set in motion, which ultimately causes death.

A mild degree of feedback can be overcome by the negative feedback control mechanisms of the body, and a vicious cycle fails to develop. For example, when a patient

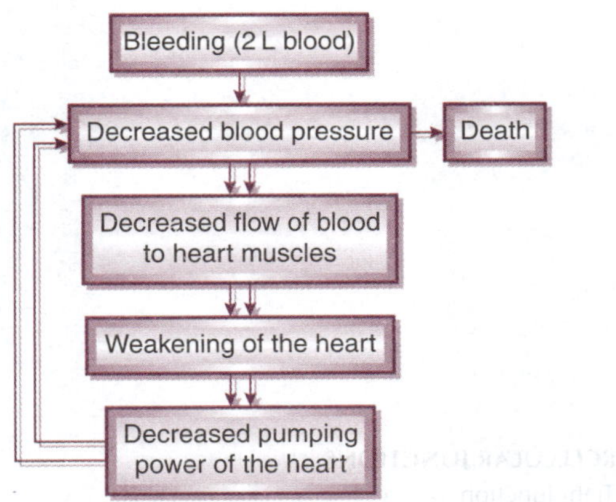

FIGURE 1.1-2 Showing how a positive feedback mechanism can cause death.

bleeds 1 L of blood instead of 2 L, the negative feedback mechanisms of controlling the blood pressure may overcome the positive feedback, and the blood pressure will return to normal, as shown in Fig. 1.1-2.

Further, sometimes positive feedback can serve useful purposes, e.g. under following circumstances:

- *Clot formation* following rupture of vessels is accelerated by a vicious cycle of thrombin formation (for details see page 212). This stops the bleeding.
- *Child birth* during labour is facilitated by progressively increasing uterine contractions due to positive feedback from stretching of cervix by head of the baby (for details see page 878).
- *Generation of nerve signals* by the vicious cycle of progressive leakage of Na^+ ions from the channels set up following stimulation of membrane of nerve fibre is due to the positive feedback.

Adaptive Control System

Adaptive control system refers to a delayed type of negative feedback mechanism. This is seen in nervous system (for details see page 930). For example, when some movements of the body occur very rapidly, there is not enough time for nerve signals to travel from the peripheral parts of the body all the way to the brain and then back to the periphery again in time to control the movements. Under such circumstances, the brain uses a principle called *feed-forward control* to cause the required muscle contraction, which retrospectively is conveyed to the brain by the sensory nerve signals from the moving part. If the movement performed is found incorrect, then the brain corrects the *feed-forward signals* that it sends to the muscle the next time the movement is required. Such a correction made by successive retrospective feedback mechanism is called *adaptive control.*

Chapter 1.2

The Cell Physiology

CELL STRUCTURE
- Cell membrane
- Cytoplasm
- Nucleus

CELL MEMBRANE
- Fluid mosaic model
- Arrangement of different molecules in cell membrane

INTERCELLULAR JUNCTIONS
- Tight junction
- Adherens junction
- Gap junction

CELL STRUCTURE

The cell is the smallest structural and functional unit of the body. The human body contains about 100 trillion cells. Different types of cells of the body possess features which distinguish one type from the other, and are specially adapted to perform one or few particular functions, e.g., the red blood cells transport oxygen from lungs to the tissues, the muscle cell is specialized for the function of contraction, the intestinal mucosal cells are specialized for absorption of foodstuffs and so on. However, most mammalian cells have an overall common structure and certain basic characteristics which are described.

Under normal conditions, cells are dynamic structures existing in fluid environment. A typical cell, as seen by the light microscope, consists of three basic components:

- Cell membrane,
- Cytoplasm and
- Nucleus.

Cell Membrane

Cell membrane or the plasma membrane is the protective sheath enveloping the cell body. It separates the contents of the cell from the external environment and controls exchange of materials between the fluid outside the cell (extracellular fluid) and the fluid inside the cell (intracellular fluid). A detailed knowledge of its structure (Fig. 1.2-1) is essential for the understanding of cell functions. Therefore, it will be discussed separately (see page 16).

Cytoplasm

Cytoplasm is an aqueous substance (cytosol) containing a variety of cell organelles and other structures. In eukaryotic cells, the nucleus and cytoplasm together form the protoplasm. The structures dispersed in the cytoplasm can be broadly divided into three groups: organelles, inclusion bodies and cytoskeleton.

A. Organelles

The organelles are the permanent components of the cells that are bounded by limiting membrane and contain enzymes, hence participating in the cellular metabolic activity. These include the mitochondria, the endoplasmic reticulum, ribosomes, the Golgi apparatus, peroxisomes, centrosomes and centrioles.

1. Mitochondria

Mitochondria are the major sites for aerobic respiration. These are oval structures about 5–12 μm in length and 0.5–1 μm in diameter, and more numerous in metabolically active cells.

Structure The mitochondria consist of:

- ***Membranes.*** There are two layers of the membrane: the outer smooth and inner folded into incomplete septa called cristae (Fig. 1.2-1A). Chemically and structurally, the membranes of mitochondria are similar to the cell membrane. The inner membrane in addition, contains lollipop-shaped globular structures present between the layers of membrane.

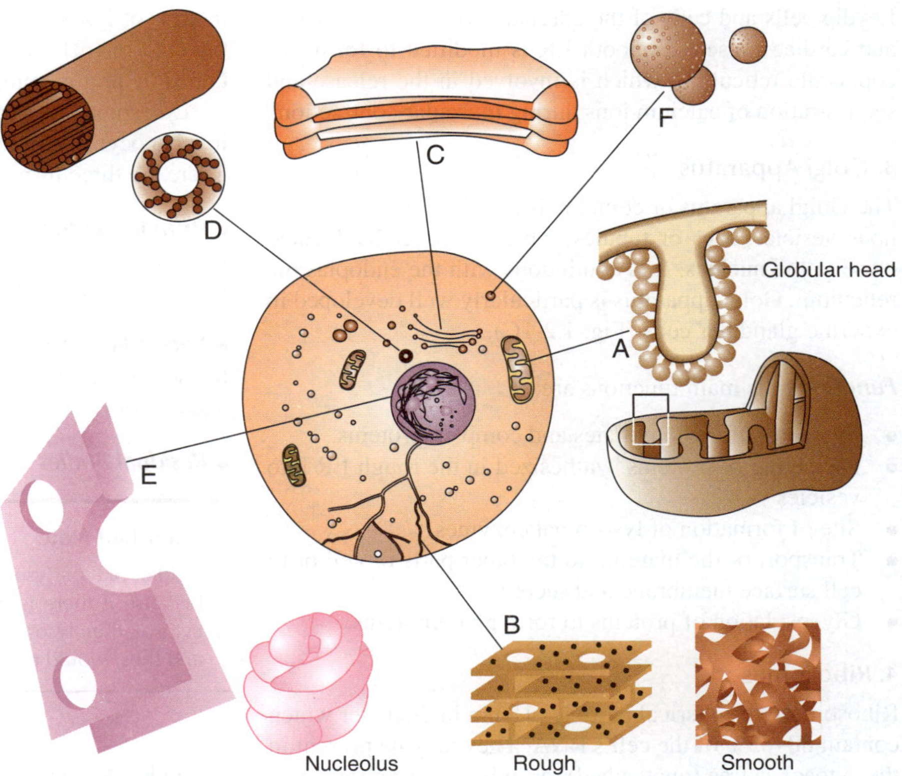

FIGURE 1.2-1 Structure of a typical cell (in the centre) showing various organelles: **A**, mitochondrion; **B**, endoplasmic reticulum (rough and smooth); **C**, Golgi apparatus; **D**, centrosome; **E**, nucleus; and **F**, secretory granules.

- ***Matrix*** of the mitochondria contains enzymes required in Krebs cycle by which products of carbohydrate, fat and protein metabolism are oxidized to produce energy, which is stored in the form of ATP in the lollipop-like globular structures.

Functions In addition to their role as power-generating units, the mitochondria may have a role in synthesizing membrane-bound proteins, since they also possess DNA and ribosomes. The mitochondria have their own genome; however, the DNA of mitochondrial genome is much less than the nuclear genome. Mitochondrial DNA encodes 13 protein subunits which are associated with proteins and are coded by nuclear genes to form enzyme complexes and ribosomal transfer RNA (needed by intramitrochondrial ribosomes for protein synthesis). The enzyme complexes responsible for oxidative phosphorylation include:

- Complex I—reduced nicotinamide adenine dinucleotide dehydrogenase (NADH)
- Complex II—succinate dehydrogenase ubiquinone oxidoreductase
- Complex III—ubiquinone-cytochrome C oxidoreductase
- Complex IV—cytochrome C oxidase

The complexes I, III and IV pump protons (H^+) into intermembranous spaces during electron transfer, and complex II along with complexes III and IV acts with complex I, coenzyme Q and cytochrome c and convert metabolites to carbon dioxide and water.

Mitochondria also have a role in apoptosis (programmed cell death).

Important Note

Mitochondrial DNA repair system is ineffective and mutation rate is higher as compared with nuclear DNA (10 times). Therefore, a large number of rare diseases due to mitochondrial DNA mutation have been traced, particularly in disorders of tissue associated with high metabolic rate.

2. Endoplasmic Reticulum

Endoplasmic reticulum (ER) is a system of flattened, membrane-bound vesicles and tubules called *cisternae* (Fig. 1.2-1B). It is continuous with the outer membrane of the nuclear envelop, Golgi apparatus and possibly with the cell membrane. Morphologically, two types of endoplasmic reticulum can be identified: rough or granular and smooth or agranular.

i. Rough Endoplasmic Reticulum The rough ER is characterized by presence of a number of ribosomes on its surface and transports proteins made by the ribosomes through the cisternae. Thus, the rough ER is especially well developed in cells active in protein synthesis, e.g. Russell's bodies of plasma cells, Nissl granules of nerve cells and acinar cells of pancreas.

ii. Smooth Endoplasmic Reticulum Smooth ER is devoid of ribosomes on its surface. It is a site of lipid and steroid synthesis. Therefore, it is found in abundance with

Leydig cells and cells of the adrenal cortex. In the skeletal and cardiac muscles, smooth ER is modified to form sarcoplasmic reticulum, which is involved in the release and sequestration of calcium ions during muscular contraction.

3. Golgi Apparatus

The Golgi apparatus or complex is a collection of membranous vesicles, sacs or tubules, which is generally located close to the nucleus. It is continuous with the endoplasmic reticulum. Golgi apparatus is particularly well developed in exocrine glandular cells (Fig. 1.2-1C).

Functions Its main functions are:

- Synthesis of carbohydrates and complex proteins.
- Packaging of proteins synthesized in the rough ER into vesicles.
- Site of formation of lysosomal enzymes.
- Transport of the material to the other parts of cell or to cell surface membrane and secretion.
- Glycosylation of proteins to form glycoproteins.

4. Ribosomes

Ribosomes are spherical particles 15 nm in diameter which contain 80–85% of the cell's RNA. They may be present in the cytosol as free (unattached), or in bound form (attached to the membrane of endoplasmic reticulum). Slightly smaller forms of ribosomes are also found in mitochondria.

Functions They are the site of protein synthesis. They synthesize all transmembrane proteins, secreted proteins and most proteins that are stored in Golgi apparatus, lysosomes and endosomes.

5. Lysosomes

Lysosomes are rounded to oval membrane-bound organelles 250–750 nm in diameter containing powerful lysosomal digestive (hydrolytic) enzymes. They are formed by the Golgi apparatus. As many as 40 different lysosomal enzymes have been synthesized. Some are listed in Table 1.2-1. These enzymes are acidic hydrolases and act best at acidic pH. The

TABLE 1.2-1 Lysosomal Enzymes and Cell Components as Their Substrates

Enzyme	Substrates
Deoxyribonuclease	DNA
Ribonuclease	RNA
Glycosidases	Glycosides and polysaccharides
Collagenases	Collagen
Arylsulphatases	Sulphate esters
Cathepsins	Proteins

interior of lysosome is acidic (pH 5) as compared to rest of the cytosol (pH 7.2). The lysosomal acidic nature is maintained by proton pump or H^+-ATPase.

Lysosomes are particularly abundant in the cells involved in phagocytic activity, e.g. neutrophils and macrophages. There are three forms of lysosomes:

- ***Primary Lysosomes or Storage Vacuoles*** are formed from the various hydrolytic enzymes synthesized by rough ER and packaged in the Golgi apparatus.
- ***Secondary Lysosomes or Autophagic Vacuoles*** are formed by fusion of primary lysosomes with parts of damaged or worn-out cell components.
- ***Residual Bodies*** are undigestible materials in the lysosomes.

Important Note

Acidic pH of lysosome is a safety feature for the cell, because if there is leakage of lysosomal contents into the cytosol, then lysosomal enzymes are not effective at pH 7.2, and thus, would not be able to digest cytosolic enzymes.

Applied Aspects

Congenital absence of lysosomal enzymes results in lysosomal storage disease, i.e. lysosomal engorgement with materials normally the enzymes degrade. Examples are:

- *Gaucher's disease* occurs due to deficiency of β-galactosidase.
- *Tay–Sachs disease* occurs due to hexoaminidase deficiency, which causes mental retardation and blindness.

6. Peroxisome

Peroxisomes, also known as microbodies, are spherical structures enclosed by a single layer of unit membrane. These are predominantly present in hepatocytes and tubular epithelial cells.

Functions They essentially contain two types of enzymes:

- *Oxidases* which are active in oxidation of lipid, and
- *Catalases* which act on hydrogen peroxide to liberate oxygen.

7. Centrosome

The centrosome consists of two short cylindrical structures called centrioles (Fig. 1.2-1D). It is situated near the centre of the cell, close to the nucleus. The centrioles are responsible for movement of chromosomes during cell division.

B. Cytoplasmic Inclusions

The cytoplasmic inclusions are the temporary components of certain cells. These may, or may not be enclosed in the membrane. A few examples of cytoplasmic inclusions are:

- *Lipid droplets.* These are seen in the cells of adipose tissue, liver and adrenal cortex.
- *Glycogen.* It is seen in the cells of liver and skeletal muscles.
- *Proteins as secretory granules* are seen in the secretory glandular cells (Fig. 1.2-1F).
- *Melanin pigment* is seen in the cells of epidermis, retina and basal ganglia.
- *Lipofuscin.* It is a yellow–brown pigment believed to be derived from secondary lysosomes and is seen in the cardiac muscle and brain cells of elderly people.

C. Cytoskeleton

The cytoskeleton is a complex network of fibres that maintains the structure of the cell and allows it to change shape and move. It primarily consists of microtubules, intermediate filaments and microfilaments, along with proteins, which anchor and tie them together (Fig. 1.2-2).

1. Microtubules

Microtubules are long hollow tubular structures without limiting membrane, about 15–25 nm in diameter. These are made up of two globular protein subunits, α- and β-tubulin. The bundles of tubulin give structural strength to the cells. Microtubules form the transport system of the cells. Some of the other organelles and protein molecules move to different parts of the cell through the microtubules. *Kinesin* and *dynein,* known as molecular motors, help in the movement of molecules through the microtubules.

The *cilia and flagella,* which project from the surface of certain cells (spermatozoa, respiratory mucosa and fallopian tubes), are also composed of microtubules enclosed in plasma membrane and are active in the locomotion of the cells.

2. Intermediate Filaments

Intermediate filaments are filamentous structures about 10 nm in diameter. Some of these filaments connect the nuclear membrane to the cell membrane. Their main function is to mechanically integrate the cell organelles within the cytoplasm. In their absence, cells rupture more easily; and when they are abnormal in humans, blistering of the skin is common.

3. Microfilaments

Microfilaments are long solid filamentous structures having a diameter of 6–8 nm. These are made up of contractile proteins, actin and myosin. Actin is the most abundant protein in the mammalian cell. It attaches to various parts of the cytoskeleton by other proteins (anchor proteins). These are identified by numbers as 4.1, 4.2, 4.9 (Fig. 1.2-2). The actin filaments interact with integrin receptors to form focal adhesion complexes (Fig. 1.2-4). The microfilaments are scattered in an unorganized network. Extension of microfilaments along with the plasma membrane on the surface of the cells forms *microvilli,* which increase the absorptive surface of the cells (e.g. intestinal epithelium). In the skeletal muscle, the presence of actin and myosin filaments is responsible for their contractile property.

Molecular Motors Molecular motors help in the movement of different proteins, organelles and other cell parts (their cargo), to all parts of the cell. Broadly, the molecular motors can be divided into two types:

1. Microtubule-Based Molecular Motors This is a superfamily of many forms of molecular motors that produce motion along the microtubules. Two important molecular motors of this family are:

i. ***Conventional kinesin.*** It is a double-headed molecule that moves its cargo towards the positive ends of microtubules.
ii. ***Dyneins.*** These have two heads with their neck pieces embedded in a complex of proteins. These include:
    - *Cytoplasmic dynein.* It moves particles and membranes towards the negative end of the microtubule.
    - *Axonemal dynein.* It can oscillate, and is thus responsible for beating of flagella and cilia which project from the surface of certain cells.

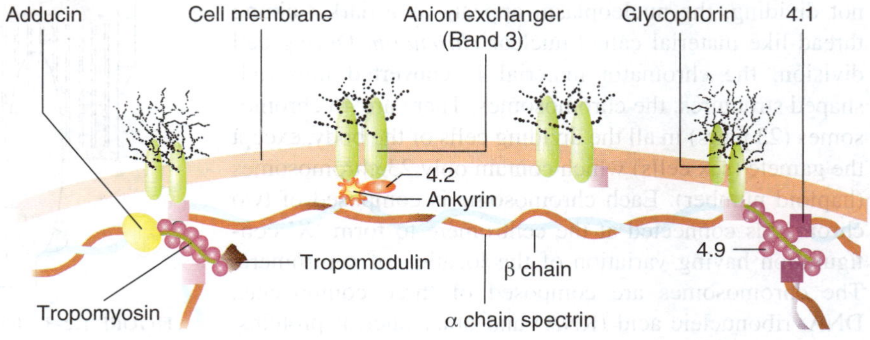

FIGURE 1.2-2 Cytoskeleton showing various proteins.

2. Actin-Based Molecular Motors This is a superfamily of many molecular motors that produce motion along the actin. The important example of this group is *myosin*.

Myosin. The superfamily is further divided into 15 classes. The two important members of this family are myosin-I and myosin-II, which are described briefly:

- *Myosin-I.* Its molecules have a single head. Myosin-I is associated with actin in many cells.
- *Myosin-II.* Its molecules have two heads, but only one head is active in a molecule. Myosin-II is associated with skeletal muscle.

Mechanism of action. The myosins form cross-bridges to the actin molecules, and the myosin heads move generating force which is responsible for movement of various cells such as:

- Contraction of intestinal villi, and
- Contraction of skeletal, cardiac and smooth muscles.

Nucleus

Nucleus is present in all eukaryotic cells. It controls all the cellular activities, including reproduction of the cell. Most of the cells are uninucleated, except a few types of cells like skeletal muscle cells, which are multinucleated. Mostly, nucleus is spherical and situated in the centre of the cell,; however, its shape and location may vary in different types of cells. The nucleus consists of an outer nuclear membrane enclosing nucleoplasm and nucleoli (Fig. 1.2-1E).

1. Nuclear Membrane

The nuclear membrane is a double-layered porous structure having a 40–70 nm wide space called *perinuclear cistern* which is continuous with the lumen of endoplasmic reticulum. The outer layer of the nuclear membrane is continuous with endoplasmic reticulum. The exchange of materials between nucleoplasm and cytoplasm occurs through the nuclear membrane.

2. Nucleoplasm

The nucleoplasm or the nuclear matrix is a gel-like ground substance containing large quantity of genetic material in the form of deoxyribonucleic acid (DNA). When a cell is not dividing, the nucleoplasm appears as a dark staining thread-like material called nuclear *chromatin.* During cell division, the chromatin material is converted into rod-shaped structures, the chromosomes. There are 46 chromosomes (23 pairs) in all the dividing cells of the body, except the gamete (sex cells) which contain only 23 chromosomes (haploid number). Each chromosome is composed of two chromatids connected at the centromere to form 'X' configuration having variation of the location of centromere. The chromosomes are composed of three components, DNA, ribonucleic acid (RNA) and other nuclear proteins. The nuclear DNA carries the genetic information which is passed via RNA into the cytoplasm for synthesis of proteins of similar composition.

3. Nucleolus

The nucleus may contain one or more rounded bodies called nucleoli. The nucleoli are the site of synthesis of ribosomal RNA. The nucleoli are more common in growing cells or in cells actively synthesizing proteins.

THE CELL MEMBRANE

An understanding of the structure and properties of the cell membrane is most essential to understand the various physiological activities of the cell, including transport across cell membrane. Electron microscopy has shown that cell membrane/plasma membrane has a *trilayer* structure having total thickness of 7–10 nm (70–100 A°) and is known as *unit membrane*. The three layers consist of *two electron dense layers* separated by an *electron-lucent layer* (clear zone). Biochemically, the cell membrane is composed of complex mixture of lipids (40%), proteins (55%) and carbohydrates (5%).

Hypothesis for Cell Membrane Structure

A few hypotheses have been proposed to explain the distribution of various biochemical components in the cell membrane. The most important hypothesis is the fluid mosaic model of Singer and Nicolson.

The Fluid Mosaic Model of Membrane Structure

In 1972, Singer and Nicolson put forward the fluid mosaic model of membrane structure (Fig. 1.2-3), which is presently most accepted. According to this model:

- *Phospholipid bilayer* is the basic continuous structure forming the cell membrane. The phospholipids are

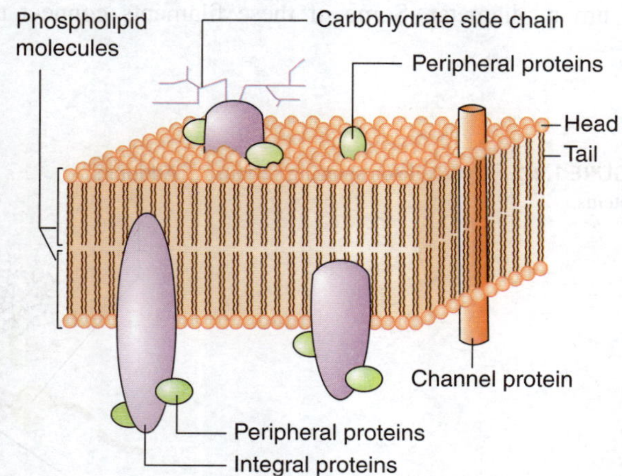

FIGURE 1.2-3 Fluid mosaic model of the cell membrane structure.

present in fluid form. This fluidity makes the membrane quite flexible, and thus allows the cells to undergo considerable changes in the shape without disruption of structural integrity.

- *The protein molecules* are present as a discontinuous mosaic of globular proteins which float about in the fluid phospholipid bilayer forming a *fluid mosaic pattern.*

Arrangement of Different Molecules in Cell Membrane

The arrangement of molecules of phospholipids, proteins and carbohydrates forming the cell membrane is as follows:

Arrangement of Lipid Bilayer of the Cell Membrane

Each lipid molecule in the lipid bilayer of the cell membrane primarily consists of phospholipid, cholesterol and glycolipids. The presence of cholesterol is responsible for the characteristic which has the consistency of olive oil. The lipid molecule is clothes' pin shape and consists of a *head end* and a *tail end.*

The head end or the globular end of the molecule contains phosphate moiety of phospholipid or hydroxyl radicle of cholesterol. It is positively charged and quite soluble in water (i.e. *polar* or *hydrophilic).* The tail end consists of two chains of fatty acids or steroid radicle of cholesterol. It is quite insoluble in water (nonpolar or hydrophobic). These lipid molecules are arranged as bilayers in such a way that their nonpolar hydrophobic tail ends are directed towards the centre of the membrane, whereas their polar hydrophilic head ends are directed outwards on either side of the membrane (Fig. 1.2-3). In this way, head ends of molecules face the aqueous phase, i.e. extracellular fluid on the outside and the intracellular fluid (cytoplasm) on the inner side. The major types of phospholipids are *phosphatidyl choline, phosphatidyl ethanolamine, glycospingolipids, sphingomyelin and cholesterol.*

Functional Significance of the Lipid Bilayer. The lipid bilayer of the cell membrane makes it a semipermeable membrane which constitutes the major barrier for the water-soluble molecules like electrolytes, urea and glucose. On the other hand, fat-soluble substances like oxygen, fatty acids and alcohol can pass through the membrane with ease.

Arrangement of Proteins in the Cell Membrane

Most protein molecules float about in the phospholipid bilayer forming a fluid mosaic pattern. The two types of proteins recognized in the cell membrane are:

- *Lipoproteins,* i.e. the proteins containing lipids which function as enzymes and ion channels, and
- *Glycoproteins,* i.e. the proteins containing carbohydrates which function as receptors for hormones and neurotransmitters.

The proteins in the cell membrane are described as:

1. Peripheral Proteins. These are present peripheral to the lipid bilayer, both inside and outside to it.

i. *Intrinsic proteins.* These are located in the inner surface of the lipid bilayer and serve mainly as enzymes. Some of these are anchored to the cytoskeleton of the cell (Fig. 1.2-2).

ii. *Extrinsic or surface proteins.* These are the proteins located on the outer surface of the lipid bilayer. These protein molecules are not associated tightly with the cell membrane, and thus can dissociate readily from the cell membrane. Some of these proteins serve as *cell adhesion molecules* (CAM) that anchor cells to neighbouring cells and to the basal lamina.

2. Integral Proteins or Transmembrane Proteins. These are the proteins that extend into the lipid bilayer. The proteins stay in the membrane because they have regions of hydrophobic amino acids which interact with fatty acid tails to exclude water. The rest of the protein is hydrophilic and faces into the cell or out into the external environment, both of which are aqueous (Fig. 1.2-3). Some proteins penetrate only part of the way into the membrane, while others penetrate all the way through. The integral proteins, on the basis of functions they serve, have been described as:

- *Channel proteins.* Some of the integral protein molecules serve as channels for water-soluble substances like glucose and electrolytes. These are also called the channel proteins.
- *Carrier proteins.* The protein molecules that help in transport of substances across the cell membrane by means of active and passive (facilitated diffusion) transport are called carrier proteins.
- *Receptor proteins.* Some of the proteins function as receptors that bind neurotransmitters and hormones, initiating physiologic changes inside the cell. The number of receptors of a cell are not constant, but keep on increasing (upregulation) or decreasing (down regulation) in response to various stimuli. Some of receptor proteins span (up and down movement) the entire thickness of the membrane several times like a sound wave and help in transport of substances.
- *Antigens.* Some proteins in the cell membrane also act as antigens. These are glycoproteins with branching carbohydrate side chains like antennae. There are an enormous number of possible shapes to these side chains, so each type of cell can have its own specific marker. This enables cells to recognize other cells and behave in an organized way, e.g. during development of tissue and organ in multicellular organisms. It also means that

foreign antigen can be recognized. Thus, these proteins help in processing the antibodies and distinguish self from nonself.

- *Pumps.* There are certain proteins in the cell membrane which act as pumps, and form the active transport system of the cell, e.g. Na^+–K^+ATPase pump, K^+–H^+ ATPase pump and Ca^{2+} pump.

Arrangement of Carbohydrates in the Cell Membrane

The carbohydrates are attached either to the proteins (glycoproteins) or the lipids (glycolipids). Throughout the surface of cell membrane, carbohydrate molecules form a thin loose covering called *glycocalyx.*

Functions of Cell Membrane Carbohydrates

- Being negatively charged, the carbohydrate molecules of the cell membrane do not allow the negatively charged particles to move out of the cell.
- The glycocalyx helps in tight fixation of the cells with one another.
- Some of the carbohydrate molecules also serve as *receptors.*

INTERCELLULAR JUNCTIONS

The cell membranes of the neighbouring cells are connected with one another through the *intercellular junctions* or the junctional complexes, which are of three types.

Before describing the types of intercellular junctions, it will be worthwhile to have some information about the cell adhesion molecules (CAMs).

Cell Adhesion Molecules

Cell adhesion molecules (CAMs) are the prominent parts of the intercellular connections by which the cells are attached to basal lamina and to each other.

Types of CAMs. CAMs have been variously classified. Most simply, they can be divided into four broad families:

1. *Integrins.* These are heterodimers that bind to various receptors.
2. *Adhesion molecules of IgG subfamily.* Through these molecules the IgG immunoglobulins bind to various antigens.
3. *Cadherins.* These are Ca^{2+}-dependent molecules that mediate cell-to-cell adhesions by haemophilic reactions.
4. *Selectins.* These are lectin-like domains that bind carbohydrates.

Mechanism of Adhesions. The CAMs act as adhesion proteins by following mechanisms:

- *Anchorage with cytoskeleton.* Many CAMs pass through the cell membrane and are anchored to the cytoskeleton inside the cell.
- *Homophilic binding,* i.e. some CAMs bind to like-molecules on the other cells.
- *Heterophilic binding,* i.e. some CAMs bind to different molecules on the other cells.
- *Binding to laminins.* Many CAMs bind to laminins, a family of large cross-shaped molecules with multiple receptor domains in the extracellular matrix.

Functions of CAMs. In addition to *binding the neighbouring cells* to each other, the CAMs perform following other functions:

- They transmit signals into and out of the cells.
- They play a role in embryonic development and formation of the nervous system and other tissue.
- They hold tissue together in adults.
- They play an important role in inflammation and wound healing.
- They also play a role in metastasis of tumours.

Types of Intercellular Junctions

1. Tight Junction. This is also called *zona occludens* or the *occluding zone* (Fig. 1.2-4A). In this type of intercellular junction, the outer layer of the cell membrane of the neighbouring cells fuse with each other, thus obliterating the space between the cells. A tight junction is composed of parallel strands of tightly packed transmembrane proteins (mainly occludin, junctional adhesion molecules and claudins). Such junctions form a barrier to the movement of ions and other

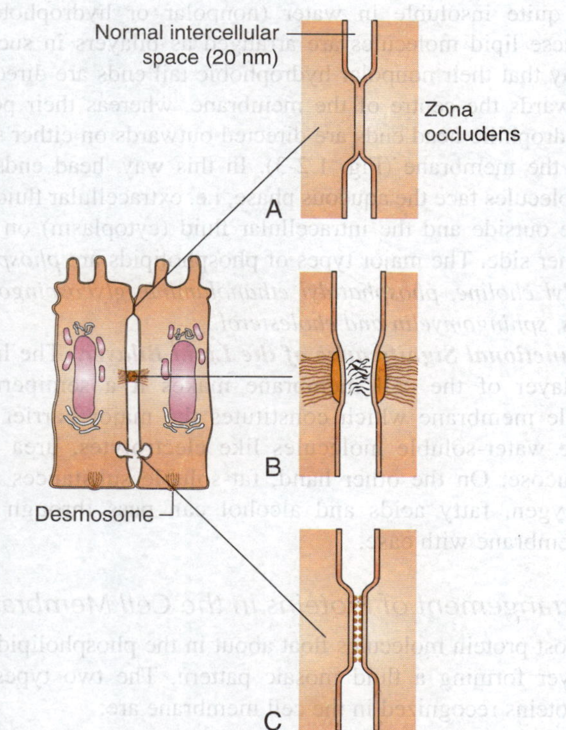

FIGURE 1.2-4 Schematic diagram of a cell showing various intercellular junctions: **A**, tight junction; **B**, adherens junction; and **C**, gap junction.

solutes from one cell to another. Following are few examples of the cells where tight junctions are present:

- Apical margins of epithelial cells, such as the intestinal mucosa.
- The renal tubular epithelial cells.
- Capillary endothelium in the brain forming the blood–brain barrier.
- Blood–aqueous barrier formed by the tight junctions between the cells of the inner non-pigmented epithelium of the ciliary body.
- Outer blood–retinal barrier formed by the tight junctions between adjacent cells of the retinal pigment epithelium.

2. Adherens Junction. This is also called *zonula adherens*. In this type of junction, cell membrane of the adjacent cells are separated by a 15–20 nm wide space which is at focal places obliterated by the dense accumulation of the proteins (cadherin and extracellular part of several transmembrane proteins) at the cell surface. Bundles of intermediate filaments project from the intercellular functional areas and radiate into the cytoplasm. This holds the adjacent cells at these focal places. These are of two types:

- *Desmosomes* are the adherens junctions where thickened focal areas are formed on both the opposing cell membranes (Fig. 1.2-4B).
- *Hemidesmosomes* are the adherens junctions where focal thickening is seen only on the membrane of one of the two adjacent cells. So, this is also known as half-desmosome. Adherens junctions are seen in the cells of epidermis. Focal adhesions attach the cell to the basal lamina and also to actin filaments present inside the cell, and thus help in cell movement.

3. Gap Junction. Gap junctions or the nexus are the channels on the lateral surfaces of the two adjacent cells through which the molecules are exchanged between the cells (Fig. 1.2-4C). Each half of the channel is surrounded by 6 subunits of proteins (the *connexins)*. The intercellular space is reduced from the usual size of 15–20 nm to 2–3 nm at such junctions. The gap junctions are seen in the heart and basal part of epithelial cells of intestinal mucous membrane. They serve the following functions:

- These permit the intercellular passage of glucose, amino acids, ions and other substances which have a molecular weight of about 1000.
- These permit rapid propagation of electrical potential changes from one cell to another as seen in cardiac muscle and other smooth muscle cells.
- These help in the exchange of chemical messengers between the cells.

Chapter 1.3

Transport through Cell Membrane

PASSIVE TRANSPORT
- Diffusion
  - Simple diffusion
  - Facilitated diffusion
  - Factors affecting diffusion
- Osmosis
  - Osmotic pressure
  - Osmole, osmolality and osmolarity
  - Tonicity of fluids

ACTIVE TRANSPORT
- Primary active transport
  - Sodium–potassium pump
  - Calcium pump
  - Potassium–hydrogen pump
- Secondary active transport
  - Sodium cotransport
  - Sodium counter-transport

VESICULAR TRANSPORT
- Endocytosis
  - Pinocytosis
  - Phagocytosis
  - Receptor-mediated endocytosis
- Exocytosis
- Transcytosis

OTHER TRANSPORT PROCESSES
- Transport across epithelial membrane
- Ultrafiltration

The physiological activities of a cell depend upon substances like nutrients, oxygen and water, which must be transported into the cell, and at the same time, metabolic waste must be transported out of the cell. Various processes involved in the transport of substances across the cell membrane may be grouped as under:

- Passive transport
- Active transport
- Vesicular transport.

PASSIVE TRANSPORT

Passive transport refers to the mechanism of transport of substances along the gradient without expenditure of any energy. It depends upon the physical factors like concentration gradient, electrical gradient and pressure gradient. Since the transport of substances occurs along the gradient, this process is also called *downhill movement.* The passive transport mechanisms operating at the cell membrane level are diffusion and osmosis.

Diffusion

Diffusion refers to passive transport of molecules from areas of higher concentration to areas of lower concentration. Diffusion through cell membrane is divided into two subtypes — simple diffusion and facilitated diffusion.

Simple Diffusion

In simple diffusion transport of atoms or molecules occurs from one place to another due to their random movement. All the molecules, whether dissolved or undissolved, are at constant random movement except at absolute zero temperature. Due to constant random movement, the molecules collide with each other and also strike with the cell membrane. The frequency of collision and the probability of striking to the cell membrane will be higher on the side of the membrane having higher concentrations of that particular molecule. In this process, there occurs a net flux of the molecules from the areas of high concentration to areas of low concentration. The net movement of the molecules ceases when the concentration of molecules are equal, and there occurs a condition of *diffusional equilibrium.* Quantitatively the net movement of the molecules across a permeable membrane where only simple diffusion is occurring is expressed by *Fick's law of diffusion,* which states that rate of diffusion (J) is directly proportional to the difference in the concentration of the substance in two regions (concentration gradient, i.e. $C_1 - C_2$) and cross-sectional area (A) and inversely proportional to the distance to be travelled (thickness of the membrane, T)

Thus $J = D\dfrac{A(C_1 - C_2)}{T}$, where D is the diffusion coefficient.

The diffusion of molecules across the biological membranes differs depending upon the lipid solubility, water solubility, type of electrical charge and size of the molecules. Further, selective permeability of the semipermeable cell membrane also affects the diffusion of different molecules. How the different molecules diffuse across a cell membrane are discussed below.

Simple Diffusion of Lipid Soluble Substances through the Cell Membrane

The rate of diffusion through the lipid bilayer of the cell membrane is directly proportional to the solubility of a substance in lipids. Therefore, molecules of substances like oxygen, nitrogen, carbon dioxide, alcohol, steroid hormones and weak organic acids and bases, being lipid soluble, diffuse very rapidly through the lipid bilayer of the cell membrane.

Simple Diffusion of Water and Other Lipid Insoluble Molecules through the Cell Membrane

Astonishingly, water and other lipid insoluble substances can also pass easily through the cell membrane. It has been shown that it is possible due to the presence of the so-called *protein channels* (made from transmembrane proteins) in the cell membrane.

Diffusion through Protein Channels

The protein channels are tube-shaped channels that extend in the cell membrane from the extracellular to the intracellular ends (Fig. 1.3-1). Therefore, even the highly lipid insoluble substances can diffuse by simple diffusion directly through these channels of the cell membrane. However, permeability of such substances depends upon their molecular size, shape and charge.

The protein channels are equipped with following characteristics:

- Selective permeability and
- Gating mechanism.

Selective Permeability of Protein Channels The protein channels are highly selective, i.e. each channel can permit only one type of ion to pass through it. This results from the characteristics of the channel itself, such as, its diameter, its shape and nature of electrical charges along its inside surfaces. Examples of some selective channels are:

- *Sodium channels* are specifically selective for the passage of sodium ions. These are 0.3 by 0.5 nm in size and their inner surfaces are *strongly negatively charged* (Fig. 1.3-2).
- *Potassium channels* are specifically selective for the passage of potassium ions. These are 0.3 by 0.3 nm in size and *not negatively charged* (Fig. 1.3-3).

Gating Mechanism in Protein Channels Some protein channels are continuously open, whereas most others are 'gated', i.e. they are equipped with actual gate-like extensions of the transport protein molecule that can open and close as per requirement. This gating mechanism is a means of controlling the permeability of the channels. The opening and closing of gates are controlled by three principal ways:

1. ***Voltage-Gated Channels.*** These respond to the electrical potential across the cell membrane. As shown in

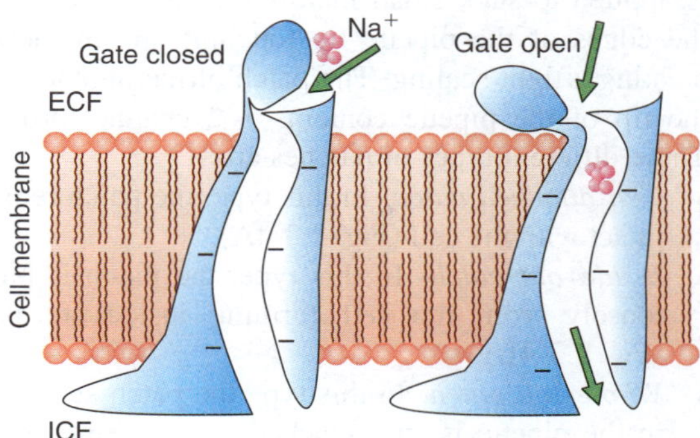

FIGURE 1.3-2 Voltage-gated sodium channels.

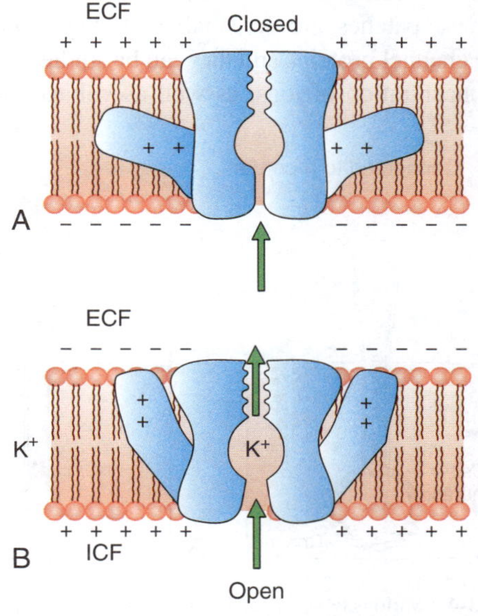

FIGURE 1.3-3 Voltage-gated potassium channels.

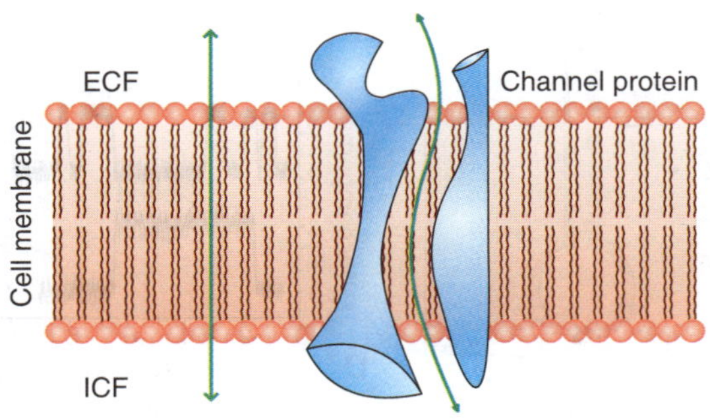

FIGURE 1.3-1 Simple diffusion.

Fig. 1.3-2, in the case of sodium channels, the gates are located at the outer end of the channels and these remain tightly closed, when there is a strong negative charge on the inside of cell membrane. When the inside of cell membrane loses its negative charge, these gates open and there occurs a tremendous inflow of sodium ions. This is the basis of occurrence of action potential in nerves that are responsible for nerve signals.

In the case of potassium channels, the gates are located at the inner end of the channel (Fig. 1.3-3) and they too open when the inside of the cell membrane loses its negative charge, but this response is much slower than that for the sodium channel. The opening of potassium channel gates is partly responsible for terminating the action potential.

The ion current flow through a single voltage-gated channel protein can be recorded by the patch clamp technique.

Patch clamp method is a simple method in which a micropipette of tip diameter 1–2 micrometre is abutted against the outer surface of the membrane and suction is applied to suck small membrane inside the pipette, the edges of the pipette tip touching the membrane, creating a tight sealing. The patch of membrane inside the tip of the pipette contains 1–2 channel proteins. Three different types of patches are:

- *Cell-attached patch:* In this type, the patch remains intact with the cell (Fig. 1.3-4A).
- *Inside–out patch:* In this type, the patch is pulled loosely from the cell forming inside–out patch (Fig. 1.3-4B).
- *Whole-cell patch:* In this type the patch sucked out in the pipette is still attached on to the rest of the cell membrane, thus providing direct access to the interior of the whole cell and is also known as whole cell recording (Fig. 1.3-4C).

These patches are so small that they contain only single channel proteins and that can be studied by varying the concentration of ions, as well as voltage, across the membrane. The transport characteristics and also the opening and closing of gates can be studied (Fig. 1.3-4D).

2. ***Ligand Gated Channels.*** Gates of these channels open when some other chemical molecule binds with the gate proteins, which is why this is also called *chemical gating.* The ligand (binding molecules) may be internal or *external.*
   - The external or extracellular ligands are also called *first messengers.* One of the most important examples of external ligand channel gating is the effect of acetylcholine on the so-called *acetylcholine channels.* This gate plays an important role in transmission of nerve signals from one nerve cell to another and from nerve cells to muscle cells.
   - The internal or the intracellular ligands are also called *second messengers.* The examples include intracellular Ca^{2+}, cAMP, or G protein produced in the cells. The second messenger generally activates protein kinases.
3. ***Mechanically Gated Channels.*** Some protein channels are opened by mechanical stretch. These mechanosensitive channels play an important role in cell movements.

Facilitated Diffusion

The water soluble substances having larger molecules, such as glucose, cannot diffuse through the protein channels by simple diffusion. Such substances diffuse through the cell membrane with the help of some carrier proteins. Therefore, this type of diffusion is called facilitated or carrier-mediated diffusion. There are many types of carrier proteins in the cell membrane, each type having binding sites that are specific for a particular substance. Among the most important substances that cross cell membranes by facilitated diffusion are *glucose* and most of the *amino acids.*

Mechanism of Facilitated Diffusion

Postulated mechanism for facilitated diffusion is shown in Fig. 1.3-5. As shown in the figure, a conformational change

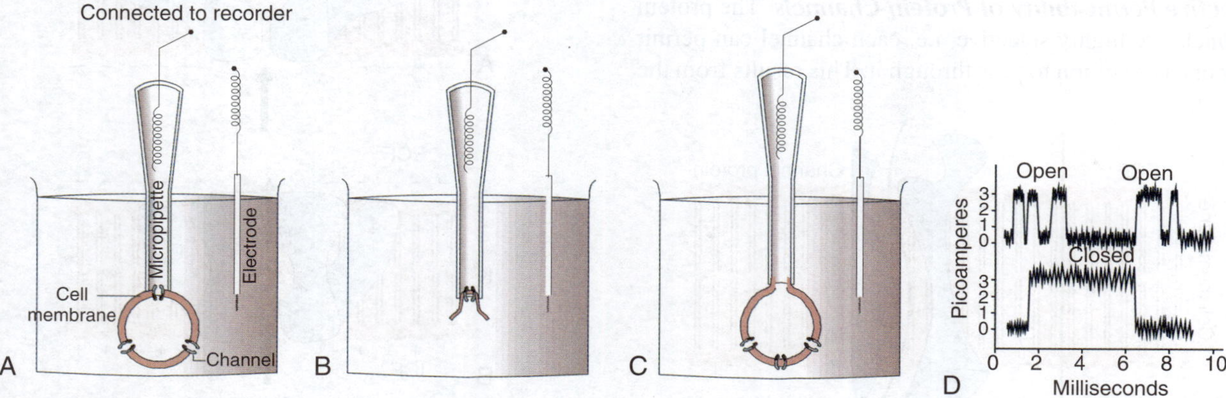

FIGURE 1.3-4 Various types of patch clamps used to study the activity of ion channels across the membrane: **A,** cell attached patch; **B,** inside out patch; **C,** whole cell patch; and **D,** note the changes in the membrane current with time and its flow through sodium channels.

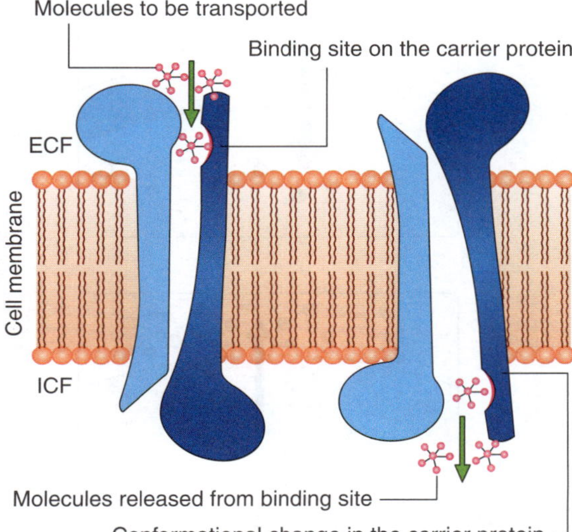

FIGURE 1.3-5 Postulated mechanism of facilitated diffusion.

occurs in the carrier protein after the molecule to be transported is bound at the receptor site. The repetitive spontaneous configurational changes allow the diffusion of the molecule. Earlier belief was that the carrier protein acts like a shuttle between the outer and inner surfaces of the cell membrane, and it has been discarded now.

Types of Carrier Protein Systems Three types of carrier protein systems are known: uniport, symport and antiport (Fig. 1.3-6). The symports and antiport are together known as cotransport.

1. ***Uniport.*** In this system, the carrier proteins transport only one type of molecules.
2. ***Symport.*** In this system, transport of one substance is linked with transfer of another substance. For example, facilitated diffusion of glucose in the renal tubular cells is linked with the transport of sodium.
3. ***Antiport.*** In this system, the carrier proteins exchange one substance for another. For example, Na^+–K^+ exchange or Na^+–H^+ exchange in the renal tubules.

Differences between Simple and Facilitated Diffusions

1. ***Specificity.*** The carrier proteins are highly specific for different molecules.
2. ***Saturation.*** As shown in Fig. 1.3-7, in simple diffusion, the rate of diffusion increases proportionately with the increase in the concentration of the substance and there is no limit to it. However, in facilitated diffusion, the rate of diffusion increases with increase in concentration gradient to reach a limit beyond which a further increase in the diffusion cannot occur. This is called *saturation* point, and here all the binding sites on the carrier proteins are occupied and the system operates at its maximum capacity.
3. ***Competition.*** When two molecules, say A and B, are carried by the same protein, there occurs a competition between the two molecules for the transport. Thus, an increase in the concentration of 'A' molecule will decrease the transport of molecule 'B', and vice versa. No such competition is known to occur in simple diffusion.

Factors Affecting Net Rate of Diffusion The mechanisms described above deal with the diffusion of substances through the cell membrane. The diffusion of the

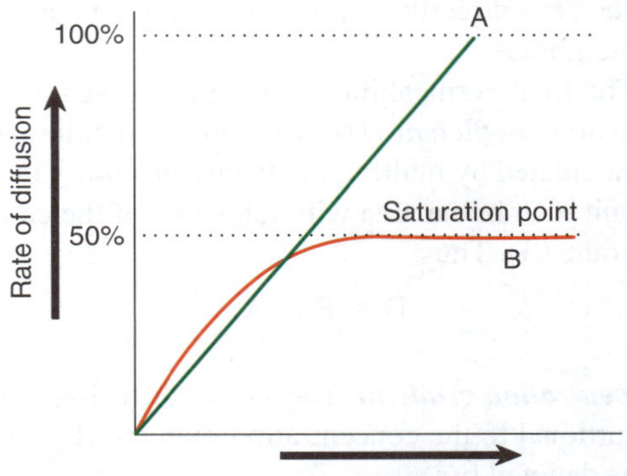

FIGURE 1.3-7 Effect of concentration of substance on rate of diffusion in: **A,** simple diffusion; and **B,** facilitated diffusion.

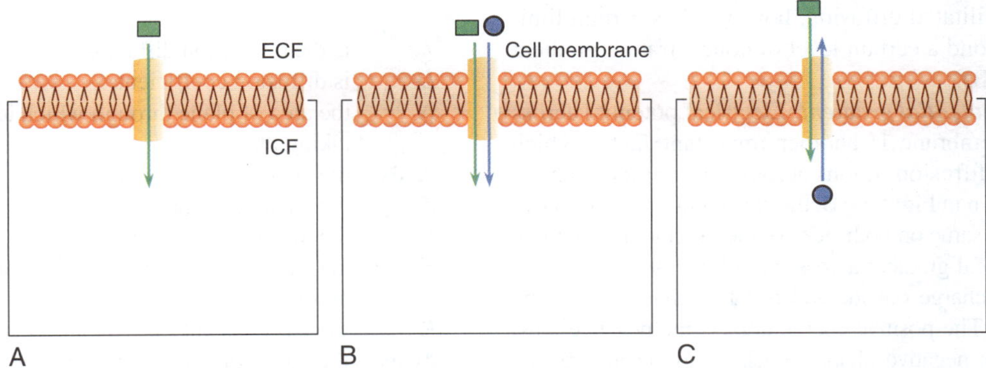

FIGURE 1.3-6 Various types of carrier protein systems: **A,** uniport; **B,** symport; and **C,** antiport.

substance can occur either way, i.e. ECF to ICF and vice versa, depending upon the prevailing environment. The factors that affect the net rate of diffusion in the desired direction are summarized:

1. ***Cell membrane permeability.*** Permeability of the cell membrane (*P*) is the major determining factor for the net diffusion, which in turn depends upon the following factors:
   - *Thickness of the membrane.* The diffusion is inversely proportional to the thickness of the cell membrane, i.e. the greater the thickness, lesser is the rate of diffusion.
   - *Lipid solubility.* Diffusion is directly proportional to the lipid solubility of the substance.
   - *Distribution of protein channels in the cell membrane.* The rate of diffusion of lipid insoluble substance is directly proportional to the number of channels per unit area of the cell membrane.
   - *Temperature.* Rate of diffusion increases with increase in the temperature. This is because of the increased motion of the molecules and ions of the solution with increase in temperature.
   - *Size of the molecules.* Rate of simple diffusion is inversely proportional to the size of molecules.
   - *Area of the membrane.* The net diffusion of the substance is directly proportional to the total area of the membrane.
   - The total permeability is often expressed as the *diffusion coefficient (D)* of the entire membrane. It is calculated by multiplying the permeability through a unit membrane area with total area of the cell membrane (*A*). Thus:

$$D = P \times A$$

2. ***Concentration gradient.*** The simple diffusion is directly proportional to the concentration gradient (Fig. 1.3-8A) and is denoted by:

   Net diffusion α D ($C_0 - C_1$), where C_0 is concentration of the substance outside, C_1 is concentration of the substance inside and D is the diffusion coefficient of the cell membrane for the substance.

   The facilitated diffusion, however, has certain limitations beyond a certain level of concentration gradient (Fig. 1.3-7B).
3. ***Electrical potential gradient.*** Electrical potential across the cell membrane is another important factor which affects the diffusion of ions across the cell membrane.

   As shown in Fig. 1.3-8B, the concentrations of negative ions are the same on both sides of the membrane, but there is an electrical gradient across the cell membrane because of positive charge outside and negative charge inside the membrane. The positive charge attracts the negative ions, whereas the negative charge repels them. Therefore, net diffusion occurs from inside to outside till the concentration gradient created balances the electrical gradient. In other words, net diffusion of any ion across the cell membrane (*J*) will be the resultant of the combined effect of concentration gradient and electrical potential gradient, and is denoted by the following equation:

$$J = -DA\left[dc/dx + \left(Z\frac{CF}{RT}\right)dv/dx\right]$$

J	is the rate of ion diffusion,
D	is diffusion coefficient,
A	the area of plane through which ion movement is taking place,
dc/dx	the concentration gradient
Z	the valency of the ion,
C	the ion concentration,
F	the Faraday constant (96,500 coulomb per mol of ion),
R	the gas constant (8.316 joules per degree),
dv/dx	the absolute temperature and the electrical potential gradient.

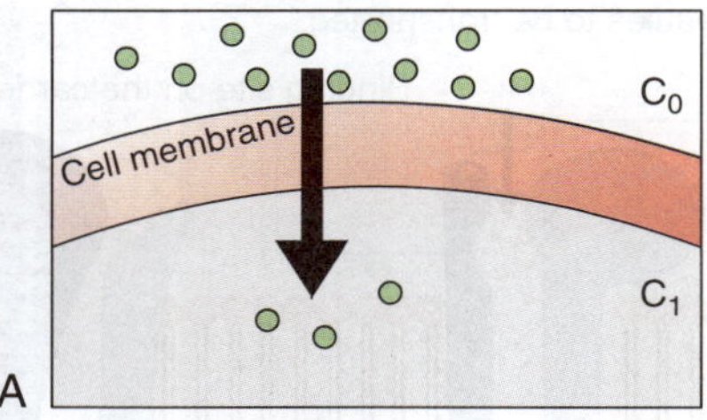

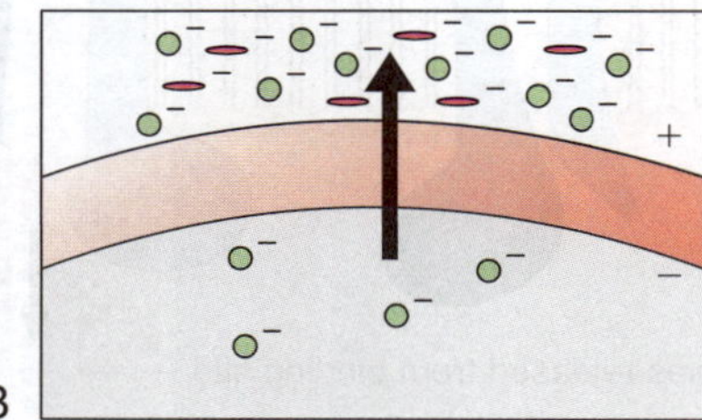

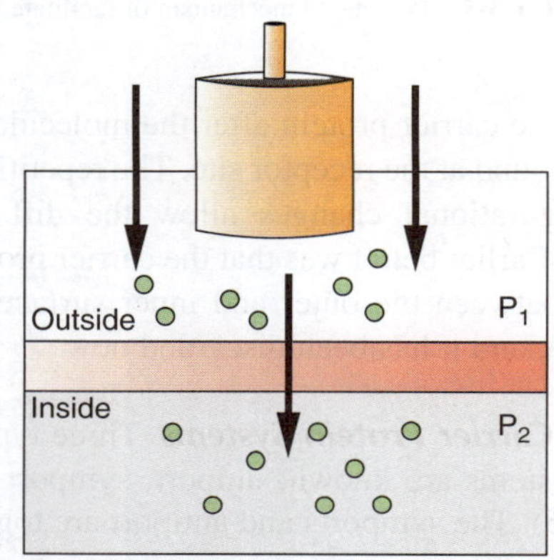

FIGURE 1.3-8 Factors affecting net rate of diffusion: **A,** concentration gradient; **B,** electrical gradient; and **C,** pressure gradient.

At normal body temperature (37°C), the electrical gradient that will balance the concentration gradient of a univalent ion can be determined by *Nernst equation:*

$$\text{EMF (in millivolts)} = \pm 61 \log \frac{C_0}{C_1}, \text{ where}$$

- EMF is the electromotive force between outside and inside of the membrane,
- C_0 is the concentration of ion outside the membrane and
- C_1 is the concentration of ion inside the membrane.

This equation is extremely important in understanding the membrane potential, hence discussed in detail in the relevant section (page 32).

4. ***Pressure gradient.*** It has been observed that the increased amounts of energy are available to cause net movements of molecules from the high pressure side towards the low pressure side. The pressure-gradient effect is demonstrated in Fig. 1.3-8C, which shows that high pressure developed by the piston on one side of the cell membrane causes greater number of molecules to strike the membrane resulting in net diffusion to the other side.

Osmosis

Osmosis refers to diffusion of water or any other solvent molecules through a semipermeable membrane, (i.e. membrane permeable to solvent but not to the solute) from a solution containing lower concentration of solutes towards the solution containing higher concentration of solutes, Fig. 1.3-9 shows osmosis across a selective permeable membrane. When a sodium chloride solution is placed on one side of the membrane and water on the other side (Fig. 1.3-9A); net movement of water occurs from the pure water into the sodium chloride solution (Fig. 1.3-9B).

Osmotic Pressure

Osmotic pressure refers to the minimum pressure which when applied on the side of higher solute concentration prevents the osmosis. Fig. 1.3-9C shows that when appropriate pressure is applied, the net diffusion of water into the sodium chloride solution is prevented.

The osmotic pressure in the body fluids refers to the pressure exerted by the solutes dissolved in water or other solvents. The osmotic pressure exerted by the colloidal substances in the body is called *colloidal osmotic pressure.* The colloidal osmotic pressure due to plasma colloids (proteins) is called *oncotic pressure.*

The osmotic pressure depends upon the number of molecules or ions dissolved in a solution rather than their size, type or chemical composition. In case of nondissociated solutes, one gram molecular weight of any substance shall contain similar number of molecules, and hence exert similar degree of osmotic pressure, i.e. equal to 22.4 atmospheres, whereas, in case of dissociated solutes, the osmotic pressure depends upon the number of ions resulting from its dissociation.

Osmole, Osmolality and Osmolarity

Osmole. is the unit used in place of grams to express the concentration in terms of number of osmotically active particles in a given solution. One osmole is equal to the molecular weight of a substance in grams divided by the number of freely moving particles liberated in solution by each molecule. Thus:

- A molar solution of glucose contains 1 mole and exerts osmotic pressure of 1 atmosphere.
- A molar solution of NaCl contains 2 osmoles (1 mole of Na^+ and 1 mole of Cl^-) and exerts osmotic pressure of 2 atmospheres.

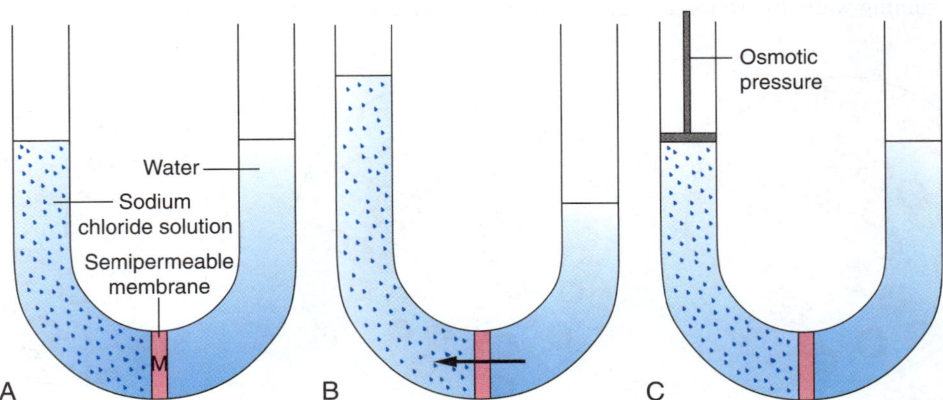

FIGURE 1.3-9 Diagrammatic representation of phenomenon of osmosis: **A,** semipermeable membrane 'M' separates sodium chloride solution from pure water; **B,** net movement of water occurs through (M) from pure water side into the sodium chloride solution side; and **C,** demonstration of osmotic pressure (net movement of water from pure water side to sodium chloride solution is prevented by applying appropriate pressure on the solution side).

- A molar solution of $CaCl_2$ contains 3 osmoles (1 mole of Ca^{2+} and 2 moles of Cl^-) and thus exerts osmotic pressure of 3 atmospheres.
- One milli osmole (mOsm) is 1/1000 of an osmole.

Osmolality. of a solution refers to the number of osmotically active particles (osmoles) per kilogram (kg) of a solution, while, ***osmolarity*** refers to the number of osmoles per litre (L) of a solution. Therefore, osmolarity is affected by the volume of the various solutes in the solution and the temperature, while osmolality is not. The osmotic pressure is determined by the osmolality and not osmolarity. However, the quantitative differences between the osmolarity and osmolality are less than 1%. In practice, *osmolarity* is more frequently used in physiological studies, since it is far easier to measure osmolarity vis-a-vis osmolality.

Normal plasma osmolality. The normal osmolality of the extracellular and intracellular fluids is 290 milliosmoles per kilogram (mOsm/kg). In the plasma of the total osmolality, 270 mOsm are contributed by Na^+, Cl^- and HCO_3^-. The remaining 20 mOsm are contributed by glucose and urea. Because of the large molecular weight and hence lesser number of particles, plasma proteins (70 g/L) contribute 2 mOsm to the total plasma osmolality.

Tonicity of Fluids

In clinical practice the word tonicity always refers to tonicity of a solution with respect to that of plasma (290 mOsm). In other words, it is the red blood cell (RBC) membrane across which the tonicity is tested. Thus:

- *Isotonic fluids* are those which have osmolality similar to plasma. RBCs neither shrink nor swell in such solution (Fig. 1.3-10A). A solution of 0.9% NaCl is isotonic with plasma.
- *Hypertonic fluids* have osmolality higher than the plasma. The RBCs shrink in such solutions by losing water by osmosis (Fig. 1.3-10B).
- *Hypotonic fluids* are those whose osmolality is lower than that of plasma. The RBCs swell up in hypotonic solutions by gaining water by osmosis (Fig. 1.3-10C).

Clinically Applied Aspects

- The total plasma osmolality may increase in patients having severe dehydration.
- Increased blood glucose levels in patients with severe diabetes also increase the plasma osmolality.
- Excessive intravenous administration of 5% glucose decreases plasma osmolality leading to swelling of the body tissues.
- Hyperosmolality can cause coma by causing water to flow out of the brain cells (hyperosmolar coma)
- Raised plasma levels of urea in patients with renal diseases also cause hyperosmolality.

ACTIVE TRANSPORT

Active transport refers to the mechanism of transport of substances against the chemical and/or electrical gradient. Active transport involves expenditure of energy which is liberated by breakdown of high energy compounds like ATP. Since the transport of substances occur against the chemico-electrical gradient, this process is also called *up-hill movement.*

Mechanism of Active Transport

The active transport is also carrier mediated, but its mechanism is different from that of facilitated diffusion. However, since the carrier proteins are involved in the transport mechanism, so like facilitated diffusion the active transport also shows specificity, saturation and competition.

Since the active transport mechanism involves the expenditure of energy, the transporting carrier protein system is also called the *'active pump mechanism'*. The substance to be transported combines with the specific carrier protein on the cell membrane. The complex so formed undergoes conformational changes and is actively pumped towards the inner surface of cell membrane where the substance is released and the carrier protein moves back to the outer surface to transport another molecule.

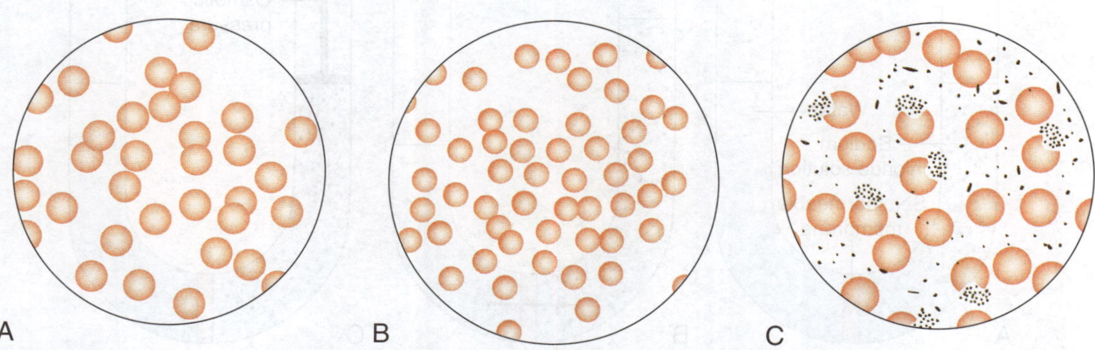

FIGURE 1.3-10 Tonicity of fluids: **A,** isotonic fluid (0.9% NaCl) has osmolarity similar to plasma, RBCs neither shrink nor swell in it; **B,** hypertonic fluid (2% NaCl) has osmolarity higher than plasma, RBCs shrink in it; and **C,** hypotonic fluid (0.3% NaCl) has osmolarity lower than plasma, RBCs swell in it and burst open.

Substances transported actively across the cell membrane include:

- ***Ionic substances*** such as Na^+, K^+, Ca^{2+}, Cl^- and I^- and
- ***Nonionic substances*** like glucose, amino acids and urea.

Types of Active Transport

The active transport is of two types:

- Primary active transport and
- Secondary active transport.

A. Primary Active Transport Processes

In primary active transport process, the energy is derived directly from the breakdown of adenosine triphosphate (ATP) or some other high-energy phosphate compound. Some of the important pumps involved in the primary active transport processes are:

- Sodium–potassium pump,
- Calcium pump and
- Potassium–hydrogen pump.

1. Sodium–Potassium Pump

Sodium–potassium (Na^+–K^+) pump is present in all the cells of the body. It is involved with the active transport of sodium ions outwards through the cell membrane and potassium ions inwards, simultaneously. Thus, this pump is responsible for maintaining the Na^+ and K^+ concentration differences across the cell membrane and for establishing a negative electrical potential inside the cells.

***Structure of Na^+–K^+ Pump** (Fig. 1.3-11).* The carrier protein involved in Na^+–K^+ pump is a complex consisting of two separate protein units, a larger the α subunit (molecular weight approximately 100,000) and a smaller β subunit (molecular weight approximately 55,000). The α subunit is mainly concerned with Na^+ –K^+ transport. It has got following binding sites:

- Three intracellular sites, one each for binding sodium ions ($3Na^+$) and ATP, and one phosphorylation site.
- Two extracellular sites, one each for binding potassium ions ($2K^+$) and ouabain.

***Mechanism of Operation of Na^+ – K^+ Pump** (Fig. 1.3-12).* The functioning of Na^+–K^+ pump involves the use of enzyme ATPase. The enzyme ATPase is activated when three sodium ions and one ATP molecule bind to their respective binding sites. The activated ATPase catalyses the hydrolysis of ATP to ADP and liberates a high-energy phosphate bond of energy (phosphorylation). The energy so liberated is believed to cause a conformational change in the carrier protein molecule extruding sodium into the extracellular fluid. This is followed by binding of two potassium ions to the receptor site on extracellular surface of the carrier protein and dephosphorylation of α subunit which returns to its previous conformation, releasing potassium into the cytoplasm.

Functions of Na^+–K^+ Pump. The Na^+–K^+ pump subserves two main functions:

1. *Controlling the cell volume.* It is the most important function of the Na^+–K^+ pump, without which most cells of the body will swell up until they burst. Inside the cells are large number of proteins and other organic compounds that cannot escape from the cell. Being negatively charged, these also collect large number of positive ions. All these substances cause osmosis of water to the interior of the cell, which is prevented by the Na^+–K^+ pump. When the Na^+–K^+ pump fails the cells swell up and burst.
2. *Electrogenic activity.* Na^+ –K^+ pump acts as electrogenic pump since it produces a net movement of positive charge out of the cell ($3Na^+$ out and $2K^+$ in); Thus

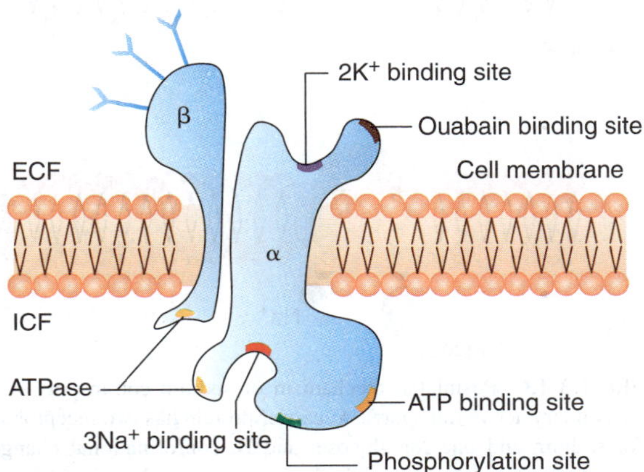

FIGURE 1.3-11 Structure of sodium-potassium ATPase pump.

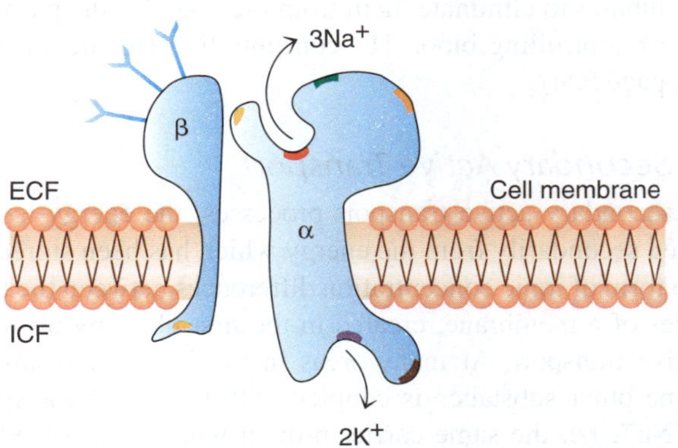

FIGURE 1.3-12 Mechanism of operation of sodium–potassium ATPase pump.

creating electrical potential across the cell membrane. This is a basic requirement in nerves and muscles to transmit the signals.

Regulation of Na^+–K^+ Pump. The activity of Na^+–K^+ pump is affected as:

- increased by cAMP, diacylglycerol (DAG), thyroid hormone, aldosterone, insulin and G actin, and
- Inhibited by low temperature, oxygen lack, dopamine, ouabain and related glycosides (digitalis) used for the treatment of heart failure.

2. Calcium Pump

The calcium pump forms another important active transport mechanism. Like Na^+–K^+ pump it also operates through a carrier protein which has ATPase activity. But the difference from Na^+–K^+ pump is that the carrier protein binds calcium ions rather than sodium and potassium ions. The calcium pump helps in maintaining extremely low concentrations of calcium in the intracellular fluid (10,000 times less than the ECF). There are two primary active transport calcium pumps. One is in the cell membrane which extrudes Ca^{2+} out of the cell, and the other calcium pump actively transports cytoplasmic calcium into the one or more of the cellular organelles like sarcoplasmic reticulum of the muscle cells and mitochondria of all the cells.

3. Potassium–Hydrogen Pump

The primary active transport system of hydrogen ion also operates through ATPase (K^+–H^+ ATPase) activity. These are present at following two places in the human body:

- *Parietal cells of gastric glands.* The K^+–H^+ pump located in these cells actively transports H^+ out of the cells into the lumen of gastric glands and K^+ into the cell from the lumen. The H^+ combines Cl^- to form HCl in the lumen of gastric glands (for details see page 591).
- *Renal tubules.* The K^+–H^+ pump is located in the intercalated cells of late distal tubules and cortical collecting ducts. Here large amounts of H^+ are secreted into the tubules to eliminate them from the body for the purpose of controlling blood H^+ concentration (for details see page 524).

B. Secondary Active Transport

In secondary active transport processes, the energy is derived secondarily from the energy which has been stored in the form of ionic concentration differences between the two sides of a membrane, created in the first place by primary active transport. At many areas in the body, transport of some other substance is coupled with the active transport of Na^+, i.e. the same carrier protein which is involved in the active transport of Na^+ also secondarily transports some other substance. The secondary active transport of substance may occur in the form of sodium cotransport or sodium counter-transport.

Sodium Cotransport

The carrier protein here acts as symport, i.e. transports some other substance along with the sodium. Substances carried by sodium cotransport include glucose, amino acids, chloride and iodine.

1. ***Sodium cotransport of glucose.*** The glucose is transported into most cells against large concentration gradient. As shown in Fig. 1.3-13A, the carrier protein has two receptor sites on the outer surface, one for sodium and other for glucose. The special feature of the carrier protein is that the conformational change in it occurs only when both the sodium and glucose molecules are attached to it. Due to conformational change in the carrier protein, both the sodium and the glucose are transported simultaneously inside the cell (Fig. 1.3-13B). The cotransport of glucose occurs during its absorption from the intestine into the blood and during the reabsorption of glucose from renal tubule in the blood (Fig. 1.3-14).
2. ***Sodium cotransport of amino acids.*** Occurs especially in the epithelial cells of intestinal tract and renal tubules during absorption of the amino acids into the blood. The mechanism of sodium cotransport of amino acids is similar to that of glucose, except that the carrier proteins involved are different. There are five sets of carrier proteins in the cell membrane, each transporting different amino acids depending upon their molecular weights.

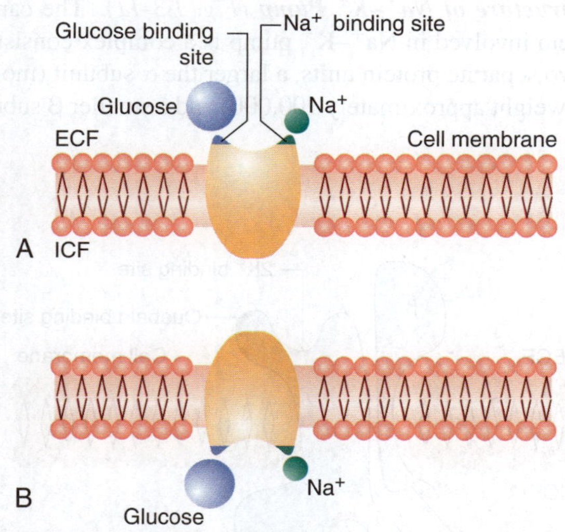

FIGURE 1.3-13 Postulated mechanism of sodium cotransport of glucose (secondary active transport): **A,** carrier protein has two receptor sites, one for sodium and one for glucose; and **B,** conformational change in carrier protein causes transport of both glucose and sodium inside the cell simultaneously.

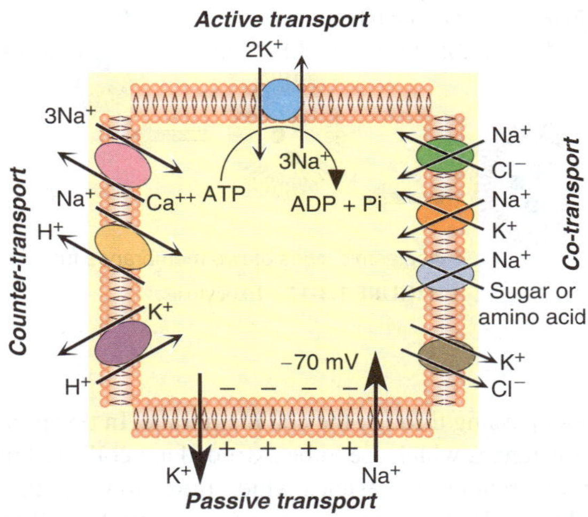

FIGURE 1.3-14 Composite diagram of the cell showing the various cotransport and counter-transport mechanisms and maintenance of membrane potential as an effect of primary active transport of Na^+ and K^+.

Sodium Counter-Transport

The carrier protein involved here acts as *antiport,* i.e. sodium ion is exchanged for some other substance. Some of the sodium counter-transport mechanisms occurring in the body are:

1. ***Sodium–calcium counter-transport*** is known to occur in almost all cell membranes with sodium ions moving inside and calcium outside the cell (Fig. 1.3-14). The transport of these ions in the opposite direction is carried by the same carrier protein.
2. ***Sodium–hydrogen counter-transport*** is especially known in the proximal tubules of kidney. Here the Na^+ ions move inside the cell and the H^+ ions move out of the cell by the same carrier protein.
3. ***Other counter-transport systems*** which exist somewhere in the body are sodium–potassium counter-transport system, sodium–magnesium counter-transport, calcium–magnesium countertransport system and chloride–bicarbonate counter-transport system.

VESICULAR TRANSPORT

Vesicular transport mechanisms are involved in the transport of macromolecules such as large protein molecules which can neither pass through the cell membrane by diffusion nor by active transport mechanisms. The vesicular transport mechanisms include endocytosis, exocytosis and transcytosis.

Endocytosis

Endocytosis is the process in which the substance is transported into the cell by infolding of the cell membrane around the substance and internalizing it (Fig. 1.3-15). It is further of three types:

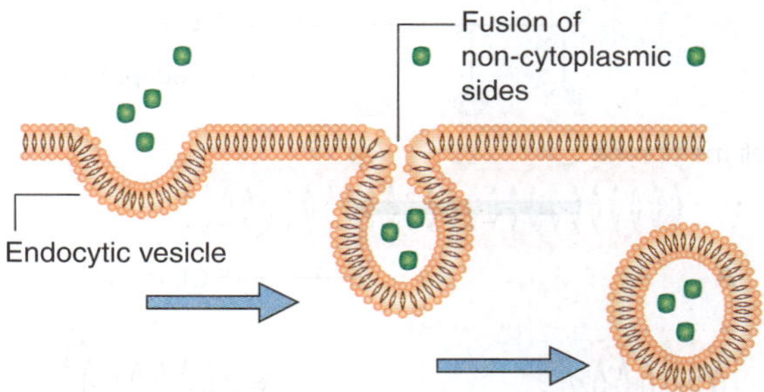

FIGURE 1.3-15 Constitutive pathway of endocytosis.

1. ***Pinocytosis,*** i.e. cell drinking refers to the process of engulfing liquid substances by the enfolding of cell membrane, e.g. reabsorption by renal tubular epithelial cells.
2. ***Phagocytosis,*** i.e. cell eating is the process of engulfing of solid particles such as bacteria, dead tissue and foreign particles by the cells. The process of phagocytosis involves three steps (i) the attachment stage, (ii) the engulfment stage and (iii) killing or degradation stage (see page 169).
3. ***Receptor-mediated endocytosis.*** In this process the substance to be transported binds with the special receptor proteins present on the cell surface. The receptor protein-substance complex is then engulfed by the cell membrane by the process of endocytosis. Transport of iron and cholesterol into the cells occurs by receptor-mediated endocytosis.

Mechanism of Endocytosis

There are two pathways by which endocytosis takes place:

1. ***Constitutive pathway (constitutive endocytosis).*** In this process the molecule (substance) first makes contact with the cell membrane, then the cell membrane invaginates to form *endocytic vesicle* followed by fusion of noncytoplasmic sides of the cell membrane and invagination is pinched off (Fig. 1.3-15).
2. ***Clathrin-mediated pathway (clathrin-mediated endocytosis).*** Clathrin-mediated endocytosis occurs at the specific sites (indentation) on the cell membrane where clathrin (a protein) accumulates (Fig. 1.3-16A–D).
   - *Structure.* Clathrin molecule is triskelion shaped with three legs radiating from the central hub.
   - *Role of clathrin.* As the endocytosis progresses, clathrin molecule forms a geometrical array and surrounds the endocytic vesicle. After complete formation of the vesicle, the clathrin molecule falls off recycle to form another vesicle. During this process another protein called *dynamin* is also involved. It helps in pinching off the vesicle at the neck region of the vesicle.
   - *Clathrin-mediated* endocytosis is responsible for internalization of substances like, nerve growth

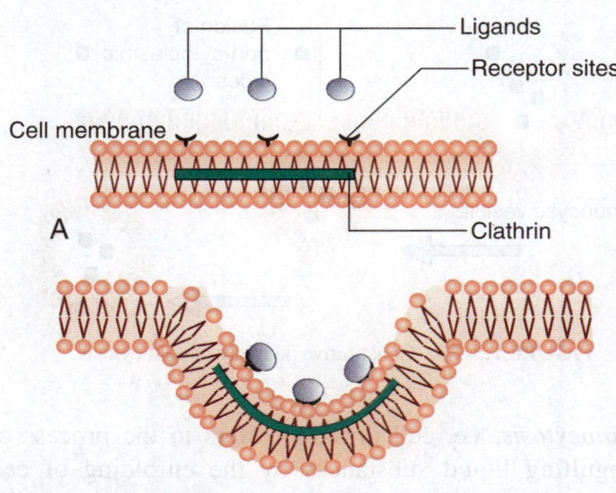

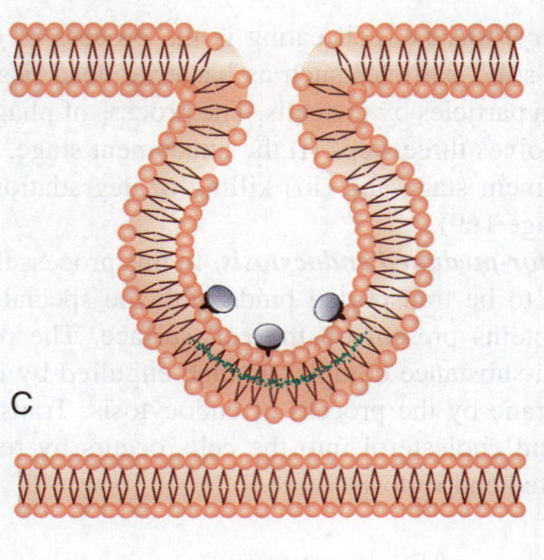

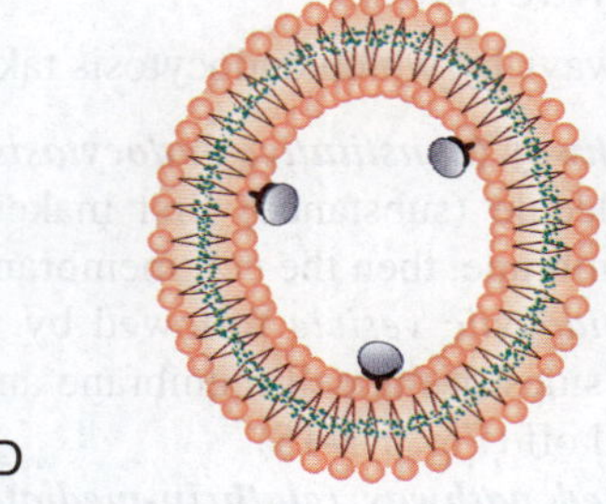

FIGURE 1.3-16 Clathrin-mediated endocytosis: **A,** the cell membrane showing receptors (to which the substance binds) and accumulation of clathrin; **B** and **C,** formation of endocytic vesicle; and **D,** complete internalization.

factor, low density lipoproteins. Receptor-mediated endocytosis also occurs by this mechanism.

The cell membrane also contains small caveolae, indentations coated with protein caveolin involved in ingestion of various amino acids and peptides.

Exocytosis

Exocytosis (Fig. 1.3-17) is reverse of endocytosis, i.e. by this process the substances are expelled from the cell

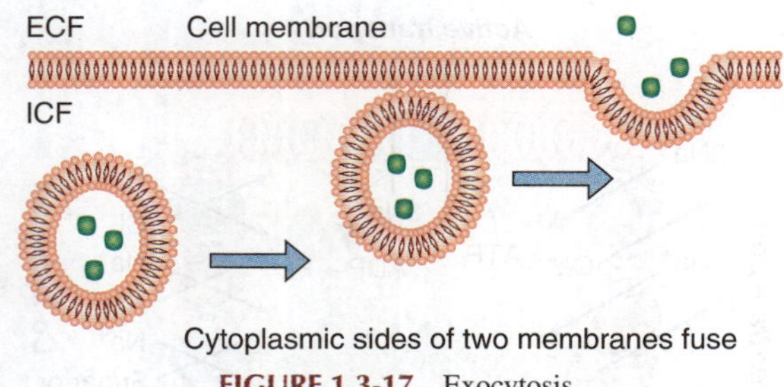

FIGURE 1.3-17 Exocytosis.

without passing through the cell membrane. In this process, the substances which are to be extruded are collected in the form of granules or vesicles which move towards the cell membrane. Their membrane then fuses with the cell membrane. The area of fusion breaks down releasing the contents to the exterior and leaving the cell membrane intact. Release of hormones and enzymes by secretory cells of the body occurs by exocytosis. The process of exocytosis requires Ca^{2+} and energy along with docking proteins. Excretion of specific hormones and granules by the cells is termed as *emiocytosis.*

There are two pathways by which secretion from the cell occurs.

1. ***Nonconstitutive pathway.*** In this process the proteins from the Golgi apparatus initially enter in the secretory granules, where processing of prohormones to mature hormones occur before exocytosis.
2. ***Constitutive pathway.*** It involves the prompt transport of proteins to the cell membrane in vesicles, with little or no processing or storage.

Transcytosis

Vesicular transport within the cell is called transcytosis or cytopemisis. It is quite similar to exocytosis and endocytosis. Three basic steps involved in this process are (i) vesicle formation, (ii) vesicle transportation and (iii) docking in the cell.

Role of Various Proteins in Vesicular Transport

The vesicles involved in the transport are coated with proteins. The different types of coating proteins have been identified which are:

- *AP-1 clathrin* present in vesicles involved in transportation from Golgi apparatus to lysosomes.
- *AP-2 clathrin* exists in endocytic vesicles involved in transportation to endosomes.
- *CO-PI and CO-PII* are coating proteins present in vesicles involved for transportation between endoplasmic reticulum and Golgi apparatus.
- *Dynamin* appears to be involved in vesicle formation from Golgi apparatus and also from cell membrane.

- *Docking protein.* Each target cell has a set of docking proteins (V snare protein) and latch proteins (T snare protein). The vesicle, when it reaches its target cell, then these proteins ensure that the vesicle will dock with the corresponding set of docking proteins.

OTHER TRANSPORT PROCESSES

So far we have considered transport across the cell membrane, i.e. movement of substances between the intracellular fluid (ICF) and extracellular fluid (ECF) through the cell membrane. In addition to it, there are many situations in the body where transport of substances occurs through the epithelia and the capillary endothelial cell membrane. Some of these processes discussed briefly are:

- Transport across epithelia and
- Ultrafiltration.

Transport Across Epithelia

Transport across epithelia involves movement of the substances from one side of the epithelium to the other. The transepithelial transport occurs in body cavities lined by continuous sheet of cells such as in gastrointestinal tract, renal tubules, pulmonary airways and other structures. For transepithelial transport to occur, the cells need to be bound by tight junctions, and have different ion channels and transport protein in different parts of their membrane. Transport across epithelia may occur in two ways:

1. ***Transport through the cells proper.*** In gastro-intestinal tract and in urinary tubules substances are transferred from the lumen into the epithelial cells at their apical borders and then from the basal borders of the cells into interstitial fluid. From the interstitial fluid the substances are finally transported into the blood through the capillaries.
2. ***Transport across the tight junctions.*** It has been identified that in the epithelia of small intestine, proximal renal tubules and gall bladder, most of the sodium chloride passes through the tight junctions (areas of tight adherence between the two adjacent cells) rather than traversing the whole length of the epithelial cells.

Ultrafiltration

When a solution of protein and salt is separated from plain water or a less concentrated salt solution by a membrane permeable to salt and water and not to the protein, there will be a net movement of water on the protein side by diffusion and a movement of salt away from the protein side. This process is called dialysis (Fig. 6.5-7).

Ultrafiltration. Refers to occurrence of dialysis under hydrostatic pressure (Fig. 4.4-26). Ultrafiltration occurs at the capillary level in the body. The capillary blood is under hydrostatic pressure. The pressure is 35 mmHg near the arteriolar end and gradually declines to 12 mmHg near the venous end of the capillary. Through the capillaries there occurs ultrafiltration of all the constituents of the plasma except the proteins into the interstitial spaces. Ultrafiltration plays an important role in the formation of body fluids. Plasma proteins, to which the capillary wall is not permeable, exert an osmotic pressure of about 25 mmHg. This osmotic pressure opposes the hydrostatic pressure, resulting in limitation of outflow of fluid from the capillaries near the arteriolar end and backflow of interstitial fluid into capillaries (by osmosis) near their venous end where osmotic pressure (25 mmHg) is greater than the hydrostatic pressure of blood (12 mmHg) (Fig. 4.4-26).

Chapter 1.4

Membrane Potential

INTRODUCTION

There exists a potential difference across the membrane of all living cells with the inside being negative in relation to the outside. This potential difference is named *membrane potential,* because the cations and anions arrange themselves along the outer and inner surfaces of the cell membrane. The magnitude of membrane potential varies from cell to cell and in a particular cell varies according to its functional status. For example, a nerve cell has a membrane potential of −70 mV (inside negative) at rest, but when it gets excited the membrane potential becomes about +30 mV (inside positive). The membrane potential at rest is called *resting membrane potential* or resting transmembrane potential or simply resting potential. The term rest does not imply that the cell is metabolically quiescent but that it is not undergoing any electrical change. The membrane potential measured during the excited state of the cell is called *action potential.* For details of action potential see page 61

GENESIS OF MEMBRANE POTENTIAL

Membrane potential is basically due to unequal distribution of ions across the cell membrane, which in turn results due to the combined effect of various forces acting on the ions. The factors involved in the genesis of membrane potential which need elaboration are:

- Selective permeability of the cell membrane,
- Gibbs–Donnan equilibrium,
- Nernst equation,
- Constant field Goldmann equation and
- Sodium–potassium ATPase pump.

Selective Permeability of the Cell Membrane

The cell membrane is selectively permeable, that is, to some ions it is freely permeable, to others impermeable and to some others it has variable permeability as:

- Ions like Na^+, K^+, Cl^- and HCO_3^- are diffusible ions. The cell membrane is freely permeable to K^+ and Cl^- and moderately permeable to Na^+.
- Though the particle size of K^+ is larger (atomic weight 39) as compared to Na^+ (atomic weight 23), the permeability for K^+ is approximately 50–100 times greater than that for Na^+. This is because hydrated K^+ is smaller than hydrated Na^+. In other words, the energy required to separate water from Na^+ is greater as compared to K^+, so the K^+ permeability is higher than Na^+.
- The cell membrane is practically impermeable to intracellular proteins and organic phosphate, which are negatively charged ions.
- The presence of gated channels in the cell membrane is responsible for the variable permeability of certain ions in different circumstances.

Gibbs–Donnan Membrane Equilibrium

According to Gibbs–Donnan membrane equilibrium, when two ionized solutions are separated by a semipermeable membrane then at equilibrium:

- Each solution shall be electrically neutral, i.e. total charges on cations will be equal to total charges on anions.
- The product of diffusible ions on one side of the membrane will be equal to the product of diffusible ions on the other side of the membrane.

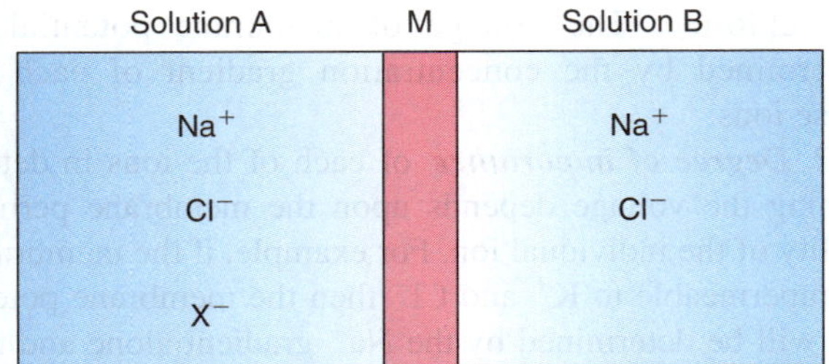

FIGURE 1.4-1 Semipermeable membrane 'M' separates ionic solutions of sodium chloride A and B.

To understand, let us consider 'M' as a semipermeable membrane separating two ionized solutions of sodium chloride A and B (Fig. 1.4-1). Then according to Gibbs–Donnan equilibrium:

1. Each solution is electrically neutral, i.e.

$$(\text{cations})_A = (\text{anions})_A, \text{ and } (\text{cations})_B = (\text{anions})_B$$

OR

$$(Na^+)_A = (Cl^-)_A \text{ and, } (Na^+)_B = (Cl^-)_B$$

2. The product of diffusible ions on both sides will be equal, i.e.

$$(\text{diffusible cations})_A \times (\text{diffusible anions})_A = (\text{diffusible cations})_B \times (\text{diffusible anions})_B$$

OR

$$[(Na^+)_A \times (Cl^-)_A] = [(Na^+)_B \times (Cl^-)_B]$$

From the above the ratio of diffusible ions will be as below:

$$\frac{(\text{diffusible cations})_A}{(\text{diffusible cations})_B} = \frac{(\text{diffusible anions})_B}{(\text{diffusible anions})_A}$$

OR

$$\frac{[Na^+]_A}{[Na^+]_B} = \frac{[Cl^-]_B}{[Cl^-]_A}$$

Thus there will be symmetrical distribution of ions at equilibrium. But if one or more nondiffusible ions 'X' are present on one side (A side) of the membrane, then according to Gibbs–Donnan, at equilibrium the distribution of diffusible ions will be as under:

1. Both solutions will be electrically neutral, i.e.

$$(Na^+)_A = (Cl^-)_A + (X^-)_A \text{ and, } (Na^+)_B = (Cl^-)_B$$

$$\text{So, } (Na^+)_A + (Cl^-)_A + (X^-) > (Na^+)_B + (Cl^-)_B \quad (1)$$

2. The product of diffusible ions on two sides will be equal, i.e.

$$(Na^+)_A \times (Cl^-)_A = (Na^+)_B \times (Cl^-)_B \quad (2)$$

From the relationship of (1) and (2), it is found that:

- $(Na^+)_A > (Na^+)_B$, and
- $(Cl^-)_A < (Cl^-)_B$

Hence there is unequal distribution of diffusible ions (asymmetrical). At equilibrium Na^+ being greater on the side which contains nondiffusible anions 'X^-' (side A) and anion Cl^- being greater on the other side (side B). However, their concentration ratios are equal.

Since the intracellular fluid (ICF) contains nondiffusible anions like proteins and organic phosphate, so, according to Gibbs–Donnan equilibrium there should be an asymmetrical distribution of diffusible ions across the cell membrane with cations being more inside than the outside. However, in reality the interior of the cell is negatively charged which will be explained in the ensuing discussion.

Nernst Equation

The asymmetrical distribution of diffusible ions across the cell membrane in the form of excess diffusible cation inside due to Gibbs–Donnan equilibrium (as explained above) results in a concentration gradient. As a result of which diffusible cations (K^+) will try to diffuse back into the ECF from ICF, but are counteracted by the electrical gradient, which will be created due to the presence of nondiffusible anions inside the cell. Thus, equilibrium will be reached between the concentration gradient and the electrical gradient resulting in diffusion potential (equilibrium potential) across the cell membrane. The magnitude of this equilibrium potential can be determined by Nernst equation as:

$$E_{(m)} = -\frac{RT}{ZF} \text{ in } \frac{(\text{Conc})i}{(\text{Conc})o}$$

where:

$E_{(m)}$	Equilibrium potential (in millivolts) of the ions at which efflux and influx of the ions are equal
R	The natural gas constant and its value is 8.316 J/degree
T	The absolute temperature
F	The Faraday constant and its value is represented as number of C/mole of charge (96,500 C/mole)
Z	The valency of the ion
ln	Symbol for natural logarithm
(Conc)i	The concentration of the ions in the intracellular fluid (inside)
(Conc)o	The concentration of the ions in the extracellular fluid (outside).

At normal body temperature (37°C), converting from the natural log to the base 10 log and replacing some of the constants with numerical values, the equation can be simplified to:

$$E_{(m)} = \pm 61 \log \frac{(\text{Conc})i}{(\text{Conc})o}$$

The equilibrium potential ($E_{(m)}$) for some of the important ions in the mammalian spinal motor neuron calculated from the simplified Nernst equation is shown in Table 1.4-1.

Goldmann–Hodgkin–Katz (GHK) Equation

The Nernst equation helps in calculating the equilibrium potential for each ion individually. However, the magnitude of the membrane potential at any given time depends on the distribution of Na^+, K^+ and Cl^- and the permeability of each of these ions. The integrated role of different ions in the generation of membrane potential can be described accurately by the *Goldmann's constant field equation* or the so-called Goldmann–Hodgkin–Katz (GHK) equation:

$$V = \frac{RT}{F} \ln \frac{P_k [K^+]_i + P_{Na^+}[Na^+]_i + P_{Cl^-}[Cl^-]_o}{P_k[K^+]_o + P_{Na^+}[Na^+]_o + P_{Cl^-}[Cl^-]_i}$$

where

V is the membrane potential,

R is the gas constant,

T is the absolute temperature,

F Faraday,

P_{k+}, P_{Na+} and P_{Cl-} are the permeabilities of the membrane to K^+, Na^+ and Cl^-, and brackets signify concentration and i and o refer to inside and outside of the cell, respectively.

Inferences of Goldmann Constant Field Equation

Following important inferences can be drawn from the Goldmann constant field equation:

1. Most Important Ions for Development of membrane potentials in nerve and muscle fibres are sodium, potassium and chloride. The voltage of membrane potential is determined by the concentration gradient of each of these ions.

2. Degree of importance of each of the ions in determining the voltage depends upon the membrane permeability of the individual ion. For example, if the membrane is impermeable to K^+ and Cl^- then the membrane potential will be determined by the Na^+ gradient alone and the resulting potential will be equal to the Nernst potential for sodium.

3. Positive ion concentration from inside the membrane to outside is responsible for electronegativity inside the membrane. This is because of the fact that due to concentration gradient, the positive ions diffuse outside leaving the nondiffusible negative ions inside the cell.

4. Signal transmission in the nerves is primarily due to change in the sodium and potassium permeability because their channels undergo rapid change during conduction of the nerve impulse and not much change is seen in the chloride channels.

TABLE 1.4-1 Equilibrium Potential ($E_{(m)}$) for Important Ions in a Mammalian Spinal Motor Neuron

Ion	Concentration (in mmol/L of H_2O)		Equilibrium potential (in mV)
	Outside the cell	*Inside the cell*	
Na^+	150	15	+60
K^+	05.5	150	−90
Cl^-	125	09	−70
Ca^{2+}	5	<1	+130

Role of Na^+–K^+ ATPase Pump

The role of Na^+–K^+ ATPase lies in building the concentration gradient. It serves to pump back the Na^+ that diffuses into the cell and K^+ that diffuses out of the cell. In the resting membrane, these diffusions are negligible, so the Na^+–K^+ pump works very feebly in this stage. Further, although the Na^+–K^+ pump is potentially electrogenic (since it pumps out three Na^+ ions for two K^+ ions), at no stage is the pump able to build up a significant membrane potential. This is because of the fact that, as soon as the pump creates a negative potential inside the cell, chloride ions rush out of the cell and restore electroneutrality. Thus, in other words, this pump, pumps out three Na^+ ions and one Cl^- ion for every two K^+ ions it pumps in.

RECORDING OF MEMBRANE POTENTIAL

Instruments Used for Recording

The essential instruments used in recording the activity of an excitable tissue are:

- Microelectrodes,
- Electronic amplifiers and
- Cathode ray oscilloscope (CRO).

Basic principles of the functioning of these instruments are described on page 70.

Technique of Recording

Technique of recording of membrane potential is described on page 71.

Chapter 1.5

Genetics: An Overview

Genetics may rightly be claimed to be one of the most important branches of biology. Foundation for the present day genetics was laid by the Mendel's work published in 1866. He demonstrated that characteristics do not blend but pass from parents to offsprings as discrete (separate) units. These units, which appear in the offspring in pairs, remain discrete and are passed on to subsequent generations by the male and female gametes each of which contain a single unit. The Danish botanist Johannied called these units genes in 1909 and the American geneticist Morgan, in 1912 demonstrated that they are carried on chromosomes. Since the early 1900, the study of genetics has made great advances. An overview of which is given here in brief.

STRUCTURAL AND FUNCTIONAL CHARACTERISTICS OF SUBSTRATE FOR GENETICS

Chromosomes

Waldeyer in 1888 coined the term chromosomes to denote the thread-like structures present in the nucleus of eukaryotic cells during division. It is now established that the chromosomes are responsible for the transmission of the hereditary information from one generation to next. There are 46 chromosomes (23 pairs) in all the dividing cells of the body except the gametes (sex cells which contain only 23 chromosomes) haploid number.

Morphology of Chromosomes

Each chromosome is composed of two chromatids connected at the *centromere.* Each chromatid consists of two *chromonemes. Telomeres* are the terminal ends of chromosomes DNA molecule.

Morphological Types of Chromosomes *Depending upon the location of the centromere, four morphological types of chromosomes are recognized (Fig. 1.5-1):*

- *Metacentric chromosomes.* The centromere divides the chromosomes into two equal arms (Fig. 1.5-1A).
- *Submetacentric chromosomes.* The centromere divides the chromosomes into two unequal arms (Fig. 1.5-1B).
- *Acrocentric chromosomes.* The centromere is located in such a way that a very short arm of chromosomes is visible (Fig. 1.5-1C).
- *Telocentric chromosomes.* The centromere is located at one end (Fig. 1.5-1D).

Functional Types of Chromosomes *There are three types of eukaryotic chromosomes:*

- *Autosomes* are the chromosomes present in somatic cells. The number of autosomes in a cell is fixed and is expressed as 2*n* or *diploid number.*
- *Sex chromosomes* are present in the sex cells and are responsible for determining the sex of an individual.
- *Supernumerary or redundant chromosomes* are also found in eukaryotic cells but their occurrence is quite uncommon.

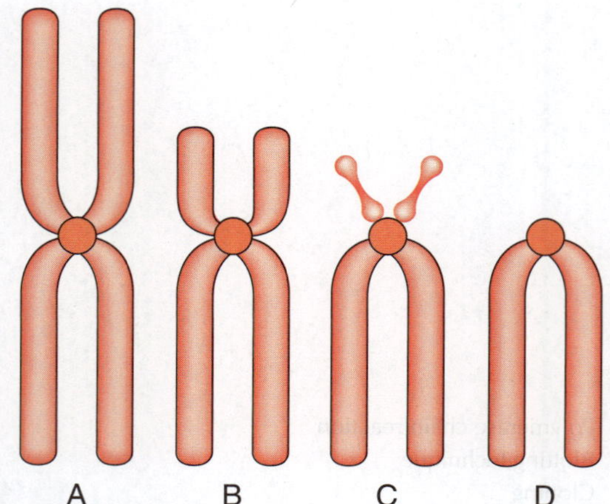

FIGURE 1.5-1 Morphological types of chromosomes: **A,** metacentric; **B,** submetacentric; **C,** acrocentric; and **D,** teleocentric.

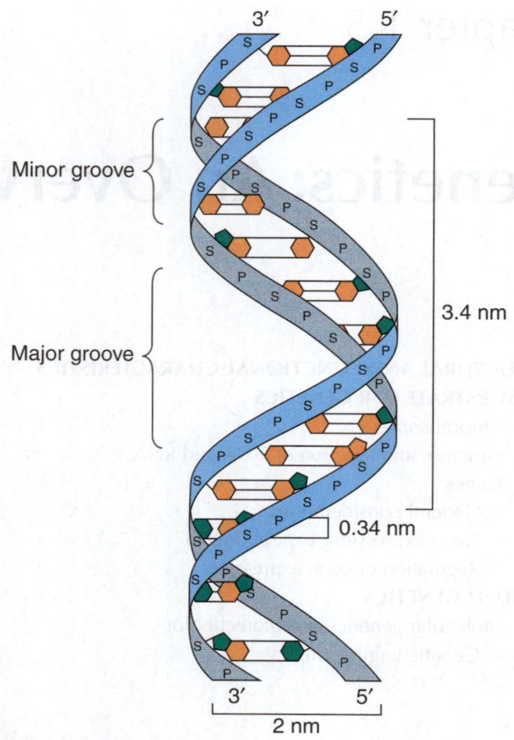

FIGURE 1.5-2 Watson–Crick model of DNA structure.

Chemical Structure of Chromosome

The chromosomes are mainly composed of DNA. The chromosome also contains RNA, basic proteins called histones, complex proteins including enzymes, some organic phosphorus compounds and inorganic salts. The amount of DNA in a haploid cell is half the amount present in a diploid cell of the same species. Further, the concentration of DNA in any cell remains constant in every circumstance. An important feature of DNA is that it is metabolically stable.

Organization of DNA in a Chromosome

See page 37.

Structure and Function of DNA and RNA

DNA

DNA, i.e. deoxyribonucleic acid, is a molecule of inheritance and thus may be regarded as the "Reserve Bank" of genetic information. It is exclusively responsible for maintaining the identity of different species of organisms for millions of years.

Structure of DNA

DNA is a polymer of four monomeric deoxyribonucleotides, namely, deoxyadenylate (dAMP), deoxyguanylate (dGMP), deoxycytidylate (dCMP) and deoxythymidylate (dTMP). Each deoxyribonucleotide in turn is composed of a nitrogenous base purines or pyrimidines (A, G, C or T), a pentose sugar, i.e. deoxyribose and a phosphate. Each molecule of DNA has equal number of adenine and thymine residues (A = T) and equal number of guanine and cytosine residues (G = C). This is known as *Chargaff's rule.*

Watson–Crick Model of DNA Structure *The salient features of Watson–Crick model of DNA (now known as B-DNA) are* (Fig. 1.5-2)*:*

- *Double helix structure.* Each DNA molecule is a right-handed double helix composed of two polydeoxyribonucleotide chains (strands) twisted around each other on a common axis.
- *Antiparallel chains.* The two chains of each DNA molecule are antiparallel, i.e. one chain runs in the 5′ to 3′ direction while the other in 3′ to 5′ direction.
- *Dimensions.* The width of a double helix is 20 Å (2 nm). Each turn (pitch) of the helix contains 10 pairs of nucleotides, each placed at distance of about 3.4 Å (0.34 nm); thus each turn is 34 Å (3.4 nm) in dimension.
- *Arrangement of base, sugar and phosphate molecule.* Each chain has a sugar–phosphate backbone with bases that project at right angles and hydrogen bond with the bases of the opposite chain across the double helix (Fig. 1.5-3).
- *Complementary chains.* The two polynucleotide chains are not identical but complementary due to base pairing.
- *Genetic information.* The genetic information resides in one of two strands known as *template strand or sense strand.* The opposite strand is antisense strand.

Types of DNA

Six forms of DNA, A to E and Z, have been identified. Among these A, B and Z forms are important.

- ***A-DNA*** is a right-handed helix. It contains 4 base pairs per turn.
- ***B-DNA*** as described by Watson and Crick (discussed above) contains 10 base pairs per turn spanning a distance

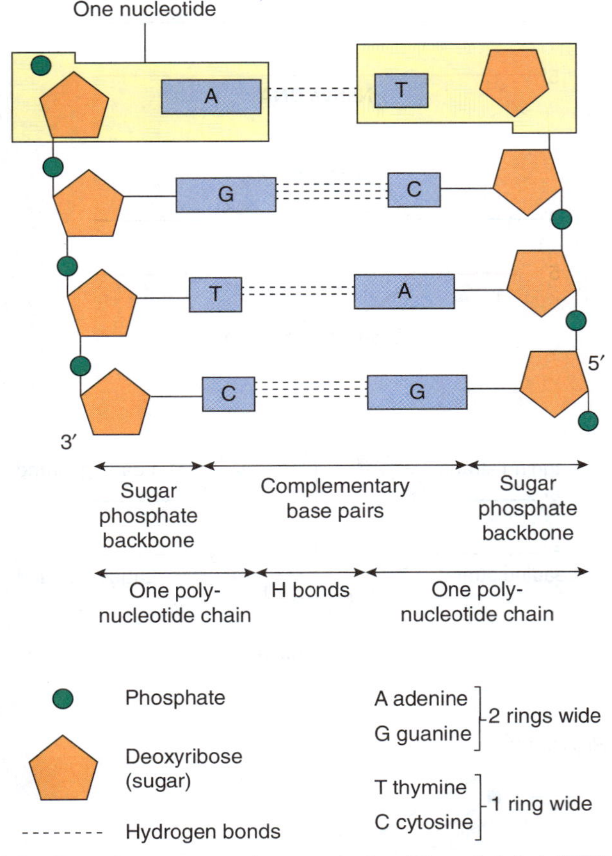

FIGURE 1.5-3 Diagrammatic structure of straightened chains of DNA.

of 3.4 nm. It is the most predominant form under physiological conditions.

- ***Z-DNA*** is a left-handed helix and contains 12 base pairs per turn. The name Z-DNA has been derived from the zigzag fashion in which the polynucleotide strands of this DNA move.

Size of DNA

DNA molecules are huge in size. The term kilobase pair (Kb = 1000 base pairs) is commonly used in DNA structure. In humans 23 haploid chromosomes have 2,900,000 Kb with a total contour length of 990 nm. Thus, a human cell contains about 2 m of DNA distributed among 46 chromosomes. Each chromosome, therefore, contains about 4.8 cm (48,000 μm) of DNA. Human chromosomes are on average about 6 μm long, with a packing ratio of 8000:1. In order to maintain the high degree of organization when DNA is folded, the histone proteins form a precise architectural scaffolding for the DNA.

Organization of DNA in the Cell

In human cells, the DNA is found in association with positively charged protein molecules called *histones.* Each DNA helix combines with a group of eight histone molecules to form structures known as *nucleosomes* which have an appearance of 'beads and string'. These nucleosomes, and the DNA strands linking them, are packed closely together to produce a 30 nm diameter helix with about six nucleosome per turn. This is known as 30 nm fibre or the *solenoid fibre.* The solenoid fibres in turn coil to form *chromatin fibres* which are further coiled and packed in the form of *chromatin* in which form DNA is present in the chromosome (Fig. 1.5-4).

RNA

Structure of RNA

RNA is a polymer of ribonucleotides held together by 3′, 5′-phosphodiester bridges. Though an RNA molecule like that of DNA is composed of nucleotides consisting of a base sugar and phosphate but it has following structural differences:

- *Single-strand.* RNA is commonly a single-stranded structure unlike DNA. However, in certain forms of RNA this strand may fold at certain places to give a double-stranded structure if complementary base pairs are in close proximity.
- *Ribose sugar.* The sugar molecule in RNA molecule is ribose in contrast to deoxyribose.
- *Base.* The pyrimidine base in a RNA molecule is uracil in place of thymine of a DNA molecule.

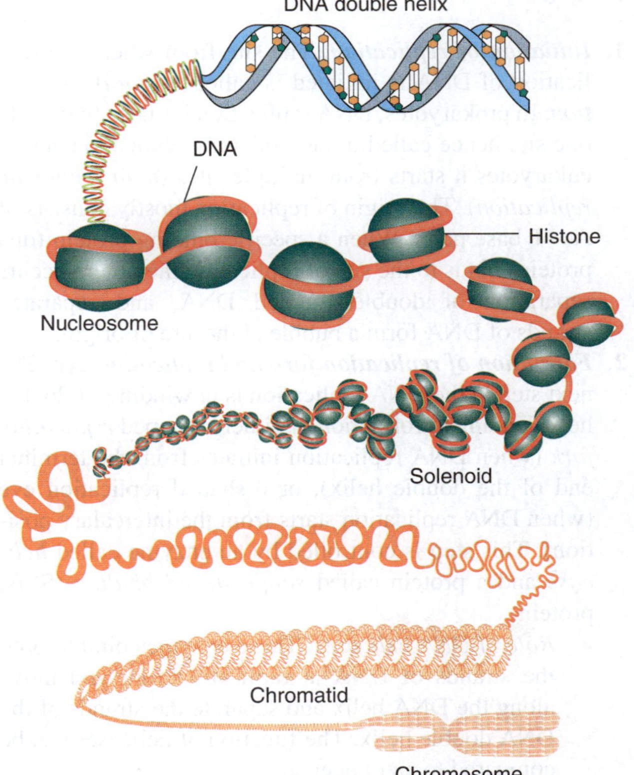

FIGURE 1.5-4 Diagrammatic organization of DNA in a chromosome of the human cell.

- *Chargaff's rule.* Due to the single-stranded structure Chargaff's rule is not obeyed, i.e. there is no specific relation between purine and pyrimidine contents.

Types of RNA

Following types of RNAs have been recognized:

- ***Messenger RNA (mRNA).*** In the human cell, it is synthesized in the nucleus and enters the cytoplasm to participate in protein synthesis.
- ***Transfer RNA (tRNA).*** There are about 20 species of tRNA corresponding to 20 amino acids present in protein structure. The structure of tRNA resembles that of clover leaf with four arms. tRNA delivers amino acids for protein synthesis.
- ***Ribosomal RNA (rRNA).*** rRNAs are present in ribosomes (factories of protein synthesis). It is believed that rRNAs play a significant role in binding of mRNA to ribosomes in protein synthesis.

DNA Replication

DNA replication is a process by which each original DNA molecule gives rise to two copies with identical structure. The method by which the DNA replicates is called *semi-conservation replication* since each new double helix retains (conserves) one of the two strands of the original DNA double helices. Steps involved in the DNA replication are (Fig. 1.5-5):

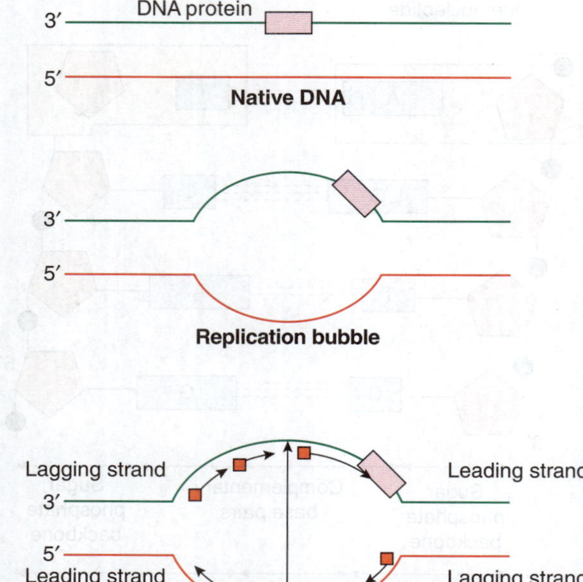

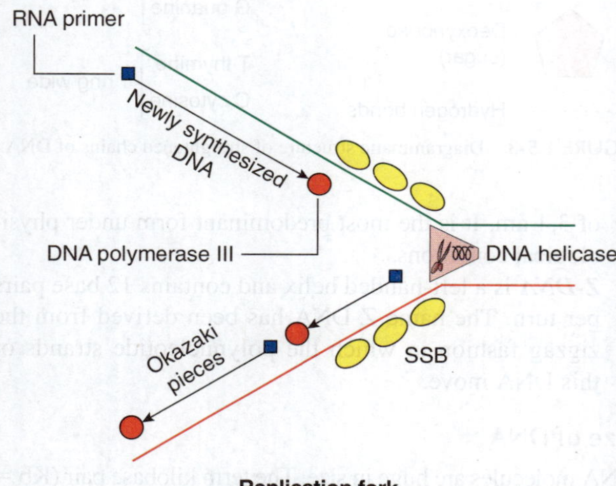

FIGURE 1.5-5 Simplified diagram showing main steps of DNA replication.

1. ***Initiation of replication.*** The site from where the replication of DNA is initiated is called *origin of replication.* In prokaryotes, DNA replication initiates from only one site hence called monorepliconic replication and in eukaryotes it starts from multiple sites (*multirepliconic replication*). The origin of replication mostly consists of A—T base pairs. When a specific binding protein (dna protein) binds to the site of replication then there occurs separation of double-stranded DNA, and separated strands of DNA form a bubble at the site of origin.
2. ***Formation of replication fork and replication eye.*** The next step in the DNA replication is unwinding of double helix leading to formation of either Y-shaped *replication fork* (when DNA replication initiates from the terminal end of the double helix), or θ-shaped replication eye (when DNA replication starts from the intercalary position). This step is controlled by an enzyme called *helicase* and a protein called *single-strand binding* (SSB) protein.
   - *Role of DNA helicases.* These enzymes bind to both the strands of DNA at replication fork and move along the DNA helix and separate the strands of the DNA double helix. The function of helicases can be compared to a zip opener.
   - *Role of single-strand DNA binding (SSB) proteins.* As the name indicates, SSB protein binds only to single-stranded DNA (separated by helicase). Main function of this protein is to keep the two DNA strands separate, hence, also called helix destabilizing protein. SSB protein also provides template for new DNA synthesis and prevent degradation of single-stranded DNA.
3. ***Formation of RNA primer.*** RNA primer consists of a short fragment of RNA (about 5–50 nucleotides). It is required for synthesis of new DNA. The RNA primer is synthesized on DNA template by specific *RNA polymerase* (primase).
4. ***DNA synthesis along the replication fork.*** DNA replication occurs simultaneously in both the leading as well

as lagging strands of Y-shaped replication fork and is of two types:

- *Continuous DNA replication.* In the leading strand, DNA polymerase III binds to the single-stranded DNA and starts to move along the strand. Each time it meets the next base on DNA, free nucleotides approach the DNA strand, and one with the correct complementary base hydrogen bonds to the base in the DNA. The free nucleotide is then in place by the enzyme until it binds to the preceding nucleotide thus extending the new strand of DNA. The enzyme continues to move along one base at time with new DNA strand growing as it does so.
- *Discontinuous DNA replication.* Occurs in the lagging strand.

Genes

General Considerations

The gene is the functional unit of DNA. A gene could therefore be defined as a piece of DNA which codes for a protein. In strictest sense, the gene can be defined as the DNA code for a single polypeptide chain. Since some proteins are made up of more than one polypeptide chains, they are therefore coded for by more than one genes.

Genome. The term genome refers to total genetic information contained in a cell.

Human genome. For humans, the genome is essentially equivalent to all of the genetic information which is present in a single set of 23 chromosomes.

Human genome project (1990–2003). The human genome project (HGP) which completed on April 14, 2003 has accomplished the following goals:

- Identified all the *approximate 30,000 genes in human DNA*.
- Determined the sequences of 3 billion chemical base pairs that make the human DNA.

Functional genomics. Understanding the functions of genes and other parts of genome is known as functional genomics.

Comparative genomics. Comparative genomics is the analysis and comparison of genome from different species.

Constitutive and inducible genes. The genes are generally considered under two categories:

- *Constitutive.* The products (proteins) of these genes are required all the time in a cell. Therefore, the constitutive genes (or housekeeping genes) are expressed more or less at a constant rate in almost all the cell and, further, they may not be subjected to regulation, e.g. enzymes of citric acid cycle.
- *Inducible genes.* The concentration of the proteins synthesized by inducible genes is regulated by various molecular signals. An inducer increases the expression of these genes while a repressor decreases, e.g. tryptophan pyrrolase of liver is induced by tryptophan.

Gene Expression: Central Dogma

As mentioned above, each cell of human body contains the entire genome, yet the genetic expression is very selective and different patterns of protein synthesis occur in different tissues. Not only this, even in the same tissue, there is wide variation in the proteins produced during the course of development.

The expression of genetic material occurs through the production of proteins. This involves two consecutive steps—transcription and translation. In transcription, the genetic information, stored in DNA, is transferred to an RNA intermediate, which in turn uses this information to direct the synthesis of proteins during translation. This unidirectional flow of information was described by FHC Crick in 1958 as the central dogma of molecular biology (Fig. 1.5-6). However, an important modification of this information flow was given by David Baltimore and H Temin, who described reversible sequence through reverse transcription or feminism in the presence of transcripts (revised central dogma).

Transcription

Transcription is a process in which RNA is synthesized from DNA. All the three types of RNAs (mRNA, tRNA and rRNA) are produced through transcription. The transcription process is selective, i.e. the entire molecule of DNA is not expressed in transcription, but the RNAs are synthesized only for selected regions of DNA. The strand of DNA that directs the synthesis of mRNA via complementary base pairing is called the *template strand* or coding or sense strand, and the other strand is known as noncoding strand or antisense strand. Transcription is accomplished by an enzyme *RNA polymerase* that gets physically associated with DNA. Only one type of such an enzyme is found in prokaryotes in contrast to eukaryotes (where three different forms of

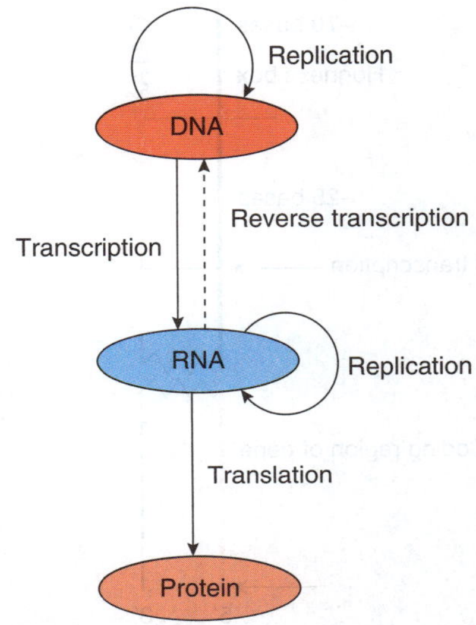

FIGURE 1.5-6 Central dogma: the flow of genetic information.

RNA polymerase are found). RNA I, II and III catalyse the synthesis of rRNA, mRNA and tRNA, respectively.

Promoter sites. RNA polymerase binds to a region of DNA called promoter site. In eukaryotes, a sequence of DNA bases has been identified. This sequence, known as Hogness box or TATA box (Fig. 1.5-7), is located on left about 25 nucleotides away (upstream) from the starting site of mRNA synthesis. There also exists another site of recognition between 70 and 80 nucleotides upstream from the start of transcription. This second site is referred to as CAAT box. One of these two sites (or sometimes both) helps RNA polymerase II to recognize requisite sequence of DNA for transcription.

Salient Features of Transcription in Eukaryotes vis-à-vis Prokaryotes are:

- Transcription in eukaryotes unlike prokaryotes occurs within the nucleus and mRNA moves out of the nucleus into the cytoplasm for translation.
- The initiation and regulation of transcription in eukaryotes is more extensive than prokaryotes.

Post-transcriptional Modifications

- The mRNA in eukaryotes is processed from the primary RNA transcript, a process called maturation which includes:
- Releases of the introns and joining with two adjacent exons to produce mature mRNA.

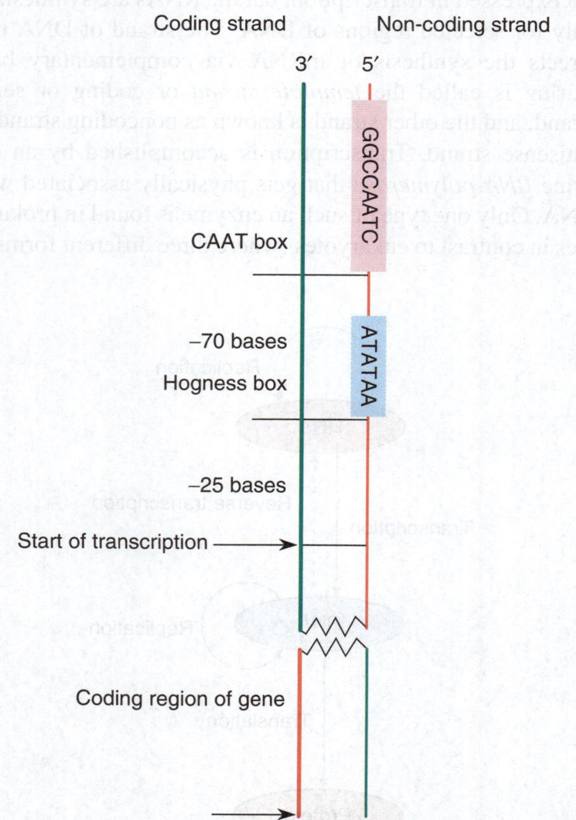

FIGURE 1.5-7 Promoter sites of DNA in eukaryotes.

- *RNA editing.* Besides, these two post-transcriptional modifications, RNA editing may also take place before translation begins.

Reverse Transcription refers to formation of DNA from RNA. The enzyme reverse transcriptase is responsible for this process. The DNA so formed is complementary (cDNA) to viral RNA can be transmitted to host DNA. Reverse transcription is known to occur in retroviruses which include human immunodeficiency virus that causes AIDS.

Translation: Biosynthesis of Proteins

Translation is the process by which genetic message carried by mRNA from the DNA is converted in the form of a polypeptide chain having specific sequence of amino acids. Before discussing the process of translation, it will be worthwhile to know something about the genetic code.

Genetic Code Process by which the information coded in the mRNA is decoded into polypeptide is referred to as *deciphering the genetic code.* Dr Hargobind Khorana shared 'Nobel Prize' in 1968 with Nirenberg and Holly for the discovery of genetic code. The genetic code (codons) is formed by three nucleotides (triplet) base sequences in mRNA. The codons are formed of four nucleotide base (A, G, C and U). These four bases produce 64 different combinations of three base codons. Of the 64 codons, the 61 codons code for 20 amino acids found in proteins and the three codons (UAA, UAG and UGA) are *termination codons* which act as stop signals in protein synthesis. The codons AUG and sometimes GUG act as *initiating codons.*

Characteristics of genetic code are:

- *Universality,* i.e. same codons are used to code for the same amino acids in all the living organisms with a few exceptions.
- *Specificity,* i.e. a particular codon always codes for the same amino acid, e.g. AUG is the codon for methionine.
- *Nonoverlapping,* i.e. the genetic code is read from a fixed point as a continuous base sequence.
- *Degenerate,* i.e. one amino acid is coded by more than one codon. The codons that designate the same amino acid are called synonyms.

Process of Protein Biosynthesis The process of protein synthesis in addition to mRNA requires amino acids tRNA, energy sources (ATP and GTP) and protein factors. Protein synthesis occurs over ribosomes which are also called *protein factories.* The protein biosynthesis involves three processes:

1. ***Activation of amino acids.*** Amino acids are activated and attached to tRNA in a two-step reaction. A group of enzymes, namely aminoacyl tRNA synthetases, is

required for this process. In the first step, an amino acid reacts with ATP in the presence of specific amino acid tRNA to form *enzyme–AMP-amino acid complex.* This complex then reacts with a specific tRNA and the amino acid is transferred to 3′ end of the tRNA to form aminoacyl tRNA.

II. ***Translation proper*** involves three steps—initiation, elongation and termination.

1. *Initiation.* The translation of mRNA begins with the formation of initiation complex.
2. *Elongation.* Ribosomes elongate the polypeptide chain by a sequential addition of amino acids to the growing carboxyl end.
   The elongation process is repeated again and again with addition of one amino acid each time till signal for termination is reached.
3. *Termination* of polypeptide synthesis is evoked by a nonsense or termination codon (UAA, UAG or UGA).

III. ***Post-translational modifications.*** The proteins synthesized in translation are as such not functional. Many changes take place in the polypeptides after the initiation of their synthesis or, most frequently, after the protein synthesis is completed. Post-translational modification includes:

- Proteolytic degradation and
- Covalent modifications (phosphorylation, hydroxylation and glycosylation).

Regulation of Gene Expression

As discussed earlier, each nucleated somatic cell in the body contains full genetic message, yet there is great differentiation and specialization in the functions of various types of adult cells. It is because of the fact that there exists a foolproof system for regulation of gene expression that maintains orderly growth in cells and prevents uncontrolled growth. The genes are controlled both spatially and temporally. The regulation of gene expression is thus absolutely essential for growth, development and differentiation of an organism. A positive regulator increases the gene expression whereas a negative regulator decreases.

Regulation of Gene Expression in Prokaryotes

In prokaryotes, gene expression is regulated by operon system. Operons are segments of genetic material which function as regulated units that can be switched on and switched off. The operon systems are of two types:

1. ***Inducible operon system*** (lac operon system). An inducible operon system is that regulated genetic material which remains switched off normally but becomes operational in the presence of an inducer. It occurs in catabolic pathway.
2. ***Repressible operon system*** (tryptophan operon system). A repressible operon system is that regulated genetic material which normally remains active/operational. It usually occurs in anabolic pathways.

Regulation of Gene Expression in Eukaryotes

The regulation of gene expression in eukaryotes is very complex and involves various mechanisms. Some of the mechanisms are:

1. ***Gene amplification.*** In this mechanism, the expression of gene is increased several folds. An example of gene amplification in humans includes development of drug resistance by the malignant cells to long-term administration of methotrexate. This occurs by amplifying the gene coding for dihydrofolate reductase.
2. ***Gene rearrangement.*** The process of gene rearrangement is responsible for the generation of 10 billion antigen-specific immunoglobulins.
3. ***Regulation of gene expression through transcription factors.*** Transcription factors are products of other genes and hence mediate transregulation by binding to specific DNA segments. This specific interaction of protein to DNA in over 80% of the nontranscription factors is brought about by one of the four DNA-binding motifs: zinc finger motif, lucine zipper motif, helix–turn–helix motif, and helix–loop–helix motif.
4. ***Regulation of gene through mRNA.*** Gene expression is also regulated by regulation of synthesis transport, processing and stability of mRNA.

APPLIED GENETICS

Applications of genetics are many more and beyond the scope of a book on physiology, only a few of interest described here include some aspects of:

- *Molecular genetics and biotechnology, and*
- *Molecular genetics and medicine.*

Molecular Genetics and Biotechnology

Biotechnology involves use of living organisms or products of living organisms for the welfare of human. Presently, molecular biology has combined with genetics to give us more powerful biotechnology. The tools of molecular genetics have provided improved way to make use of living organisms for the benefit of humans. The subject of molecular genetics and biotechnology is expanding fast and has already become very vast. The present discussion includes only a few important aspects viz.

- Genetic engineering,
  - Stages of recombinant DNA technology
  - Application of recombinant DNA technology,
- Polymerase chain reaction
- Blotting techniques
- Cloning
- Apoptosis.

Genetic Engineering/Recombinant DNA Technology

The terms genetic engineering/recombinant DNA technology/DNA cloning/molecular cloning/gene cloning all refer to the process of transfer of a DNA fragment of interest from one organism to a self-replicating genetic element such as a bacterial plasmid. In other words, this technology involves cutting, modifying and joining DNA molecules using enzymes such as restriction enzymes and DNA ligase.

Stages of Recombinant Technology

Stages of recombinant technology are:

Stage 1: Generation of a Copy of Gene Required. This is the most difficult part of the process. Three methods are used to get a copy of a gene:

- Making a copy of the gene from its mRNA, using reverse transcriptase,
- Synthesizing the gene artificially and
- Using a *shotgun approach* which involves chopping up the DNA with *restriction enzymes* and searching for the piece with the required gene (Fig. 1.5-8).

Stage 2: Joining the Gene to a Vector or Carrier Molecule. A vector is a carrier of a DNA molecule to which the generated gene is attached for cloning. Three commonly used vectors in recombinant DNA technology are (Fig. 1.5-8):

- Plasmids,
- Bacteriophages and
- Cosmids.

Stage 3: Introduction of Vector DNA into the Host Cell to Produce Chimeric DNA. The main aim of genetic engineering is to insert a DNA of interest (generated gene) into a vector DNA so that the DNA fragment replicates along with the vector after annealing. This hybrid combination of two fragments of DNA is referred to as *chimeric DNA* or *hybrid DNA* or *recombinant DNA*.

Stage 4: Cloning of Chimeric DNA (Fig. 1.5-9). A clone is a large population of identical molecules, bacteria or cells that arise from a common ancestor. The chimeric DNA contained in a plasma (vector) can be introduced into bacterial cells by a process called *transfection*. The replicating bacterial cell (host cell) permits the amplification of the chimeric DNA of the vector. In this way, cloning results in the production of large number of identical target DNA molecules. The cloned target DNA is released from the vector by cleavage (using appropriate restriction endonucleases), isolated, characterized and used for various purposes.

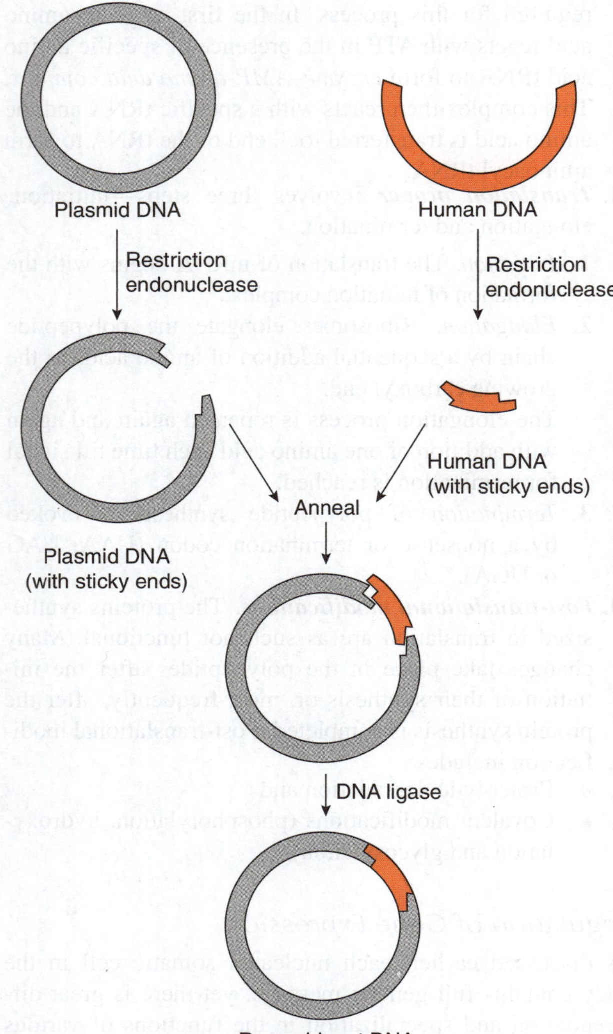

FIGURE 1.5-8 Stages of recombinant DNA technology.

Applications of Genetic Engineering

Genetic engineering has revolutionized the application of molecular biology to medical/agricultural sciences that has immensely benefitted the mankind. A few important applications are:

1. ***Production of proteins/hormones.*** It is possible to produce proteins/hormones in large amount for therapeutic purposes. These include insulin, growth hormone, erythropoietin, interferons, vaccines and blood clotting factors.
2. ***Molecular analysis of diseases*** such as sickle cell anaemia, thalassaemia, cystic fibrosis using recombinant DNA technology has led to better understanding of these diseases.
3. ***Laboratory diagnostic applications.*** Using this technique, the diagnosis of diseases like AIDS has become simple and rapid.
4. ***Gene therapy*** for correcting a genetic defect is very useful application of RBT (see page 48).
5. ***Prenatal diagnosis of genetic diseases*** such as sickle cell anaemia is possible from the DNA collected from the amniotic fluid by using DNA probes.

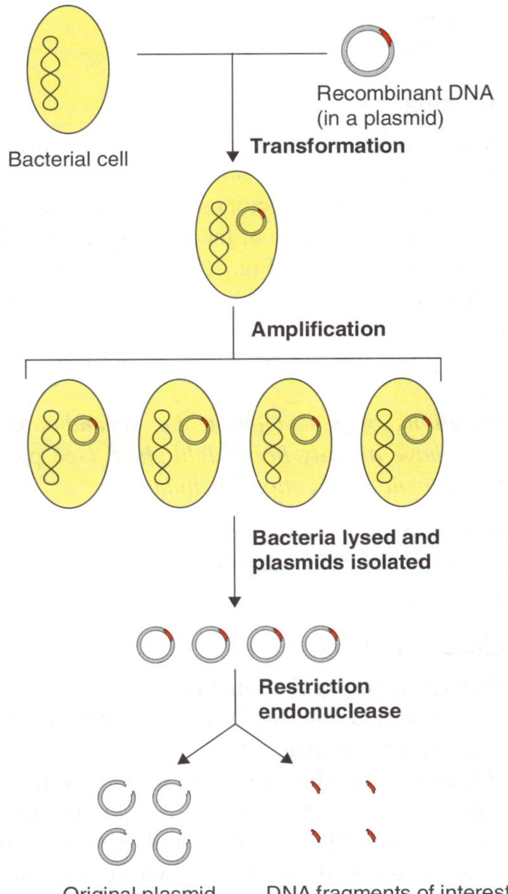

FIGURE 1.5-9 Cloning of a recombinant DNA.

6. ***Transgenesis*** refers to transfer of genes into the fertilized ovum which will be found in somatic as well as germ cells and passed on to successive generation.
7. ***Application in forensic medicine:*** *DNA fingerprinting* applying southern blot technique is useful in identifying criminals and settling the disputes of parenthood of children.
8. ***Industrial applications.*** Enzymes synthesized by this technology are used to produce sugar, cheese and detergents.
9. ***Agricultural applications*** include development of genetically engineered plants to increase the yield of crops, to resist draught and to resist diseases.
10. ***Evolution.*** This technique helps in bridging several missing links in the evolution by amplifying the DNA by PCRs from the archaeological sample of extinct animals.

Polymerase Chain Reaction

Polymerase chain reaction (PCR) is a sensitive, selective and extremely rapid method of amplifying a target sequence of DNA.

Technique *of PCR involves following steps:*

- *Denaturation of DNA* refers to separation of double-stranded target DNA into single strand by heating.
- *Annealing with two primers* (one for each strand) is allowed to occur after cooling the single DNA strand.
- *DNA amplification* occurs by synthesis of new DNA strand in the presence of enzyme DNA polymerase and the substrates deoxyribonucleotide triphosphates. These strands are compliments to the target DNA. The cycle of DNA amplification is repeated again and again. The Taq DNA polymerase is *heat resistant;* this special feature makes it suitable for automation of PCR. PCR results in the amplification of target DNA by about a million (10^6) fold with high specificity.

Application of PCR. PCR is highly sensitive; it can detect even the presence of a single molecule of DNA. PCR amplification of sequences of human genomic DNA produces an amount of target DNA (up to 1 mg) which is sufficient for direct application in any one of a wide range of molecular biological procedures, including direct DNA sequencing.

PCR has several applications:

- Rapid diagnosis of AIDS;
- DNA fingerprinting is useful in kinship analysis and in the identification of crime suspects;
- Prenatal diagnosis of genetic diseases;
- Study of evolution from DNA of archaeological samples and
- Sex identification.

Blotting Techniques

Blotting techniques refer to the analytical techniques used for the identification of a special DNA, or RNA or a protein. These include:

- Southern blotting (for DNA),
- Northern blotting (for RNA) and
- Western blotting (for protein).

Southern Blotting

Southern blotting technique is named after the scientist who identified it while the northern and western blot techniques are the laboratory jargons which are now accepted.

Steps of southern blotting are:

- *Extraction of DNA* from the cells (say leucocytes).
- *Cleavage of DNA* into fragments by restriction endonucleases.
- *Separation of the fragments* of DNA is done by gold electrophoresis.
- *Denaturation of DNA* is done either prior to or during transfer by placing the gel in an alkaline solution (NaOH).
- *Transfer of DNA fragments to a sheet of nitrocellular paper* from the agarose gel is done by blotting (hence the name blot).

- *Fixation of DNA fragments to the membrane* is then done by any of the following methods:
  - oven baking 80°C, or
  - ultraviolet cross-linking.
- *Formation of labelled DNA hybrid complexes.* After fixing the DNA fragments, the membrane is placed in a solution of labelled DNA probe. This leads to hybridization reaction forming labelled DNA hybrid complexes.
- *Identification of labelled DNA hybrid complex.* After the hybridization reaction has been carried out, the membrane is washed to remove unbounded radioactivity and regions of hybridization are identified *by autoradiography* by placing the membrane in contact with X-ray film.

Applications. *Important applications of southern blotting are:*

- DNA fingerprinting, and
- Detection of mutant gene causing cystic fibrosis.

Northern Blotting

Northern blotting is similar to southern blotting except that it is for RNA instead of DNA.

Applications. *Important applications of northern blotting are analysis of the expression of a gene in a particular tissue.*

Western Blotting

Western blotting is the technique for identification of a specific protein. It involves the transfer of electrophoresed protein bands from SDS polyacryl amide gel onto a nitrocellulose membrane followed by probing using a labelled antibody probe.

Applications. *Western blot test is widely used as confirmatory test of HIV. In combination with a positive enzyme-linked immunosorbent assay (ELISA), a positive western blot is 99.9% accurate in detecting HIV infection.*

Cloning

Cloning refers to making many identical copies of a molecule.

Certain terms *which need to be defined before discussing the different types of cloning include:*

- *Transformation* refers to introduction of any DNA molecule into any living cell.
- *Transfection* refers to introduction of purified DNA molecules into cultured cells.
- *Transduction* is the transfer of genetic material or DNA from one cell to another with the help of a virus.
- *Microinjection* is a method of introducing new DNA into a cell by injecting it directly into the nucleus.
- *Biolistics* refers to the means of introducing DNA into cells that involves bombardment with high-velocity microprojectiles located with DNA.

Types of cloning. *Some important types of cloning are:*

- Gene cloning/DNA cloning,
- Reproductive cloning,
- Therapeutic cloning and
- Tissue culture.

Gene Cloning

Gene cloning refers to the process of transfer of a DNA fragment of interest from one organism to a self-replicating genetic element (cloning vector) such as bacterial plasmid and subsequent propagation of the recombinant DNA molecule in the host organism (Fig. 1.5-9). Other terms used to denote gene cloning are DNA cloning and recombinant DNA technology (RDT).

Details of this process have already been described on page 42.

Applications *of gene cloning, i.e. recombinant DNA technology have already been highlighted* (see page 42). *Important genetic applications include:*

- Gene therapy,
- Gene engineering of organisms and
- Sequencing genomes.

Reproductive Cloning

Reproductive cloning is a technology used to generate an animal that has same nuclear DNA as another currently or previously existing animal.

Technique. Reproductive cloning uses the technique of somatic cell nuclear transfer (SCNT). In this technique, genetic material is transferred from the nucleus of a donor adult cell to an egg whose nucleus, and thus its genetic material, has been removed. The reconstructed egg containing the DNA from a donor cell is then treated with chemicals or electric current to stimulate cell division. Once the cloned embryo reaches a suitable stage, it is transferred to the uterus of a female host where it continues to develop until birth. A sheep (Dolly) was created by somatic cell nuclear transfer process from a cell taken from the parent's udder by the research team at the Roslin Institute in Edinburgh (Scotland) in February 1997.

Applications. *Reproductive cloning can be used to repopulate endangered animals or animals that are difficult to breed. Examples are:*

- In 2001, the first clone of an endangered animal, a wild ox called a *gaur* was born. The young gaur died from an infection about 48 hours after its birth.
- In Italy (2001), a successful cloning of a healthy baby *mouflon,* an endangered wild sheep was reported. The cloned mouflon is living at a wild centre in Sardinia.

Embryo Cloning (Therapeutic Cloning)

- Therapeutic cloning refers to the production of human embryos for use in research.
- This process is aimed at harvesting stem cells that can be used to study human development and to treat diseases rather than to create a cloned human being.

- Stem cells are extracted from the egg at the blastocysts stage of development and can be used to generate virtually any type of specialized cells in the human body.
- First human embryo for the purpose of therapeutic research was cloned in November, 2001 by the scientists from Advanced Cell Technologies (ACT), a biotech company in Massachusetts.

Applications. *Stem cells can be used to serve as replacement cells to treat heart disease, Alzheimer's disease, cancer and other diseases.*

Tissue Culture

Cells may also be cloned for special purposes. This technique is called *tissue culture.* Certain cells when placed in a suitable medium can be cultured indefinitely.

Applications. *The use of cloned cells allows the study of the action of such chemicals as hormones, drugs, antibiotics, cosmetics and pharmaceutical products to be made on cells. Such a technique is a useful substitute for laboratory animals such as rats, cats and dogs.*

Apoptosis

Apoptosis versus cell necrosis. Apoptosis, also called as programmed cell death (PCD), occurs under genetic control. Since the cell's own genes play an active role in its demise, so apoptosis can also be called *cell suicide.* It should be distinguished from necrosis in which the healthy cells are destroyed by some injury inflicted on the cells, e.g. inflammation. Since necrosis is caused by some external process, it can be also called *cell murder*. Thus, apoptosis is a natural process while necrosis is an unnatural process. Consequently, apoptosis does not induce a local inflammatory response while cell necrosis does.

Need and examples of apoptosis. *Apoptosis is a very common process during development as well as adulthood, the need of which is highlighted with some examples:*

1. ***Apoptosis for proper development of tissues***
   - *In the central nervous system,* large number of neurons are produced and then die during the remodelling that occurs during development and synapse formation.
   - *During formation of the fingers and toes* of the fetus, the apoptosis plays an important role of removing the web tissue between the finger and toes.
   - *During sexual development* in fetal life, apoptosis is responsible for regression of duct systems.
2. ***Apoptosis for normal functioning of adult tissues***. Examples are:
   - *Cyclic breakdown of endometrium* that leads to start of menstruation is caused by apoptosis.
   - *Epithelial cells* that lose their connection to the basal lamina and surrounding cells undergo apoptosis.
   - *Enterocytes sloughed off* the tips of intestinal villi undergo apoptosis.
3. ***Apoptosis to destroy the cells that represent a threat to the integrity of the organism***. Examples are:
   - Apoptosis of the cells infected with virus;
   - Apoptosis of the cells of the immune system to prevent them from attacking body constituents;
   - Apoptosis of the cells with DNA damage and
   - Apoptosis of the cancer cells.

Mechanism of Apoptosis

The final common pathway leading to apoptosis is the activation of a group of cysteine proteases called *caspases* which exist in cells as inactive proenzymes (Fig. 1.5-10).

Triggering stimuli. Apoptosis can be triggered by external and internal stimuli (Fig. 1.5-10).

- *Internal stimuli.* One of the important pathways goes through the mitochondria, which release *cytochrome* and a protein called smac/DIABL0, causing activation of the *caspase 9.*
- *Apoptosis-inducing factor (AIF)* located in the intermembrane space of mitochondria migrates to nucleus and destroys DNA after binding leading to cell death.
- *External stimuli.* One ligand that activates receptors triggering apoptosis is FAS (a transmembrane protein that projects from natural killer cells and T lymphocytes but also exists in circulating form). Another ligand is tumour necrosis factor (TNF). These activate the enzyme caspase 8 followed by cascade of caspase activation.

Net result of caspase activation *is DNA fragmentation, cytoplasmic and chromatin condensation and eventually membrane bleb formation with cell breakup and removal of the debris by phagocytosis (Fig. 1.5-10).*

Molecular Genetics and Medicine

Clinical applications of molecular genetics in medicine are rapidly increasing owing to research and advances in the molecular aspect of genetics, regulation of gene expression and protein synthesis. Some of the aspects in relation to molecular genetics and medicine described here are:

- Mutations and genetic human diseases;
- Detecting human genetic variations (genetic screening);
- Genetics and cancer and
- Gene therapy.

Mutations and Genetic Human Diseases

Mutations

Mutation refers to a change in the DNA structure of a gene. The substances or factors that are responsible for the mutations are called *mutagens,* e.g. X-rays, ultraviolet light, certain chemicals, etc.

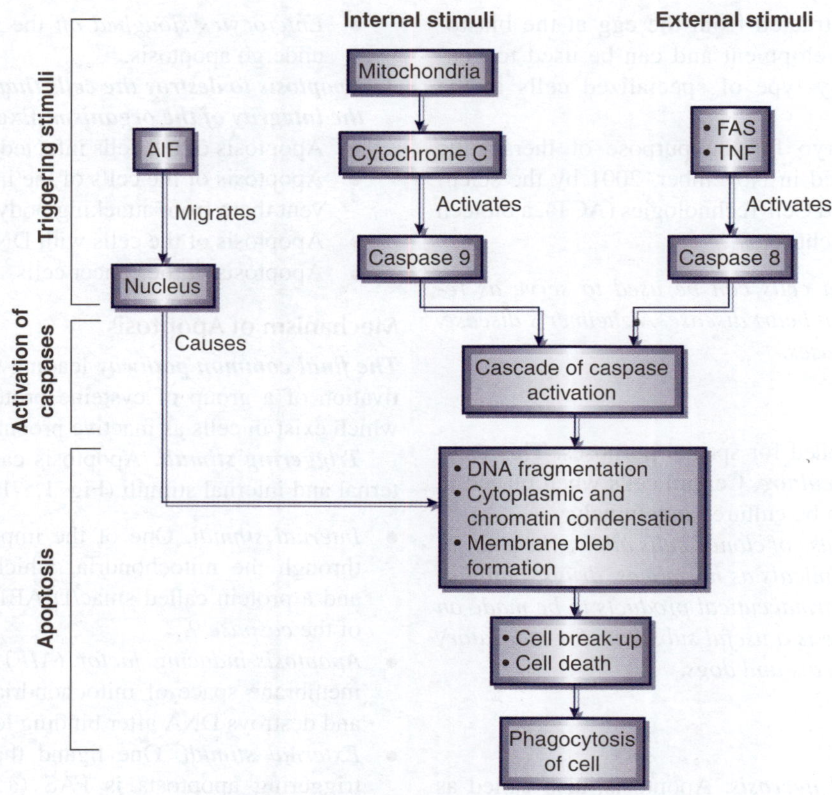

FIGURE 1.5-10 Steps involved in apoptosis.

There are two major types of mutations:

1. ***Point mutations.*** In this type, one base pair of DNA is replaced by another. Point mutations are further of two subtypes: transitions and transversions.
   - *Transitions.* In this type of mutation, purine or pyrimidine is replaced by another purine or pyrimidine, respectively.
   - *Transversions.* In this type of mutation, a purine is replaced by pyrimidine or pyrimidine is replaced by purine.

   Effects of point mutations. Point mutations can lead to one of the following effects:

   a. *Silent mutation.* No detectable effect is produced when the codon (of mRNA) containing change base codes for same amino acid. For example, UCA codes for serine but when there is change in third base (UCU) still it codes for serine. Therefore, when no effect is detected it is called *silent mutation.*

   b. *Missense mutation.* This occurs when altered base codes for different amino acid and that amino acid in a protein molecule may be acceptable or partially acceptable or not acceptable as far as the action of protein molecule is concerned. The amino acid so formed is called *mistaken* or *missense amino acid.* The classical example of effect of missense mutation is sickle cell anaemia.

   c. *Nonsense mutation.* When the codon with changed base may become the *termination codon* and acts as stop signal and thus causes termination of protein synthesis at that point, the effect produced is called nonsense mutation.

2. ***Frame shift mutations.*** This occurs when one or more than one base pairs are either deleted or inserted into the DNA of gene. Therefore, frame shift mutations are also called deletion or insertional mutations.

   Effects of frame shift mutations. *The consequences as a result of insertion or deletion of a base in a gene cause altered reading frame of the mRNA. Thus, the machinery of mRNA (containing codon) is unable to recognize that a new base is added or missing. Since there is no punctuation in reading of codons, translation continues and as a result of that the proteins synthesized will have many altered amino acids and/or premature terminated proteins.*

Genetic Human Diseases

Salient aspects of some common genetic human diseases associated with mutations are summarized in Table 1.5-1.

Genetic Screening

Genetic screening refers to detection of mutant genes in an individual (detecting human genetic variations). Modern genetics is making this much earlier than it was in the past.

TABLE 1.5-1 Some Common Genetic Diseases

Genetic disease/ disorder	Chromosome affected	Type of mutation	Expression of gene	Main symptoms	Defect	Frequency at birth
Gene Mutations						
Sickle cell anaemia	11	Substitution	Codominant (sometimes described as recessive) autosomal	Anaemia and interference with circulation	Abnormal haemoglobin molecule	1 in 1600 among black people
Cystic fibrosis	7	In 70% of cases is a deletion of three bases	Recessive autosomal	Unusually thick mucus clogs lungs, liver and pancreas	Failure of chloride ion transport mechanism in cell surface membranes of epithelial cells	1 in 1800 among white people
PKU (phenylketonuria)	12	Substitution	Recessive autosomal	Brain fails to develop normally	Enzyme phenylalanine hydroxylase defective	1 in 18,000
Huntington's chorea (disease)	4	A newly discovered type of mutation—the normal gene has 10–34 repeats of CAG at one end, the HC gene has 42–100 repeats of CAG	Dominant autosomal	Gradual deterioration of brain tissue starting on an average in middle age	Brain cell metabolism is inhibited	1 in 10,000 to 1 in 20,000 worldwide
Haemophilia	X	Substitution	Recessive sex linked	Blood does not clot	Factor VIII or IX protein defective	1 in 7000
Chromosome Mutations						
Down's syndrome	21	Extra chromosome (trisomy 21)		Reduced intelligence, characteristic facial features		1 in 750
Klinefelter's syndrome (XXY)	Sex	Extra X chromosome in male (trisomy)		Feminized male		1 in 500
Turner's syndrome (XO)	Sex	Missing X chromosome in female (monosomy)		Sterile female		1 in 2500

Autosomal – affecting nonsex chromosome (autosome).
Monosomy – one chromosome missing ($2n - 1$).
Trisomy – one extra chromosome ($2n + 1$).
Monosomy and trisomy are examples of **aneuploidy,** where the total number of chromosomes is not an exact multiple of the haploid number.

Field of Genetic Screening

There are three situations where genetic screening is of particular relevance:

1. ***Prenatal diagnosis.*** Prenatal diagnosis aims at identifying the health problems of unborn babies. Parents can be provided counselling and option for abortion as per situation.
   Techniques of prenatal diagnosis include:
   - Chorionic villus sampling (CVS),
   - Amniocentesis and
   - Preimplantation diagnosis.
2. ***Carrier diagnosis.*** This is the identification of people who carry a particular genetic disease, usually with no visible symptom or harm to themselves. Examples include sickle cell anaemia, cystic fibrosis and phenylketonuria (PKU).
3. ***Predictive diagnosis.*** This is the prediction of a future disease from which one is likely to suffer. The classic example of this 'genetic time bomb' is Huntington's chorea where the onset of disease occurs in middle age.

Genetics and Cancer

Cancer is a disease characterized by uncontrolled cell growth.

Points Favouring Genetic Basis for Cancer

- *Hereditary predisposition* is noted in some cancers like colon cancer and retinoblastoma.
- *Chromosomal abnormalities* are noted in many forms of cancers like Burkitt's lymphoma and acute myeloid leukaemia.
- *Defective DNA repair mechanisms* have been associated with occurrence of cancers.
- *Genetic damages* (mutagenesis) by the action of various agents like ionizing radiations and UV rays are associated with occurrence of cancer.

Genes and Molecular Factor Involved in Pathogenesis of Cancer

1. Oncogenes. Over 100 oncogenes (cancer-causing genes) have been described. These genes are derived by somatic mutations from the closely related *proto-oncogenes* (normal genes that encode proteins having a role in cell's normal activities).

Genetic changes converting proto-oncogenes into oncogenes are:

- *Missense mutation,* i.e. change in the amino acid sequence of proto-oncogene protein converts it into oncogene.
- *Gene amplification,* e.g. Myc genes have been amplified in human leukaemia, breast, stomach, lung and colon cancer.
- *Chromosomal translocations,* e.g. in Burkitt's lymphoma, a region of chromosome 8 is translocated to either chromosome 2, 14 or 22. The breakpoint in chromosome 8 causes the overexpression of c-myc gene.
- *Retroviral integration,* e.g. in avian lymphomas, the integration of the avian leucosis virus can enhance the transcription of the c-myc gene.

2. Tumour Suppressor Gene (Antioncogenes). Over 10 tumour suppressor genes have been described which produce proteins that suppress a tumour. When a tumour suppressor gene becomes inactivated by mutation, it becomes more likely that cancer will occur. It is important to note that for causing cancer, both alleles of tumour suppressor genes should be mutated. The most studied of these genes are RB gene (retinoblastoma gene) and P^{53} gene.

- ***RB gene.*** Retinoblastoma (RB) gene functions as cancer suppressor. After two mutations (Knudson's two-hit hypothesis) when both copies of the gene at the retinoblastoma locus (14.1 band on the long arm of chromosome 13, i.e. 13q 14.1) are lost, deleted or inactivated, retinoblastoma (tumour of retina occurring in early childhood) develops.
- ***P^{53} gene.*** About 50% of all human cancer are associated with defects in P^{53} gene.

  Induction of the P^{53} gene leads to the synthesis of P^{53} protein that functions as a transcription factor and can:
  - Activate genes that promote DNA repair,
  - Activate genes that arrest cell division and may generally repress other genes that are required for cell division.
  - Activate genes that promote apoptosis.

  Mutation in P^{53} gene leads to production of P^{53} protein that fails to perform the aforementioned functions and permit other mutations in DNA to persist. The accumulated mutations eventually cause cancer.

3. Mutator Genes. Normal cells have caretaker genes that regulate DNA repair, i.e. they prevent faulty DNA transcription and regulation. The mutated version or mutator gene is characterized by loss of normal surveillance function that renders DNA susceptible to accumulation of mutation, and therefore progression of cancer.

4. Telomeres in Cancer. Telomeres take care of the terminal tips of the chromosomes, which progressively shorten due to repetitive cell division. Telomerase is the enzyme required for continued recognition of telomere in successive cell divisions. Cancer cell expresses telomerase with consequent telomerase lengthening and this helps the transformed cells to maintain their cancerous state.

Conclusion. *To conclude, cancer is a multistep phenomenon where series of genetic changes with or without virus infection cause the development of final cancerous state (Fig. 1.5-11). These genetic changes can be produced by:*

- Ionizing radiations,
- Chemic carcinogens,
- Radioactive material,
- Spontaneous mutations and
- Inherited mutations.

Gene Therapy

Gene therapy is the name given to methods that aim to cure an inherited disease by providing the patient with a correct copy of the defective gene. Gene therapy has now been extended to include the attempts to cure any disease by introduction of a cloned gene into the patient.

Basic Principles

Basic principles involved in correcting a genetic defect are:

- ***Gene replacement,*** i.e. replacement of a mutant gene with a normal gene.
- ***Gene correction,*** i.e. correction of the mutated area (specific bases) of DNA leaving the rest of DNA unchanged.
- ***Gene augmentation,*** i.e. insertion of a foreign DNA into the genome of a cell to rectify the genetic defect.

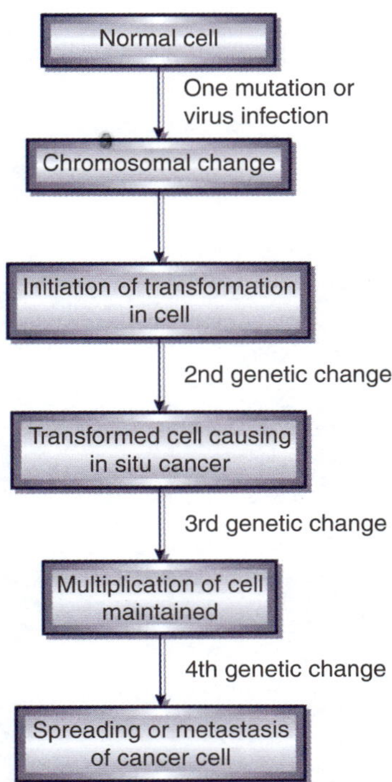

FIGURE 1.5-11 Multistep phenomena of series of genetic changes leading to development of cancer.

Basic approaches *to gene therapy are:*

- ***Germ line therapy*** can be carried out by microinjection of DNA into the isolated egg cell that is reimplanted into the mother. If successful, the gene is present and expressed in all cells of the resulting individual. Thus, theoretically the germ line therapy can be used to treat any inherited disease. At the moment such treatment is regarded as unethical in humans because the gene would be passed on to future generations.
- ***Somatic cell therapy.*** In humans, at the moment the focus is on somatic cell therapy. This involves changing some, though not all, of the somatic cells which are nonsex cells of the body. Changes in these cells cannot be inherited. The patients treated will therefore be cured but they will still be able to pass the faulty gene on to their offspring. Steps involved in this therapy are:
  - Isolation of the cells with the gene defect from a patient;
  - Growing the isolated cells in culture;
  - Transfecting the isolated cell with a remedial gene construct;
  - Selecting, growing and testing the transfecting cells and
  - Either transplanting or transfusing the transfecting cells back into the patients.

Examples of Successful Trials of Gene Therapy

Somatic cell therapy in cystic fibrosis of the lung. The gene (cDNA) cloned in adenovirus vectors or contained in liposomes, when introduced into the respiratory tract via an inhaler, is taken up by the epithelial cells. These epithelial cells then synthesize normal protein called CFTR. Probably, 10% of the cells need to be corrected to eliminate the problem.

Somatic cell therapy in severe combined immunodeficiency disease (SCID). In this disease, the mutated gene is unable to synthesize the enzyme ADA adenosine deaminase. ADA is needed by the white blood cells (lymphocytes) responsible for immunity against infection. Without ADA, the child develops SCID and dies of infection in the early childhood.

Two children, aged 4 and 9, suffering from SCID were selected for gene therapy in USA in 1990. Lymphocytes were isolated from the children, then a normal gene was introduced by means of a retrovirus vector and the cells were replaced. These children had shown significant improvement after 1 year of therapy, repeated every 1 to 2 month.

Gene therapy in cancer may have great potentiality:

- Inactivation of oncogenic gene by introduction of a gene or an antisense RNA of an oncogenic gene;
- Introduction of an active version of tumour suppressor gene;
- Introduction of a gene that will selectively kill the cancer cells and
- Gene therapy to improve the natural killing of cancer cells by the patient's immune system.

Part II

Systemic Physiology

Section

Section 2

Nerve Muscle Physiology

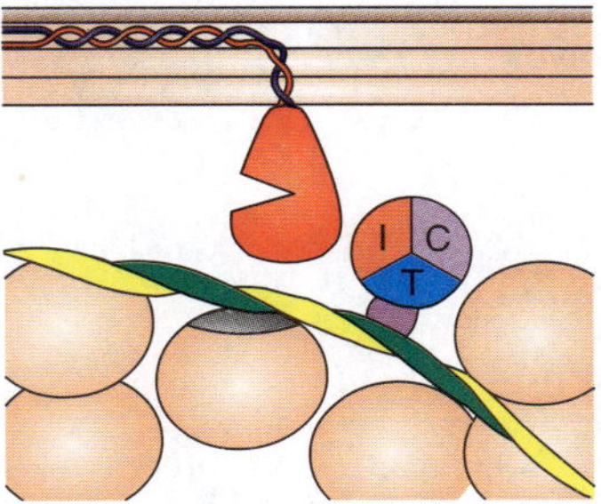

The nerve and muscle cells are *excitable*, that is, capable of generation of electrical impulses at their membranes. For this very reason, the physiological aspects of these excitable tissues are discussed together in this section.

The electrical impulses generated in the excitable tissues, in most instances, can be used to transmit signals along the membranes. A neuron is the basic unit of nervous tissue. It is specialized for the function of reception, integration and transmission of information in the body. Muscles, like neurons, are excitable tissues but are characterized by the fact that a mechanical contraction follows an action potential.

To understand the physiological aspects, it is imperative to have knowledge about the *functional anatomy* and physiological properties of the nerve, the muscle and the neuromuscular junction. Further, to understand the fundamental aspects of generation of the electrical impulses by the excitable tissues, it will be worthwhile to revise the basics of membrane potential which have been described in Chapter 1.4 (page 32).

Chapter 2.1

The Nerve

FUNCTIONAL ANATOMY

Neuron

Neuron or the nerve cell is the structural and functional unit of the nervous system. An aggregation of the neuronal cell bodies located inside the central nervous system (CNS) is called a *nucleus* and that located outside the CNS is called a *ganglion.* The nervous system of humans is made up of innumerable neurons. The total number of estimated neurons in the human brain is more than 10^{12}. The neurons are linked together in a highly intricate manner. It is through these connections that the body is made aware of changes in the environment or of those inside the body itself; and appropriate responses to such changes are produced.

Structure

Neurons vary considerably in size, shape and other features. However, most of them have some major features in common. The neuron is like any other cell in the body except that it has processes. The basic structure of a neuron is best studied in a spinal motor neuron. A neuron primarily consists of the cell body and processes called *neurites,* which are of two kinds, the dendrites and the axon (Fig. 2.1-1).

Cell Body The cell body of a neuron is also called the *soma* or *perikaryon* and may be round, stellate, pyramidal or fusiform in shape. Like any other cell it consists of a mass of cytoplasm with all its principal constituents surrounded by a cell membrane. The cell body contains a large nucleus with one or two nucleoli but there is no centrosome. The absence of centrosome indicates that the neuron has lost ability for division. Thus, neurons once destroyed are replaced by neuroglia only. In addition to the general features of a typical cell (page 12), the cytoplasm of a neuron has following distinctive characteristics (Fig. 2.1-1):

Nissl Granules/Bodies. These are basophilic granules, and when seen under electron microscope these bodies seem to be composed of rough-surfaced endoplasmic reticulum. The presence of abundant granular endoplasmic reticulum is an indication of the high level of protein synthesis in neurons. The proteins are needed for the maintenance and repair and for the production of neurotransmitters and enzymes. The Nissl bodies are present in the dendrites as well, but are usually absent from axon hillock and the axon. These bodies disintegrate into fine dust and finally disappear (*chromatolysis*) on fatigue, due to the effect of certain poisons and on sectioning of the axon.

Neurofibrillae. The presence of a network of neurofibrillae in the cytoplasm of the neuron is another distinctive feature. These consist of microfilaments and microtubules. In certain degenerative diseases like Alzheimer's disease, the neurofilament protein gets altered, resulting in the formation of characteristic lesions called *neurofibrillary tangles.*

Pigment Granules. These are seen in some neurons. For example, *neuromelanin* is present in the neurons of substantia nigra. Aging neurons contain the pigment *lipofuscin.*

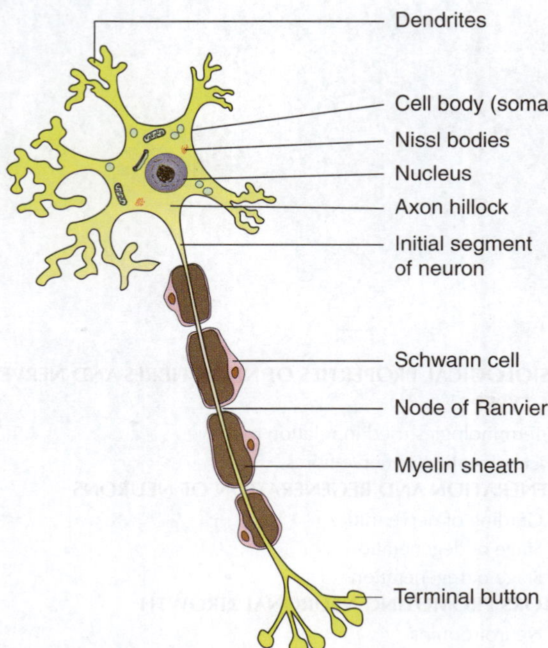

FIGURE 2.1-1 Structure of a typical neuron.

Dendrites

The dendrites are multiple small branched processes. Dendrites contain Nissl bodies and neurofibres. These often look thorny due to numerous minute projections called *spines* present on their surface. The spines are the site of synaptic contact.

Dendrites are the *receptive processes* of the neuron receiving signals from other neurons via their synapses with axon terminals. The synaptic inputs produce *graded local potentials* which get algebraically summated on the surface of dendrites. Dendrites usually do not produce action potentials. They mostly conduct graded potentials. Some very long dendrites like axons may conduct action potentials.

Axon

The axon is the single longer process of the nerve cell. It varies in length from a few microns to one metre. It arises from the conical extension of the cell body called *axon hillock,* which is devoid of Nissl bodies. The part of the axon between the axon hillock and the beginning of the myelin sheath is called the *initial segment.* In the axon, the cell membrane continues as *axolemma* and the cytoplasm as *axoplasm.* The axon terminates by dividing into a number of branches, each ending in a number of *synaptic knobs* also known as *terminal buttons* or axon telodendria. Synaptic knobs contain microvesicles in which chemical neurotransmitters are stored. *Myelin sheath* is present around the axons in the so-called myelinated nerve fibres (Fig. 2.1-2A). Myelin sheath, which consists of protein–lipid complex is produced by glial cells called *Schwann cells* which encircle the axon, forming around it a thin sleeve (Fig. 2.1-2B). The Schwann cell wraps its membranes about 100 times around an axon and then the myelin is compacted by an extracellular membrane protein called protein zero (Po). Each Schwann cell provides the myelin sheath for a short segment of the axon. At the junction of any two such segments, there is a short gap, i.e. (periodic 1 μm constrictions at about 1 mm distance). These gaps are the *nodes of Ranvier.* In the central nervous system of mammals myelin sheath is formed by oligodendrocytes rather than Schwann cells. There are some axons which are devoid of myelin sheath. These *unmyelinated axons* invaginate into the cytoplasm of Schwann cells (Fig. 2.1-2C).

Myelination of axons increases the speed of conduction and greatly increases their diameter. In motor nerves, speed is important. Hence motor neurons to muscles and sensory (proprioceptive) fibres from muscles are heavily myelinated.

Axons perform the specialized function of conducting impulses away from the cell body. They transmit propagated impulses (all or none transmission).

Applied Aspects

In demyelinating disorders such as *multiple sclerosis* there occurs patchy destruction of myelin sheath in the central nervous system.

Multiple sclerosis is an autoimmune disease in which antibodies and white blood cells attack the myelin sheath leading to inflammation and injury to myelin sheath. Due to loss of myelin sheath there is leakage of K^+ through voltage-gated channels resulting in hyperpolarization and thus failure of action potential conduction.

Sign and symptoms: In patients with multiple sclerosis the physiological deficit ranges from muscle weakness, fatigue, diminished motor function & sensory disturbances. The diagnosis of these patients are based on following tests:

i. *Nerve conduction tests* which detect slow conduction in motor and sensory pathways.

ii. *Cerebrospinal fluid analysis* which detects oligoclonal bands indicative of an abnormal autoimmune response against myelin sheath.

iii. *Magnetic resonance imaging (MRI) assessment* visualizes multiple sclerotic area in the brain .

Treatment: Although there is no specific treatment of multiple sclerosis, drugs like *interferon* can suppress autoimmune response.

Types of Neurons

Neurons have been variously classified as:

I. Depending Upon the Number of Poles Depending upon the number of poles from which processes arise, neurons are divided into unipolar, bipolar and multipolar (Fig. 2.1-3).

1. Unipolar Neurons have a single pole, from which both the processes—axons and dendrites arise (Fig. 2.1-3A). True unipolar cells are present only in embryonic stage in human beings. However, the primary sensory neurons

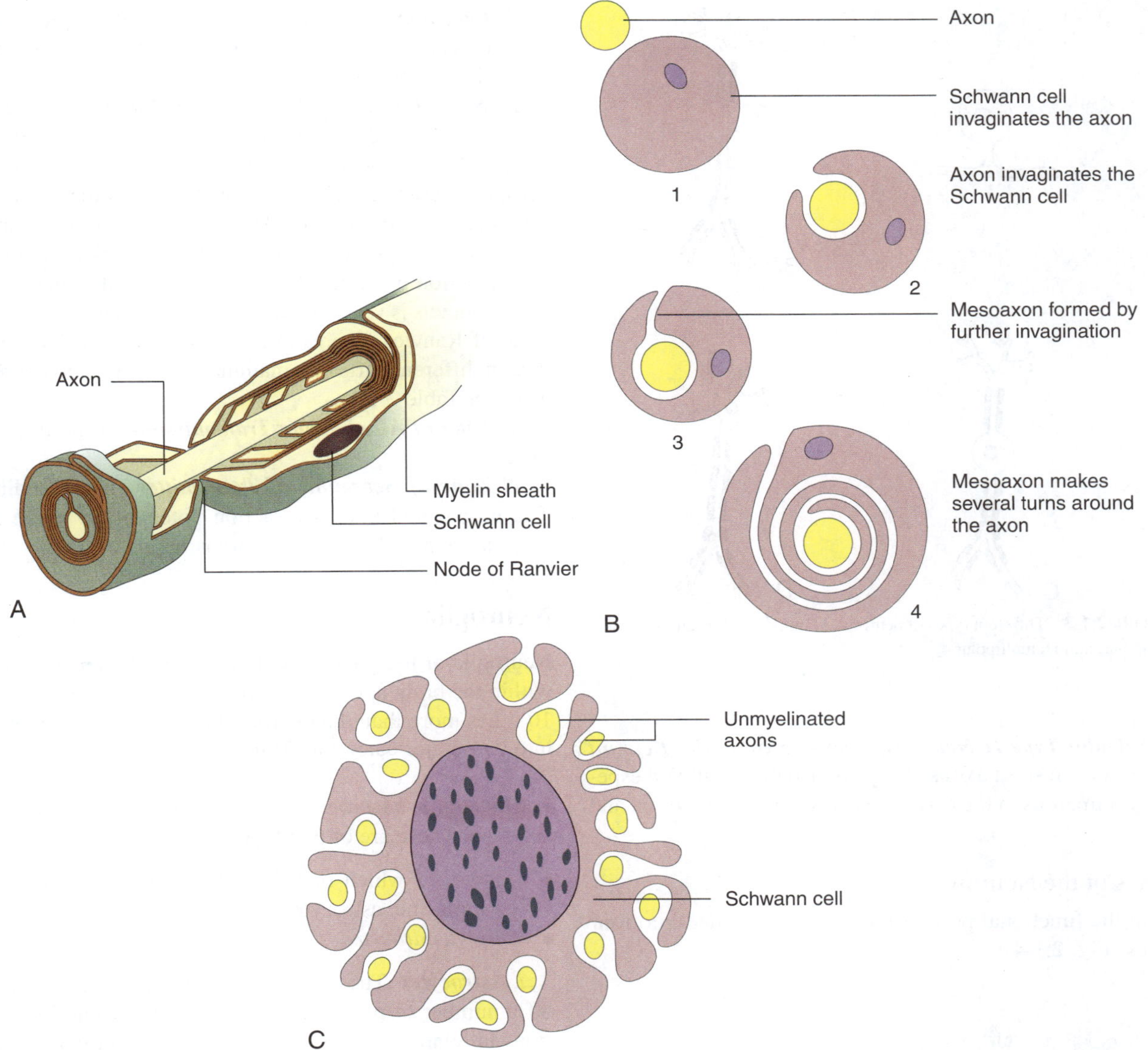

FIGURE 2.1-2 Structure of a myelinated neuron: **A,** Schwann cell encircles the axon to form myelin sheath; **B,** stages of myelination; and **C,** structure of an unmyelinated neuron. **Note:** Unmyelinated axons invaginate cytoplasm of Schwann cell.

(neurons conveying impulses from a sensory receptor to spinal cord) are *pseudounipolar* (Fig. 2.1-3B).

2. Bipolar Neurons have two poles, one for axons and the other for dendrites (Fig. 2.1-3C). Bipolar neurons are found in the vestibular and cochlear ganglia and in the nasal olfactory epithelium and as bipolar cells in the retina.

3. Multipolar neurons have many poles. One of the poles gives rise to axons and all others to dendrites (Fig. 2.1-3D). Most vertebrate neurons, especially in the CNS are multipolar. The dendrites branch profusely to form the dendritic tree.

II. Depending Upon the Function Depending upon the functions, the neurons are of two types–motor and sensory.

1. Motor Neurons, also known as efferent nerve cells, carry the motor impulses from CNS to the peripheral effector organs like muscles, glands and blood vessels. These neurons have very long axons and short dendrites.

2. Sensory Neurons, also known as afferent nerve cells, carry sensory impulses from periphery to the CNS. These neurons have short axons and long dendrites.

III. Depending Upon the Length of Axons Depending upon the length of axons the neurons are divided into Golgi type I and Golgi type II.

1. Golgi Type I Neurons also known as projection neurons, have long axons. Their cell body lies in the CNS and axons reach the remote peripheral organs. They include the neuron forming peripheral nerves and long tracts of brain and spinal cord.

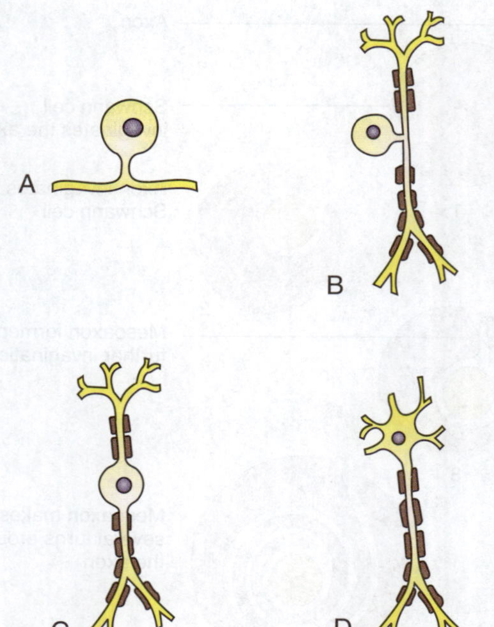

FIGURE 2.1-3 Different types of neurons: **A,** unipolar; **B,** pseudounipolar; **C,** bipolar; and **D,** multipolar.

2. Golgi Type II Neurons, also known as *short circuit neurons* have short axons. They are usually small and especially numerous in the cerebral cortex, cerebellar cortex and retina.

Zones of the Neuron

From the functional point each neuron is divided into four zones (Fig. 2.1-4):

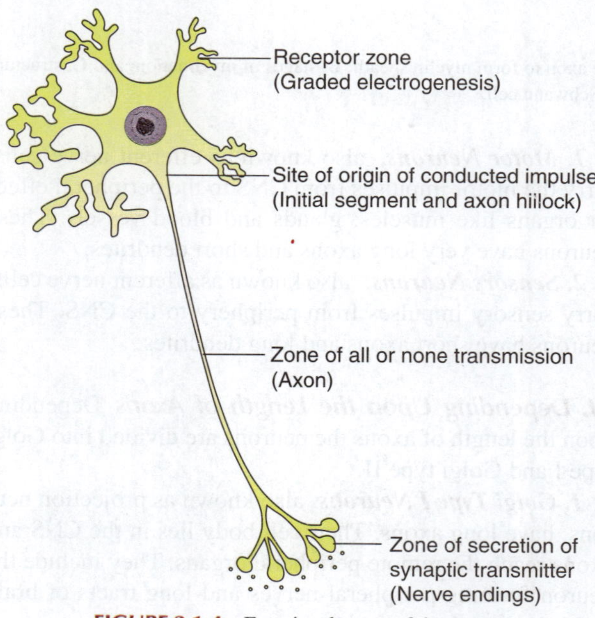

FIGURE 2.1-4 Functional zones of the neuron.

1. Receptor Zone (dendritic zone) is the region where local potential changes are generated by integration of the synaptic connections.

2. Site of Origin of Conducted Impulse is the site where propagated action potentials are generated. In case of spinal motor neurons, *initial segment* and in cutaneous sensory neurons the *first node* of Ranvier is the site of origin of conducted impulses. The distribution of ion channels along the axon plays an important role in initiation of propagated action potential. The concentration of voltage-gated Na^+ channels is very high in the initial segment and the first node of Ranvier. The estimated distribution of Na^+ channels in different parts of a mammalian myelinated neuron is as under Table 2.1-1.

3. Zone of All or None Transmission in the neuron is the axon.

4. Zone of Secretion of Transmitter (nerve endings). The propagated impulses (action potential) to nerve endings cause the release of neurotransmitter.

Neuroglia

Neuroglia or the glial cells are the supporting cells present within the brain and spinal cord. They are numerous, about 10 times more than the neurons. Glial cells may be divided into two major categories (Fig. 2.1-5):

1. Macroglia Macroglia or large glial cells are ectodermal in origin. These are of two types:

- *Astrocytes* which may be subdivided into fibrous and protoplasmic astrocytes; and
- *Oligodendrocytes.*

i. Astrocytes These are small star-shaped cells that give off a number of processes which frequently end in expansions in relation to blood vessels and in relation to the surface of brain. *Fibrous astrocytes* (Fig. 2.1-5A) are seen mainly in the white matter and *protoplasmic astrocytes* (Fig. 2.1-5B) in the grey matter.

TABLE 2.1-1 Distribution of Sodium Channels in Human Myelinated Neuron

Part of the neuron	Number/μm^2
Cell body	50–75
Initial segment	350–500
Surface of myelin sheath	<25
Node of Ranvier	2000–12,000
Axon terminals	20–50
Unmyelinated axon	~110

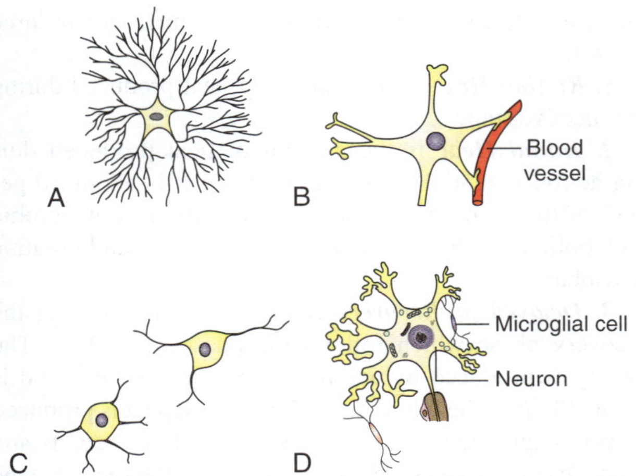

FIGURE 2.1-5 Different types of glial cells: **A,** fibrous astrocyte; **B,** protoplasmic astrocyte; **C,** oligodendrocyte; and **D,** microglial cells.

Functions. In addition to supportive function, the astrocytes play a role in:

- Regulation of synaptic activity,
- Metabolism of neurotransmitters and of neuromodulators and
- Maintenance of blood–brain barrier.

ii. Oligodendrocytes Oligodendrocytes have rounded or pear-shaped bodies with scanty processes (Fig. 2.1-5C). These cells provide myelin sheath to nerve fibres that lie within the brain and spinal cord. Oligodendrocytes give off multiple processes which form myelin sheath on many neighbouring axons.

2. Microglia Microglia or the small glial cells are mesodermal in origin. These are the smallest neuroglial cells having flattened cell bodies and short processes (Fig. 2.1-5D). They are more numerous in grey matter than in white matter. These act as phagocytes and become active after damage to nervous tissue by trauma or disease.

Peripheral Nerve

A compact bundle of axons located outside the CNS is called a nerve. In a nerve the axons are arranged in different bundles called fasciculi (Fig. 2.1-6).

- Each axon or nerve fibre is covered by *endoneurium* which is bounded internally by basal lamina around the Schwann cells and externally by the relatively impermeable inner basal lamina of the perineurium.
- Each fasciculus is covered by *perineurium.* The cells of perineurium are tightly adherent and act as a barrier to passage of particulate traces, dye molecules or toxins into the endoneurium.
- The whole nerve is covered by *epineurium* which is a tubular sheath formed by areolar membrane. It limits the extent to which the nerve can be stretched by body movements or external pressure, thereby protecting the fragile axons inside the nerve.

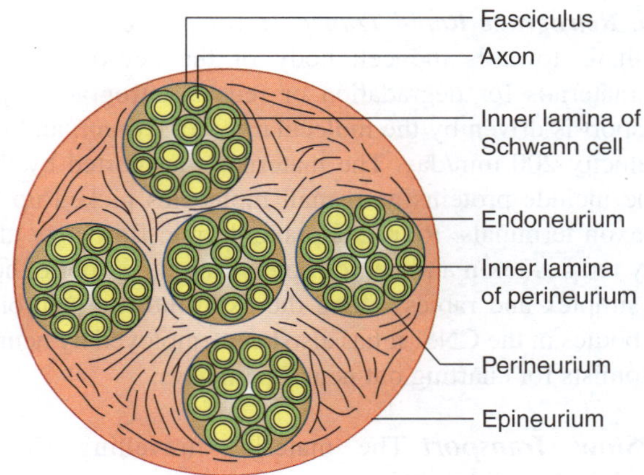

FIGURE 2.1-6 Cross-section of a peripheral nerve.

BIOLOGICAL ACTIVITIES

Protein Synthesis

The cell bodies (soma) of all the neurons contain cellular apparatus required for protein synthesis, i.e. the ribosomes and the Golgi apparatus. Since the axons do not have these organelles, all the proteins including the neurotransmitters are synthesized in the cell body and then transported along the axon to the synaptic knobs by the process of *axoplasmic flow,* as discussed below. Thus, the cell body maintains the functional and anatomic integrity of the axon. Therefore, if the axon is cut, the part distal to cut degenerates (Wallerian degeneration).

Axoplasmic Transport

Axoplasm, the cytoplasm of the neurons is in constant motion. The axoplasmic transport is vital to nerve cell functions, since movement of various materials occur through it. The axoplasmic transport is of two types: rapid and slow.

1. Rapid Transport Some materials travel 100–400 mm a day along the axoplasm and constitute the rapid transport. Microtubules play an important role in this form of transport. Rapid transport is bidirectional, i.e. both away from and towards the cell body.

i. Anterograde or Orthograde Rapid Transport occurs from the neuron cell body to the axon terminal. It is driven by the molecular motors *kinesin* and *dynein.* The materials transported by anterograde rapid transport include membrane-bounded organelles like short tubules of reticulum, mitochondria, small vesicles, actin, myosin and the clathrin used in recycling of synaptic vesicle membrane.

*ii. **Retrograde Rapid Transport*** occurs from the nerve terminals towards the cell body of the neuron, returning materials for degradation or reuse. Retrograde rapid transport is driven by the molecular motor *dynein*, and has a velocity 200 mm/day. The materials transported by this mode include proteins and small molecules picked up by the axon terminals. Retrograde axoplasmic flow may also carry tetanus toxin and neurotropic viruses (e.g. polio, herpes simplex and rabies) along the axon into the neuronal cell bodies in the CNS. It has also been employed by neuroanatomists for charting out neural pathways.

2. Slow Transport The materials travelling slowly (0.1–2 mm in a day) in the axoplasm constitute the slow transport. Slow transport is only unidirectional, away from the cell body (anterograde). It is responsible for flow of axoplasm containing protein subunits of neurofilaments, tubulins of the microtubules and soluble enzymes.

The exact mechanism of slow axonal transport is not known. Probably, axoplasmic matrix moves with the cytoskeleton which moves as a whole due to the continual polymerization at the leading end and depolymerization at the trailing end.

Metabolism and Heat Production in the Nerve Fibres

Like other cells of the body, the metabolic activities occur in the nerve fibres as well; but the metabolism in nerve fibres occurs at a very low level. About 70% of the total energy required is used to maintain polarization of the membrane by the action of Na^+–K^+ATPase pump. The energy required to maintain polarization of the resting membrane is supplied mainly by combustion of sugars and phospholipids.

During nerve activity, the ATP and creatine phosphate breakdown, i.e. undergo hydrolysis and supply energy for the propagation of the nerve impulse. At maximum activity, the metabolic rate of nerve fibres just doubles the metabolic rate at resting stage. Whereas, in skeletal muscles the metabolic activity rate may increase by 100 times than the metabolic rate at rest. However, the chemical changes during metabolic activity are almost the same in a nerve and a muscle, i.e. if oxygen supply is deficient, pyruvic acid and lactic acids are formed and accumulate. The nerve fibres are rich in vitamin B_1, which is essential for complete oxidation of pyruvic acid and lactic acids. Further, unlike muscles, even in the absence of oxygen, processes like excitability, conductivity and recovery can go on in a nerve for a considerable period.

Heat Production in the Nerve Fibres As discussed above, the metabolism in the nerve fibre is very slow; therefore, during resting phase only a small amount of heat is produced, which increases to some extent during phase of activity. In a nerve fibre, heat is produced in three phases:

1. Resting Heat is the amount of heat produced during the inactive stage.

2. Initial Heat is the amount of heat produced during action potential (stage of activity). It is about 10 per cent of the total heat produced. It results from anaerobic metabolic activity due to breakdown of ATP and creatine phosphate.

3. Delayed or Recovery Heat is produced during the recovery phase which follows the phase of activity. The energy is produced by aerobic metabolic activities and is about 30 times the initial heat. The delayed heat is produced in two stages: the first stage lasts for a few seconds and produces only a small amount of heat, and the second stage lasts for 10–30 min and contributes the major amount of the total heat produced. The energy produced during recovery stage is used for resynthesis of ATP and creatine phosphate and as such for restoring the normal excitability of the nerve fibre.

ELECTRICAL PROPERTIES OF NERVE FIBRE

The main electrical properties of the nerve fibres are:

- *excitability,* i.e. the capability of generating electrical impulses (action potential), and
- *conductivity,* i.e. the ability of propagating the electrical impulses generated along the entire length of nerve fibres.

Excitability

Excitability is that property of the nerve fibre by virtue of which it responds by generating a nerve signal (electrical impulses or the so-called action potentials) when it is stimulated by a suitable stimulus which may be mechanical, thermal, chemical or electrical. In experimental studies, electrical stimulus is more frequently employed since its strength and frequency can be accurately controlled.

Before discussing the excitability (production of action potential), it will be useful to know about the electrical potential in the nerve fibre at rest, i.e. before it is stimulated (resting membrane potential). Further, when the stimulus is subthreshold it does not produce action potential but it causes some change in the resting membrane potential termed as electrotonic potential. After discussing the production of action potential, various characteristics of the stimulus which can affect the production of action potential will be discussed.

Resting Membrane Potential

There exists a membrane potential of −70 mV (inside negative) across the membrane of nerve fibre at rest. This is called *resting membrane potential.* The study of electrical activity of a tissue has been made possible due to advances in the method of the recording electrical potentials, especially the development of microelectrodes and 'cathode ray oscilloscope (CRO)' (for details see page 70).

As shown in Fig. 2.1-7A, when two electrodes are placed on the surface of a nerve fibre and connected to a CRO, no potential difference is observed. However, if one of the microelectrodes is inserted inside the nerve fibre (Fig. 2.1-7B), a steady potential difference of −70 mV (inside negative) is observed on the CRO. This is resting membrane potential (RMP) and indicates the resting state of cell also called *state of polarization.*

Ionic Basis of Resting Membrane Potential (RMP)

The details of the processes concerned with the ionic basis of RMP, i.e. selective permeability of cell membrane, Gibbs–Donnan equilibrium, Nernst equation, Goldman's constant field equation and role of Na^+–K^+ pump have been discussed in Chapter 1.4 on *membrane potentials* (page 32). However, the ionic basis of RMP is summarized here.

In a nutshell, the distribution of ions across the cell membrane and the nature of cell membrane are responsible for the RMP. Basically, RMP is diffusion potential modified to some extent by the activity of Na^+–K^+ pump as:

- Because of large concentration gradient the K^+ ions diffuse out of the membrane via K^+ channels, but the *electrical gradient* created opposes it.

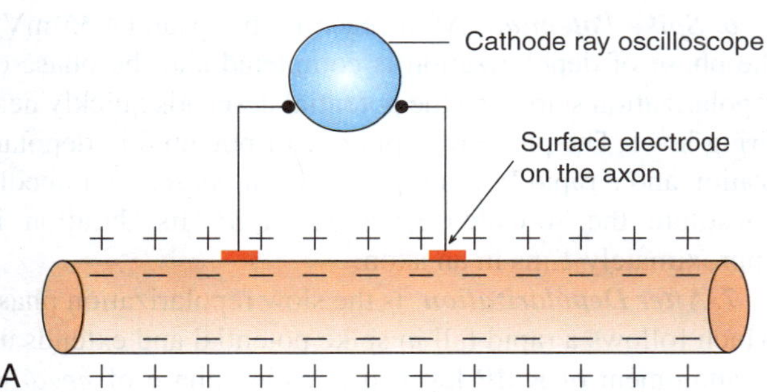

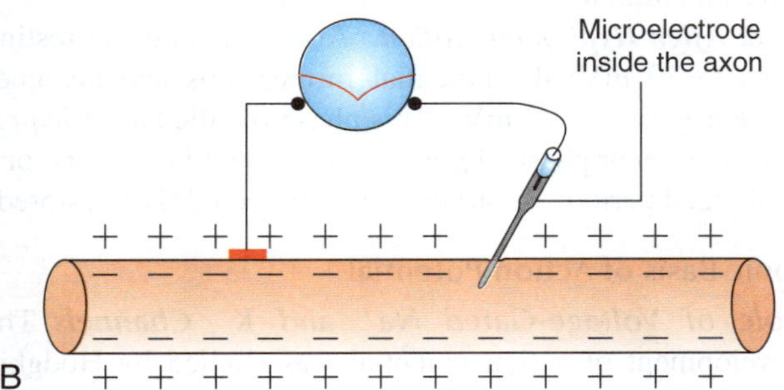

FIGURE 2.1-7 Recording of resting membrane potential: **A,** both electrodes are on the surface of axon, no potential difference is recorded; and **B,** one electrode on the surface and other inserted inside the axon, potential difference (−70 mV) is recorded.

- Consequently, equilibrium is reached where the potential difference is such that it effectively balances the outward diffusion of K^+ due to concentration gradient.
- At the equilibrium, there is slight excess of cations on the outside and anions on the inside. This condition is maintained by Na^+–K^+ pump, which pumps Na^+ back and keep the intracellular concentration of Na^+ low.
- Na^+–K^+ pump being electrogenic (because it pumps 3 Na^+ ions out of the cell for every $2K^+$ ions it pumps in), it also contributes a small amount to the membrane potential by itself.

At rest, membrane permeability to K^+ is greater due to more opened K^+ channels than the Na^+ channels. Therefore, the intracellular and extracellular K^+ concentration is the main determinant of resting membrane potential and that is why RMP is closed to equilibrium potential for K^+.

Action Potential

When the stimulus is subminimal or subthreshold, it does not produce action potential, but does produce some changes in the RMP. There is slight depolarization for about 7 mV which cannot be propagated, since propagation occurs only if the depolarization reaches a firing level of 15 mV (−55 mV). Therefore, this is a local response or phenomenon termed the *electrotonic potential.* As depicted in Fig. 2.1-8, the electrotonic potential does not obey all or none law. As is clear from Fig. 2.1-8, when the intensity of stimulus is increased gradually, every time there is an increase in the amplitude of the local response till firing level of 15 mV is reached. Once the firing level is reached, there occurs action potential, i.e. there occurs abrupt depolarization with propagation (action potential) of the cell membrane which was in a polarized state. The adequate strength of stimulus necessary for producing the action potential in a nerve fibre is known as *threshold* or *minimal stimulus.* In other words, the *action potential* may be defined as the brief sequence of changes which occur in the resting membrane potential when stimulated by a threshold stimulus.

Phases of Action Potential

The action potential basically occurs in two phases: depolarization and repolarization. When the nerve is stimulated, the polarized state (−70 mV) is altered, i.e. RMP is abolished and the interior of the nerve becomes positive (+35 mV) as compared to the exterior. This is called *depolarization phase.* Within no time there occurs a reverse to the nearly original potential and this second phase of action potential is called *repolarization phase.*

Action Potential Curve obtained when resting membrane potential is being recorded on a CRO and the nerve fibre is stimulated at a short distance away from the

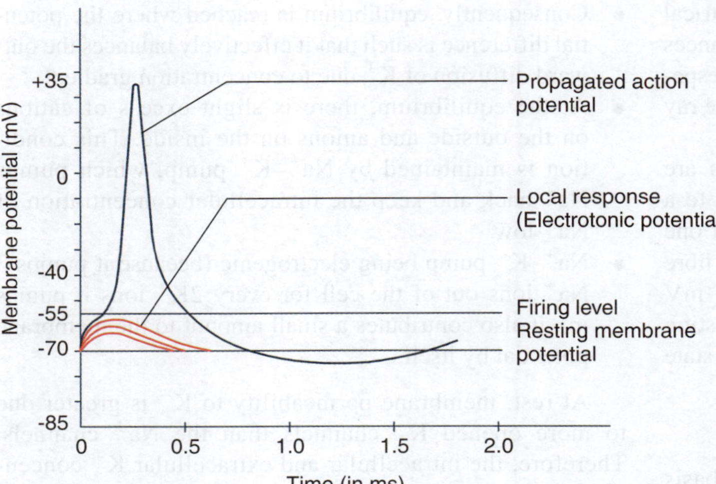

FIGURE 2.1-8 Electrotonic potentials (local response).

recording electrode (Fig. 2.1-9A), has the following components (Fig. 2.1-9B):

1. Resting Membrane Potential is recorded as a straight baseline at 270 mV.

2. Stimulus Artefact is recorded as mild deflection of the baseline as soon as the stimulus is applied. The stimulus artefact occurs due to leakage of current from the stimulating electrode to the recording electrode.

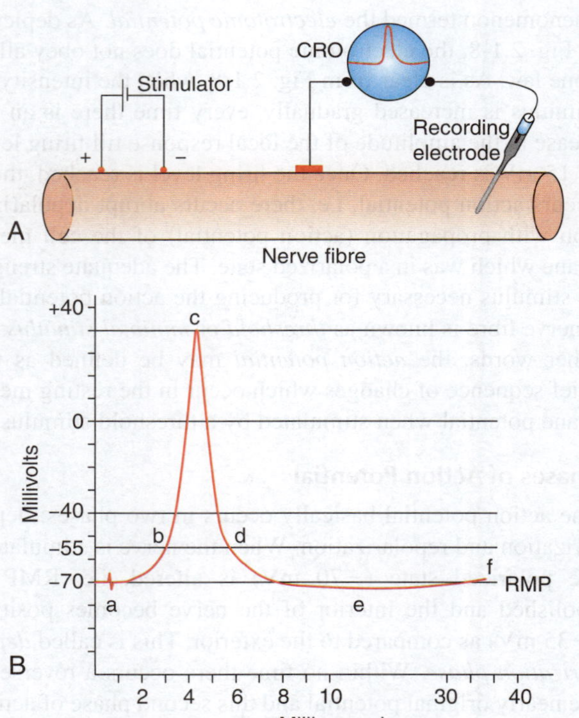

FIGURE 2.1-9 Recording of action potential of a large mammalian myelinated nerve fibre: **A,** arrangement for recording action potential; and **B,** various phases (components) of action potential. (a = stimulus artefact, b = firing level, b to c = depolarization, c to d = repolarization, d to e = after depolarization and e to f = after hyperpolarization).

3. Latent Period is recorded as short isoelectric period (0.5–1 ms) following the stimulus artefact. It represents the interval between the application of stimulus and the onset of action potential. It depends upon the distance between the site of stimulation and the point of recording and the velocity of action potential along the particular axon.

4. Firing Level. After the latent period, phase of depolarization starts. To begin with depolarization proceeds relatively slow up to a level called the *firing level* (255 mV), at which depolarization occurs very rapidly.

5. Overshoot. From the firing level, the curve reaches the zero potential rapidly and then *overshoots* the zero line up to +35 mV.

6. Spike Potential. After reaching the peak (+35 mV), the phase of depolarization is completed and the phase of repolarization starts and the potential descends quickly near firing level. The phase of rapid rise of potential in depolarization and a rapid fall in repolarization phase, combinedly constitute the so-called *spike potential.* Its duration is approximately 1 ms in an axon.

7. After Depolarization is the slow repolarization phase which follows a rapid fall in spike potential and extends up to attainment of RMP level. It is called phase of *negative after potential* and lasts for about 4 ms.

8. After Hyperpolarization. After reaching the resting level (−70 mV) the potential further falls and becomes more negative (−72 mV). This phase is called *after hyperpolarization* or phase of *positive* after potential. It lasts for a prolonged period (35–40 ms). Finally the RMP is restored.

Ionic Basis of Action Potential

Role of Voltage-Gated Na^+ and K^+ Channels The development of action potential was studied by Hodgkin and Huxley using the *voltage clamp technique.* According to *Hodgkin–Huxley theory,* the sequence of events is:

Polarization Phase. Resting membrane potential (−70 mV) is due to distribution of more cations outside the cell membrane and more anions inside the cell membrane. At this point, though Na^+ is more in ECF, it cannot enter the cell due to the impermeability of the membrane.

Depolarization Phase. When threshold stimulus is applied to the cell membrane, at the point of stimulation (Fig. 2.1-10) the permeability of the membrane for Na^+ ions increases. At first the rise of permeability for Na^+ is slow till it reaches *firing level.* When the membrane potential depolarizes, the Na^+ channels start opening up. The opening of the Na^+ channels depolarizes the membrane further, leading to the opening of greater numbers of Na^+ channels. Thus, there is *positive feedback spiral,* the so-called Hodgkin cycle (Fig. 2.1-11), resulting in rapid change in membrane potential. Once firing level is reached, the voltage-gated Na^+ channels open massively and as the concentration gradient and electrical gradient of this ion are directed inward, there occurs a rapid influx of Na^+ ions into the cell (Fig. 2.1-12A). This rapid entry of Na^+ is sufficient to overwhelm the repolarizing forces and the membrane potential seems to be carried towards the equilibrium potential of Na^+ (+60 mV). However, the depolarization does not reach a value greater than +35 mV because of following reasons:

- Na^+ channels are inactivated in a fraction of ms and the gates close again.
- Due to rapid influx of Na^+, the concentration gradient diminishes and during overshoot phase the electrical gradient for Na^+ also reverses.
- Change in the membrane potential during depolarization results in opening of voltage-gated K^+ channels (Fig. 2.1-12B). Therefore, within a fraction of ms of the threshold excitation K^+ leaves the cell along its concentration gradient.

Repolarization Phase. Repolarization occurs due to decrease in further Na^+ influx and K^+ efflux through the voltage-gated K^+ channels which open later than Na^+ channels but remain activated for a prolonged period (Fig. 2.1-10, 2.1-12B).

Decrease in Na^+ influx and efflux of K^+ causes net transfer of positive charge out of the cell that serves to complete the repolarization.

After Depolarization. After the rapid initial repolarization (spike potential), further repolarization occurs slowly. This is due to the fact that rate of K^+ efflux slows down as the electrical gradient responsible for initial rapid diffusion declines. This last phase of slow repolarization due to slow efflux of K^+ is called *after depolarization* (Fig. 2.1-12C).

After Hyperpolarization. The slow efflux of K^+ continues even after the resting membrane potential is reached, resulting in a prolonged phase of *hyperpolarization* during which the membrane potential falls up to −72 mV. However, little after, the voltage-gated K^+ channels also shut down. The final ionic distribution is brought to the resting state by the action of Na^+–K^+ pump and the leak channels (K^+ and Cl^-) (Fig. 2.1-12D).

Role of Calcium Ions In addition to Na^+ and K^+ ions, the Ca^{2+} ions also play some role in the development of action potential. The concentration of Ca^{2+} in ICF is very low as compared to ECF. Therefore, when Na^+ channels are open, some Ca^{2+} ions also move inside the cell through these opened up Na^+ channels. Further, a separate class of channels known as *slow calcium channels* also exists in the cell membrane. These calcium channels also open up admitting Ca^{2+} during development of action potential.

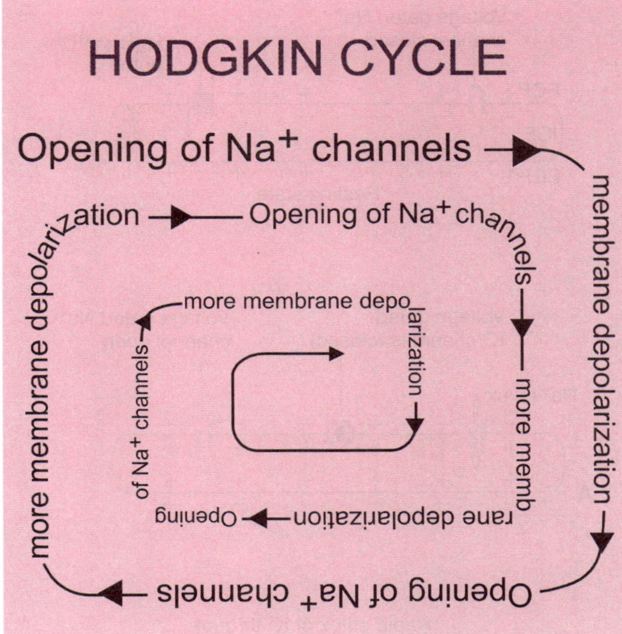

FIGURE 2.1-11 Positive feedback spiral (Hodgkin cycle).

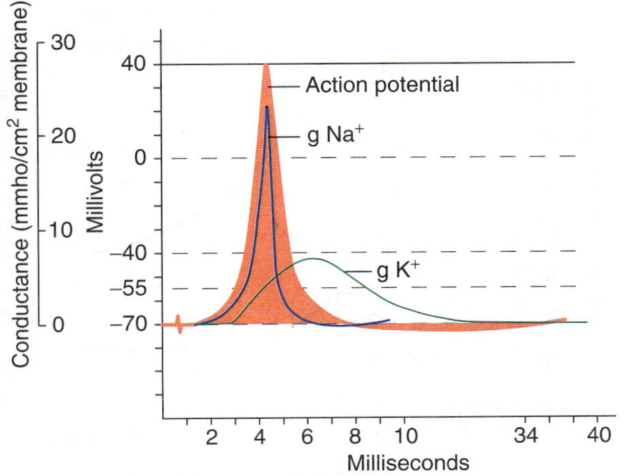

FIGURE 2.1-10 Changes in sodium (Na^+) and potassium (K^+) conductance during action potential.

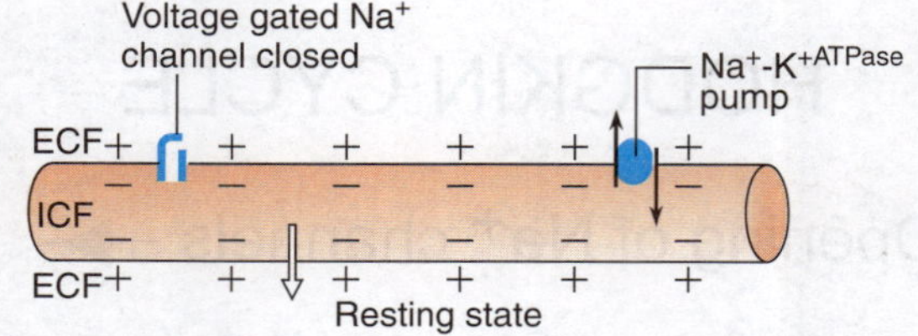

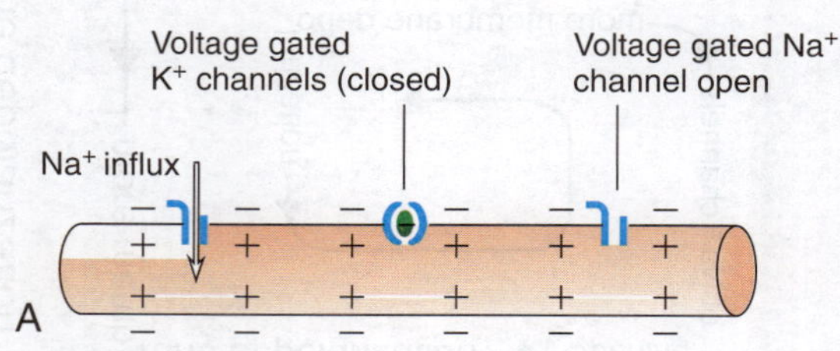

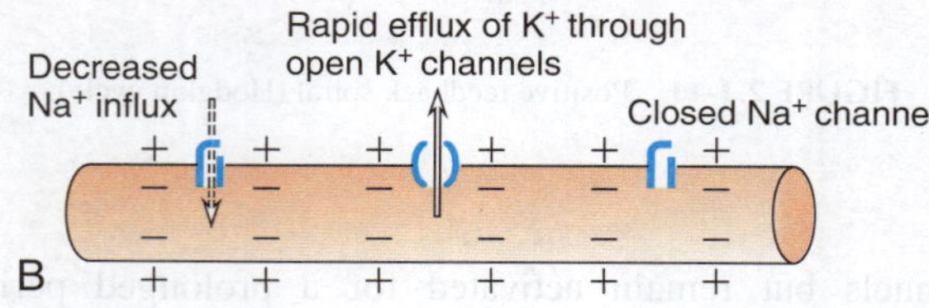

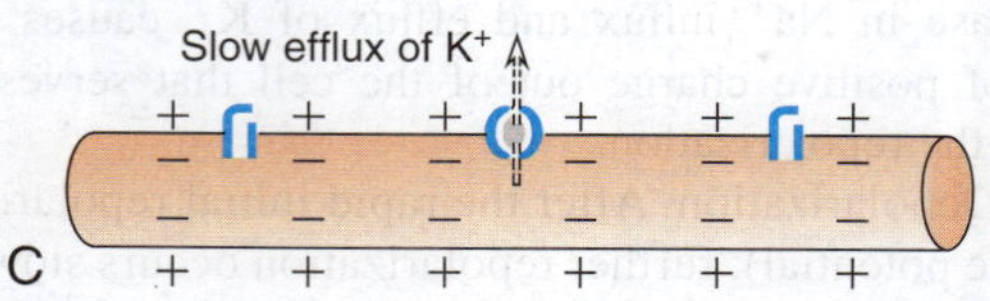

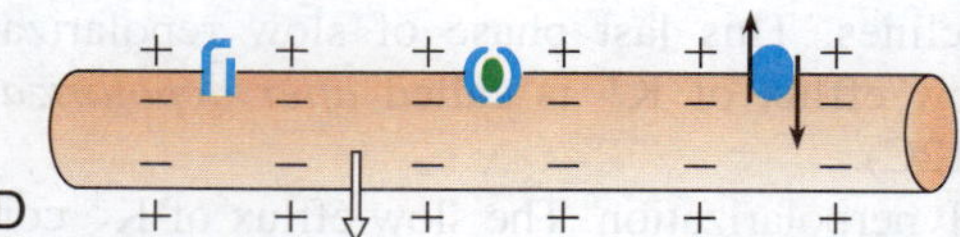

FIGURE 2.1-12 Schematic diagram to show the role of voltage-gated ion channels in resting state and during action potential: in resting state (Na^+–K^+ ATPase pump active); **A,** during depolarization phase (Na^+ channels open up and K^+ channels remain closed); **B,** during rapid repolarization phase (K^+channels open up resulting rapid efflux of K^+ and Na^+ influx decreases); **C,** during after depolarization and hyperpolarization phases, (Na^+channels get closed, K^+ efflux slows down); and **D,** restoration of resting membrane potential by activation of Na^+–K^+ ATPase pump (resulting efflux of **three** Na^+ and influx of **two** K^+).

Important Note

- Low extracellular Ca^{2+} concentration increases the excitability of nerve and muscle by decreasing the amount of depolarization necessary for initiating changes in Na^+ and K^+ conductance required for action potential, and
- Increase in Ca^{2+} concentration stabilizes the membrane by decreasing excitability.

The *calcium channels* are especially important in cardiac and smooth muscles where these are in abundance. In fact, in some types of smooth muscles, the fast sodium channels are hardly present, so the action potentials then are caused almost entirely by activation of the slow calcium channels.

Characteristics of Nerve Excitability Vis-à-Vis Characteristics of the Stimulus

The excitable nerve fibre exhibits some peculiar characteristics of the excitability depending upon the strength and duration of the stimulus used and the electrogenic state of the nerve fibre when stimulus is applied. Some of the important excitability characteristics are described.

1. Strength–Duration Curve

It has been observed experimentally that an action potential is produced if the nerve fibre is stimulated by a stimulus of adequate strength (intensity) and duration. The minimal intensity of stimulating current acting for a given duration producing an action potential is called *threshold intensity.* The relationship between the strength and duration of a stimulus has been studied by varying the duration of a stimulus and finding out the threshold strength for each duration. The record of results plotted on a semilog-graph paper gives the *strength–duration curve* (Fig. 2.1-13). Following inferences can be drawn from the strength–duration curve:

- ***Rheobase (R)*** refers to the minimum intensity of stimulus which if applied for adequate time (utilization time) produces a response.
- ***Chronaxie (C)*** refers to the minimum duration for which the stimulus of double the rheobase intensity must be applied to produce a response. Within limits, chronaxie of a given excitable tissue is constant, In other words,

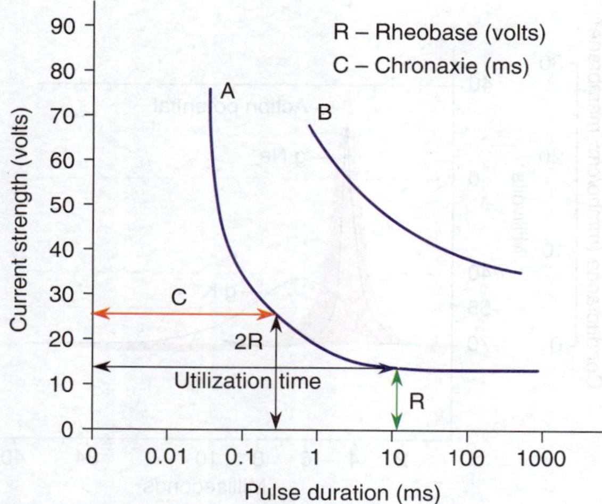

FIGURE 2.1-13 Strength–duration curves: **A,** for nerve; and **B,** for muscle.

the chronaxie is an index of the excitability of a tissue and can be used to compare the excitability of various tissues. For example, a nerve fibre has far shorter chronaxie value than a muscle fibre indicating greater excitability of the former.

- When a stimulus of weaker intensity than the rheobase is applied, it will not produce a response, no matter how long the stimulus is applied.
- Stimulus of extremely short duration will not produce any response, no matter how intense that may be.

Important Note

Plotting of strength–duration curve has significance in following situations:

- Nerve injury: Following an injury the affected nerve fibres become inexcitable after a few days. If only most excitable fibres get injured then the strength–duration curve will represent the response of intact less excitable fibres.
- If there is complete injury to the motor nerve, then all the fibres completely degenerate. In this situation, denervated muscle will respond only on direct stimulation.
- When denervated muscle fibres completely degenerate, then no response will be obtained on direct stimulation.
- On resuturing the nerve, if motor nerve fibre regenerate later, then strength–duration curve gradually returns to normal.
- If the motor neurons are destroyed, then no regeneration occurs; therefore, no recovery can occur and functional loss is purely motor.

2. All or None Response

A single nerve fibre always obeys 'all or none law', that is, when a stimulus is applied, either the axon does not respond with a spike production of action potential or it responds to the maximum of its ability. In other words:

- When a stimulus of subthreshold intensity is applied to the axon, then no action potential is produced *(none response);*
- A response in the form of spike of action potential is observed when the stimulus is of threshold intensity; and
- There occurs no increase in the magnitude of action potential when the strength of stimulus is more than the threshold level (all response).

This all or none relationship observed between the strength of stimulus and the response achieved is known as 'All or None Law' (Fig. 2.1-14).

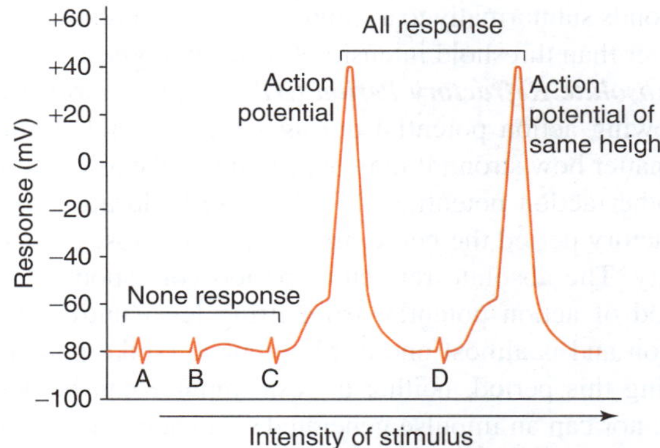

FIGURE 2.1-14 All or none response in a single nerve fibre: **A** and **B**, represent subthreshold; **C,** threshold; and **D,** suprathreshold stimuli.

Membrane Excitability during Action Potential

When a stimulus is applied to the nerve fibre membrane during the stage of action potential (produced by a previous threshold stimulus) the response elicited depends upon the stage of action potential. Depending upon the response elicited to the stimulus the period of action potential can be divided into: refractory period, supernormal period and subnormal period (Fig. 2.1-15).

i. Refractory Period Refractory period refers to the period following action potential (produced by a threshold stimulus) during which a nerve fibre either does not respond or

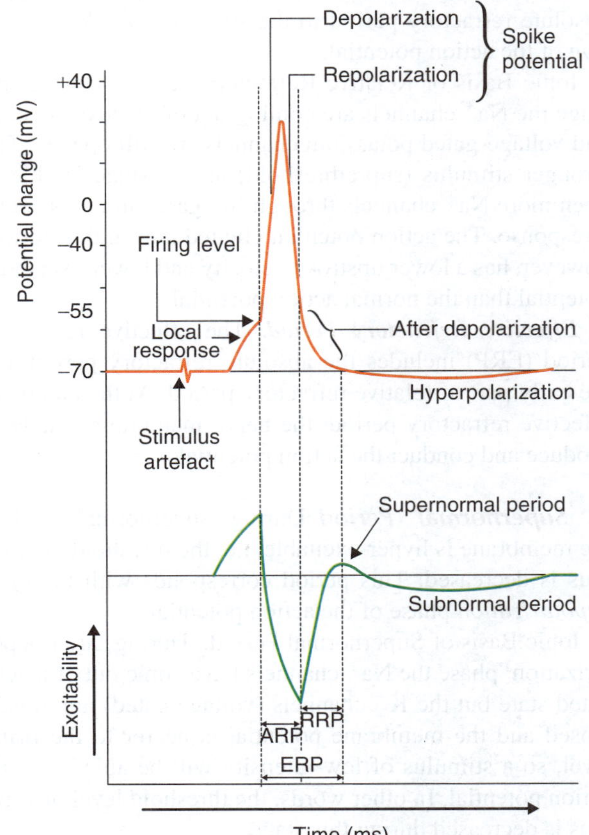

FIGURE 2.1-15 Membrane excitability during different phases of action potential: ARP (absolute refractory period), RRP (relative refractory period) and ERP (effective refractory period).

responds subnormally to a stimulus of threshold intensity or greater than threshold intensity. It is of two types:

Absolute Refractory Period (ARP). It is a short period following action potential during which second stimulus, no matter how strong it may be, cannot evoke any response (another action potential). In other words during absolute refractory period the nerve fibre completely loses its excitability. The absolute refractory period corresponds to the period of action potential from firing level until repolarization and is almost one-third complete (spike potential). During this period, neither a fresh impulse can be generated, nor can an impulse generated elsewhere pass through this area.

Ionic Basis of Absolute Refractory Period. During upstroke of action potential (depolarization), the *m gates* of sodium channels in the membrane of nerves are opened rapidly. During downstroke (early repolarization), the channels are closed by closure of inactivation *(h) gates* of the sodium channel and slow potassium channels are not yet opened. These sodium channel gates do not open unless potential comes back to resting level. Therefore, during this period (absolute refractory period) the nerve fibre is not stimulated at all.

Relative Refractory Period (RRP). It is a short period during which the nerve fibre shows response, if the strength of stimulus is more than normal. It extends from the end of absolute refractory period to the start of *after depolarization* of the action potential.

Ionic Basis of Relative Refractory Period. During this stage the Na^+ channels are coming out of inactivated stage and voltage-gated potassium channels are still opened. The stronger stimulus (suprathreshold) at this stage is able to open more Na^+ channels through 'm' gates and thus excite a response. The action potential elicited during this period, however, has a lower upstroke velocity and lower overshoot potential than the normal action potential.

Effective Refractory Period. The effective refractory period (ERP) includes the absolute refractory period and the early part of relative refractory period. At the end of an effective refractory period, the nerve membrane is able to produce and conduct the action potential.

ii. Supernormal Period During supernormal period, the membrane is hyper-excitable, i.e. the threshold of stimulus is decreased. This period corresponds with the *after depolarization* phase of the action potential.

Ionic Basis of Supernormal Period. During 'after depolarization' phase the Na^+ channels have come out of inactivated state but the K^+ channels (voltage gated) are mostly closed and the membrane potential is nearer to the firing level, so a stimulus of low intensity will be able to excite action potential. In other words, the threshold level of stimulus is decreased during this stage.

iii. Subnormal Period During this period the membrane excitability is low, i.e. the threshold of stimulus is increased. This period corresponds with the *after hyperpolarization* stage of the action potential.

Basis of Subnormal Period. During *after hyperpolarization* phase the intracellular negativity further increases (approximately −72 mV). Thus the membrane potential goes farther away from the firing level and so the threshold of stimulus increases. This phase of subnormal period lasts for about 40 ms.

3. Accommodation

We have studied that when a stimulus of sufficient strength (threshold level) is applied quickly, then the action potential is produced. However, when the stimulus strength is increased slowly to the firing level (during constant application), no *action potential is produced.* This is because of the fact that firing level of depolarization of the nerve fibre is not reached as the membrane adapts to the applied stimulus. This phenomenon of adaptation to the stimuli is called *accommodation.* Therefore, a *square pulse stimulus* (Fig. 2.1-16A) which rises sharply to its peak level effectively triggers an action potential. Whereas, a *saw-tooth pulse* stimulus (Fig. 2.1-16B), which rises to its peak slowly, often fails to trigger an action potential.

Ionic Basis of Accommodation. When the membrane depolarizes, both Na^+ and K^+ channels open up. If depolarization occurs rapidly, the opening of the Na^+ channels overwhelm the repolarizing forces and the typical action potential is produced. However, when the induced depolarization is produced slowly, more and more Na^+ channels open up, only to get inactivated after 1 ms, while the K^+ channels remain open which tend to restore the membrane potential. Thus, the repolarizing forces overwhelm the depolarizing forces and so the action potential is not produced.

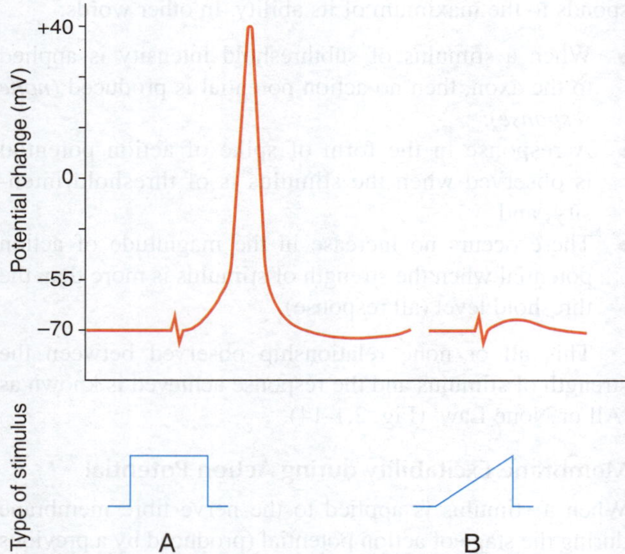

FIGURE 2.1-16 Single nerve fibre response to: **A,** square pulse stimulus; and **B,** saw tooth pulse stimulus.

4. Infatiguability

A nerve fibre cannot be fatigued, even if it is stimulated for a long time. This property of infatiguability is due to the fact that during action potential neither a fresh impulse (action potential) can be generated nor the action potential can be conducted through the nerve fibre. In other words, once stimulated, the nerve cannot be stimulated immediately again due to absolute refractory period (see page 66) and thus cannot be fatigued.

Electrotonic Potential and Local Response

When a nerve fibre is stimulated by subminimal or subthreshold stimuli, the action potential is not produced, but there do occur some changes in the resting membrane potential. These local nonpropagated changes are called *electrotonic potentials or acute subthreshold potentials.*

Types of Electrotonic Potentials Depending upon the nature (negative or positive) of subthreshold level current used to stimulate, (Fig. 2.1-17) the electrotonic potentials are of two types:

Catelectrotonic Potential. Catelectrotonic potentials are localized depolarizing potential changes in the membrane potential produced when the stimulus of subthreshold strength is applied with cathode. This potential change rises sharply and then decays exponentially with time.

Anelectrotonic Potential. Anelectrotonic potentials are the localized hyperpolarizing potential changes in the membrane potential when anodal subthreshold current is applied.

Production of Electrotonic Potentials

The electrotonic potentials are produced due to passive changes in the membrane polarization caused by addition or subtraction of the charge by the particular electrode.

Graded Potentials As shown in Fig. 2.1-17, the electrotonic potentials produced by varying intensities of stimuli are proportionate to the magnitude of stimulation. Therefore, these are also known as *graded potentials.* The graded response is achieved both at cathode and anode up to 7 mV of depolarization or hyperpolarization. At anode, the graded response is achieved even with stronger stimuli. However, the cathodal responses become greater than the proportionate increase in the stimulus intensities to produce depolarization 7–15 mV. This disproportionate response at cathode occurs due to opening of more voltage-gated Na^+ channels, and is called *local response* A further increase in the intensity of cathodal stimulus may produce *firing level* (15 mV) initiating the action potential (Fig. 2.1-17B).

Differences between graded potentials and action potential are summarized in Table 2.1-2.

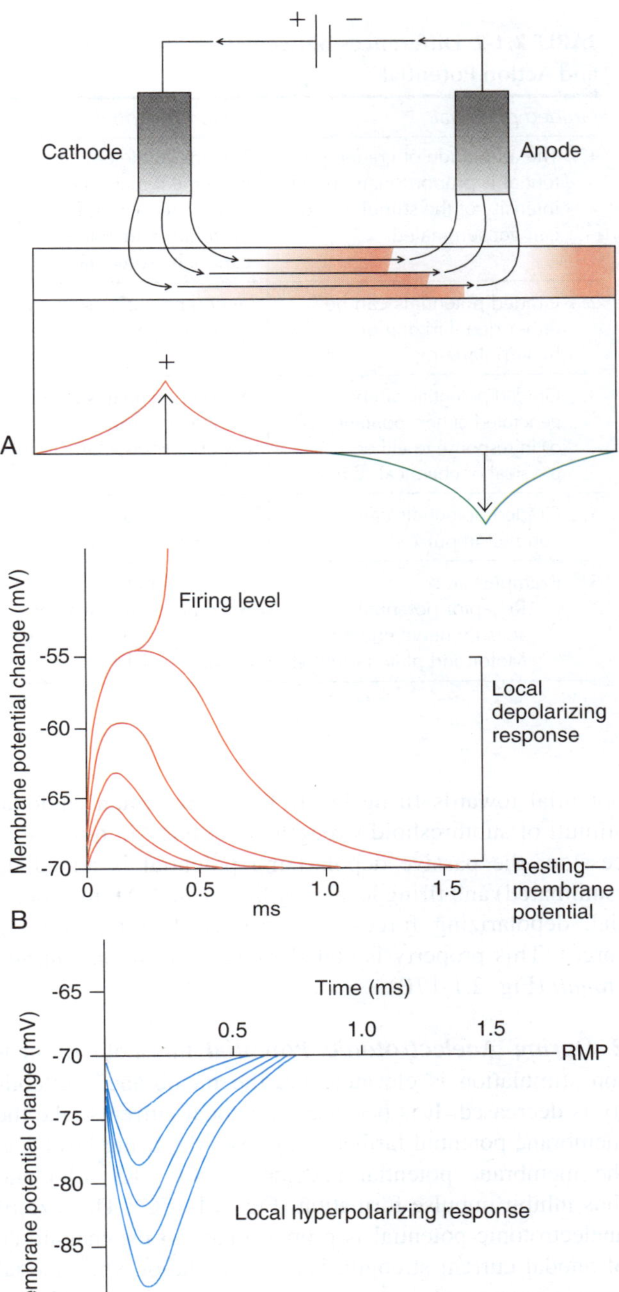

FIGURE 2.1-17 Electrotonic potential: **A,** arrangement of recording electrotonic potentials; **B,** catelectrotonic potential recorded by application of subthreshold stimuli (varying intensities) at cathode; and **C,** anelectrotonic potential recorded by application of stimuli (varying intensities) at anode.

Changes in Excitability During Electrotonic Potential

1. During Catelectrotonic Potential, the threshold of neuron to stimulation decreases, i.e. the excitability increases. The cathodal currents move the membrane

TABLE 2.1-2 Differences between Graded Potential and Action Potential

Graded potential	Action potential
1. The amplitude of graded potential is proportionate to the intensity of the stimulus and can get summated.	The amplitude of action potential remains constant with increasing intensity of stimulus, therefore it cannot be summated.
2. Graded potentials can be either depolarizing or hyperpolarizing	Action potential is always depolarizing.
3. Graded potential can be generated either spontaneously or in response to either physical or chemical stimuli.	Action potential is generated only in response to membrane depolarization.
4. Graded potentials cannot conduct impulse	Action potential can conduct impulses
5. Examples are: • Receptor potential at sensory nerve endings • Motor end plate potential	Examples are: Action potential of a nerve fibre, skeletal muscle and cardiac muscle

potential towards firing level. Therefore, when cathodal stimuli of subthreshold strength are applied in quick succession, the passive depolarizing potential is added up (summated) and firing level may be reached. At this potential, depolarizing forces are stronger than repolarizing forces. This property is called *summation of subminimal stimuli* (Fig. 2.1-17B).

2 During Anelectrotonic Potential threshold of neuron stimulation is elevated, i.e. the membrane excitability is decreased. It is because the anodal currents take the membrane potential farther away from the firing level (i.e. the membrane potential becomes about −85 mV) and thus inhibit impulse formation (Fig. 2.1-17C). The size of anelectrotonic potential is proportionate to the magnitude of anodal current strength. When stimulation with anodal current is stopped, it may lead to overshoot of membrane potential towards depolarization direction. This *rebound depolarization* response is sometimes so large that the firing level may be reached producing the action potential.

Inhibition of Excitability

There are certain factors which inhibit the excitability of the nerve fibres. These factors are called *membrane-stabilizing factors.* Some of the factors or the conditions which lead to inhibition or decrease in excitability are:

1. High Extracellular Calcium Concentration. A high extracellular Ca^{2+} concentration decreases membrane permeability to Na^+ ions thereby decreasing the membrane excitability.

2. Local Anaesthetics. Local anaesthetic agents like *procaine, tetracaine* and *lidocaine* act directly by binding to the activation gates of the Na^+ channels. These agents block the Na^+ channels thus reducing the membrane excitability. Therefore, effect of local anaesthetics on membrane excitability depends upon the distribution or density of Na^+ channels. For example, in myelinated nerves, the density of Na^+ channels is high at *node* of Ranvier. The local anaesthetics are unable to block all the Na^+ channels, hence myelinated nerve fibres are less sensitive to local anaesthetics, whereas unmyelinated nerve fibres are highly susceptible to local anaesthesia.

Recording of Resting Membrane Potential and Action Potential

See page 70.

Conductivity

Conductivity refers to propagation of nerve impulse (action potential) in the form of a wave of depolarization through the nerve fibre. Normally in the body, the action potential is transmitted through nerve fibre in one direction, but in experimental conditions when nerve fibre is stimulated in the middle, the action potential initiated is conducted equally in either direction (Fig. 2.1-18B). Mechanism of conduction of action potential along an unmyelinated nerve fibre and a myelinated nerve fibre is described below.

Propagation of Action Potential in an Unmyelinated Axon

The steps of propagation of action potential along an unmyelinated axon are summarized:

- In the resting phase (polarized state) the axonal membrane is outside positive and inside negative (Fig. 2.1-18A).
- When an unmyelinated axon is stimulated at one site by a threshold stimulus, there occurs action potential at that site, i.e. that site is depolarized. In other words, that site's outside becomes negative and inside positive (reversal of polarity) but the neighbouring areas up to now remain in polarized state (Fig. 2.1-18C).
- As ECF and ICF are both conductive to electricity, a current will flow from positive polarized area to negative activated area through ECF and in the reverse direction in ICF (Fig. 2.1-18C). Thus, a *local circuit current* flows between the resting polarized site to the depolarized site of the membrane (current sink).
- This circular current flow depolarizes the neighbouring area of the membrane upto firing level and a new action potential is produced which in turn depolarizes the neighbouring area ahead. Thus, due to successive depolarization of the neighbouring area, the action potential is propagated along the entire length of the axon (Fig. 2.1-18D).

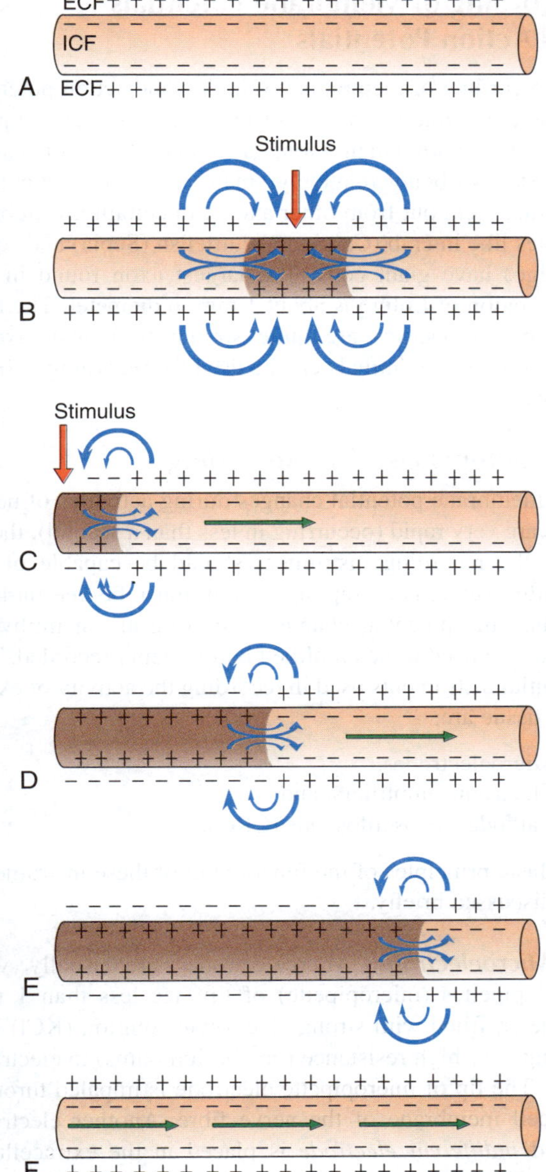

FIGURE 2.1-18 Electrotonic conduction of impulse in an unmyelinated nerve fibre: **A,** resting phase (polarized state); **B,** conduction of impulse in both directions when stimulus applied at the middle of nerve fibre; **C,** when stimulus applied at one end of the nerve fibre; **D** and **E,** propagation of impulse in one direction along the nerve fibre; and **F,** repolarization (occurs in same direction).

This type of conduction is known as *electrotonic conduction*. Once initiated, the moving impulse cannot spread to reverse direction because the proximal site is in *refractory state* and thus the distal sites being in polarized state keep on getting depolarized. Thus, the direction of propagation of impulse is that of current flow inside the nerve fibre (Fig. 2.1-18E).

- The depolarization remains at any site for some length of time, therefore, portion which depolarizes first also repolarizes first. Thus, the repolarization is also propagated following the depolarization (Fig. 2.1-18F).
- The magnitude of action potential does not change as it is conducted along the membrane, because the new action potentials are being generated constantly. However, the speed of propagation of action potential varies in different tissues.

Propagation of Action Potential in a Myelinated Axon

As discussed in the functional anatomy of nerves, the myelinated nerve fibres have a wrapping of myelin sheath with gaps at regular intervals which are devoid of myelin sheath (nodes of Ranvier). The axonal membrane in the naked area (nodes of Ranvier) bears densely packed ion channels. The myelin sheath acts as an insulator and does not allow the current flow. Therefore, in myelinated nerve fibres, the *local circuit of current flow* only occurs from one node of Ranvier to the adjacent node (Fig. 2.1-19). That is, the impulse (action potential) jumps from one node of Ranvier to next. This is known as *saltatory conduction*. Since the impulse jumps from one node to other, the speed of conduction in myelinated fibres is rapid (50 to 100 times faster) than the unmyelinated fibre.

Orthodromic Versus Antidromic Conduction

Normally, the action potential is propagated in one direction. That is, usually the nerve impulse from the receptors or synaptic junctions travels along the entire length of the axon to their termination. This type of conduction is called *orthodromic conduction*. The conduction of nerve impulse in the opposite direction, as seen in the sensory nerve supplying the blood vessels, is called *antidromic conduction*.

Conduction Velocity

Factors Affecting Conduction Velocity

The velocity of conduction in nerve fibres varies from as little as 0.25 m/s in very small unmyelinated fibres to as high as 100 m/s in very large myelinated fibres. In general, the factors affecting conduction velocity are:

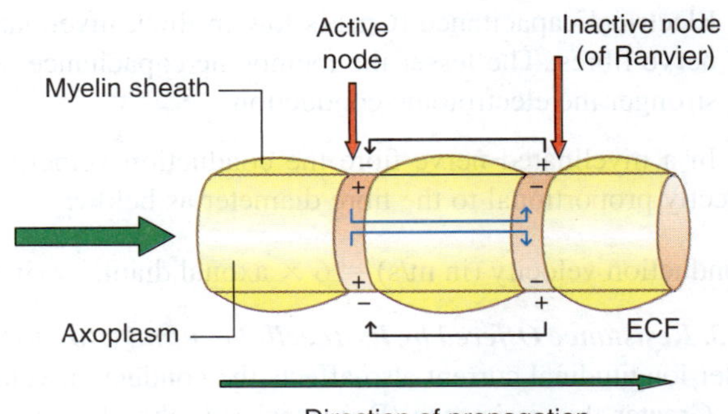

FIGURE 2.1-19 Saltatory conduction along a myelinated nerve fibre.

A. Factors Attributable to Action Potential Generation

1. Temperature affects conduction velocity by its effect on the duration of the action potential. A decrease in temperature causes a marked increase in the duration of action potential (specially the spike) and thus delays conduction, i.e. slows down the conduction velocity.

2. Level of Resting Membrane Potential (RMP) affects the conduction velocity variably. Where the RMP is less negative, it slows down both generation of action potential and electrotonic conduction. When RMP is more negative, it slows down the generation of action potential but speeds up electrotonic conduction. The resultant effect on conduction velocity is variable but usually a decrease.

3. Level of Threshold Potential (Firing Level) if it is low the conduction velocity is increased. It is due to the fact that at low firing level one action potential can trigger a second action potential a distance away where the local currents are feeble. A decrease in the firing level occurs when the concentration of divalent ion in the extracellular fluid (ECF) decreases.

B. Factors Attributable to Electrotonic Conduction

1. Axon Diameter affects the conduction velocity through the *resistance offered by the axoplasm* (Ri) to the flow of axoplasmic current. Greater this resistance, weaker is the electrotonic conduction. If the diameter of the axon is greater, the axoplasmic resistance (Ri) is lesser and hence the velocity of conduction is higher.

- In an unmyelinated nerve fibre, the conduction velocity is directly proportional to the square root of the fibre diameter (D), i.e.

$$\text{Conduction velocity} \propto \sqrt{D}$$

2. Myelination increases conduction velocity by its following effects:

- By increasing the axon diameter.
- By the saltatory conduction produced due to its insulating effect (as discussed above).
- *Resistance offered by the membrane* (Rm) is high in thick myelinated nerve fibres. When Rm is high, the membrane current falls resulting in higher axoplasmic current and stronger electrotonic conduction.
- Electrical capacitance (Cm) is low in thick myelinated nerve fibres. The lesser the membrane capacitance, the stronger the electrotonic conduction.

In a myelinated nerve fibre the conduction velocity is directly proportional to the fibre diameter as below:

$$\text{Conduction velocity (in m/s)} = 6 \times \text{axonal diameter (in } \mu)$$

3. Resistance Offered by Extracellular Fluid (Ro) to the outer longitudinal current also affects the conduction velocity. Greater this resistance (Ro), weaker is the electrotonic conduction. However, Ro usually remains constant.

Recording of Membrane Potentials and Action Potentials

The recording of membrane excitation and action potential is made possible by the use of highly sophisticated equipment. The mammalian axons are about 20 μm or less in diameter, so being relatively small, it is very difficult to separate them out from other axons. In certain invertebrate species like in crab (Carcinus), cuttlefish (Sepia) and squid (Loligo) have giant cells. The largest axon found in the neck region of Loligo is about 1 mm in diameter. The fundamental properties are quite similar to human axons. Therefore, these animals can be used for recording various events.

Instruments Used for Recording

The membrane potential changes during activities of nerve fibre are very rapid (occurring in less than a second); therefore, the recording instrument should be capable of responding extremely rapidly, i.e. it must be inertia-less. Further, the potential changes occurring are in millivolts and hence need to be amplified before being recorded. The essential instruments used in recording the activity of excitable tissue are:

- Microelectrodes,
- Electronic amplifiers, and
- Cathode-ray oscilloscope (CRO).

Basic principles of the functioning of these instruments are discussed briefly.

1. Microelectrodes Microelectrodes are usually very small pipettes (micropipette) of tip size less than 1 mm diameter, filled with strong electrolyte solution (KCl) and having very high resistance (one billion ohms) to electrical flow. The tip of micropipette electrode is impaled through the cell membrane of the nerve fibre. Another electrode called *indifferent electrode* is placed in the extracellular fluid (Fig. 2.1-20).

The microelectrode can be connected to cathode-ray oscilloscope through a suitable amplifier for recording rapid changes in membrane potential during nerve impulse transmission.

2. Electronic Amplifier This device can magnify the potential changes of the tissue to more than thousand times so that these can be recorded on the oscilloscope screen.

3. Cathode-Ray Oscilloscope Cathode-ray oscilloscope (CRO) is almost an inertialess instrument which can record and measure the electrical events of living tissues instantaneously. The CRO primarily consists of a glass tube with a cathode, fluorescent surface (screen) and two sets of electrically charged plates (Fig. 2.1-20).

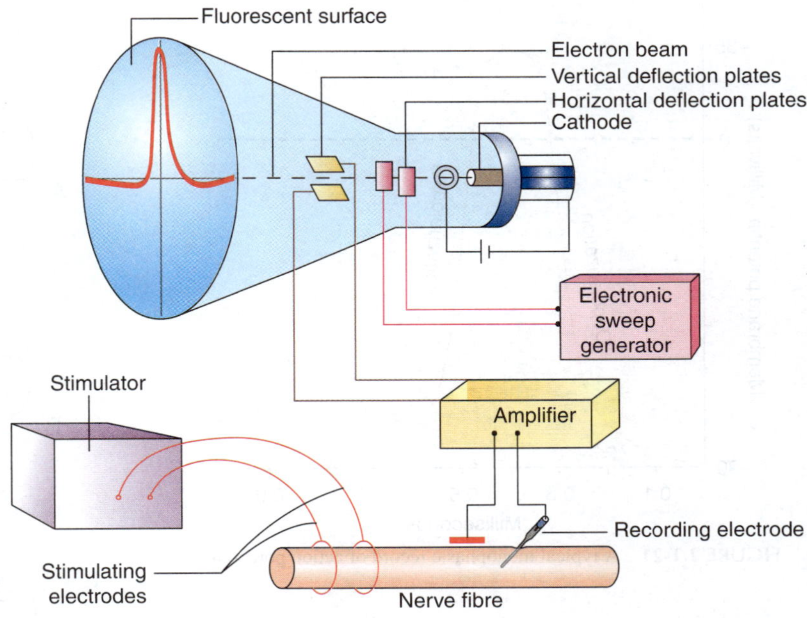

FIGURE 2.1-20 Cathode ray oscilloscope and simplified diagram to record action potential from a nerve fibre.

Cathode is in the form of an electronic gun. When connected to a suitable anode and electric current is passed, the electronic gun emits electrons.

Fluorescent Surface (the face of glass tube coated with fluorescent material) acts as a screen. The electrons emitted from the cathode are directed into a beam which hits this screen.

Electrically Charged Plates are arranged in two sets: vertical and horizontal

- Horizontal Deflection Plates are placed on either side of the electron beam. These are connected to sweep generator (*electronic sweep circuit*). When a voltage is applied across these plates, the beam of electrons (being negatively charged) is attracted towards the positively charged plate and repelled away by the negatively charged plate. If 'saw-tooth voltage' (i.e. voltage increased slowly, then suddenly reduced, and again slowly increased) is applied, the electron beam will steadily move towards the positively charged plate (with slowly increasing voltage), than back to its original position (with sudden reduction in the voltage), and again move towards the positively charged plate. In this way the electron beam is made to sweep across the fluorescent screen horizontally, which will give a continuous marking of line of glowing light.
- Vertical Deflection Plates are placed above and below the electron beam. These are connected to recording electrodes placed on the nerve through an electronic amplifier. The potential change occurring in the nerve will charge these plates which will cause vertical (upward and downward) deflection of the electron beam. The magnitude of deflection will be proportional to the potential difference between the two plates. Thus, action potential is recorded as vertical deflection of the beam as it moves across the fluorescent screen of the cathode ray oscilloscope.

Recording of Resting Membrane Potential

The arrangement of electrodes for recording membrane potential is shown in Fig. 2.1-7. The electrical potential is recorded at the surface of the membrane (exterior) and inside the membrane at each point in a nerve fibre. Starting from one end of the nerve fibre (left side of the figure) and passing to the other end (right side) and when both the electrodes (indifferent and microelectrodes) are on the surface (outside) of the nerve fibre membrane, then no potential difference was recorded (zero potential), which is potential of extracellular fluid. However, when microelectrode is made to penetrate into the interior of cell, a constant potential difference (−70 mV) is observed. This is known as resting membrane potential (Fig. 2.1-7).

Recording of Action Potential

Monophasic Recording of Action Potential For monophasic recording of action potential, one microelectrode is placed inside the nerve fibre and the other electrode on the outside surface. These electrodes are then connected to the cathode-ray oscilloscope (Fig. 2.1-20). When the nerve is stimulated, as shown in Fig. 2.1-21, a typical monophasic record of action potential obtained has the following components:

- Depolarization
- Repolarization

It has been described in detail on page 61.

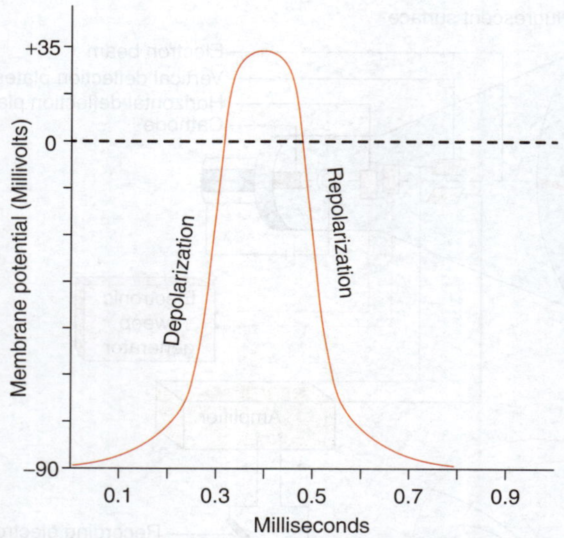

FIGURE 2.1-21 A typical monophasic record of action potential.

Biphasic Recording of Action Potential For biphasic recording of action potential, both the exploring electrodes (x and y) are placed on the outside surface of nerve fibre, and they are connected to a cathode-ray oscilloscope (Fig. 2.1-22). When the nerve is stimulated, the excitation of one electrode will cause deflection opposite to that of another during the passage of impulse. Record of this alternate deflection (one negative below the baseline and one positive above the baseline (called *biphasic action potential)* is depicted:

- During *resting state* only baseline is recorded as both electrodes are equipotential (Fig. 2.1-22A).
- When a threshold stimulus is applied, an action potential is initiated and first the membrane under electrode x gets depolarized (outside −ve) but the membrane under electrode y is still polarized (outside +ve). Because of the potential difference between the two electrodes, a downstroke is recorded by CRO (Fig. 2.1-22B).
- When impulse passes beyond 'x' but has not reached 'y', and membrane under electrode x is repolarized (outside +ve), then the record comes back to a baseline as again the membrane under the two electrodes becomes equipotential (Fig. 2.1-22C).
- As shown in Fig. 2.1-22D, when the impulse reaches y electrode, the membrane under it gets depolarized (outside −ve). Since at x the membrane is repolarized (outside +ve), the potential difference between the two electrodes is recorded as upstroke by CRO.
- When impulse passes beyond 'y', and membrane under it is repolarized (outside +ve); once again the record comes to baseline as both electrodes are again equipotential (Fig. 2.1-22A).
- A typical complete record of biphasic action potential is shown in Fig. 2.1-23.

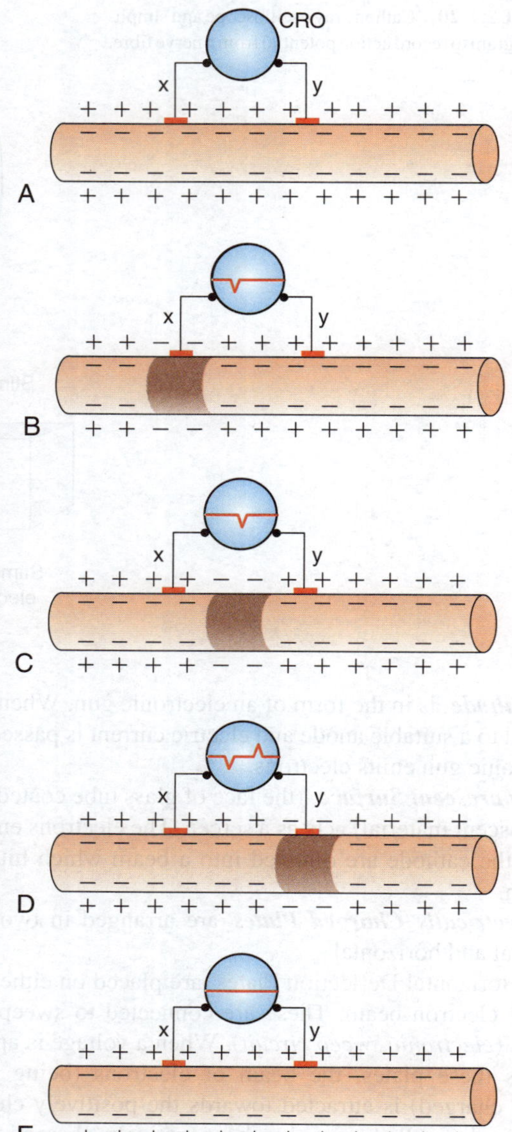

FIGURE 2.1-22 Arrangement for recording biphasic action potential (recording electrodes x and y are on the surface of nerve fibre connected to cathode-ray oscilloscope): **A,** resting state; **B,** on stimulation when wave of excitation reaches at electrode 'x'; **C,** when impulse passes beyond electrode 'x'; **D,** when impulse reaches at electrode 'y', and **E,** when impulse passes away from electrode 'y'.

Advantages of Biphasic Recording

1. Comparatively easy process, since both the electrodes are placed on the outside surface of the nerve.
2. Propagation of action potential can also be recorded.

Disadvantages of Biphasic Recording

1. Graph obtained is variable depending upon the distance between the electrodes and the rate of conduction of impulse in the nerve fibre.
2. Proper analysis of action potential cannot be done as can be done in monophasic recording.

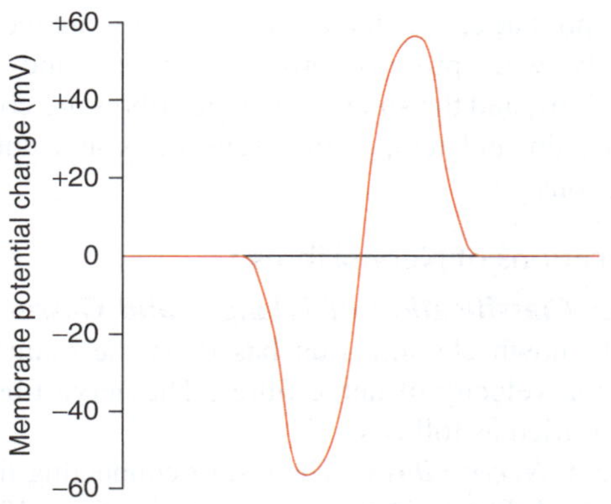

FIGURE 2.1-23 A typical complete record of biphasic action potential.

3. Potential difference recorded is somewhat smaller than actual, as nerve fibre has to be kept in a solution to prevent drying.

Compound Action Potential and its Recording

Compound action potential is the monophasic recording of action potential from a *mixed* nerve which contains different types of nerve fibres with varying diameter. Therefore, the compound action potential represents an algebraic summation of the all or none action potentials of many axons.

Response of a Mixed Nerve to Stimulus Response of a mixed nerve to a stimulus will depend upon the thresholds of the individual axon in the nerve and their distance from the stimulating electrode as below (Fig. 2.1-24):

• ***Subthreshold Stimulus*** stimulates none of the axons and thus no response is observed.

• ***Threshold Intensity Stimulus*** makes the axons with low threshold to fire and thus a small potential change is observed.

• ***With Further Increase in the Intensity of Stimulus,*** the axons with higher thresholds also fire. The electrical response increases proportionately until the stimulus is strong enough to excite all of the axons in the nerve. The stimulus which excites all the axons is called *maximal stimulus.*

• ***Supramaximal Stimulus*** does not produce any further increase in the potential.

Features of a Compound Action Potential

- It has a unique shape (multiple peaks), because a mixed nerve is made up of different fibres with various speeds of conduction.
- The number and size of the peaks vary with the types of fibres in the particular nerve being studied.
- When less than maximal stimuli are used, the shape of compound action will depend upon the number and type of fibres stimulated.
- Thus, a typical record of compound action potential will contain three different curves labelled as α, β and γ (Fig. 2.1-24).

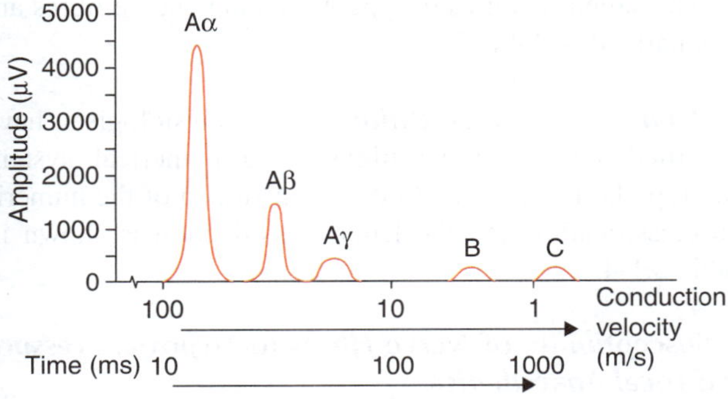

FIGURE 2.1-24 Typical record of compound action potential (recorded from a mixed nerve) showing multiple peaks.

PHYSIOLOGICAL PROPERTIES OF NERVE FIBRES

The properties of the nerve fibres are mainly because of the nerve cells being excitable tissue, i.e. having a low threshold for excitation. Therefore, the main properties of the nervous tissue are excitability and conductivity and all other properties are secondary to these. After studying the electrical activities of the nerve fibres in detail, their important physiological properties can be summarized as:

1. Excitability, i.e. the nerve fibres when stimulated produce waves of depolarization, called *excitation impulse* (for details see page 60).

2. All and none Response, i.e. when stimulated, the nerve fibre either shows no excitation or responds to the maximum of its ability (for details see page 65).

3. Refractory Period, i.e. when the nerve fibre is stimulated by two successive stimuli of more than threshold intensity:

- it responds to the first stimulus, but
- is unable to respond to the second stimulus for quite some time, called the refractory period (for details see page 65).

4. Summation, i.e. response to the successive subthreshold stimuli can be summated. When one subthreshold stimulus is applied, the nerve fibre does not respond. However, if two or more subthreshold stimuli are applied within a short interval of about 0.5 ms, the response may be produced. This is because the subthreshold stimuli are summed up. This property is called summation (also see page 68).

5. Accommodation, i.e. the excitability of the nerve fibre is decreased when a constant current is passed through it. A similar feature of the nerve endings is called adaptation. That is, the nerve fibres accommodate and the nerve endings adapt when a constant current is passed (for details see page 66).

6. Infatiguability, i.e. a nerve fibre cannot be fatigued, even if it is stimulated continuously for a long time (also see page 67).

7. Conductivity, i.e. the nerve fibres possess the ability to transmit the excitation impulse along its entire length (for details see page 68).

NERVE FIBRE TYPES

Various schemes for classification of nerve fibres on the basis of their diameter and their conduction velocity have been proposed. The best known classification is of Erlanger and Gasser. Before discussing this important classification it will be useful to be familiar with the various terminologies used in relation to nerve fibres and certain facts about the conduction velocity in nerve fibres.

Terminology Used in Relation to Nerve Fibres

- *Myelinated versus nonmyelinated fibres.* The myelinated nerve fibres are covered by a myelin sheath while the nonmyelinated nerve fibres have no such sheath.
- *Somatic versus visceral nerve fibres.* Somatic nerve fibres supply the skeletal muscles of the body while visceral nerve fibres supply the various internal organs (viscera).
- *Cranial versus spinal nerves.* Nerve fibres arising from the brain form the cranial nerves while those arising from the spinal cord form the spinal nerves.
- *Motor versus sensory nerve fibres.* Motor nerve fibres, also known as *efferent fibres* carry motor impulses from CNS to different parts of the body. The sensory nerve fibres, also known as *afferent fibres* carry sensory impulses from different parts of the body to CNS.
- *Adrenergic versus cholinergic nerve fibres.* Adrenergic nerve fibres secrete noradrenaline while cholinergic fibres secrete acetylcholine as neurotransmitter.

Certain Facts about the Conduction Velocity in Nerve Fibres

- Fibres of larger diameter conduct impulses more rapidly than those of smaller diameter.
- The impulse conducted through larger diameter nerve fibres will have greater magnitude and lesser duration of spike, lesser threshold of excitation and lesser refractory period, as compared to the impulses conducted through nerve fibres of smaller diameter.
- The speed of conduction is about 6 times the diameter of a myelinated nerve fibres. Since the diameter of myelinated nerve fibres varies from 1 to 20 μm, the conduction velocity will vary from 6 to 120 m/s.
- In unmyelinated nerve fibres the speed of conduction is proportional to the square root of the diameter of the nerve fibre. Since the largest unmyelinated nerve fibres have a diameter of 1 μm, their maximum conduction velocity will be 1 m/s.
- By and large, the larger nerve fibres are concerned mainly with proprioceptive sensations and somatic functions, and the smaller diameter fibres are concerned with pain and temperature sensations and autonomic functions.

Classifications of Nerve Fibres

1. Letter Classification of Erlanger and Gasser This is the best known classification based on the diameter and conduction velocity of nerve fibres. The nerve fibres have been classified as follows:

'Type A' Nerve Fibres. The fastest conducting fibres are called type A fibres. Their diameter varies from 12–20 μm and conduction velocity from 70 to 120 m/s. They are myelinated fibres.

Type A fibres have been further subdivided into α, β, γ and δ fibres. Type A fibres subserve both motor and sensory functions:

Motor 'type A' fibres

- ***Aα fibres*** supply extrafusal fibres in skeletal muscles.
- ***Aγ fibres*** supply intrafusalfibres in muscle spindles.
- ***Aδ fibres*** are collaterals of Aα fibres (to extrafusal fibres) that innervate some intrafusal fibres.

Sensory 'type A' fibres

- ***Aα sensory fibres*** carry impulses from encapsulated receptors in skin, joints and muscles. Some of them carry impulses from the gut.
- ***Aδ sensory fibres*** are afferents from thermoreceptors and nociceptors (pain receptors).

'Type B' Nerve Fibres. These fibres are myelinated, have a diameter of less than 3 μm and their conduction velocity varies from 4 to 30 m/s. They form preganglionic autonomic efferent fibres and afferent fibres from skin and viscera, and free nerve ending in connective tissue of muscle.

'Type C' Nerve Fibres. These are unmyelinated, have a diameter of 0.4–1.2 μm and their conduction velocity varies from 0.5 to 4 m/s. These form the postganglionic autonomic fibres, some sensory fibres carrying pain sensations, some fibres from thermoreceptors and some from viscera.

The salient features of type A, B and C nerve fibres are summarized in Table 2.1-3.

2. Numerical Classification Some physiologists have classified sensory nerve fibres by a numerical system into type Ia, Ib, II, III and IV. A comparison of the numerical classification and the letter classification is shown in Table 2.1-4.

3. Susceptibility of Nerve Fibres to Hypoxia, Pressure and Local Anaesthetics

Hypoxia. As shown in Table 2.1-5, the type B fibres are most susceptible to hypoxia. Since, the preganglionic

TABLE 2.1-3 Salient Features of Type A, B and C Nerve Fibres

Fibre	Type	Myelinated/ nonmyelinated	Fibre diameter (μm)	Conduction velocity (m/s)	Spike duration (ms)	Absolute refractory period (ms)	Function: Efferent	Function: Afferent
A	α	Myelinated	12–20	70–120	0.4–0.5	0.4–1	Somatic motor	Proprioception
	β	Myelinated	5–12	30–70	0.4–0.5	0.4–1	—	Touch and pressure
	γ	Myelinated	3–6	15–30	0.4–0.5	0.4–1	Motor to muscle spindles	—
	δ	Myelinated	2–5	12–30	0.4–0.5	0.4–1	—	Pain, cold and touch
B	–	Myelinated	<3	3–15	1.2	1.2	Preganglionic autonomic	—
C	–	Nonmyelinated	0.4–1.2	0.5–2	2	2	Postganglionic autonomic (sympathetic)	Pain, temperature some mechanoreceptors and reflex responses

TABLE 2.1-4 Numerical vis-à-vis Letter Classification of Sensory Nerve Fibres

Types of nerve fibre: Numerical classification	Letter classification	Origin
Ia	A α	Muscle spindle (annulospiral endings)
Ib	A α	Golgi tendon organ
II	A β	Muscle spindle, (flower spray endings), touch and pressure
III	A δ	Pain and cold receptors, some touch receptors
IV	C	Pain, temperature and other receptors.

TABLE 2.1-5 Susceptibility of Nerve Fibres to Hypoxia, Pressure and Local Anaesthetics

Sensitivity to	Type of nerve fibre: Most susceptible	Intermediate susceptible	Least susceptible
Hypoxia	B	A	C
Pressure	A	B	C
Local anaesthetics	C	B	A

autonomic fibres are of type B, therefore, hypoxia is associated with alteration of the autonomic functions in the body such as rise in heart rate, blood pressure and respiration.

Pressure. Type A fibres are most susceptible to pressure and type C least. Therefore, pressure on a nerve can produce temporary paralysis due to loss of conduction in motor, touch and pressure fibres (type A), while pain sensation (carried by type C fibres) remain relatively intact. This is a common observation after sitting cross-legged for long periods and after sleeping with arms under the head.

Local Anaesthetics. Type C fibres (conducting pain, touch and temperature sensations generated by cutaneous receptors) are most susceptible to local anaesthetics. This fact is useful for surgical interventions under local anaesthesia.

DEGENERATION AND REGENERATION OF NEURONS

When the axon of neuron is injured, a series of degenerative changes are seen at three levels:

- In the axon distal to injury,
- In the axon proximal to injury and
- In the cell body.

Along with the degenerative changes, the reparative process (regeneration) also starts soon if the circumstances are favourable. The effects of injury to a nerve and the occurrence of regenerative changes thereafter will depend upon the degree and type of damage.

Grading of Nerve Injury

Common causes of nerve injury are: transection (through and through cut), crushing of nerve fibres, local injection of toxic substances, ischaemia due to obstruction of blood flow and effects of hyperpyrexia on the neurons. Sunderland had graded the injury to nerve fibres in order of severity into the following degrees:

- ***First Degree Injury*** involves only transient loss of function resulting from a mild pressure on the nerve. The temporary loss of function is caused by local anoxia produced by ischaemia following obstruction to the blood flow. The lost function of the nerve fibres returns within few hours to few weeks of the removal of the causative pressure, since the axon is not destroyed.

- ***Second Degree Injury*** includes severe nerve damage with intact endoneural tube. It results from a severe and prolonged pressure on the nerve. The nerve fibre is severely damaged at the pressure point and is followed by degenerative changes. However, the regeneration and restoration of the function of the nerve are facilitated as the endoneural tube remains intact.

- ***Third Degree Injury*** includes severe damage to the nerve fibre with interruption of the endoneural tube.

- ***Fourth Degree Injury*** refers to a severe damage to the nerve fibres associated with disorganization of nerve fasciculi.

- ***Fifth Degree Injury*** is labelled when there occurs complete transection, i.e. the nerve fibres are cut through and through. Degenerative changes are initiated very early following fifth degree injury to the nerve fibres.

Stage of Degeneration

The degenerative changes which occur in the part of axon distal to the site of injury are referred to as *anterograde degeneration* or Wallerian degeneration (after the discoverer A Waller, 1862). The degenerative changes occurring in the neuron proximal to the injury are referred to as *retrograde degeneration.* These changes take place in the cell body and in the axon proximal to injury.

Changes in the Part of Axon Distal to Injury

Degenerative changes in the part of axon distal to injury, also known as anterograde degeneration or Wallerian degeneration occur within few hours of injury. The changes take place in the entire length of this part of the axon simultaneously. The degeneration changes start within few hours of injury and continue for about 3 months and include the following (Fig. 2.1-25).

Axis Cylinder Axis cylinder becomes swollen and irregular in shape within a few hours of injury. After a few days it breaks up into small fragments, the neurofibrils within it break down into granular debris and are seen in the space occupied by axis cylinder.

Myelin Sheath shows slow disintegration which starts on the 8th day and continues up to the 32nd to 35th day. In fact myelin sheath is converted into fat droplets containing cholesterol esters.

Neurilemmal Sheath is usually unaffected but the Schwann cells start multiplying rapidly.

Macrophages invade the region and remove degenerating axons, myelin and cellular debris and thus the neurilemmal tube becomes empty.

Schwann Cell's cytoplasm proliferates rapidly and fills up the empty neurilemmal tube. These cells produce a large series of membranes that help to form numerous tubes which play a vital role in the regeneration of nerve fibres.

Changes in the Cell Body of Neuron Changes in the cell body of the injured neuron start within 48 h and continue up to 15–20 days. The changes are (Fig. 2.1-26):

Nissl Substances undergo disintegration and dissolution (*chromatolysis).* The process of chromatolysis starts around the nucleus and spreads in the periphery.

Golgi Apparatus, Mitochondria and Neurofibrils are fragmented and eventually disappear.

Cell Body draws in more fluid, enlarges and becomes spherical.

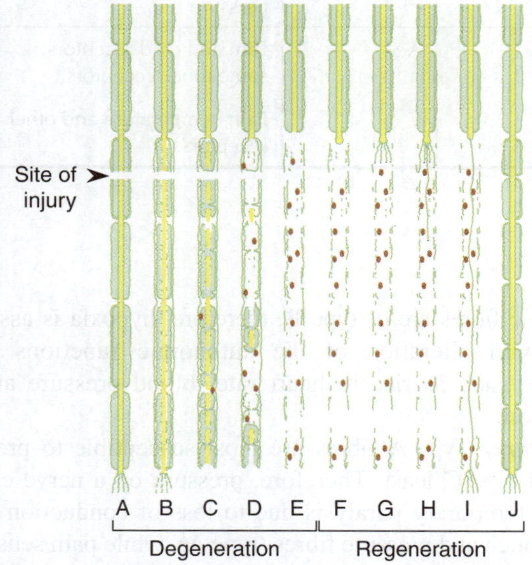

FIGURE 2.1-25 Degenerative changes (Wallerian degeneration) in distal part of a nerve fibre after injury (A–E) and subsequent regenerative changes (F–J).

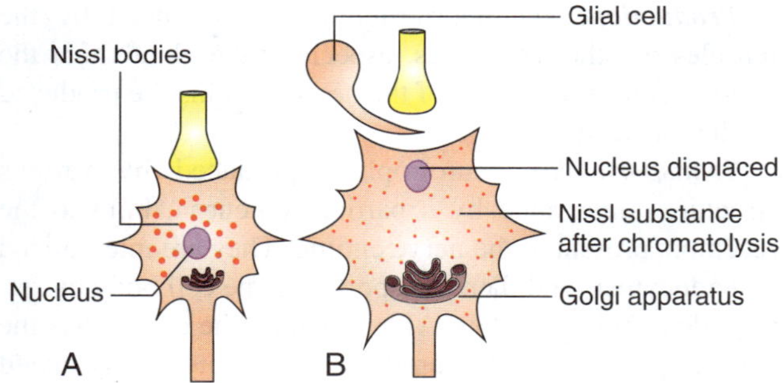

FIGURE 2.1-26 Changes in cell body of a neuron after injury (**B**) and normal cell body of a neuron (**A**).

Nucleus is displaced to the periphery (towards cell membrane). Sometimes, the nucleus is extruded out of the cell, in which case the neuron atrophies and finally disappears completely.

Severity of Degenerative Changes in the Cell Body

Severity of degenerative changes in the cell body is variable. The changes are more severe when the injury to the axon is near the cell body, and when the injury is caused by a forcible tear rather than a sharp cut. In some cases, the chromatolysis ends in cell death followed by degeneration of all its processes. If the cell survives, the changes described above are reversed after a period of time.

Changes in the Part of Axon Proximal to Injury

Changes in the part of axon proximal to injury occur only up to the first or second node of Ranvier near the injury and are similar to the changes seen in the distal part of the axon. Changes seen in the proximal part of axon along with those seen in the cell body of neuron constitute the *retrograde degeneration.*

Transneuronal Degeneration It is sometimes observed that changes resulting from axonal injury are not confined to the injured neuron, but extend to other neurons with which the injured neuron synapses. This phenomenon is referred to as *transneuronal degeneration.* The degeneration can extend through several synapses (as demonstrated in the visual pathway).

Stage of Regeneration

The stage of degeneration is followed by stage of regeneration under favourable circumstances (listed below). It starts within 4 days of injury but becomes more active after 30 days and may take several months to one year for complete recovery.

Factors Affecting Regeneration

- Regeneration occurs more rapidly when a nerve is crushed than when it is severed and the cut ends are separated.
- Chances of regeneration of a cut nerve are considerably increased if the two cut ends are near each other (gap does not exceed 3 mm); and if scar tissue does not intervene between them.
- Chances of regeneration are more if the two cut ends remain in the same line, and are not moved away from each other.
- Presence of neurilemma is a must for regeneration to occur. Therefore, axons in CNS once degenerated never regenerate as these nerve fibres have no neurilemma.
- Presence of nucleus in the neuron cell body is also a must for regeneration to occur. If it is extruded, the neuron is atrophied and the regeneration does not occur.

Regenerative Changes

Anatomical Regeneration

1. Changes in the Axon

• Stage of Fibres Formation. Axis cylinder from the proximal cut end of the axon elongates and gives out fibrils up to 100 in number in all directions. These branches grow into the connective tissue at the site of injury in an effort to reach the distal cut end of the nerve fibre (Fig. 2.1-25F and G).

• Stage of Entry of Fibrils into Endoneural Tube. Strands of Schwann cells from the distal cut end of axon guide the regenerating fibrils to enter their axon endoneural tube and once the fibril enters the endoneural tube it grows rapidly within it. The rate of growth which is initially low (0.25 mm/day) increases rapidly once the regenerating axon enters the endoneural tube (3–4 mm/day). The axonal fibrils that fail to enter any one of the tubes degenerate. It often happens that more than one fibril (1–25) enters the same tube. Under such circumstances, the largest fibril survives and the rest degenerate.

• Stage of Active Growth. The axonal fibril growing through the endoneural tube enlarges and establishes contact with an appropriate peripheral end organ. The new axon formed in this way is devoid of myelin sheath (Fig. 2.1-25H and I). The process of regeneration up to this stage takes about 3 months.

• Stage of Myelination. The myelin sheath is then formed by the cells of Schwann slowly. The myelination is completed in one year. Thus, there occurs a progressive increase in the thickness of nerve fibre. The regenerated nerve fibre, however, obtains only 80% of the original diameter.

2. Changes in the Cell Body of Neuron

- Nissl granules followed by Golgi apparatus appear in the cell body.
- The cell loses excess fluid and regains its normal size.
- The nucleus occupies the central position.

Important Note

Axonal regeneration is promoted by growth promoting factor secreted by Schwann cell & adhesion molecules of immunoglobulin family (e.g. NgCAMK).

- In CNS the neurons do not require a growth promoting factor for regeneration.
- Events such as astrocyte proliferation, microglial activation, scar formation, inflammatory reaction following CNS injury are unfavourable for degeneration.

The above changes in some of the neurons start within 20 days of injury and are completed in 80 days. Regenerative changes in the cell body may occur, even when the axon does not regenerate.

Functional Regeneration The above-described regenerative changes constitute anatomical regeneration. The functional (physiological) recovery, however, occurs after a long period.

Complications Following Nerve Injury

1. Complete Atrophy of the nerve fibre occurs in severe injuries where regeneration does not occur due to absence of favourable circumstances.

2. Functional Complications in the form of misinterpretation of sensations occur when the fibrils do not enter the appropriate tubes and thus there are faulty connections.

3. Neuroma Formation occurs if during regeneration the nerve fibrils growing from the proximal cut end of axon, do not find their way if the gap between two cut ends is too large. Under such circumstances, the fibrils turn round in search of the endoneural tube in a whorl-like mass known as *neuroma*, which may be quite painful.

Phantom Limb is a feeling sometimes perceived by a patient following amputation of the limb. Neuroma, developed at the site of amputation, when excited, causes the patient to feel like the lost limb is present (a feeling of phantom limb).

FACTORS PROMOTING NEURONAL GROWTH

Various factors affecting neuronal development, growth and survival have been isolated and studied. These can be broadly arranged into two groups:

- Neurotrophins, and
- Other factors affecting neuronal growth.

Neurotrophins

Neurotrophins are the proteins which provide trophic support to the neurons, i.e. they promote nerve growth and survival. They also have a role in neuronal plasticity.

Production. The neurotrophins are produced by the muscles or other structures, especially the glands that the neurons innervate. Some of the neurotrophins are produced by the astrocytes.

Transport. The neurotrophins produced by various structures innervated by a particular neuron, bind to the receptors present at the nerve ending. They are internalized by endocytosis and then transported to the cell body by retrograde axoplasmic flow. After reaching the cell bodies the neurotrophins foster the production of proteins associated with neuronal development, growth and survival.

Established Neurotrophins Include:

- Nerve growth factor (NGF),
- Brain-derived neurotrophic factor (BDNF),
- Neurotrophin-3 (NT-3) and
- Neurotrophin 4/5 (NT-4/5).

1. Nerve Growth Factor. Nerve growth (NGF) is probably the first neurotrophin recognized. It promotes the growth of *sympathetic nerves and* some sensory nerves.

- It is found in various tissues in human beings and many species of animals. NGF is particularly found in high concentration in the submaxillary salivary glands of the male mice.
- NGF is made up of 2α, 2β and 2γ subunits.
  - The a subunits have trypsin-like activity.
  - The β subunits are similar in structure to insulin and possess all the nerve-growth promoting activities.
  - The γ subunits are serine proteases. Their functions are unknown.
- Receptor of NGF is TrkA (tyrosine kinase activity A)
- A low affinity NGF receptor called P 75 ^{NTR} forms a heterodimer with TrkA receptors, and increase the affinity and specificity for NGF. However, in absence of Trk receptors, it forms homodimer, that causes apoptosis.
- NGF is also present in the brain and appears to be responsible for the growth and maintenance of cholinergic neurons in the basal forebrain and striatum.
- Immunosympathectomy, i.e. complete destruction of the sympathetic ganglia is produced when antiserum against NGF is injected in a newborn animal.

2. Brain-derived Neurotrophic Factor

- It has a growth promoting role for peripheral sensory nerves, since it has been seen that BDNF-deficient mice lose peripheral sensory nerves and have severe degenerative changes in their vestibular ganglia.
- Receptor for BDNF is TrkB.

3. Neurotrophin-3

- The neurotrophin-3 (NT-3), plays a growth promoting role in cutaneous mechanoreceptors, since its disruption by gene knockout gives rise to marked loss of these receptors.
- Receptors for NT-3 are TrkC (mainly) and TrkA and B (to some extent).

4. Neurotrophin-4/5
- Receptors for neurotrophin-4/5 is TrkB.

Other Growth-Promoting Factors

Factors, other than neurotrophins, which promote nerve growth include:

- ***Ciliary Neurotrophic Factor (CNTF).*** It is produced by Schwann cells and astrocytes and plays a growth promoting role in lesioned and embryonic spinal cord neurons. It is believed that it may be of some value in treating human diseases in which motor neurons degenerate.
- *Leukaemia inhibitory factor (LIF),*
- *Insulin-like growth factor-I (IGF-I),*
- *Transforming growth factor (TGF),*
- *Fibroblast growth factor (FGF) and*
- *Platelet-derived growth factor (PDGF).*

Chapter 2.2

Neuromuscular Junction

STRUCTURE AT NEUROMUSCULAR JUNCTION
- Terminal button
- Presynaptic membrane
- Synaptic cleft
- Postsynaptic membrane

NEUROMUSCULAR TRANSMISSION
- Release of acetylcholine
- Effect of acetylcholine
- End plate potential
- Removal of acetylcholine

DRUGS AFFECTING AND DISORDERS OF NEUROMUSCULAR JUNCTION
- Drugs affecting neuromuscular junction
  - Neuromuscular blockers
  - Neuromuscular stimulators
- Disorders of neuromuscular junction
  - Myasthenia gravis
  - Lambert–Eaton syndrome

STRUCTURE OF NEUROMUSCULAR JUNCTION

Neuromuscular junction refers to the intimate contact of the nerve endings with the muscle fibre to which they innervate. Characteristics of the nerve and muscle fibre at and near the neuromuscular junction are given in Fig. 2.2-1.

Terminal Button. The axon of a neuron supplying a skeletal muscle loses its myelin sheath and divides into a number of fine branches that end in small swellings (knobs) called *terminal buttons* or end feet, which forms a neuromuscular junction at the centre of muscle fibre (Fig. 2.2-1A). The nerve terminal or the so-called synaptic knob contains large number of vesicles (about three lakh) containing acetylcholine. Mitochondria are also present in the nerve terminal. The acetylcholine is synthesized by the mitochondria and is stored in the vesicles (Fig. 2.2-1B). The mitochondria contain adenosine triphosphate (ATP) which is the source of energy for synthesis of acetylcholine.

Presynaptic Membrane. This refers to the axonal membrane lining the *terminal buttons* of the nerve endings.

Synaptic Cleft. It is a 50–100 nm wide space between the presynaptic membrane and the postsynaptic membrane. It is filled by extracellular fluid with reticular fibres forming the matrix.

Postsynaptic Membrane (Fig. 2.2-1B). This is the name given to the muscle fibre membrane (sarcolemma) in the region of neuromuscular junction. The muscle membrane in this region is thickened and depressed to form the *synaptic trough* in which the terminal button fits. This thickened portion of the muscle membrane is also called *motor end plate.* On each end plate only one nerve fibre ends (like other synapses there is no convergence of multiple inputs). Further, the postsynaptic membrane is thrown into large number of folds called *subneural clefts* or pallisades. These increase the surface area. The postsynaptic membrane, near the junction folds, contains *receptor sites* for acetylcholine called the *nicotinic–acetylcholine (ACh) receptors.* The matrix of subneural cleft contains the enzyme cholinesterase which can degrade acetylcholine.

NEUROMUSCULAR TRANSMISSION

The skeletal muscle is stimulated only through its nerve. The neuromuscular junction transmits the impulses from the nerve to muscle. The *sequence of events* which causes transmission of impulse through neuromuscular junction are:

- Release of acetylcholine by the nerve terminals
- Effect of acetylcholine on postsynaptic membrane
- Development of end plate potential
- Miniature end plate potential
- Removal of acetylcholine by cholinesterase
- Initiation of the action potential in muscle fibre.

Release of Acetylcholine by the Nerve Terminals. When the nerve impulse (action potential) travelling in the nerve fibre (axon) reaches the terminal buttons, the voltage-gated Ca^{2+} channels present on the presynaptic membrane open up increasing its permeability to Ca^{2+} ions. Consequently, the Ca^{2+} ions present in the ECF of synaptic cleft enter the terminal buttons.

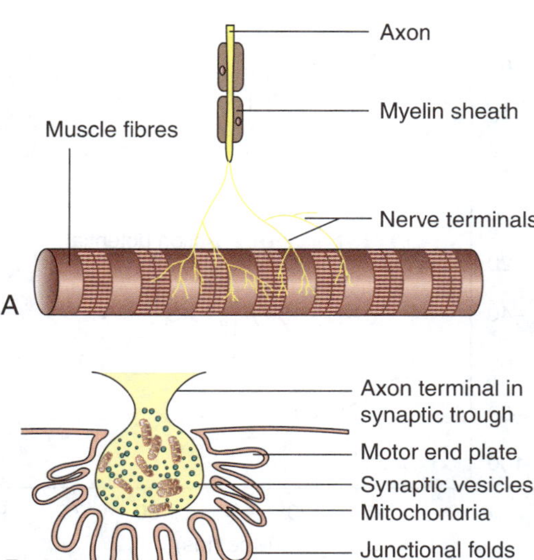

FIGURE 2.2-1 Structure of neuromuscular junction: **A,** the axon of the neuron loses its myelin sheath and divides into fine branches; and **B,** structure of terminal button and motor end plate.

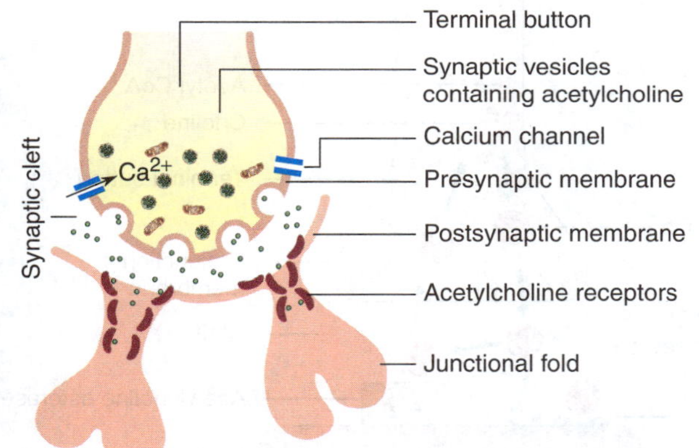

FIGURE 2.2-2 Detailed structure of neuromuscular junction showing Ca^{2+} channels on presynaptic membrane and ACh receptors on postsynaptic membrane.

The elevated Ca^{2+} levels in the cytosol of terminal buttons bring about a fusion of vesicles (containing acetylcholine) with the presynaptic membrane and trigger a marked increase in exocytosis of vesicles releasing acetylcholine in the synaptic cleft..Each vesicle contains about 10,000 molecules of acetylcholine, and, at a time about 125 vesicles burst by exocytosis (Fig. 2.2-2).

Effect of Acetylcholine on the Postsynaptic Membrane. The acetylcholine so released diffuses in the synaptic cleft and binds to the nicotinic–ACh receptors located mainly on the junctional folds of the motor end plate (postsynaptic membrane).

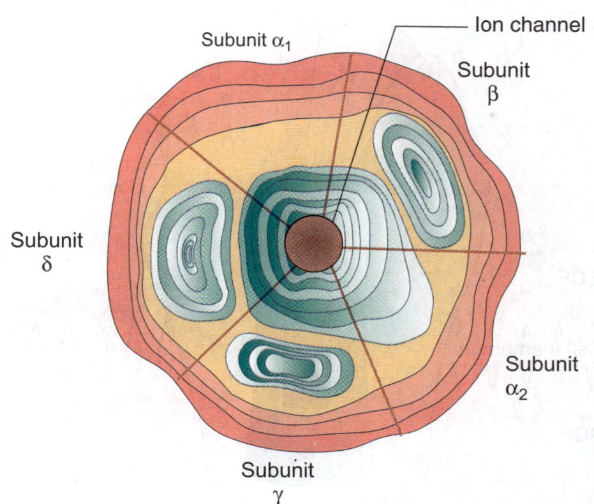

FIGURE 2.2-3 Structure of acetylcholine receptor from below.

Each receptor is actually *an acetylcholine-gated ion channel* (Fig. 2.2-3) made of a protein complex having molecular weight of 275,000 and is composed of five subunits (two alpha and one each of beta, delta and gamma). This protein complex penetrates all the way through the membrane forming a tubular channel which is kept closed (Fig. 2.2-4A).

When two molecules of acetylcholine get attached to the binding site of the receptors (i.e. two alpha units), there occurs a conformational change in the protein complex leading to opening up of the tubular channels (Fig. 2.2-4B). In other words, conductance to Na^+ and Ca^{2+} ions is increased at the motor end plate.

Development of End Plate Potential. Due to opening of the acetylcholine-gated channels in the end plate membrane, a large number of Na^+ ions from the ECF enter inside the muscle fibre following the electrochemical gradient.

The resting membrane potential at the postsynaptic membrane is about −80 to −90 mV. When sodium ions enter inside carrying with them large numbers of positive charges, there occurs depolarization causing a local positive potential change inside the muscle fibre membrane called the *end plate potential.*

End Plate Potential (EPP) is not the action potential. It is localized, nonpropagated, does not obey the all-or-none law and decays exponentially away from the plate.

The end plate potential is nonpropagative, but when a critical level of −60 mV is reached, it triggers the development of action potential in the muscle fibre (Fig. 2.2-5). The action potentials are generated on either side of the end plate and are conducted away from the end plate in both the

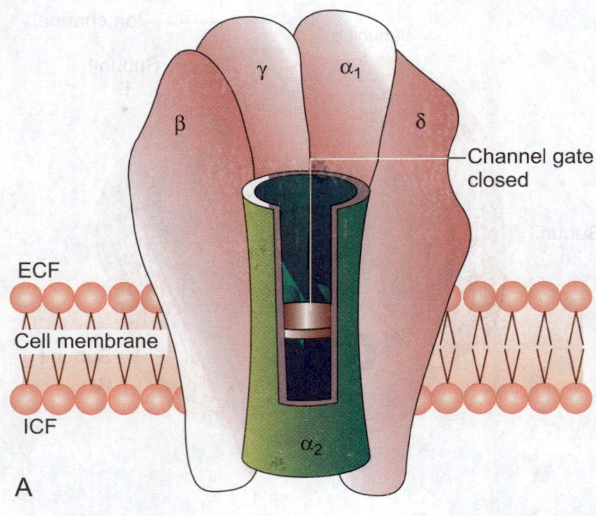

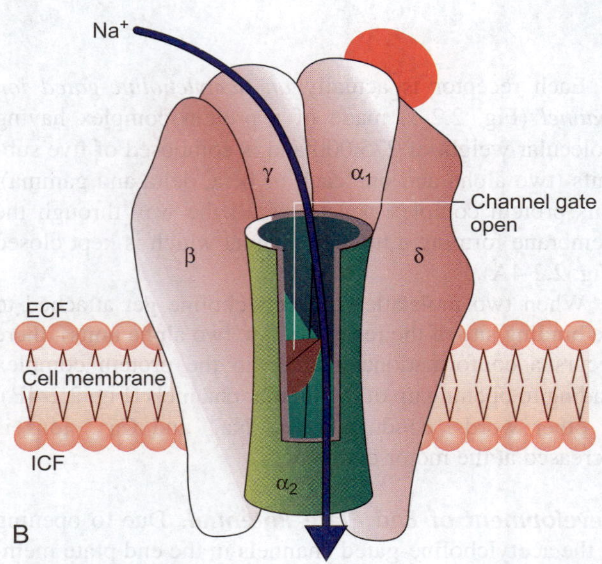

FIGURE 2.2-4 Acetylcholine-gated ion channels: **A,** closed state; and **B,** open state (conformational change occurred due to binding of two molecules of ACh to the binding sites).

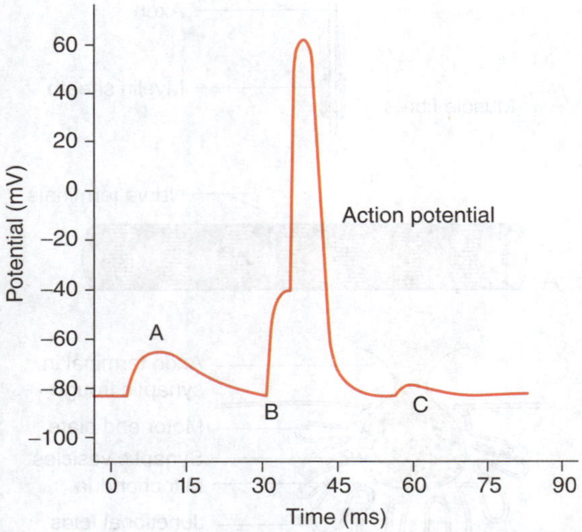

FIGURE 2.2-5 End plate potential and development of action potential in muscle fibre: **A,** weak end plate potential (<60 mV); **B,** end plate potential triggers propagating action potential (>−60 mV); and **C,** miniature end plate potential.

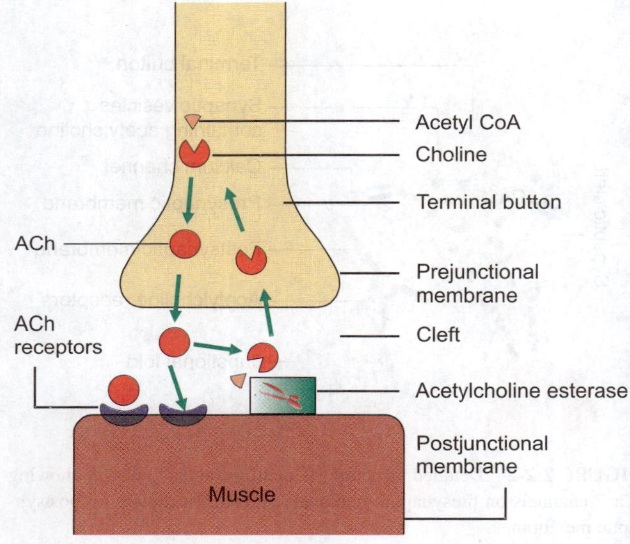

FIGURE 2.2-6 Removal of acetylcholine from the synaptic cleft of neuromuscular junction.

directions along the muscle fibres thus causing muscle contraction.

Miniature End Plate Potential. Even at rest, small quanta of acetylcholine are released randomly from the nerve terminal. Each quantum of acetylcholine produces a weak end plate potential about 0.5 mV in magnitude. This is called *miniature end plate potential.* The size of the quanta of acetylcholine released in this way varies directly with the Ca^{2+} concentration and inversely with the Mg^{2+} concentration at the end plate. The miniature end plate potential similar to that seen at the myoneural junction has been observed at other cholinergic synapses as well.

Removal of Acetylcholine. Acetylcholine released in the synaptic cleft is removed within 1 ms by two means (Fig. 2.2-6):

- Most of the acetylcholine is destroyed by the enzyme acetylcholinesterase which is present in the matrix of synaptic cleft.
- A small amount of the acetylcholine diffuses out of the synaptic space and is then no longer available to act on the muscle fibre membrane.

The acetylcholine is so potent that its stay in the synaptic space even for this short period of 1 ms is sufficient to excite the muscle fibre. It is important to note that the rapid removal of acetylcholine prevents the repeated excitation of muscle fibre.

DRUGS AFFECTING AND DISORDERS OF NEUROMUSCULAR JUNCTION

Drugs Affecting Neuromuscular Junction

Neuromuscular Blockers. Neuromuscular blockers are the drugs that block transmission at the neuromuscular junction. Some of the common neuromuscular blockers, which are commonly used, in clinical practice and in research are:

*1. **Curare*** or the active principle of D-tubocurarine prevents the neuromuscular transmission by combining with acetylcholine receptors. The acetylcholine released thus cannot combine with the receptors and so the end plate potential does not develop. The curariform drugs are called *receptor blockers* since they block the neuromuscular transmission by acting on acetylcholine receptors.

*2. **Bungarotoxin*** found in the venom of deadly snakes also blocks neuromuscular transmission by binding with acetylcholine receptors.

*3. **Succinylcholine and Carbamylcholine*** act like acetylcholine and cause depolarization of the postsynaptic membrane. But these are not destroyed by cholinesterase and so the muscle remains in a depolarized state for a long time. Thus, these drugs block the myoneural junction by keeping the muscle in a depolarized state.

*4. **Botulinum Toxin*** is derived from the bacteria *Clostridium botulinum*. It blocks the transmission across the myoneural junction by preventing the release of acetylcholine from the terminal buttons of the nerve endings.

Neuromuscular Stimulators

Drugs Having Acetylcholine-Like Action. The drugs methacholine, carbachol and nicotine act like acetylcholine and produce end plate potential exciting the muscle fibre. However, these drugs are either not destroyed or are destroyed very slowly by the enzyme acetylcholineesterase. So they cause repeated stimulation and continuous action of muscle, thereby causing a state of muscle spasm.

Drugs That Inactivate the Enzyme Cholinesterase (Anticholinesterase). The drugs like neostigmine, physostigmine and disopropylfluorophosphate (DFP) stimulate the neuromuscular junction by inactivating the enzyme acetylcholinesterase. Once this enzyme is inactivated, the acetylcholine released at the nerve terminal cannot be hydrolysed, this leads to repeated stimulation and continuous action of muscle.

The effect of neostigmine and physostigmine lasts for several hours while that of DFP lasts for several weeks. The DFP is thus a lethal poison which can cause death due to laryngeal spasm.

Disorders of Neuromuscular Junction

Myasthenia Gravis. Myasthenia gravis is a disorder in which the myoneural junction is unable to transmit signals from the nerve fibre to muscle fibres, thereby causing paralysis of the involved muscles. The worldwide incidence of this disease is 25–125 out of hundred million people. The disease is more common in females than in males. Myasthenia is probably an autoimmune disease. In this disease, antibodies are produced against the acetylcholine-gated channels (receptors) present on the motor end plate which destroy these channels. Thus, the acetylcholine released at the nerve terminal is not able to produce adequate end plate potential to excite the muscle fibre.

Clinical Features. The main clinical feature of the disease is muscle fatigue with sustained or repeated activity. It is usually presented in following forms:

- In one form, mainly extraocular, muscles are involved and in other form there is generalized weakness of skeletal muscles.
- In severe cases of myasthenia gravis, thymus may play a role by supplying helper T-cells sensitized against thymic protein that cross react with nicotinic–ACh-receptors and destroy them. Studies show that the number of receptors on motor end plates of affected muscle is reduced by 70–90%.

If the disease is intense enough, the patient dies of paralysis, particularly of respiratory muscles.

Treatment. Weakness of the muscles improves after a period of rest or administration of ACh–esterase inhibitor. Thymectomy may also improve the symptoms.

Lambert–Eaton Syndrome. In this disease, antibodies are produced against the calcium channels present on the presynaptic membrane, which destroy the channels. Consequently, Ca^{2+} influx into the nerve terminal is markedly decreased and thereby release of acetylcholine is also reduced. Scanty amount of acetylcholine is not able to produce adequate end plate potential to excite muscle fibres, producing muscular weakness. A similar type of syndrome can also occur after the use of aminoglycoside antibiotics which impair the functioning of Ca^{2+} at nerve terminals.

Chapter 2.3

Skeletal Muscle

INTRODUCTION

The muscle cell, like the neuron, is an excitable tissue, i.e. an action potential is generated when it is stimulated either chemically, electrically or mechanically. Further, the muscle is a contractile tissue with a chemically stored energy which can be transformed into mechanical energy.

There are three different types of muscles in the body: skeletal muscles, cardiac muscles and smooth muscles. Based on certain distinctive features the muscles can be grouped as:

Striated Versus Nonstriated Muscles *Striated muscle* cells show large number of cross striations at regular intervals when seen under a light microscope. Skeletal and cardiac muscles are striated.

Nonstriated muscle cells do not show any striations. Smooth muscles or the so-called plain muscles are nonstriated.

Voluntary Versus Involuntary Muscles *Voluntary muscles* can be made to contract under our will to perform the movements we desire. All skeletal muscles are voluntary muscles. These are supplied by somatic motor nerves.

Involuntary muscle's activities cannot be controlled at will. Cardiac and all smooth muscles are involuntary muscles. These are innervated by autonomic nerves.

Skeletal Muscles The skeletal muscles, as the name indicates, are attached with the bones of the body skeleton and their contraction results in the body movements. They constitute about 40% of the total body mass.

FUNCTIONAL ANATOMY AND ORGANIZATION

Structural Organization of Muscle

Structurally, the skeletal muscle consists of a large number of muscle fibres and a connective tissue framework organized as (Figs. 2.3-1, 2.3-2):

- Each *muscle fibre* is surrounded by delicate connective tissue called *endomysium* which contains large quantity of elastic tissue arranged longitudinally.

- The muscle fibres are grouped into a number of bundles called *fasciculi.* Each fasciculus is surrounded by a stronger sheath of connective tissue called *perimysium.*
- All the fasciculi collectively form the *muscle belly.* The connective tissue that surrounds the entire muscle belly is called *epimysium.*
- At the junction of the muscle with its tendon, the fibres of endomysium, perimysium and epimysium become continuous with the fibres of the tendon.
- *Tendons* are fibrous terminal ends of the muscles made up of collagen fibres.

Structure of a Muscle Fibre

Each muscle fibre is basically a long (1–4 cm), cylindrical (10–100 micron in diameter) multinucleated cell. Its cell membrane is called *sarcolemma* and the cytoplasm is called *sarcoplasm.* Like any other cell, in the sarcoplasm are embedded many structures, the nuclei, Golgi apparatus, mitochondria, sarcoplasmic reticulum, ribosomes and glycogen and occasional lipid droplets. In addition, the sarcoplasm mainly contains number of *myofibrils* which form the main structure of a muscle fibre. The sarcolemma along with the sarcoplasmic reticulum forms the so-called *sarcotubular system* which will be described in detail later.

Myofibril

Each muscle fibre consists of a large number of myofibrils which are arranged parallel to each other and run along the entire length of the muscle fibre. Myofibril is about 1–2 μm in diameter and 1–4 cm in length depending upon the length of the muscle fibre.

Each myofibril consists of many thick and thin filaments (myofilaments) made up of a number of contractile proteins. Thick filaments are made up of myosin and are about 1500, while thin filaments are made of actin and about 3000 in number in each myofibril. The peculiar arrangement of these myofilaments when seen under a *light microscope* gives an appearance of alternate dark and light bands (striations) as described:

Striations of Muscle Fibres

The dark and light bands result from a difference in the refractive index of its different parts. The arrangement is as follows (Fig. 2.3-2D):

- The dark band is called *A band* (anisometropic to polarized light). It is 1.5 μm in length. In the area of A band, the thick (myosin) filaments line up the thin filaments.
- In the centre of each A band there is a lighter H-zone where thin filaments do not overlap the thick filaments (the word H either represents the discoverer, Henson or the hell which in German means light).
- In the centre of each H-zone is seen an M line, which is more pronounced during muscle contraction.

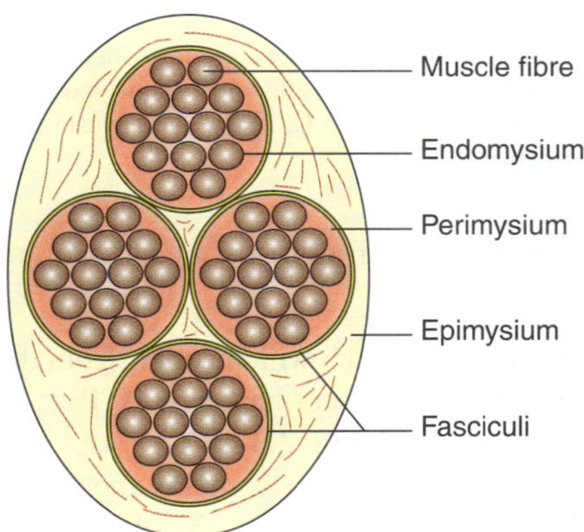

FIGURE 2.3-1 Transverse section of skeletal muscle seen under light microscope.

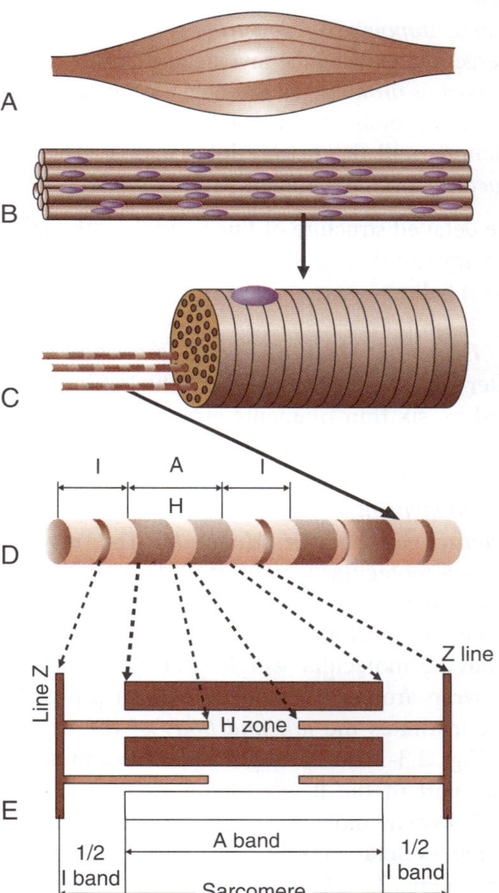

FIGURE 2.3-2 Schematic diagram showing structural organization of skeletal muscle: **A,** muscle belly; **B,** muscle fibres grouped into fasciculi; **C,** muscle fibre; **D,** myofibril; and **E,** arrangement of thick and thin filaments.

- The light band is called *I band*, because it is isotropic to polarized light. It is about 1 µm in length. This area contains only thin (actin) filaments.
- Each I band is bisected by a narrow dark *Z line* (the word Z has been taken from Z Wischenscheibe which in German means between discs).
- The portion of myofibril between two successive Z lines is called a *sarcomere*. Thus, a sarcomere includes ½ I band + A band + ½ I band and is about 2.5 µm in length at rest. The sarcomere is the structural and functional unit of the muscle fibre. During muscle contraction, the sarcomere reduces in length to 1.5 µm and during stretching of the muscle it increases in length to 3.5 µm.

Thick and Thin Filaments

The thick and thin filaments (Fig. 2.3-2E) form the *contractile apparatus* of a striated muscle. These are made up of three types of proteins:

- *Contractile proteins* are *myosin* and *actin* which interact to generate the contractile force in a muscle.
- *Regulatory proteins,* also called relaxation proteins, include *tropomyosin and troponin.* These regulate the interaction between the myosin and actin.
- *Anchoring proteins,* as the name indicates, anchor the different proteins to each other as well as to the sarcolemma and the extracellular matrix. These include *α-actinin, titin, nebulin* and *dystrophin.*

The detailed structure of thick and thin filaments forming the myofibril as revealed by *electron microscopy* is described below:

Thick Filament Thick filaments are about twice the diameter of thin filaments. Each thick filament is surrounded by six thin filaments arranged in a regular hexagonal manner. A thick filament is made up of hundreds of molecules of a complex actin-binding contractile protein called *myosin.*

Structure of Myosin Molecule. The myosin molecule has a molecular weight of 480,000 and is made up of six polypeptide chains, two heavy chains (each having molecular weight 200,000) and four light chains (each having molecular weight 20,000). The two heavy chains wrap around each other to form a double helix, which constitutes the *tail and body* of the myosin molecule (Fig. 2.3-3B). The light chains combine with the terminal part of the heavy chains to form the globular *head* of myosin molecule. The myosin molecule present in the skeletal muscle has two heads and is called *myosin-II* (Fig. 2.3-3C) (single-headed myosin present in some other cells of the body is called myosin-I). These heads contain an *actin-binding site* and a *catalytic site* that hydrolyses ATP. During muscle contraction, the head forms the *cross-bridging* (described later). Digestion with trypsin generates two fragments of myosin molecules (Fig. 2.3-4):

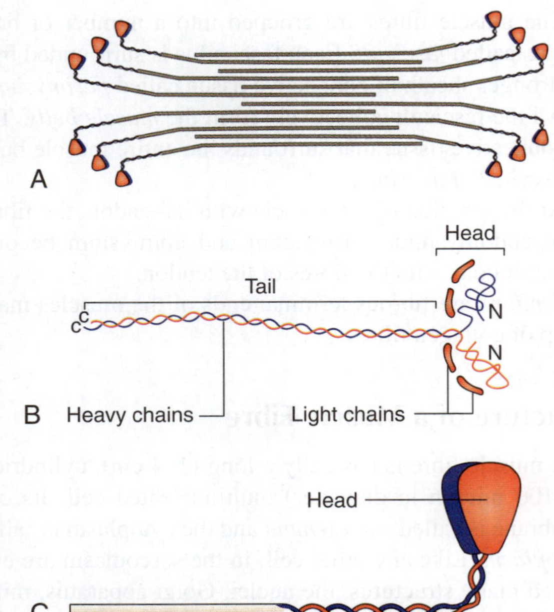

FIGURE 2.3-3 Myosin molecules: **A,** arrangement of myosin molecules in thick filament; **B,** structure of myosin molecule; and **C,** molecule of myosin II (with two heads).

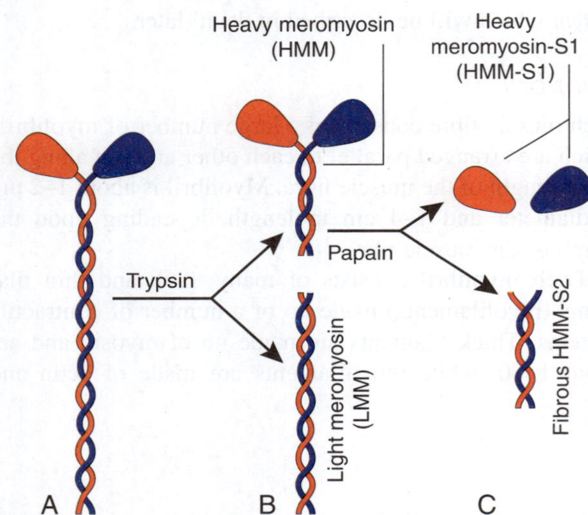

FIGURE 2.3-4 Myosin molecule after digestion with trypsin and papain: **A,** before digestion with trypsin; **B,** after digestion with trypsin (form two fragments LMM and HMM); and **C,** heavy meromyosin fragment after digestion with papain.

- *Light meromysin (LMM)* which comes from the tail part of the myosin. It does not have any ATPase activity or actin-binding ability (Fig. 2.3-4B).
- *Heavy meromysin (HMM)* contains the globular head as well as part of the tail (Fig. 2.3-4B). HMM can be further split by papain into two parts (Fig. 2.3-4C): the *globular HMM-SI,* which has all the ATPase activity and

actin-binding ability, and the fibrous, HMM-S2, which has none of it.

Arrangement of myosin molecules in a thick filament

In a thick filament, half of the myosin molecules are oriented with their heads in one direction and the remaining half in the opposite direction (Fig. 2.3-3A). Because of this arrangement, the central portion of a thick filament is devoid of the head portions of the myosin molecules. This accounts for the comparatively lighter H-zone seen in the centre of dark A band. The central overlapping of the myosin molecules of each side creates a central bulge in each of thick filaments which accounts for the M line seen on light microscopy.

Thin Filament The thin filament has a head end (that extends into the A band) and a tail end that is anchored to the Z line (through a protein called α-actinin). Each thin filament is made up of contractile protein molecules (actin) and two types of regulatory protein molecules (tropomyosin and troponin) (Fig. 2.3-5).

Actin. About 300–400 actin molecules are present in each thin filament. The actin molecules form a long double helix consisting of two chains of globular units. The globular molecules are *G-actin*, and the chain formed by them is designated as *F-actin*.

Tropomyosin. About 40–60 tropomyosin molecules are present in each thin filament. Tropomyosin are long filaments that lie in the groove between the two chains of actin molecules. It covers the binding site of actin where the myosin head comes in contact with actin. Thus, it is a regulatory protein that prevents the interaction between actin and myosin filaments.

Troponin. Troponin molecules are small globular units located at intervals along the tropomyosin molecule. The troponin molecule has three subunits:

- ***Troponin-T*** binds the other troponin components to tropomyosin.
- ***Troponin-I*** prevents the interaction of myosin heads with active sites on actin.
- ***Troponin-C*** contains binding site for Ca^{2+} that initiates muscle contraction. Each molecule of troponin-C binds to four molecules of Ca^{2+} ions.

Arrangement of Anchoring Proteins of Contractile Apparatus The anchoring proteins of the contractile apparatus include α-actinin, titin, nebulin and dystrophin-associated glycoproteins. These are arranged as:

- α-actinin cross links the actin filaments in the area of Z line (Fig. 2.3-6A).

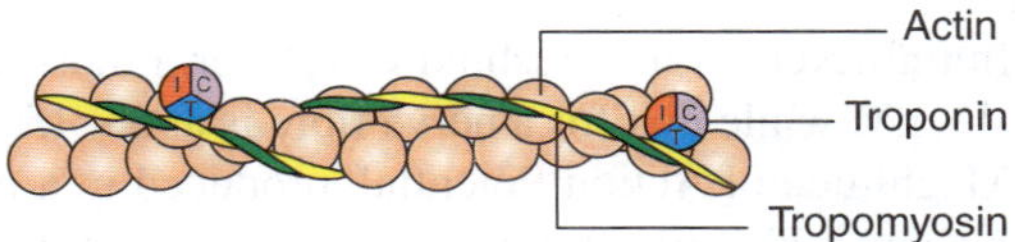

FIGURE 2.3-5 Structure of a thin filament.

- Titin earlier called as *connectin* or gap filament is a large elastic filament which interconnects the Z lines. It forms the *series elastic components* of the muscle.
- Nebulin is an inextensible filament which is connected at one end to the α-actinin in the area of Z line and at another end to the tropomyosin–troponin complex of thin filaments at regular intervals.
- Dystrophin–glycoprotein Complex. The dystrophin–glycoprotein complex (Fig. 2.3-6B) forms the best known anchor protein complex, which provides structural support and strength to myofibril. As shown in Fig. 2.3-6B, the *dystrophin* molecule forms a rod that connects the thin actin filament to the two proteins (a and b dystroglycan) present in the sarcolemma which in turn are connected to the merosin subunit of *laminin* molecule present in the basal lamina matrix. The dystroglycans in turn associated with transmembrane glycoprotein complex made up of a, b, g and d sarcoglycans.

Important Note

The dystrophin–glycoprotein complex is of special importance because genetic defects in it are associated with many of the different forms of *muscular dystrophy.*

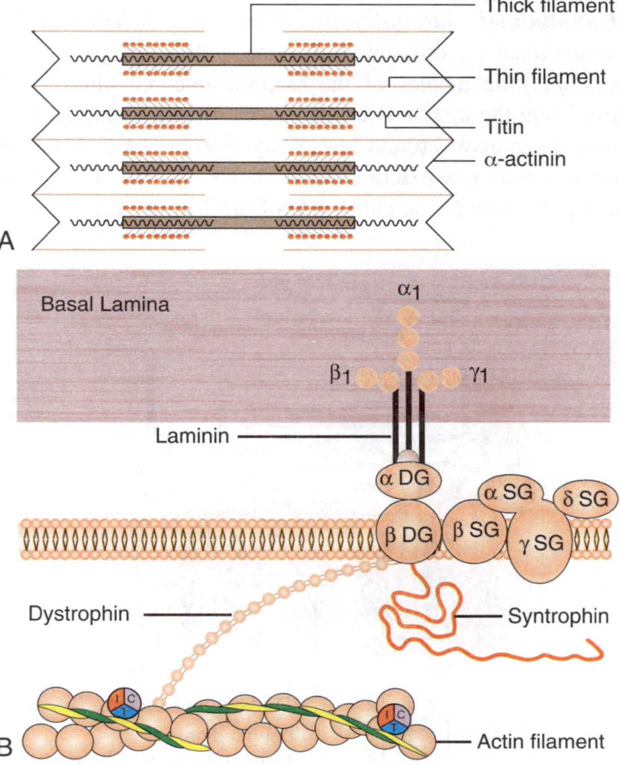

FIGURE 2.3-6 Arrangement of anchoring proteins of the contractile apparatus: **A,** α-actinin (which cross link the thin filament in area of Z lines) and titin (interconnects two Z lines), and **B,** dystrophin–glycoprotein (DG) complex associated with sarcoglycan (SG) complex of four glycoproteins α, β, γ and δ.

Sarcotubular System

The sarcolemma (cell membrane of muscle cell) along with the sarcoplasmic reticulum (the endoplasmic reticulum of muscle cell) forms a highly specialized system called sarcotubular system. This plays an important role in the internal conduction of depolarization within the muscle fibre. The sarcotubular system (which under an electron microscope appears as vesicles and tubules) is primarily formed by a transverse tubular system (T-system) and a longitudinal sarcoplasmic reticulum (Fig. 2.3-7).

Transverse Tubular System (T-System) The T-system of transverse tubules is formed by the through and through invagination of sarcolemma into the muscle fibre in the region of junction of A and I bands (Fig. 2.3-7). Since the T-tubules are formed by the invagination of sarcolemma, their lumen contains ECF which surrounds the muscle cell. These T-tubules facilitate the rapid transmission of the impulse in the form of action potential from sarcolemma to the myofibrils. The membrane of T-tubules contains voltage-gated Ca^{2+} channels called *dihydropyridine* receptors (as they get blocked by the drug dihydropyridine), through which they activate the longitudinal sarcoplasmic reticulum.

Longitudinal Sarcoplasmic Reticulum (L-Tubules) The longitudinal sarcoplasmic reticulum is the name given to the *sarcoplasmic* tubules of the sarcoplasmic reticulum which run along the long axis of the muscle fibre forming a closed tubular system around each myofibril. These L-tubules do not open to the exterior like T-tubules. The longitudinal sarcoplasmic tubules on either side of the T-tubule are dilated to form the so-called *terminal cisterns.* A T-tubule with the two terminal cisterns lying in close proximity (contiguity) constitutes a *triad* which is found at the junction of A and I bands. Thus, there are two triads in each sarcomere (Fig. 2.3-7).

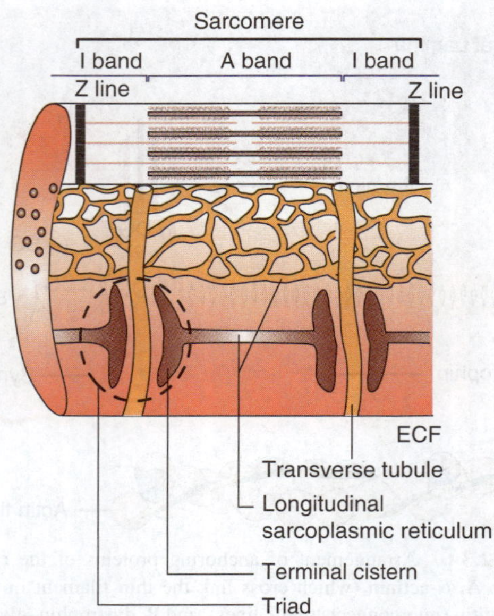

FIGURE 2.3-7 Sarcotubular system showing transverse tubules and longitudinal sarcoplasmic reticulum.

The longitudinal tubules store a large quantity of calcium ions. When the action potential reaches the cisterns of L-tubules, these Ca^{2+} ions released are into the sarcoplasm through the calcium channels present on their membrane. The calcium channels are not voltage gated. These are called *ryanodine receptors,* as they are kept in open position by ryanodine alkaloid.

PROCESS OF MUSCLE EXCITABILITY AND CONTRACTILITY

As we know, the muscle is an excitable tissue, i.e. when stimulated an action potential is produced (*electrical phenomenon*). The skeletal muscle responds to stimulus by contracting (*mechanical phenomenon*). The events that link the electrical phenomenon with the mechanical phenomenon is called *excitation–contraction coupling phenomenon.* These three phenomena which mark the excitability and contractility of the muscle when stimulated by the nerve innervating it are discussed.

Process of Muscle Excitation

It refers to electrical phenomenon and ionic fluxes in skeletal muscle fibres. As discussed in the transmission across neuromuscular junction (page 80), an end plate potential (EPP) is developed at the motor end plate by the nerve impulse travelling across the innervating axon. The end plate potential, as discussed earlier (page 81), is localized and nonpropagated. However, when EPP reaches a threshold level, it produces an *action potential* which propagates over muscle fibre surface and into the muscle fibre along the transverse tubules.

Essential Features of Electrical Phenomena Essential features of electrical phenomena which occur in the muscle fibre (resting membrane potential and action potential) are similar to those occurring in a nerve fibre. These have been described on page 60 (students are advised to revise them). However, there are some quantitative differences between the electrical phenomenon occurring in a skeletal muscle fibre and a nerve fibre which are summarized below:

1. Resting Membrane Potential in a skeletal muscle fibre is about 290mV, while in a nerve fibre it is about −70 mV.

2. Initial Excitation Threshold Level for a muscle fibre is 30–40 mV, while that for a nerve fibre is about 15 mV.

3. Magnitude of Action Potential produced in a muscle fibre is about 120–130 mV while that produced in the nerve fibre is about 100–105 mV.

4. Duration of Spike Potential is longer in a muscle fibre (5 ms) than in a nerve fibre (0.4–2 ms).

5. Absolute Refractory Period is also longer in a muscle fibre (1–3 ms) than in a nerve fibre (0.4–2 ms).

6. Maximum Number of Impulses which can pass through a muscle fibre are much less (100–200/s) than the nerve fibre (1000/s).

7. The Excitability of the muscle is far less than that of the neuron, that is, *chronaxie* in a muscle fibre is longer while in a nerve fibre it is shorter.

8. Conduction Velocity of Action Potentials in a skeletal muscle fibre is low, 3–5 m/s. In a nerve fibre, the conduction velocity of an action potential is variable, being directly proportional to its diameter. In a myelinated nerve fibre, the conduction velocity can be as high as 120 m/s.

9. Equilibrium Potential for different ions in a skeletal muscle fibre and a nerve fibre is as shown in Table 2.3-1.

Process of Excitation–Contraction Coupling

The process by which depolarization of a muscle fibre initiates contraction is called excitation–contraction coupling. The sequence of events by which an action potential in the plasma membrane of a muscle fibre leads to cross-bridge activity (excitation–contraction coupling) is as:

- Action potential initiated in the plasma membrane of a muscle fibre spreads rapidly on the surface as well as into the interior of the muscle fibre through the T-tubules.
- When the action potential reaches the tip of the T-tubule, it activates the voltage-gated channels called dihydropyridine receptors (DHP) which are located in the T-tubule membrane (Fig. 2.3-8).
- Activated DHP receptors in turn trigger the opening of Ca^{2+}-release channels located on the terminal cisterns, the so-called *ryanodine receptor (RYR)*. This is possible because the lateral cisterns are located very close to the tips of T-tubules and the protein channels of the cisterns (DHP and RYR) are mechanically interlocked. Thus, in short, when the DHP is activated by the depolarization of T-tubules, it undergoes conformational changes which result in the opening of RYR (being actually pulled open).
- Due to opening of calcium-release channels (RYR), calcium ions diffuse into the cytoplasm. The concentration of Ca^{2+} in the ICF is increased by some 2000 times, i.e. from 10^{-7} moles/L to 2×10^{-4} moles /L.
- The Ca^{2+} ions get attached to troponin-C and start a chain of events (discussed below) which produces contraction. Thus, the calcium ions act as a linking or coupling material between the excitation and the contraction of the muscle. Hence, the calcium ions are said to form the basis of excitation–contraction coupling.

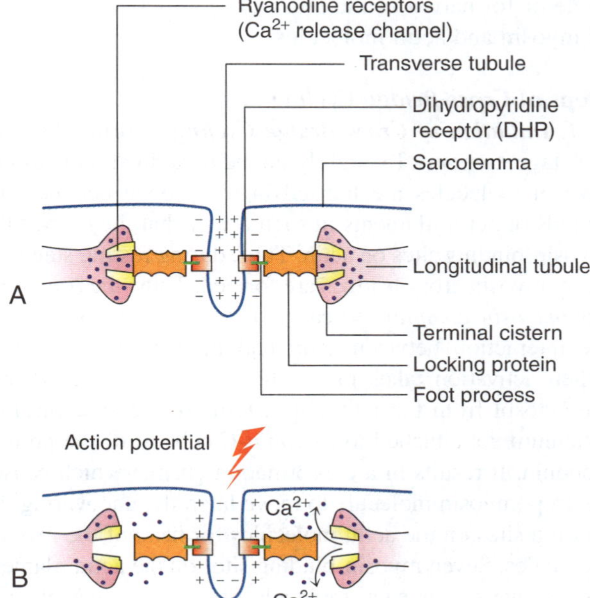

FIGURE 2.3-8 Mechanism of release of calcium ions from terminal cistern of longitudinal tubules: **A,** in resting state Ca^{2+}-release channels (RYR) remain closed due to mechanical interlocking between DHP and RYR; and **B,** during activation state (depolarization of T-tubule). Conformational change in DHP results in opening of RYR and release of Ca^{2+}.

TABLE 2.3-1 Equilibrium Potential of Different Ions in Skeletal Muscle Fibre and Nerve Fibre

Ion	Equilibrium potential (mV)	
	Skeletal muscle fibre	*Nerve fibre*
Na^+	+65	+60
K^+	− 95	−90
H^+	−32	−25
Cl^-	−90	−70
HCO^-_3	−32	−25

Process of Muscle Contraction

Molecular Basis of Muscle Contraction

The process of muscle contraction is initiated by the calcium ions as discussed above. The molecular basis of muscle contraction describes the role of the contractile molecules myosin and actin play in the process of muscle contraction. AF Huxley and HE Huxley in 1954 put forward the *sliding theory* or *ratchet theory* to explain how the actin filaments slide over myosin filaments forming the actin–myosin complex during muscular contraction. This theory is called *walk-along theory* or the modern theory of muscular contraction. This theory explains that the sliding of filaments is brought about by a repeated cycle of formation of the *cross-bridges* between the head of myosin and actin molecules.

Steps of Cross-Bridge Cycling

1. Initiation of Cross-Bridge Cycling. During the resting stage, troponin-I is lightly bound to actin and the tropomyosin molecules are located in the groove between the strands of actin filaments in such a way that they block the myosin-binding sites on actin. Thus, during resting stage, no actin–myosin cross-bridges are formed. Thus, the *troponin–tropomyosin complex,* so-called *relaxing proteins,* inhibits the interaction between actin and myosin (Fig. 2.3-9A). When activation takes place, the Ca^{2+} ions released into the cytosol from the terminal cisterns of the sarcoplasmic reticulum get attached to *troponin-C* subunit of the protein troponin. It results in a conformation change which causes the tropomyosin molecule to move laterally, uncovering the binding sites on the actin molecules for head of the myosin molecules. Seven myosin-binding sites on the actin filament are uncovered for each molecule of troponin that binds a Ca^{2+} ion. Thus, the cross-bridge cycle is switched on (initiated) by the lateral movement of tropomyosin (Fig. 2.3-9B).

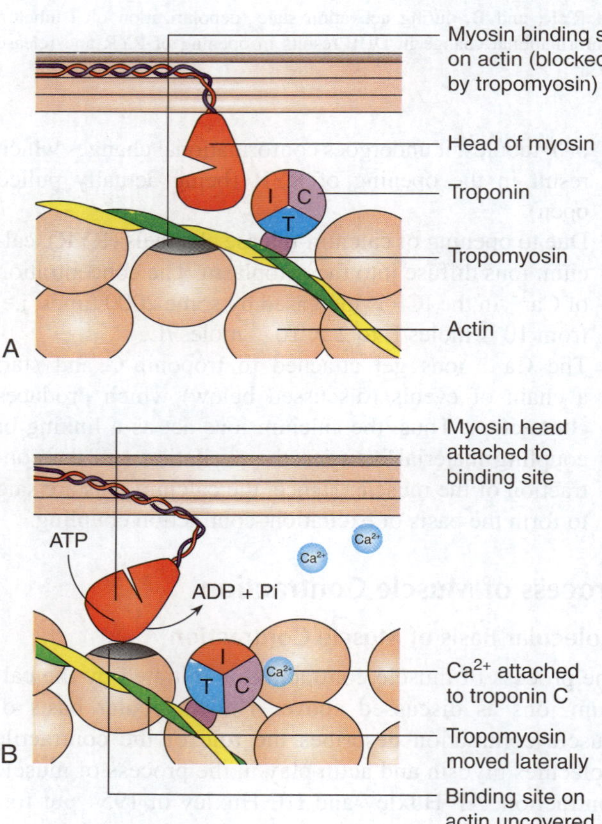

FIGURE 2.3-9 Initiation of cross-bridge cycling: **A,** resting state (myosin-binding site on actin is covered by troponin–tropomyosin complex); and **B,** on activation, Ca^{2+} binds to troponin-C subunit and this results in conformational change and lateral displacement of tropomyosin (causing uncovering of binding site for myosin (head of myosin) on actin (initiation of cross-bridge cycle).

2. Formation of Actin–Myosin Complex (i.e. Attachment of Myosin Head to Active Site of Actin Filament). The head of myosin molecule binds with ATP. The ATPase activity of myosin head immediately causes breaking of ATP to ADP and Pi cleavage products which remain bound to myosin head. The head of myosin therefore becomes energized. The activated myosin head extends perpendicularly (at 90° conformation) towards the actin filament and gets attached to the actin filament (Fig. 2.3-10) (Stages I and II). The reaction occurs as:

$$\text{A} + \text{M. ADP.Pi} \xrightarrow{\textit{actin binding}} \text{A.M.ADP.Pi}$$

3. The Power Stroke. Formation of the *actin–myosin-ADP Pi* complex triggers simultaneously the following two events:

- Release of the Pi and ADP from the complex, and
- A conformational change in the myosin head causing it to flex towards the arm of the cross-bridge. The flexion of the myosin head from the high-energy 90° conformation to low-energy 45° conformation generates mechanical force (the power stroke). The power stroke has either or both of the following effects:
  - *If the load on the muscle is small,* then the actin filament slides over the myosin filament, producing muscle shortening (Fig. 2.3-10) (Stage III).

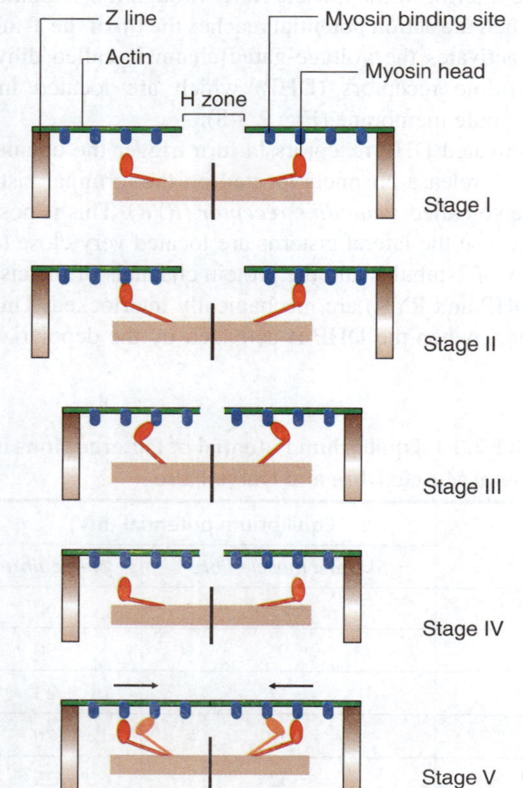

FIGURE 2.3-10 Stages of cross-bridge cycling (for details see text).

- *If the load on muscle is large,* then the actin filaments are unable to slide over the myosin filament; under such circumstances, the flexion of the myosin head will produce stretching of the elastic neck of myosin molecule.

Thus, the energy stored in head of myosin cross-bridge is utilized for the power stroke. The reaction occurs as:

A.M. ADP. Pi $\xrightarrow{\textit{bridge movement}}$ A.M. + ADP + Pi myosin head still remains attached to active site of actin filament at 45° position but stops sliding.

4. Detachment of Head of a Cross-Bridge from Active Site of Actin Filament. The release of ADP and Pi allows a fresh ATP molecule to bind to the myosin head. The *myosin ATP complex* has a low affinity for actin, and therefore, it results in the dissociation of myosin head from the actin filament (Fig. 2.3-10) (stage IV). The reaction is as:

A.M. + ATP.→ A + M.ATP

5. Reactivation of Myosin Head. The freshly bound ATP molecule splits again, and the myosin head is reactivated for the next cycle to begin. The energized head extends perpendicularly towards the actin filament and gets attached to the new active site for repeating the cycle. This reaction occurs as:

M.ATP $\xrightarrow{\textit{energized cross-bridge}}$ M.ADP. Pi

Thus with each cross-bridge cycle, there is movement of the actin filament towards the centre of myosin to a small degree. Repeated cross-bridge cycling causes the movement of actin filaments of either side towards the centre of myosin filament of the sarcomere leading to muscle contraction (Fig. 2.3-10) (stage V).

Steps in Muscle Relaxation. Within a few milliseconds of the action potential, the calcium pump transports Ca^{2+} ions present in sarcoplasm during contraction back into the longitudinal portion of the sarcoplasmic reticulum, from where the Ca^{2+} ions are discharged into the terminal cistern for storage (Fig. 2.3-11).

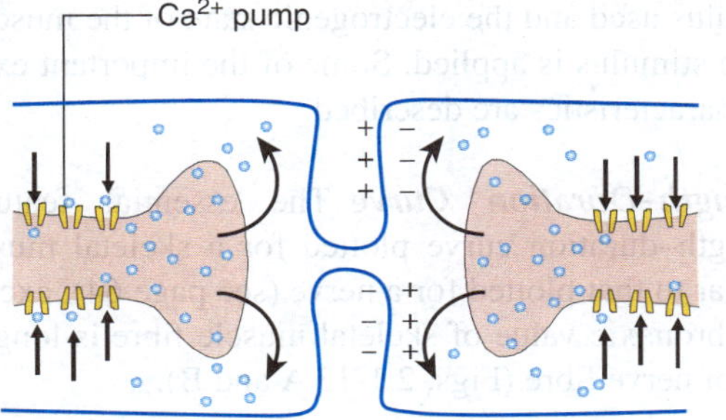

FIGURE 2.3-11 Transport of Ca^{2+} from sarcoplasm into longitudinal tubules by Ca^{2+} pump.

Removal of calcium from troponin restores blocking action of troponin–tropomyosin complex. Myosin cross-bridge cycle closes and muscle relaxes.

Functions of ATP in Skeletal Muscle Contraction and Relaxation

1. *Hydrolysis of ATP* by myosin energizes the cross-bridges providing the energy for force generation.
2. *Binding of ATP to myosin* causes dissociation of cross-bridges, allowing the bridges to repeat their cycle of activity.
3. *Hydrolysis of ATP by Ca^{2+}* ATPase in the sarcoplasmic reticulum provides the energy for active transport of calcium back into the cisternae, lowering cytoplasmic calcium, ending the contraction and allowing muscle fibre to relax.

Applied Aspects

Rigor mortis refers to shortening and rigidity of all the body muscles which occurs some hours after death. The rigidity occurs because of fixation of cross-bridges of myosin head to actin filaments in an abnormal and resistant manner due to loss of all the ATP (which is normally required for detachment of cross-bridges of myosin heads from the actin filaments cause relaxation). Depending upon the environmental temperature and other factors, the rigidity disappears after some hours due to destruction of the muscle proteins by enzymes released from cellular lysosomes. The appearance and disappearance of rigor mortis is used by the forensic experts in fixing the time of death.

Changes Produced by Sliding of Thin Filaments over Thick Filaments during Muscle Contraction Fig. 2.3-12 shows the following changes produced by sliding of thin filaments over thick filaments during muscle contraction.

1. The width of A band remains constant,
2. H-zone disappears,
3. I band width decreases,
4. The Z lines move closer,
5. The sarcomere shortens and
6. The actin filaments from the opposite end of the sarcomere approach each other, and when the muscle shortening is marked, these filaments apparently overlap.

Sequence of Events During Muscle Contraction and Relaxation when Stimulated by a Nerve

The events that occur during contraction and relaxation in a skeletal muscle when excited by a nerve are summarized sequence wise:

Nerve excitation
- Stimulation of motor neuron

↓
- Initiation of action potential in motor neuron's axon

↓

Nerve conduction
- Propagation of action potential in the motor nerve

↓
- Impulse reaching at nerve ending (at synaptic button)

Neuromuscular transmission
- Increased permeability of presynaptic membrane to Ca^{2+} ions

↓
- Inflow of Ca^{2+} ions from ECF into the nerve terminals

↓
- Release of ACh from micro vesicles present at nerve terminal

↓
- Diffusion of ACh into synaptic cleft

↓
- Binding of ACh to receptors on the motor end plate (postsynaptic membrane)

↓
- Opening of ACh-gated channels in the motor end plate membrane

↓
- Entry of mainly Na^+ ions and to a lesser extent Ca^{2+} ions through these channels into the muscle fibre

↓
- Development of end plate potential (EPP)

Muscle excitation
- Local EPP when reaches a threshold magnitude, voltage-gated Na^+ channels are opened up at the site

↓
- Generation of action potential (AP) in the muscle fibre by end plate depolarization

↓
- Propagation of AP in muscle fibre along the surface and into the fibre along the T-tubules

↓

Excitation–contraction coupling
- Release of Ca^{2+} ions from terminal cistern

↓
- Diffusion of Ca^{2+} ions into the sarcoplasm

↓
- Binding of Ca^{2+} ions to troponin-C

↓

Muscle contraction (molecular theory)
- Uncovering of binding sites for myosin on actin

↓
- Cross-bridge formation between myosin head and actin

↓
- Angular movement of cross-bridges (power stroke)

↓
- Sliding of thin filaments over thick filaments

↓
- Initiation of muscle contraction

↓

Muscle relaxation
- Active transport of Ca^{2+} into sarcoplasmic reticulum

↓
- Decreased concentration of Ca^{2+} in sarcoplasm

↓
- Removal of Ca^{2+} ions from troponin-C

↓
- Cessation of cross-bridge cycling

↓
- Relaxation of muscle fibre

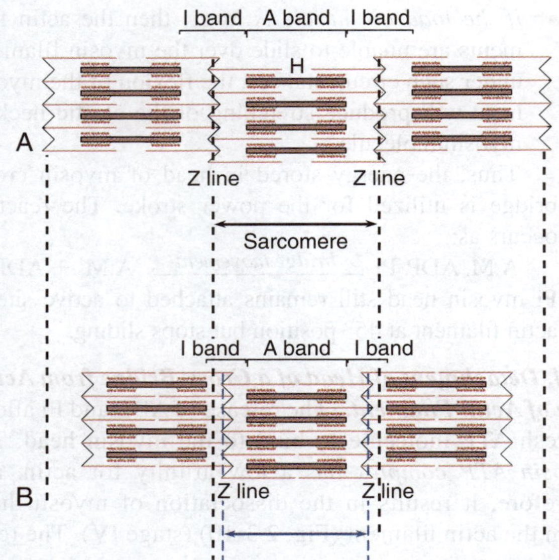

FIGURE 2.3-12 Changes produced in a sarcomere by sliding of thin filament (actin) over thick filament (myosin) during muscle contraction: **A,** relaxed state; and **B,** contracted state.

CHARACTERISTICS OF MUSCLE EXCITABILITY AND CONTRACTILITY

Excitability

Excitability is the property by which tissues respond to stimuli. The skeletal muscles respond by undergoing depolarization (development of action potential).

Characteristics of Electrical Phenomenon in a Skeletal Muscle The essential features of the resting membrane potential (RMP) and action potential (AP) of skeletal muscles are similar to those of a nerve (see page 60). The quantitative differences between the electrical phenomenon occurring in a skeletal muscle fibre and a nerve fibre are summarized on page 88.

Characteristics of Skeletal Muscle Fibre Excitability vis-à-vis Characteristics of the Stimulus The skeletal muscle fibres exhibit some peculiar characteristics of the excitability depending upon the strength and duration of the stimulus used and the electrogenic state of the muscle fibre when stimulus is applied. Some of the important excitability characteristics are described:

Strength–Duration Curve The essential features of strength–duration curve plotted for a skeletal muscle are similar to that plotted for a nerve (see page 64), except that the chronaxie value of skeletal muscle fibre is longer than that of nerve fibre (Figs. 2.1-13 A and B).

- Chronaxie value in frog's skeletal muscle is about 3 ms.

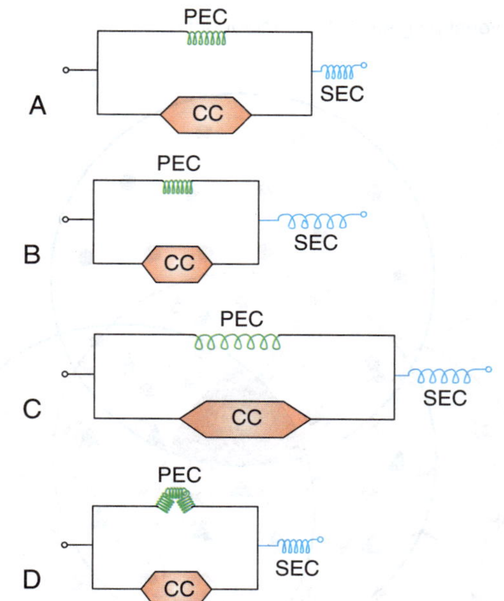

FIGURE 2.3-13 Three-component model of skeletal muscle consisting of contractile component (CC), series elastic component (SEC) and parallel elastic component (PEC): **A,** when muscle is at normal length; **B,** during isometric contraction; **C,** when muscle is passively stretched; and **D,** in isotonic contraction.

- Normal value of chronaxie in human skeletal muscles varies from 0.08 to 0.32 ms.
- Chronaxie is 10 times more in skeletal muscles of infants than in adults.

Contractility

To understand contractile response and its characteristics after discussing the process of muscle excitability and contraction, it is essential to have a knowledge about the following elementary aspects in relation to skeletal muscle:

- Contractile and elastic components of a muscle,
- Muscle length,
- Type of muscle fibres and
- Motor unit.

Contractile and Elastic Components of a Muscle

To understand certain facts associated with muscle contraction such as shortening, contraction without shortening and effect of passive stretch, a *three-component model* has been proposed. According to this model, the skeletal muscle as a whole consists of three components (Fig. 2.3-13A):

- Contractile component,
- Series elastic component and
- Parallel elastic component.

1. Contractile Component The contractile component (CC) represents the thick (myosin) and thin (actin) filaments present in the myofibrils. It is considered to be viscous in nature, i.e. it offers no resistance to stretch and is unable to return to its original length after it has shortened. The contractile component comprises 60% (3/5th) of the total muscle proteins.

2. Series Elastic Component The series elastic component (SEC) refers to that elastic tissue of the muscle which is present in series with the contractile component (CC) of the muscle. It consists of the elastic tendon of the muscle. In resting condition, the SEC offers resistance to passive stretch and explains how muscle is able to contract even when its external length does not change, i.e. isometric contraction (Fig. 2.3-13B). It also explains how the muscle regains its original length after contracting isometrically.

3. Parallel Elastic Component The parallel elastic component (PEC) refers to the elastic tissue of the muscle which is attached parallel to the CC. The PEC is represented by the structural elastic tissue of the muscle such as connective tissue sheaths of the muscle, sarcolemma and gap filaments. Presence of this component explains why the muscle regains its original length after it is passively stretched (Fig. 2.3-13C and D). In an isotonic contraction, this component gets folded up. It also offers some resistance to passive stretch.

The SEC and PEC combinedly form 40% (2/5th) of total muscle proteins.

Concepts about Muscle Length

The following concepts about muscle length will be useful in understanding certain characteristics about muscle contraction:

- ***Optimum length*** refers to that length of the muscle at which it will develop *maximum active tension.*
- ***Resting length*** of a muscle represents the length of the muscle during relaxed state under natural conditions in the body. The resting length of many muscles in the body is optimum length.
- ***Equilibrium length*** refers to the length of a relaxed muscle cut free from its bony attachments.
- ***Initial length*** is the length of the muscle before it contracts.

Motor Unit

Motor unit is the functional unit of muscle contraction in the intact body. It consists of the single motor neuron cell body, its axon fibres, and the muscle fibres innervated by it (Fig. 2.3-14). The cell bodies of the motor neurons (α motor neuron) supplying the skeletal muscle fibres lie in the ventral horn of the spinal cord or the motor cranial nerve nuclei.

Characteristic Features of Motor Unit

Innervation Ratio. The number of muscle fibres supplied by single neuron constitutes the innervation ratio or

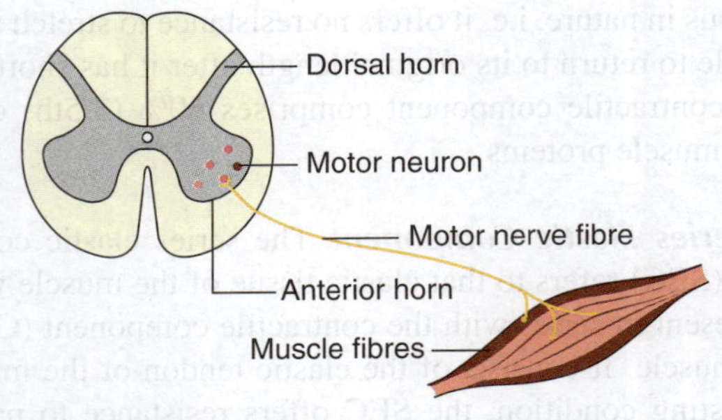

FIGURE 2.3-14 Structure of a motor unit.

the size of the motor unit. The innervation ratio of a motor unit varies with the precision of the movement to be produced by the muscle supplied. For example, in extraocular muscles (concerned with the eye movements) and hand muscles (for fine movements) the innervation ratio is only 3–6 muscle fibres per motor unit. Whereas in gastrocnemius muscle and in muscles of the back (concerned with posture maintenance), the innervation ratio is up to 2000 muscle fibres per motor unit.

Motor Neuron Pool. All the motor neurons for a given muscle make up the motor neuron pool.

Recruitment of Motor Units. The force of contraction is graded by recruitment of additional motor units (size principle). The *size principle* states that as additional motor units are recruited, more motor neurons are involved and more tension is generated.

Motor Unit Territory. The motor unit territory is the term used for the area occupied by a single motor unit in a transverse section of a muscle. For example, in biceps muscle, the motor unit territory ranges from 2 to 5 mm in diameter. The muscle fibres of each motor unit are not bunched together in the muscle, but are scattered and overlap with other motor units. In other words, there is overlapping of motor units territories (Fig. 2.3-15). The intermingling of motor fibres from different motor units results in smooth muscle movements. The importance of overlapping of motor units will be discussed later in detail.

Type of Motor Units. Each motor neuron innervates only one type of muscle fibre. In other words, in a single motor unit the muscle fibres supplied by it are of the same type. Therefore, depending on the type of muscle fibres, the (fast or slow type) motor units are also of two types:

- ***Type I*** (red or slow) motor units, and
- ***Type II*** (white or fast) motor units. The characteristic features of each type of motor units are given in Table 2.3-2.

Contractile Response

Contractile response is the characteristic feature of a skeletal muscle. When stimulated, an action potential is developed in the muscle fibres, which is followed by the muscle contraction. The muscle contraction is manifested by either

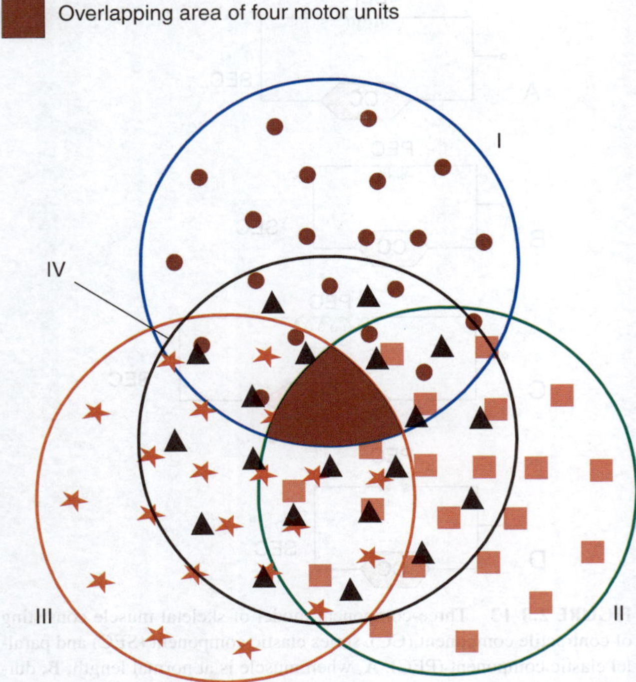

FIGURE 2.3-15 Motor unit territory of four motor units (I to IV) along with their central overlapping area seen in a schematic cross-section.

shortening (*isotonic contraction*) or development of tension (*isometric contraction*) or both. The contractile response can be studied in an *isolated nerve muscle preparation.* In experimental studies, frog's gastrocnemius-sciatic nerve preparation is used to demonstrate the different characteristics of the contractile response. The contractile response of a muscle to a single stimulus through its nerve can be recorded using a suitable lever system on kymograph or physiograph.

A typical contractile response consists of a brief contraction followed by relaxation, and is referred to as *single muscle twitch.* The contractile response of a skeletal muscle can be discussed under the following headings:

- Isometric versus isotonic contraction,
- Single muscle twitch and
- Factors affecting force of contraction.

Isometric Versus Isotonic Contraction

Isometric Contraction. As the name indicates (iso = same, metric = measure, i.e. length), in this type of contraction, the length of muscle remains same but tension is developed in the muscle. Thus, there is no movement of the object. Since work done is the product of *force* × *distance*, therefore, in isometric contraction *no external work is done.*

How the muscle length remains same in isometric contraction is depicted in Fig. 2.3-13B. As shown in this figure, the shortening produced by *contractile component (CC)* of the muscle is compensated by the stretching of the series elastic component (SEC).

TABLE 2.3-2 Characteristic Features of Type I and Type II Motor Units

Characteristics	Motor unit type I	Motor unit type II
1. Muscle fibre type:	The muscle fibres of type I motor unit are: slow, red and involved in tonic activity	The muscle fibres of type II motor units are: fast, white and involved in phasic activity
2. Motor unit innervation ratio:	High (120–160 muscle fibres/axon), e.g. postural muscles	Low (<6 muscle fibres/axon), e.g. extraocular muscles
3. Metabolism	Aerobic, low glycolytic and high oxidative capacity	Anaerobic, high glycolytic and low oxidative capacity.
• Mitochondria number	High	Low
• Glycogen contents	Low	High
• Capillary density	High	Low
• Blood supply	High	Normal
• Myoglobin content	High	Low
• Enzymes: NADH dehydrogenase	High	Low
Phosphorylase activity	Low	High
Myosin ATPase activity	Low	High
4. Axon diameter	Small	Large
5. Axon conduction velocity	Slow	Fast
6. Twitch duration of the muscle	Long	Brief
7. Tetanic tension	Small	Large
8. Type of movements	These are adapted for tonic contraction, i.e. for posture maintenance and are first to be recruited during muscle contraction	These are adapted for phasic contractions, e.g. fine and skilled movements, and these remain inactive during contraction and are recruited only when brief and powerful contraction is required
9. Fatiguability	Fatigue resistant	Easily fatiguable
10. Further types	–	Type II motor units are further of four types: IIa, IIb, IIc and IIm. IIa: are fast, fatigue resistant and glycolytic. IIb: are fast, fatiguable and glycolytic. IIc: contain muscle fibres found in fetal stage. IIm: are superfast, having unique myosin structure and present mainly in the jaw muscles.

Examples of Isometric Contraction of Muscles

- Contraction of muscles which help in maintaining posture against gravity, and
- Contraction of arm muscles when trying to push a wall.

Isotonic Contraction. As the name indicates (iso = same, and tonic = tone or tension), in this type of contraction, the tension in the muscle remains same whereas its length decreases. Since the muscle length is shortened, so the *external work is done* in isotonic contraction. As shown in Fig. 2.3-13D, in isotonic contraction, the contractile component (CC) and parallel elastic component (PEC) are shortened, but the series elastic component (SEC) does not stretch further, producing a visible shortening of the muscle.

Examples of Isotonic Muscle Contraction

- Contraction of leg muscles during walking and running,
- Contractions of muscles while lifting a weight and
- Contraction of muscles during flexion of arm.

Single Muscle Twitch

As mentioned earlier, the single muscle twitch or also known as the simple muscle twitch refers to the typical contractile response of a skeletal muscle to the single stimulus.

Recording of Single Muscle Twitch. For experimental demonstration, the single muscle twitch is recorded using frog's *gastrocnemius-sciatic nerve preparation.* Ideally, the single muscle twitch should be recorded in isotonic conditions. Technically speaking, to get a perfect isotonic contraction is impossible, but practically near isotonic contraction can be recorded by using a very light isotonic lever. Fig. 2.3-16 shows the arrangement for recording the isotonic contraction. In this, one end of the muscle is tied and the other end is kept free to allow shortening and is connected to the isotonic lever which is moved easily by the muscle.

Phases of Single Muscle Twitch. A single muscle twitch recorded under isotonic conditions from a frog's gastrocnemius-sciatic preparation. It shows (Fig. 2.3-17):

- *Point of stimulation (PS)* denotes the time when the stimulus is applied,
- *Point of contraction (PC)* refers to the starting point of muscle contraction,
- *Point of maximum contraction (PMC)* denotes the highest point of muscle contraction and
- *Point of maximum relaxation (PMR)* refers to the point where relaxation is completed.

The total duration of the muscle twitch is 0.1 s and it shows three phases: latent period, contraction phase and relaxation phase.

1. Latent Period (LP). As shown in Fig. 2.3-17, the contraction occurs after a brief gap of stimulation. This time interval of 0.01 s between the point of stimulation (PS) and the point of start of contraction (PC) is called the latent period.

The latent period includes:

- Time taken by the impulse to travel from point of stimulation on the nerve to the neuromuscular junction,
- Time taken by the impulse for neuromuscular transmission,
- Time taken by excitation–contraction coupling phenomenon,
- Time taken by chemical events to cause muscle contraction (sliding phenomenon),
- Time taken for development of tension in the muscle and
- Time taken by inertia of recording lever.

Factors Affecting Latent Period

- Latent period is longer when the distance between the point of stimulation on nerve and the neuromuscular junction is more and vice versa.
- Latent period is more if the load on muscle is heavier.
- It decreases with increase in temperature and vice versa.

2. Contraction Phase (CP). Contraction phase of about 0.04 s extends from the point of start of contraction (PC) to the point of maximum contraction (PMC) and is recorded as upward movement of the lever. During this phase, the muscle shortens by about 20% of its resting length. The magnitude of contraction is affected by many factors (see factors affecting force of contraction at page 97).

3. Relaxation Phase. The contraction phase is followed by the relaxation phase of about 0.05 s during which the muscle is stretched back to its original length by the deadweight suspended from the recording lever. It is recorded as downward movement of the recording lever system. The relaxation period is prolonged when the dead-weight is lighter. In general, the relaxation phase is longer than the contraction phase.

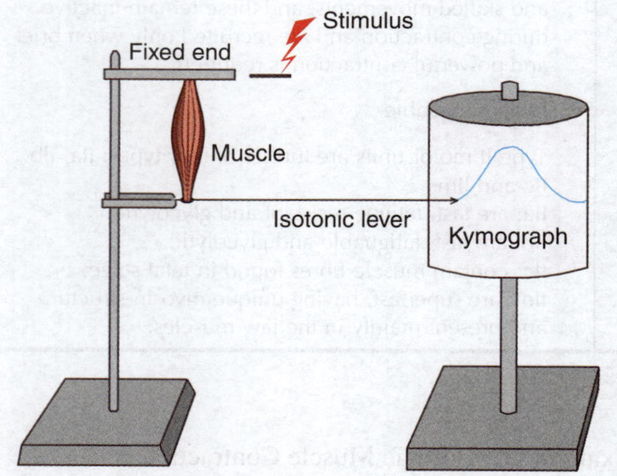

FIGURE 2.3-16 Arrangement for recording isotonic contraction.

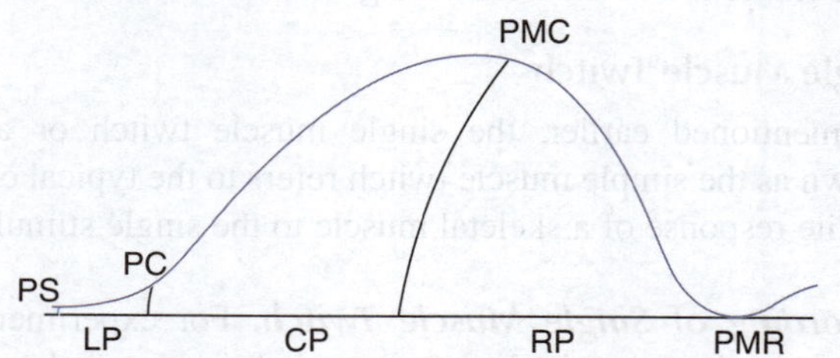

FIGURE 2.3-17 Typical single muscle curve recorded from frog's gastrocnemius-sciatic nerve preparation. PS: point of stimulation, PC: point of contraction, PMC: point of maximum contraction, PMR: point of maximum relaxation, CP: contraction period and RP: relaxation period.

Duration of twitch. The total duration of twitch (*contraction time*) varies with the *type of muscle fibres:*

- *Fast (white) muscle fibres* (e.g. extraocular muscles and muscle of hands for fine movements) have shorter contraction time (about 0.025 s).
- *Slow (red) muscle fibres* (e.g. back muscles) have longer contraction time (0.1 s).

The total duration of twitch also varies from species to species. In human skeletal muscle, the duration of twitch is 30–50 ms in comparison to 100 ms in frog's (amphibian's) muscle.

Relation between Electrical and Mechanical Events of Single Muscle Twitch. Fig. 2.3-18 shows the electrical events (action potential) and mechanical response (simple muscle twitch curve) plotted on the same time scale after

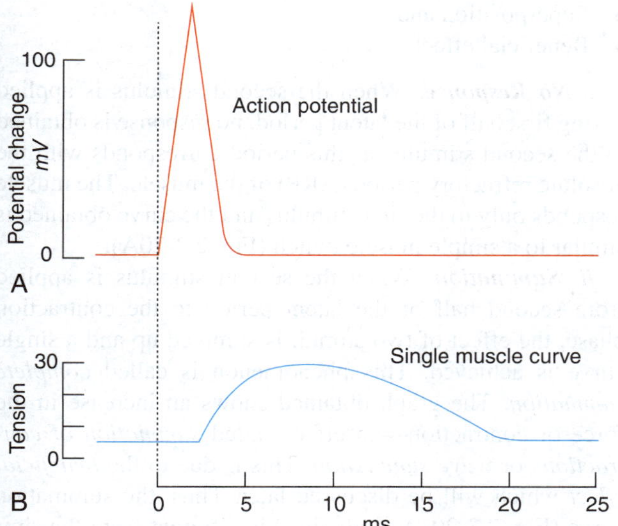

FIGURE 2.3-18 Electrical (**A**) and mechanical (**B**) responses of mammalian skeletal muscle fibre to a single maximum stimulus plotted on same time scale.

being recorded separately. From this relationship graph, it can be concluded that:

- The twitch starts about 2 ms after the start of depolarization of the membrane but always before the repolarization is completed, and that
- The refractory period (absolute refractory period) is very short and lies in the first half of the latent period of the single muscle twitch.

Factors Affecting Contractile Response

The factors that can affect the contractile response (force of contraction) of a skeletal muscle are:

- Strength of stimulus,
- Frequency of stimulus,
- Load on the muscle (preload and after-load),
- Initial length of muscle and
- Temperature.

Strength of Stimulus.

A Single Muscle Fibre obeys the all or none law, i.e.

- A subthreshold stimulus evokes no response, and
- With threshold, maximal and supramaximal stimuli the contractile response remains constant.

The Whole Muscle, however, when stimulated with different intensity stimuli the response obtained (force of contraction) is a graded one. This fact can be well demonstrated in an isolated nerve muscle preparation.

In the Isolated Nerve-Muscle Preparation. The graded response is obtained when stimuli of different intensities were applied through the nerve in a nerve-muscle preparation (Fig. 2.3-19). The whole muscle responds to the stimuli as:

- *Subthreshold stimuli* do not evoke any response.
- *Threshold stimulus,* i.e. a stimulus just sufficient to elicit response and produces minimal contraction.
- *Suprathreshold stimuli* produce a graded response (i.e. the force of contraction goes on increasing with the increase in strength of stimulus till a maximum limit

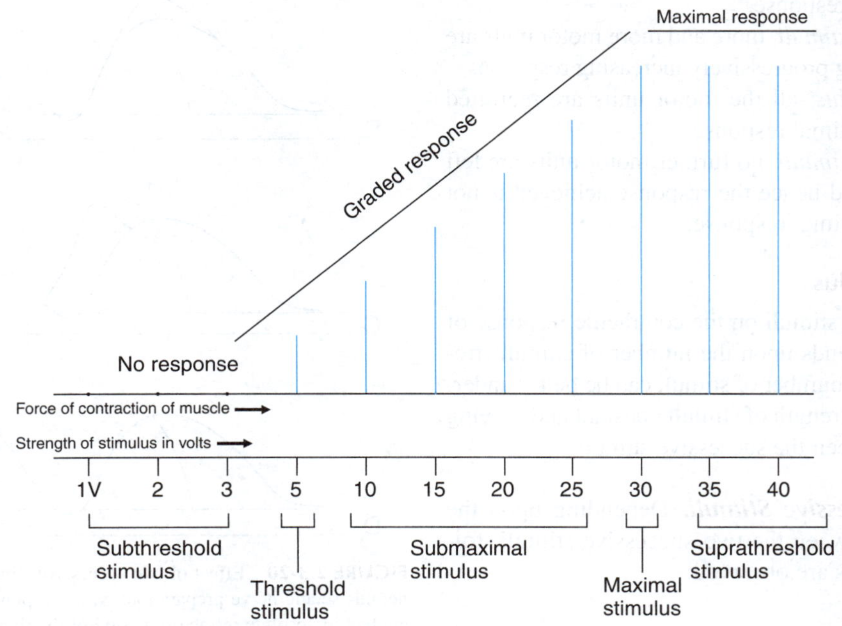

FIGURE 2.3-19 Effect of strength (intensity) of stimulus on an isolated nerve muscle preparation of frog.

is reached). This is because, as the strength of stimuli is increased, more and more muscle fibres are recruited into activity. This phenomenon is called *quantal* or *multi fibre summation.* The graded response achieved by suprathreshold stimuli is called *submaximal response.*

- *Maximal stimulus* is that stimulus which produces the maximal response (i.e. the maximal stimulus excites all the motor units).
- *Supramaximal stimulus* refers to the stimulus which exceeds the maximal value. Supramaximal stimuli do not increase the response beyond the maximal response. This is because, at the maximal stimulus, all the motor units are already contracting to their maximum extent and thus any further increase in the strength of stimuli (supramaximal stimulus) has no effect in increasing the force of contraction.

In the Intact Body. In the intact body, the whole muscle gets stimulus from the activity of anterior horn cells through their axons to the muscle fibres supplied by that particular neuron, i.e. by *recruitment of motor units.* With minimum activity, only a few motor units are recruited for activity. With increasing activity, more and more motor units (from the motor neuron pool of a muscle) are recruited into activity. This phenomenon is called *multiple motor unit summation.*

Thus, in an intact body, the relationship between the number of motor units recruited and the mechanical response achieved in terms of type of stimulus can be interpreted as below:

- *At subthreshold stimulus*, no motor units are recruited and hence no response is achieved.
- *At threshold stimulus*, the minimum number of motor units (say 1 or 2) are recruited which are just sufficient to excite minimal response.
- *At suprathreshold stimuli,* more and more motor units are recruited producing progressively increasing response.
- *At maximal stimulus,* all the motor units are recruited producing the maximal response.
- *At supramaximal stimuli,* no further motor units are left to be recruited, and hence the response achieved is not more than the maximal response.

Frequency of Stimulus

The effect of repeated stimuli on the contractile response of a skeletal muscle depends upon the number of stimuli (frequency). The effect of number of stimuli can be better understood by keeping the strength of stimuli constant and varying the time interval between the successive stimuli.

Effect of Two Successive Stimuli. Depending upon the length of interval between the two successive stimuli, following types of effects are observed:

- No response,
- Summation,
- Superposition and
- Beneficial effect.

i. No Response. When the second stimulus is applied during first half of the latent period, no response is obtained to the second stimulus as this period corresponds with the absolute refractory period (ARP) of the muscle. The muscle responds only to the first stimulus and the curve obtained is similar to a simple muscle twitch (Fig. 2.3-20A).

ii. Summation. When the second stimulus is applied from second half of the latent period to the contraction phase, the effect of two stimuli is summed up and a single curve is achieved. This phenomenon is called *complete summation.* The graph obtained shows an increase in the force of contraction—an effect called *summation of contractions* or *wave summation.* This is due to the *beneficial effect* which will be discussed later. Thus, the summation curve (Fig. 2.3-20B) so obtained is different from the simple muscle curve by having:

- A greater amplitude, and
- A broader base.

iii. Superposition. When the second stimulus is applied during relaxation phase of the curve due to first stimulus, the relaxation phase is cut short and another contraction occurs. The second curve is superimposed over

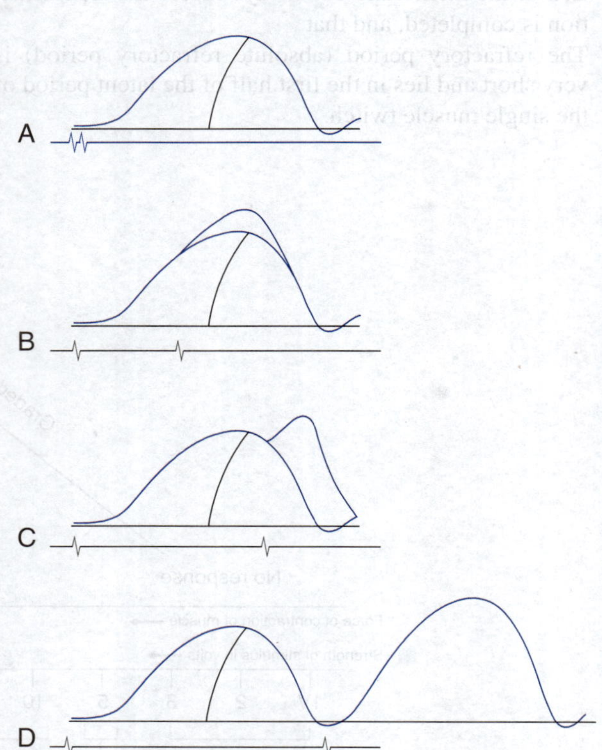

FIGURE 2.3-20 Effect of two successive stimuli in an isolated gastrocnemius-sciatic nerve preparation: **A,** no response (when second stimulus applied in absolute refractory period of the first response); **B,** summation effect; **C,** superposition (incomplete summation); and **D,** beneficial effect.

the first curve (Fig. 2.3-20C). This is called phenomenon of *superposition* or *incomplete summation* of waves. The amplitude of the second curve is more than that of the first curve. This is also due to the beneficial effect, which is explained below.

iv. Two separate curves with beneficial effect. When the second stimulus is applied soon after the relaxation phase of the curve due to first stimulus, another complete curve is obtained. However, the force of second contraction is greater than that of the first contraction (Fig. 2.3-20D). The increase in the force of contraction of second curve is due to the beneficial effect.

Beneficial Effect and its Causes. As discussed above, when second stimulus is applied at any stage after the first half of the latent period (i.e. at any time after the absolute refractory period), the force of second contraction is more than that of the first one. In other words, the contraction produced by first stimulus proves beneficial for the second one. This is called *beneficial effect.*

Causes. of beneficial effect are:

- Some of the *calcium ions* released from the terminal cisterns into the sarcoplasm during first contraction are also available in addition to those released by the second stimulus when the two stimuli are applied successively. These additional Ca^{2+} ions increase the duration of active state of second stimulus. The prolonged active state in turn increases the amount of stretch on the series elastic component of the muscle and so more force is transmitted to the recording lever (or to the bones in the intact body), thus increasing the height of the curve.
- *Viscosity of the muscle* and thus the elastic inertia of the muscle is decreased to some extent by the first contraction, which contributes to the beneficial effect for the second contraction.
- *Increase in H^+* ion concentration due to the first contraction also adds to the beneficial effect for the second contraction.
- *Increase in the temperature* due to first contraction decreases the viscosity of the muscle and thus contributes to the beneficial effect.

Effect of Multiple Stimuli. The effect of multiple successive stimuli on the contractile response of a skeletal muscle depends upon the total duration of twitch and the frequency of stimuli. The basic principle that governs the effect of multiple stimuli is the same that explains the effect of two successive stimuli. That is the response obtained will depend upon whether the next stimulus falls:

- After the first twitch, or
- On relaxation phase of first twitch or
- On contraction phase or to second half of latent period of first twitch.

Based on the above facts, following types of responses are observed due to multiple stimuli:

- Discrete responses,
- Incomplete tetanus and
- Complete tetanus.

i. Discrete Responses. If the frequency of stimulation is such that the next successive stimulus falls after completion of relaxation phase of the previous twitch, then the succeeding contractions obtained, with brief intervals between them, are complete individual twitches (with contraction and relaxation phases). Such a response is called a *discrete response.* Further, each successive twitch has increased force of contraction (due to beneficial effect of previous twitch) till a maximal beneficial effect is achieved (Fig. 2.3-21A). This phenomenon is called the *staircase effect* or *treppe* (a German word for staircase).

Thus, if the total duration of a twitch is 100 ms, then frequencies less than 10/s (i.e. each stimulus coming after every 100 ms) will produce discrete responses with a staircase effect.

ii. Incomplete Tetanus or Clonus. When the frequency of multiple stimuli is such that the next successive stimulus falls on the relaxation phase of the previous twitch, then the succeeding contraction obtained will be superposed over the previous twitch due to incomplete summation of waves. The record so obtained shows a progressive increase in amplitude up to a certain level beyond which there is no further increase. This phenomenon, as already mentioned, is called *staircase effect* or *treppe*. On stoppage of stimulation, the lever returns to normal (Fig. 2.3-21B). The series of jerky contractions of the muscle, with period of incomplete relaxation in between, so obtained is referred to as state of *subtetanus* or *incomplete tetanus* or *clonus.*

Thus, when the total duration of a twitch is 100 ms, then frequencies between 10 and 20/s (i.e. each stimulus coming after every 50 ms but before 100 ms) will fall on the relaxation phase of previous twitch and produce incomplete tetanus.

iii. Complete Tetanus. When the frequency of multiple stimuli is such that the next successive stimulus falls in the second half of latent period to the contraction phase of the previous twitch (i.e. before relaxation begins), then due to complete summation effect, the muscle will remain in a state of sustained, smooth and forceful contraction called *tetanus* or tetanic contraction (Fig. 2.3-21C). The graph shows an increasing slope of the uninterrupted tracing, which exceeds the peaks of single twitches. When the stimulation is stopped, the muscle relaxes immediately. However, if the stimulation is continued further, a plateau is maintained until the muscle begins to fatigue, after which it relaxes gradually. During complete tetanus, the tension developed in the muscle is four times greater than that developed during the individual muscle twitch.

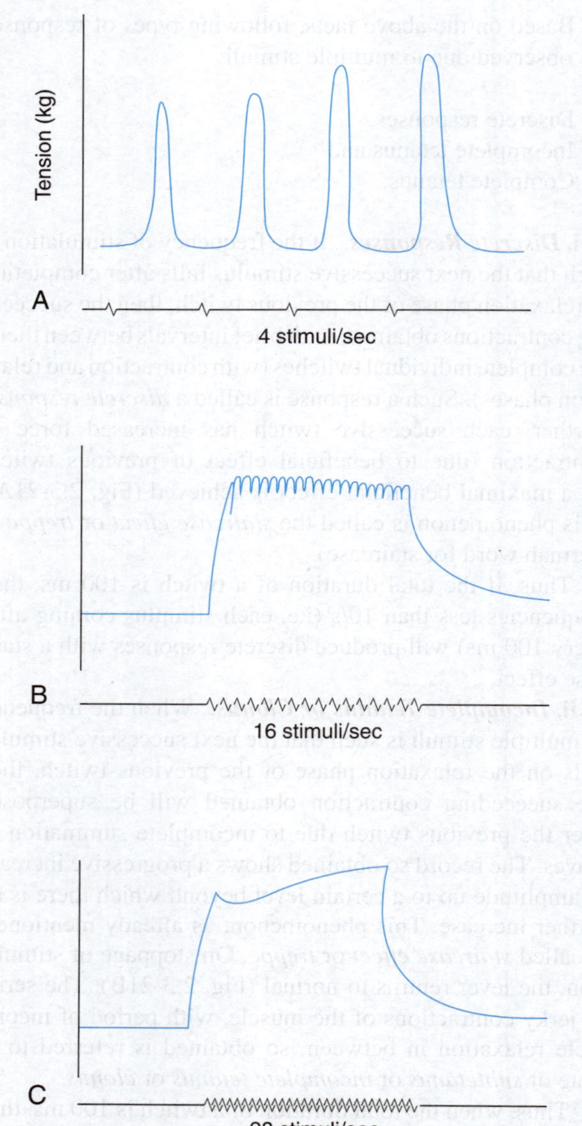

FIGURE 2.3-21 Effect of multiple stimuli in an isolated gastrocnemius-sciatic nerve preparation: **A,** discrete responses; **B,** incomplete tetanus (clonus); and C, complete tetanus (sustained contraction).

Thus, when the total duration of twitch is 100 ms, then frequencies more than 20/s (i.e. each stimulus coming before 50 ms) will fall on the contraction phase of previous twitch and produce complete tetanus. The rate of stimulation at which there is complete fusion of individual contraction to produce tetanus is called the *tetanizing* or *fusion* frequency.

Ionic Basis of Tetanus. The Ca^{2+} ions released in sarcoplasm during single twitch are removed quickly and relaxation occurs. When the muscle is stimulated in rapid succession, there occurs a progressive accumulation of Ca^{2+} ions in the sarcoplasm. The longer stay of Ca^{2+} ions in the sarcoplasm increases the duration of active state (due to continuous recycling of myosin heads). This increases the amount of stretch on the series elastic component (SEC) and the tension developed rises to tetanic levels.

Effect of Load

Load is the force exerted by the weight of an object on the muscle. The force exerted by the contracting muscle on the object is known as *muscle tension.* Thus, muscle load and muscle tension are two opposing forces. The load acting on the muscle is of two types: free-load (or preload) and after-load.

Effect of Free-Load. A load that starts acting on a muscle before it starts to contract is called free-load (or preload). Example of a free-load on the muscles in an intact body is filling water from a tap by holding a bucket in the hand. The free-load increases the force of contraction and work efficiency of the muscle. The free-load stretches the muscle passively producing a *passive tension* across the muscle. This passive tension increases the force of muscle contraction in two ways:

- By increasing the initial length of the muscle to its resting length at which maximum force is generated, and
- By adding an elastic recoil force to the muscle during its contraction.

Effect of Initial Length on Force of Contraction. According to Starling's law, the force of contraction is a function of the initial length of muscle fibres. Therefore, up to physiological limits, the greater the initial length, greater is the force of contraction.

Length–tension Relationship. When a muscle is removed from the body, it shortens because muscles in the body are in a state of slight stretch. The length of the muscle when it is detached from its bony attachments is called *equilibrium length.*

The *length–tension relationship graph* can be plotted by measuring isometric tension at different muscle lengths in an isolated muscle preparation. For this, the isolated muscle is attached to an *isometric lever,* which does not allow the shortening of muscle to occur. The tension developed is recorded through the force transducer (Fig. 2.3-22). The length of the muscle is varied by changing the distance between its two attachments and the recording is made as:

- First, at each length, the *passive tension* is measured. The passive tension is due to stretching of parallel and series elastic components of the muscle (PEC and SEC).
- The muscle is then electrically stimulated at each length and the tension developed is recorded. The *total tension* so recorded includes both the passive tension and the active tension developed due to contraction of the contractile component (CC) of the muscle.
- The *active tension* is thus denoted by the difference between the total tension and passive tension at any length.

Length–tension relationship graph is then plotted with increase in muscle length (in cm) along horizontal axis and

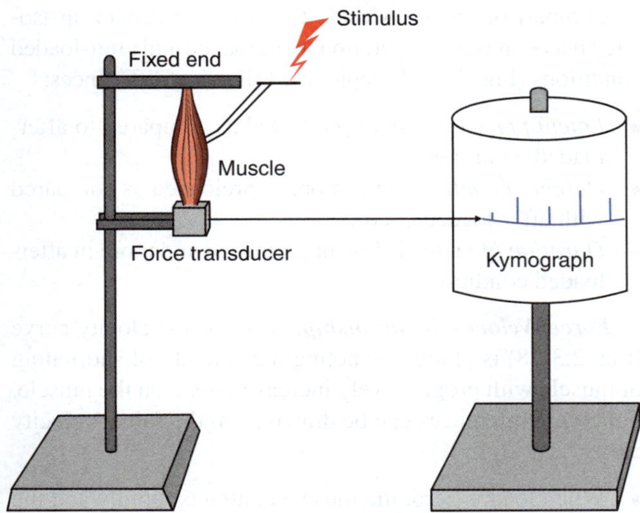

FIGURE 2.3-22 Arrangement for recording isometric contraction in an isolated nerve-muscle preparation.

tension (in kg) along the vertical axis (Fig. 2.3-23). The following inferences can be drawn from this graph:

- *Passive tension* due to elastic components (PEC and SEC) of the muscle increases with the passively increased muscle length.
- *Active tension* developed is maximum at the *optimum length* of the muscle (position B in Fig. 2.3-23) which is equivalent to the *resting length* in intact body.
- *Total tension* is contributed by active tension and passive tension at different muscle lengths as below:
  - At muscle length less than optimal level, the total tension is mainly due to active tension (position A in Fig. 2.3-23). Because at such a lower initial length there is no stretch on the muscle and so passive tension fails to develop.
  - At a muscle length twice the optimal length, the total tension is mainly due to passive tension (position D in Fig. 2.3-23). Because at this muscle length the contractile tissue cannot contract and so the active tension is at zero level.
  - At a muscle length one and a half times the optimal length, the total tension is equally contributed by the active and passive tension (position C in Fig. 2.3-23).

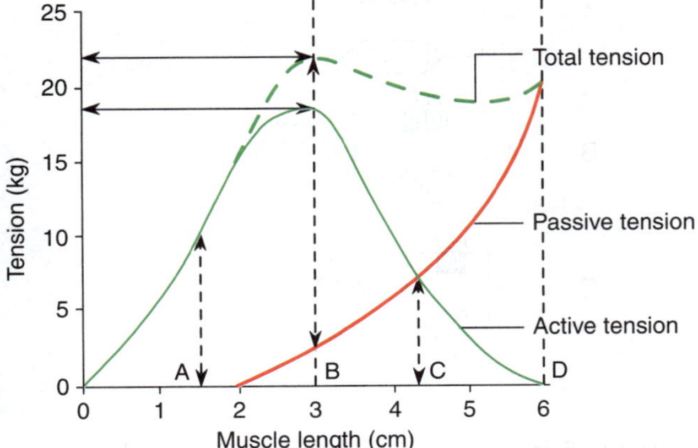

FIGURE 2.3-23 Length–tension relationship graph.

Molecular Basis of Length–Tension Relationship. During isometric contraction, the tension developed in the muscle is proportional to the cross-bridges formed between actin and myosin filaments. The effect of muscle length on the tension produced during contraction can be explained by the sliding filament theory of muscle contraction as:

- *At optimum length* (position B in Fig. 2.3-24), there is optimum overlapping between the actin and myosin filaments, so maximum cross-bridges are formed between them.
- *At muscle length shorter than optimum* length (at position A in Fig. 2.3-24), the thin filaments overlap each other and thus reduce the cross-bridges between actin and myosin filaments and so the active tension produced is less.
- *When the muscle is overstretched* (position C in Fig. 2.3-24), the Z lines are pulled apart and the overlapping between the actin and myosin filaments is markedly reduced and so no active tension is developed at this level.

Effect of After-Load. After-load refers to the load which acts on the muscle after the beginning of muscular contraction. Thus, the after-load opposes the force produced by muscle contraction. The work done in an after-loaded muscle is less than that of a free-loaded muscle. An example of after-load in an intact body is lifting any object from the ground. The load acts on the muscles of arm only after

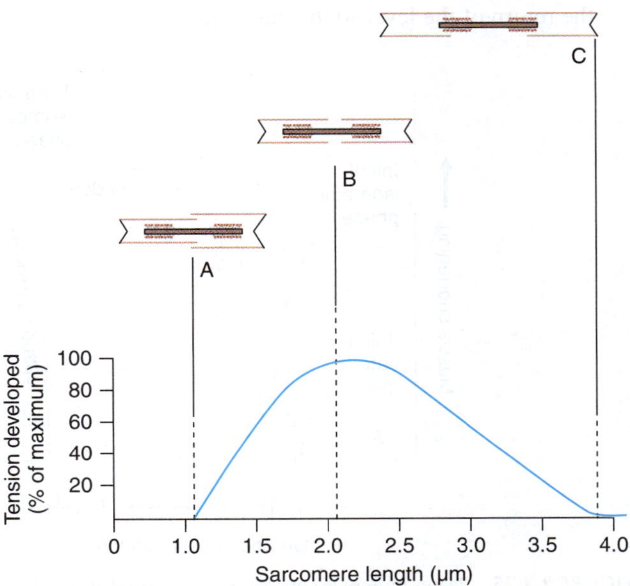

FIGURE 2.3-24 Molecular basis of length–tension relationship.

lifting the object off the ground, i.e. only after beginning of the muscular contraction.

Phases of Muscle Contraction with After-load. *Experimentally,* the effect of after-load can be studied by subjecting the muscle to *after-load preparation;* when a muscle contracts against a load it shows three phases:

i. *Initial isometric contraction phase.* In this phase of muscular contraction, as the name indicates, there occurs no shortening of the muscle. The contraction of contractile components (CC) stretches the series elastic component (SEC) and there occurs a rise in the tension (Fig. 2.3-25B). The rise in tension continues till it equals the load. This is the end point of isometric phase.
ii. *Intermediate isotonic contraction phase* starts when the muscle tension exceeds the load and load starts moving. There occurs shortening of the muscle without further stretching of SEC (Fig. 2.3-25C).
iii. *Terminal isometric phase.* After the muscle becomes shorter than the resting length, any further shortening is associated with a decrease in the tension. And, when the tension generated equals the load, the muscle once again starts contracting isometrically.

Effect of Increasing Load in after-loaded Condition. Fig. 2.3-26 is the graph depicting effect of progressively increasing weight in after-loaded muscle preparation. It shows that:

- As the load increases, the latent period increases due to lever inertia.
- The amplitude of contraction decreases progressively as the muscle has to lift greater load.
- Contraction period decreases due to decrease in the duration of active state.
- Relaxation period also decreases, since the load hastens the return of the lever to the baseline.

Comparison of the Muscle Curves recorded in an isolated nerve-muscle preparation in preloaded and after-loaded conditions (Fig. 2.3-27) depict the following differences:

- *Latent period* is less in preloaded as compared to after-loaded condition.
- *Height of contraction* is more in preloaded as compared with after-loaded curve.
- *Duration of twitch* is less in preloaded and more in after-loaded condition.

Force–Velocity Relationship. The force–velocity curve (Fig. 2.3-28) is plotted by noting the velocity of shortening of muscle with progressively increasing load on the muscle. Following inferences can be drawn from the force–velocity curve:

- When load is zero, the muscle contracts rapidly and the velocity of muscle shortening is maximum (V_{max}).
- As the load increases, the velocity of shortening decreases. With further increase in the load, a stage comes when the muscle is unable to lift the load. At this point, the muscle contracts isometrically.
- Between the two extremes of zero load and immovable load, all contractions have variable durations of isometric and isotonic contractions.
- In the force–velocity curve, mt is the point of maximum efficiency of the muscle. It lies about 1/3rd of the abscissa and 1/3rd from the ordinate.

Calculation of Work Done by Muscle

The work done by the muscle is calculated in both the free-loaded and after-loaded contractions, utilizing the following data (Fig. 2.3-29A):

- Height of the muscle contraction curve for each weight (*H*),
- Length of long arm of the lever between fulcrum and the writing point (*L*),

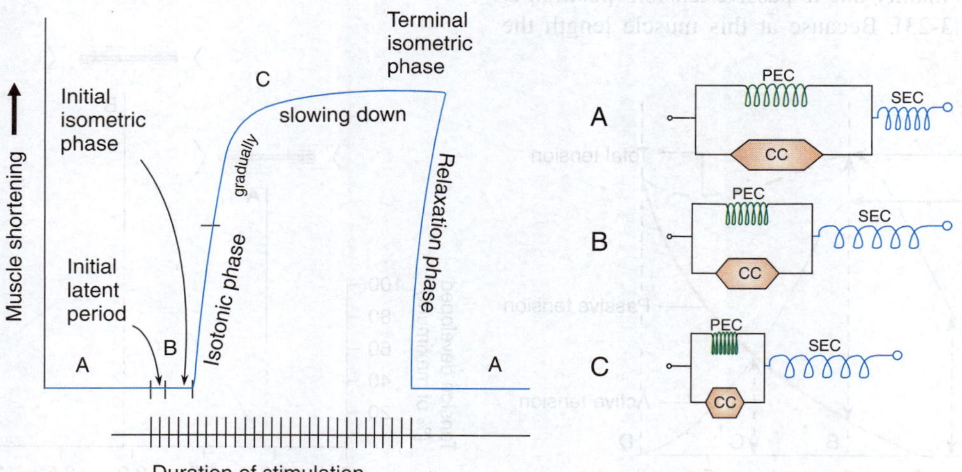

FIGURE 2.3-25 Phases of muscle contraction in after-loaded condition: **A,** resting state; **B,** initial isometric contraction; and **C,** intermediate isotonic contraction which gradually slows down and tension decreases and becomes equal to load and no further shortening (terminal isometric phase).

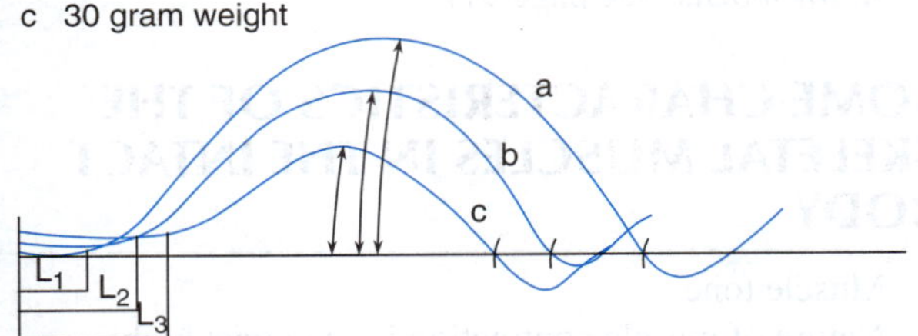

FIGURE 2.3-26 Effect of increasing load in after-loaded condition in an isolated muscle-nerve preparation.

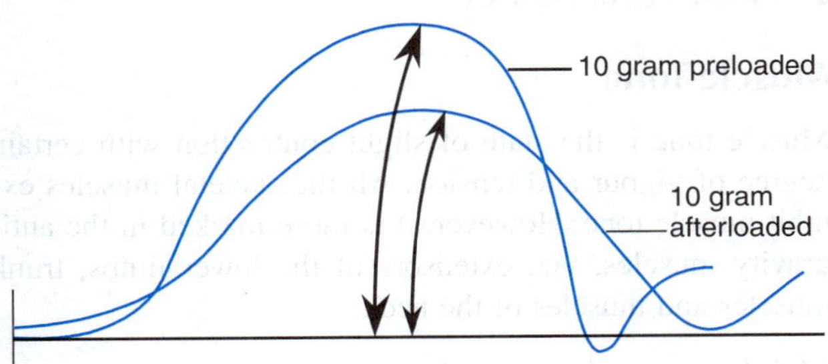

FIGURE 2.3-27 Comparison of muscle curves recorded during pre-loaded and after-loaded conditions using 10 g weight.

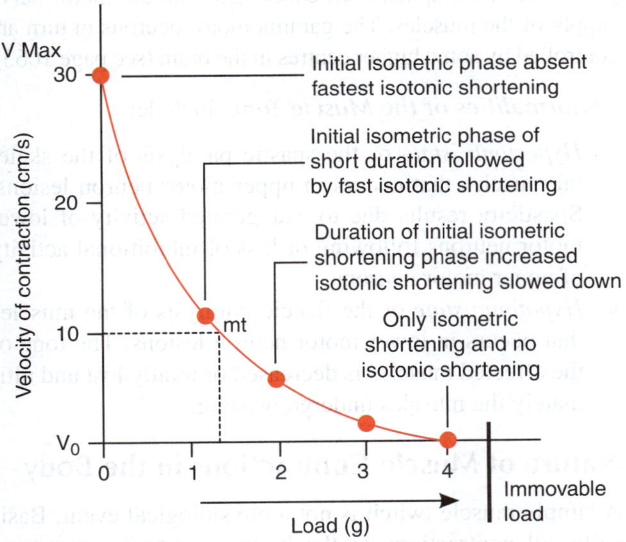

FIGURE 2.3-28 Force–velocity curve plotted by recording velocity of shortening of skeletal muscle with progressively increasing load.

- Length of short arm of the lever between fulcrum and point where weight is added (l) and
- Actual height up to which the weight is lifted (h).

Calculations

- Actual height (h) is calculated taking into consideration the magnification factor (which is equal to L/l):

$$\frac{h}{H} = \frac{1}{L}, h = H \times \frac{1}{L}$$

Work done is then calculated as:
Work done $W = w$ (weight in g) $\times$ h (actual height in cm)

$$W\ (gm/cm) = w \times \frac{1}{L} \times H$$

- To express the work done in ergs, the above reading is multiplied by 981.
- A graph is then plotted, indicating the weight on the abscissa and the work done on the ordinate (Fig. 2.3-29B).

Effect of Temperature

The contractile response is altered due to the effect of temperature. The effect of temperature can be studied by changing the temperature of the Ringer's solution in which muscle-nerve preparation is immersed. The effect of temperature noted on the amplitude of contraction, and its various periods is given below:

At room Temperature, a normal simple muscle is recorded as shown in Fig. 2.3-30A.

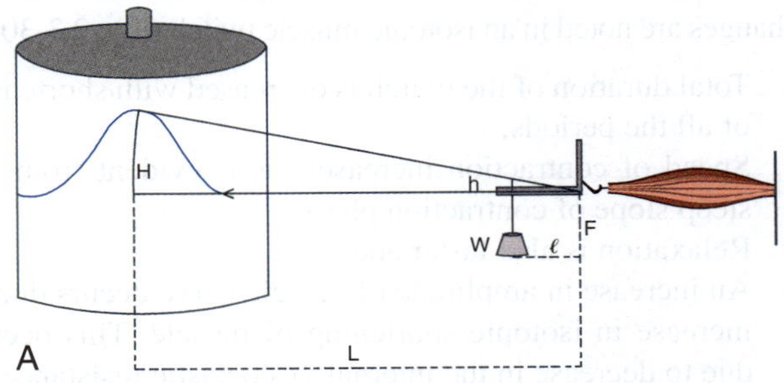

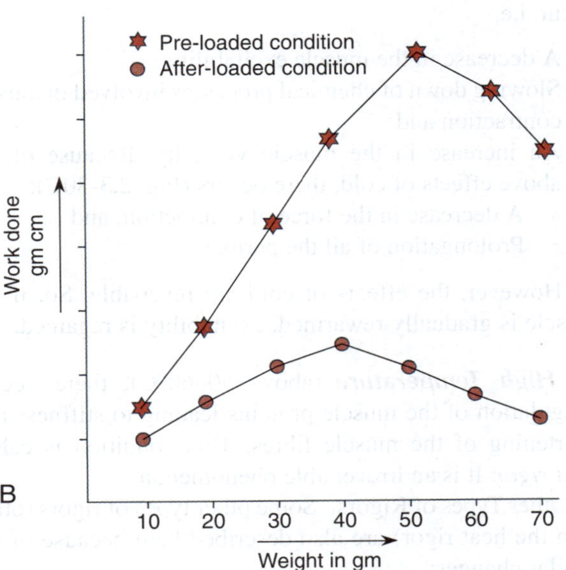

FIGURE 2.3-29 Work done by the muscle: **A,** calculation of work done by finding actual height of contraction; and **B,** graphical representation of work done by the muscle in preloaded and after-loaded conditions.

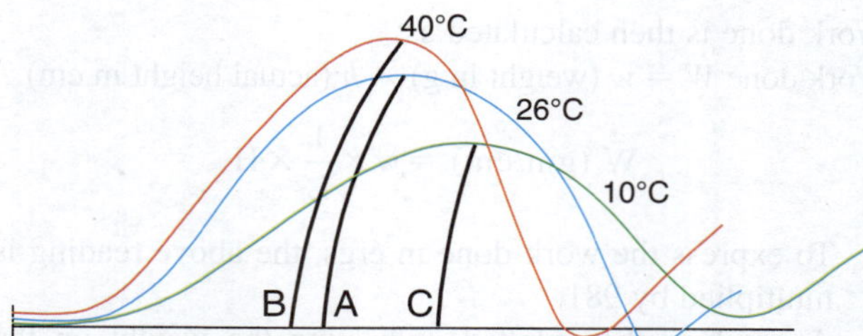

FIGURE 2.3-30 Effect of temperature in an isolated nerve-muscle preparation: A, at room temperature (26°C); B, at moderately high temperature (40°C); and C, at cold temperature (10°C).

At Moderately High Temperature (say 40°C), there occurs:

- Faster diffusion of Ca^{2+} ions from sarcoplasmic reticulum to sarcoplasm leading to:
  - An increase in the muscle excitability,
  - Acceleration of the chemical processes involved in muscle contraction and
- A decrease in muscle viscosity.

Because of the above effects of temperature, the following changes are noted in an isotonic muscle twitch (Fig. 2.3-30B):

- Total duration of the twitch is decreased with shortening of all the periods,
- Speed of contraction increases, as is evident from the steep slope of contraction phase,
- Relaxation is also faster and
- An increase in amplitude of muscle curve occurs due to increase in isotonic shortening of muscle. This occurs due to decrease in the internal viscoelastic resistance.

At Low Temperature (say 5–10°C), the reverse changes occur, i.e.

- A decrease in the muscle excitability,
- Slowing down of chemical processes involved in muscle contraction and
- An increase in the muscle viscosity. Because of the above effects of cold, there occurs (Fig. 2.3-30C):
  - A decrease in the force of contraction, and
  - Prolongation of all the periods.

However, the effects of cold are reversible. So, if the muscle is gradually rewarmed, excitability is regained.

At High Temperature (above 50–60°C), there occurs coagulation of the muscle proteins leading to stiffness and shortening of the muscle fibres. This condition is called *heat rigor.* It is an irreversible phenomenon.

Other Types of Rigors. Some other types of rigors (other than the heat rigor) are also described here because of the similar changes:

- *Cold rigor.* It occurs following exposure to severe cold. It is a reversible phenomenon.
- *Calcium rigor.* It occurs due to increased calcium content. It is also a reversible phenomenon.
- *Rigor mortis* (see page 91).

SOME CHARACTERISTICS OF THE SKELETAL MUSCLES IN THE INTACT BODY

- Muscle tone
- Nature of muscle contraction in the intact body
- Gradation of muscular activity
- Muscle fatigue
- Mechanics of muscles

Muscle Tone

Muscle tone is the state of slight contraction with certain degree of vigour and tension. All the skeletal muscles exhibit muscle tone. However, it is more marked in the antigravity muscles, viz. extensors of the lower limbs, trunk muscles and muscles of the neck.

Maintenance of Muscle Tone. Muscle tone is a state of partial tetanus of the muscle maintained by asynchronous discharge of impulses from gamma motor neurons in the anterior grey horn of the spinal cord concerned with the motor nerve supply of the muscles. The gamma motor neurons in turn are controlled by some higher centres in the brain (see page 1063).

Abnormalities of the Muscle Tone include:

- *Hypertonic state* or the spastic paralysis of the skeletal muscles that occurs in upper motor neuron lesions. Spasticity results due to exaggerated activity of lower motor neurons following or loss of inhibitional activity of upper motor neurons.
- *Hypotonic state* or the flaccid paralysis of the muscles that occurs in lower motor neuron lesions. The tone of the affected muscles is decreased or totally lost and ultimately the muscles undergo wasting.

Nature of Muscle Contractions in the Body

A simple muscle twitch is not a physiological event. Basically, all contractions in the body are tetanic in nature. Weak contractions result from low frequency of firing (5–10/s) of the motor units. The expected jerkiness and the disadvantage of incomplete tetanus are overcome by the asynchronous discharge (out of step firing) of groups of motor units. When one group is firing, the others are silent, and vice versa. Algebraic summation occurs, the individual variations are evened out and a smooth contraction results. The degree to which the motor neuron discharge is asynchronous is related both to the force and duration of contraction. (In a subtetanus experiment, the muscle fibres contract and relax at the same time in response to the low-frequency stimulation). Such a situation does not occur in the body.

With increasing firing rates and, of course, with more recruitment of motor units, contractions become stronger until, at and beyond the tetanizing rate, sustained and powerful contractions result.

Gradation of Force of Muscle Contraction in the Intact Body

For performing different kinds of work, e.g. picking up a pen from the table, or lifting a 10 kg weight, same muscles are involved but in these different situations, muscles can generate different degree of power. This property of skeletal muscles is known as gradation of force of contraction. Gradation of muscle power in muscles is made possible by certain factors which affect the force of contraction. These are:

1. Recruitment of Motor Units. The force of contraction produced in a muscle depends upon the number of motor units recruited. When minimal activity is required, only a few motor units are recruited. With increasing effort, more and more motor units from the *motor neuron pool* of a muscle are recruited into activity. This phenomenon is called multiple motor unit summation.

2. Frequency of Nerve Impulses. The motor control system in the brain can vary the force of contraction by varying the frequency of nerve impulses stimulating the muscle. As the impulse frequency increases, its effects are summated (*wave summation*) and the muscle tension increases.

3. Synchronization of Impulses. At any one time, the motor units are in different phases of activity, i.e. some are contracting and others are relaxing. Due to algebraic summation, the muscle gives a steady but weak pull. With increasing synchronization of the motor units, the force of contraction increases.

4. Effect of Initial Length of Muscle Fibre. According to Starling's law, up to an optimal limit, the greater the initial length of the muscle fibres, greater is the force of contraction. This, however, is not the usual method of varying the force of contraction in the intact body.

5. Warming Up. Warming up is the term used in the parlour of sports persons for the exercises performed before actually participating in any game event. These pregame 'warm up' due to beneficial effects of the exercise increase the muscle performance when the person takes part in the actual event.

Muscle Fatigue

Failure of a muscle to maintain tension as a result of previous contractile activity is known as muscle fatigue. If the muscle is allowed to rest after the onset of fatigue it recovers its ability to contract. Muscle fatigue is discussed under two separate situations:

- Fatigue in an isolated muscle, and
- General fatigue.

Fatigue in Isolated Nerve-Muscle Preparation

In an isolated nerve-muscle preparation, when the muscle is repeatedly stimulated through its nerve, the graph (Fig. 2.3-31) obtained shows the following features:

- The first few contractions increase in amplitude due to beneficial effect.
- As stimulation is continued, there occurs a progressive increase in the latent period, and a decrease in the amplitude. The rise of tension becomes slower, relaxation becomes more gradual and incomplete, and finally the muscle fails to contract altogether, and the recording lever does not return to the base line, i.e. the muscle remains in a state of partial contraction called *contraction remainder or contracture*. This failure of response, after repeated stimuli, is called fatigue.

Site and Cause of Fatigue. The *site of fatigue,* when the muscle has undergone fatigue through stimulation of its nerve, is *neuromuscular junction,* because the muscle responds briskly on direct stimulation. The *cause of fatigue* is depletion of acetylcholine from the motor nerve endings and interference with neuromuscular transmission by substances like pyruvic and lactic acids, and breakdown products of ATP.

The repeated stimulation of muscle itself leads to actual muscle fatigue and is due to depletion of muscle glycogen.

General Fatigue

General fatigue refers to the fatigue of most of the muscles that develops after prolonged general exercise such as marathon running and competitive football match playing.

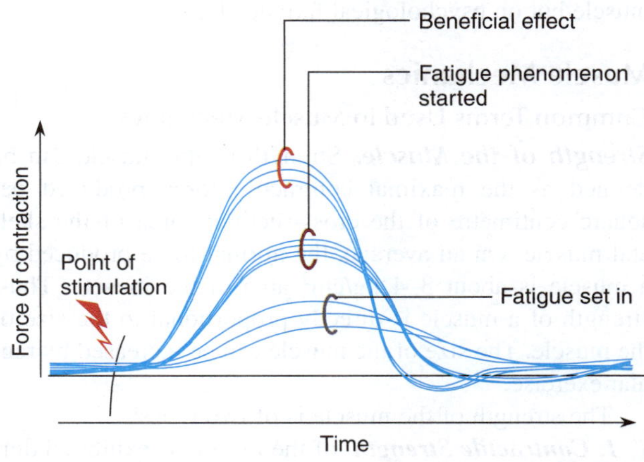

FIGURE 2.3-31 Phenomenon of fatigue in an isolated muscle-nerve preparation.

Onset and Recovery of Fatigue Depends on:

- Intensity and duration of exercise, and
- Type of muscle fibres. Fast glycolytic fibres fatigue early and also recover rapidly from fatigue. Slow oxidative fibres do not fatigue early but they also require longer time of rest (up to 24 h) for complete recovery.

Site, Causes and Mechanism of Fatigue. In the human body, the sites of fatigue are in the following order:

- Fatigue of *synapses of central nervous* system due to slight hypoxia occurs first of all. It is particularly of so high intensity in short-duration exercises.
- The second site of fatigue is *motor neurons* (anterior grey horn cells) of spinal cord.
- *Motor end plate* in the neuromuscular junction may also be fatigued.
- Changes in muscles also contribute to development of fatigue:
  - In short-duration high-intensity exercises such as weight lifting and short distance running, there occurs increased acidity in the muscle cells which accompanies rise in lactic acid (formed due to anaerobic glycolysis). H^+ ion concentration directly inhibits cross-bridge cycles and therefore force generated by them. The second cause is decrease in release of Ca^{2+} ions from the sarcoplasmic reticulum.
  - In long-duration low-intensity exercises such as marathon race, depletion of muscle glycogen is an important contributing factor.

Psychological Fatigue

Lack of motivation due to failure of cerebral cortex to send excitatory signals to motor neurons causes an individual to stop exercising. The psychological fatigue (feeling of weariness) is different from *physiological fatigue* of the muscles. The muscles are actually not fatigued (therefore, it is not a true muscle fatigue). An athlete's performance, therefore, depends not only on the physical status of appropriate muscle but on psychological fatigue also.

Muscle Mechanics

Common Terms Used in Muscle Mechanics

Strength of the Muscle. Strength of the muscle can be defined as the maximal contractile force produced per square centimetre of the cross-sectional area of the skeletal muscle. On an average, the normal force produced by a muscle is about 3–4 kg/cm^2 area of the muscle. Thus, strength of a muscle is directly proportional to the size of the muscle. The size of the muscle can be increased by regular exercise.

The strength of the muscle is of two types:

1. Contractile Strength of the muscle is exhibited during actual shortening (isotonic contraction) of the muscle. For example, the strength developed in the leg muscles during taking off the body from the ground while jumping is the contractile strength.

2. Holding Strength refers to the force produced while stretching the contracted muscles. For example, the force developed in the leg muscles while landing after jumping is the holding force. The holding strength of a muscle is greater than the contractile strength.

Power of the Muscle. Power of the muscle refers to the amount of work done by the muscle in a given unit of time. It is expressed in kilogram-metre per minute (kg-m/min). Thus, the muscle power is the product of strength and speed. The power output of a muscle is determined by the energy input per second and its mechanical efficiency.

Endurance of the Muscle. Endurance of the muscle refers to its capacity to withstand the power produced during activity. In other words, it is the ability of the muscle to contract repeatedly over time. The muscle endurance depends mostly on the nutrition to the muscle.

Muscle Tension and Excursion. When a muscle contracts, the external work done is observable as the force generated by the muscle, which is known as *muscle tension,* and/or a change in the muscle length, which is known as *muscle excursion.* Muscle length usually shortens during isotonic contraction. However, due to simultaneous passive stretching the muscle length may increase under certain circumstances. In such situations the work done is negative.

Muscle Action. When a muscle or group of muscle contracts, a movement is produced in the associated part of the skeletal lever system of the body; such a resultant movement is referred to as the action of that muscle. For example, flexion or extension produced at some joint in the body is the action of the concerned muscles.

Certain Facts about Muscle Mechanics

Certain facts about the muscle mechanics in human body are as follows:

1. Skeletal Lever System. In our body, the muscle, bones and joints form a system of lever. At most places in the body, the anatomical system provides third class levers. According to principles of physics, with third class levers, much greater force is required to lift the same load, although the speed of lifting is faster. Therefore, speed of action with human muscle is fast but requires greater force.

2. Advantage of Resting Length. Attachments of most of the muscles in the body are such that many of them are normally at or near their resting length when they start to contract, and thus force of contraction produced is more.

3. Situations for Isometric Contractions. In muscles that extend over more than one joint, movement at one joint may compensate for movement at another in such a way that relatively little shortening of the muscle occurs during contraction. Such situations, for nearly isometric contraction, permit development of maximal tension per contraction. For example, in the case of hamstrings muscles which extend over the hip as well as knee joint, the lengthening of the muscles across the hip joint compensates the shortening across the knee joint.

4. Peculiar Integration of Momentum and Balance into the Body Movements. This makes a possible maximal motion with minimal muscular exertion. Due to such integration, the stress put on the tendon and bones is rarely over 50% of their failure strength, protecting them from damage. For example, during walking each limb passes rhythmically through two phases: the support or *stance phase* (when the foot is on the ground) and the *swing phase* (when the foot is off the ground). The support phases of the two legs overlap, so that there are two periods of double support during each cycle. There is a brief burst of activity in the leg flexors at the start of each step, and then the leg is swung forward with little more active muscular contraction. Thus, in this way, the muscles are active for only a fraction of each step. Therefore, walking for long periods causes relatively little fatigue.

5. Integrated Muscle Action. The muscles may play a functional role as an agonist, antagonist or synergist during a particular movement. These relationships are not absolute, but vary with the activity, position of the body and the direction of the resistance that the muscle must overcome.

- Agonist refers to a muscle (or group of muscles) which on contraction acts as the principal muscle producing a joint motion.
- Antagonists refer to those muscles which have actions opposite to the agonist. Antagonists do not contract during a particular movement, but passively elongate or shorten to permit the motion to occur.
- Synergists refer to those muscles which contract along with the agonist to produce a motion. The synergist may act as an assistant mover, neutralizer or a stabilizer.
- Assistant mover is the muscle which aids the prime mover (agonist) in performing a particular motion.
- Neutralizers are the muscles which neutralize the action of those muscles which prevent the agonist to produce a particular movement. For example, the extensors of the wrist neutralize the wrist flexors and these allow the long flexors of the fingers to contract and close the fist.
- Stabilizers refer to those muscles which stabilize a proximal joint so that another muscle may act effectively at a distal joint. For example, the wrist extensors stabilize the wrist joint, so that the hand can be used effectively.

6. Active and Passive Insufficiency. This phenomenon is seen in muscles which extend over two joints. Failure to produce a tight fist by the finger flexors when the wrist is in flexion is an example of active insufficiency. Passive insufficiency of rectus femoris occurs due to excessive stretching when there is knee flexion with hip extension.

ELECTROMYOGRAPHY AND COMMON DISORDERS OF MUSCLES

Electromyography

Electromyography refers to the technique of recording the total electrical activity of the motor nerve and the muscle under study. The machine used to record the said electrical activity is called *electromyograph* and the record obtained is called the *electromyogram.*

Recording Technique

The basic recording unit of the electromyograph is a cathode ray oscilloscope. The electromyography can be recorded using two types of electrodes:

1. ***Surface electrodes*** or skin electrodes are placed on the skin above the surface of the muscle to be studied. They are convenient but are not precise, so they are not commonly used.
2. ***Needle electrodes*** are inserted into the muscle under study. The commonest inserted electrode used in EMG is the *bipolar concentric needle electrode.* It consists of an insulated stainless steel hypodermic needle which contains an insulated fine wire in its barrel: the wire and the needle have bared tips. With needle electrodes, it is usually possible to pick up the activity of a single muscle fibre.

Protocol for Recording EMG

For recording of EMG, the patient is made to lie comfortably in a quiet room. The needle electrode is inserted into the muscle and a ground lead is attached to the same limb to which the muscle under study belongs. The recordings are then taken as:

- ***At rest,*** the muscle is explored systematically for presence of any *spontaneous activity.*
- ***During slight muscle contraction,*** the recording is made from different sites to assess the size and duration of activity of different motor units (*motor unit potentials*).
- ***During maximal muscle contraction (against resistance)*** to record the *interference pattern,* which helps in determining the abnormal recruitment of motor units, if any. Observations made help in differentiating whether the problem is myogenic or neurogenic.

Electromyogram

Components of a normal electromyogram along with the common abnormalities which can be detected are given:

Spontaneous Activity at Rest Normally, at rest, there is complete electrical silence and no spontaneous activity is recorded, except for:

1. The Insertion Activity. When a needle electrode is inserted into a muscle it evokes a discharge of action potentials (due to mechanical stimulus). These potentials are of short duration and small amplitude (Fig. 2.3-32A). The insertion activity is:

- Prolonged in denervated muscle, and
- Absent when muscle tissue is not viable.

2. End Plate Noise. After the cessation of insertion activity, no other spontaneous activity is seen but for a monophasic negative potential in the end plate region called *end plate noise* (Fig. 2.3-32B). These potentials correspond to the miniature end plate potential (MEP) of the neuromuscular junction.

Voluntary Activity during Muscle Contraction

The potential change recorded during muscle contraction is called *motor unit potential* (MUP). The motor unit potential is the compound potential which represents the sum of the individual action potentials generated in the few muscle fibres of the motor unit that are within the pick-up range of the recording electrode. Since fibres of several motor units intermingle singly, each EMG electrode records the activity of more than one motor units. The electromyographic records obtained *during different grades of muscle* contraction have the following characteristics:

1. On minimal Voluntary Contraction. only a single or two smaller motor units in the vicinity of needle electrode give off electrical discharge. The MUP recorded has the following features (Fig. 2.3-33A):

- It has a regular rhythmic fashion.
- Frequency is low (5–10/s).
- Amplitude of MUP is usually between 200 μV and 3 mV and is determined largely by the distance between the recording electrode and the active fibres that are closest to it.
- Duration of each spike of MUP normally varies between 2 and 15 ms and is related to the anatomic scatter of end plates of these muscle fibres in the motor units that are within the pick-up zone of the recording electrode.

2. With the Progressive Increase in the Voluntary Contraction. the firing rate of small units increases until it reaches a certain frequency, when larger units are recruited. Fig. 2.3-33B shows the recruitment pattern with moderate force of contraction.

3. During Maximal Contraction. so many motor units are recruited and thus the so many rhythmically recurring motor unit potentials become superimposed upon one another on the oscilloscope screen that it is impossible to determine their individual characteristics. The resulting appearance of the EMG is designated as *normal interference pattern* (Fig. 2.3-33C).

Interpretation of EMG Record Taken during Muscle Contraction Features to be noted while analysing the

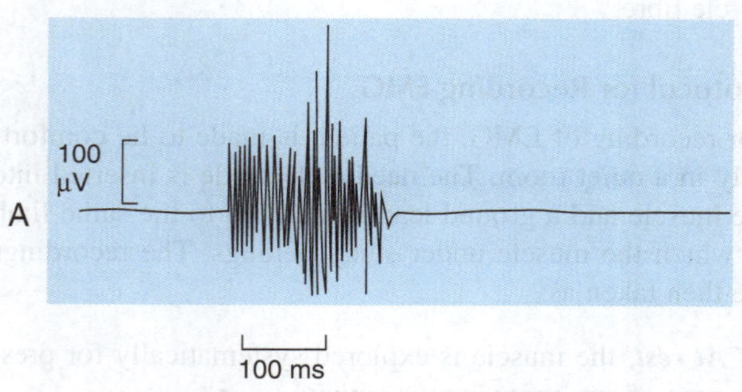

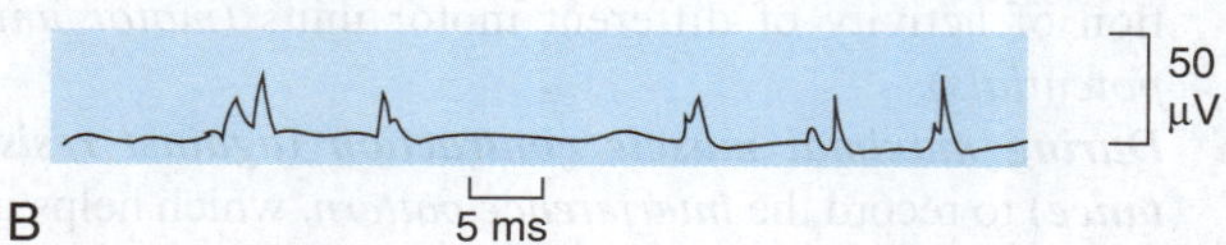

FIGURE 2.3-32 Electromyogram showing spontaneous activity at rest: **A,** complete silence followed by insertion activity; and **B,** end plate potential noise.

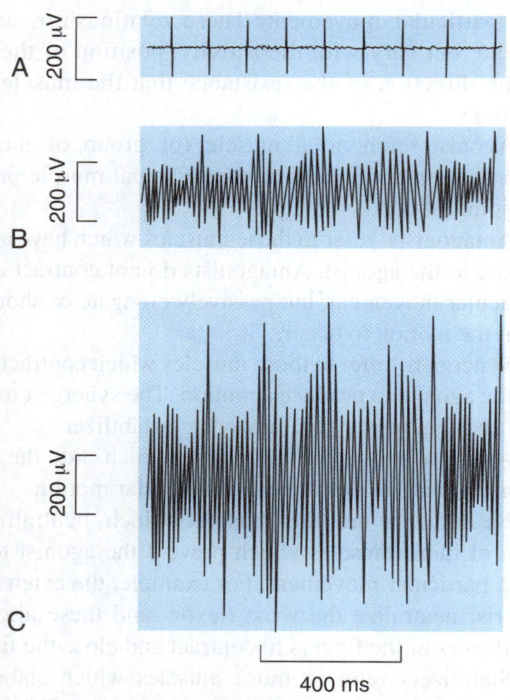

FIGURE 2.3-33 Electromyogram during voluntary muscle activity: **A,** on minimal contraction, **B,** on moderate contraction (recruitment pattern); and **C,** on maximum contraction (normal interference pattern).

EMG record taken during voluntary muscle contraction include:

- *Onset frequency,* i.e. the frequency when the MUPs first appear,
- *Recruitment frequency,* i.e. the frequency at which a particular unit must fire before another is recruited and
- *Density of the interference pattern,* i.e. the frequency of MUPs at maximal contraction.

Abnormal Spontaneous Activities Abnormal spontaneous activities which can be recorded during resting phase are:

*1. **Fasciculation Potentials*** resemble MUPs and represent the involuntary contraction of muscle fibres of a single motor unit. The fasciculation (jerky, visible twitching of a group of muscle fibres) occurs in patients with chronic partial denervation especially due to spinal cord lesions.

*2. **Fibrillation Potentials*** are of very short duration (0.5–2 ms) and low amplitude (25 and 100 μV). They occur at a regular rhythm (2–10/s) and always have an initial positive phase and a secondary negative phase (Fig. 2.3-34).

The fibrillation potentials are produced due to involuntary contraction of the single muscle cells which have been dissociated from nervous control following denervation.

Abnormalities during Voluntary Activity Abnormalities of MUP frequency and amplitude detected during voluntary activity are as follows:

*1. **Decrease in the Density of the Interference*** or the so-called *sparse interference pattern* is seen in patients with *neurogenic weakness* of the muscle when the number of functional motor units is reduced and thus the MUP frequency during maximal contraction is decreased. The amplitude of MUP record is however normal, since the number of muscle fibres in each unit are normal. In severe cases, the interference pattern may be completely lost.

*2. **Low Amplitude of MUP*** is observed in patients with *myogenic causes* of muscle weakness due to reduction in the number of muscle fibres per motor unit. However, the interference pattern during maximal contraction remains normal since the number of motor units available for recruitment is not reduced.

*3. **High Amplitude of MUP*** is recorded from the denervated muscles that have subsequently got reinnervated. It is because of the fact that during reinnervation, the number of muscle fibres in each motor unit is increased (since the muscle fibres which have lost their innervation get innervated by the axonal branches of the neighbouring motor unit).

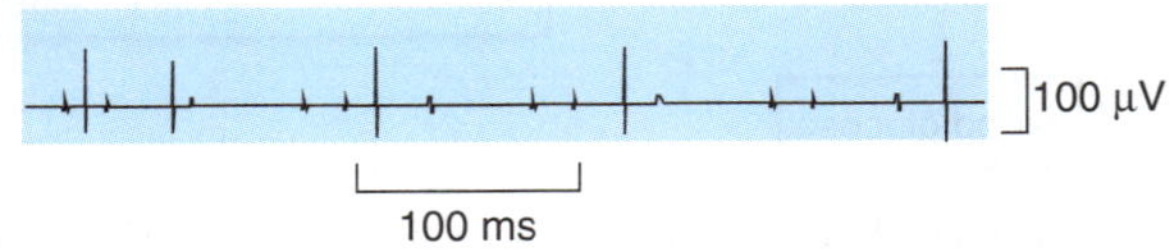

FIGURE 2.3-34 Fibrillation potential recorded from denervated muscle.

Disorders of Skeletal Muscles

1. Muscular Dystrophy Muscular dystrophy is a syndrome which occurs due to genetic mutation and is characterized by progressive muscle weakness.

Duchenne's Muscular Dystrophy is caused by mutations of the dystrophic gene that cause dystrophin to be absent from the muscles. It is an X-linked disorder occurring in about 1 of every 3000 male infants. It causes great disability and eventually proves fatal by the age of 30 years.

Becker's Muscular Dystrophy is an autosomal recessive disorder occurring due to a mutation in the gene for sarcoglycan or other components of dystrophin–glycoprotein complex. It is a milder form of the disease in which the dystrophin is present but is either altered or reduced in amount.

Malignant Hyperthermia is also related to dysfunction of muscle ion channels due to mutation in gene for ryanodine receptors for Ca^{2+}-release channels in the sarcoplasmic reticulum. This mutation results in dysfunction of Ca^{2+} channel to shut down after stimulation, thus more availability of Ca^{2+} causes increase in contractility of muscles leading to more production of heat.

2. Myotonia Myotonia is a disorder that occurs due to abnormalities of the sodium and chloride channels caused by abnormal genes on chromosomes 7, 17 or 19. It is characterized by an abnormally prolonged muscle relaxation after voluntary contraction.

3. Myasthenia Gravis It is a disorder of the neuromuscular junction, characterized by a grave weakness of the muscles (see page 83).

4. Abnormal Muscle Tone The normal muscle tone of a muscle may be increased or decreased constituting an abnormal muscle tone (see page 104).

5. Metabolic Myopathies Metabolic myopathies occur due to mutation of genes that code enzymes involved in carbohydrate and protein metabolism of the muscles for the production of ATP (McArdle syndrome). Metabolic myopathies usually present as intolerance to exercise.

6. Fibrillation and Denervation Hypersensitivity The denervation of skeletal muscles in lower motor neuron lesions causes flaccid paralysis of the muscle, fibrillation and denervation hypersensitivity.

- ***Fibrillation*** is characterized by fine, irregular contractions of individual muscle fibres.
- ***Denervation Hypersensitivity*** refers to when the muscle becomes highly sensitive to acetylcholine.

SOURCE OF ENERGY AND METABOLIC PHENOMENON DURING MUSCLE CONTRACTION

- Chemical composition of muscle
- Energy source for muscle contraction
- Oxygen consumption, demand and debt
- Changes in pH during muscle contraction
- Thermal changes during muscle contraction

Chemical Composition of Muscle

Chemical composition of a skeletal muscle is as follows:

1. *Water.* It constitutes the major bulk of (75%) the muscle weight.
2. ***Muscle proteins*** form 20% of the muscle mass. These include the contractile proteins (actin, myosin, troponin and tropomyosin), myogen and myoglobin. Myoglobin is a conjugated protein. Like haemoglobin, its main function is to carry oxygen.
3. ***Organic substances other than proteins*** present in the muscle fibre include:
   - *Carbohydrates:* glycogen and hexaphosphate.
   - *Lipids:* neutral fat, cholesterol, lecithin and steroids.
   - *Nitrogenous substances:* ATP, adenylic acid, creatine, phosphocreatine, urea, uric acid, xanthine and hypoxanthine.
4. ***Inorganic substances*** present in the muscle are:
   - *Cations:* potassium, sodium, calcium, magnesium and
   - *Anions:* chloride, phosphate and sulphate.

Energy Source for Muscle Contraction

The muscle contraction requires lot of energy. In fact, the muscle has been labelled as a *machine for converting chemical energy into mechanical work.* The immediate source of energy is ATP and the ultimate source is the intermediary metabolism of carbohydrate and lipids.

Hydrolysis of ATP The hydrolysis of ATP provides energy for muscle contraction (for details see molecular basis of muscle contraction page 89). ATP stored in the muscle initiates the contractile activity but is consumed after a few twitches. In about 3 s, all the ATP stored in the muscle cell is depleted. Thus, there is need for resynthesis of ATP.

Resynthesis of ATP There are three ways in which a muscle fibre can resynthesize ATP from ADP during contractile activity:

1. Phosphorylation of ADP by Creatine Phosphate. Immediately after the depletion of ATP stores of the muscle, ATP is regenerated using the energy released by the dephosphorylation of creatine phosphate (CP) reserves of the muscle fibre.

$$\text{Creatine phosphate} + \text{ADP} \Leftrightarrow \text{creatine} + \text{ATP}.$$

The above reaction, known as *Lohman's reaction,* is rapid and requires only single enzyme. It is reversible and obeys law of mass action. Since the amount of creatine phosphate is limited, the amount of ATP formed by this mechanism is only sufficient for contraction of the muscle for next about 5 s. Therefore, the next mechanism comes into play immediately.

[At rest, the muscle contains large quantities of ATP, therefore, the reaction proceeds from right to left forming creatine phosphate, and thus the store is built up.]

2. Glycolysis. After depletion of creatine phosphate reserves, the next important source of energy which is used to reconstitute both ATP and phosphocreatine, is glycogen (previously stored in the muscle cell) by the process of glycolysis which can sustain muscle contraction for about 1 min. As shown in Fig. 2.3-35, each molecule of glycogen after glycolysis produces two molecules of pyruvic acid and two molecules of ATP. Further changes in pyruvic acid depend upon the availability of oxygen.

- In the absence of oxygen, the pyruvic acid is converted into lactic acid which is released into the blood. From the blood, lactic acid is taken up by the kidney and liver where it is reconverted into glucose and released back into circulation (Cori cycle).
- If oxygen is available, the pyruvic acid enters into *Krebs' cycle.*

A total of 38 ATP molecules are formed during breakdown of each glycogen molecule as below:

- 2 molecules of ATP are formed during glycolysis,
- 2 molecules of ATP are formed during Krebs' cycle and
- 34 molecules of ATP are formed utilizing the hydrogen ions produced during breakdown of a glycogen molecule.

Importance of glycolysis is two fold:

- First, the glycolytic reactions occur even in the absence of oxygen, so that muscle contraction can be

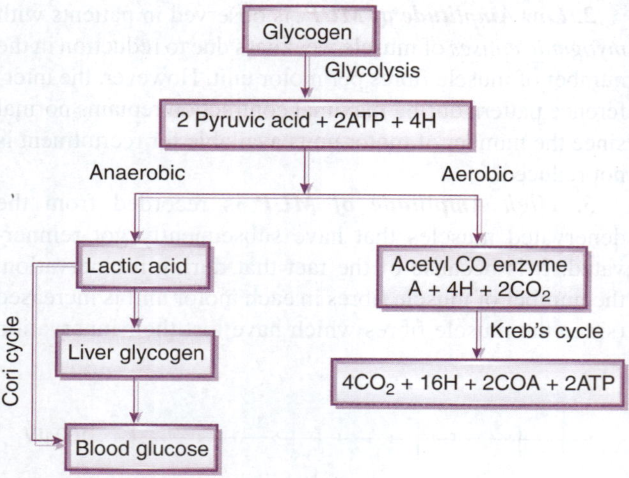

FIGURE 2.3-35 Schematic diagram showing breakdown of glycogen stored in a muscle cell.

sustained for a short time even when oxygen is not available.

- Second, the rate of formation of ATP by glycolysis process is about 2½ times as rapid as ATP formation when the cellular foodstuffs react with oxygen.

3. Oxidative metabolism. Oxidative metabolism, i.e. combining of oxygen with various cellular foodstuffs to liberate ATP is the final source of energy during muscle contraction. This source contributes more than 95% of all energy used by the muscles for sustained long-term contraction. Foodstuffs used in oxidative metabolism include fats, carbohydrates and proteins as:

- *Fatty acids* are used for resynthesis of most of the ATP during prolonged muscle contraction lasting over a period of many hours.
- *Glycogen* contributes about half of the energy required for muscle contraction lasting for 2–4 h.

Important Note

- During intense but short lasting exercise, e.g. in a 100m race that takes 10 s, 85% of the energy consumed is derived anaerobically.
- During moderate intensity exercise, e.g. in a 3 km race that takes 16 min, 20% of the energy consumed is derived anaerobically.
- During mild intensity prolonged exercise, e.g. in a long distance race that takes about an hour, only 5% of the energy comes from anaerobic metabolism.

Oxygen Demand, Consumption and Debt ***Oxygen demand*** increases with the intensity of exercise (i.e. intensity of muscle contraction). It has been reported that in a sprint lasting for ½ min, the oxygen demand is around 20 L/min.

Oxygen Consumption or oxygen utilization is the volume of oxygen which has been actually consumed during the exercise. The maximum amount of oxygen that can be consumed by a person while performing severe exercise (irrespective of the demand) is VO_2 max. A world-class sprinter is expected to have a VO_2 max around 75 ml/kg/min (about 4 L/min).

Oxygen Debt. During intense exercise, the maximum oxygen consumed is much less than the oxygen demand. So the energy requirement is met with by the *anaerobic pathway.* After the period of exercise, extra O_2 is consumed to remove the excess lactate collected due to anaerobic glucose breakdown, replenish the ATP and phosphoryl creatine store, and replace the small amounts of oxygen that have come from myoglobin. This amount of extra oxygen consumed is called O_2 debt and is proportionate to the extent to which energy demands during exercise exceeded the capacity of aerobic synthesis of energy store, i.e. extent to which *oxygen deficit occurred* during exercise. Oxygen debt can be measured experimentally by determining oxygen consumption after exercise until constant basal consumption is reached and then subtracting the basal oxygen consumption from total oxygen consumed during this period (Fig. 2.3-36).

Applied Aspect

To avoid excessive O_2 debt early in the race, the experienced long-distance runners begin the race very slowly to allow the cardiorespiratory system to gear up to the energy demands of muscular activity; once a steady state is attained due to cardiorespiratory readjustment, the oxygen supply balances the oxygen requirements of the muscles. This state of oxidative metabolism to provide energy for the muscles can continue for several hours without producing excessive oxygen debt. This prevents too much anaerobic metabolism and accumulation of lactic acid which hamper the efficiency.

Mechanical Efficiency of Muscle During contraction, the efficiency of muscle is about 25%. Mechanical efficiency is equal to output/input. Therefore, mechanical efficiency is equal to

$$\frac{\text{Work done by the muscle (W)}}{\text{Oxygen consumption } (VO_2)}$$

OR

$$\frac{W \text{ (kilopond metre/min/426.7)}}{VO_2\text{(L/min)} \times 5}$$

(Since 426.7 kilopond metre/min = 1 kcal, and 1 L/min VO_2 at STPD produces 5 kcal of energy;STPD means standard temperature (0°C) pressure (760 mmHg) and dry)

- Therefore, mechanical efficiency in isotonic contraction is approximately 25% of the energy expenditure and rest 75% is degraded as heat and

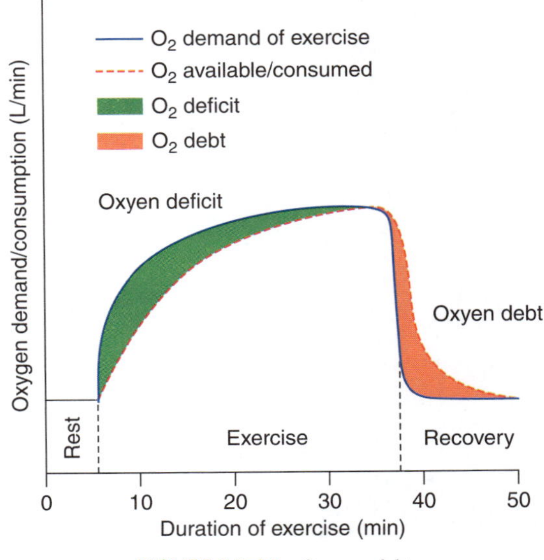

FIGURE 2.3-36 Oxygen debt.

- During isometric contraction as no external work is done, therefore, mechanical efficiency is nil and 100% energy expenditure disappears as heat

Changes in pH During Muscle Contraction

Changes occurring in the pH and reaction of the muscle during contraction are as follows:

- *During resting condition*, the reaction of muscle is alkaline with a pH of 7.3.
- *During onset of muscle contraction,* due to dephosphorylation of ATP to ADP, the pH of muscles becomes acidic.
- *During later part of muscle contraction,* due to resynthesis of ATP from creatine phosphate, the muscle reaction again becomes alkaline.
- *At the end of muscle contraction,* due to formation of pyruvic acid and/or lactic acid, the muscle reaction once again becomes acidic.

Thermal Changes during Muscle Contraction

Thermal changes in the muscle during contraction can be accurately measured using suitable thermocouple. The different phases of heat production during muscle contraction are:

1. Resting Heat. Resting heat is in the heat generated when the muscle is at rest, i.e. not contracting. It is the external manifestation of the basal metabolic process of the muscle.

2. Initial Heat. Initial heat refers to the heat generated in excess of resting heat during muscular contraction. It is made up of the following components:

- ***Activation heat*** refers to initial rapid liberation of energy before the actual contraction of the muscle. It is mostly due to the heat liberated while calcium ions are released from the L-tubules of sarcoplasmic reticulum and the myosin ATPase is activated.
- ***Shortening heat*** is produced when the muscle contracts isotonically. It is produced due to various structural changes in the muscle fibre like movement of cross-bridges and myosin heads and breakdown of glycogen. It is absent during isometric contraction.
- ***Maintenance heat*** is generated during isometric contraction when no actual shortening of the muscle fibre takes place. Its cause is complicated and mostly obscure.

3. Recovery Heat. Recovery heat refers to the heat produced in excess of resting heat, following muscle contraction. It continues for about 30 min after the cessation of muscle contraction. This heat is generated by the metabolic processes that restore the muscle to its precontraction state. These include calcium ATPase activity which pumps back calcium into the sarcoplasmic reticulum and also regeneration of ATP and other energy substrates. The recovery heat is approximately equal to initial heat (heat produced during contraction).

4. Relaxation heat. This is the extra heat, in addition to the recovery heat, which is produced during relaxation of the isotonically contracted muscle. It is the external manifestation of the extra work done on the muscle to stretch it back to its original length.

Important Note

Fenn effect

Fenn effect states that the heat produced is directly proportional to the work done. When the work done is more, the expenditure of ATP will also be more; therefore, Fenn effect can be considered to state that more work done causes more expenditure of energy.

Chapter 2.4

Smooth Muscle and Cardiac Muscle

SMOOTH MUSCLE

Functional Anatomy and Organization

Smooth muscles (nonstriated muscles), as the name indicates, are characterized by the absence of the typical cross-striated patterns seen in skeletal muscles. Because of their spontaneous activity or activity through the autonomic nervous system, they are also called *involuntary muscles.*

The smooth muscle cells are long fusiform in shape and are aggregated to form bundles or *fasciculi*. The fasciculi are aggregated to form layers of variable thickness. Thus, smooth muscles exist either in sheet or bundles of fibres. In each layer, the cells are so arranged that the thick central part of one cell is opposite the thin tapering ends of adjoining cells (Fig. 2.4-1.)

Types of Smooth Muscles

Smooth muscles are of two types: single-unit or unitary and multiunit smooth muscles.

1. Single-unit Smooth Muscles Single-unit smooth muscles are also called *visceral smooth muscles* since they are present in the walls of hollow viscera such as gastrointestinal tract, uterus, ureters, urinary bladder and respiratory tract. ***Salient features of single-unit smooth muscles*** are:

- These are arranged in the form of large sheets and have low-resistance bridges between individual muscle cells and function in a *syncytial fashion* and that is why they are called single-unit muscles (Fig. 2.4-2). The low-resistance intercellular bridges or the so-called *gap junctions* are in abundance and have high conductance for the ions. Therefore, the syncytium contracts as a single unit in many large areas.
- These muscles have their own rhythmic contractility *myogenic tone* that is independent of the nerve supply. The rate of contraction may be determined by the *pacemaker regions* present within the muscles. The nervous influence only modulates their activity, i.e. the role of the nerves is to increase or decrease the rate of rhythmic contraction.
- Contraction of this kind of smooth muscles is also stimulated by *stretching*. The muscles of smaller blood vessels are mainly of this kind and their contraction

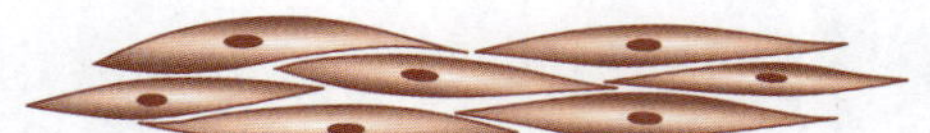

FIGURE 2.4-1 Arrangement of smooth muscle fibres.

in response to stretch is involved in autoregulation of blood flow.

- In addition to the autonomic nervous system, their contractile activity is also influenced by some non-neural stimuli, e.g. hormones and local tissue factors (such as temperature and pH).

2. Multiunit Smooth Muscles Multiunit smooth muscles, as the name indicates, are made up of multiple individual units without interconnecting bridges, i.e. *non-syncytial in* character (Fig. 2.4-1). These are *located* in most blood vessels, epididymis, vas deferens, iris, ciliary body and piloerector muscles.

Salient Features. of Multiunit Smooth Muscles are:

- These muscles are made up of multiple individual units of muscle fibres, each innervated by a single nerve ending.
- Each muscle fibre has got an outer membrane made up of glycoproteins which help to insulate and separate the muscle fibres from each other. These muscles contract when an appropriate nerve stimulus reaches, i.e. contraction is *neurogenic.* Here, a single stimulus to the nerve causes repeated firing of action potential which produces *irregular tetanic contraction* (rather than a single muscle twitch produced by a single action potential as seen in skeletal muscle).
- These fibres do not exhibit spontaneous contraction, i.e. *no pacemaker activity.*
- Since the *gap junctions* are not present, the excitation remains localized within the motor unit.
- These muscles do not respond to stretch.

Innervation and Neuromuscular Junction of Smooth Muscles

Nerve Supply Smooth muscles are innervated by autonomic nerves, both sympathetic as well as parasympathetic. The two have opposite effects. In some organs, sympathetic stimulation causes contraction and parasympathetic stimulation causes relaxation of smooth muscles. While in some other organs, a reverse action is seen. The autonomic nerves supplying the smooth muscles emerge out as *preganglionic fibres* which relay in a ganglion. Postganglionic fibres run along the length of muscle fibres and groove them.

Neuromuscular Junction The postganglionic nerve fibres, approach the smooth muscles, branch extensively and come in close contact with large number of smooth muscle fibres (Fig. 2.4-3). The neuronal network so formed has a beaded appearance due to the large enlargements called *varicosities* (Fig. 2.4-4). These varicosities contain the chemical neurotransmitter (acetylcholine or norepinephrine).

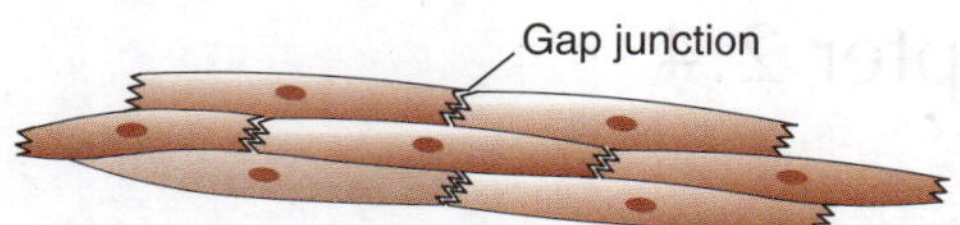

FIGURE 2.4-2 Single-unit smooth muscle fibre showing gap junctions between two adjacent cells.

In the smooth muscle, the nerve fibres are not ending in *motor end plates* (as seen in skeletal muscles), i.e. the nerve fibres do not make any direct contact with the muscle fibres. Instead, the nerve fibres release its neurotransmitter from each varicosity into the interstitial fluid close to the muscle fibres. The neurotransmitter so released diffuses into a large number of cells and causes activation of all muscle fibres up to where it is forming a syncytium. Therefore, here a single stimulus does not cause stimulation of all muscle fibres in the whole organ. Thus, repeated stimuli are needed to cause release of more chemical transmitter to stimulate the remaining cells. Further, in a sheet of smooth muscle cells, often only the cells on the surface are innervated. The deeper cells are stimulated by spread of action potentials through the gap junctions.

Excitatory Junctional Potential (EJP) or Inhibitory Junctional Potential (IJP), i.e. either a depolarizing or a hyperpolarizing response may be recorded from a smooth muscle, in response to an appropriate nerve stimulus. These potentials summate with repeated stimuli. The EJP and IJP are *local responses* like those seen in a synapse (excitatory and inhibitory postsynaptic potential, EPSP and IPSP).

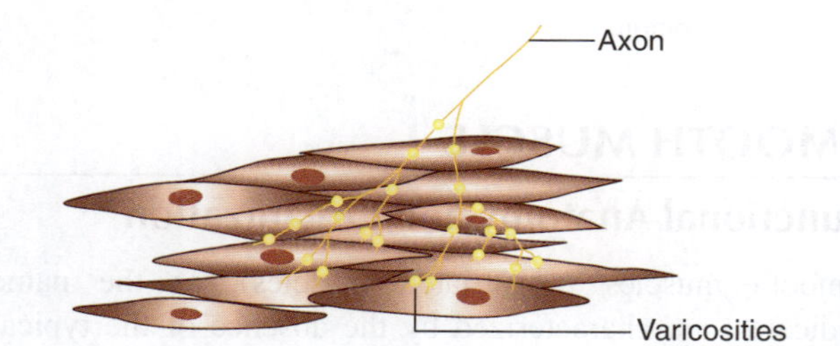

FIGURE 2.4-3 The nerve supplying to smooth muscle showing varicosities (beaded appearance).

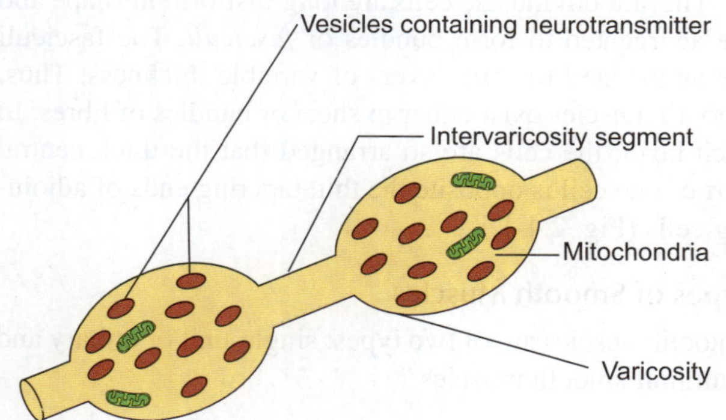

FIGURE 2.4-4 Detailed structure of postganglionic nerve ending innervating smooth muscle cells.

Structure of Smooth Muscle Fibre

Each smooth muscle fibre is a long spindle-shaped cell (myocyte) having a broad central part and tapering ends (Fig. 2.4-5A). The length of smooth muscle fibre is highly variable (15–500 μm) depending upon the organ in which they are present. For example,

- *Digestive tract* fibres are 30–40 μm long and 5 μm in diameter,
- Fibres in *blood vessels* are 15–20 μm long and 2–3 μm in diameter and
- Fibres in *uterus* are 300 μm long and 10 μm in diameter.

Salient Features of Structure of a Smooth Muscle Fibre

Plasma Membrane. which binds the smooth muscle is surrounded by an external lamina. Adjacent smooth muscle cells communicate through gap junctions.

Nucleus. is oval or elongated and lies in the central part of the cell.

Sarcoplasm, in addition to a single nucleus, contains other cell organelles like mitochondria (source of energy), a Golgi complex, some granular endoplasmic reticulum and free ribosomes. Apart from these, it also contains myofibrils and intermediate filaments.

Sarcoplasmic Reticulum similar to that in skeletal muscle is present, but is not as developed.

Myofibrils are made up of contractile proteins, myosin and actin filaments. The *longitudinal striations* seen on light microscopy are due to these myofibrils. Since the thick and thin filaments do not have the highly ordered arrangement as seen in striated muscles, no cross striations are seen. Other salient differences from the skeletal muscle are:

- The *sarcotubular system* and *triads* encountered in striated muscles are not well developed in smooth muscles.
- Smooth muscles contain relatively less *thick filaments* and more *thin filaments.*
- Z-line is not well defined in smooth muscles.
- *Myosin-II* present in smooth muscle is chemically different from that seen in skeletal muscles. It binds to actin only if its light chain is phosphorylated. Thus, phosphorylation of myosin is necessary for the contraction of smooth muscles.
- *Thin actin filaments* are also different from those in skeletal muscle due to absence of the troponin protein molecules.
- *Dense bodies* are bounded by α-actinin, (Fig. 2.4-5B) and attached to the cell membrane through α-actinin. The actin filaments are attached to these dense bodies. In between actin filaments, the thick myosin filaments are situated. There are cross-bridges between actin and myosin, which help in the sliding mechanism of muscle contraction. When the muscle contracts, the points on the cell membrane where dense bodies are attached, are drawn closer to each other. This converts an oblongated smooth muscle into one that is oval (Fig. 2.4-5C).

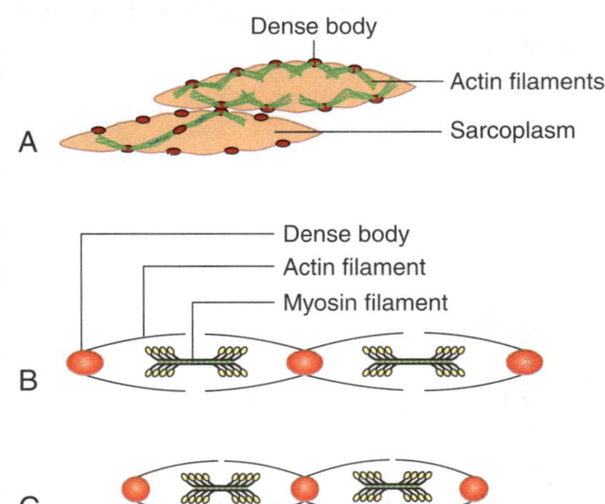

FIGURE 2.4-5 Structure of smooth muscle: **A,** arrangement of thin (actin filaments attached to dense bodies) and thick (myosin) filaments; **B,** position of dense bodies in relaxed state; and C, the dense bodies are drawn closer to each other in contracted state.

Process of Excitability and Contractility

- Process of muscle excitation
- Process of excitation–contraction coupling
- Process of muscle contraction

Process of Muscle Excitation

Process of muscle excitation basically includes the electrical activity in smooth muscle which differs in a multiunit smooth muscle from that of in a single-unit muscle, and so is discussed separately.

Electrical Activity in Single-Unit (Visceral) Smooth Muscles

Resting Membrane Potential. The resting membrane potential in a visceral smooth muscle ranges between −50 and −75 mV. Sometimes it may reach as low as −25 mV. Thus, the peculiarity of the resting membrane potential is its *unstability,* i.e. there is no true resting value, rather it keeps

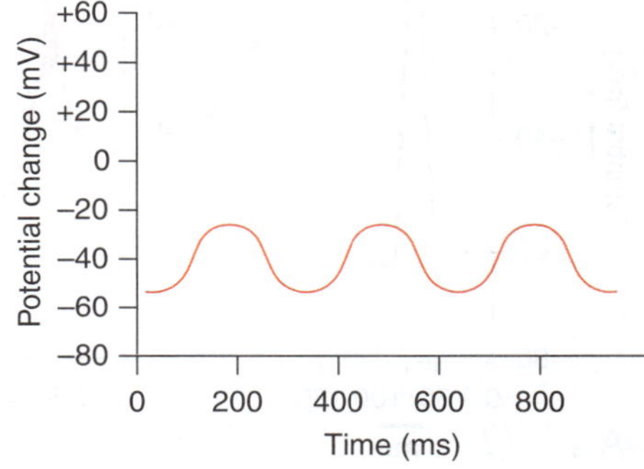

FIGURE 2.4-6 Resting membrane potential (fluctuating type) in visceral smooth muscle.

on oscillating between −55 and −35 mV (Fig. 2.4-6). These oscillations in the RMP occur due to superimposition by the *pacemaker potentials* which in turn occur due to rhythmic changes in either Ca^{2+} channel permeability and/or the activity of Na^{+}–K^{+} pump.

Action Potential. When depolarization reaches threshold potential, an action potential is generated, which is transmitted to the adjacent muscle cells through the gap junction. Three types of action potentials are known to occur in the visceral smooth muscle fibres, viz. spike potential, spike potential superimposed over pacemaker potential and action potential with plateau.

1. Spike Potential. A typical spike potential, similar to that seen in skeletal muscles, is also observed in most, if not all, single-unit smooth muscles. However, it differs from the spike potential of skeletal muscle in many ways: (i) its average duration varies between 10 and 50 ms; (ii) its amplitude is very low and (iii) it does not reach the isoelectric base (Fig. 2.4-7A). The spike action potential, in a smooth muscle, can occur due to following modes of stimulations:

- Electrical stimulation,
- Effect of hormones on the smooth muscle,
- Action of neurotransmitters from the nerve fibre and
- By stretch of a smooth muscle as seen in gut wall.

For example, when the gut is overfilled by intestinal contents, due to stretch there occurs local automatic contraction which sets up a peristaltic wave that moves the contents away from the overfilled intestine.

2. Spike Potential Superimposed Over Slow Wave Potentials. The slow wave rhythms, also called as pacemaker waves, are seen in many visceral smooth muscles such as muscles of gut. These waves themselves cannot cause muscle contraction. However, in self-excitatory smooth muscles, the slow waves can initiate action potential. When the potential of slow waves rises above the level of about −35 mV (the approximate threshold for eliciting action potential in most visceral smooth muscles), an action potential develops and spreads over the muscle mass. Such a spike potential appears rhythmically at a rate of about one or two spikes superimposed at the peak of each slow wave (Fig. 2.4-7B) and causes rhythmic contractions of the self-excitatory smooth muscles.

3. Action Potential with Plateau is seen in some tissues such as in the ureter, the uterus under some conditions and some types of vascular smooth muscles. As shown in Fig. 2.4-7C, this type of action potential starts with rapid depolarizatioin as is seen in the skeletal muscles. However, like skeletal muscles, the repolarization does not occur immediately, but is delayed by 100–1000 ms. This prolonged depolarization accounts for the sustained contraction of certain smooth muscle fibres.

Ionic Basis of Action Potential. In smooth muscles, the depolarization occurs due to entry of Ca^{2+} ions from ECF to the inside of the cell rather than Na^{+} ions (as seen in skeletal muscles). The smooth cell membrane has far more *voltage-gated calcium channels* than does skeletal muscle but few voltage-gated sodium channels. Unlike sodium channels, the calcium channels open and close slowly. This accounts for the prolonged action potential observed in smooth muscles. The calcium ions, in addition to causing depolarization, also produce contraction of smooth muscles by directly acting on the contractile mechanism.

Electrical Activity in Multiunit Smooth Muscles

The multiunit smooth muscles (such as the muscles of iris and piloerector muscles) usually respond to nerve stimuli. The nerve endings secrete the neurotransmitter (acetylcholine or norepinephrine), which causes depolarization of the smooth muscle membrane. Since fibres are too small, they do not generate an action potential. The local depolarization is called the *excitatory junctional potential (EJP)*. However, the EJP spreads electrotonically over the entire fibre and is sufficient to cause the muscle contraction.

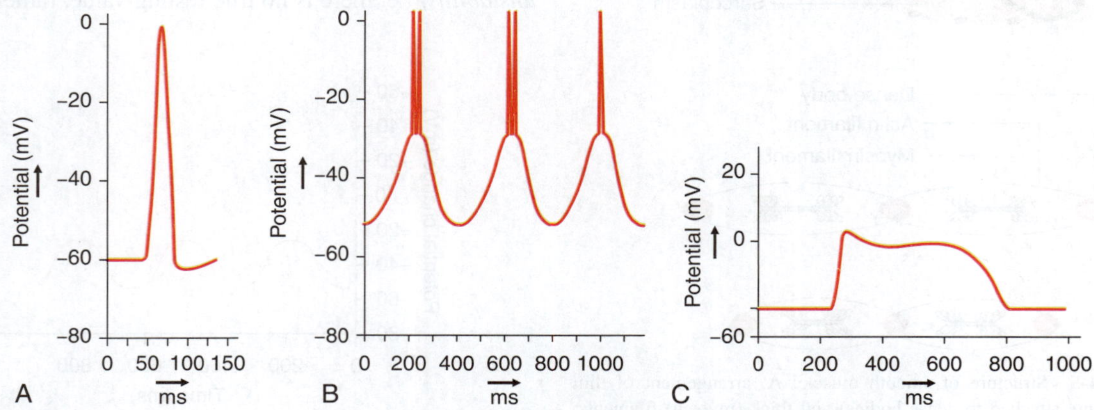

FIGURE 2.4-7 Three types of action potentials recorded from smooth muscles: **A,** spike potential; **B,** spike potential superimposed over slow wave potentials; and **C,** action potential with plateau.

Process of Excitation–Contraction Coupling

Excitation–contraction coupling refers to the sequence of events by which an excited plasma membrane of a muscle fibre leads to cross-bridge activity by increasing cytosolic (sarcoplasmic) calcium concentration. Since a smooth muscle can be excited by so many possible ways, there are different ways of excitation–contraction coupling as well. Three different mechanisms of excitation–contraction coupling known in smooth muscles are described below:

1. Electromechanical Coupling occurs when the smooth muscle is excited through sarcolemmal depolarization. Due to depolarization of the membrane, the *voltage-gated* Ca^{2+} channels present on it are opened and the Ca^{2+} ions from the ECF move into the sarcoplasm. These Ca^{2+} ions in turn stimulate the release of more Ca^{2+} from the sarcoplasmic reticulum. This process is called Ca^{2+}*-induced* Ca^{2+} release (CICR). The raised sarcoplasmic Ca^{2+} level brings about the excitation–contraction coupling.

2. Pharmaco-mechanical Coupling occurs when the smooth muscle is excited by some chemical agent and not by membrane depolarization. Two mechanisms of pharmaco-mechanical coupling known are:

- The chemical agents (neurotransmitters and hormones) bind to the *ligand-gated* Ca^{2+} channels present on the sarcolemma and open them up resulting in influx of Ca^{2+} from the ECF.
- The chemical agents bind to the *membrane receptors* and activate the second messenger system of G-protein → generation of inositol triphosphate (IP_3) from the membrane phospholipids → release of calcium ions from the *intracellular* Ca^{2+} stores, i.e. from the sarcoplasmic reticulum.

3. Mechano-mechanical Coupling occurs when the muscle is excited by stretch. Due to stretching, the *stretch-sensitive* Ca^{2+} channels present on the sarcolemma open up resulting in influx of Ca^{2+} from the ECF.

The excitation–contraction coupling in smooth muscle is a slow process. Calcium initiates this process by binding with calmodulin. The *calcium–calmodulin complex* so formed triggers muscle contraction by a sequence of events discussed below.

Process of Smooth Muscle Contraction

The molecular mechanism of smooth muscle contraction by cross-bridge cycling and sliding of filaments is similar to the skeletal muscle. However, since the smooth muscle does not contain the regulatory proteins tropomyosin and troponin, its regulation is different. In a smooth muscle, one of the light chains of the myosin filament located in the neck region serves the function of tropomyosin and thus is called the *regulatory chain of myosin.* Similarly, the Ca^{2+}-binding protein *calmodulin* plays the role of troponin.

Steps of Cross-Bridge Cycling Steps of cross-bridge cycling in a smooth muscle are summarized (Fig. 2.4-8):

1. Activation of the Enzyme Myosin Light Chain Kinase (MLCK). The enzyme MLCK is activated by the Ca^{2+}–calmodulin complex.

2. Phosphorylation of the Myosin Regulatory Chain. The activated enzyme MLCK uses ATP to phosphorylate the myosin regulatory chain.

3. Cross-bridging. When the myosin regulatory chain is phosphorylated, the head of myosin filament acquires the capability to bind with actin filament to form the cross-bridge (Fig. 2.4-8B).

4. Power Stroke. Formation of the actin–myosin ADP-Pi complex triggers a conformational change in the myosin head causing it to flex towards the arm of the cross-bridge. The flexion of the myosin head generates mechanical force (*the power stroke*) (Fig. 2.4-8C).

Due to power stroke, the actin filament slides over the myosin filament producing contraction. As shown in Fig. 2.4-5C, the *dense bodies* play a role in the contraction of a smooth muscle fibre. In fact, the dense bodies of smooth muscles serve the same role as the Z-disc (Z-line) in skeletal muscle.

5. Relaxation of Smooth Muscle. To cause relaxation of the smooth muscle contraction, it is necessary to remove the calcium ions from the sarcoplasm. This is accomplished by the calcium pump which pumps the calcium from ICF to ECF and also from ICF into the sarcoplasmic reticulum. When the cytoplasmic Ca^{2+} falls to the resting level, the processes involved in the contraction of smooth muscle automatically reverse except for the phosphorylation of the myosin head. Reversal of this occurs when the enzyme *myosin phosphatase* causes dephosphorylation of the myosin regulatory chain. After this, the cross-bridge cycling stops and the contraction ceases (Fig. 2.4-8D). The time required for relaxation of contracted muscle, therefore, is determined to a great extent by the amount of active myosin phosphatase in the cell.

The calcium pumps operating in the smooth muscles are slow acting in comparison with the fast-acting sarcoplasmic reticulum pump in skeletal muscles. Therefore, the duration of smooth muscle contraction is prolonged (in seconds) as compared to skeletal muscles (from 1/100th to 1/10th of a second).

Characteristics of Smooth Muscle Excitation and Contraction

Certain characteristic features of smooth muscle excitation and contraction are as follows:

1. Slow excitation–Contraction Coupling As shown in Fig. 2.4-9, a smooth muscle starts contracting approximately 200 ms after the start of the spike potential (i.e. 150 ms after the spike is over). The peak of contraction is reached after

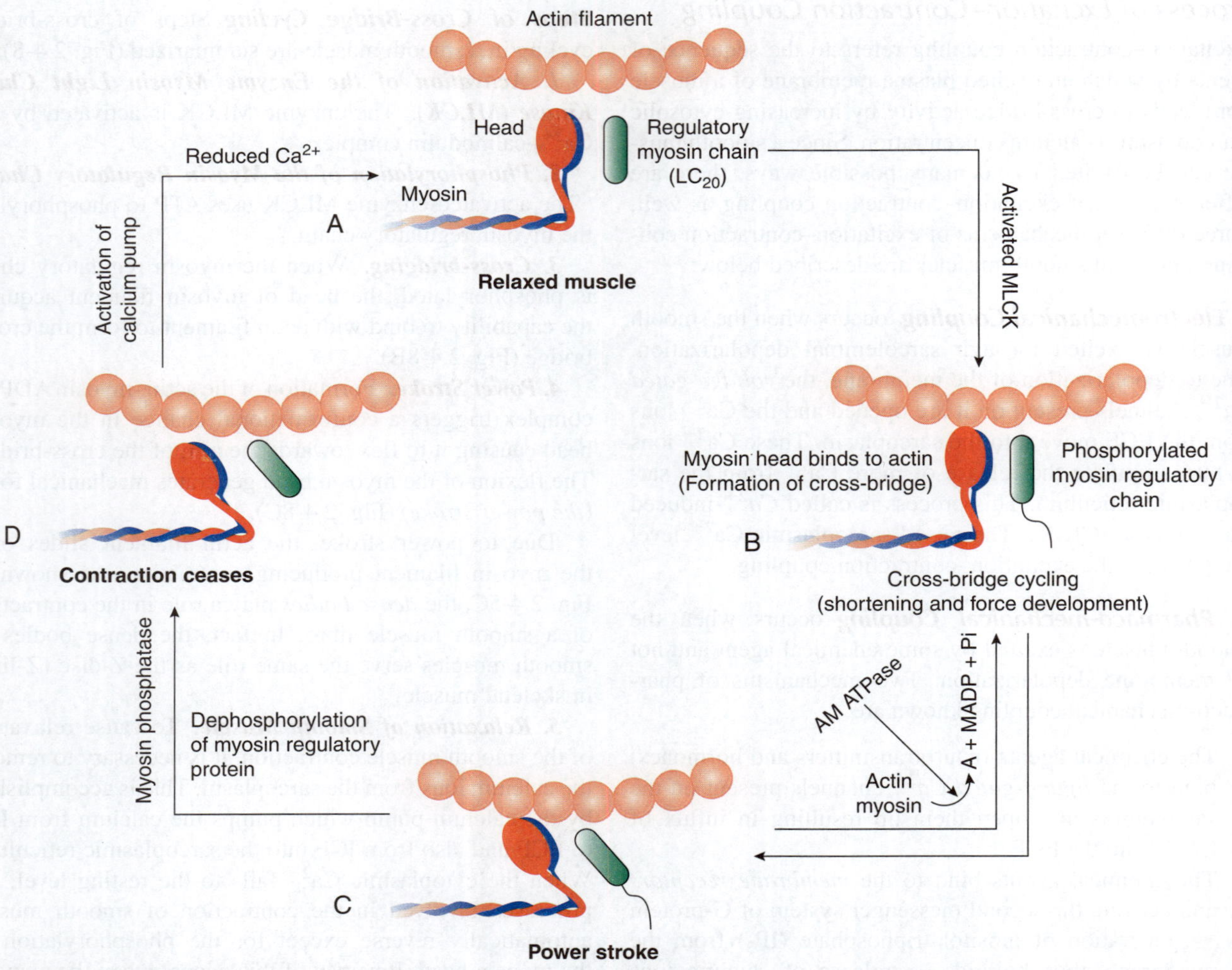

FIGURE 2.4-8 Steps of cross-bridge cycling in smooth muscle: **A,** relaxed muscle; **B,** activation of myosin light chain kinase (MLCK) catalyses phosphorylation of myosin regulatory chain and initiates cross-bridging between myosin head and actin filament; **C,** power stroke, triggered by conformational change in myosin head due to formation of actin–myosin ADP-Pi complex; and **D,** dephosphorylation of myosin regulatory protein resulting in cessation of cross-bridging.

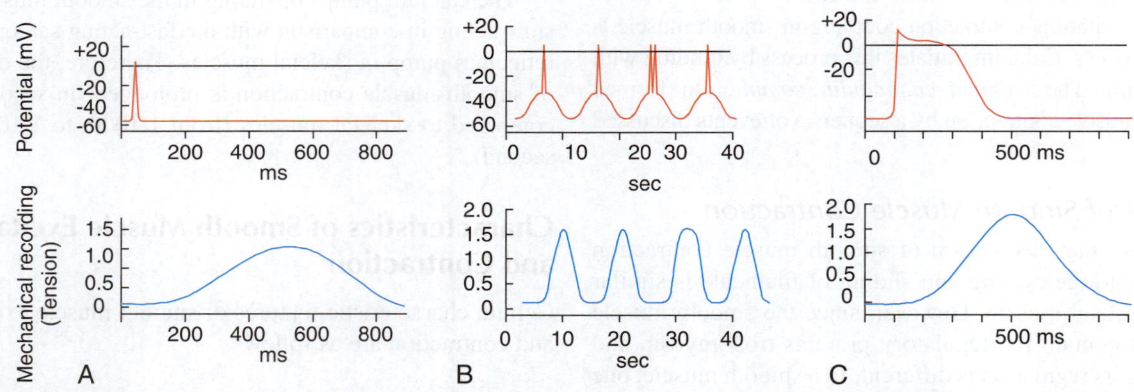

FIGURE 2.4-9 Record of mechanical activity of smooth muscle following various types of potential: **A,** spike potential; **B,** spike potential superimposed over slow wave potential; and **C,** action potential with plateau.

500 ms of the spike. Thus, the excitation–contraction coupling is very slow in smooth muscles compared with the skeletal muscles.

2. Plasticity A smooth muscle exhibits the property of plasticity, i.e. it can readjust its resting length (the length at which a muscle generates maximum active tension). Thus, the smooth muscle defies the usual *length–tension relationship* that is valid for striated muscles (skeletal as well cardiac muscles); when a smooth muscle is passively stretched, it first exerts increased tension, which gradually reduces to prestretch level (even when the stretch is maintained). Therefore, the *length–tension relationship curve* in a smooth muscle is not a smooth curve but a jagged line (Fig. 2.4-10).

It has been explained by the observation that at longer fibre lengths, the thick filaments are disposed in series (Fig. 2.4-11A) while at shorter length, the thick filaments are disposed in *parallel* (Fig. 2.4-11B).

3. Latch Phenomenon Latch phenomenon is another characteristic exhibited by smooth muscles. It refers to the mechanism by which a smooth muscle can maintain a high tension without actively contracting. This phenomenon allows long-term maintenance of tone in many smooth muscle organs. In such a state, the muscle cannot generate active tension but can effectively resist passive stretching. This phenomenon appropriately suits the function of smooth muscles, since in most instances, it has to resist stretch rather than actively move a load. These smooth muscles are mostly found in the walls of hollow viscera that must resist excessive stretching. The latch phenomenon can be explained by the fact that when the myosin kinase and myosin phosphatase enzyme are both strongly activated, the cycling frequency of the myosin heads and the velocity of contraction are great. Then, as the activation of the enzymes decreases, the cycling frequency decreases, but at the same time, the lower activation of the enzymes causes the myosin heads to remain attached to the actin filaments for a larger and longer proportion of the cycling period. Therefore, the number of heads attached to the thin filament at any given time remains large. Because the number of heads attached to the actin determines the static force of contraction, tension is maintained, yet little energy is used by the muscle, because ATP is not degraded to ADP, except on the rare occasion when head detaches.

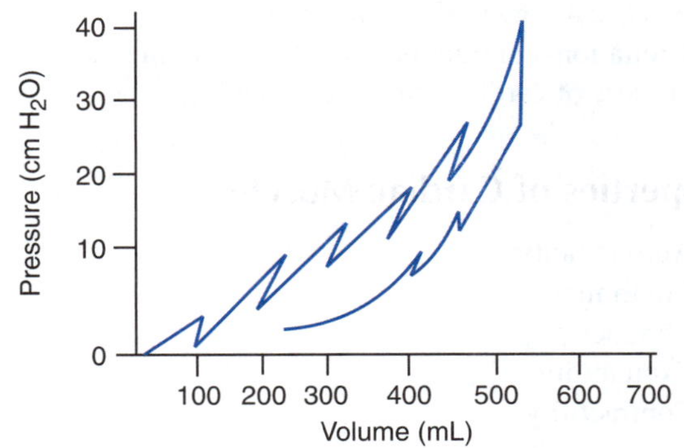

FIGURE 2.4-10 Plasticity in smooth muscle fibre.

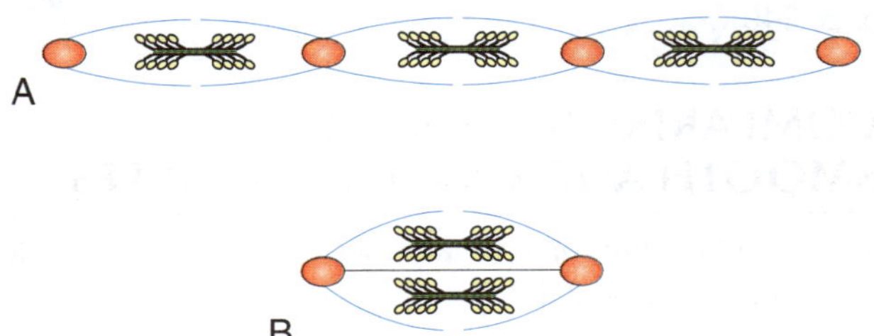

FIGURE 2.4-11 **A,** At longer fibre length, myosin filaments are disposed in series; and **B,** at shorter fibre length, thick filaments are disposed in parallel.

4. Marked Shortening of Smooth Muscle during Contraction Marked shortening of smooth muscle during contraction is another characteristic of smooth muscle that makes it different from the skeletal muscle. A smooth muscle can contract more than two thirds its stretched length, while a skeletal muscle can contract up to one third its stretched length. This property allows the smooth muscle to perform, especially important, functions in the hollow viscera, allowing the gut, bladder, blood vessels and other internal bodily structures to change their lumen diameters from very large down to almost zero.

5. Energy Required to Sustain Smooth Muscle Contraction Energy required to sustain smooth muscle contraction is much less that required by a skeletal muscle. It is because of the fact that the attachment cycling of the cross-bridges is slow in smooth muscles and that only one molecule of ATP is required for each cycle, regardless of its duration.

Excitation and Inhibition of Smooth Muscles

Excitation of Smooth Muscles

Multiunit Smooth Muscles are stimulated only through nerves.

Single-unit Smooth Muscles can be excited by several ways:

- Through nerves (i.e. by neurotransmitter such as ACh),
- By hormones (Fig. 2.4-12A and B),
- Through pacemaker (spontaneous excitation),
- Stretching (due to stretch receptor) and
- Cold temperature.

Functions. After excitations, smooth muscles perform following functions:

- Control the movement of material through most of the hollow organs.

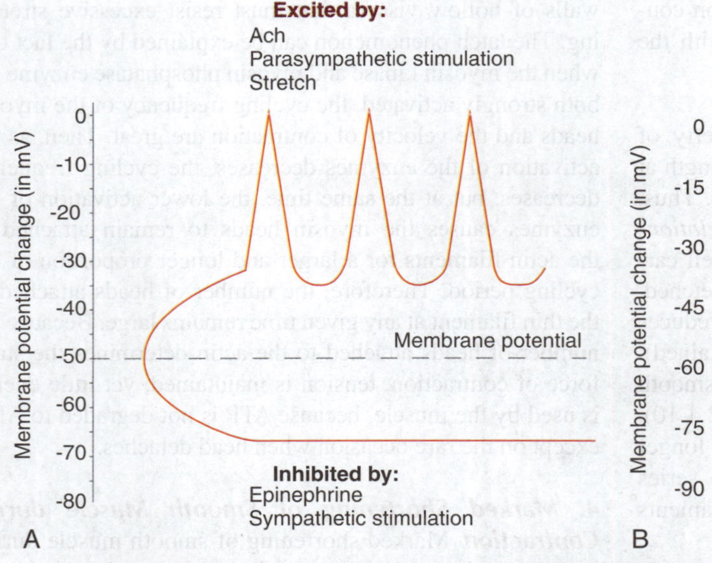

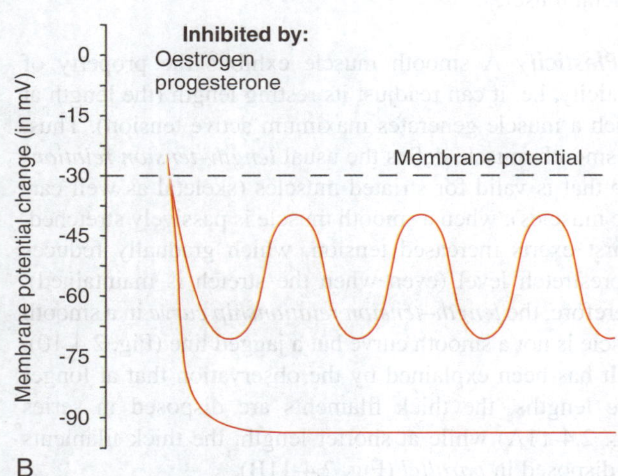

FIGURE 2.4-12 Effect of various agents on the membrane potential of smooth muscles: **A,** intestinal wall; and **B,** uterus.

- Propel material in the gastrointestinal tract.
- Control flow of blood in the arterioles.
- Expel material from the bladder and vas deferens.
- Control piloerection.
- Muscles of iris control the amount of light reaching the retina.

Inhibition of Smooth Muscles

- ***Through Nerves*** (i.e. by neurotransmitter epinephrine) by sympathetic stimulation, e.g. in case of intestinal smooth muscle.

- ***Through Hormones,*** e.g. progesterone decreases the activity of the uterus by acting on pacemaker potential (Fig. 2.4-12A and B).

Applied Aspects

- In ***Bronchial asthma,*** over excitation of airway's smooth muscles leads to bronchial constriction, therefore, for quick relief, inhalers are commonly used because they deliver β-adrenergic agonist (e.g. ventoline, albuterol and sambutirol).
- ***To increase blood flow,*** *nitric oxide (NO)* is a natural molecule that relaxes smooth muscles of the blood vessels. Its mechanism of action through enzyme phosphodiesterase (PDE), which transforms cyclic guanosine monophosphate (c GMP) into GMP. The specific inhibitors of PDE V (an isoform found in corpora cavernosa of penis) like sildenafil, tadalafil and vardenafil are used for increasing blood flow to offset erectile dysfunction. For details see page 351.

CARDIAC MUSCLE

Functional Anatomy

- Structural organization of cardiac muscle
- Structure of a cardiac muscle fibre
- Sarcotubular system.

Process of Excitability and Contractility

- Electrical potentials in cardiac muscle
- Excitation–contraction coupling phenomenon
- Process of cardiac muscle contraction.

Properties of Cardiac Muscle

- Automaticity
- Rhythmicity
- Conductivity
- Excitability
- Contractility.

Functional anatomy and physiology of cardiac muscle is discussed in Chapter 4.1 of 'Cardiovascular System' (see page 240).

COMPARISON OF SKELETAL, SMOOTH AND CARDIAC MUSCLES

The salient features of skeletal, smooth and cardiac muscles are shown in Table 2.4-1.

TABLE 2.4-1 Comparison of Skeletal, Smooth and Cardiac Muscles

Feature	Skeletal muscle	Cardiac muscle	Smooth muscle
Structural Features			
• Striations	Present	Present	Absent
• Size of fibres			
• length	1–40 mm	80–100 μm	50–500 μm
• diameter	50–500 μm	15 μm	2–10 μm
• Shape of the muscle fibre	Cylindrical	Cylindrical	Spindle shaped
• Branching of fibres	Absent	Present	Absent
• Connection between fibres	Absent	Functional connections present forming functional syncytium	In single-unit muscle, functional connections are present. In multiunit muscles, no connections
• Nucleus	Single or multiple at periphery	Single, central with many nuclei	Single
• Sarcoplasmic reticulum (SR)	Very well developed	Well developed but not as in skeletal muscles	Moderately developed
• Sarcotubular system	Well developed, two triads present at A-I junction	Present, one triad per sarcomere, T-tubule present at Z-line	Present, but not well developed
• Thick and thin filaments	Arranged regularly	Arranged regularly	Not arranged regularly
• Sarcomere	Present	Present	Not present
• Regulating protein	Troponin	Troponin	Calmodulin
• Calcium store and calcium pump in SR	High	Moderate	Low
• Sodium channels in the membrane	Fast voltage-gated Na^+ channels	Fast voltage-gated Na^+ channels with slow voltage-gated Na^+–Ca^{2+} channels	Mainly slow voltage-gated Na^+–Ca^{2+} channels. Very few fast voltage-gated Na^+ channels
• Mitochondria	Few	Many	Few
Nerve Supply and Control			
• Nerve supply	Somatic nerves	Autonomic nerves – Sympathetic: excitatory (transmitter—norepinephrine) – Parasympathatic: inhibitory (transmitter—acetylcholine)	Autonomic nerves – Sympathetic: inhibitory – Parasympathatic: excitatory
• Control	Voluntary	Involuntary	Involuntary
Electrical Features			
• Resting membrane potential	−90 mV	−90 mV	−55 mV
• Action potential shape and duration	Spike potential of 5 ms	Plateau potential of 100–300 ms	– Single-unit muscle: variable, plateau potential of 100–1000 ms and spike potential also seen of 10–50 ms duration – Multiunit muscle: spike potential
• Stimulated by	Somatic nerves	Autonomic nerves	Autonomic nerves, hormones and local tissue factors
• Excitability	High	Moderate	Low
• Conductivity	Fast	Slow	Slow
• Absolute refractory period	1–3 ms	180–200 ms	Not defined
• Autorhythmicity	Not present	Present	Present in single-unit muscle

Continued

TABLE 2.4-1 Comparison of Skeletal, Smooth and Cardiac Muscles—cont'd

Feature	Skeletal muscle	Cardiac muscle	Smooth muscle
Excitation–contraction Coupling			
• Speed of phenomenon	Rapid	Very rapid	Very slow
• Site of calcium attachment	Troponin	Troponin	Myosin
• Mechanism of Ca^{2+} mobilization	T-tubule is depolarized	Ca^{2+}-induced Ca^{2+} release	Inositol triphosphate increases release of Ca^{2+}
• Dependence on concentration of ECF calcium concentration	Not dependent	Partly dependent	Almost totally dependent
Contractility Characteristics			
• Rate of contraction	Fast	Fast	Slow
• Rate of relaxation	Fast	Fast	Slow
• Duration of muscle twitch	– In fast fibres: 7.5 ms – In slow fibres: 100 ms	1½ times the total duration of action potential	About 1000 ms
• All or none law	Obeyed by single muscle fibre	Obeyed by whole muscle	– Single-unit muscle: obeyed by whole muscle – Multiunit muscle: obeyed by single muscle fibre
• Multiple fibre (quantal) summations	Possible	Not possible, as it is a functional syncytium	Not possible
• Tetanus (wave summation)	Possible	Not possible due to long refractory period	Not possible, as the process of contraction is long
• Fatigue	Possible	None, since long refractory period ensures recovery and also due to presence of more blood supply	Possible but difficult to demonstrate
• Length–tension relationship	Maximum tension is developed at optimal length	Maximum tension developed at optimal length	Shows property of plasticity
Chemical Composition, Blood Supply, Oxygen Consumption and Muscle Energetics			
• Protein	Maximum	Less	Less
• Glycogen	Less	More	Less
• ATP and phosphogen	Present	Present	Present
• Fats	Mainly neutral fats	More phospholipids and cholesterol than others	Mainly neutral fats
• Blood supply	840 ml/min (3–4 ml/100 g/min)	Abundant, 250 ml/min (80 ml/100 g/min)	350 ml/min (1.4 ml/100 g/min)
• Oxygen consumption	Moderate	High	Low
Energy Utilization Under Basal State by			
• Fats	20%	60%	Mainly
• Carbohydrates	60%	35%	Very few
• Proteins	20%	5%	Very few

Section 3

Blood and Immune System

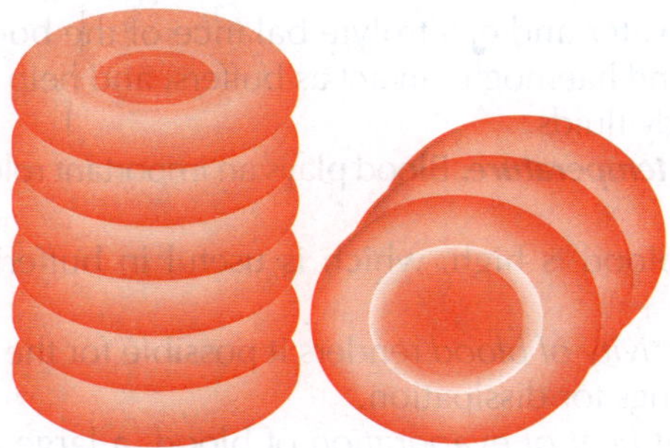

Blood is a fluid connective tissue which transports substances from one part of the body to another. It provides nutrients and hormones to the tissues and removes their waste products. Blood, confined in the cardiovascular system, constitutes a major part of the extracellular fluid of the body.

Some of the important physical characteristics of blood are:

- ***Colour*** of blood is opaque red due to the pigment haemoglobin in the RBCs. The arterial blood is bright red and venous blood is dark red in colour.
- ***Volume*** of blood in an average adult is about 5–6 L (8% of the body weight or 80 ml/kg body weight).
- ***Viscosity*** of blood is five times more than that of water.
- ***Specific gravity*** of blood is 1.050–1.060. Specific gravity of RBC is greater (1.090) than that of plasma (1.030).
- ***pH of blood*** is about 7.4 (ranges from 7.38 to 7.42), i.e. it is alkaline in nature. In acidosis, pH of blood falls below 7.38 and in alkalosis pH is more than 7.42.

Blood is composed of two main components, plasma and cellular elements.

Plasma constitutes about 55% of the blood volume. It is a clear straw-coloured fluid portion of blood. ***Plasma proteins,*** an important constituent of plasma, form about 7% of its volume.

Cellular elements of blood are about 45% of the total blood volume and constitute the so-called packed cell volume (PCV).

Blood cells are:

- Erythrocytes or red blood cells (5 million/mm^3),
- Leucocytes or white blood cells (4000–11,000/mm^3) and
- Platelets or thrombocytes (1.5–4 lakh/mm^3).

Functions of Blood

1. ***Nutritive function.*** Blood carries the nutritive substances like glucose, amino acids, fatty acids, vitamins, electrolytes and others, from the gut to the tissues where they are utilized.
2. ***Respiratory functions.*** Blood picks up oxygen from the lungs and delivers it to the various tissues. The most important function of blood is the uninterrupted delivery of O_2 to the heart and brain. It also carries away CO_2 from the tissues to the lungs, from where it is expelled out in the expired air.
3. ***Excretory function.*** Blood transports various metabolic waste products, such as urea, uric acid and creatinine, to the excretory organs (kidney, skin, intestine and lungs) for their disposal.
4. ***Transport function.*** The various hormones produced by the endocrine glands, the biological enzymes and antibodies are transported by the blood to the target tissue, to modulate metabolic process.
5. ***Protective function.*** Blood plays an important role in the defence mechanism of the body:
   - Neutrophils and monocytes engulf the microorganisms entering the body by phagocytosis.
   - Lymphocytes and gamma globulins initiate an immune response.
   - Eosinophils accomplish detoxification, disintegration and removal of foreign proteins.
6. ***Homeostatic function.*** Blood plays an important role in maintaining the internal environment of the body (homeostatic function):
   - The water content of blood is freely interchangeable with the interstitial fluid and helps in maintaining the water and electrolyte balance of the body.
   - Plasma proteins and haemoglobin act as buffers, and help in maintaining the acid–base balance and pH of the body fluids.
7. ***Maintenance of body temperature.*** Blood plays an important role in regulation of the body temperature, as described:
   - *Specific heat* of blood is high, which is useful in buffering the sudden changes in the body temperature.
   - *High heat conductivity of blood* renders it possible for the distribution of heat from deep organs to the skin and lungs for dissipation.
   - Due to *high latent heat of evaporation* of blood, a large amount of heat is lost from the body by evaporation of water from the lungs and skin.
8. ***Storage function.*** Blood serves as a ready-made source of substances stored in it (such as glucose, water, proteins and electrolytes for use in emergency conditions like starvation, fluid loss and electrolyte loss).

Immune System

The immune system that constitutes the body's defence system consists of immunological cells distributed in two main components: mononuclear phagocytic system and lymphoid component. The immune system of the body responds to an antigen by two ways:

- ***Humoral or antibody-mediated immunity (AMI)*** which is mediated by antibodies produced by plasma cells.
- ***Cell-mediated immunity (CMI)*** which is mediated directly by the sensitized lymphocytes.

Chapter 3.1

Plasma and Plasma Proteins

PLASMA

Plasma is the clear straw-coloured fluid (with dissolved solid substances) portion of the blood minus its cellular elements. It constitutes about 55% of the blood volume.

Composition

Plasma contains the following constituents:

Water. Water is the main constituent of plasma, forming 91% of it.

Solids. The solids dissolved in the plasma constitute a total of 9% of the plasma. The solid constituents of the plasma are given below.

- ***Plasma proteins*** form 7% of the solids in plasma. Their normal value ranges from 6.4 to 8.3 g/dL. They include albumin, globulins, fibrinogen and others.
- ***Other organic molecules*** which form 1% of the solids include the following:
  - *Carbohydrates,* mainly glucose (100–120 mg/dL).
  - *Fats* are neutral fats (30–150 mg/dL), phospholipids (150–300 mg/dL) and cholesterol (150–240 mg/dL).
  - *Nonprotein nitrogenous (NPN) substances* (28–40 mg/dL) are ammonia (traces), amino acids, creatine (1–2 mg/dL), creatinine (0.6–1.2 mg/dL), xanthine (traces), hypoxanthine (traces), urea (20–40 mg/dL) and uric acid (2–4 mg/dL).
  - *Hormones, enzymes and antibodies.*
- ***Inorganic substances*** which constitute 1% of the solids in plasma include sodium, potassium, calcium, magnesium, chloride, iodide, iron, phosphates and copper.

Gases. Gases present in the plasma are oxygen, carbon dioxide and nitrogen.

Serum

Plasma from which fibrinogen and clotting factors (II, V and VIII) have been removed is called serum. Serum is formed when the blood is allowed to clot in a test tube and clot is retracted. Serum has a higher serotonin (5HT) content because of the breakdown of platelets during clotting.

PLASMA PROTEINS

Classification of Plasma Proteins

Plasma proteins form the major solid constituent of the plasma. The total plasma protein concentration is 7.4 g/dL (ranges from 6.4 to 8.3 g/dL). The major forms of plasma proteins are albumin, globulins and fibrinogen. Since serum is plasma minus clotting protein (fibrinogen), therefore, the albumin and globulins are usually referred to as serum albumin and serum globulins. Presently, more than 100 types of plasma proteins have been identified. The original classification is based on the classical method of precipitation of salts as described by Howe (1922). By electrophoretic techniques, the globulins have been further subclassified. Based on these, the important fractions of plasma proteins are given below:

- Albumin (4.8 g/dL),
- Globulins (2.3 g/dL) include:
  - Alpha 1 (α_1) globulin,
  - Alpha 2 (α_2) globulin,
  - Beta (β) globulin and
  - Gamma (γ) globulin.
- Fibrinogen (0.3 g/dL).

Methods of Separation of Plasma Proteins

1. Precipitation by Salting out Different fractions of the plasma proteins are precipitated out by using different concentrations of the salts as described below.

Sodium sulphate solution was used by Howe in 1922. He fractionized the plasma proteins in three major fractions:

- *Fibrinogen* is removed with clot converting plasma into serum,
- *Globulins* are precipitated out by 22% sodium sulphate solution from the serum and
- *Albumin* remains in the serum.

Ammonium sulphate solution is utilized to precipitate the plasma protein fractions in different strengths:

- *Albumin* is precipitated by full saturation.
- *Globulins* are precipitated by half saturation. Among the globulins, there is a fraction which can be precipitated by one-third saturation with ammonium sulphate and is termed *euglobulin.* The rest is called *pseudoglobulin.*
- *Fibrinogen* is separated by one-fifth saturation with ammonium sulphate.

2. Cohn's Fractional Precipitation Method Varying concentrations of *ethanol* solution are used at low temperature to fractionalize the plasma proteins. Each fraction, so obtained, though being a mixture of proteins, it contains one of the proteins predominantly as given below.

- *Fraction I* is rich in fibrinogen,
- *Fraction II* mainly contains gamma globulins,
- *Fraction III* contains alpha and beta globulins, including isoagglutinins and prothrombin,
- *Fraction IV* mainly consists of alpha and beta globulins and
- *Fraction V* is rich in albumin.

3. Electrophoresis Separation of Protein Fractions The electrophoresis method separates the plasma proteins into different fractions, depending upon the electric charge of each fraction due to a difference in their migration rates. Serum should be used for electrophoresis, as the fibrinogen of plasma gives a discrete band which can easily be mistaken for a paraprotein.

Technique. Various techniques of electrophoresis have been developed. Depending upon the support medium used, common methods are:

- Tiselius or free boundary electrophoresis,
- Paper electrophoresis,
- Cellulose acetate strip electrophoresis and
- Agar gel electrophoresis.

Electrophoretic protein patterns. Mostly in clinical laboratories, cellulose acetate is used as a supporting medium. After resolution and staining, five bands of plasma proteins are identified. The amount of these bands can be quantified using densitometric staining techniques. On the basis of paper electrophoresis, the following classes of serum proteins (Fig. 3.1-1) are identified:

- Albumin (55%),
- Alpha-1 globulins (5%),
- Alpha-2 globulins (9%),

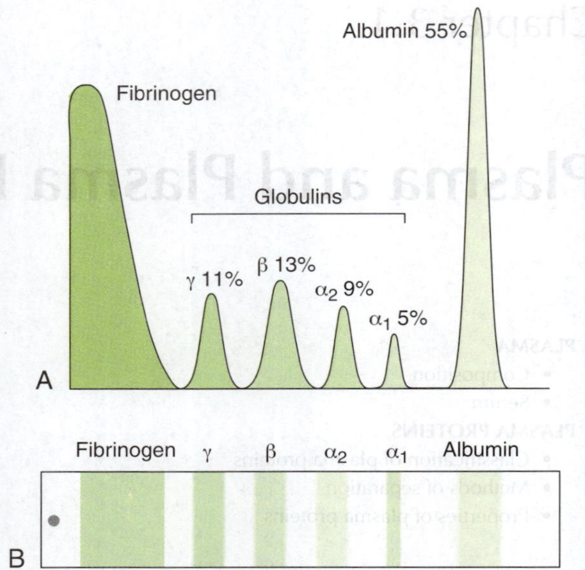

FIGURE 3.1-1 Paper electrophoresis showing: **A,** relative amount of plasma proteins and **B,** bands of different plasma proteins.

- Beta globulins (13%) and
- Gamma globulins (11%).

Clinical use. Electrophoretic separation is very useful in clinical diagnosis. It helps in knowing:

- The change in relative concentration of different proteins,
- The presence of abnormal proteins and
- The absence of normal proteins.

4. Immunoelectrophoresis Technique This technique makes use of the antigenicity and electric charge of protein to separate them. The proteins are separated on the basis of electrophoretic patterns formed by precipitation at the site of antigen–antibody reaction. This technique is more specific and the number of fractions obtained is much more than the ordinary electrophoresis.

5. Ultracentrifugation Technique In this technique, a suitable preparation of plasma in buffered solution is centrifuged at a speed up to 60,000 rpm and a force up to 160,000 g. The proteins are separated into fractions depending upon their *sedimentation constant,* which is the property of weight, shape and density of the protein molecules.

Three different sediments, albumin, globulin and fibrinogen, are formed. This method is also useful in determining the molecular weight of these proteins.

Properties of Plasma Proteins

1. Molecular Weight Plasma proteins are large molecules with the following molecular weight:

- Albumin: 69,000,
- Globulins: From 90,000 to 156,000 and
- Fibrinogen: 500,000.

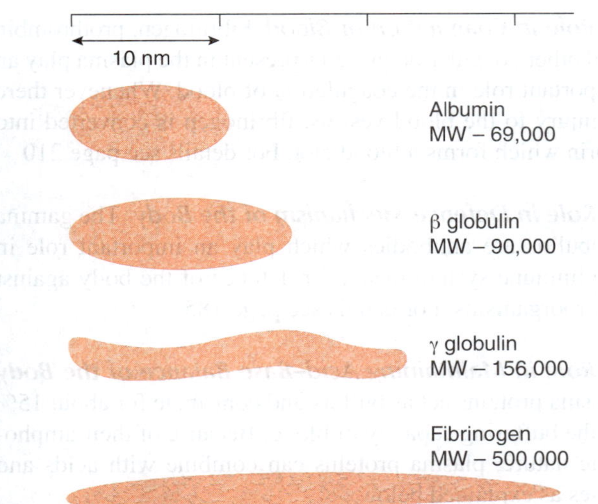

FIGURE 3.1-2 Relative dimensions, molecular weights and shapes of different plasma proteins.

Thus, fibrinogen has the highest molecular weight. Relative size and shape of different plasma proteins are shown in Fig. 3.1-2.

2. Osmotic Pressure The plasma proteins exert an oncotic pressure of about 25 mmHg.

3. Specific Gravity The specific gravity of the plasma proteins is 1.026.

4. Isoelectric Point Proteins can ionize either as acids or as bases owing to the fact that the side chains of their constituent amino acids contain a selection of amino group (NH_2) and carboxyl groups (–COOH). At an intermediate pH (specific for each protein), the protein molecules carry an equal number of positive and negative charges and hence, have a zero net charge. This pH value for electrical neutrality of the molecule is known as the *isoelectric point.*

5. Electrophoretic Mobility Proteins act as *anions* in alkaline solutions and as *cations* in acidic solutions. Because of this property, they possess electrophoretic mobility.

6. Precipitation by Salts Proteins can be precipitated by different concentrations of salts. This property of proteins is utilized for their separation by the precipitation method.

7. Water Solubility Protein molecules are soluble in water because of the presence of polar residues like NH_2 and COOH.

8. Amphoteric Nature Protein molecules are amphoteric in nature because of the presence of NH_2 and COOH groups. By virtue of their amphoteric nature, the plasma proteins act as efficient buffers.

Features of Individual Fractions of Plasma Proteins

1. Albumin.

- ***Plasma levels*** are 4.8 g/dL (range 3–5 g/dL).
- ***Molecular weight*** of prealbumin is 60,000 and that of albumin is 69,000.
- ***Synthesized*** in liver.
- ***Half-life*** is about 10 days.

2. Globulins.

- ***Plasma levels*** are 2.3 g/dL (range 2–3 g/dL).
- ***Molecular weight*** varies from 90,000 to 15,600.
- ***Types*** include alpha-1, alpha-2, beta-1, beta-2 and gamma globulins.
- ***Forms of globulins*** are described below:
  i. *Glycoproteins* consist of carbohydrates and protein.
  ii. *Lipoproteins* consist of alpha-2 globulin and lipids. It has got the following subtypes:
     - *High-density lipoproteins (HDL).* These are alpha lipoproteins which contain 50% protein with large amount of cholesterol and phospholipids.
     - *Low-density lipoproteins (LDL).* These are beta lipoproteins and contain large amount of glycerides.
     - *Very low-density lipoproteins (VLDL).* These are also beta lipoproteins and have higher proportion of fat in the form of triglycerides or cholesterol.
     - *Chylomicron (CM)* contains 98% triglycerides. It is synthesized in the intestine following a meal.

Important Notes

The HDL level is decreased by smoking, sedentary habits and obesity, whereas exercise and moderate intake of alcohol increase the level of HDL.

  iii. *Transferrin* is an alpha 2-beta globulin having a molecular weight of 90,000. It has the specific property of iron binding, and thus helps in its transport and storage. Each molecule of transferrin binds two atoms of ferric iron.
  iv. *Haptoglobin (Hb–Hp)* is an alpha-2 globulin having a molecular weight of 90,000. It forms stable complexes with free haemoglobin. However, the Hb–Hp complex is too large to pass through glomerulus; thus the function of Hb–Hp is to prevent the loss of free Hb into the urine, thereby conserving valuable iron present in the haemoglobin.
     - Haptoglobin is an acute phase protein and its level is elevated in many inflammatory states.
  v. *Ceruloplasmin* is an alpha 2-beta globulin having a molecular weight of 16,000. It binds with copper and helps in its transport and storage. Its deficiency causes Wilson's disease (hepatolenticular degeneration), a disease caused due to abnormal copper metabolism

in which the liver and brain are damaged due to high levels of free copper.

Menkes disease is another disorder of copper metabolism that occurs due to mutation in the gene for copper binding P-Type of ATPase. It is a sex-linked disease, which affects only the male infants mainly involve the nervous system, connective tissue and vasculature, and is usually fatal in infancy. This disease is also called '*Kinky or Steely hair disease*'.

vi. *Fetuin* is a growth-promoting protein seen in infants and newborns.

vii. *Immunoglobulins* are gamma globulins which play a role in immunity.

viii. *Angiotensinogen* is an alpha-2 globulin.

ix. *Haemagglutinins* are antibodies against the red blood cells antigens.

3. Fibrinogen

- ***Plasma levels*** are 0.3 g/dL.
- ***Molecular weight*** varies from 400,000 to 500,000.
- ***Synthesized*** in the liver.
- ***Chemical structure***. Protein part of the molecule is made up of six polypeptide chains (α_2, β_2 and γ_2) joined by disulphide bonds.
- ***Functions*** as a clotting protein.

4. Prothrombin

- ***Plasma levels*** are 40 mg/dL.
- ***Molecular weight*** is 68,000.
- ***Synthesized*** in the liver. Synthesis is promoted by vitamin K.

Functions of Plasma Proteins

1. Exert Osmotic Pressure Protein molecules are unable to pass across the capillary membrane and consequently exert colloid osmotic pressure of about 25 mmHg on the capillary membrane. About 70–80% of the osmotic pressure is contributed by the albumin fraction. The colloid osmotic pressure plays an important role in the exchange of water between the blood and tissue fluid as explained below:

- At the *arterial end of capillaries*, due to higher hydrostatic pressure than the colloid osmotic pressure, filtration of fluid out from vessels to tissue spaces occurs.
- At the *venous end of capillaries*, due to lower hydrostatic pressure than the colloid osmotic pressure, absorption of fluid from the tissue spaces into the vessels occurs (see page 318).

2. Contribution to Blood Viscosity Plasma proteins, owing to their size and particularly their shape, greatly contribute to the blood viscosity. Fibrinogen and globulins are significant contributors to blood viscosity because of their asymmetrical shape. The blood viscosity plays an important role in the maintenance of blood pressure by providing resistance to the flow of blood in blood vessels.

3. Role in Coagulation of Blood Fibrinogen, prothrombin and other coagulation proteins present in the plasma play an important role in the coagulation of blood. Whenever there is injury to the blood vessels, fibrinogen is converted into fibrin which forms a blood clot. For details see page 210

4. Role in Defence Mechanism of the Body The gamma globulins are antibodies which play an important role in the immune system meant for defence of the body against microorganisms. For details see page 185

5. Role in Maintaining Acid–Base Balance of the Body Plasma proteins act as buffers and contribute for about 15% of the buffering capacity of blood. Because of their amphoteric nature, plasma proteins can combine with acids and bases as explained below:

- *In acidic pH,* the NH_2 group of the proteins acts as a base and accepts proton and is converted to NH_4.
- *In alkaline pH,* the COOH group of the proteins acts as an acid and can donate a proton and thus becomes COO^- and
- *At normal pH* of blood, proteins act as acids and combine with cations (mainly sodium).

6. Transport Function Plasma proteins combine easily with many substances and play an essential role in their transport as explained below:

- *Carbon dioxide* is transported by plasma proteins in the form of carbamino compound.
- *Thyroxine* is transported by an alpha globulin called thyroxine-binding protein (TBP).
- *Cortisol* is transported by transcortin which is a mucoprotein.
- *Vitamin A, D and E* are transported by the high- and low-density lipoproteins (HDL and LDL).
- *Vitamin B*12 is bound to transcobalamin for transport.
- *Bilirubin* is associated with albumin and also with fractions of the alpha globulin.
- *Drugs* of various types are transported after combining with albumin.
- *Calcium* present in the plasma is partly (50%) bound to the proteins for transport.
- *Copper* is bound to ceruloplasmin (alpha-2 globulin) for transport.
- *Free haemoglobin* in the vessels is bound by haptoglobin and carried to the reticuloendothelial system.

7. Role as Reserve Proteins Plasma proteins serve as reserve proteins and are utilized by the body tissues during conditions like:

- Fasting,
- Inadequate protein intake and
- Excessive catabolism of body proteins.

8. Role in the Suspension Stability of the Red Blood Cells Suspension stability refers to the property of red blood cells by the virtue of which they remain uniformly suspended in the blood. Globulins and fibrinogen accelerate this property.

9. Fibrinolytic Function The enzymes of the fibrinolytic system digest the intravascular clot (thrombus) and thus save from the disastrous effects of thrombosis.

10. Role of Nourishment of Tissue Cells Plasma proteins are utilized by the leucocytes to produce substances known as *trephones* or *carrel,* which are essential for the nourishment of tissue cells.

11. Role in Genetic Information Many plasma proteins exhibit *polymorphism.* Polymorphism is a Mendelian trait that exists in the population with differing prevalence. They serve as a valuable tool for the studies of population genetics. Plasma proteins that show polymorphism are haptoglobin, transferrin, ceruloplasmin and immunoglobulins.

Synthesis of Plasma Proteins

Site of Synthesis *In an embryo,* plasma proteins are synthesized by the mesenchymal cells through a process of secretion or dissolution of their substances. First, albumin is produced and then other proteins are synthesized.

In adults, plasma proteins are synthesized as described below:

- Albumin and fibrinogen are synthesized mostly by reticuloendothelial cells of the liver.
- Alpha and beta globulins are synthesized by the liver, spleen and bone marrow.
- Gamma globulins are synthesized by B lymphocytes.

Plasma proteins are generally synthesized on the membrane-bound polyribosomes. They traverse the major secretory route in the cell (rough ER membrane → smooth ER membrane → Golgi apparatus → secretory vesicle) before entering into the plasma. Thus, most plasma proteins are synthesized as preprotein form.

Factors Affecting Synthesis of Plasma Proteins

1. Dietary Proteins. Dietary proteins play the most essential role in the synthesis of plasma proteins. The relation of plasma proteins to diet was studied in plasma protein-depleted dogs first by Whipple George H in 1956 by an experiment procedure called *plasmapheresis.*

Plasmapheresis. In this experiment, the dog is rendered hypoproteinaemic by repeatedly withdrawing whole blood and injecting back the cellular elements of the blood (suspended in Ringer–Locke solution). This process is repeated daily till the level of plasma proteins falls to 4 g/100 ml. Thereafter, different standard diets are given and their effects on protein synthesis are studied. Following conclusions have been drawn from these experiments:

- *Dietary proteins* are essential for the synthesis of plasma proteins.
- *Chemical resemblance* of food protein amino acid with those of the plasma proteins to be synthesized determines their efficacy to synthesize a particular protein.
- *Essential amino acids* must be present in the diet for the satisfactory synthesis of plasma proteins.
- *Dietary proteins of animal origin* favour albumin synthesis.
- *Dietary proteins of plant origin* favour globulin synthesis.
- *Regeneration period.* Regeneration of plasma proteins occurs within 14 days.
- *Rate of regeneration* of plasma proteins is very fast, within first 24 h.

2. Other Factors. Other factors which effect plasma protein synthesis in the body are as follows:

- *Presence of infection* in the body reduces plasma protein synthesis.
- *Exposure to some antigen* stimulates formation of antibodies.
- *Inflammatory conditions* promote the synthesis of a number of other proteins.
- *Variation in colloid oncotic pressure* influences the albumin synthesis.
- *Interleukin-1,* a material released by the activated macrophages in the body, stimulates the synthesis of many acute phase proteins in the liver.
- *Prostaglandins* are also reported to increase the synthesis of acute phase proteins, possibly through stimulation of macrophage release of interleukin-1.

Changes in Plasma Proteins in Health and Disease

Normal Levels

- ***Total proteins:*** 7.4 g/dL (range 6.4–8.3 g/dL),
- ***Albumin:*** 4.8 g/dL (range 3.5–5.5 g/dL),
- ***Globulin:*** 2.3 g/dL (range 2–3.5 g/dL) and
- ***Albumin: globulin ratio*** *(A/G ratio)* is 1.7:1.

Physiological Variations

- ***In infants,*** the total protein level is low (about 5.5 g/dL) due to low gamma globulins.
- ***In old age,*** there is a tendency for the albumin level to fall and the total globulin level to rise.
- ***In pregnancy,*** during first 6 months, the albumin and globulin levels decrease while the fibrinogen level increases.

Abnormalities of Plasma Protein Levels

Hypoproteinaemia. Hypoproteinaemia refers to generalized decrease in the levels of plasma proteins.

Causes of Hypoproteinaemia include the following:

- ***Dietary deficiency*** and starvation are associated with hypoproteinaemia after the body's reserve proteins are depleted.
- ***Malabsorption syndrome*** due to intestinal diseases, such as sprue, is associated with hypoproteinaemia.
- ***Liver diseases*** like hepatitis and cirrhosis cause hypoproteinaemia due to reduced synthesis of proteins in the liver.
- ***Renal diseases*** like nephrotic syndrome cause hypoproteinaemia due to more loss of proteins in the urine.
- ***Haemorrhage and extensive burns*** are associated with acute hypoproteinaemia.
- ***Hereditary analbuminaemia*** is an inborn defect in the genetic level, where there is no synthesis of albumin.
- ***Congenital afibrinogenaemia*** is a rare condition characterized by defective blood clotting.

Effects of Hypoproteinaemia Low levels of plasma proteins are associated with a decrease in the plasma osmotic pressure, which causes water retention and oedema of the body tissue.

Hyperproteinaemia. Hyperproteinaemia, i.e. increase in the plasma protein levels, is seen in the following conditions:

- *Acute inflammatory conditions* are associated with increased synthesis of the so-called *acute phase proteins,* which include C-reactive proteins, alpha antitrypsin, haptoglobin, fibrinogen and ceruloplasmin.
- *Acute tissue destruction* as in myocardial infarction is also associated with raised levels of acute phase proteins.
- *Chronic inflammation and malignancies* are also associated with raised levels of C-reactive proteins.
- *Multiple myeloma* is associated with the increased levels of the so-called *Bence–Jones* proteins and myeloma globulin due to their abnormal formation in the bone marrow.

Reversal of Normal A/G Ratio The normal albumin: globulin (A/G) ratio (1.7:1) is reversed in the following conditions:

- When albumin synthesis is decreased as it occurs in liver diseases (globulin levels being normal because many globulins are synthesized by B lymphocytes).
- When globulin levels are increased (as occurs in most of the conditions) associated with hyperproteinaemia.

Chapter 3.2

Red Blood Cells and Anaemias

CHARACTERISTIC FEATURES OF RED BLOOD CELLS

Functional Morphology

The red blood cells (mature erythrocytes) form one of the important constituents of the cellular elements of the blood. Each red blood cell (RBC), like any other cell in the body is bounded by a *cell membrane* but is *non-nucleated* and lacks the usual cell organelles. The cytoplasm of the RBC contains a special pigmented protein called the *haemoglobin* which forms 90% of the weight of the erythrocyte. The red colour of the RBCs, and thus of the blood, is due to the presence of haemoglobin.

Normal Size, Shape and Counts of RBCs

Normal Size

- *Diameter* of each RBC is 7.2 μm (range 6.9–7.4 μm),
- *Thickness* in the periphery is 2 μm and in the centre 1 μm,
- *Surface area* of each RBC is about 120–140 μm^2 and
- *Volume* is about 80 μm^3 (range 78–86 μm^3).

Normal Shape

The red blood cells are circular, biconcave discs (Fig. 3.2-1).

Advantages of biconcave shape are:

- It renders the red cells quite flexible so that they can pass through capillaries whose minimum diameter is 3.5 μm (Fig. 3.2-2).
- The biconcavity provides greater surface area as compared to volume which allows considerable alterations in the cell volume. Thus, the RBC can withstand considerable changes of osmotic pressure or minimum tension is offered on the membrane when changes in volume of cells occur. In this way, the RBCs can resist haemolysis to a certain extent when placed in hypotonic solutions.
- Greater surface area allows easy exchange of O_2 and CO_2 and rapid diffusion of other substances.

Normal Counts

- *At birth,* normal RBC count is 6–7 million/mm^3.
- *In adult males,* the normal count varies from 5 to 6.5 million/mm^3 (average 5.5 million/mm^3).

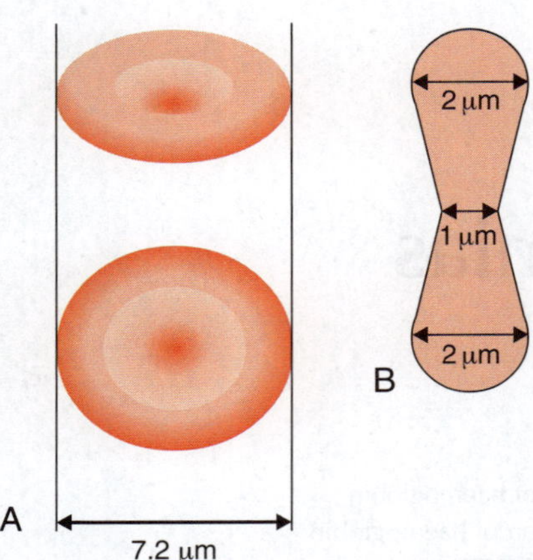

FIGURE 3.2-1 Size and shape of a normal red blood cell: **A,** biconcave disc (diameter 7.2 µm); and **B,** thickness (2 µm at the periphery and 1 µm in the centre).

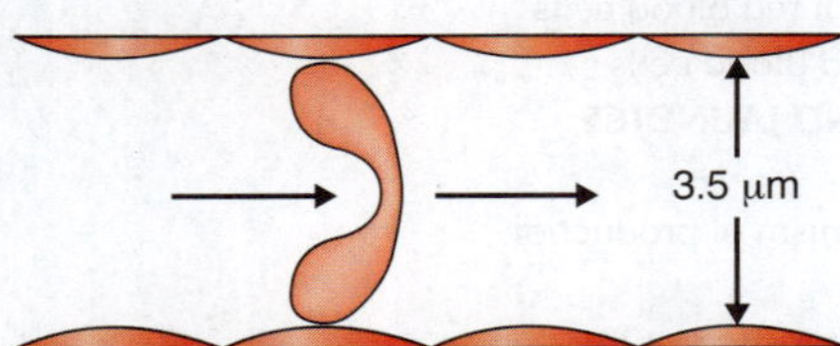

FIGURE 3.2-2 Showing how flexibility of red blood cell allows it to pass through smaller capillaries (diameter 3.5 µm).

- *In females,* it varies from 4.5 to 5.5 million/mm^3 (average 4.8 million/mm^3).
- *Clinically,* a count of 5 million/mm^3 is considered as 100%.

Variations in Size, Shape and Counts of RBCs

Variations in Size. Variation in size is called *anisocytosis:*

- ***Microcytosis,*** i.e. decrease in the size of red blood cells occurs:
  - In iron deficiency anaemia,
  - During prolonged forced breathing and
  - When osmotic pressure of blood is increased.
- ***Macrocytosis,*** i.e. increase in the size of red blood cells occurs:
  - In megaloblastic anaemia,
  - During muscular exercise and
  - When osmotic pressure of blood is decreased.

Variations in Shape. Variation in shape is called *poikilocytosis.* Abnormal shapes of the RBCs are (Fig. 3.2-3) given below:

- *Crenation or shrinkage* of RBCs is seen when they are suspended in hypertonic solution. This occurs because of the outward diffusion of water from the red blood cells.
- *Spherocyte* is a globular-shaped RBC. It is seen in a hereditary disease called spherocytosis. These cells are more fragile. Similar changes in the shape of RBCs are observed when they are suspended in hypotonic solutions.
- *Elliptocytes,* i.e. elliptical shape of the RBCs is seen in certain anaemias.

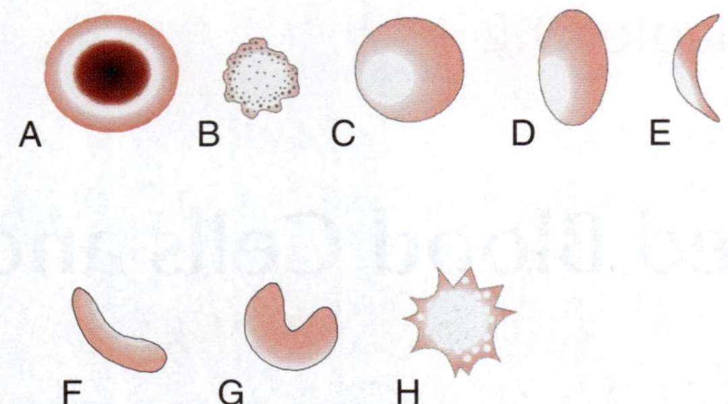

FIGURE 3.2-3 Variations in the shapes of red blood cells: **A,** normal; **B,** crenation; **C,** spherocyte; **D,** elliptocyte; **E,** sickle cell; **F,** discocyte; **G,** stomatocyte; and **H,** echinocyte.

- *Sickle cell,* i.e. crescent shape of the RBCs occurs in sickle cell anaemia because of the presence of abnormal haemoglobin (haemoglobin S).
- *Poikilocytes,* i.e. unusual shapes of RBCs such as flask-shaped, hammer-shaped or other abnormal shapes occur due to deformed cell membrane.

Variations in Counts ***Physiological increase in the RBC count (physiological polycythaemia)*** is seen in the following circumstances:

- *Age.* At birth, the RBC count is 6–7 million/mm^3 of blood. After about 10 days of birth, the count decreases due to destruction of cells. This is the cause of *physiological jaundice* in the newborn. In infants, the RBC count is slightly more than that in the adults.
- *Sex.* RBC count in adult females (average 4.8 million/mm^3) is lower than adult males (average 5.5 million/mm^3).
- *High altitude.* RBC count of the individuals residing in high-altitude areas (above 10,000 feet from the sea level) have high RBC count (7 million/mm^3) because of hypoxic stimulation of erythropoiesis.
- *Excessive exercise.* Mild hypoxia and spleen contraction cause temporary increase in the RBC count.
- *Emotional conditions* like anxiety are associated with temporary increase in the RBC count due to sympathetic stimulation.
- *Increase in atmospheric temperature* causes a temporary elevation of RBC count.
- *After meals,* the RBC count is raised slightly.

Polycythaemia *or pathological increases in RBC count (above 7 million/mm^3)* is of two types:

- ***Primary polycythaemia*** or polycythaemia vera is also called erythema, and occurs in myeloproliferative disorders, like malignancies of the bone marrow. The RBC count is persistently above 14 million/mm^3 and is always associated with high WBC count.
- ***Secondary polycythaemia*** occurs due to certain conditions producing a state of chronic hypoxia in the body, such as:
  - Congenital heart disease,
  - Chronic respiratory disorders like emphysema,

- Repeated mild haemorrhages and
- Phosphorus and arsenic poisoning.

In polycythaemia, haematocrit may be raised up to 60–70% and total blood volume also increases. As a result, there is engorgement of the entire vascular system. Blood viscosity also increases (three times as that of normal).

Effects of Polycythaemia Greater increase in blood viscosity is responsible for:

i. *Thrombosis:* The incidence of thrombosis increases because the blood flow through peripheral vessels becomes sluggish.
ii. *Increase in arterial pressure* due to rise in total peripheral resistance.
iii. *Ruddy complexion:* A person with polycythaemia vera has a ruddy complexion due to increased RBC count with a blueish tint (cyanotic) to the skin due to increased deoxygenated Hb, as a result of the sluggish blood flow through the skin capillaries.

Physiological Decrease in RBC Count *is seen in the following conditions.*

- *At high barometric pressure,* the RBC count is decreased slightly due to high O_2 tension of the blood.
- *After sleep,* the RBC count is decreased slightly.
- *In pregnancy,* there occurs relative reduction in RBC count due to haemodilution caused by increase in the plasma volume.

Anaemia. In anaemia, there may occur marked reduction in the RBC count, or the haemoglobin level, or both (see page 156).

Packed Cell Volume and Red Cell Indices

The red cell indices or absolute values (blood standards) include the entities mean corpuscular volume (MCV), mean corpuscular haemoglobin (MCH) and the mean corpuscular haemoglobin concentration (MCHC). These indices are quite helpful in diagnosing the type of anaemia. These indices are calculated from the values of packed cell volume, the haemoglobin concentration and the red cell count.

Packed Cell Volume

Packed cell volume (PCV) refers to the percentage of the cellular elements (RBCs, WBCs and platelets) in the whole blood. Since the volume of WBCs and platelets is very less, so for all practical purposes the PCV is considered equivalent to the volume of packed red cells (VPRC), or the so-called *haematocrit value.* However, in conditions where the number of WBCs is markedly increased, the values of PCV differ from that of the VPRC (haematocrit values). The normal values of PCV in males are about 45% and in females about 42%. The VPRC is increased in polycythaemia and decreased in anaemia.

Determination of PCV. The blood is mixed with anticoagulant oxalate and is centrifuged in a graduated tube called the *haematocrit tube* or the Wintrobe tube (Fig. 3.2-4) at a speed of 3000 rpm for about 30 min. The heavier red blood cells settle at the bottom leaving clear plasma above. The white blood cells and platelets which constitute only about 1% of the volume of blood are seen as a thin white layer called *buffy coat* on the top of the red cell mass.

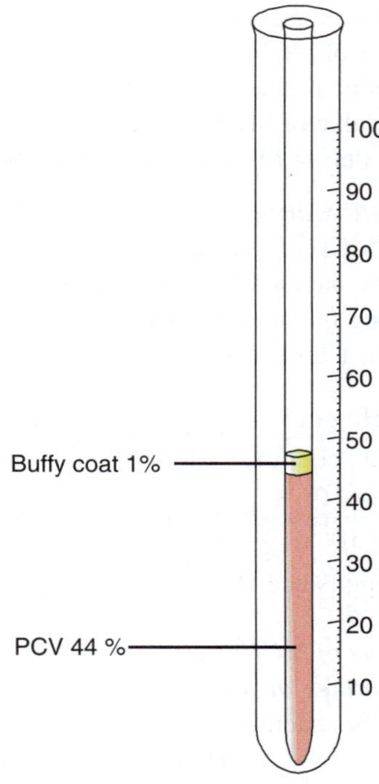

FIGURE 3.2-4 Wintrobe's tube showing packed cell volume.

- *Observed haematocrit* is the value of haematocrit obtained by the above described method.
- *True haematocrit* is calculated by multiplying observed haematocrit by 0.98. It is calculated because even if the red cells are fully packed, about 2% of plasma is trapped in between the cells.
- *Body haematocrit* is present in large and small blood vessels. It is calculated by multiplying the observed haematocrit with 0.87. It is calculated because the haematocrit is estimated from the venous blood whose haematocrit is greater than the whole body. In general, haematocrit in larger vessels is more than in the smaller vessels.

Red Cell Indices

The red cell indices defined below are calculated taking normal values of RBC count 5 million/mm^3, PCV 45% and haemoglobin (Hb) level of 15 g/dL.

1. Mean Corpuscular Volume. The mean corpuscular volume (MCV) refers to the average volume of a single red blood cell. It is calculated by dividing the packed cell volume (PCV) by the red cell count.

$$\text{MCV} = \frac{\text{PCV in 1000 ml of blood, i.e. (PCV} \times 10)}{\text{RBC count/mm}^3}$$

$$= \frac{45 \times 10}{5} = 90\ \mu\text{m}^3$$

- One cubic micrometer (mm^3) is equal to one femtolitre (fL).
- Normal value of MCV is 90 μm^3 (range 78–94 μm^3) when the MCV value is normal is referred as *normocytosis*.
- Decreased value of MCV occurs in *microcytosis*.
- Increased value of MCV occurs in *macrocytosis*.

2. Mean Cell (Corpuscular) Haemoglobin. Mean cell haemoglobin (MCH) refers to the average weight of haemoglobin (Hb) contained in each red blood cell. It is calculated by dividing the amount of Hb in 1 L of blood by the red cell count in 1 L of blood.

$$\text{MCH} = \frac{\text{Hb gm/L}}{\text{RBC count/L}} = \frac{\text{Hb g/dL} \times 10}{\text{RBC count/mm}^3 \times 10^{12}}$$

$$= \frac{15 \times 10}{5 \times 10^{12}} = 30 \times 10^{-12} \text{ gm.}$$

$$= 30 \text{ pg [since } 10^{-12} \text{ gm} = \text{one picogram (pg)]}$$

- *Normal value of MCH* is 30 pg (range 27–33).
- *Increased values of MCH* occur in spherocytosis and megaloblastic anaemia.
- MCH is not used to find out the type of anaemia.

3. Mean Cell (Corpuscular) Haemoglobin Concentration. The mean cell haemoglobin concentration (MCHC) refers to the amount of Hb expressed as percentage of the volume of a RBC. It is calculated by dividing the amount of Hb in g/dL by the volume of packed cells in 100 ml of blood and then multiplying by 100.

$$\text{MCHC} = \frac{\text{Hb g/dL}}{\text{PCV/100 ml}} \times 100 = \frac{15}{45} \times 100 = 33.3\%$$

- *Normal values of MCHC* are 33.3% (range 30–38%). RBCs with normal value of MCHC are called *normochromic*.
- *In hypochromic RBCs,* the values of MCHC are less than the normal, as is seen in iron deficiency anaemia.
- *Hyperchromia* is very rare, high levels of MCHC (>38%) cannot occur, since the RBCs cannot hold Hb beyond the saturation point.
- Since MCHC is independent of RBC count and size of RBCs, it is considered to be of greater clinical significance compared with other absolute values.

4. Colour Index. The colour index (CI) refers to the ratio of haemoglobin to RBC. For calculating CI, Hb of 14.8 g/dL is taken as 100% and RBC count of 5 million/mm^3 is taken as 100%.

$$\text{CI} = \frac{\text{Percentage of normal Hb}}{\text{Percentage of normal RBC count}} = \frac{100}{100} = 1$$

For example, if the Hb level is 14.8 g/dL, i.e. 100% of normal values and RBC count is 4.5 million, i.e. $4.5 \times 100 = 90\%$ of the normal values, then CI = 100/90 = 1.11.

- Normal values of colour index vary from 0.85 to 1.15.
- Colour index is insignificant because normal range of RBC is very wide. Therefore, it has been long abandoned and is not used for any diagnostic purposes.

Rouleaux Formation and Erythrocyte Sedimentation Rate

Rouleaux Formation

- Rouleaux formation refers to the tendency of RBCs to pile-up one over the other like a pile of coins (Fig. 3.2-5). The discoid shape and protein coating of red cells play a major role in Rouleaux formation. Rouleaux formation does not occur in normal circulation under physiological conditions, as the moving cells show little or no tendency to adhere. However, within a blood vessel, in the absence of significant flow and when the blood is taken out, the red cells tend to form Rouleaux.
- This is a reversible phenomenon, but it promotes sedimentation of RBCs. It should not be confused with agglutination where the cells are irreversibly clumped.
- Albumin decreases the Rouleaux formation, while fibrinogen, globulin and other products of tissue destruction increase Rouleaux formation.

Erythrocyte Sedimentation Rate

Erythrocyte sedimentation rate (ESR) is the rate at which the red blood cells sediment (settle down) when the blood containing an anticoagulant is allowed to stand in a vertically placed tube. It is expressed in millimetre at the end of the first hour.

Methods of Determination of ESR

1. Westergren's Method. A total of 1.6 ml of blood diluted with 0.4 ml of 3.8% sodium citrate (making a total of 2 ml) is loaded in the Westergren pipette which is then fitted to stand vertically. The reading is taken after 1 h. The Westergren tube is 30 cm long and is open at both the ends (Fig. 3.2-6A).

2. Wintrobe's Method. About 1 ml of blood mixed with anticoagulant EDTA is loaded in a Wintrobe tube up to '0' mark and the reading is taken after 1 h. The Wintrobe tube is 11 cm long and is open only at one end (Fig. 3.2-6B).

Note. *Since the Westergren pipette is longer, chances of an error in measurement of ESR is reduced. Therefore, Westergren's method is preferred over Wintrobe's method for estimation of ESR.*

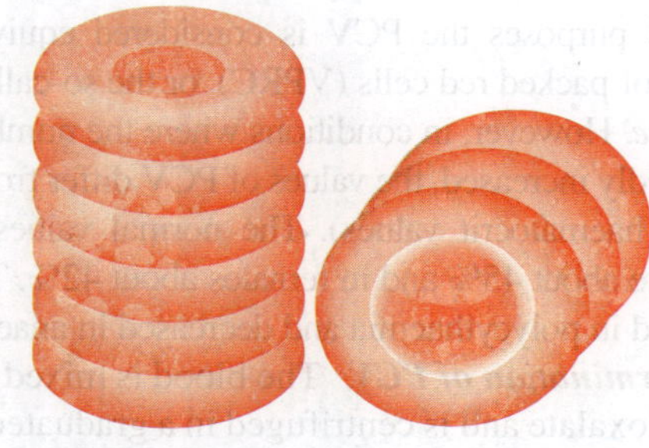

FIGURE 3.2-5 Rouleaux formation.

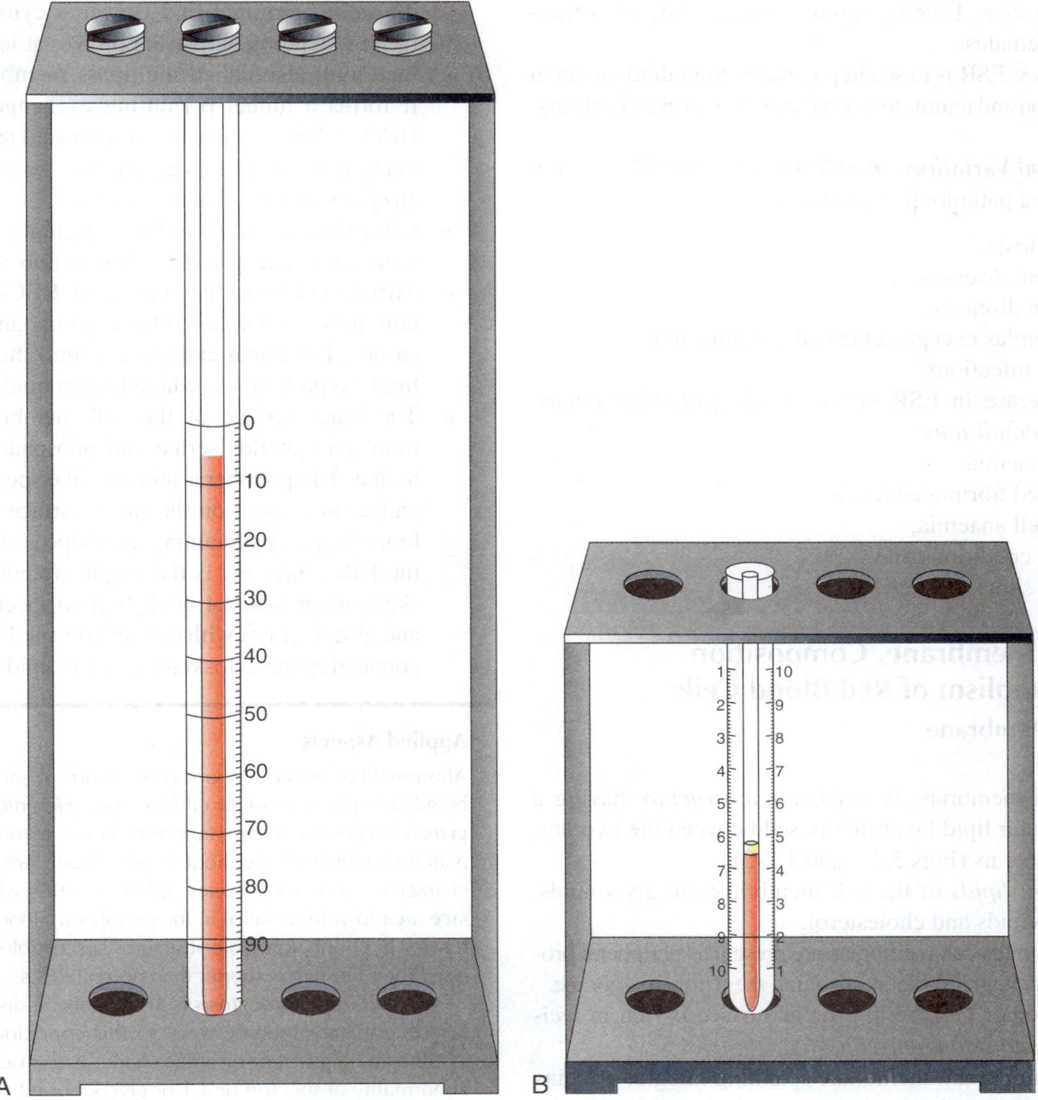

FIGURE 3.2-6 Westergren's pipette (A) and Wintrobe's tube (B) used for determining erythrocyte sedimentation rate (ESR).

Clinical Significance of ESR

- *Normal values* of ESR by Westergren's method in males vary from 3 to7 mm and in females from 5 to 9 mm in the first hour.
- Values of ESR are raised in a large number of pathological conditions, so it has got no specific diagnostic value. However, raised levels of ESR do suggest presence of some chronic inflammatory condition in the body.
- Estimation of ESR is more useful as a *prognostic test*, i.e. to judge the progress of the disease in patients under treatment.

Factors Affecting ESR

- *Rouleaux formation*. Increased tendency of Rouleaux formation raises the erythrocyte sedimentation rate. Fibrinogen and the proteins, which enter the plasma in inflammatory (globulins) and neoplastic diseases, favour Rouleaux formation and thus increase ESR. Increase in MCV, decrease in MCH and spherocytosis retard Rouleaux formation and thus decrease ESR.
- *Size of the red blood cells*. Increase in the size of the RBCs (macrocytosis) raises the ESR.
- *Number of red blood cells*. When the number of RBCs increased, the ESR is decreased and when the number of RBCs is decreased (as in anaemia), the ESR is increased.
- *Viscosity of blood*. ESR is increased when the viscosity of blood is decreased and vice versa.

Physiological Variations in ESR

- *Age*. ESR is less in infants and old people compared with young adults.
- *Sex*. ESR is greater in females (5–9 mm) than males (3–7 mm).

- *Menstruation.* ESR is slightly raised during menstruation in females.
- *Pregnancy.* ESR is raised in pregnancy from third month to parturition and returns to normal after 3–4 weeks of delivery.

Pathological Variations in ESR *Increase in ESR* is seen in the following pathological conditions:

- Tuberculosis,
- Malignant diseases,
- Collagen diseases,
- All anaemias except sickle cell anaemia and
- Chronic infections.

Decrease in ESR *occurs in the following pathological conditions:*

- Polycythaemia
- Decreased fibrinogen levels,
- Sickle cell anaemia,
- Allergic conditions and
- Peptone shock.

Red Cell Membrane, Composition and Metabolism of Red Blood Cells

Red Cell Membrane

Structure

- Red cell membrane is a *trilaminar structure* having a bimolecular lipid layer interposed between the two layers of proteins (Figs 3.2-7 and 1.2-2).
- *Important lipids* of the cell membrane are glycolipids, phospholipids and cholesterol.
- *Proteins* in the cell membrane are present as peripheral proteins and integral proteins spanning the whole membrane.
  - The outer peripheral protein surface is rich in *lecithin and sphingomyelin.*
  - The important membrane spanning integral proteins include an anion exchange protein (*band 3*) and *glycophorins* which contain a number of polysaccharide *blood group antigens.*
  - *Band-3* is a transmembrane glycoprotein with its carboxyl terminal end (towards external surface) and its amino terminal end (towards cytoplasmic surface), extending across the bilayer at least 10 times, therefore, also called multipass membrane protein. It forms a tunnel permitting exchange of Cl^- for HCO_3^-. The cytoplasmic amino acid terminal binds many proteins (4.1, 4.2, ankyrin, several glycolytic enzymes and also haemoglobin).
  - *Glycophorins A, B and C* are single pass type at transmembrane proteins. The amino acid terminal extrude out from the surface of RBCs which contain polysaccharides (blood group antigens). The carboxyl terminal end extends into the cytosol and binds to protein 4.1, which in turn binds to spectrin.
  - The inner surface of the cell membrane contains more phosphatidylserine and phosphatidyl ethanolamine. The peripheral proteins like spectrin, ankyrin and actin present on the inner surface of the membrane help in maintaining the shape and flexibility of the RBC. *Spectrin* is the major protein of the cytoskeleton; protein 4.1 binds both to spectrin and actin and also interacts with certain phospholipids (thereby connecting the cytoskeleton to the lipid layer).

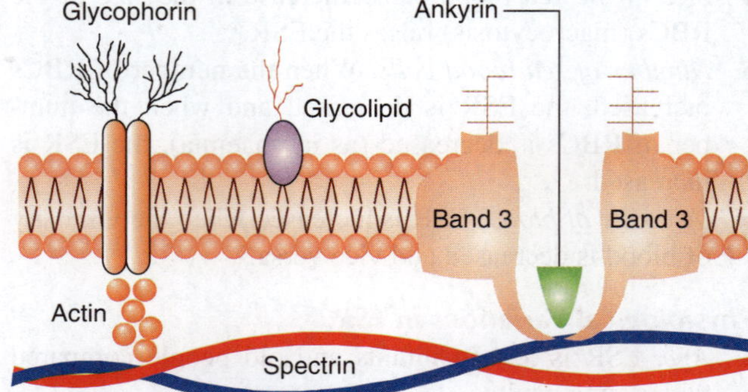

FIGURE 3.2-7 Schematic diagram showing ultra-structure of red cell membrane.

Applied Aspects

Abnormalities in the amount or structure of spectrin cause hereditary spherocytosis or elliptocytosis. ***Hereditary spherocytosis*** is a genetic disease transmitted as an autosomal dominant trait, which affects about 1: 5000 North Americans. It is characterized by spherocytes (spherical RBCs with low surface area to volume ratio) in the peripheral blood. The spherocytes are nondeformable structures susceptible to osmotic lysis. Their lifespan is shorter than normal RBCs.

Hereditary elliptocytosis is also a genetic disorder similar to hereditary spherocytosis. In this condition, red cells assume an elliptical or disc-like shape. It also occurs due to abnormality of spectrin or 4.1 or glycophorin C.

Permeability. The red cell membrane is a *semi-permeable membrane,* allowing some substances to pass through and preventing some.

- *Impermeable* to sodium, calcium and barium ions, to fats and sugars;
- *Slightly impermeable* to amino acids; and
- *Freely permeable* to all anions like Cl^-, SO_4^- and HCO_3^-, and to urea, ammonia, aldehyde, alcohol and bile salts.

Composition of Red Blood Cells

The body of RBCs bounded by the cell membrane contains a sponge-like stroma which is composed of the following structures:

- *Water* constitutes 60% of the wet weight of RBC.
- *Haemoglobin,* held in the meshes of stroma, constitutes 35% of the wet weight and 90% of the dry weight of RBC.

- *Lipids* form the major constituents of the rest of 5% of stroma. These include cephalin, lecithin and cholesterol.
- *Proteins* include glutathiones and an albumin-like insoluble protein. These act as reducing agents preventing damage to the haemoglobin.
- *Lipoproteins.* Almost half of the lipids are bounded to the protein forming a lipoprotein complex known as *elenin (Calvin).*
- *Enzymes* of the glycolytic system, catalase, carbonic anhydrase and other enzymes and inorganic salts are also present in the RBC.
- *Glucose and amino acids* are present in small amounts.
- *Ions.* Anions of the plasma (Cl^-, PO_4^-, HCO_3^-) are present often in large amounts. The cations Na^+ and Ca^{2+} are either present in very small amount or are absent. Cation K^+ is present in sufficient amount inside the RBC.
- *Nonprotein nitrogenous (NPN) substances.* Urea, NH_4, creatine and uric acid have a higher concentration inside the RBC than the plasma.

Metabolism of Red Blood Cells

Glucose, taken up by facilitated diffusion, is the only fuel utilized by the RBC. The mature RBC has a low respiratory quotient and consumes very little oxygen. The glucose metabolism and its special significance in RBC are described below:

Embden–Meyerhof Pathway *is responsible for 90% of the glycolysis. Two molecules of ATP are generated from each molecule of glucose. Special significance of this pathway is given below.*

2,3-Biphosphoglycerate (2,3-BPG) *synthesized in a side reaction in this pathway influences the oxygen affinity of haemoglobin and thus plays an important role in the red cell physiology. Factors affecting 2,3-BPG concentration in RBC include the following:*

- Acidaemia hinders glycolysis and thereby decreases 2,3-BPG synthesis.
- Hypoxia prevents Krebs' cycle and thereby increases 2,3-BPG synthesis.
- Thyroid hormone, androgens and growth hormone increase 2,3-BPG concentration.

Hexose Monophosphate (HMP) Shunt *oxidizes about 10% of glucose. Special significance of this pathway in RBC metabolism is given below:*

- NADPH generated by this pathway keeps the glutathione in reduced form. Reduced glutathione, in turn protects sulphydryl groups in haemoglobin and RBC membrane from oxidation by peroxides, superoxide, drugs and toxins.
- *Glucose-6 phosphate dehydrogenase (G6PD)* is the key enzyme in the HMP shunt. Inherited deficiency of this enzyme leads to compromise of RBC function and viability in the face of such oxidant stress; thus causing a number of disorders characterized by susceptibility to haemolysis (see page152).

Utilization of ATP

- A major portion of ATP obtained through glycolysis is utilized in maintaining the Na^+/K^+ ATPase pump.
- Some of the energy is utilized in maintaining the integrity of the red cell membrane.
- Some of the energy is spent in maintaining the haemoglobin iron in reduced form (Fe^{2+}).

FORMATION OF RED BLOOD CELLS

Formation of red blood cells is a part of the process of development of blood cells (RBCs, WBCs and platelets) called *haemopoiesis* which includes:

- Erythropoiesis, i.e. development of RBCs,
- Leucopoiesis, i.e. development of WBCs and
- Thrombopoiesis or megakaryocytopoiesis, i.e. development of platelets.

Sites of Haemopoiesis

- ***In the first 2 months of gestation,*** the *yolk sac* is the main site of haemopoiesis *(mesoblastic stage)* (Fig. 3.2-8).
- ***From the third month of gestation,*** the liver and spleen become the main sites of blood formation and continue to do so till birth. The spleen makes a small contribution as compared to the liver *(hepatic stage).*
- ***From the 20th week of gestation,*** haemopoiesis begins in the bone marrow and by the seventh or eighth month, it becomes the main site *(myeloid stage).*
- ***At birth*** (in normal full-term), almost whole of the haemopoiesis occurs in the bone marrow.

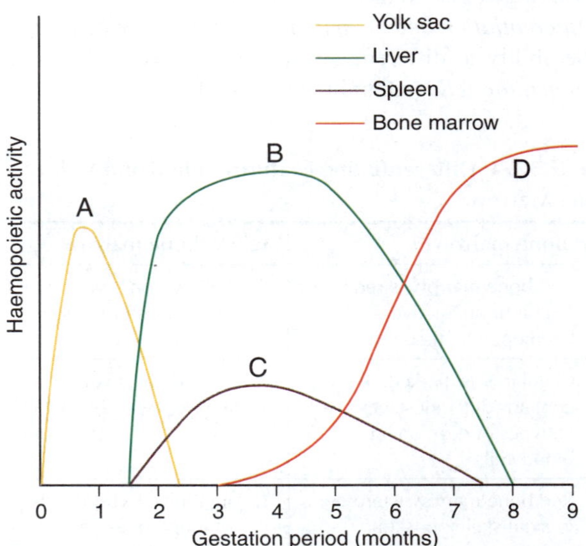

FIGURE 3.2-8 Sites of haemopoiesis during different periods in human life: **A,** yolk sac; **B,** liver; **C,** spleen; and **D,** bone marrow.

- *In young children,* active haemopoietic bone marrow is found in both axial skeleton and bones of extremities. The active haemopoietic bone marrow is red in colour due to marked cellularity and hence is called *red bone marrow.* However, during this period, there occurs a progressive fatty replacement throughout the long bones converting red bone marrow into the so-called *yellow bone marrow.*
- *In adults,* therefore, haemopoietic (red) bone marrow is confined to *axial skeleton* (skull, vertebrae, sternum, ribs, sacrum and pelvis) and *proximal ends of long bones* (humerus, femur and tibia). Even in these haemopoietic areas, about 50% of the bone marrow consists of fat. The differences between red and yellow bone marrow are summarized in Table 3.2-1.
- *In adults, during pathological conditions,* when there is an increased demand of blood cells, the *nonhaemopoietic (yellow) marrow* is capable of reverting back to active haemopoiesis.
- *During pathological conditions,* when the increased demand of blood cells cannot be met by the hyperactivity of bone marrow alone, even the liver and spleen resume their fetal role of haemopoiesis, as the stem cell retains its potential haemopoietic activity. Such a situation is referred to as *extra medullary haemopoiesis.*

Blood Cell Precursors

The Stem Cells. The *monophyletic theory* of haemopoiesis is now widely accepted, according to which all blood cells originate from a single ancestral cell called *pluripotent* or *multipotent stem cell.* The stem cells have the appearance of small or intermediate-sized lymphocytes. Stem cells possess two *fundamental properties:*

- *Self-replication,* i.e. stem cells are capable of cell division to give rise to more stem cells, and
- *Differentiation and commitment,* i.e. the stem cells have the ability to differentiate into specialized cells called *progenitor cells* (committed stem cell).

TABLE 3.2-1 Differentiating Features of Red and Yellow Bone Marrow

Red bone marrow	Yellow bone marrow
1. Red bone marrow is red in colour and active haemopoietic tissue.	1. Yellow bone marrow is yellowish in colour and inactive.
2. Cellularity is marked. It contains different stages of all types of developing blood cells.	2. Cellularity is very less and replaced by fatty tissue.
3. Red bone marrow is present in axial skeleton (skull, vertebrae, sacrum, sternum and pelvis) and long bones in children.	3. In adults, except ends of long bones and axial skeleton, all other bones contain yellow bone marrow.

Progenitor Cells. The stem cells, after a series of divisions differentiate into progenitor cells:

- ***Pluripotent progenitor cells*** which can give rise to any type of blood cells,
- ***Lymphoid (immune system)*** stem cells which ultimately develop into lymphocytes, and
- ***Myeloid (trilineage) stem cells*** which later differentiate into three types of cell lines:
  - *Granulocyte–monocyte progenitors* which produce all leucocytes except the lymphocytes,
  - *Erythroid progenitors* which produce red blood cells, and
  - Megakaryocyte progenitors which produce platelets.

Features of Progenitor Cells. Morphologically, the progenitor cells present in the bone marrow cannot be differentiated from the stem cells, as they both lookalike. However, they can be differentiated by immunological techniques, taking advantage of the different types of molecules present on their cell membrane.

Progenitor cells possess ability to give rise to clones *(group of cells), so they are also called* colony-forming cells *(CFC) or* colony-forming units *(CFU). The three types of progenitor cells are given:*

- ***CFU-GEMM*** (colony-forming unit–granulocyte, erythroid, megakaryocyte, macrophage) refers to a multipotent progenitor cell, i.e. *myeloid progenitor cells.*
- ***BFU-E*** (burst-forming unit–erythroid) form large colonies of erythroid series.
- ***CFU-E*** (colony-forming unit–erythroid) develops into erythrocytes.
- ***Ba-CFU*** refers to basophil colony-forming units.
- ***Eo-CFU*** are eosinophil colony-forming units.
- ***M-CFU*** refers to monocyte colony-forming units.
- ***G-CFU*** are neutrophil-forming units.

The broad outlines of haemopoiesis discussed above are summarized in Fig. 3.2-9. Further details of erythropoiesis are discussed in this chapter and details of development of other blood cells are discussed in the relevant chapters.

Bone Marrow Examination. The red bone marrow contains the stem cells, progenitor cells, colony-forming cells and various types of blood cells in different stages of development, which can be observed in a stained smear of red marrow obtained from the iliac bone or sternum (Fig. 3.2-10). Normally, in the red marrow the haemopoietic stem cells comprise only 0.01–0.5% of the total marrow population. About 75% of the cells are immature white cells and about 25% of the cells are immature red cells, thus forming a ratio of 3:1; while in peripheral blood the ratio of white and red cells is 1:600. This vast difference is because the lifespan of red cells is far greater than that of the white cells.

Control of Haemopoiesis

The growth of different blood cells from the stem cells is controlled and regulated by the haemopoietic growth factors,

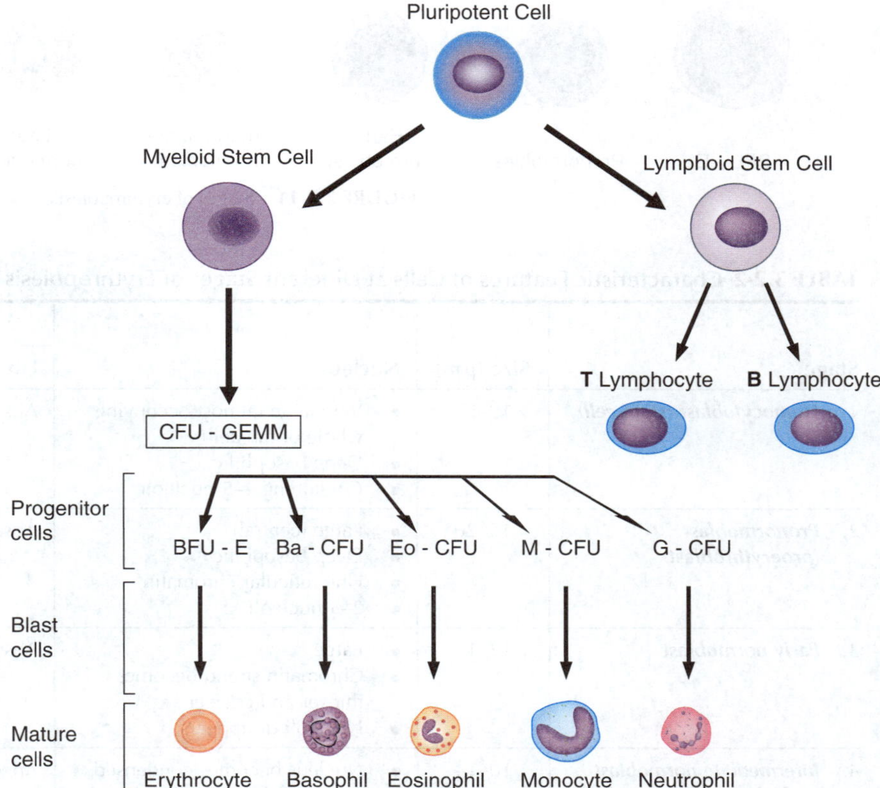

FIGURE 3.2-9 Schematic broad outline of haemopoiesis.

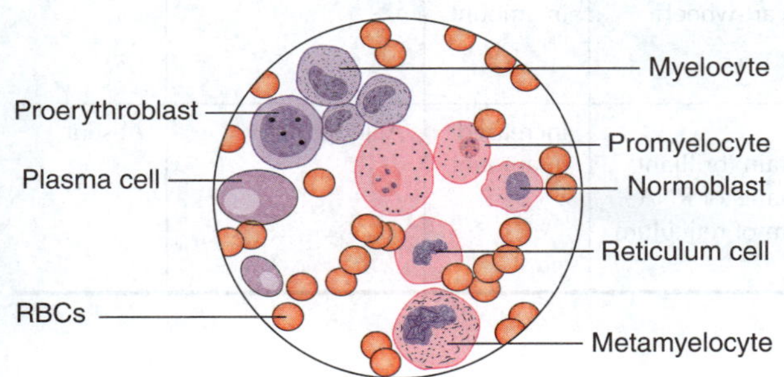

FIGURE 3.2-10 Smear from red bone marrow showing various types of cells at different stages of development.

which in general are called *cytokines.* Cytokine is a general term used to denote the proteins released by cells that act as intercellular mediators. The cytokines which control the formation of different types of blood cells are called *colony stimulating factors (CSF),* which are given below:

- *G-CSF* stimulates granulocytic precursors,
- *M-CSF* stimulates monocytic precursors,
- *GM-CSF* stimulates both the granulocytic and monocytic precursors.
- *Interleukins (1L)* refer to the cytokine stimulating lymphocytic precursor, for example, IL-1, IL-3, etc.
- *Erythropoietin* refers to the cytokine stimulating the erythroid series of cells.

Stages of Erythropoiesis

The red blood cells develop from the burst-forming unit-erythrocyte (BFU-E) and colony-forming unit-erythrocyte (CFU-E) which are derived from the committed progenitor cells.

The well-defined and readily recognizable lineages of nucleated red cells (erythroid series) which form different stages of erythropoiesis (Fig. 3.2-11, Table 3.2-2) are as under:

1. Pronormoblast or Proerythroblast is the earliest recognizable cell of the erythroid series seen in the red bone marrow. Its features are the following:

- *Size* is large with a diameter of 15–20 μm.
- *Cytoplasm* is scanty and deeply basophilic. The deep blue colour of cytoplasm is due to high content of RNA which is associated with active protein synthesis.
- *Nucleus* is large, central with a fine reticular chromatin and contains many nucleoli.
- *Haemoglobin* is absent at this stage.
- *Mitosis* is seen in these cells.

2. Early (Basophilic) Normoblast (basophilic early erythroblast). The pronormoblast progresses into the early normoblast, which is a round cell having the following features:

- *Size* is large with a diameter of 12–16 μm.
- *Cytoplasm* is scanty and still basophilic.

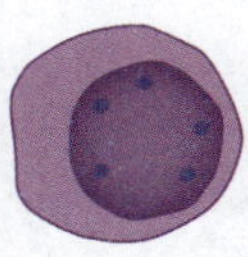
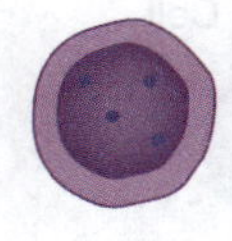
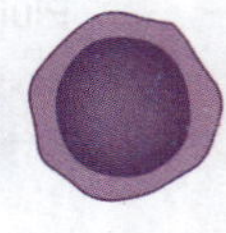
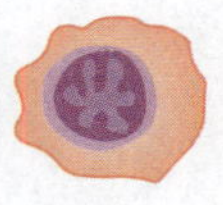
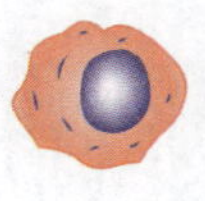
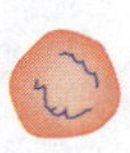
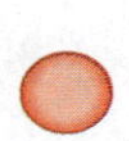

FIGURE 3.2-11 Stages of erythropoiesis.

TABLE 3.2-2 Characteristic Features of Cells at Different Stages of Erythropoiesis

Stage	Size (μm)	Nucleus	Cytoplasm		Mitosis
			Hb	Staining	
1. ***Homocytoblast (stem cell)***	19–23	• Very large (almost occupying whole of the cell) • Deep basophilic • Containing 4–5 nucleoli	Absent	Deep basophilic	Present++
2. ***Pronormoblast (proerythroblast)***	15–20	• Large (central) • Deep basophilic • Fine reticular chromatin • 2–3 nucleoli	Absent	Scanty and deep basophilic	++
3. ***Early normoblast***	12–16	• Large • Chromatin strand becomes thicker and coarser • Nucleoli disappears	Absent	Still basophilic	++
4. ***Intermediate normoblast (polychromatic normoblast)***	10–14	• Nucleus becomes condensed, coarse and basophilic • Nucleoli absent	Appears	Acidophilic with basophilic hue (polychromatic)	+
5. ***Late normoblast (orthochromaticnormoblast)***	8–10	• Nucleus small, pyknotic with dark chromatin (cart-wheel appearance) • Nucleoli absent	Increased in amount	Acidophilic	Absent
6. ***Reticulocyte***	7–7.5	• Nucleus absent • With supravital stain (brilliant cresyl blue) remnants of RNA appear in the form of reticulum in the cytoplasm	Increased in amount	Acidophilic	Absent

- *Nucleus* is large, chromatin strands are thicker and coarse and nucleoli have disappeared.
- *Haemoglobin* is not present.
- *Mitosis* is seen. The basophilic normoblasts undergo rapid proliferation.

3. *Intermediate (Polychromatic) Normoblast* (polychromatic erythroblast) is the next maturation stage in the erythroid series. Its features are the following:

- *Size* is about 10–14 μm.
- *Cytoplasm* becomes polychromatic, i.e. contains admixture of basophilic RNA and acidophilic haemoglobin.
- *Nucleus* becomes condensed, coarse and deeply basophilic with no nucleoli.
- *Haemoglobin* appears.
- *Mitosis* is still present.

4. *Late (Orthochromatic) Normoblast* (orthochromatic erythroblast) is the last nucleated cell of the erythroid series. Its features are the following:

- *Size* is reduced to 8–10 μm.
- *Cytoplasm* is characteristically acidophilic with diffuse basophilic hue.
- *Nucleus* at this stage is small, pyknotic with dark chromatin.
- *Haemoglobin* increases in amount.
- *Mitosis* is absent at this stage.

5. *Reticulocyte* is the last stage in the formation of erythrocytes, which is why it is also called young red cell. Its features are the following:

- *Size and shape.* The reticulocyte is a flat, disc-shaped, slightly larger (7–7.5 μm) than the mature erythrocytes.

- *Cytoplasm* still contains small amounts of RNA. With supervital stain such as brilliant cresyl blue, the RNA appears in the form of a reticulum (net-like structure) and because of this character the cell is called a reticulocyte. With Romanowsky stain, the cytoplasm gives a faint polychromatic tint.
- *Nucleus* is absent, the reticulocyte results when the nucleus is extruded from the late normoblast within the marrow.
- *Haemoglobin* increases in amount equal to that present in a mature erythrocyte.
- *Mitosis* is absent.

Maturation of Reticulocyte into Erythrocyte. The reticulocytes are juvenile red cells devoid of nucleus but contain ribosomal RNA so that they are still able to synthesize haemoglobin. A reticulocyte spends 1–2 days in marrow and circulates for 1–2 days in the peripheral blood before maturing in the spleen, to become a biconcave red cell. The mature red cell has lost its nucleus, as well as the ribosomes and mitochondria. It thus cannot synthesize haemoglobin and any other protein. The immature cells in various stages of development are found outside (around) the blood sinusoids of the bone marrow. Normally, only mature blood cells are able to enter the circulation. The reticulocytes are also found normally in the peripheral blood. Normal range of reticulocytes in healthy adults is 0.5–2% and in infants is 2–6%. Abnormal increase in circulating reticulocytes is called *reticulocytosis.* This is seen when the rate of erythropoiesis is very high, as occurs in haemolytic anaemia and following the treatment of deficiency anaemias.

The reticulocytes in the peripheral blood are distinguished from mature red cells by a slightly basophilic hue in the cytoplasm, similar to that of an orthochromatic normoblast. Reticulocytes can be counted in the laboratory by vital staining with dyes, such as new methylene blue or brilliant cresyl blue.

Summary of Changes Occurring in Cells of Erythroid Series during Maturation. It takes 7 days for the formation and maturation of red blood cells. Till the reticulocyte stage,, it takes 5 days and to become a matured red cell from the reticulocyte, it takes 2 days. Various changes which occur during maturation from the pronormoblast to the erythrocyte stage are summarized below:

- ***Size*** of the cell (from 15–20 μm of pronormoblast) goes on decreasing with subsequent stages till it reaches about 7 μm.
- ***Nucleus*** first condenses, then becomes pyknotic and finally disappears at the stage of reticulocyte formation.
- ***Haemoglobin synthesis*** starts at the stage of intermediate normoblast and then its content increases progressively.
- ***Cytoplasm staining.*** Initially, before the appearance of haemoglobin, the cytoplasm is basophilic. When haemoglobin starts appearing cytoplasm becomes polychromatic, i.e. stained both by acidic and basic dyes. In the stage of late normoblast when haemoglobin synthesis is almost completed, cytoplasm is stained by acidic dye.
- ***Mitosis*** is seen up to the stage of intermediate normoblast. During these stages, 3–5 cell divisions occur. In this way, each pronormoblast gives rise to 8–320 late normoblasts. From the stage of late normoblast onwards, the mitosis ceases and the cell only matures.

Regulation of Erythropoiesis

Erythropoietin. *Erythropoietin* is a hormone which regulates the process of erythropoiesis. It is a glycoprotein having a molecular weight of 34,000.

Site of Formation. Erythropoietin is mainly (85%) produced by the juxtaglomerular apparatus of the kidney. Extrarenal sources like the liver and cells of the tissue macrophage system produce about 15% of erythropoietin, especially when hypoxia is marked.

Stimulus for Secretion. A certain basal level of the hormone is necessary for the normal rate of erythropoiesis. The main function of the red blood cells is to supply oxygen to the tissues. Therefore, whenever, there is hypoxia or a decrease in the number of red blood cells (e.g. after haemorrhage or in haemolytic anaemia), there occurs a release of renal erythropoietic factor from juxtaglomerular cells of the kidney. The renal erythropoietic factor acts on the plasma alpha globulin called erythropoietinogen to form the erythropoietin (Fig. 3.2-12). Thus, the levels of erythropoietin vary with degree of hypoxia or the number of circulating red blood cells. This explains how polycythaemia (increased red blood cell count) is observed in hypoxic states such as in normal individuals residing at high altitude or in patients suffering from cardiopulmonary disorder. On the other hand, if the number of red blood cells in circulation is more, e.g. after transfusion of blood in a normal person, the erythropoietin formation is decreased. For details see page 796.

Actions of Erythropoietin. Erythropoietin increases erythropoiesis by acting at the site of erythropoiesis (It may be yolk sac, liver, spleen and bone marrow depending upon the age). Erythropoietin, along with co-operation of other factors (e.g. interleukin-3 and insulin-like growth factor) promotes erythropoiesis because of its following actions:

- Erythropoietin exerts its chief effect on the stem cells causing them to differentiate into burst-forming units (BFU-E).
- It promotes haemoglobin synthesis by increasing globin synthesis and potentiating δ-aminolevulinic acid synthetase.

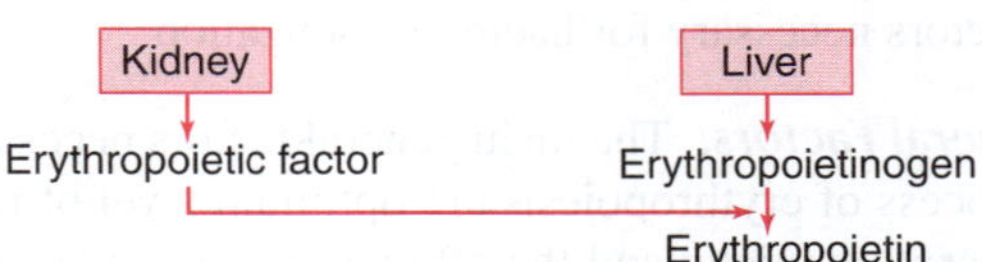

FIGURE 3.2-12 Mechanism of erythropoietin secretion.

- It also promotes every stage of maturation from pronormoblast to the mature red cells.
- Erythropoietin also promotes release of RBCs from bone marrow into the peripheral circulation.

Mechanism of Action. Erythropoietin (EPO) acts by binding to specific receptors present on the surface of erythroid precursor cells. For further details see page 796.

Factors Increasing Erythropoietin Secretion. The degree of oxygenation and number of RBCs in circulation act as feedback mechanisms to control the secretion of erythropoietin, i.e. depending upon the condition, they either increase or decrease erythropoietin secretion to normalize the erythropoiesis. Other factors which increase secretion of erythropoietin are:

1. Hormones which increase erythropoietin secretion are:

- *Androgens* (male sex hormones) enhance erythropoietin secretion. This explains the greater RBC counts in males compared with females.
- *Thyroxine* also promotes erythropoiesis. This explains the occurrence of polycythaemia in hyperthyroidism.
- *Other hormones* which increase erythropoietin secretion are growth hormone, prolactin, ACTH and adrenocortical steroids.

2. Haemolysates, i.e. the products released following RBC destruction, also increase erythropoietin secretion.

3. Nucleotides which enhance erythropoietin secretion include cAMP, NAD and NADP.

4. Vasoconstrictor drugs produce renal hypoxia, which in turn increases erythropoietin secretion.

Factors Decreasing Erythropoietin Secretion are the following:

- Adenosine antagonists, e.g. theophylline and
- Oestrogen decreases erythropoietin secretion by:

- Decreasing synthesis of globin in liver, and
- Depressing the erythropoietic response to hypoxia.

Important Notes

For therapeutic purpose (in anaemic state due to renal failure) recombinant erythropoietin (rEPO) is available as epoetin α.

Factors Necessary for Erythropoiesis

Factors necessary for erythropoiesis can be divided in three groups:

- General factors,
- Special maturation factors and
- Factors necessary for haemoglobinization.

I. General Factors. The main general factors necessary for the process of erythropoiesis are optimum level of the hormone *erythropoietin* and the efficient *feedback mechanism* controlling the secretion of *erythropoietin*.

All the factors (including hypoxia) affecting erythropoietin and feedback mechanism have been discussed in the regulation of erythropoiesis.

II. Special Maturation Factors. Special factors which are essential for maturation of a red blood cell include vitamin B_{12}, intrinsic factor of Castle and folic acid.

Vitamin B_{12}. Vitamin B_{12} (cyanocobalamin), also known as extrinsic factor is essential for maturation of red cells.

- ***Daily requirement*** of vitamin B_{12} in adults is 1–2 μg. Since its deficiency causes pernicious anaemia, it is also called antipernicious factor.
- ***Sources of vitamin B_{12}.*** There is no plant source for vitamin B_{12}. Dietary sources of vitamin B_{12} are milk, meat and liver of animals. It is present in the normal diet and is also synthesized by the bacterial flora of the colon. The colonic cobalamins are unabsorbable in humans.
- ***Absorption of vitamin B_{12}.*** is not possible in the absence of the intrinsic factor. The *intrinsic factor of Castle* is a glycoprotein secreted by the parietal cells of gastric mucosa. It combines with dietary vitamin B_{12} present in

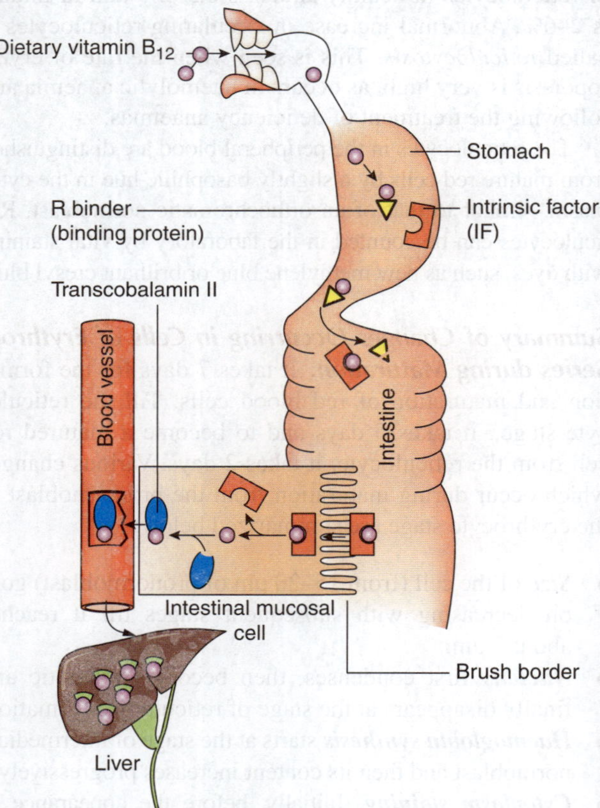

FIGURE 3.2-13 Schematic diagram showing absorption and transport of vitamin B_{12}.

the stomach to form the intrinsic factor—cyanocobalamin complex which then becomes bound to specific receptors in the ileum and is absorbed by endocytosis (Fig. 3.2-13).

- ***Transport of vitamin B_{12}.*** Inside the mucosal cells, the cobalamin is transferred from the intrinsic factor to transcobalamin II, another binding protein which transports vitamin B_{12} in the blood (Fig. 3.2-13).
- ***Storage of vitamin B_{12}.*** It is stored in large amounts in liver (there may be up to 3 years supply) and also to some extent in the muscles. Whenever required, it is transported from the liver into the bone marrow.
- ***Role of vitamin B_{12}.*** It is required for the synthesis of DNA and maturation of nucleus and cell. Its interaction with folic acid is shown in Fig. 3.2-14. Deficiency of vitamin B_{12} leads to:
  - Failure of maturation of nucleus.
  - Cells remain large (megaloblasts) and become more fragile. Normally, during maturation, cell size decreases progressively.
  - There occurs a reduction in the cell division.

Folic Acid. Folic acid (pteroylglutamic acid) and related compounds are known as folates—play an important role in the synthesis of DNA.

- Daily requirement of folates for a normal healthy adult is 100 μg.
- Sources of folates are leafy vegetables, yeasts, pulses and liver. The body obtains folates by the breakdown of food polyglutamates to monoglutamates in the small intestine or mucosal cells. Folic acid, as such, is available only as a medicinal compound.
- Role of folic acid in DNA synthesis. In the plasma, folate appears as methyl tetrahydrofolate, which is changed to tetrahydrofolate (THF) by a pathway for which vitamin B_{12} is essential (Fig. 3.2-14). Without this, active folate co-enzymes are poorly formed. For synthesis of DNA, 5,10 methylene THF is the essential form. Dihydrofolate from this step is reconverted to the THF by dihydrofolate reductase, an enzyme inhibited by the folate antagonist (methotrexate). Formyl THF (folinic acid) will bypass both the metabolic blocks created by vitamin B_{12} deficiency or methotrexate and acts as an antidote to this drug.
- Folate deficiency causes megaloblastic anaemia (see page 162).

III. Factors Necessary for Haemoglobinization. Various factors necessary for haemoglobin formation in the red blood cells are described on page 150.

HAEMOGLOBIN

The cytoplasm of erythrocytes (red blood cells) contains an *oxygen-binding protein* called haemoglobin. Erythrocyte precursors synthesize haemoglobin, while the mature erythrocytes lose the property of synthesizing haemoglobin. The inclusion of haemoglobin within the erythrocytes is most effective for functional purposes, since it avoids the following *disadvantages* which would have occurred if the haemoglobin was present in the plasma as free haemoglobin:

- Increase in blood viscosity causing a rise in blood pressure,
- Increase in the osmotic pressure,

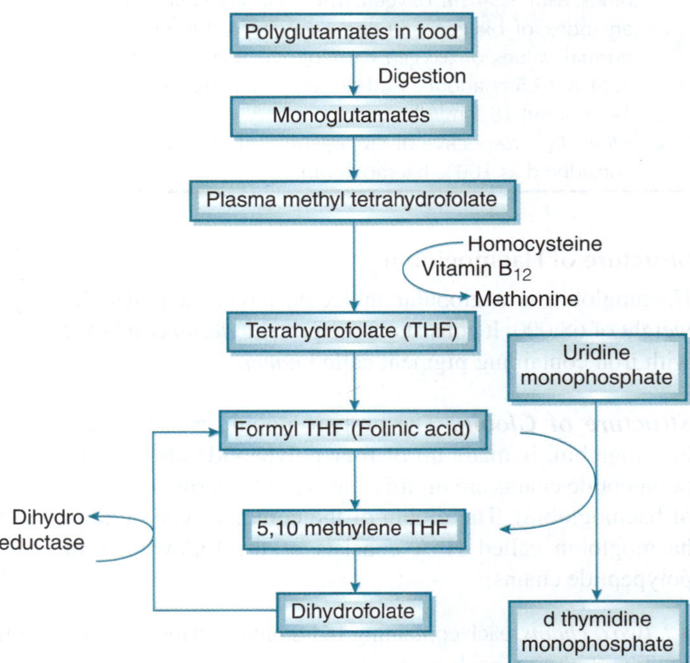

FIGURE 3.2.14 Metabolic pathway showing interaction of vitamin B_{12} and folate in the synthesis of DNA.

- Rapid destruction of haemoglobin by the reticulo–endothelial system and
- Excretion of haemoglobin by kidney (haemoglobin urea).

In pathologic states, e.g. acute haemolytic disorder, Hb appears in the plasma and may lead to above-mentioned consequences.

Normal Blood Haemoglobin

The normal blood haemoglobin concentration at different ages is given below (Fig. 3.2-15).

- ***In Fetus,*** just before birth, the haemoglobin concentration of blood from the umbilical cord ranges from 16.5 to 18.5 g/dL.
- ***After Birth,*** the haemoglobin concentration increases rapidly and may reach up to 23 g/dL. This occurs due to:
  - the transfusion of cells from the placenta to infant, and
  - haemoconcentration by reduction of plasma volume.
- ***At the end of 3 months.*** After 2 days of birth, the haemoglobin levels start falling and stabilize at the end of 3 months to 10.5 g/dL.
- ***At 1 year of age.*** The concentration then rises gradually to reach 12 g/dL.
- ***In Adult Males,*** the mean blood haemoglobin (Hb) concentration is 15.5 g/dL (range 14–18 g/dL) and
- ***In Adult Females,*** the mean Hb concentration is 14 g/dL (range 12–15.5 g/dL).

Important Notes

- The normal haemoglobin becomes 100% saturated when blood is equilibrated with 100% oxygen (PO_2, 760 mmHg).
- One gram of haemoglobin when fully saturated combines with 1.34 ml oxygen. Thus, Hb concentration is an index of oxygen carrying capacity of blood. Thus, normal values of oxygen carrying capacity in males is 1.34 × 15.5 = about 21 ml/dL, and in females is 1.34 × 14 = about 18.5 ml/dL.
- *Clinically,* irrespective of the age, a level of 14.8 g/dL is considered as 100% haemoglobin.

Structure of Haemoglobin

Haemoglobin is a globular molecule having a molecular weight of 68,000. It consists of the protein *globin* combined with iron containing pigment called *haem.*

Structure of Globin. The protein globin, present in the haemoglobin, is made up of four polypeptide chains. The polypeptide chains are of different types (described in types of haemoglobin). The globin of the common type of adult haemoglobin called HbA consists of the following four polypeptide chains:

- *Two α chains,* each containing 141 amino acid residues and
- *Two β chains,* each containing 146 amino acid residues.

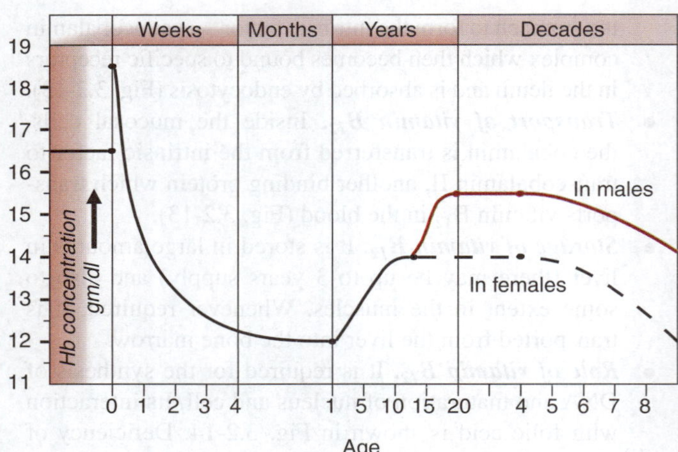

FIGURE 3.2-15 Normal blood haemoglobin concentration at different ages.

Therefore, the normal adult haemoglobin A is written as HbA ($\alpha^2\beta^2$).

Structure of Haem. The haem is an iron–porphyrin complex called *iron–protoporphyrin IX,* i.e. it consists of a porphyrin nucleus and iron. The structural characteristics of the haem (iron–protoporphyrin IX) are given below (Fig. 3.2-16A, B and C).

Porphyrin Nucleus

- The porphyrin nucleus consists of four *pyrrole rings* numbered I, II, III and IV, i.e. porphyrins are tetrapyrroles.
- The pyrrole rings are joined together by four *methine bridges* (=CH—). The carbon atoms of methine bridges are labelled α, β, γ and δ.
- Eight *side chains* are attached to the pyrrole ring at positions labelled 1 to 8. These are:
  - Four *methyl* (H_3C) side chains at positions 1, 3, 5 and 8,
  - Two *vinyl* ($CH.CH_2$) side chains at positions 2 and 4 and
  - Two *propionic acid* ($CH_2.CH_2.COOH$) side chains at positions 6 and 7.

The Iron

- The iron in the haem is in *ferrous* (Fe^{2+}) form.
- The iron is attached to the nitrogen atom of each pyrrole ring.
- On the iron (Fe^{2+}) a bond is available for loose union, where:
  - In oxyhaemoglobin, O_2 is attached,
  - In carboxyhaemoglobin, CO is attached, and so on (see derivatives of haemoglobin).

Attachment of Haem to Globin. One molecule of haemoglobin contains four units of haem, each attached to one of the four polypeptide chains constituting globin (Fig. 3.2-16D). As there are four units of haem in one molecule of haemoglobin, so there are four iron atoms in one molecule of Hb which can carry four molecules (eight atoms) of oxygen.

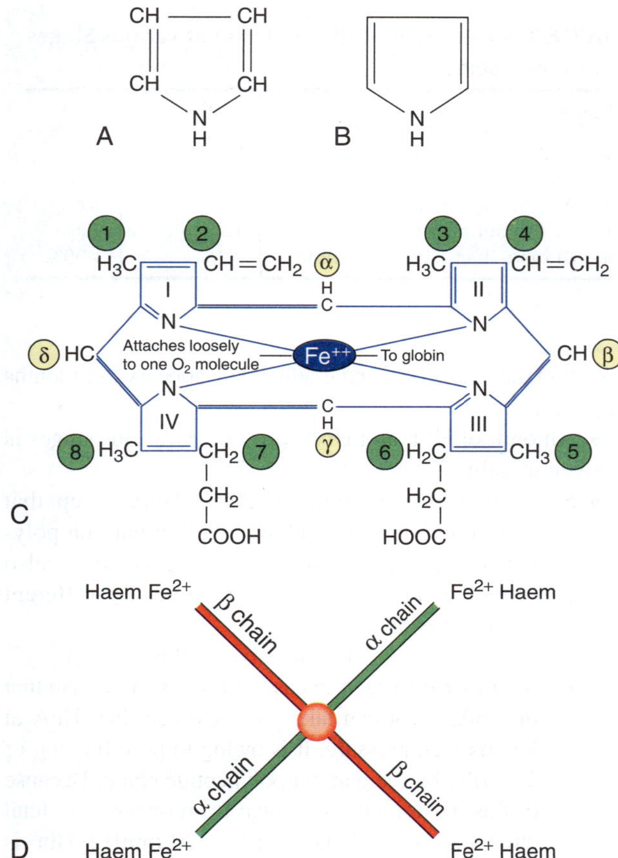

FIGURE 3.2-16 Chemistry of haemoglobin: **A,** structure of a pyrrole ring; **B,** conventional outline of a pyrrole ring; **C,** arrangement of pyrrole rings in one unit of haem (iron protoporphyrin X); and **D,** arrangement of four units of haem in one molecule of haemoglobin.

Functions of Haemoglobin

1. Transport of O_2 from Lungs to Tissues

- *In the lungs,* one molecule of O_2 is attached loosely and reversibly at the sixth covalent bond of each iron atom of the haemoglobin to form *oxyhaemoglobin* represented as HbO_2:

Hb	+	O_2	→	HbO_2
Deoxygenated (reduced) haemoglobin				Oxygenated haemoglobin

- Oxygenation of the 1st haem molecule in the haemoglobin increases the affinity of the 2nd haem for oxygen, which in turn increases the affinity of the 3rd haem and so on. In this way, affinity of haemoglobin for the 4th oxygen molecule is many times that for the 1st molecule. Because of this:
  - Haemoglobin reacts with oxygen very rapidly taking less than 0.01 s. Similarly, deoxygenation of haemoglobin is also very rapid, and
  - The oxygen–haemoglobin dissociation curve becomes sigmoid shaped (see page 430).
- The affinity of haemoglobin for oxygen is influenced by pH, temperature and concentration of 2,3-diphosphoglycerate or biphosphoglycerate, i.e. 2,3-BPG (a product of metabolism of glucose) in the RBCs.
- As the concentration of 2,3-BPG rises, the affinity of Hb for oxygen falls and the oxygen–haemoglobin dissociation curve is shifted to the right (see page 432) and as a result more oxygen is released by blood to the tissues. *It is important to note that:*
  - *At high altitude* (e.g. 5000 m above the sea level) 2,3-BPG concentration in red cells increases by 50% and thus more oxygen is available to the tissues.
  - *As 2,3-BPG accumulates,* it depresses hexokinase and 2,3-BPG mutase activity by negative feedback control. Glucose metabolism in this way is related to oxygen transport via intracorpuscular 2,3-BPG concentration.
  - *Stored blood* loses its 2,3-BPG concentration and oxygen affinity increases resulting in less release of oxygen. The addition of inosine and adenosine to stored blood increases 2,3-BPG formation and restores the normal affinity of haemoglobin for oxygen.

2. Transport of CO_2 from the Tissues to the Lungs. Haemoglobin also transports CO_2 from the tissues to the lungs.

- It is important to note that CO_2 from the tissues is transported by combining with amino acids of the globin part as shown below and not in combination with Fe^{2+} atom like O_2.

$$\underset{\text{Haemoglobin}}{R-N\begin{matrix}H\\H\end{matrix}} + CO_2 \rightarrow \underset{\text{Carbamino-haemoglobin}}{R-N\begin{matrix}H\\COOH\end{matrix}}$$

- Deoxygenated Hb forms carbamino-haemoglobin more readily than oxygenated Hb. That is why venous blood becomes more suitable for transport of CO_2 from the tissues to the lungs.

3. Control pH of the Blood. The haemoglobin constitutes the most important acid–base buffer system of blood. Although, the concentration of Hb is roughly twice the concentration of plasma proteins, Hb has six times the buffering capacity compared with plasma proteins.

Development of Haemoglobin

- The human haemoglobin first appears at about six weeks after gestation. The red cells contain embryonic haemoglobin Portland ($\zeta_2\gamma_2$),Hb Gower I ($\zeta_2\epsilon_2$) and Hb Gower II ($\alpha_2\epsilon_2$) (Fig. 3.2-17)
- At about 10–11 weeks, fetal Hb [HbF($\alpha_2\gamma_2$)] becomes prominent.

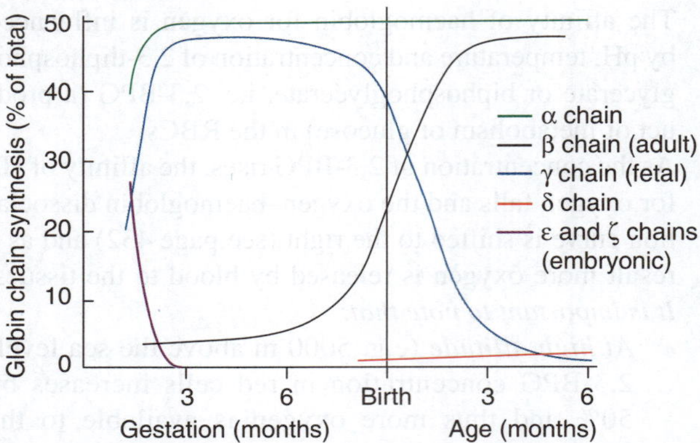

FIGURE 3.2-17 Development of human haemoglobin chains.

- At about 38 weeks, there is synthesis of adult Hb [HbA ($\alpha_2\beta_2$)], a small amount of HbF is produced during postnatal life because few red cell clones called F cells (small pool of immature committed erythrocyte precursor) retain the ability to produce Hb F.

The human haemoglobin is encoded by gene clusters (α and β). The α-like gene clusters are located on chromosome 16 and β-like on chromosome 11. The locus control region (LCR) element is located in the upstream control expression of each cluster. Therefore, normal red blood cells differentiation requires co-ordinated expression of the globin genes, genes responsible for haem and Fe metabolism.

Varieties of Haemoglobin

Apart from species differences, several varieties of haemoglobin occur in human beings. In all varieties of haemoglobin, the haem moiety remains the same. It is the composition of polypeptide chains of the globin part of the haemoglobin which differs in various varieties of haemoglobin. Various varieties of haemoglobin can be grouped as under:

- Physiological varieties of haemoglobin, and
- Haemoglobinopathies.

Physiological Varieties of Haemoglobin

Adult Haemoglobin. Adult haemoglobin is of two types.

i. ***Haemoglobin A*** [HbA ($\alpha_2\beta_2$)]. It is the main form of normal adult haemoglobin. As described on page 144, its globin part consists of two alpha and two beta polypeptide chains. It is a spheroidal molecule with a molecular weight of 68,000.

ii. ***Haemoglobin A2*** [HbA_2 ($\alpha_2\delta_2$)]. It is a minor component (about 2.5% of the total Hb) in normal adults. Its globin part consists of two alpha and two delta polypeptide chains. Delta chains have slightly different amino acid composition (out of 146, 10 amino acids are different) compared with β chains.

Fetal Haemoglobin. Fetal haemoglobin, or haemoglobin F [HbF $\alpha_2\gamma_2$] as the name indicates, refers to the haemoglobin present in the fetal RBCs and gradually disappears 2–3 months after birth.

TABLE 3.2-3 Amount of HbF and HbA at Various Stages in Human Beings

Stage	HbF	HbA
• At 20 weeks of intrauterine	94%	6%
• At birth	80%	20%
• At 2 months after birth	50%	50%
• At 4 months after birth	10%	90%
• At more than 1 year after birth	<1%	>99%

- **Amount of HbF and HbA** present at various stages is as given in Table 3.2-3.
- **Structure of HbF** is similar to that of HbA, except that its globin part consists of two alpha and two gamma polypeptide chains (in place of beta chains). Gamma chains also have 146 amino acids, but its 37 amino acids are different than that of beta chains.
- **Special features** of HbF are given below.
  - ***Affinity for oxygen*** in case of HbF is more than that of HbA, i.e. it can take more oxygen than HbA at low oxygen pressure. It is owing to poor binding of 2,3-BPG by the gamma polypeptide chain. Because of this, movement of oxygen from maternal to fetal circulation is facilitated. At PO_2 20 mmHg, HbF is 70% saturated while HbA is only 30–35% saturated. For details see page 433.
  - ***Resistance to action of alkalies*** is more in HbF than HbA. This property is used in a photoelectric colorimetric method to estimate HbF in the presence of HbA.
  - ***Lifespan*** of HbF is much less (1–2 weeks) compared with that of HbA (120 days).

Haemoglobinopathies. Haemoglobinopathies, i.e. abnormal formation of haemoglobin occurs due to disorders of globin synthesis, haem synthesis being normal.

Classification: There are five major classes of haemoglobinopathies. Structural haemoglobinopathies occur due to gene mutation resulting in alteration in amino acid sequence in the globin chain include:

i. *Sickle cell anaemia* occurs due to HbS and is an example of structural haemoglobinopathy.
ii. *Thalassaemia syndromes* occur due to mutation that impairs the production of globin mRNA resulting in deficient or absent globin biosynthesis.
iii. *Thalassaemic haemoglobin variants*: when there are combined features of thalassaemia and structural haemoglobinopathies, e.g. Hb E, Hb C, Hb L and Hb J.
iv. *Hereditary persistence of fetal haemoglobin (HPFH)*: due to increased levels of fetal haemoglobin in adult life.
v. *Acquired Haemoglobinopathies* occur due to modification of Hb molecule by toxins, e.g. methaemoglobin,

sulfhaemoglobin, carboxyhaemoglobin and haemoglobin H in leukaemia.

1. Sickle Cell Haemoglobin or haemoglobin S (HbS)

- HbS is the most important haemoglobinopathy.
- It occurs in 10–20% of Negroes. Sickle cell gene originated in the black population in Africa.
- HbS is formed due to substitution of valine for glutamic acid at position 6 in the beta chain of HbA.
- When HbS is reduced (e.g. in low O_2 tension or when pH at tissue level is low), it becomes much less soluble and precipitates into crystals within the RBCs. The crystals elongate producing changes in shape of the cells from biconcave to sickle-shaped cells (sickling), (Fig. 3.2-18).

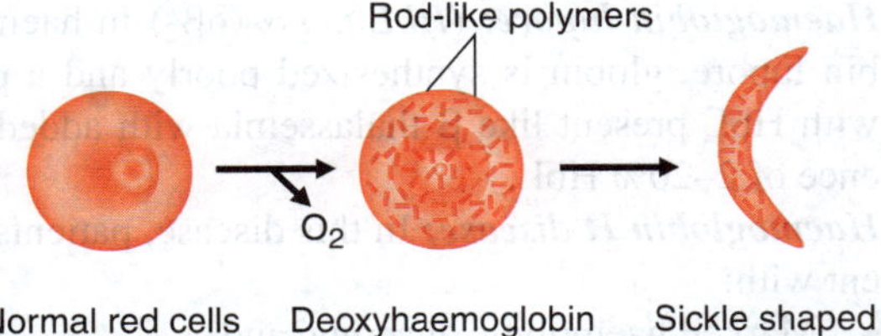

FIGURE 3.2-18 Mechanism of sickling of red blood cell containing haemoglobin S (HbS).

- The cells containing HbS are less flexible compared with RBCs containing HbA, hence leading to blockade of microcirculation.
- Sickle-shaped cells greatly increase blood viscosity thereby decreasing the blood flow to tissues.
- Sickle-shaped cells are more fragile and are very liable to undergo haemolysis producing the so-called sickle cell anaemia.
- Sickle trait is inherited as Mendelian dominant, but the full-blown disease is autosomally recessive. Heterozygous individual with sickle cell trait rarely has severe symptoms, but homozygous develop full-blown disease.
- The individual with the sickle cell trait has resistance to one type of malaria.

Pathophysiology of sickle cell crisis *has been depicted in* Fig. 3.2-19.

Treatment of sickle cell anaemia

- Presence of HbF in RBCs decreases the polymerization of deoxygenated HbS. There are two drugs: 5-*azacytidine* and *hydroxyurea,* which lead to formation of HbF in children and adults. These drugs have been tried in patients with sickle cell anaemia and have shown good preliminary results.

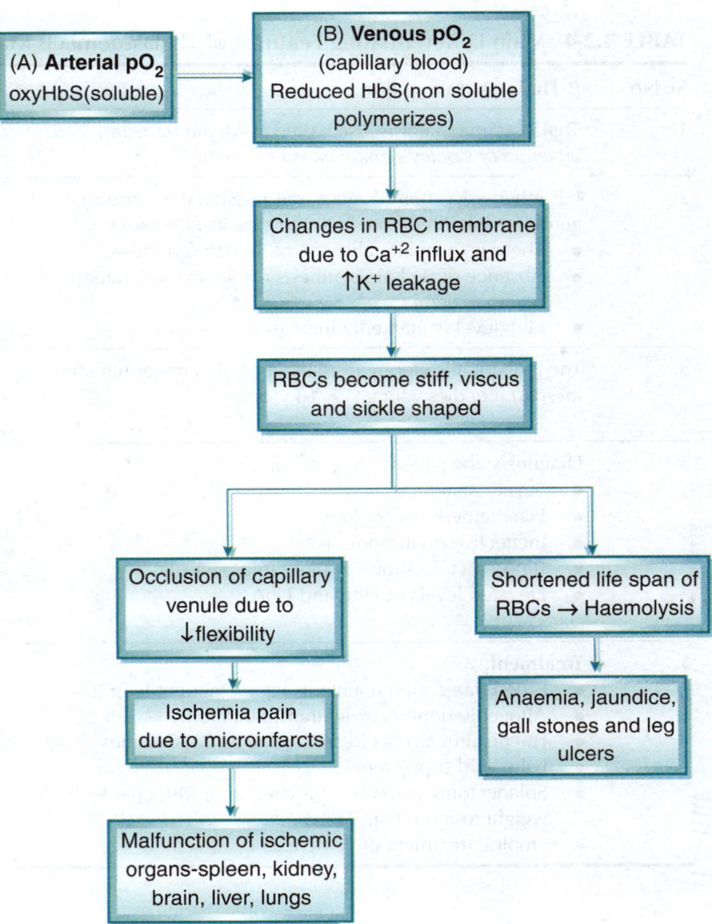

FIGURE 3.2-19 Pathophysiology of sickle cell crisis.

- Bone marrow transplantation has cured the disease in some cases.

2. Thalassaemia (Mediterranean anaemia) is a haemoglobinopathy characterized by the following features:

- ***Cause.*** Thalassaemia results due to defect in the synthesis of polypeptide chain α and β of HbA.
- ***Types.*** Depending upon whether α or β chains are not synthesized, α thalassaemia or β thalassaemia may occur, respectively. *α thalassemia syndrome* may present in the following forms depending on deletion on α globin loci:
  - **i.** *The* α thalassaemia trait: May be asymptomatic or silent carrier state or may resemble β thalassemia minor .
  - **ii.** The homozygous state of α thalassemia: In this condition there is excess of γ globin form, i.e. Hb Barts (Υ_4) which has very high oxygen affinity. Hence, there is no delivery of the oxygen to fetal tissues leading to asphyxia, oedema (Hydrops foetalis), congestive heart failure and death in utero.
- ***β Thalassaemia*** is more common and is further of two types: thalassaemia major and thalassaemia minor.
- ***Features*** of thalassaemia major and minor are depicted in Table 3.2-4.

3. Hemoglobin variants include:

i. ***Haemoglobin E(HbE),*** *i.e.* $\alpha_2\beta^{2(26glu\ lys)}$ is the most common variant of Hb detected in the United States. Hb E homozygous are asymptomatic. Blood picture shows that microcytosis, hypochromia and Hb levels are rarely less than 10 g/dL.

ii. ***Haemoglobin C (HbC).*** Hb C, like Hb S is formed by substitution of lysine for glutamic acid at β 6 position. In Hb C type of variant there is no sickling of RBCs, but HbC may precipitate in polymer formation in association with Hb S. Homozygous HbC disease presents with mild haemolytic anaemia, splenomegaly, mild jaundice and pigment gall stones (Ca-bilirubinate stones).

iii. ***Haemoglobin lupore:*** *(HbL i.e.* $\alpha_2(\delta\beta_2)$ In haemoglobin lupore, globin is synthesized poorly and a person with HbL present like β thalassemia with added presence of 2–20% HbL.

iv. ***Haemoglobin H disease:*** In this disease, patients present with:

- Marked haemolytic anaemia, and
- Haematocrit is 22–32%

TABLE 3.2-4 Main Differentiating Features of Thalassaemia β Major and Minor

Sr. No.	β Thalassaemia major	β Thalassaemia minor
1.	Thalassaemia major is also called as *Mediterranean anaemia or Cooley's anaemia* is less common.	Thalassaemia minor is more common.
2.	It is inherited as homozygous transmission (i.e. abnormal genes are inherited from both the parents), therefore, • There is complete absence of β chain synthesis. • Absence of β chain synthesis results in moderate to severe anaemia. • HbF level is markedly increased.	It is inherited as heterozygous transmission (i.e. abnormal gene is inherited from one parent), Therefore, • The synthesis of β chain is not completely absent (partial). • Anaemia is of mild type. • HbF level is either normal or slightly elevated.
3.	The individual suffering from thalassaemia major has short lifespan, i.e. dies young (17–18 years)	The individuals suffering from thalassaemia minor comparatively survive longer (up to adult) and transmit abnormal gene to their offspring.
4.	**Diagnosis**: the patient presents with: • Severe anaemia. • Haematocrit is very low. • Ineffective erythropoiesis. • Blood picture shows marked microcytosis. • Elevated levels of HbF and HbA_2.	• β thalassemia minor usually presents with microcytosis and hypochromia but with minimal or mild anaemia. • Hepatosplenomegaly. • Haematocrit 28–40%. • Blood picture as of iron deficiency anaemia. • HbA_2 levels are usually normal or may be elevated to 4–8%.
5.	**Treatment:** • Blood transfusion maintains haematocrit at least 27–30%. • Allogenic bone marrow transplantation. • Fe-chelating agents (defroxamine to avoid hemosidrosis). • Folic acid supplements. • Splenectomy increases the volume of RBCs per/kg body weight to more than 50%. • Employ treatment of Fe deficiency anaemia.	• Usually requires no treatment, but genetic counselling and parent education about the effect of the disease is important.

- MCV is markedly low (60–70 μm^3)
- Peripheral blood smear shows abnormal cells with hypochromia, microcytosis, target cells and poikilocytosis. Peripheral smear stained with supravital stain detects HbH.

v. *Other haemoglobin variants are:* Hb J and HbM disease, cause haemolytic anaemia.

Detection and Characterization of Haemoglobinopathies

Detection and characterization of haemoglobinopathies can be made by the following tests:

- *Routine investigations* include complete haemogram and examination of peripheral blood smear.
- *Screening and Quantification* can be done by haemoglobin electrophoresis and also by using specialized technique like isoelectric focusing and high-pressure liquid chromatography (HPLC).
- *Function assays* for HbS include sickling test, solubility test, precipitation test and oxygen affinity (P_{50}) to detect low/high affinity of oxygen.
- *Spectrophotometry* to detect % of abnormal Hb, e.g. methaemoglobin and carboxyhaemoglobin.
- *For complete characterization of haemoglobinopathy, the following tests should be done:*
  - Amino acid sequencing,
  - Polymerase chain reaction (PCR),
  - Allele specific oligomerotyde hybridization, automated DNA hybridization and
  - Automated DNA sequencing.

Derivatives of Haemoglobin (Reactions of Haemoglobin)

Haemoglobin has the property to readily react with any gas or other substance to form the so-called derivatives of haemoglobin. These include:

1. *Oxyhaemoglobin.* As described on page 145, haemoglobin reacts readily with oxygen to form oxyhaemoglobin which is an unstable and reversible compound, i.e. oxygen can be released from this compound. In this compound iron remains in ferrous state.

2. *Reduced Haemoglobin* or deoxygenated haemoglobin is formed when oxygen is released from the oxyhaemoglobin.

HbO_2	→	Hb	+ O_2
Oxyhaemoglobin	→	reduced haemoglobin	

3. *Carbamino-haemoglobin* is a compound of Hb with carbon dioxide

$$HbNH_2 + CO_2 \rightarrow HbNHCOOH$$

4. *Carboxyhaemoglobin* or carbon monoxy haemoglobin is a compound of Hb with carbon monoxide (CO):

$$Hb + CO \rightarrow COHb$$

The affinity of haemoglobin for CO is much more (200–250 times) than its affinity for oxygen. Because of this, the CO displaces oxygen from haemoglobin, thereby reducing the oxygen carrying capacity of blood. For details see page 433.

5. Methaemoglobin. When reduced or oxygenated haemoglobin is treated with an oxidizing agent, e.g. potassium ferricyanide, the ferrous (Fe^{2+}) is oxidized to ferric (Fe^{3+}); the sixth bond is attached to OH to form the compound methaemoglobin. Methaemoglobin is represented as HbOH.

Disadvantages *of methaemoglobin are:*

- It cannot unite reversibly with gaseous oxygen; the O_2 of the attached OH is not given off in a vacuum.
- When present in large amount, it produces blue colour of skin (cyanosis) because of its dark colour.

Normally, some oxidation of haemoglobin to methaemoglobin (HbOH) does occur; but the methaemoglobin formed is soon converted back to haemoglobin by the enzyme NADH – methaemoglobin reductase present in the RBCs. Hereditary methaemoglobinaemia may result due to congenital absence of this enzyme.

6. Sulphaemoglobin is formed by a combination of haemoglobin with hydrogen sulphide (H_2S).

7. Nitrous Oxide Haemoglobin is formed when haemoglobin combines with nitrous oxide.

8. Glycosylated Haemoglobin is a derivative of haemoglobin A present in very small amounts, e.g. ***haemoglobin A_{1C} (HbA_{1C}),*** in which glucose is attached to terminal valine in the β chains. The level of glycosylated haemoglobin in the blood increases in poorly controlled patients of diabetes mellitus.

Important Note

Normally the fraction of Hb glycosylated is approximately 5% and is proportionately blood glucose level. Since half-life of an erythrocyte is 60 days (lifespan 120 days), therefore level of HbA_{1C} reflects the mean blood glucose concentration over preceding 6–8 weeks. Therefore, estimation of HbA_{1C} provides valuable information of management of diabetes mellitus.

Derived Products of Haemoglobin. Derived products of haemoglobin are of two types: iron containing and iron free.

1. Iron-Containing Derived Products of Haemoglobin are:

- *Acid haematin* or *alkali haematin* is formed by the action of acid or alkali with haemoglobin.
- *Haemochromogen* is obtained by reduction of alkali haematin.
- *Cathaemoglobin* is a compound of haemoglobin containing ferric ion with denatured globin.
- *Haem*

2. Iron-Free Derived Products of Haemoglobin are:

- Haematoporphyrin,
- Haempyrrole,
- Haematoidin and
- Bilirubin.

Synthesis of Haemoglobin

Haemoglobin is synthesized in the cytoplasm of intermediate normoblasts. Four haem units join with one molecule of globin to form one unit of haemoglobin.

Synthesis of Haem. Haem is synthesized in the mitochondria. Steps of synthesis are (Fig. 3.2-20):

- Succinyl-CoA (derived from the citric acid cycle in mitochondria) and glycine are the starting substances in the synthesis of haem. These condense to form α-amino-β-ketoadipic acid. The condensation requires pyridoxal phosphate for activation of glycine.
- The α-amino-β-ketoadipic acid gets rapidly decarboxylated to δ-aminolaevulinic acid (ALA) in the presence of enzyme ALA synthetase in the mitochondria.
- The *protoporphyrin IX* is then formed after a series of reactions promoted by other enzymes.
- Finally, ferrous ion is introduced into the protoporphyrin-IX molecule to form *haem* in a reaction catalysed by the enzyme haem synthetase.

Synthesis of Globin. Globin, the protein part of the haemoglobin is synthesized in ribosomes.

Factors Controlling Haemoglobin Formation. Whipple's standard anaemic dog studies show that iron as well as dietary proteins, both play a very important role in the synthesis of haemoglobin. In addition, certain other minerals and vitamins also control the haemoglobin formation.

1. Role of Proteins. First class proteins provide amino acids required for synthesis of globin part of the haemoglobin. A low protein intake retards haemoglobin regeneration even in the presence of excess iron; the limiting factor being lack of globin. The relative values of various foods in providing the required amino acids are:

- *Most valuable* food is of animal origin and consists of liver, spleen, kidney and heart.
- *Foodstuffs of intermediate value* are again of animal origin and include the muscles.
- *Foodstuffs of least* value include bread and other cereals, dairy products, most vegetables and fruits and salmon.

2. Role of Iron. Iron is necessary for formation of haem part of haemoglobin. In addition to dietary iron, the iron released by degradation of RBCs is also reused for synthesis of haemoglobin. Various aspects of iron metabolism are discussed on page 158.

3. Role of Other Metals.

- *Copper.* Copper is essential for haemoglobin synthesis, as it promotes the absorption, mobilization and utilization of iron. Usually, copper deficiency seldom occurs, since requirement of copper is very little and that it occurs in adequate amounts in the diet and most iron preparations contain traces of copper.
- *Cobalt.* Cobalt is required for synthesis of vitamin B_{12} by bacterial action in the lumen of gut of sheep and other cattle. However, its role in humans is not evidenced. Further, in some species, cobalt increases the production of erythropoietin which in turn stimulates RBC formation.
- *Calcium.* Calcium is reported to help indirectly by conserving iron and its subsequent utilization.

4. Role of Vitamins. Vitamin B_{12}, folic acid and vitamin C help in synthesis of nucleic acid which in turn, is required for the development of RBCs. Vitamin C also helps in absorption of iron from the gut.

5. Role of Bile Salts. Presence of bile salts in the intestine is necessary for proper absorption of metals like copper and nickel, which in turn are essential factors for synthesis of haemoglobin.

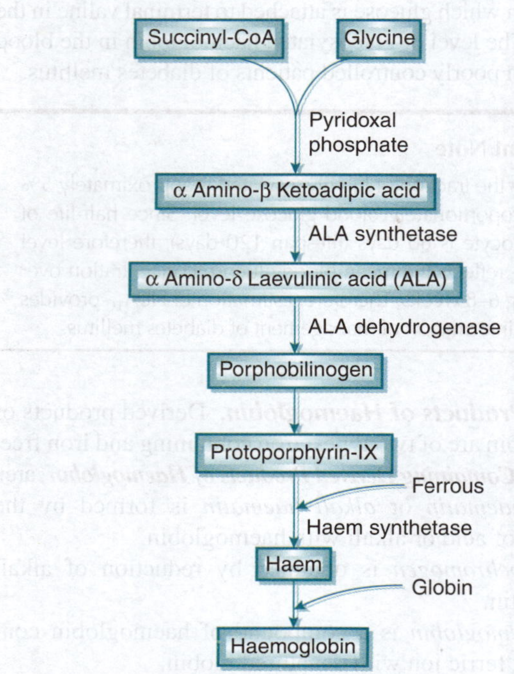

FIGURE 3.2-20 Steps of synthesis of haemoglobin.

Degradation of Haemoglobin

Tissue macrophages (reticuloendothelial system), especially those lining the hepatic and splenic sinusoids phagocytize the old RBCs. Haemoglobin is broken down and bilirubin is formed within the macrophages. The iron released from degraded haemoglobin enters the plasma and the bilirubin enters into the bile canaliculi. For details see page 151.

RED CELL FRAGILITY

Red cell fragility refers to the susceptibility of red cell membrane to break or burst. The process of breaking of RBCs and release of haemoglobin into the plasma is called haemolysis. Red cell fragility, depending upon the underlying mechanism, is of two types:

- Osmotic red cell fragility, and
- Mechanical red cell fragility.

Osmotic Red Cell Fragility

Osmotic red cell fragility refers to the susceptibility of the red cell membrane to get lysed due to changes in the osmotic pressure of the solution in which they are suspended.

Effect of Osmotic Pressure of Solution on the RBCs

- ***Isotonic solutions*** have tonicity as that of plasma. These include 0.9% NaCl, 5% glucose, 10% mannitol and 20% urea. When RBCs are placed in these solutions, they remain suspended in them, i.e. neither swell nor shrink. This is because the osmotic pressure of the isotonic solutions is equal to the osmotic pressure within the RBCs.
- ***Hypertonic solutions*** (e.g. >0.9% NaCl, 20% mannitol) have osmotic pressure more than the osmotic pressure within the RBCs. Therefore, when the RBCs are placed in such solutions, fluid goes out of the cells and they shrink.
- ***Hypotonic solutions*** (e.g. <0.9% NaCl) have osmotic pressure less than the osmotic pressure within the RBCs. Therefore, when the RBCs are placed in such solutions, they swell up by absorbing water from outside and finally burst, i.e. get haemolyzed.

Osmotic Red Cell Fragility Test. To perform the osmotic red cell fragility test, the NaCl solutions of different concentrations (from 0.2 to 0.9%) are taken in series of Cohn's tubes. One or two drops of blood are added in each tube, mixed gently and left undisturbed for 1 h. Following observations may be made:

- ***No haemolysis.*** The RBCs settle down as red dots at the bottom of the tube with clear saline solution above.
- ***Onset of haemolysis.*** A few RBCs rupture and the saline is tinged red with the released haemoglobin. The RBCs which have not ruptured are seen as red dots at the bottom of tube with red-tinged saline solution above.
- ***Completion of haemolysis.*** All the RBCs rupture and make the whole saline solution uniformly red with no red dots at the bottom of the tube.

Normal values (index of fragility)

- *Onset of haemolysis* (fragility) in normal RBCs occurs in 0.48% NaCl, and
- *Completion of haemolysis* (ending of fragility) occurs in 0.35% NaCl.
- *Explanation*. Normally, only the older red cells with comparative fragile membrane are haemolyzed in around 0.48% of NaCl solution, since these cells cannot withstand this hypotonicity. But, younger cells are not affected. In 0.35% NaCl, even the youngest cells are haemolyzed and so haemolysis is completed.

Abnormal Osmotic Fragility. ***Increase in osmotic fragility index*** occurs in following conditions:

- *Congenital spherocytosis,* i.e. when the RBCs are spherical. In this condition onset of haemolysis occurs at 0.7% NaCl and it is completed at 0.45% NaCl solution.
- *Autoimmune haemolytic anaemia* in which the autoantibodies damage the structure proteins and render the red cells more fragile.
- *Deficiency of glucose 6-phosphate dehydrogenase (G6PD)* increases the tendency of red cells to get haemolyzed by antimalarial drugs and other agents.
- *Venom of cobra and other insects* contains lecithinase, which dissolves lecithin from red cell membranes making them more fragile.

Decrease in osmotic fragility index occurs when the RBCs become slender, e.g. in iron deficiency anaemia. In this condition, the onset of haemolysis occurs at 0.36% NaCl and is completed at 0.24% NaCl solution.

Mechanical Red Cell Fragility

The red cells are subjected to mechanical stress and trauma as they pass through the capillaries and trabeculae of the spleen some 300,000 times during their lifespan of 120 days. They are made more brittle due to unusual mechanical stress. The red cells can become more rigid as a result of pathological changes in the membrane or in the cell contents caused by a number of red cell disorders. The cells thus become mechanically more fragile, i.e. less liable to tolerate deforming stresses, than the normal healthy red cell.

A normal or less osmotic fragility does not rule out the possibility of high mechanical fragility. For example, in sickle cell anaemia, the RBCs are sickle-shaped and have a high mechanical fragility, but the osmotic fragility of the sickled cells is normal or even low.

Mechanical Fragility Test. Mechanical fragility test can be performed by placing blood in a flask containing glass beads, and vigorously rotating the flask. The haemoglobin concentration of the supernatant is then measured, which provides an idea about the degree of haemolysis.

LIFESPAN AND FATE OF RED BLOOD CELLS

LifeSpan of Red Blood Cells

Normally, the average lifespan of red blood cells is 120 days.

Determination of Lifespan of Red Blood Cells

1. Differential Agglutination Method. In this method, an individual is transfused with red blood cells of a different but compatible group. For example, 'O' group blood is transfused to an 'A' group individual. About one litre of blood should be transfused so that substantial number of donor cells can be obtained to count. Then, a small quantity of blood is withdrawn from the recipient. The red cells are separated and treated with anti-A serum. The 'A' cells agglutinate and 'O' cells remain dispersed, which are counted. The procedure is repeated every day till the group 'O' cells are seen. The experiments show that some of the transfused cells can be seen surviving for about 120 days.

2. Radioactive Isotope Method. In this method, about 15–20 ml of blood is withdrawn from an individual and then put RBCs are tagged with radioactive substances like radioactive iron or radioactive chromium. These RBCs are injected back into the same individual. Blood samples are then collected from the individual every day and radioactivity is determined. The isotope survival curve is plotted by plotting the radioactivity of blood as a function of time and the mean lifespan of red blood cells is calculated. If the curve for loss of radioactivity is suitably corrected, it is found to be almost linear, falling to zero at about 120 days. The half-life of the cells (50% destruction) being about 60 days, the curve gives the maximum survival time of the youngest cells, the mean survival time, and the average destruction of the cells in a heterogeneous sample.

Causes of Reduction in the Lifespan of Red Blood Cells

I. Defects in Red Blood Cells (Corpuscular Defects)

1. Hereditary spherocytosis. It is an autosomal dominant disorder characterized by small and spherical red blood cells. These cells cannot be compressed; therefore, they get easily ruptured while passing through pulp of spleen. They show increased osmotic fragility so that haemolysis may commence at 0.7% NaCl and be completed at 0.4% NaCl solution, lifespan of such RBCs is reduced to 15–20 days. In this condition, the spleen is enlarged and serum bilirubin level may be raised to 20–50 mmol/L.

2. Sickle cell anaemia. In this condition, RBCs contain abnormal haemoglobin, called haemoglobin-S. The cell membrane of sickle-shaped red blood cells is more fragile and gets easily haemolyzed and their lifespan is reduced. For details see page 147.

3. Thalassaemias. In this condition, the red blood cells are abnormal in having reduced amount of HbA, to compensate for which there are increased amounts of HbA_2 ($\alpha_2\delta_2$) and HbF ($\alpha_2\gamma_2$). The red cells are rapidly haemolyzed and thus their lifespan is reduced. Children with thalassaemia get hypochromic anaemia, fail to thrive and die young. For details see page 148.

4. Deficiency of red cell enzymes. The red blood cells deficient in certain enzymes become more susceptible to haemolysis and their lifespan is decreased. Some of such conditions are:

- *Glucose 6-phosphate-dehydrogenase deficiency.* It is inherited as sex-linked character. Glucose-6 phosphate dehydrogenase catalyses the reaction in pentose phosphate pathway and produces NADPH. NADPH plays a key role as a reducing agent in RBCs and other cells.

NADPH in RBCs serves as a cofactor for glutathione reductase in generating reduced glutathione, which detoxifies hydrogen peroxide (H_2O_2). In absence of reduced glutathione,

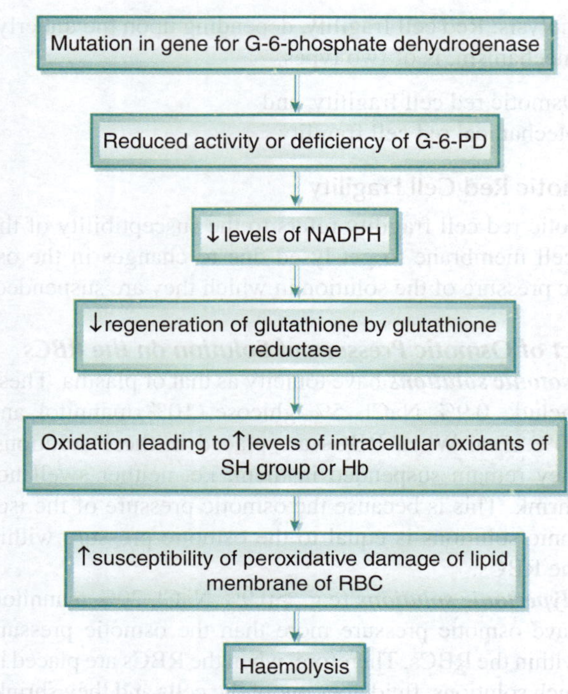

FIGURE 3.2-21 Flow diagram depicting effects of deficiency of G-6 phosphate dehydronase.

Hb is oxidized and gets denatured and forms precipitates called *Hienz*'s *bodies*, which causes membrane damage. Therefore, deficiency of G6PD results in oxidative damage to RBCs due to impaired production of NADPH (Fig. 3.2-21).

In this condition, as reducing power of the red cells is decreased and they become more vulnerable to damage by oxidizing agents such as primaquine and other antimalarial drugs.

- *Pyruvate kinase deficiency* may also produce haemolytic anaemia with reduction in lifespan of RBCs.
- *Paroxysmal nocturnal haemoglobin urea* is a rare condition in which red cells are hypersensitive to lysis by complement.

II. Extracorpuscular Defects

1. Transfusion of mismatched blood produces haemolysis, drastically reducing lifespan of RBCs.

2. Autoimmune haemolytic disorders. In such conditions, antibodies are formed against the patient's own red blood cells. These autoantibodies may be of IgG or IgM class and they may be bound to red cell membrane or occur in serum. Some react maximally at 37°C (warm type) and others at 20°C (cold type).

3. Hypersplenism, due to any cause, may enhance destruction of red blood cells, leucocytes and platelets.

Fate of Red Blood Cells

The cell membrane of old RBCs (after about 120 days) becomes more fragile due to decreased NADPH activity. The younger RBCs can easily pass through the capillaries which have a diameter smaller than the red cells. The older cells with fragile membranes are destroyed while trying to squeeze through the capillaries. The destruction of red cells occurs mostly in the capillaries of spleen because they have very thin lumen. Because of this, the spleen is also called the graveyard of red blood cells. The haemoglobin released after haemolysis of red cells is taken up by the tissue macrophages.

The tissue macrophage system (reticuloendothelial system) includes the following phagocytic cells:

- *In the bone marrow,* these cells form part of the lining of the blood sinuses (littoral cells);
- *In the liver,* they lie at intervals along the vascular capillaries (Kupffer cells),
- *In the spleen,* they are found in the pulp, and
- *In the lymph nodes,* they line the lymphatic paths.

Fate of Haemoglobin (Fig. 3.2-22)

- In the macrophages, the haem part of the haemoglobin molecule is altered by oxidation of one of its methine (=CH) bridges. The tetrapyrrole ring structure is thus broken and four pyrrole groups become arranged as a straight chain. As a result of this chemical change, the green iron-containing compound *choleglobin is formed.* As the name implies, the choleglobin molecule still contains the original globin.
- Next, the *choleglobin splits off* into globin, iron and biliverdin (tetrapyrrole straight chain free from globin and iron).
- *Globin* is degraded into amino acids and joins the amino acid pool of plasma and is released.
- *Iron* released into the circulation is:
  - carried into the bone marrow for reutilization, and
  - in the other tissues it combines with apoferritin to form the ferritin (storage form of iron).
- *Biliverdin* (tetrapyrrole straight chain free from globin and iron) is converted into bilirubin (by the enzyme biliverdin reductase) and is released into the blood.

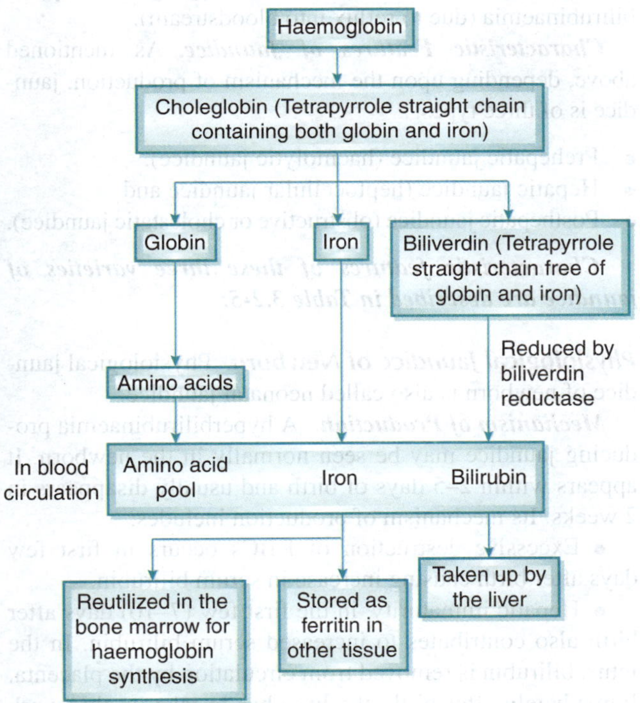

FIGURE 3.2-22 Fate of haemoglobin.

BILIRUBIN AND JAUNDICE

Bilirubin Formation and Its Fate

As discussed above, the bilirubin is formed in the macrophages after degradation of haemoglobin. It undergoes the following changes (Fig. 3.2-23):

1. Uptake of Bilirubin. Macrophages release the bilirubin into circulation. This bilirubin is called free or *unconjugated bilirubin.* It is a lipid soluble and in the plasma it is bound to the albumin (protein-conjugated). It is this protein conjugation of bilirubin which is responsible for solubility of the bilirubin complex in the plasma and which prevents its excretion by the kidneys.

2. Conjugation of Bilirubin. The unconjugated bilirubin (bound to albumin) from the circulation is taken up by the liver.

- In the liver, the bilirubin is removed from the albumin and taken up at sinusoidal surface of hepatocytes by carrier-mediated transport system (facilitated diffusion).
- Once bilirubin enters the hepatocytes, it binds to certain cytosolic proteins (ligandin and protein Y). These

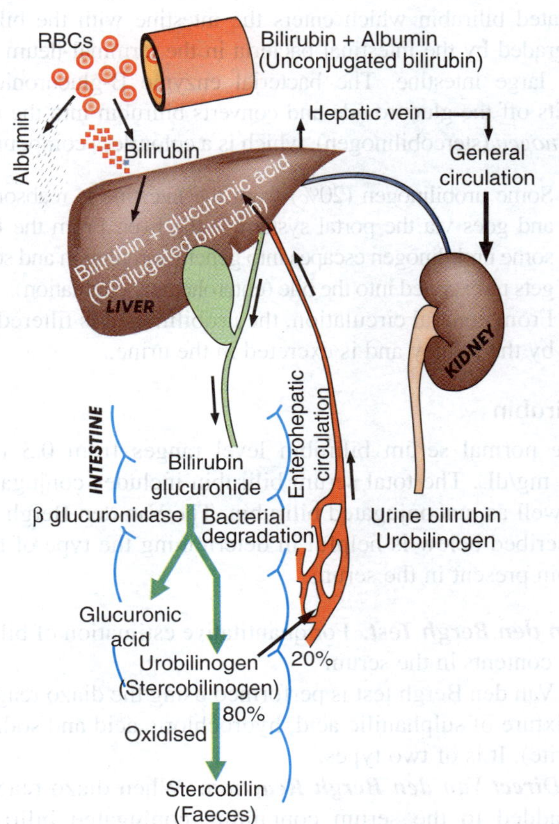

FIGURE 3.2-23 State of bilirubin in the body (details in the text).

proteins help to keep the bilirubin in solubilized form before conjugation, and also prevent efflux of bilirubin back into blood stream.

- In the hepatic cells it is conjugated with uridine diphosphate glucuronic acid (UDP-glucuronic acid) making it a water soluble conjugated *bilirubin.* The reaction is catalyzed by the enzyme *glucuronyl transferase* present in the hepatic microsomes (smooth endoplasmic reticulum of liver cells). The reaction occurs in two stages:

- Bilirubin + UDP – glucuronic acid $\xrightarrow{\text{UDP–glucuronyl transferase}}$ Bilirubin monoglucuronide + UDP
- Bilirubin monoglucuronide + UDP – glucuronic acid $\xrightarrow{\text{UDP–glucuronyl transferase}}$ Bilirubin diglucuronide +UDP

3. Excretion of Bilirubin. The conjugated bilirubin from the hepatic cells is excreted into the bile canaliculi through active transport, i.e. it is excreted against a concentration gradient into the bile canaliculi. This active transport is the rate-limiting step in the entire process of bilirubin excretion and needs energy. The protein involved is MRP-2 (multidrug resistance like protein-2) also called multispecific organic anion transporter (MOAT). It is located on the plasma membrane of bile canaliculi. Most of the conjugated bilirubin is excreted into the bile and enters the intestine. Some of it escapes into general circulation and is excreted by the kidneys in urine as *urine bilirubin.*

4. Formation and Excretion of Urobilinogen. The conjugated bilirubin which enters the intestine with the bile is degraded by the intestinal bacteria in the terminal ileum and the large intestine. The bacterial enzyme β-glucuronidase splits off the glucuronide and converts bilirubin into the *urobilinogen* (stercobilinogen), which is a colourless compound.

- Some urobilinogen (20%) from the intestine is reabsorbed and goes via the portal system to the liver. From the liver some urobilinogen escapes into general circulation and some gets re-excreted into the bile (enterohepatic circulation).
- From general circulation, the urobilinogen is filtered off by the kidney and is excreted in the urine.

Bilirubin

The normal serum bilirubin level ranges from 0.3 mg–1.0 mg/dL. The total serum bilirubin includes conjugated, as well as, unconjugated bilirubin. The Van den Bergh test described below is helpful in determining the type of bilirubin present in the serum.

Van den Bergh Test. For quantitative estimation of bilirubin contents in the serum

Van den Bergh test is performed using the diazo reagent (mixture of sulphanilic acid, hydrochloric acid and sodium nitrite). It is of two types:

Direct Van den Bergh Reaction. When diazo reagent is added to the serum containing conjugated bilirubin (water soluble), a reddish-brown colouration is obtained within 30 s. This is called direct positive Van den Bergh reaction.

Indirect Van den Bergh Reaction. When diazo reagent is added to the serum mainly containing unconjugated bilirubin (water insoluble), no colour is obtained. However, if some solvent like methanol (which dissolves the unconjugated bilirubin) is added, the reddish-brown colouration is obtained. This is called indirect positive Van den Bergh reaction.

Hyperbilirubinaemia (Jaundice)

Jaundice (icterus) refers to the yellow appearance of the skin, sclera and mucous membranes resulting from an increased bilirubin concentration (*hyperbilirubinaemia)* in the body fluids. Clinically, jaundice is detectable when the plasma bilirubin exceeds 2–3 mg/dL. Internal tissues and body fluids are coloured yellow, but not the brain, as bilirubin does not cross the blood–brain barrier other than in the immediate neonatal period.

Mechanisms Producing Jaundice. Hyperbilirubinaemia producing jaundice can result from the following mechanisms:

1. Excessive Breakdown (haemolysis) of Red Blood Cells produces the so-called haemolytic jaundice or prehepatic jaundice or retention hyperbilirubinaemia due to over production.

2. Damage to the Liver Cells (infective or toxic) produces the so-called hepatic or hepatocellular jaundice.

3. Obstruction to Bile Ducts produces the obstructive or posthepatic or cholestatic jaundice or regurgitation hyperbilirubinaemia (due to reflux into bloodstream).

Characteristic Features of Jaundice. As mentioned above, depending upon the mechanism of production, jaundice is of three types:

- Prehepatic jaundice (haemolytic jaundice),
- Hepatic jaundice (heptocellular jaundice and
- Posthepatic jaundice (obstructive or cholestatic jaundice).

Characteristic features of these three varieties of jaundice are described in Table 3.2-5:

Physiological Jaundice of Newborn. Physiological jaundice of newborn is also called neonatal jaundice.

Mechanism of Production. A hyperbilirubinaemia producing jaundice may be seen normally in the newborn. It appears within 2–5 days of birth and usually disappears in 2 weeks. Its mechanism of production includes:

- Excessive destruction of RBCs occurs in first few days after birth causing increase in serum bilirubin.
- Hepatic immaturity in the first few (7–10) days after birth also contributes to increased serum bilirubin. In the fetus, bilirubin is removed from circulation by the placenta. Immediately after birth, the liver has to take up this work

TABLE 3.2-5 Characteristic Features of Three Types of Jaundice

Haemolytic jaundice (prehepatic jaundice)	Hepatocellular jaundice (hepatic jaundice)	Cholestatic or obstructive jaundice (posthepatic jaundice)
1. Mechanism of production		
Excessive breakdown of RBCs producing unconjugated bilirubin in amounts more than the healthy liver can conjugate and excrete.	*Inability of the liver* to efficiently conjugate as well as transport bilirubin into the bile due to liver cell damage caused by some infective or toxic agent.	*Obstruction to the bile flow* due to any cause from hepatocytes to duodenum.
2. Types of serum bilirubin accumulated		
Unconjugated hyperbilirubinaemia occurs since it is being produced in excess of what can be conjugated by the liver.	*Both unconjugated* as well as *conjugated* bilirubin is increased in serum.	*Conjugated hyper*bilirubinaemia results due to impaired flow of bile.
3. Van den Bergh test		
Indirect positive reaction (because unconjugated bilirubin is present in blood).	*Biphasic reaction* (because conjugated and unconjugated bilirubin are present.	*Direct positive reaction* (because only conjugated bilirubin is present.
4. Urine bilirubin		
Absent (Unconjugated bilirubin is insoluble in water. It is transported in plasma in bound form with albumin. Since albumin is not filtered into urine, unconjugated bilirubin too is not filtered in urine. Because of this haemolytic jaundice is also called *acholuric jaundice* (no bile pigment in urine).	***Present*** Conjugated bilirubin is water soluble and is present in plasma in dissolved form. It gets easily filtered in urine. This type of jaundice is also called *choluric jaundice*, i.e. (bile pigment present in urine).	***Present*** (Since conjugated bilirubin is filtered in urine).
5. Urine urobilinogen		
Increases (Because liver is excreting lot of conjugated bilirubin in the intestine with the bile, so, more urobilinogen is formed. Part of it is reabsorbed and goes to general circulation and thus urine urobilinogen is increased).	***Decreases*** (Because, damaged liver cells are producing and excreting less of conjugated bilirubin and thus less urobilinogen is formed).	***Markedly decreased or absent*** (Because of obstruction the conjugated bilirubin is not released into the intestine and thus no urobilinogen is formed).
6. Faecal stercobilinogen (normal 25–250 mg/day).		
• *Markedly increased* (because of more formation as described above). • So faeces are *dark brown* in colour.	• *Reduced* (because of less formation as described above). • So stools are *pale* in colour.	• *Absent* (when obstruction is complete). • So stools are *clay* coloured.
7. Faecal fat level		
Normal, i.e. 5–6% of total intake/day (as bile is present in gut for normal digestion of fats).	*Increased* up to 40–50% (because of deficiency of bile in the intestine, emulsification and absorption of fat is inadequate. This produces bulky, pale, greasy and foul smelling faeces, called steatorrhoea).	*Increased*
8. Specific blood tests		
• *Peripheral blood film* shows signs of haemolysis, i.e. anaemia, reticulocytosis and abnormal RBCs.	Normal	Normal
• *Plasma albumin, globulin and A/G ratio:* normal.	Albumin is decreased due to less synthesis by damaged liver, globulin increases and A/G ratio decreases.	Normal
• *Serum alkaline phosphatase*: normal, i.e. 5–13 KA units/100 ml (because excreted in bile).	Increased (because less excretion in bile)	Markedly increased (because not excreted in bile).
• *Liver function tests* *Normal* (as liver is healthy).	*Impaired* (as liver is damaged).	*Normal or* mildly impaired.

which takes 7–10 days to mature and fully conjugate the bilirubin.

Prevention and Treatment.

• Prevention. Neonatal jaundice can be prevented by administration of hepatic microsomal enzyme inducers (e.g. phenobarbital) to the pregnant mother or newborn. The microsomal enzyme inducers increase the activity of glucuronyl transferase in liver.

• Treatment. Normal jaundice can be effectively treated by *phototherapy.* Exposure of the skin to white light causes photoisomerization of bilirubin to water-soluble *lumirubin* which can be rapidly excreted in bile without requiring any conjugation. Thus, phototherapy is of value in treating infants with jaundice, irrespective of its cause.

Applied Aspects

Kernicterus

Unconjugated bilirubin because of its hydrophobic property can cross the blood–brain barrier. When concentration of unconjugated bilirubin in plasma exceeds that which can be tightly bound to albumin (20–25 mg/dL), it enters into the central nervous system and thus results in kernicterus or encephalopathy. The basal ganglia of CNS are mainly affected. For details see page 947

Congenital Nonhaemolytic Jaundice (Crigler–Najjar Syndrome Type I and II):

Crigler–Najjar syndrome type I is a rare autosomal recessive disorder which occurs due to mutation of gene encoding bilirubin UGT activity. The disease is characterized by raised serum bilirubin levels (usually exceed 20 mg/dL). The disease is fatal and phenobarbitol has no effect on formation of bilirubin. Liver transplantation is the only treatment.

Crigler–Najjar syndrome type II. In this, some activity of the enzyme is retained, therefore in these patients, serum bilirubin level does not exceed 20 mg/dL and responds to phototherapy and phenobarbitol.

- **Gilbert syndrome** is also caused by mutation in genes encoding bilirubin-UGT, but 30% enzyme activity persists. Therefore no harmful effects.
- **Dubin–Johnson syndrome** is a benign autosomal recessive disorder with conjugated hyperbilirubinaemia either in childhood or in adult. It occurs due to mutation in the gene encoding MRP-2 (the protein involved in secretion of bilirubin in the bile).
- **Rotor syndrome** is a rare benign condition which may be occurring due to abnormality in hepatic storage of bilirubin, characterized by chronic conjugate hyperbilirubinaemia.
- **Toxic hyperbilirubinaemia** occurs due to toxin-induced liver dysfunctions, caused by chloroform, aceta-aminophen, viral hepatitis and mushroom poisoning.

ANAEMIAS

Definition and Classification

Definition

Anaemia is not a single disease but a group of disorders in which haemoglobin concentration of blood is below the normal range for the age and sex of the subject. Therefore, anaemia is labelled when haemoglobin concentration is less than:

- 13 g/dL in adult males,
- 11.5 g/dL in adult females,
- 15 g/dL in newborn, and
- 9.5 g/dL at 3 months of age.

Low RBC count *(less than 4 million/mm^3) is usually, but not always associated with low haemoglobin levels in anaemia.*

Grading of anaemia, *depending upon the level of haemoglobin, has somewhat arbitrarily been made as:*

- Mild anaemia—Hb 8–10 g/dL
- Moderate anaemia—Hb 6–8 g/dL and
- Severe anaemia—Hb below 6 g/dL.

Classification

Aetiological (Whitby's) Classification. Types of anaemia depending upon the causative mechanism are:

A. Deficiency Anaemias

- Iron deficiency anaemia,
- Megaloblastic anaemia (pernicious anaemia) due to deficiency of vitamin B_{12},
- Megaloblastic anaemia due to deficiency of folic acid and
- Protein and vitamin C deficiency can also cause anaemia.

B. Blood Loss Anaemias. or haemorrhagic anaemias are commonly known and can be:

- *Acute posthaemorrhagic anaemia* as in accidents, and
- *Chronic posthaemorrhagic anaemia*

C. Haemolytic Anaemias. These are relatively uncommon and occur in conditions associated with increased destruction of red blood cells. These can be:

1. Hereditary haemolytic anaemias, e.g. as seen in:

- Thalassaemia (see page 148),
- Sickle cell anaemia (see page 147),
- Hereditary spherocytosis (see page 151) and
- Glucose 6-phosphate dehydrogenase (G6PD) deficiency (see page 152).

2. Acquired haemolytic anaemias such as:

Immunohaemolytic anaemia (due to antibodies against RBCs),

- Microangiopathic haemolytic anaemia (due to mechanical damage to RBCs,
- Haemolytic anaemia due to direct toxic effects (e.g. in malaria, snake venom, toxic effects of drugs and chemicals),
- Haemolytic anaemia in splenomegaly and

- Haemolytic anaemia in paroxysmal nocturnal haemoglobinuria (PNH).

D. Aplastic Anaemia. It occurs due to failure of bone marrow to produce RBCs. It is of two main types:

- Primary aplastic anaemia, and
- Secondary aplastic anaemia.

E. Anaemia Due to Chronic Diseases. It is seen in tuberculosis, chronic infections, malignancies, chronic lung diseases. The mechanism of causation of anaemia is complex. The tissue macrophages are believed to become activated so that RBCs are removed from the blood faster than they can be formed in bone marrow.

Morphological (Wintrobe's) Classification. Based on the mean cell volume (MCV), i.e. cell size and the mean corpuscular haemoglobin concentration (MCHC), i.e. haemoglobin saturation of RBCs, the anaemias can be classified as:

1. Normocytic Normochromic Anaemias. These are characterized by normal MCV (78–94 μm^3) and normal MCHC (30–38%). Such a morphological picture is seen in:

- Acute posthaemorrhagic anaemia,
- Haemolytic anaemias and
- Aplastic anaemias.

2. Microcytic Hypochromic Anaemias. These are characterized by reduced MCV (<78 μm^3) and reduced MCHC (<30%). Examples of such anaemias are:

- Iron deficiency anaemia,
- Chronic posthaemorrhagic anaemia,
- Sideroblastic anaemia and
- Thalassaemia.

3. Macrocytic Normochromic Anaemia is characterized by increased MCV (>94 μm^3) and normal MCHC (30–38%). Examples are:

- Megaloblastic anaemia (pernicious anaemia) is due to deficiency of vitamin. B_{12}, and
- Megaloblastic anaemia due to deficiency of folic acid.

General Clinical Features of Anaemia

Anaemic Hypoxia results due to decreased O_2-carrying capacity of blood in anaemia owing to reduced haemoglobin concentration. The hypoxia brings about several cardiorespiratory compensatory responses. So, general clinical features (symptoms and signs) in patients with anaemia are due to those caused by:

- Resulting tissue hypoxia, and
- Resulting compensatory mechanisms.
  Haemoglobin level at which symptoms and signs of anaemia develop *depends upon three main factors:*
- *Speed of onset of anaemia.* Rapidly progressive anaemia causes more symptoms than anaemia of slow onset.
- *Severity of anaemia.* Mild anaemia usually produces no symptoms. Severe anaemia (Hb < 6 g/dL) of rapid onset produces significant clinical features.
- *Age of the patient.* Young patients tolerate anaemia quite well vis-à-viselderly patients and develop less marked features.

General Clinical Manifestations of Anaemia which occur either due to tissue hypoxia or due to compensatory mechanisms are:

- ***Generalized muscular weakness,*** tiredness and easy fatigability occur due to muscle hypoxia.
- ***Pallorness of skin and mucous membranes*** (buccal and pharyngeal mucous membrane, conjunctiva, lips, ear lobes, palm and nail bed) occurs due to deficiency of red coloured haemoglobin in the blood.
- ***Respiratory symptoms*** such as breathlessness with increased rate and force of respiration occur due to compensatory stimulation of respiratory centre.
- ***Cardiovascular manifestations*** such as palpitation, tachycardia and cardiac murmurs occur as a result of compensatory mechanisms increasing the cardiac output. In very severe cases of anaemia, features of cardiac failure and angina pectoris may also occur.
- ***Central nervous system (CNS) manifestations*** due to cerebral hypoxia include lethargy, headache, faintness especially on exertion, tinnitus, restlessness, confusion and drowsiness.
- ***Ocular manifestations*** include visual disturbances and retinal haemorrhages and cotton wool spots.
- ***Gastrointestinal system symptoms*** include anorexia, flatulence, nausea, constipation. In pernicious anaemia, there occurs atrophy of papillae on the tongue.
- ***Reproductive system*** involvement occurs in females in the form of menstrual disturbances such as amenorrhoea and menorrhagia and loss of libido.
- ***Renal system*** involvement may occur in severe anaemia causing disturbances of renal function and albumin urea.
- ***Basal metabolic rate (BMR)*** is increased in severe anaemia.

Description of Different Types of Anaemias

Deficiency Anaemias

Deficiency anaemias are quite common and occur due to deficiency of factors necessary for erythropoiesis. These include:

- Iron deficiency anaemia,
- Megaloblastic anaemia due to vitamin B_{12} deficiency (pernicious anaemia),
- Megaloblastic anaemia due to folic acid deficiency,
- Anaemia due to protein deficiency and
- Anaemia due to vitamin C deficiency.

Iron Deficiency Anaemia

Iron deficiency anaemia is the commonest nutritional deficiency disorder present throughout the world, but its prevalence is higher in the developing countries. In India, iron deficiency is the commonest cause of anaemia. Iron deficiency anaemia is much more common:

- In women between 20–45 years than in men.
- At periods of active growth in infancy, childhood and adolescence.

Before discussing the different aspects of iron deficiency anaemia, it will be worthwhile to discuss about normal iron metabolism.

Iron Metabolism

Iron is one of important metals present in the human body. The body of a healthy adult contains 4–5 g (72–90 mmol) of iron in the following forms:

- *Haemoglobin* contains about 70% of the total body iron (2.5 g or 45 mmol).
- *Storage iron* amounts to about 20–23% of total body iron (1.5 g, i.e. 18–27 mmol). Two-third of the iron is stored as ferritin and one-third as haemosiderin.
- *Myoglobin* (myohaemoglobin) present in the red muscles contain about 5% of the total body iron (0.2 g or 3.6 mmol)
- *Intracellular enzymes* account for less than 0.1 g (1.8 mmol), i.e. about 2–3% of total body iron. The iron containing enzymes include cytochrome oxidase, catalase and peroxidase cytochrome.

Daily Requirement and Dietary Sources of Iron

Daily requirement. Only 10% of the dietary intake of iron is absorbed. Therefore, daily requirement in adult males is 5–10 mg/day and in females is 20 mg/day (to compensate the menstrual loss). Pregnant and lactating women require about 40 mg of iron per day.

Dietary sources. Foodstuffs vary both in their iron content and availability of iron for absorption into the body. The dietary sources of iron are meat, liver, egg, leafy vegetables, whole wheat and jaggery. The iron in foods of animal origin is better absorbed than iron in foods of vegetable origin.

Absorption of Iron

- Absorption occurs mainly in the duodenum and upper jejunum.
- Normally, about 10% of the 15–20 mg iron ingested each day is actually absorbed in healthy adult male. This absorption is more in menstruating women.

Mechanism of Iron Absorption. Mechanism of iron absorption for the purpose of understanding can be described under three headings:

A. Transport of iron across the brush border of enterocyte
B. Fate of iron in the enterocyte, and
C. Transport of iron in the plasma.

A. Transport of Iron Across Brush Border of Enterocyte. In the diet, iron may be present as haem (derived from meat) or nonhaem iron.

1. ***Absorption of haem iron.*** Haem iron is the iron present in myoglobin, haemoglobin and related compounds. From these compounds, the haem is released by proteolytic enzymes in the gut. From the lumen, the haem is transported inside the enterocyte across the brush-border membrane by an unidentified *haem transport* protein. Inside the cell, the ferrous iron (Fe^{2+}) is released from the haem by the enzyme haemoxygenase. The fate of Fe^{2+} so released is as that of nonhaem Fe^{2+} as given (Fig. 3.2-24). Haem iron absorption is not affected by other dietary constituents.
2. ***Absorption of nonhaem iron.*** Most of the dietary nonhaem iron is present in ferric form (Fe^{3+}), whereas iron can be absorbed more efficiently in ferrous form (Fe^{2+}).
   - Iron has got tendency to form insoluble complexes with dietary phytates, phosphates and dietary fibres. These complexes are more soluble at low pH. Gastric HCl tends to break insoluble iron complex apart and thus facilitates iron absorption. This explains the occurrence of iron deficiency anaemia in patients with deficient gastric acid secretion (achlorhydria).
   - Ascorbic acid and other reducing agents promote iron absorption by reducing ferric iron to ferrous form and also by preventing iron from forming insoluble iron complexes within the chyme.
   - Ferrous iron (Fe^{2+}) is transported across the brush border by the *iron transport protein, i.e.* proton coupled divalent metal transporter (DMT-1) present on the cell membrane (Fig. 3.2-24). This protein is not specific for iron, as it can transport a large variety of divalent cations. Once inside the enterocyte, the fate of nonhaem ferrous iron is the same as that of haem iron.

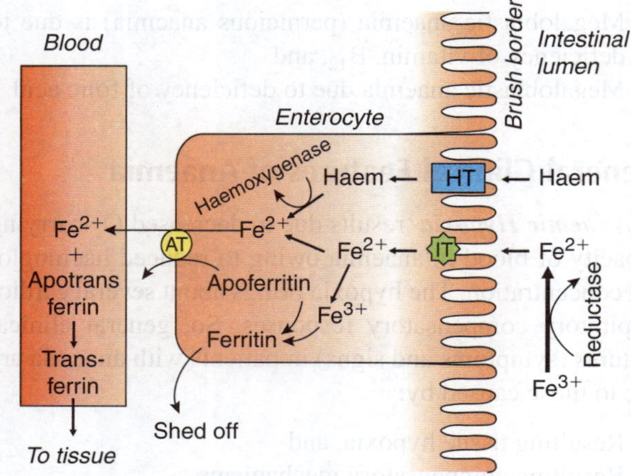

FIGURE 3.2-24 Absorption of iron. Haem is carried across brush border of enterocyte by a haem transport protein (HT), and Fe^{2+} of nonhaem iron by iron transport protein (IT). Inside the enterocyte, some iron binds to ferritin and some crosses the basolateral membrane by active transport process (AT). In the blood, iron binds to the transport protein transferrin (TF).

B. Fate of iron in the enterocyte. As shown in Fig. 3.2-24, in the cytosol of enterocyte, the free ferrous iron (Fe^{2+}) has two fates:

- A part of Fe^{2+}, depending upon the body's requirement, is actively transported across the basolateral membranes of the enterocytes into the interstitium, from where it enters the blood. Across the basolateral membrane of enterocytes the transport is carried out by another protein called iron regulating protein-I (IREG-I) .
- Rest of the ferrous iron is oxidized to ferric form and bound to apoferritin forming ferritin. It is difficult to release iron from this storage form, and in general the ferritin stays in the enterocyte until the cell is sloughed off at the tip of villus.

C. Transport of iron in the blood. Normally, the iron absorbed into the blood binds with a beta globulin (apotransferrin) to form the transferrin and is transported in this form in the plasma. Iron combines loosely in the globulin apotransferrin and can be released easily to enter any of the tissue cells at any point in the body.

Factors Affecting Absorption of Iron. Factors affecting absorption of iron from the gut are:

1. ***Form of dietary iron***
   - *Haem iron.* Iron may be present as haem iron or nonhaem iron forming about 10–15% of the iron present in diet of animal origin, is relatively unaffected by the composition of diet. Haem is absorbed directly, i.e. without splitting off of iron *from protoporphyrin.*
   - In *nonhaem iron* the ferrous (Fe^{2+}) form is better absorbed than ferric (Fe^{3+}) form. Therefore, reducing agents such as vitamin C enhance iron absorption by converting ferric into ferrous.
2. ***Meat and fish*** in the diet considerably enhance absorption of nonhaem iron. The exact mechanism is, however, unknown.
3. ***Human breast milk*** improves the iron absorption.
4. ***The acid gastric juice*** (HCl from stomach) favours absorption of nonhaem iron by causing its solubilization and reduction. Therefore, absorption of ferric iron is impaired in subjects with gastrectomy or achlorhydria.
5. ***Dietary factors inhibiting nonhaem iron*** absorption are:
   - *Phytates* in foods (cereals) reduce iron absorption by forming insoluble iron salts.
   - *Phosphates,* calcium, egg white and bovine milk proteins inhibit iron absorption.
   - *Phenols* present in legumes, tea, coffee and wine cause poor absorption of iron.
6. ***Iron stores in the body*** affect iron absorption as:
   - *Decrease* in iron store of the body (e.g. in iron deficiency anaemia or when erythropoiesis is increased due to hypoxia) enhance iron absorption.
   - *An increase in iron storage* in the body reduces iron absorption by the gut mucosa.

Storage of Iron in the Body. In the body, iron is stored in two forms, the ferritin and the haemosiderin.

Storage of iron as ferritin. The iron released into the tissues by apotransferrin combines with the protein apoferritin to form the *ferritin*. Thus, iron is stored as ferritin in the cells of the body. Maximum amount of iron is stored in the hepatocytes of liver and cells of reticuloendothelial system. In other cells of the body only a small amount of iron is stored.

Storage of iron as haemosiderin. When the intake of iron in the diet is in extremely large quantities, some amount of iron is also stored as a compound *haemosiderin* in reticuloendothelial cells. The haemosiderin is highly insoluble and thus represents a more stable form of storage iron than the ferritin. Therefore, iron exchanges mostly with the ferritin, since exchange with haemosiderin is very slow.

Regulation of Body Iron. Regulation of body iron, i.e. iron balance in the body is unique in that it is achieved by control of absorption rather than by control of excretion. Regulation of mucosal absorption has been explained by mucosal block theory.

Mucosal Block Theory of Absorption. This theory states that:

- Iron absorption is increased when body iron stores are depleted or when erythropoiesis is increased, and decreased under the reverse conditions.
- As compared to normal conditions (Fig. 3.2-25A), in iron deficiency states, a larger percentage of dietary iron enters the circulation and a smaller amount forms ferritin in the epithelial cells (Fig. 3.2-25B).
- In the presence of iron overload, more ferritin is formed in the enterocytes and shed with these cells in the stools (Fig. 3.2-25C).

The details of the regulatory processes involved remain obscure. However, following views have been put forward to explain the mucosal block theory.

1. ***Saturation of apoferritin and apotransferrin.*** Most of the iron in the body is stored as ferritin, which is formed by a combination of iron with the protein apoferritin present in the cytoplasm of the body cells. When essentially all apoferritin in the body is saturated with iron, it becomes difficult for the transferrin to release its iron to the tissue cells. Consequently the whole of the apotransferrin is saturated with iron and thus the mucosal cells are loaded with the transferrin. Because of the unavailability of the apotransferrin, the mucosal cells are not able to take up any more luminal iron. Mucosal cells have a lifespan of 3–4 days, at the end of which they get sloughed off into the intestine. Mucosal transferrin (containing iron) is also lost with it and the body gets rid of excess of iron.
2. ***Decreased rate of apoferritin synthesis.*** When body has excess of iron, due to feedback mechanism, the rate of

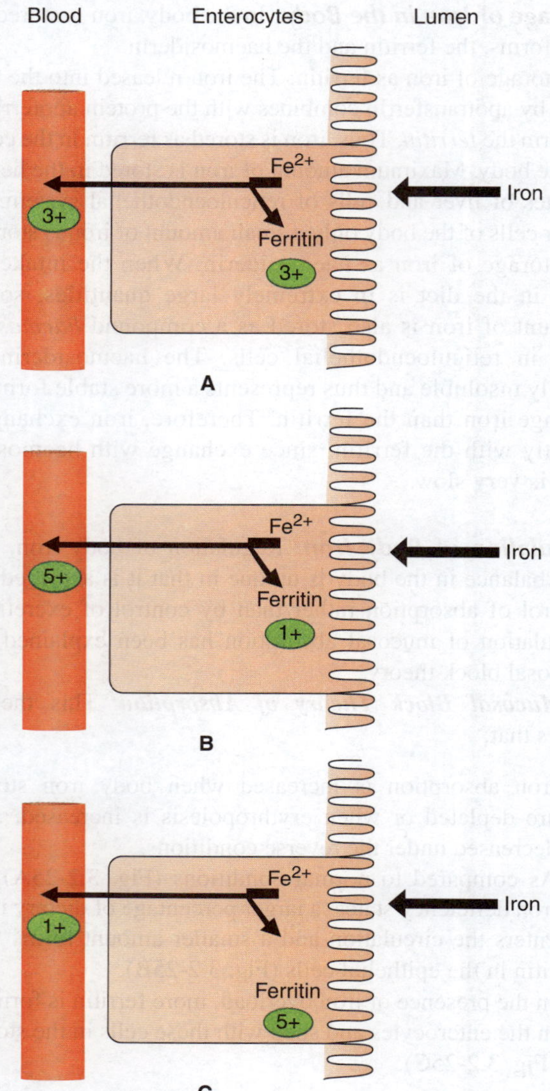

FIGURE 3.2-25 Mucosal block theory of regulation of iron absorption: **A,** normally (say, e.g. equal amount (3^+) of iron is bound to form ferritin and enters the blood across basolateral membrane; **B,** in iron deficiency states, less iron forms ferritin (e.g. 1^+) and more enters the blood, e.g. 5^+; and **C,** in iron overload, more ferritin is formed (5^+) and less enters the blood 1^+.

apoferritin synthesis in the liver is also decreased and thus less iron is absorbed by the intestinal cells.

3. ***Role of specific iron receptors in the brush border.*** Recently it has been proposed that the absorption of iron by the enterocytes is determined by the presence of receptors on the brush border. Iron receptors in brush border preparations of the small intestine are inversely related to the level of body iron stores. Iron deficient animals show an increase in the number of receptor population, which can be reversed by iron loading.

Conclusion. *The current understanding of the regulation of body iron is still in a state of fix with following conclusions:*

- The control seems to reside primarily in the need-based transfer of iron from the enterocyte to the portal blood.
- Some control is also exerted at the level of uptake of iron from the intestinal lumen.
- In cases of iron overload, some iron can be transported from the plasma to the enterocytes. This iron is lost when the enterocytes are shed into the lumen. In this way, the intestine serves to excrete excess iron in a bid to prevent accumulation of excessive iron in the body.

  Thus, the statement that iron content of the body is regulated only by absorption is also true, only to a limited extent.

The Iron Cycle. The iron cycle refers to the continuous exchange of iron between the plasma and RBCs. The steps of iron cycles are (Fig. 3.2-26):

- From the plasma, the iron is transported into bone marrow as transferrin.
- In the bone marrow, the transferrin binds to the specific transferrin receptors present on the surface of intermediate normoblasts.
- In the intermediate normoblasts, the iron is incorporated into the haemoglobin. The mature RBCs containing haemoglobin are then released into the plasma.
- RBCs, after their death (on completion of lifespan), are engulfed by macrophages.
- After phagocytosis, the red cell membrane is lysed and haem is released from the haemoglobin. By the haemoxy genase reaction, iron is liberated from the haem.
- Macrophages lining the sinuses of liver and spleen release iron back into the plasma where it binds with the apotransferrin to form transferrin, thus completing the iron cycle. Each day, about 30 mg of iron goes through this cycle. In addition, about 2 mg iron enters the plasma from the diet also.

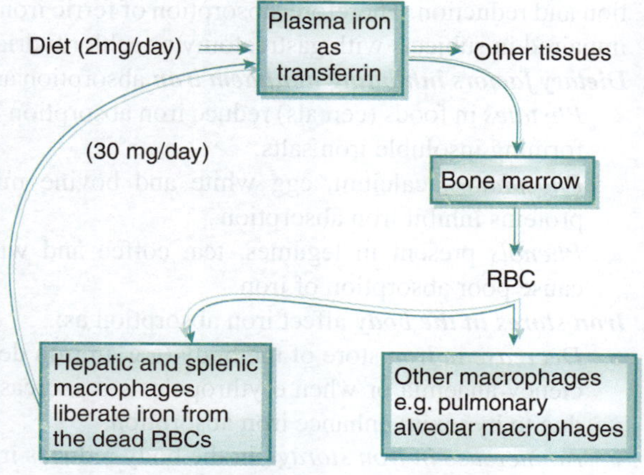

FIGURE 3.2-26 Iron cycle.

Role of Iron in the Body. Iron is utilized in the synthesis of:

- *Haemoglobin* in the RBCs (main role),
- *Myoglobin* in the muscles, and
- *Cytochromes* the intracellular enzymes.
  Uptake of the iron by tissues
- *RBCs* are the main takers of iron (about 30 mg/day)
- *Other tissues* take up about less than 2 mg iron each day as follows:
- *Liver.* Out of the tissues other than RBCs, liver takes up the largest amount of iron.
- *Intestinal mucosal cells.* Iron is stored as transferrin in the intestinal mucosal cells which regulate the iron absorption as discussed above.
- *Skeletal muscles.* Iron is utilized to produce myoglobin by the muscles.
- *Proliferating cells of the body.* Iron is utilized for synthesis of enzymes cytochrome and catalases, which are required in excess by the proliferating cells of the body.

Applied Aspects

Iron deficiency results in iron deficiency anaemia.

Iron excess. Iron overload may occur when its absorption exceeds its excretion. Such a condition occurs due to:

- *Excessive intake* of iron, and
- *Idiopathic* or congenital failure of mucosal feedback mechanism controlling iron absorption.
- *Excessive* destruction of erythrocytes may also be associated with siderosis.

The excess of iron in the body results in accumulation of hemosiderin in the tissues producing the so-called *haemosiderosis*. Excess of haemosiderin damages the tissues and produces the condition of ***haemochromatosis.***

Haemochromatosis may be hereditary or acquired.

The hereditary or primary haemochromatosis occurs due to mutation of HFE gene located on chromosome-6. The individual with homogeneous mutated HFE gene absorbs excess amounts of iron because normally the HFE gene inhibits expression of the transporter responsible for iron intake. Haemochromatosis is characterized by:

- Pigmentation of the skin,
- Diabetes due to pancreatic damage (bronze diabetes),
- Cirrhosis of liver,
- Carcinoma of the liver and
- Atrophy of gonads.

Causes of Iron Deficiency Anaemia

Causes of iron deficiency vary with age, sex and country of residence of patient. In general, the causes of iron deficiency anaemia can be grouped as:

1. Inadequate Dietary Intake of Iron as in:

- Milk fed infants,
- Poor economic status individuals,
- Anorexia, e.g. in pregnancy and.
- Elderly individuals due to atrophy and poor dentition

2. Increased loss of Iron (as blood loss) from the body, e.g.

- *Uterine bleeding in females* in the form of excessive menstruation, repeated miscarriages, postmenopausal bleeding, etc.
- *Gastrointestinal bleeding* due to peptic ulcer, haemorrhoids, ulcerative colitis, etc.
- *Renal tract bleeding,* e.g. haematuria.
- *Nasal bleeding,* i.e. repeated epistaxis.
- *Bleeding from lungs* as haemoptysis.

3. Increased Demand of Iron as in:

- Infancy, childhood and adolescence,
- Menstruating females and
- Pregnant females.

4. Decreased Absorption of iron, as seen in:

- Partial or total gastrectomy,
- Achlorhydria and
- Intestinal malabsorption diseases.

Clinical Features, Laboratory Findings and Treatment

Clinical Features of Anaemia

1. ***General features of anaemia***
   See page 157.
2. ***Characteristic features of iron deficiency anaemia*** are in the form of the following epithelial tissue changes:
   - *Nails* become dry, soft and spoon shaped (koilonychia).
   - *Tongue* becomes angry red (atrophic glossitis).
   - *Mouth* may show angular stomatitis.
   - *Oesophagus* may develop their membranous webs at the postcricoid area leading to dysphagia (Plummer–Vinson syndrome).

Laboratory Findings

1. Blood Picture and Red Cell Indices

- *Haemoglobin* concentration is decreased.
- RBCs are hypochromic (deficient in haemoglobin) and microcytic (smaller in size). They show anisocytosis and poikilocytosis.
- *Red cell indices* like MCV, MCH and MCHC are decreased.

2. Bone Marrow Findings are:

- Marrow cellularity: erythroid hyperplasia,
- Erythropoiesis: normoblastic and
- Marrow iron: deficient reticuloendothelial iron stores and absence of siderotic iron granules.

3. Biochemical Findings

- Serum iron decreases, often under 50 μg/dL (normal 60–160 μg/dL).
- Serum bilirubin less than 0.4 mg/dL.
- Serum ferritin is less than 30 μg/dL indicating poor tissue iron stores.
- Total iron-binding capacity (TIBC) is increased.

Treatment. Treatment of iron deficiency anaemia consists of:

- Oral administration of Fe^{2+} salts, and
- Correction of causative factor if possible.

Megaloblastic Anaemia

Megaloblastic anaemias are characterized by abnormally large cells of erythrocyte series. These are caused by defective DNA synthesis due to deficiency of vitamin B_{12} and/or folic acid (folate).

Aetiological Types

I. Megaloblastic Anaemia due to Vitamin B_{12} Deficiency. Salient features of vitamin B_{12} and intrinsic factor of Castle should be understood before discussing other aspects of anaemia due to vitamin B_{12} deficiency (see page 142).

Causes of Vitamin B_{12} Deficiency are:

1. *Inadequate dietary intake* may occur in:
   - Strict vegetarians, and
   - Breast-fed infants.
2. *Malabsorption of vitamin B^{12}* is more often the cause of deficiency and may be due to:
   - *Gastric causes* leading to deficiency of intrinsic factors such as an autoimmune cause of failure of secretion of intrinsic factor (Addisonian pernicious anaemia), gastrectomy and congenital lack of intrinsic factor.
   - *Intestinal causes* which are associated with decreased vitamin B_{12} absorption are tropical sprue, ileal resection, Crohn's disease, fish tapeworm infestation and intestinal blind loop syndrome.

Addisonian Pernicious Anaemia. Aetiology. Addisonian pernicious anaemia is the term which is used specifically for the megaloblastic anaemia due to vitamin B_{12} deficiency occurring as a result of failure of secretion of intrinsic factor by the stomach owing to an autoimmune atrophy of gastric mucosa. Thus, pernicious anaemia is an autoimmune disease and in about 50% of patients, antibodies to intrinsic factor can be demonstrated. The disease is rare before the age of 30 years, occurs mainly between 45 and 65 years and affects females more frequently than males.

Features of Pernicious Anaemia include:

- *Features of megaloblastic anaemia* (described on page 162), and
- ***Specific features*** of pernicious anaemia are:
  - Anti-intrinsic factor antibodies in serum (present in 50% cases) and
  - Abnormal vitamin B_{12} absorption test corrected by addition of intrinsic factor (Schilling test).

Treatment of pernicious anaemia consists of regular administration of vitamin B_{12} by intramuscular route:

II. Megaloblastic Anaemia due to Folate Deficiency

Salient features of folic acid. and its role in erythropoiesis (see page 143).

Causes of folate deficiency. are:

1. *Inadequate dietary intake* due to poor intake of vegetables as seen in poor people, infants and alcoholics.
2. *Malabsorption,* e.g. in coeliac disease, tropical sprue and Crohn's disease.
3. *Increased demand* as occurs in:
   - Physiological conditions such as pregnancy, lactation and infancy and
   - Pathological conditions of cell proliferation, such as increased haematopoiesis (as in haemolysis) and malignancies.
4. *Effect of drugs* such as: certain anticonvulsants (e.g. phenytoin), contraceptive pills and certain cytotoxic drugs (e.g. methotrexate).
5. *Excess urinary folate loss,* e.g. in active liver disease and congestive heart failure.

Features of folate deficiency anaemia. include:

- *Features of megaloblastic anaemia*, and
- *Specific features of folate deficiency* are:
  - Low serum folate levels and
  - Low red cell folate levels.

Clinical Features of Megaloblastic Anaemia

A. General Features of Anaemia See page 157.

B. Characteristic Features of Megaloblastic Anaemia

1. Blood Picture and Red Cell Indices

- *Haemoglobin* level is low.
- RBCs are larger in size (macrocytosis) but contain a normal concentration of haemoglobin (normochromia).
- *MCV* increases to 95–160 μm^3 (normal 78–94 μm^3).
- *MCH* increases to 50 pg (normal 28–32 pg).
- *MCHC* usually normal (35 ± 3%) because both MCV and MCH increase. In late stages, MCHC may decrease.
- *Peripheral smear* shows nucleated RBCs with marked anisocytosis and poikilocytosis.
- *Reticulocyte count* increases to more than 5% (normal less than 1%).
- *Lifespan of RBCs* is decreased.
- *WBCs and platelets* decrease because of encroachment of megaloblastic tissue.

2. Bone Marrow Picture

- Bone marrow shows *megaloblastic hyperplasia* characterized by presence of:
  - 70% proerythroblasts and early normoblasts (normal 30%), and
  - 30% intermediate and late normoblasts (normal 70%).
- *Marrow iron.* Prussian blue staining for iron in the marrow shows an increase in the number and size of iron granules in the erythroid precursors.

3. Biochemical Finding

- *Serum bilirubin* increases more than 1 mg/dL (normal 0.2–0.8 mg/dL) due to excessive destruction of RBCs in spleen, liver and bone marrow.

- *Urine urobilinogen* excretion may increase due to increased serum bilirubin.
- *Serum iron and* ferritin is usually increased because iron is not utilized by immature RBCs.
- *Serum vitamin B_{12}* levels are decreased (normal 150–350 pg/ml) in patients with megaloblastic anaemia due to vitamin B_{12} deficiency.
- *Serum folate levels* are decreased in patients with megaloblastic anaemia due to folic acid deficiency.
- *Red cell folate levels* are a more reliable indicator of tissue stores of folate than serum. In folic acid deficiency, red cell folate levels are decreased.

4. Schilling Test is performed in two stages:

In the first stage, a large intramuscular dose of vitamin B_{12} is given to saturate the plasma transport protein. Thereafter, radiolabelled vitamin B_{12} is administered orally, and 24 h urine samples are collected to detect vitamin B_{12}. Normally more than 7% of the dose is present in the urine and patients with impaired absorption will have less than 3% of the dose.

The second stage of Schilling test is performed to detect pernicious anaemia due to lack of intrinsic factor. Radiolabelled vitamin B_{12} along with intrinsic factor is administered. Combined use of vitamin B_{12} and intrinsic factor should correct abnormally low absorption due to lack of intrinsic factor. Therefore, urine vitamin B_{12} level will be improved.

Chapter 3.3

White Blood Cells

WHITE BLOOD CELLS TYPES AND THEIR COUNTS

White blood cells (WBCs) or leucocytes are so named since they are colourless in contrast to the red colour of the RBCs. These are nucleated cells which play an important role in the defence mechanism of the body.

The leucocytes of the peripheral blood are of two main varieties, distinguished by the presence or absence of granules. These are: granulocytes and nongranulocytes.

Types of White Blood Cells

Granulocytes White blood cells with granules in their cytoplasm are called granulocytes. Depending upon the colour of granules, granulocytes are further divided into three types:

Neutrophils. They contain granules which take both acidic and basic stain.

Eosinophils. They contain granules which take acidic stain.

Basophils. They contain granules which take basic stain.

Agranulocytes White blood cells that do not contain granules in their cytoplasm are called agranulocytes. These are of two types:

- Lymphocytes and
- Monocytes.

Normal WBC Counts

Total Leucocyte Count Total leucocyte count (TLC) varies with age as:

- ***Adults:*** 4000–11,000/mm^3 of blood.
- ***At birth,*** in full-term infant: 10,000–25,000/mm^3 of blood.
- ***Infants*** up to 1 year of age: 6000–16,000/mm^3 of blood.
- ***Children***, 4–7 years of age: 5000–15,000/mm^3 of blood.
- ***Children,*** 8–12 years of age: 4500–13,500/mm^3 of blood.

Differential and Absolute Leucocyte Count Differential leucocyte count (DLC) and absolute count in normal adults are shown in Table 3.3-1.

Clinical Significance of Differential and Absolute Counts The differential leucocyte count (DLC) tells us if there is an increase or decrease in a particular type of leucocyte, because in different diseases, one or the other type of cells shows an increase or decrease in its numbers. The differential count is done in 100–200 cells, and tells only a relative increase or decrease in a particular variety of cells, with a corresponding decrease or increase in the other types of cells. For example, an increase in the percentage of neutrophils would be associated with a decrease in percentage of lymphocytes, thus giving an impression of lymphocytopenia. But if the TLC is taken into account, the

TABLE 3.3-1 Differential Leucocytes Count and Absolute Count in Normal Adults

WBCs	Differential count (%)	Absolute count (per mm^3)
Granulocytes		
• Neutrophils	40–75	2000–7500
• Eosinophils	1–6	40–440
• Basophils	0–1	0–100
Agranulocytes		
• Lymphocytes	20–40	1500–4000
• Monocytes	2–10	500–800

absolute lymphocyte count could be within a normal range. Therefore, DLC alone is not of much importance and so is never done as an isolated test, but always it is part of full blood counts, including TLC and then calculating absolute count.

Variations in WBCs Count

Leucocytosis Leucocytosis refers to increase in total WBC count above 11,000/mm^3.

Physiological Causes of Leucocytosis are:

1. ***Age.*** In newborn babies up to the age of 1 year, the WBC count is higher. At birth, the WBC count is about 18,000/mm^3, which drops gradually to the adult level.
2. ***Exercise.*** The WBC count is increased after exercise.
3. ***After food intake,*** the WBC count is raised.
4. ***Mental stress*** and emotional conditions like anxiety are associated with raised WBC count.
5. ***Pregnancy.*** At full-term pregnancy, the WBC count is 12,000–15,000 mm^3.
6. ***Exposure to low temperature*** also causes leucocytosis.

Pathological Causes of Leucocytosis are:

1. Acute bacterial infections especially by pyogenic organisms,
2. Acute haemorrhage,
3. Burns,
4. Postoperative period,
5. Tuberculosis and
6. Glandular fever.

Leucopenia Leucopenia refers to decrease in the total WBC count below 4000/mm^3.

Causes of Leucopenia are:

1. Infections by nonpyogenic bacteria, especially typhoid fever and paratyphoid fever,
2. Viral infections such as influenza, smallpox, mumps, etc.,
3. Protozoal infections,
4. Starvation and malnutrition,
5. Aplasia of bone marrow and
6. Bone marrow depression due to:
   - Drugs such as chloromycetin and cytotoxic drugs used in malignant diseases.
   - Repeated exposure to X-rays or radiations.
   - Chemical poisons like arsenic, dinitrophenol and antimony.

Leukaemia Leukaemia is a malignant disease of the blood in which there occurs an increase in the total WBC count associated with the presence of immature WBCs in the peripheral blood. Total WBC count is usually above 50,000/mm^3, and may be as high as 100,000–300,000/ mm^3 (see page 177).

FORMATION OF WHITE BLOOD CELLS

The process of development and maturation of white blood cells (leucocytes), called *leucopoiesis,* is a part of haemopoiesis (formation of blood cells). All the blood cells develop from the so-called pluripotent *haemopoietic stem cells (PHSCs).* The stem cells after a series of divisions differentiate into *progenitor cells,* which are also called as colony-forming units (CFU) (for details see page 138).

Leucopoiesis can be discussed under two headings:

- Formation of granulocytes (granulopoiesis) and monocytes and
- Formation of lymphocytes (lymphopoiesis).

Formation of Granulocytes and Monocytes

The granulocytes and monocytes are formed in the bone marrow from the colony-forming unit called CFU-GM (colony-forming unit granulocytes and monocytes): The progenitor cells (CFU-GM) forming different cells are further named as:

- CFU-G are neutrophil-forming units,
- CFU-EO refers to eosinophil-forming units,
- CFU-Ba are basophil-forming units and
- CFU-M refers to monocyte-forming units.

The development of granulocytes through various stages is called *myeloid series* and development of monocytes through various stages is called *monocyte–macrophage series.*

Myeloid Series

Some Facts About Granulopoiesis

- The cells of myeloid series include myeloblast (most primitive precursor), promyelocytes, myelocytes, metamyelocytes, band forms and segmented granulocyte (mature form). These cells can be grouped together in two pools:
  - *Proliferative or mitotic pool* is formed by the myeloblast, promyelocyte and myelocyte; and

- *Mature or postmitotic pool* includes the metamyelocytes, band forms and segmented granulocytes.
- The process of granulopoiesis takes about 12 days.
- Granulocytes are formed and stored in the bone marrow. When need arises, they are released in circulation. Normally, about three times as many granulocytes are stored in the bone marrow as circulated in the peripheral blood.

Features of the Cells of Myeloid Series (Fig. 3.3-1)

1. Myeloblast. It is the earliest recognizable cell of the granulocyte series. Myeloblasts form about 2% of the total marrow cells. Its features are:

- *Size.* Myeloblast varies in diameter from 16 to 20 μm.
- *Cytoplasm* is basophilic, present as thin rim around the nucleus and is devoid of granules.
- *Nucleus* is large (nearly filling the cells), round to oval, has fine chromatin and contains 2–5 well-defined pale nucleoli.
- *Mitosis* is marked (+++).

2. Promyelocytes. Myeloblasts progress into the promyelocyte which has following features:

- *Size* varies from 14 to 18 μm.

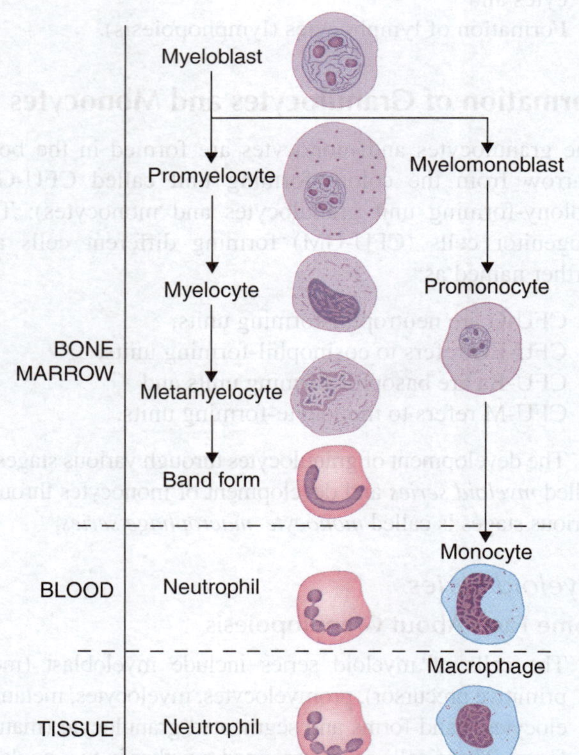

FIGURE 3.3-1 Granulopoiesis and features of the cells of myeloid series and monocyte–macrophage series.

- *Cytoplasm* increases in amount and is characterized by the presence of *azurophil granules.* These granules are also called *primary nonspecific granules* and these give a positive reaction with the peroxidase stain.
- *Nucleus* is round or oval, slightly small than the nucleus of myeloblast and having fine chromatin, which is condensed. The nucleoli are present but are less prominent and fewer than those in the myeloblast.
- *Mitosis* is a characteristic feature (+++).

3. Myelocyte, also called myelocyte proper, is the next cell in myeloid series. Its features are:

- *Size* varies from 12 to 16 μm.
- *Cytoplasm* is characterized by the presence of *specific (secondary) granules* and accordingly the cell can be identified at this stage as:
  - Neutrophil myelocyte,
  - Eosinophil myelocyte and
  - Basophil myelocyte.

  The primary granules are also present at this stage but their formation is stopped.
  - *Nucleus* is eccentric, round to oval, having coarse nuclear chromatin and no nucleoli.
  - *Mitosis* continues up to this stage. Multiplication of these cells is maximum.

4. Metamyelocyte has the following features:

- *Size* varies from 10 to 14 μm.
- *Cytoplasm* increases in amount and becomes more liquid. Both primary and secondary granules are present. Depending upon the features of secondary granules, the metamyelocytes are distinguished as:
  - Neutrophil metamyelocyte,
  - Eosinophil metamyelocyte and
  - Basophil metamyelocyte.
- *Nucleus* decreases in size becomes indented and lobed (horseshoe shape). The nuclear chromatin is dense and clumped. Nucleoli are absent.
- *Mitosis* stops at this stage.

5. Band or Stab Form refers to juvenile granulocytes which has the following features:

- *Size* is slightly smaller than metamyelocyte.
- *Cytoplasm* is pink and contains fine evenly distributed granules.
- *Nucleus* is characterized by further condensation of chromatin and transformation of nucleus shape into a band configuration (deeply indented V-shaped) of uniform thickness which may be twisted.

6. Mature Granulocytes ultimately formed are neutrophils, eosinophils and basophils. Their morphological features are described on page 168.

Monocyte–Macrophage Series (Fig. 3.3-1)

The monocyte–macrophage series of cells basically form a part of myeloid series along with the granulocytes and are thus formed in the bone marrow. These are described separately because of the different morphological stages which include: monoblast, promonocytes and monocyte.

1. Monoblast. It is a large cell similar in structure to the myeloblast from which it cannot be distinguished on morphological grounds alone. Therefore, it is preferable to call the earliest precursor of granulocytic series as *myelomonoblast.*

2. Promonocyte. It is a young monocyte about 20 µm in diameter. Its *nucleus* is large, indented (often kidney shaped) and contains one nucleolus. The nuclear chromatin is arranged in a loose network. The *cytoplasm* is basophilic and contains *no azurophilic granules,* but may have fine granules which are larger than those in mature monocyte.

3. Monocyte. Morphological features of a mature monocyte are described on page 176. These resemble metamyelocytes and are best distinguished by the presence of fine chromatin. In metamyelocytes, the chromatin is dense and clumped.

From the bone marrow, the monocytes migrate into the spleen and the lymphoid tissues in considerable numbers. The transformed stages of these cells in various tissues are called *tissue macrophages* and form a part of *tissue–macrophage system,* which was previously known as *reticuloendothelial system.*

Formation of Lymphocytes

Lymphocytes are formed from the *lymphocyte stem cells,* which are formed from the pluripotent haemopoietic stem cells (PHSC) in the bone marrow (Fig. 3.2-9). The lymphocyte stem cells migrate into the thymus and peripheral lymphoid tissues, where they proliferate and mature into lymphocytes. In humans, the bone marrow and thymus form the primary lymphopoietic *organs,* where lymphoid stem cells undergo spontaneous division independent of antigenic stimulation. The tissues that actively produce lymphocytes from the germinal centres of lymphoid follicles as a response to antigenic stimulation constitute the so-called *secondary or reactive lymphoid tissue.* It is comprised by the:

- Lymph nodes,
- Spleen and
- Gut-associated lymphoid tissue (GALT).

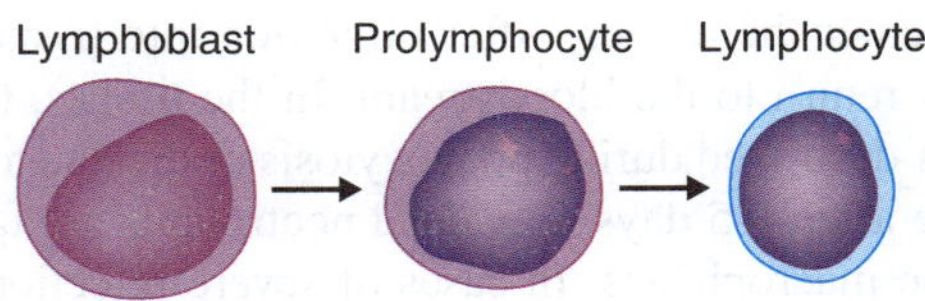

FIGURE 3.3-2 Formation of lymphoid series cells.

Lymphoid Series

The maturation stages of lymphoid series are (Fig. 3.3-2):

1. Lymphoblast. It is the earliest recognizable cell of the lymphoid series. It is an actively dividing cell and resembles the myeloblast morphologically, except for the following minor differences:

- The nucleus contains fewer nucleoli (1–2) compared with the myeloblast (2–5),
- Nuclear chromatin is slightly clumped and stippled compared with fine meshwork in myeloblast and
- Nuclear membrane is fairly dense compared with that of the myeloblast.

2. Prolymphocyte is the intermediate stage between the lymphoblast and mature lymphocyte. Its features are:

- *Diameter* is 9–18 µm.
- *Nucleus* is round to indented, with slightly stippled or coarse chromatin and may have 0–1 nucleoli.
- *Cytoplasm* is scanty and nongranular.

3. Lymphocytes. Prolymphocytes mature successively into large lymphocyte and small lymphocyte, both of which are found in the circulation.

- Then some lymphocytes enter thymus, where they are processed and come out as T lymphocytes. In thymus, a factor called *thymosin* plays an important role in the processing.
- Some lymphocytes are processed in the liver (in fetal life) and bone marrow (after birth). These come out as B *lymphocytes.* The word B comes from 'bursa of Fabricius', which is the site of B cell processing in birds. Morphological features of large and small lymphocytes are described on page 175.

Regulation of Leucopoiesis

The constancy of leucocyte count suggests an efficient feedback mechanism to control their production and release (Fig. 3.3-3). During tissue injury and inflammation, bacterial toxins, products of injury, etc. cause a great increase in the rate of production and release of leucocytes. Thus, unlike erythropoiesis, the products of dead and dying white cells themselves control leucopoiesis. The substances that stimulate or inhibit the process of leucopoiesis are complex and include the following:

Role of Cytokines The cytokines that control the formation of different types of granulocytes are called *colony-stimulating factors (CSFs).* The CSFs are glycoproteins formed by monocytes and T lymphocytes and include:

- *G-CSF* which stimulates granulocyte precursors,
- *M-CSF* which stimulates monocytic precursors and

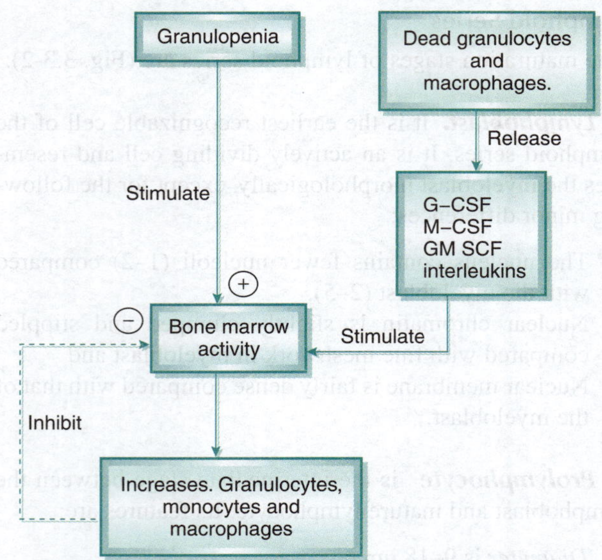

FIGURE 3.3-3 Schematic diagram of regulation of leucopoiesis.

- *GM-CSF* which stimulates both the granulocyte and monocytic precursors.
- The cytokines that control lymphocyte formation are called *interleukins*, e.g. IL-I, IL-3, etc. Interleukins are formed by monocytes, macrophages and endothelial cells (see page 196).

Role of Prostaglandins ***Prostaglandins*** formed by monocytes, *lactoferrin* and possibly some other agents also play a role in control of leucopoiesis.

MORPHOLOGY, FUNCTIONS, LIFESPAN AND VARIATIONS IN COUNTS OF WBCs

Morphological features of various types of WBCs, as studied under microscope with Leishman's staining and haematoxylin-eosin stain (Fig. 3.3-4), are summarized below along with their functions and variations in their counts.

Neutrophils

Morphological Features

The polymorphonuclear neutrophils, commonly called polymorphs or neutrophils, have the following morphological features (Fig. 3.3-4A):

- ***Diameter.*** Diameter of a neutrophil varies from 10 to 14 μm.
- ***Nucleus.*** A young neutrophil has a single horseshoe-shaped nucleus, which becomes lobed as the cell grows. Nucleus of a mature neutrophil is purple in colour and multilobed (2–6 lobes), that is why a neutrophil is also called polymorphonuclear leucocyte. The lobes of the nucleus are connected by chromatin filaments, seen clearly through the cytoplasm.

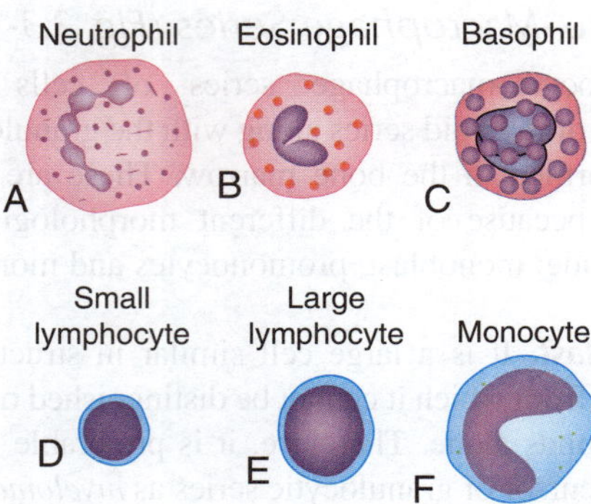

FIGURE 3.3-4 Morphological features of white blood cells: **A,** neutrophil; **B,** eosinophil; **C,** basophil; **D,** small lymphocyte; **E,** large lymphocyte; and **F,** monocyte.

- ***Cytoplasm.*** Cytoplasm of neutrophil is pale bluish in colour and full of fine (pinpoint) granules.
  - Granules take both acidic and basic stain and look violet–pink in colour.
  - Granules are *lysosomal* in origin and contain a variety of enzymes that include glycosidases, sulphatases, phosphatases, nucleases and proteolytic enzymes. They can thus lyse any type of substance.
  - In addition, the granules liberate histamine and peroxidase enzyme which help in killing the ingested bacteria.

Kinetics, Lifespan and Fate of Neutrophils

- The neutrophils released from the bone marrow enter the circulation. In blood, they exist in two equal populations:
  - The *circulating pool* comprises 50% cells, which are circulating in the blood at any instant, and
  - The *marginal pool* is constituted by the rest of 50% of cells, which remain marginated or sidelined, i.e. sticking to the endothelial cells of closed capillaries, venules, small veins and sinusoids.

  There is a rapid exchange between the two pools.
- For every neutrophil in blood, there are about a 100 mature neutrophils held in the bone marrow as reserve. These are released in the circulation when required. The stimulus for their release comes from the dead leucocytes, which release a granulocyte-inducing factor, and also by the hormone cortisol.
- Following their release from the bone marrow, granulocytes remain in circulating blood for 8–10 h and then they enter the tissues. After migration into tissues, they never return to the bloodstream. In the tissues, they are either destroyed during phagocytosis or die due to senescence after 4–5 days. The dead neutrophils are taken up by the macrophages. In cases of severe infection, lifespan of neutrophils may become as short as few hours.

- A huge number of neutrophils is also eliminated daily, mainly into the intestine and out via faeces and to some extent into the respiratory secretions.
- *Old senile neutrophils* are characterized by:
  - Loss of motility,
  - Poorly stained granules,
  - Increased nuclear lobulation and
  - Easy breakability while making blood smear.

Functions

The neutrophils along with monocytes constitute the first line of defence against microorganisms, viruses and other injurious agents that enter the body. Neutrophils subserve this role by the following mechanisms:

1. ***Phagocytosis.*** The neutrophils engulf the foreign particles or bacteria, digest them and ultimately may kill them by a process called phagocytosis. Various steps of phagocytosis are described below in detail.
2. ***Reaction of Inflammation.*** The neutrophils also release leucotrienes, prostaglandins, thromboxanes, etc. that bring about the reactions of inflammation like vasodilatation and oedema.
3. ***Febrile Response.*** The neutrophils contain a fever-producing substance called *endogenous pyrogen,* which is an important mediator of febrile response to the bacterial pyrogens.

Phagocytosis Phagocytosis (cell eating) refers to the process of engulfment and destruction of solid particulate material by the cells. The cells performing this function are called phagocytes. In addition to neutrophils, the monocytes and fixed tissue macrophages also work as phagocytes. The process of phagocytosis involves the following steps:

*1. **Margination.*** The normal axial blood flow consists of central stream of cells (leucocytes and RBCs) and peripheral cell-free layer of plasma close to vessel walls. In the area of infection, the neutrophils get *marginated,* i.e. get attached towards the capillary endothelium and start rolling along its surface. This process is called *margination* or *pavementing.* The margination is caused by binding of the *selectins* (cell adhesion molecules) present on the endothelial cells with the carbohydrate molecules present on the surface of neutrophils. The endothelial selectins are markedly increased in the areas where there is inflammation (Fig. 3.3-5A).

*2. **Emigration and Diapedesis.*** The marginated neutrophils are emigrated in a large number from the blood at the site of *infection* caused by the foreign microorganism. They are motile and move by diapedesis into the tissues by passing through the junction between the endothelial cells of the blood vessels (Fig. 3.3-5B). The diapedesis of neutrophils is brought about by microtubules, microfilaments and interaction of actin with myosin-I on the inner side of the cell membrane.

*3. **Chemotaxis.*** Chemotaxis refers to the process by which the neutrophils are attracted towards bacteria at the site of inflammation. The process of chemotaxis is mediated by the chemotactic agents called *chemokines,* which

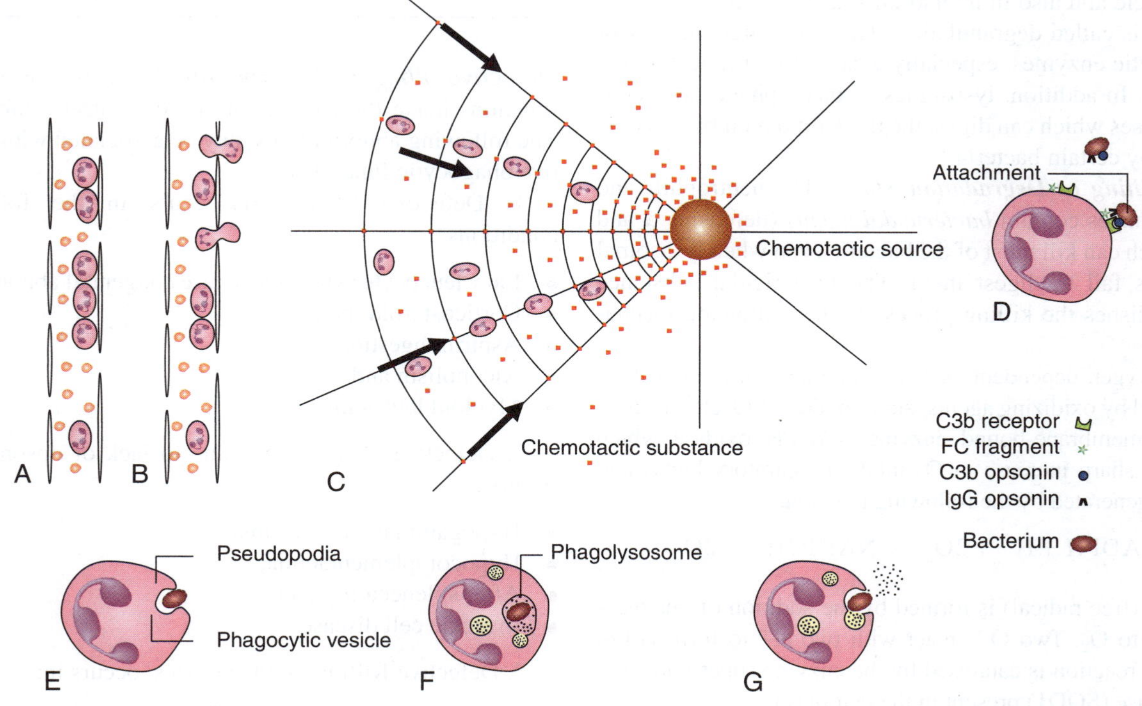

FIGURE 3.3-5 Stages of phagocytosis: **A,** margination; **B,** diapedesis; **C,** chemotaxis; **D,** opsonization; **E,** engulfment; **F,** formation of phagolysosome; and **G,** degranulation.

are released at the infected area. There are various types of chemokines, and they include:

- Leukotriene B_4 (LTB_4) and
- Components of the complement system (C_{5a}) and cytokines (polypeptides from lymphocytes and monocytes).

The chemoattractants increase the adhesive nature of neutrophils, which form clumps surrounding the infected area (Fig. 3.3-5C).

4. Opsonization (Attachment Stage). Opsonization refers to the process of coating of bacteria by the *opsonins* by which bacteria become tasty to the phagocytes. The principal opsonins are naturally acting factors in the serum and include IgG opsonin and opsonin fragment of complement protein. As shown in Fig. 3.3-5D, the opsonized bacteria are easily bound to the surface of phagocyte (attachment stage). This process triggers G protein-mediated responses, increases motor activity of the cell, exocytosis and respiratory bursts.

5. Engulfment Stage. The increased motor activity of neutrophils leads to prompt ingestion of bacteria by endocytosis. The neutrophils project *pseudopodia* in all directions around the opsonized particle, which is bound to the surface of neutrophil (Fig. 3.3-5E). Pseudopodia meet each other on opposite side and fuse. This creates an enclosed chamber with engulfed material. It breaks away from the membrane forming a *phagocytic vesicle*. Then the lysosomes of the cell fuse with the phagocytic vesicle to form a *phagolysosome* or phagosome (Fig. 3.3-5F).

6. Secretion (Degranulation) Stage. Once the bacteria are engulfed, the lysosomes pour their enzymes into the vesicle and also in interstitial space (Fig. 3.3-5G). This process is called degranulation. There are large number of proteolytic enzymes, especially geared up for digesting the bacteria. In addition, lysosomes of macrophages also contain lipases which can digest the thick lipid membranes possessed by certain bacteria.

7. Killing or Degradation Stage. The neutrophils and macrophages contain *bactericidal agents* (defensins α and β), which can kill most of the bacteria even when lysosomal enzymes fail to digest them. The bactericidal substance accomplishes the killing process by the following mechanisms:

- Oxygen-dependent bactericidal mechanism, which is mediated by oxidizing agents (superoxides, H_2O, etc.) formed by the membrane-bound enzyme NADPH oxidase which leads to sharp increase in O_2 intake (respiratory burst) and $O^-{}_2$, is generated by the following reaction:

$$NADPH + H^+ + 2O_2 \rightarrow NADP2H^+ + 2O^-{}_2$$

$O^-{}_2$ (free radical) is formed by the addition of one electron to O_2. Two $O^-{}_2$ react with two H^+ to form H_2O_2. This reaction is catalysed by the enzyme superoxide dismutase (SOD1) present in the cytoplasm.

$$O^-{}_2 + O_2{}^- + H^+ + H^+ \xrightarrow{SODI} H_2O_2 + O_2$$

$O^-{}_2$ and H_2O_2 (oxidants) both are bactericidal agents, but H_2O_2 is converted by the enzyme catalase into H_2O and O_2.

$$H_2O_2 \xrightarrow{catalase} H_2O + O_2$$

- Neutrophils also discharge another enzyme known as myeloperoxidase, which converts Cl^-, Br^-, I^- and CN^- to their corresponding acids (HOCl, HOBr, HOI, etc). These acids are also potent oxidants.

- Oxygen-independent bactericidal mechanism works through lysosomal hydrolases, defensins and cationic protein. Elastases. and metaloproteinases attack directly the collagen, and other proteinases destroy the membrane of invading bacteria.

Note: In congenital myeloperoxidase deficiency, there is reduction of microbial killing power of neutrophils due to nonformation of hypochlorous acid.

Important Notes

- Phagocytosis is completed after the stage of killing is over.
- A neutrophil can usually phagocytose 5–20 bacteria, before it itself becomes inactivated or dead.
- Neutrophils are not capable of phagocytosing particles much larger than bacteria.
- Neutrophils killed by the toxins released from the bacteria are collected in the centre of infected area. These are called pus cells and together with plasma leaked from the blood vessels, liquefied tissue cells and red blood cells escaped from the damaged capillaries constitute the pus.

Defective Phagocytic Functions Defective phagocytic functions make the patients prone to recurrent infections. The following abnormalities may be associated with defective phagocytic functions.

1. Defective Chemotaxis occurs in the following conditions:

- Lazy leucocyte syndrome, a rare congenital abnormality.
- Corticosteroid therapy,
- Aspirin ingestion,
- Alcoholism and
- Myeloid leukaemia

2. Defective Phagocytosis due to lack of opsonization occurs in:

- Hypogammaglobulinaemia,
- Hypocomplementaemia,
- After splenectomy and
- In sickle cell disease.

3. Defective Killing by Phagocytes occurs in:

- ***Chronic granulomatous diseases of childhood.*** In this condition, there is failure to generate superoxide radical

($O^-{}_2$) in both neutrophils and monocytes, leading to inability to kill the phagocytosed bacteria.

- ***Chediak–Higashi syndrome*** is an autosomal recessive disorder associated with reduced chemotaxis and phagolysosomal fusion.
- ***Congenital myeloperoxidase deficiency.*** During phagocytosis, enzyme NADPH oxidase and myeloperoxidase are mainly responsible for killing of invading organism. Myeloperoxidase helps catalysing the formation of oxidants. Therefore, due to its deficiency, microbial killing power is reduced but not absent, because most of the oxygen-dependent bactericidal mechanism remain intact.
- ***Rheumatoid arthritis:*** In this disease, the enzyme NADPH in the neutrophils may cause local destruction of the host tissue.
- ***Severe congenital glucose-6-phosphate deficiency*** leads to failure in NADPH production, thus O_2^- generation. Multiple infections occur in this condition due to defective killing of organisms.
- ***Amyotrophic lateral sclerosis,*** mutation of SOD-encoding gene, results in defective absence of SOD. In this disease, there is accumulation of O_2^- molecule in motor neurons which destroy them.

4. Neutrophil Hypomotility is associated with decreased phagocytosis. In this condition, actin present in the neutrophils do not polymerize normally; therefore, neutrophils move slowly.

Inflammation

Inflammation is a reaction or tissue change complex brought about by the substances released from the injured tissue or in response to foreign substances such as bacteria. Inflammation is characterized by redness, swelling and tenderness or pain. It includes sequence of reactions (Fig. 3.3-6):

- Vasodilatation of local blood vessels,
- Leakage of large quantity of fluid into the interstitial spaces (due to increased capillary permeability and its clotting due to leakage of fibrinogen and other clotting factors),

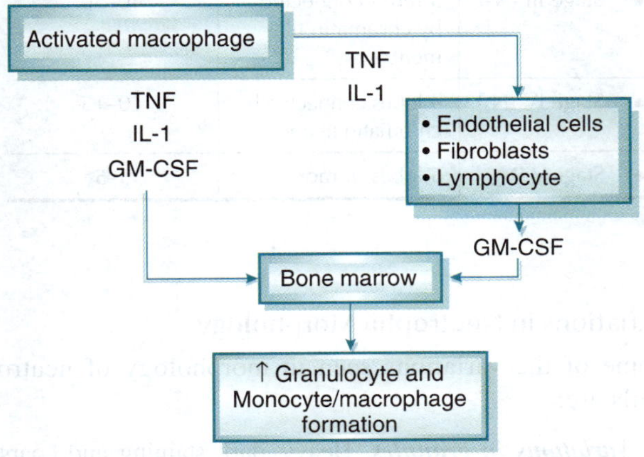

FIGURE 3.3-6 Sequence of events during inflammation.

- Migration of large number of granulocytes and monocytes into the tissue and
- Swelling of the tissue.

The substances released from the injured tissues include histamine, serotonin, prostaglandins, lymphokines, reaction products of complement and clotting system.

In inflammation, tissue macrophages are the first line of defence against infection. Within an hour or so, neutrophil from the blood invade the inflamed area. Therefore,

- Within few hours, there is an acute increase in neutrophil count (neutrophilia) that may go up to 4000–5000/μL.
- Along with neutrophils, monocytes also enter into inflamed tissue and enlarge to become macrophages. As pointed out earlier, macrophages can phagocytize about five times more bacteria and larger particles (including even neutrophil and necrotic tissue).
- The next reaction is increased production of granulocytes and monocytes in the bone marrow as a result of stimulation of GM-progenitor cells, due to the release of colony-stimulating factors (GM-CSF). A powerful feedback mechanism to remove the cause of inflammation is provided by GM-CSF, along with TNF and interlukin-1.

Walling-off Effect of Inflammation is to wall off the area of injury from remaining tissue. This effect is brought about by blockage of tissue spaces and lymphatics by clotting of tissue fluid by fibrinogen. The walling-off process is important for delaying the spread of infection.

Important Note

- **Nuclear factor-kB (NF-kB) is** a transcription factor that plays a key role in the inflammatory response. *NF-kB normally exists as bound form to* $I_{kB\alpha}$ (inactive state) in the cytoplasm of the cell. The stimuli such as cytokines, oxidants, viruses, etc. separate NF-kB from $I_{kB\alpha}$. Free NF-kB enters into the nucleus and gets bound to DNA of genes, responsible for inflammatory mediators and causing increase in their production and secretion.
- **Glucocorticoids:** *The anti-inflammatory action of* glucocorticoids is by increasing the production of $I_{kB\alpha}$ to inhibit NF-kB activity.

Variations in Counts

Neutrophilia Neutrophilia refers to increase in the circulating neutrophil counts (absolute count > 10,000/mm^3). It is the commonest cause of leucocytosis.

Causes

Physiological causes of neutrophilia are:

- Newborn babies,
- After exercise,
- After meals,
- Pregnancy,

- Menstruation,
- Parturition,
- Lactation,
- Mental stress and emotional stress and
- After injection of epinephrine.

Pathological causes of neutrophilia are:

- Acute pyogenic bacterial infections,
- Noninfective inflammatory conditions like gout and acute rheumatic fever,
- Acute tissue destruction as in:
  - Burns,
  - Postoperatively and
  - Myocardial infarction.
- Acute haemorrhage,
- Myoproliferative disorders like polycythaemia vera,
- Poisoning by chemicals and drugs like lead, mercury, etc..
- Poisoning by insect venom and
- Intoxicating conditions like uraemia and diabetic ketoacidosis.

Neutropenia Decrease in neutrophil count is known as neutropenia (absolute count < 2500/ mm^3).

Causes of Neutropenia

- Typhoid and paratyphoid fever,
- Malaria,
- Aplasia of bone marrow and
- Bone marrow depression due to:
  - Drugs such as chloromycetin and cytotoxic drugs used in malignant diseases,
  - Repeated exposure to X-rays and radiations and
  - Chemical poisons like arsenic.

Arneth Count

Counting the number of neutrophils with different nuclear lobes and expressing the count as percentage of cells with different number of nuclear lobes is called Arneth or Cooke's–Arneth count. Different stages with normal count are shown in Fig. 3.3-7 and Table 3.3-2.

Clinical Significance. The Arneth count is useful in judging the rate of formation of neutrophils. The neutrophils enter the bloodstream mostly as bilobed cells, but the number of lobes increases to 5 or more by the end of their short lifespan of 8–10 h. The three-lobed cells are fully mature and functionally the most efficient. Thus, the presence of younger cells (shift to the left) and more mature cells (shift to the right) in the blood can provide important information about the rate of formation and release of neutrophils from the bone marrow.

- ***In left shift*** (more younger cells), $N_1 + N_2 + N_3$ is more than 80%. It indicates hyperactive bone marrow (high rate of formation).
- ***In right shift*** (more mature cells), $N_4 + N_5$ is more than 20%. It indicates hypoactive bone marrow (slow rate of formation).

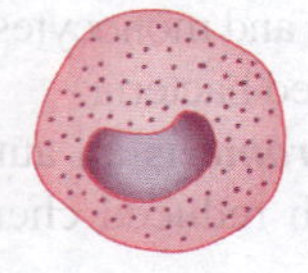

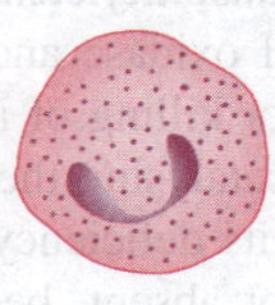

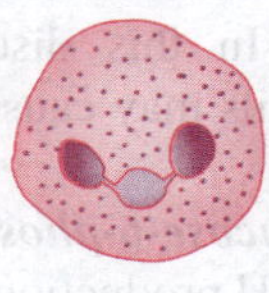

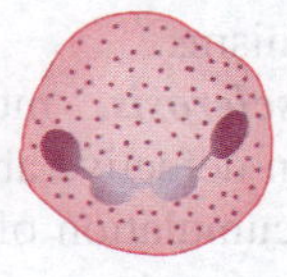

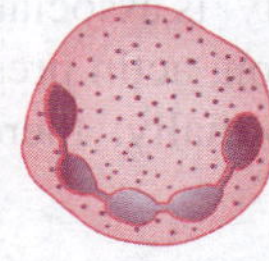

FIGURE 3.3-7 Stages of Cooke's–Arneth count.

TABLE 3.3-2 Cooke's–Arneth Count

Stage	Nuclear lobes	Normal count (%)
• Stage I (N_1)	1 (the nucleus is C-shaped)	5–10
• Stage II (N_2)	2 lobes are connected by a filament	20–30
• Stage III (N_3)	3 lobes connected by chromatin filament	40–50
• Stage IV (N_4)	4 lobes connected by chromatin filament	10–15
• Stage V (N_5)	5 lobes or more	3–5

Variations in Neutrophil Morphology

Some of the variations seen in morphology of neutrophils are:

1. ***Variations in granules.*** Heavy, dark staining and coarse toxic granules are the characteristics of bacterial infections.

2. ***Formation of vacuoles in cytoplasm.*** Cytoplasmic vacuolation may develop in bacterial infections such as in septicaemia.
3. ***Formation of dohle bodies in cytoplasm.*** Dohle bodies are small, round or oval patches, 2–3 μm in size seen in the cytoplasm of neutrophils (Fig. 3.3-8A) in patients with bacterial infections.
4. ***Presence of sex chromatin with nuclear lobes.*** Sex chromatin is a normal finding seen in 2–3% of neutrophils in females. It consists of a drumstick appendage of chromatin about 1 μm across, and attached to one of the nuclear lobes by a thin chromatin strand (Fig. 3.3-8B). Their presence is indicative of 2X chromosomes.
5. ***Hypersegmented neutrophils.*** Presence of hypersegmented (more than 5 nuclear lobes) neutrophils in the peripheral blood (Fig. 3.3-8C) is called a *shift-to-right*. It is indicative of a hypoactive bone marrow, as seen in megaloblastic anaemia and uraemia.
6. ***Band and star form neutrophil.*** Presence of band and star form neutrophils, i.e. premature neutrophils with decreased nuclear lobes (Fig. 3.3-1) in the peripheral blood is called *shift-to-left*. It is indicative of hyperactive bone marrow, as seen in severe infections and leukaemias.
7. ***Pelger–Huet Anomaly.*** It is an inherited disorder in which majority of the neutrophils have decreased number of nuclear segments (1–2) and coarsely staining chromatin. The nuclei appear rod-like, dumb-bell or spectacle-like (Fig. 3.3-8D).

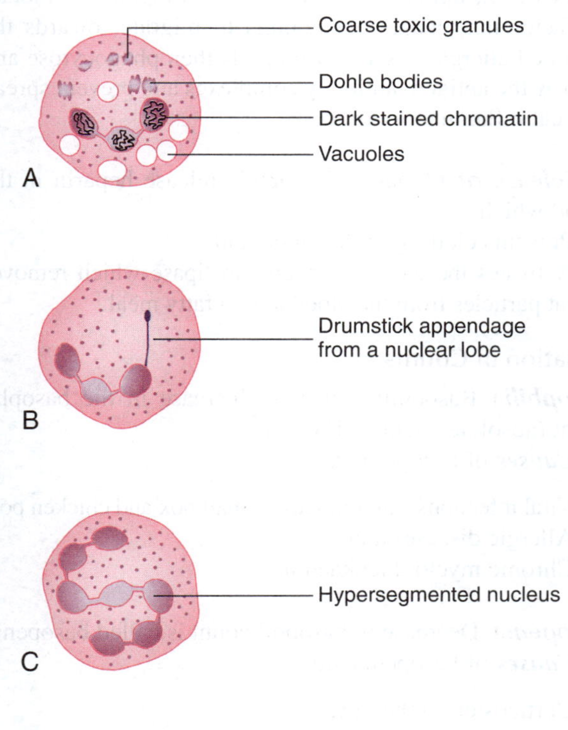

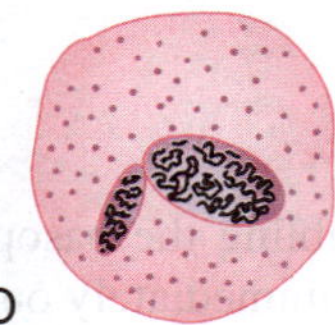

FIGURE 3.3-8 Some variations in neutrophil morphology: **A,** Dohle bodies; **B,** female sex chromatin; **C,** hypersegmented neutrophil; and **D,** hereditary Pelger–Huet anomaly.

Eosinophils

Morphological Features

Morphological features of eosinophils (Fig. 3.3-4B) are:

- ***Diameter.*** Diameter of eosinophils is similar to neutrophils, i.e. 10–14 μm.
- ***Nucleus.*** Nucleus is purple in colour and is bilobed in 85% of the cells. The two lobes are connected by the chromatin strands and thus look *spectacle shaped.* The remaining 15% of the eosinophils have trilobed nucleus.
- ***Cytoplasm.*** Cytoplasm is acidophilic and appears bright pink in colour.
  - It contains coarse, deep red-staining granules which do not cover the nucleus.
  - The granules in eosinophils contain basic protein and stain more intensely for peroxidase than granules in the neutrophils.
  - The granules contain histamine, lysosomal enzymes and eosinophil chemotactic factor of anaphylaxis (ECF-A).

Functions of Eosinophils

1. Mild Phagocytosis. Eosinophils are not very motile and thus have very mild phagocytic activity. Like neutrophils, eosinophils are attracted towards the endothelial cells by selectins and enter the tissue by diapedesis.

2. Role in Parasitic Infestations. They play an important role in the defence mechanism of body, especially in *parasitic infestations.* Eosinophils act through the following lethal substances present in their granules:

- ***Major basic protein (MBP)*** makes up about 50%of the mass of large granules. It is a highly *larvicidal* polypeptide. Because of this, eosinophils are able to damage the parasitic *larvae,* which are large to be engulfed by phagocytosis.
- ***Eosinophil cationic protein (ECP)*** is a potent bactericidal and major destroyer of helminths. It is about 10 times more potent than MBP in destroying helminths by means of complete disintegration. It is also a neurotoxin.
- ***Eosinophil peroxidase*** is capable of destroying helminths, bacteria and tumour cells.

- ***Eosinophil-derived neurotoxin*** is capable of destroying the nerve fibres.

3. Role in Allergic Reaction. The eosinophils increase in number in allergic conditions like bronchial asthma and hay fever.

- They are capable of *detoxifying* inflammation-inducing substances (released by mast cells and basophils) like histamine and bradykinin.
- They inhibit mast cell degranulation.
- They phagocytose and destroy antigen–antibody complexes and thus prevent spread of local inflammatory process.
- *Arylsulphatase B*, present in the fine granules of eosinophils, has the ability of inactivating sulphur-containing leukotrienes that tissue mast cells liberate in immediate hypersensitivity reactions.
- *Lysophospholipase* is an unusual membrane-bound protein present in the eosinophils, which forms crystals called *Charcot-Leyden crystals* in the pulmonary secretions of patients with bronchial asthma.

4. Role in Immunity. The eosinophils are present in abundance in the mucosa of respiratory tract, gastrointestinal tract and urinary tract, where they probably provide mucosal immunity.

Variation in Counts

Eosinophilia Eosinophilia refers to increase in the eosinophil count (absolute count $> 500/mm^3$).

Causes of eosinophilia are:

- Allergic conditions like bronchial asthma and hay fever,
- Tropical pulmonary eosinophilia,
- Parasitic infestation, e.g. intestinal worms like hookworm, roundworm and tapeworm,
- Skin diseases like urticarial and
- Scarlet fever.

Eosinopenia Eosinopenia is the decrease in eosinophil count (absolute count $< 50/mm^3$).

Causes of eosinopenia are:

- ACTH and steroid therapy,
- Stressful conditions and
- Acute pyogenic infections.

Basophils

Morphological Features (Fig. 3.3-4C)

- ***Diameter.*** Diameter of a basophil is similar to neutrophil and eosinophil, i.e. 10–14 μm.
- ***Nucleus.*** Nucleus of basophils is irregular, may be bilobed or trilobed, and its boundary is not clearly defined because of overcrowding with coarse granules.
- ***Cytoplasm.*** Cytoplasm of basophils is slightly basophilic and appears blue. It is full of granules.
  - Granules of basophils are very coarse and stain deep purple or blue with basic (methylene) dye.
  - Granules are in plenty and completely fill the cell and overload the nucleus.
  - The granules of basophils contain heparin, histamine and 5-HT.

Functions

1. Mild Phagocytosis. Basophils have very mild phagocytic function.

2. Role in Allergic Reaction. Basophils also enter into the tissue and release cytokine and inflammatory mediators such as histamine, bradykinin, slow-reacting substances of anaphylaxis (SRS-A) and serotonin (5HT). These substances, in turn cause local vascular and tissue reactions that cause allergic manifestations by binding of specific antigen to cell-fixed IgE molecules (for details see page 201).

3. Role In Preventing Spread of Allergic Inflammatory Process. Basophils also release eosinophil chemotactic factor that causes eosinophils to migrate towards the inflamed allergic tissue. Eosinophils then phagocytose and destroy the antigen–antibody complexes and prevent spread of local inflammatory process.

4. Release of Heparin. Basophils release heparin in the blood which:

- Prevents clotting of the blood and
- Activates the enzyme lipoprotein lipase which removes fat particles from the blood after a fatty meal.

Variation in Counts

Basophilia Basophilia refers to increase in the basophil count (absolute count $> 100/mm^3$).

Causes of basophilia are:

- Viral infections, e.g. influenza, small pox and chicken pox,
- Allergic diseases and
- Chronic myeloid leukaemia.

Basopenia Decrease in basophil count is called basopenia

Causes of basopenia are:

- Corticosteroid therapy,
- Drug-induced reactions and
- Acute pyogenic infections.

Mast Cells

Mast cells are large tissue cells resembling the basophils. These are present in bone marrow and immediately outside the capillaries in the skin. Mast cells are granulated cells of connective tissue; their granules contain proteoglycans, histamine and many proteases.

Functions. Mast cells play role in allergic reactions similar to the basophils.

- When allergens bind to the surface of mast cell coated with Ig G molecules, the degranulation of mast cells occurs and thus involved in inflammatory responses.
- Mast cells also play an important role in acquired immunity; they release TNF-α in response to bacterial product by antibody-independent mechanism.

Lymphocytes

Morphological Features

There are two types of lymphocytes large and small having almost similar structure. Majority of lymphocytes in peripheral blood are small, but large lymphocytes are also found. Morphological features of lymphocytes are:

- ***Diameter.*** Diameter of large lymphocytes varies from 12 to 16 μm and that of small lymphocytes from 7 to 10 μm (Figs. 3.3-4D and E).
- ***Nucleus.*** Lymphocytes have a large, round and single nucleus, which almost completely fills the cell. It stains deeply blue, giving an *ink-spot appearance.* Nuclear chromatin is coarsely clumped and shapeless.
- ***Cytoplasm.*** The cytoplasm is scanty, i.e. its amount is always less than that of nucleus. It is seen as a crescent of clear light blue colour around the nucleus. Cytoplasm does not contain visible granules.

Functional Subtypes Based on their developmental background, lifespan and functions, the small lymphocytes have been broadly classified into three subtypes (Fig. 3.3-9):

1. ***B lymphocytes,*** which are processed in the bone marrow, are concerned with the humoral immunity.
2. ***T lymphocytes,*** which are processed in the thymus and concerned with the cellular immunity.
3. ***Natural killer (NK) cells*** are lymphocyte-like cells that nonspecifically kill any cell that is coated with immunoglobulin IgG. This phenomenon is called *antigen-dependent cell-mediated cytotoxicity (ADCC).* Thus, NK cells provide *innate immunity*. They are highly cytotoxic against tumour cells and virus-infected cells.

The aforementioned functional subtypes of lymphocytes are not morphologically distinguishable, but they have distinctive surface molecules that are identifiable by immunochemical methods. The NK cells lack identifying surface markers.

Kinetics, Lifespan and Fate of Lymphocytes

- After processing, the T lymphocytes (processed in the thymus) and B lymphocytes (processed in the bone marrow; B stands for 'bursa of Fabricius', the site of B cell processing in birds) enter the circulation where they are present in an approximately 70:30 ratio.

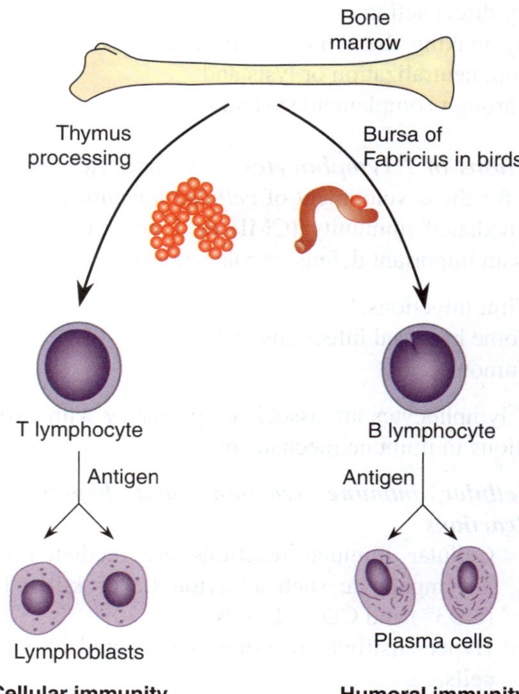

FIGURE 3.3-9 Processing of stem cells in thymus and bone marrow to become immunocompetent T and B lymphocytes.

- Many of the lymphocytes remain in circulation for a few hours, then leak out through the venules and settle in the *peripheral lymphoid tissues,* which include lymph nodes, spleen, gut-associated lymphoid tissue (GALT) and lymphoid tissue associated with respiratory and urinary tracts. At any given time, only about 2% of the body lymphocytes are in the peripheral lymphoid tissue.
- Some of the lymphocytes re-enter the blood circulation through the lymphatics, draining the peripheral lymphoid tissues. In this manner, they recirculate for months or years. Thus, the lymphocytes have a lifespan of months or a year depending upon body's need for these cells.

Functions

Lymphocytes play an important role in immunity. *Immunity* is the capacity of human body to resist all types of microorganisms and toxins that tend to damage the tissue or organ. Functionally, the lymphocytes are classified into two types: the B lymphocytes and T lymphocytes.

Functions of B Lymphocytes B lymphocytes as well as their derivatives, the plasma cells, are responsible for the development of *humoral immunity* also called antibody-mediated immunity (AMI). B lymphocytes produce antibodies (gamma globulins), which circulate in the blood and constitute the humoral immunity. Humoral immunity is the major mechanism of defence against the invading organisms, especially the bacteria. Antibodies fight against the invading organisms:

- By direct action,
- By making them inactive by agglutination, precipitation, neutralization or lysis and
- Through complement system.

Functions of T Lymphocytes T lymphocytes are responsible for the development of *cellular immunity,* also called cell-mediated immunity (CMI) or T cell immunity. CMI plays an important defensive role against:

- Viral infections,
- Some bacterial infections and
- Tumour cells.

T lymphocytes are associated primarily with two main functions in immune mechanism:

1. ***Cellular immune reactions and hypersensitivity Reactions***
   - Cellular immune reactions are mediated by the T lymphocyte such as cytotoxic or killer T cells ($CD3^+$) and $CD8^+$ T cells.
   - Hypersensitivity reaction is mediated by $CD4^+$ T cells.
2. ***Immunoregulatory function.*** The $CD4^+$ helper cells regulate the immune mechanism by regulating the function of other T cells, B cells and haemopoietic stem cells.

For details of the role of lymphocytes in immunity, see page 182.

Variations in Count

Lymphocytosis Lymphocytosis refers to increase in the lymphocyte count (absolute count > 4000/mm^3).

Physiological causes of lymphocytosis are:

- *In healthy infants and young children,* the lymphocytes count is usually high (about 60% in DLC) while the TLC is normal (relative lymphocytosis).
- *In females,* during menstruation lymphocytes are increased.

Pathological causes of lymphocytosis are:

- Chronic infections like tuberculosis, hepatitis and whooping cough.
- Viral infections like chicken pox,
- Autoimmune diseases like thyrotoxicosis,
- Infectious mononucleosis and
- Lymphatic leukaemia (most common cause of lymphocytes > 10,000/mm^3).

Lymphopenia Lymphopenia or lymphocytopenia refers to decrease in the lymphocyte count (absolute count below 1500/mm^3).

Causes of lymphopenia are:

- Patients on corticosteroid and immunosuppressive therapy,
- Hypoplastic bone marrow,
- Widespread irradiation and
- Acquired immunodeficiency syndrome (AIDS, see page 203).

Monocytes

Morphological Features (Fig. 3.3-4F)

Diameter. The monocyte is the largest mature leucocyte in the peripheral blood measuring some 12–20 μm in diameter.

Nucleus. The nucleus of monocyte is large, single and eccentric in position, i.e. present on one side of the cell. It may be notched, or indented, i.e. horseshoe or kidney shaped. It may appear oval or rounded in side view. Nucleus has characteristically fine reticulated chromatin network.

Cytoplasm. The cytoplasms is abundant, pale blue and usually clear (no granules); sometimes, it may contain fine purple, dust-like granules called *azur granules* which may be few or numerous.

Kinetics, Lifespan and Fate of Monocytes

- The kinetics of monocytes is less well understood than that of granulocytes.
- After release from the bone marrow, the monocytes remain in circulation for 10–20 to over 40 h and then they leave the blood to enter the extravascular tissues.
- In the tissues, the monocytes get converted to macrophages and form the part of so-called *tissue macrophage system* (reticuloendothelial system). In the tissues, they can live for months or even years unless destroyed while performing the phagocytic function.

Functions

1. Role in Defence Mechanism. Monocytes along with neutrophils play important role in the body's defence mechanism. Their main function is *phagocytosis.* Monocytes after entering in the tissue get converted to macrophages. These are more powerful phagocytes than neutrophils and are capable of phagocytosing as many as 100 bacteria. They also have the ability to engulf large particles such as red blood cells and malarial parasites.

The process of phagocytosis by monocytes is similar to that described in neutrophils (see page 169).

2. Precursor of Tissue Macrophages. Monocytes are the precursors of tissue macrophages. The mature monocytes stay in the blood only for few (10–20) hours. Then they leave the blood to enter the extravascular tissue and get converted into tissue macrophages (for details see page 179).

3. Role in Tumour Immunity. Monocytes may also kill tumour cells after sensitization by lymphocytes.

4. Synthesis of Biological Substances. Monocytes synthesize complement and other biologically important substances.

Variations in Count

Monocytosis A rise in the blood monocytes above 800/mm^3 is termed as monocytosis.

Causes of monocytosis are:

1. *Certain bacterial infections* such as tuberculosis, syphilis and subacute bacterial endocarditis,
2. *Infectious mononucleosis* or the so-called glandular fever,
3. *Viral infections,*
4. *Protozoal* and rickettsial infections, e.g. malaria and kala-azar,
5. *Haemopoietic disorders* like monocytic leukaemia and myeloproliferative disorders and
6. *Collagen vascular disorder.*

Monocytopenia Monocytopenia refers to decrease in the monocyte count.

Causes. Monocytopenia is rare. It may be seen in hypoplastic bone marrow.

APPLIED ASPECTS

Leukaemoid Reactions

Leukaemoid reaction refers to a reactive excessive leukocytosis in the peripheral blood resembling that of leukaemia in a subject who does not have leukaemia. In spite of confusing blood picture, the leukaemoid reactions are characterized by:

- Absence of the clinical features of leukaemia such as splenomegaly, lymphadenopathy and haemorrhages and
- Presence of the features of underlying disorders causing leukaemoid reaction, such as infections, intoxication and malignant diseases.

Types of Leukaemoid Reactions

Leukaemoid reaction may be myeloid or lymphoid.

1. Myeloid Leukaemoid Reaction is characterized by *leucocytosis,* usually moderate, not exceeding 100,000/mm^3. In majority of the cases, the granulocyte series is involved.

2. Lymphoid Leukaemoid Reaction is also characterized by moderate leucocytosis. TLC usually does not exceed 100,000/mm^3. The DLC reveals mostly mature lymphocytes simulating the blood picture seen in the chronic lymphoid leukaemia.

Leukaemias

Leukaemias constitute a group of malignant diseases of the blood in which there occurs an increase in the total WBC count associated with the presence of immature WBCs in the peripheral blood. The total WBC count is usually above 50,000/mm^3 and may be as high as 100,000–300,000/mm^3.

- The proliferation of leukaemic cells takes place primarily in the bone marrow and in certain form in the lymphoid tissues.
- There are associated features of:
  - Bone marrow failure (e.g. anaemia and thrombocytopenia) and
  - Involvement of other organs (e.g. liver, spleen, lymph nodes, meninges, brain, skin, etc.)

Types of Leukaemias Leukaemias account for 4% of all cancer deaths. Leukaemias are classified on the basis of cell types predominantly into *myeloid* (involving cells derived from the myeloid stem cells) and *lymphoid* (involving the cells derived from lymphoid stem cells). On the basis of natural history of disease each variety can be divided into *acute* and *chronic* types. In this way, the main types of leukaemias are:

1. *Acute myeloblastic leukaemia (AML),*
2. *Acute lymphoblastic leukaemia (ALL),*
3. *Chronic myeloid leukaemia (CML),*
4. *Chronic lymphoid leukaemia (CLL) and*
5. *Hairy cell leukaemia (HCL) which is an unusual variant of lymphoid neoplasia.*

Chapter 3.4

Immune Mechanisms

INTRODUCTION

Immunity refers to resistance of the body to pathogens and their toxic products. Various aspects in relation to the immune mechanisms which need detailed discussion are introduced briefly:

Types of Immunity. Immunity primarily is of two types: innate immunity which is present by birth, and acquired or adaptive immunity which is achieved during the lifetime by the individual.

Antigens. Antigens are substances that can stimulate an immune response in the body.

Antibodies. Antibodies or immunoglobulins (Igs) are gamma globulins which are produced in response to antigenic stimulation.

Immune System. The immune system that constitutes the body's defence system consists of lymphoid organs, reticuloendothelial components and the various types of immunological cells distributed throughout the body.

Immune Response. The immune system of the body responds to an antigen by two ways:

- *Humoral or antibody-mediated immunity (AMI)* which is mediated by antibodies produced by plasma cells, and
- *Cell-mediated immunity (CMI)* which is mediated directly by the sensitized lymphocytes.

Immune Tolerance. Immune tolerance refers to the inability of a host to express a specific immunological response to an antigen.

Autoimmunity. Refers to the condition when the body's immune response gets directed towards its own tissues which are normally exempted as self.

Immunomodulation. Refers to process of modifying the body's immune response. It may be in the form of:

- *Immunoenhancement (immunopotentiation),* i.e. to enhance the antibody or cell-mediated immune response against an antigen, and
- *Immunosuppression,* i.e. to reduce the body's immune response against the antigens.

Hypersensitivity. Refers to an abnormal immune response which produces physiological or histopathological damage in the host.

ARCHITECTURE (COMPONENTS) OF IMMUNE SYSTEM

The immune system which constitutes the body's defence system consists of immunological cells distributed in to two main components:

1. Mononuclear phagocytic system, and
2. Lymphoid component.

Mononuclear Phagocytic System

Mononuclear phagocytic system (MPS), also known as *tissue-macrophage system,* is the new name given to the system previously called as *reticuloendothelial system* (*RES*).

Formation of Mononuclear Phagocytic System. The monocytes enter the blood from the bone marrow and circulate for about 3 days. From the blood, the monocytes migrate into the tissue where they attain maturity, i.e. they increase in size and a large number of lysosomes and mitochondria develop in their cytoplasm. In this way, they acquire the ability to phagocytose and thus get converted to macrophages. The macrophages wander through tissues (*mobile macrophages*) and perform scavenger functions of eliminating microorganisms and other foreign particles that invade the tissues. Some of these macrophages become attached to certain tissues in the body (*fixed macrophages*) and remain there for several months. These tissue macrophages scattered in different parts of the body combinedly constitute the *tissue macrophage system* or the so-called *mononuclear phagocytic system (MPS).* The tissue macrophage system includes the macrophages present at the following sites in the body:

- Macrophages lining the sinusoids of liver (Kupffer cells),
- Spleen,
- Bone marrow (littoral cells),
- Lymph nodes,
- Lungs (pulmonary alveolar macrophages or PAM, also called dust cells),
- Connective tissue (histiocytes),
- Pleura and peritoneum,
- Subcutaneous tissue,
- Bones (osteoclasts) and
- Central nervous system (microglial cells).

Constituent Cells of Mononuclear Phagocytic System. The term mononuclear phagocytic system was coined in 1960 to include the following constituents:

- Precursor cells of the monocyte series from bone marrow,
- Promonocytes from the bone marrow,
- Monocytes from the bone marrow and blood and
- Tissue macrophages present in the above-cited sites in the body.

The MPS does not include the following cells which were included in the reticuloendothelial system (RES):

- Reticulum cells of the spleen and lymph nodes,
- Endothelial cells and
- Fibroblasts.

Functions of Mononuclear Phagocytic System. The MPS functions as a physiological unit, i.e. if any part of it is put out of action, the rest of the system undergoes compensatory hypertrophy and makes up the deficiency. The MPS plays the following roles in the body:

1. Role in Inflammation and Healing. The cells of MPS ingest cell debris, broken down RBCs, fibrin and bacteria from the inflamed area and promote healing process.

2. Role in Defence Against the Bacteria Invading the Body Tissues. These cells ingest the invading bacteria and are thus concerned with the defence of the body against the bacteria. During infection, these cells rapidly increase in number resulting in enlargement of the organs which are rich in these cells, e.g. spleen, lymph nodes, etc.

3. Role in the Immune Response played by MPS:

- The cells of MPS ingest and process the antigen entering the body. The processing of antigen is essential before an antigen can evoke cell-mediated immunity (CMI) or stimulate antibody formation in plasma cells.
- The cells of MPS have receptors for immunoglobulins and complements, so these are very efficient in phagocytosing the antigen–antibody complement complexes.

4. Role in Removal of Old RBCs. The aged RBCs or those damaged by the action of antibodies are removed by the cells of MPS in different organs like spleen, bone marrow, liver, etc.

5. Role in Removal of Old WBCs and Platelets. Like RBCs, WBCs and platelets are also removed by the cells of MPS system.

6. Storage Function. The cells of MPS store excess lipids and mucoprotein and become swollen.

Lymphoid Organs

The lymphoid component of the immune system consists of a network of lymphoid organs, tissues and cells and the product of these cells. Lymphoid organs can be classified into:

A. *Central or primary lymphoid organs*, which include:
  - **I.** Thymus, and
  - **II.** Bursa equivalent (fetal liver and bone marrow); and

B. *Peripheral lymphoid organs*, which include:
  - **I.** Lymph nodes,
  - **II.** Spleen and
  - **III.** Mucosa-associated lymphoid tissues (MALT).

Primary (Central) Lymphoid Tissues

Thymus

The thymus gland is a complex lymphoreticular organ located in mediastinum just above the heart. It consists of two (right and left) encapsulated lobes joined together by a fibrous connective tissue. Each lobe is divided into many lobules. Histologically, each lobule consists of outer *cortex* and inner *medulla.* Both cortex and medulla consist of two types of cells:

- ***Epithelial cells.*** These cells form a network in which thymocytes and macrophages are found.
- ***Thymocytes*** refer to the immature lymphocytes predominantly present in the cortex and mature lymphocytes mainly present in the medulla. Lymphocytes produced in the thymus are called thymus-derived lymphocytes or T lymphocytes or simply T cells. Lymphocyte proliferation in thymus is not dependent on antigenic stimulation.

Role of Thymus in the Immune System

- The main function of the thymus is development of cell-mediated immunity. The stem cells destined to form T lymphocytes leave the bone marrow and migrate to the thymus where they further differentiate.
- The thymus confers immunological competence on the lymphocytes during their stay in the organ. In the thymus, T lymphocytes are educated so that they become capable of mounting a cell-mediated immune response against an appropriate antigen. This is affected under the influence of the thymic microenvironment and several hormones, such as *thymosin* and *thymopoietin* produced by the thymic epithelium.
- The *immunologically competent lymphocytes* migrate from thymus into peripheral lymphoid organs as mature T lymphocytes which are precommitted to their function and antigen specificity. These are selectively seeded into paracortical areas of peripheral lymph nodes and into the white pulp of the spleen around the central arterioles. These regions are known as *thymus-dependent* areas.

Effects of Thymectomy

1. ***Thymectomy in newborn animals*** produces:
   - Lymphopenia and atrophy of peripheral lymphoid tissue,
   - Suppression of delayed hypersensitivity reactions,
   - Failure to reject foreign tissue grafts and
   - Markedly increased susceptibility to infections.
2. ***Thymectomy in adult animals*** produces immune deficiency after a few months, i.e. after the existing pool of immunologically competent lymphocytes is depleted.

The above observations 1 and 2 prove that:

- The thymus is responsible for development of immunologically competent T lymphocytes, and
- The thymus is also responsible for maintenance of an adequate pool of T lymphocytes in adult life.

Bursa Equivalent

In humans, the fetal liver and bone marrow appear to be the equivalent of avian bursa of Fabricius. *Bursa of Fabricius* in birds is also a site of lymphocytic proliferation and differentiation. Immunocompetent lymphocytes produced in the bursa are called bursa lymphocytes or B lymphocytes or B cells. The mature B cells migrate from the bursa into outer or superficial cortex of the germinal follicles and medullary cords of lymph nodes and lymphoid follicles of spleen. These sites are known as *bursa-dependent* or *thymus-independent* areas. Following appropriate antigenic stimulation, B lymphocytes transform into plasma cells and secrete antibodies which constitute the *humoral immunity* or *antibody-mediated immunity (AMI)*. Surgical removal of bursa (bursectomy) from newly hatched birds destroys their subsequent ability to produce antibodies but does not affect their ability to produce cell-mediated immunity (CMI).

Since fetal liver and bone marrow appear to be the mammalian equivalent of the avian bursa of Fabricius, so the bone marrow is the site not only of haemopoiesis but also of initial differentiation of stem cells to B lymphocytes.

Peripheral Lymphoid Organs

Lymph Nodes

The lymph nodes are small bean-shaped or oval structures which form part of the lymphatic network distributed throughout the body.

Structural Characteristics of Lymph Node (Fig. 3.4-1)

- ***Capsule*** of connective tissue covers each lymph node. From the capsule trabeculae penetrate into the lymph node.
- ***Afferent lymphatics*** enter into each lymph node at its convex surface and drain into the peripheral subcapsular sinus.
- ***Efferent lymphatics*** leave the lymph node at the concavity (hilum) as a single large lymph vessel.
- ***Microscopically,*** the lymph node consists of two parts—peripheral cortex and central medulla.

  Cortex of the lymph node consists of several rounded aggregates of lymphocytes called *lymphoid follicles.* Each follicle has a pale-staining germinal centre surrounded by small dark-staining area of lymphocytes representing *B-cell area* of the node. Besides proliferating lymphocytes, the follicles contain dendritic macrophages which capture and process the antigens.

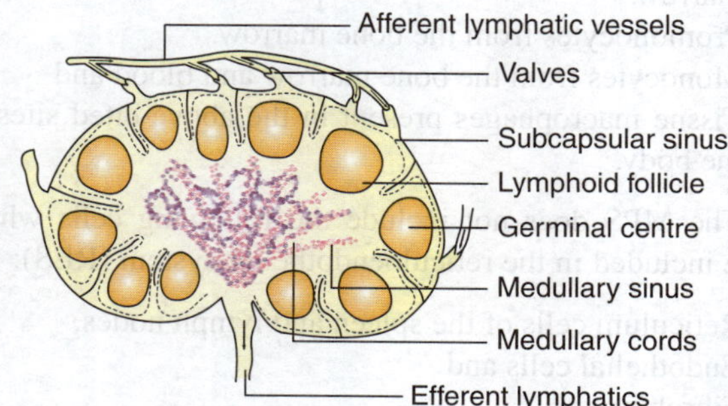

FIGURE 3.4-1 Structure of a lymph node.

- *Paracortex* is the deeper part of cortex, i.e. the zone between the peripheral cortex and the inner medulla and represents the *T-cell area (the bursa-independent area).*
- *Medulla* is predominantly composed of cords of plasma cells and some lymphocytes *(medullary cords).* The medullary cords contain B lymphocytes and along with the lymphoid follicles constitute the *bursa-dependent areas* of the lymph node.

Functions of Lymph Nodes

1. ***To mount immune response in the body.*** It is the main function of lymph nodes. A bulk of antigens is processed and antibody production occurs in the lymphoid follicles (for details see page 189).
2. ***To perform the function of active phagocytosis*** for particulate material is another main function of the lymph nodes. The lymph nodes constitute a series of inline filters. Lymph must pass through at least one lymph node before mixing with the bloodstream. Over 99% of the lymph passes through the lymph sinuses, and only 1% penetrates the lymphoid follicles.

Spleen

The spleen is the largest lymphoid organ of the body. Under normal conditions, the average weight of the spleen is about 150 g.

Structural Characteristics *(Fig. 3.4-2)*

- ***Capsule*** of connective tissue surrounds the spleen. From the capsule extend connective tissue *trabeculae* into the pulp of the organ and serve as a supportive network. Unlike some animals like cats and dogs, the capsule of human spleen contains very few smooth muscle fibres; hence, it is not capable of marked contraction.
- ***Grossly*** on a cut section, the spleen consists of a homogeneous, soft, dark red mass called *red pulp.* In the red pulp are seen scattered white nodules called *white pulp* (malpighian bodies).

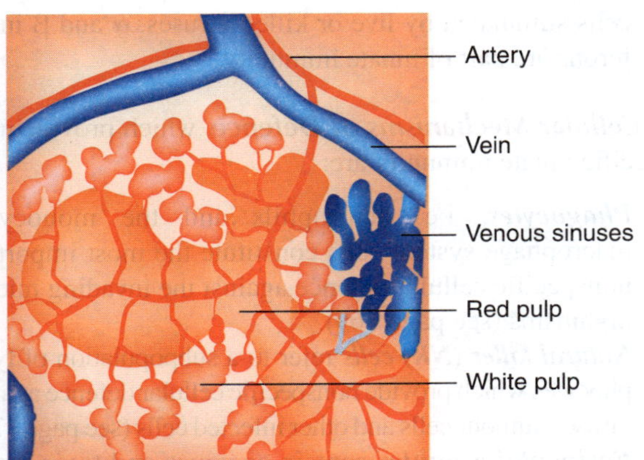

FIGURE 3.4-2 Structure of spleen.

- ***Microscopically,*** the structural characteristics are:
  - ***Red pulp*** consists of the thin-walled *blood sinuses* with *splenic cords* between them. The splenic cords consist of a collection of lymphocytes and macrophages arranged in cords in the fine network of reticular cells and fibres. This finer network forms a filtering bed that filters out red cells, white cells and platelets passing through the red pulp.
  - ***White pulp*** consists of lymphocytes surrounding an eccentrically placed central artery. These periarteriolar lymphocytes are mainly *T lymphocytes.* In addition, the white pulp also contains the lymphoid follicles composed principally of *B lymphocytes.*

Blood circulation. Blood enters the spleen by the *splenic artery* which divides into branches that penetrate the splenic tissue via trabeculae. From the trabeculae arise small branches called *central arteries.* Each central artery gives off a number of *penicillar arterioles* which open into large, thin-walled blood *sinusoids.* From the sinusoids the blood is drained into the venous channels. This pattern of circulation is called the *closed circulation.* According to another view, the spleen has an open circulation, i.e. the penicillar arterioles open into the fine network of red pulp. Ultimately, blood is drained into sinusoids and venous channels.

Functions of Spleen

1. ***Role in immune response.*** The spleen constitutes an important component of the defence system. It is an active site for production of T and B lymphocytes and antibodies. Blood-borne antigens entering the spleen are phagocytosed and processed by macrophages and fixed phagocytic mononuclear cells. Presentation of antigens, on the surface of such cells, to the splenic lymphocytes results in the formation of secondary follicles containing germinal centres of dividing and differentiating B cells which ultimately form antibodies. After splenectomy, antibody production continues to occur in other lymphoid organs but the antibody response is delayed and the antibody titre does not rise as high as in normal individuals.
2. ***Role in removal of old RBCs, WBCs and platelets.*** Tissue macrophages present in the spleen like other components of the *mononuclear phagocytic system (MPS)* play an important role in the removal of old RBCs, WBCs and platelets. The spleen seems to possess a special capability of trapping even mildly damaged erythrocytes. This ability has been attributed to the uniquely slow circulation of RBCs along the splenic cords where RBCs come in close contact with the splenic macrophages. This ability of spleen to detect and destroy abnormal type of blood cells is called *cutting action of spleen.*
3. ***Role in haematopoiesis.*** During the 4th and 5th month of fetal life, erythropoiesis occurs in spleen. In postnatal life, under pathological conditions when the entire bone marrow is exhausted, the spleen may become the site of *extramedullary erythropoiesis.*

4. ***Role in iron metabolism.*** Spleen macrophages have a special ability to recycle iron liberated from the phagocytosed RBCs, for synthesis of fresh haemoglobin in the bone marrow. Other tissue macrophages have this ability much less, and the lung macrophages (PAM) do not have this ability at all.
5. ***Role as a reservoir.*** Spleen serves as a reservoir for mobilization of RBCs in some animals like cats and dogs. In humans, this function is not important since the splenic capsule lacks smooth muscles and thus cannot contract to any significant degree. However, spleen serves as reservoir for *platelets*. About 30% of the total circulating platelets may be present in the spleen adhering to the reticular cells in the red pulp or endothelial cells of the sinusoids.
6. ***Role in regulating portal blood flow.*** The vasculature of spleen also plays a role in regulating the portal blood flow.

Mucosa-Associated Lymphoid Tissue

Mucosa-associated lymphoid tissue (MALT) refers to the lymphoid tissue distributed along the mucosa lining the alimentary, respiratory, genitourinary and other surfaces which are constantly exposed to numerous antigens. Tonsils, adenoids and Peyer's patches of small intestine are known as gut-associated lymphoid tissue (GALT). Peyer's patches are small patches of organized lymphoid tissue along the intestine containing B lymphocytes (in germinal centre) and T lymphocytes. They play a primary role in defence against infectious organisms entering via the gastrointestinal tract (GIT).

IMMUNITY

Immunity refers to resistance of the body to pathogens and their toxic products. It can be classified as:

I. *Innate immunity*
  1. Nonspecific and
  2. Specific innate immunity:
     - Species.
     - Racial and
     - Individual.

II. *Acquired (adaptive) immunity*
  1. Active acquired (adaptive) immunity,
     - Natural and
     - Artificial.
  2. Passive acquired (adaptive) immunity
     - Natural and
     - Artificial.

Innate Immunity

- *Innate or natural immunity* is the inborn capacity of the body to offer resistance to pathogens and their toxic products. It is due to genetic and constitutional make up of an individual.
- It may be *specific* (against a particular organism) or *nonspecific*.
- Innate immunity may be:
  - *Species immunity,* i.e. resistance to a pathogen shown by all members of a species.
  - *Racial immunity,* i.e. resistance to a pathogen shown by only a particular race within a species.
  - *Individual immunity,* i.e. resistance to a pathogen shown by a particular individual within a race.

Mechanisms of Innate Immunity

1. Mechanical Barrier against invading microorganisms is provided by the intact skin and mucosa in the body.

2. Surface Secretions constitute one of the important mechanisms of innate immunity. These include:

- ***Secretions*** from the sebaceous glands of skin, which contain both saturated and unsaturated fatty acids that kill many bacteria and fungi.
- ***Saliva,*** constantly produced in the mouth cavity, has an inhibitory effect on many microorganisms.
- ***Gastric juice*** and highly acidic environment of stomach may hydrolyse microbial invaders.
- ***Tears*** poured in the conjunctival sac mechanically wash away the particles and a hydrolytic enzyme, lysozyme present in the tears, can destroy most of the microorganisms.

3. Humoral Defence Mechanisms provide innate immunity by the nonspecific microbicidal substances present in the body fluids. A few examples are:

- ***Lysozyme*** is found in high concentration in most tissue fluids except CSF, sweat and urine. It is a mucolytic enzyme which kills microorganisms by splitting sugars of the structural mucopeptide of their cell wall.
- ***Basic polypeptides*** containing nonspecific microbicidal activity include leukins, arginine- and lysine-containing proteins protamine and histone.
- ***Complements*** have lytic and several other effects on foreign substances (see page 192).
- ***Interferons*** are antiviral substances produced by the cells stimulated by live or killed viruses. α and β interferons are part of innate immunity.

4. Cellular Mechanisms of Defence which provide nonspecific innate immunity are:

- ***Phagocytes,*** i.e. neutrophils and the monocyte–macrophage system cells constitute the most important nonspecific cellular defence against the invading microorganisms (see page 169).
- ***Natural killer (NK) cells*** refer to a subpopulation of lymphocytes which provide nonspecific cellular defence against viruses, tumour cells and other infected cells (see page 175).
- ***Eosinophil granules*** contain enzymes and toxic molecules that act against larvae of helminths (see page 173).

Acquired (Adaptive) Immunity

The resistance that an individual acquires during his lifetime is known as acquired or adaptive immunity. It is antigen specific and may be antibody- or cell mediated. It is of two types: active and passive.

1. Active Immunity

Active immunity is acquired by the synthesis of antibodies (humoral immunity) and production of immunocompetent cells (cell-mediated immunity) by the individual's own immune system in response to an antigenic stimulation.

Natural and Artificial Active Immunity. Active immunity can be induced naturally or artificially.

i. Natural Active Immunity. Natural active immunity results either from a subclinical or clinical infection. For example, a large majority of adults in the developing countries possess natural active immunity to poliomyelitis due to repeated subclinical infections with polio virus during childhood.

ii. Artificial Active Immunity. Artificially, active immunity is induced by introducing antigens in the body in the form of vaccines and this process is called *active immunization.* The vaccines are preparations of live or killed microorganisms or their products. Examples of vaccines are:

- Bacterial vaccines
  - Live: BCG vaccine for tuberculosis and
  - Killed: TAB vaccine for typhoid.
- Bacterial product vaccines
  - Tetanus toxoid and
  - Diphtheria toxoid.
- Viral vaccines
  - Live: Sabin vaccine for poliomyelitis, MMR vaccine for measles, mumps and rubella, and 17 D vaccine for yellow fever.
  - Killed: Salk vaccine for poliomyelitis, neural and non-neural vaccines for rabies.

2. Passive Immunity

Passive immunity refers to the immunity that is transferred to a recipient in a ready-made form. Here, the individual's immune system does not play an active role.

Natural and Artificial Passive Immunity

i. Natural Passive Immunity is the transfer of ready-made antibodies from the mother as:

- *In a fetus,* the IgG antibodies are transferred from the mother through the placenta.
- *After birth,* immunoglobulins are passed to the newborn through breast milk. Human colostrum is rich in IgA antibodies which are resistant to digestion in stomach and small intestine.

Passively transferred antibodies are generally against all common infectious diseases in the locality. These confer immunity on the neonate up to 3 months of age. Therefore, most paediatric infections are more common after the age of 3 months when maternal immunoglobulins disappear. By active immunization of mother during pregnancy, the immune status of the neonate can be improved. Therefore, immunization of pregnant women with tetanus toxoid is recommended in countries where neonatal tetanus is common.

ii. Artificial Passive Immunity. Artificially, passive immunity can be transferred to the recipients by injecting ready-made antibodies. This is done by administration of hyperimmune sera of men or animals.

Examples of artificial passive immunity include injection of:

- Antitetanus serum (ATS),
- Antidiphtheric serum (ADS) and
- Antigas gangrene serum (AGS).

After first administration, the passively administered antibodies are removed by metabolism and following subsequent injections by metabolism and immune elimination. Therefore, immunity conferred is short lived.

Differences between Active and Passive Immunity

Differences between active and passive immunity are summarized in Table 3.4-1.

ANTIGENS

Definition

Antigen. Antigens are substances that can stimulate an immune response in the body. Most antigens are proteins, but some are carbohydrates, lipids and nucleic acids. The specificity of an antigen is due to specific areas of its molecule called *determinant sites* or *epitopes.* The epitopes can bind to specific binding sites called *paratopes* of the antibody molecule (Fig. 3.4-3). A pure protein can have several epitopes and thus can stimulate formation of many distinct antibodies.

Hapten or incomplete Antigen is a chemical substance of low molecular weight that cannot induce an immune response by itself. Nevertheless, haptens can produce the immune response when combined with larger molecules (usually proteins), which serve as carriers. For example, the atropine molecule is a hapten and does not produce an immune response, but when it combines with tear proteins it can excite immune response.

In contrast to complete antigens, haptens contain a single epitope.

Some Facts about Antigenicity

Immunogenicity. Immunogenicity, i.e. ability of an antigen to stimulate an immune response is determined by:

- Size of molecule,
- Foreignness of molecule,

TABLE 3.4-1 Differences between Active and Passive Immunity

Active immunity	Passive immunity
1. Production	
Antibodies are produced by the body's own immune system in response to antigens introduced naturally or artificially in the body.	Received passively by the host. No participation of host's immune system. It is conferred by administration of ready-made antibodies naturally or artificially in the body.
2. Negative phase	
Negative phase is present in development of active immunity during which the immunity is transiently lowered. This is due to an antigen combining with the pre-existing antibodies and lowering their level.	There is no negative phase in passive immunity, as antigens are not injected.
3. Latent period	
Active immunity develops after a latent period varying from 4 days to 4 weeks. This is the time required for generation of antibodies and immunocompetent cells.	There is no latent period. Passive immunity is effective immediately.
4. Secondary response	
Due to immunological memory, the secondary response, i.e. response to antigen introduced second time, is more enhanced.	There is no immunological memory. Rather subsequent administration of antibodies is less effective due to immune elimination.
5. Duration	
Active immunity is long lasting.	Passive immunity is short lasting.
6. Effectivity	
Active immunity is more effective and confers better protection.	Passive immunity is less effective and provides inferior immunity.
7. Applicability in immunodeficient individuals	
Active immunity is not applicable in immunodeficient individuals.	Passive immunity is applicable in immunodeficient hosts.

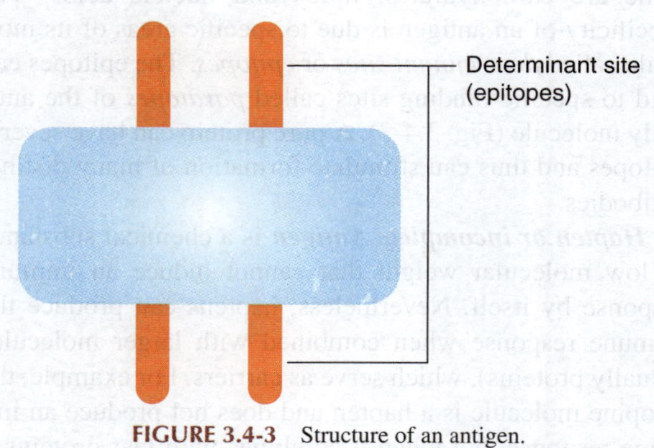

FIGURE 3.4-3 Structure of an antigen.

- Chemical structure of molecule,
- Susceptibility of the substance to the tissue enzymes,
- Genetic constitution of the host and
- Dosage, route and timing of administration.

Antigen Specificity. Antigen specificity is determined by chemical grouping and acid radicals. The antigen specificity is not absolute, i.e. some cross-reactions can occur between antigens which bear stereochemical similarities.

Species Specificity. Tissues of all individuals in a species contain species-specific antigens. However, some degree of cross-reactivity is seen between antigens from related species.

Isospecificity. Isoantigens are the antigens which are found in some but not all members of a species. On the basis of isoantigens, a species may be divided into different groups. The best example of isoantigens is human blood group antigens on the basis of which all humans can be divided into blood groups A, B, AB and O. Each of these groups may be further divided into Rh-positive and Rh-negative. This carries clinical importance in blood transfusion, isoimmunization during pregnancy and disputed paternity.

Histocompatibility Antigens

Histocompatibility antigens refer to the antigens present on the plasma membrane of cells of each individual of a species. These antigens are encoded by genes known as histocompatibility genes which collectively constitute the major histocompatibility complex (MHC). These are located on the short arm of chromosome 6. MHCs present on the surface of leucocytes were previously known as human leucocyte-associated antigens (HLA) and now known as histocompatibility lymphocyte antigen (HLA). These have been studied extensively in organ transplantation. The major histocompatibility antigens in man and mouse are known as HLA and H_2, respectively. No two persons, except identical twins, have the same MHC proteins. No two persons can have the same MHC proteins on plasma membranes of their cells.

Classes of MHC genes- There are three subclasses of MHC genes: class I, II and III.

- ***MHC class I*** molecules are found on the surface of virtually all the cells of the body excluding red blood cells. The MHC class I refers to the products of HLA-A, HLA-B and HLA-C loci (Fig. 3.4-4).
- ***MHC class II*** antigens are encoded by the HLA-DP, HLA-DQ and HLA-DR loci, all of which reside within HLA-D region of HLA complex (Fig. 3.4-4). In man, MHC class II antigens are only found on immunologically reactive cells such as B lymphocytes, macrophages, monocytes and activated T lymphocytes.
- ***MHC class III.*** The genes coding for the complement components of the classical (C_2 and C_4) and the alternative (properdin factor B) pathways also reside in the MHC genes complex located between MHC class I and class II regions (Fig. 3.4-4).

HLA Tissue Typing. Histocompatibility typing or the so-called HLA tissue typing refers to detection of MHC class I and MHC class II antigens. HLA typing is used:

1. To determine HLA compatibility prior to organ/tissue transplantation from one individual to another within a species.
2. For paternity testing.
3. For anthropologic studies.
4. For establishing HLA disease association.

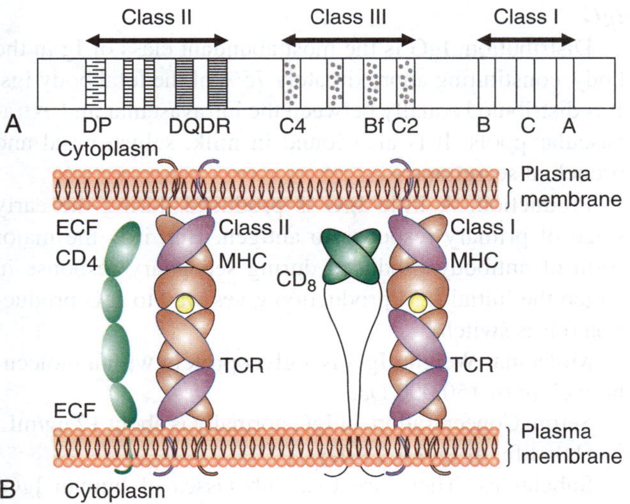

FIGURE 3.4-4 HLA complex: **A,** showing the location of MHC class I, II and III antigen proteins in HLA complex; and **B,** structure of MHC proteins and their relation to CD_4 and CD_8.

ANTIBODIES

Antibodies or immunoglobulins (Igs) are gamma globulins which are produced in response to antigenic stimulation. These react specifically with the antigens which stimulated their production. All antibodies are immunoglobulins but all immunoglobulins are not antibodies. Immunoglobulins (Igs) have been divided into five distinct classes or isotypes, namely, IgG, IgA, IgM, IgD and IgE.

Structure of Antibody

IgG has been studied extensively and serves as a model of basic structural unit of all Igs. An immunoglobulin is a Y-shaped molecule made of four polypeptide chains: two heavy (H) and two light (L). These are held together by disulphide bonds (Fig. 3.4-5).

Heavy Chains

- Heavy (H) chains have a molecular weight of 50,000 Da.
- H chains are structurally and antigenically distinct for each class of Ig and are named as:
  - α (alpha) in IgA,
  - δ (delta) in IgD,
  - ϵ (epsilon) in IgE,
  - γ (gamma) in IgG and
  - μ (mu) in IgM.
- The NH_2 terminal half of each chain has a variable sequence of amino acids and is called the *variable region.* In the heavy chain, it is designated as VH.
- The COOH terminal of each chain has a relatively constant sequence and is called the *constant region.* In the heavy chain, it is designated as CH.
- Two H chains are always identical in a given molecule. In IgG, each H chain contains 440 amino acids.

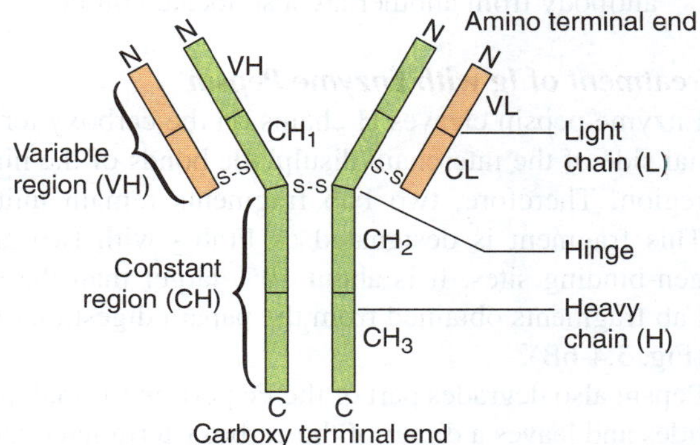

FIGURE 3.4-5 Basic structure of an antibody showing the arrangement of heavy and light chains and its variable and constant domains.

- Intrachain sulphide bonds fold each chain into incomplete loops. In the heavy chains, there are four loops of 110 amino acids, and each loop forms a globular domain. One domain designated as VH lies in the variable region and CH_1, CH_2 and CH_3 lie in the constant region (Fig. 3.4-5).

Light Chains

- Molecular weight of light (L) chains is 25,000 Da.
- L chains are of two types: k (Kappa) and λ (lambda). A molecule of Ig may have either k or λ chains but never both together. k and λ chains occur in a ratio of about 2:1 in human serum.
- Similar to H chains, the variable region of L chains is designated as VL and constant region is designated as CL.
- Like H chains, the L chains are also always identical in a given molecule. In IgG, each L chain contains 220 amino acids.
- In the light chain, there are two loops each containing 110 amino acids. Each loop forms a globular domain. One domain in variable region is designated as VL and the other in the constant region is designated as CL (Fig. 3.4-5).

Fragments of Immunoglobulins

1. When Treated with Enzyme Papain. When treated with enzyme papain, each immunoglobulin splits into three fragments (Fig. 3.4-6A):

- ***Fab (fragment antigen binding)*** are two identical fragments. Each Fab bears all the variable regions and thus possesses the antigen-binding sites. The portion of the H chains present in the Fab is called Fd piece.
- ***Fc (fragment crystallizable)*** is the third fragment having a molecular weight of 5000 Da. As the name indicates, it can be crystallized. It lacks the ability to bind to antigen and it serves the following functions:
  - Binds complements leading to complement fixation.
  - Binds to cell receptors (FcRs).
  - Determines placental transfer of Ig.
  - Determines skin fixation and catabolic rate.
  - Antigenic determinants that distinguish one class of antibody from another are also located on Fc.

2. Treatment of Ig with Enzyme Pepsin

- Enzyme pepsin cleaves H chains on the carboxy terminal side of the interchain disulphide bonds of the hinge region. Therefore, two Fab fragments remain united. This fragment is designated as $F(ab)_2$ with two antigen-binding sites. It is about 10% larger than the two Fab fragments obtained from the papain digestion of Ig (Fig. 3.4-6B).
- Pepsin also degrades part of the Fc portion to small peptides and leaves a dimer of the carboxy terminal quarter of the chain, termed pFc (Fig. 3.4-6B).

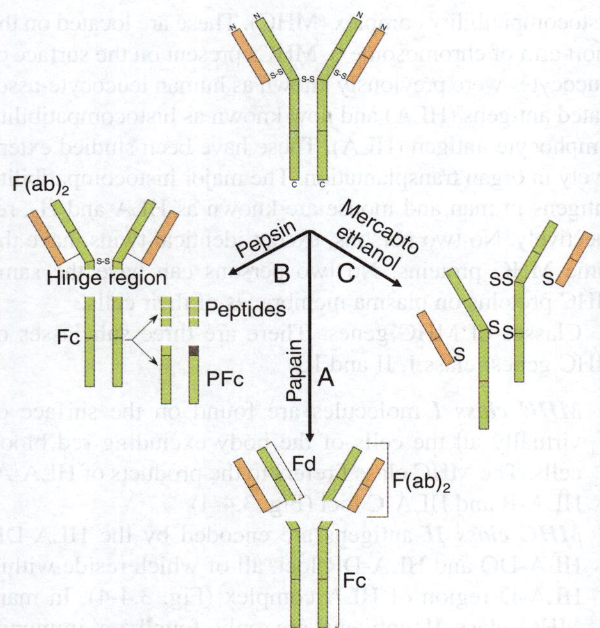

FIGURE 3.4-6 Various fragments of an antibody when treated with: A, enzyme papain; B, enzyme pepsin; and C, a reducing agent (mercaptoethanol).

3. Treatment of Ig with Reducing Agent. Treatment of Ig with a reducing agent such as mercaptoethanol, in the presence of urea, reduces disulphide bonds releasing the four peptide chains, two heavy and two light (Fig. 3.4-6C).

Types of Immunoglobulins

On the basis of physiochemical and antigenic structure, five distinct classes of immunoglobulins are identified in human serum. These are IgG, IgA, IgM, IgD and IgE.

IgG

Distribution. IgG is the most abundant class of Ig in the body, constituting approximately 75% of the total body Igs. It is distributed equally between the intravascular and extravascular pools. It is also found in milk, saliva, nasal and bronchial secretions.

Production. A little IgG is produced during the early stage of primary response to antigen. But, it is the major form of antibody produced during secondary response in which the initial IgM production gives way to IgG production (class switch).

Molecular Weight. IgG is a glycoprotein with a molecular weight of 150,000 Da.

Serum Concentration. of IgG normally is about 12 ng/mL.

Half-life. of IgG is 21 days.

Subclasses. There are four subclasses of human IgG: IgG1, IgG2, IgG3 and IgG4, possessing distinct types of heavy chains known as γ1, γ2, γ3 and γ4, respectively.

Placental Transfer. IgG is the only class of Igs that can cross the placenta and is responsible for protection of the infant during the first few months of life. IgG is also found along with IgA, in milk during the first few weeks after birth, providing additional protection if the infant is breast-fed.

Binding Characteristics of IgG are:

- Macrophages and monocytes bear Fc receptors (FcRs) which bind to the Fc portion of IgG1 and IgG3 in CH_3 domain. Such binding permits these cells to exhibit antibody-dependent cellular toxicity (ADCC).
- IgG usually exhibits high affinity for antigens leading to efficient neutralization of toxins.
- Among NK null cells, a distinct subpopulation of cytotoxic cells has been recognized which also possess FcRs for Fc part of IgG; they are capable of lysing or killing target cells sensitized with IgG and are called killer cells.
- Platelets also possess FcRs for Fc portion of IgG leading to aggregation, degranulation and release of histamine.
- IgG is the only Ig which has the property to fixing guinea pig's skin. Thus, IgG participates in most immunological reactions such as complement fixation, precipitation and neutralization of toxins and viruses.

Catabolism of IgG is unique in that it varies with its serum concentration, that is, when its level is raised catabolism is rapid.

IgM

Distribution. IgM constitutes about 10% of the total serum immunoglobulins. In contrast to IgG, IgM, because of its large size, remains almost exclusively in the serum and is not usually found extravascularly in body cavities or secretions.

Production. Phylogenetically, IgM is the oldest Ig class. It is the only Ig which is produced before birth. It is the predominant Ig produced during primary response. It appears early in the secondary response but its level does not rise significantly thereafter.

Structure. IgM normally exists as a pentamer consisting of five Ig subunits (Fig. 3.4-7).

- Its heavy chain μ type and light chain k or λ.
- The Hμ chain has four CH domains rather than three as seen in H chains of IgG.
- H chains are held together by disulphide bonds between CH_3 domains.
- There is an additional peptide chain called the joining (J) chain. The J chain may be largely responsible for the polymerization process, which occurs shortly before the molecule is secreted by plasma cells.

Molecular Weight. IgM is a glycoprotein with a molecular weight of 9,000,000 Da.

Serum concentration of IgM is 1.2 ng/mL.

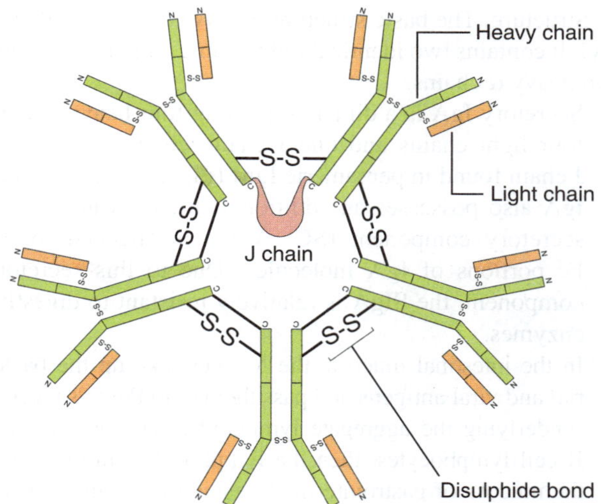

FIGURE 3.4-7 Structure of IgM immunoglobulin.

Half-life of IgM is about 5 days. Since they are relatively short-lived, their demonstration in the serum indicates recent infection.

Placental Transfer. Pentamer IgM is apparently too large to cross the placenta. As it cannot cross the placental barrier, the presence of IgM in a fetus or newborn indicates intrauterine infection. Its detection is therefore useful for the diagnosis of congenital syphilis, rubella and toxoplasmosis.

Binding Characteristics. IgM contains 10 Fab fragments, and thus 10 antigen-binding sites. Therefore, theoretically, it can bind to 10 antigen molecules. However, practically, IgM is capable of binding to as few as five molecules of antigen.

- IgM is much more efficient than IgG in its ability to fix complement by the classical pathway promoting lysis and death of most Gram-negative bacteria. This greater efficiency is due to the fact that the complement may bind to several Fc regions of pentameric IgM simultaneously, thus initiating a complement cascade and target cell lysis with a single molecule.
- IgM causes effective agglutination but its opsonizing power is rather weak.

IgA

Distribution. IgA is the second-most abundant class constituting about 15% of human serum Igs where it exists as a *monomeric* Ig. Its more important form is the *dimeric* form, known as *secretory* IgA (SIgA). It is the predominant class of Igs in secretions such as milk, tears, nasal secretions, saliva, lung secretions, genitourinary and gastrointestinal fluids.

Production. Secretory IgA is synthesized by plasma cells in the subepithelial tissues of the body.

Structure. The basic structure of IgA is similar to that of IgG. It contains two identical light chains (either k or λ) and two heavy α chains.

- Secretory IgA is a dimer containing four heavy chains, four light chains and one J chain which is similar to J chain found in pentameric IgM (Fig. 3.4-8). Secretory IgA also possesses an additional structural unit called secretory component (SC) which is attached to the Fc portions of IgA molecules. Due to this secretory component, the SIgA is relatively resistant to digestive enzymes.
- In the intestinal mucosa, the M cells take up the bacterial and viral antigens and pass them onto Peyer's patches (underlying the aggregate lymphoid tissue) and activate B cell lymphocytes, then the lymphocytes infiltrate into the mucosa of gastrointestinal, respiratory, genitourinary, female reproductive tract and also the breast tissue. There these B cells secrete Ig as when exposed to an antigen that initially activates them. The Sc component of IgA antibodies is secreted by epithelial cells that acts as a receptor for binding to IgA. This thus provides secretory immunity.

Molecular weight of IgA is 160,000 Da; while that of SIgA is 385,000 Da.

Serum concentration of IgA is 2 ng/mL.

Half-life of IgA is about 6 days.

Binding Characteristics. IgA does not fix complement in the classical pathway but can activate the alternative pathway. It promotes phagocytosis and intracellular killing of microorganisms.

Important Note

- SIgA coats the microbes and inhibits their adherence to the mucosal cells thereby preventing the entry into the body tissues. *Nisseria gonorrhoeae* which produces IgA protease can penetrate the mucosal barrier even in an immune person.

IgD

Structure. Like other monomeric antibodies, IgD is composed of two light chains (either k or λ) and two heavy chains designated as δ chains.

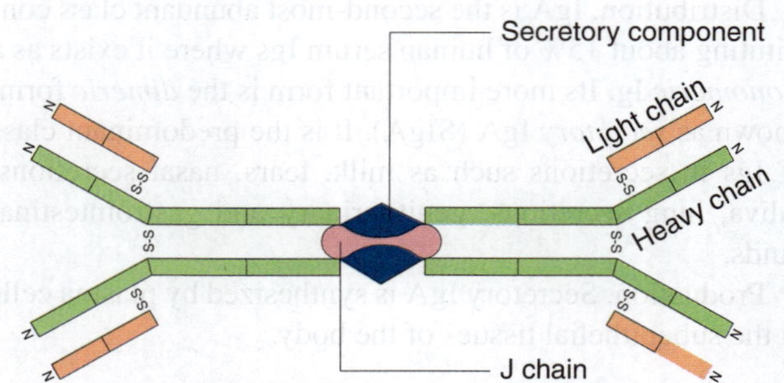

FIGURE 3.4-8 Structure of secretory IgA molecule.

Molecular weight of IgD is 180,000 Da.

Distribution. IgD is present on the surface of B lymphocytes (which are destined to differentiate into antibody-producing plasma cells) and are known to act as antigen receptors for the B cells.

Serum concentration of IgD is 0.03 ng/mL.

Half-life of IgD is about 3 days.

Placental Transfer. It does not cross the placenta.

Binding Characteristics. IgD does not bind complement. Since it is present on the surface of B lymphocytes, it is involved in antigen recognition. Reaction of an antigen with surface immunoglobulin may lead to cell differentiation and antibody synthesis.

IgE

Structure. Structure of IgE is similar to that of IgG. It consists of two light chains (either k or λ) and two heavy chains designated as ϵ (epsilon) chain.

Molecular weight of IgE is 190,000 Da.

Production. IgE is chiefly produced in the lining of the respiratory and intestinal tracts.

Distribution and Serum Concentration. Mostly a person's IgE is fixed to the surface of mast cells and basophils. It is present in extremely low concentration (0.00004 ng/mL) in the serum. However, the serum IgE levels are raised in atopic (type I hypersensitivity) conditions like asthma and hay fever.

Half-life of IgE is about 2 days.

Heat Stability. In contrast to other Igs, IgE is heat labile and gets inactivated by heating at 56°C for 30 min.

Placental Transfer. It does not cross the placental barrier.

Binding Characteristics. It does not fix complement.

- The Fc portion of IgE binds to the Fc receptors present on the surface of mast cells and basophils leaving antigen-binding sites free to react with specific antigen. When a specific antigen binds with such IgE, the reaction results in the degranulation of mast or basophil cells with the release of pharmacologically active substances such as histamine, slow-reacting substances of anaphylaxis (SRS-A), mast cell chemotactic factor, eosinophil chemotactic factor, etc.
- IgE production is particularly known to be stimulated in parasitic infestation. It has been suggested that mast cell-bound IgE reacts with antigens on the parasite followed by release of histamine. This results in increased vascular permeability followed by influx of plasma and cells (particularly eosinophils) and destruction of parasite.

Summary of Characteristic Features and Functions of Immunoglobulins

The characteristic differentiating features of various immunoglobulins are summarized in Table 3.4-2.

TABLE 3.4-2 Characteristic Differentiating Features of Various Immunoglobulins

Feature	IgG	IgA	IgM	IgD	IgE
• ***Structure characteristics*** - Structural unit - Heavy chain class - Light chain class	Monomer γ1, γ2, γ3, γ4 k or λ	Monomer SIgA is dimer α1, α2 k or λ	Pentamer μ k or λ	Monomer δ k or λ	Monomer ε
• ***Additional chain***	–	J, SC	J	–	–
• ***Molecular weight*** (in kDa)	150	160-385	900	180	190
• ***Carbohydrate content*** (%)	3	8	12	13	12
• ***Serum concentration*** (ng/mL)	12	2	1.2	0.03	0.00004
• ***Half-life*** (days)	21	6	5	3	2
• ***Secretion from serousmembranes***	No	Yes (SIgA)	No	No	Yes
• ***Placental transfer***	Yes	No	No	No	No
• ***Heat stability*** (56°C)	Yes	Yes	Yes	Yes	No
• ***Complement fixation***	Classical	Alternative	Classical	None	None
	Pathway		pathway	pathway	pathway
• ***Binding to tissue***	Heterogeneous	None	None	None	Heterogeneous
• ***Role in the body***	Protects the body fluids	Protects the body surfaces	Protects the bloodstream	Role not known	Mediate type I hypersensitivity

From the available information, the specific functions of various immunoglobulins appear as:

- ***IgG*** protects the body fluids,
- ***IgA*** protects the body surfaces,
- ***IgM*** protects the bloodstream,
- ***IgE*** mediates type I hypersensitivity and
- ***IgD's*** role is not clearly known.

DEVELOPMENT OF IMMUNE RESPONSE

Development of an immune response implies *development of acquired active immunity* in the body. The immune system of the body responds to an antigen by two ways:

1. Humoral or antibody-mediated immunity (AMI), and
2. Cell-mediated immunity (CMI).

Development of Humoral Immunity

The humoral immunity is mediated by antibodies and so is also called antibody-mediated immunity (AMI). The antibodies are produced by plasma cells which in turn are produced by B lymphocytes.

Role of Humoral Immunity

1. The humoral immunity provides defence against most extracellular bacterial pathogens and viruses that infect through the respiratory and intestinal tract.
2. It participates in immediate hypersensitivity reactions of type I, II and III.
3. Humoral immunity is also associated with certain autoimmune diseases.

Types of Humoral Immune Responses

The antibody response to stimulation by an antigen is of two types (Fig. 3.4-9):

- Primary humoral response, and
- Secondary humoral response.

Primary Response refers to the response of the body's immune system to an antigen which is introduced into the body for the first time. Always there is a latent period varying from 4 days to 4 weeks before the primary response in the form of a rise in the serum antibodies titre can be detected.

Secondary Response refers to the response of the body's immune system to an antigen which is introduced into the body on a second occasion. Such a response occurs more quickly and more abundantly. This is because of the fact that the immune system is liable to retain the memory of a prior antigenic exposure for long periods (immunological memory) and produce enhanced response when encountered with the same antigen for the second time.

Immune Response Arch. The development of immune response can be subdivided using the concept of "Immune

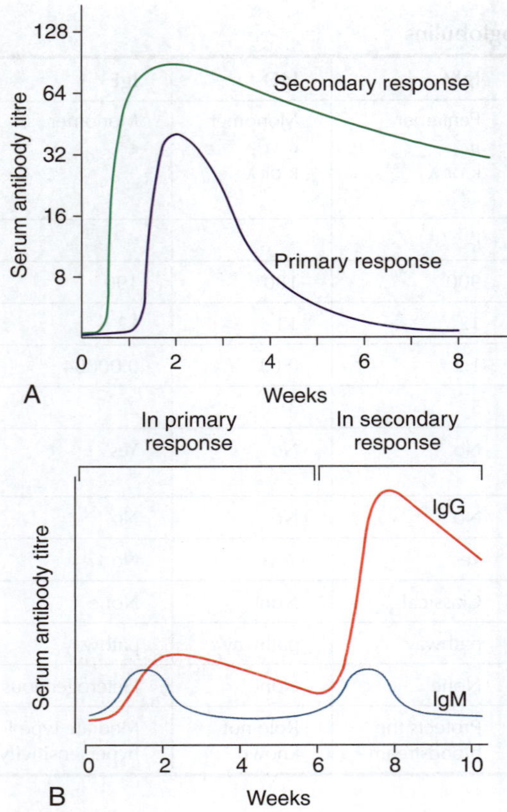

FIGURE 3.4-9 Response of body immune system to an antigen: **A,** time course of antibody production in primary versus/secondary response; and **B,** serum levels of IgM and IgG antibodies in primary and secondary response.

Response Arch" into three phases—afferent, processing and effector.

Phases of Humoral Immune Response (Figs. 3.4-10, 3.4-11)

1. Antigen Processing and Presentation Once the antigen enters the body, it is phagocytosed by the macrophages (nonspecific response). Phagocytosed material is broken down into polypeptide fragments. The antigen polypeptide fragments then combine with the MHC II present in the macrophages and move to the cell surface. This is called *processing of antigen.* The processed antigen is then presented to immunocompetent lymphocytes by the macrophages. So, the macrophages are also called *antigen-presenting cells (APCs).* Other antigen-presenting cells which can process and present the antigen to lymphocytes are:

- B lymphocytes themselves and
- Dendritic cells present in the skin (Langerhans cells), thymus (medulla), lymph nodes (cortex and paracortex), spleen and other secondary lymphoid organs.

2. Recognition of Antigen by Lymphocytes. The lymphocytes possess the antigen recognition receptors. These include the membrane-bound (surface) immunoglobulins (mIgs or sIgs) in B lymphocytes and T cell receptors (TCRs) in the T lymphocytes. These receptors serve as specific surface receptors, recognizing and interacting with only a single antigenic determinant on the antigen presented to the lymphocytes. This process of binding of processed antigen to specific receptors on the surface of lymphocytes in technical terms is called *recognition of antigen by lymphocytes.* Thus, many million different T and B lymphocytes, each with the ability to respond to particular antigen, are present in the body.

Important Note

The receptors on circulating T cell (TCRs) are mainly made of α and β polypeptide units, hence called α and β T cells. About 10% of T cell receptors (TCRs) have γ and δ polypeptide units, and they are designated as γδ T cells.

3. Lymphocyte Activation. The lymphocytes that have combined with antigen are activated, i.e. the lymphocytes become larger and look like a lymphoblast. This is known as *blast transformation.* Activated B lympocytes and helper T cells (CD_4 cells) play a major role in humoral immunity. The macrophages liberate IL-1 and cause further activation of B lymphocytes and helper (CD_4T) cells.

Activation of T Lymphocytes. Activation of helper T cells by the processed antigen complex is essential for humoral immunity. The activated helper T cells secrete two substances: interleukins 2 (IL2) and B cell growth factor which further promote proliferation of B lymphocytes and their transformation into plasma cells. This phenomenon is called *T–B cooperation.*

Activation of B Lymphocytes. After receiving cooperation from T helper cells (T–B cooperation), B lymphoblasts proliferate forming clones of cells that respond to this antigen (*clonal selection*). A clone is the population of cells descended by asexual reproduction from a single cell. The B lymphocytes proliferate and transform into two types:

- Plasma cells, and
- Memory B cells.

Role of plasma cells. When a B lymphocyte is converted to a plasma cell, its cytoplasm expands. It is filled with granular endoplasmic reticulum. The plasma cells secrete antibodies.

Role of memory B cells. A small portion of the activated B lymphocytes do not enlarge or undergo blast transformation. Instead, they only proliferate and transform into small-sized memory B cells, which occupy the lymphoid tissue throughout the body. Memory B cells have a long lifespan and remain inactive. When the body is exposed to the same antigen for the second time, they are able to recognize it become active, i.e. they are responsible for secondary response of antibodies.

4. Production of Antibodies. The plasma cells so formed secrete antibodies which are also called

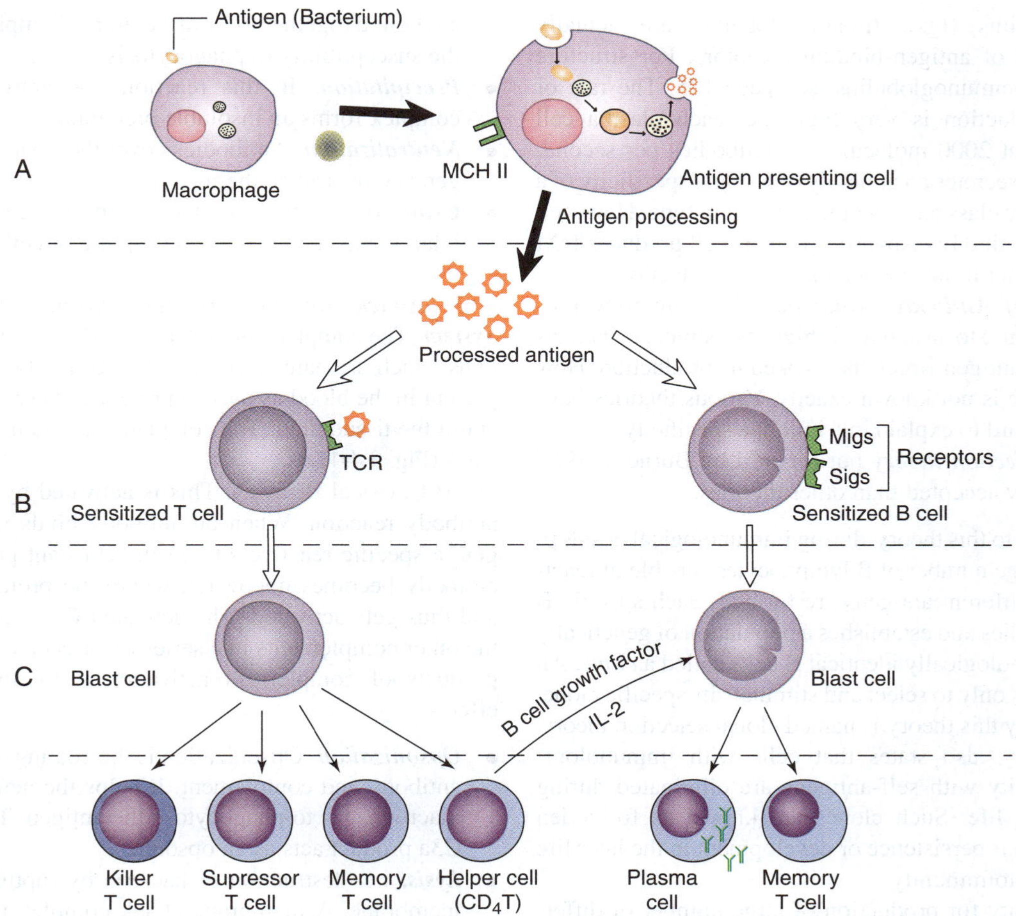

FIGURE 3.4-10 Broad outline of development of humoral immune response: **A,** antigen processing and presentation to immunocompetent cells; **B,** recognition of antigen by the lymphocytes; and **C,** activation of lymphocytes (blast transformation).

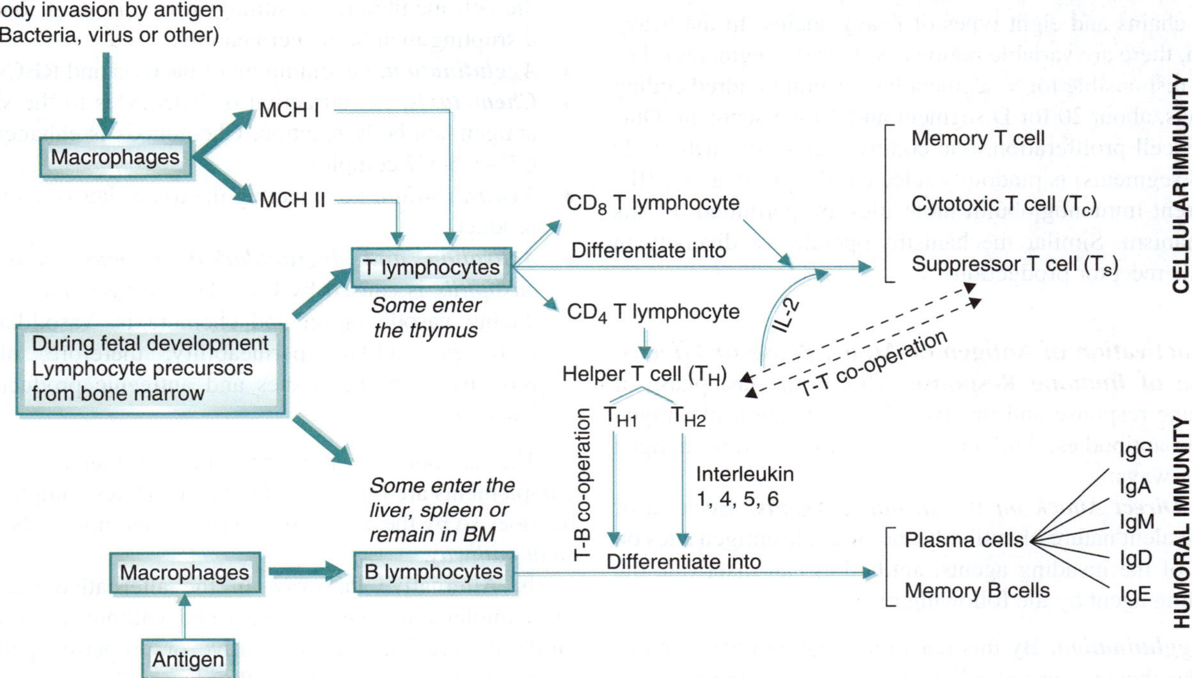

FIGURE 3.4-11 Summary of immune response.

immunoglobulins (Igs). Immunoglobulins are actually secreted form of antigen-binding receptors. For structure and class of immunoglobulins, see page 185. The rate of antibody production is very high, i.e. each plasma cell produces about 2000 molecules of antibodies per second. A plasma cell secretes an antibody of a single specificity of a single antibody class and a single light chain type. However, in a primary antibody response, a plasma cell produces IgM initially and later it may switch onto IgG production.

Theories of Antibody Production. The antibody produced in response to an antigen is highly specific, i.e. it reacts only with the antigen which has evoked its production. How this is possible is not known exactly. Various theories have been put forward to explain this immune specificity.

Clonal selection theory put forward by Burne in 1957 is more widely accepted than other theories.

- According to this theory, during immunological development, a large number of B lymphocytes capable of reacting with different antigens are formed. Each specific B cell multiplies and establishes a population of genetically and immunologically identical B cells called a *clone.* An antigen has only to select and stimulate its specific clone. That is why this theory is named clonal selection theory.
- This theory also states that cells with immunological reactivity with self-antigens are eliminated during embryonic life. Such clones are known as forbidden clones. Their persistence or development in the later life leads to autoimmunity.
- The diversity for production of large number of different types of immunoglobulins by human B cells has a genetic basis.

The immunoglobulin molecules possess two types of light chains and eight types of heavy chains. In the heavy chain, there are variable regions (V, D and J segments). The gene responsible for V segment has several hundred coding regions, about 20 for D segment and 4 for J segment. During B cell proliferation, one coding region for each (V, D and J segments) is randomly selected; therefore, about 10^{15} different immunoglobulin molecules are permitted by this mechanism. Similar mechanisms operate for diversity in T cells receptor production.

5. Inactivation of Antigen or Attack Phase or Effector Phase of Immune Response. This is the last phase of immune response and involves the inactivation of antigen by the antibodies. Antibodies act on the invading antigen in two ways:

1. Direct Attack on the Invading Agents. Because of the bivalent nature of antibody and multiple antigen sites on most of the invading agents, antibodies can inactivate the invading agent by the following reactions:

- ***Agglutination.*** By this reaction, large number of particles (bacteria or red cells) with antigens on their surface are bound together to form a clump. Clumping increases the susceptibility to phagocytosis.
- ***Precipitation.*** In this reaction, the antigen–antibody complex forms an insoluble precipitate.
- ***Neutralization***. Antibodies cover the toxic sites of antigen and neutralize them.
- ***Cytolysis.*** Antibodies attach to the membranes of cellular agents thereby causing rupture of cells.

2. Attack on the Antigen through Complement System The complement system includes 11 enzymatic proteins which are named as C1 to C9, B and D. All these are present in the blood as plasma proteins. These are also present in the tissue fluid. The complement system acts in three ways (Fig. 3.4-12):

(a) Classical Pathway. This is activated by an antigen–antibody reaction. When an antibody binds with an antigen, a specific reactive site on the constant portion of the antibody becomes uncovered where the protein C1 binds and thus gets activated. The activated C1 in turn activates the other complements in a series of cascade reactions. The products of complement activation cause the following effects:

- ***Opsonization.*** Opsonization is the coating of antigen by antibody and complement. It helps the neutrophils and macrophages to phagocytose the antigen. The activated C3a product acts as an opsonin.
- ***Lysis,*** i.e. destruction of bacteria by rupturing the cell membrane. A membrane attack complex is formed by C5b–C6–C7–C8–C9.The cell lysis is brought about by the complement system by inserting proteins called *perforins* into the cell membrane. Perforins make holes in the cell membranes, resulting in free flow of ions and disrupting membrane permeability.
- ***Agglutination,*** i.e. clumping of bacteria and RBCs.
- ***Chemotaxis,*** i.e. attraction of leucocytes to the site of antigen–antibody reaction. Chemotaxis is enhanced by C5b–C6–C7 complex.
- ***Neutralization,*** i.e. covering the toxic sites of antigenic products.
- ***Activation and degranulation of mast cells and basophils*** is caused by C4b. This releases factors producing vasodilatation and chemotaxis. Vasodilatation increases capillary permeability; therefore, plasma proteins enter the tissues and antigenic products are inactivated.

The antibodies which can fix and thereby activate complements are IgM and IgG. IgA also fixes complements but does so by the *alternative pathway* and not by the *classical pathway.*

(b) Alternative Pathway. In the alternative pathway, the complement system is activated without an antigen–antibody reaction. The alternative or properdin pathway is initiated by binding of the factor I (a protein in

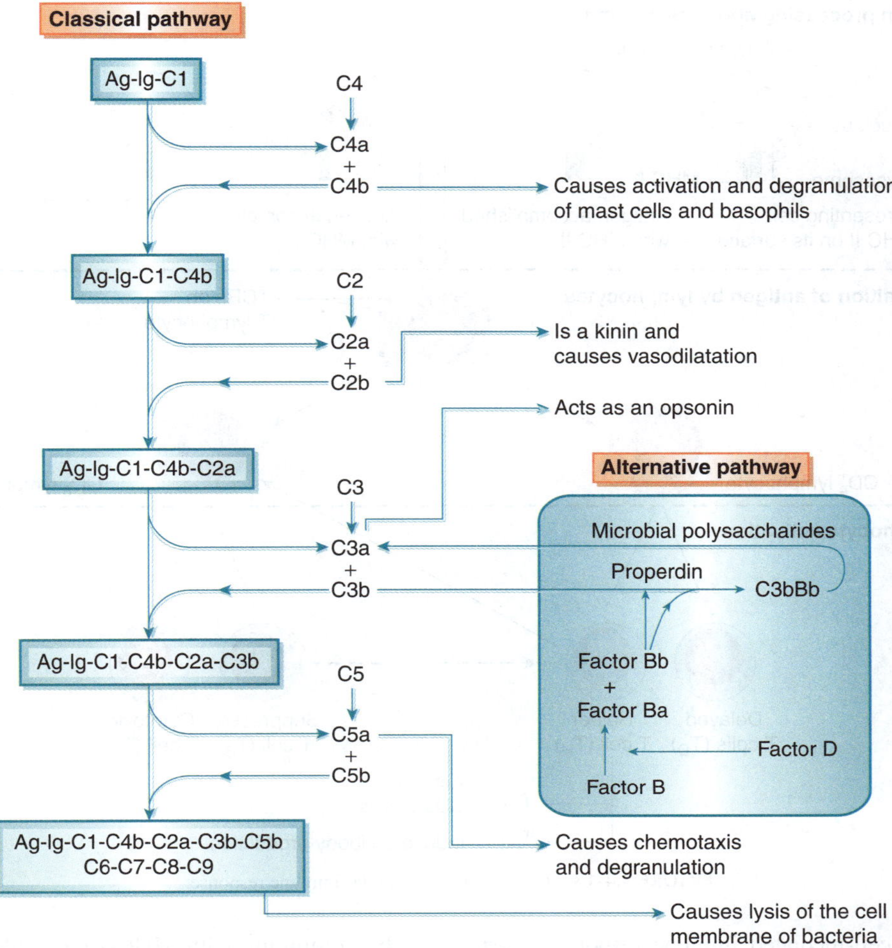

FIGURE 3.4-12 Broad outline of classical and alternative pathway of complement system.

circulation) with polysaccharide present in the cell wall of invading organism, i.e. bacteria (endotoxin) and yeast cell wall (zymogen). This binding triggers reactions that activate C3 and C5 which ultimately attack the antigenic products of invading organisms. *Properdin* (a circulating protein) stabilizes the activating enzyme complex that is why the alternative pathway is also called properdin pathway. Because this pathway does not involve an antigen–antibody reaction, it is one of the first line of defence against invading organisms.

(c) Mannose-binding Lectin Pathway of complement system is triggered when lectin binds to mannose groups in bacteria.

Development of Cellular Immune Response

The cellular immunity refers to specific acquired immunity which is accomplished by effector T cells and macrophages (Figs. 3.4-11, 3.4-13). It is also called cell-mediated immunity (CMI).

Role of Cellular Immunity

1. Cellular immunity protects the host against fungi, most of the viruses and intracellular bacterial pathogens like *Mycobacterium tuberculosis, M. leprae* and *Brucella*.
2. It participates in allograft rejection and graft versus host reaction.
3. CMI participates in delayed hypersensitivity reaction.
4. CMI is also associated with certain autoimmune diseases.
5. It provides immunological surveillance and immunity against cancer (tumour immunity).

Types of Cellular Immune Response

Like humoral immune response, the cellular immune response is also of two types:

- ***Primary cellular response*** which is produced by initial contact with a foreign antigen, and
- ***Secondary cellular response*** which is produced when the host is subsequently exposed to the same antigen.

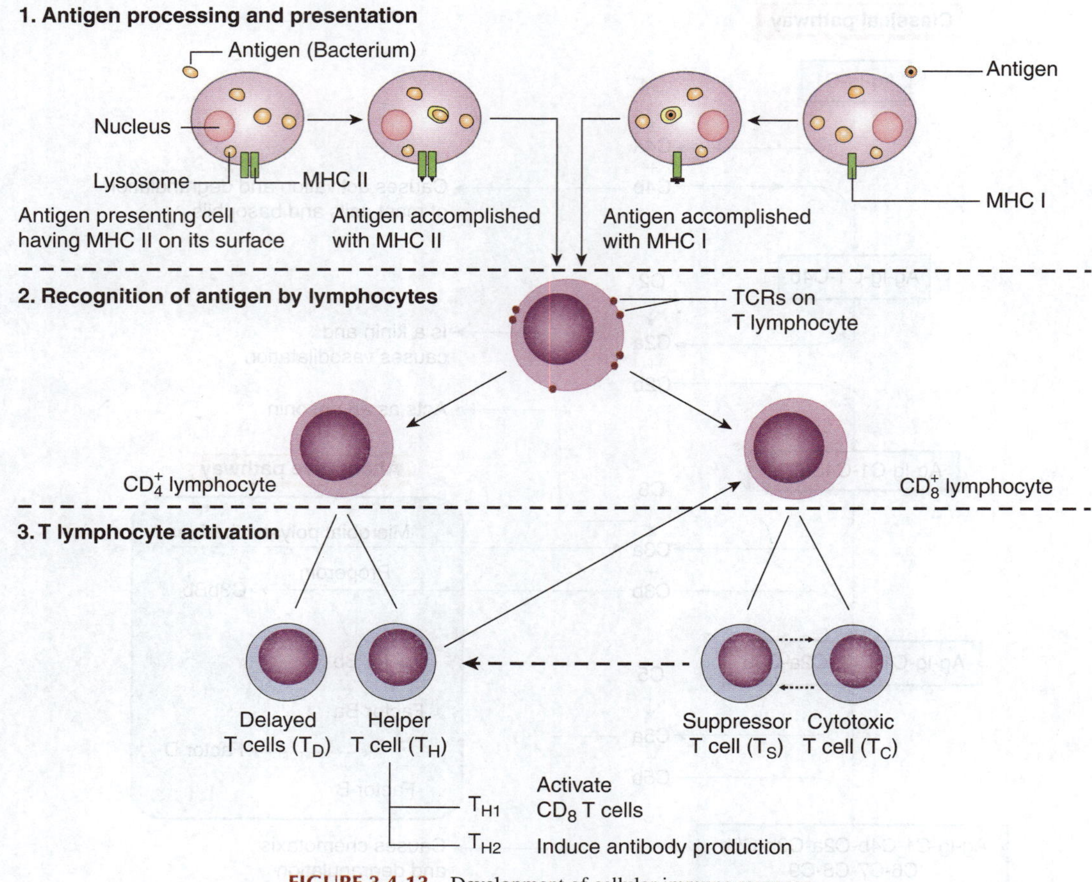

FIGURE 3.4-13 Development of cellular immune response.

The secondary cell-mediated immune response is usually more pronounced and occurs more rapidly. Further, because of the availability of specific memory cells, an increased number of effector cells are produced in secondary response.

Phases of Cellular Immune Response

The development of cellular immune response can be subdivided, using, the concept of immune response arch in three phases—afferent phase, processing phase and effector phase.

1. Antigen Processing and Presentation. An antigen entering the host body is phagocytosed and degraded into polypeptide fragments by the antigen-processing cells (APCs) which include macrophages and dendritic cells present in the peripheral lymphoid tissue. The antigen polypeptide fragments then become associated with MHC antigen and are expressed on the surface of APC. Two modes of antigen processing are known:

- Processing of Phagocytosed Material, e.g. bacterial antigen, is accomplished by combining with MHC-II molecules, and
- Processing of Antigen Derived Within the Cell, e.g. viral antigens synthesized in infected cell, is accomplished by combining with MHC-I molecules (probably in the endoplasmic reticulum).

2. Recognition of Antigen by Lymphocytes. T lymphocytes possess the antigenic recognition receptors known as *T cell receptors* (TCRs). These receptors serve as specific surface receptors recognizing and interacting with only single antigenic determinant on the antigen presented to lymphocytes. Further, the mature T lymphocytes can be differentiated into two antigenic subtypes depending on the ensemble of their surface antigens: CD4+ cells and CD8+ cells.

- CD8+ cells recognize the combination of foreign antigen and class I MHC antigen, and
- CD4+ cells recognize the combination of foreign antigen and class II MHC antigen.

T Lymphocyte Differentiation (Activation).

CD8+ Type of T Lymphocytes. after combining with foreign antigen–MHC-I complex are activated and differentiate into:

- Cytotoxic T cells (Tc cells), and
- Suppressor T cells (Ts cells).

CD4+ Type of T Lymphocytes after combining with foreign antigen–MHC-II complex are activated and differentiate into:

- Helper T cells (T_H cells), and
- Delayed type hypersensitivity T cells (TD cells).

T–T Cooperation. The differentiation of T lymphocytes into T_H, T_C, T_S and T_D cells is interdependent. This interdependence is called T–T cooperation.

Release of Differentiated T cells. The differentiated T lymphocytes so formed are released into the lymph and then enter the blood through which they are distributed throughout the body. They also pass out through capillary walls and enter in tissue fluid. From the tissue fluid they enter back into the lymph, and then to lymphoid tissue and once again into blood. Thus, T lymphocytes circulate again and again throughout the body, sometimes lasting for months or years.

T Lymphocyte Memory Cells. are also formed. These spread throughout the lymphoid tissues of entire body. Therefore, on subsequent exposure to the same antigen, release of T cells occurs far more rapidly and much more powerfully than in the first response (secondary response).

4. Attack Phase of Cell-Mediated Immunity.

Role of Cytotoxic T Cells. ***Cytotoxic T cells*** (Tc cells) and natural killer cells (NK cells) are responsible for the attack phase of cell-mediated immunity.

Cytotoxic T cells have some receptor protein on their outer membrane. On the basis of their receptors and functions, cytotoxic T cells are divided into αβ and γδ ($\alpha\beta T_c$ and $\gamma\delta T_c$) cells. Cytotoxic T cells bind antigen-bearing cells (target cells) tightly and destroy them by the following mechanisms:

i. ***Perforin-mediated killing.*** The Tc cells after binding with the target cell secrete a hole-forming protein called *perforin*. The perforins literally punch round holes in the membrane of target cells in the presence of extracellular calcium (calcium-dependent lysis). The pores so formed cause cell death by disrupting cell homeostasis.
ii. ***Lysis through cytotoxic substances.*** After binding with target cells, the Tc cells enlarge and release cytotoxic substances.
iii. ***Induction of apoptosis.*** Tc cells secrete tumour necrosis factor B (TNF-B) which increases the Ca^{2+} permeability of antigen-bearing cell. The increased intracellular calcium activates enzymes that cause degradation of nucleus producing apoptosis.

Role of Helper T Cells (TH Cells). Helper T cells are of two types: T_H^1 and T_H^2.

i. ***Helper T^1 (T_H^1) cells*** play their roles by secreting three cytokines:
   - *Interleukin 2 (IL-2)* secreted by helper T_1 cells activates the CD8+ cells to differentiate into cytotoxic T cells and suppressor T cells (T–T cooperation).
   - γ *Interferon (IFN-γ)* has the direct ability to kill antigen-bearing cells.
   - *Tumour necrosis factor-B (TNF-B)* can induce apoptosis in antigen-bearing cells.
ii. ***Helper T_2 (T_H^2) cells*** secrete interleukins 4, 5, 6, 10 and 13 and primarily with activation of B lymphocytes produce antibodies (T–B cooperation).

Role of Suppressor T Lymphocytes (T_S Cells)

- Suppressor T cells regulate the activity of cytotoxic T cells. Thus, the cellular immune response is a balance between T_C cells and Ts cells.
- Suppressor T cells also play an important role in preventing the cytotoxic T cells from destroying the body's own tissue along with the invading organism.
- Suppressor T cells also suppress the activities of helper T cells.

Cytokines

Cytokines are small protein molecules which act like hormones to regulate immune response.

Types, Cell Source and Effects. Types, cell source and effects of various cytokines are summarized in Table 3.4-3. As shown in Table 3.4-3, the cytokines are secreted not only by lymphocytes and macrophages but also by endothelial cells, neuroglial cells and other types of cells. Broadly, cytokines can be grouped as:

- ***Interleukins (IL).*** These are the principal cytokines and include IL-1 to IL-13 (Table 3.4-3).
- ***Other cytokines*** include:
  - Chemokines,
  - Growth factors,
  - Colony-stimulating factors (CSF),
  - Tumour necrotic factors (TNF α and TNF β) and
  - Interferons (IFN).

  Chemokines are the substances that attract neutrophils and other white blood cells to the area of immune response or inflammation. About 40 chemokines have been identified. The receptors of chemokines are serpentine and act via G proteins. Chemokines also play role in cell growth and angiogenesis.

Mechanism of Action

1. Local Effects. Cytokines act in an *autocrine* (i.e. on the cell that produced them) or *paracrine* (i.e. on the cell close by) manner through their specific receptors.

Receptors of Cytokines have been grouped under the superfamily. The *superfamily* includes receptors of:

- Cytokines,
- Haematopoietic growth factors,
- Prolactin and
- Growth hormone.

TABLE 3.4-3 Main Characteristics of Human Interleukins and Other Immunoregulatory Cytokines

Type of cytokine	Cell source	Effects
I. Interleukins (IL)		
IL-1 α and β	Macrophages and other antigen-processing cells (APCs)	i. B cell proliferation, ii. Igs production, iii. Stimulation of T cells and iv. Inflammation fever.
IL-2	Activated helper cells (TH[1]), cytotoxic cells (Tc) and natural killer cells (NK)	i. Proliferation of activated T cell. ii. B cell proliferation, Igs expression.
IL-3	T lymphocytes	Growth of early progenitor cell
IL-4	TH[2] and mast cells	i. Eosinophil growth and its function, ii. B cell proliferation, iii. Igs expression, iv. MHC class II expression, v. Proliferation of TH[2] and Tc cells and vi. Inhibition of production of inflammatory cytokines.
IL-5	TH[2] and mast cells	Growth of eosinophils and its function.
IL-6	Activated TH[2] cells APC and other somatic cells	i. Act with IL-I and TNF to stimulate T cells, ii. Proliferation of B cells and Igs production and iii. Stimulates thrombopoiesis.
IL-7	Thymic and bone marrow stromal cells	Lymphopoiesis (T and B cells)
IL-8	Macrophages	Stimulates neutrophil activity and promote their accumulation.
IL-9	From cultured T cells	Stimulates haematopoietic and thymopoietic factors.
IL-10	Activated helper cells (TH[2]), TCD8, B lymphocyte and macrophages	i. Inhibition of cytokine production, ii. Stimulates B cells and antibodies production and its functions, iii. Suppresses cell-mediated immunity and iv. Causes growth of mast cells.
IL-11	Stroma cells	Stimulates haematopoiesis and thrombopoiesis
IL-12	Macrophages and B cells	Stimulates proliferation of cytotoxic T cells and killer cells (Tc and NK).
IL-13	TH[2] cells	Promotes cell-mediated immune response. i. B cell proliferation, IgG expression, class II MHC expression, ii. Proliferation of TH[2], Tc cells and their function and iii. Inhibition of production of inflammatory cytokines
II. Other cytokines	Activated macrophages	i. IL-I type effects and
TNF α		ii. Causes vascular thrombosis and necrosis of tumour cells.
TNF β	Activated TH[1] cells	Vascular thrombosis and tumour cell necrosis
Interferon (IFN α and β)	Macrophages, neutrophils and other somatic cells	i. Antiviral effects, ii. Stimulates class II MHC cells and iii. Activation of macrophages and NK cells.
IFN-γ	Activated TH[1] and NK cells	i. Antiviral effect, ii. Activation of class I MHC cells and class II MHC cells and iii. Promotes cell-mediated immunity.
TGFβ	Activated T lymphocytes, platelets, macrophages and somatic cells	i. Anti-inflammatory effect by suppressing cytokine production and MHC-II cells, ii. Inhibits proliferation of macrophages and lymphocytes, iii. Proliferation of B cells and iv. Healing (by stimulating fibroblast cells).

The superfamily of receptors has been divided into three *subfamilies:*

- Subfamily I includes receptors for IL-4 and IL-7.
- Subfamily II includes receptors for IL-3, IL-5 and IL-6.
- Subfamily III includes receptors of IL-2 and other cytokines and related proteins, e.g. IL-2R and Tac antigen.

Systemic Effects. Interleukin-1 (IL-1) affects the various body systems:

- ***Central nervous system effect.*** It causes fever, slow wave sleep, secretion of CRH and anorexia.
- ***Metabolic effects.*** It increases hepatic protein synthesis, excretion of sodium and decreases plasma zinc and iron level and also cytochrome P_{450}. It also causes lactic acidosis.
- ***Haematological effects.*** It increases number of circulating neutrophils, colony-stimulating factors and nonspecific resistance.
- ***Vascular system effect.*** It stimulates leucocyte adherence to the vessel wall, increases synthesis of prostaglandins, releases platelet-activating factor and increases the capillary permeability.

OTHER IMMUNE MECHANISM-RELATED ASPECTS

Some other aspects related to immune mechanisms which need to be elaborated are:

- Immune tolerance,
- Immune modulation,
- Autoimmunity,
- Hypersensitivity and
- Immunodeficiency diseases.

Immune Tolerance

Types of Immune Tolerance. Immune tolerance may be defined as a state of unresponsiveness to an antigen. It occurs in two forms: natural and acquired.

1. Natural Tolerance refers to nonresponsiveness to a self-antigen. During embryonic development, when the immune system is immature, any antigen which comes in contact with the immature immune system is recognized as self-antigen. Therefore, it does not evoke any response in later life when body is exposed to the same antigen.

2. Acquired Tolerance means unresponsiveness to a potential antigen. It is of further two types: general and specific.

(i) ***General immunological tolerance*** results due to impairment of the immune system; hence, there is lack of responsiveness to potential antigens.

(ii) ***Specific immunological tolerance*** arises when a potential antigen induces a state of unresponsiveness to itself and not to other antigens. This happens when an antigen becomes tolerogenic (tolerogen).

- In some instances, when an antigen is presented at particular concentration, it might induce specific immunological tolerance or unresponsiveness, whereas when presented at some other concentration, it promotes immunity. Therefore, an antigen that induces tolerance is referred to as *tolerogen.*
- Specific acquired tolerance has consequences for the host defences. Presence of tolerogenic epitopes on the pathogens compromises with the ability of the body to resist infections.

Mechanism of Tolerance. Immunotolerance can arise by three possible mechanisms:

- Clonal deletion,
- Clonal anergy and
- Suppression.

1. Clonal Deletion. During embryonic life, clones of B and T cells are formed. These B and T cells possess receptors which recognize the antigens and are selectively deleted or eliminated and therefore, not available to respond on subsequent exposure to that antigen in later life.

2. Clonal Anergy. Clones of B and T cell receptors which recognize self-antigen might remain, but cannot be activated. This is referred as clonal anergy.

3. Suppression. Clones of B and T cells expressing receptors that recognize self-antigen are preserved and capable for recognition of an antigen when activated. However, an immune response might be inhibited through active suppression.

Factors Influencing Induction of Tolerance. A number of factors influence induction of immunological tolerance. These are: species, competency of the host, antigen and age of the host.

1. Species. Immunological tolerance varies from species to species. For example, species like rabbits and mice can be rendered tolerant more rapidly as compared to guinea pigs and chickens.

2. Immunological Competency of the Host also effects induction of tolerance. If degree of immunological competency of the host is high, then induction of tolerance is very difficult. On the other hand, newborns and embryos are particularly susceptible for induction of tolerance because their immune system is immature and not very competent.

3. Antigen. Induction of tolerance also depends upon the antigen (i.e. its physical nature, dose and its route of administration).

i. ***Physical nature of an antigen*** refers to the form of an antigen, i.e.

- Aggregated form, or
- Soluble (free form).

For example, human gamma globulin is *heat aggregated* and it is highly immunogenic in mice. But when deaggregated, it becomes tolerogenic. This is probably due to the fact that antigens in the aggregated form are easily phagocytosed by the macrophages and then presented to antibody-forming cells. On the other hand, soluble antigens or deaggregated antigens or free antigens escape phagocytization by the macrophages; therefore, they are not so easily processed and are tolerogenic.

ii. ***Dose***. The induction of tolerance is also dose dependent. It has been observed that high doses of antigen tolerize the B cells and minute doses of an antigen when introduced repeatedly tolerize the T cells, but a moderate dose of the same antigen is immunogenic. Dose-dependent tolerance occurs by two ways:
   - *Immune paralysis* or *high zone tolerance* occurs when high doses of antigen are introduced. It may be because of depletion of specific clone cells.
   - *Low zone tolerance* occurs when a subimmunogenic dose of some thymus-dependent antigen is repeatedly introduced.

iii. ***Route of administration*** of an antigen also effects the induction of tolerance. An antigen when introduced intravenously, even at its highest concentration, can cause tolerance. This is due to the fact that the antigen has a fast contact with more number of cells and also reaches the spleen, to which the suppressor cells Ts migrate leading to tolerance.

4. Age of the Host. As mentioned above, the immune system competency is related to the age of the host. Therefore, embryo and newborns can develop immune tolerance easily.

Tolerance to Fetus. Fetus is genetically different from the mother and thus it should evoke an immune response in the mother. However, it usually never happens and it is considered to be the best example of immune tolerance. **Various factors which prevent an immunological response in a mother against its fetus are described:**

1. Placenta. Placenta plays an important role by different ways:

- Immediately after implantation, the trophoblast cells lose their immunogenic capacity due to decrease in MHC antigen density.
- There is formation of mucoprotein coating on the cell surface.
- Anti-MHC antibodies which are produced in the mother get absorbed into the placenta and their entry into fetal circulation is prevented. Thereby, the placenta acts as a shield against the immunological response.

2. Alpha Fetoprotein. During embryonic development, α fetoprotein (AFP) is produced which acts as an immunosuppressive agent.

3. Progesterone. During pregnancy, high levels of progesterone have an immunosuppressive effect.

4. Fetal T Cells. get activated when the fetus is exposed to mother T cells through the placenta and suppress the mother's T cells.

Immune Modulation

Immune modulation refers to modification of the immunological response. It can be either enhanced or suppressed.

Immune Enhancement. Immune enhancement means there is increase in the response in terms of rate, intensity, duration and even induction of response to substances which were earlier nonimmunogenic.

Immunological response can be potentiated by use of certain substances referred to as adjuvants.

Adjuvants. Adjuvants are the compounds which when introduced along with or mixed with an antigen, nonspecifically enhance or modify the immune response to that antigen. The first adjuvant was discovered by Freund hence known as Freund's adjuvant. Their contribution in enhancement of response is basically achieved by two ways:

i. *More and prolonged production* of antibodies, and
ii. *Increasing the number of effector* cells.

Mechanism of action. Adjuvants act by the following ways:

- They alter the distribution and persistence of an antigen in the host.
- They stimulate lymphocyte number nonspecifically.
- They activate macrophages.

Types. Adjuvants are of two main types:

i. *Incomplete adjuvants.* Substances like aluminium hydroxide, aluminium phosphate and certain mineral oils (lanolin oil) act as incomplete adjuvants. When an aqueous solution of an antigen is mixed with mineral oil, an emulsion is formed, which serves as a depot for that antigen causing slow and prolonged release of the antigen.
ii. *Complete adjuvant.* The cell walls of certain bacteria like tubercular bacilli and Gram-negative bacilli (e.g. diphtheria and of whooping cough) act as complete adjuvants because the constituents of the cell wall convert the soluble antigen into insoluble and particulate form which can be easily phagocytosed by macrophages. A typical example of a complete adjuvant is *killed mycobacterium bacilli*.

Adverse effects of adjuvants are delayed hypersensitivity reactions in human beings (see page 202) and formation of local granuloma (inflammatory reaction, at the site of inoculation).

Immune Suppression. Immune suppression refers to reduction in the immunological response. It is of two types:

1. Specific Immune Suppression or Immune Tolerance. (See page 197).

2. NonSpecific Immune Suppression. It is caused by immunosuppressive agents which inhibit the immune response of macrophages and B and T cells leading to either lowered phagocytosing capacity of the macrophages or production of antibodies and lymphokines.

Immunosuppressive Agents refer to methods or substances causing immunosuppression. These have been grouped as physical, chemical and biological agents.

A. *Physical Immunosuppressive Agents* (methods):

1. ***Irradiations.*** This is the most common method for prolonged survival of transplants. Irradiations cause breakage in the nucleic acid chains of replicating cells.
2. ***Surgical procedures*** like thymectomy, splenectomy and thoracic duct drainage.
   - *Thymectomy.* Removal of fetal thymus gland ensures absolute depletion of mature T cells but the effect of thymectomy decreases with age. Therefore, this method is not usually applicable.
   - *Splenectomy.* Though most of the antibodies are formed in the spleen, but splenectomy has little effect in adult life (because other peripheral organs—lymph nodes—can compensate for absence of spleen).
   - *Thoracic duct drainage* is another method of immune suppression first used in humans during heart transplant. In this, the thoracic duct is cannulated and lymph is drained for many days, leading to decrease in size and weight of lymph node and depletion of lymphocyte (lymphopaenia).

B. Chemical Methods are nonspecific suppressants and have limited effectiveness. This group includes the following drugs:

1. ***Corticosteroids*** suppress the immune response by the following ways:
   - They impair the maturation of activated cells.
   - They suppress the production of antibodies.
   - Have an anti-inflammatory effect and diminish the responsiveness of B and T lymphocytes.
   - They also inhibit production of IL-1 and IL-2.

   Corticoids, though commonly used, have limited effectiveness due to their side effects, as prolonged use leads to hypertension, bone necrosis, cataract and mental disturbances.
2. ***Cyclosporin or tacrolimus (FK-506)*** has been widely used as an immunosuppressive drug in organ transplants. This acts by inhibiting the production of IL-2. Normally, activation of T cell receptor increases intracellular calcium (Ca^{2+}) that activates calcineurin via calmodulin. Calcineurin in turn dephosphorylates the transcription factor NF-AT that moves into the nucleus and increases the gene coding activity for IL-2. The drugs cyclosporin (Csp) and tacrolimus (Tcl) prevent dephosphorylation of NF-AT (Fig. 3.4-14). It also has adverse effects on the liver and kidney.
3. ***Cytotoxic drugs*** such as *azathioprine* and *cyclophosphamide* act on various stages of nucleic acid synthesis and

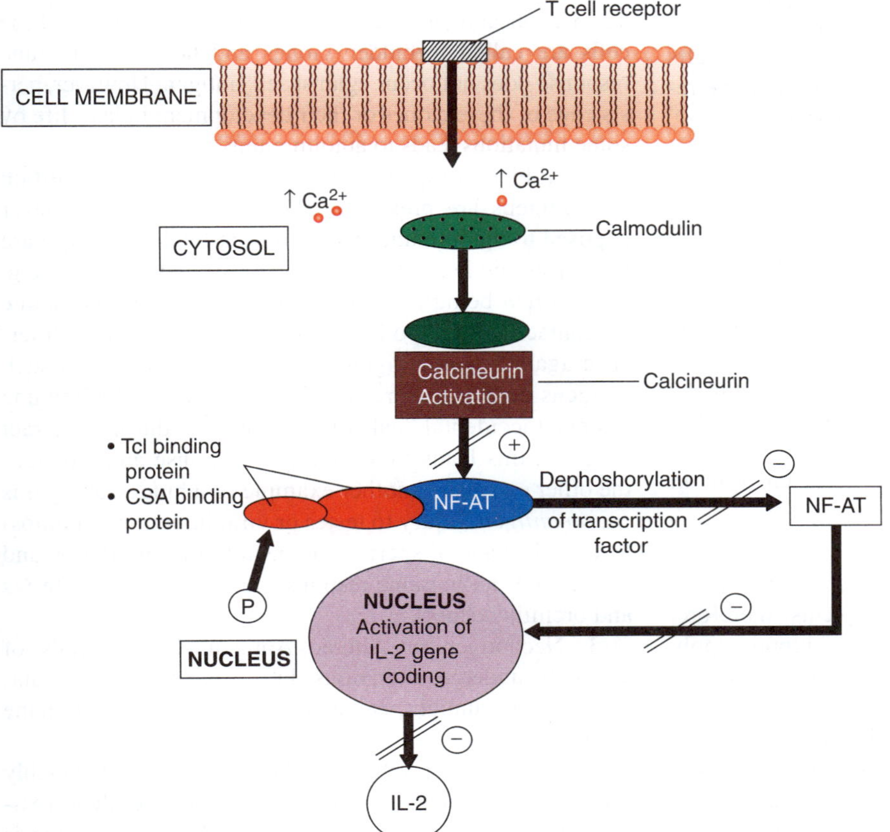

FIGURE 3.4-14 Mechanism of action of cyclosporine C and tacrolimus in T lymphocytes.

thus prevent replication of lymphocyte. *Methotrexate*, an antagonist of folic acid, produces competitive inhibition of an enzyme reductase (essential for synthesis of DNA). This drug is a known anticancer drug.

C. Biological Methods include:

1. *Antigen-induced suppression.* This method is used for desensitization against an allergen. In this method, if the body is exposed to small doses of antigen for long time, then it can develop resistance to that antigen.
2. *Antibody-induced suppression.* This method of immunosuppression is used in pregnant mothers (Rh −ve) to prevent sensitization against Rh antigen (from fetus) by injecting anti-D after expulsion of placenta.
3. *Antilymphocytic serum* is used for depletion of T cell population. In this method, antilymphocytic serum is prepared from horse by injecting human lymphocytes. The antibodies present in the horse serum destroy body T cell pool, but antibody production remains normal. The main drawback of this method is that the ability to fight against viral infection is tremendously decreased.

Tissue Transplantation

Tissue transplantation refers to the transplant of a tissue or whole organ from one part of same individual to another part or to another individual. When tissues such as skin and kidney are transplanted from a donor to a recipient of the same species, the transplant is usually taken up for some time, but then becomes necrotic and is rejected. The grafts are rejected because the recipient produces an immune reaction against the grafted tissue (foreign tissue).

Types of Grafts Different types of grafts are:

- ***Autografts.*** When a graft tissue is taken from one part of the body and transplanted to another part of the body of same individual.
- ***Isograft.*** When transplanted tissue is taken from the identical twins.
- ***Allograft.*** When transplanted tissue is taken from an individual and grafted to another person of same species.
- ***Xenograft.*** When the transplanted tissue is taken from an individual of a different species (i.e taken from an animal and grafted to human).

Rejection of Grafts. In autografts and isografts, the antigens are of the same type as in recepients; therefore, the transplanted tissue is taken up easily if blood supply is adequate. On the other hand, in xenografts, an immune response always occurs and within few weeks the graft is rejected. The organs or tissue like skin, kidney, liver, heart, bone marrow and lung transplanted as allografts are taken up safely if proper matching is done and after transplantation proper immunosuppressive therapy is carried out.

Tissue Typing. The human leucocyte antigen (HLA) complex is mainly responsible for graft rejection. Six of these antigens are present on the cell membrane of each person. There are more than trillion possible combinations. Therefore, development of significant immunity against any one of these antigens can cause graft rejection. The tissue type matching between siblings, parent of a recipient is more successful for transplantation.

Prevention of Graft Rejection can be achieved by suppressing the immune system of the recipient. For details see page 199.

Autoimmunity

During fetal life, when many antigens are presented to the immune system, they are recognized as self-antigens and antibodies and cytotoxic T cells are not produced.

Therefore, tolerance to self-antigen is produced. However, sometimes body starts producing antibodies or T cells against self-antigen (own cells or tissue) leading to an autoimmune disease. Therefore autoimmunity may be defined as immune response to self-antigen.

Mechanism of Autoimmunity. The possible mechanisms involved in development of autoimmunity are:

1. Forbidden Clones. According to clonal selection theory, antibody-forming lymphocytes are formed against different antigens. In fetal life, lymphocytes are also formed against self-antigens, but get depleted. The clones of these cells are called forbidden clones and hence an immune response does not occur against self-antigen. However, persistence of these clones or their development in later life by some mutations leads to autoimmunity.

2. Hidden Antigen or Sequestrated Antigen. Certain self-antigens are present in the close system and never exposed to the immune system during fetal life. These are known as hidden antigens or sequestrated antigens, e.g. *lens protein* being enclosed by its capsule does not come in contact with blood; therefore, immunological tolerance against such antigens does not develop. When such antigens in later life are somehow exposed to the immune system (accidental leak of lens protein during cataract surgery), this leads to an immune response and damages the other eye also. Another example of a hidden antigen is *sperm antigen*. Injury to testes or viral infections (mumps) leads to leakage of sperm proteins into the circulation and thus evokes an immune response against one's own testes and orchitis occurs.

3. Neoantigen or Altered Antigen. Certain cells of the body undergo alterations due to exposure to irradiations, drugs, sunlight, etc. and start producing an immune response.

4. Cross-reacting Antigen. Although antibodies are highly specific for a particular antigen, but in some cases they cross-react with other cells or body tissue. This phenomenon is

called as *molecular mimicry* and these antigens are called cross-reacting antigens. For example, in rheumatic heart disease, the heart is damaged by antibodies formed against streptococci.

5. Mutations. The body immune system becomes competent for self-antigen by certain mutations.

6. Unbalanced Activity of Helper and Suppressor T Cells. It has been observed that optimum antibody response always depends upon the balance activity of helper (TH) and suppressor T cells. If somehow the activity of these cells is altered, i.e. overactivity of TH cells and underactivity of Ts cells, then it may result in autoimmunity.

Autoimmune Diseases. Common autoimmune diseases include:

1. ***Autoimmune anaemia.*** For example:
   - Haemolytic anaemia. Antibodies react with one's own RBCs.
   - Pernicious anaemia. Antibodies react against gastric mucosa.
2. ***Thrombocytopenic purpura.*** Autoantibodies react with self-platelets.
3. ***Graves' disease.*** Autoantibodies bind to thyroid cells and stimulate them.
4. ***Hashimoto's disease.*** T cells react against the antigen on the thyroid cells.
5. ***Insulin-dependent diabetes mellitus.*** Antibodies damage the β cells (insulin producing cells) of the pancreas.
6. ***Rheumatoid arthritis.*** Antibodies damage the joints.
7. ***Rheumatic fever.*** Antibodies cross-react with valves of the heart.

Hypersensitivity

Hypersensitivity is an abnormal response which produces physiological or histopathological damage in the host. There are five types of hypersensitivity reactions:

- Type I (anaphylaxis or IgE mediated)
- Type II (antibody-mediated cytotoxicity),
- Type III (immune complex-mediated disorders) and
- Type IV (delayed type or T cell-mediated hypersensitivity).
- Type V (stimulatory).

The characteristic features of each hypersensitivity reaction are given in Table 3.4-4.

Type I Hypersensitivity or Anaphylaxis. It is mediated by IgE antibodies and occurs due to mast cells degranulation resulting in release of histamine and many other vasoactive substances. Type I reaction (anaphylaxis) depends on the amount of histamine release and route of stimulating antigen. It occurs in two forms: local anaphylaxis and generalized anaphylaxis.

- ***Local anaphylaxis*** occurs when an antigen called as allergen is administered locally in smaller dose. Examples of local anaphylaxis are asthma and hay fever.
- ***Systemic or generalized anaphylaxis*** is a shock-like condition. It occurs in individuals who are intensely allergic and when an antigen is administered in large amount or through systemic route.

Mechanism of Type I Hypersensitivity. In type I hypersensitivity reaction, the individual first comes in contact with an antigen and antibodies (IgE) are produced which get bound to mast cells or to fixed basophils. The specific

TABLE 3.4-4 Characteristics of Hypersensitivity Reactions

Characteristics	Type I	Type II	Type III	Type IV
1. Time of onset of reaction	1/2–8 h	5–12 h	3–8 h (peak 48–72 h)	24–48 h
2. Reaction mediators	IgE, histamine, serotonin, SRS-A, etc.	IgG, IgM and complement	IgG, IgM, neutrophils, eosinophils, lysosomal enzymes	T lymphocytes, macrophages and lymphokines
3. Response to intradermal injection of antigen (allergen)	Wheal and flare	–	Erythema and oedema	Erythema and induration
4. Passive transfer with	Serum	Serum	Serum	T cells
5. Samples	• Anaphylaxis, • Asthma • Hay fever • Allergic with food and insect bite	• Transfusion reactions (incompatibility reaction) • Haemolytic disease of newborn • Drug-induced allergies	• Arthus reaction • Serum sickness	• Tuberculin test • Contact dermatitis • Graft rejection

IgE antibodies are fixed to mast cell surface by its Fc portion. After second exposure, the allergen passes on to these sensitized cells (IgE-fixed mast cells) and get attached onto the Fab site of IgE molecule attached to mast cell. Antigen–antibody binding triggers the degranulation of mast cells and releases pharmacologically active chemicals (histamine, serotonin, bradykinin and slow-reacting substances of anaphylaxis) causing vasodilatation, sensory nerve ending stimulation, etc. The individuals susceptible to type I hypersensitivity reaction are called *atopic* and reaction is known as *atopy*. Example of type I hypersensitivity includes allergic rhinitis and atopic dermatitis.

Type II Hypersensitivity or Antibody-Mediated Autotoxicity. It is an immediate reaction in which antigen-bearing cells are damaged. The mechanism involved in this reaction is either complement- or antibody-mediated cytotoxicity.

Examples. Type II hypersensitivity is most commonly seen in:

- Incompatible blood transfusion.
- Autoimmune haemolytic anaemia and
- Haemolytic disease of the newborn. When antibodies react with the cells on which these antigens are present, i.e. RBCs get damaged.

Type III Hypersensitivity (Immune Complex-Mediated Hypersensitivity). Monocytes and macrophages are efficient in binding and removal of antigen–antibody complexes. When the body is exposed repeatedly to an antigen, which is not cell bound (free, small and soluble), then the body faces great difficulty, because the antigen–antibody complexes formation occurs in the serum and subsequently get deposited in the normal body tissue. Complement system is also activated (particularly C3a and C5a), which is cytotoxic for monocytes, macrophages and even nearby normal tissue where the antigen–antibody complexes are deposited. *Glomerulonephritis* is the best example of type III hypersensitivity reaction.

Type IV or Delayed Hypersensitivity. Delayed hypersensitivity is the cell-mediated reaction in tissues of a sensitized individual. The reaction is due to sensitization of T lymphocytes and not by antibodies or by B lymphocytes. The reaction starts after several hours (48–72 h). Two types of delayed hypersensitivity reactions are recognized: tuberculin (infection) type and contact dermatitis.

Tuberculin Test. In this test, a small dose of tuberculin, or purified protein derivative from *Mycobacterium tuberculosis*, is injected intradermally in an individual sensitized earlier by tubercular protein by infection or by immunization.

Within 48–72 h an inflammatory reaction of 5 mm diameter appears at the site of injection. The inflammatory reaction is recognized by erythema (increased blood flow) and induration (due to infiltration with large number of T lymphocytes and macrophages).

Contact Dermatitis. is type IV hypersensitivity reaction. Hypersensitivity against various chemicals in the forms of ointments, dyes, cosmetics, etc. is tested by *patch test*.

- ***Patch test.*** In this test, a patch of an allergen is applied to the skin under a dressing. If itching occurs within 4–5 h and local reaction in the form of redness and induration appears within 24 h, then the test is positive.

Type V or Stimulatory Hypersensitivity. Over the last few years, type V hypersensitivity has been added to the original four types. In this reaction, an antibiotic can act as a stimulant to target cell or organ. An example is long- acting thyrostimulatory (LATS) antibody, a feature of Grave's disease. The LATS antibody is directed towards a portion of TSH receptor in the thyroid and mimics the function of thyroid stimulatory hormone.

Immunodeficiency Diseases

Immunodeficiency diseases occur when the body defence mechanisms are impaired. The defect may lie in one or more of the following components of the immune system:

- Lymphocytes (B and T) and natural killer (NK) cells,
- Phagocytic cells and
- Complement proteins.

Immunodeficiency diseases may be classified as primary or secondary.

Primary Immunodeficiency Primary immunodeficiency occurs due to defect in the development of the immune system. Various primary immunodeficiency syndromes are as under:

1. Humoral Immune Deficiency (due to B cell defect) may manifest as:

X-linked agammaglobulinaemia is the first immune deficiency disorder recognized by Bruton in 1952, hence also known as Bruton's disease. It is seen in males but sporadic cases are found in females. The basic defect in this disorder is failure of premature B cells to differentiate into mature B cells. The disease is characterized by:

- Recurrent infections with pyogenic bacteria.
- Tonsils and adenoids are atrophied.
- Lymph node biopsy reveals depletion of bursa-dependent areas.
- B cells are either absent or remarkably decreased.
- Serum immunoglobulins (all the five classes) are absent.

2. Cellular Immunodeficiencies occur due to defect in T cells and manifest as:

- Thymic hypoplasia (Di George syndrome), and
- Purine nucleoside phosphorylase (PNP) deficiency.

i. ***Thymic hypoplasia or Di George syndrome*** results due to a congenital malformation affecting third and fourth pharyngeal pouches from where thymus develops.

Defective or nondevelopment of thymus T cells are deficient or absent in circulation. The disease is characterized by:

- Thymus is hypoplastic.
- In lymph nodes and in spleen, thymus-dependent areas are absent.
- Infants with this defect are susceptible to viral and intracellular bacterial infections.
- B cells are normal.
- Immunoglobulin levels are normal.

ii. ***Purine nucleoside phosphorylase (PNP) deficiency.*** Due to gene defect in chromosome 14, PNP enzyme is lacking resulting in defective metabolism of cytosine and inosine to purine which is essential for T cell proliferation. Therefore, a patient with this disorder shows decreased cell-mediated immunity.

3. Combined Immunodeficiencies occur due to defect in both B and T cells. This defect may manifest as *severe combined immunodeficiency diseases* (SCID). Many distinct patterns have been described:

- Agammaglobulinaemia,
- Adenosine deaminase deficiency and
- Reticular dysgenesis.

4. Complement Immune Deficiency Disorder. In this disorder, complement proteins are deficient due to genetic defect resulting in lack of various complement functions like phagocytosis, antibody killing of bacteria, lysis of virus, tumour cells and histamine release by mast cells.

5. Phagocytic Disorders lead to increased susceptibility to infections.

Secondary Immunodeficiency Disease. Acquired deficiencies of immunological response mechanisms can occur secondarily to number of diseases. Secondary immunodeficiency is more common than the primary immunodeficiency. Acquired immune deficiency syndrome (AIDS) is the most important.

AIDS, i.e. acquired immune deficiency syndrome is characterized by reduction in the number of helper T cells because of infection by human immunodeficiency virus (HIV). AIDS was first of all detected in the USA in 1981. HIV is of two types, HIV-1 and HIV-2.

Spread of Disease. AIDS is a major worldwide life-threatening disease spreading rapidly. Daily about 8500 persons get infected with HIV. The high-risk groups include: sex workers, drug addicts, homosexual males, persons with extramarital relations and recipients of unscreened blood transfusion.

Transmission. There are mainly three routes of transmission:

1. ***Parenteral route*** is through blood contact involving:
   - Unscreened blood transfusion,
   - Tattooing,
   - Use of infected razors, syringes, needles, etc.,

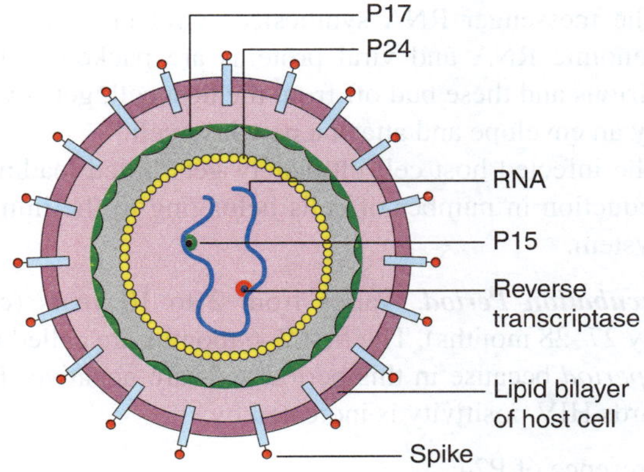

FIGURE 3.4-15 Schematic diagram of structure of HIV.

   - Use of poorly sterilized dental instruments and
   - Organ transplants.
2. ***Sexual route*** accounts for about 85% of HIV infection due to multiple sex partners, sex workers, homosexuality and artificial insemination. The virus is present in sufficient concentration in the semen and vaginal secretions of the infected person.
3. ***Transplacental route.*** Infection can be transmitted from infected mother to her fetus (vertical transmission) across the placenta and also to the infant through breast milk (perinatal transmission).

AIDS does not spread through mosquito bites, hugging, kissing and sharing meals.

Structure of HIV. HIV is a retrovirus having rounded outline and consists of (Fig. 3.4-15):

- ***The core*** has two single strands of genomic RNA, enzyme reverse transcriptase and protein P-15 associated with genomic RNA. Genomic RNA is surrounded by two coverings:
  - Inner covering is cone shaped consisting of P-24, and
  - Outer covering of P-17.
- ***Genome*** has two types of genes—overlapping and split genes (8 in HIV-1 and 9 in HIV-II). Virus is surrounded by *host-derived envelop with spikes containing* protein components complementary to CD_4 or T_4 receptors present on the surface of helper T cells, monocytes, macrophages and some other nerve cells.

Virus Multiplication. When virus comes in contact with the cells having receptors of T_4 antigen (helper T cells, monocytes, macrophages and some nerve cells), it sticks to the receptor site and then passes into the cell. Then free genomic RNA synthesizes a copy DNA with help of enzyme reverse transcriptase and biochemicals of the host.

- The copy DNA forms complement strand and the duplex attaches to the host DNA in the form of *provirus.* Provirus may multiply with host cell and ultimately forms *genomic RNA* and messenger RNA.

- The messenger RNA synthesizes viral proteins. Then genomic RNA and viral proteins are packed to form virions and these bud off from the host cell, get covered by an envelope and attack a new host cell.
- The infected host cell ultimately gets killed leading to reduction in number of cells belonging to the immune system.

Incubation Period. Varies from 2 to 10 years (commonly 27–28 months). The first 2–6 months are called *window period* because in this period tests are negative. Then onwards HIV positivity is indicated by:

- Presence of P24,
- Antiviral antibodies and
- Reduction in number of T cells.

Signs and Symptoms are mostly of opportunistic infections due to decreased immunity. They include:

- Repeated episodes of diarrhoea,
- Unexplained weight loss,
- Prolonged cough, night sweating, continuous fever for more than 1 month,
- Tuberculosis, candidiasis of mouth and oesophagus,
- Brain damage and
- Ulcers, Kaposi sarcoma (cancer of skin and lymph nodes).

HIV Tests. Laboratory tests employed for diagnosis of HIV infection may be classified into three groups:

A. ***Screening tests*** are used to screen antibodies against HIV. The most commonly used test is ELISA (enzyme-linked immune sorbent assay) test. It is highly sensitive. For negativity, it is 100% correct but for a positive test there is a 5–6% chance of false positive.

B. ***Supplement tests.*** These tests also detect antibodies against HIV and are recommended for validation of positive tests on screening. The commonly employed test is *western blot assay.* It is a highly sensitive and specific assay for culturing blood and testing plasma for virus.

C. ***Confirmatory tests.*** These tests confirm HIV infection in an individual who is seropositive. These tests include:

- Virus isolation,
- Detection of P24 antigen and
- Detection of viral nucleic acid by polymerase chain reaction.

Treatment. Triple drug treatment is employed which includes:

- Protease inhibitor,
- Reverse transcriptase inhibitor, and
- AZT (azidothymidine).
- Interleukins are added to make the treatment more effective.

Prevention. Preventive measures against HIV infection include:

- ***Education.*** National AIDS Control Organization (NACO) has been set up under the Ministry of Health and Family Welfare. Awareness is being imparted through all means of publicity and by NGOs in schools, colleges, factories, farms, etc.
- ***Screening*** is compulsorily carried out in case of blood donors, organ donors, semen donors, foreigners and sex workers.
- ***AIDS-positive*** persons are advised to prevent sexual contacts and pregnancy.
- Ban on prostitution.
- ***Safer sex*** with single partner, use of condoms and barrier creams.
- Use of disposable syringes, needles, blood bags and I/V sets.
- ***Proper sterilization*** of razors, blades and dental equipment by using 70% alcohol, 35% sodium hypochloride, 5% formaldehyde, boiling for 15 min or autoclaving.

Chapter 3.5

Platelets, Haemostasis and Blood Coagulation

PLATELETS

Structure and Composition

Platelets (small plates), also known as thrombocytes (thrombo = clot; cytes = cells), are the third types of blood cells having the following features:

- *Size.* Platelets are the smallest blood cells varying in diameter from 2 to 4 μm, with an average volume of 5.8 μm^3.
- *Shape and colour.* Platelets are colourless, spherical or oval discoid structures.
- *Leishman staining* shows a platelet consists of a faint bluish cytoplasm containing reddish-purple granules.
- *Nucleus* is absent in the platelets, and therefore, these cannot reproduce.

Electron Microscopic Structure. Under an electron microscope, a platelet shows the following structural and compositional characteristics (Fig 3.5-1):

1. Cell Membrane. Each platelet is enclosed in a 6 nm thick trilaminar membrane identical to plasma membrane of tissue cells. It consists of lipids (phospholipids, cholesterol and glycolipids), carbohydrates, proteins and glycoproteins. Its salient features are:

- ***Glycoproteins*** forming the surface coat of the platelet membrane prevent adherence of platelets to normal endothelium, but accelerate the adherence of platelets to collagen and damaged endothelium in injured blood vessels.
- ***Phospholipids*** of the platelet membrane contain platelet factor-3, which plays an activating role at several points in the blood clotting process.
- ***Invagination*** of the surface membrane forms the so-called *canalicular system* or the *surface connecting system.*
- ***Receptors*** present on the platelet membrane are meant for combining with specific substances like collagen, fibrinogen ADP and the von Willebrand factor in vessel walls.
- ***Precursors*** of various substances like thromboxane A_2, prostaglandins, leukotrienes and platelet factors 3 and 4 are also present in the platelet membrane.

2. Microtubules. Microtubules are made up of polymerized proteins called tubulins. These form a compact bundle which is present immediately beneath the platelet membrane and encircles the whole cytoplasm. These are responsible for maintenance of the discoid shape of circulating platelets.

3. Cytoplasm. Cytoplasm of the platelets contains Golgi apparatus, endoplasmic reticulum, few mitochondria, microtubules, microvesicles, filaments, granules, glycogen, lysosomes, proteins, enzymes and hormonal substances. The role of some of the active factors is described:

- ***Endoplasmic reticulum and Golgi apparatus.*** These structures synthesize various enzymes and store large quantities of calcium.

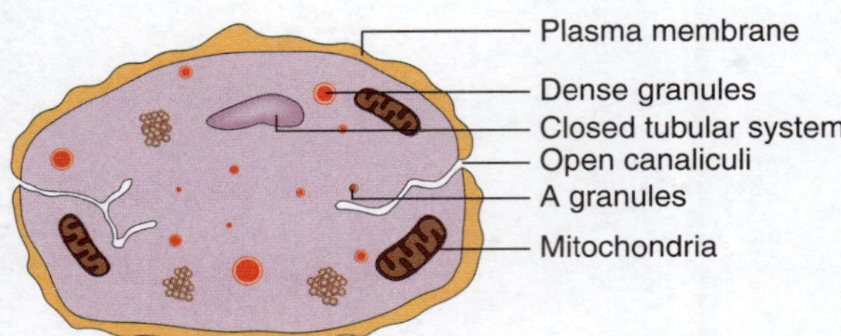

FIGURE 3.5-1 Ultra structure of a platelet.

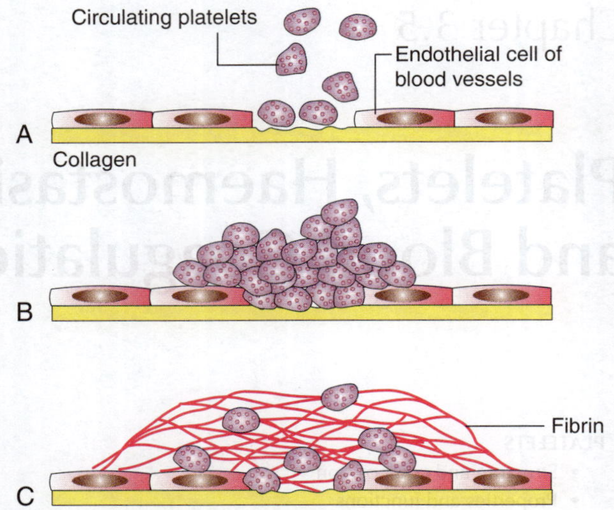

FIGURE 3.5-2 Properties of platelets: **A,** adhesiveness; **B,** aggregation; and **C,** formation of haemostatic plug.

- ***Mitochondria.*** These are capable of forming ATP and ADP.
- ***Contractile proteins*** include actin, myosin and thrombosthenin. Actin and myosin molecules are similar to those of contractile proteins of the muscles. Contractile proteins can cause the platelet to contract and are thus responsible for the clot retraction.
- ***Other proteins*** present in the cytoplasm are:
  - *Fibrin stabilizing factor.* It is an important protein having a role in blood coagulation.
  - *Platelet-derived growth factor.* It causes growth of vascular endothelial cells, vascular smooth muscle cells and fibroblasts; and thus is involved in the repair of damaged blood vessels.
  - *Von Willebrand factor (VWF)* is a large, circulating protein molecule produced by the endothelial cells of the vessel wall. It plays an important role in platelet adherence.
- ***Granules.*** Two types of granules are present in the cytoplasm of platelets.
  - *Dense granules* contain substances (like phospholipids, triglycerides, cholesterol) ATP, ADP and serotonin (5HT). Platelets cannot synthesize 5HT, so they obtain their 5HT while passing through GIT.
  - *α-granules* contain secreted proteins such as clotting factors and platelet-derived growth factor (PDGF).
- ***Enzymes*** present in the cytoplasm of platelets include adenosine triphosphatase and the enzyme necessary for synthesis of prostaglandins. Prostaglandins act as local hormones and have local vascular and tissue reactions.

Properties and Functions

Properties of Platelets (Fig 3.5-2)

1. Adhesiveness. Platelets possess the property of adhesiveness, i.e. when they come in contact with any wet or rough surface, they are activated and stick to the surface. Factors responsible for adhesiveness are collagen, thrombin, ADP, thromboxane A_2, calcium ions and the von Willebrand factor. Whenever there is injury to the vessel wall, platelets adhere to the exposed collagen and the von Willebrand factor, to their receptors present on the platelet membrane.

2. Aggregation. Platelets have the property to aggregate, i.e. they stick to each other. This is due to ADP and thromboxane A_2. Platelet binding causes their activation which results in release of contents of the granules. The released ADP acts on ADP receptors on the platelet membrane and produces further accumulation of platelets (platelet aggregation). Platelet aggregation is also fostered by the platelet-activating factor (PAF), cytokines (secreted by platelets), neutrophils and monocytes. The platelet-activating factor acts via a G protein–coupled receptor (GPCR).

Note: In human beings, there are different types of ADP receptors (P_2Y_1, P_2Y_2 and P_2X_1).

3. Agglutination. Clumping together of platelets is called agglutination. This occurs due to the action of some platelet agglutinins.

Functions of Platelets. When activated, platelets perform the following functions:

1. Role in Haemostasis. Haemostasis refers to spontaneous arrest of bleeding from an injured blood vessel. Process of haemostasis is discussed in detail on page 208. Platelets play following roles in haemostasis:

- *Vasoconstriction* is induced by the serotonin (5HT) and other vasoconstrictors secreted by the platelets.
- *Temporary haemostatic plug* is formed by the platelets due to their properties of adhesiveness and aggregation.
- *Definitive haemostatic plug* formation process is also initiated by platelets.

2. Role in Clot Formation. Process of clot formation involves a complex series of events (described on page 209). Platelets play an important role in the formation of the intrinsic prothrombin activator which is responsible for the onset of blood clotting.

3. Role in Clot Retraction. Process of clot retraction is described on page 213. Contractions of contractile proteins (actin, myosin and thrombosthenin) present in the platelets play an important role in clot retraction.

4. Role in Repair of Injured Blood Vessels. The platelet-derived growth factor (PDGF) present in the cytoplasm of platelets plays an important role in the repair of endothelium and other structures of the injured/damaged blood vessels.

Important Note

- Platelet-derived growth factor (PDGF) is also produced by macrophages and endothelial cells. It is made up of two subunits α and β.

5. Role in Defence Mechanism. Platelets, due to their property of agglutination are capable of phagocytosis. These are particularly helpful in phagocytosis of carbon particles, viruses and immune complexes.

6. Transport and Storage Function. Platelets can take up 5HT against the concentration gradient when they pass from the GIT. The 5HT is stored in the platelets and transported to the site of injury, where it is released.

Normal Count and Variations

Normal Count. Normal platelet count ranges from 1.5 to 4.5 lakh/μL with an average count of 2.5 lakh/μL.

Physiological Variations

1. ***Age.*** Platelet count is less in infants (1–2 lakh/μL). Adult levels are reached by the third month after birth.
2. ***Sex.*** Normally there is no difference in the platelet counts of males and females. However, during menstruation the count is reduced in females.
3. ***After meals*** the platelet count is slightly increased.
4. ***After strenuous muscular exercise*** platelets may increase.
5. ***At high altitude*** the platelet count increases.

Pathological Variations

A. Thrombocytosis. An increase in the number of platelets more than 4.5 lakh/μL is called thrombocytosis.

Causes of thrombocytosis. Platelet count is increased:

1. After splenectomy,
2. After:
   - Haemorrhage,
   - Severe injury,
   - Major surgical operation and
   - Parturition.
3. In myeloproliferative disorders such as:
   - Chronic myeloid leukaemia,
   - Polycythemia vera and
   - Myelofibrosis.

B. Thrombocytopenia. Decrease in the number of platelets below 1.5 lakh/μL is called thrombocytopenia.

Causes of thrombocytopenia are:

1. Idiopathic thrombocytopenic purpura
2. Bone marrow depression due to:
   - Effects of various cytotoxic drugs,
   - Whole body irradiation and
   - Hypoplastic and aplastic anaemia.
3. Acute leukaemia or secondary deposits of malignancy in the bone marrow.
4. In infections like smallpox, chicken pox, scarlet fever, typhoid and dengue fever.
5. In hypersplenism.
6. Intoxaemia, septicaemia and uraemia.

Formation of Platelets

Formation or development of platelets is called *thrombopoiesis.* The platelets are produced in the bone marrow. The pluripotent stem cell destined to form platelets is converted into colony forming units called Meg-CFU, which develop into platelets after passing through various stages.

Stages in Platelet Production (Fig 3.5-3)

1. Megakaryoblast. The earliest recognizable precursor of platelets in the bone marrow is megakaryoblast. It arises from Meg-CFU by a process of differentiation.

- *Diameter* of megakaryoblast is about 20–30 μm,
- *Cytoplasm* is small, blue and nongranular, and
- *Nucleus* is large, oval or kidney-shaped with several nucleoli.

2. Promegakaryocyte. Promegakaryocyte is formed from the megakaryoblast. A megakaryoblast undergoes endoreduplication of nuclear chromatin, i.e. nuclear chromatin replicates repeatedly in multiples of two without division of

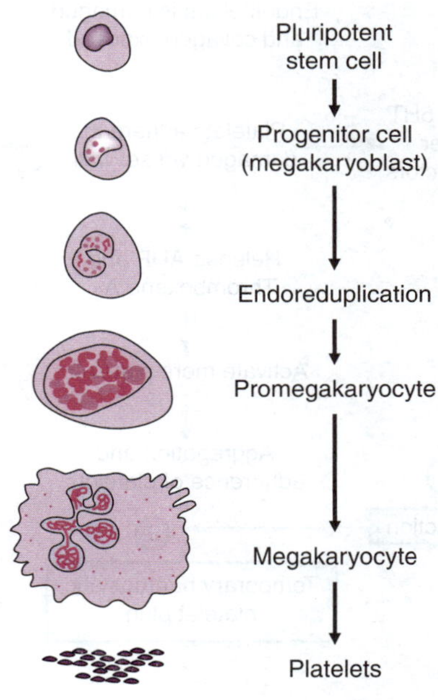

FIGURE 3.5-3 Stages of thrombopoiesis.

the cell. Ultimately, a large cell containing up to 32 times the normal diploid content of nuclear DNA is formed when further nuclear replication ceases and the cytoplasm becomes granular. The granules are intensely basophilic.

3. Megakaryocyte. A promegakaryocyte matures into a megakaryocyte with the following features:

- *Diameter.* Mature megakaryocyte is a large cell, 30–90 µm in diameter.
- *Nucleus.* Megakaryocyte has single multilobed (4–16 lobes) nucleus with coarsely clumped chromatin.
- *Cytoplasm* is abundant, light blue in colour and contains red–purple granules.
- *Cell margin* is irregular and shows many pseudopodia. Platelets are formed from pseudopodia of megakaryocyte cytoplasm which get detached into the blood stream. Each megakaryocyte may form upto 4000 platelets. The formation of platelets from the stem cell takes about 10 days.

Control of Thrombopoiesis. Thrombopoiesis seems to be regulated by the following humoral factors:

- Thrombopoietin, and
- Megakaryocyte-colony stimulating activity (Meg-CSA).

Thrombopoietin promotes maturation of megakaryocytes and is a circulating protein produced by the liver and kidney. Thrombopoeitin acts through its receptors present on platelets and controls the platelet production by feedback mechanism, i.e. when the number of platelet count is low, less will bind to the platelets and more will be available for platelet production. On the other hand, when the number of platelets is high, more will bind to the receptors and less will be available for stimulation of platelet production.

Megakaryocyte colony-stimulating factor (Meg-CSF) controls the production of megakaryocytes.

Lifespan and Fate of Platelets. Lifespan of platelets varies from 8 to 12 days with an average of 10 days. Platelets are destroyed by the tissue macrophage system in the spleen. Therefore:

- *Splenomegaly* causes reduction in the platelet count, and
- *Splenectomy* is followed by an increase in platelet count.

HAEMOSTASIS

Haemostasis refers to spontaneous arrest or prevention of bleeding from injured/damaged vessels by the physiological process. The process of haemostasis is initiated immediately following an injury/damage to the blood vessel. It involves three main steps (Fig 3.5-4):

- Vasoconstriction,
- Formation of temporary haemostatic plug and
- Formation of the definitive haemostatic clot.

1. Vasoconstriction. Vasoconstriction plays an important role in the process of haemostasis. It is induced as:

Initial Vasoconstriction. affects several centimetres in both the directions from the site of injury and occurs immediately

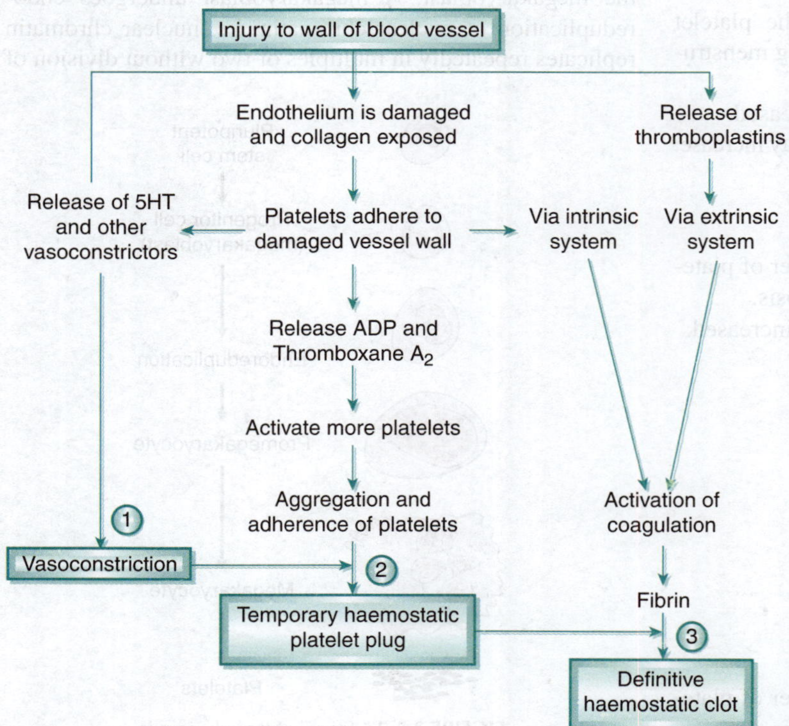

FIGURE 3.5-4 Steps of haemostasis.

following injury to the vessels. The degree of spasm is proportionate to the degree of trauma to the blood vessel. The vasoconstriction may be intense enough to stop the bleeding from small vessels. Initial vasoconstriction is caused by the direct effect of injury on the vascular smooth muscles. It is transient and is maintained for several minutes or even hours by humoral facilitation.

Humoral Facilitation of Vasoconstriction. Following an injury/damage to the wall of blood vessel, the platelets get adhered to the damaged endothelium and exposed collagen. These platelets immediately release 5HT and other vasoconstrictors which augment the initial vasoconstriction. The vasoconstriction so induced is, thus, purely a local phenomenon. Usually arterioles and small arteries respond by vasoconstriction and decrease the loss of blood from the damaged blood vessel.

2. Formation of Temporary Haemostatic Plug. Formation of a temporary haemostatic plug by the platelets at the site of injury involves following steps:

Platelet Adhesion. Following injury, platelets come in contact with damaged collagen fibres and endothelial cells of the vessel wall and change their characteristics. That is, they begin to swell and assume irregular forms with large numbers of pseudopodia protruding from the surface. The contractile proteins of the platelets contract forcibly and cause release of granules that contain multiple factors. They become sticky and therefore adhere to the collagen of damaged cell walls and to the damaged endothelium.

Platelets Activation. The platelets secrete large quantities of ADP and thromboxane A_2 which act on the nearby platelets and cause their activation. Stickiness of these additional platelets causes them to adhere to originally activated platelets. In this way, a vicious cycle is initiated which leads to activation and adherence of a large number of platelets.

Platelets Aggregation. The large numbers of activated sticky platelets stick to each other forming platelets aggregation. Platelets aggregation is also increased by *platelet-activating factor* (PAF), a cytokine secreted by neutrophils, monocytes and platelet cell membrane lipids.

Platelet aggregation initiates a series of reactions which result in the formation of thromboxane A_2 and prostacyclin from the platelet membrane phospholipids.

Formation of Temporary Haemostatic Plug. The platelets adherence and aggregation ultimately leads to the formation of the platelet plug. At first, it is a fairly loose plug, but is successful in blocking the blood loss if the vascular opening is small.

Inhibition of Further Plug Formation. Prostacyclin formed from the membrane phospholipids inhibit thromboxane formation, and thus curtail the process of further plug formation. This reaction keeps the platelets plug localized, i.e. prevents intravascular spread of plug.

3. Formation of Definitive Haemostatic Plug. The temporary platelet plug is converted into the definitive haemostatic plug by the process of clot formation (blood coagulation), which involves a complex series of events (see page 210). Platelets play an important role in the formation of the intrinsic prothrombin activator which is responsible for initiating the process of clot formation (page 211). The blood clot formed at the site of injury results in a tight unyielding seal or the so-called definitive haemostatic plug.

BLOOD COAGULATION

Blood remains in a fluid condition within the blood vessels throughout life. But, when the blood is shed from the blood vessels or collected in a container, it loses its fluidity within a few minutes and gets converted into a jelly-like mass, which is called a *clot*. This phenomenon is called *coagulation* or clotting of blood. Both these properties of blood are essential for life:

- ***Fluidity*** is essential for circulation, and
- ***Coagulation*** provides an indispensable defence against excessive bleeding from the wounds. Thus, coagulation of the blood is one of the mechanisms involved in the process of haemostasis (prevention of blood loss).

The process of blood coagulation consists of a complex cascade of reactions. The final step in the process of coagulation is transformation of plasma protein *fibrinogen* into *fibrin* forming a sort of network within which the cellular elements of the blood are arrested. Before discussing the mechanism of blood coagulation in detail, it will be worthwhile to study the essential features of the various clotting factors involved in this process.

CLOTTING FACTORS

The process of coagulation essentially involves a stepwise activation of certain substances, mostly proteins, present in the blood and/or tissue fluids. These substances are called clotting factors and have been given Roman numerals:

- Factor I (fibrinogen),
- Factor II (prothrombin),
- Factor III (thromboplastin),
- Factor IV (calcium),
- Factor V (labile factor or proaccelerin or accelerator globulin),
- Factor VI (nonexistent),
- Factor VII (stable factor or proconvertin),
- Factor VIII (antihaemophilic factor A (AHF) or antihaemophilic globulin (AHG)),
- Factor IX (Christmas factor or plasma thromboplastic component (PTC or antihaemophilic factor B))
- Factor X (Stuart–Prower factor),
- Factor XI (plasma thromboplastin antecedent, i.e. PTA or antihaemophilic factor C),
- Factor XII (Hageman factor or glass factor or contact factor),
- Factor XIII (fibrin-stabilizing factor or fibrinase or Laki–Lorand factor),

- HMW-K (high molecular weight kininogen or Fitzgerald factor),
- Pre-Ka (Prekallikrein or Fletcher factor),
- Ka-(kallikrein) and
- PL-(platelet phospholipid).

Factor I (Fibrinogen). It is a soluble plasma protein globulin in nature. Its molecular weight is 340,000 Da and is synthesized in the liver. It has 6 polypeptide chains, with its plasma concentration about 0.3 g/dL. It is converted into fibrin in the presence of the enzyme thrombin.

Factor II (Prothrombin). It is an inactive precursor of thrombin. Its features are described on page 212.

Factor III (Thromboplastin). It is also called tissue factor or tissue thromboplastins. It is released in the extrinsic pathway formation of prothrombin activator (see page 211).

Factor IV (Calcium). Ionic calcium is essential for blood coagulation. Its role in coagulation is described on page 213.

Factor V (Labile Factor). It is also called proaccelerin. It is a protein and as the name indicates, it is the labile or unstable factor of the plasma. It is required for the formation of the prothrombin activator and thus conversion of prothrombin to thrombin in both, extrinsic as well as intrinsic mechanisms of blood coagulation. Factor V is consumed during clotting and is therefore absent from serum. Its deficiency occasionally occurs as a congenital anomaly simulating haemophilia.

Factor VII (Stable Factor or Autoprothrombin I). It is a stable protein synthesized in liver in the presence of vitamin K. It is required for activation of factor X in the extrinsic pathway. It is not consumed during clotting and therefore is present in serum, as well as plasma. Deficiency of factor VII is a rare natural occurrence, but is frequently induced by oral anticoagulant drugs of the coumarin type, overdosage of which may lead to bleeding.

Factor VIII (Antihaemophilic Globulin). It is a protein of β_2 globulin type synthesized in the liver. It is required for the activation of factor X, and thus formation of the prothrombin activator in intrinsic pathway. It is consumed during clotting and is therefore absent from the serum. Its congenital deficiency causes classical haemophilia (haemophilia A), which is an inherited disease in which the clotting time is prolonged.

Factor IX (Christmas Factor). It is also called plasma thromboplastic component (PTC) or autoprothrombin II. It is a protein synthesized in the liver independent of vitamin K. It is activated by the active factor XI in the presence of Ca^{2+}, and is essential for the formation of prothrombin activator in the intrinsic pathway. Its absence or deficiency causes haemophilia B, which is an inherited disease and is similar to haemophilia A. This disease was first discovered in a patient named Christmas and hence the factor was termed as *Christmas factor*.

Factor X (Stuart–Prower Factor). It is a protein present in plasma and is synthesized in the liver. It is activated by active factor IX in the presence of factor VIII, Ca^{2+} and phospholipids. Activated factor X, along with active factor V, Ca^{2+} and phospholipids forms a complex which is called *prothrombin activator,* both in extrinsic as well as intrinsic pathways.

Factor XI (Plasma Thromboplastin Antecedent). It is activated by active factor XII. It is required for the activation of factor IX in the presence of Ca^{2+} in intrinsic pathway. Its deficiency causes a haemorrhagic state.

Factor XII (Hageman Factor). Factor XII is activated to XIIa when it comes in contact with negatively charged surfaces, foreign substances or rough surfaces. Its activation in the blood initiates intrinsic pathway by activating factor XI (PTA) to XIa. Activated factor XII also activates prekallikrein to kallikrein, which in turn activates XII to XIIa (*feedback activations*). In deficiency of factor XII, blood clots very slowly in glass but there is no haemorrhagic state.

Factor XIII (Fibrin-Stabilizing Factor). This is a plasma protein which is required for stabilization of fibrin polymers in the presence of Ca^{2+}.

HMW-K (High Molecular Weight Kininogen). It is responsible for attracting prekallikrein and factor XI to the site of reaction with factor XII. This is possible because HMW-K, like factor XII, is attracted towards the negatively charged surfaces which provide the site of reactions.

Prekallikrein and Kallikrein. Prekallikrein is activated to kallekrein by XIIa, which in turn activates XII to XIIa. This phenomenon is called feedback activation of XII and is shown as:

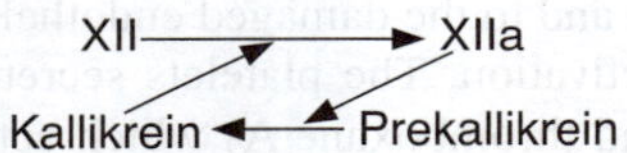

Platelet Phospholipids (PPL). Platelets contain phospholipids which are essential for clotting in the absence of tissue extract, i.e. in intrinsic pathway of coagulation. *Arabic* numerals are sometimes used for platelet activities affecting blood coagulation. For example, the term:

- *Platelet factor 3 (PF-3)* is used for platelet phospholipid procoagulant activity.
- *Platelet factor 4 (PF-4)* is used for heparin neutralizing activity of platelets.

MECHANISM OF COAGULATION

Normally, blood circulates in the blood vessels and does not clot spontaneously. Factors responsible for this will be discussed later. Clot formation is initiated under the following situations:

- Trauma to the vascular wall and adjacent tissues,
- Trauma to blood,
- Contact of blood with damaged endothelial cells or collagen or other tissue elements outside the vessel.

The process of coagulation involves a *cascade* of reactions in which activation of one factor leads to activation of the next clotting factor (Fig 3.5-5). This enzyme cascade reaction is also called waterfall *sequence*. It is important to note that each factor activates (compared to its own amount) a huge quantity of the other factor, i.e. at each stage amplification of result is obtained. Thus, the process can be viewed as a *bioamplifier.* The process of coagulation can be divided into three main steps:

A. Formation of prothrombin activator,
B. Conversion of prothrombin to thrombin, and
C. Conversion of fibrinogen into fibrin.

A. Formation of Prothrombin Activator

Process of coagulation is initiated by formation of a complex substance called prothrombin activator. Two different mechanisms involved in the formation of the prothrombin activator are:

1. Extrinsic pathway, and
2. Intrinsic pathway.

Extrinsic Pathway

The extrinsic pathway of formation of prothrombin activator begins with trauma to the vascular wall or the tissues outside the blood vessel. It includes the following three basic steps (Fig 3.5-5).

1. Release of Tissue Thromboplastins. The traumatized tissues release several substances which are together known as *tissue thomboplastin (factor III).* This includes phospholipids of cell membranes of the tissues and lipoprotein complex containing glycoprotein which acts as an enzyme.

2. Activation of Factor X to Form Activated Factor X. Tissue thromboplastin combines with factor VII (stable factor) to form the tissue thromboplastin factor VII complex, which in the presence of Ca^{2+} activates factor X to form activated factor X (Xa).

3. Effect of Activated Factor X to form Prothrombin Activator. The activated factor X, along with tissue phospholipids or phospholipids released from platelets, factor V (labile factor) and Ca^{2+} forms a complex which is called prothrombin activator.

Intrinsic Pathway

The intrinsic pathway of formation of prothrombin activator begins in the blood itself following trauma to the blood or exposure of blood to collagen in a traumatized vascular wall. The steps of intrinsic pathway are summarized in Fig 3.5-5:

• ***Activation of Factor XII.*** Trauma to blood or exposure to collagen fibres underlying damaged vascular endothelium (or electronegatively charged wettable surface such as

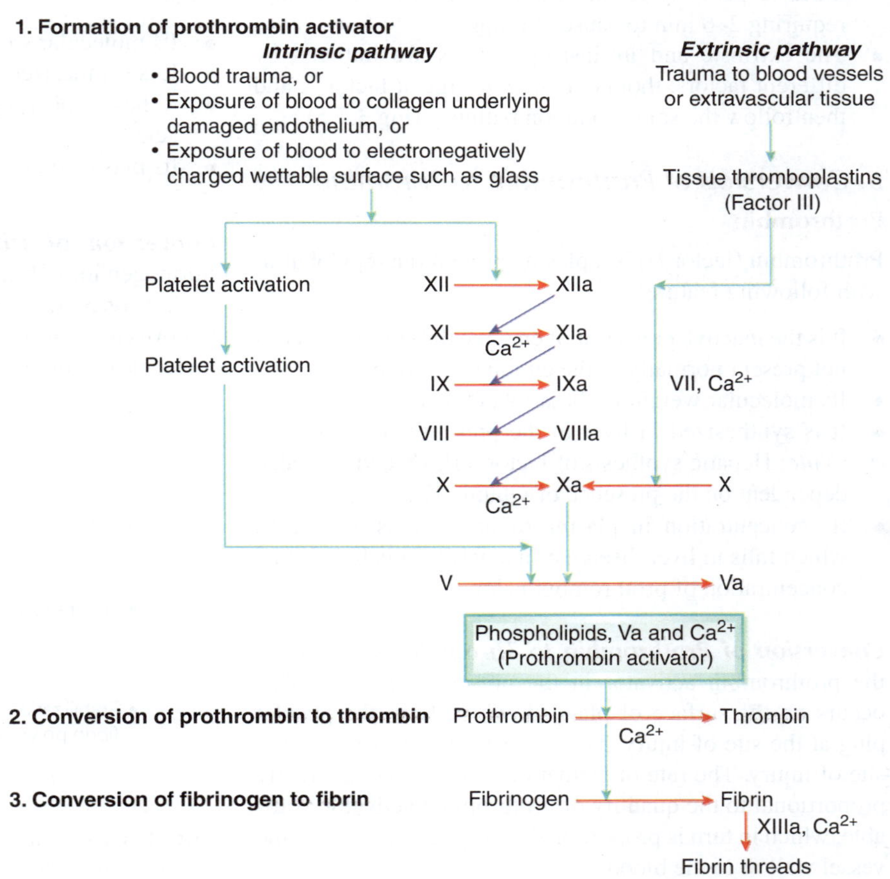

FIGURE 3.5-5 Mechanism of blood coagulation.

glass, in vitro) activates plasma factor XII to form XIIa and initiates the intrinsic pathway. Platelets are also activated.

- ***Activation of Factor XI*** to form XIa is caused by the activated factor XII. High molecular weight (HMW), kininogen and prekallikrin accelerate this reaction.

- ***Activation of Factor IX*** to form IXa is in turn caused by the activated factor XI in the presence of Ca^{2+}.

- ***Activation of Factor X.*** Factor IXa in the presence of activated factor VIII, Ca^{2+} and phospholipids (released by activated platelets) activate factor X to form Xa. In thrombocytopenia and deficiency of factor VIII (classical haemophilia), this reaction is deficient.

- ***Formation of Prothrombin Activator.*** The activated factor X, along with the phospholipids released by activated platelets, activated factor V and Ca^{2+} forms a complex which is called prothrombin activator.

Extrinsic Versus Intrinsic Pathway

- Extrinsic pathway begins with trauma to the vascular wall or the tissue outside the vessel wall, while intrinsic pathway begins in the blood itself.
- Extrinsic pathway is explosive in nature, with severe tissue trauma clotting occurring in as little as 15 s, while intrinsic pathway is much slower to proceed, usually requiring 2–6 min to cause clotting.
- The extrinsic and intrinsic pathways are initiated by different factors, though, both converge at factor X and then follow the same common pathway (Fig 3.5-5).

B. Conversion of Prothrombin to Thrombin

Prothrombin

Prothrombin (factor II) is a plasma protein (an α_2 globulin) with following features:

- It is the inactive precursor of enzyme thrombin (which is not present normally in the circulating blood).
- Its molecular weight is about 69,000 Da.
- It is synthesized in liver in the presence of vitamin K (***Note***: Hepatic synthesis of factor VII, IX and X is also dependent on the presence of vitamin K).
- Its concentration in plasma of an adult is 40 mg/dL which falls in liver diseases: In a newborn baby, plasma concentration of prothrombin is lower.

Conversion of Prothrombin to Thrombin is caused by the prothrombin activator in the presence of Ca^{2+}. This occurs on the surface of platelets which form the platelet plug at the site of injury. Thus, clot formation starts at the site of injury. The rate of formation of thrombin is directly proportional to the quantity of prothrombin activator available, which in turn is proportional to degree of trauma to the vessel wall or to the blood.

Thrombin

Thrombin so formed acts as proteolytic enzyme. Its molecular weight is 34,000 Da, exactly half of prothrombin. The amount of thrombin produced is in excess of the need. It has been estimated that the amount of thrombin produced during clotting of only 1 mL of blood is sufficient to coagulate 3 litres of blood. Thus, this presents a dangerous possibility of extensive intravascular clotting whenever the haemorrhage mechanism is in operation (even in a trivial cut). However, practically it does not occur so, since there exist adequate mechanisms in the body to prevent it (see page 214).

Roles Played by Thrombin are:

- *Conversion of fibrinogen to fibrin* (discussed below).
- *Positive feedback role of thrombin*: It accelerates the rate of formation of prothrombin activator by activating factors VIII, V and XIII. The cascade mechanism of enzyme activation acts in such a way that small amounts of activated factor XII ultimately generate large amounts of prothrombin activator. In this way, thrombin itself can cause further conversion of prothrombin into thrombin (amplification effect).
- It also activates protein-C (which is an anticoagulant).

C. Conversion of Fibrinogen to Fibrin

Fibrinogen

Fibrinogen (Factor I) is a soluble plasma protein globulin in nature.

- Its molecular weight is 340,000.
- It is synthesized in the liver.
- It has 6 polypeptide chains each having 450 amino acids.
- Its plasma concentration is about 0.3 g/dL.

Conversion of Fibrinogen into Fibrin Conversion of fibrinogen into fibrin involves three reactions (Fig 3.5-6):

1. Proteolysis. Thrombin acting as proteolytic enzyme removes four low molecular weight peptide chains from each molecule of fibrinogen to convert it into fibrin monomer.

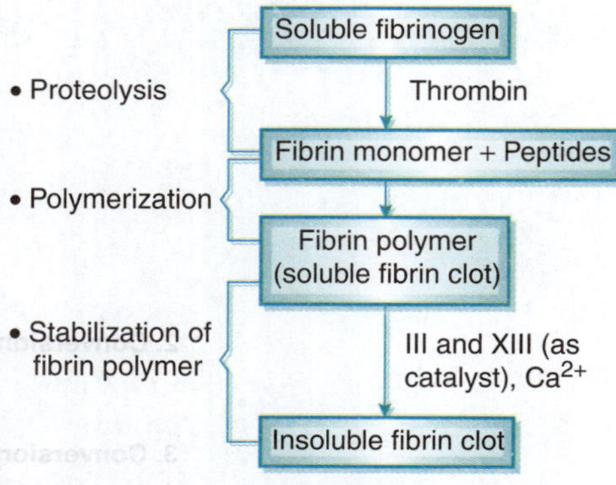

FIGURE 3.5-6 Types of reactions involved in conversion of soluble fibrinogen into insoluble fibrin clot.

2. *Polymerization.* Fibrin monomer polymerizes with another monomer to form *long fibrin* threads which form reticulum of the clot. Initially, the clot is weak because the fibrin threads are not cross-linked with each other.

3. *Stabilization of Fibrin Polymers.* Fibrin stabilizing factor (factor XIII), which is normally present in the plasma and also released from the activated platelets is activated by the thrombin to form XIIIa, but XIIIa in the presence of Ca^{2+} causes formation of covalent cross-linkages between fibrin threads, thus adding tremendous strength to the fibrin meshwork. The fibrin meshwork traps the remaining components of plasma and blood cells to form a solid mass called clot.

Blood Clot Retraction

The blood clot formed at the end of the coagulation process is composed of a meshwork of fibrin threads running in all directions along with the entrapped blood cells, platelets and plasma. The fibrin threads adhere to the damaged surface of blood vessels.

At this juncture, it is important to note that *coagulation is the property of plasma alone.* The RBCs and WBCs do not take part in it. They only become caught up in the meshwork of the clot.

- Within a few minutes after a clot is formed, it begins to contract and usually squeezes out most of the fluid called *serum* (plasma without fibrinogen and other clotting factors) within 30–60 min.
- *Platelets are essential* for clot retraction. Platelets are attached to fibrin fibres of the clot in such a way that they actually bind different fibres together. The contractile proteins (platelet thrombosthenin, actin and myosin) present in the cytoplasm of platelets cause strong contraction of platelet spicules attached to fibrin fibres. This helps to compress the fibrin meshwork, i.e. cause clot contraction. This contraction is activated by thrombin and calcium ions. The process of contraction of blood clot and oozing of serum is called *clot retraction.*
- If a blood clot is kept for several hours, the clot retracts to about 40% of its original volume.
- Clot retraction is impaired if blood platelets have been removed.

Role of Calcium in Blood Coagulation

From the study of mechanism of blood coagulation, it is quite clear that except for the first two steps in the intrinsic pathway, calcium ions are required for promotion of all the reactions. Therefore, in the absence of calcium ions, blood clotting will not occur. Thus, coagulation of blood can be prevented in vitro (e.g. for storage in the blood bank or for separation of plasma) by removal of calcium ions. The use of oxalates and citrates as in vitro anticoagulants is based on this principle. However, in vivo the degree of hypocalcaemia (e.g. due to deficiency of vitamin D or hypoparathyroidism) is compatible with life and does not cause bleeding disorder.

Role of Vitamin K, Liver and Vascular Wall in Haemostasis and Coagulation

Vitamin K

Chemical Structure. Vitamin K is a complex naphthoquinone derivative. There are at least two fractions present in natural vitamin K, of which it (1.4-naphtho-quinone) is more active. It is soluble in fat solvents and insoluble in water. Therefore, it can only be administered orally or intramuscularly. However, for intravenous administration it has to be specially prepared by being very finely emulsified.

Sources. Vitamin K is obtained from food, as well as synthesized by bacterial flora in the gut.

- *Food source.* Vitamin K is found in traces in green vegetables, cereals and animal tissues.
- *Synthesis by bacterial flora.* Vitamin K can be synthesized by many bacteria including those normally present in the human intestine (e.g. *E. coli*). In humans, the bacterial flora can provide an adequate supply of vitamin K and thus its deficiency from dietary abnormalities is very rare.

Dietary vitamin K and that synthesized by the bacterial flora is absorbed from the gut and reaches the liver. Its absorption from the small intestine only occurs in the presence of adequate amounts of bile salts. In the liver, synthesis of following factors is dependent upon vitamin K:

- Coagulant like prothrombin,
- Factor VII, IX and X, and
- Circulatory anticoagulant protein.

Vitamin K Deficiency.

Effects. In the deficiency of vitamin K prothrombin, time and blood clotting time is prolonged and serious haemorrhages may occur.

Causes. As mentioned above, vitamin K deficiency is unlikely to develop in dietary deficiency alone. Deficiency of vitamin K is seen in following clinical conditions:

1. *Obstructive jaundice.* In this condition, bile salts do not reach the gut and thus vitamin K cannot be absorbed.
2. *Newborn babies* are likely to develop vitamin K deficiency and thus haemorrhagic disorders because gut bacterial flora which synthesizes vitamin K is not developed satisfactorily in the early infancy. Therefore, it is recommended that the newborn babies should be routinely given injection of vitamin K to prevent its deficiency.
3. *Chronic diarrhoea.* The syndrome of vitamin K deficiency has been reported in chronic diarrhoea. The cause may be failure of absorption or an abnormal state of the intestinal bacteria leading to defective synthesis of vitamin K. This syndrome may also occur with defective fat absorption in sprue.

4. *Side effect of antibiotics.* Vitamins K deficiency has also been reported in morbid patients living on glucose–saline transfusion and receiving heavy amounts of broad spectrum antibiotics particularly *cephalosporin.* Antibiotics kill the bacterial flora of the gut leading to deficient synthesis of vitamin K.

Role of Liver. Liver plays following significant role in the coagulation mechanism:

1. ***Synthesis of procoagulants.*** It is the site of synthesis of factor V, VII, IX, X, prothrombin and fibrinogen.
2. ***Removal of activated procoagulants.*** Liver also removes the activated procoagulants from the blood.
3. ***Synthesis of anticoagulants.*** Liver also synthesizes anticoagulants like heparin, antithrombin III and protein-C.

Liver failure can cause both:

- *Bleeding disorders* due to hypocoagulability of the blood; and
- *Uncontrolled extensive clotting* inside the blood vessels where clotting is not only unwanted, but dangerous as well.

Role of Blood Vessels. Role played by endothelium, subendothelial tissue and smooth muscles of the media of the blood vessels in coagulation and haemostasis mechanisms is summarized.

Endothelium. Endothelium plays both an anticoagulatory as well as a coagulatory role.

Anticoagulatory Roles Played by Endothelium

- It acts as a barrier between the thrombogenic subendothelial tissue and the blood.
- It produces heparin and α_2 macroglobulin which are coagulation inhibitors.
- Smoothness of uninjured endothelial cells prevent platelet aggregation.
- Endothelial cells produce PGI_2 (a prostaglandin), which opposes platelet aggregation.

Roles in Clotting Mechanism

- ***Endothelium secretes von Willebrand's factor (VWF).*** The plasma VWF acts as a connecting bridge between the platelets and the subendothelial tissue (exposed after injury) and thus initiates platelet aggregation and haemostasis.
- ***Tissue factor (TF)*** is released by endothelial cells following trauma. The TF initiates the process of extrinsic pathway of clotting mechanism.
- ***Plasminogen activator*** which activates plasminogen to plasmin is also released by endothelial cells.

Subendothelial Tissue. Subendothelial tissue, which chiefly consists of collagen fibres, plays the following roles in coagulation:

- *Platelet aggregation* is initiated when blood comes in contact with the subendothelial collagenous tissue; and
- *Intrinsic coagulation pathway* is initiated when factor XII is activated following contact of blood with subendothelial collagenous tissue.

Vascular Smooth Muscle. Smooth muscles of the vascular wall play a role in haemostasis by causing vasoconstriction. Vasoconstriction is initiated by mechanical injury to muscles and is later facilitated by the vasoconstrictors such as serotonin, prostaglandins and noradrenaline released by the platelets which adhere at the site of injury.

Why Circulating Blood Does Not Clot

We all know that blood circulating in the blood vessels does not clot and that fluidity of the blood is essential for life. By now we have discussed most of the factors responsible for fluidity of the blood. They are summarized below.

1. Velocity of Circulation. Blood is pumped into the vessels and circulated at a constant velocity which contributes to its fluidity. That is why, a decrease in circulation velocity in certain conditions is associated with intravascular clotting.

2. Surface Effects of Endothelium

- Smoothness of endothelial lining inhibits platelet adhesion and thus prevents initiation of intrinsic clotting mechanism.
- A layer of glycocalyx (mucopolysaccharide) adsorbed to the inner surface of endothelium being negatively charged repels clotting factors (anion proteins) and platelets and thereby prevents clotting.
- Intact endothelium acts as a barrier between the thrombogenic subendothelial collagenous tissue and the blood.
- Endothelial cells also produce thrombin-binding protein (thrombomodulin), which slows the process of clotting by removing thrombin (see page 216)

3. Circulatory Anticoagulants or the so-called natural anticoagulants present in the blood, which prevent clotting, are:

- Heparin,
- Antithrombin III,
- Alpha 2 macroglobulin and
- Protein-C (for details see page 216).

4. Fibrinolytic Mechanism. Protein-C is a naturally occurring anticoagulant which inactivates factor V and VIII, and also inactivates an inhibitor of tissue plasminogen activator increasing the formation of plasmin which acts fibrinolytic.

- Further, whenever there is trauma, along with activation of clotting mechanism, the fibrinolytic system is also activated, which prevents spread of intravascular clotting.

5. Removal of Activated Clotting Factors. Liver plays a role in preventing the intravascular clotting by removing activated clotting factors in the event of onset of spontaneous clot formation.

Thrombosis

We have studied that physiologically under normal conditions the circulating blood does not clot and that clotting of blood occurs only extravascularly when a vessel has been injured and bleeding has occurred. However, under certain pathological conditions, intravascular clotting may occur. The intravascular clotting is called *thrombosis,* and the clot so formed is called thrombus. Thus, *thrombus* may be defined as a solid mass formed in the living heart or blood vessels from the constituents of blood. Intravascular thrombosis can be distinguished from extravascular clotting or clotting in wounds, and also from clotting which occurs in blood vessels after death.

Predisposing Factors. Virchow described three primary events which predispose to thrombus formation (*Virchow's triad).* These are:

1. Endothelial Injury. We have studied how an intact endothelium prevents coagulation (page 214). Endothelial injury may occur in many conditions, of which a few important ones are: ulcerated plaques in advanced atherosclerosis, haemodynamic stress in hypertension, arterial disease, diabetes mellitus and hypercholesterolaemia.

2. Alterations in Flow of Blood. Both, in turbulence as well as stasis of blood, normal axial flow of blood is disturbed and platelets come in contact with endothelium initiating thrombus formation. Stasis of blood is commonly associated with venous thrombosis especially in leg veins after major operations on the abdomen (postoperative thrombosis), or otherwise bedridden patients in which muscular contraction in legs and trunk (responsible for normal venous blood flow) is decreased.

3. Hypercoagulability of Blood which predisposes to thrombosis may occur due to:

- Increase in coagulation factors such as fibrinogen, prothrombin, factors VIa, VIIa and Xa.
- Increase in platelet count and their adhesiveness, and
- Decreased levels of coagulation inhibitors such as antithrombin III and fibrinogen degradation products.

Sequence of Events in Thrombogenesis. Sequence of events which lead on the formation of a thrombus are:

- ***Adherence of Platelets*** to endothelium (in the individuals having any of the above listed predisposing factors) is the first step in thrombogenesis. The mass of platelets grows by adhesion of other platelets as they pass by. The laminae of platelets (which fuse together and lose their identity) stand out as layers running transversely to the blood stream. Passing leucocytes adhere to their borders (like flies on sheets of sticky flypaper).
- ***Activation of Coagulation System.*** The platelets liberate thromboplastin and activate coagulation system; thus filaments of fibrin spread out from them on all sides. Fibrin filaments from one lamellae meet with filaments from the next lamellae. The lamellae of platelets are thus braced together by fibrin filaments.
- ***Entanglement of Red Blood Cells and White Blood Cells*** then occurs in the fibrin network, and finally a solid mass of a peculiarly constructed clot called thrombus is formed. The red cells disintegrate and lose their haemoglobin; the initial red thrombus as it ages becomes yellowish-grey; but newly formed thrombi added to it will be red.

Types of Thrombi. Grossly, there are three types of thrombi:

- ***Red Thrombi.*** Venous thrombi are usually red and occlusive. Red thrombi are soft, red and gelatinous. Red thrombi closely resemble blood clots in vitro.
- ***White Thrombi.*** Arterial thrombi usually tend to be white and mural, whereas white thrombi are pale and firm.
- ***Mixed or Laminated Thrombi*** are also common and consist of alternate white and red layers called *lines of Zahn.*

Effects of Thrombi. Intravascular thrombi may cause variable effects (may be even life-threatening) depending upon their size and site. Thrombi cause harmful effects by one of the following mechanisms:

1. Ischaemia and Infarction. Thrombi may decrease or stop the blood supply to part of an organ and cause ischaemia, which may subsequently result in infarction. *Arterial thrombi* usually produce ischaemia and infarction. For example, thrombus formation in coronary arteries may cause myocardial ischaemia and infarction.

2. Thromboembolism. The thrombus or its part may get dislodged and be carried along in the blood stream as *embolus* to lodge in a distant vessel. Cardiac and venous thrombi produce emboli more frequently than arterial thrombi. Examples of emboli formation are:

- *Pulmonary embolism,* i.e. blockage of pulmonary artery may be caused by an embolus arising from the calf veins.
- *Cerebral embolism,* i.e. blockage of cerebral artery may be caused by an embolus arising from the heart or carotid artery.

Prevention of Thrombi. Formation and/or extension of a thrombus can be prevented by administration of:

- *Drugs which decrease platelet adhesiveness* such as aspirin, dextran or dipyridamole, and
- *Anticoagulants* such as low doses of heparin and dicoumarol
- *Intermittent compression* or electrical stimulation of the calf muscles is necessary in addition to above drugs for preventing postoperative venous thrombosis.

ANTIHAEMOSTATIC MECHANISMS

The factors which balance the tendency of the blood to clot in vivo constitute the *antihaemostatic factors.* These can be grouped as:

- Factors preventing platelet aggregation,
- Factors preventing coagulation (circulatory anticoagulants) and
- Factors causing fibrinolysis (fibrinolytic mechanism).

A. Factors Preventing Platelet Aggregation

Prostacyclin. Prostacyclin is an endogenous factor which prevents platelet aggregation by inhibiting the thromboxane A_2 formation (which promotes platelet aggregation). Normally, there is a delicate balance between thromboxane A_2 and prostacyclin, which keeps the platelet plug localized, i.e. prevents intravascular spread of plug. For details see page 799

Note. The drug *aspirin* also inhibits the formation of thromboxane A2 and thus can prevent platelet plug formation. This makes aspirin a valuable drug for the prevention of thrombosis in patients prone to myocardial infraction and stroke.

B. Circulatory Anticoagulants

The natural anticoagulants circulating in the blood constitute the anticoagulant mechanism of the body. These include:

- Heparin,
- Antithrombin III or heparin cofactor II, and
- Protein-C.

1. Heparin. Heparin is a powerful, naturally acting anticoagulant since it was first isolated from the liver, and so it is named heparin (hepar = liver). However, it is also present in many other organs. It is a polysaccharide (glycosaminoglycan) containing many sulphate groups. Its molecular weight is 15,000–18,000 Da.

- ***Secretion.*** Heparin is secreted by the basophils and mast *cells* (present in various tissues such as liver, lungs and tissues rich is connective tissue).
- ***Destruction.*** Heparin is destroyed by the enzyme *heparinase* present in the liver.
- ***Functions.*** Heparin is one of the factors, which maintains fluidity of the circulating blood and prevents spread of intravascular thrombosis postoperatively and after trauma to vessels.
- ***Mechanism of Action.*** Heparin is present on the luminal surface of vascular endothelium. Heparin by itself has little or no anticoagulant properties, but it acts as cofactor with antithrombin III (antithrombin–heparin cofactor) and increases the effectiveness of antithrombin III by hundredfold for removing thrombin. During clot formation, most of the thrombin formed from prothrombin gets adsorbed onto fibrin threads, heparins thus prevent further excessive spreading of the clot. The remaining thrombin that does not get adsorbed on fibrin, soon combines with antithrombin III and blocks the effect of thrombin on fibrinogen. Therefore, heparin acts as an anticoagulant by the following mechanisms:

  - Prevents activation of prothrombin to thrombin.
  - Inhibits the action of thrombin on fibrinogen.
  - Facilitates the action of antithrombin III, i.e. acts as its cofactor and thereby inhibits the active forms of clotting factors IX, X, XI and XII.

2. Antithrombin III. Antithrombin III is present in plasma as well as vascular endothelium. It is a protease inhibitor, which inactivates a number of coagulation factors (active from of IX, X, XI and XII) including thrombin. Its action is greatly facilitated by heparin as mentioned above.

3. Protein C. Protein C is a plasma protein synthesized in liver. It, along with *thrombomodulin* and protein-S constitute an important negative feedback pathway that keeps the coagulatory process under control. The steps of protein-C pathway are given in Fig 3.5-7.

- ***Thrombomodulin*** is a thrombin-binding protein produced by all endothelial cells except those in the cerebral microcirculation. It converts thrombin into *protein C* activator.
- ***Protein C*** is activated by the protein C activator. For the formation of activated protein C (APC), a cofactor protein-S is required.
- ***Activated Protein C (APC)*** inactivates factors VIIIa and Va and thus inhibits the clotting mechanism. It also increases fibrinolysis by promoting plasmin formation.

C. Fibrinolytic Mechanism

Fibrinolysis refers to the process that brings about the dissolution of fibrin. The important component of the fibrinolytic system is *plasmin* or fibrinolysin, which is present in the blood in an inactive form called *plasminogen* or profibrinolysin. The fibrinolytic or the so-called plasmin system causes lysis of blood clot allowing slow cleaning of extraneous blood clots in the tissue. It also allows reopening of clotted blood vessels. Especially, it removes minute clots which are formed in many tiny peripheral vessels, which would eventually occlude if there was no plasmin system.

Plasminogen. Plasminogen is a β-globulin produced by the liver. Structurally, human plasminogen consists of a

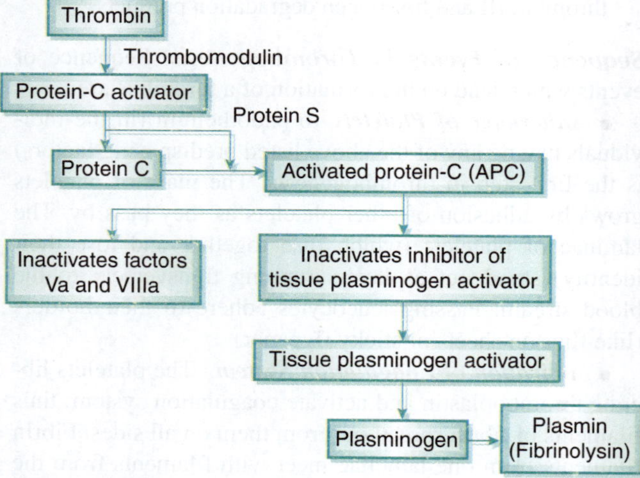

FIGURE 3.5-7 Steps of protein C pathway in inhibiting coagulation and promoting fibrinolysis.

heavy chain of 560 amino acids and a light chain of 241 amino acids. The heavy chain at its amino terminal is folded into five loops, which are held together by disulphide bonds. These loops are called *kringles*. The kringles are the binding sites by which the molecule attaches to fibrin and to other clotting proteins (clotting factors) and also to prothrombin. During clotting or purification of fibrinogen, it is associated closely with the fibrinogen molecule. It is extremely difficult to prepare fibrinogen free of plasminogen. A normal clot usually contains sufficient amounts of plasminogen to ensure clot dissolution if it is activated. Plasminogen is activated by plasminogen activator systems to produce plasmin.

The receptors of plasminogen are located mainly on the surface of endothelial cells and also on different types of cells. When plasminogen binds to its receptors it gets activated

Plasmin. Plasmin is a powerful protease formed from its precursor, the plasminogen. It lyses fibrin and fibrinogen into fragments known as *fibrin degradation products (FDP)* that inhibit thrombin. Thus, there is a negative feedback which controls plasmin generation. There are two plasminogen activator systems in the body: intrinsic and extrinsic.

Extrinsic Plasminogen Activator System. It seems to be the predominant mechanism of plasminogen activation since, in its absence, there is extensive spontaneous fibrin deposition. Wound healing is delayed and there are also defects in growth and fertility; since plasminogen system not only lyses clots but also plays a role in the cell movement and in ovulation.

The extrinsic activator system (Fig 3.5-8) operates through the following agents:

1. Tissue plasminogen activator (TPA) also called as vascular plasminogen activator is released from the vascular endothelium. The release of TPA from the vessel wall depends upon the release of serotonin from platelets and also release of adrenaline. When there is physical/mental stress or exercise or liberation of adrenaline on sympathetic stimulation, the TPA is released vigorously and thus removes fibrin so that bleeding tends to prolong. In violent deaths (e.g. of a soldier in the battlefield), the blood is fluid and incoagulable due to fibrinolysis. This is due to a large amount of adrenaline released into the blood before death. The adrenaline causes rapid release of TPA from endothelial cells causing massive fibrinolysis. Another factor which regulates release of TPA is fibrin itself (autoinactivation).

   Mechanism of action: Tissue plasminogen activator binds to fibrin via lysine-binding sites and activates plasminogen to plasmin.

   Note. It is important to note that TPA is now produced by recombinant DNA techniques and is available for clinical use. It lyses clots in the coronary arteries if given to patients soon after the onset of myocardial infarction.

2. Urokinase-type plasminogen activator (UPA). The UPA is found in a number of tissues including endothelial cells, renal cells and tumour cells. Urokinase is isolated from cultured human kidney cells and induces a systemic lytic state like TPA.

   Note: *Streptokinase and staphylokinase* are bacterial enzymes known to produce activation of plasmin-like TPA and UPA. Streptokinase (Streptase) is a protein produced by β-haemolytic streptococci. It forms streptokinase–plasminogen complex which produces a conformational change that exposes active sites on plasminogen molecule and lyse to form plasmin. Therefore, they are used in the treatment of early myocardial infarction to lyse thrombi.

Intrinsic Plasminogen Activator System. Contact factors (factor XIIa and kallikrein) that initiate clotting mechanism also stimulate the dissolution of clots by activating plasminogen and constitute the intrinsic plasminogen activator system (Fig 3.5-9).

Fibrinolysis Inhibitors. The rate of fibrinolysis is influenced by the promotors (i.e. plasminogen activators) and inhibitors. Fibrinolysis inhibitors are present in plasma, blood cells, tissues and extracellular matrix. These can inhibit plasmin (antiplasmin) or prevent the activation of plasminogen. The various inhibitors are:

- *Antiplasmins* such as α_2-antiplasmin,
- *Drugs* like aprotinin (a trypsin inhibitor) and epsilon–aminocaproic acid (EACA) inhibit fibrinolysis.

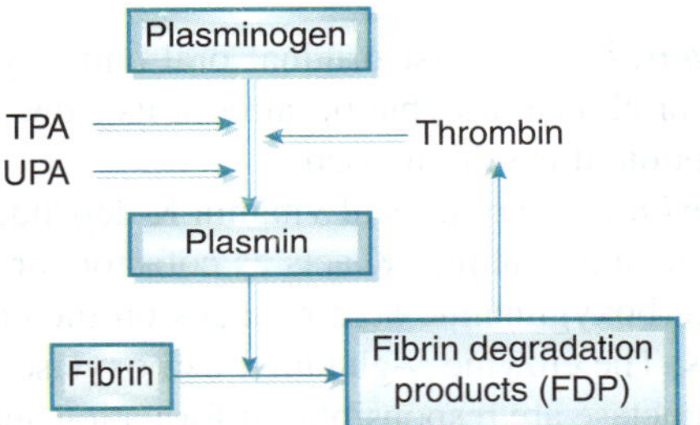

FIGURE 3.5-8 Fibrinolytic mechanism operating through extrinsic plasminogen activator system.

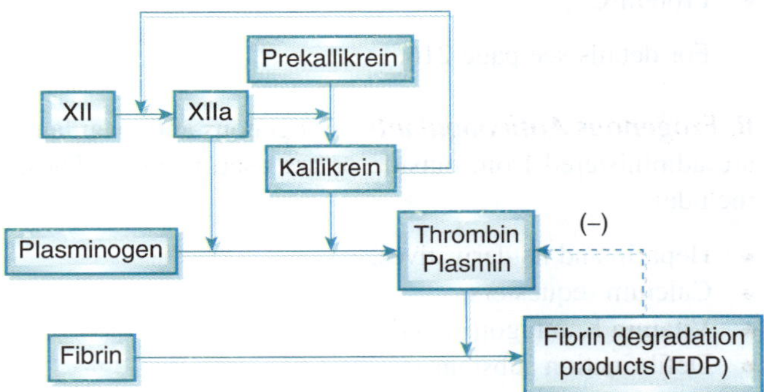

FIGURE 3.5-9 Fibrinolytic mechanism operating through intrinsic plasminogen activator system.

Physiological Role of Fibrinolysis System. Plasmin of the fibrinolysis system plays the following physiological roles:

1. Cleaning the Minute Clots of Tiny Vessels. It has been suggested that in physiological conditions the clotting system of the plasma is continually forming small amounts of fibrin, which are deposited to form a thin layer on vascular endothelium and that the fibrinolytic system is constantly in action to prevent excessive fibrin formation.

2. Promote Normal Healing Process. Lysis of clot formed as a result of tissue injury helps to promote normal healing process.

3. Liquefaction of Menstrual Clot in the vagina is carried out by fibrinolytic system.

4. Liquefaction of Sperms in the Epididymis when seminal ejaculation does not occur is caused by the fibrinolysin system.

5. Role in Inflammatory Response. In addition to its fibrinolytic activity, plasmin can form plasma kinins (bradykinins and kallidin) and thus contribute to the vascular and sensory features (pain) of the inflammatory response to injury.

Anticoagulants

Anticoagulants refer to the substances which delay or prevent the process of coagulation of blood. In vitro, blood clotting can be prevented by substances which sequester calcium, e.g. sodium citrate or oxalate, sodium edetate (EDTA).

In vivo, the tendency of thrombosis can be inhibited by:

- Antagonizing clotting factors (e.g. heparin),
- By destruction of the key substance fibrinogen or
- By inhibiting the synthesis of factors II, VII, IX and X (vitamin-K antagonists).

Types. Anticoagulants may be divided into endogenous and exogenous anticoagulants.

A. Endogenous Anticoagulants. Endogenous anticoagulants are those which are present inside the blood naturally:

- Heparin,
- Antithrombin III, and
- Protein-C.

For details see page 216.

B. Exogenous Anticoagulants. Exogenous anticoagulants are administered from outside or are used in vitro. These include:

- Heparin and its derivatives,
- Calcium sequesters,
- Vitamin K antagonist and
- Defibrination substances.

1. Heparin. Heparin, a naturally acting anticoagulant can also be synthesized. It inhibits blood coagulation both in vivo and in vitro (see page 216). For commercial use, heparin is extracted from certain animal tissue, and is prepared in pure form. Synthesized form has longer life; therefore, its action lasts for 4–5 h. It mainly inhibits activated factors of intrinsic and common pathway including thrombin, Xa and IXa. This effect results in prolongation of platelet thromboplastin time (PTT) and thrombin time (TT). See page 224.

Clinical use: Due to its rapid action heparin can be used:

- To treat thrombosis and pulmonary emboli.
- Initial management of patient with unstable angina, acute myocardial infarction (MI) and during cardiac bypass surgery.
- In selected patients with disseminated intravascular coagulation (DIC).

  Note: Protamine. The basic protein is used as an antidote to neutralize the effect of heparin, because it forms an irreversible complex with heparin.
- ***Danaparoid*** is a mixture of nonheparin glycosamine glycan isolated from porcine intestinal mucosa cells (84% heparin, 12% dermatan sulphate and 4% chondroitin sulphate). It mainly causes inhibition of factor Xa by antithrombin, but does not prolong PTT.
- ***Lepirudin*** is a recombinant derivative of hirudin present in salivary gland secretion of medicinal leech. It is a direct inhibitor of thrombin.

2. Calcium Sequesters or Decalcifying Agents. In vitro, blood clotting can be prevented by substances which sequester (remove) calcium from the blood. These include two types of agents:

- Substances which form insoluble salts with calcium such as sodium citrate and sodium oxalate, and
- Calcium chelators which bind calcium such as ethylenediaminetetraacetic acid (EDTA).

3. Vitamin K Antagonists. These are used orally and thus can prevent coagulation in vivo effectively. These agents occupy vitamin K receptor sites in the liver and prevent vitamin K from carrying out its normal physiological function, hence the name vitamin K antagonists. Thus, these substances inhibit synthesis of vitamin K-dependent factors, i.e. factors VII, IX and X. These include coumarin derivatives (e.g. dicoumarol), warfarin, phenindione and nicoumalone.

i. ***Dicumarol*** is the first original oral anticoagulant isolated for clinical use, but because of its slow and erratic absorption, it is seldom used.

ii. ***Warfarin.*** For synthesis of vitamin K-dependent coagulation factors, vitamin K acts as cofactor for formation of γ carboxyglutamic acid residues on the coagulation factors. The enzyme γ-glutamyl carboxylase and epoxide reductase are responsible for formation and metabolism of vitamin K. Warfarin acts by inhibiting enzyme epoxide reductase complex-1 (VKOR-1). This enzyme

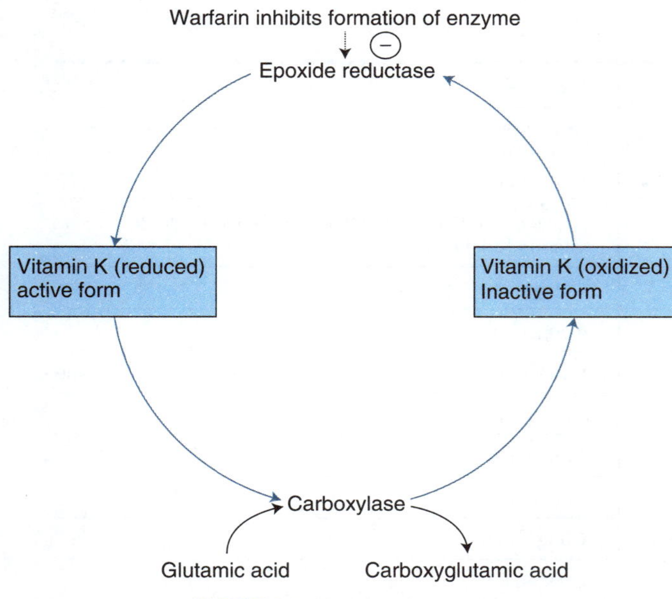

FIGURE 3.5-10 Vitamin K cycle.

converts inactive (oxidized) form of vitamin K into active (reduced) form (Fig 3.5-10). The anticoagulant function of warfarin begins after 24 h and lasts longer.

4. Thrombolytic Drugs include tissue plasminogen activator (TPA), streptokinase and urokinase. For details see page 217.

5. Antiplatelet Drugs like aspirin prevent platelet plug formation (For details see page 209).

6. Defibrination Substances. Defibrination substances are those which cause destruction of fibrinogen. These include:

- *Malaysian pit viper venom.* It is a type of snake venom which in vivo acts as anticoagulant by causing defibrination and also by stimulating the fibrinolytic system. In vitro, it has a direct anticoagulant effect on fibrinogen by forming imperfect fibrin polymer.
- *Arvin or Ancord.* It is a purified preparation of snake venom. It is glycoprotein in nature and is administered by injection. It acts as an anticoagulant by causing defibrination and thus producing fibrinogenpenia.

7. Cold. Keeping blood cold (at 5–10°C) can retard the process of coagulation but cannot absolutely prevent it. Because of this reason, blood is stored in blood banks at low temperature but some anticoagulant agent is always used. Further, it looks paradoxical that whenever bleeding occurs, ice is applied to arrest the haemorrhage (while cold delays coagulation); in fact, when ice is applied on the surface it prevents bleeding by inducing reflex vasoconstriction.

BLEEDING DISORDERS

Bleeding disorders are characterized by spontaneous escape of blood from blood vessels (in the tissues, inside the body cavities or on few surfaces like (skin and mucous membrane) or persistent and/or excessive bleeding following minor injuries like tooth extraction, etc.

Classification of Bleeding Disorders

I. Platelet Disorders

A. *Deficiency of blood platelets. Thrombocytopenic purpura.*
   1. Essential or idiopathic thrombocytopenic purpura and
   2. Secondary thrombocytopenic purpura.

B. *Functional disorder of platelets*

II. Coagulation Disorder or Defective Coagulation Mechanism

1. Deficiency of clotting factors (see Table 3.5-1),
2. Vitamin K deficiency (see page 213),
3. Anticoagulant overdose and
4. Disseminated intravascular clotting (DIC).

III. Vascular Disorders. DAMAGE of Capillary Endothelium (nonThrombocytopenic Purpura)

- Due to infection by bacteria and their toxins,
- Due to toxic effects of drugs and chemicals,
- Due to avitaminosis C,
- Allergic purpura and
- Connective tissue diseases.

Only a few important bleeding disorders are described briefly.

Purpura

Purpura is a group of bleeding disorder occurring due to various causes. The term purpura is derived from purple-coloured petechial haemorrhages and bruises in the skin. The blood that leaks out changes colour from red to blue to dark blue and green over a period of time.

Causes and Types of Purpura

I. Platelet Disorders. Platelets play an important role in haemostasis and coagulation (see functions of platelets page 206); therefore, platelet disorders are associated with bleeding disorders. Platelet disorders include:

1. Deficiency of platelets (thrombocytopenic purpura). Normal platelet count ranges from 1.5 to 4.5 lakh/mm^3 average, count of 2.5 lakh/μL. Decrease in the platelet count below 1.5 lakh/μL is called thrombocytopenia. Thrombocytopenic purpura may be:

- ***Primary thrombocytopenic purpura*** (idiopathic, cause not known). In many of the idiopathic cases, antibodies develop against platelets (immune thrombocytopenic purpura, ITP).

TABLE 3.5-1 Deficiency of Clotting Factors

Deficiency of factor	Clinical syndrome	Cause
• Factor I	Fibrinogenopenia Afibrinogenaemia	Depletion during pregnancy with premature separation of placenta Congenital (rare)
• Factor II	Hypoprothrombinaemia (Haemorrhagic tendency in liver disease)	Decreased hepatic synthesis, usually secondary to vitamin K deficiency
• Factor V	Parahaemophilia	Congenital
• Factor VII	Hypoconvertinaemia	Congenital
• Factor VIII	Haemophilia A or classical haemophilia	Congenital defect due to abnormal gene on X chromosome
• Factor IX	Haemophilia B or Christmas disease	Congenital
• Factor X	Stuart–Prower factor deficiency	Congenital
• Factor XI	PTA deficiency	Congenital
• Factor XII	Hageman trait (does not produce bleeding)	Congenital
• Von Willebrand's factor	Von Willebrand's disease	Congenital

- ***Secondary causes of platelet deficiency*** (secondary thrombocytopenic purpura) are:
  - Bone-marrow depression due to effects of various cytotoxic drugs. Whole-body irradiation and hypoplastic and aplastic anaemia.
  - Leukaemia and secondary deposits of malignancies in the bone marrow,
  - Acute septicaemia, toxaemia, uraemia, and
  - Hypersplenism.

Relation between platelet count and bleeding is as follows:

Platelet count	Bleeding
• Above 100,000/μL	No clinical symptoms; bleeding is rare.
• From 50,000–100,000/μL	Bleeding may occur after major surgery.
• From 20,000–50,000/μL	Bleeding occurs with minor trauma in everyday life.
• Below 20,000/μL	Spontaneous haemorrhage in urinary tract, G1 tract, nosebleeds, etc.
• At very low counts	Fatal haemorrhage may occur in the brain.

Treatment

- In thrombocytopenic purpura, bleeding can be effectively stopped for few days by transfusing either fresh blood or platelets only.
- Splenectomy is also helpful because the spleen removes large numbers of platelets from the blood.

2. Functional disorders of platelets (thrombocytopenic purpura). Functional disorders of platelets (defects in platelet adhesion or aggregation) are characterized by prolonged bleeding time with normal platelet counts. Functional disorders of platelets include:

- ***Drug-induced defects*** occur with aspirin, large doses of penicillin and other drugs.
- ***Von Willebrand's disease.*** It is inherited as an autosomal dominant trait. This condition is associated with a deficiency of factor VIII-related antigen (VIII R:Ag) also called as von Willebrand factor (VWF). This factor acts as a carrier of factor VIII, so its deficiency results in diminished adherence of platelets to collagen fibres in a damaged vessel.

  Treatment

  Von Willebrand disease can be treated by injecting 1-deamino-8D arginine vasopressin (DDAVP) or desmopressin intravenously. DDAVP releases VWF and Factor VIII from endothelial stores.

  Antifibrinolytic agents like epsilon-aminocaproic acid (EACA) or Tranexamic acid is an important therapy either alone or with DDAVP, particularly during dental procedures (e.g. tooth extraction).
- ***Other diseases*** in which platelet functions become defective are uraemia, cirrhosis and leukaemia.

II. Vascular Disorders. Bleeding tendencies seen in patients with vascular disorders (damage to capillary endothelium) are referred to as *nonthrombocytopenic purpura.* In all cases of purpura due to vessel wall defects, the platelet counts are normal, but bleeding time is prolonged and capillary fragility test is positive.

Causes of Nonthrombocytopenic Purpura

1. ***Drug-induced damage to capillary wall*** is seen in patients with prolonged treatment with corticosteroids, penicillin, sulpha drugs and aspirin.

2. ***Deficiency of vitamin C (scurvy)*** causes failure of collagen formation and associated with impaired hydroxyproline synthesis. Petechiae and bleeding from gums occur due to decreased intercellular substance and less stable capillary basement membrane.
3. ***Allergic purpura*** occurs due to damage to capillary walls by antibodies.
4. ***Infections*** such as typhus, bacterial endocarditis and haemolytic streptococcus may be associated with capillary wall damage.
5. ***Senile purpura*** refers to purpuric haemorrhagic spots seen on the back of hands and forearms due to prolonged pressure or mild trauma. Small vessels in old age rupture due to increased mobility of skin resulting from loss of elastic and connective tissues around the blood vessels.
6. ***Connective tissue diseases*** are also sometimes associated with damage to capillary walls and purpuric haemorrhages.

Haemophilia

Haemophilia is the name given to a group of disorders occurring due to *hereditary deficiency of coagulation* and characterized by bleeding tendencies hardly distinguishable from one another, associated with increased clotting time (CT). The haemophilia includes:

- Haemophilia A (83% cases),
- Haemophilia B (15% cases) and
- Haemophilia C (2% cases).

1. Haemophilia A

- Haemophilia A, also known as true or classical haemophilia occurs due to *deficiency of factor VIII, i.e.* antihaemophilic globulin (AHG).
- It is the most common hereditary coagulation disorder. Being a sex linked recessive disease, it affects males exclusively and females act as carriers (Fig 3.5-11). The carrier female shows no symptoms due to the presence of the X chromosome, which is dominant over recessive chromosome (X*) X. Only mating of a haemophilic male with a carrier female will produce a haemophilic female, which is a very rare occurrence.

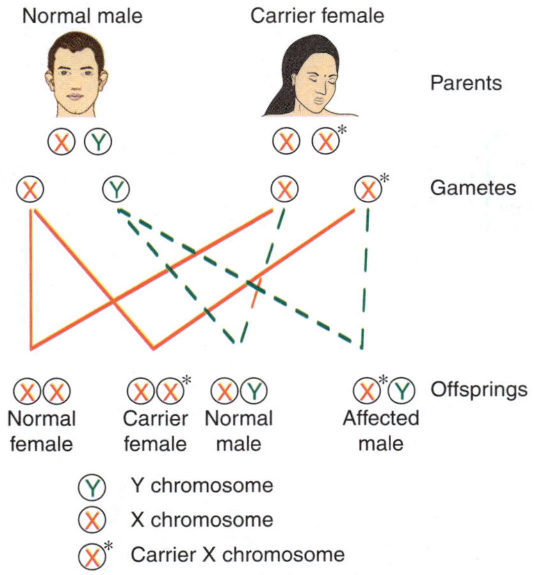

  The majority of patients with haemophilia A have blood levels of factor VIII below 5%, and so usually bleed severely on minor trauma. Relationships of levels of factor VIII with status of haemostasis are as:

Factor VIII activity	Status of haemostasis
>50%	Normal haemostasis
25–50%	Excessive bleeding after Severe trauma
5–25%	Excessive bleeding after Minor trauma
1–5%	Severe bleeding on minor trauma
<1%	Spontaneous bleeding

- Clinical features (bleeding tendency) are not apparent since birth but generally start early in life (within first three years).
- The haemophilics have the tendency to bleed into soft tissues, muscles, joints, GI tract, urinary tract and from the nose.
- Joints of haemophilic patients become severely damaged due to repeated joint haemorrhage.
- Haemorrhage into the soft tissue around the floor of the mouth may cause respiratory obstruction and death by suffocation.
- Haemophilics have normal bleeding time, platelet count and prothrombin time. Coagulation time (CT) is increased and typically, the patients have prolonged PTT.
- Hemophilia A can be treated by transfusion of:
  - Repeated small fresh blood, within 30 min of collection from the donor (because factor VIII is lost rapidly on storage), or
  - Fresh plasma or
  - Factor VIII concentrate commercially available as cryoprecipitated antihaemophilic factor for intravenous infusion.

FIGURE 3.5.11 Sex-linked inheritance of haemophilia A.

2. Haemophilia B

- Haemophilia B, also known as *Christmas disease,* occurs due to deficiency of factor IX (Christmas factor or plasma thromboplastin component (PTC). It was discovered in a family with the surname Christmas.
- Like haemophilia A, haemophilia B is also a recessive X-linked disease that occurs in males and is transmitted by females.
- Since factor IX is more stable on storage, it is not necessary to use fresh blood for treatment.

3. Haemophilia C

- Haemophilia C refers to a deficiency of PTA (factor XI).

- It is inherited as *Mendelian dominant* and affects both males and females.
- This condition may occur without bleeding tendency.
- Clotting time in this condition may be prolonged or may be within normal limits.

Disseminated Intravascular Coagulation

- Disseminated intravascular coagulation (DIC), as the name indicates, refers to the condition when clotting mechanism becomes activated in widespread areas of the circulation (Fig 3.5-12).
- Due to widespread intravascular coagulation, there occurs plugging of small vessels with clots resulting in decreased O_2 and nutrient supply to its tissues causing multiple organ damage.
- The widespread intravascular coagulation uses up most of the coagulation factors and platelets present in the blood resulting in failure of haemostatic mechanism. The patient thus develops bleeding tendencies and hence, the condition is also called *consumption coagulopathy.*
- The fibrin degradation products (FDP) that are formed as a result of fibrinolysis of the clot have antihaemostatic effect and further aggravate the bleeding tendency.
- DIC, is thus a grave condition. It can result as a consequence of an adverse condition in which there occur large amounts of traumatized or dying tissue in the body, which release thromboplastin, or toxins accumulate in the body, which stimulate many coagulation factors. DIC is associated with conditions like septicaemic shock, metastatic malignancies, prolonged postpartum haemorrhage, snake bite, etc.

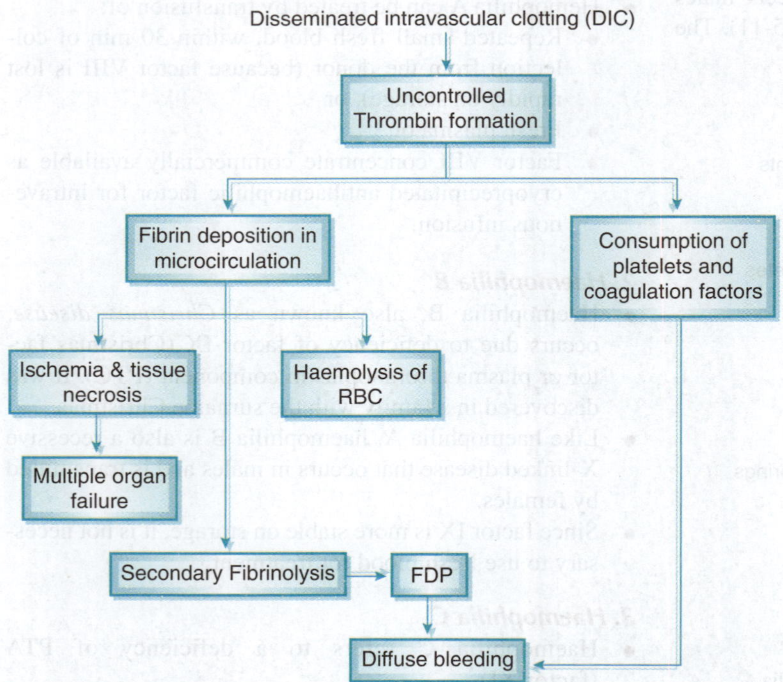

FIGURE 3.5-12 Interaction between coagulation and fibrinolytic pathway results in thrombosis and bleeding in disseminated intravascular coagulation.

Treatment: The main basis of DIC treatment is:

- To control or elimination of underlying primary cause.
- Management of hemorrhagic symptoms due to thrombocytopenia by platelet concentrate (dose 1–2U/kg body weight)
- Drugs to control coagulation; such as heparin, antithrombin III or fibrinolytic agents (EACA or tranexamic acid in low doses)

Laboratory Tests in Bleeding Disorders

Bleeding Time (BT)

Definition. Bleeding occurs from the skin when it is pricked with a needle, which normally stops of its own within a few minutes. The time lapse between the skin prick and the arrest of bleeding is called *bleeding time* (BT).

Procedure. ***(i) Duke's method***. To estimate BT, the tip of a finger or ear lobe is pricked with a sharp needle. A stopwatch is run and blood is wiped away with a clean filter paper every 15 s till bleeding stops. The time taken for the arrest of bleeding is BT.

Normal BT by Duke's method varies from 1 to 6 min. Normal BT indicates that platelets count and their function, as well as health of capillaries is normal.

(ii) Ivy's method. In this method, a pressure of 40 mmHg is applied to the upper arm with a blood pressure cuff and then a skin deep prick is made on the anterior surface of the forearm. Rest of procedure is same as above. *Normal BT by Ivy's method is 3–6 min at 37°C.*

Note: Bleeding time depends on the depth of the prick. Specified depth of prick in Duke's method for ear lobe is 4 mm and for IVY method for forearm is 2.5 mm.

Prolonged BT occurs in purpura, while it is normal in haemophilia.

Important Note

- A clean or straight cut with a blade or knife bleeds longer than an irregular injury. In an irregular cut, bleeding time is less because collagen gets exposed and a rough surface available for platelet aggregation and factor XII can get activated.

Capillary Fragility Test of Hess or Tourniquet Test

Tourniquet test is performed to assess the mechanical fragility of the capillaries by raising pressure within them. It may demonstrate latent purpura.

Procedure. A circle of 1-inch diameter is marked on the front of the forearm. Any purple spots present in the circle are marked with blue ink. Then a pressure midway between systolic and diastolic blood pressure is applied on the upper arm for 15 min using the blood pressure cuff. Appearance of 10 or more new petechiae is a positive test. *Positive tourniquet test* occurs in various types of purpurae and vessel wall defects.

Platelet Count

Normal Platelet Count varies from 1.5–4.5 lakh/μL with an average 2.5 lakh/μL. Platelet count is decreased in primary and secondary thrombocytopenic purpura (pages 207 and 220).

Procedure *(i) Direct method.* Fresh blood should be diluted in a RBC pipette with Reese-E kar fluid and the stained platelets should then be counted in a haemocytometer. *(ii) Indirect method.* In this method, platelet count is calculated from the RBC count and platelet:RBC ratio. Normally there is 1 platelet to 16–18 red cells.

Coagulation Time (CT)

Definition. Coagulation time (CT) refers to the time taken by the fresh fluid blood to get coagulated (demonstrated by formation of fibrin threads). It is an insensitive measure in the assessment of coagulation defects and is abnormally prolonged when the coagulation factors are seriously deficient.

Procedure. (i) Capillary tube method. In this method, a capillary tube is filled with fresh blood from the finger prick and 1 cm bits of the tube are broken from one end every 30 s. The end point is reached when fibrin threads span a gap of 5 mm between the broken ends (*rope formation*). *Normal CT* by capillary method is 3–6 min.

Comments. It is important to note that clotting of blood with this method involves both the intrinsic and extrinsic systems, as there is injury to the blood, as well as to the tissue.

(ii) Modified Lee–White test tube method (whole blood coagulation time). Presently, this method is considered the standard method to estimate CT. Principle of this method is to collect blood with a clean nontraumatic venipuncture and put it in an 8 mm diameter test tube at 37°C and see how long it requires to clot. The end point is reached when test tube can be tilted through an angle greater than 90° without spilling the blood. *Normal value of CT* by Lee–White method is 8–12 min for a glass tube and 20–60 min for a siliconized tube. Clotting time is more because siliconized tubes are smooth surfaced, and therefore, activation of factor XII becomes slow or difficult.

Comments. This method tests the intrinsic system of blood clotting as there is no admixture of blood with tissue fluid. Therefore, this method is considered more reliable than the capillary tube method.

Importance of Clotting Time. The CT is prolonged in haemophilia and other clotting disorders, because thrombin cannot be normally generated; however, the bleeding time (BT), which reflects vasoconstriction and platelet plug formation independently of clot formation, is normal since CT can increase due to deficiency of any of the factors so it is a nonspecific test. More specific tests include *prothrombin time, partial thromboplastin time, thromboplastin generation test, thrombin time,* etc. Specific tests can pinpoint the particular deficient factor.

- *Physiologically,* clotting time is reduced during menstruation and before and during parturition.
- *Pathologically CT is prolonged in* haemophilia, liver diseases, afibrinogenaemia, Christmas disease, vitamin K deficiency and disseminated intravascular coagulation (DIC).

Prothrombin Time (PT)

Procedure. *Quick's one-stage method* now is the standard method to measure prothrombin time (PT). In this method, tissue thromboplastin (commercially available) and calcium chloride solution (to provide calcium ion) are added to the oxalated or citrated plasma of the patient; and the mixture is incubated at 37°C. The end point is conversion of fluid plasma into a gel (due to formation of fibrin). Normal PT is 11–16 s.

Plasma from a normal person is used as a control and the result is expressed as prothrombin ratio (PTR). Normal PTR varies from 0.9–1.2.

Note: International normalized ratio. Prothrombin time may vary even in the same individual depending on the difference in the tissue factor activity and analytical system. International normalized ratio (INR) is devised for standardized measurement of prothrombin time. For each type and batch of tissue factor, the manufacturing company assigns an international sensitivity index (ISI), which indicates the tissue factor activity with the standardized sample. The INR is the ratio of prothrombin time of person to normal control sample raised to the power of ISI:

$$INR = [PT\ test/PT\ control]^{ISI}$$

The normal range of INR is 0.9–1.3.

Short prothrombin time or low INR (e.g. 0.5) is mainly determined by prothrombin concentration. The curve relating prothrombin time to prothrombin concentration is used to quantify the concentration of prothrombin in the blood (Fig 3.5-13).

Comments. Intrinsic system is not involved in this test since plasma does not contain platelets. Obviously it is extrinsic system which is tested. In this test, calcium nullifies the effect of oxalate or citrate and tissue thromboplastin acts as the prothrombin activator, i.e. it initiates extrinsic pathway. Though originally introduced as a test for prothrombin activity (hence its name), it is also sensitive to deficiency of factor I, V, VII and X.

Importance of PT. *PT is increased* in patients on oral anticoagulants, liver failure, vitamin K deficiency, abnormally low fibrinogen concentration, deficiency of factors II, V, VII and X.

- *PT is normal* in haemophilia and Christmas disease.

It is used to monitor patients receiving anticoagulant therapy (e.g. warfarin) to adjust its dose.

Partial Thromboplastin Time (PTT)

Partial thromboplastin time (PTT), also known as kaolin cephalin clotting time (KCCT), detects coagulation defects too small to lead to prolongation of the whole blood clotting time.

Procedure. To the oxalated or citrated plasma of the patient are added kaolin (to provide surface contact), cephalin (to provide phospholipids) and calcium chloride (to provide calcium ions), and the mixture is incubated at 37°C. The end point is formation of plasma gel. Normal PTT is about 40 s.

Comments. Since the mixture so formed lacks tissue thromboplastins, so extrinsic pathway is not involved in this test. Thus, it measures the intrinsic pathway, i.e. factors XII, XI, X, IX, VIII, V, II and I.

Importance of PTT. It is used to monitor the heparin therapy.

PTT is prolonged in haemophilia, von Willebrand's disease, liver failure, deficiency of contact factor XII, anticoagulant therapy and intravascular clotting.

Thromboplastin Generation Test (TGT)

This test measures generation of thromboplastin, i.e. the efficiency of a part of the intrinsic mechanism of coagulation. Normal value of TGT is 12 s or less. Prolonged TGT indicates deficiency of factors needed to form prothrombin activator by the intrinsic mechanism, i.e. factor VIII, IX, X and V.

Comments. From values of prothrombin time (PT) and thromboplastin generation test (TGT), following inferences can be drawn:

- In haemophilia, PT is normal but TGT is prolonged.
- In pure factor VII deficiency, PT is prolonged, but TGT will remain normal.
- In factor X deficiency, both PT and TGT will be abnormal.

Thrombin Time (TT)

This test measures the final step in coagulation, i.e. functional fibrinogen available. In this test, thrombin is added to plasma, which will convert fibrinogen present in the plasma to fibrin. Normally, a clot is formed in about 10 s, which is the end point. *TT is prolonged* in hypofibrinogenaemia, dysfibrinogenaemia, DIC and heparin treatment.

Clot Retraction Test

Clot retraction test measures time needed for contraction of an undisturbed clot. It indicates the function and number of platelets. Normally, clot retraction begins within 2 h and is completed within 24 h.

- *Clot retraction is retarded* in thrombocytopenia.
- Clot is small and soft in thromboasthenia, i.e. functional disturbance of platelets.

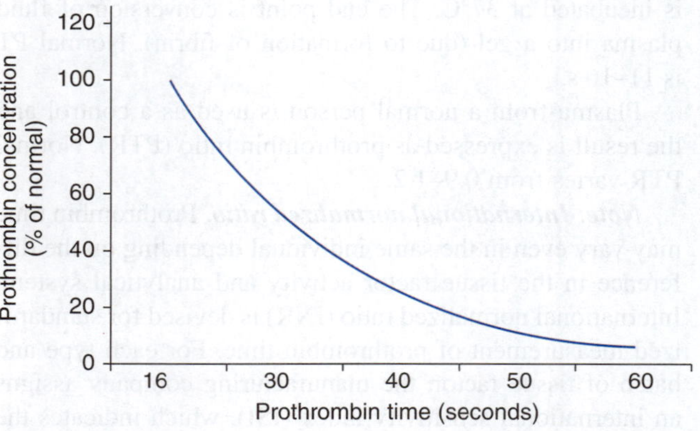

FIGURE 3.5-13 Prothrombin concentration in blood in relation to prothrombin time.

Chapter 3.6

Blood Groups and Blood Transfusion

BLOOD GROUPS

Introduction

Agglutinogens and Agglutinins

- ***Agglutinogens*** refer to the antigens present on the cell membranes of RBCs. A variety of antigens are present on the cell membrane, but only a few of them are of practical significance.
- ***Agglutinins*** refer to the antibodies against the agglutinogens. These are present in the plasma.
- ***Agglutination*** of RBCs can be caused by the antigens present on their cell membrane in the presence of suitable agglutinins (antibodies). That is why, these antigens are called agglutinogens.

Blood Grouping Systems. Depending upon the type of agglutinogen present or absent on the red cell membranes, various blood grouping systems are known, which can be classified as:

- ***Major blood group systems*** are based on the presence of agglutinogens which are widely prevalent in the population and are known to cause the worst transfusion reactions. These include:
  - The classical ABO blood grouping system and
  - Rh (CDE) blood grouping system.
- ***Minor blood group systems*** are based on the presence of agglutinogens which are found only in a small proportion of the population and occasionally produce mild transfusion reactions. These include:
  - MNS blood group system and
  - P blood group system.
- ***Familial blood group systems*** are based on the presence of agglutinogens which are found only in a few families. Examples of familial blood group systems are Kell, Duffy, Lutheran, Lewis, Deigo, Kidd and many others.

Note: From a clinical point of view, only major blood group systems, i.e. classical ABO and Rh (CDE) blood grouping systems are important and so will be discussed in detail.

Landsteiner Law. Karl Landsteiner, in 1900, framed a law in relation to agglutinogens and agglutinins, which states that:

1. ***If an agglutinogen is present*** on the red cell membrane of an individual, the corresponding agglutinin must be absent in the plasma; and
2. ***If an agglutinogen is absent*** from the cell membrane of RBCs of an individual, the corresponding agglutinin must be present in the plasma.

   It is important to note that:
   - The Landsteiner law is applicable to ABO blood group system only and

- The law is not applicable to other blood group systems, because there are no naturally occurring agglutinins in these systems.

Classical ABO Blood Grouping System

A and B Agglutinogens

- The classical ABO blood grouping system is based on the presence of antigens called A and B agglutinogens on the cell membrane of RBCs.
- A and B agglutinogens are complex oligosaccharides differing in their terminal sugars. In antigen A, the terminal sugar is N-acetylgalactosamine while in B antigen, the terminal sugar is galactose. Basically, these antigens are carbohydrates present on the backbone of the cell membrane of RBCs, either as glycosphingolipids or glycoproteins, and are secreted into plasma and body fluids as glycoproteins. H substance is the precursor on which A and B antigens are added, and H substance is formed by addition of fructose to glycoprotein or glycolipid backbone. Then, addition of N-acetyl galactosamine produces A antigen and galactose the B antigen.
- The A and B antigens present on the membranes of RBCs are also present in many other tissues, like salivary glands, pancreas, kidney, liver, lungs and testis, and also in body fluids like saliva, semen and amniotic fluid. The antigens on RBC membrane are glycolipids, while in the tissues and body fluids they are soluble glycoproteins.
- In addition to A and B antigens, H antigen is also present usually in all individuals. H antigen is not antigenic, so there is no corresponding antibody.

Anti-A and Anti-B Agglutinins

All individuals produce antibodies to ABH carbohydrate antigen that they lack; thus, A blood group individual produces anti-B, 'B' blood group anti-A, 'AB' blood group-neither A nor B and O blood group produces both anti A and B.

- The individuals with rare *Bombay blood group* produce antibodies to H substance as well as to A and B antigens.
- The naturally occurring antibodies are termed as isoagglutinins and demonstrable agglutinins are present in 50% of newborns only that have been filtered across the placenta.
- The specific agglutinins start appearing at 10 days; reach a peak at 10 years and then decline.
- Anti-A (or α) agglutinin and anti-B (or β) agglutinin refer to the antibody, i.e. which reacts with or acts on antigen A, and antigen B, respectively.
- The α and β agglutinins are globulins of the IgM type and *cannot cross the placenta.*
- There are two types of α agglutinins: the α_1 and α proper.
- Presence or absence of a and b agglutinins is determined by Landsteiner law as described above.
- The α and β agglutinins act best at low temperature (5–20°C) and are therefore also called cold antibodies.

However, the production of anti-A and anti-B has been explained by the fact that the blood group substance (antigen) has similarity with substances present in food and bacterial antigens. They enter the body along with food, bacteria and other ways. The bacterial antigens that belong to intestinal flora get absorbed and induce antibody production, because they are recognized as nonself antigens.

Types of ABO Blood Groups

Depending upon the presence or absence of A and B agglutinogens and α and β agglutinins, there are four types of blood groups.

Blood Group A is characterized by:

- Presence of A agglutinogen and absence of B agglutinogen on the cell membrane of RBCs.
- Presence of anti-B (or β) agglutinin and absence of anti-A (or α) agglutinin from the plasma.
- Group A has two subgroups: A_1 and A_2. The α_1-agglutinin agglutinates with subgroup A_1 only, while α-proper agglutinin agglutinates with both A_1 and A_2 subgroups.

Blood Group B is characterized by:

- Presence of B agglutinogen and absence of A agglutinogen on the membrane of RBCs, and
- Presence of anti-A (or α) agglutinin and absence of anti-B (or β) agglutinin from the plasma.

Blood Group AB is characterized by:

- Presence of both A and B agglutinogens on the cell membrane of RBCs, and
- Absence of both anti-A (or α) and anti-B or (β) agglutinins from the plasma.
- Blood group AB has two subgroups, namely A_1B and A_2B.

Blood Group O is characterized by:

- Absence of both A and B agglutinogens on the red cell membrane, and
- Presence of both anti-A and anti-B agglutinins in the plasma.

Population Distribution of ABO Blood Groups (Table 3.6-1)

Inheritance of ABO Blood Groups

Agglutinogens A and B or the nonantigenic substances which determine the blood groups are genetically inherited as Mendelian dominant in the classical Mendelian pattern.

The genes that determine A and B phenotypes are located on chromosome 9P. The enzymes glycosyltransferases are the gene products which confer enzymatic ability for addition of specific antigenic carbohydrates. Therefore,

TABLE 3.6-1 Population Distribution of ABO Blood Groups in India vis-à-vis in Britain

Blood group	India (%)	Britain (%)
A	20	42
B	40	09
AB	08	03
O	32	46

individuals who lack 'A' and 'B' transferases are 'O' type, while those who inherit both 'A' and 'B' are 'AB' type, and

Individuals who lack the H gene (responsible for coding fructose transferase) cannot produce H substance. Such individuals are homozygous for silent h allele (hh) and are known as Bombay phenotype, i.e. (Oh), but are rare. The ABO phenotype and possible genotype have been listed in Table 3.6-2. ***If the blood group of the father is B and that of the mother is A, then the blood group of the offspring*** will be as shown in Table 3.6-3:

The various possibilities of inheritance of antigen A, B or nonantigenic substance O from the mother and father will determine the blood group of the offspring as shown in Table 3.6-4:

- ***Agglutinogens A and B First Appear in the Sixth Week of Fetal Life.*** Their concentration at birth is 1/5th of adult level and it progressively rises during puberty and adolescence.
- ***Anti-A (or α) and Anti-B (or β) Agglutinins*** (specific blood group antibodies) are absent at birth, but they appear 10–15 days after birth and reach a maximum concentration by the age of 10 years.
- ***Origin of Agglutinins.*** Agglutinins A and B are of gamma globulins (mainly IgM and IgG types) produced by the bone marrow and lymph nodes. As we know, the antibodies are produced in response to an antigen. In case of ABO blood groups, the antibodies (i.e. agglutinins A or B are produced in persons who do not possess the corresponding antigen A or B on the surface of RBCs. The probable mechanism of appearance of α and β agglutinins is described. Antigens very similar to A and B antigens are commonly present in the intestinal bacteria and foods. When the newborn is exposed to these antigens, these are absorbed into the blood and stimulate the formation of antibodies against the antigens recognized as nonself (i.e. not present in their own body) by the immune system.

Note: The gut of an infant is relatively permeable to larger protein molecules compared with adults; therefore, the bacterial antigens get absorbed intact from the gut and induce antibody production.

- ***Agglutinin Titre.*** The quantity of agglutinin is practically nil immediately after birth. The titre of agglutinin starts rising after 2 months as the infant begins to produce agglutinins and maximum titre is attained by the age of 8–10 years and then starts declining throughout the life (Fig. 3.6-1). The relative concentration of agglutinins in saliva and semen is 600, amniotic fluid 175, tears 5, urine 3, cerebrospinal fluid 0 and red blood cells 8.32.

Note. The figures indicate the dilution factor before losing the agglutinating potency.

TABLE 3.6-2 The ABO Phenotypes and Possible Genotypes

Phenotype	Genotypes
Blood group A	AA, AO
Blood group B	BB, BO
Blood group AB	AB
Blood group O	OO

TABLE 3.6-3 The Possible Blood Groups (Genotype and Phenotype) of Offspring when the Blood Group of Father is B and That of Mother is A

	Father				Mother				
Phenotype	*B*				*A*				
Genotype	*BB*		*BO*		*AA*		*AO*		
Inherited gene	*B*	*B*	*B*	*O*	*A*	*A*	*A*	*O*	
	I	*II*	*III*	*IV*	*1*	*2*	*3*	*4*	
Offspring	1	2	3	4					
I	AB	AB	AB	BO					Genotype
	AB	AB	AB	B					Phenotype
II	AB	AB	AB	BO					Genotype
	AB	AB	AB	B					Phenotype
III	AB	AB	AB	BO					Genotype
	AB	AB	AB	B					Phenotype
IV	AO	AO	AO	OO					Genotype
	A	A	A	O					Phenotype

Determination of ABO Blood Groups

The ABO blood group of an individual can be determined by mixing one drop of suspension of his/her red cells (in isotonic saline) with a drop each of antiserum A (containing α agglutinins) and antiserum B (containing β agglutinins) separately on a glass slide. The antiserum A will cause agglutination (clumping of RBCs having A antigens and antiserum B will cause agglutination of RBCs having B antigens). The blood group of the individual will be shown

TABLE 3.6-4 Possible Blood Groups of Offspring Depending upon the Blood Group of Father and Mother

Mother		Father					
Phenotype →		A		B		AB	O
↓	Genotype→ ↓	AA	AO	BB	BO	AB	OO
A	AA AO	A, O	AB, B, A, O			B, AB O	B,O
B	BB BO	A,B,AB,O		B, O		A,B,AB	B, O
AB	AB	A, B, AB		A,B,AB		A,B,AB	A,B
O	OO	A, O		B, O		A, B	O

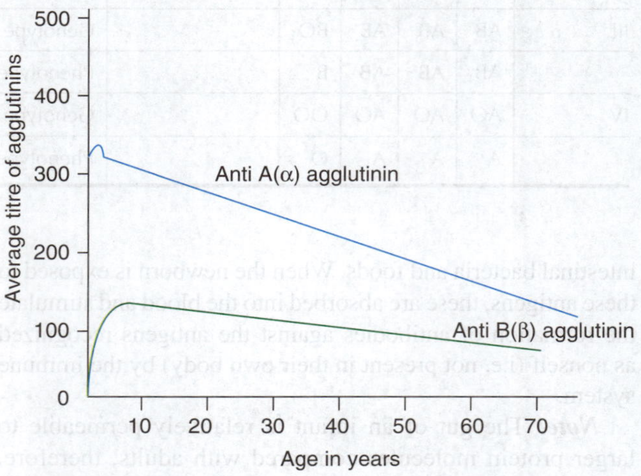

FIGURE 3.6-1 Titre of agglutinins with age. The figure indicates the dilution factor before losing its agglutinating potency.

TABLE 3.6-5 Determination of Blood Group of an Individual

Blood group of RBCs suspension	Agglutination with	
	Antiserum A (containing α agglutinins)	*Antiserum B (containing β agglutinins)*
A	+	–
B	–	+
AB	+	+
O	–	–

by the presence of agglutination with one, both or none of the sera (Table 3.6-5 and Fig. 3.6-2).

Note: The antisera A and B are available commercially. For a quick identification, the anti-A serum is tinted blue and anti-B serum is tinted yellow.

Rh (Rhesus) Blood Grouping System

Rh Antigens

- The antigens responsible for this blood grouping system are called Rh antigens or Rh agglutinogens or Rh factor because these were first discovered in the RBCs of rhesus monkeys. Based on the presence of Rh antigen, two types of blood groups are described:
  - Rh positive blood group and
  - Rh negative blood group.
- The Rh antigens were discovered by Landsteiner and Weiner in 1940. They noticed that when RBCs of the rhesus monkey (monkey with red ischial callosity) were injected into a rabbit, antibodies were formed against these RBCs. When this rabbit's serum was tested against human red cells, agglutination occurred in 85% of the cases, i.e. this person's RBCs contained antigens which reacted with antibodies formed against the rhesus monkey's RBCs. They labelled this antigen as Rh antigen and such persons as Rh +ve. The remaining 15% were labelled as Rh –ve.
- Three types of Rh antigens, viz. C, D and E have been recognized. However, D antigen is the commonest and produces the worst transfusion reactions. Therefore, for all practical purposes, the term Rh antigen refers to D antigen. Consequently, the Rh +ve and Rh –ve individuals are also sometimes called D +ve and D –ve individuals, respectively.
- Rh antigens are integral membrane proteins. These are *not found* in tissues other than RBCs (e.g. ABO antigens, which are also found in some other tissues).

Rh Antibodies

- There are no natural antibodies of Rh antigens, while in the ABO system of blood grouping α or β antibodies

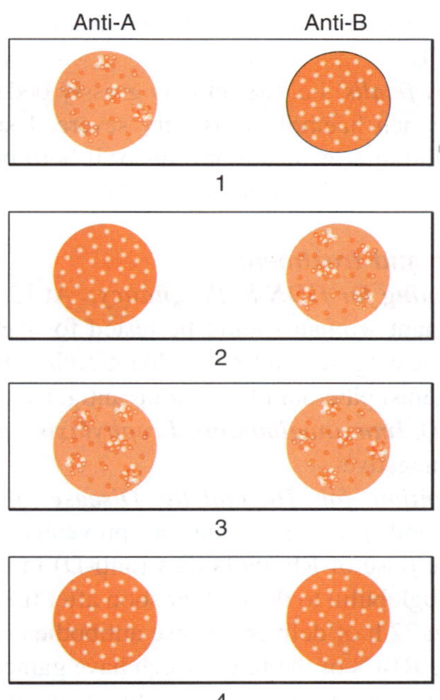

FIGURE 3.6-2 Determination of blood groups—the RBCs showing agglutination with antisera are: **1,** of blood group 'A' with antisera A; **2,** of blood group B with antisera B; **3,** of blood group 'AB' with antisera A and B (both); and **4,** of blood group 'O' with none.

are always present naturally if the appropriate antigen is absent.

- Rh antibodies (also called anti-D) are produced only when an Rh −ve individual is transfused with Rh +blood or when an Rh −ve mother gives birth to an Rh +ve baby (Rh +ve RBCs of fetus enter into the maternal circulation), Rh antibodies of IgG type and can cross the placenta. Since these react best at body temperature, they are also called warm antibodies.
- Once produced, the Rh antibodies persist in the blood for years and can produce serious reactions during the second transfusion. Because of the same reason during second pregnancy in an Rh −ve mother with Rh +ve fetus, severe incompatibility reactions occur causing the so-called haemolytic disease of newborns (because Rh antibodies present in the mother can cross the placenta).

Inheritance of Rh Antigens

- The Rh antigen (D antigen) is inherited as the dominant gene D. When gene D is absent from a chromosome, its place is occupied by the alternate form (allelomorph) called 'd' Rh gene, which is inherited from both the father and the mother.
- An Rh +ve individual may have two genotypes, DD (homozygous) or Dd (heterozygous). Out of 85% Rh +ve individuals, about 35% have DD genotype and 50% have Dd genotype.
- The genotype of Rh −ve individuals is dd.
- Therefore, the genotype (gene composition) of the offspring will be:
  - DD when gene D is carried by both sperm and ovum,
  - Dd, when one gamete carries D and the other d and
  - dd, when both the gametes carry gene d.

Inheritance of Rh antigen is summarized in Fig. 3.6-3.

Haemolytic Disease of Newborn

Haemolytic disease of newborn (HDN) occurs as a result of incompatibility of Rh blood groups between the mother and fetus. The mechanism is described below. It is important to note that incompatibility of ABO blood groups between the mother and fetus is very common, but there is seldom any complication because the α and β agglutinins, i.e. antibodies against antigen A and B are of IgM type, which cannot cross the placental barrier.

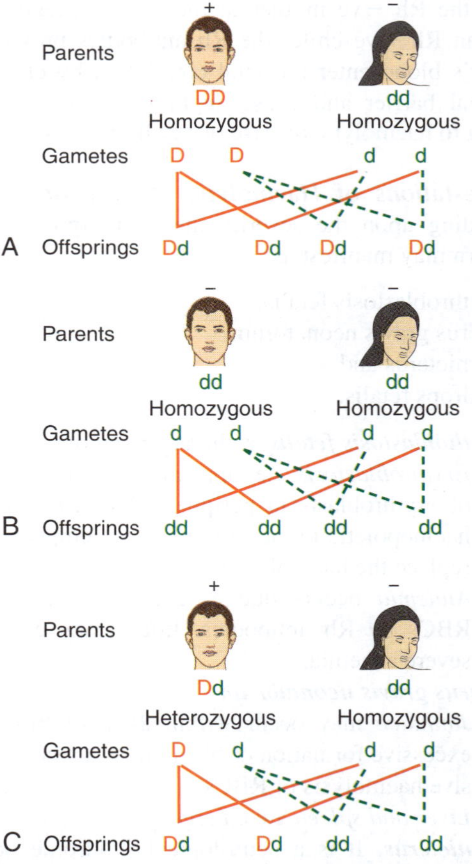

FIGURE 3.6-3 Inheritance of Rh antigen: **A,** when father is homozygous Rh +ve and mother is homozygous Rh −ve; then all the offspring are heterozygous Rh +ve; **B,** when father and mother both are homozygous Rh –ve, then all the offspring are homozygous Rh −ve; and **C,** when father is heterozygous Rh +ve and mother is homozygous Rh −ve, then 50% of offspring are Rh +ve (heterozygous) and other 50% are Rh −ve (homozygous).

Mechanism of Haemolytic Disease of Newborn in Rh Incompatibility. Mechanism of development of haemolytic disease of the newborn can be described under the following steps:

1. Entrance of Rh +ve Fetal RBCs into Rh −ve Mother's Circulation during First Pregnancy. When an Rh −ve mother (genotype dd) bears an Rh +ve child (genotype Dd) with father being Rh +ve (genotype DD or Dd), at the time of delivery the fetal RBCs enter maternal circulation because of severance of umbilical cord. Before delivery, usually the fetal and maternal circulation do not mix. Since the Rh +ve RBCs enter maternal circulation during delivery, so the first child is usually normal.

2. Production of Rh Antibodies (anti-D) in Mother. During postpartum period, i.e. within a month after delivery, the mother develops Rh antibodies in her blood. As mentioned earlier, the Rh antibodies are of IgG type and are able to cross the placental barrier. Once formed, the Rh antibodies persist for a long period in the mother's blood.

3. Rh Incompatibility Reaction during Second Pregnancy. When the Rh −ve mother in the second pregnancy also bears an Rh +ve child, the Rh antibodies present in the mother's blood enter the fetal circulation by crossing the placental barrier and cause agglutination of fetal RBCs leading to haemolytic disease of newborn.

Manifestations of Haemolytic Disease of Newborn. Depending upon the severity the haemolytic disease of newborn may manifest as:

- Erythroblastosis fetalis,
- Icterus gravis neonatorum,
- Kernicterus and
- Hydrops fetalis.

1. ***Erythoblastosis fetalis*** is characterized by:
   - *Erythroblastosis,* i.e. appearance of a large number of erythroblasts in peripheral blood occurs as the haemopoietic tissue of the baby attempts to rapidly replace the haemolysed RBCs.
   - *Anaemia* occurs due to excessive haemolysis of RBCs by Rh antibodies. Infant may even die of severe anaemia.
2. ***Icterus gravis neonatorum***
   - *Jaundice* may occur within 24 h of birth due to excessive formation of bilirubin as a result of excessive haemolysis of RBCs.
   - *Liver and spleen* are enlarged.
3. ***Kernicterus.*** It is a neurological syndrome occurring in newborns with severe haemolysis. The excessive bilirubin formed may enter the brain tissue as the blood–brain barrier is not well developed in infants and cause damage. The bilirubin mostly affects the basal ganglia, producing disturbance of motor activities. It usually develops when the serum bilirubin level exceeds 18 mg/dL.
4. ***Hydrops fetalis,*** i.e. the fetus is grossly oedematous. It occurs when haemolysis is very severe. Usually there occurs intrauterine death of fetus or if born prematurely or even at term, the infant dies within a few hours.

Prevention and Treatment

- ***Screening for HDN in Pregnancy:*** At 12–16 weeks, every pregnant woman should be tested for ABO and Rh group and testing for red cell alloantibodies that maybe directed against paternal blood group antigens.
- ***Anti-D Immunoglobulins Prophylaxis*** in a mother who is Rh negative
- ***Prevention for Haemolytic Disease of Newborn*** during second pregnancy can be prevented by injecting a single dose of Rh antibodies (anti-D) in the form of Rh-immunoglobulin to the mother soon after the first childbirth within 72 h of delivery. These antibodies will destroy the Rh +ve RBCs of the fetus which have gained access to maternal circulation. In this way, active antibodies will not be formed by the mother.

Note: Maternal blood sample is checked for remaining fetal RBCs and extra anti-D should be given if indicated.

Treatment of Haemolytic Disease of Newborn. Treatment of haemolytic disease of the newborn is replacement of baby's Rh +ve blood with Rh −ve blood. The baby's own blood is removed slowly with the help of a polyethylene catheter into the inferior vena cava along the umbilical vein, and is replaced by an equal amount of Rh −ve blood. This is called exchange transfusion.

About 400 ml of Rh −ve blood is infused in 1.5–2 h. The procedure may be repeated many times during the few weeks of neonatal period to maintain low-levels of bilirubin to prevent Kernicterus.

By this time (6–18 weeks), the infant's own Rh +ve RBCs replace the Rh −ve infused RBCs, the time required for formation of RBCs (erythropoiesis)

Clinical Applications of Blood Grouping

1. In Blood Transfusion. Though before blood transfusion cross-matching is always done (for details see page 231); blood grouping, however does help in narrowing down the choice of compatible blood.

2. In Preventing Haemolytic Disease in newborns due to Rh incompatibility (as discussed above).

3. In Paternity Disputes. The ABO, Rh and MNS blood grouping is helpful in settling cases of disputed paternity. Antigens A and B are dominant, whereas O is recessive. It is possible to prove that a person could not have been the father, but not that he was or is father, e.g.

- If the child's blood group is O, whatever the blood group of the mother, a person with blood group AB cannot be the father,
- If the child's blood group is AB, whatever the blood group of the mother, a person with blood group O cannot be the father (Table 3.6-6). The predictive value of such a test is strengthened further if several blood group systems are considered. DNA fingerprinting can prove or disprove fatherhood with 100% certainty.

4. In Medicolegal Cases. Any red stain on a clothing may be claimed to be blood by a supposed victim. Therefore, it is first confirmed that it really is blood by preparing hemin crystals from the stain extract. Blood grouping of the extracted sample can then prove or disprove the claims of victim.

5. In Knowing Susceptibility to Diseases. The incidence of certain diseases is related to blood groups, e.g.

- Individuals with blood group O (nonsecretors) are said to be more susceptible to duodenal ulcer (peptic ulcer) than the individuals with blood group A and B (secretors).
- Individuals with blood group A are more susceptible to carcinoma of stomach, pancreas and salivary glands.
- To some extent, incidence of diabetes mellitus is more in individuals with blood group A.

Other Blood Group System

More than 100 blood group systems are recognized, which are composed of more than 500 antigens. These include:

- ***Lewis system (Le):*** In this system, carbohydrate antigen is not the integral part of the red cell membrane but is adsorbed on RBC membrane from the plasma. The antibodies to Lewis are IgM type and cannot cross the placenta.
- ***I system:*** In this system, the antigens are oligosaccharides related to H, A, B and Le, but differ in their branching system. The antibodies produced are cold agglutinins, and their binding is low at body temperature.
- ***P system*** is another blood group in which the carbohydrate antigen is controlled by specific glycotransferases, and its clinical significance is in rare cases.
- ***MNSsU system*** is regulated by genes located on chromosome 4. M and N are determinants of an RBC membrane protein (i.e., glycophorin A_1) and Ss are of glycophorin B.

BLOOD TRANSFUSION

Indications

Blood transfusion is a life-saving measure and should be carried out when it is absolutely essential. Common situations in which blood transfusion is indicated are:

1. Blood Loss. Severe blood loss is the most important indication for blood transfusion. It may occur in:

- Accidents,
- Major operations,
- Ruptured peptic ulcer,
- Ruptured aortic aneurysm and
- Ruptured ectopic pregnancy.

2. For Quick Restoration of Haemoglobin in patients with severe anaemia it is required in situations like pregnancy and emergency surgery.

3. Exchange Transfusion is required in haemolytic disease of newborn.

4. Blood Diseases like aplastic anaemia, agranulocytosis, leukaemias, haemophilia, purpurae and clotting defects may require blood transfusion.

5. Acute Poisoning, e.g. carbon monoxide poisoning.

Donor and Recipient

Donor refers to a person who donates the blood and the person who receives blood is a recipient.

Precautions to be taken while selecting a donor are:

- Donor should be healthy, and aged between 18 and 60 years.
- Pregnant and lactating mothers preferably should not donate blood.

TABLE 3.6-6 Predictive Blood Groups of Parents in Paternity Disputes

Blood group of child	Parents must have given blood group	Mother's blood group	Father not have been of blood group
O	O + O	No matter which	AB
AB	A + B	No matter which	O
A	A + O or A + A	B or O	B or O
B	B + O or B + B	A or O	A or O

Note. The child's true ABO typing may not be set until 1 year of age.

- Donor should be screened to exclude the diseases which are spread through blood such as AIDS, viral hepatitis, malaria and syphilis.
- Haemoglobin and PCV of the donor should be within normal range. Its approximate concentration is tested using the Tallquist method or the specific gravity method.

Universal Donor. Blood of the individuals with blood group O does not contain any agglutinogen. So, when this blood is transfused to a person with any blood group (A, B, AB or O), theoretically its RBCs will not be agglutinated. Because of this fact, an individual with blood group O is called universal donor. However, practically this term is no longer valid, as it ignores the complications produced by existence of the Rh factor and other blood group systems.

Universal Recipient. Blood of an individual with blood group AB does not contain any agglutinins. So, theoretically when such an individual receives blood from an individual with any blood group (A, B, AB or O), there should be no transfusion reaction. Because of this fact, an individual with AB blood group is called universal recipient. However, practically this term is also no more valid because it ignores the complications produced by the existence of Rh factor and other blood group systems.

Precautions to be Observed during Blood Transfusion

1. Absolute Indication should always be there for the transfusion of blood.

2. Cross-matching should always be done before the blood transfusion. For it blood is collected from donor as well as recipient. Plasma and RBCs are separated in each. The cross-matching involves two steps: major and minor cross-matching.

- ***Major cross-matching** (direct cross-matching) will reveal the presence of anti-ABO agglutinin in the serum of recipient and also complete anti-D. Major cross-matching involves mixing of donor's cells with recipient's plasma.* This is called major cross-matching because of the fact that when mismatched blood is transfused in a recipient, the donor cells get agglutinated as against their agglutinogen there is sufficiently high concentration of agglutinins in the recipient's plasma.
- ***Minor cross-matching.** Involves mixing of recipient's cells with donor's plasma.* This is called a minor cross-match due to the fact that reaction of donor's plasma and recipient's cells usually does not occur or is very mild on giving mismatched blood transfusion because:
  - Firstly, the donor's plasma in the transfusion (about 250 ml) is usually so diluted by the much larger volume of recipient's blood (about 5 L) that it rarely causes agglutination even when the titre of agglutinins against the recipient's cell is high and
  - Secondly, donor's agglutinins are also neutralized by soluble agglutinogens which are found free in the recipient's body fluid.

Coomb's test detects incomplete anti-D. It is carried out in two stages:

- Direct Coomb's test: Suspension of donor is when red cells in 20% albumin are tested against the recipient's plasma. Direct Coomb's test reveals presence of incomplete antibodies present on the RBCs.
- Indirect Coomb's test: This test is supplemented on washed red blood cells and recipient plasma to detect incomplete anti–D, which are not present on the RBCs.

Important Notes

- *For all practical purposes,* if there is no agglutination in either of the cases (major as well as minor cross-matching) described above, only then the recipient can safely receive donor's blood.
- *In extreme emergencies* like war casualties and massive train accidents, where time does not permit the grouping and cross-matching, O-Rh negative blood (universal donor) may be used.

---

3. Rh +ve Blood Should Never be Transfused to Rh −ve Person. It is particularly a must for females at any age before menopause, because once she is sensitized by the Rh antigen, the anti-D antibodies are formed and she will not be able to bear an Rh +ve fetus. In other words, Rh + transfusion may make a woman permanently childless.

4. Donor's Blood Should Always be Screened for diseases which are spread through blood such as AIDS, hepatitis B, malaria and syphilis.

5. Blood Bag/Bottle Should be Checked for the name of recipient and blood group on the label before starting the blood transfusion.

6. Blood Transfusion Should be given at Slow Rate (not more than 20 drops/min). If rapid transfusion is given, citrate present in stored blood may cause chelation of calcium ions leading to decreased serum calcium level and tetany.

7. Proper Aseptic Measures must be taken during transfusion of blood.

8. Careful Watch on Recipient's Condition is a must for the first 10–15 min of starting the transfusion, and from time to time, later. The transfusion must be stopped if there is a rapid rise of temperature (>40°C), or any other reaction.

Hazards of Blood Transfusion

1. Mismatched Transfusion Reactions. Mismatched transfusion reaction is the most serious and potentially fatal hazard of blood transfusion. It is characterized by:

- *Agglutination* of donor's red blood cells in the recipient's circulation.
- *Tissue ischaemia* occurs due to blockage of certain vessels by agglutinated cells. Soon, the patient complains of violent pain in the back or elsewhere and tightness of chest.

- *Haemolysis* of agglutinated red cells occurs rapidly releasing large amounts of haemoglobin in circulation (haemoglobinaemia)
- *Haemolytic jaundice* may occur due to excessive formation of bilirubin from haemoglobin released by haemolyzed RBCs.
- *Renal vasoconstriction* is caused by toxic substances released from the haemolyzed RBCs.
- *Circulatory shock* occurs due to loss of circulating red cells and release of toxic substances leading to fall in arterial blood pressure and decreased renal blood flow.
- *Haemoglobinuria* occurs when total free haemoglobin becomes more than that can bind with haptoglobin (plasma protein binding haemoglobin). The extra free haemoglobin leaks through glomerular membrane and is passed in urine producing haemoglobinuria.
- *Renal tubular damage.* If urine is acidic and glomerular filtration is slow, the free haemoglobin passing through glomeruli is precipitated in the tubules as acid haematin. This obstructs the lumen of tubules producing renal tubular damage.
- *Acute renal shutdown (anuria)* sets in ultimately due to the combined effects of renal vasoconstriction, circulatory shock, hypotension and renal tubular damage. Acute renal shutdown usually occurs within a few minutes to few hours after transfusion of mismatched blood and continues.
- *Uraemia* (increased nitrogenous substances and potassium in the body) results due to acute renal failure, soon producing coma and death.

2. Circulatory Overload due to hypervolaemia may occur following blood transfusion when the transfusion is rapid, especially in patients with cardiac diseases, chronic anaemia and kidney diseases. The rate of transfusion therefore, should not exceed 1 ml/kg body weight 1 h.

3. Transmission of Blood-Borne Infections such as AIDS, viral hepatitis, malaria, syphilis, etc. maybe transmitted to recipient from the infected donor.

4. Pyrogenic Reaction characterized by fever and chills may occur probably due to destruction of leucocytes and platelets by antibodies against them.

5. Allergic Reactions such as skin rashes and asthma may occur if donor blood contains substances to which patient is allergic.

6. Hyperkalaemia may occur after excessive transfusion because K^+ concentration in stored blood is high. Owing to leakage of K^+ from the RBCs into the plasma.

7. Hypocalcaemia producing tetany may occur following massive transfusion of citrated blood. Following rapid and massive transfusion, the citrate cannot be metabolized fully. The extra citrate chelates calcium ions leading to decreased serum calcium levels and tetany. That is why, intravenous calcium gluconate is given with citrated blood transfusion.

8. Reduced Tissue Oxygenation may occur in patients receiving large amounts of transfusion. Red cells in stored blood have very low amounts of 2,3-BPG in them and thus have high affinity for O_2 and consequently tend to give off less O_2 to the tissues. The reduced release of O_2 to tissues can cause serious problems.

9. Haemosiderosis due to iron overload may occur following repeated transfusions, as in thalassaemic patients. The excessive iron is deposited in liver, heart and endocrine organs and produces damage.

10. Thrombophlebitis at the venepuncture site may develop if the needle remains in the same site for many hours.

11. Air embolism, i.e. entry of air into the blood is much less likely to occur because of the use of plastic bags which collapse down as they empty out of blood.

Autologous Blood Transfusion

Autologous blood transfusion refers to transfusion of an individual's own blood which has been withdrawn and stored. Autologous transfusion is done under following situations:

- ***For Elective Surgery,*** a self-predonation is a common practice in some hospitals. After starting a course of iron tablets, two units of blood are collected, one 16 days and another 8 days before surgery. This practice avoids the hazards of transfusion of blood donated by some other individual.

- ***During Surgery,*** the cell-saver machine when used sucks up blood from the wound, recycles it, and returns it to the patient's body.

- ***Some Sportspersons*** are also known to use autologous transfusion a few days before an important event to enhance their performance.

Storage of Blood for Transfusion

Some facts about the storage of donated blood are:

- *One unit of blood* (420 ml) can be collected from a donor at a time under all aseptic measures. An individual can safely donate one unit of blood every 6 months. ACD mixture (120 ml) is added to the blood and stored in a sterile container.
- *Contents of ACD mixture* are:
  - Acid citrate (monohydrous), 0.48 g,
  - Trisodium citrate, 1.32 g and
  - Dextrose 1.47 g
  - Distilled water 100 ml.
- *Dextrose (glucose) present in ACD mixture provides* energy for maintenance of sodium–potassium pump activity. The pump activity is essential for maintaining the size of cells. Therefore, if the glucose is not added to stored blood, the RBCs swell up and haemolyze rapidly. Further, glucose liberates lactic acid, which by decreasing the pH helps in survival of RBCs, both in vitro and in vivo.
- *Anticoagulant activity* is provided by the citrates present in the ACD mixture, which also decreases the pH of blood.

- *Up to 21 days* the blood can be stored under above conditions.
- *The RBCs in the stored blood* swell up due to following changes as a result of decreased cell metabolism in cold storage.
  - *Loss of intracellular* K^+, which increases plasma K^+ concentration from 4–5 to 20–30 mEq/L,
  - *Increase in intracellular* Na^+ from 12 to 30–40 mEq/L,
  - *Increase in intracellular water content.* Because of the above changes, the RBCs become more spherocytic and their haemoglobin in hypotonic solution increases. Such cells may rupture in vitro even in 0.8% NaCl solution. With reference to Na^+ and K^+ content, volume, shape and saline fragility, the RBCs become normal within 48 h of transfusion.
- *WBCs and platelets in stored blood* are virtually absent after 24 h of storage. Therefore, stored blood is not a suitable medium for transferring WBCs and platelets to a recipient.
- *After transfusion of stored blood,* 80% RBCs survive for 24 h, and thereafter, surviving cells are destroyed at a rate of 1% per day.

BLOOD COMPONENTS

The whole blood is routinely collected for transfusion. The most donated blood is processed into its various components:

- Packed Red blood Cells (PRBCs)
- Platelets
- Fresh frozen plasma (FFP)
- Cryoprecipitates
- Plasma derivatives
- WBC concentrates

Whole blood: The whole blood provides oxygen-carrying capacity and volume expansion. Therefore, it is an ideal for patients of acute haemorrhage (> 25% of total volume loss). The whole blood is separated into RBCs and platelet-rich plasma by slow centrifugation. The platelet-rich plasma is then centrifuged at high speed to yield one unit platelets and one unit of fresh frozen plasma (FFP). The cryoprecipitate is produced by thawing FFP to precipitate the plasma proteins and then separated by centrifugation.

Apheresis is technology which is used for collection of multiple units of platelets from single donor and for preparation of various plasma derivatives such as albumin, immunoglobulin, antithrombin and coagulation factor concentrates from pooled plasma from many donors.

1. ***Packed red blood cells (PRBC)*** increase oxygen-carrying capacity. Therefore, used in severely anaemic patients to maintain adequate oxygenation (especially hypoplastic and haemolytic anaemia). The advantage of PRBC over whole blood is:
   a) Circulatory overloading is prevented.
   b) Extra burden of sodium, potassium and other electrolytes on the body system can be prevented.
   c) Plasma can be used for other patients (example: burns).
2. ***Platelets*** are collected either as pools prepared from five to eight random donors (RDs) or as single donor apheresis (SDAPs). These are transfused in patients with thrombocytopenia to reduce the incidence of bleeding. The threshold for prophylactic platelet concentrate transfusion is 5000/μL. Other indications for platelet concentrate transfusion are:
   - Prolonged surgical procedure in which patients' platelets are consumed to stop bleeding.
   - Massive blood transfusions of stored blood (platelets and leucocytes have short life).
   - Leukaemia and lymphoma, because of less production of platelets.
   - Patients receiving chemotherapy/radiotherapy as a treatment for malignancy because anticancer drugs suppress the bone marrow activity.

   Note: Grouping and cross-matching should be done because platelet concentrate is not absolutely free from RBCs.
3. ***Fresh frozen plasma (FFP)*** contains plasma proteins (fibrinogen, albumin, protein C, protein S and antithrombin) and stable factors. Therefore, indications for fresh frozen plasma may be used as plasma for replacement therapy to expand blood volume in conditions where fluid lost from the body (e.g. burns) is massive. The indications for FFP are:
   - For correction of coagulation disorders,
   - In cases of deficient plasma proteins (hypoalbuminemia),
   - Reversal of warfarin effects and
   - Treatment for thrombotic–thrombocytopenic purpura.
4. ***Cryoprecipitate:*** Cryoprecipitate is an ideal source of fibrinogen, factor VIII, and von Willebrand factor (VWF).
5. ***Plasma derivatives:*** Pooled plasma from multiple donors provide specific protein derivatives:
   - Albumin solution is used as a plasma substitute for replacing fluid volume. Also, it acts as volume expander because it stays longer in the circulation due to its high molecular weight.
   - Immunoglobulin preparations are used in:
     - Immunodeficient patients to prevent infections,
     - Anti-D immunoglobulins to prevent the development of endogenous response to Rh antigen (see page 230) and
     - Antisera containing immunoglobulins against Hepatitis B, C, etc.
6. ***WBC concentrates:*** WBC concentrate is prepared from fresh whole blood by leukapheresis. WBC concentrate is used in patients with granulocytopenia and immunodeficiency (occurs due to chemo and radiotherapy) or any other cause where infection becomes unresponsive to antibiotic therapy.

Section 4

Cardiovascular System

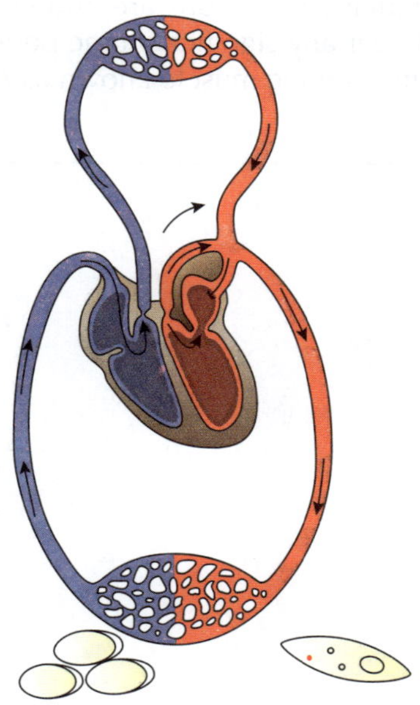

The cardiovascular system (CVS) consists of the heart and the blood vessels. The *heart* acts as a system of two pumps working in series and forms the driving force for blood flow. The blood vessels that take blood from the heart to various tissues are called *arteries*. The smallest arteries are called *arterioles*. Arterioles open into a network of *capillaries*, which constitute the microcirculation. The most important function of blood vessels, i.e. the rapid exchange of materials between the blood and extracellular fluid, bathing the tissue cells is served by the capillaries. In other words, capillaries serve as the *exchange region*. In some situations, capillaries are replaced by slightly different vessels called *sinusoids*. Blood from capillaries (or from sinusoids) is collected by small *venules* which join to form *veins*. Veins serve as the blood reservoir and return the collected blood to the heart.

Functions of CVS

Primary functions of the CVS as a transport system are carried out by *convection* (i.e. the mass movement of fluid caused by a difference in pressure between two points). These functions are:

- Distribution of nutrients and oxygen (O_2) to all body cells and
- Collection of waste products and CO_2 from different body cells and to carry them to excretory organs for excretion.

Secondary functions that are subserved by the CVS are:

1. Thermoregulation by control of blood flow to the skin and extremities to enhance or retard heat loss,
2. Distribution of hormones to the target tissues and
3. Delivery of antibodies, platelets and leucocytes to aid body defence mechanism.

Physiology of CVS

Physiology of CVS includes various aspects of physiology of heart as a pump and physiology of two main divisions of blood circulation – the pulmonary and systemic circulation.

- The heart consists of two pumps in series (right and left halves) that are connected by pulmonary and systemic circulation.
- In systemic circulation, the various systemic organs receive blood through parallel distribution channels. The parallel arrangement of vessels supply the body organs with blood of the same arterial composition (i.e. same O_2 and CO_2 tension, pH, glucose level) and essentially the same arterial pressure.
- Since the pulmonary and systemic circulation divisions are arranged in series, both ventricles must pump the same amount of blood over any significant time period. Such a balanced output is achieved by an intrinsic property of the cardiac muscle known as *Frank–Starling mechanism*.

Chapter 4.1

Functional Anatomy of Heart and Physiology of Cardiac Muscle

FUNCTIONAL ANATOMY OF HEART

The heart is a muscular pump designed to ensure the circulation of blood through the tissues of the body. The human heart weighs approximately 300 g and it consists of two halves, right and left, both structurally and functionally. The right half circulates blood through the lungs for the purpose of oxygenation (i.e. through pulmonary circulation). The left heart circulates blood to tissues of the entire body (i.e. through the systemic circulation).

Chambers of Heart

Each half of the heart consists of an inflow chamber called the *atrium* and an outflow chamber called the *ventricle* (Fig. 4.1-1). Thus, there are four chambers in the heart.

Atria

- ***Interatrial septum*** separates the right and left atria which are thin-walled chambers.
- ***Right atrium*** receives deoxygenated blood from tissues of the entire body through the *superior and inferior venae cavae.* This blood passes into the right ventricle through the right *atrioventricular orifice* which is guarded by *tricuspid valve.* The right atrium has got the pacemaker known as *sinoatrial node* that produces cardiac impulses and *atrioventricular (AV)* node that conducts these impulses to the ventricles.
- ***Left atrium*** receives oxygenated blood from the lungs through the four *pulmonary veins* (two rights and two lefts). This blood passes into left ventricle through the *left AV orifice* which is guarded by the mitral valve.

Ventricles

- ***Interventricular septum*** separates the right ventricle from left ventricle.
- ***Interior of each ventricle*** has an inflow part and an outflow part. The inflow part of each ventricle is a rough inner surface because of the presence of numerous bundles of cardiac muscles called *trabeculae carnae. Papillary muscles* are finger-like processes attached to the ventricular wall at one end, but free at the other. They are functionally related to the AV valves.
- ***Right ventricle*** receives blood from the right atrium and pumps through the pulmonary trunk (which divides into right and left pulmonary arteries) into the lungs. The *pulmonary valve* is present at the junction of right ventricle and pulmonary trunk.
- ***Left ventricle*** receives blood from the left atrium and pumps out into systemic circulation through the aorta. *Aortic* valve is present at the junction of left ventricle and the *ascending aorta.*

Valves of Heart

There are four valves in human heart, two AV valves and two semilunar valves. Valves allow unidirectional flow of blood.

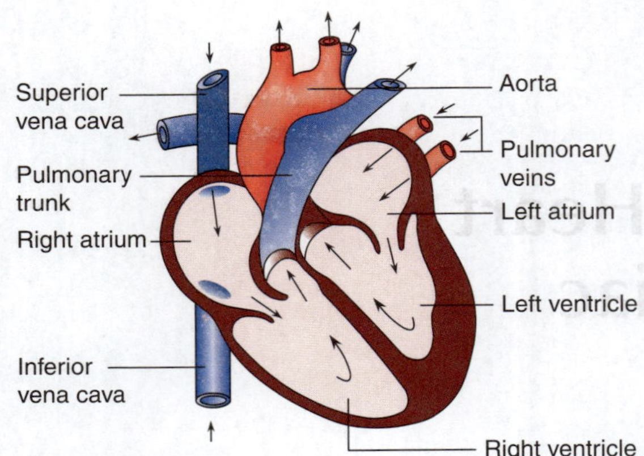

FIGURE 4.1-1 Schematic diagram of the heart to show its chambers.

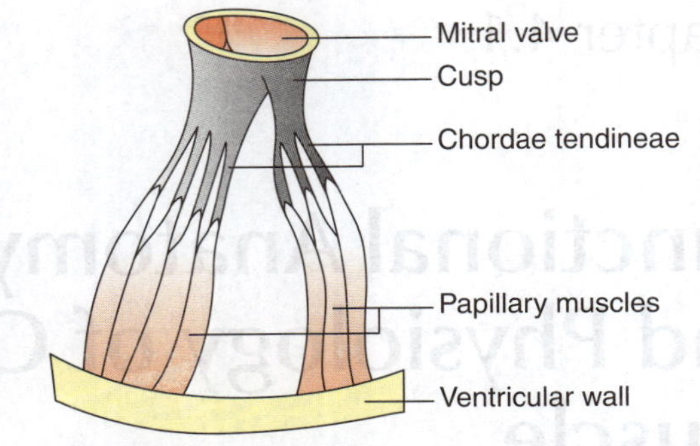

FIGURE 4.1-3 Bicuspid valve attached with papillary muscles and chordae tendineae.

AV Valves The AV valves open towards the ventricles and close towards the atria. They allow blood to flow from atria to ventricles. But when ventricles contract, they are closed, and thus prevent backflow of blood from ventricles to atria.

- ***Right AV valve*** is known as *tricuspid valve* and is made of 3 cusps: anterior, posterior and septal (Fig. 4.1-2).
- ***The left AV valve*** is called *mitral valve* or *bicuspid valve* and is made of 2 cusps: anterior and posterior (Figs. 4.1-2, 4.1-3).
- At the periphery, the cusps (flaps) of the AV valves are attached to the *AV ring,* which is a fibrous connection between the atria and ventricles. The free edges of the cusps are attached to *papillary muscles* through the cord-like structures called the *chordae tendineae* (Fig. 4.1-3).
- ***Papillary muscles*** arise from the inner surface of ventricles and contract when the ventricular walls contract. They do not help the valves to close but prevent the bulging of the valves into the atria when ventricles contract. Therefore, in the event of paralysis of papillary muscles or rupture of chordae tendineae the AV valve bulges (into the atria), and there occurs regurgitation of blood into the atria during systole when ventricles contract.

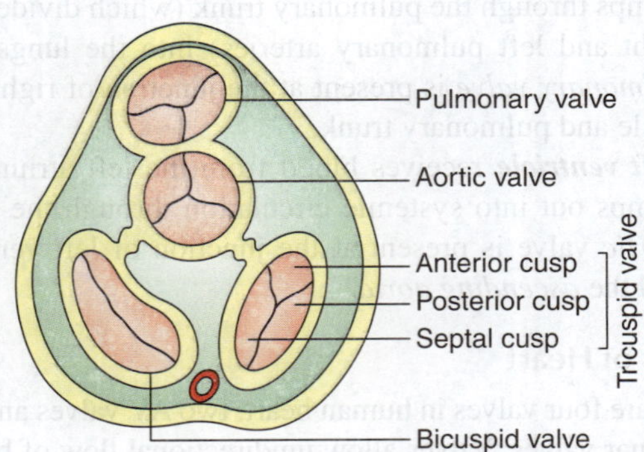

FIGURE 4.1-2 Valves of the heart.

Semilunar Valves

- ***Aortic valve*** is the semilunar valve present at the opening of aorta in left ventricle. It is made of three semilunar cusps: one anterior and two posterior (Figs. 4.1-4, 4.1-5).
- ***Pulmonary valve*** is the semilunar valve present at the opening of pulmonary trunk into the right ventricle. It is also made of three semilunar cusps: one posterior and two anterior (Fig. 4.1-4).
- ***Semilunar valves open*** away from ventricles and close towards the ventricles. These valves open when ventricles contract allowing the blood to flow from left ventricle to aorta and from right ventricle to pulmonary trunk.
- ***Semilunar valves close*** when ventricles relax, thus preventing backflow of blood from aorta or pulmonary trunk into the ventricles.

Structure of the Walls of Heart

Walls of the heart are composed of a thick layer of cardiac muscles, the *myocardium* (see page 240), covered

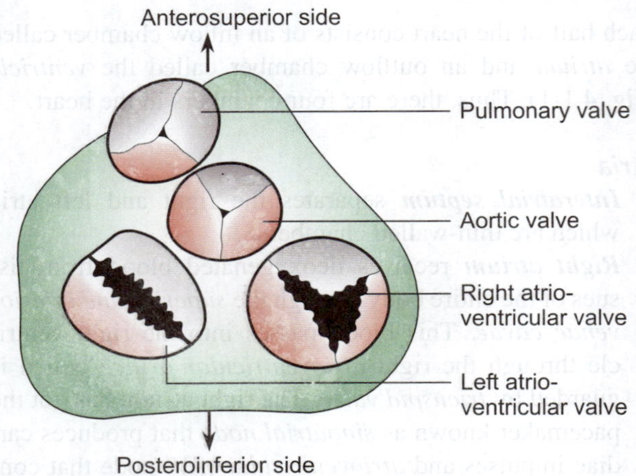

FIGURE 4.1-4 Semilunar valves and atrioventricular valves viewed from the posterosuperior aspect after removing the atria.

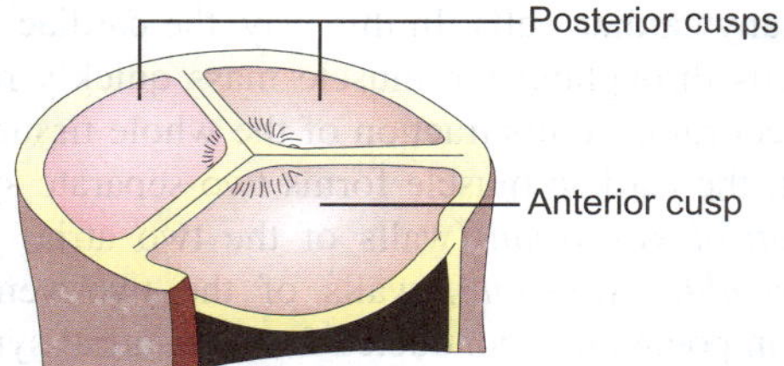

FIGURE 4.1-5 Aortic valve.

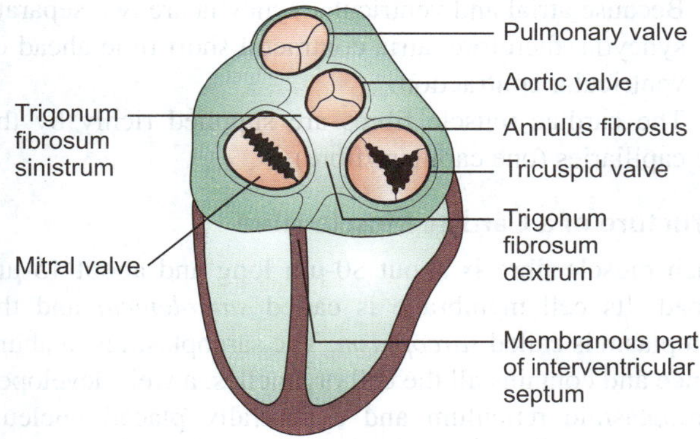

FIGURE 4.1-6 Skeleton of the heart.

externally by the epicardium and lined internally by the *endocardium*.

- Walls of the atrial portion of the heart are thin.
- Walls of the ventricular portion of the heart are thick.

Skeleton of the heart (Fig. 4.1-6) consists of fibrous rings that surround the AV, pulmonary and aortic orifices and are continuous with the membranous part of the ventricular septum. The fibrous rings around the AV orifices separate the muscular walls of the atria from those of the ventricles but provide attachment for the muscle fibres. The fibrous rings support the bases of the valve cusps and prevent the valves from stretching and becoming incompetent.

Pericardium. The heart and roots of the great vessels are enclosed by a fibroserous sac called pericardium. Its function is to restrict excessive movements of the heart as a whole and to serve as a lubricated container in which different parts of the heart can contract. Pericardium consists of two layers: outer fibrous and inner serous (Fig. 4.1-7A and B).

- ***Fibrous pericardium*** surrounds the heart like a bag and is attached with the surrounding structures.
- ***Serous pericardium*** has parietal and visceral layers. The *parietal layer* of serous pericardium lines the fibrous pericardium and is reflected around the roots of the great vessels to become continuous with the *visceral layer of serous pericardium* that closely cover the heart and is often called the *epicardium.* The slit-like space between the parietal and visceral layers of the serous pericardium is called *pericardial cavity* which contains small amount of *pericardial fluid* that acts as a lubricant to facilitate the movement of the heart.

Myocardium The myocardium (muscular tissue of the heart) is the main tissue constituting the walls of the heart. It consists of three types of muscle fibres:

- *Cardiac muscles* forming the walls of the atria and ventricles – contractile unit of the heart (see page 240),
- Muscle fibres forming the *pacemaker* which is the site of origin of cardiac impulse (see page 252) and
- Muscle fibres forming the conducting system which transmits the impulse to the various parts of the heart (see page 253).

Endocardium Endocardium is a thin, smooth and glistening membrane lining the myocardium internally. It consists of a single layer of endothelial cells. The endocardium continues as the endothelium of great vessels opening in the heart.

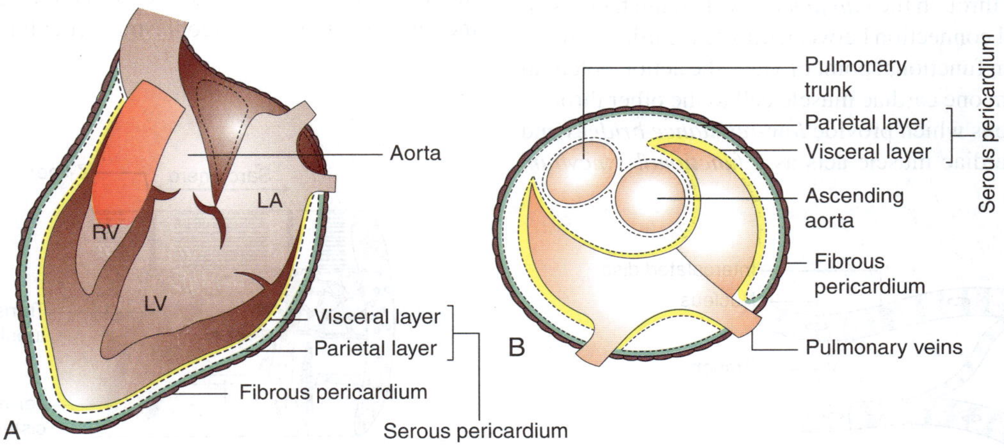

FIGURE 4.1-7 Schematic sagittal section of the heart showing fibrous and serous pericardium (**A**) and transverse section through upper part of the heart and pericardium (**B**).

PHYSIOLOGY OF CARDIAC MUSCLE

Functional Anatomy

The myocardium consists of three types of muscle fibres:

- *Cardiac muscles* forming the walls of atria and ventricles (contractile unit of the heart),
- Muscle fibres forming the *pacemaker* which is the site of origin of cardiac impulse and
- Muscle fibres forming the *conductive system* which transmits the impulse to the various parts of the heart.

This chapter is mainly devoted to physiology of cardiac muscles forming the walls of atria and ventricles.

Structural Organization of Cardiac Muscle

- The cardiac muscle fibres are *striated* and resemble quite a lot to skeletal muscle fibres in structure. However, unlike the skeletal muscles, the cardiac muscles are *involuntary* (like smooth muscles). Thus cardiac muscles share some characteristics with skeletal muscles and some with smooth muscles.
- The cardiac muscle fibres are *ribbon like* rather than cylindrical. These are *branched* and interdigitate freely with each other, but each fibre is a complete separate unit. The branches from the neighbouring fibres join together. At the point of contact of two muscle fibres, the membranes of both muscle fibres are fused together and thrown into extensive infolding forming the so-called *intercalated disc* (Fig. 4.1-8). These discs form tight junctions between the muscle fibres and do not allow the ions to pass through. However, the intercalated discs provide a strong union between fibres and thus play an important role during contraction of muscle fibres by transmitting the pull of one contractile unit along its axis to the next, thereby increasing the force of contraction.
- Along the sides near the outer border of intercalated disc, the two adjacent muscle fibres are connected with each other through the *gap junctions.* Though there is no anatomical connection between different cardiac muscle fibres, from functional point of view, the action potential passes from one cardiac muscle cell to the other through gap junctions which provide *low-resistance bridges* and thus the cardiac muscle acts as a *functional syncytium* of many cardiac cells. In this way, the cardiac impulse spreads throughout the muscle mass quickly resulting in a coordinated contraction of the whole tissue. In the heart, the cardiac muscle forms two separate syncytia, the *atrial syncytium* (walls of the two atria) and the *ventricular syncytium* (walls of the two ventricles). Action potential is conducted from the atrial syncytium to ventricular syncytium by way of specialized conducting system. Each syncytium obeys all or none of the law. Because atrial and ventricular syncytia are two separate syncytia, therefore, atria contract a short time ahead of ventricular contraction.
- The cardiac muscle fibres are supplied richly by the capillaries (one capillary/fibre).

Structure of a Cardiac Muscle Fibre

Each muscle fibre is about 80-μm long and about 15-μm broad. Its cell membrane is called *sarcolemma* and the cytoplasm is called *sarcoplasm.* The sarcoplasm is in abundance and contains all the cell organelles, a well-developed sarcoplasmic reticulum and a centrally placed nucleus. Each muscle fibre is made up of a number of *myofibrils* which lie parallel to each other. Each myofibril is 2 μm in diameter.

Myofibril. Each myofibril consists of thick and thin filaments. Essentially the structure and striations seen under a light microscope and a detailed electron microscope is similar to that of a skeletal muscle (see page 85).

Sarcotubular System

The sarcotubular system in cardiac muscles is well developed like that of skeletal muscles (page 88). However, the tubules of the T-system penetrate the sarcomere at Z-line (Fig. 4.1-9) and not at the junction of A and I bands (as in skeletal muscles). Therefore, in cardiac muscles, there is only one triad per sarcomere as compared to two in skeletal muscles (page 88). Further, the tubules are much wider than in skeletal muscles and typical triads are not always present. They are often replaced by dyads having one T-tubule and one cistern of the sarcoplasmic reticulum (L-tubule).

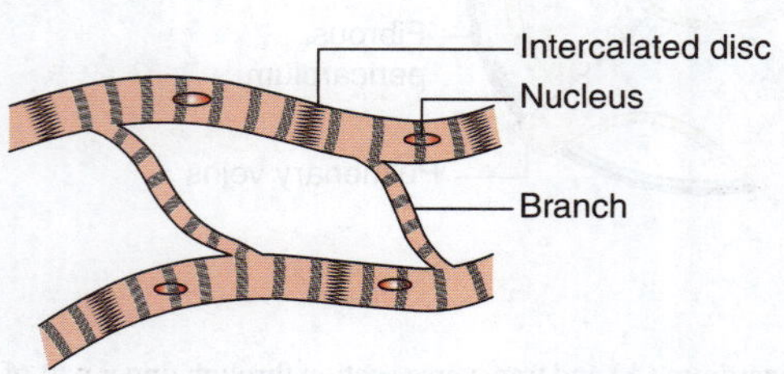

FIGURE 4.1-8 Structure of cardiac muscle.

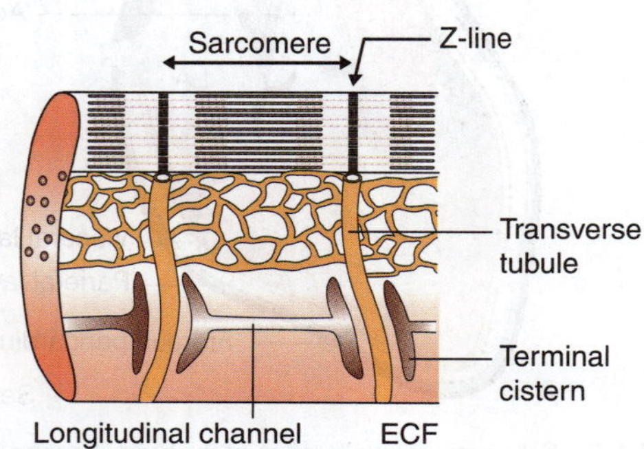

FIGURE 4.1-9 Sarcotubular system in the cardiac muscle.

Process of Excitability and Contractility: An Electromechanical Phenomenon

The cardiac muscle being an excitable tissue produces an action potential (*electrical phenomenon*) when stimulated and responds by contracting (*mechanical phenomenon*). The events which link the electrical phenomenon with mechanical phenomenon constitute the *excitation–contraction coupling phenomenon.* These three phenomena are discussed separately. As discussed earlier, the cardiac muscles comprise working myocardial cells or the contractile myocardial cells (CMC), pacemaker and conducting tissue. The present discussion is limited to activities in the CMC.

Electrical Potentials in Cardiac Muscle

Resting Membrane Potential The resting membrane potential (RMP) of a normal cardiac muscle fibre is −85 to −95 mV (negative interior with reference to exterior).

Action Potential When stimulated, each cardiac muscle fibre shows an electrical activity known as propagated action potential. It is different from the electrocardiogram, which refers to extracellular recording of the summed electrical events of all the cardiac muscle fibres generated with each heart beat (see page 253).

The action potential recorded from a single cardiac muscle fibre is unusually long and can be divided into five distinct phases (Fig. 4.1-10) as follows:

- ***Phase 0: Rapid Depolarization.*** The phase 0 (upstroke) is characterized by the depolarization which proceeds rapidly, an overshoot is present, as in skeletal muscle and nerve. In mammalian heart, depolarization lasts about 2 ms. In this phase, amplitude of potential reaches up to +20 to +30 mV (positive interior with reference to exterior).

  Ionic basis. The initial rapid depolarization and the overshoot are due to the rapid opening of voltage-gated Na^+ channels and rapid influx of Na^+ ions similar to that occurring in nerve and skeletal muscle.
  At −30- to −40-mV membrane potential, the calcium channels also open up and influx of Ca^{2+} ions also contributes in this phase.
  Note: Tetradotoxin (TT_X) is a specific blocker of sodium channels, acts as a very potent poison, because it blocks the influx of sodium ions, hence no excitation of cardiac muscle fibres and therefore, no contraction.

- ***Phase 1: Initial Rapid Repolarization.*** Rapid depolarization is followed by a very short-lived slight rapid repolarization. The membrane potential reaches from +30 mV to −10 mV during this phase.

  Ionic basis. The initial rapid repolarization is due to closure of Na^+ channels and opening of K^+ channels resulting in transient outward current.

- ***Phase 2: Plateau.*** During plateau phase, the cardiac muscle fibre remains in the depolarized state. The membrane potential falls very slowly only to −40 mV during this phase. The plateau lasts for about 100–200 ms. This plateau in action potential explains the 5–15 times longer contraction time of the cardiac muscle as compared to the skeletal muscle.

  Ionic basis. Very slow repolarization during the plateau phase is due to:
  - Slow influx of Ca^{2+} ions resulting from opening of sarcolemmal *L-type Ca^{2+}* channels, and
  - Closure of a distinct set of K^+ channels called the inward-rectifying K^+ channels.

- ***Phase 3: Repolarization.*** During this phase, complete repolarization occurs and the membrane potential falls to the approximate resting value of −80 mV. This phase lasts for about 50 ms.

  Ionic basis. The slow repolarization results from closing of Ca^{2+} channels and opening of following two types of K^+ channels.
  - *Delayed outward rectifying K^+ channels,* which are voltage-gated and are activated slowly and
  - *Ca^{2+}-activated channels* which are activated by the elevated sarcoplasmic Ca^{2+} levels.

- ***Phase 4: Resting Potential.*** In this phase of RMP (also called as polarized state), the potential is maintained at −90 mV.

  Ionic basis. The RMP is maintained by a resting K^+ current, the largest contributor to which is the inward rectifying K^+ current.

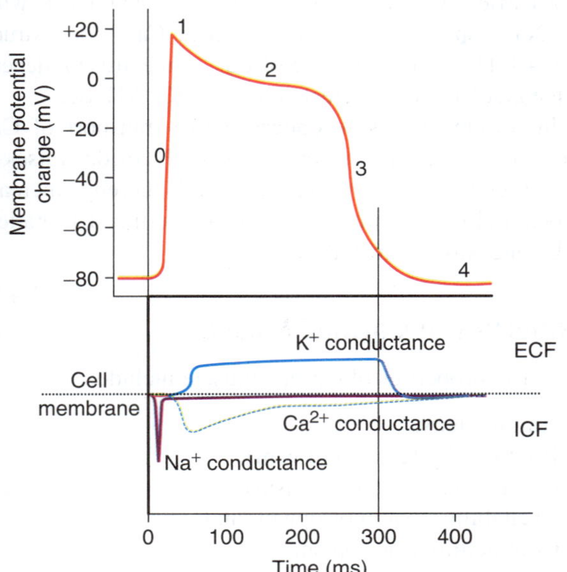

FIGURE 4.1-10 Various phases of action potential and ion conductance: Phase 0 = depolarization; Phase 1 = rapid repolarization; Phase 2 = plateau phase; Phase 3 = late rapid repolarization and Phase 4 = resting potential.

Duration of Action Potential. The duration of action potential (primarily repolarization is about 250 ms) at a heart rate of 75 beats/min. The duration of action potential decreases with increased heart rate (150 ms at a heart rate of 200 beats/min). It is shorter in the atrial muscle. This type of action potential found in CMCs of the ventricles is referred to as *fast response*.

Spread of Action Potential through Cardiac Muscles. As discussed in functional anatomy, the cardiac muscle acts as a physiological syncytium due to the presence of gap junctions amongst the cardiac muscle fibres. Because of this, the action potential spreads through the cardiac muscles very rapidly. Further, as there are two syncytia (the atrial and the ventricular) in the heart, the action potential is transmitted from atria to ventricles only through the fibres of specialized conductive system.

Excitation–Contraction Coupling Phenomenon in Cardiac Muscles Excitation–contraction coupling refers to the sequence of events by which an excited plasma membrane of a muscle fibre leads to cross-bridge activity by increasing sarcoplasmic calcium concentration.

The sequence of events during excitation–contraction coupling in the cardiac muscles is similar to those observed in a skeletal muscle (see page 89), with the following exception:

In cardiac muscles (as against that in skeletal muscles), extra calcium ions diffuse into the sarcoplasm from T-tubules without which the contraction strength would be considerably reduced. The T-tubules of cardiac muscle contain mucopolysaccharides which are negatively charged and bind an abundant store of calcium ions. T-tubules open directly to the exterior and therefore, Ca^{2+} ions in them directly come from extracellular fluid. These Ca^{2+} ions diffuse into the sarcoplasm when action potential propagates along the T-tubules (Fig. 4.1-11A and B). Because of this, strength of cardiac muscle contraction depends to a great extent on Ca^{2+} concentration in ECF. Whereas, skeletal muscle contraction is hardly affected by the calcium concentration in ECF.

Process of Cardiac Muscle Contraction

The molecular mechanism of cardiac muscle contraction by cross-bridge cycling and sliding of filaments is primarily similar to that of skeletal muscles (page 89) and smooth muscles (page 117). However, its regulation shows features of both the skeletal and smooth muscles.

- Troponin–tropomyosin complex controls the onset and offset of cross-bridge cycling, similar to that in the skeletal muscles and
- Like smooth muscles, the contractility of cardiac muscle is sensitive to *phosphorylation*.

Relaxation of Cardiac Muscle

Relaxation of cardiac muscle (diastole) occurs when levels of Ca^{2+} ions fall in the cardiac muscle fibres. During diastole,

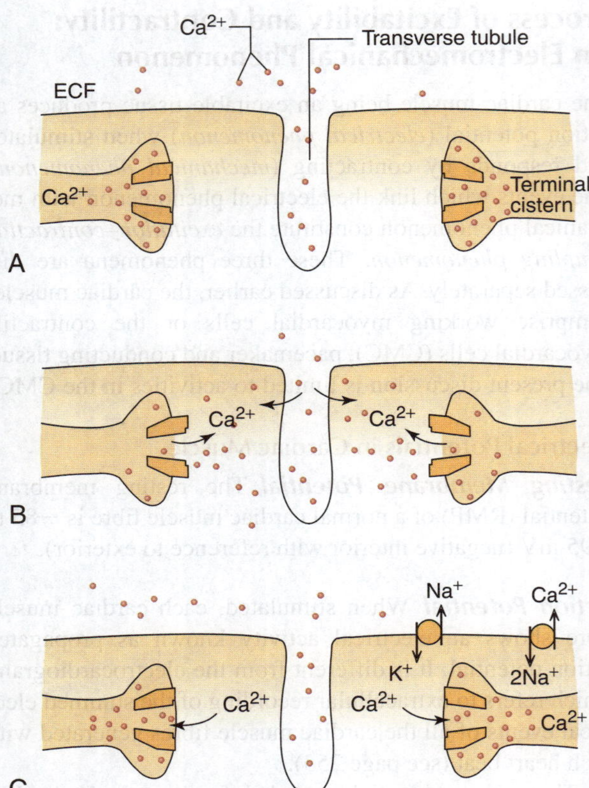

FIGURE 4.1-11 Dynamics of Ca^{2+} during excitation–contraction coupling phenomenon and relaxation in cardiac muscle. **A,** in resting state; **B,** calcium-induced calcium release during excitation and contraction state; **C,** during relaxation state.

the Ca^{2+} ions are extruded out of the cardiac muscle fibre by a carrier system operating at the sarcolemma in which two Na^+ ions are exchanged for each Ca^{2+} ion extruded (Fig. 4.1-11C). Thus, the rate of Ca^{2+} ion extrusion depends on the gradient of Na^+ created by Na^+-K^+ ATPase.

Inhibition of this secondary active transport of Ca^{2+} ions, e.g. by digitalis or other cardiac glycosides raises the intracellular Ca^{2+} concentration and thereby increases myocardial contractility. This effect is utilized in patients with congestive heart failure.

Properties of Cardiac Muscle

The basic properties of cardiac muscle include:

- Automaticity,
- Rhythmicity (chronotropism),
- Conductivity (dromotropism),
- Excitability (bathmotropism) and
- Contractility (inotropism).

Some of the properties of cardiac muscle, viz automaticity, rhythmicity and conductivity are discussed in Chapter 4.2 (see page 248).

The characteristics of excitability and contractility are described here.

Excitability

Excitability (bathmotropism) is the property by which tissues respond to stimuli. The cardiac muscle responds by depolarization (development of action potential). The essential features of the RMP and action potential of cardiac muscle have been discussed on page 241.

One of the characteristics of cardiac muscle excitability which needs a special emphasis is its refractory period.

Refractory Period Refractory period refers to the period following action potential during which the cardiac muscle does not respond to a stimulus. Cardiac muscle has a long refractory period (250–300 ms in ventricles and about 150 ms in atria). It is of two types as follows.

1. Absolute Refractory Period (ARP). During this period the cardiac muscle does not show any response at all. It extends from phase 0 to half of phase 3 of action potential, i.e. until the membrane potential reaches approximately 50 mV during repolarization (Fig. 4.1-12). Normal duration of ARP in ventricles is about 180–200 ms.

2. Relative Refractory Period (RRP). During this period the muscle shows response if the strength of stimulus is increased to maximum. It extends from second half of the phase 3 to phase 4 of the action potential. Normal duration of RRP in ventricles is about 50 ms.

Significance of Long Refractory Period in Cardiac Muscle. As shown in Fig. 4.1-12, the cardiac muscle is refractory to any stimulus during the contraction phase (systole), therefore, the complete summation of contractions and thus tetanus cannot be produced in the cardiac muscle. This property is very useful. Since the heart has to function as a pump, it must relax, get filled up with blood and then contract to pump out the blood. A tetanized heart would be useless as a pump.

Experimental Demonstration of Refractory Period in Heart. Experimental demonstration of refractory period in heart can be done both in a beating heart as well as in a quiescent heart.

Refractory period in a beating heart of a pithed frog can be demonstrated during recording of a cardiogram. As shown in Fig. 4.1-13, *when the electrical stimulus is applied to the base of ventricle during systole,* no response is seen, depicting thereby that the heart is in ARP during systole.

- *When the stimulus is applied during diastole*, the heart responds by premature contraction producing *extra systole* followed by a *compensatory pause.* The total duration of the extra systole and the compensatory pause is equivalent to the duration of two cardiac cycles. These events can be explained as:
  - When the stimulus is applied during diastole, the premature contraction occurs since the heart is in the phase of *RRP.*
  - The natural impulse from the sinus venosus arrives at the time of premature contraction (ARP) and cannot produce contraction and thus the heart has to wait for the arrival of the next natural impulse. The heart stops during this period in relaxation producing the so-called *compensatory pause.*

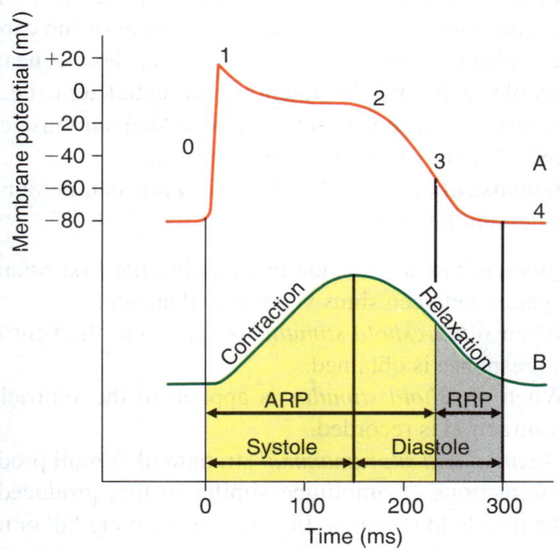

FIGURE 4.1-12 Record of action potential (A) and mechanical response (B) from the cardiac muscle fibre shown on same time scale depicting the significance of long refractory period. ARP, absolute refractory period; RRP, relative refractory period.

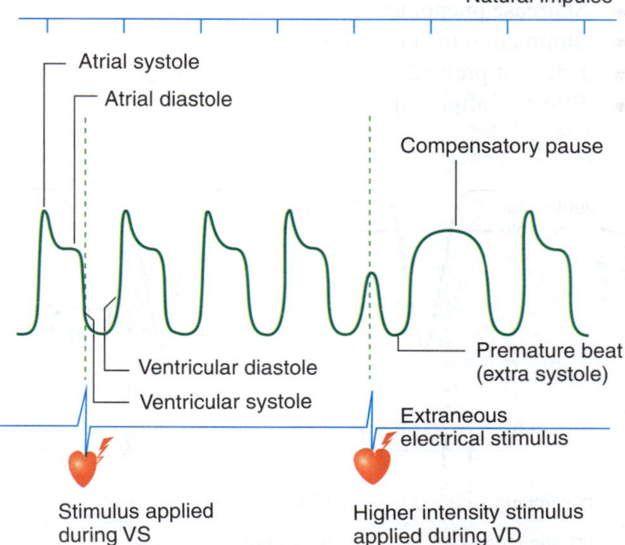

FIGURE 4.1-13 Demonstration of refractory period in beating heart of a frog. VS, ventricular systole; VD: ventricular diastole.

Refractory period in a quiescent heart can be demonstrated as:

- The heart is made quiescent by applying the first *Stannius ligature* between the sinus venosus and the right auricle.
- An electrical stimulus is applied at the base of the ventricle to stimulate the heart which starts contracting. When another stimulus is applied immediately after the first (i.e. during systole phase), the heart does not show any response, indicating that during contraction (systole), heart is in ARP (Fig. 4.1-14).
- When the second stimulus is applied during diastole the heart responds producing extra systole and the compensatory pause (Fig. 4.1-14), indicating that heart is in the state of *RRP* during diastole.

Contractility

Contractility is the ability of the cardiac muscle to actively generate force to shorten and thicken to do work when sufficient stimulus is applied.

Process of myocardial contractility is discussed on page 246.

Mechanical response in cardiac muscle fibre begins just after the start of depolarization and lasts about 1.5 times as long as the action potential (Fig. 4.1-15B). Thus the mechanical response (300 ms) overlaps the electrical response (200 ms) for the whole period. This is in contrast to skeletal muscle, where the mechanical response begins a few milliseconds after the end of repolarization and lasts for 30–50 ms in mammalian skeletal muscle and 100 ms in amphibian skeletal muscle (Fig. 4.1-15A).

Characteristic features of myocardial contractility and factors affecting are:

- All or none law,
- Staircase phenomenon,
- Summation of subminimal stimuli,
- Effect of preload,
- Effect of afterload,

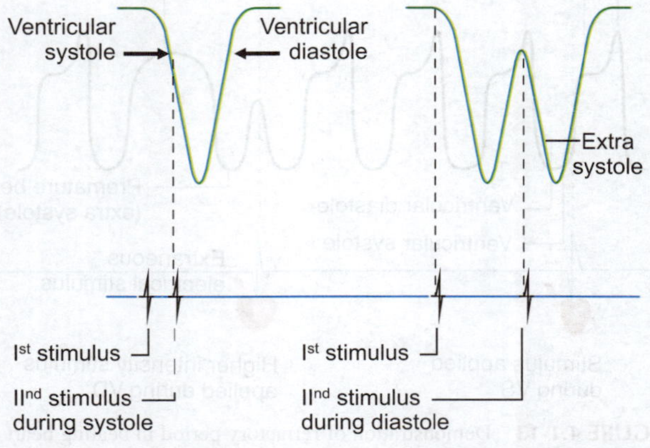

FIGURE 4.1-14 Refractory period in quiescent heart of a frog.

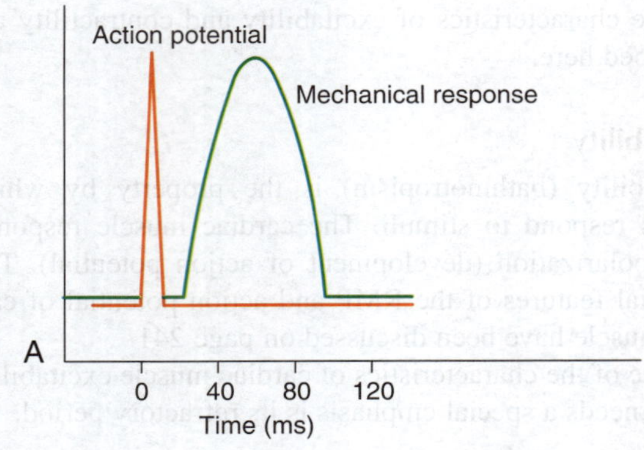

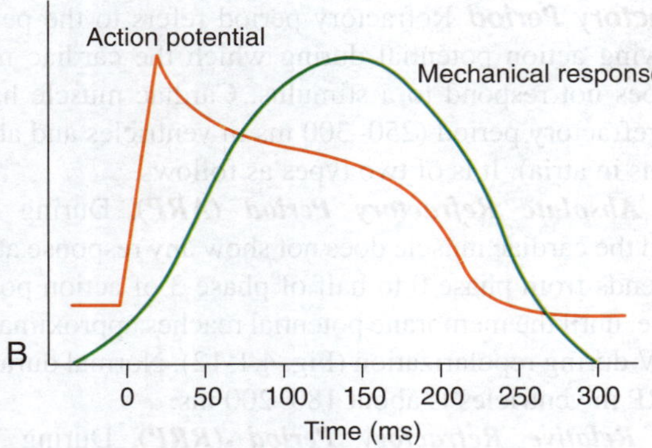

FIGURE 4.1-15 Relationship of action potential and mechanical response (A) in skeletal muscle and (B) in cardiac muscle.

- Effect of ions (see page 271) and
- Effect of temperature (see page 104).

1. All or None Law The response of the cardiac muscle to a stimulus is all or none in character, i.e. when a stimulus is applied, either the heart does not contract at all (none response) or contracts to its maximum ability (all response). This is because of the syncytial arrangement of the cardiac muscle fibres. Therefore, the 'all or none' law in heart is applicable to the whole functional syncytial unit, i.e. the entire atria or entire ventricle. While in skeletal muscles, it is applicable only to a single muscle fibre.

Demonstration of 'All and None' Law can be done in the quiescent heart of frog as:

- *Quiescent heart* is made by applying the first Stannius ligature between sinus venosus and atrium.
- When *subthreshold stimulus* is applied to the ventricle, no response is obtained.
- When *threshold stimulus* is applied to the ventricle, a contraction is recorded.
- *Maximal and supramaximal* strength of stimuli produce contractions of amplitude similar to that produced by the threshold stimulus (Fig. 4.1-16), proving 'all or none law' property of the cardiac muscle.

2. Staircase Phenomenon (Treppe) Staircase phenomenon or effect refers to the successive increase in the force of

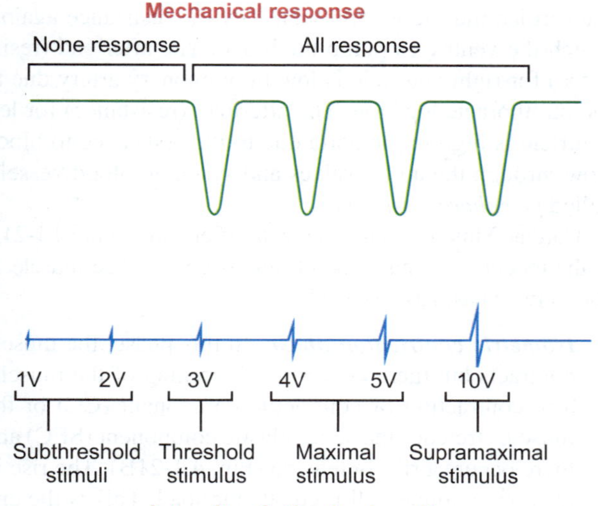

FIGURE 4.1-16 Demonstration of all or none law in quiescent heart of a frog.

cardiac contractions in the first few (4–5) contractions after the quiescent heart starts beating, e.g. as seen after vagal stimulation (Fig. 4.1-17). This is because of the beneficial effect.

Cause of Beneficial Effect. When the heart stops, there occurs an increase in Na^+ and a decrease in K^+ concentration inside the cell, which increases Ca^{2+} influx. Thus, there occurs a progressive increase in the Ca^{2+} concentration in sarcoplasm due to the increase in Ca^{2+} influx with each action potential. This produces a progressive increase in the strength of the few (4–5) cardiac muscle contractions.

Demonstration of Staircase Phenomenon can be done in the quiescent heart of frog as:

- *Quiescent heart* is made by applying the first Stannius ligature between sinus venosus and atria.
- *Ventricle is stimulated* repeatedly at intervals of 2 s without changing the strength of the stimulus.
- *Graph obtained* (Fig. 4.1-18) will show that in the first few contractions, the force of contraction is increased and then it remains constant. This is called staircase phenomenon or treppe (German word for staircase).

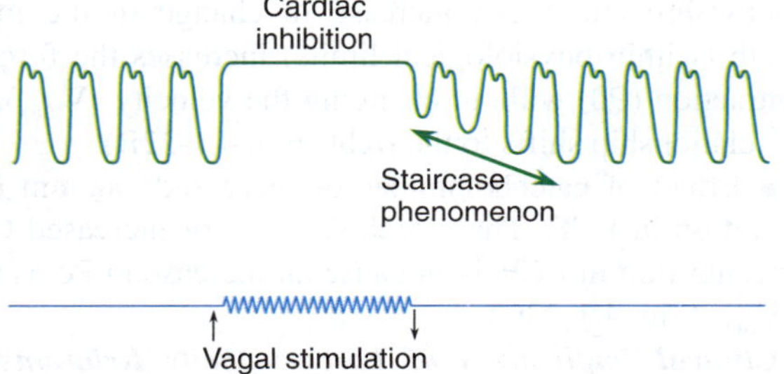

FIGURE 4.1-17 Staircase phenomenon (treppe) in cardiac muscle after vagal stimulation in frog.

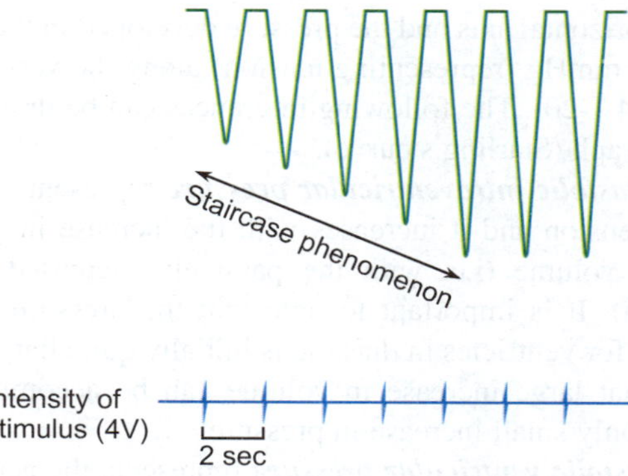

FIGURE 4.1-18 Demonstration of staircase phenomenon in quiescent heart of a frog.

3. Summation of Subminimal Stimuli When a subthreshold stimulus is applied to the quiescent heart, there occurs no response. However, when subthreshold stimuli are applied repeatedly at an interval of one half to one second, there occurs a contraction of the heart after about 10 to 20 stimuli. This phenomenon is called *temporal summation* of subminimal stimuli (Fig. 4.1-19).

4. Effect of Preload A load which starts acting on a muscle before it starts to contract is called *preload.* The preload increases the initial length of the muscle. According to Starling's law, the force of contraction is the function of the initial length of the muscle fibres; and up to physiological limits the greater the initial length, greater is the force of contraction. In the case of heart muscles, the end diastolic volume forms the preload. The effect of changing end diastolic volume on force of cardiac contraction has been studied by Frank and Starling in 1910. *The Frank–Starling law of heart* states that within physiological limits the force of cardiac contraction is proportional to its end diastolic volume.

Length–Tension Relationship. Length–tension relationship, i.e. the relation between initial fibre length and total tension in cardiac muscle is basically similar to that in skeletal muscle (see page 101). In cardiac muscles, the length–tension relationship graph is plotted with the end diastolic volume in ml (representing initial length) along

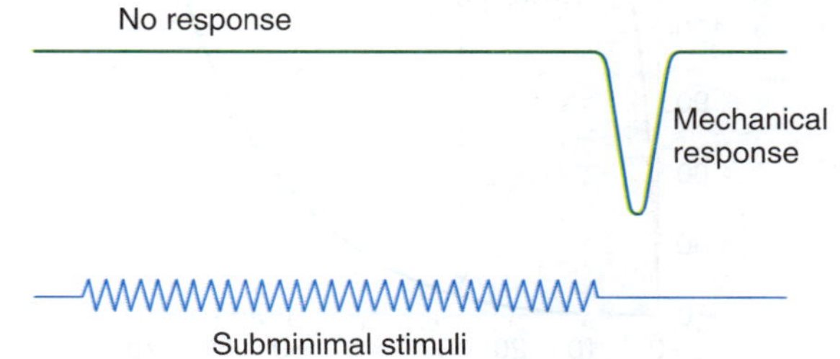

FIGURE 4.1-19 Temporal summation of subminimal stimuli in quiescent heart of a frog.

the horizontal axis and the pressure developed in the ventricle in mmHg (representing tension) along the vertical axis (Fig. 4.1-20). The following inferences can be drawn from this graph (Starling's curve).

Diastolic intraventricular pressure represents the passive tension and it increases with the increase in end diastolic volume (i.e. with the passively increased muscle length). It is important to note that the pressure–volume curve for ventricles in diastole is initially quite flat, indicating that large increase in volume can be accommodated with only small increase in pressure.

Systolic ventricular pressure represents the active tension developed (isometric tension) which is proportionate to the degree of diastolic filling of the heart (initial length of muscle fibres). The graph (Fig. 4.1-20) shows that the developed tension increases as the diastolic volume increases until it reaches a maximum (ascending limb of Starling curve), then tends to decrease (descending limb of Starling's curve). However, unlike skeletal muscle, the decrease in developed tension at high degrees of stretch is not due to decreased number of cross-bridges between actin and myosin, because even severely dilated hearts are not stretched to this degree. The descending limb is instead due to beginning of disruption of the myocardial fibres.

Clinical Significance of Frank–Starling Law of Heart and its role in control of cardiac output is discussed in Chapter 4.3 (see page 290).

5. Effect of Afterload Afterload refers to the load which acts on the muscle after the beginning of muscular contraction. The afterload affecting the force of contraction of

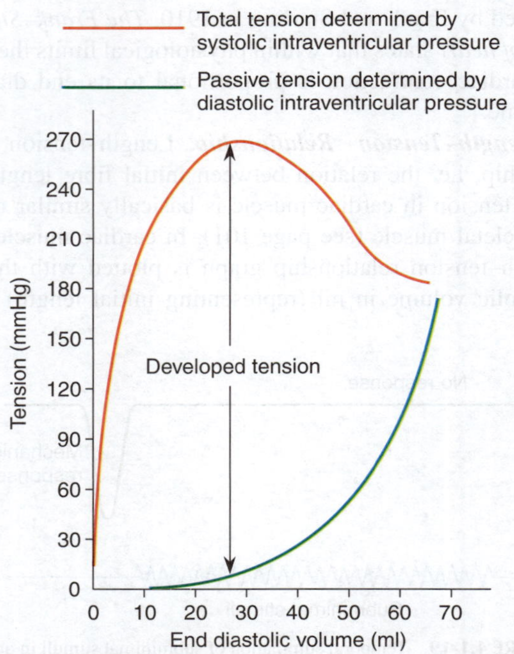

FIGURE 4.1-20 Length–tension relationship in cardiac muscle.

the cardiac muscle is represented by the resistance against which the ventricles pump the blood. The afterload (resistance) for right ventricle is low in pulmonary artery due to its intrathoracic location. The afterload (resistance) for left ventricle is high in the aorta due to the resistance to blood flow through the aortic valves and systemic blood vessels, called *peripheral resistance*.

Cardiac Muscle Contraction with Afterload. Figure 4.1-21A is the model for contraction of afterloaded cardiac muscle. It shows two phases as given below.

- ***Isometric contraction phase.*** In this phase, the muscle contracts but there occurs no shortening of the muscle. The contraction of contractile component (CC) of the muscle stretches the series elastic component (SEC) and there occurs a rise in tension (Fig. 4.1-21B). The rise in tension continues till it equals the load. This is the end point of isometric contraction.
  Isotonic contraction phase starts when the muscle tension exceeds the load starts moving. There occurs shortening of the muscle without further stretching of SEC (Fig. 4.1-21C). The performance of CC is given by the force–velocity relationship.

• ***Force–Velocity Relationship.*** The force–velocity curve is plotted by noting the velocity of muscle contraction with progressively increasing the load on the muscle. In the heart, the load is represented by the resistance against which the ventricles pump the blood and velocity of muscle contraction is represented by the stroke output. Following inferences can be drawn from the force–velocity curve (Fig. 4.1-22A).

- When the load is zero, the muscle contracts rapidly and the velocity of muscle shortening is maximum (V_{max}).
- As the load increases progressively, the velocity of shortening decreases till it reaches zero. At this point, the force developed is called maximum isometric force and is represented by Po. Therefore, during muscle contraction, the velocity of shortening and force developed are inversely related. The force–velocity relationship curve is influenced by change in initial length of the muscle and the effect of catecholamines.

• **Effects of change in initial length on force–velocity relationship curve.** An increase in change in the initial length (within physiological limits) increases the force of contraction (Po) without changing the velocity (V_{max}), i.e. the relationship shifts to the right (Fig. 4.1-22B).

• **Effect of catecholamines or increased calcium concentration in ECF.** The catecholamines or increased Ca^{2+} concentration in ECF, both cause an increase in Po as well as V_{max} (Fig. 4.1-22C).

Clinical Implication of Force–velocity Relationship. The cardiac muscle can alter its work and power (rate of working) at any given load and muscle length by nature of

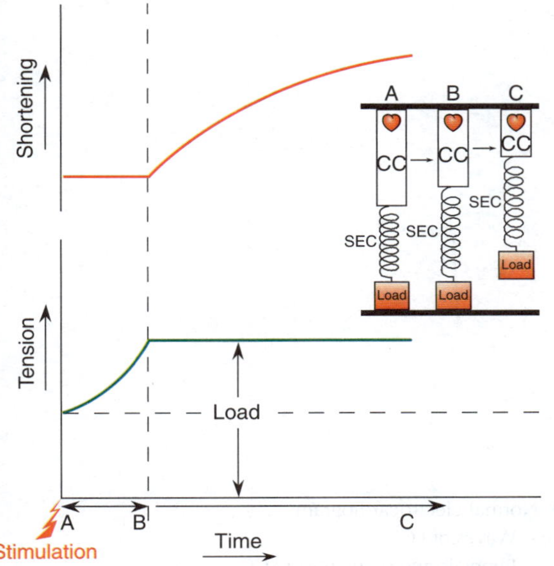

FIGURE 4.1-21 Model of contraction of cardiac muscle in afterloaded condition. **A,** resting phase; **B,** isometric contraction, phase; **C,** in isotonic contraction phase.

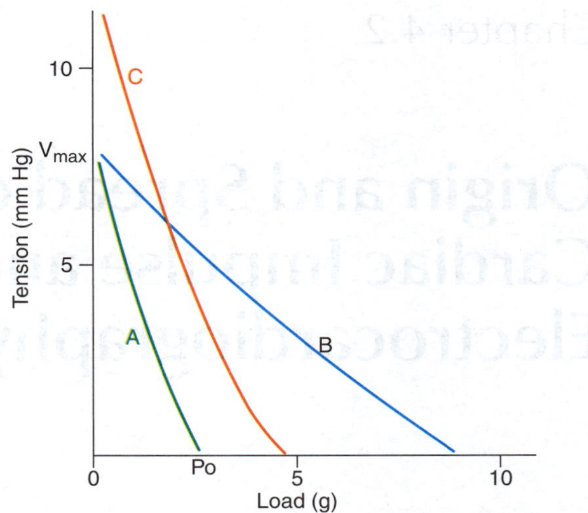

FIGURE 4.1-22 Force–velocity curve in cardiac muscle **(A)**, and effect of change of initial length **(B)** and effect of catecholamines or increased Ca^{2+} concentration in ECF(C) on it.

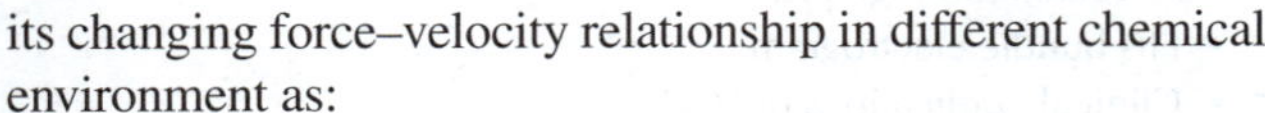

its changing force–velocity relationship in different chemical environment as:

- When the pressure against which the heart is pumping the blood is raised, the heart strokes out less blood than it receives for several beats. Consequently, blood accumulates in the ventricle increasing the end-diastolic volume which increases the initial length of muscle fibres (i.e. size of the heart). The distended heart beats more forcefully and output returns to its previous level, i.e. by an increase in the initial length of cardiac muscle the Po is increased and the V_{max} is achieved.
- Conversely, when the pressure against which the heart is pumping the blood is reduced, the stroke output rises transiently but the size of heart decreases and the stroke output falls to the previous constant level.

Chapter 4.2

Origin and Spread of Cardiac Impulse and Electrocardiography

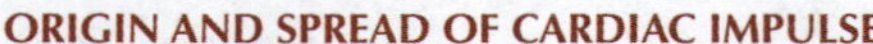

ORIGIN AND SPREAD OF CARDIAC IMPULSE

- Introduction
- Anatomic consideration
  - Conducting system of the heart
  - Innervational characteristics of the heart
- Mechanism of origin of rhythmic cardiac impulse
  - Pacemaker
  - Electrical potential in pacemaker tissue
  - Role of autonomic nervous system in controlling heart rhythm
- Spread of cardiac impulse
  - Conduction from SA node and atria
  - Conduction through AV node
  - Conduction through ventricles

ELECTROCARDIOGRAPHY

- Introduction
- Recording of ECG
  - ECG leads
  - Electrocardiograph
- Normal electrocardiogram
  - Waves of ECG
  - Intervals and segments of ECG
- Vectorial analysis of electrocardiogram and vector cardiography
  - Concept of cardiac vectors
  - Mean electrical axis
  - Vector cardiography
- His bundle electrogram
- Clinical applications of ECG
  - Cardiac arrhythmias
  - Myocardial infarction
  - Hypertrophy of various chambers of heart
  - Effects on ECG of changes in the ionic composition of blood

ORIGIN AND SPREAD OF CARDIAC IMPULSE

Introduction

The cardiac muscle possesses special properties which include autorhythmicity, conductivity, excitability and contractility. The heart is able to perform its action as a unique pump because of these properties interacting in the same sequence as enumerated above.

Autorhythmicity, refers to the property of cardiac muscle which enables the heart to initiate its own impulse at constant rhythmical intervals. Because of this property, the heart continues to beat even after all nerves to it are sectioned or even if the heart is cut into pieces, the pieces continue to beat. This is one of the earliest properties manifested during development even before the muscle fibres acquire the typical histological features. This is because of the presence of the specialized *pacemaker tissue* in the heart that can initiate repetitive action potentials. The pacemaker tissue makes a *conduction system* that normally spreads impulses through the heart.

Anatomic Consideration

Conducting System of the Heart

The conducting system of the heart consists of specialized fibres of the heart muscle present as the sinoatrial node, interatrial tract, internodal tracts, the atrioventricular (AV) node, the AV bundle of His and its right and left terminal branches, and the subendocardial plexuses of Purkinje fibres (Fig. 4.2-1).

1. Sinoatrial Node. Sinoatrial (SA) node is located in the wall of right atrium, just to the right of the opening of superior vena cava. Spontaneous rhythmical electrical impulses arise from the SA node and spread in all directions to

- Cardiac muscles of atria,
- Interatrial tract to left atrium and
- Internodal tracts to AV node.

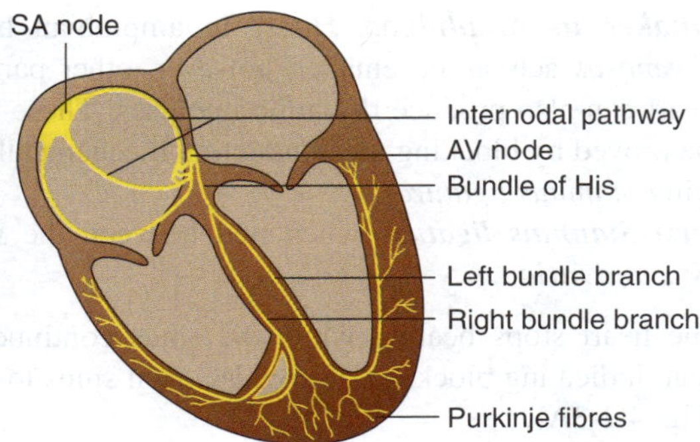

FIGURE 4.2-1 Specialized conducting tissues of the heart.

2. Interatrial tract (Bachman's Bundle). It is a band of specialized muscle fibres that run from SA node to left atrium. It causes simultaneous depolarization of the atria, since the velocity of conduction of impulse in this tract is faster than the rest of the atrial muscles.

3. Internodal Conduction Pathway. Impulses from the SA node have been shown to travel to the AV node more rapidly than they can travel by passing along the ordinary myocardium. This phenomenon has been explained by the description of special pathways in the atrial wall (Fig. 4.2-2), having a structure consisting of a mixture of Purkinje fibres and ordinary cardiac muscle cells. Three internodal conduction paths have been described:

- ***Anterior internodal pathway of Bachman*** leaves the anterior end of SA node and passes anterior to the superior vena cava opening. It then descends on the atrial septum and ends in the AV node.
- ***Middle internodal pathway of Wenckebach*** leaves the posterior end of SA node and passes posterior to superior vena cava opening. It then descends on the atrial septum to end in the AV node.
- ***Posterior internodal pathway of Thorel*** leaves the posterior part of the SA node and descends through the crista terminalis and the valve of inferior vena cava to the AV node.

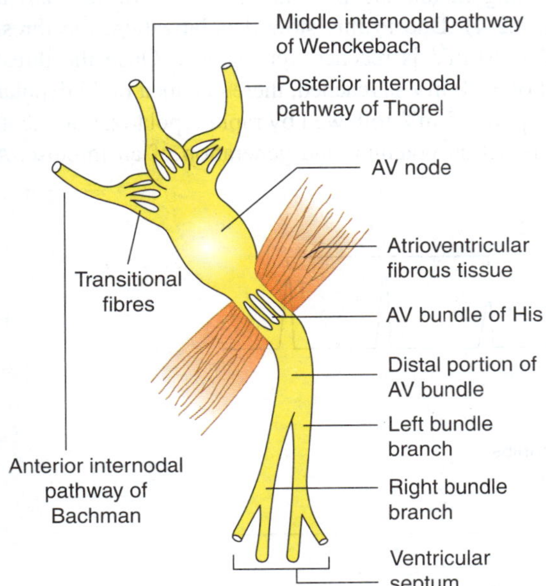

FIGURE 4.2-2 Internodal conduction pathways.

4. AV Node. The AV node is strategically located just beneath the endocardium on the right side of lower part of atrial septum, near the tricuspid valve. It is stimulated by the excitation wave that travels through internodal tracts and atrial myocardium. From it, the cardiac impulse is conducted to ventricles by the AV bundle.

5. AV Bundle of His. The AV bundle arises from the AV node, descends through the fibrous skeleton of the heart and divides into right bundle branch (RBB) for right ventricle and left bundle branch (LBB) for the left ventricle. The branches break up and become continuous with the plexus of Purkinje fibres.

6. Purkinje Fibres. These are spread out deep to the endocardium and reach all parts of the ventricles, including the bases of papillary muscles.

Characteristic Histological Features of Conducting System

- The conduction system of the heart is composed of modified cardiac muscle that has *fewer striations* and *indistinct boundaries.*
- The SA node and, to a lesser extent the AV node, also contains *small round cells* with few organelles, which are connected by *gap junctions.* These are probably the actual pacemaker cells, and therefore they are called *P cells.*
- The atrial muscle fibres are separated from those of the ventricles by a fibrous ring. Normally, the AV bundle is the only pathway of cardiac muscle that connects the myocardium of the atria and myocardium of ventricles and is thus the only route along which the cardiac impulse can travel from the atria to the ventricles.

Innervational Characteristics of Heart

- Both SA node and AV node are richly supplied by the sympathetic as well as parasympathetic nerves. Parasympathetic fibres come from the vagus nerve and most sympathetic fibres come from the stellate ganglion.
- SA node develops from the structures on the right side of the embryo and that is why it is supplied by right vagus nerve and right-sided sympathetics.
- AV node develops from the structures on the left side of the embryo and that is why it is supplied by left vagus and left-sided sympathetic nerves.
- Noradrenergic fibres are epicardial, whereas the vagal fibres are endocardial.
- Connections exist for reciprocal inhibitory effects of sympathetic and parasympathetic innervation of the heart on

each. Thus, acetylcholine acts presynaptically to reduce norepinephrine release from the sympathetic nerves, and conversely, neuropeptide Y released from the noradrenergic endings may inhibit the release of acetylcholine.

Mechanism of Origin of Rhythmic Cardiac Impulse

Pacemaker

The part of the heart from which rhythmic impulses for heart beat are produced is called *pacemaker.* In mammalian heart, though the other parts of the heart like AV node, atria and ventricle can also produce the impulse, but *SA node acts as a pacemaker* because the rate of impulse generation by SA node is the highest. However, when there occurs blockage of transmission of impulse from SA node to AV node, the pacemaker activity may shift from SA node to other sites, e.g. AV node. When pacemaker is other than SA node, it is called as *ectopic pacemaker.* Ectopic pacemaker causes abnormal sequence of contraction of different parts of the heart.

Rate of production of rhythmic impulses by different parts of the heart is:

- SA node: 70–80/min,
- AV node: 40–60/min,
- Atrial muscle: 40–60/min and
- Ventricular muscles: 20–40/min.

Experimental evidences to prove that SA node acts as a pacemaker in mammalian heart are:

- SA node becomes electrically negative before any other part of the atria thereby indicating that it is the first region to become active.
- Stimulation of SA node accelerates the heart rate.
- Local cooling of SA node reduces and warming increases the heart rate.
- When SA node is destroyed artificially, there occurs immediate stoppage of heart followed by an altered rhythm of heart beats (due to ectopic pacemaker taking over the function).

Pacemaker in Amphibian Heart In amphibian heart, *sinus venosus* acts as pacemaker, however, other parts of the heart can also produce rhythmic impulses. These facts can be proved by blocking the conduction mechanically by applying *Stannius ligatures.*

First Stannius ligature when tied between the *sinus venosus and atria*:

- The heart stops beating while the sinus continues to beat, indicating blockage of impulse from sinus to atria (Fig. 4.2-3A).
- After sometime, the atria start generating their own impulse which is also transmitted to ventricles and the atrial and ventricular segment starts beating independent of the sinus rhythm but at a slower rate (Fig. 4.2-3B).

Second Stannius ligature is then tied between the atria and ventricle around the AV groove. After this ligature:

- The atria continue to beat with its own rhythm while the ventricle stops beating indicating blockage of the impulse from the atria to the ventricle (Fig. 4.2-3C).
- After sometime, the ventricle generates its own impulse and starts beating independent of atria at much slower rate than the atrial rate. This is referred to as idioventricular rhythm (Fig. 4.2-3D).

Electrical Potential in Pacemaker Tissue

The electrical potential in cardiac muscle (contractile myocardial cells (CMC)) has been described on page 241. As shown in Figure 4.1-10 in phase 4 of action potential of cardiac muscle (CMC), there exists a constant resting membrane potential of −85 to −90 mV. In pacemaker (SA node) fibres, however, the resting membrane potential is only of −55 to −60 mV; and that this is not steady, i.e. it shows a slow rise in resting membrane potential due to slow depolarization (Fig. 4.2-4). Due to this slow depolarization, the threshold level −40 mV is reached very slowly. Once the threshold level of −40 mV is reached, there occurs a rapid depolarization up to +5 mV followed by rapid repolarization, i.e. there occurs action potential and generation of an impulse. After

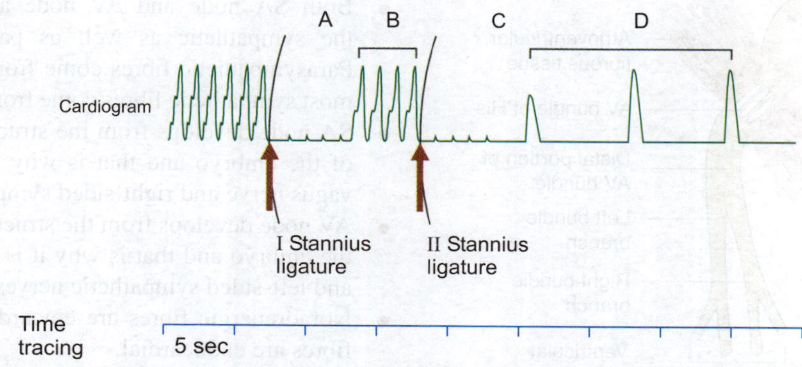

FIGURE 4.2-3 Effect of Stannius ligature I and II on frog's heart: **A,** blockage of impulse from sinus venosus to atria; **B,** atrialrhythm; **C,** blockage of impulse from atria to ventricle; and **D,** idioventricular rhythm.

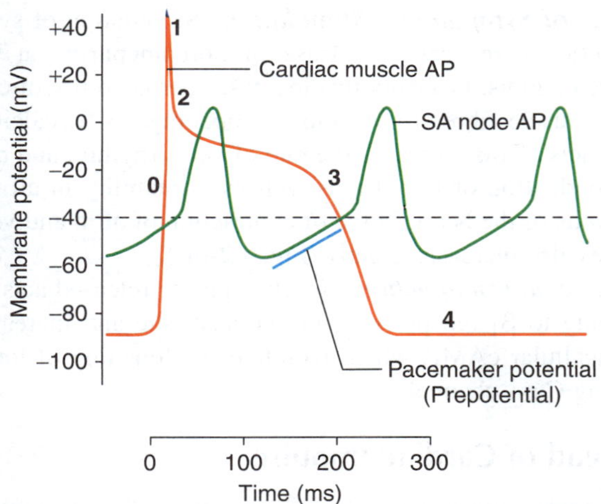

FIGURE 4.2-4 Phases of action potential in cardiac muscle fibre (0, 1, 2, 3, 4) and SA node showing pacemaker potential. AP = Action potential.

rapid repolarization (phase 3 of action potential), once again the resting membrane potential (phase 4 of action potential) is reached which is not stable and starts rising slowly to again reach at threshold level to produce the second impulse. This slow rising resting membrane potential in between the action potentials is called *prepotential* or *pacemaker potential* (Fig. 4.2-4). Ionic basis of pacemaker potential is explained below. Presence of this unique feature in the cells of pacemaker tissue is the underlying mechanism responsible for self-generation of rhythmic impulses (autorhythmicity).

Ionic Basis of Pacemaker Potential and Action Potential in SA Node The myocardial cells present in the SA node and AV node are called *slow fibres* and the other myocardial cells are called *fast fibres* depending on the membrane potential and the shape and conduction velocity of the action potential (Fig. 4.2-5).

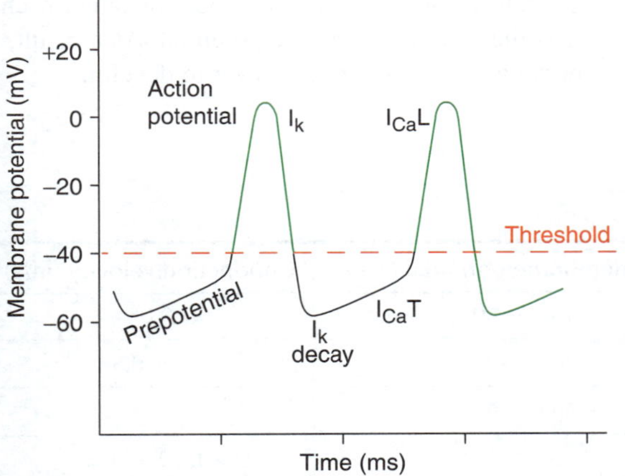

FIGURE 4.2-5 Pacemaker potential and its ionic basis. IcaT: Ca^{2+} conductance through transient calcium channels; IcaL: Ca^{2+} conductance through long lasting channels; Ik: potassium conductance.

- The slow fibres of the pacemaker tissue have a unique feature, i.e. leakage of resting membrane for sodium (while the resting membrane of fast fibres is relatively impermeable to Na^+). This causes *slow diffusion of Na^+ into the SA nodal fibres under resting condition. This slow entry of Na^+ in the cells slowly raises the potential to −55 mV* (i.e. causes slow depolarization) due to the presence of non selective channels. This slow depolarization forms the initial part of pacemaker potential (Fig. 4.2-5). Nodal tissues also possess certain funny (f) channels because of their unusual activation following hyperpolarization, associated with increased permeability to both sodium and potassium but dominant effect is that of sodium conductance. These channels are also called 'h' channels, because of their activation during hyperpolarization of the membrane (−40 to −60 mV)
- Then the 'T' (transient) calcium channels open up and there is slow influx of Ca^{2+} causing further depolarization in the same at slower rate till a threshold level of −40 mV is reached. Thus calcium current (Ica) due to the opening of 'T calcium channels' forms the later part of pacemaker potential.
- At the threshold level (−40 mV) the 'long lasting calcium channels' open up and the action potential starts with rapid depolarization due to influx of Ca^{2+}. Thus, it is important to note that the depolarization in SA node is mainly due to influx of Ca^{2+} rather than Na^+. Consequently, the depolarization is not as sharp as in the other myocardial fibres.
- At the end of depolarization, potassium channels open up and calcium channels close. This causes K^+ to diffuse out of the fibres resulting in rapid repolarization to −55 to −60 mV.
- Again, due to the unique feature of slow fibres of the SA node (i.e. *leakage of resting membrane to Na^+) the resting potential does not become stable but slow depolarization starts due to slow influx of Na^+ making initial part of prepotential.* And ultimately due to repetition of the above described steps another action potential is initiated. In this way, impulses are generated at regular intervals of time (*autorhythmicity*).

Role of Autonomic Nervous System in Controlling Heart Rhythm

Vagal Tone. SA node is richly innervated by parasympathetic fibres from the right vagus. Normal activity of vagus liberates acetylcholine from its nerve endings which increases the permeability of SA nodal fibres for potassium producing hyperpolarization (due to rapid efflux of K^+). This hyperpolarization slows the firing rate of SA node from its automatic rate of 90–120 impulses/min to the actual heart rate of about 72 beats/min. The normal vagal activity is called vagal tone.

Effect of Parasympathetic Stimulation. Parasympathetic stimulation causes release of acetylcholine at vagal nerve

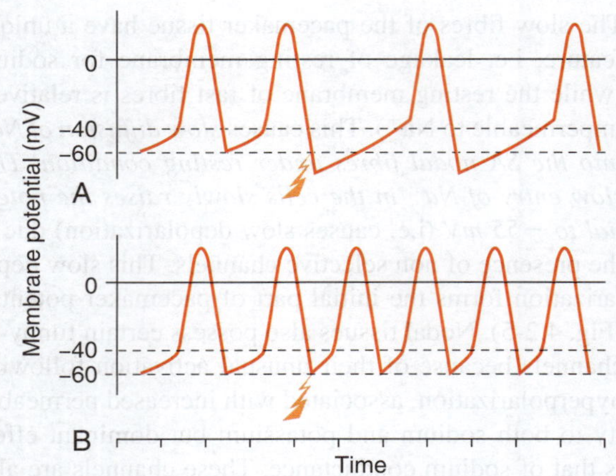

FIGURE 4.2-6 Effect of parasympathetic (A) and sympathetic (B) stimulations on pacemaker potential.

endings and by the above described mechanism causes (Fig. 4.2-6A):

- Decrease in heart rate by decrease in the rate of sinus rhythm. The acetylcholine released at the cholinergic nerve endings to nodal tissue causes hyperpolarization of the membrane by increasing permeability to K^+. The increase in conductance (efflux) of K^+, decreases the slope of prepotential.

  Mechanism of action: This action of Ach is mediated by M_2 receptors via βγ subunit of G protein, which opens the special set of K^+ channels and slows the depolarizing effect of Na^+ channels (I_h).

  Activation of M_2 receptors also decreases cyclic adenosine 3'5' monophosphate in the pacemaker cells and slows the Ca^{2+} channels opening, thus decreasing the firing rate.
- Decrease in the rate of transmission of impulses to ventricles due to decreased excitation of the conducting system. Strong parasympathetic stimulation may even completely block the transmission and ventricles may stop beating for 4–10 s. If it happens, Purkinje system initiates the rhythm causing ventricular contraction at a rate of 15–40/min. This phenomenon is called *vagal escape.*

Effect of Sympathetic Stimulation. Stimulation of sympathetic nerves causes release of norepinephrine at the nerve endings. Probably this increases permeability of cardiac muscle fibres to calcium by opening up 'L calcium channels'. This increases the rate of sinus rhythm, and rate of conduction of impulse as well as excitability in all the portions of the heart. Force of contraction of atria and ventricles also increases greatly (Fig. 4.2-6B).

Mechanism of action: Norepinephrine released acts by binding to β_1 receptors on the nodal tissue and increases intracellular cAMP, which facilitates the opening of long-lasting Ca^{2+} channels.

Spread of Cardiac Impulse

The cardiac impulse which originates in the SA node in the form of action potential spreads throughout the heart through the conduction system (properties of which are summarized in Table 4.2-1) in the sequence given below.

- ***SA Node and atria.*** The impulse travels over the muscle fibres of atria with which the ends of SA nodal fibres are fused, and through the interatrial tract to the left atrium. Conduction through these fibres causes simultaneous depolarization of both the atria. Atrial depolarization is completed in about 0.1 s. Through the internodal tracts (anterior, middle and posterior) the impulse reaches to AV node from SA node within 0.03 s after its origin.
- ***AV Node.*** *Conduction through AV node* is slow; there is a delay of about 0.1 sec. *The causes of AV nodal delay are:*
  - Transitional fibres connecting internodal tracts and AV node are very small and conduct the impulse at a very slow rate, i.e. 0.02–0.05 m/s. AV nodal fibres also conduct the impulse at a very slow rate (0.02–0.05 m/s).
  - Resting membrane potential of transitional fibres and AV nodal fibres (− 50 mV) is much less negative than rest of the cardiac muscle fibres (−90 mV). At this level of −50 to −55mV potential, the fast Na^+ channels get closed due to inactivation gates. Therefore, opening of slow sodium–calcium channels thereby causes action potential. As a result, AV nodal action potential is slower to develop.

TABLE 4.2-1 Properties of the Conduction System

Tissue	Fibres diameter (μm)	Resting membrane potential (mV)	Conduction velocity (m/s)
SA node	–	−40 to −50	0.05
Atrial muscle	8–10	−70 to −80	0.3–0.5
Interatrial and internodal tract	15–20	−80 to −90	1.0
AV node	Variable	−50	0.02–0.05
Purkinje fibres	70–80	−70	2.0–4.0
Ventricular muscle	10–16	−80	<1.0

- There are very few gap junctions connecting successive fibres in the pathway.

The ability of the AV node to slow and to block the rapid impulse is called *detrimental contraction.* This *AV nodal delay is useful*, for it provides time for completion of atrial contraction and their emptying, (i.e. ventricular filling) before the ventricles contract. This delay is shortened by stimulation of the sympathetic nerves to the heart and lengthened by stimulation of the vagii.

- ***Ventricular conduction.*** The impulses conducted through the AV node are distributed to ventricles through bundle of His, its branches, and Purkinje fibres in 0.08–0.15 s. In humans, depolarization of the ventricular muscle proceeds as follows (Fig. 4.2-7):
  - Starts at the left side of interventricular septum,
  - Moves first to the right across the mid portion of the septum,
  - The wave of depolarization then spreads down the septum to apex of heart.
  - It, then, returns along the ventricular walls to the AV groove, proceeding from the endocardial to the epicardial surface.
  - The last parts of the heart to be depolarized are the posterobasal portion of the left ventricles, the pulmonary conus, and the upper most portion of the septum.

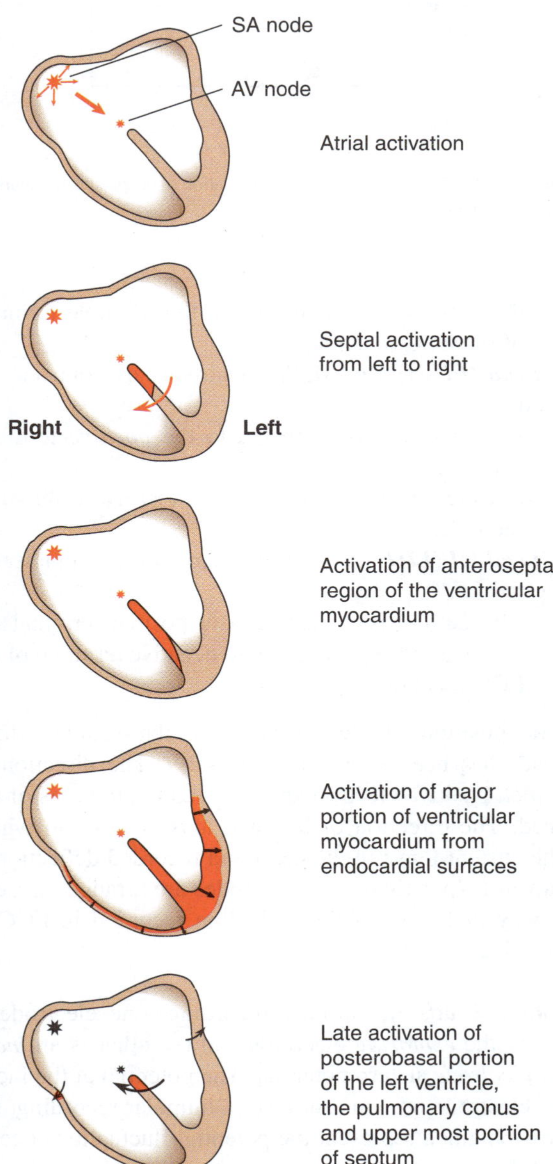

FIGURE 4.2-7 Spread of cardiac impulse.

Time taken for impulse to travel through different tissue is depicted below:

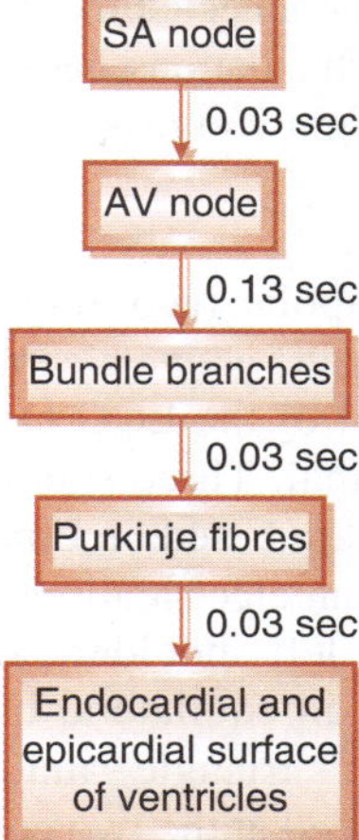

Thus, total time required for conduction from SA node to endocardial surface is 0.22 s.

Important Note

The AV bundle is the only connecting tissue between atria and ventricles. Therefore, if there is destruction of the AV node, then atria and ventricles beat independent of one another, i.e. atria at the rate of 72 beats/min and ventricles at a slower rate (30–40 beats/min). There is a complete dissociation of atrial and ventricular beating and is called *idioventricular rhythm.*

ELECTROCARDIOGRAPHY

Introduction

William Einthoven, a Dutch physiologist, originally developed the technique of electrocardiography. He was awarded the Nobel prize in 1924 for his contribution and is called the father of modern electrocardiography.

Electrocardiography (ECG) refers to extracellular recording of the summed-up electrical events of all the cardiac muscle fibres generated with each heart beat. Electrically, heart behaves as a *dipole,* i.e. a two-terminal battery in which the excited part (depolarized segment) forms a negative pole and the nonexcited part forms the positive pole (Fig. 4.2-8). Thus, ECG is nothing but the surface recording of the potential difference between the two poles of the heart dipole at a given time. The record of the potential fluctuations during the cardiac cycle is called the *electrocardiography*. The machine used to record these potential fluctuations is called *electrocardiograph,* which is essentially a sensitive galvanometer.

Recording of ECG

ECG Leads

ECG leads refer to the two electrodes which are placed on the body surface and connected to ECG machine for measuring the potential fluctuations between only two points. ECG is recorded using two types of leads, the bipolar and unipolar leads.

Bipolar Leads In bipolar recording, *both the electrodes are active* and one of the active electrodes is connected to the negative terminal of the ECG machine and the other to the positive terminal. Three standard limb leads used in bipolar recording are based on Einthoven's assumption that the body is like an electrically homogeneous plate in which the right and left shoulders and the pubic region form the corners of an equilateral triangle with heart in its centre (Einthoven's triangle) and that two active electrodes need to be placed at the two corners of this triangle (Fig. 4.2-9). However, for convenience, the electrodes are connected to the left arm (LA), right arm (RA) and left foot (LF) instead of the shoulders and the pubic region (Fig. 4.2-9). Practically, it does not make any difference whether the electrodes are placed in proximal or distal part of the extremities, because the current flows in the body fluids and so the records obtained are similar.

In three standard limb leads, the two active electrodes are connected as:

- ***Lead I (LI).*** In LI, the two active electrodes are connected to LA and RA.
  - LA electrode is connected to the positive terminal and

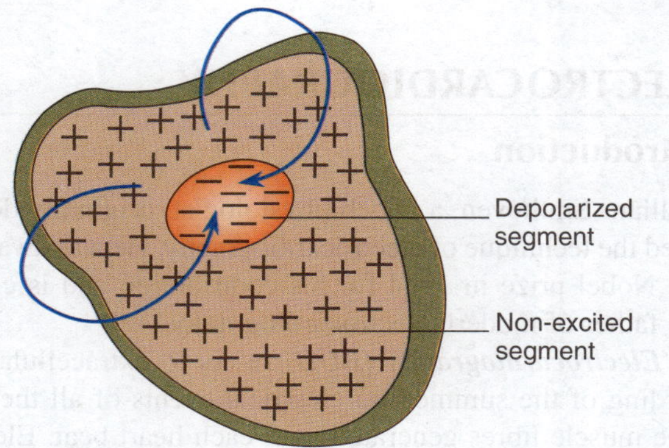

FIGURE 4.2-8 The heart as a dipole.

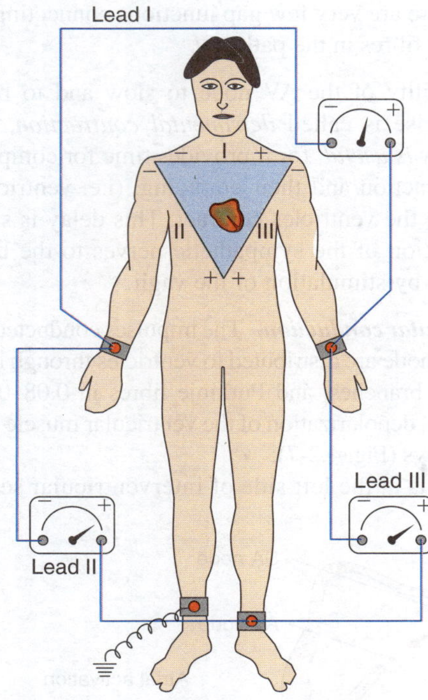

FIGURE 4.2-9 Einthoven's triangle and position of electrodes for standard limb leads (I, II and III).

  - RA electrode is connected to the negative terminal of the ECG machine.
- ***Lead II (LII).*** In LII, the electrodes are connected to RA and LF.
  - LF electrode is connected to the *positive* terminal and
  - RA electrode is connected to *negative* terminal of the ECG machine.
- ***Lead III (LIII).*** In LIII, the electrodes are connected to LA and LF.
  - LF electrode is connected to the positive terminal and
  - LA electrode is connected to negative terminal of the ECG machine.

The position of electrodes in bipolar standard limb leads has been shown in Fig. 4.2-9. The direction in which positive electrode points is called the axis of the lead. The direction of the lead axis is same in which the current flows in the heart and recorded deflection is upwards (positive). The electrodes are arranged in such a way that most of the deflection recorded in ECG is positive.

Unipolar Leads In unipolar recording, one electrode is *active* or the *exploring* electrode and the other is an *indifferent electrode* at zero potential. The potential at the indifferent electrode remains zero, so in unipolar recording, the records obtained represent the potential fluctuations occurring at the site of exploring electrode.

In a volume conductor, the sum of potentials at the points of an equilateral triangle with a current source at the centre is zero at all times. Therefore, if the three electrodes (placed on LA, RA and LF) are connected to a common terminal, through a resistance, an indifferent electrode that stays near zero potential is obtained. In clinical electrocardiography, two types of unipolar leads are used.

Unipolar Chest Leads. There are six unipolar chest leads (precordial leads) designated V_1 to V_6. The indifferent electrode is obtained as described above and the active electrode is placed on six points on the chest as given below (Fig. 4.2-10).

- *Lead V_1*: In the right fourth intercostal space, just near the sternum.
- *Lead V_2*: In the left fourth intercostal space, just near the sternum.
- *Lead V_3*: Halfway between V_2 and V_4.
- *Lead V_4*: In the left fifth intercostal space at midclavicular line.
- *Lead V_5*: In the left fifth intercostal space at anterior axillary line.
- *Lead V_6*: In the left fifth intercostal space at mid axillary line.

Unipolar Limb Leads. These include lead VL, VF and VR. In unipolar limb leads, one *exploring* (active) *electrode* is placed over a limb (In lead VL over the left arm, in VF over the left foot and in lead VR over the right arm), and is connected to the positive terminal of the electrocardiograph. The *indifferent electrode* is obtained as described above and is connected to the negative terminal of the electrocardiograph. These leads are not used and have been replaced by augmented limb leads.

Augmented Unipolar Limb Leads. Generally augmented unipolar limb leads designated as aVR, aVL and aVF are used. In augmented leads, the size of potential is increased by 50% without any change in the configuration from the nonaugmented record. The *active electrode* is from one of the limbs, and the indifferent electrode is obtained by connecting the other two limbs through 5000 ohms resistance as:

- Lead aVR: Active electrode is from right arm (RA) and indifferent electrode is from left arm (LA) + left leg (LF).

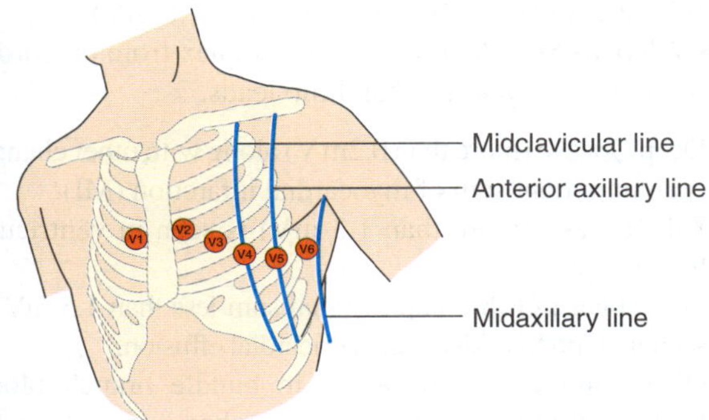

FIGURE 4.2-10 Position of electrodes for chest leads (V_1–V_6).

- Lead aVL: Active electrode is from LA and indifferent electrode is from RA + LF.
- Lead aVF: Active electrode is from LF and indifferent electrode is from RA + LA.

Why these leads are called augmented leads is explained below.

Suppose in non augmented unipolar limb leads, the potential at left arm (VL) = right arm (VR) = left foot (VF)

Then,

$$\text{aVF} = \text{VL} - (\text{VR} + \text{VF})/2$$

Or

$$2\ \text{aVF} = 2\text{VL} - (\text{VR} + \text{VF}) \qquad \text{...... equation I}$$

In Einthoven triangle, if electrodes are connected to three limbs through a high resistance, then

$$\text{VL} + \text{VR} + \text{VF} = 0$$

Or

$$\text{VL} = -(\text{VR} + \text{VF}) \qquad \text{...... equation II}$$

Substituting value of $-(\text{VR} + \text{VF})$ in equation I, then

$$2\text{aVL} = 2\text{VL} + \text{VL}$$

Or

$$\text{aVL} = 3/2\ \text{VL}$$

Thus potential recorded in aVL is one and half times as that of recorded in VL.

Electrocardiograph

The electrocardiograph (ECG machine) is essentially a sophisticated string galvanometer. A modern electro-cardiograph amplifies and records the potential fluctuations on a moving strip of paper. Following recording mechanisms are used:

- Some machines have a writing ink pen that records directly on the moving sheet of paper.
- In other machines instead of ink pen, special paper is used which turns black on exposure to heat. The stylus (recording pen) is made hot by electrical current flowing through its tip.

Calibration of Time and Voltage on ECG Paper

- The special ECG paper having 1 mm and 5 mm squares (Fig. 4.2-11) is used. The tracing is usually made at a standard recording speed of 25 mm/s.
- On horizontal axis, therefore, each millimetre represents 0.04 s (1/25).
- The sensitivity of electrocardiograph is adjusted in such a way that a potential fluctuation of 1 mV causes a vertical deflection of 1 cm. Thus, on vertical axis each millimetre represents 0.1 mV magnitude of potential.

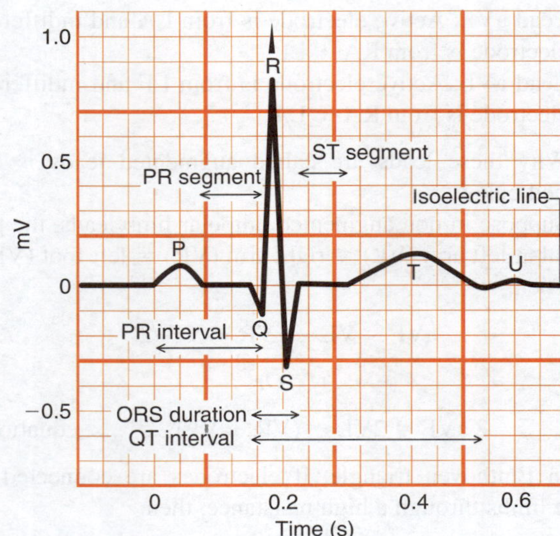

FIGURE 4.2-11 Calibration of time and voltage (amplitude) on special ECG paper.

Normal Electrocardiogram

Electrocardiogram (ECG) refers to the record of the potential fluctuations during the cardiac cycle. As a result of sequential spread of the excitation in the atria, the interventricular septum and the ventricular walls (Fig. 4.2-7) and finally repolarization of the myocardium, a series of positive and negative waves designated as P, Q, R, S and T are recorded during each cardiac cycle. Depolarization moving towards an active electrode in a volume conductor produces a positive deflection, whereas depolarization moving in the opposite direction produces a negative deflection.

Therefore, the shape and polarity of P, Q, R,S and T waves will vary in different leads due to differences in the orientation of each lead with respect to the heart (Fig. 4.2-12). *Configuration of a typical electrocardiogram* from a bipolar limb lead II (LII) is described below (Fig. 4.2-11).

Waves of ECG

P Wave

• ***Configuration.*** P wave is the positive (upright rounded deflection.

• ***Cause.*** It is produced by the depolarization of atrial musculature so also called atrial complex.

• ***Duration*** of P wave is not more than 0.1 s.

• ***Amplitude*** of P wave is from 0.1 to 0.12 mV.

• ***Clinical Significance.*** Magnitude of P wave is a guide to the functional activity of atria.

- In mitral stenosis the left atrium is hypertrophied and P wave becomes larger and prolonged.
- In tricuspid stenosis right atrium is hypertrophied and P wave becomes tall (0.5 mV) and peaked with normal duration.

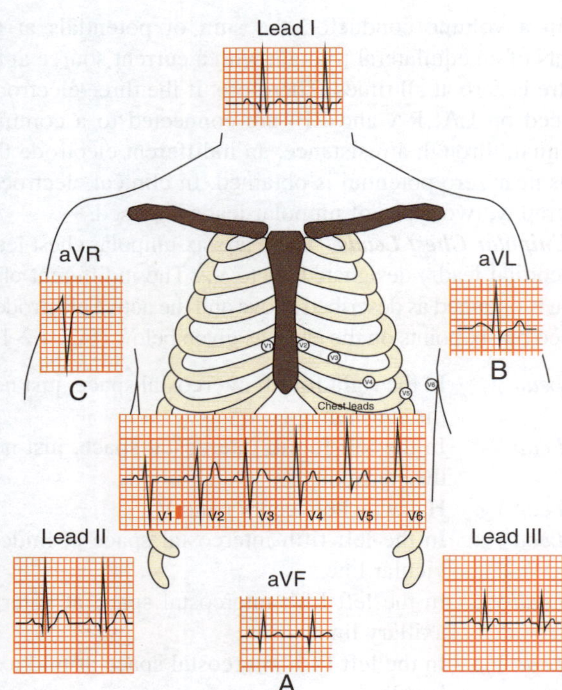

FIGURE 4.2-12 The electrocardiographic complexes recorded from different leads.

- In atrial fibrillation P wave disappears and replaced by fine irregular oscillations.
- When the cardiac impulse arises from an ectopic pacemaker, the P wave is altered or even inverted.

QRS Complex

• ***Configuration.*** QRS complex consists of three consecutive waves. Q wave is a small negative wave which may be absent normally quite often. It is continued as a tall positive R wave which is followed by a small negative S wave.

• ***Cause.*** The QRS complex is caused by ventricular depolarization.

• ***Duration*** of QRS Complex is Normally less than 0.08 s. It is a Measure of Intraventricular Conduction Time.

• ***Amplitude*** of Q Wave is 0.1–0.2 mV, R wave is 1.0 mV, and S wave is 0.4 mV (total 1.5–1.6 mV).

• ***Clinical Significance.*** QRS complex from precordial leads are more important than limb leads.

- Deep Q wave (more than 0.2m V) along with other changes is an important sign of myocardial infarction (MI).
- Tall R wave (more than 1.3 mV) is seen in ventricular hypertrophy.
- Low-voltage QRS complex (total sum less than 1.5 mV) is seen in hypothyroidism and pericardial effusion.
- QRS complex is prolonged in bundle branch block. Prolonged QRS complex is seen when one or both the ventricles are hypertrophied or dilated.

In blockage of Purkinje system, the QRS complex is abnormally prolonged (>0.12 s) due to decrease in impulse conduction.

Bizarre pattern of QRS complex is caused by destruction of cardiac muscle in ventricular region, and local blockages in the Purkinje system resulting in irregular impulse conduction, rapid shifts in voltages and axis deviations.

T Wave

- ***Configuration.*** T wave is the last, positive, dome-shaped deflection. Normally it is in the same direction as QRS complex, because ventricular repolarization follows a path opposite to depolarization.
- ***Cause.*** T wave represents ventricular repolarization.
- ***Duration*** of T wave is approximately 0.27 s.
- ***Amplitude*** of T wave is about 0.3 mV.
- ***Clinical Significance***

- In old age, T wave is flattened.
- Exercise increases its amplitude in healthy hearts.
- Inverted T wave is an important sign of myocardial ischaemia or infarction.
- Tall and peaked T wave occurs in hyperkalaemia.

Important Note

Digitalis toxicity – Digitalis is a drug used for increasing the strength of cardiac muscle (glycoside). Nonspecific changes in T wave (inversion of T wave, biphasic T wave) may occur, biphasic T wave is the earliest sign of digitalis toxicity.

U Wave

- ***Configuration.*** It is a small round positive wave.
- ***Cause.*** It occurs due to slow repolarization of papillary muscle.
- ***Duration*** of U wave when present is 0.08 s.
- ***Amplitude*** of U wave is about 0.2 mV.
- ***Significance.*** It is rarely seen normally. It becomes prominent in hypokalemia.

Note: Since atrial repolarization coincides ventricular depolarization, so it is merged with QRS complex and thus not recorded as a separate wave.

Intervals and Segments of ECG

P–R Interval It is measured from the onset of P wave to the onset of the QRS complex. Actually it is PQ interval but Q wave is frequently absent therefore it is called P–R interval.

- It measures the *AV conduction time,* including the AV nodal delay.
- Its *duration* varies from 0.12 to 0.21 sec depending on the heart rate.
- *Clinical significance.* Prolonged PR interval indicates AV conduction block. First degree block is produced when PR interval is between 0.2 and 0.3 s and second degree block is produced when PR interval is increased (0.3–0.45 s).

J Point J point refers to the point on ECG which coincides with the end of depolarization and start of repolarization of ventricles, i.e. it occurs at the end of QRS complex. At this point, since all parts of the ventricles are depolarized no current flows around the heart. Therefore, at J point the potential of ECG is exactly zero voltage.

QT Interval It is the time from the start of the QRS complex to the end of T wave.

- It indicates total *systolic time of ventricles,* i.e. ventricular depolarization and repolarization.
- *Duration* of QT interval is about 0.4 s (QRS duration and ST segment duration).
- *Clinical significance.* Ischaemia and any ventricular conduction defects prolong the QT interval. In hypocalcaemia also QT interval is prolonged.

TP Interval It is measured from the end of T wave to the beginning of P wave.

- It measures the *diastolic period* of the heart.
- Variable TP interval indicates AV dissociation.

P–P Interval P–P interval is the interval between two successive P waves. Equal P–P intervals indicate rhythmic depolarization of the atria.

ST Segment It is an isoelectric period between the end of QRS complex and beginning of T wave.

- Its *duration* is about 0.32 s.
- It corresponds with *ventricular repolarization.*
- *Clinical significance.* ST segment is elevated in patients with MI. In fact, whenever there is current of injury the TP segment shifts away from the zero and so it does not remain at the same potential level as ST segment. However, since in ECG, TP is considered as reference potential level, so whenever a current of injury is evident in ECG, it is called ST segment shift.

Characteristic Features of ECG Complex in Unipolar Chest Leads

The ECG complex produced in unipolar chest leads (V_1–V_6) represents the electrical activity of the part of the heart which lies nearest to the active electrode (Fig. 4.2-13).

P Wave is positive in all the leads because the excitation wave moves from SA node to AV node, i.e. posterior to anterior.

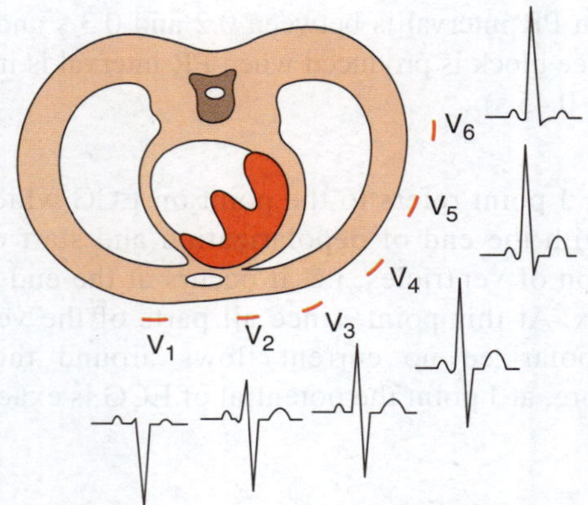

FIGURE 4.2-13 Pattern of QRS complex in chest leads (V_1–V_6).

QRS Complex represents the electrical activity of ventricles and so its configuration changes in different leads are as below.

- *In V_1* and V_2 (which reflect right ventricular activity), the main QRS complex is *negative*.
- *In V_3* and V_4 (which reflect activity of both ventricles including interventricular septum), the main QRS complex is *biphasic*.
- *In V_5* and V_6 (which reflect left ventricular activity), mainly the main QRS complex is *positive*.

Thus as shown in Fig. 4.2-13,

- ***R Wave*** gradually increases in size from V_1 to V_6 leads. In leads V_1, R wave represents activity of right ventricle and in V_6 of left ventricle.
- ***S Wave*** gradually decreases in size from lead V_1 to V_6. In lead V_1, S wave represents activity of left ventricle and in lead V_6 of right ventricle.

Characteristic Features of ECG Complex in Unipolar Limb Leads and Augmented Limb Leads

The ECG complex in unipolar limb leads and augmented limb leads is characterized by the electrical activity of that part of the heart which faces the active electrode of that particular unipolar limb lead as:

Lead VF and aVF. These leads reflect the electrical activity of inferior surface of the heart which is formed by parts of both right and left ventricles and interventricular septum. Therefore, QRS complex in these leads like that of V_3 and V_4 is predominantly *biphasic* (Fig. 4.2-12A).

Lead VL and aVL. These leads reflect the electrical activity of left outer side of the heart which is mainly formed by the left ventricle. Therefore, QRS complex in these leads like that of V_6 is predominantly *positive* (Fig. 4.2-12B).

Lead VR and aVR. These leads reflect the activity of the cavity of the ventricles, irrespective of the position of heart. Therefore, *P wave, QRS complex and T wave* all are *negative deflection* (Fig. 4.2-12C).

Vectorial Analysis of Electrocardiogram and Vector Cardiography

In the discussion until this point, we have studied the configuration of various positive and negative waves of the ECG complex and their clinical significance. In addition to the information gained from the changes in the configuration of various waves, the vectorial analysis of the electrocardiogram also provides many useful information pertaining to cardiac abnormalities. The concept of cardiac vector, methods of vector analysis and their clinical significance are discussed.

Concept of Cardiac Vectors

- During cardiac cycle (depolarization and repolarization of heart), current flows in the heart at every instant. The magnitude and direction of the potential generated can be represented in the form of an arrow which is called a vector. By convention, the arrow head points towards the direction and the length of the arrow is drawn proportional to the voltage of the potential.
- During most of the cycle of ventricular depolarization, direction of electrical potential (negative to positive) is from the base of ventricles towards the apex. This preponderant direction of potential during depolarization is called the *mean QRS vector* (mean electrical axis (MEA) of the heart) and is drawn through the centre of the ventricles in a direction from the base of the heart toward the apex (Fig. 4.2-14).
- The *instant vector,* however, represents the magnitude and direction of potential at a particular instant during the cardiac cycle. The instantaneous vectors of 5 different instants during the process of ventricular depolarization are shown in Figure 4.2-15.

Calculating the MEA from Standard Lead Electrocardiogram

As discussed earlier, the MEA refers to the *mean vector* produced during a cardiac cycle (i.e. by P, QRS and TP, ECG complex).

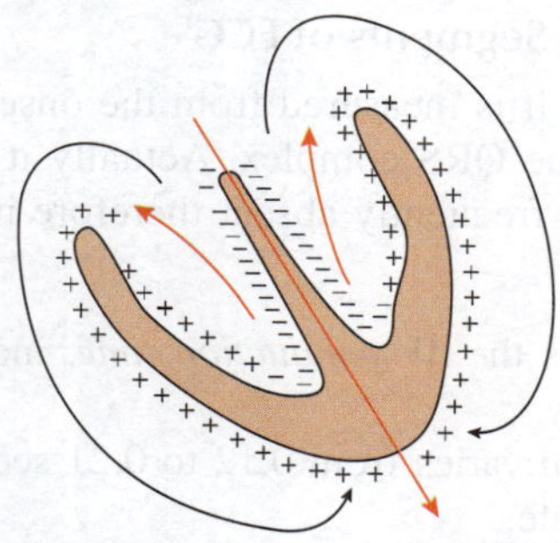

FIGURE 4.2-14 Instantaneous mean vector during ventricular depolarization.

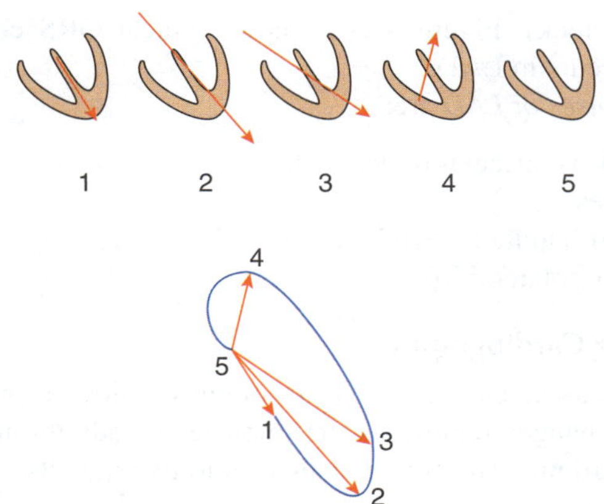

FIGURE 4.2-15 The instantaneous mean vector of five different instants during process of ventricular depolarization and construction of QRS vector cardiogram.

- In the frontal plane, MEA can be calculated from any two standard (i.e. bipolar) limb leads (using Einthoven's triangle or triaxial reference system) or any two augmented limb leads (using hexa-axial reference system).
- The MEA in the horizontal plane is derived using the precordial (chest) leads.

Triaxial Reference System involves moving the sides of Einthoven's triangle so that they intersect at the centre of triangle. Lead I then divides the system into an upper (negative) and a lower (positive) hemisphere. The triaxial system of representation reveals that (Fig. 4.2-16B):

- The axis of lead I is 0°, because the electrodes lie in the horizontal direction with positive electrode to the left,
- The axis of lead II is about 60° as the electrodes are placed on the right arm (negative) and left leg (positive) and
- The axis of lead III is about 120°, as the electrodes are placed on the left arm (negative) and left leg (positive).

The Hexa-axial Reference System involves superimposition of the axis of augmented limb leads on the triaxial system. The hexa-axial system of vector representation reveals that (Fig. 4.2-16C):

- The axis of lead aVF is 190°,
- The axis of lead aVR is 210° and
- The axis of lead aVL is −30°.
- *Clinically the frontal MEA of the QRS complex* is more useful and is determined from the two standard limb leads as:
  - The Q and S waves (negative values) are added algebraically to the R wave (positive value) for each of two leads. The result gives the magnitude and the direction of the QRS vector (+ or −) in each lead. For example:

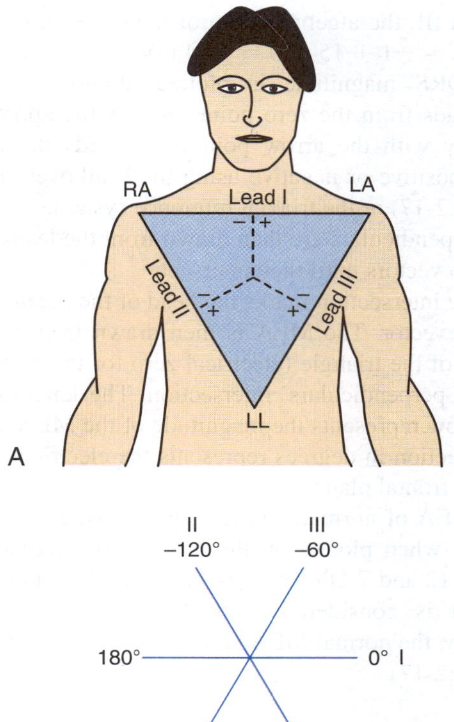

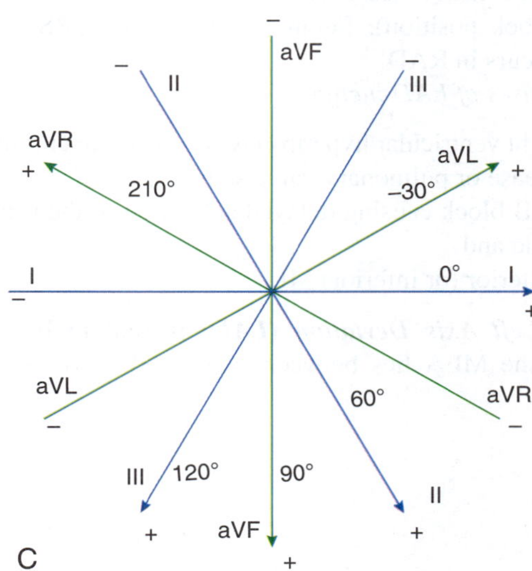

FIGURE 4.2-16 Schematic drawing for calculating the mean electrical axis (MEA): **A,** Einthoven triangle and connections of bipolar limb leads; **B,** the triaxial reference system in which lead I, II and III collapsed into their respective zero points and **C,** the hexa-axial reference system obtained by adding augmented unipolar limb leads (aVR, aVL and aVF) to triaxial system.

- In lead I, the algebraic sum of Q (−3), R (+13), S (−5) = −3 + 13 − 5 = 5 mV and

- In lead III, the algebraic sum of the Q (−1), R (+15), S (−0) = −1 + 15 − 0 = +14 mV.
- The QRS magnitude is plotted along the respective leads from the zero point towards the appropriate polarity with the arrow pointing towards the correct pole (positive or negative using the Einthoven triangle (Fig. 4.2-17) or the triaxial reference system.
  - Perpendiculars are then drawn from the leads of the two vectors until they intersect.
  - The intersection marks the head of the mean electrical vector. The MEA is then drawn from the centre of the triangle (electrical zero for the system) to the perpendiculars' intersection. The length of this arrow represents the magnitude of the MEA, and its direction in degrees represents the electrical axis in the frontal plane.
- The MEA of normal ventricles lies between −30° and +120° when plotted on the hexa-axial reference system or (2 and 7 O'clock, respectively, if the hexa-axial system is considered a clock face Fig. 4.2-18A). Usually, the normal MEA is 59°, i.e. 5 O'clock positive (Fig. 4.2-17).

Abnormalities of MEA

1. Right Axis Deviation (RAD) is said to be present when the MEA lies between +120° and +180° (7 and 9 O'clock position). Figure 4.2-18 shows QRS complex that occurs in RAD.

Causes of RAD include:

- Right ventricular hypertrophy secondary to chronic lung disease or pulmonary valve stenosis.
- RBB block causing delayed activation of the right ventricle and
- Posterior (or inferior) MI.

2. Left Axis Deviation (LAD) is said to be present when the MEA lies between −30° and −90° (or 2 and 12 O'clock). Figure 4.2-18 shows typical QRS complex that occurs in LAD.

Causes of LAD are:

- Left ventricular hypertrophy,
- Obesity,
- Left bundle branch block and
- Anterolateral MI.

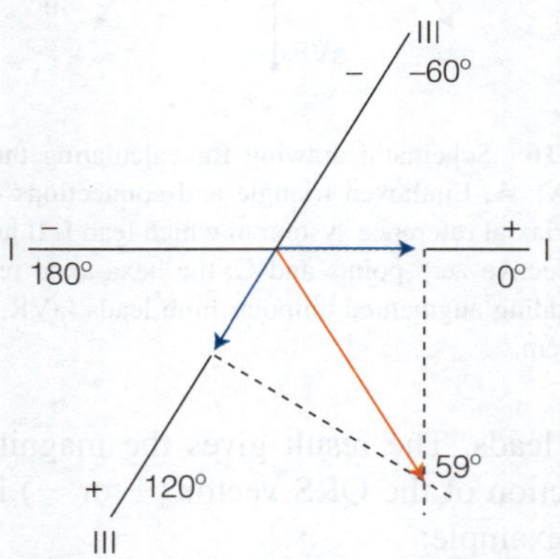

FIGURE 4.2-17 Plotting the mean electrical axis (MEA) of the ventricles from two electrocardiographic leads (leads I and III).

Vector Cardiography

As discussed earlier, the vector of current flow through the heart changes rapidly as the impulse spreads through the myocardium. The vector changes into two aspects:

- Increase or decrease in length corresponding to change in voltage (magnitude) and

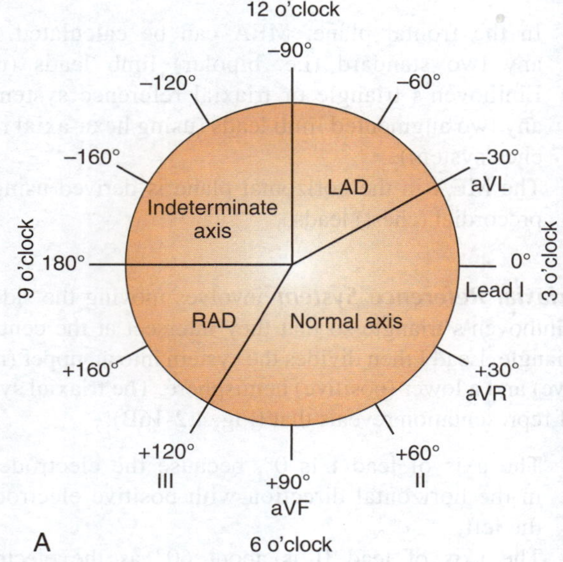

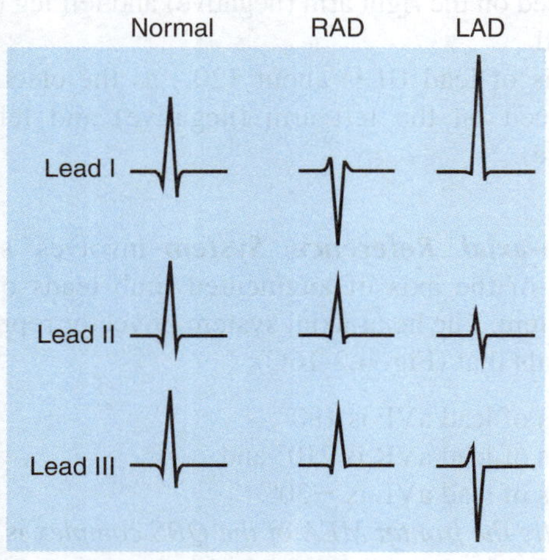

FIGURE 4.2-18 **A,** Mean electrical axis (MEA) in the frontal plane (using hexa-axial system) showing normal axis, right axis deviation (RAD) and left axis deviation (LAD); and **B,** QRS complexes (normal in RAD and in LAD) seen in leads I, II and III.

- Changes its direction because of changes in the average direction of the electrical potential of the heart.

Figures 4.2-15 and 4.2-19 show the instant vectors of 8 different successive instants during the process of ventricular depolarization (i.e. in a normal QRS complex). On joining the positive ends of the vectors a loop is obtained which is called *vector cardiogram.*

A continuous record of all the vectors is made using an *oscilloscope*. The procedure is called vector cardiography and the record obtained in the form of a loop called vector cardiogram (similar to P, QRS and T that described above). Three loops can be recorded during one cardiac cycle (Fig. 4.2-20). Atrial depolarization cannot be recorded with standard technique of vector cardiography because of the prolonged time course and small voltages involved.

1. P Loop. It is caused by atrial depolarization. It is small and is directed leftward and inferiorly, resulting in a positive P wave in three bipolar limb leads.

2. QRS Loop. It is caused by ventricular depolarization. The normal QRS loop is inscribed counterclockwise and is directed leftward, inferior and posterior. Figure 4.2-19 shows, how the QRS loop generates the QRS complex in three limb leads.

3. T Loop. It results from ventricular repolarization, which is roughly opposite in direction to the depolarization. This reversal of direction results in T wave that normally is in the same direction as the QRS complex.

His Bundle Electrogram

- His bundle electrogram (HBE) refers to recording the electrical activity of the heart obtained through the intracardiac ring electrodes placed near the tricuspid valve.

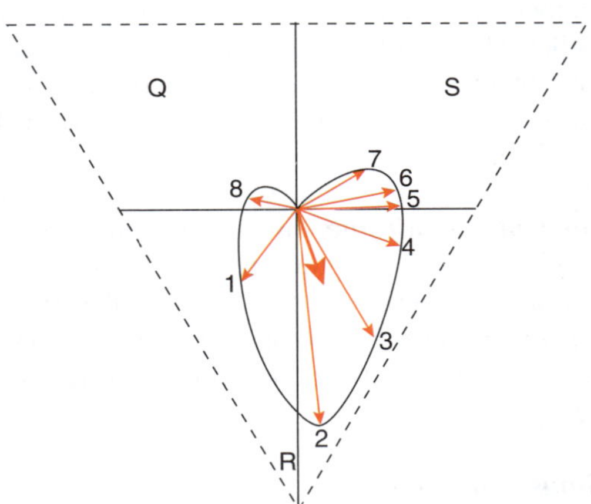

FIGURE 4.2-19 Instant vector of eight arbitrary stages of ventricular depolarization and reconstruction of QRS complex from QRS loop for three bipolar limb leads. Arrows indicate the direction of loop recording.

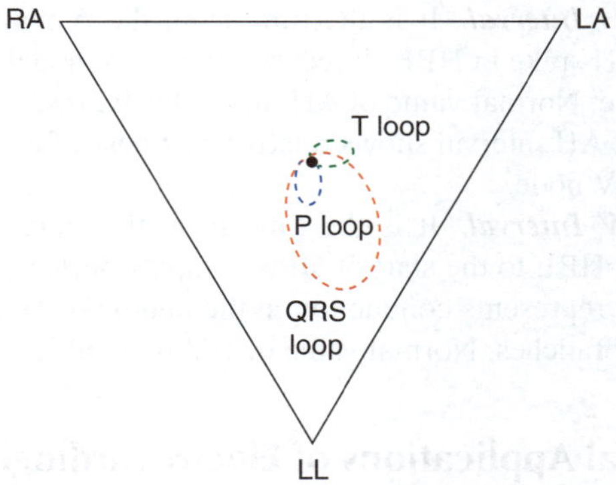

FIGURE 4.2-20 The vector cardiographic loops P, QRS and T.

- It is accomplished with a catheter containing ring electrodes at its tip that is passed through a vein to the right side of heart and manipulated into a position close to the tricuspid valve. Three or more standard electrocardiographic leads are recorded simultaneously.
- Normal HBE shows the following deflections (Fig. 4.2-21).
  - *A deflection,* which corresponds to activation of AV node,
  - *H spike,* is due to transmission of impulse through the His bundle and
  - *V deflection* is produced during ventricular depolarization.

Uses of HBE It is especially useful in patients with heart blocks. From the HBE and ECG from standard leads it is possible to accurately time the following three intervals:

- ***PA Interval.*** It is the time from the first appearance of atrial depolarization to the A wave in HBE. It represents conduction time from the SA node to AV node. Normal value of PA interval is 27 ms.

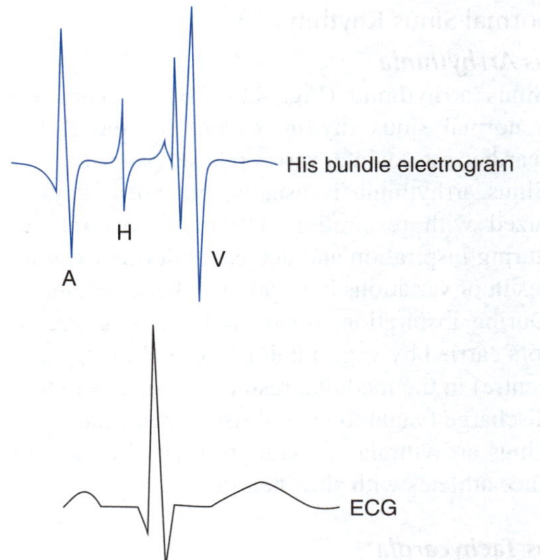

FIGURE 4.2-21 Normal His bundle electrogram (HBE) with simultaneously recorded ECG.

• ***AH Interval.*** It is the time from the A wave to the start of H spike in HBE. It represents the AV nodal conduction time. Normal value of AH interval is 92 ms; the higher value of AH interval shows relative slowness of conduction in the AV node.

• ***HV Interval.*** It is the time from the start of the H spike in HBE to the start of QRS complex deflection in the ECG. It represents conduction in the bundle of His and the bundle branches. Normal value of HV interval is 43 ms.

Clinical Applications of Electrocardiography

ECG is an indispensable tool in the diagnosis, prognosis and planning treatment in most of the cardiac disorders. The important applied aspects which need special mention are:

- Cardiac arrhythmias,
- Myocardial infarction,
- Hypertrophy of various cardiac chambers and
- Effects on ECG of changes in the ionic composition of blood.

Cardiac Arrhythmias

Cardiac arrhythmias refers to disruption of the normal cardiac rhythm. The normal cardiac rhythm implies a regular sinus rhythm with a normal cardiac rate, between 60 and 100 beats/min (average 72 beats/min). *Sinus rhythm* is said to be present when the SA node is pacemaker, and each P wave is followed by a normal QRS complex, the P–R and Q–T intervals are normal, and R–R interval is regular. Cardiac arrhythmias may be discussed as:

- Abnormal sinus rhythm,
- Conduction disturbances (heart blocks) and
- Ectopic cardiac rhythm.

Abnormal Sinus Rhythm

Sinus Arrhythmia

- Sinus arrhythmia (Fig. 4.2-22B) is characterized by a normal sinus rhythm except for the R–R interval (cardiac rate) which varies in a set pattern.
- Sinus arrhythmia is usually, but not always synchronized with respiration. Usually, heart rate increases during inspiration and decreases during expiration, as a result of variations in vagal tone that affect the SA node. During inspiration, impulses from lung stretch receptors carried by vagii inhibit cardioinhibitory area (vagal centre) in the medulla, resulting decrease in tonic vagal discharge (vagal tone) and rise in heart rate.
- Sinus arrhythmia is common in children and in endurance athletes with slow heart rates.

Sinus Tachycardia

- Sinus tachycardia (Fig. 4.2-22C) is characterized by a normal sinus rhythm except for increased heart rate (i.e. decreased but regular R–R interval). Tachycardia is labelled when heart rate is more than 100 beats/min.

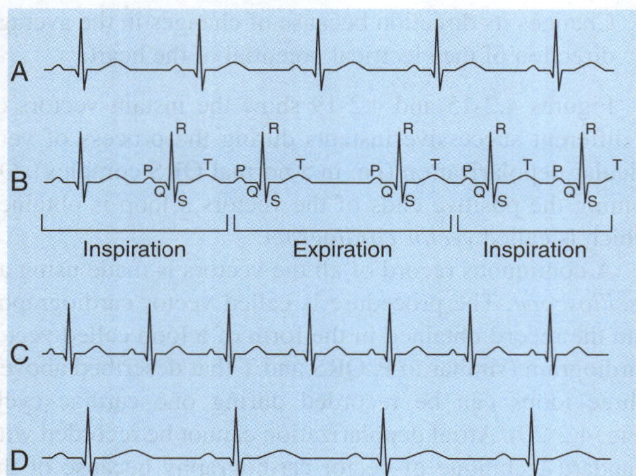

FIGURE 4.2-22 Electrocardiogram tracings showing: **A,** normal sinus rhythm; **B,** sinus arrhythmia; **C,** sinus tachycardia; and **D,** sinus bradycardia.

- Sinus tachycardia is a normal response to exercise and is also associated with fever, hyperthyroidism and as a reflex response to low arterial pressure.

Fever. The heart rate increases by 10 beats/min for each degree Fahrenheit (18 beats/min/°C) rise in body temperature up to 105 °F (40.5 °C); with further rise in body temperature, heart rate may decrease due to debility of heart muscle. Tachycardia in fever occurs due to increase in metabolic rate of SA node which directly increases its excitability.

Sympathetic activity. Factors which increase sympathetic activity also lead to tachycardia, e.g. hypovolemic shock (as a reflex response to low arterial pressure), exercise, hyperthyroidism. For details see page 256.

Sinus Bradycardia

- Sinus bradycardia (Fig. 4.2-22D) is characterized by a normal sinus rhythm except for decreased heart rate (i.e. increased but regular R–R interval). Bradycardia is labelled when heart rate becomes less than 60 beats/min.
- Sinus bradycardia is more commonly seen in highly trained endurance athletes due to increased vagal lone, sometimes it may be abnormal.

Carotid Sinus Syndrome. In patients with carotid sinus syndrome, the baroreceptors present in carotid sinus are very sensitive, even mild pressure on the neck elicits strong baroreceptor reflex to cause bradycardia, sometimes heart may stop for 5–10 s. For baroreceptor reflex details see page 340.

Sick Sinus Syndrome

- Sick sinus syndrome refers to a condition characterized by marked bradycardia accompanied by dizziness and syncope.

- ***Causes*** of sick sinus syndrome include:
  - Sinus bradycardia that does not improve with sympathetic stimulation or vagal inhibition.
  - SA nodal block (see below) and
  - Sinus arrest, i.e. complete stoppage of sinus discharge.
- ***Treatment,*** when the condition causes severe symptoms, consists of implantation of artificial pacemaker. Sinus node dysfunction accounts for over half of the pacemaker implants.

Pacemakers are the electronic devices that sense and pace the activity of the chambers of the heart by programming in most physiological way to maintain the cardiac output. The artificial pacemakers are the stimulators planted underneath the skin and electrodes are usually connected to right ventricles to provide rhythmical impulses to ventricles.

Conduction Disturbances (Heart Blocks)

Heart blocks refer to slowing down or blockage of cardiac impulse (generated from SA node) along the cardiac conductive pathway. Conduction blockage may occur as:

- SA nodal block,
- AV nodal block and
- Bundle branch block.

SA Nodal Block

- SA nodal block or the so-called SA block is characterized by the blockage of impulse conduction from SA node to atria.
- It occurs in the elderly and in patients recovering from coronary artery occlusion.
- It occurs suddenly and initially the heart stops (i.e. neither atria nor ventricles contract for a while). After an interval of approximately two cardiac cycles, the AV node becomes the pacemaker, and the heart starts functioning again. This is called *AV nodal rhythm.*
- SA block may manifest as *sick sinus syndrome* (described above).
- AV nodal rhythm also called *junctional rhythm* (Fig. 4.2-23) is characterized by inverted P wave and normal QRS complex, and the rate is slower than sinus rhythm.

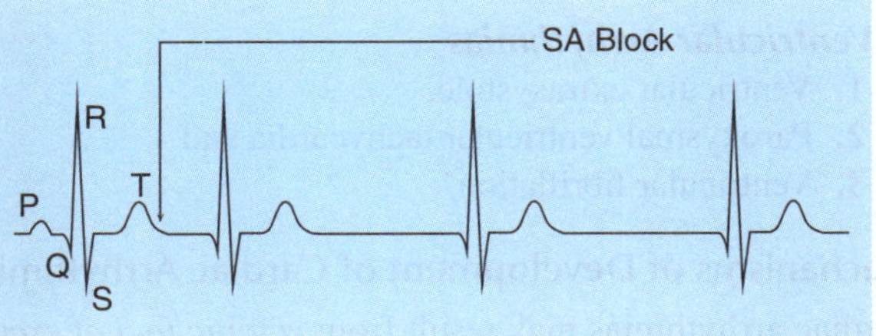

FIGURE 4.2-23 AV nodal rhythm seen in SA node blockage.

AV Nodal Block. AV nodal blockage may occur as *incomplete heart* block (which includes first-degree and second-degree heart blocks) or complete heart block (third-degree heart block). AV nodal blockages are associated with following conditions:

- *Coronary insufficiency* can cause AV nodal ischaemia.
- *Compression of AV node* by scar tissue or by calcification.
- *Inflammation of AV node* results due to myocarditis can depress conduction of impulse from atria to ventricles.
- *Vagal excitation* results due to strong stimulation of baroreceptors in carotid sinus syndrome.

First-Degree AV Nodal Block. First-degree AV nodal (or heart) block is characterized by slowing of conduction at the level of AV node. Though all the atrial impulses reach the ventricles but the PR interval is abnormally long, i.e. more than 0.21 s (Fig. 4.2-24B), but seldom increases more than 0.30 s.

Second-Degree AV Nodal Block. In second-degree AV nodal block (Fig. 4.2-24C and D), not all atrial impulses are conducted to ventricles. It is usually associated with organic heart diseases. Consequently, there may be one ventricular contraction after every 2, 3 or 4 atrial contractions producing the so-called 2:1, 3:1 or 4:1 block (*constant block*). Other forms of second degree heart blocks are:

- Wenckebach phenomenon (Mobitz type I block). It is characterized by a progressive lengthening of the P–R interval in successive beats and finally a failure of one impulse to be transmitted.
- Periodic block (Mobitz type II). It is characterized by an occasional failure of conduction that results in an atrial to ventricular rate of for example 6:5 or 8:7. The P–R interval is constant.

Third-Degree (Complete) AV Nodal Block.

- In third-degree complete AV block, no impulse from atria can pass to the ventricles.
- Therefore, ventricles start beating at their own rhythm (about 40 beats/min) called idioventricular rhythm.
- The atria, however, continues to beat at the normal sinus rhythm of about 72 beats/min. Thus, ECG shows that there is complete dissociation between P waves and QRS complexes called *atrioventricular dissociation.* (Fig. 4.2-24E).
- Third-degree block is *caused* by organic heart diseases, septal myocardial infarction and damage to bundle of His during surgical repair of congenital interventricular septal defects.
- Third-degree block may be associated with prolonged ventricular standstill (asystole) until a ventricular focus begins firing. The asystole, lasting for a minute may result in cerebral ischaemia producing dizziness and fainting (syncope), the condition is termed *Stokes–Adams' syndrome.* Even death may also occur due to prolonged cerebral ischaemia.

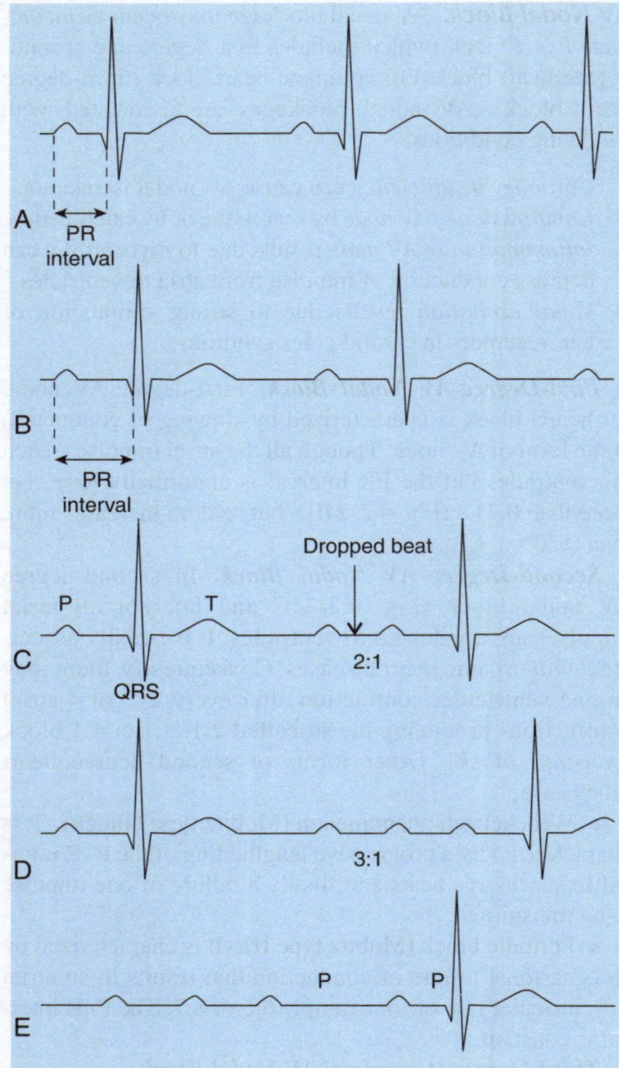

FIGURE 4.2-24 Various types of AV nodal blocks: **A,** normal sinus rhythm; **B,** first-degree AV block; **C,** second-degree AV block (2:1); **D,** 3:1 block; and **E,** complete AV block (third degree).

Treatment. Mostly these patients are provided with artificial pacemakers.

Bundle Branch Block

- Bundle branch block refers to conduction blocks in one or more branches of the bundle of His.
- In this condition, excitation passes normally down the bundle on the intact side and then sweeps back through the muscle to activate the ventricle on the blocked side.
- Therefore, the ventricular rate is normal, but the QRS complexes are prolonged (beyond 0.12 s) and deformed (Fig. 4.2-25). The characteristic features of the branch involved are:

• ***Right Bundle Branch Block (RBBB)*** may occur in otherwise healthy individuals or secondary to chronic pulmonary disease. The activation of right ventricle is delayed and ECG may show features of RAD (Fig. 4.2-25A).

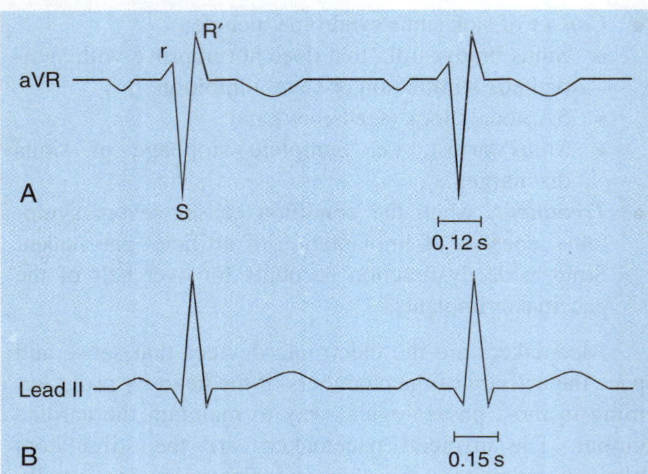

FIGURE 4.2-25 Electrocardiogram characteristics in bundle branch blocks: **A,** right bundle branch block; and **B,** left bundle branch block.

• ***Left Bundle Branch Block (LBBB)*** is usually associated with organic heart disease. It is best diagnosed using left precordial leads (Fig. 4.2-25B).

• ***Hemiblock or Fascicular Block*** refers to block in either anterior or posterior fascicle of LBB. Left anterior hemiblock (LAH) produces abnormal LAD in ECG, whereas left posterior hemiblock (LPH) produces abnormal RAD.

• ***Bifascicular Block,*** i.e. RBBB with LAH or LPH is not uncommon.

• ***Trifascicular Block,*** i.e. RBBB with LAH and LPH may also occur.

Note: HBE is useful for detailed analysis of the site of block when there is a defect in the conduction system.

Ectopic Cardiac Rhythm

Ectopic cardiac rhythm refers to abnormal cardiac excitation produced either by an ectopic focus or a re-entry phenomenon. Ectopic cardiac rhythm includes the following conditions:

A. Atrial Arrhythmias

1. Atrial extra systole,
2. Paroxysmal atrial tachycardia,
3. Atrial flutter and
4. Atrial fibrillation.

B. Ventricular Arrhythmias

1. Ventricular extrasystole,
2. Paroxysmal ventricular tachycardia and
3. Ventricular fibrillation.

Mechanisms of Development of Cardiac Arrhythmias

Cardiac arrhythmias may result from *ectopic foci of excitation* and/or re-entry mechanism.

1. Ectopic Foci of Excitation Under normal circumstances, SA node acts as a pacemaker since its rate of rhythmic discharge is more rapid than the rate of discharge of other parts of conduction system and myocardium of heart. However, in certain abnormal conditions, the His–Purkinje fibres or the myocardial fibres become hyperexcitable and discharge spontaneously. In these conditions, increased automaticity of the heart is said to be present. The site in the heart which becomes hyperexcitable is called an *ectopic focus* which may behave as:

- ***Single discharge.*** When the irritable ectopic focus discharges once, an *extra systole* or *premature* beat is caused before the next normal beat. Depending upon the site of ectopic focus the premature beat may be atrial, nodal or ventricular.
- ***Repetitive discharge.*** If the ectopic focus discharge impulses repeatedly at a rate higher than that of SA node, the tachycardia with very high rate (tachyarrhythmias) results. Depending upon the rate and rhythm and the site of ectopic focus, the tachyarrhythmias are named as:
  - Paroxysmal tachycardia (atrial, nodal and ventricular),
  - Atrial flutter,
  - Atrial fibrillation and
  - Ventricular fibrillation.

2. Re-entry Mechanism Re-entry mechanism or the circus movement refers to a phenomenon in which the wave of excitation propagates repeatedly (continuously) within a closed circuit. It is a more common cause of tachyarrhythmias. Re-entry of excitation wave is known to occur under two situations: (1) in the presence of transient block in the conduction pathway and (2) in the presence of an abnormal extra bundle of conducting tissue called bundle of Kent.

Re-entry due to Transient Block in the Conduction System

- Normally, during depolarization of a ring of cardiac tissue, the impulse spreads in both directions of the ring (Fig. 4.2-26A) and the tissue behind each branch of the impulse is refractory and thus the impulse cannot go down the other side.
- When there is a transient block on one side, the impulse can go down on the other side of ring (Fig. 4.2-26B), because this portion is not depolarized and so not refractory.
- If the transient block is worn off, the impulse from retrograde direction is conducted through this (previously blocked) area and then continues to circle indefinitely. This phenomenon is called circus movement or re-entry phenomenon (Fig. 4.2-26C).
- The site of re-entry keeps on producing impulses continuously. If the re-entry is in AV node, the re-entrant activity depolarizes the atrium and the resulting atrial beat is called an *echo beat.* In addition, the re-entrant activity in the node propagates back down to ventricles producing paroxysmal nodal tachycardia. The re-entrant activity can also become established in atrial muscle fibres (producing atrial tachycardias, flutter or fibrillation) and in ventricular muscle fibres (producing ventricular tachycardia or ventricular fibrillation).

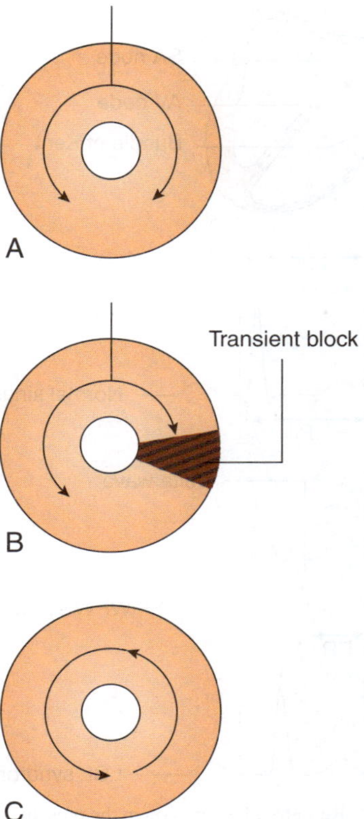

FIGURE 4.2-26 Re-entry phenomenon or circus movements, a cause of cardiac arrhythmias; **A,** normal depolarization of a ring cardiac tissue; **B,** spread of wave of excitation in presence of transient block; and **C,** circus movement.

Re-Entrant Activity in the Presence of Bundle of Kent

- Bundle of Kent is an abnormal extra bundle of conducting tissues present in some individuals. This bundle connects the atria and ventricles directly, so the conduction is very rapid than through the regular conductive system.
- If a transient block develops in the normal conductive system, the impulse from SA node reaches the ventricle through the bundle of Kent and produces excitation. If the blockage in the normal conduction system wears off, then the excitation wave from the ventricle travels in the opposite direction and re-enter the AV node and a circus movement is established (Fig. 4.2-27).
- This re-entrant activity produces echo beat in atria and nodal paroxysmal tachycardia or the so-called supraventricular tachycardia.
- The nodal paroxysmal tachycardia occurring in patients with bundle of Kent is called *Wolff–Parkinson–White syndrome*, producing short PR interval, prolonged slurred

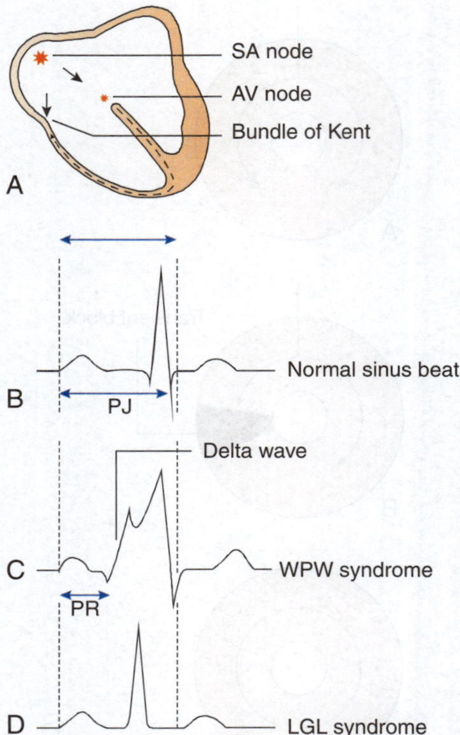

FIGURE 4.2-27 Re-entry phenomenon in the presence of bundle of Kent (**A**) and electrocardiogram record in a patient with bundle of Kent showing short PR interval, wide and slurred. QRS complex with normal PJ interval (Wolff-Parkinson-White (WPW) syndrome) (**C**) and Lown-Ganong-Levine (LGL) syndrome (**D**).

QRS deflection but normal PJ interval (start of P wave to end of QRS complex).

Salient Features of Cardiac Arrhythmias

Extra Systole Extra systole (premature beat, premature contraction or ectopic beat) refers to the contraction of the heart prior to the time that normal contraction would have been expected. It is caused by some ectopic focus in the atria or ventricles and thus the premature beat may be atrial or ventricular.

Causes of extra systole: The main cause of ectopic foci is mechanical irritation, which occurs due to ischaemia of local area of heart, calcified plaques, cardiac catheterization and local toxic irritation caused by drugs, nicotine, caffeine, etc.

Atrial Extra Systole (Premature Beat)

Cause. Atrial premature beat is caused by an ectopic focus in the atrium which becomes pacemaker for one beat. Atrial premature beats may occur frequently in healthy persons. In athletes, lack of sleep, increased consumption of coffee, smoking etc.

ECG appearance (Fig. 4.2-28B) of atrial premature beat is characterized by:

- A premature P wave occurs early and has an aberrant configuration and an abnormal short PR interval because of the different path of atrial depolarization.
- QRS complex and T wave are normal.
- Interval between premature beat and next succeeding beat is slightly prolonged called compensatory pause.
- The subsequent cardiac rhythm is shifted and reset, because the premature beat discharges the SA node, which then repolarizes and fires after the normal interval.

Significance. Since atrial extra systole occurs normally, the patient may or may not be aware of an occasional irregularity in the cardiac rhythm.

Ventricular Extra Systole

Cause. Ventricular extra systoles can arise from any portion of the ventricular myocardium and occasionally occur in otherwise healthy individuals. Frequently ventricular premature beats occur with many forms of heart disease, especially coronary artery disease (because ischaemia increases the irritability of the myocardium).

ECG appearance of ventricular premature beat is characterized by (Fig. 4.2-28C):

- Absence of P wave preceding the QRS complex.
- QRS complex is prolonged and bizarre shaped because of the slow spread of the impulse from the ectopic focus through the ventricular muscle to the rest of the ventricle.
- T wave is usually appositely directed from the QRS complex.
- Compensatory pause is often long. Since retrograde transmission of depolarization to the atria usually

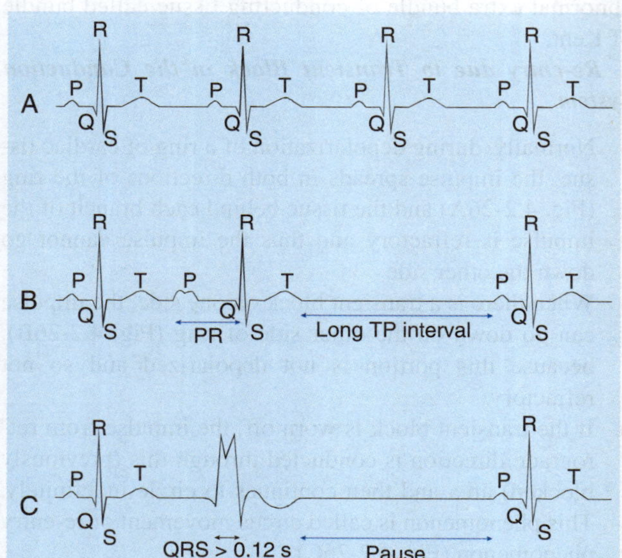

FIGURE 4.2-28 Electrocardiographic record in extra systole: **A,** normal ECG; **B,** ECG with atrial premature beat (atrial extra systole); and **C,** ECG with ventricular premature beat.

does not occur with premature ventricular beat, so, the atrial rate remains unaltered. The atrial depolarization that follows the premature ventricular beat arrives while the AV node is still refractory and, therefore, it is not conducted to the ventricles, creating a pause in the ventricular rhythm. This pause is usually fully compensatory so that R–R interval of the beat preceding the premature ventricular beat interval together equals two normal cycle lengths. Thus, the ventricular premature beats do not interrupt the regular discharge of the SA node, whereas atrial premature beats often interrupt and "reset" the normal rhythm.

The beat following ventricular premature beat is usually stronger than the normal because of the added stroke volume and thus usually detected by the patient.

Interpolated beats. When the patient's sinus rhythm is slow, in that case a premature ventricular beat may occur without altering the normal R–R interval. Such a premature ventricular beat is termed an interpolated beat.

Pulse Deficit. Ventricles contract ahead of time in atrial and ventricular premature beats. Sometimes by that time ventricles are not filled with blood and stroke volume output during the contraction is therefore decreased or even absent. During such a contraction, pulse wave passing to periphery may be so weak that it is not felt at the radial artery. A deficit in the number of pulses felt in the radial pulse in relation to the number of contraction in the heart is called pulse deficit.

Atrial Arrhythmias

• ***Atrial Tachycardia*** (Fig. 4.2-29A) occurs when an atrial site (outside the SA node) becomes the dominant pacemaker. It is characterized by very regular rates ranging from 140 to 220 beats/min. Atrial tachycardia may be caused by overindulgence in caffeine, nicotine or alcohol and may also occur during anxiety attack.

• ***Paroxysmal Atrial Tachycardia (PAT)*** as the name indicates occurs in paroxysms, which usually begin suddenly and lasts for few seconds. PAT may result from discharge of a single *ectopic site* or a *re-entry phenomenon* (described on page 265).

ECG appearance of PAT is characterized by an inverted P wave before each QRS complex, and this P wave is partially superimposed on to the normal T wave of the preceding beat (Fig. 4.2-29B)

• ***Atrial Flutter*** is said to occur with atrial rates of 220–350 beats/min. During atrial flutter, AV node is unable to transmit all of the atrial impulses and therefore the ventricular rate may be half, one-third or one-fourth of the atrial rates. Like atrial tachycardia, atrial flutter may result either from a single ectopic focus or a re-entry phenomenon.

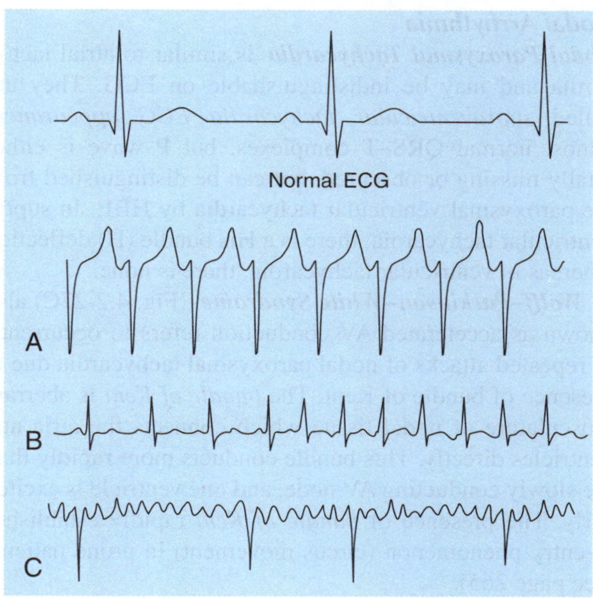

FIGURE 4.2-29 Electrocardiographic record in atrial arrhythmia: **A,** atrial tachycardia; **B,** paroxysmal atrial tachycardia – onset in middle of record (lead I); and **C,** atrial fibrillation.

ECG appearance in atrial flutter: the P wave is strong and QRS-T complex follows once after two P waves or three P waves (2:1 or 3:1 rhythm).

• ***Atrial Fibrillation*** (Fig. 4.2-29C) is characterized by a totally irregular, rapid rate (350–500 beats/min). In it, there occurs contraction of only small portion of the atrial musculature at one time because large portion of the atria are still in refractory period. *Ventricular rate* is completely irregular because only a fraction of the atrial impulses that reach the AV node are transmitted to the ventricles.

ECG appearance is characterized by:

- Small irregular oscillations called F waves. There are no recognizable P waves
- R–R interval is irregularly irregular
- QRS complex and T wave are normal because the impulses that are transmitted through the AV node are conducted normally through the ventricles.

Causes. Atrial fibrillations are frequently associated with enlarged atria secondary to AV valve diseases.

Treatment. Atrial fibrillations can be converted back to normal rhythm by cardioversion/defibrillation. A strong single electric shock of alternating current is passed through the heart for a fraction of second. All action potential stop and heart remains quiescent for few seconds (3–5 s) or refractoriness of heart. After that it begins to beat with normal rhythm.

Complications. Long-term fibrillation is associated with *thrombi* in the atrial appendages.

Nodal Arrhythmia

Nodal Paroxysmal Tachycardia is similar to atrial tachycardia and may be indistinguishable on ECG. They are called *supraventricular tachycardia ECG appearance:* almost normal QRS–T complexes, but P wave is either totally missing or obscured, but can be distinguished from the paroxysmal ventricular tachycardia by HBE. In supraventricular tachycardia, there is a His bundle (H) deflection whereas in ventricular tachycardia, there is none.

Wolff–Parkinson–White Syndrome (Fig. 4.2-27C) also known as accelerated AV conduction refers to occurrence of repeated attacks of nodal paroxysmal tachycardia due to presence of bundle of Kent. The *bundle of Kent* is aberrant musculature or nodal tissue which connects the atria and ventricles directly. This bundle conducts more rapidly than the slowly conducting AV node, and one ventricle is excited early. The presence of *bundle of Kent* rapidly establishes re-entry phenomenon (circus movement) in prone patients (see page 265).

Lown–Ganong–Levine Syndrome (Fig. 4.2-27D). It is characterized by attacks of paroxysmal supraventricular tachycardia, usual nodal tachycardia in individuals with short PR intervals and normal QRS complexes. In this condition, depolarization presumably passes from the atria to the ventricles via an *aberrant bundle* that bypasses the AV node but enters the intraventricular conducting system distal to node.

Ventricular Arrhythmias

Paroxysmal Ventricular Tachycardia occurs when a ventricular site discharges rapidly and repetitively, usually as a result of *re-entry phenomenon.* Alterations in vagal tone (by carotid sinus massage or Valsalva manoeuvre) do not affect ventricular tachycardia because the ventricles do not receive any efferent vagal innervation.

Causes. Ventricular tachycardias are usually associated with serious heart disease or drug toxicity.

ECG appearance is characterized by (Fig. 4.2-30B):

- Wide, bizarre QRS complexes that occur at rapid rate and
- P waves are usually indistinguishable.

Significance. Ventricular tachycardia is more serious because cardiac output is decreased, sustained ventricular tachycardia can be a life-threatening when it degenerates into ventricular fibrillation.

Ventricular Fibrillation occurs when small segments of ventricular myocardium show rapid, irregular ineffective contractions. In this condition, cardiac output is zero and so the peripheral pulse is absent. ECG is must to differentiate ventricular fibrillation from the cardiac standstill.

Causes. Ventricular fibrillation is very common during electric shock and during ischaemia of conductive system. Other causes are coronary occlusion, trauma to heart, chloroform anaesthesia and improper handling of heart during cardiac surgery.

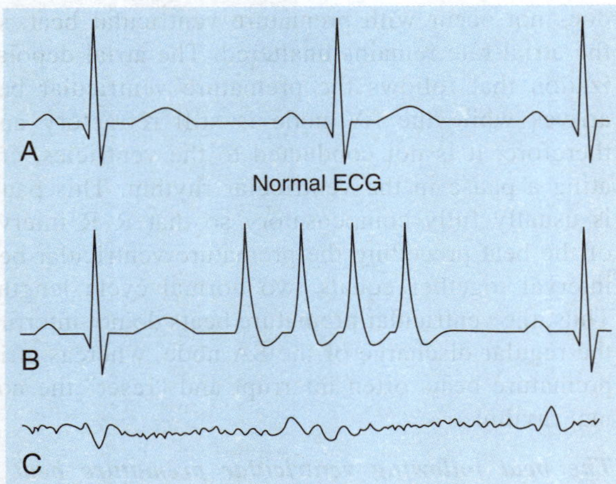

FIGURE 4.2-30 Electrocardiographic record in ventricular arrhythmias: **A,** normal; **B,** paroxysmal ventricular tachycardia; and **C,** ventricular fibrillation.

ECG appearance (Fig. 4.2-30C) is characterized by:

- Undulating waves of varying frequency and amplitude. The voltage of the ECG waves in ventricular fibrillation is about 0.2-0.5 mV or less.
- Ventricular premature beats are usually seen as the precipitating cause, one of which falls on the *vulnerable period* of the T wave (i.e. the interval near the peak of T wave when the ventricle is partially repolarized). A premature beat during the vulnerable period produces fibrillation because the chances of re-entry occurring are more.

Significance. Ventricular fibrillation is the most common cause of sudden death in patients with myocardial infarcts.

Treatment. Cardiopulmonary resuscitation must be started immediately to prevent tissue death. For details see page 471.

Immediate electric or electronic defibrillation (cardioversion) should be performed.

- *T* cardioversion/defibrillation is done by applying electrodes directly to two sides of the heart or on the chest wall using 110 volts of 60 cycles at alternating current for 0.1 s or 1000 volts of direct current for thousandth of a second.

Techniques for Evaluation of Arrhythmia

1. Electrocardiographic monitoring is the ideal way of establishing a correlation between symptoms and a rhythm disturbance, but this is not always easy because symptoms are usually sporadic.

- When episodes of arrhythmia are infrequent, then continuous 24-h monitoring may be helpful.

- Exercise testing may be helpful if symptoms are associated with stress or exertion.

2. Heart Rate Variability (HRV) refers to beat to beat variation of heart rate. The R–R interval variations during resting condition represents a fine tuning of beat to beat control mechanisms. HRV reflects fluctuations rather than absolute levels of sympathetic and parasympathetic impulse. The analysis of beat to beat variation in heart rate is used to investigate sympathovagal imbalance, i.e. integrity of autonomic activity and vulnerability to various cardiovascular disorder resulting from autonomic imbalance. HRV is recorded by ECG lead II on Polyrite D system and its time domain and frequency domain variables are analyzed. Details of HRV are beyond the scope of the book.

3. Electrophysiological Testing is intracardiac, electrocardiographic recordings is useful in diagnosis and management of complex arrhythmia.

4. Autonomic Testing is an important component of evaluation in patients with recurrent syncope. Autonomic testing can be done by simple Head up tilt test (HUT), also called as Tilt Table Test.

5. Tilt Table Testing is based on the fact that in upright posture, there is venous pooling in lower limbs that reflexly increases heart rate and vasoconstriction (compensatory mechanism). Head-up-tilt-testing can identify the syncope due to vasovagal /autonomic imbalance.

Treatment of Arrhythmia

1. Mechanical Measures are used to interrupt the attack. These include: Valsalva manoeuver and carotid sinus massage. These manoeuvers stimulate the vagus nerve, delays A–V conduction and block the re-entry mechanism, and ultimately terminating arrhythmia.

2. Anti Arrhythmic Drugs have limited efficiency due to frequent side effects. Broadly antiarrhythmic drugs are divided into four classes based on their electropharmacological actions:

- ***Class I agents*** block membrane sodium channels, thus slowing conduction and prolonging the refractoriness. These include: Quinine and procainamide.
- ***Class II agents*** are beta adrenergic blockers, which decrease automaticity, prolong AV conduction. Examples are propranolol and metaprolol.
- ***Class III*** agents block K^+ channels and prolong repolarization and prolonging QT interval.
- ***Class IV*** agents are calcium channel blockers, which decrease automaticity and A–V conduction, e.g. Verapamil.

3. Radiofrequency Ablation: Cardiac catheter with electrodes attached to its tip is passed into the chambers of the heart, and exact location of ectopic focus or accessory bundle responsible for arrhythmia is identified. The ablation can be done by applying radiofrequency band (300–3000 kHz) with catheter tip. Radiofrequency is particularly useful in conditions that cause supraventricular tachycardias, Wolff–Parkinson–White syndrome and atrial flutter.

The radiofrequency generates energy for biomedical applications like coagulation and cauterization of the tissue.

Myocardial Infarction

Myocardial infarction refers to the ischaemic necrosis of a part of myocardium which occurs when coronary blood flow ceases or is reached below a critical level (see page 360). The ECG is very useful for diagnosing and localizing areas of myocardial infarction.

ECG Appearance. The ECG undergoes a series of changes following the myocardial infarction. These changes must be recorded daily with ECG tracing for diagnostic purpose. The *hallmark of acute myocardial infarction* is:

- *Elevation of ST segment* (Fig. 4.2-31 LI) in the leads overlying the area of infarct and
- *Depression of ST segment* (Fig. 4.2-31 LII) in the leads on the opposite side of area of infarct.

ECG appearance in old cases of myocardial infarct is characterized by:

- ST segment returns to normal,
- Appearance of Q wave (Fig. 4.2-31 LI and LII) in some of the leads in which it was not previously present and
- An increase in the size of normal Q wave in some of the other leads.

Physiological Basis of ECG Changes in Acute Myocardial Infarction The alterations in ECG pattern seen in acute myocardial infarction are attributed to *injury current* which flows from the affected to the unaffected part of myocardium. This happens because of the fact that the affected part of myocardium gets depolarized partly or completely but does not get repolarized rapidly. The three major abnormalities that cause

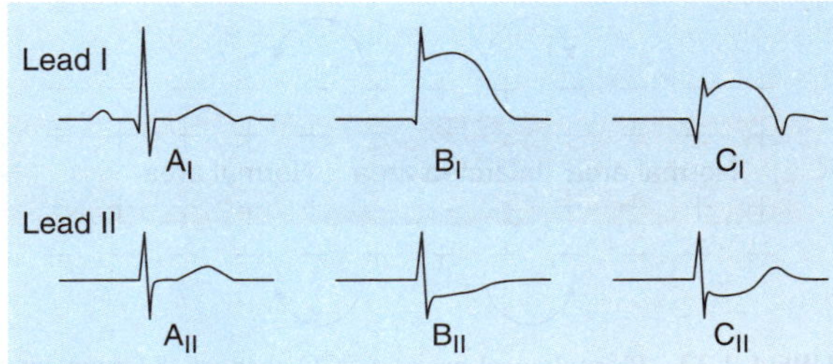

FIGURE 4.2-31 Electrocardiographic record in anterior wall ischaemia in lead I and II respectively: AI and AII, normal ECG; BI and BII, ECG within few hours of ischaemia, note ST segment elevation in lead I and depression in lead II (reciprocal); and CI and CII, ECG after several weeks, note ST segment returns to normal and Q wave appears.

ECG changes (ST segment elevation) in acute myocardial infarction are:

1. Decline in Resting Membrane Potential. The ischaemic necrosis of the myocardial fibres results in breakdown of cell membrane producing increased K^+ efflux and increase in Na^+ influx. Therefore, inside of the infarcted cells becomes less negative as compared to the unaffected area. Therefore, during ventricular diastole, the *zcurrent flows into the infarct* from the unaffected area (Fig. 4.2-32B). This results in a depression of TQ segment of the ECG in the leads overlying the infarcted area. However, the electronic arrangement in electrocardiographic recorders is such that TQ segment depression is recorded as ST segment elevation.

2. Delayed Depolarization of infarcted cells causes the infarcted area to be positive relative to the unaffected area. Therefore, current flows out of infarcted area into the unaffected area (Fig. 4.2-32C).

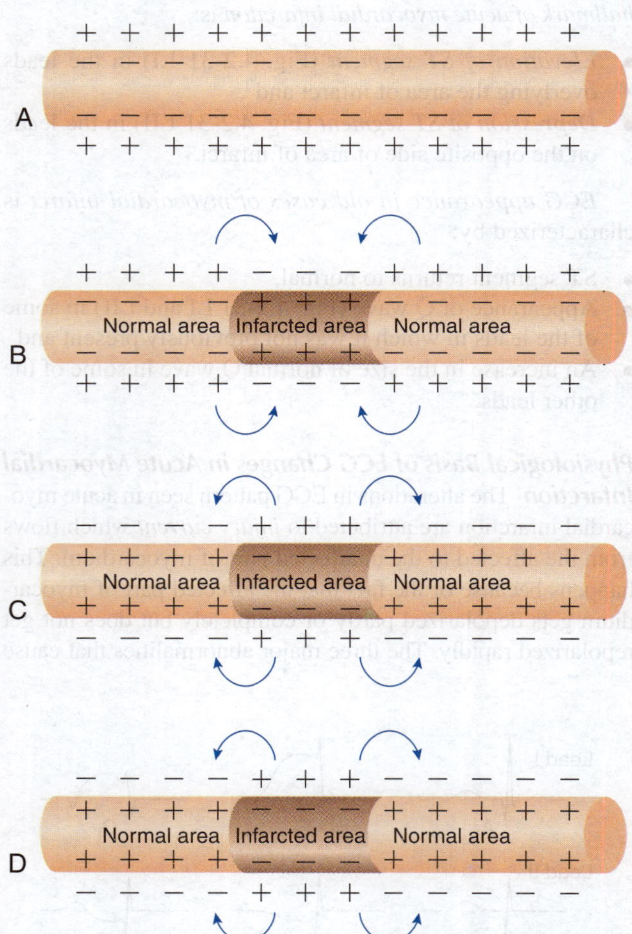

FIGURE 4.2-32 Physiological basis of ECG changes (ST segment elevation) in acute myocardial infarction: **A,** normal resting state; **B,** decline in resting membrane potential in infarct area as compared to normal neighbouring (unaffected) region; **C,** delayed depolarization of infarct area as compared to neighbouring areas; and **D,** rapid repolarization of infarct area in comparison to normal neighbouring areas.

3. Rapid Repolarization. The repolarization in infarcted cells occurs rapidly as compared to unaffected area due to accelerated opening of K^+ channels. Because of the rapid repolarization in the infarct, the membrane potential of the affected area becomes greater than that of the unaffected area. Extracellularly, current therefore flows out of the infarct into normal unaffected area (Fig. 4.2-32D). This current flow toward electrodes over the injured area, causing increased positivity between the S and T waves of ECG. Consequently, leads on the opposite side of the heart show ST segment depression.

Physiological Basis of ECG Changes in Old Cases of Myocardial Infarction After some days or weeks of infarction, the dead myocardium and scar tissue become electrically silent. Therefore, the affected area becomes negative relative to the unaffected normal myocardium during systole, and it fails to contribute its share of positivity to the electrocardiographic complexes. The occurrence of Q wave in some leads (which normally lack) and deepening of Q wave in other leads is one of the manifestations of this negativity.

Localization of Area of Myocardial Infarction

1. ***Anterior myocardial infarction***
- Leads showing changes of MI are LI, aVL and V_3–V_5
- Leads showing reciprocal changes are LII, LIII and aVF.

2. ***Posterior (inferior) myocardial infarction***
- Leads showing changes of MI include LII, LIII and aVF.
- Leads showing reciprocal changes are LI, aVR, aVL and V_1–V_6.

3. ***Lateral myocardial infarction***
- Leads showing changes of MI include LI, aVL and V_6 and
- Leads showing reciprocal change are LII, LIII, aVF and V_1.

4. ***Septal myocardial infarction***
- Leads showing changes of MI are V_1–V_3.

Complications Complications of myocardial infarction are ventricular arrhythmias which mainly occur due to reentrant activity during the first 30 min of infarction, and increased automaticity after 12 h.

Important Note
- The infarcts which affect epicardial part of myocardium damages the sympathetic nerves resulting in denervation hypersensitivity to catecholamines in the area beyond the infarct.
- On the other hand, endocardial lesions interrupt vagal activity, therefore unopposed sympathetic fibres activity results.

Ventricular Hypertrophy

Ventricular hypertrophy occurs when the work of the ventricle is increased sufficiently. In ventricular hypertrophy, the number of myocardial cells remains the same, but the diameter of the individual cells increases, raising the diffusion distance for O_2 and other metabolites.

Left Ventricular Hypertrophy (LVH) occurs in patients with systemic hypertension or aortic valve stenosis. Right ventricular hypertrophy (RVH) occurs in patients with pulmonary hypertension, pulmonary valve stenosis and some congenital heart disease.

ECG Appearance is characterized by (Fig. 4.2-18B) the following.

1. ***R wave.*** There is direct correlation between the thickness of ventricular wall and the height of R wave in the overlying leads. Therefore:
   - In LVH, the R wave is tall in leads I, aVL, V_5 and V_6 and
   - In RVH, the R wave is tall in lead III, aVR, V_1 and V_2.
2. ***QRS duration*** is increased slightly due to the increased muscle mass. It is usually less than 0.12 s, but occasionally may exceed this value.
3. ***Mean electric axis (MEA)*** shows (Fig. 4.2-18A):
   - LAD in LVH and
   - RAD in RVH.

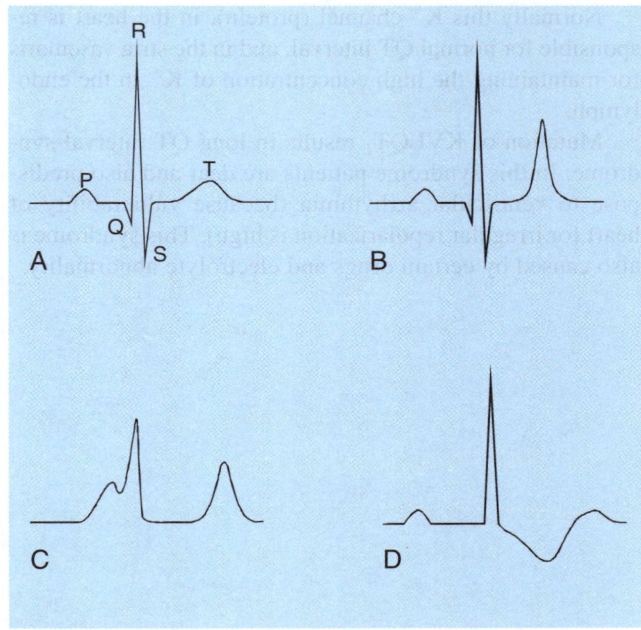

FIGURE 4.2-33 Electrocardiographic changes in relation to plasma levels of potassium: **A,** normal tracing (plasma K + 4–5.5 mEq/L); **B,** hyperkalaemia (plasma K + 7.0 mEq/L); **C,** hyperkalaemia (plasma K + 8.0 mEq/L); and **D,** hypokalemia (plasma K + 2.5–3.5 mEq/L).

Effect of Changes in the Ionic Composition of Blood on Electrical Activity of Heart

The electrical activity of the heart depends upon the distribution of ions like Na^+, K^+ and Ca^{2+} in the ECF. Therefore, changes in the ECF concentration of these ions will affect the potentials of myocardial fibres and produce changes in the ECG as described:

Plasma Level of Sodium Low plasma (ECF) levels of Na^+ may be associated with low voltage ECG complexes.

Plasma Levels of Potassium Depending upon the levels of plasma K^+ following ECG changes are seen:

1. ***With normal plasma levels of K^+ (4–5.5 mEq/L).*** The normal ECG tracings (Fig. 4.2-33A) are produced with PR interval = 0.16 s; QRS interval = 0.06 s, QT interval = 0.4 s.
2. ***Hyperkalaemia,*** i.e. increase in plasma K^+ is very dangerous and potentially lethal condition because of its effects on heart.

Hyperkalaemia with plasma K^+ ± 7.0 mEq/L, the PR and QRS intervals are within normal limits. The T wave become tall and peaked (Fig. 4.2-33B), which is a manifestation of altered repolarization.

- *In hyperkalaemia* with plasma K^+ levels, 8.5 mEq/L the ECG shows (Fig. 4.2-33C).
  - Broad and slurred QRS complex with a QRS interval of 0.2 s occurs due to paralysis of atria.
  - T wave remains tall and slender.
- A further increase in plasma K^+ levels may result in ventricular tachycardia and ventricular fibrillation.
- As the extracellular K^+ concentration increases, the resting membrane potential of the muscle fibres decreases. Eventually the fibres become unexcitable, and the heart stops in diastole.

3. ***Hypokalaemia,*** i.e. decrease in the plasma levels of potassium is a serious condition but it is not as rapidly fatal as hyperkalaemia. It produces the following changes in ECG (Fig. 4.2-33D):
   - PR interval is prolonged,
   - U waves become prominent,
   - ST segment is depressed,
   - Late T wave inversion may occur in the precordial leads and
   - If the T and U waves merge, the apparent QT interval is often prolonged, but if the T and U waves are separated, the true QT interval is of normal duration.

Long QT syndrome. Long QT syndrome occurs due to genetic abnormality which blocks one type of K^+ channels $KVLQT_1$ resulting in slow K^+ efflux, prolonging cardiac action potential and hence QT interval. The incidence of ventricular arrhythmia and sudden death is more with prolonged QT interval.

Normally this K^+ channel (protein), in the heart is responsible for normal QT interval, and in the stria vascularis for maintaining the high concentration of K^+ in the endolymph.

Mutation of $KVLQT_1$ results in long QT interval syndrome. In this syndrome patients are deaf and also predispose to ventricular arrhythmia (because vulnerability of heart for irregular repolarization is high). This syndrome is also caused by certain drugs and electrolyte abnormality.

Plasma Levels of Calcium

- ***Hypercalcaemia,*** i.e. increased in extracellular Ca^{2+}, clinically is rare if ever high enough to affect the heart. However, when large amounts of calcium are infused into experimental animals, the heart relaxes less during diastole and eventually stops in systole (*calcium rigor*).
- ***Hypocalcaemia,*** i.e. decreased plasma level of Ca^{2+} produces prolongation of the ST segment and consequently the QT interval is also increased.

Chapter 4.3

Heart as a Pump: Cardiac Cycle, Cardiac Output, and Venous Return

CARDIAC CYCLE
- Introduction
- Phases of cardiac cycle
  - Atrial systole
  - Atrial diastole
  - Ventricular systole
  - Ventricular diastole
- Events during cardiac cycle
  - Pressure changes in the ventricles
  - Pressure changes in the atria
  - Pressure changes in the pulmonary artery
  - Volume changes in the ventricles
  - Valvular events (heart sounds)
  - Pressure-volume loop
- Duration of systole and diastole vis-a-vis heart rate
  - Effect of heart rate
  - Clinical indices
- Arterial pulse

CARDIAC OUTPUT AND VENOUS RETURN
- Definition
- Measurement of cardiac output
- Variations in cardiac output
- Regulation of cardiac output
  - Cardiac output control mechanisms
  - Role of heart rate in control of cardiac output
  - Integrated control of cardiac output
- Heart-lung preparation
- Cardiac and vascular function curves

CARDIAC CYCLE

Introduction

The heart as a pump can be considered actually comprising of two separate pumps in the series: a *right heart* that pumps the blood through the lungs and a *left heart* that pumps the blood through the peripheral organs. Further, each sided pump consists of an atrium and a ventricle. The atria act as *primary pumps* for the ventricles, helping to move the blood into the ventricles. The ventricles in turn provide the major force that propels the blood through pulmonary and systemic circulations. To act as a pump, the heart contracts and relaxes rhythmically. The terms *systole* (contractile phase) and *diastole* (relaxation phase) usually refer to ventricular events but may be prefixed by 'atrial' to refer to atrial contraction and relaxation, respectively. The heart has an *intrinsic contraction rate* because it contains its own pacemaker normally located in the SA node. As discussed in Chapter 4.2, the cardiac impulse arising from the SA node spreads in the whole heart. The electrocardiogram records the *electrical events* that precede and initiate the corresponding *mechanical events* as:

- *P wave* is caused by spread of depolarization through the atria, and this is followed by *atrial contraction.*
- *QRS waves* which appear 0.16 s after the onset of P wave are caused by depolarization of the ventricles which initiates *contraction of the ventricles.*
- *T wave* represents the stage of repolarization of the ventricles at which time the ventricular muscle fibres begin to relax. Therefore, T wave occurs slightly before the end of ventricular contraction.

The cardiac cycle, thus includes both electrical and mechanical events that occur from the beginning of one heart beat to the beginning of the next.

Cardiodynamics is the study of the mechanical events associated with the contraction and relaxation of the heart. These include:

- pressure changes in the ventricles,
- pressure changes in the atria,
- pressure changes in the aorta,

- volume changes in the ventricles and
- valvular events, i.e. production of heart sounds.

Phases of Cardiac Cycle

Duration of each cardiac cycle at a normal heart rate of 75 beats/min, is 60/75 = 0.8 s.

During each cardiac cycle, both atria contract (*atrial systole*) and relax (*atrial diastole*), and both ventricles contract (*ventricular systole*) and relax (*ventricular diastole*).

Therefore, each cardiac cycle can be considered to consist of simultaneously occurring atrial and ventricular cycles with following phases (Figs 4.3-1 and 4.3-2).

Atrial Cycle

1. Atrial systole or atrial contraction phase (0.1 s)
2. Atrial diastole (0.7 s).

Ventricular Cycle

Ventricular systole (0.3 s) consisting of:

1. Isovolumic (isometric) contraction phase (0.05 s) and
2. Phase of ventricular ejection which can be further divided into rapid ejection phase (0.1 s) and slow ejection phase (0.15 s).

Ventricular diastole (0.5 s) consisting of:

1. Protodiastole (0.04 s),
2. Isovolumic (isometric) relaxation phase (0.06 s),
3. Rapid passive filling phase (0.11 s),
4. Reduced filling phase or diastasis (0.19 s) and
5. Last rapid filling phase which coincides with the atrial systole (0.1 s).

Atrial Cycle

Atrial Systole

- Atrial systole or the atrial contraction phase lasts for 0.1 s and coincides with the last rapid filling phase of ventricular diastole (Figs 4.3-1 and 4.3-2).

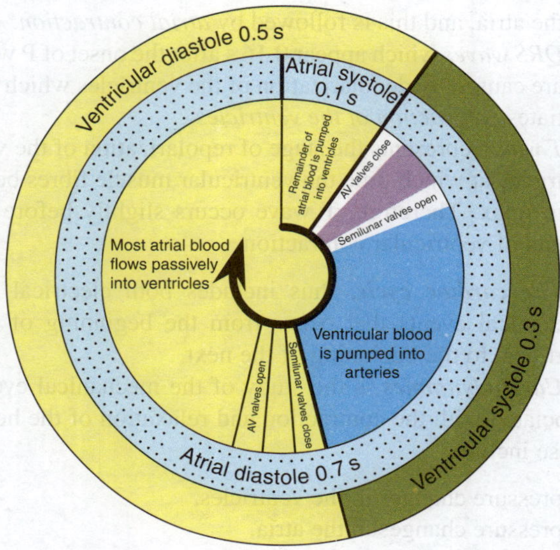

FIGURE 4.3-1 Duration of phases of cardiac cycle.

- Before the beginning of atrial systole, the ventricles are relaxing, AV valves are open and blood is flowing from the great veins into the atria and from the atria into the ventricles. Thus the atria and ventricles are forming a continuous cavity.
- When the atrial contraction begins, about 75% of the blood has already flown into the ventricles. Thus, atrial contraction usually causes an additional 25% filling of the ventricles. Therefore, even if the atria fail to function, it is unlikely to be noticed unless a person exercises.

The contraction of atria causes:

- *Increase in intra-atrial pressure* by 4–6 mmHg in right atrium and 7–8 mmHg in left atrium. The pressure rise in right atrium is reflected into the veins and is recorded as *a-wave* from the jugular vein.
- *Increase in the ventricular pressure* occurs slightly due to pumping of blood in the ventricles.
- *Narrowing of great veins* at the origin (inferior vena cava and superior vena cava opening in right atrium, and pulmonary veins opening in left atrium) decreasing venous return to the heart. Some regurgitation of the blood occurs into the great veins as no valves are present at their entrance into the atria.

Atrial Diastole

After the atrial systole, there occurs atrial diastole (0.7 s). This period coincides with the ventricular systole and most of the ventricular diastole (Fig. 4.3-1).

- During atrial diastole, atrial muscles relax and there occurs gradual filling of the atria due to continuous venous return and the pressure gradually increases in the atria and drops down to almost zero with the opening of AV valves (Fig. 4.3-3). Then the pressure again rises and follows the ventricular pressure during the rest of atrial diastole.

Ventricular Cycle

Ventricular Systole

After the atrial contraction phase is over, the ventricles get excited by the impulse travelling along the conduction system and the ventricles start contracting. The ventricular systole lasts to 0.3 s, and has the following phases.

1. Phase of Isovolumic (Isometric) Contraction

- With the beginning of ventricular contraction, the ventricular pressure exceeds atrial pressure very rapidly causing closure of AV valves (this event is responsible for production of first heart sound).
- Since the AV valves have closed and semilunar valves have not opened, the ventricles contract as a closed chamber and the pressure inside the ventricles rises rapidly to a high level.

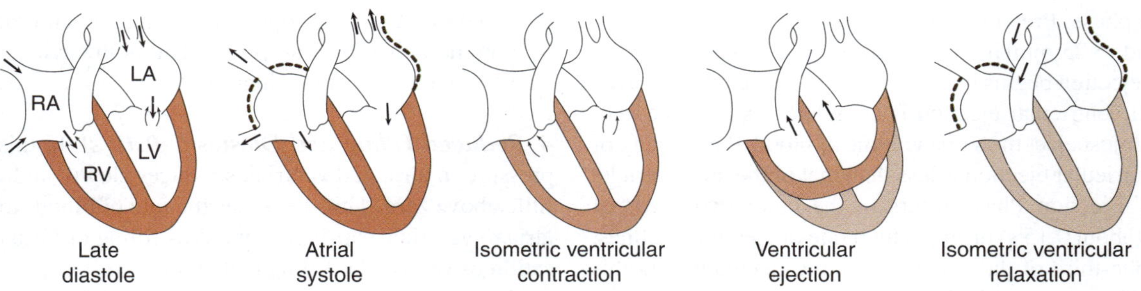

FIGURE 4.3-2 Phases of cardiac cycle.

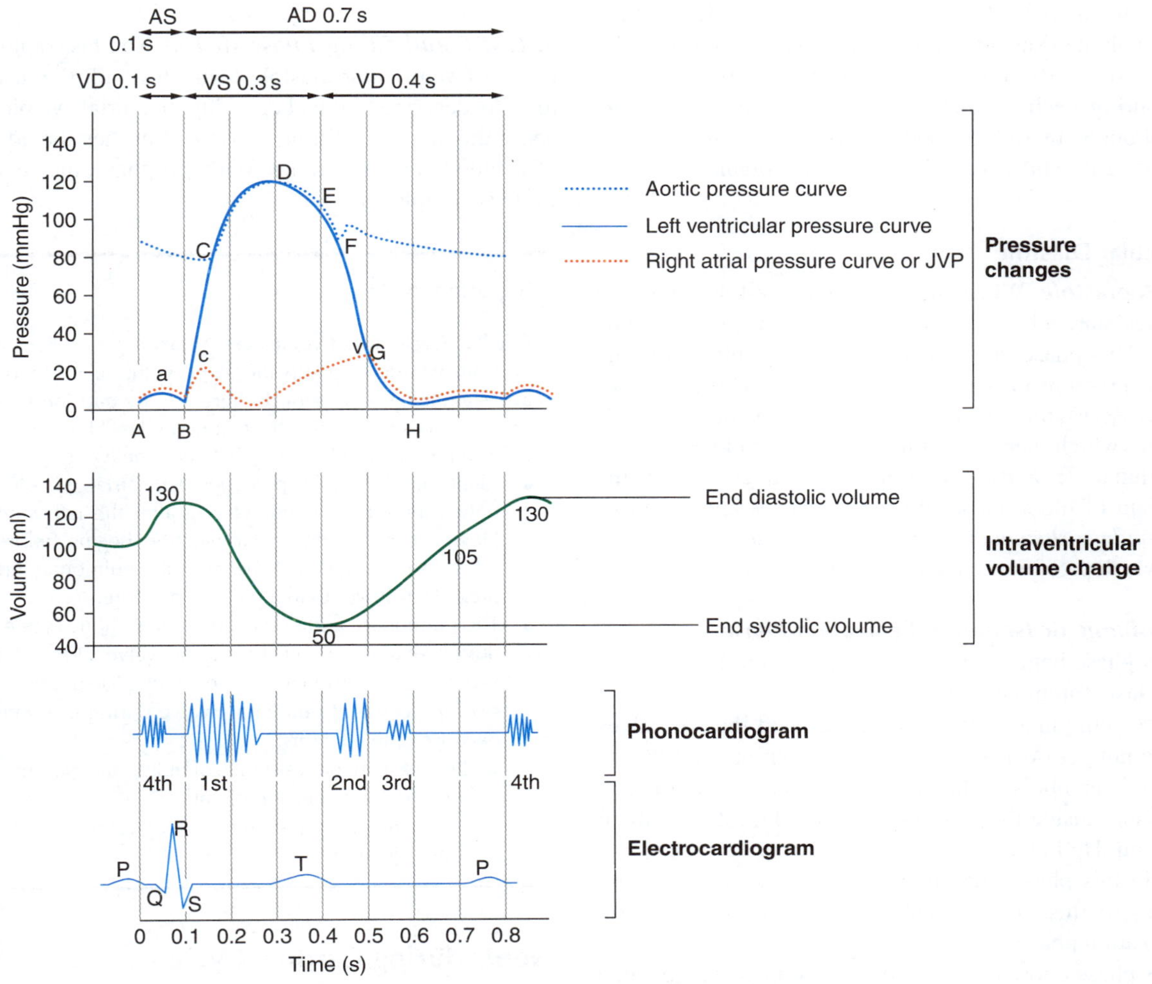

FIGURE 4.3-3 Phases and events during cardiac cycle.

- As the ventricles contract, the volume of blood in the ventricles does not change; hence this phase is called *isovolumic contraction phase.*
- During this phase, due to sharp rise in ventricular pressure, there occurs bulging of AV valves into the atria producing a small but sharp rise in intra-atrial pressure called *c-wave*.
- This phase lasts for 0.05 s, until the pressure in the left and right ventricles exceeds the pressure in the aorta (80 mmHg) and pulmonary artery (10 mmHg) and the aortic and pulmonary valves open.

2. Phase of Ventricular Ejection The ventricular ejection phase begins with the opening of semilunar valves and lasts for about 0.25 s. It can be further divided into two phases.

Rapid Ejection Phase. As soon as the semilunar valves open, the blood is rapidly ejected out for about 0.1 s. About two-thirds of the stroke volume is ejected in this rapid ejection phase. Pressure rises to 120 mmHg in the left ventricle and to 25 mmHg in the right ventricle. The right ventricular ejection begins before that of left and continued even after left ventricular ejection is complete. As both the ventricles almost eject the same volume of blood, the velocity of right ventricular ejection is less than that of the left ventricle.

Slow Ejection Phase refers to the latter two-thirds of systole (about 0.15 s) during which rate of ejection declines. About one-third of the stroke volume is ejected during this phase. The intraventricular pressure starts declining and falls to a value slightly lower than in aorta, but for a short period momentum keeps the blood flowing forward.

Volume changes. At the end of each diastole the ventricular volume is about 130 ml. This is called end-diastolic volume. About 80 ml of blood is ejected out by each ventricle during each systole. This is called *stroke volume.* Thus, about 50 ml of the blood is left in each ventricle at the end of systole. This is called *end-systolic volume.*

Ventricular Diastole

1. Protodiastole When the ventricular systole ends, the ventricles start relaxing and intraventricular pressure falls rapidly. This phase lasts for 0.04 s. During this phase, the elevated pressure in the distended arteries (aorta and pulmonary artery) immediately pushes the blood back towards ventricles which snaps the semilunar valves to close. Closure of semilunar (i.e. aortic and pulmonary) valves prevents the movement of blood back into the ventricles and produces the *second heart sound* (S_2). It also causes *dicrotic notch* in the down slope of aortic pressure called the *incisura.*

2. Isovolumic or Isometric Relaxation Phase

- This phase begins with the closure of semilunar valves and lasts for about 0.06 s.
- Since semilunar valves have closed and the AV valves have not yet opened, the ventricles continue to relax as closed chambers in this phase. This causes rapid fall of pressure inside the ventricles (from 80 mmHg to about 2–3 mmHg in left ventricle.
- As in this phase, the ventricular volume remains constant, so this phase is called isovolumic or isometric relaxation phase.
- This phase ends when the AV valves open, as indicated by the peak of *v-wave* on the atrial pressure tracing (Figs 4.3-2 and 4.3-3).

3. Rapid Passive Filling Phase (0.11 s)

- During ventricular systole, the atria are in diastole and venous return continues so that the atrial pressure is high when the AV valves open. The high atrial pressure causes a rapid, initial flow of blood into the ventricles. The rapid passive filling phase produces the *third heart sound (S_3)*, which is not normally audible in adults but may be heard in children.
- Once the AV valves open, the atria and ventricles are a common chamber and pressure in both cavities falls as ventricular relaxation continues.

4. Reduced Filling and Diastasis (0.19 s) In this phase, pressure in atria and ventricles reduces slowly and remains little above zero. This decreases the rate of blood flow from atria to ventricle causing a very slow filling or virtually cessation of ventricular filling called *diastasis.*

Note. It is important to note that about 75% blood passes from atria to ventricles during rapid filling and reduced filling phases of ventricular diastole.

5. Last Rapid Filling Phase (0.1 s) The last rapid filling phase of ventricular diastole coincides with the atrial systole. As described in the beginning, the atrial systole brings about the last rapid filling phase and pushes the additional 25% blood in the ventricles. With this phase, the ventricular cycle is completed.

Important Note

Cardiac Cycle: Right versus Left Heart

Both ventricles pump the same volume of blood over any significant time period; therefore, by and large events on the two sides of the heart are similar. However, there exists a minor asynchronicity between the two sides as:

- Right atrial systole precedes left atrial systole, but right ventricle starts contracting after the left ventricle. However, right ventricular ejection begins before the left ventricular ejection, because the pulmonary arterial pressure is lower than the aortic pressure.
- The pulmonary and aortic valves close at the same time during expiration, but the aortic valve closes slightly before the pulmonary valve during inspiration. The slower closure of pulmonary valve during inspiration is because of two factors:
  - Decrease in the resistance of pulmonary vascular tree with prolonged ejection, and
  - An increase in systemic venous return which prolongs ejection.

Events during Cardiac Cycle

The events associated with contraction and relaxation of the heart during a cardiac cycle include pressure changes in the ventricles, atria and aorta; volume changes in the ventricles and valvular events. Most of these have been described during various phases of the cardiac cycle; however, they are once again repeated to highlight them.

Pressure Changes in the Ventricles

Pressure changes in the ventricles during cardiac cycle are consistent with the maintenance of systemic and pulmonary circulation. The intraventricular pressure can be measured with the help of cardiac catheterization. Pressure changes observed during various phases of cardiac cycle are as depicted in Figs 4.3-2 and 4.3-3.

During Atrial Systole Before the onset of atrial systole, i.e. during diastasis the pressure inside the ventricles is a little above zero. During atrial systole, there occurs a slight increase in the intraventricular pressure (about 6–7 mmHg in right ventricle and about 7–8 mmHg in left ventricle) due to pumping of blood in the ventricles. In the intraventricular pressure curve (Fig. 4.3-3), the segment AB represents the pressure changes during atrial systole. The point A denotes the onset of atrial systole and the point B denotes the closure of AV valve.

During Ventricular Systole

During Phase of Isovolumic (Isometric) Contraction, since the AV valves have closed and semilunar valves have not opened, so the ventricles contract as a closed chamber and pressure inside them rises rapidly to a high level. In the intraventricular pressure curve (Fig. 4.3-3), this phase is represented by the segment BC. The point C denotes the opening of semilunar valves and commencement of ventricular ejection phase.

During Rapid Ejection Phase the ventricles contract at a rate greater than the rate at which blood is ejected so a great rise in the pressure occurs. Pressure rises to maximum of 120 mmHg in the left ventricle and 25 mmHg in the right ventricle. The maximum pressure in the left ventricle is 4–5 times more than in the right ventricle. This is because of the thick wall of the left ventricle. In the intraventricular pressure curve (Fig. 4.3-3), this phase is denoted by the segment CD. The point D denotes the peak point of intraventricular pressure after which it starts declining.

During Slow Ejection Phase there is no further ventricular contraction and the pressure starts declining (Fig. 4.3-3, segment DE).

During Ventricular Diastole

During Protodiastole, the intraventricular pressure drops rapidly as the ventricles start relaxing. When the intraventricular pressure falls below that of aorta and pulmonary artery, the semilunar valves are closed due to back flow of blood. In the intraventricular pressure curve (Fig. 4.3-3) this phase is represented by segment EF, and the point F denoted the closure of semilunar valves.

During Isovolumic (Isometric) Relaxation Phase, since the semilunar valves have closed and AV valves have not yet opened up so the ventricles relax as closed chamber and there occurs a rapid fall in the intraventricular pressure (from 80 mmHg to about 2–3 mmHg in left ventricle). When the pressure inside the ventricles fall below the pressure in atria, the AV valves open up and the phase of rapid passive filling commences. In the intraventricular pressure curve (Fig. 4.3-3), the segment FG represents this phase and the point G coincides with the opening of AV valve.

During Rapid Passive Filling Phase, the intraventricular pressure further falls since the ventricles are relaxing though blood is being filled in them (segment GH in Fig. 4.3-3).

During Reduced Passive Filling Phase, there is no turbulence and the blood flows very slowly and smoothly and virtually there occurs cessation of ventricular filling (*diastasis*). The ventricular pressure remains a little above zero.

Pressure Changes in the Atria

The intra-atrial pressure can be studied by recording with the help of intracardiac catheterization. The left atrial pressure can also be determined indirectly by measuring the pulmonary capillary wedge pressure. The tracing of the jugular venous pulse is also similar to the intra-atrial pressure curve, and it has three positive waves called a, c and v and two descents namely x, z and y (Fig. 4.3-3). Relationship of intra-atrial pressure changes with the phases of cardiac cycle is:

During Atrial Systole Before the onset of atrial systole, the intra-atrial pressure is slightly above zero and is slightly greater than the ventricular pressure. During atrial systole there occurs a sharp rise in intra-atrial pressure (by 4–6 mmHg) in right atrium and by 7–8 mmHg in left atrium) and causes a pressure wave recorded as *a wave* from the jugular vein ('a' stands for atrial systole). Immediately after atrial systole the intra-atrial pressure falls due to start of atrial relaxation in atrial diastole. 'a' wave becomes prominent during inspiration due to decreased intrathoracic pressure (Fig. 4.3-3).

During Ventricular Systole

During Phase of Isovolumic (Isometric) Contraction, due to sharp rise in intraventricular pressure, AV valves bulge into the atria producing a small but sharp rise in atrial pressure producing the so-called *c wave* ('c' stands for contraction of the ventricle).

During Ventricular Ejection Phase, the intra-atrial pressure drops sharply in rapid ejection phase. This happens so, because the papillary muscles (attached to the cusps of AV valves by chordae tendineae) contract when the ventricular walls contract and pull down the fibrous AV ring causing enlargement of atrial lumen and thus decreasing the intra-atrial pressure. This drop in the intra-atrial pressure produces the *X descent*. The 'x' descent occurs due to both relaxation of atria and downward pull of tricuspid valve during ventricular systole (ejection phase). Therefore, as the ventricles contract, the atria get slowly filled with blood flowing in from the great veins and the atrial pressure starts rising.

During Ventricular Diastole

During Isovolumic (Isometric) Relaxation Phase, the atrial pressure continues to rise as long as AV valves remain closed, i.e. till the end of isovolumic relaxation. This results in the third positive wave called *v wave* ('v' stands for venous filling). This shows a gradual increase in atrial pressure.

During Rapid Passive Filling Phase, the AV valves open allowing rapid flow of blood from atria to ventricles. So, the atrial pressure drops sharply to a little above zero level and remains so till the beginning of next atrial systole. This fall in atrial pressure produces the 'y' descent.

Important Note

Clinical significance of jugular vein pulsations: A careful inspection of the pulsations of jugular vein may give useful information in following clinical conditions:

- Large 'a' wave occurs in tricuspid stenosis.
- *Giant a-wave* (cannon wave) may be observed in patients with complete heart block and
- Differentiation between atrial and ventricular premature beats may be made by inspection of jugular pulse. It will show *a wave* in atrial premature beats and not in ventricular premature beats.
- 'a' wave is absent in atrial fibrillations.
- Prominent 'v' wave is observed in tricuspid regurgitation.

Pressure Changes in the Aorta

Pressure in the aorta varies between 80 to 120 mmHg during the cardiac cycle and can be recorded by using catheter. Aortic pressure changes during various phases of cardiac cycle (Fig. 4.3-3) are explained below.

During Atrial Systole During atrial systole, the pressure in the aorta is about 80 mmHg.

During Ventricular Systole During ventricular systole the intraventricular pressure rises and reaches above that of the aorta during beginning of the *ventricular ejection phase* when the aortic semilunar valve opens and blood starts flowing from the left ventricle into the aorta. Hence, the aortic pressure starts rising along with the intraventricular pressure during rapid ejection phase and reaches maximum (120 mmHg) at the end of rapid ejection phase. It is important to note that during most of the rapid ejection phase, the aortic pressure remains slightly lesser than the ventricular pressure *during reduced ejection phase* and the aortic pressure starts falling along with the ventricular pressure.

During Ventricular Diastole

During Protodiastole, aortic pressure is slightly higher than that in the left ventricle. This causes backward flow of blood and closure of aortic semilunar valve. Due to sudden closure of semilunar valve, the back flowing blood collides against the closed aortic valve. This collision causes a small but sharp rise in aortic pressure. This small rise produces a notch called *incisura.* This sharp pressure rise is recordable even from peripheral arteries and is called *dicrotic notch.*

During Rest of the Diastole, the aortic pressure smoothly declines. By the time the aortic pressure declines to about 80 mmHg, another ventricular systole boosts the aortic pressure again.

Pressure Changes in Pulmonary Artery

Pressure curve in the pulmonary artery is similar to that of aorta but pressures are low (about one-sixth of that in aorta). Pulmonary artery systolic pressure averages 15–18 mmHg and its pressure during diastole is 8–10 mmHg.

Volume Changes in the Ventricles during Cardiac Cycle

During Atrial Systole Atrial systole coincides with the last rapid filling phase of ventricular diastole. When the atrial contraction begins about 105 ml (75%), the blood has already flown into the ventricles. The atrial contraction causes additional 25 ml (25%) filling of the ventricles. In the ventricular volume curve (Fig. 4.3-3), this phase is represented by the AB segment. Thus at the end of atrial systole, i.e. at the end of ventricular diastole, the ventricular volume is about 130 ml. This is called *end-diastolic volume.*

During Ventricular Systole

During Isovolumic Contraction Phase, as the name suggests, there occurs no change in the ventricular volume (Fig. 4.3-3, segment BC).

During Ventricular Ejection Phase, about 80 ml of the blood is ejected out by each ventricle. This is called *stroke volume* (Fig. 4.3-3, segment CD). The percentage of the end-diastolic volume that is ejected out with each stroke during systole (about 65%) is called *ejection fraction.* Thus, about 50 ml of the blood in each ventricle at the end of ventricular systole is called *end-systolic volume.*

During Protodiastole and Phase of Isovolumic Relaxation, there occurs no change in the ventricular volume (Fig.4.3-3, segments DE and EF).

During Rapid Filling Phase and Slow Filling Phase, the ventricular volume changes rapidly and then slowly, respectively. About 75% of the ventricular filling (105 ml of blood) occurs during these phases (Fig. 4.3-3, segment FG and GH).

Valvular Events (Heart Sounds)

A total four heart sounds (first, second, third and fourth) are produced by certain mechanical activities during each cardiac cycle. The study of heart sounds has important diagnostic value in many heart diseases. There are three methods to study the heart sounds:

1. *Auscultation with stethoscope.* The first and second heart sound can be heard normally with the help of stethoscope.

2. *By using microphone*, the amplified heart sounds (first, second and third) can be heard using a loudspeaker.
3. *Phonocardiogram* is the graphical record of all the four heart sounds. This is achieved by placing an electronic sound transducer over the chest and connecting it to a recording device like polygraph. The four heart sounds are described below.

First Heart Sound (HS_1)

Cause. First heart sound is produced by vibrations set up by the sudden closure of AV valves at the start of ventricular systole, during phase of isovolumic contraction (Fig. 4.3-3).

Characteristics. The first heart sound is long and soft when heart rate is low, and loud when the heart rate is high. Its duration is about 0.15 s and frequency is 25–45 Hz. It sounds like the spoken word 'LUBB'.

Site for Auscultation. It can be heard by auscultation of the chest with stethoscope. It is best heard over mitral and tricuspid areas. *Mitral area* is located in the fifth intercostal space just internal to mid clavicular line. *Tricuspid area* is located in the fifth intercostal space near the sternum (Fig. 4.3-4).

In Phonocardiogram, the first heart sound is recorded as a single group of 9–13 waves. The amplitude of the waves is small to start with but later rapidly rises to fall to form *crescendo and diminuendo* series of waves (Fig. 4.3-3).

Correlation with ECG. First heart sound coincides with peak of R wave in ECG.

Second Heart Sound (HS_2)

Cause. It is caused by vibrations associated with closure of the semilunar valves just at the onset of ventricular diastole.

Characteristics. The second heart sound is a short, loud, high pitched sound. Its duration is 0.12 s and frequency is 50 Hz. It sounds like the spoken word 'DUBB'.

Site for Auscultation. It can be heard by auscultation of the chest with stethoscope. It is best heard over the aortic and pulmonary areas. *Aortic area* lies in the right second intercostal space near the sternum, *pulmonary area* is in the left second intercostal space close to sternum (Fig. 4.3-4).

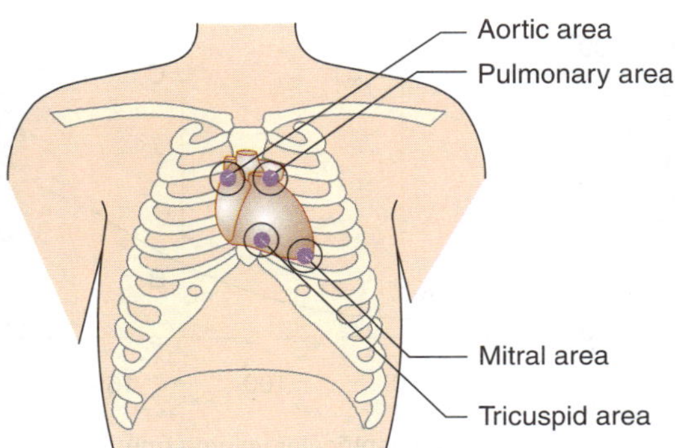

FIGURE 4.3-4 Auscultatory areas over the chest.

In Phonocardiogram, second heart sound is recorded as a single group of 4–6 waves having same amplitude (Fig. 4.3-3).

Correlation with ECG. Second heart sound usually coincides with end of T wave in ECG.

Note I: During inspiration, time interval between closure of aortic and pulmonary valve is prolonged. Therefore second heart sound is to be reduplicated, which is called *physiological splitting of second heart sound.*

Third Heart Sound (HS_3)

Cause. Third heart sound is caused by vibrations set up in the cardiac wall by the inrush of blood during *rapid filling phase* of ventricular diastole.

Characteristics. Third heart sound is a short, soft and low pitched sound. Its duration is 0.1 s. Normally, it cannot be heard by auscultation with stethoscope.

In Phonocardiogram, the third heart sound is found with only 1–4 waves grouped together (Fig. 4.3-3).

Correlation with ECG. The third heart sound appears between T and P waves of ECG.

Fourth Heart Sound (HS_4)

Cause. It is caused by vibrations set up during atrial systole which coincides with last rapid filling phase of ventricular diastole.

Characteristics. It is normally not audible. Sometimes it can be heard immediately before the first sound when atrial pressure is high or when ventricle is stiff in condition such as ventricular hypertrophy. It is a short and low pitched sound. Its duration is about 0.03 s and frequency about 3 Hz.

In Phonocardiogram, the fourth heart sound merges with first heart sound many times. When it appears as a separate entity, it has 1–2 waves with very low amplitude (Fig. 4.3-3).

Correlation with ECG. Fourth heart sound coincides with the interval between the end of P wave and onset of Q wave.

Note II: Heart sound HS_3 and HS_4 are comparatively less important, because normally they are inaudible.

Cardiac Murmurs Cardiac murmurs are the abnormal heart sounds produced during the cardiac cycle.

Mechanism of Production. Cardiac murmurs are produced by a turbulent blood flow or by change in the direction of blood flow. Normally, the blood flows through the heart and blood vessels as *laminar flow* which is streamlined and silent. The *turbulent flow,* on the other hand, produces vibrations in the tissues that are heard as murmurs.

Causes. Murmurs are caused in following conditions:

- ***Valvular stenosis,*** i.e. narrowing of any of the cardiac valve (mitral, tricuspid, aortic or pulmonary valve).
- ***Valvular insufficiency,*** i.e. regurgitation of any of the cardiac valve.

- ***Ventricular septal defect (VSD),*** i.e. a congenital hole in the ventricular septum.
- ***Atrial septal defect (ASD),*** i.e. a congenital hole in the interatrial septum.
- ***Coarctation of aorta,*** i.e. congenital narrowing of systemic aorta.
- ***Patent ductus arteriosus (PDA),*** i.e. a congenital disorder in which there is backward flow of blood from aorta into the pulmonary artery.

Types. Depending upon the timing of appearance these have been classified as (Fig. 4.3-5).

- *Systolic murmur,* which is produced during systole,
- *Diastolic murmur,* which is produced during diastole and
- *Continuous murmur,* which is produced continuously.

The types of murmur produced depend upon the site and type of abnormality (Table 4.3-1).

Site of Auscultation. The murmurs are best heard by placing the stethoscope on the chest wall closest to their origin, e.g. aortic area, pulmonary area, mitral area or tricuspid area.

Note: Abnormal vascular sounds heard over blood vessels are called *bruit*. Bruits can be heard in the following conditions.

- In case of highly vascular goiter.
- In atherosclerosis, bruit can be heard over carotid artery when its lumen gets narrowed or distorted.
- Over an aneurysm (dilation of a large artery).

TABLE 4.3-1 Types of Murmurs Depending on Site and Type of Abnormality

Site of abnormality	Type of abnormality	Type of murmur
• Aortic or pulmonary valve	Stenosis	Systolic
	Insufficiency	Diastolic
• Mitral or tricuspid valve	Stenosis	Diastolic
	Insufficiency	Systolic
• Interventricular septum	Congenital hole	Systolic
• Aorta	Coarctation	Systolic
• Ductus arteriosus	Patent	Continuous
• Blood	Anaemia	Systolic

Pressure–Volume Loop Ventricular pressure–volume loop refers to the graph obtained in the form of a loop by plotting pressure along the ordinate and volume along the abscissa at various stages of cardiac cycle. Thus, the pressure–volume loop is an alternate method of representing the cardiac cycle. Normal ventricular pressure–volume loop is shown in Fig. 4.3-6.

- ***Segment AB*** represents the rapid, passive filling phase, reduced filling phase and last rapid filling phase (atrial systole) of the ventricular diastole. This segment reveals that:
  - Ventricular volume at the end of diastole (at point B) is about 130 ml (end-diastolic volume). Point B marks the closure of AV valves.
  - Ventricular pressure rises from 2–3 mmHg point A to about 6–7 mmHg at point B (end of atrial systole).
- ***Segment BC*** represents the isovolumic contraction phase of ventricular systole. This segment reveals that during this phase:
  - Volume remains same, i.e. about 130 ml, but the pressure rises from 6–7 mmHg to about 80 mmHg.

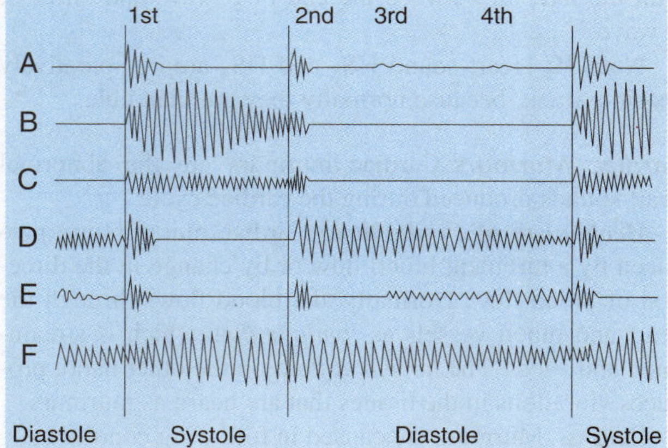

FIGURE 4.3-5 Cardiac murmurs on phonocardiography: A, normal phonocardiogram; B, systolic murmur (in aortic stenosis); C, systolic murmur (in mitral regurgitation); D, diastolic murmur (in aortic regurgitation); E, diastolic murmur (in mitral stenosis); and F, continuous murmur (in patent ductus arteriosus).

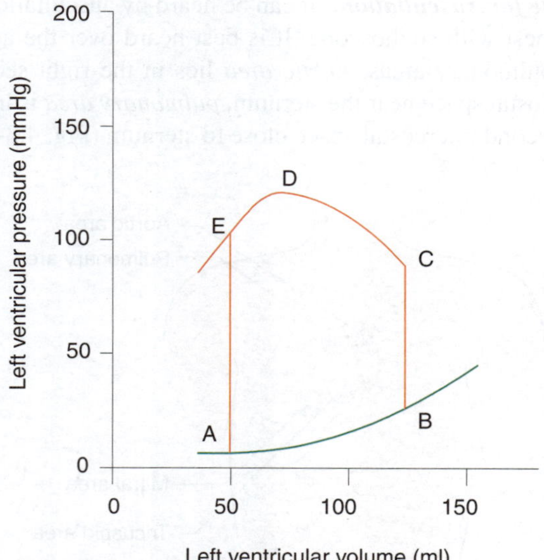

FIGURE 4.3-6 Pressure–volume loop of left ventricle.

- ***Segment CE*** represents the ventricular ejection phase of ventricular systole. Point C marks the opening of semilunar valves. The segment CD represents the rapid ejection phase and segment DE represents the *slow ejection phase.* The segment CE reveals that:
  - During rapid ejection phase (segment CD), the ventricular pressure increases rapidly up to a maximum of 120 mmHg and then falls during slow ejection phase (segment DE) to about 80 mmHg.
  - During ventricular ejection phase (segment CE), the ventricular volume decreases from about 130 ml to about 50 ml, called as *end-systolic volume.*
- ***Segment EA*** of the pressure–volume loop represents the phase of *isovolumic relaxation.* Point E marks the closure of semilunar valves. This segment reveals that:
  - Ventricular pressure falls rapidly from about 80 mmHg to about 2–3 mmHg.
  - Ventricular volume remains unchanged.

Disadvantage of Pressure–Volume Loop. In this, the time dimension is eliminated and therefore it is not possible to tell from this loop how fast the events are occurring.

Advantage of Pressure–Volume Loop is that the work done by the heart is instantly apparent from the area enclosed by the loop.

Clinical Significance. The pressure–volume loop can be utilized in changed haemodynamic state like exercise, heart failure, etc. to understand pressure–volume events during cardiac cycle.

Duration of Systole and Diastole vis-a-vis Heart Rate

Normal Duration

- Duration of each cardiac cycle at a normal heart rate of 75 beats/min is 60/75 = 0.8 s,
- Duration of ventricular systole is 0.3 s and
- Duration of ventricular diastole is 0.5 s.

Effect of Heart Rate

- Cardiac muscle has the unique property of contracting and repolarizing faster when the heart rate is high.
- Therefore, when the heart rate increases, the total duration of cardiac cycle decreases, e.g. at a heart rate of 200 beats/min the total duration of cardiac cycle is 60/200 =0.3 s.
- It is important to note that though the duration of all phases of the cardiac cycle decreases at high heart rate, but the *duration of diastole* decreases much more than the duration of systole. For example, when the heart rate increases from 75 to 200 beats/min, the duration of systole decreases from 0.3 to 0.16 s while that of diastole decreases from 0.5 to 0.14 s (Table 4.3-2).

This fact has following important physiologic and *clinical implications:*

- It is during diastole that the heart muscle rests, and coronary blood flow to the subendocardial portion of the left ventricle occurs only during diastole. Therefore, at very high rate, there occurs reduction in cardiac perfusion and there are chances of myocardial ischaemia.
- Furthermore, most of the ventricular filling occurs in diastole. At heart rate up to 180 beats/min, filling is adequate as long as there is ample venous return and cardiac output per minute is increased by an increase in heart rate. However, at very high heart rate, filling may be compromised to such a degree that cardiac output per minute falls and symptoms of heart failure develop.

Clinical Indices

Information about the duration of isovolumic ventricular contraction is of considerable clinical importance in many cardiac disorders. However, exact measurement of the duration of isovolumic ventricular contraction is difficult in clinical situations. Therefore, certain other indices have been evolved from which indirectly required information can be obtained. These indices given below are relatively easy to measure from the recording of ECG, phono-cardiogram and carotid pulse simultaneously (Fig. 4.3-7).

- ***Total electromechanical systole (QS_2)*** is the period from the onset of QRS complex to the closure of the aortic valve, as determined by the onset of second heart sound.
- ***Left ventricular ejection time (LVET)*** is the period from the beginning of the carotid pressure rise to the dicrotic notch.
- ***Pre-ejection period (PEP)*** is the difference between QS_2 and LVET and represents the time for the electrical as well as the mechanical events that precede systolic ejection.
- ***Ratio of PEP/LVET*** is normally about 0.35, and it increases without a change in QS_2, when left ventricular performance is compromised in many cardiac diseases.

TABLE 4.3-2 Change in Duration of Various Events of Cardiac Cycle with Increase in Heart Rate

	Duration in seconds	
Event	*At heart rate of 75 beats/min*	*At heart rate of 200 beats/min*
Cardiac cycle	0.8	0.3
Systole	0.3	0.16
Diastole	0.5	0.14

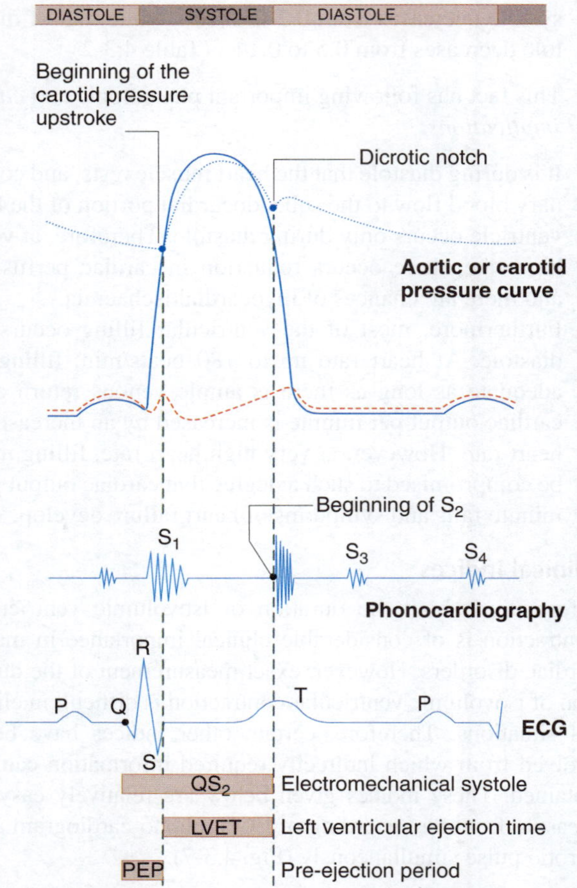

FIGURE 4.3-7 Durations of systolic time interval.

Arterial Pulse

Arterial pulse is also an event related to cardiac cycle. The blood forced into the aorta during systole not only moves the blood in the vessels forward but also sets up a pressure wave that is transmitted along the *arteries to the* periphery. The pressure wave expands the arterial walls as it travels, and expansion is palpable as the *pulse.*

Velocity of Transmission of Pulse Wave Velocity of transmission of pulse wave is independent of and much higher than the velocity of blood flow, the maximum value of which in larger arteries is only 50 cm/s. The rate of travel of pulse wave is about:

- 4 m/s in the aorta and its branches,
- 8 m/s in the large arteries and
- 16 m/s in the small arteries of young adults.

Consequently, the pulse is felt at the arteries after short interval of the peak of systolic ejection into the aorta (Fig. 4.3-8). This interval can be measured accurately by recording and is directly proportional to the distance of artery from the heart. For the common carotid artery, this period is about 0.02 s while for the radial artery at the wrist, it is about 0.1 s. With the advancing age, the arteries become more rigid and the pulse wave moves faster.

Methods of Recording Arterial Pulse The tracings of arterial pulse can be made by following techniques of recording:

1. Manometric Technique. It is used in animals. In this technique, a cannula is inserted into the dissected artery and is connected to manometer or any other recording device to obtain the arterial pulse tracing.

2. Dudgeon's Sphygmograph Method. In this method arterial pulse is recorded from the radial artery with the help of Dudgeon's sphygmograph which is tied to the wrist in such a way that a small plate rests on the skin overlying the artery. A series of levers used in this instrument magnify the movements of arterial wall and record on a moving strip of smoked paper.

3. Electronic Transducer Method. The electronic transducer is placed on the skin overlying any artery. The transducer throws light on the artery and the light reflected from the flowing blood is deducted by the sensor of the transducer. The arterial pulse in the form alterations in the frequency of reflected light rays are amplified and recorded by connecting the transducer to a recording device like polygraph.

Interpretation of Arterial Pulse Tracing The pulse tracing recorded from the carotid artery shows following characteristics (Fig. 4.3-9).

- *Ascending limb,* also known as *anacrotic limb* or primary limb, is due to the rise in pressure during systole.
- *Descending limb,* also known as *catacrotic limb* represents the fall in pressure during diastole.
- *Percussion wave (P)* corresponds to ejection phase of ventricular systole.
- *Tidal wave (T)* is due to falling blood column during slow ejection phase.
- *Dicrotic notch (N)* is due to closure of aortic valve and marks end of ventricular systole.
- *Dicrotic wave (D)* is due to rebound of blood column from closed aortic valve.

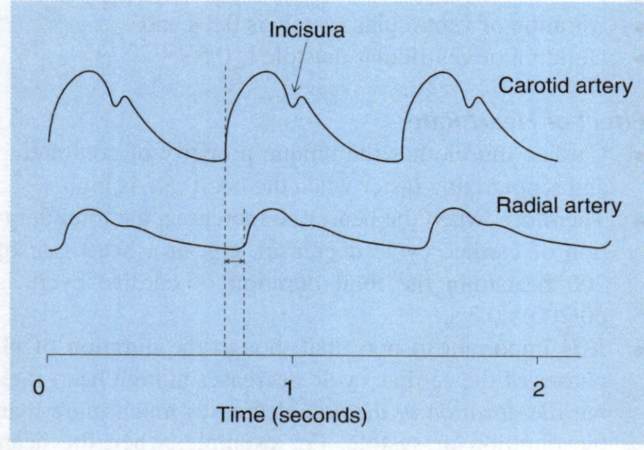

FIGURE 4.3-8 Velocity of transmission of pulse wave.

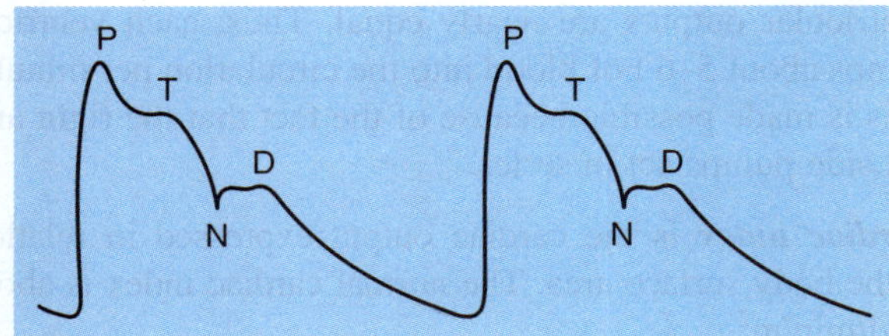

FIGURE 4.3-9 Record of arterial pulse from carotid artery: (P) percussion wave; (T) tidal wave; (N) dicrotic notch; and (D) dicrotic wave.

When the record is taken from peripheral arteries at a distant place from the heart, e.g. femoral or radial arteries, the contour or shape of record changes. In arterioles and capillaries the waves disappear.

Examination of Arterial Pulse Examination of the arterial pulse is an essential feature of clinical examination. Arterial pulse can be palpated from any superficial artery, e.g. radial, femoral, dorsalis pedis, carotid, etc. Most frequently, pulse is examined from the radial artery because It is conveniently approached without exposing the body, and can be easily palpated as it is placed superficially against the bone.

Examination of the pulse should include following aspects:

1. Pulse Rate refers to the number of pulses per minute. It is a convenient method of determining heart rate.

- *Normal pulse rate* varies with age being 150–180 min in fetus, 130–140 min at birth, about 90 min at the age of 10 years and about 72/min in adults.
- *Increased pulse rate* represents tachycardia and occurs during exercise, in anxiety, in fever, in hyperthyroidism and in atrial and ventricular tachycardias.
- *Decreased pulse rate* represents bradycardia and is seen in hypothyroidism and incomplete heart blocks.

2. Volume of Pulse also known as strength of arterial pulse or amplitude or impact can be felt. It represents stroke volume or the pulse pressure (i.e. systolic–diastolic pressure). Pulse pressure is mainly affected by stroke output, compliance (distensibility) of the arterial tree, and to some extent by the character of ejection of blood from the heart. Therefore pulse pressure is determined by the ratio of stroke output to compliance of arterial tree. For details see page 323.

- *Rapid and thready pulse* occurs in hypovolaemia as in severe haemorrhage and there is marked reflex vasoconstriction.
- *Increased volume pulse* is seen during exercise and in ventricular hypertrophy.

3. Rhythm of Pulse is noted as regular or irregular. Under normal conditions and during sinus bradycardia or sinus tachycardia pulse appears at regular intervals.

- *Irregular pulse rhythm* is a feature of extra systole, atrial fibrillation and other cardiac arrhythmias, type of arrhythmia is confirmed only on ECG (see page 269). The irregular pulse rhythm may be regularly irregular or irregularly irregular.

4. Character of Pulse is felt on palpation. It denotes the tension and waves in the pulse. Feeling of different characters of the pulse can be learnt by subjective experience.

- ***Normal character*** (Fig. 4.3-10A) of the pulse is sinuous on examination, i.e. an upstroke is followed by downstroke. Normally, it is not possible to feel the different waves of the pulse or slight variations in the character. However, in certain heart diseases and valvular defects, the normal character is altered and can be easily felt while palpating the peripheral arterial pulse.

A few *abnormal characters* of the pulse are described as:

- ***Water hammer pulse*** (Fig. 4.3-10B) also known as collapsing pulse is characterized by a sudden upstroke followed by a sudden downstroke without insuria. It is best felt by raising the patient's arm and holding it by grasping the wrist with palm of the observer. Sometimes the upstroke is so strong that it leads to head nodding with each heart beat, called as Corrigan sign or Corrigan pulse.

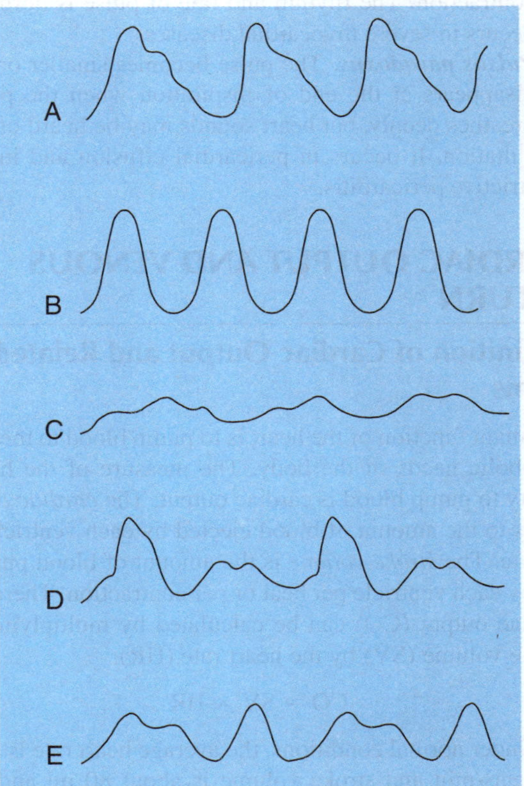

FIGURE 4.3-10 Character of arterial pulse: **A,** normal character; **B,** water hammer pulse; **C,** anacrotic pulse; **D,** pulsus alternans; and E, pulsusbisferiens.

Cause of water hammer pulse is aortic insufficiency or regurgitation.

Mechanism of water hammer pulse in aortic regurgitation is as follows:

- When the aortic valve closes, blood regurgitates from the aorta into the left ventricle. So, aorta empties earlier and this is the cause of sudden downstroke.
- Due to regurgitation of blood from aorta into left ventricle, the end-diastolic volume is increased. So next beat is forceful (due to Frank–Starling mechanism), and this is the cause of sudden upstroke of next beat.

- ***Anacrotic pulse*** (Fig. 4.3-10C). Normally, there is a single upstroke in the arterial pulse. In anacrotic pulse, there are two upstrokes. It occurs in patients with aortic stenosis. First upstroke in anacrotic pulse is due to slow rise in ventricular systole owing to aortic stenosis and second is due to dicrotic wave which normally occurs on the downstroke.
- ***Bisferiens pulse*** (Fig. 4.3-10E). This a combination of anacrotic and collapsing pulses, both can be felt distinctly. It is found in conditions when aortic stenosis and incompetency are combined.
- ***Pulsus alternans*** (Fig. 4.3-10D*).* In this condition, every normal pulse alternates with a weak pulse. This is because of alternate variation in the force of ventricular contraction. The rhythm and rate of pulse is normal. It occurs in severe myocardial diseases.
- ***Pulsus paradoxus.*** The pulse becomes smaller or even disappears at the end of inspiration when the patient breathes deeply, but heart sounds may be heard on auscultation. It occurs in pericardial effusion and in constrictive pericarditis.

CARDIAC OUTPUT AND VENOUS RETURN

Definition of Cardiac Output and Related Terms

The main function of the heart is to pump blood to meet the metabolic needs of the body. The measure of the heart's ability to pump blood is cardiac output. The *cardiac output* refers to the amount of blood ejected by each ventricle per minute. The *stroke volume* is the amount of blood pumped out by each ventricle per beat or per contraction. Therefore, cardiac output (CO) can be calculated by multiplying the stroke volume (SV) by the heart rate (HR):

$$CO = SV \times HR$$

Under normal conditions, the average heart rate is about 70 beats/min and stroke volume is about 80 ml and thus cardiac output is $80 \times 70 = 5.6$ l.

The cardiac output is expressed in litres per minute and normally varies from 5–6 l/min. In health, the right and left ventricular outputs are nearly equal. Thus, each ventricle pumps about 5–6 l of blood into the circulation per minute. This is made possible because of the fact that the right and left side pumps act in series.

Cardiac index is the cardiac output expressed in relation to the body surface area. The normal cardiac index is about 3.2 l/min/m^2.

Distribution of the Cardiac Output Of the total cardiac output, about 75% is distributed to the vital organs of the body and rest 25% to the skeletal muscle, other organs of the body and skin. The distribution of the cardiac output to various organs of the body is shown in Table 4.3-3.

Cardiac Reserve

- The cardiac reserve refers to the maximum increase in the cardiac output above the normal value. It is usually expressed in percentage.
- Value of cardiac reserve observed are:
  - In healthy young adults : 300–400%
  - In old age : 200–250%
  - In athletes : 500–600%
- The cardiac reserve is:
  - Maximum during heavy exercise and
  - Minimum or nil in cardiac diseases.

Measurement of Cardiac Output

Cardiac output, in experimental animals, can be measured directly with the help of an electromagnetic flowmeter placed on the ascending aorta. However, in human, only indirect methods are possible and include:

- Methods based on Fick's principle,
- Indicator or dye dilution method,
- Thermodilution method,

TABLE 4.3-3 Distribution of Cardiac Output to Various Organs

Body organ	Amount of blood flow (ml/min)		Percentage of total cardiac output	
Liver	1500		25	
Kidney	1300		about 25	75
Brain	750			
Heart	250	1500	25	
Lungs	500			
Skeletal muscles and other body organs	1000	1500	25	
Skin	500			

- Method employing inhalation of inert gases and
- Physical methods such as:
  - Doppler technique echocardiography,
  - Ballistocardiography and
  - Cineradiographic technique.

Methods Based on Fick's Principle

Fick's Principle The Fick's principle states that the amount of a substance taken up by an organ (or by the whole body) per unit of time is equal to the arterial level of the substance (A) minus the venous level (V) times the blood flow (F), i.e.

$$Q = (A - V)\,F$$

or

$$F = \frac{Q}{(A-V)}$$

This principle can be of course, only in situations in which the arterial blood is the sole source of the substance taken up. The Fick's principle can be used to measure cardiac output by two methods:

- Fick's principle direct method and
- Fick's principle indirect method.

Fick's Principle (Direct Method) In this method (Fig. 4.3-11), cardiac output is determined by measuring the pulmonary blood flow. As we know:

- Pulmonary blood flow/min = right ventricular output and
- Right ventricular output 5 left ventricular output (cardiac output).

Measurement of pulmonary blood flow can be made by measuring the amount of O_2 taken by the blood from the lungs, O2 concentration of the venous blood from

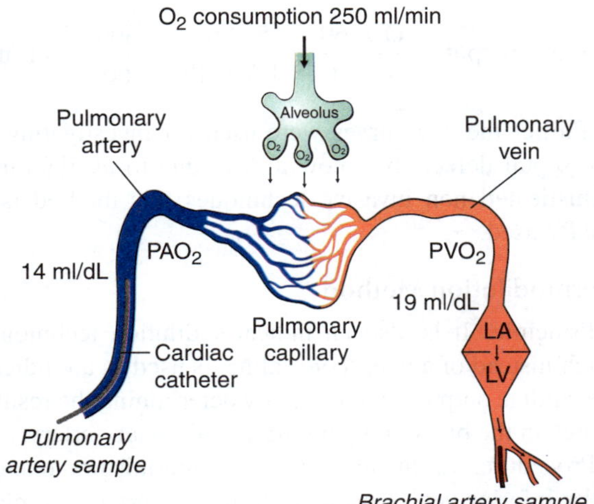

FIGURE 4.3-11 Estimation of cardiac output by Fick's principle. PAO2, oxygen content of pulmonary artery blood and PVO2, oxygen content of pulmonary vein blood.

pulmonary artery (PAO_2) and O_2 concentration of the arterial blood from the pulmonary vein (PVO_2).

- Amount of O_2 uptake/min is determined with the help of a spirometer,
- PAO_2 is measured from the venous blood sample taken from the pulmonary artery directly with the help of a cardiac catheter. The cardiac catheter is inserted into a vein at the forearm and is then guided up under fluoroscopic control through the venous channels into the right atrium, right ventricle and pulmonary artery.
- PVO_2 because of practical difficulty in taking sample from pulmonary vein, is measured from the arterial blood sample taken from any peripheral artery, e.g. brachial artery (the O_2 content of all the major arteries is same as that of pulmonary veins). According to Fick's principle:

$$\text{Pulmonary blood flow} = \frac{\text{Amount of } O_2 \text{ taken by the lungs/min}}{PVO_2 - PAO_2}$$

or

$$\text{Cardiac output} = \frac{O_2 \text{ taken by the lungs/min}}{PVO_2 - PAO_2}$$

For example, if O_2 uptake is 250 ml/min, PVO_2 is 19 ml/100 ml and PAO_2 is 14 ml/100 ml, then

$$\text{Cardiac output} = \frac{250 \times 100}{19 - 14} = \frac{25000 \text{ ml/min}}{5} = 5000 \text{ ml/min} = 5 \text{ l/min.}$$

Disadvantages of Fick's Principle (Direct Method)

- It is an invasive technique, so there are risks of infection and haemorrhage.
- The cardiac output estimated may be somewhat higher than normal as the patient becomes conscious of the whole technique.
- A fatal complication like ventricular fibrillation may occur if the indwelling catheter irritates the ventricular walls, especially when the cardiac output is being measured during heavy exercise.

Fick's Principle (Indirect Method) In this method, arterial puncture and right heart catheterization are avoided and CO_2 excretion by the lungs is used instead of O_2 uptake:

- CO_2 excretion by the lungs is measured by spirometry,
- Arterial CO_2 ($PACO_2$) is estimated from alveolar air and
- Mixed venous blood CO_2 ($PVCO_2$) is estimated by rebreathing into a closed bag. With rebreathing, the CO_2 in the bag will come into equilibrium with the venous blood in lungs. The breathing should be done in an interrupted manner so that the blood level of CO_2 is not increased.

According to Fick's principle:

$$\text{Cardiac output} = \frac{CO_2 \text{ output/min}}{PACO_2 - PVCO_2}$$

Indicator or Dye Dilution Method

Principle In this method, a known amount of the dye is injected into a large vein or preferably into right atrium by cardiac catheterization. By its passage through heart and pulmonary circulation it will be evenly distributed in the blood stream. Its mean concentration during the first passage through an artery can be determined from successive samples of blood taken from artery. The blood flow in l/min (F) is given by the following formula:

$$F = \frac{Q}{Ct}, \text{ where:}$$

F = Blood flow in l/min,
Q = Quantity of the dye injected,
C = Mean concentration of dye and
t = Time duration in seconds of the first passage of dye through the artery.

Prerequisites for an Ideal Indicator The indicator (dye) used should have following characteristics:

- It should be nontoxic.
- It must mix evenly in the blood.
- It should be relatively easy to measure its concentration.
- It should not alter the cardiac output or haemodynamics of blood flow.
- Either it must not be changed by the body during mixing period or the amount changed must be known.
- The dye commonly used in humans for determining the cardiac output is *Evans blue* (T-1824) or radioactive isotopes.

Procedure

Injection of Dye. A few millilitre of venous blood is withdrawn from the antecubital vein and it is mixed with 5 mg Evans blue dye. The blood containing dye is then injected rapidly into the vein.

Estimation of Duration of First Passage of Dye (t) and Mean Concentration (C) of Dye in Arterial Blood. Serial samples of arterial blood from the brachial artery are taken every 2 s and the dye concentration is determined.

- When the dye concentration is plotted as a function of time, a curve shown in Fig. 4.3-12 as A, B, C and D is obtained. The curve shows that the dye concentration reaches a peak and then steadily declines only to rise again (CD part of the curve) owing to recirculation of the dye.
- *Time duration of first passage of dye through the artery (t)* is determined by extrapolation of the descending limb (BC) of the curve to time scale axis. The point (E) on the time scale where the extrapolated limb meets it, tells the time (AE) of first circulation of dye in seconds.
- *The mean concentration (C)* of the dye is determined by representing the triangle area ABE as a rectangle AEFG with same area and one of its arm being AE. The height of the rectangle (AG) tells the mean concentration (C) of dye.
- *Calculation of cardiac output* is then made using the formula described above. For example, when:
  - Amount of dye injected (Q) is 5 mg,
  - Time duration for first circulation is 40 s and
  - Mean concentration of dye (C) = 15 mg/l, then

$$\text{Cardiac output} = \frac{Q \times 60}{C \times t} = \frac{5 \times 60}{1.5 \times 40} = \frac{300}{60} = 5 \text{ L/min}$$

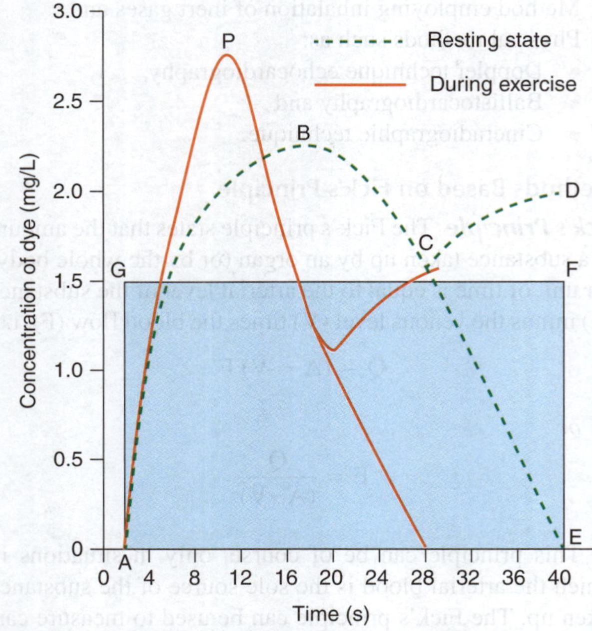

FIGURE 4.3-12 Estimation of cardiac output by indicator (dye) dilution method.

Earlier the dye curves were used for investigating cardiac septal defects but, now a days due to availability of sophisticated non invasive techniques this method is not usually used.

Thermodilution Method

Principle. It is also an indicator dilution technique in which instead of a dye, 'cold saline' is used as an indicator. The cardiac output is measured by determining the resultant change in the blood temperature in pulmonary artery.

Procedure. In this technique, two thermistors, one each in the inferior vena cava and pulmonary artery are placed with the help of cardiac catheter.

- A known volume of sterile cold saline is then injected into the inferior vena cava.

- Temperature of the blood entering the heart from inferior vena cava and that of the blood leaving the heart via pulmonary artery is determined by the thermistors.
- The cardiac output is then measured from the values of temperature by applying the principle of indicator dilution technique.

$$F = V_I \times (T_B - T_I)/\Delta T_B \times t$$

where:
F – blood flow in litre per second,
V_I – volume of the injectate,
T_B and T_I – temperature of blood and injectate, respectively,
ΔT_B – mean change in the pulmonary artery blood,
t – duration of first passage of injectate in seconds.

Note: The advantage of thermal dilution over dye dilution method is that withdrawal of blood for sampling is not required. Therefore, this method is useful for estimating cardiac output in infants and small children in whom the blood volume is limited.

Method Employing Inhalation of Inert Gases

- In this technique, an inert gas which dissolves in plasma but does not combine with Hb or other constituents of the blood is used as an indicator. Such gases include nitrous oxide and acetylene; the last one gives more accurate results.
- The pulmonary blood flow (which is equal to the cardiac output) in then determined from the following values:
  - The quantity of gas absorbed in the given time,
  - The partial pressure of the gas in the alveolar air,
  - The solubility of the gas (a known factor).

Physical Methods

Physical methods developed to measure the cardiac output include the following.

Echocardiography Echocardiography refers to ultrasonic evaluation of cardiac functions. It is a noninvasive technique that does not involve injections or insertion of a catheter. It involves B-scan ultrasound at a frequency of 2.25 MHz using a transducer which also acts as receiver of the reflected waves. The recording of the echoes displayed against time on an oscilloscope provides a record of:

- The movement of the ventricular wall and septum, and valves during the cardiac cycle.
- When combined with Doppler techniques, echocardiography can be used to measure velocity and volume of flow through the valves.
- Thus, it is particularly useful in evaluating end-diastolic volume (EDV), end-systolic volume (ESV), cardiac output (CO) and valvular defects.

Ballistocardiography Method This method is not used practically. Ballistocardiography refers to graphical record of the pulsations created due to ballistic recoil of the pumping heart. The ballistic recoil occurs in accordance with Newton's third law of motion, i.e. when heart pumps blood into aorta and pulmonary artery, recoil is given to the heart and the body in the opposite direction. This is similar to that of ballistic recoil when a bullet is fired from the rifle.

The ballistic recoil pulsations can be recorded graphically by making the subject to lie on a suspended bed movable in the long axis of the body. The cardiac output is determined by analyzing the graph obtained.

Variations in Cardiac Output

Physiological Causes of Variations in Cardiac Output

- ***Age.*** Because of less body surface area, children have more cardiac index than adults.
- ***Sex.*** Since the body surface area is less in females, they have more cardiac index than the males.
- ***Diurnal variation.*** In the early morning, cardiac output is low which increases in the day time depending upon the basal condition of the individual.
- ***Environmental temperature.*** Moderate change in environmental temperature does not cause any change in cardiac output. A high environmental temperature is associated with an increase in the cardiac output.
- ***Anxiety and excitement*** are reported to increase the cardiac output by 50–100%.
- ***Eating*** is associated with an increase in cardiac output approximately by 30%.
- ***Exercise*** may increase the cardiac output up to 700% depending upon the vigorousness of exercise.
- ***Pregnancy.*** An increase in cardiac output to the tune of 45–60% is reported during the later months of the pregnancy.
- ***High altitude.*** The cardiac output is increased at high altitude due to release of adrenaline as a consequence to hypoxia.
- ***Posture change.*** Sitting or standing from lying down position may decrease the cardiac output by 20–30% because of pooling of blood in lower limbs.

Pathological Causes of Variations in Cardiac Output

- ***Increase in cardiac output*** is seen in following conditions:
  - *Fever,* due to increased oxidative processes,
  - *Anaemia*, due to hypoxia and
  - *Hyperthyroidism*, due to increased metabolism.
- ***Decrease in cardiac output*** may occur in following conditions:
  - *Rapid arrhythmias,* due to incomplete filling,
  - *Congestive cardiac failure,* due to weak contractions of heart,
  - *Cardiac shock,* due to poor pumping and circulation,

- *Incomplete heart block,* owing to defective pumping action of the heart,
- *Haemorrhage,* because of decreased blood volume and
- *Hypothyroidism,* due to decreased basal metabolism.

Regulation of Cardiac Output

The cardiac output increases or decreases in various physiological and pathological conditions as described above. The variations in the cardiac output are brought out by certain factors operating through certain mechanisms by an integrated role.

The cardiac output (CO), as we know, is the product of stroke volume (SV) and heart rate (HR), i.e. CO = SV × HR. Therefore, variations in the cardiac output can be produced by the factors that change stroke volume or heart rate, or both. The main factors affecting cardiac output are venous return, myocardial contractility, peripheral resistance and heart rate (Fig. 4.3-13).

Cardiac Output Control Mechanisms

The cardiac output is regulated by two mechanisms: intrinsic and extrinsic.

1. Intrinsic Autoregulation (Frank–Starling Mechanism)

The force of contraction of cardiac muscle fibres like that of skeletal muscle fibres depends upon its preload. The preload determines the initial length (resting length) of the muscle fibres. According to *Frank–Starling law* of heart, 'within physiological limits' the force of contraction

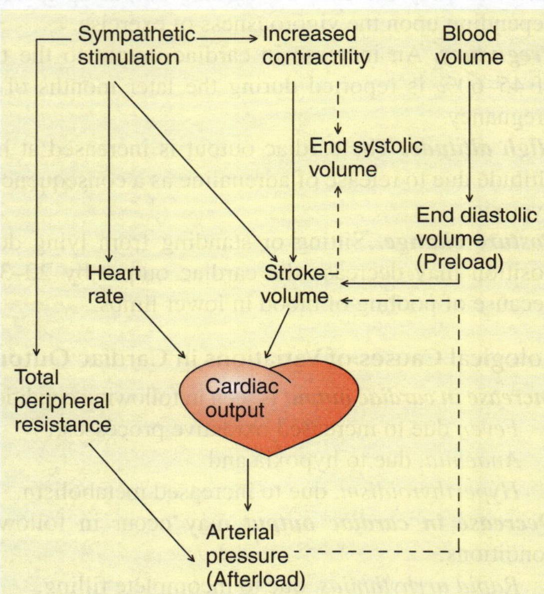

FIGURE 4.3-13 Interaction between the factors that regulate cardiac output and arterial pressure. Solid lines indicate increase and dotted lines indicate a decrease.

of *cardiac muscle* is proportionate to the initial length of muscle fibres. In the heart, end-diastolic volume forms the preload. Thus, the stretching of the cardiac muscle fibres to increase their initial length depends upon the end-diastolic volume. Therefore, precisely, the Frank–Starling law of heart can be stated as, within physiological limits the force of cardiac contraction is proportional to its end-diastolic volume (EDV). This fact was demonstrated about a century ago by Frank and Starling on the heart–lung preparation in a dog described on page 293. Since, in this intrinsic regulation mechanism, cardiac muscle fibres are stretched to increase their initial length, it is also termed as *heterometric mechanism.*

The relationship between ventricular stroke volume and end-diastolic volume is called the *Frank–Starling curve (Fig. 4.3-14).* Details of the effect of preload on force of myocardial contraction including the *length–tension relationship* are described in detail on page 245.

Factors Affecting End-diastolic Volume The end-diastolic volume refers to the *venous return* to the heart during diastole. Therefore, the factors that normally operate to regulate end-diastolic volume, i.e. the degree to which cardiac muscle is stretched are the same which affect the venous return.

Up to physiological limits the cardiac output is directly proportional to the venous return. Thus, over any significant period of time, venous return must equal cardiac output. For individual at rest, the cardiac output and venous return are approximately 5 l/min. A complicated interaction of neural, humoural and physical factors determine the flow rate. Factors affecting venous return (Fig. 4.3-14) are:

1. Respiratory Pump. Normally the intrapleural (intrathoracic) pressure at the end of expiration is about −2 mmHg. During inspiration, the intrathoracic pressure becomes more negative (about −5 mmHg) due to which the diameter of inferior vena cava is increased and pressure inside it is reduced; and there occurs descent of diaphragm which increases the intra-abdominal pressure. The decreased pressure inside the inferior vena cava coupled with increased intra-abdominal pressure during inspiration results in increased flow of blood into the right atrium. This mechanism of increased blood flow during inspiration is called *respiratory pump.* This respiratory pump operates strongly in forced respiration and in severe muscular exercise increasing the venous return.

2. Cardiac Pump. The cardiac pump influences the venous return by two kinds of forces: 'vis-a-tergo' and 'vis-a-fronte'.

- ***Vis-a-tergo*** refers to the forward push from behind, i.e. the propelling force which pushes the blood from veins into the right atrium. Vis-a-tergo results from the myocardial contraction during systole and is supplemented by the elastic recoil of the arterial wall (windkessel effect, see page 314).

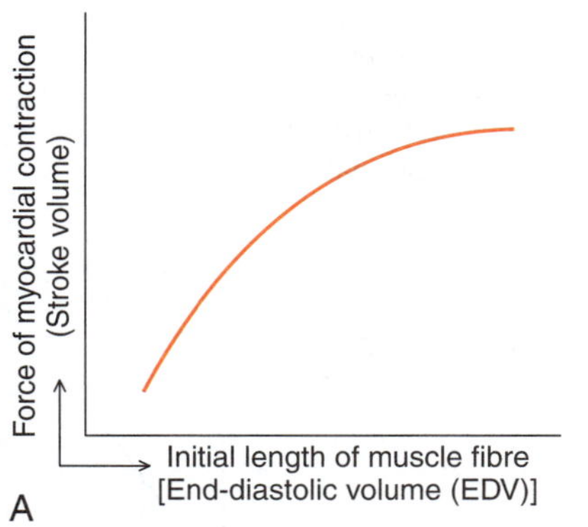

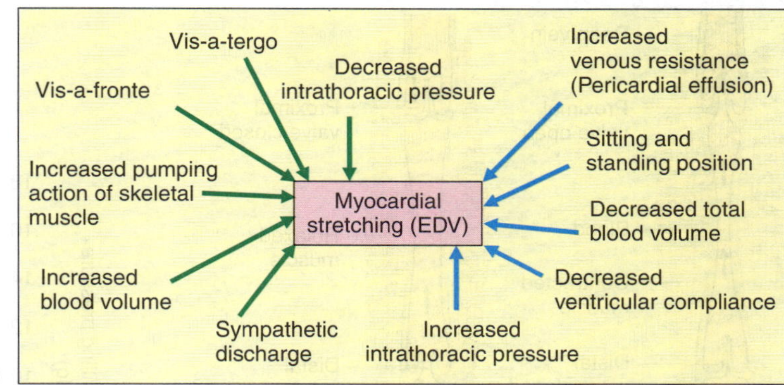

FIGURE 4.3-14 Frank–Starling curve **(A)** and factors affecting end-diastolic volume. Arrows on the left (green) indicate increase and arrows on right (blue) indicate decrease **(B)**.

- ***Vis-a-fronte*** refers to the suction force acting from the front which basically pulls the blood from the great veins into the right atrium. This suction force is created by ventricular contraction and has following two components:
  - *Ventricular systolic suction* results from pulling down of the fibrous AV ring causing enlargement of atrial lumen and thus decreasing the intra-atrial pressure which sucks blood from the inferior vena cava and superior vena cava. The fibrous AV ring is pulled down due to contraction of papillary muscles.
  - *Ventricular diastolic suction* results from the opening of AV valves allowing rapid flow of blood from atria to ventricles. The sudden decrease in atrial pressure in turn sucks blood from the great veins.
  - So, a decrease in ventricular compliance, i.e. an increase in the ventricular stiffness produced by myocardial infarction, infiltrative diseases and other abnormalities will decrease the venous return.

3. Muscle Pump. The muscle pump mechanism is responsible for flow of blood from the veins of the limbs to the heart. Therefore, increased pumping action of skeletal muscles will increase the venous return and decreased pumping of skeletal muscles will decrease the venous return.

Working of muscle pump is now explained. Two types of veins are present in the limbs: superficial and deep veins. Blood flows from the superficial veins into deep veins through communicating veins. Due to the presence of valves in the limb veins the blood flows in one direction, i.e. from periphery towards heart and not in reverse direction.

- *When the skeletal muscles contract*, the deep veins present in between the muscles are compressed and due to increased pressure the valve present proximal to the contracting muscle is opened up while the valve present on distal end is tightly closed and in this way the blood is propelled up towards the heart (Fig. 4.3-15A).
- *When the skeletal muscle relaxes*, a negative pressure is created in the segment of veins. So, due to back flow the proximal valve is closed and the distal valve is opened and blood is sucked up (Fig. 4.3-15B).
- *With rhythmic contractions of skeletal muscles* in this way, the blood is squeezed out of the limbs towards the heart.

Applied Aspect

In certain professions (e.g. nurses, traffic police, etc.) the individuals have to keep standing for a long time of a day. In such persons, sometimes the excessive venous pressure stretches the veins of the legs to such an extent that their diameter increases and the venous valves become incompetent. The venous pressure further increases and gradually the veins of lower limbs become large, tortuous and bulbous. This condition is called *varicose veins*.

4. Blood Volume. The mean circulating filling pressure (MCFP) which is equivalent to mean systemic filling pressure (MSFP) refers to the equilibrated pressure measured everywhere as a result of stoppage of blood flow in systemic circulation when heart stops pumping. The level of MSFP influences the venous return. Greater the MSFP more the venous return and lower the MSFP lesser the venous return (Fig. 4.3-16).

The MCFP in turn depends upon the level of blood volume. When relationship of blood volume and MCFP is plotted, the graph (Fig. 4.3-17) shows that:

- At blood volume of 4 l the MCFP is nearly zero because the veins are unstressed,
- At blood volume of 5 l the MCFP raises to 7 mmHg and
- At higher blood volume there is linear increase in MCFP.

Thus, the increased blood volume increases the venous return and a decreased blood volume decreases the venous return.

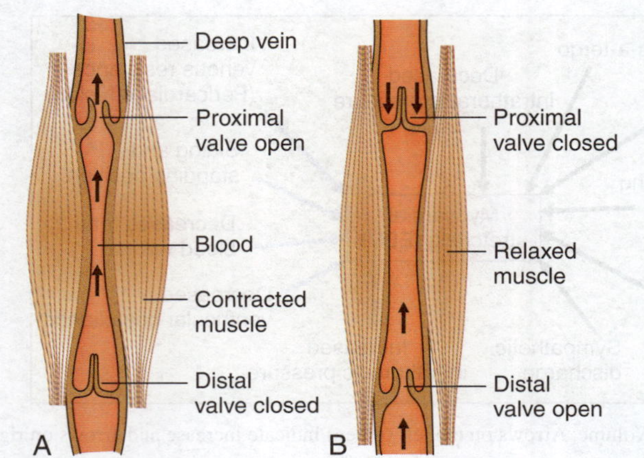

FIGURE 4.3-15 Mechanism of muscle pump: **A,** during contraction of muscles; and **B,** during relaxation of muscles.

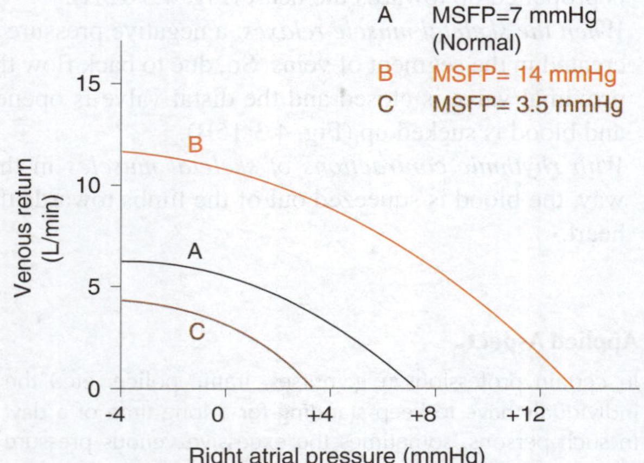

FIGURE 4.3-16 Venous return curve showing relationship with mean systemic filling pressure.

5. Sympathetic Discharge. On sympathetic stimulation, there occurs increase in the venous tone which decreases the capacity of the venous system (veins are capacitance vessels). Due to decrease in the venous capacity the MCFP rises which increases the venous return. At normal blood volume, a strong sympathetic stimulation raises the MCFP from 7 to 17 mmHg. And inhibition of sympathetics decreases the MCFP from 7 to 4 mmHg (due to venous dilatation) and thus decreases the venous return.

6. Standing Body Position is associated with a decreased venous return due to peripheral pooling of the blood.

7. Resistance to Venous Return. Normally, 2/3rd resistance to venous flow is offered by veins and 1/3rd by the arteries. Resistance decreases the venous return. The venous resistance is considered to be more important regarding venous return, as the veins being capacitance vessels, rise in the venous pressure is less effective to push the blood towards the heart. On the other hand, as with increased resistance in arterioles or small arteries, with little accumulation of blood in the arteries there is great increase in the pressure (30 times as compared to veins) which overcomes

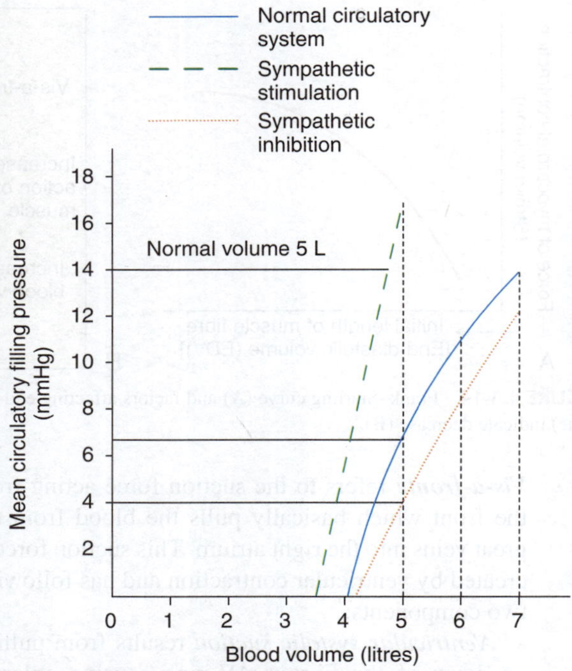

FIGURE 4.3-17 Relationship between mean circulatory filling pressure and blood volume.

the effect of increase in resistance. As shown in Fig. 4.3-18, decrease in the resistance to venous return to one half of the normal increases the venous return two times and rotates the curve upwards (Fig. 4.3-18B); while an increase in the resistance to venous flow twice the normal decreases the venous return to half and rotates the curve downwards (Fig. 4.3-18C).

Clinical Significance of Frank–Starling Mechanism

For Small, Momentary Adjustments Necessary for Keeping the Outputs of Two Ventricles Equal and adjusting them to match the venous return the intrinsic regulation works

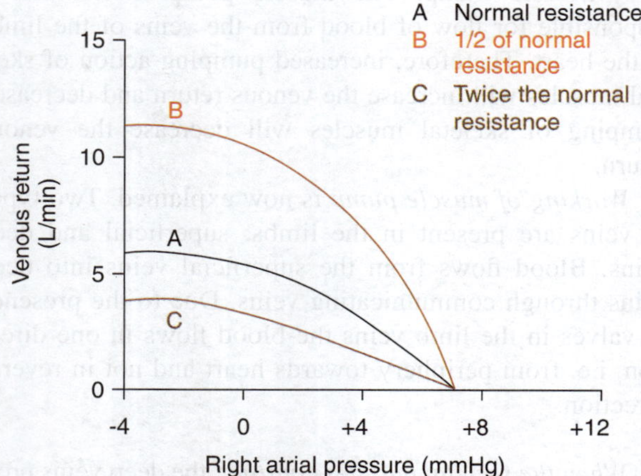

FIGURE 4.3-18 Venous return curve showing relationship between venous return and resistance to it: A, at normal resistance; B, at resistance one half of the normal; and C, at resistance twice as that of normal.

continuously. For example, if the output of the right ventricle increases momentarily, the venous return to left heart will increase, which in turn will increases the output of the right ventricle. The accuracy with which this adjustment is made can be understood by considering what would happen if the right ventricular output exceeds left ventricular output by as little as 0.1 ml/beat, i.e. 7 ml/min. Then, in a period of 3 h, the pulmonary blood volume will be increased by more than 1 l (7 $\times$ 60 $\times$ 3 = 1260 ml). This will prevent the optimal exchange of gases across the lungs and result in severe pulmonary insufficiency.

Maintenance of Constant Stroke Volume When the Peripheral Resistance is Increased is Carried Out by Intrinsic Mechanism. When the peripheral resistance (blood pressure) is increased, initially the heart is unable to pump all the blood it normally does. The accumulated blood in the ventricle stretches the muscle fibres leading to great force of contraction and thus the stroke volume is restored to normal in spite of greater resistance to the outflow.

Intrinsic Control Mechanism Serves as a Life-saving Device in Cardiac Failure. Left ventricular failure causes accumulation of blood within left ventricle, thereby decreases blood supply to vital organs. Soon, accumulation of blood in the left ventricle, increases the initial length of muscle fibres leading to greater cardiac output according to Frank–Starling mechanism. However, when accumulation of blood is too great, the Frank–Starling law will fail to operate leading to decrease in blood supply to the vital organs and ultimately death may occur.

2. Extrinsic Regulation (Autonomic Neural Mechanism)

In this mechanism, stroke volume increases due to *increased myocardial contractility* without any increase in the initial muscle length. Therefore, it is also called *homometric mechanism*. The homometric regulation is governed by autonomic neural mechanism as:

Sympathetic Activity

Stimulation of the sympathetic nerves to the heart results in increased myocardial contractility and is known as *positive inotropic effect*. The positive inotropic effect of the norepinephrine liberated at the sympathetic nerve endings is augmented by circulating norepinephrine.

Positive inotropic effect also can be defined as an increase in the *maximal velocity* of shortening (V'max) when it is plotted as a function of afterload. For the ventricles, the afterload is the arterial pressure during the ejection phase. During any muscle contraction, the velocity of shortening and the force developed are inversely related. For details of the effect of afterload and the *force velocity curve*, see page 253.

Inhibition of sympathetic system has opposite effects. Under normal conditions, there is continuous slow rate of discharge through sympathetic fibres to the heart which maintains pumping 30% above with no sympathetic stimulation. Therefore, when sympathetic activity is inhibited, the ventricular force of contraction decreases.

In intact animals, stimulation of sympathetic nerves produces a marked increase in the heart rate and a moderate increase in the stroke volume leading to a manifold increase in the cardiac output.

Characteristics of Increased Myocardial Contractility

Characteristics of Homometric Regulation. The increased myocardial contractility achieved by homometric regulation differs from the increase in force of contraction of myocardium achieved by heterometric regulation. Its characteristic features are:

- The ventricles contract more forcefully and more rapidly, i.e. velocity of shortening of muscle is increased. As a result, the ventricles are able to do more work per stroke, i.e. ejection fraction increases at the same end-diastolic volume (without increase in venous return).
- Due to more complete emptying of ventricles during each systole, the *end-systolic volume is decreased.*
- Due to increased stroke output, *arterial pressure is increased.*

Mechanism of Effects of Sympathetic Stimulation. Sympathetic stimulation increases the myocardial contractility by causing *activation of* β1 adrenergic receptors and Gs. Activation of β_1 receptors results in activation of adenylyl cyclase and increased intracellular cyclic AMP, which in turn:

- Increases the concentration of Ca^{2+} within the myocardial cells causing a more rapid and forceful contraction and
- Via protein kinase causes more rapid intake of Ca^{2+} by sarcoplasmic reticulum (SR), which shortens the duration of both the action potential and contraction.

Parasympathetic Activity. There is a negative inotropic effect of parasympathetic (vagal) stimulation. This effect, however, is not much because vagal fibres are mainly distributed to the atria and not much to the ventricles.

Role of Heart Rate in Control of Cardiac Output

The cardiac output and heart rate both are increased during exercise, proportionate to its severity. Since, cardiac output is the product of stroke volume and heart rate, it is tempting to attribute the increase in cardiac output to increase in the heart rate. However, in fact it is not so. It has been seen that when heart rate alone is increased, e.g. by change in the frequency of discharge of an artificial cardiac pacemaker, the cardiac output does not increase at all. As shown in Fig. 4.3-19, the progressive increase in the heart rate is associated with a proportionate decrease in stroke volume because of reduced diastole time and thus reduced end-diastolic volume. Conversely, when the heart rate is reduced the ventricular diastole is prolonged leading to more ventricular filling and thus an increased stroke volume.

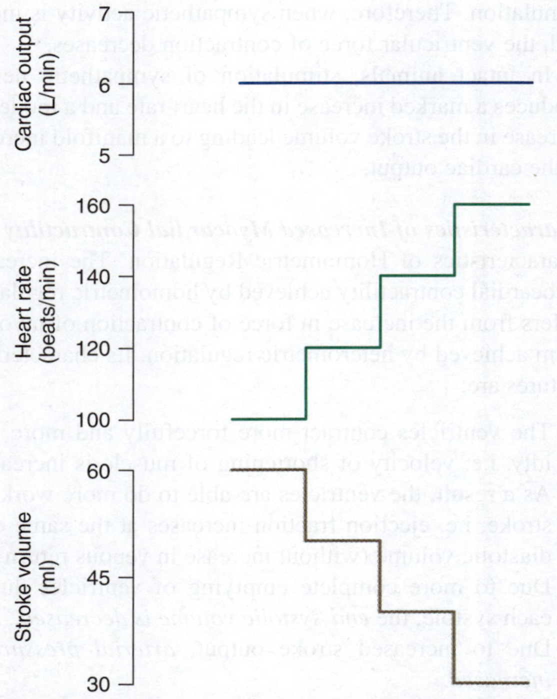

FIGURE 4.3-19 Effect of increase in heart rate through an artificial pacemaker on stroke volume and cardiac output.

During exercise, the sympathetic stimulation produces a marked increase in the heart rate (200–300%) due to positive chronotropism and moderate increase (50–60%) in the stroke volume due to positive inotropism leading to manifold increase in cardiac output.

Integrated Control of Cardiac Output

In intact animals and humans, the intrinsic and extrinsic mechanisms described above operate simultaneously in an integrated way to maintain cardiac output. Therefore, in a given situation, depending upon the status of end-diastolic volume and status of myocardial contractility, the individual will have one of the curves from the 'family of Frank–Starling curves'.

Interaction of Frank–Starling Mechanism and Myocardial Contractility

Factors causing increased myocardial contractility shift the Frank–Starling curve to the left (Fig. 4.3-20). Increased contractility (positive inotropism) refers to greater contraction force at a given preload or end-diastolic volume. Factors increasing myocardial contractility are:

1. *Sympathetic stimulation* increases myocardial contractility by causing activation of β_1 adrenergic receptors, as discussed above.
2. *Catecholamines* also exert their positive inotropic effect via their action on cardiac β_1 adrenergic receptors by a mechanism similar to that of sympathetic stimulation.
3. *Xanthines* such as caffeine and theophylline exert their positive inotropic effect by inhibiting the breakdown of cyclic AMP.
4. *Glucagon* causes positive inotropic effect by increasing the formation of cyclic AMP.
5. *Digitalis and related drugs* exert their positive inotropic effect by their inhibitory effect on Na^+–K^+ ATPase in the myocardium. The inhibition causes an increase in intracellular Na^+, which in turn increases the availability of Ca^{2+} in the cell. Digitalis which was initially prepared from the plant *Digitalis purpurea* has been used for centuries to treat heart failure.

Factors Causing Decreased Myocardial Contractility shift the Frank–Starling curve to the right (Fig. 4.3-20). The decreased contractility (negative inotropism) represents a decrease in the force of contraction at any fibre length or ventricular volume. Its causes are:

1. *Parasympathetic (vagal) stimulation.* Since the vagal fibres are distributed mainly to atria and not to ventricles, vagal stimulation causes negative inotropic effect on the atrial muscles and indirectly mild negative inotropic effect on the ventricles reducing strength of heart contraction by 20–30%.

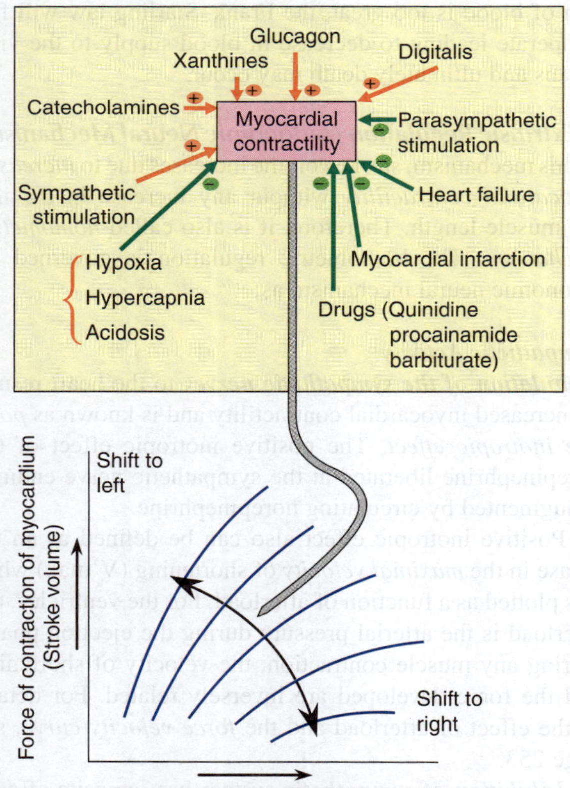

FIGURE 4.3-20 Effect of changes in myocardial contractility on Frank–Starling curve. The factors which increase the contractility shift the curve to left and those decrease the contractility shift the curve to right.

2. *Heart failure* is also associated with reduced myocardial contractility due to intrinsic depression. The cause of this depression is not known.
3. *Myocardial infarction* may result in fibrotic and non-functional area in myocardium resulting in reduction of total ventricular performance.
4. *Hypercapnia, hypoxia and acidosis* produce negative inotropic effect by causing a decrease in the formation of cyclic AMP.
5. *Drugs* such as quinidine, procainamide and barbiturates depress myocardial contractility.

Relative Contribution of Intrinsic and Extrinsic Mechanism in Controlling Cardiac Output under some common situations are given below.

- ***During rest in a normal person***, an equilibrium is maintained between the intrinsic and extrinsic control mechanisms of stroke volume and the sinus rhythm (heart rate). In this way, about 5–6 l blood is received by the heart (venous return) and the same amount is ejected out (cardiac output) in a minute at a normal heart rate of about 70–80 beats/min.

  Regulation of cardiac output when venous return increases in the absence of stimulation of heart (e.g. as occurs immediately after a change of posture from standing to lying) is carried out by the Frank–Starling mechanism.
- ***During exercise in normal persons***, both intrinsic and extrinsic mechanisms are geared up. Actual measurements of end-diastolic and end-systolic volumes have revealed no change or even a decrease in the end-diastolic volume in mild to moderate exercise. At the same time, there is evidence of increased sympathetic discharge to heart in the form of decreased end-systolic volume and tachycardia. It has been explained that the increased venous return produced by skeletal muscle pump action and increased respiration is tackled by improved pumping of the heart. Therefore, it can be concluded that, in mild to moderate exercise, the pumping ability of the heart is enhanced mainly by greater sympathetic discharge. In severe exercise, when the venous return is large enough to raise the end-diastolic volume, Frank–Starling mechanism also comes into play over and above the increased sympathetic discharge thus result in very high cardiac output.
- ***In patients with transplanted hearts.*** Frank–Starling mechanism is practically the only mechanism regulating the cardiac output since there is absence of cardiac innervation (Fig. 4.3-21). During exercise, the increase in cardiac output seen in these patients is not so rapid, and their maximal increase is smaller than in normal individuals but is appreciable.

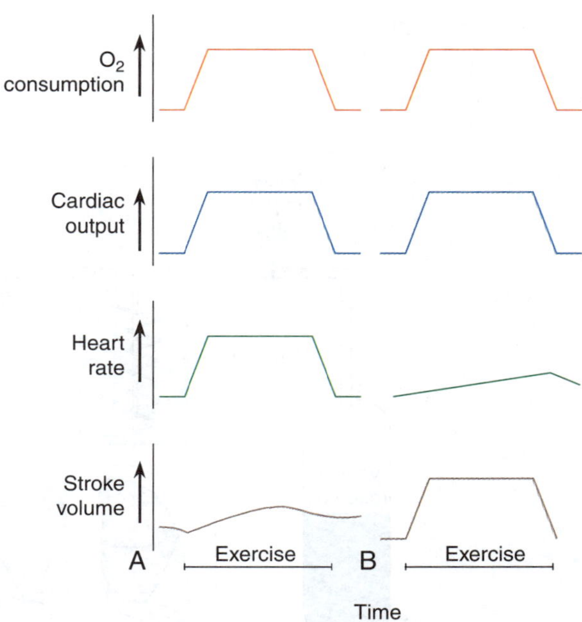

FIGURE 4.3-21 Cardiac response to moderate exercise: A, in normal human; and B, in patients with transplanted heart.

Heart–Lung Preparation

The Frank–Starling's heart–lung preparation is an experimental set up in a dog, devised to demonstrate the effects of various factors on the activities of heart. In this preparation, as the name suggests, blood does not flow to any part of the body except the heart and lungs. The animal is actually dead and heart is functionally denervated.

Experimental Set-up Experimental set up (Fig. 4.3-22) of the heart–lung preparation includes following essential steps:

- ***Trachea*** is cannulated and lungs are artificially ventilated.
- ***Aorta*** is ligated beyond the origin of innominate artery so that systemic circulation of the body is blocked.
- ***Innominate artery*** is cannulated and connected to mercury manometer to measure the arterial blood pressure and also through a series of tubes to:
  - *Elastic vessel,* which provides elasticity artificially similar to that of arterial wall,
  - *Resistance vessel,* which is used to provide resistance artificially. The resistance applied can be measured through the attached manometer.
  - *Warming glass coil,* which is kept inside a water bath with a heater. The temperature of the water bath is controlled, so that the temperature of blood can be maintained.
  - *Flowmeter* which determines the amount of blood flowing through it (cardiac output).
  - *Venous reservoir* which represents the peripheral venous system. It is connected through a tube to the

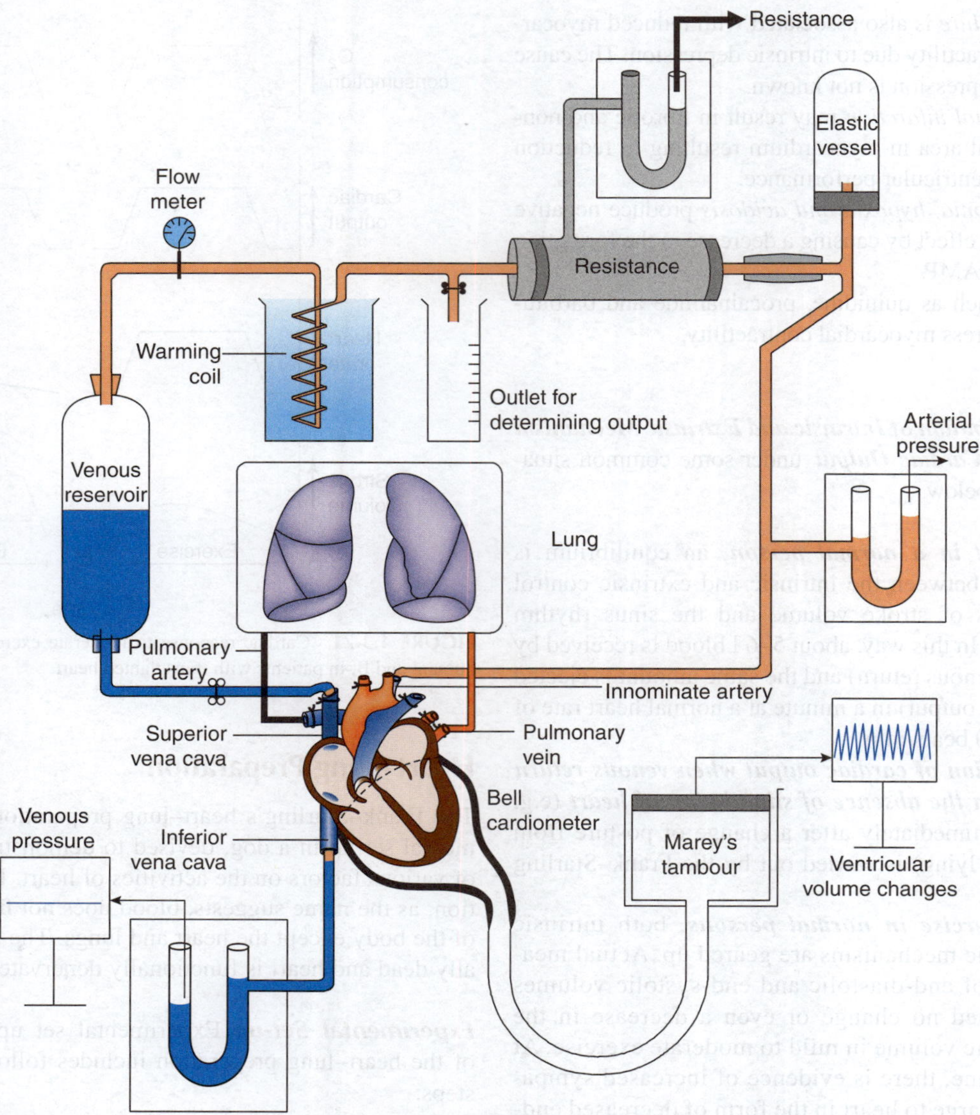

FIGURE 4.3-22 Heart–lung preparation.

superior vena cava. A screw type clamp is fitted to the rubber tube. It is used to adjust the amount of blood returning to heart (venous return).

Thus, the blood ejected from the left ventricle after passing through the above attachment ultimately reaches the right atrium. From there the blood flows to the right ventricle, pulmonary artery, lungs and back to heart through the pulmonary veins.

- ***Inferior vena cava*** is attached to manometer to record the right atrial pressure.
- ***Bell's cardiometer*** is fitted to the ventricle for measuring the stroke volume of the heart. The recording is made through *Marey's tambour* connected to the cardiometer.

Uses of Heart–Lung Preparation In the heart–lung preparation, heart works as an isolated organ. It can be used to demonstrate the effect of various factors on the heart's activities as:

1. Effect of Venous Return on Stroke Volume (Frank–Starling Mechanism). Venous return to the heart is changed through the venous reservoir and stroke volume at different levels of venous return is recorded through the cardiometer. The record shows:

- An increase in stroke volume with increase in venous return, (Fig. 4.3-23) and
- A decrease in stroke volume with decrease in venous return.

These observations demonstrate the Frank–Starling's law (intrinsic mechanism controlling stroke volume).

2. Effect of Sympathetic Stimulation on Stroke Volume when the stellate ganglion (cardiosympathetic nerve) is stimulated without any change in the venous return, the stroke

volume is increased but with lower end-systolic and end-diastolic volume (Fig. 4.3-24). This activity demonstrates the extrinsic control mechanism of stroke volume. Right atrial pressure is also reduced. It is due to increased suction of blood from the atria by the vigorously contracting ventricle.

3. Combined Effect of Increase in End-diastolic Volume and Sympathetic Stimulation on Stroke Volume. At a given rate of sympathetic stimulation, the end-diastolic volume is gradually increased and the resulting stroke volume is plotted against the end-diastolic volume, to give a Frank–Starling curve with different rates of sympathetic stimulation (0/S–10/S) a family of such curves is obtained (Fig. 4.3-25). From these curves, it can be inferred that even during sympathetic stimulation an increase in end-diastolic volume increases the stroke volume of heart.

4. To Demonstrate the Effect of Peripheral Resistance on Cardiac Output. Resistance is increased through the resistance vessel and its effect on cardiac output is recorded:

- With increase in the peripheral resistance cardiac output is increased and
- With decrease in the peripheral resistance the cardiac output is decreased.

5. Cardiac Function Curves can also be recorded using a heart–lung preparation. These include:

- The cardiac output curves,
- The venous return curves and
- The cardiovascular curves.

Cardiac and Vascular Function Curves

The cardiac and vascular function curves provide the graphic analysis of cardiac output, capacity of the ventricles to pump and relationship between cardiac output and central venous pressure (CVP). Such a graphical analysis provides useful information in patients with cardiac failure. Most of the curves are obtained from animal experiments by using heart–lung preparation. However, they do represent the function of ventricles in human heart. These curves include:

- Cardiac function curves,
- Vascular function curves and
- Cardiovascular function curves.

Cardiac Function Curves The cardiac function curves reflect the relationship between CVP, i.e. right atrial pressure and the cardiac output (Frank–Starling curve). Three types of cardiac function curves are:

1. Normal Cardiac Function Curve. As shown in Fig. 4.3-26A, the plateau level of normal cardiac function curve is about 13 l/min, i.e. 2.5 times the normal cardiac output (5 l). This means that the normal heart, functioning without any excess nervous stimulation can pump an amount of venous return up to about 2.5 times the normal venous return before the heart becomes a limiting factor in the control of cardiac output.

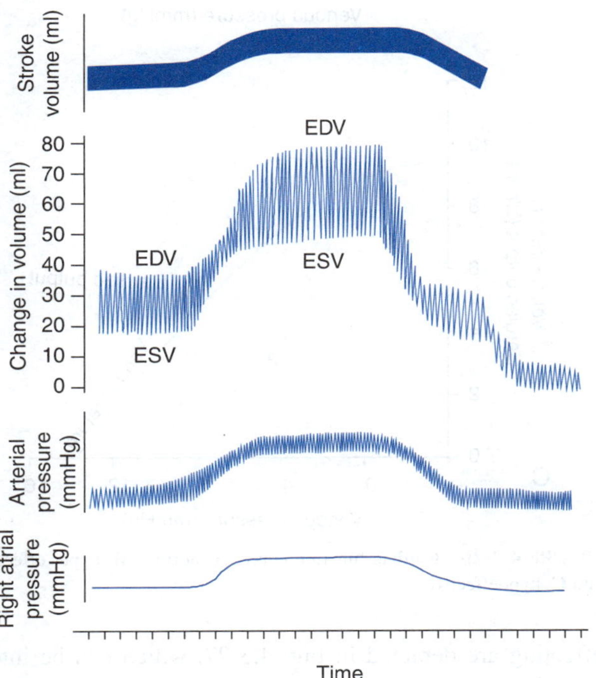

FIGURE 4.3-23 Tracings from heart–lung preparation demonstrating the effect of venous return on stroke volume, end-diastolic volume, end-systolic volume, arterial pressure and venous pressure.

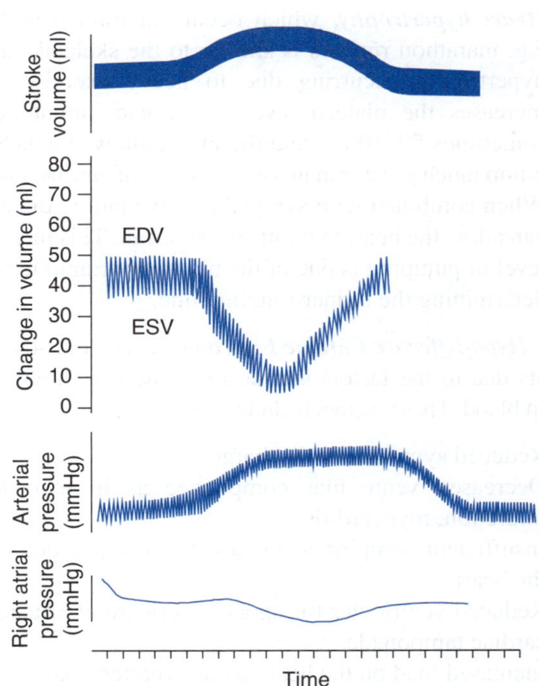

FIGURE 4.3-24 Tracings from heart–lung preparation demonstrating the effect of sympathetic nerve stimulation on stroke volume, end-diastolic volume, end-systolic volume, arterial pressure and venous pressure.

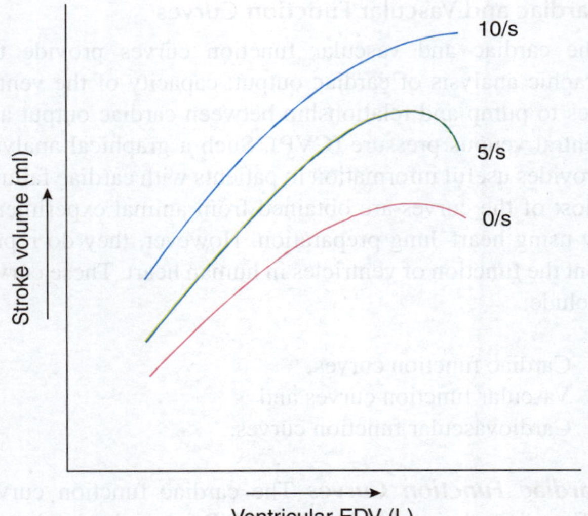

FIGURE 4.3-25 Family of Frank–Starling curves obtained by combined effect to increase in end-diastolic volume and sympathetic stimulation on stroke volume on heart–lung preparation.

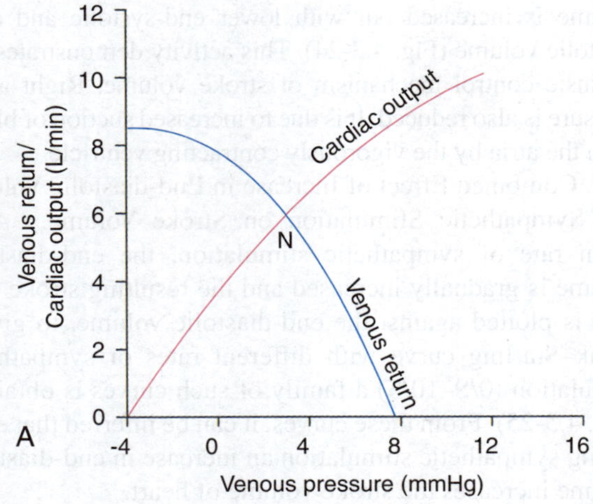

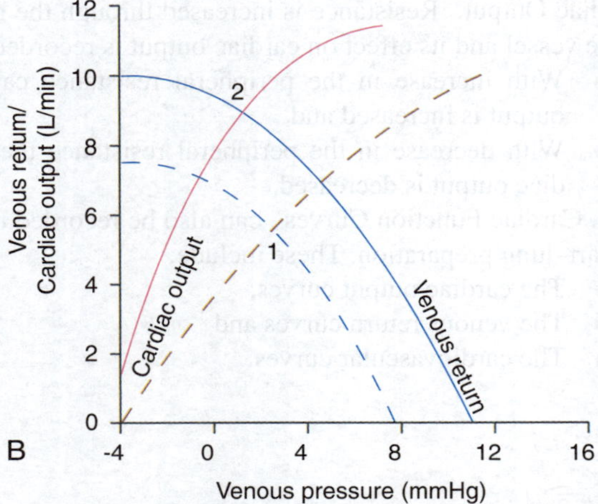

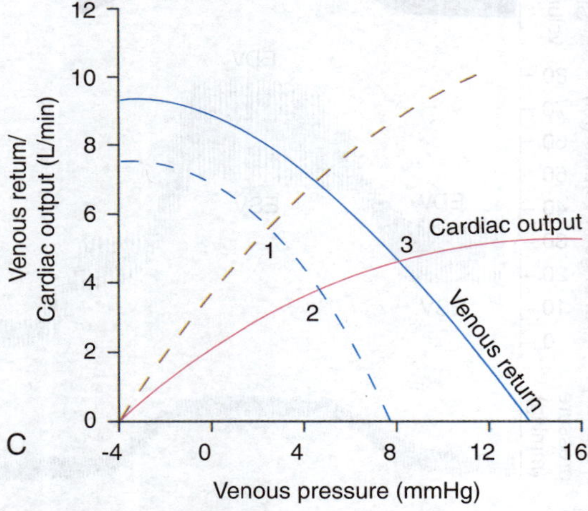

FIGURE 4.3-26 Cardiac function curve: **A,** normal; **B,** hyper effective and **C,** hypoeffective.

2. Hyper-Effective Cardiac Function Curve. As shown in Fig. 4.3-26B, the hyper-effective heart pumps better than normal. Factors resulting in a hyper-effective heart are:

- ***Sympathetic stimulation of heart,*** which can raise the plateau level of the cardiac output curve to almost twice the plateau of normal curve.
- ***Heart hypertrophy,*** which occurs in trained athletes, e.g. marathon runners is similar to the skeletal muscle hypertrophy occurring due to heavy exercise. This increases the plateau level of cardiac output curve, sometimes 50–100%, and therefore, allows the heart to pump much greater than usual amount of cardiac output. When combined with sympathetic excitation, the effect can allow the heart to pump 30–40 l/min. This increased level of pumping is one of the most important factors in determining the runner running time.

3. Hypo-Effective Cardiac Function Curve (Fig. 4.3-26C) results due to the factors that decrease the heart's ability to pump blood. These factors include:

- Reduced sympathetic discharge,
- Decreased ventricular compliance as in myocardial infarction, myocarditis,
- Insufficient pumping as in valvular or septal defects of the heart,
- Reduced ventricular filling as in pericardial effusion or cardiac tamponade,
- Increased load on the heart, as in hypertension.

Vascular Function Curves The vascular function curves reflect the relationship between venous return and venous pressure. Normal vascular function curve and the factors affecting are depicted in Fig. 4.3-27, which can be interpreted as:

- As shown in Fig. 4.3-27A, in a *normal curve,* the venous pressure decreases as venous return increases because the transfer of blood from the venous to the arterial system increases. When venous return is zero, venous pressure is maximum and is referred to as the mean circulatory filling pressure (MCFP).

- The MCFP increases with increase in blood volume (Fig. 4.3-17) and also increases with increase in sympathetic stimulation (which increases venous tone). These factors, which increase the MCFP, cause the vascular function curve to shift to the right (Fig. 4.3-27B).
- *Changes in arteriolar resistance* alter the slope of the vascular function curve. An increased resistance reduces the cardiac output (venous return) and a decreased resistance increases the venous return (Fig. 4.3-27C).

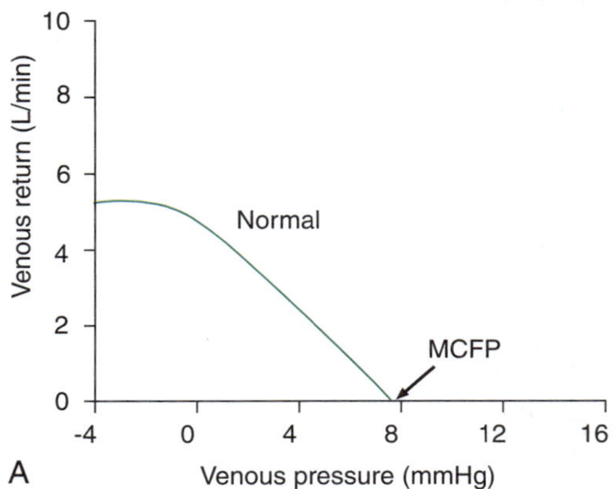

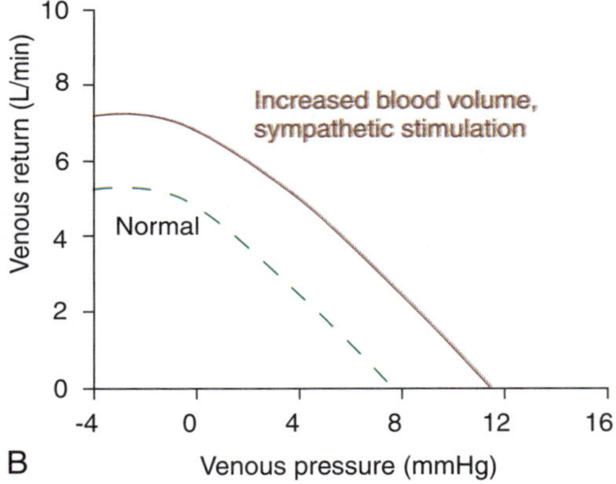

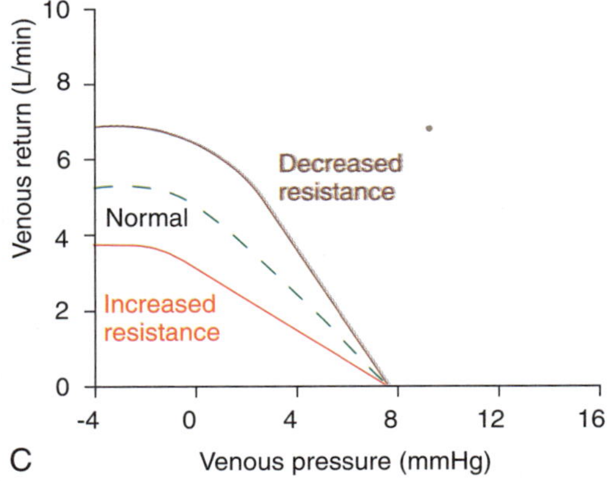

FIGURE 4.3-27 Vascular function curves: **A,** normal; **B,** effect of increased blood volume and sympathetic stimulation; and **C,** effect of change in arterial resistance.

Cardiovascular Function Curves The cardiovascular function curves refer to the coupled cardiac and vascular function curves. Since both venous return and cardiac output depend on the venous pressure, the cardiac and vascular function curves can be combined into a single group. The intersection of the two curves gives the operant value of cardiac output and venous pressure (Fig. 4.3-26A and 4.3-28). Any change in cardiac contractility, blood volume or vascular resistance will cause the operating point to shift, but *cardiac output and venous return will always be equal.* Exercise and congestive heart failure (described below) are just two of many conditions that can alter the operating point of the system.

Effect of Exercise on Cardiovascular Function Curve. The overall effect of exercise is an increase in cardiac output that is proportional to the exercise intensity as shown in Fig. 4.3-28B.

- *Activation of sympathetic system* increases ventricular contractility and heart rate causing the *cardiac output curve to shift to left* (i.e. upward) and *vasodilation,* which occurs in the skeletal muscles, reduces the total peripheral resistance or afterload, causing the *vascular function curve to shift to right.* Thus, the operating point shifts from 1 to 2 (Fig. 4.3-26B) depicting thereby that with increase in venous return the cardiac output is increased proportionately.

Cardiovascular Function Curve in Congestive Heart Failure. In congestive heart failure, the output of one or both ventricles is not sufficient to supply the needs of the body (Fig. 4.3-28C).

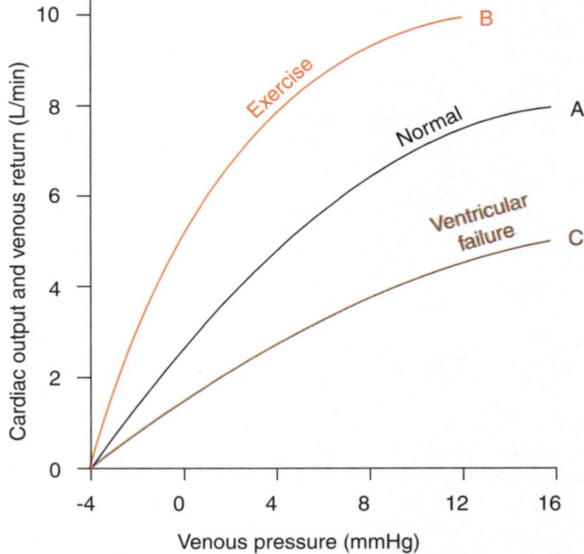

FIGURE 4.3-28 Cardiovascular function curves: A, normal; B, during exercise; and C, in congestive heart failure.

- ***Decreased contractility of the heart*** is the primary defect in the congestive heart failure (e.g. in myocarditis and valvular heart disease), reducing cardiac output and thus shifting the cardiac function curve downwards. Point 2 in Fig. 4.3-26C and 4.3-28C reflects the reduction in cardiac output from the normal level (Point 1).
- ***Increase in blood volume,*** due to retention of fluids and electrolytes by the kidneys in response to renin–angiotensin–aldosterone axis, increases the venous return (shifting the vascular function curve to right) and raises the venous pressure. The cardiac output, thus, returns toward normal (Point 3 in Fig. 4.3-26C), but it is at the expense of an enlarged ventricle.
- High venous pressure produces oedema. Left ventricular failure results in pulmonary oedema and right ventricular failure may lead to ankle swelling and fluid accumulation in viscera.

Chapter 4.4

Dynamics of Circulation: Pressure and Flow of Blood and Lymph

INTRODUCTION

Dynamics of circulation is concerned with flow of blood and lymph and also the pressure in the various segments of the vascular system of the body. For descriptive purposes, the 'dynamics of circulation' is discussed under the following headings:

- Functional organization and structure of vascular system,
- Haemodynamics,
- Blood flow and pressure in different segments of circulatory system and
- Blood pressure

FUNCTIONAL ORGANIZATION AND STRUCTURE OF VASCULAR SYSTEM

Organization of Vascular System

The vascular system, which consists of different types of blood vessels, constitutes the transport system of the body whose *primary functions* are: (i) distribution of nutrients and oxygen to all body cells, and (ii) collection of waste products and CO_2 from different body cells and to carry them to excretory organs for excretion. *Secondary functions* subserved by the vascular system are thermoregulation, distribution of hormones to the target tissues and distribution of antibodies and cells concerned with defence mechanism to various parts of the body.

To perform the above functions, the vascular system is organized into two separate circulations, systemic and pulmonary, arranged in series (Fig. 4.4-1). In addition, parallel to the circulation of blood is the disposed circulation of lymph which helps the blood circulation to perform its various functions.

Systemic Circulation supplies blood to various systemic organs through parallel distribution channels (Fig. 4.4-1). This parallel arrangement of vessels ensures the supply of blood of the same arterial composition (i.e. same O_2 and CO_2 tension, pH, glucose level and essentially the same arterial pressure) to various body organs. In systemic circulation, from the left ventricle, blood is pumped through the

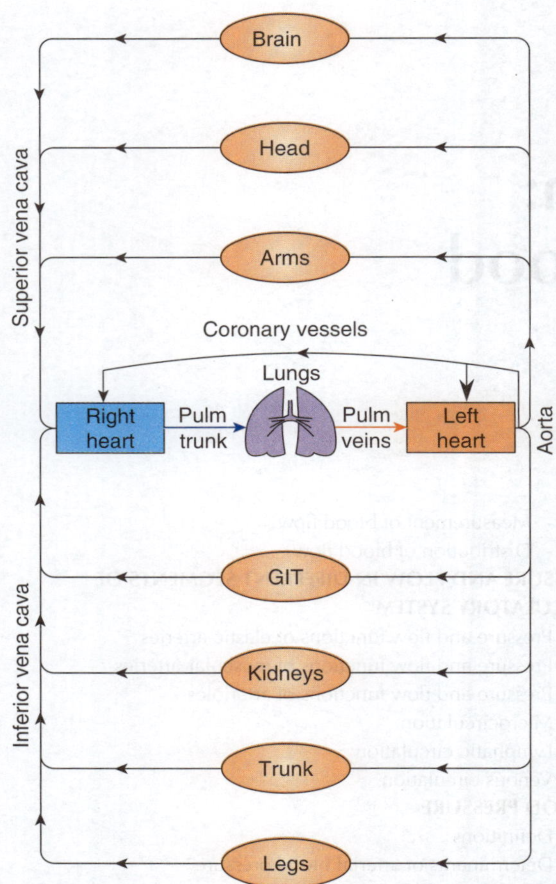

FIGURE 4.4-1 A schematic illustration of the organization of cardiovascular system depicting the series arrangement of pulmonary and systemic circulation and parallel arrangement of vessels supplying blood to organs.

arteries and arterioles to the capillaries, where it equilibrates with the interstitial fluid. The capillaries drain through the venules into the veins and ultimately to the right atrium.

Pulmonary Circulation is meant for oxygenation of blood. Since pulmonary circulation is arranged in series with systemic circulation, it receives the same amount of blood over any significant time period. Such a balanced output is achieved by the intrinsic property of the cardiac muscle known as Frank–Starling mechanism which has been described in the section on cardiac output (page 288). In pulmonary circulation, from the right ventricle, blood is pumped through the pulmonary arteries to the pulmonary capillaries. In the pulmonary capillaries, the blood equilibrates with the O_2 and CO_2 of alveolar air. The capillaries then drain the oxygenated blood through venules and then through pulmonary veins into the left atrium.

Lymphatic Circulation which is disposed in parallel to the circulation of blood can be considered a third type of circulation. Some tissue fluid enters the lymphatic channels as lymph, which is ultimately drained into the venous system via the thoracic lymphatic duct and the right lymphatic duct.

Systemic Vascular Tree The arrangement of systemic circulation permits wide variations in regional distribution of blood. For descriptive purposes and from a functional point of view, the systemic vascular tree can be divided into the following types of blood vessels:

- *Large elastic arteries* (Windkessel vessels) include aorta and its main branches such as carotid, iliac and axillary arteries,
- *Large muscular* arteries (distribution vessels) which include most of the arteries of the body, e.g. arteries like radial, ulnar and popliteal,
- Arterioles and precapillary sphincters (resistance vessels),
- Meta-arterioles and capillaries (exchange vessels),
- Venules (postcapillary resistance vessels),
- Veins (capacitance vessels) and
- Arteriovenous anastomoses (shunt or thoroughfare vessels).

Structure of Blood Vessels

Structural Characteristics

General Structural Characteristics Histologically, walls of most of the blood vessels except the capillaries consist of three coats. General structural characteristics of a large artery are (Fig. 4.4-2):

1. Tunica Intima. It is the innermost coat of the vessel wall. In large arteries, from inside-out, it consists of:

    - *Endothelial lining,* which is very smooth and silky, and consists of single layer of cells. It lies in contact with blood.
    - *Basal lamina* is a thin layer of glycoprotein which lines the external aspect of the endothelium.
    - *Subendothelial connective tissue* is a delicate layer of connective tissue which lies outside the basal lamina.
    - *Internal elastic lamina* is a thin membrane formed by elastic fibres.

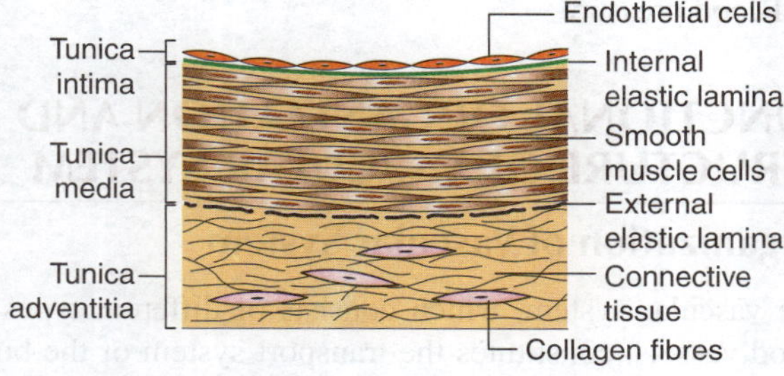

FIGURE 4.4-2 Histological structure of an artery.

2. Tunica Media. It is the middle, thickest coat of the vessel wall. It consists of smooth muscles and elastic tissue. The ratio of these two tissues varies from vessel to vessel. On the outside, tunica media is limited by a membrane formed by elastic fibres called the *external elastic lamina.*

3. Tunica Adventitia. It is the outermost coat of the vessel wall. It is made of connective tissue in which collagen fibres are prominent. This layer prevents undue stretching or distension of the blood vessel.

Important points to be noted are:

- Fibrous elements in the intima and adventitia (mainly collagen) run longitudinally (i.e. along the length of the vessel).
- Elastic tissue and smooth muscles forming tunica media run circularly.
- Elastic fibres forming internal and external elastic laminae are often in the form of fenestrated sheets.

Specific Structural Characteristics

- ***Large (elastic) arteries,*** in their tunica media, have dominant elastic tissue which provides them property of distensibility and elastic recoil.
- ***Medium size arteries.*** In these arteries, the elastic tissue, both in intima and media, is much less and thus the proportion of smooth muscles increases.
- ***Arterioles*** have characteristically no elastic tissue. Their media consists of a thick layer of smooth muscles and they have a *relatively narrow lumen.* Because of their structural characteristics, they act as resistance vessels.
- ***Meta-arterioles*** are relatively high-resistance conduits between arterioles and veins.
- ***Capillaries*** arise directly from arterioles or meta-arterioles. A cuff of smooth muscle cells called the *precapillary sphincter* surrounds the origin of capillaries in some region. The capillary wall does not contain any tunica media and adventitia. It is formed essentially by endothelial cells which are lined on the outside by a basal lamina (glycoproteins), branching perivascular cells called *pericytes.* Further details of capillaries are described in the section on microcirculation.
- ***Postcapillary venules,*** which measure 20–60 μm in diameter, are the *most permeable part* of microcirculation.
- ***Veins*** are relatively thin-walled structures that contain very small amount of elastic tissue and smooth muscles compared with arteries. These are highly distensible part of the vascular system and that is why also form the so-called *reservoir vessels.*

Essential Characteristics Essential characteristics of blood vessels like lumen diameter, wall thickness, approximate total cross-sectional area and percentage of blood volume contained are shown in Table 4.4-1.

Vascular Smooth Muscle

Vascular smooth muscle (VSM) is a key structure in the physiology of vascular system and thus needs special emphasis.

Arrangement in Tunica Media of the Vessels

Vascular smooth muscle is found in all segments of vascular tree, except the capillaries. Arrangement of vascular smooth muscles, however, varies in different segments:

- *In the* Windkessel *vessels*, they are disposed in a spiral fashion.
- *In the arterioles,* they are arranged more circularly and so on contraction may cause complete obliteration of the lumen.

Types of VSM. From a functional point of view, VSM is of two types: single unit (visceral type) and multiunit. The visceral type VSM fibres have inherent property of myogenic activity to stretch and are mainly present in small arteries, arterioles and meta-arterioles. The multiunit smooth muscle fibres are not excited by stretch.

TABLE 4.4-1 Essential Characteristics of Various Types of Blood Vessels

Types of blood vessels	Lumen diameter	Cross-sectional area (cm^2)	Velocity of blood flow	Pressure as cumulative blood volume %
• Aorta	2.5 cm	4.5	20 cm/s	2
• Arteries	0.4 cm	20	4 cm/s	8
• Arterioles	30 μm	400	2 mm/s	1
• Capillaries	05 μm	4500	0.2 mm/s	5
• Venules	20 μm	4000	0.2 mm/se	54
• Vein	0.5 cm	40	2 cm/s	
• Vena cava	3 cm	18	4.5 cm/s	

Innervational Characteristics

- Smooth muscles of the blood vessels are innervated by sympathetic fibres. These muscles contain α-adrenergic receptors. Therefore, noradrenaline causes contraction of muscle fibres leading to vasoconstriction.
- Sympathetic fibres exert tonic effect even at rest, resulting in the existence of vasomotor tone in the blood vessels.
- Stimulation of sympathetics increases the vasomotor tone, as a result the vessels are constricted and narrowed.
- Inhibition of sympathetic discharge results in decreased vasomotor tone and hence vasodilation.
- Skeletal muscle arterioles also contain β_2 receptors in addition to the α receptors; therefore, adrenaline causes dilation of these vessels.
- Besides α-adrenergic receptors, smooth muscles of the blood vessels are also stimulated by other agents like O_2 tension, lactic acid, etc. which are described in local control (page 349).

Excitation and Contraction Characteristics of VSM

- *Resting membrane potential (RMP)* is rather low in VSM compared with cardiac and skeletal muscles.
- *Typical action potential (AP)* is absent in VSM, nevertheless, with activity, some changes in membrane potential, resembling action potential, are seen.
- *Cause of development of AP* in VSM is entry of Ca^{2+} from ECF to ICF; therefore, calcium channel blockers like *nifedipine* powerfully prevent VSM contraction. That is why these drugs are extremely popular in the treatment of hypertension.
- *Contraction,* once developed in the VSM, takes long time to relax again, i.e. there occurs *sustained contraction.* Thus, sympathetic stimulation elevates blood pressure which tends to stay for some time.

HAEMODYNAMICS

Haemodynamics, which refers to study of blood flow in various segments of the vascular system, can be discussed under the following headings:

- General principles governing (factors affecting) blood flow,
- Circulation time,
- Types of blood flow,
- Measurement of blood flow,
- Distribution of blood flow to various regions of the body and
- Regulation of blood flow in different situations.

General Principles Governing (Factors Affecting) Blood Flow

Flow- Pressure-–Resistance Relationship

Relationship between flow of a fluid with the pressure and resistance offered to it through a rigid tube was studied by a French physiologist Poiseuille in 1842. Hagen, a contemporary of Poiseuille, worked further with the problem and found out the mathematical expression. Poiseuille's results (and their mathematical expression) were based on the measurement of the flow of a Newtonian fluid, i.e. a fluid that showed a viscosity which was unaffected by flow rate, through rigid tubes under the influence of steady head of pressure. The relationship studied is known as Poiseuille's law or Poiseuille–Hagen law.

Poiseuille's Law

Poiseuille's law expressing the relation between the flow (Q) and pressure gradient (ΔP) in a long narrow tube of length L, viscosity of fluid η and radius r of the tube is as:

$$Q = \frac{\Delta P \pi r^4}{8 \eta l}$$

Thus, according to Poiseuille's law, the flow (Q) of a Newtonian fluid through a rigid tube is determined by:

1. Pressure Gradient (ΔP), i.e. difference in the pressure between the two ends of the tube. In other words, fluid always flows from an area of high pressure (P_1) to one of lower pressure (P_2), and rate of flow (Q) is determined by the pressure gradient ($P_1 - P_2$), i.e. $Q \propto \Delta P$ or ($P_1 - P_2$).

2. Radius of Tube. The flow of fluid varies directly as the fourth power of radius (r^4). Thus, if the radius is halved, the flow will decrease by 16 times and vice versa. Thus, this factor is very important for flow of blood through the blood vessels.

3. Viscosity of Fluid (η). The flow of fluid varies inversely with the viscosity of fluid, i.e. greater the viscosity, lesser the flow and vice versa.

4. Length of the Tube (L). The flow is inversely proportional to the length of the tube. This is easily understandable, as every segment of the tube is offering resistance to the flow; therefore, longer the length, greater will be the total resistance offered.

Resistance (R). According to mathematical calculation in principles of physics, resistance (R) is represented by 8 $L\eta/\pi r^4$. By replacing 8 $L\eta/\pi r^4$ with R in Poiseuille's law, it becomes:

$$Q = \frac{\Delta P}{R}$$

Thus, Poiseuille's law can be considered analogous to Ohm's law of current in which:

$$\text{Current (flow)} = \frac{\text{Voltage (Pressure gradient)}}{\text{Resistance}}$$

Hence, the rate of flow (Q) is inversely proportional to the resistance (R).

The Poiseuille's law is valid for straight rigid tubes with Newtonian fluid flowing through them. Since blood vessels are not rigid and blood is not a Newtonian fluid; therefore, strictly speaking the Poiseuille's law does not apply to flow of blood through the vascular system. Nevertheless, the important principles relating flow, pressure gradient and resistance remain applicable, so they are discussed in relation to blood flow as:

- Blood flow and pressure gradient relationship, and
- Blood flow and resistance relationship.

Blood Flow and Pressure Gradient Relationship

According to Poiseuille's law, fluid always moves from an area of higher pressure to one of lower pressure. This downhill movement of blood (i.e. along the pressure gradient) occurs in the vascular system. Fig. 4.4-3 depicts the mean lateral pressure and blood flow in various components of the cardiovascular system (represented as cumulative blood volume in per cent). In systemic circulation, pressure at the beginning of aorta is about 100 mmHg and near the terminal portion of inferior vena cava it is nearly zero. Therefore, $P_1 - P_2 = (100 - 0) = 100$ mmHg. Note the progressive decrease in pressure from the left ventricle through the systemic circulation until blood enters the right ventricle. It is important to note that the greatest pressure drop occurs in the arterioles, which represent the highest resistance segment of the systemic circulation. Further, according to Poiseuille's law, at constant length and radius of a tube and viscosity of the fluid, the relationship between pressure and flow through a rigid tube is linear, i.e. as pressure increases, flow of fluid also increases (Fig. 4.4-4A). The relationship between flow of blood and pressure in the blood vessels is however not linear:

- In distensible vessels (e.g. aorta), the increase in flow as a result of a rising pressure head is initially less than that occurring in rigid tube, as due to elastic recoil they are slightly collapsed. However, later the flow in such vessels is greater than the rigid tubes (Fig. 4.4-4B), as they distend. At further higher pressure, the flow becomes linear as the vessels cannot distend any more due to the presence of fibrous tissue in the adventitia.

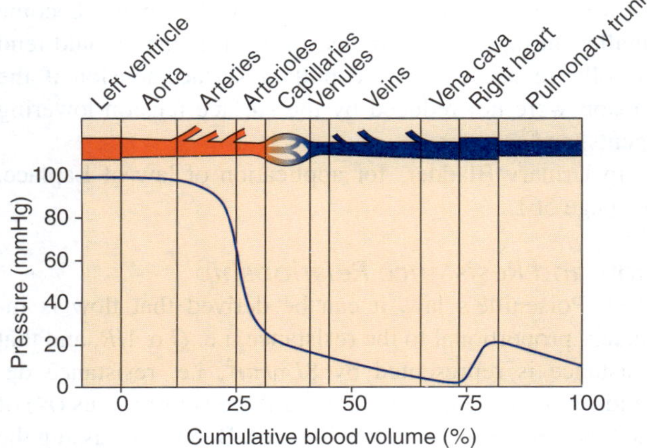

FIGURE 4.4-3 Mean lateral pressure in various components of vascular system and cumulative blood volume.

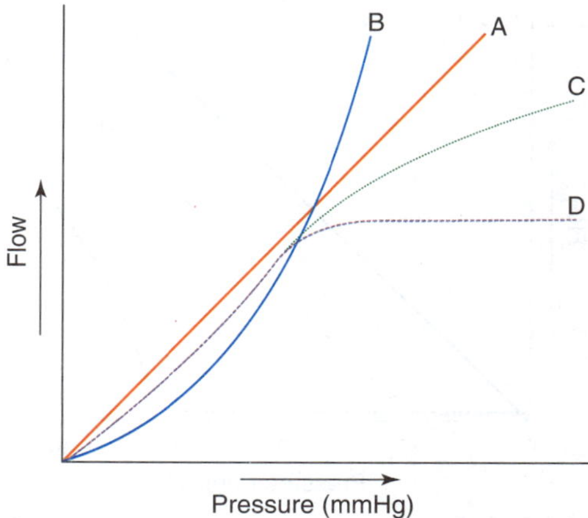

FIGURE 4.4-4 Relationship of pressure to flow: A, in a rigid tube; B, in a distensible blood vessel (aorta); C, in a distensible blood vessel containing active myogenic contractile element, whose contraction affects the distensible effects of raised pressure; and D, in a distensible vessel containing myogenic contractile element, which serves to stabilize flow over a wide range of pressure (80–200 mmHg), such vessels would show autoregulation.

- In resistance vessels, i.e. arterioles, the distension in the absence of other influences, at a given pressure head, would increase their internal radius and would correspondingly cause a raised flow at the pressure. However, in real life, it does not occur so because smooth muscles present in the media of arterioles when distended react actively to stretch by contracting. This myogenic contractile response to stretch offsets the elastic effect and so the flow in these vessels becomes less than the rigid tubes, i.e. the curve becomes concave to the pressure axis (Fig. 4.4-4C).
- In the arterioles where the myogenic contractile response even exceeds the elastic effect of raised pressure, the blood flow is maintained and does not increase with the further increase in the pressure (Fig. 4.4-4D). Thus, as shown in Fig. 4.4-4D, such arterioles serve to stabilize the blood flow over a wide range of pressure (80–200 mmHg). This phenomenon is called *autoregulation.*

Critical Closing Pressure

Since the flow–pressure relationship in a rigid tube is linear, the flow will cease only if the pressure is zero (Fig. 4.4-5A). However, in a blood vessel, the flow ceases when the blood pressure is 20 mmHg or even more (Fig. 4.4-5B). The pressure value at which the vessel collapses, its lumen closes and flow ceases is called *critical closing pressure (CCP).* The blood flow ceases when the blood pressure falls below the CCP because:

- Certain amount of intramural pressure is essentially required to push the RBCs (with average diameter of 7.5 μm) through the capillaries (average diameter 5 μm).
- Further, the tissue pressure exerted over the vessels also causes their collapse. So, a certain amount of intramural pressure is a must to counteract the tissue pressure and thus to keep the vessels patent and to maintain the blood flow.

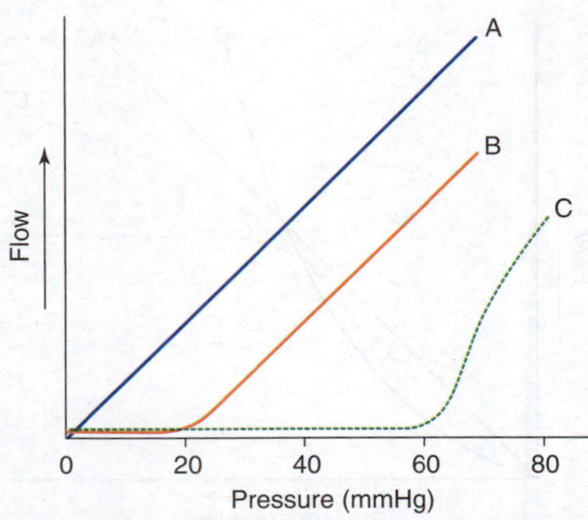

FIGURE 4.4-5 Relationship of pressure and flow in a rigid tube (A) and a blood vessel (B) and on sympathetic stimulation (C), depicting critical closing pressure (CCP).

Values of Critical Closing Pressure

- When whole blood is flowing through the vessels, the average value of critical closing pressure (CCP) is 20 mmHg (Fig. 4.4-5B).
- When plasma is flowing, the value of CCP is about 5–10 mmHg.
- On sympathetic stimulation, the value of CCP increases to 60 mmHg (Fig. 4.4-5C)
- On sympathetic inhibition, the value of CCP falls to 0 mmHg.

Equilibrium of Factors at Critical Closing Pressure

- In general, vasomotor tone of the blood vessels tries to constrict the vessels. This tone is increased by sympathetic stimulation and decreased by sympathetic inhibition.
- Intramural pressure tries to dilate the blood vessels up to a certain limit. When a point is reached where the intramural pressure (*P*) is not able to maintain an equilibrium with tension (*T*) in the vessel wall, at this point the blood vessel closes and the pressure at which it occurs is called critical closing pressure. Laplace law described below helps to explain this equilibrium relationship.

Law of Laplace Law of Laplace governs relation between the distending pressure and tension in the wall of a distensible viscus including blood vessels (Fig. 4.4-6). According to this law, the distending pressure (*P*) in a distensible hollow object is equal at equilibrium to the tension in wall (*T*) divided by the two principal radii of curvature of the object (r_1 and r_2):

$$P = T\left(\frac{1}{r_1} + \frac{1}{r_2}\right), \text{ where}$$

T is expressed in dynes/cm, r_1 and r_2 are in cm, and so *P* is expressed in dynes/cm^2.

- *In a sphere*, $r_1 = r_2$. Therefore,

$$P = \frac{T}{r}$$

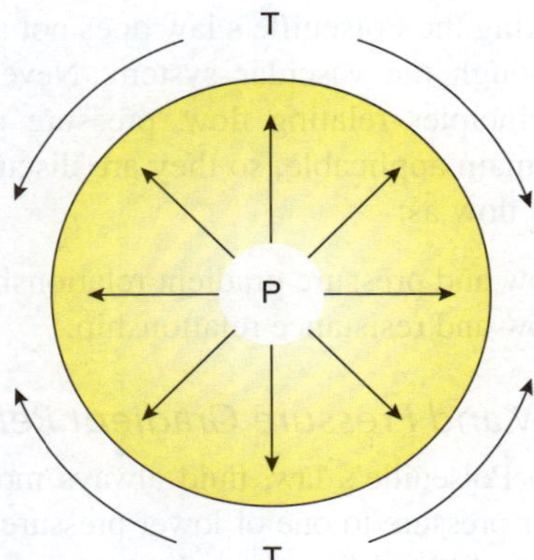

FIGURE 4.4-6 Relationship between distending pressure (P) and wall tension (T) in a hollow viscus.

- *In a cylinder* such as a blood vessel, one radius is infinite. Therefore,

$$P = \frac{T}{r}$$

Physiological Applications of Law of Laplace. This law applies to all the hollow viscous structures in the body. Some of its important applications are:

In Vascular System. As described above, for blood vessels, Laplace equation is $P = T/r$. This equation shows that smaller is the radius of a blood vessel, lesser is the tension (*T*) on the walls of the blood vessel required to balance the distending pressure or force (*P*). For example,

- In aorta, the tension at normal pressure is 170,000 dynes/cm.
- In inferior vena cava, it is about 21,000 dynes/cm.
- But in the capillaries, it is approximately 16 dynes/cm. This explains why capillaries being so thin walled and delicate are not prone to rupture.

In Heart. *Law of Laplace also explains* the disadvantage faced by a dilated heart. When the radius of a cardiac chamber is increased, a greater tension must be developed in the myocardium to produce any given pressure; consequently, a dilated heart must do more work than a nondilated heart.

In Lungs, the radii of curvature of the alveoli become smaller during expiration, and these structures would tend to collapse because of the pull of surface tension if the tension were not reduced by the surface tension-lowering agents (surfactants).

In Urinary Bladder, for application of law of Laplace, see page 561.

Flow and Resistance Relationship

From Poiseuille's law, it can be derived that flow is inversely proportional to the resistance, i.e. $Q \propto 1/R$, and that resistance is represented by $8L\eta/\pi r^4$, i.e. resistance depends upon the length (*L*) and fourth power of radius (r^4) of the tube and viscosity of the fluid (η). Before discussing the effect of these factors on the blood flow, it will be worthwhile to know about the *peripheral resistance unit* (PRU), i.e. unit of peripheral resistance in vascular system and concept of total peripheral resistance (TPR) in the body.

Peripheral Resistance Unit (PRU) As discussed above, Poiseuille's law can be considered analogous to Ohm's law, so:

$$\text{Flow, i.e. Q(ml/s)} = \frac{P_1 - P_2\text{(mm of Hg)}}{\text{Resistance (R)}}$$

$$\text{Thus, R} = \frac{P_1 - P_2\text{ (mm of Hg)}}{\text{Q (ml/s)}}$$

As flow is in ml/sec, therefore, in vascular system, *peripheral resistance unit (PRU)* is mm of Hg/mL/s.

Total Peripheral Resistance (TPR) At rest, in the systemic circulation, pressure at the beginning of aorta (P) is 100 mmHg and near the terminal portion of inferior vena cava (P_2) is 0 mmHg. Therefore, pressure gradient ($P_1 - P_2$) = (100 − 0) = 100 mmHg; and rate of blood flow (Q) through circulatory system is 100 ml/s. Thus at rest, the resistance (R) of the entire systemic circulation is called 'total peripheral resistance' (TPR), which can be calculated from the formula:

$$R = \frac{P_1 - P_2\text{ (mm of Hg)}}{\text{Flow (ml/s)}}$$

$$\text{TPR at rest} = \frac{100\text{ mmHg}}{100\text{ ml/s}} = 1\text{ mm of Hg/ml/s} = 1\text{PRU},$$

- TPR during maximum vasoconstriction may increase to 4 PRU, and
- TPR during maximum vasodilation may decrease to 0.2 PRU.
- Pulmonary vascular resistance is about 0.1–0.2 PRU.

Factors that Affect Resistance to Blood Flow According to Poiseuille's law, resistance (R) depends upon the length of tube (L), fourth power of radius of tube (r^4) and viscosity of the fluid (η). Since in an intact body the length of the blood vessels does not change, i.e. remains constant, the major factors that determine the resistance to flood flow are:

I. The viscosity of blood and
II. The radius of vessels.

Blood Viscosity and Resistance. Resistance (R) to blood flow is directly proportional to viscosity (η) of blood.

Definition and Unit of Viscosity. ***Viscosity*** was described by Isaac Newton in 1713 as internal friction to flow in a fluid or lack of slipperiness. These terms emphasize that when a fluid moves along a tube, laminae in the fluid slip on one another and move at different speeds thereby causing a velocity gradient in a direction perpendicular to the wall of the tube. This velocity gradient is called the *rate of shear*. A simple viscous fluid known as *Newtonian fluid* is defined as one whose viscosity does not vary with the rate of shear and remains constant at different rates of laminar flow. Therefore, resistance met by the fluid moving through a tube in a streamlined flow is due to the friction between adjacent laminae and not due to the friction between vessel wall and fluid. Thus, greater the internal friction, greater is the difference in velocity (shear rate) between two laminae and greater the coefficient of viscosity.

- ***Unit of viscosity*** is *Poise* (after Poiseuille). A fluid of 1 poise viscosity has a force of 1 dyne/cm^2 of contact between layers when flowing with a velocity gradient of 1 cm/s. 1 Poise is considered to be consisting of 100 centipoise (CP). *Viscosity of water* at 21°C is 0.01 poise or 1 centipoise.
- ***Relative viscosity*** is a more often used term, and refers to the viscosity of a fluid relative to the viscosity of water at body temperature (37°C).
  - Water has a viscosity of 0.695 centipoise at body temperature.
  - Plasma, which has a viscosity of 1.2 CP at 37°C, thus has a relative viscosity of 1.7.
  - Blood (plasma plus cells), which has a viscosity of 2.8–3 CP at 37°C, thus has a relative viscosity of about 4–5.

Factors Affecting Blood Viscosity

1. *Shear rate or velocity gradient.* Viscosity of the blood decreases as the shear rate or velocity gradient increases and vice versa.
   - *At high shear rate,* the RBCs occupy the central axis of the tube and move with their long axis parallel to the direction of flow where the flow rate is fastest, leaving the cell-free zone of plasma at periphery. This process is called *plasma skimming* (Fig. 4.4-7A). This causes least friction between the cells and plasma and

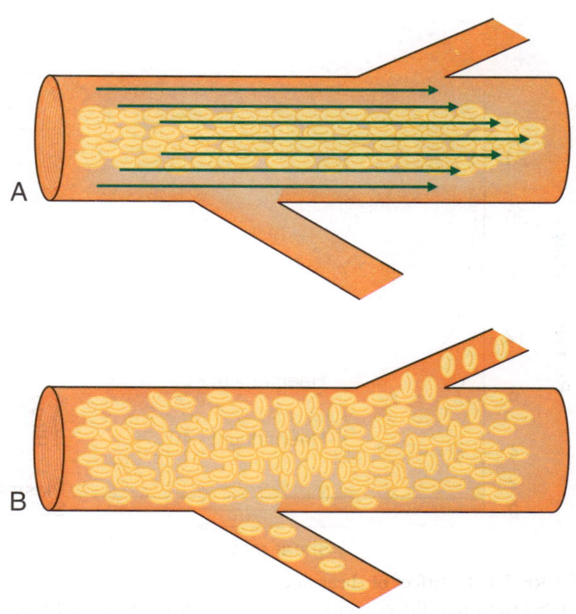

FIGURE 4.4-7 Features of streamlined flow at high flow rate (**A**) and at slow flow rate (**B**).

thus viscosity decreases. At high rates of flow, blood behaves almost like a Newtonian fluid with constant viscosity (Fig. 4.4-8).

Note. The phenomenon of plasma skimming is responsible for low value of haematocrit in capillary blood. The haematocrit of capillary blood is about 25% lower than that of venous blood.

- *When shear rate is low* (at low flow rate), tendency of RBCs to occupy central axis decreases (Fig. 4.4-7B). The suspended RBCs in plasma increase internal friction due to collision among these suspended particles. So, with slow shear rate the viscosity increases.

2. ***Haematocrit.*** In general, variation in the haematocrit is the major factor that changes the viscosity of blood. An increase in haematocrit tends to reduce flow rate because of increased viscosity. The normal haematocrit for men is 40–45%, whereas the normal value for premenopausal women is 35–40%. Viscosity of blood with a haematocrit of 40% is approximately three times that of water.
   - *In vitro,* the relative viscosity of blood increases proportionally with increase in haematocrit (above 45%).
   - *In vivo,* the effect of increased haematocrit on viscosity is affected by the diameter of the vessels as discussed:
     - In large vessels, increase in haematocrit causes appreciable increase in the viscosity. However, in small vessels (<10 µm diameter), i.e. arterioles, capillaries and venules, change in viscosity per unit change in haematocrit is much less compared with large vessels (Fig. 4.4-9). How it happens, is explained here.

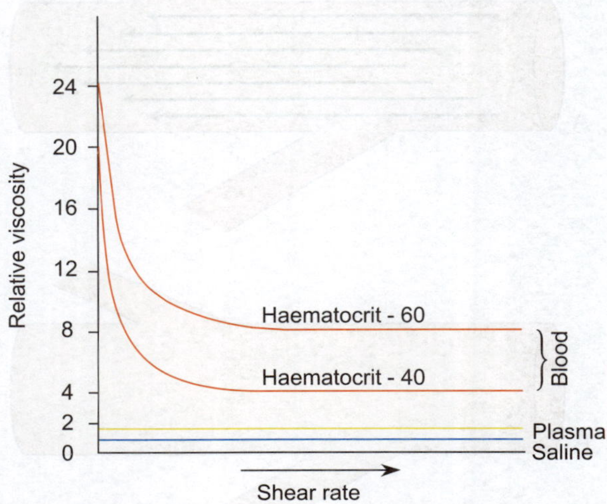

FIGURE 4.4-8 Effect of shear rate on relative viscosity of blood. Note, at higher shear rate, the viscosity of blood becomes constant and it behaves like a Newtonian fluid such as plasma or saline.

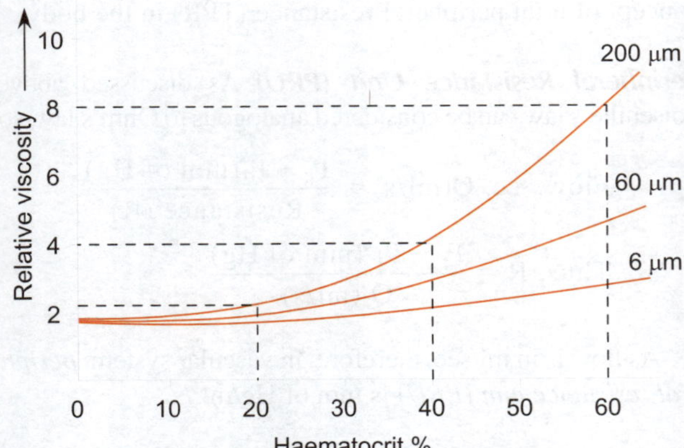

FIGURE 4.4-9 Relationship between the haematocrit and relative viscosity when blood flows through a tube of diameter 200, 60 and 6µm.

3. ***Diameter of blood vessels.*** The relationship between viscosity and diameter of the vessels is expressed as *Fahraeus–Lindquist effect* after the name of the workers. According to their experimental observations, the viscosity of blood in vessels with diameter less than 300 µm is less than the viscosity of blood in larger diameter vessels. These workers reported that in a tube of 40 µm diameter, the relative viscosity of blood was only 70% of that through a tube of 150 µm. Further, studies have also shown that in a tube of 14 µm diameter the, viscosity was only 47% of that through a tube of 150 µm.
   Explanation for Fahraeus–Lindquist effect. This effect was observed only when the experiments were performed using blood and not when studied with water and plasma. Factors responsible for this effect are:
   - The RBCs present in the blood are deformable in nature, so that apparent viscosity of blood does not change while passing through a tube of smaller diameter.
   - Due to the phenomenon of plasma skimming in large- and moderate-sized vessels, blood that enters the small vessels such as capillaries is of lesser haematocrit (25% less than the whole blood haematocrit). The width of cell-free zone at the periphery is constant whatever may be the tube diameter and correspondingly occupies a bigger proportion in narrow tubes. As a result, the total relative viscosity is less in smaller diameter vessels. Because of this effect, a satisfactory flow rate exists even in the blood vessels whose diameters are small.
   - In addition, there is a suggestion that capillary endothelial cells secrete a substance (mucopolysaccharide) which further helps to lower the viscosity of the blood in the capillaries.

   Applied aspect of Fahraeus–Lindquist effect. Because of this effect, haematocrit changes have relatively little effect on the *resistance* except when the changes are large.

4. ***Temperature.*** Cooling increases the viscosity of blood. In an intact body, though there is no variation in the body temperature normally, the cutaneous and subcutaneous vessels and even those of deeper regions in the limbs are subjected to considerable alteration of temperature due to atmospheric temperature. Thus, when the hand is kept in ice water, regional viscosity of the blood shows a threefold increase.
   Pathological conditions associated with high blood viscosity are:
   - Severe polycythaemia,
   - Abnormal shaped RBCs (congenital spherocytosis),
   - Abnormally high immunoglobulin level and
   - Lowered body temperature (in frost bite).

   To summarize. Viscosity of blood is *inversely proportional to:*
   - Flow rate (shear rate) and
   - Temperature within limit.

   Directly proportional to:
   - Haematocrit, i.e. packed cell volume (PCV),
   - Concentration of plasma proteins, especially immunoglobulins and
   - Diameter of vessel wall.

Radius of Blood Vessels and Resistance. As mentioned earlier, the rate of flow is proportional to the fourth power of the radius (r^4) of the blood vessels. Thus, even a small change in the calibre of the blood vessels will produce a marked change in blood flow. For example, at a pressure head of 100 mmHg, the change in flow rate with change in the radius is:

Radius	*Flow rate*
1 mm	1 ml/min
2 mm	16 ml/min
4 mm	256 ml/min.

Among the blood vessels, in aorta and large arteries, there is little resistance. Arterioles are the major seat of vascular resistance because of the following facts:

- These are small bored vessels (30 μm in diameter).
- Presence of large amount of smooth muscles in their wall. Thus, constriction of arterioles increases the resistance and decreases blood flow while dilation of arterioles decreases the resistance and increases the blood flow.

Control of blood flow to organs or tissues is thus regulated primarily by altering the radius of the arterioles. Because the arterioles control the flow to various vascular beds, they are considered the *stopcocks* of the circulation. In our body, arterioles are in large bulk in splanchnic region and skeletal muscles, and constitute the major site of peripheral resistance. Because of their characteristics, arterioles play an important role in the following functions:

- Control of blood flow during alteration in arterial blood pressure, i.e. autoregulation (see page 315),
- Control of blood flow following occlusive ischaemia, i.e. reactive hyperaemia (see page 315),
- Control of blood flow during exercise (see page 315) and
- Conversion of pulsatile flow from heart to a steady flow, in association with elastic vessels (see page 314).

Velocity of Blood Flow

The velocity of blood flow refers to displacement of blood per unit time, i.e. cm/s, while the rate of blood flow is the amount of blood flowing per unit time, i.e. cm^3/s. The physiologically important aspects to be considered in relation to velocity of blood flow are:

- Velocity and cross-sectional area relationship, and
- Velocity–pressure relationship.

Velocity and Cross-sectional Area Relationship

- The relationship between velocity (V), quantity of blood flow (Q) and cross-sectional area (A) of the blood vessel is:

$$V = \frac{Q}{A}$$

- Thus, if quantity of blood flow (Q) remains constant and the cross-sectional area (A) increases, then the velocity of blood flow will decrease.
- Since cross-sectional area of capillaries is 1000 times as that of aorta, the velocity of blood flow in capillaries is approximately 1 mm/s as compared to 40 cm/s in aorta.
- The total cross-sectional area of various types of blood vessels, the velocity of blood flow and pressure in the various segments of the cardiovascular system plotted as a function of the cumulative blood volume are shown in Fig. 4.4-10 and Table 4.4-1.

Thus, Fig. 4.4-10 depicts that to keep the flow rate equal, the velocity of flow must vary inversely with the cross-sectional area of each vascular segment. This is in accordance with the continuity principle, according to which in any system arranged in series, the flow through each vascular segment must be equal to the flow through every other, unless one segment becomes progressively distended.

Velocity–Pressure Relationship

To understand the effect of velocity of blood flow on pressure, it is important to understand the concept of total energy (total pressure), potential energy and kinetic energy put forward by Burton in 1965.

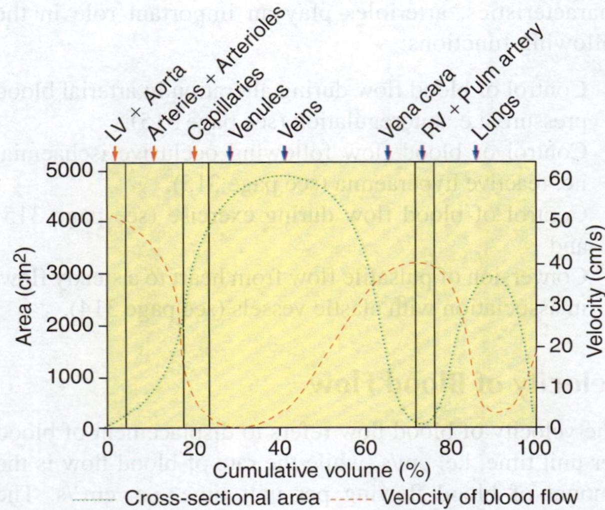

FIGURE 4.4-10 Relationship between cross-sectional area, velocity of blood flow and pressure as a function of cumulative blood volume.

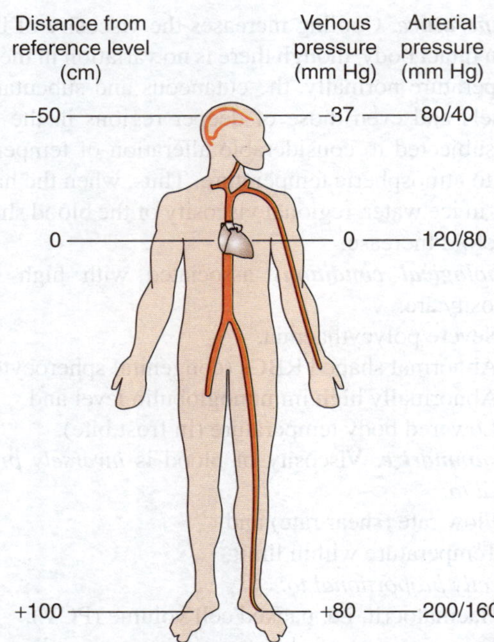

FIGURE 4.4-11 Effect of hydrostatic pressure of blood on arterial and venous pressure in an upright position.

Total energy (total pressure) of a fluid in a tube at any point equals the sum of the potential energy and kinetic energy.

Potential energy of a fluid in a tube comprises hydrostatic pressure and lateral (static) pressure.

1. Hydrostatic Pressure (Ph) results from a difference in vertical height in a fluid-filled system. Because of gravity, fluid has weight that generates force, which is proportional to its vertical height:

$$Ph = \delta \cdot h \cdot g,$$

where δ = fluid density, h = height of fluid column above or below a reference level and g = gravitational constant.

Some facts about effects of hydrostatic pressure on human vascular system are:

- The zero reference level is at the right atrium, so vascular segments higher than reference point will have negative gravity effect and vascular segments below reference point will have positive gravitational effect.
- Both arteries and veins at any given horizontal level are affected by the same hydrostatic pressure of blood so that the pressure gradient between arteries and veins is same (about 100 mmHg), i.e. it is not altered (Fig. 4.4-11).
- As shown in Fig. 4.4-11, in an upright person, assuming that foot is 100 cm below the heart, the pressure in the vessels (arteries as well as veins) of foot is 100 cm H_2O (77 mmHg) higher than the pressure at the root of aorta.
- In a supine position, the hydrostatic effect is eliminated because the entire cardiovascular system is essentially at the same horizontal level.

2. Lateral (Static) Pressure represents the pressure in the cardiovascular system that is usually measured with a strain gauge or transducer after eliminating the hydrostatic pressure effect. To eliminate hydrostatic pressure effect, it is essential to place the gauge or the sphygmomanometer cuff at the *zero reference* (phlebostatic) level, which is equivalent to the level of right atrium.

Kinetic energy is the momentum that blood gains because of its mass and velocity:

$$\text{Kinetic energy} = \frac{mV^2}{2}$$

where m = mass and V = velocity.

Thus, when velocity of flow is very low, kinetic energy is negligible.

Total energy (total pressure), as stated above according to Burton, at any point equals the sum of potential energy and the kinetic energy. Therefore, when velocity of flow is very low (i.e. with negligible kinetic energy), the magnitude of total energy (i.e. total pressure or perfusion pressure) is almost equal to the lateral pressure. However, when the velocity of flow is high, the lateral pressure exerted by the flowing fluid is much less than the total pressure exerted. This is because of the fact that at high velocity of flow some potential energy is *converted into kinetic energy.* The effect of velocity of flow on total pressure exerted is expressed mathematically by:

Bernoulli's principle which states that in a supine position (i.e. when the effect of gravity or hydrostatic pressure effect is removed), the total energy or pressure (E) of flowing blood in a vessel is:

$E = P + ½\rho V^2$, where

P = lateral pressure, ρ (Rho) = the density of blood and V = Velocity of blood in the vessel.

Experimental Demonstration of Velocity–pressure Relationship. The velocity–pressure relationship expressed above in *Bernoulli's principle* can be demonstrated experimentally by a system of pilot tubes (Fig. 4.4-12) as:

- AB is a tube through which fluid is flowing from direction A to B.
- The tube AB has central narrow segment S_2 where velocity of flow is higher. On each side of the narrow segment are wide segments S_1 and S_3, where velocity of flow is low. The length of arrows represents relative velocity of flow.
- Six tubes (a_1, a_2, a_3, b_1, b_2 and b_3) are inserted in the tube AB. Lower ends of tubes a_1, a_2 and a_3 are so constructed that they face upstream and hence record the total energy (total pressure), while tubes b_1, b_2 and b_3 record lateral pressure only.
- *In segment S_1 of the tube AB,* where velocity of the flow is low (because the diameter is big), there is little difference in the height of fluid level in a_1 (representing total energy) and b_1 (representing lateral pressure).
- *In segment S_2 of the tube AB,* where velocity of the flow is very high (due to smaller diameter), there is marked difference in the height of fluid level in a_2 (representing total energy) and b_2 (representing lateral pressure). This shows that when velocity of flow is high, potential energy is converted into kinetic energy and the potential energy (lateral pressure) becomes much less than the total pressure (potential energy plus kinetic energy).
- *In segment S_3 of the tube AB,* where velocity of the flow slows again (due to bigger diameter), part of the kinetic energy is transformed into potential energy and consequently lateral pressure is increased, and the difference between the height of fluid level in a_3 (representing total energy and b_3 (representing lateral pressure) decreases.

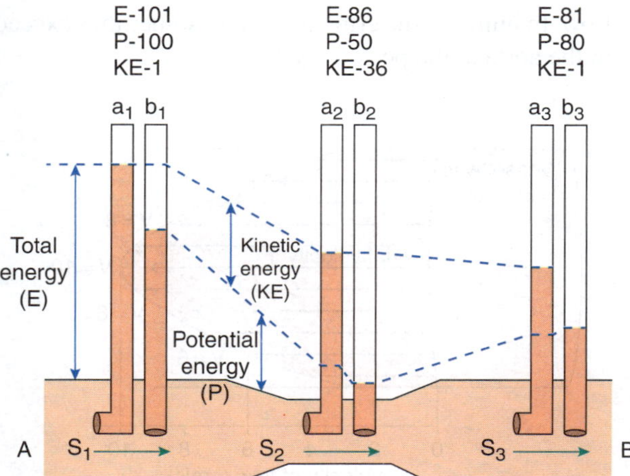

FIGURE 4.4-12 Experimental set-up demonstrating the effect of velocity on pressure and also effect of resistance on pressure (for explanation see text).

Conversion of Energy and Loss of Energy. Considering the values of total pressure (*E*), lateral pressure (*P*) and kinetic energy (KE) in tubes a_1, a_2, a_3 and b_1, b_2, b_3, the following conclusions can be drawn:

- *Energy can be converted* between potential and kinetic energy ($P \Leftrightarrow$ KE); as:
    - In segment S_1, *P* is 100 and KE is 1;
    - In segment S_2, *P* falls to 50 and KE increases to 36 and
    - In segment S_3, *P* increases to 80 and KE falls to 1.
- *Energy in a moving fluid is progressively lost* due to resistance offered by the walls of the tubes as E which in segments S_1 is 101, falls to 86 in S_2 and in S_3 is 81. Further, the energy loss (pressure drops) occurs more where the resistance is high (narrow S_2 segment).

Physiological Significance of Velocity–pressure Relationship The values of *E*, *P* and KE in Fig. 4.4-12 clearly reveal that flow is a down gradient of total energy, and not of lateral pressure. Therefore, Burton pointed out that the kinetic energy factor has to be borne in mind when pressures are measured by catheterizing blood vessels (discussed below). The relative importance of kinetic energy factor in various segments of the vascular system is:

- In the arterial system, the kinetic energy factor is negligible, except in the aorta in heavy exercise.
- In the vena cava, kinetic energy is important only during exercise.
- In the atria and pulmonary artery, kinetic energy is not inconsiderable at rest and is very important when the cardiac output is increased.
- It has been calculated (Burton, 1965) that the kinetic energy factor is 50–55% of the total energy in the vena cavae, atria and pulmonary artery.
- Thus, in the circulation at rest, the kinetic energy factor is of little importance on the systemic arterial side and of only moderate significance in the systemic veins. Flow, therefore can be regarded as occurring between the root of aorta and the right atrium by virtue of a pressure gradient ($P_1 - P_2$).

Significance of Kinetic Energy Factor While Measuring Pressure by Catheterizing Blood Vessels

- When measuring pressure, unless the top of the catheter has its opening at right angles to the stream (Fig. 4.4-13A) (measuring 'side pressure'), the pressure recorded is not accurate at that point. If the catheter faces the oncoming bloodstream or if an end cannula is tied into the artery, the flow of blood is prevented and the manometer registers a pressure higher than that by the factor $\frac{1}{2}\rho V^2$ (Fig. 4.4-13B).

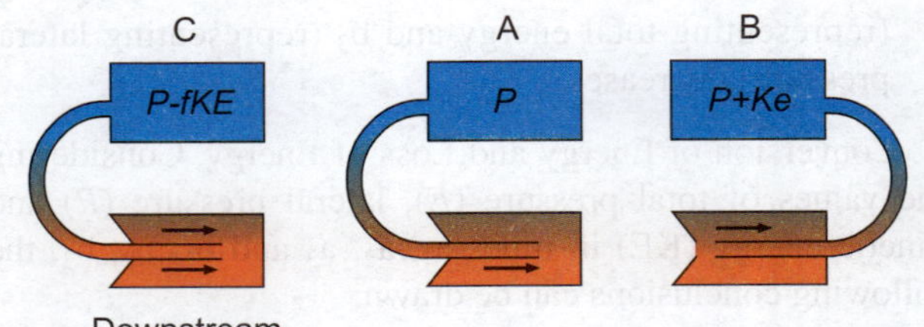

FIGURE 4.4-13 Experimental set-up demonstrating significance of kinetic energy factor while measuring pressure by catheterizing a blood vessel.

- If the catheter opening faces downstream (Fig. 4.4-13C), the pressure recorded is lower than the pressure in the fluid by slightly less by the factor $\frac{1}{2}\rho V^2$ (flow is distorted by streaming round the catheter tip and this reduces the correction required). Such a catheter placement is the accepted technique for recording of pulmonary arterial pressure.

Circulation Time

Circulation time refers to the time taken by the particles in blood in reaching from one point to another. It measures average linear velocity of blood. Calculation of circulation time in different regions of the body has clinical importance in circulation disorders of that particular region. The circulation time between two points can be estimated by injecting a substance into one segment of the circulation and of noting the time lapse when it can be detected at another point. Example of estimation of circulation time in certain regions is:

- ***Arm to retina circulation time*** is estimated by injecting fluorescein dye in the vein of arm and detecting its appearance with the fundus camera on retina (procedure is called fundus fluorescein angiography).
- ***Arm to tongue circulation time*** can be estimated by injection of bile salts in the vein of arm and appearance of bitter taste of bile salts. Average normal arm to tongue circulation time is 15 s.
- ***Arm to face circulation time*** is estimated by injecting histamine in the arm vein and noting the time taken for causing flushing of face. Average arm to face time is 24 s.
- ***Arm to lung circulation time*** can be estimated by noting the interval between the injection of a bolus of ether into the vein of arm and the appearance of coughing produced by its arrival in the lungs. Average arm to lung time is 6 s.
- ***Foot to foot circulation time.*** A dye injected into the vein of a foot reaches the other foot after circulation through the heart within 80 s. It indicates total circulation time.
- ***Factors affecting circulation time*** are:
  - Increased cardiac output,
  - Exercise,
  - Excitement,
  - Adrenaline and
  - Basal metabolic rate.

Blood Flow: Types, Measurement and Distribution

Types of Blood Flow

Blood flow in the vascular system is of two types:

- Laminar blood flow and
- Turbulent blood flow.

Laminar Blood Flow Blood flow in the blood vessels is normally in streamline, like the flow of liquids in narrow rigid tubes. Such a blood flow is called laminar blood flow and is considered to consist of a series of thin laminae slipping over one another.

- The outermost lamina, i.e. an infinitely thin layer of blood in contact with the wall of the blood vessel, does not move and the next lamina has some velocity. The subsequent inner layers have progressively increasing velocity, and thus the innermost lamina, i.e. the core of the bloodstream, has the maximum velocity (Fig. 4.4-14).
- The laminar blood flow being streamlined is noiseless and within physiological limits shows a linear relationship with pressure.

Turbulent Blood Flow The above-described laminar blood flow occurs up to a certain velocity, at or above which the blood flow becomes turbulent. The velocity of flow at which blood flow becomes turbulent is called critical velocity.

- In turbulent blood flow, the blood moves in irregular varying paths continuously mixing within the vessel and colliding with the vessel wall. This causes a greater energy loss compared with laminar flow.
- Turbulent blood flow is noisy and does not show a typical linear relationship with the pressure.
- Normally, none of the small vessels show turbulent flow. In humans, the critical velocity sometimes exceeds in the aorta at the peak of systole.

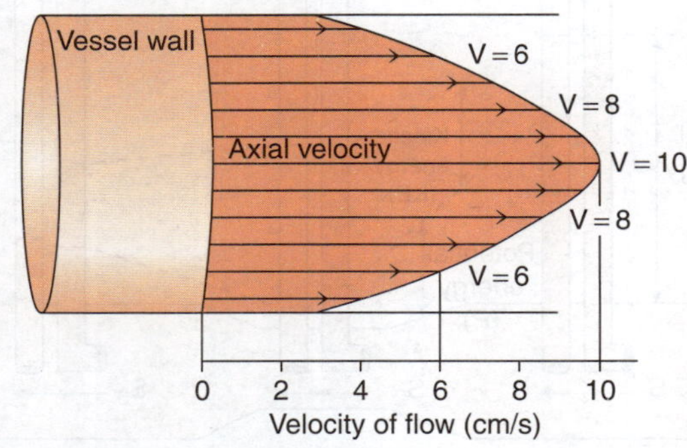

FIGURE 4.4-14 Laminar blood flow showing different velocities of the different laminae resulting in parabolic distribution of velocities. Note the central core of bloodstream has greatest velocity.

Probability of Turbulence. The chances of blood flow becoming turbulent are determined by the *probability of turbulence,* which is denoted as Re (Reynolds number), named for the man who described it. According to Reynold, the probability of turbulence (Re) is:

- Directly proportional to the:
  - Density of blood (ρ) equal to 1,
  - Diameter of the vessel (D) in cm,
  - Velocity of blood flow (V) in cm/s and is
- Indirectly proportional to:
  - Viscosity of the blood (η) in poises.

$$\text{thus Re} = \frac{\rho DV}{\eta}$$

- Blood flow is usually not turbulent when *Re* is less than 2000.
- Chances of blood flow becoming turbulent are increased when Re exceeds 2000.

  When *Re* is more than 3000, turbulence is almost always present.

Conditions Associated with Turbulent Blood Flow

- ***Constriction of the artery*** by an atherosclerotic plaque (Fig. 4.4-15) or by any other cause, e.g. application of external pressure while measuring the blood pressure with sphygmomanometer, is associated with a blood flow velocity which exceeds critical velocity and thus causes the turbulent blood flow. The turbulent flow generates vibrations (sounds) which can be heard over the artery by a stethoscope, e.g. *Korotkoff sounds* heard while recording the blood pressure or the *murmur* heard over a constricted artery.
- ***Anaemia*** is frequently associated with turbulence, because of *lowered blood viscosity.* This may be the explanation of the systolic murmurs that are common in anaemia.
- ***Large diameter vessels,*** e.g. ascending aorta, as mentioned above, may have turbulent flow at the peak of systolic ejection which may cause *ejection systolic murmur.*

Measurement of Blood Flow

Following methods are known for measurement of blood flow in various parts of the body:

1. Methods Based on Fick's Principle Methods based on Fick's principle can be used to measure blood flow through some of the organs like the lungs, the heart and the brain. The methods are similar to those described for measurement of cardiac output (page 285).

2. Para-Amino-Hippuric (PAH) Acid Clearance Method Para-amino-hippuric acid clearance method is used to determine the renal blood flow and thus study the renal physiology (see page 553).

3. Venous Occlusion Plethysmography Venous occlusion plethysmography is a simple but crude method of measuring blood flow through the limbs.

Principle. It is based on the principle that if venous return of a region (part) is suddenly obstructed, that part increases in size due to arterial flow. The increase in size is equivalent to the blood flow to that part.

Procedure. To measure blood flow through a limb (say a forearm), the part is enclosed in a watertight chamber (plethysmograph) connected to a volume recorder. The venous drainage from the limb is occluded for a few seconds by inflating the sphygmomanometer cuff to 60 mmHg. The increase in the size of the arm will displace the water in the plethysmograph, which will be recorded with a volume recorder (Fig. 4.4-16). The displacement is equal to the blood flow to the part during that period.

4. Electromagnetic Flowmeter The electromagnetic flowmeter is based on the principle that when a vessel containing blood (a conductor) is placed between the two poles of a magnet, voltage is generated in the blood flowing through the magnetic field. The magnitude of the voltage is proportionate to the volume of flow and can be measured with an appropriately placed electrode on the surface of the vessel (Fig. 4.4-17).

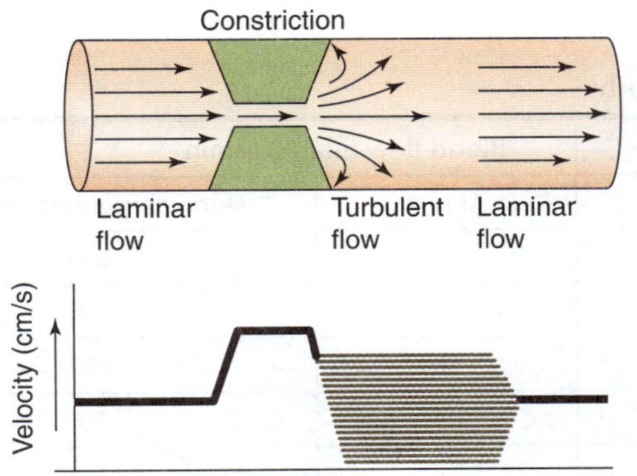

FIGURE 4.4-15 Turbulent blood flow caused by constriction of the lumen of blood vessel.

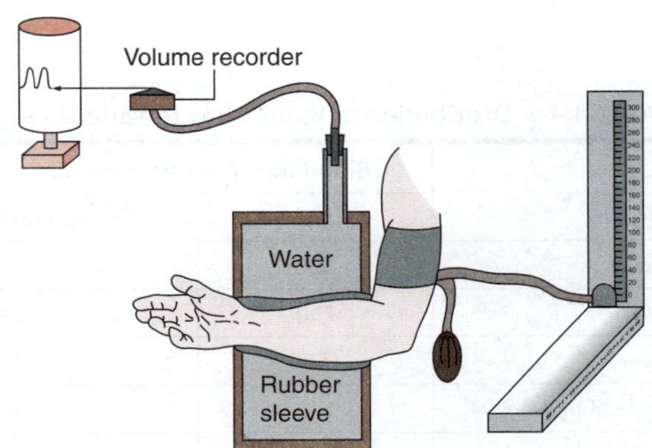

FIGURE 4.4-16 Plethysmography showing measurement of blood flow in forearm.

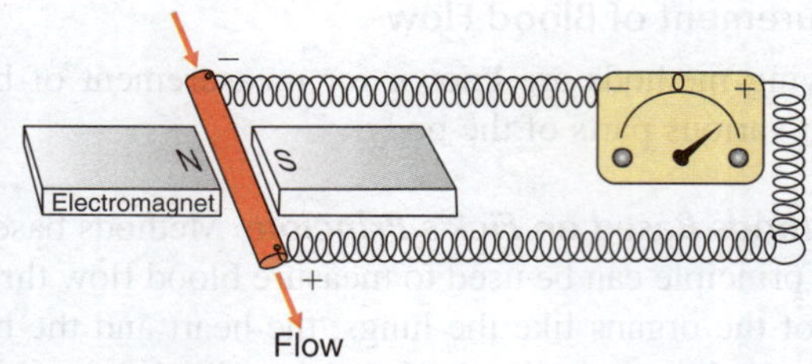

FIGURE 4.4-17 Principle of electromagnetic flowmeter.

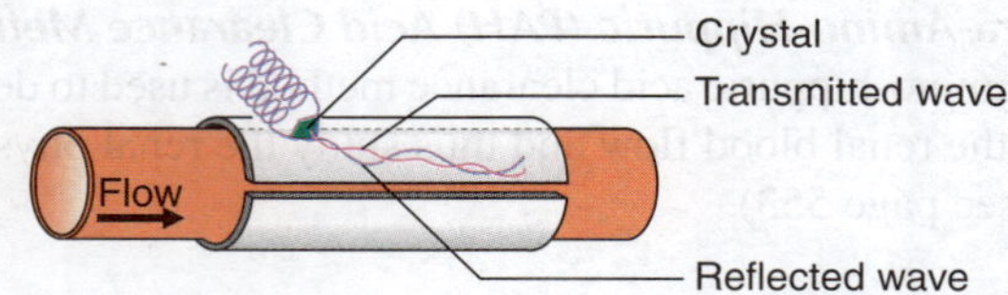

FIGURE 4.4-18 Principle of ultrasonic flowmeter.

5. Doppler Flowmeter (Ultrasonic Flowmeter) Ultrasonic flowmeter is based on the principle of Doppler effect. In this instrument, ultrasonic waves are sent into a vessel diagonally from one crystal, and the waves reflected from the red and white blood cells are picked up by a second downstream crystal (Fig. 4.4-18). The frequency of the reflected waves is higher by an amount that is proportionate to the rate of flow toward the second crystal because of the Doppler effect.

Distribution of Blood Flow to Various Regions of the Body

At rest, about 5 L of blood enters aorta per minute. In terms of tissue weight, blood flow to liver, brain and heart is very high. Kidney has high blood flow because it is related to excretory function rather than metabolic requirement. The distribution of blood flow to various organs and regions of the body during resting conditions and during maximum activity conditions is shown in Table 4.4-2.

- At rest, at least 50% of the circulating blood volume is in the systemic veins, 12% is in the heart cavities, and 18% in the lower pressure pulmonary circulation; only 2% is in the aorta, 8% in the arteries, 1% in the arterioles and 5% in the capillaries.
- When extra blood is administered by transfusion, less than 1% of it is distributed in the arterial system (the high pressure system) and all the rest in the systemic veins, pulmonary circulation and heart chambers other than the left ventricle (the 'low-pressure system').

PRESSURE AND FLOW IN VARIOUS FUNCTIONAL SEGMENTS OF SYSTEMIC VASCULAR TREE

Pressure and velocity of flow of blood in the various parts of systemic circulation along with the pulmonary circulation summarized in Table 4.4-1 and Fig. 4.4-19 show that:

- ***Pressure*** in the left ventricle, aorta and large arteries is *pulsatile* (i.e. rises to a peak value during systole and decreases to minimum during diastole) and becomes continuous in the capillaries. Based on the pressure changes, the whole of the vascular system is broadly divided into:
  - *High-pressure system* which includes left ventricle, arteries and arterioles. This system controls the blood pressure and blood flow in the body.
  - *Low-pressure system* includes capillaries, venules, veins, right atrium, pulmonary vessels and left atrium. The low-pressure system is responsible for the control of blood volume and venous return.
- ***Velocity*** of blood flow in proximal part of aorta averages 40 cm/s. However, the flow in aorta is phasic, and velocity ranges from 120 cm/s during systole to even a negative value at the time of transient backflow before the aortic valve closes in diastole.
- ***Total cross-sectional area (TA)*** of the vessels increases from 4.5 cm^2 in the aorta to 4500 cm^2 in the capillaries.
- ***Relative resistance (RR)*** is highest in the arterioles. As mentioned in the beginning of chapter, from functional

TABLE 4.4-2 Distribution of Blood Flow to Various Organs of the Body

Organs	Blood flow per organ ml/min		Blood flow ml/100 g/min	
	At rest	*During maximum activity*	*At rest*	*During maximum activity*
Heart	250	1200	80	400
Brain	750	2100	55	150
Liver	1500	3000	58	120
Skeletal muscles	150	1800	04	70
Kidney	1200	1400	400	450
Skin	200	3500	08	150

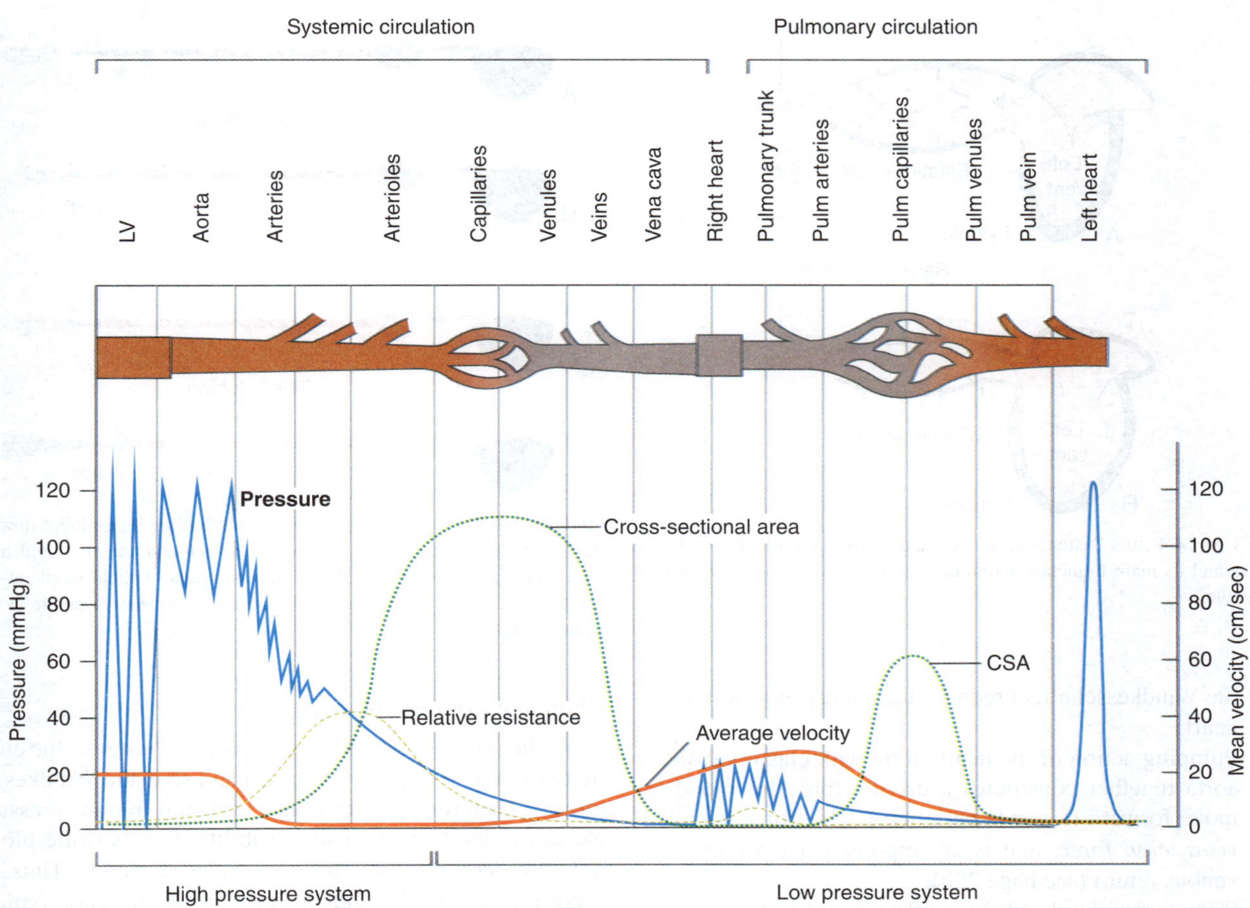

FIGURE 4.4-19 Diagram showing pressure changes, velocity of blood flow through systemic circulation, total cross-sectional area of the blood vessels and relative resistance in the vessels (which is highest in the arterioles).

point of view, the systemic vascular tree has been divided into various functional segments. Pressure and flow functions of the following functional segments of systemic vascular tree are:

- Elastic arteries,
- Muscular arteries,
- Arterioles,
- Microcirculation,
- Venous circulation and
- Lymphatic circulation.

Pressure and Flow Functions of Elastic Arteries

The large elastic arteries (Windkessel vessels) include aorta and its main branches such as carotid, iliac and axillary arteries. These vessels contain elastic tissue in their walls in abundance which provides them two properties of distensibility and elastic recoil. The effect of these two properties of the elastic arteries on pressure and flow of blood is distensibility and elastic recoil.

Distensibility

As we know, the heart acts as a pump and ejects about 70 ml of blood into the aorta with each systole. The distensibility (compliance) of the elastic arteries allows them to accommodate the stroke volume of heart with only a moderate increase in pressure (from 80 to 120 mmHg) (Fig. 4.4-20A). Due to distension of these vessels, a part of energy released from the heart is stored as potential energy in the wall of aorta.

Elastic Recoil

During diastole, the stretched elastic wall of the aorta recoils and the potential energy stored in the wall is released onto the blood. This causes the blood to flow during diastole also; in this way, the pressure in the aorta does not fall below 80 mmHg (Fig. 4.4-20B). In other words, the elastic recoil of big arteries acts as a subsidiary pump for a continuous blood flow. This recoil effect is called Windkessel *effect.* Windkessel is a German word meaning elastic reservoir.

Functions of Elastic Vessels

1. They reduce velocity of blood flow to some extent during ventricular contraction (systole) due to property of distensibility.
2. They cause increase in velocity of blood flow to some extent during ventricular diastole by elastic recoil. Thus,

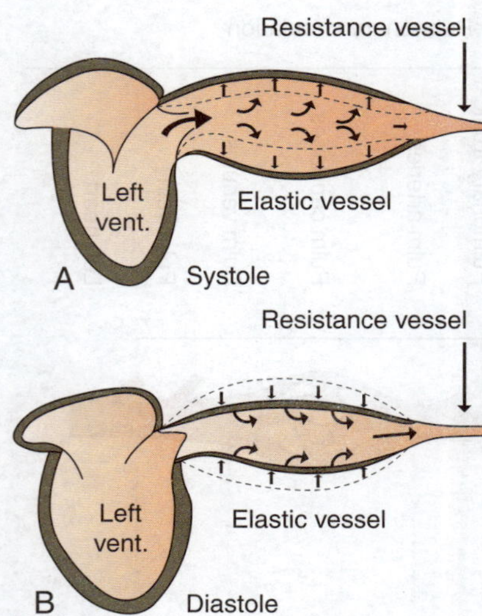

FIGURE 4.4-20 Distensibility **(A)** and elastic recoil **(B)** seen in aorta and its main branches maintain arterial pressure and flow during diastole.

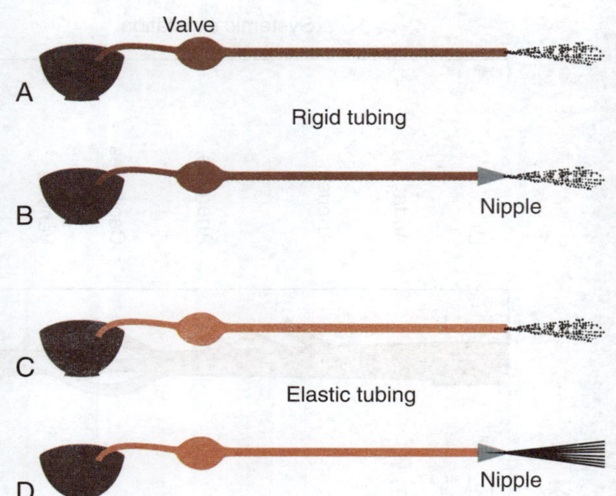

FIGURE 4.4-21 The Borelli's experiment showing intermittent flow of fluid in a rigid tube without nipple at the open end **(A)**,in a rigid tube with nipple at the open end **(B)**, in an elastic tube without nipple at the open end **(C)** and continuous flow in an elastic tube with nipple at the openend **(D)**.

the Windkessel effect reduces the energy expenditure of heart.

3. Pumping action of the heart along with elastic recoil of aorta together constitutes a driving force for blood to move forward (towards periphery). This force is called *vis-a-tergo force,* and is an important determinant for venous return (see page 288).
4. Conversion of pulsatile blood flow from heart to a steady continuous flow. Since the heart contracts intermittently, therefore, the pressure and flow from the heart into large arteries is pulsatile. The elastic vessels act together with arterioles (resistance vessels) to convert this pulsatile flow into a steady continuous flow in the tissue capillaries, which allows maximum exchange between the blood and tissues. This role of elastic vessels and the arterioles can be explained by a simple experiment performed by Borelli.

Borelli's Experiment. In this experiment, one end of a rubber bulb having a one-way valve is dipped into a beaker of pure water and its other end is attached to a tube (Fig. 4.4-21). When the bulb is squeezed repeatedly, the water flow in different situations is as follows:

- ***Intermittent flow*** is seen when the tube is rigid whether without (Fig. 4.4.21A) or with (Fig. 4.4-21B) a narrow nipple attached to the outlet (open end), and also when the tube is elastic but without a narrow nipple attached (Fig. 4.4-21C).
- ***Continuous flow*** is, however, seen when a narrow nipple is attached to the outlet of an elastic tube (Fig. 4.4-21D). This set-up can be compared to combined effect of the aorta (elastic tubes and arterioles (narrow nipples producing resistance) which produce a continuous and streamlined flow of blood.

Clinically Applied Aspects

1. Due to Age-Related Degenerative Changes, the elasticity of large vessels is decreased and so is the Windkessel effect. Therefore, in old age, systolic blood pressure increases due to loss of distensibility and diastolic blood pressure decreases (due to loss of elastic recoil). Thus, in a normal healthy individual aged about 70 years, typical blood pressure is 160/70 mmHg. That is, there occurs *systolic hypertension* with *increased pulse pressure* (SBP – DBP).

2. Atherosclerotic Changes in Small Blood Vessels are also common in old age. These produce *essential hypertension, i.e.* an increase in systolic as well as diastolic blood pressure.

Pressure and Flow Functions of Muscular Arteries

The muscular arteries comprise most of the named arteries in the body such as radial artery, facial artery, ophthalmic artery and so on. These arteries serve as the *distributing channels* to the organs. Their relatively large lumen minimizes the pressure drop that occurs as a result of resistance.

Pressure and Flow Functions of Arterioles

Structural Characteristics

Each arteriole is only a few millimetre long and branches many a times to supply about 10–100 capillaries. The characteristic features of arterioles are:

- A thick muscular wall having profuse vasomotor (sympathetic) innervation; and

- A relatively narrow lumen (30 μm), because of which these vessels are considered the major site of peripheral resistance. The arterial pressure drops by about 50 mmHg while passing through few millimetre long arterioles (Fig. 4.4-19).

Functions of Arterioles

1. Control of Blood Flow to the Organs The arterioles play a major role in the control of blood flow to organs or tissues. So, they are considered *stopcocks (valves) of circulation.* The constriction of arterioles increases the resistance and decreases the blood flow while dilation of arterioles decreases the resistance and increases the blood flow. Thus, blood flow is primarily regulated by altering the radius of arterioles, since according to Poiseuille's law rate of flow, it is proportional to the fourth power of the radius, i.e. r^4 (see page 302). The arterioles control blood flow to organs by the following two mechanisms:

Control of Blood Flow during Alterations in Blood Pressure (Autoregulation)

Autoregulation. It is the ability of an organ or tissue to adjust its vascular resistance and maintain a relatively constant blood flow over a wide range of arterial pressure (Fig. 4.4-22). This is accomplished by a change in the resistance (due to change in lumen as above) proportionate to change in the arterial pressure. Autoregulation is well developed in the kidney, brain, heart, skeletal muscle and mesentery. Two theories have been put forward to explain the phenomenon of autoregulation.

- ***Metabolic theory*** proposed that an increased arterial blood pressure initially increases blood flow to a tissue or organ. This increased blood flow washes out the vasodilator substances such as CO_2, H^+, nitric oxide, adenosine, prostaglandins, K^+, phosphate ions and low oxygen levels in the area. As a result, the arterioles constrict, vascular resistance increases and blood flow returns to normal. However, it has been reported that changes in the concentration of any of the above-mentioned substances cannot explain autoregulation.
- ***Myogenic theory.*** According to this theory, the vascular smooth muscle (VSM) responds to wall tension, which is a function of pressure and wall radius according to the law of Laplace (see page 304). An increase in arterial pressure initially stretches the smooth muscle fibres, in response to which the VSM contracts and returns the wall tension to control levels that can only be achieved with vessels of smaller radius. The narrowed lumen increases the resistance and compensates for the higher arterial pressure, returning the blood flow to control levels.

Control of Blood Flow after Occlusive Ischaemia (Reactive Hyperaemia). Reactive hyperaemia is a phenomenon by which the vessels control blood flow to the organ after a period of ischaemia following occlusion of the artery to an organ or tissue. Due to this phenomenon, the blood flow exceeds the control level when the occlusion is resolved. The magnitude and duration of reactive hyperaemia depends on the duration of occlusion (Fig. 4.4-23). It has been proposed that reactive hyperaemia occurs due to a metabolic mechanism that controls blood flow to tissues.

Control of Blood Flow during Exercise. The arteriolar smooth muscles respond not only to sympathetic discharge, but also to products of local metabolism. So, by these two mechanisms, regional blood flow is controlled in such a way that it is almost exactly proportional to the metabolic requirements of the tissues. For example, during muscular exercise, strong sympathetic discharge causes constriction of arterioles of the splanchnic region (where blood is not immediately required). Also, in the skeletal muscles, metabolites like CO_2, H^+, lactic acid, etc. cause marked arteriolar dilation and consequently blood flow is diverted from the splanchnic region to the skeletal muscles and heart to meet the elevated demand due to metabolic activity.

2. Conversion of Pulsatile Flow from Heart to a Steady Continuous Flow As described in function of the elastic vessels, the arterioles along with the elastic vessels convert the pulsatile flow in the arteries to a steady flow in capillaries. For explanation, see Borelli's experiment (see page 324).

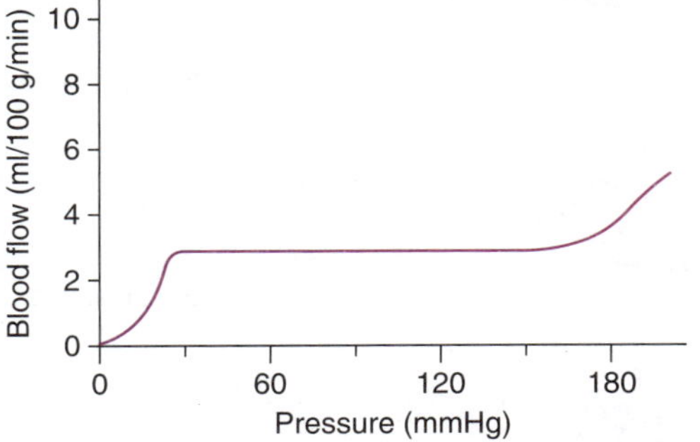

FIGURE 4.4-22 Autoregulation of blood flow. Note the blood flow remains relatively constant over a wide range of arterial pressure. This is accomplished by change in resistance proportionate to change in arterial pressure.

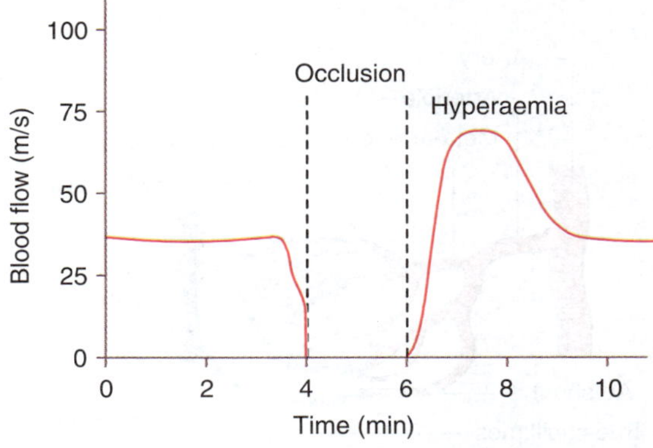

FIGURE 4.4-23 Phenomenon of reactive hyperaemia, which increases blood flow after a period of ischaemia.

Microcirculation

Architecture of Microcirculation

The microcirculation involves a meshwork of vessels less than 100 μm in diameter. These include small arterioles, meta-arterioles, capillaries, postcapillary venules and arteriovenous shunts (Fig. 4.4-24):

- ***Meta-arterioles.*** The arterioles divide into smaller muscle walled vessels, sometimes called meta-arterioles and these in turn feed into capillaries.
- ***Precapillary sphincters*** refer to a cuff of smooth muscle cells that surround the origin of capillaries. These determine the size of capillary exchange area at one particular moment in the tissue. For example, increase in the sphincter patency increases number of open capillaries. It is unsettled whether the meta-arterioles are innervated, and it appears that the precapillary sphincters are not. However, they can of course respond to local or circulating vasoconstrictor substances.
- ***Capillaries*** arise directly from arterioles or meta-arterioles. These vessels allow easy exchange of gases and nutritive substances across them and so are also called as *exchange vessels*. Capillaries constitute the most important segment of the circulatory system. Their structure and functions will be discussed in detail.
- ***Postcapillary venules,*** which measure 20-60 μm in diameter, are the *most permeable part* of the microcirculation.
- ***Arteriovenous anastomosis (shunt or thoroughfare vessels).*** These are short, low-resistance connections between the arterioles and veins, bypassing the capillaries. These are abundantly innervated by vasomotor sympathetic fibres. These vessels are especially found in the skin of fingers, toes and earlobes, where they are involved in the regulation of body temperature.

Structural Characteristics of Capillaries

Each capillary has an average diameter of 5 μm, length of 50 μm, wall thickness of 1 μm and cross-sectional area of 40 μm^2.

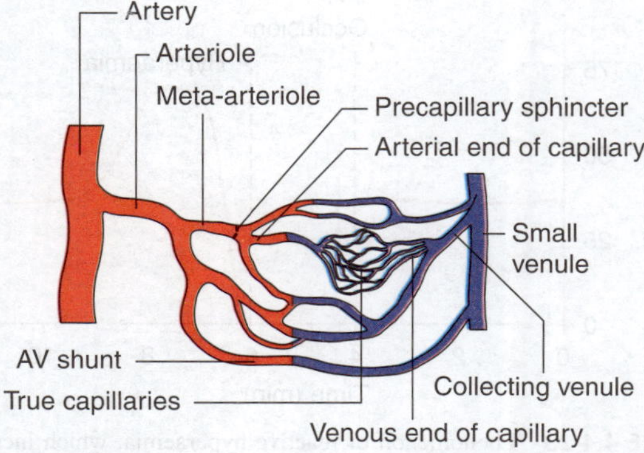

FIGURE 4.4-24 Architecture of microcirculation.

The capillary wall essentially consists of a single layer of endothelial cells which are lined on the outside by a basal lamina (glycoprotein); overlying the basal lamina there may be isolated branching perivascular cells called *pericytes*.

The endothelial structure of capillaries varies in different organs depending on the function of the particular tissue. Under electron microscope, three types of capillaries have been identified: continuous or nonfenestrated capillaries, fenestrated capillaries and discontinuous capillaries or sinusoids.

1. Continuous Capillaries are characterized by a single layer of endothelial cells which are almost continuous, except for small clefts of 6–7 nm in size in between the cells. It is believed that most of water-soluble ions (Fig. 4.4.25A) and molecules pass across the capillary through these clefts (or *slit pores*). These are the most common type of capillaries and are found in most of the body tissues viz. skeletal muscle, adipose tissue, connective tissue, pulmonary circulation and so on.

The junction between endothelial cells of capillaries of the brain and retina are tight and possess a complete basement membrane that retards or prevents the transfer of many substances and constitutes the so-called *blood–brain barrier and blood–retinal barrier,* respectively.

2. Fenestrated Capillaries consist of thin endothelial cells with large fenestrations (20–100 nm in diameter) in between which are bridged by a thin basement membrane which surrounds the endothelial cells (Fig. 4.4-25B). The fenestrations permit the passage of relatively large molecules and make the capillaries porous. Fenestrated capillaries are found in organs where transport of fluid is paramount, e.g. renal glomeruli, intestinal villi, most endocrinal glands, ciliary processes in the eye, choroid plexus and so on.

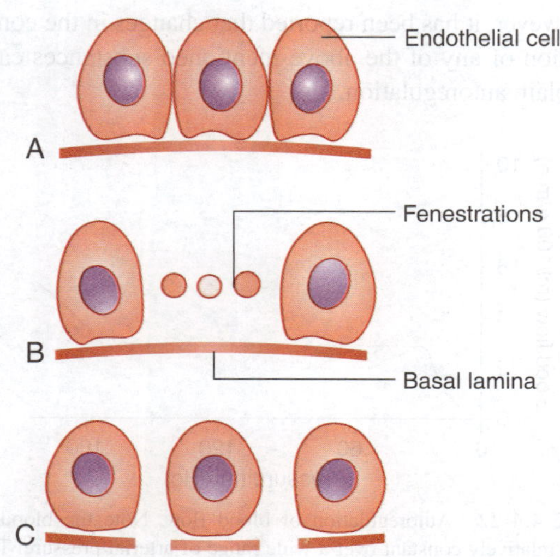

FIGURE 4.4-25 Structure of different types of capillaries: **A,** continuous; **B,** fenestrated; and **C,** discontinuous.

3. Discontinuous Capillaries are characterized by large gaps (600–3000 nm in diameter) between endothelial cells that are not closed by basement membrane (Fig. 4.4-25C). Through these gaps, even formed elements of blood can pass freely. Such capillaries are also called sinusoids and are found in bone marrow, liver and spleen.

Functional Characteristics of Capillaries

The primary function of circulation is to transport nutrients to the tissues and remove waste products—occurs in the capillaries. About 10 billion capillaries, which have a total surface area of 500–700 m^2, provide this function for the body. The cross-sectional area of capillary bed when fully patent is 2800 times that of aorta.

Active and Inactive Capillaries

- ***In Resting Tissues,*** most of the capillaries (75%) are collapsed (inactive capillaries) and blood bypasses them to flow through the *thoroughfare vessels* connecting arterioles to the venules.
- ***In Active Tissues,*** the meta-arterioles and the precapillary sphincters dilate. The intracapillary pressure rises, overcoming the critical closing pressure and blood flows through all the capillaries (active capillaries).

The opening and closing of the precapillary sphincters is controlled mostly by the local metabolic vasodilators and possibly also through sympathetic innervation.

Capillary Pressure and Flow

Capillary Pressure varies considerably; therefore, it is difficult to describe a generalized picture of capillary pressure and flow. However, typical values in human nail bed capillaries are 35 mmHg at the arteriolar end and 15 mmHg at the venous end, and thus vary over the length of capillary (average being 25 mmHg). The pulse pressure is approximately 5 mmHg at the arteriolar end and 0 at the venous end. Average capillary pressure is less than 10 mmHg in pulmonary capillaries and hepatic sinusoids.

Blood Flow Velocity. The capillaries are short, but blood moves slowly (average velocity being 0.3–0.4 mm/s) because of a large cross-sectional area. The velocity varies widely—within short periods of time; it can range from 0–1 mm/s within the same capillary. The transit time of blood between the arteriolar end to the venular end of an average-sized capillary is 1–2 s.

Blood Flows into the capillaries intermittently because of the phenomenon of vasomotion, i.e. intermittent contraction of meta-arterioles and precapillary sphincters. This in turn is mainly controlled by concentration of oxygen and waste products of tissue metabolism.

Transcapillary Exchange

The capillary blood brings oxygen, electrolytes and nutrients to the tissues and removes the waste products of cellular metabolism. The exchange of these substances occurs across the thin membrane formed by the endothelial cells. Before discussing the chief mechanism of transcapillary exchange, it will be worthwhile to know about interstitium and interstitial fluid.

Interstitium and Interstitial Fluid

Spaces between the cells in the body are collectively known as *interstitium,* which constitutes about one-sixth of the body. The fluid present in the interstitium is called *interstitial fluid.* The interstitium also contains two major types of solid structures: collagen fibre bundles and proteoglycan filaments. *Collagen fibres* are strong and therefore they provide most of the tensional strength to the tissues. *Proteoglycan filaments* consist of 98% hyaluronic acid and 2% protein, and form fine reticular filaments described as *brush file.* Most of the interstitial fluid is entrapped in the proteoglycan filaments and the two combinedly constitute the *tissue gel.* Rest of the interstitial fluid (<1%) forms the *free fluid.* Free fluid and gel are continuously interchanging with each other. Fluid can pass through the tissue gel very slowly but diffusion can occur through it as rapidly as in free fluid. Gases, nutrients and cellular waste products diffuse through the tissue gel very freely. *Oedema* results due to increased free fluid in the tissues.

Mechanisms of Transcapillary Exchange Exchange of substances occurs primarily in the capillaries and postcapillary venules. The major mechanisms of exchange are diffusion and filtration (bulk flow). Some substances also pass through the cells by *vesicular transport*.

Diffusion across Microvascular Endothelium. Diffusion is the principal mechanism of microvascular exchange of materials between the plasma and the interstitial fluid against their concentration gradient.

- ***Lipid-soluble substances*** like O_2 and CO_2 diffuse most freely across the cell membrane.
- ***Water and water-soluble micromolecules*** (molecular weight less than 69,000) like Na^+, Cl^-, K^+, glucose, urea, etc. diffuse almost freely through the intercellular clefts and intracellular pores in the capillary membrane.
- ***Large molecules*** (molecular weight more than 69,000) such as albumin and other plasma proteins cannot cross the endothelial barrier. However, some amount of albumin does enter the interstitial fluid.

Factors Affecting Rate of Diffusion across the capillary wall thus are pore size of the capillary, molecular size of the diffusing substance and the concentration difference of the substances between two sides of the membrane.

For details about the 'diffusion', see page 23.

Filtration and Reabsorption across Microvascular Endothelium. The backflow or ultrafiltration of protein free plasma determines the distribution of fluid across the capillaries. The rate of filtration and absorption at any point along the capillary wall depends on the balance of forces known as *Starling forces.* According to Starling's hypothesis, the filtration absorption is expressed as:

$$K(Pc + \pi i) - (Pi + \pi c)$$

K = the permeability-surface area coefficient
Pc = the hydrostatic capillary pressure,
Pi = the hydrostatic interstitial pressure,
πc = oncotic pressure of blood and
πi = oncotic pressure of the interstitium.
Thus, Pc − Pi, represents the hydrostatic pressure gradient, and $\pi c - \pi i$ represents the oncotic pressure gradient. *Starling forces* are defined:

1. **Hydrostatic capillary pressure (Pc)** tends to force the fluid out through the capillary membrane. The values of hydrostatic capillary pressure in most of the tissues are:

- At the arterial end = 30–40 mmHg,
- At the venous end = 10–15 mmHg and
- In the middle = 25 mmHg.

It is important to note that in the kidneys, the glomerular capillary pressure is 50–60 mmHg (see page 492). The hydrostatic capillary pressure depends on:

- The arterial blood pressure,
- Pre- and postcapillary resistance and
- Venous pressure (most important).

2. **Hydrostatic interstitial pressure (Pi)** tends to force fluid inward through the capillary membrane. It is about −2 mmHg in subcutaneous tissue but is positive in the liver and kidneys, and as high as +6 mmHg in the brain.

3. **Oncotic pressure of blood or plasma colloid osmotic pressure (πc)** results from the osmotic pressure of plasma proteins. It tends to pull fluid inward through the capillary membrane. It is about 25–27 mmHg.

4. **Oncotic pressure of the interstitium (πi)** is due to the presence of proteins in the interstitial space. It tends to pull fluid out of the capillary membrane. The effective oncotic pressure in the interstitium is estimated to range between 5 and 10 mmHg (average 8 mmHg).

Calculation of Net Filtration at the Capillaries From the above description, the net forces acting on the fluid at the arteriolar and venous end of a typical muscle *capillary* can be calculated (Table 4.4-3):

- Thus, at arteriolar end, the filtering force of 15 mmHg moves the fluid out of capillary (filtration) into the interstitium, while at venous end the filtering force of −10 mmHg moves the fluid into the capillary (reabsorption) from the interstitium.
- The net filtering force for the whole capillary is 5 mmHg.

In the example given above, we have studied the balance of Starling forces at the arteriolar and venous end of the capillary only. However, over the length of the capillary, the hydrostatic pressure gradually declines to zero near the middle of capillary. From here, the inward forces become dominant and reabsorption process starts to reach its maximum at the venular end (Fig. 4.4-26).

TABLE 4.4-3 Calculation of Net Filtration Force at the Capillaries

	At the arteriolar end (mmHg)	At the venous end (mmHg)
• **Forces tending to move fluid outward**		
• Capillary hydrostatic pressure (P_c)	35	10
• Interstitial oncotic pressure (π_i)	3	3
Total outward force ($P_c+\pi_i$)	**38**	**13**
• **Forces tending to move fluid inward**		
• Oncotic pressure of blood (π_c)	25	25
• Interstitial hydrostatic pressure (P_i)	−2	−2
Total inward force ($\pi_c + P_i$)	**23**	**23**
• **Filtering force**	38-23 =15	13–23 =−10
• **Net filtering force of the whole capillary**	= (15 − 10) = 5	

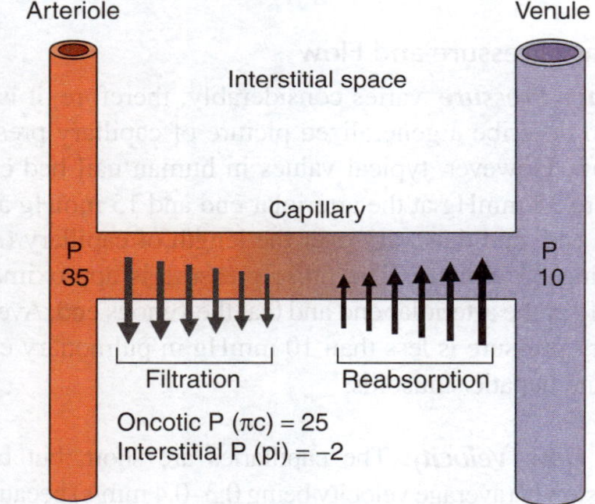

FIGURE 4.4-26 Filtration and reabsorption in a capillary due to balance of Starling forces.

Capillary Filtration and Reabsorption in Different Tissues In above example, we have calculated *net filtration forces.* However, the net filtration in the capillaries varies in the different tissues not only on the balance of Starling forces (net filtration force), but also by the capillary filtration coefficient (K).

Capillary Filtration Coefficient or the so-called permeability–surface area coefficient (K) of a tissue depends on the number of capillaries receiving blood flow and the permeability of capillaries (i.e. type of capillaries). Because of the extreme difference in the permeabilities and surface areas of the capillary systems in different tissues, the capillary filtration coefficient (*K*) may vary more than 100-fold among the different tissues. For example,

- In subcutaneous tissues, '*K*' is −0.01 ml/min/mmHg/100 g tissue and
- In kidney, '*K*' is –4.2 ml/min/mmHg/100 g tissues, which is almost 400 times as great as '*K*' of many other tissues. This obviously causes a much greater rate of filtration in the glomerular capillaries of the kidney.

Thus, depending upon the balance of Starling forces and capillary filtration coefficient (*K*), the capillary exchange in some important tissues is:

- *In renal glomerular capillaries,* fluid moves out of almost the entire length of the capillaries.
- *In interstitial capillaries,* fluid moves out of the capillaries from the arteriolar end up to the middle part and then moves into the capillaries.
- *In pulmonary capillaries,* filtration does not occur at all.

Flow-limited and Diffusion-limited Capillary Exchange

Flow-limited Exchange. It is worth noting that small molecules often equilibrate with the interstitial fluid of the tissues near the arteriolar end of each capillary. In such situations, the total diffusion can be increased by increasing the blood flow. Therefore, exchange of such substances is called flow limited (Fig. 4.4-27).

Diffusion-limited Exchange. The transfer of substances that do not reach equilibrium with the tissues during their passage through the capillaries is called diffusion-limited exchange (Fig. 4.4-27). Therefore, exchange of such substances cannot be increased by increasing the blood flow.

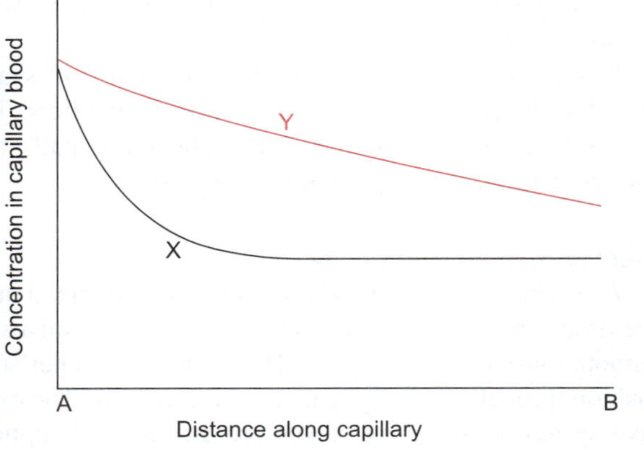

FIGURE 4.4-27 Flow-limited (X) and diffusion-limited (Y) capillary exchange. A and B indicate arteriolar and venous ends of the capillary.

Exudate versus Transudate

Exudate refers to the protein-rich fluid that comes out of the capillaries with marked increase in their permeability under conditions of inflammation due to any cause.

Transudate refers to the fluid that enters the interstitial fluid through normal capillaries. It does not have appreciable amount of proteins.

Total Capillary Exchange in the Body

It has been observed that in the whole body (leaving aside the glomerular capillary filtration), approximately 24 L of fluid is transferred per day from the capillaries to the interstitial spaces of the body. Of this, about 85–90% is reabsorbed back to the capillaries and the rest is returned to the circulation via the lymphatics. Since the capillaries are said to be impermeable to plasma proteins, the filtered fluid should contain all the constituents of plasma except proteins. However, a small amount of albumin does pass out of the capillary membrane. And practically whole of it is returned to the circulation through the lymphatics.

Lymphatic Circulation

Lymph: Formation and Composition

Formation. As discussed in capillary exchange, most (90%) of the fluid filtered at arterial end of the capillary is reabsorbed at its venous end, and the remaining 10% enters the circulation through lymphatics and is called lymph. Thus, the lymph is a transudate formed from blood in the tissue spaces, i.e. it is derived from the interstitial fluid.

Composition of lymph is similar to plasma except that its protein content is usually lower than that of plasma.

- ***Protein content*** of the lymph varies with the region it drains:
  - In most of the tissues, protein concentration of the interstitial fluid is 2 g/100 ml, so lymph also has the same content of protein.
  - Lymph from liver has protein concentration of 6 g/100 ml and that from the intestine 3–4 g/100 ml.
  - Since about two-third of the lymph is derived from liver and intestine, the thoracic duct lymph (mixture of lymph from different areas) has usually a protein content of 3–5 g/100 ml.
- ***Fat content.*** Since the lymphatic system also provides a route of absorption of long-chained fatty acids and cholesterol from the intestine (in the form of *chylomicrons*), the lymph from the intestine contains these large molecules of fat. After a fatty meal, these fat globules may be so numerous that the lymph becomes milky and is then called *chyle*.
- ***Cellular content.*** Suspended in the lymph are cells that are chiefly lymphocytes. Most of these lymphocytes are added to the lymph as it passes through lymph nodes, but some are derived from the tissues drained by the nodes.

Lymphatic Vessels

The lymphatic system constitutes an accessory route for the removal of interstitial fluid. The small lymph vessels are called lymph capillaries and the large lymph vessels are called lymphatic trunks and the largest lymph vessel is thoracic duct.

Lymph Capillaries The lymph capillaries are *present* in most tissues of the body except brain, cartilage, splenic pulp, bone marrow and avascular structures (e.g. cornea and nails).

The lymph capillaries *originate* as closed endothelial tubes that are permeable to fluid and high molecular weight compounds.

The *structure* of lymph capillaries (Fig. 4.4-28) is basically similar to that of blood capillaries with the following differences:

- The basal lamina around the endothelial cells is absent or poorly developed.
- Pericytes or connective tissue is not present around the lymph capillaries.
- There are no visible fenestrations in the endothelium.
- The junctions between endothelial cells are open, with no tight intercellular connections. In fact, the edges of the endothelial cells overlap in such a way that they form minute flap valves. So, through the lymph capillary, the substances that can pass are larger molecules such as proteins, fat droplets and particulate matter like bacteria. But once inside, the fluid particles cannot move out of capillary wall, since the tendency to backflow closes the flap valve (Fig. 4.4-28).

Larger Lymph Vessels The lymphatic capillaries join to form larger lymph vessels which ultimately form lymphatic trunks and lymphatic ducts as:

- ***Thoracic duct*** is the largest lymph vessel in the body. It carries lymph from both sides of the body below the diaphragm and from the left side above the diaphragm. Near its termination, it receives the *left subclavian lymphatic trunks* carrying lymph from left upper limb, the *left jugular lymphatic trunk* carrying lymph from left half of head and neck, and sometimes the *left bronchomediastinal lymphatic trunk* carrying lymph from left half of thorax (usually this trunk enters the subclavian vein independently).

  The thoracic duct ends by opening into the junction of the left subclavian vein and the internal jugular vein.
- ***Right lymphatic duct*** drains lymph from the right half of the body above the diaphragm. It is formed by the *right bronchomediastinal trunk* carrying lymph from the right half of thorax, *right jugular trunk* draining lymph from the right half of head and neck, and *right subclavian trunk* carrying lymph from the right upper limb. The right lymphatic duct ends by opening into the right subclavian vein.

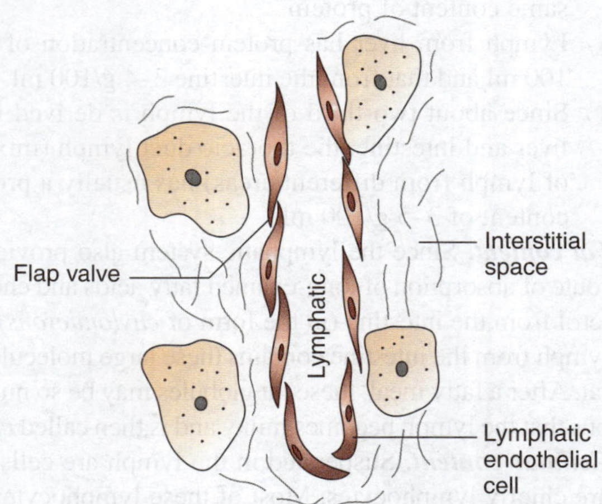

FIGURE 4.4-28 Structure of lymphatic capillary.

Structure of larger lymph vessels is similar to that of veins:

- *Three coats,* i.e. tunica intima, tunica media and tunica adventitia, can be distinguished.
- *Valves* similar to those in veins are present in abundance in small as well as large lymphatic vessels. The valves often give lymph vessels a beaded appearance.

Lymph Flow

Functions of Lymph Flow

1. Returns Proteins from Tissue Spaces to Blood. Lymph flow represents the only mechanism for returning albumin and other interstitial macromolecules to the circulatory system. The lymphatic system recovers approximately 200 g of protein daily that has been lost from the microcirculation. In addition, excess fluid is removed from the interstitium to maintain a gel state.

2. Absorption of Nutrients, especially fats from the gastrointestinal tract.

3. Acts a Transport Mechanism to remove red blood cells that have lost into the tissues as a result of haemorrhage.

4. Supplies Nutrients and Oxygen to those parts where blood cannot reach.

5. Role in Defence Mechanism. Lymph nodes associated with lymphatic system act as efficient filters. They have sinuses lined with phagocytic cells that engulf bacteria, red cells and other particulate material.

Mechanism of Lymph Flow

1. Intrinsic Lymphatic Pump. Lymph is pumped out of the tissues by the lymphatic vessels which have valves and smooth muscles in their walls. They contract in a peristaltic fashion, propelling the lymph along the vessels. The extensive system of one-way valves present in the lymphatics maintains lymph flow towards the heart.

2. Pumping by External Compression of the Lymphatics. Though the contractions of lymphatics are the principal factor propelling the lymph, the lymph is also pumped by the external compression of the lymphatics by:

- Contraction of the skeletal muscles,
- Movements of different body parts,
- Arterial pulsations and
- Compression of tissue by objects outside the body.

3. Negative Intrathoracic Pressure during inspiration increases the rate of lymph flow.

4. Suction Effect of High-velocity Blood Flow in the veins in which the lymphatics terminate also promotes lymph flow.

5. Interstitial Fluid Pressure. An increase in the interstitial fluid pressure increases the lymph flow up to a certain limit.

6. Increase In Capillary Surface Area by capillary distension is associated with increased lymph flow under the following conditions:

- Increased capillary pressure,
- Increase in local temperature and
- Infusion of fluid.

7. Increase in Capillary Permeability under the following conditions is also associated with increased lymph flow:

- Increase in temperature,
- Effect of toxins and
- Decreased oxygen (hypoxia).

8. Increase in Functional Activity of the Tissue also increases the lymph flow.

Normal Lymph Flow

- ***Normal Lymph Flow*** is 2–4 L/day (80–150 ml/h) for the entire body.
- ***Rate of Lymph Flow*** varies in different organs and is highest in the gastrointestinal tract and the liver.
- ***In Lymphatics,*** rate of lymph flow is 100 ml/h through thoracic duct and about 20 ml/h through other lymphatic channels.

Rate of formation of lymph is somewhat accelerated by regional venous obstruction (which leads to decreased absorption of tissue fluids into blood capillaries) and also by arteriolar dilations (which leads to increased tissue fluid formation).

Venous Circulation

Structural Characteristics of Veins

Walls of veins, compared with arteries, at equivalent levels in the vascular tree are thin walled and contain small amount of elastic tissue and smooth muscle, and have larger lumen. Because of their structural characteristics, they are more distensible and collapsible.

Lumen of the veins is larger than the equivalent arteries. In comparable vessels, the veins provide a larger cross-sectional area than do the arteries.

Valves are present in the veins of the dependent parts of the body (Fig. 4.3-15) that prevent the backflow of venous blood. The valves also support the column of blood so that increase in capillary pressure in the dependent parts of the body (caused by hydrostatic pressure) is minimized.

Functions of the Veins

1. Blood Reservoirs Because of their feature of *distensibility and collapsibility,* the veins serve as blood reservoirs. About 60–70% of the circulating blood is present in the venous system. When their blood content decreases, the veins assume an elliptical profile because of their *collapsibility*. As the venous blood content increases, they assume more and more circular profile to accommodate progressively greater amount of blood per unit length. Further increase in the volume of blood is accommodated by distension of the walls without any significant increase in venous pressure. In other words, small changes in pressure can cause large changes in volume (Fig. 4.4-29). Due to this property, veins are also called *capacitance vessels.*

Certain portions of the circulatory system are highly compliant and are especially important as blood reservoirs. These include:

- ***Spleen*** can sometimes decrease in size and release as much as 100 ml of blood into the reservoir of circulation.
- ***Liver*** sinuses can also release several hundred millilitres of blood into the rest of circulation.
- ***Large abdominal veins*** can contribute as much as 300 ml.
- ***Venous plexuses beneath the skin*** can also contribute several hundred millilitres of blood.

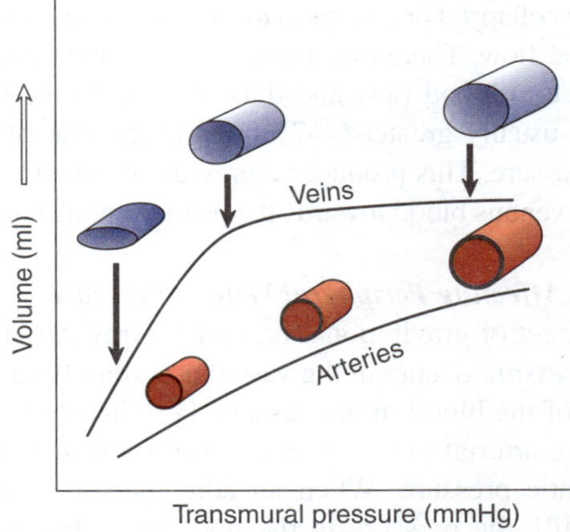

FIGURE 4.4-29 Pressure–volume relationship of arteries and veins. The slope of each line at any point represents compliance (distensibility). Note that the veins are much more compliant than the arteries at low pressure because veins are not completely distended at these pressures.

2. Conduits The systemic veins carry blood from the tissues to the right atrium, and the pulmonary veins collect blood from the lungs and return it to the left atrium.

3. Maintenance of Cardiac Output Veins help to maintain the cardiac output whenever there is loss of blood. After blood loss from an external or internal injury, reflex increase in sympathetic discharge produces contraction of the smooth muscles in the walls of the veins. As a result of venular contraction, there occurs a decrease in their capacity leading to increased venous return to heart. In this way, veins help to maintain cardiac output by maintaining normal venous return in spite of blood loss.

Venous Pressure and Flow

The venous system is a low-resistance, low-pressure and highly distensible part of the vascular system. At normal pressures, the veins are approximately 20 times more compliant than the arteries.

Central Venous Pressure Central venous pressure refers to the pressure in the right atrium because all the systemic veins open into the right atrium. The normal right atrial pressure is about 0 mmHg (i.e. equal to atmospheric pressure), but it can rise to as high as 20–30 mmHg under abnormal conditions such as heart failure and massive blood transfusion. The right atrial pressure can decrease to as low as −3 to −5 mmHg when the heart (right atrium) is pumping with vigour or when venous return is greatly depressed.

Peripheral Venous Pressure The pressure in the venules is about 10 mmHg. As the veins approach the heart, there is a gradual decrease in the venous pressure. In the great veins, near the heart, venous pressure is approximately 5 mmHg. Large veins do not offer any resistance when they are distended. However, many of the large veins entering the thorax are compressed by the surrounding tissues, so they are at least partially collapsed or collapsed to an ovoid state. This impedes the blood flow. Therefore, large veins do offer considerable resistance to blood flow and thus pressure in the peripheral veins is usually greater (4–7 mmHg) than that of the right atrial pressure. This produces a pressure gradient which propels the venous blood towards the heart (venous return).

Factors Affecting Peripheral Venous Pressure

1. Effect of gravitational pressure. Gravitational *hydrostatic pressure* occurs in the vascular system because of the weight of the blood in the vessels. Peripheral venous pressure, like arterial pressure, is affected by this gravitational hydrostatic pressure. When an adult person stands absolutely still, the pressure in the body veins because of the effect of hydrostatic pressure is (Fig. 4.4-11):

- At the level of heart, it is 0 mmHg.
- At the level of ankles, it is approximately +80 mmHg.
- At other levels in the body, from heart to feet, the venous pressure varies between 0 and 80 mmHg. It increases by 0.77 mmHg for each centimetre below the right atrium. Therefore, if the venous valves are incompetent, as in *varicose veins,* it results in venous pooling, i.e. accumulation of blood in the lower parts of the body.
- Pressure in the veins above the right atrium decreases by 0.77 mmHg for each centimetre. Therefore, *neck veins* completely collapse due to atmospheric pressure on the outside of neck, and pressure inside the vein almost remains zero.
- *Subdural venous sinuses in the skull* cannot collapse because of the tough noncollapsible nature of dura mater; therefore, a negative hydrostatic pressure (−10 mmHg) exists in them. Because of this reason, if a dural sinus is opened during a neurosurgical procedure with the patient seated, air is sucked into the sinus, resulting in *air embolism.*

2. Effect of venous resistance. Increased venous resistance can raise peripheral venous pressure to some extent. Like arterioles, myogenic tone of the veins induced by sympathetic constrictor nerves helps to adjust the capacity of vascular system. This is especially useful in postural changes. For example, sudden change of posture from lying down to standing position results in peripheral pooling of the blood in veins of legs and feet due to effect of gravity. Therefore, venous return to heart decreases, systemic blood pressure falls and may cause dizziness. However, normally, the compensatory mechanism operated via baroreceptor reflex prevents any fall in blood pressure (see page 335). Increase in venous resistance due to compression of peripheral veins within or without causes an increase in peripheral venous pressure.

3. Effect of central venous pressure. Peripheral venous pressure, to a great extent, depends upon the central venous pressure. Therefore, any factor that increases central venous pressure (i.e. right atrial pressure) will also increase the peripheral venous pressure. Common causes associated with rise in right atrial pressure are:

- Increased blood volume (massive blood transfusion,
- Heart failure and
- Arteriolar dilation decreases peripheral resistance causing rapid flow of blood from arterioles thus increasing the central venous pressure.

4. Effect of venous valves and venous pump. The venous pressure in feet is approximately +90 mmHg in a standing position because of hydrostatic pressure effect. However, movements of legs and muscle contractions (*muscle pump or venous pump)* squeeze the blood out of veins; the *valves* in the veins are arranged in such a way that the direction of blood can only be towards the heart. Thus, lowers the pressure in the veins. Therefore, in walking adults, venous pressure remains less than

25 mmHg due to combined effect of 'venous pump' and venous valves.

Measurement of Peripheral and Central Venous Pressure

- ***Clinical assessment of venous pressure*** is made by observing the degree of distension of neck veins. When right atrial pressure is increased up to 10 mmHg, the lower neck veins begin to protrude in sitting position (in normal person, in this position, the neck veins are never distended).
- ***Peripheral venous pressure measurement with a manometer*** can be made easily by connecting it to cannula inserted into a superficial vein.
- ***Central venous pressure measurement using a cardiac catheter*** whose tip is led up to superior vena cava through a superficial vein can be made accurately. The other end of the catheter is connected to a pressure transducer.

Venous Flow and Venous Return

As we know, the blood flows in the veins towards the heart due to a pressure gradient which exists between the right atrial pressure (0 mmHg) and the peripheral veins (6–7 mmHg). The *velocity of blood flow* in the veins increases with increase in the size of vein. In inferior vena cava, the average velocity of blood flow is 10 cm/s.

Venous return has been discussed in detail on page 288.

BLOOD PRESSURE

Definitions (Terminology)

Blood Pressure

Blood pressure is the lateral pressure exerted by the flowing blood on the walls of the vessels. It is usually measured in mmHg. Without any further qualification, the term blood pressure denotes the *arterial pressure*. While describing the pressure exerted by the blood column in other types of blood vessels, the type of vessels is also mentioned, e.g. *capillary pressure* and *venous pressure*.

As described in *Bernoulli's experiment* (page 309), the lateral pressure exerted on the vessel wall by the flowing blood represents the *potential energy* (PE) and the *end on pressure* (perfusion pressure) represents the total energy, i.e. kinetic energy (KE) plus potential energy (PE). Kinetic energy (KE) depends on the velocity of blood flow. Therefore, with velocity of flowing blood remaining constant, a rise in lateral pressure (potential energy) indicates a rise in perfusion pressure (total energy) and vice versa.

Systolic Blood Pressure

- The arterial pressure varies with phases of cardiac cycle. The maximum arterial pressure during systole is called *systolic blood pressure,* and occurs during ventricular ejection.
- The systolic blood pressure is a function of the cardiac output (CO), i.e. it represents the extent of work done by the heart.
- Normal systolic blood pressure in a young adult is 120 mmHg (range: 105–135 mmHg).
- Systolic blood pressure undergoes considerable fluctuations, e.g. it is increased during excitement, exercise and meals, and is decreased during sleep and rest.

Diastolic Blood Pressure

- Diastolic blood pressure refers to the minimum arterial pressure during diastole and occurs just before the onset of ventricular ejection.
- Normal diastolic blood pressure in a young adult is 80 mmHg (range 60–90 mmHg).
- The diastolic pressure is the function of total peripheral resistance (TPR) and indicates the constant load against which the heart has to work. It undergoes much less fluctuations.

Conventional Expression of Blood Pressure Conventionally, systolic and diastolic blood pressures are denoted as numerator and denominator, respectively. For example, blood pressure of a normal person is written as 120/80 mmHg.

Pulse Pressure

- Pulse pressure is the arithmetic difference between systolic and diastolic blood pressures.
- Normally, average pulse pressure is 40 mmHg.
- It determines the pulse volume.
- It depends upon three factors: arterial volume, stroke volume and arterial elastic constant. Thus, according to Young's elastic modules, the pulse

$$\text{pressure (PP)} = \frac{\Delta V}{V} - \frac{1}{Ka}, \text{ where}$$

  - ΔV is arterial uptake volume (approximately equal to but not less than the stroke volume),
  - V is arterial volume (proportional to the mean arterial pressure) and
  - Ka is arterial elastic constant.
- The high pulse pressure is indicative of systolic hypertension and indirectly determines decrease in elasticity of blood vessels.

Mean Arterial Pressure

- Mean arterial pressure (MAP) is the average of all pressure measured millisecond by millisecond throughout the cardiac cycle.
- Since the duration of cardiac systole is shorter than the duration of diastole, the MAP is not equal to the algebraic mean of the systolic and diastolic blood pressures, i.e. it is not equal to (systolic pressure + diastolic pressure).½

- A mathematically precise method for finding out MAP is to find the area under the arterial pressure curve and divide it by the duration of curve (Fig. 4.4-30). However, it is a time-consuming and cumbersome method.
- Practically, MAP is roughly equal to diastolic pressure (DP) plus one-third of pulse pressure (PP), i.e.

$$DP + \frac{1}{3}pp$$

- MAP, in fact equals total peripheral resistance (TPR) divided by cardiac output (CO), i.e.

$$MAP = \frac{TPR}{CO}$$

- MAP is same for each organ and determines the pressure head. Thus, regional blood flow through an organ depends on it.
- All cardiovascular reflexes are sensitive to mean arterial pressure.
- Normal value of MAP is 93 mmHg (range: 90–100 mmHg).

Determinants of (Factors affecting) Arterial Blood Pressure

- The arterial blood pressure (BP) is a function of the product of cardiac output (CO) and total peripheral resistance (PR), i.e.

$$\text{Arterial BP} = CO \times PR$$

- Therefore, arterial blood pressure is affected by conditions that affect either cardiac output or peripheral resistance.
- Changes in cardiac output affect the systolic pressure more than diastolic pressure, while changes in peripheral resistance affect diastolic pressure more than the systolic pressure.
- As discussed in the section on cardiac output (page 284), the cardiac output is a function of *heart rate* and *stroke volume*, so these two are important determinants of the blood pressure.
- The peripheral resistance (page 305) depends upon the viscosity of blood, elasticity of the vessel wall and velocity of the blood flow. Thus, these factors are also important determinants of the blood pressure.

Effect of some of the important determinants of the blood pressure is shown in Fig. 4.3-13 and described here briefly:

1. Heart Rate. An increase in heart rate usually increases the cardiac output and decreases the duration of cardiac cycle and thus raises the blood pressure. The increase in cardiac output due to increase in heart rate increases diastolic pressure more than the systolic pressure (because increased heart rate duration of diastole decreases more than systole and the tendency of fall in pressure during diastole decreases).

After an increase in heart rate, the arterial pressure rises, increasing the driving pressure for flow, until the amount of blood exiting the arterial system equals the amount entering. At this time, the transfer of blood from the venous to the arterial system has raised the arterial pressure and lowered the venous pressure.

Conversely, reduction in heart rate decreases the arterial blood pressure.

2. Stroke Volume. An increase in stroke volume increases the cardiac output and raises the arterial pressure, and the

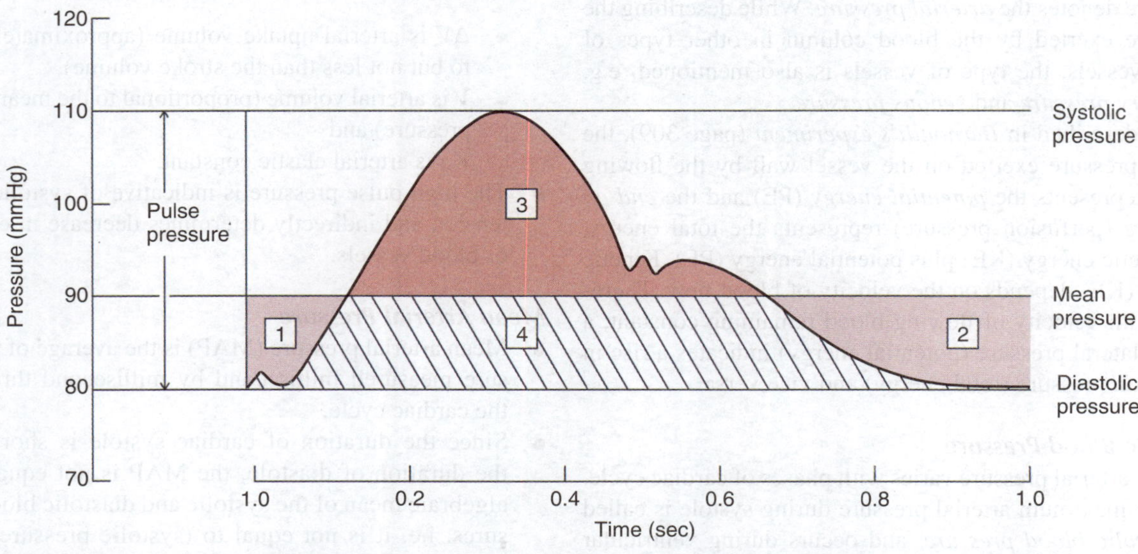

FIGURE 4.4-30 Arterial pressure curve. The line for MAP is drawn in such a way indicating that area (1 + 2) = area 3.

reverse effect occurs due to decrease in the stroke volume. When increase in cardiac output is primarily due to increase in stroke volume, it mainly increases systolic blood pressure. While an increase in cardiac output due to increase in both the stroke volume and heart rate increases systolic as well as diastolic pressure.

3. Arterial Elastic Constant. It refers to stiffness of the arterial system which progressively increases from birth until death (Fig. 4.4-31). An increase in arterial elastic constant (or loss of elasticity of vessel wall) with advancing age results in decreased stretching of the elastic vessels during systole. This results in increased pressure during systole (*systolic hypertension*) with normal diastolic blood pressure. It is characterized by high pulse pressure. When stiffness occurs in small vessels, the diastolic blood pressure is also increased.

4. Arterial Blood Volume. An increase in total blood volume increases both systolic and diastolic blood pressures by increased quantity of blood in the arterial system and greater stretching of the vessel wall.

Conversely, *haemorrhage* and *blood pooling* reduces the arterial pressure by reducing the circulating blood volume. Gravity or marked vasodilation by neural, chemical or mechanical factors may lead to blood pooling in dependent portions of the body and decrease circulating blood volume.

5. Peripheral Resistance (PR). Peripheral resistance is an important determinant of arterial pressure. An increase in PR increases and a decrease in PR decreases the arterial pressure. Increased PR raises the arterial pressure by raising the arterial volume due to reduction in the amount of blood that leaves the arterial system. The arterial pressure rises until the new pressure is sufficient to overcome the additional resistance to flow, and arterial outflow again equals inflow.

Peripheral resistance in turn is determined by radius of vessels (arterioles), velocity of blood flow and viscosity of blood. For details, see page 305.

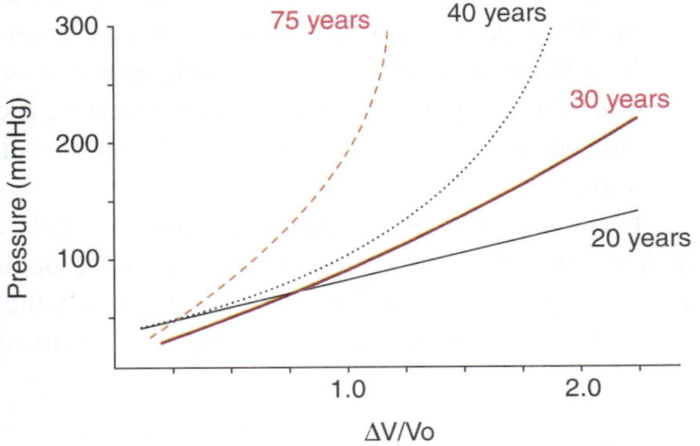

FIGURE 4.4-31 The average pressure–volume relationship of arterial system in 20-, 30-, 40-year-old individuals. Note the increasing elastance (decreased distensibility) that occurs with aging. V = volume change, VO = unstressed arterial volume.

Variations in Blood Pressure

Physiological Factors Affecting Blood Pressure

1. Age. In healthy humans, both systolic and diastolic pressures rise with age.

- *At birth,* systolic blood pressure is 40 mmHg (range: 20–60 mmHg). It then rises rapidly up to 1 month of age.
- *At 1 month* of age, the systolic blood pressure becomes about 80 mmHg and then rises slowly.
- *At about 17 years* of age, normal adult level of blood pressure 120/80 mmHg is reached, which remains almost constant up to 40 years of age and then very slowly rises.
- *At about 70 years of age,* the normal value of blood pressure is 160/90 mmHg. The increase in blood pressure associated with advancing age is due to increase in rigidity of vessel wall owing to arteriosclerotic changes.
- *A convenient empirical formula* as to what should be considered as normal blood pressure at various ages (after 10 years of age) is:
  - Systolic blood pressure: 110 + 3/5 of age in years.
  - Diastolic blood pressure: 70 + 2/5 of age in years.

2. Sex. *Before menopause,* females have little lower (4–6 mmHg) systolic blood pressure than males of corresponding age. This may be because of effect of oestrogen, while *after menopause,* systolic blood pressure in females is little higher (4–6 mmHg) than males of same age group.

3. Effect of Meals. *Systolic blood pressure* increases by 4–6 mmHg after meals and this effect lasts for about 1 h. This occurs due to two reasons:

- *Increase in heart rate* due to pressure over the heart by distended abdomen and
- *Increased epinephrine release* from adrenal medulla. *Diastolic blood pressure* either remains unchanged or decreases slightly due to vasodilation in splanchnic vessels.

4. Emotions. Increased sympathetic activity during emotional situations such as excitement, fear and worry leads to increase in systolic blood pressure due to increase in the cardiac output.

5. Climatic Temperature. *Exposure to cold* produces rise in the blood pressure by increase in peripheral resistance due to cutaneous vasoconstriction through hypothalamic stimulation. Conversely, *exposure to hot temperature* lowers the blood pressure by decreasing peripheral resistance due to cutaneous vasodilation, again through hypothalamic pathway.

6. Diurnal Variation. Systolic blood pressure shows a diurnal variation of about 6–10 mmHg, the values being

lower in the morning and higher in the afternoon. In night workers, however, a reverse rhythm is observed.

7. Exercise. In muscular exercise, generally systolic blood pressure rises and diastolic blood pressure falls. However, the effect of exercise is different in trained individuals (regular exerciser) than the untrained individuals (occasional exerciser). Further, the effect also varies depending upon the severity of exercise, whether mild, moderate or severe. However, blood pressure returns to normal levels within 5 min of stoppage of exercise due to sudden relaxation of muscles which produces vasodilation (for details, see page 1213).

8. Effect of Gravity. In standing position, due to hydrostatic (gravitational) effect of the blood column, the pressure in the vessels below heart level is increased and in the vessels above heart level, it is decreased (Fig. 4.4-11). For every centimetre below or above the heart level, the pressure increases or decreases by 0.77 mmHg, respectively. Therefore, in an individual having 120/80 mmHg blood pressure in brachial artery, the blood pressure in the dorsalis pedis artery (which is about 100 cm below heart level) will be about 200/160 mmHg, i.e. about 80 mmHg more ($0.77 \times 100 = 77$ mmHg = about 80 mmHg). Therefore, for clinical recording, blood pressure should always be checked at the heart level.

9. Effect of Change in Posture. Sudden change in posture from lying down to standing initiates some momentary changes in blood pressure which in normal humans are immediately rectified by baroreceptor reflexes, and practically such changes are not experienced. However, in patients with autonomic disturbances, these changes become symptomatic. A chain of physiological changes in blood pressure during change of posture is:

- Immediately on standing, there occurs peripheral pooling of blood in dependent parts leading to decreased venous return and decreased cardiac output, and momentary fall in systolic blood pressure. Fall in systolic pressure immediately decreases baroreceptor discharge via vasomotor centre leading to increased *diastolic blood pressure*. On standing, there also occurs an increase in peripheral resistance and momentary increase in diastolic blood pressure.

Thus, immediately after standing from lying down posture, a rise in diastolic blood pressure can be recorded for about 30–60 s. Later on, due to decrease in baroreceptor discharge, blood pressure comes back to normal and no symptoms are experienced by the normal individuals.

10. Sleep. In complete relaxed state, during early hours of sleep, there occurs general vasodilation leading to fall in blood pressure up to 15–20 mmHg. However, in disturbed sleep, blood pressure increases due to increased sympathetic discharge.

11. Body Built. Systolic blood pressure is slightly higher in obese individuals compared with thin-built individuals. Further, falsely higher values are obtained in obese individuals while testing brachial artery blood pressure using standard arm cuff. This occurs because there is more tissue between the cuff and artery and so, some of the cuff pressure is dissipated. Therefore, use of a cuff that is wider than the standard arm cuff is recommended for accurate record of blood pressure in obese individuals.

Measurement of Blood Pressure

Direct Method

Direct method of measuring blood pressure is used in experimental studies. In it, a cannula or T-tube is inserted into an artery and connected to either:

- ***Mercury manometer*** and pressure is recorded on the kymograph or
- ***Pressure transducer*** (strain gauge) which in turn is connected to Polyrite for recording.

The record will show fluctuations as depicted in Fig. 4.4-32, upper level of which indicates systolic blood pressure and lower level indicates diastolic blood pressure.

Indirect Method

In humans, blood pressure is measured indirectly by using a sphygmomanometer.

Sphygmomanometer Commonly called blood pressure apparatus, a sphygmomanometer is the instrument used to measure blood pressure. It consists of the following parts:

1. Manometer. Two types of manometers are used:

- *Aneroid manometer* (Fig. 4.4-33) in which metal bellows, mechanical rings and a dial replaces the glass tube mercury manometer. It is also very commonly used nowadays. However, it needs calibration against a mercury manometer from time to time.
- *Mercury manometer* is commonly used in a classical sphygmomanometer (Fig. 4.4-34). It consists of a *graduated narrow glass tube* having markings 0–300. Upper end of the tube is closed and lower end is connected to lower end of a wide lumen *mercury reservoir.* Upper end of the mercury reservoir is connected to an inflatable rubber bag through a rubber tube.

2. The Cuff. The blood pressure apparatus cuff also known as 'armlet' or 'Riva-Rocci cuff' (after the name of discoverer) consists of an inflatable rubber bag which is enclosed in a cotton bag having a long strip of inelastic

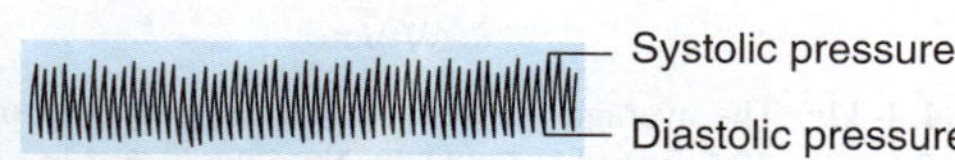

FIGURE 4.4-32 Record of arterial blood pressure obtained by direct arterial cannulation method.

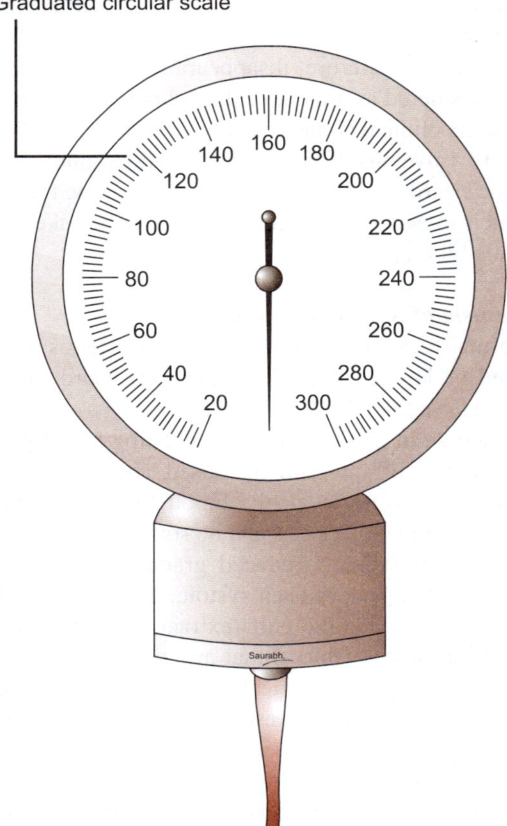

FIGURE 4.4-33 Aneroid sphygmomanometer.

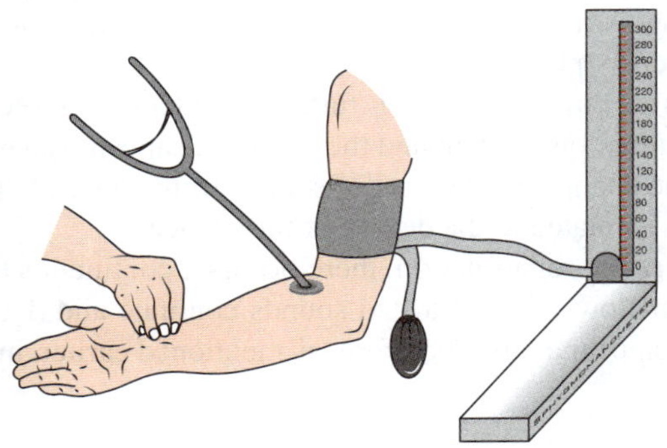

FIGURE 4.4-34 Procedure of recording blood pressure by auscultatory method.

cloth. The dimensions of the commonly used rubber bag are 24 cm × 12 cm. It should be at least as wide as half the upper arm's circumference. The bag width (12 cm) should be more in obese adults, about 4-5 cm for children and 2–3 cm for the newborns.

3. Air Pump. It is a rubber bulb with a one-way valve at its free end, and a 'leaky valve' and a knurled screw at the other end where the rubber tube leading to the cuff is attached. The cuff can be inflated by turning the leak-valve screw clockwise and alternately compressing and releasing the bulb. Deflation is achieved by turning the screw anti-clockwise.

Procedure. The blood pressure may be tested with the subject lying supine or sitting, but should be physically and mentally relaxed and free from excitation. The cuff of the blood pressure apparatus is applied on the upper arm with the centre of the rubber bag lying over the brachial artery which lies medially, and its lower edge should be about 3 cm above the elbow (Fig. 4.4-34).

The blood pressure can be measured using palpatory method, oscillatory method or auscultatory method.

1. Palpatory Method. Palpatory method described by Riva-Rocci in 1896 includes the following steps:

- Palpate and feel pulsations of the radial artery with the tips of finger of left hand.
- Keeping fingers of left hand on the pulse, slowly inflate the cuff using air pump with the right hand until the pulse disappears. Then raise the pressure further by 30–40 mm in the manometer.
- Open the leak valve of air pump and control it so that the pressure gradually falls in steps of 2–4 mm. Note the reading at which pulse just reappears. This reading corresponds to *systolic blood pressure.* After this, deflate the cuff quickly to zero pressure.
- Take three readings in each arm, fully deflating the cuff a few minutes between each reading. Mean of the three readings should be taken as systolic blood pressure. The actual pressure is usually 4–6 mm higher than the recorded value, since initial 2–3 beats are often missed while feeling the pulse.
- *Disadvantage* of the palpatory method is that the diastolic blood pressure cannot be measured by this method.

2. Oscillatory Method. Oscillatory method is not preferred.

- In this method, initial steps up to raising the pressure in the cuff by 30–40 mm after the pulse disappears are same.
- Then the mercury column in the graduated glass tube of manometer is carefully watched while slowly lowering the cuff pressure. The *oscillations* will appear and become prominent once the pressure in the cuff is roughly equal to the systolic pressure.

3. Auscultatory Method. Auscultatory method, described by Korotkoff in 1905, is the most useful technique.

- Initial steps up to raising the pressure in the cuff by 30–40 mm above the level where the radial artery pulse disappears are similar to palpatory method. However, before inflating the cuff, the point just before the brachial artery bifurcating the cubital space, just medial to the tendon of biceps muscle, is marked.

- Then the diaphragm of stethoscope is placed on the mark in cubital space and is kept in position with the help of thumb and fingers of left hand.
- Pressure in the cuff is lowered slowly by opening the leak valve of the air pump with right hand. While doing so, initially no sound is heard. However, when mercury column is lowered further, a tap sound is heard. The character and quality of sound go on changing while further lowering the mercury column by deflating the cuff, and ultimately the sound disappears. These sounds are called Korotkoff sounds and from these the levels of systolic and diastolic blood pressure are noted as described below. When the sounds disappear, the cuff should be deflated quickly.

Korotkoff Sounds

Phases of Korotkoff Sounds. Depending upon the characteristic features, the Korotkoff sounds have been described in five phases (Fig. 4.4-35):

- ***Phase I sounds*** start with a *clear tap* which indicates the *systolic blood pressure*. The clear, tapping and sharp sounds last for 10–12 mmHg fall in mercury column.
- ***Phase II sounds*** are *murmurish,* i.e. soft and swishing and last for next 14–15 mmHg fall in mercury column.
- ***Phase III sounds*** are clear, knocking and banging in character and last for next 14–15 mmHg fall in mercury column.
- ***Phase IV sounds*** start with *sudden muffling* and mark the *diastolic blood pressure*. The muffled sounds are indistinct, dull and faint, as if coming from a distance and last for next 4–5 mmHg fall in mercury column.

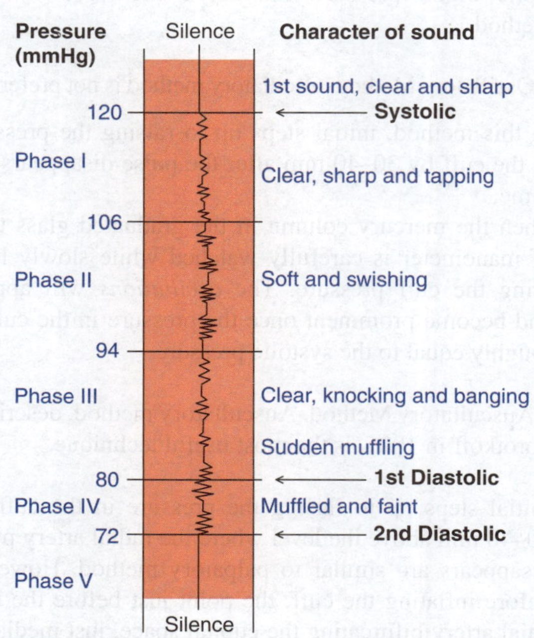

FIGURE 4.4-35 Phases of Korotkoff sounds.

- ***Phase V*** is labelled when no sound is heard. Since the beginners may not appreciate beginning of muffling of sounds and therefore, disappearance of the sound may be considered as a mark of diastolic pressure. However, in some clinical situations such as hyperthyroidism and aortic valve insufficiency where the sounds continue to be heard even when the pressure is low, the level at which muffling of sounds starts is to be taken as diastolic blood pressure.

Mechanism of Korotkoff Sounds

- Normally, the blood flow through the arteries is streamlined or laminar, and no sounds are heard over them when auscultated.
- As shown in Fig. 4.4-36, while testing blood pressure, when the cuff pressure is raised above the expected systolic pressure level, the blood flow in the brachial artery completely ceases and no sounds are heard. When the cuff pressure is reduced gradually, a time comes when, at the peak of each systole, the intraarterial pressure just exceeds the cuff (extraarterial) pressure. The small amounts of blood that are ejected at high velocity (exceeding the critical velocity) through the partially narrowed artery result in *intermittent turbulence* which produces the sounds. Also, the blood column in the distal part of the artery, i.e. below the cuff, is set into vibrations by the jets of blood striking against it, which contributes to the sounds. These sounds are called *Korotkoff sounds.*
- When the cuff pressure nears the diastolic pressure level, the artery is still partially constricted, but the turbulent flow is now continuous and the sounds have a *muffled quality* (phase IV).
- As the cuff pressure falls further, the blood flow becomes laminar once again and the sounds disappear (phase V).
- The change in character of sounds from phase I to phase IV is related to the degree of turbulence.
- In aortic regurgitation, there occurs a continuous turbulent flow so the muffled sounds continue and does not disappear at all. Therefore, as mentioned earlier, in such

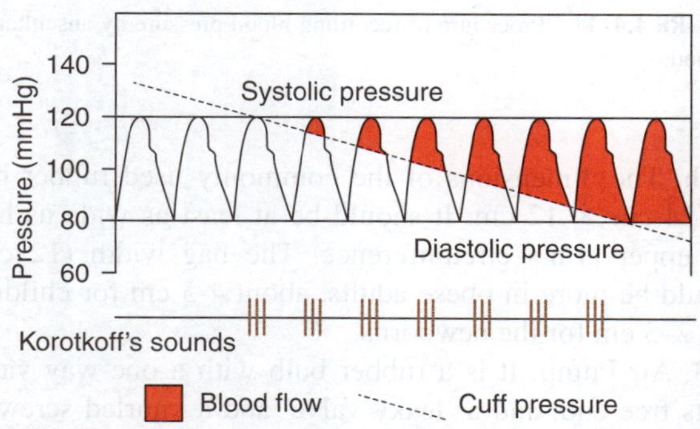

FIGURE 4.4-36 Change in blood flow and production of Korotkoff sounds with change in cuff pressure.

cases, the start of muffling of sounds should be considered a mark of diastolic pressure. In fact in this condition, a slight pressure with a stethoscope alone (without the cuff) may produce clear, sharp, snapping sounds, called the *pistol-shot sounds.*

Auscultatory gap. In some patients of hypertension, there may be a gap in the Korotkoff sounds. As the mercury is lowered, a few faint sounds are heard which soon disappear only to reappear once again at a much lower pressure. This brief interruption in the sounds is called the *aucultatory or silent gap.* If the mercury column is raised to this gap only, one may miss the first appearance of sounds, which indicates systolic pressure, and thus record a false low systolic pressure. To avoid this mistake, the mercury column must always be raised 50-60 mm above the level at which the radial pulse disappears. One can then be sure the cuff pressure is well above the systolic level.

Precautions to be Taken While Recording Blood Pressure

1. Basal arterial pressure should always be recorded in the lying down (recumbent) position. This will avoid effect of gravity on blood pressure (page 326) and for this reason the arterial pressure will be same if recorded from any artery.
2. The position of the arm and sphygmomanometer should be at the heart level, again to avoid the effect of gravity.
3. The cuff size should always be appropriate for accurate measurement of blood pressure (see page 327).
4. The palpatory method must always be employed first to avoid auscultatory gap.
5. The cuff pressure should never be kept high for any length of time because the discomfort may cause generalized reflex vasoconstriction, thus raising the blood pressure.
6. It is a good practice to compare the pressure in the two arms when measuring the pressure for the first time.
7. Last but not the least, the subject should be physically relaxed and free from tension and anxiety.

Note. The systolic blood pressure as measured by sphygmomanometer is usually 10–20 mmHg lower and diastolic pressure is higher by about 8 mmHg than direct arterial cannulation method.

Regulation of Blood Pressure

Arterial blood pressure is controlled by several mechanisms which under physiological conditions maintain the normal mean arterial pressure (MAP) within a narrow range of 95–100 mmHg. The different mechanisms concerned with regulation of blood pressure have been discussed in detail in Chapter 4.5 on Cardiovascular Regulation and have been briefed here just for orientation about control of blood pressure. Each mechanism performs a specific function. Various mechanisms controlling arterial pressure can be grouped as:

A. Rapid blood pressure control mechanism,
B. Intermediate blood pressure control mechanisms and
C. Long-term blood pressure control mechanisms.

Rapid Blood Pressure Control Mechanism (Nervous Regulating Mechanism)

Rapid blood pressure control mechanism or the so-called short-term control mechanism primarily includes the following three nervous reflexes:

1. Baroreceptor reflexes (see page 340),
2. Central nervous system ischaemic response (see page 347) and
3. Chemoreceptor reflexes (see page 346).

Salient Features. The nervous reflexes that rapidly control the blood pressure are described in detail elsewhere. Their salient features are:

- These *act very rapidly,* i.e. within seconds to few minutes of alterations in the blood pressure.
- These are *short-term mechanisms,* i.e. these act for few hours to few days and are thus insignificant in long-term regulation of blood pressure.
- These are useful in preventing *acute decreases in blood pressure* (e.g. during severe haemorrhage) as well as in preventing *excessive increases in blood pressure* (e.g. as might occur in response to excessive blood transfusion).

Intermediate Blood Pressure Control Mechanisms

The intermediate blood pressure control mechanisms that are important in blood pressure control after several minutes of acute pressure changes are:

1. Renin–angiotensin vasoconstrictor mechanism (for details see page 348),
2. Stress relaxation and reverse stress relaxation mechanism and
3. Capillary fluid shift mechanism.

   Salient features of intermediate blood pressure control mechanisms are:
   - These mechanisms come into play after several minutes of acute pressure changes and reach full function within a few hours.
   - These mechanisms play their role from few days to few weeks.
   - All these mechanisms basically try to control the alterations in blood pressure by altering the blood volume.

Stress Relaxation and Reverse Stress Relaxation Mechanisms

- ***Stress Relaxation Mechanism*** refers to vasodilation occurring due to stress on the vascular smooth muscles.

When pressure in the vessels become too high (e.g. following massive slow intravenous transfusion), the vessels become stretched and continue to stretch for minutes or hours. This causes relaxation of blood vessels simply by vascular tone adjustment. This leads to an increase in the capacity of the arterial system with a concomitant fall in blood pressure.

- ***Reverse Stress Relaxation Mechanism*** operates when the blood pressure is low due to less stress on the vessels walls and tries to restore it back to normal. For example, when blood pressure falls due to prolonged slow bleeding, there occurs tightening of blood vessel walls by vascular tone adjustment secondary to less stress on the vessel wall (reverse stress relaxation mechanism). This mechanism tries to restore the blood pressure back to normal. This mechanism can correct up to 15% change in blood volume below normal.

Capillary Fluid Shift Mechanism Capillary fluid shift mechanism helps in restoring both low and high blood pressure back to normal:

- ***When blood pressure is raised,*** the mean capillary pressure is also high, resulting in shift of fluid from circulation to the interstitial fluid compartments. This reduces the blood volume to restore the arterial pressure (Fig. 4.4-26).
- ***When blood pressure is lowered,*** the mean capillary pressure is also low, resulting in absorption of fluid from the interstitial compartments to circulation. Thus, the blood volume is increased which helps to return the blood pressure back to normal.

The capillary fluid shift mechanism is about two times more effective than baroreceptor reflex mechanism in controlling the blood pressure, but it acts much more slowly (intermediate-acting mechanism) than baroreceptor mechanism (rapid-acting mechanism).

Long-term Blood Pressure Control Mechanisms

Kidneys play main role in the long-term control of blood pressure by the following mechanisms:

1. ***Direct mechanism,*** i.e. 'renal body fluid feedback mechanism'.
2. ***Indirect mechanisms*** control kidney functions indirectly via following hormonal mechanisms:
   i. Aldosterone system and
   ii. Renin–angiotensin system (see page 348).

Renal–Body Fluid System for Arterial Pressure Control The most important mechanism for the long-term control of blood pressure is linked to control of circulatory volume by the kidney, a mechanism known as the *renal–body fluid feedback system.* In fact, it is similar to the capillary fluid shift mechanism except that only the renal glomerular capillaries are involved in the process.

Modes of Operation of Renal–Body Fluid Feedback System. The renal–body fluid system corrects blood pressure by causing appropriate changes in blood volume through *diuresis* and *natriuresis*:

- ***When blood pressure rises too high,*** the kidneys excrete increased quantities of sodium and water because of *pressure natriuresis* and *pressure diuresis,* respectively. As a result of increased renal excretion, the extracellular fluid volume and blood volume both decrease until blood pressure returns to normal and the kidneys excrete normal amounts of sodium and water.
- ***When the blood pressure falls too low,*** the kidneys reduce the rate of sodium and water excretion, and over a period of hours to days, if the person drinks enough water and eats enough salt to increase blood volume, the blood pressure will return to its previous level. This mechanism being very slow to act is not of major importance in the acute control of arterial pressure. However, it is by far the most potent of all long-term arterial pressure controllers.

The sequence of events in order of occurrence during control of blood pressure by this mechanism is summarized as:

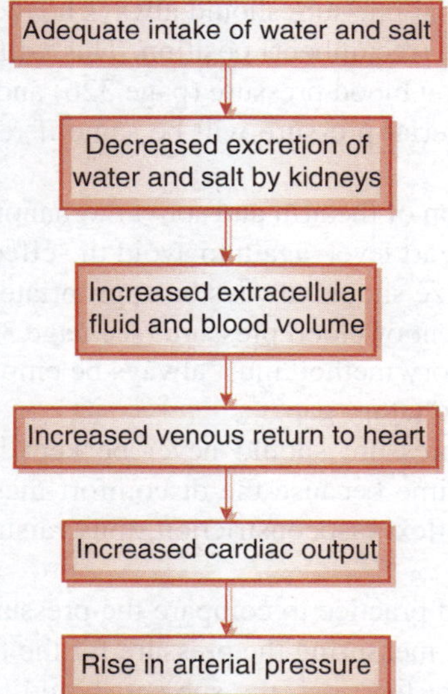

Determinants of the Renal-Body Fluid Feedback Mechanism. The two factors that determine the long-term control of arterial pressure by renal–body fluid mechanism are: renal output curve for salt and water and level of salt and water intake. As long as these two factors remain constant, the mean arterial pressure will also remain exactly at the normal level of 100 mmHg. For arterial pressure to deviate from the normal level for long periods of time, one of these two factors must be altered.

Fig. 4.4-37 shows the effect of different arterial pressures on urine volume output by an isolated kidney. The figure demonstrates that:

- As arterial pressure rises, there occurs a marked increase in the output of volume (pressure diuresis) and sodium (pressure natriuresis).

- As long as the arterial pressure will remain above the normal equilibrium point, renal output will exceed the intake of salt and water resulting in a progressive decline in extracellular fluid volume.
- When blood pressure falls below the equilibrium point, the renal output of water and salt will be lower than the intake resulting in a progressive increase in extracellular volume.
- At the normal arterial pressure, a balance between renal output and intake of salt and water occurs at so-called the *equilibrium point.*
- As shown in Fig. 4.4-37B, due to an abnormality of the kidney, the renal output curve is shifted and the equilibrium point is obtained at a level of high blood pressure (150 mmHg).
- The renal output and salt and water intake demonstrate that theoretically arterial pressure will be raised with increase in salt and water intake. However, in reality, the blood pressure does not rise every time the sodium intake is increased. This is accomplished mainly by decreasing the formation of angiotensin II and aldosterone, which increases the ability of kidney to excrete salt and water, and results in compensatory *left shift of the pressure natriuresis curve.*

Salient Features of Renal–Body Fluid Feedback Mechanism. The salient features of the renal–body fluid feedback mechanism can be summarized as:

- The renal–body fluid feedback mechanism takes several hours to show any significant response.
- These mechanisms operate very powerfully to control arterial pressure over days, weeks and months.
- The effectiveness of these mechanisms becomes steadily greater with time.

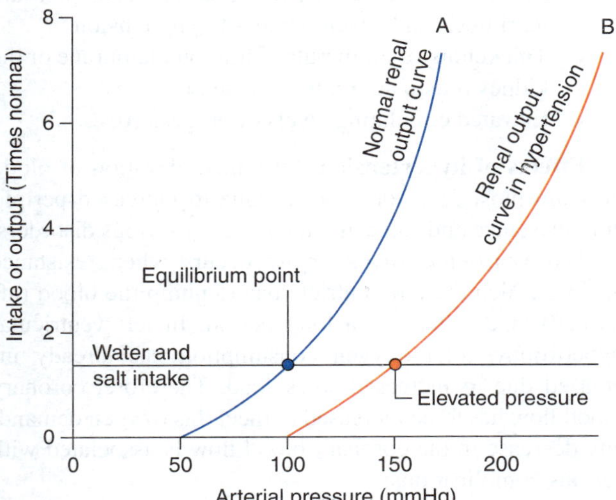

FIGURE 4.4-37 Analysis of arterial blood pressure regulation by equating the renal output curve with salt and water intake. The equilibrium point describes the level at which arterial pressure will be regulated.

- These mechanisms, if given sufficient time, control arterial pressure at the level that provides normal output of salt and water by the kidneys.
- As long as kidney function is unaltered, these mechanisms overcome the disturbances that tend to alter arterial pressure such as increased total peripheral resistance over a long period and thus are able to control the blood pressure.

Conclusion

To conclude, it can be stated that *rapid control* of arterial pressure begins with life-saving measures of the *nervous reflexes,* continues with sustaining characteristics of the *intermediate pressure controls* and finally is stabilized at the *long-term pressure level by the renal–body fluid feedback mechanism.*

Pathological Variations in Blood Pressure

Hypertension

Definition. Hypertension (HT) refers to a condition in which value of systolic blood pressure is persistently more than 140 mmHg and/or that of diastolic blood pressure is above 90 mmHg. If there is an increase only in systolic blood pressure, it is called *systolic hypertension* in which the pulse pressure is raised.

Types of hypertension. It is of two types : primary and secondary hypertension.

1. ***Primary hypertension,*** also known as *essential hypertension,* is characterized by a raised blood pressure without any underlying disease. Risk factors for primary HT include: heredity, obesity, mental tension and smoking. Blood pressure is raised due to increased peripheral resistance. Primary HT presents in two clinical forms:
   - *Benign hypertension,* in which blood pressure is moderately raised. Untreated hypertension over the years may cause cardiac, vascular and renal complication.
   - *Malignant hypertension* or accelerated hypertension refers to a sudden marked rise in blood pressure (e.g. systolic up to 250 mmHg and diastolic up to 150 mmHg). Malignant hypertension is an emergency and may sometimes be even fatal.
2. ***Secondary hypertension*** refers to a condition in which blood pressure is raised due to some other underlying disease. Common causes of secondary hypertension are:
   - *Cardiovascular diseases* producing secondary hypertension are atherosclerosis and coarctation of aorta.
   - *Renal diseases* causing secondary hypertension are stenosis of renal artery, glomerulonephritis and tumour of juxtaglomerular cells leading to formation of excess of angiotensin II.

Goldblatt's hypertension, also known as renovascular hypertension, refers to the hypertension due to compression of renal artery or its branches. It can be of two types:

- *One-kidney Goldblatt hypertension.* This happens when one kidney is already removed and the renal artery of other kidney is constricted due to any reason.
- *Two-kidney Goldblatt hypertension.* This occurs when the artery to one kidney is constricted while the artery to other kidney is normal.

Mechanism. Due to occlusion of renal artery, there occurs renal ischaemia, which triggers release of renin causing rapid elevation of blood pressure for the first hour or so. This is followed by a slower additional rise in blood pressure during next several days. This happens because the hypereninaemia increases angiotensin II levels (for details, see causing severe vasoconstriction and aldosterone release leading on to sodium and water retention.

- *Endocrinal disorders* associated with secondary hypertension are: Cushing's syndrome (excessive secretion of glucocorticoids from adrenal cortex).
- *Hyperaldosteronism* (excessive secretion of aldosterone or other mineralocorticoids from adrenal cortex) causes renal Na^+ and water retention, consequently leading to expansion of ECF volume and blood pressure rises. Hyperaldosteronism occurs due to mutations in number of genes. In humans, different gene mutations have been identified which are responsible for hypertension.
  - i. Hypertension caused by mutation of a single gene is referred to as monogenic hypertension that is a rare entity (<1%).
  - ii. A hybrid gene encodes adrenocorticotropic-sensitive aldosterone synthetase enzyme that causes hyperaldosteronism, this condition is known as *glucocorticoid-remediable hyperaldosteronism (GRA).* Normally, glucocorticoids do not suppress aldosterone secretion, but in this autosomal dominant disorder, hypertension can be remedied by administering glucocorticoids that suppress ACTH secretion.
  - iii. The genes coding aldosterone synthase and 11 β-hydroxylase are identical and close to each other on chromosome 8. Therefore, mutation of hybrid gene in GRA also results in 11 β-hydroxylase deficiency, which causes hypertension by increasing the secretion of deoxycorticosterone.
  - iv. In deficiency of 11-β hydroxysteriod type-2 enzyme due to gene mutation, the cortisol has marked mineralocorticoid effect and the syndrome is known as *apparent mineralocorticoid excess (AMI).* In this condition, there is loss of specificity for mineraloreceptors. Therefore, clinical picture resembles as of hyperaldosteronism because cortisol acts on minrealocorticoid receptors. The plasma level of aldosterone and renin is low in this syndrome.
  - v. Mutations of genes for ENaCs (epithelial sodium channels) in *Liddle syndrome* cause increased activity of ENaCs due to reduced degradation of β and γ subunits in collecting ducts, thereby causing an increase in renal Na^+ reabsorption by mineralocorticoids leading to renal Na^+ retention and hypertension.
- *Pheochromocytoma* (tumour of adrenal medulla) secretes adrenaline/noradrenaline/both, causing sustained hypertension (see page 766).
- *Pill hypertension* is produced due to contraceptive pills containing large amount of estrogen that causes increased secretion of angiotensinogen.
- *Neurologic disorders* which may produce secondary hypertension include raised intracranial pressure, tractus solitarius and sectioning of nerve fibres from carotid sinus.
- *Pregnancy-induced hypertension (PIH)* is noticed in some of the pregnant women. Its exact cause is not known. It may be because of some autoimmune processes during pregnancy or the release of some vasoconstrictor agents from placenta or due to excessive secretion of hormones causing rise in blood pressure.

- ***Hypertension in preeclampsia (toxaemia of pregnancy).*** Preeclampsia or toxaemia of pregnancy is a syndrome that occurs in approximately 5–10% of expectant mother. Hypertension is one of the major manifestations of this syndrome. The precise cause is not clearly known, but ischaemia of placenta and subsequently release of toxic factors are believed to play role in manifestations of preeclampsia.
- Hypertension occurs due to endothelial dysfunction of vasculature resulting in decreased release of nitrous oxide and other substances causing vasoconstriction, decreased GFR, impaired renal pressure natriuresis and development of hypertension.
- Thickening of glomerular filtration membrane of the kidney due to autoimmune diseases.
- Elevated circulating levels of progesterone.

Effects of hypertension. Sustained elevation of blood pressure most commonly occurs due to increased peripheral resistance and can cause a number of serious disorders.

Left ventricular hypertrophy occurs when resistance against which the left ventricle has to pump the blood (afterload) is elevated for a long period. In left ventricular hypertrophy, total oxygen consumption has already increased due to increased work load. Therefore, coronary blood flow has to be increased to meet this oxygen demand; any decrease in the coronary blood flow is associated with serious complications:

- *Myocardial infarction.* Incidence of myocardial infarction is higher in hypertensive individuals. For details, see page 360.

- *Atherosclerosis.* The incidence of atherosclerosis increases in hypertensives.
- *Thrombosis.* Hypertensive individuals are predisposed to cerebral thrombosis resulting in stroke and haemorrhage.
- *Renal failure* is an additional complication of hypertension.
- *Heart failure* occurs due to increase in the after load. For details, see page 384.

Treatment. The incidence of heart failure, stroke and renal failure can be avoided by active treatment. Blood pressure can be lowered effectively by use of the following drugs:

- α-adrenergic receptor blockers,
- β-adrenergic receptor blockers,
- Inhibitors of angiotensin converting enzyme and
- Calcium channel blockers.

Details of treatment are beyond the scope of this book. Therefore, for mechanism of action, doses, etc., students are advised to consult pharmacology and medicine books.

Hypotension Hypotension refers to a condition in which values of blood pressure are below the normal range. Clinically, when the systolic blood pressure is less than 90 mmHg, it is considered hypotension. It is of the following types:

- *Primary hypotension,* also known as essential hypotension, is a disorder of unknown aetiology.
- *Secondary hypotension,* as the name indicates, occurs secondary to some other underlying diseases such as myocardial infarction, neurogenic shock, haemorrhagic shock, hypoactivity of pituitary gland and hypoactivity of adrenal glands.
- *Postural hypotension* refers to sudden fall in blood pressure when patients stand up from lying down posture. It occurs due to some dysfunction of autonomic nervous system.

Chapter 4.5

Cardiovascular Regulation

INTRODUCTION

Cardiovascular control makes *circulatory adjustments* which are essential to cope up with the timely needs of each and every organ of the body and is thus of fundamental importance for survival.

Need for Cardiovascular Control

Functions served by cardiovascular control are:

- *To increase the blood supply* to active tissues, e.g. during exercise to skeletal and cardiac muscles.
- *Redistribution of blood* to increase or decrease the heat loss from the body as per requirements.
- *Circulatory adjustments* during routine cardiovascular stresses like change in posture, hours of excitement, fear, anxiety, meals, sleep, etc.
- *Maintenance of adequate flow to vital organs* such as brain, heart, and kidney all the times including emergencies such as shock and haemorrhage, even at the expense of the circulation to the rest of the body, as the vital organs may develop irreversible changes in no time. For example, the brain is irreversibly damaged within 3 min of ischaemia, while skin, skeletal muscle, and gastrointestinal tract can tolerate reduction of blood for longer duration. The earlier described functions sub served by the cardiovascular control system, in other words, qualify the need for cardio-vascular control.

Circulatory Adjustments

Circulatory adjustments which ensure that all of the organs receive sufficient blood flow are: (1) control of blood volume and (2) control of arterial pressure. These circulatory adjustments are made by the cardiovascular control mechanisms primarily by regulating following parameters.

A. Regulation of Cardiac Performance, i.e. alterations in the activities of heart which include:

1. *Chronotropic action,* i.e. effect on heart rate which may be in the form of:
   - Increased heart rate (tachycardia) or positive chronotropic effect.
   - Decreased heart rate (bradycardia) or negative chronotropic effect.
2. *Inotropic action,* i.e. effect on force of contraction which may be in the form of:
   - Increase in the force of contraction (positive inotropic effect) or
   - Decrease in the force of contraction (negative inotropic effect.
3. *Dromotropic action,* i.e. effect on conduction of impulse through the heart, which may be in the form of:
   - Increase in the velocity of impulse conduction (positive dromotropic effect) or
   - Decrease in the velocity of impulse conduction (negative dromotropic effect).
4. *Bathmotropic action,* i.e. effect on the excitability of the cardiac muscle, which may be in the form of:
   - Increased excitability of cardiac muscle (positive bathmotropic effect) or
   - Decreased excitability of cardiac muscle (negative bathmotropic effect).

B. Regulation of performance of blood vessels which primarily includes:

1. *Alterations in diameter of arterioles* which change the peripheral resistance and also the hydrostatic pressure in the capillaries and
2. *Alteration in diameter of veins* which changes the venous pressure and thus venous return and the cardiac output.

Cardiovascular Control Mechanisms

The cardiovascular control mechanisms which play their role in making circulatory adjustments during the routine and emergency cardiovascular stresses can be grouped as:

- Neural control mechanism
- Humoral control mechanism and
- Local control mechanisms.

NEURAL CONTROL MECHANISM

Neural regulation of circulation is of fundamental importance since it responds within seconds. However, neural mechanism has little to do with local adjustments of blood flow to the tissues, except for certain tissues such as skin.

Main Role of Neural Control Mechanism

The nervous regulation mainly controls systemic functions of the circulatory system (whenever required) such as:

- Redistribution of blood flow to different parts of the body,
- Increasing pumping activity of heart and
- Rapid control of arterial pressure.

Components of Neural Control Mechanism The neural cardiovascular regulating mechanism consists of:

A. Medullary Cardiovascular Control Centres. These are the prime centres concerned with neural control of circulation. These include:

- Medullary sympathetic centre (vasomotor centre),
- Medullary parasympathetic centre (nucleus ambiguus) and
- Medullary relay centre for cardiorespiratory and afferents (nucleus of tractussolitarius, i.e. NTS).

B. Autonomic Nervous System Supplying the Heart and Blood Vessels. The regulation of circulation by medullary control centres is exerted almost entirely through the autonomic nervous system (ANS). The sympathetic component of ANS is most important for controlling circulation, and the parasympathetic component mainly contributes to regulation of heart functions.

C. Afferent Impulses to Medullary Centres. The vasomotor centre (VMC) is influenced by afferent impulses from the higher centres and a large number of other areas.

D. Role of Skeletal Nerves and Muscles in Controlling Blood Pressure.

Medullary Cardiovascular Control Centres

1. Vasomotor Centre

Though popularly known as VMC, more appropriately it should be called *medullary sympathetic centre.* It is the primary cardiovascular regulatory centre located in the medulla oblongata of brainstem. It consists of groups of neurons situated bilaterally in the reticular substance of medulla at the floor of fourth ventricle. The medullary cardiovascular centre is constituted by following different areas (Fig. 4.5-1):

Pressor Area Pressor area is located in the rostral ventrolateral medulla (RVLM). It contains glutaminergic neurons which exert *excitatory* effect on thoracolumbar spinal sympathetic neurons.

- ***Continuous sympathetic vasoconstrictor tone.*** Normally, the neurons forming the pressor area of the VMC show *inherent tonic activity,* i.e. they discharge rhythmically (at a rate of about 1 impulse per second) in a tonic fashion to excite sympathetic preganglionic neurons present in the intermediolateral (IML) grey column of the spinal cord. In this way, the continuous signals are passed to the sympathetic vasoconstrictor nerves fibres over the entire body. This *sympathetic vasconstrictor tone* maintains a partial state of contraction of blood vessels. When this tone is blocked, for example, by spinal anaesthesia, the blood vessels throughout the body dilate and arterial pressure may fall to as low as 50 mmHg.
- ***Stimulation of pressor area*** produces:
  - *Arteriolar constriction* which increases the systemic blood pressure,
  - *Venoconstriction* which decreases blood stored in the venous reservoir and increases venous return,
  - *Increase in heart rate* or positive chronotropic effect and
  - *Increase in force of contraction* or positive inotropic effect.

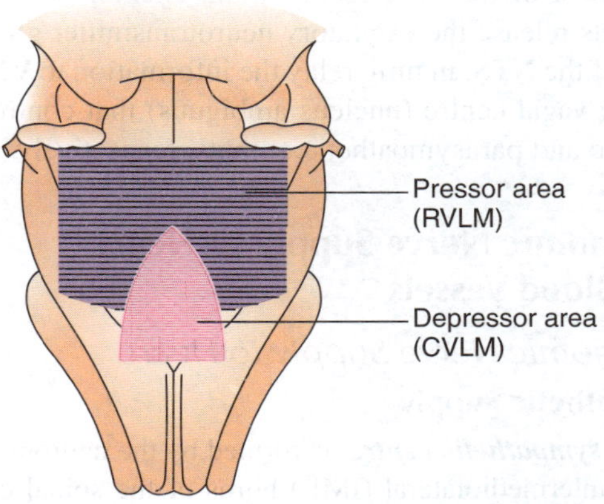

FIGURE 4.5-1 Medullary cardiovascular control centres.

Important Note

Cases of essential hypertension are associated with neurovascular compression of RVLM. Magnetic resonance angiography (MRA) in patients with schwannoma or meningiomas lying nearer to RVLM has indicated higher incidence of co existence of hypertension and neurovascular compression due to increased sympathetic activity. For details of hypertension see page 331.

Depressor Area Depressor area is situated bilaterally in the *caudal ventrolateral medulla* (CVLM). Stimulation of neurons forming the depressor area produces decrease in the sympathetic activity due to inhibition of the tonically discharging impulses of the pressor area causing:

- *Arteriolar dilation* which decreases systemic blood pressure,
- *Venodilatation* which increases storage of blood in venous reservoir and decreases venous return and cardiac output,
- *Decrease in the heart rate* or negative chronotropic effect and
- *Decrease in force of contraction* or negative inotropic effect.

2. Medullary Parasympathetic Centre

Medullary parasympathetic centre or *cardiac vagal centre* (earlier also called cardioinhibitory centre) is now called by its specific name, i.e. the *nucleus ambiguus.* It is located lateral to the medullary reticular formation (the neurons located in this centre are not tonically active). Nucleus ambiguus receives afferents via nucleus tractus solitarius (NTS) and in turn sends inhibitory pathway in the form of vagal fibres to: *heart* to decrease heart rate and force of cardiac contraction.

3. Medullary Relay Station for Cardio-Respiratory Afferents

NTS of the vagus nerve forms the so-called medullary relay station for cardiorespiratory afferents. It receives afferents from most of the baroreceptors and chemoreceptors. The afferents release the excitatory neurotransmitter glutamate. Cells of the NTS, in turn, relay the information to VMC and cardiac vagal centre (nucleus ambiguus) that control sympathetic and parasympathetic outputs, respectively.

Autonomic Nerve Supply to Heart and Blood Vessels

Autonomic Nerve Supply to Heart

Sympathetic Supply

Spinal sympathetic centre is formed by the neurons located in the intermediolateral (IML) horns of the spinal cord extending from T_1 to L_2 spinal segments.

The IML cells are neurons from which the sympathetic fibres actually originate,

- ***Preganglionic sympathetic fibres*** (small, myelinated) supplying the heart arise from the neurons lying in the IML horns of the T_1 to T_5-*spinal segments* and pass into the sympathetic trunk to superior, middle and inferior cervical ganglia and upper thoracic ganglia where they synapse (Fig. 4.5-2).
- ***Postganglionic fibres*** (long, unmyelinated) leave the ganglia and pass via superior, middle and inferior *cardiac sympathetic nerves* and supply to nodal tissues (SA node and AV node) and cardiac muscles (of atria and ventricles Fig.4.5-2). It is important to note that:
  - Sympathetics from right side are primarily distributed to SA node.
  - Sympathetics from left side are primarily distributed to AV node.

Stimulation of cardiac sympathetic nerves causes:

- *Increased heart rate* (positive chronotropic effect) by increasing rhythmicity of SA node see page 252,
- *Increase in the conduction of impulse* through heart (positive dromotropic action see page 252),
- *Increase in the excitability* of myocardium (positive bathmotropic effect), and
- *Increase in the force of contraction* of myocardium (positive inotropic effect see page 252).

Parasympathetic Supply Parasympathetic fibres to the heart are carried through two vagii (Fig. 4.5-3).

- ***Preganglionic fibres*** (long, myelinated) arise from the *nucleus ambiguous* located in the medulla and travel along the vagii to reach the heart through their cardiac branches to synapse in the *ganglia* located within the superficial and deep cardiac plexuses and also in the walls of atria.
- ***Postganglionic fibres*** (small, unmyelinated) are distributed to the atria, SA node, AV node and AV bundle. It is important to note that:
  - The right vagus is distributed mainly to SA node,
  - The left vagus is distributed mainly to AV node,
  - No vagal motor fibres are distributed to the ventricles,
  - Parasympathetic fibres to the heart are *endocardiac.*

Stimulation of parasympathic fibres to heart causes:

- *Decrease in heart rate* by decreasing rate of impulse generation by SA node (negative chronotropic effect). For details see page 251.
- *Decrease in conduction of impulse* through the conduction tissue (negative dromotropic effect).
- *Decrease in the excitability of atria* only (negative bathmotropic effect) see page 251.
- *Decrease in the force of contraction* of atria only (negative inotropic effect). There is no effect on force of contraction of ventricles.

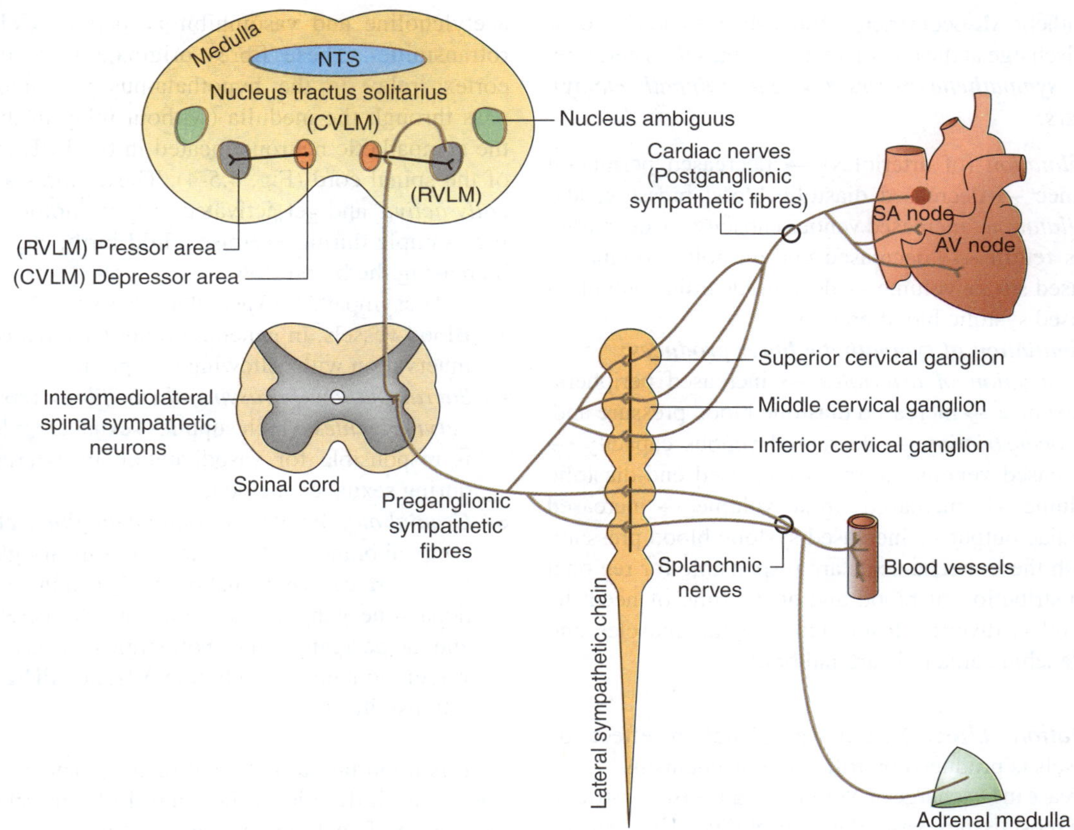

FIGURE 4.5-2 Sympathetic innervation to heart and blood vessels.

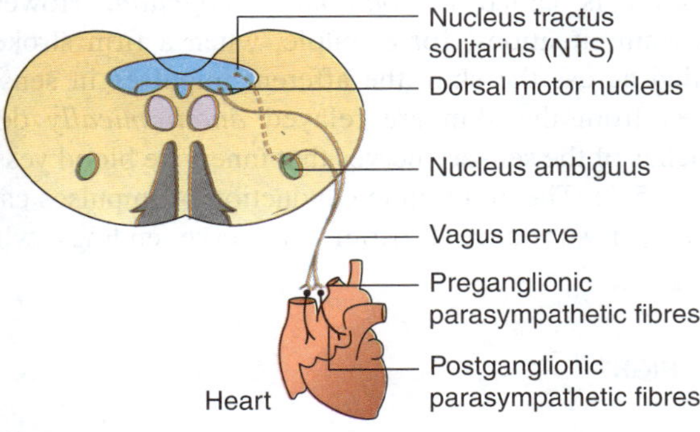

FIGURE 4.5-3 Parasympathetic innervation of the heart.

Vagal Tone. There is a moderate amount of tonic discharge in the cardiac sympathetic nerves at rest, but there is a good deal of tonic vagal discharge, called the *vagal tone,* in humans and other large animals. Therefore, when vagii are cut in the experimental animals, the heart rate rises. Similarly, in adult humans the resting heart rate which is about 72 beats/min rises to 150–180 beats/min after the administration of vagolytic drugs such as atropine, because of the unopposed sympathetic tone. When both adrenergic and cholinergic systems are blocked in humans, the heart rate is approximately 100 beats/min. Since the resting heart rate is about 72/min, it confirms that at rest, the vagal tone is greater than the sympathetic tone (see page 251).

Autonomic Nerve Supply to Blood Vessels

The autonomic efferents supplying the blood vessels produce two types of effects:

- Vasoconstriction and
- Vasodilatation.

Vasoconstriction Effect Vasoconstriction effect is produced by the sympathetic fibres supplying the blood vessels which originate from the IML horns in T_1 to L_2 spinal segments.

Vasoconstrictor fibres have norepinephrine and sometimes neuropeptide Y as neurotransmitter and are called *noradrenergic fibres.*

These noradrenergic fibres innervate all the blood vessels of the body except the *true capillaries* and cerebral regional circulation. The small arteries and arterioles are more richly innervated as compared to large vessels. Furthermore, arterioles of skin, skeletal muscles and splanchnic arterioles have more supply as compared to those of brain and myocardium.

Sympathetic vasoconstrictor fibres show tonic (i.e. continuous) discharge at the rate of about 1 impulse/s. Therefore, ***when the sympathetic nerves are cut (sympathectomy), there occurs:***

- *Vasodilatation* (of arterioles) → decreased peripheral resistance → decreased diastolic blood pressure, and *Venodilatation*– increased venous capacity → decreased venous return → decreased end-diastolic volume → decreased stroke volume → decreasedcardiac output → decreased systolic blood pressure.

Stimulation of sympathetic fibres produces:

- *Constriction of arterioles* → increased peripheral resistance → increased diastolic blood pressure and
- *Venoconstriction* → decreased venous capacity → increased venous return → increased end-diastolic volume → increased stroke volume → increased cardiac output → increased systolic blood pressure. Both these mechanisms are responsible for regional redistribution of blood and at the time of need the blood is diverted from skin, skeletal muscles and splanchnic area to heart and brain.

Vasodilatation Effect Neural vasodilatation effect on blood vessels is produced by following mechanisms:

1. Decrease in Discharge of Noradrenergic Vasoconstrictor Nerves. In most tissues, vasodilation is produced by decreasing the rate of tonic discharge in the vasoconstrictor nerves. When the blood pressure is increased, the increased carotid sinus nerve activity causes central reflexes that inhibit vasoconstriction (producing vasodilation) and tonic effect on heart (producing bradycardia).

2. Sympathetic Cholinergic Vasodilator Nerves. Some of the organs of the body such as skeletal muscles, heart, lungs, liver, kidney and uterus in addition to adrenergic vasoconstrictor sympathetic fibres also receive innervation by *cholinergic vasodilator sympathetic* fibres having acetylcholine and vasoinhibitory peptide (VIP) as neurotransmitter. These fibres originate from the cerebral cortex, relay in the hypothalamus and midbrain, and pass through the medulla (without relay in the VMC) to the sympathetic neurons located in the IML grey column of the spinal cord (Fig. 4.5-4). These fibres are not *tonically active,* and get activated only in biological stresses, for example during exercise, child birth, etc. and help in increasing the blood flow.

3. Parasympathetic Vasodilator Nerves.

- Blood vessels, in general, do not have parasympathetic innervation with following exceptions:
- *Sacral outflow parasympathetic fibres* represented by *nervi erigentes* which supplies sexual erectile tissue and is responsible for vasodilatation in external genitalia during sexual excitement.
- *Cranial outflow of parasympathetic fibres* along chorda tympani branch of facial nerve to salivary glands.
- *Cholinergic neurons* that probably originate in the sphenopalatine ganglia also innervate the cerebral vessels and the postganglionic cholinergic neurons on the blood vessels contain acetylcholine, VIP, and PHM- 27 as neurotransmitters.

It is important to note that parasympathetic vasodilator fibres play little role in the control of general circulation. Activation of such nerves only contributes to pleasure and fulfilling important biological functions.

4. Vasodilation by Axon Reflex. Conduction of normal sensory afferent impulses from the skin to spinal cord is called *orthodromic conduction*. However, in certain situations, for example, when a firm stroke is applied across the skin, the afferent impulses in sensory nerves from the skin are relayed *antidromically* down branches of the sensory nerves that innervate blood vessels (Fig. 4.5-5). The antidromic conduction of impulses cause release of substance P from the nerve endings which

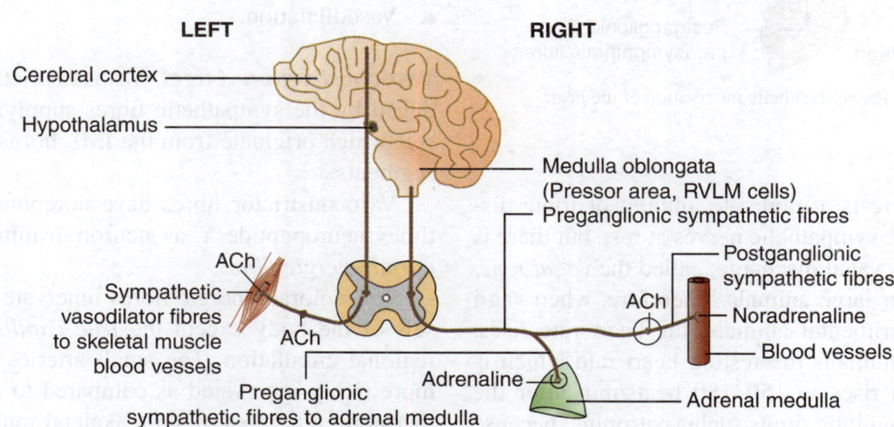

FIGURE 4.5-4 Pathway of sympathetic vasodilator fibres (on left side), and sympathetic vasoconstrictor system (on right side).

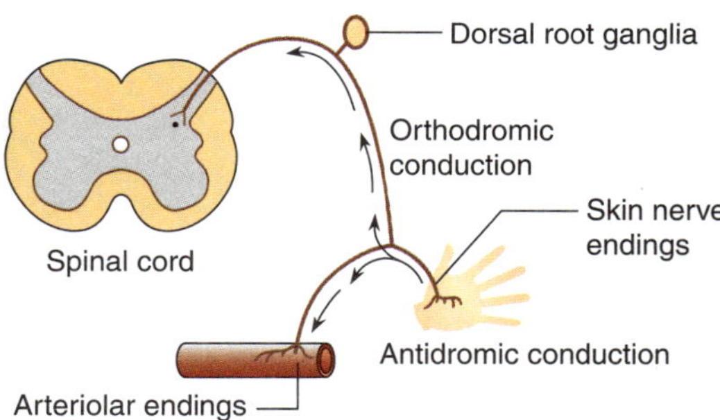

FIGURE 4.5-5 Pathway of axon reflex.

produces vasodilation and increases capillary permeability. This local neural mechanism (which does not involve the CNS) is called *axon reflex*. It is responsible for local vasodilation and does not contribute in the systemic control of circulation.

Afferent Impulses to Medullary Cardiovascular Control Centres

The medullary control centres are influenced by afferent control impulses from the higher centres and a large number of other areas (Fig. 4.5-6). These include:

- Afferent impulses from higher centres controlling VMC,
- Afferent impulses from respiratory centres,
- Cardiovascular reflex mechanisms operating through medullary control centres
  - Baroreceptor reflex,
  - Chemoreceptor reflexes,
- Direct effects on vasomotor area
  - Central nervous system ischaemic response,
  - Cushing reflex,
- Afferents from nociceptive stimuli.

Afferent Impulses from Higher Centres Controlling Vasomotor Centre and Cardiacvagal Centre

Cerebral Cortex

Stimulation of various areas of motor cortex leads to complex motor responses that include appropriate cardiovascular adjustments. There are descending tracts to the vasomotor area from cerebral cortex (particularly the limbic cortex) that relay in the hypothalamus. Some examples of the influence of limbic system on the VMC are:

- *Tachycardia and hypertension* produced by emotions such as sexual excitement and anger,
- *Bradycardia and fainting* occurring during sudden emotional shock,
- *Fight or flight response* is a complex set of responses which increases cardiac output and raises blood pressure in anticipation of flight or physical defence.

Hypothalamus

The connections between the hypothalamus and vasomotor area are reciprocal, with afferents from the brainstem closing the loop. The hypothalamus serves to integrate many somatic and autonomic responses. Examples are:

- *Temperature regulation.* The effect of temperature changes on the hypothalamic centres are relayed to the medulla, which causes the vessels of skin to constrict (heat conservation) or to dilate (heat dissipation).
- *Emotional stresses* influence the heart rate and blood pressure by impulses relayed from hypothalamus to stimulate or inhibit the medullary centres.

Reticular Formation

Reticular formation of pons, mesencephalon and diencephalon also influences the vasomotor area, for example:

- Pain usually causes rise in blood pressure via afferent impulses in the reticular formation converging on the vasomotor area. However, prolonged severe pain may cause vasodilation and fainting.

Afferent Impulses from Respiratory Centres

Impulses arising from the respiratory centres affect the heart rate by changing the vagal tone and the alterations produced are known as *sinus arrhythmia* which occurs during forced breathing. Sinus arrhythmia is common in some children and in some adults even during quiet breathing.

- *During inspiration,* the impulses arising from the respiratory centres during inspiration inhibit the cardiac vagal centre causing reduced vagal tone and *sinus tachycardia.*
- *During expiration,* the respiratory centres stop sending inhibitory impulses to the cardiac vagal centre causing increased vagal tone and sinus bradycardia.

Cardiovascular Reflex Mechanisms Affecting Medullary Control Centres

Cardiovascular reflex mechanisms are multiple subconscious special nervous control mechanisms that operate through medullary control centres all the time to maintain the arterial pressure within the normal range. Almost all of these are *negative feedback reflex mechanisms* and include:

- Baroreceptor reflex mechanisms and
- Chemoreceptor reflex mechanism.

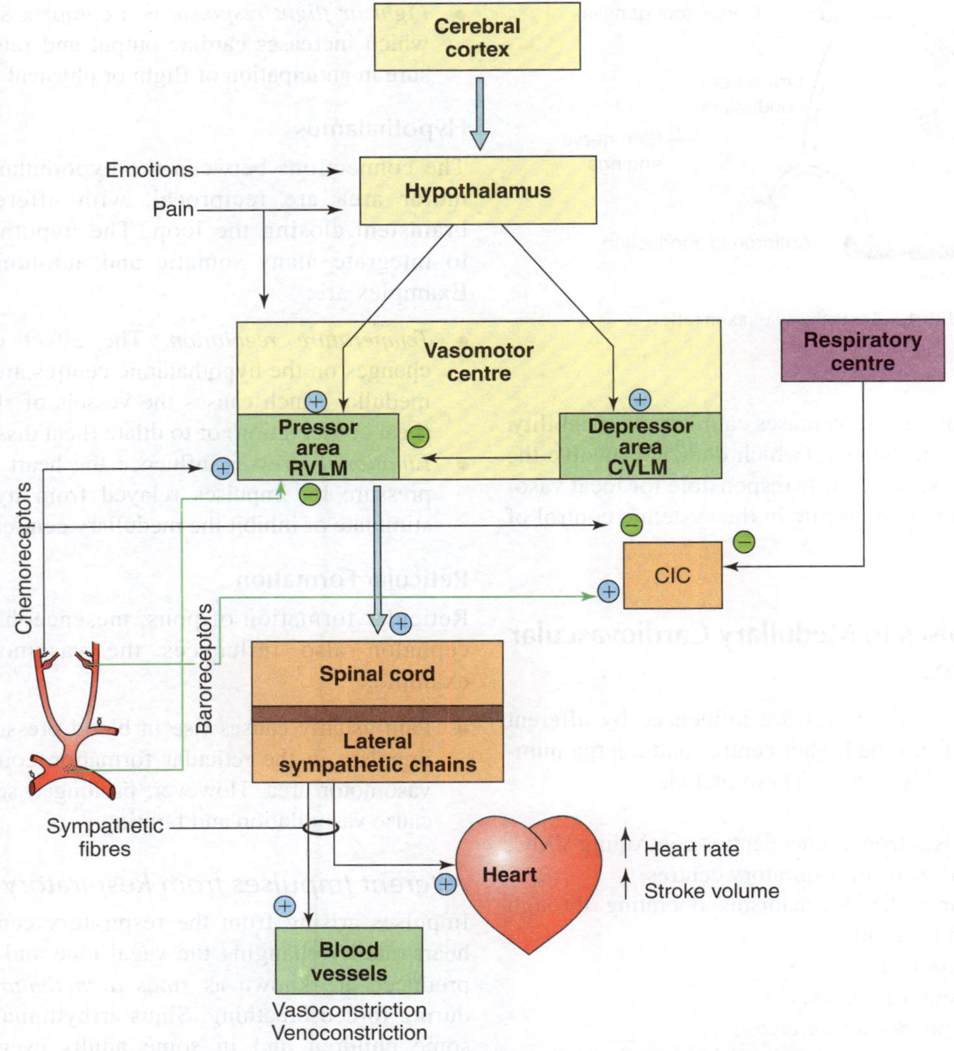

FIGURE 4.5-6 Scheme to show afferent impulses affecting medullary cardiovascular control centres.

Baroreceptor Reflex Mechanisms

Baroreceptors also known as mechanoreceptors or pressure receptors and are the stretch receptors located in the walls of heart and large blood vessels. These are spray type nerve endings, i.e. they are extensively branched, knobby, coiled and intertwined ends of myelinated nerve fibres that resemble golgi tendon organs. These are stimulated by distension of the structures in which they are located, and so they discharge at an increased rate when the pressure in these structures rises. The increased baroreceptor discharge leads to *inhibition* of tonic discharge of vasoconstrictor nerves and *excitation* of vagal innervation of heart and thereby produces: vasodilation, venodilation, bradycardia, decrease in cardiac output and decrease in blood pressure.

With this definition of baroreceptor reflex mechanism, the baroreceptors will be discussed in detail as under following headings:

Classification and Location of Baroreceptors

Functional Classification Functionally, baroreceptors can be grouped as:

1. ***High-pressure baroreceptors,*** which monitor the arterial circulation. These include the baroreceptors located at:
   - Carotid sinus,
   - Aortic arch,
   - Wall of left ventricle,
   - Root of right subclavian artery and
   - Junction of the thyroid artery with common carotid artery.
2. ***Low-pressure baroreceptors*** are located in the low-pressure area of circulation and are collectively referred to as *cardiopulmonary receptors.* These include:
   - Atrial receptors scattered in the wall of right and left atrium.

- Baroreceptors located in the right atrium at the entrance of the superior and inferior vena cave and in the left atrium at the entrance of pulmonary veins.
- Pulmonary receptors located in the wall of pulmonary trunk and its divisions into right and left pulmonary artery.

Anatomical Classification Anatomically, baroreceptors can be grouped as:

1. ***Arterial baroreceptors,*** which are located in the walls of the arteries, distributed mainly in adventitial layer. These can be further divided into two groups:
   - i. *Systemic arterial baroreceptors* which include the following and these are located at:
     - Carotid sinus,
     - Aortic arch,
     - Root of right subclavian artery and
     - Junction of thyroid artery and common carotid artery.
   - ii. *Pulmonary baroreceptors,* which are located in the wall of pulmonary trunk and its divisions into right and left pulmonary artery.
2. ***Cardiac baroreceptors*** are located in the walls of heart subendocardially and can be divided into atrial and ventricular receptors which include:
   - i. *Atrial receptors*
     - Atrial stretch receptors with nonmyelinated afferent fibres which are scattered throughout the wall of atria and interatrial septum.
     - *Pulmonary venoatrial receptors,* which are located in the left atrium just at the entrance of pulmonary veins.
   - ii. *Ventricular receptors,* which are scattered throughout the left ventricle and interventricular septum.

Carotid and Aortic Arch Baroreceptors

Location of Carotid and Aortic Arch Baroreceptors

- ***Carotid baroreceptors*** are located in carotid sinus which is a small dilatation of the internal carotid artery just above the bifurcation of the common carotid artery into external and internal carotid branches (Fig. 4.5-7).
- ***Aortic arch baroreceptors*** are located in the wall of arch of aorta (Fig. 4.5-7).
- ***Other systemic arterial baroreceptors*** (similar to carotid and aortic baroreceptors) are also found at the root of right subclavian artery and junction of thyroid artery and in the common carotid artery.

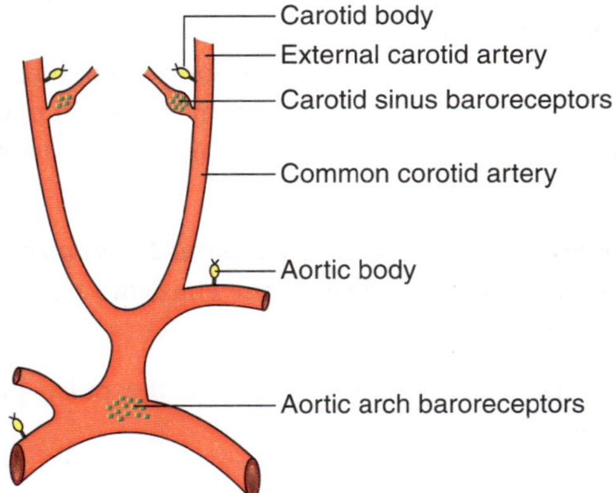

FIGURE 4.5-7 Location of baroreceptors (carotid sinus and aortic arch) and chemorecepters (carotid bodies and aortic bodies.

Innervation of Baroreceptors (Fig. 4.5-8)

- ***Carotid sinus baroreceptors*** are innervated by carotid sinus nerve (Hering's nerve) which is a branch of glossopharyngeal nerve.
- ***All other baroreceptors*** are supplied by the vagus nerve.
- ***Afferent fibres*** from the baroreceptors pass via the glossopharyngeal and vagus nerves to the medulla. Most of them end in the nucleus of the tractus solitarius (NTS), where they secrete an excitatory transmitter, presumably, glutamate.
- ***Buffer nerves.*** The carotid sinus nerve and vagal fibres from the carotid sinus and aortic arch baroreceptors, respectively, are commonly called buffer nerves, as these are involved in buffering the blood pressure, i.e. preventing sudden rise and fall in blood pressure.
- ***Projections from NTS*** (excitatory glutaminergic projections) terminate on to the:

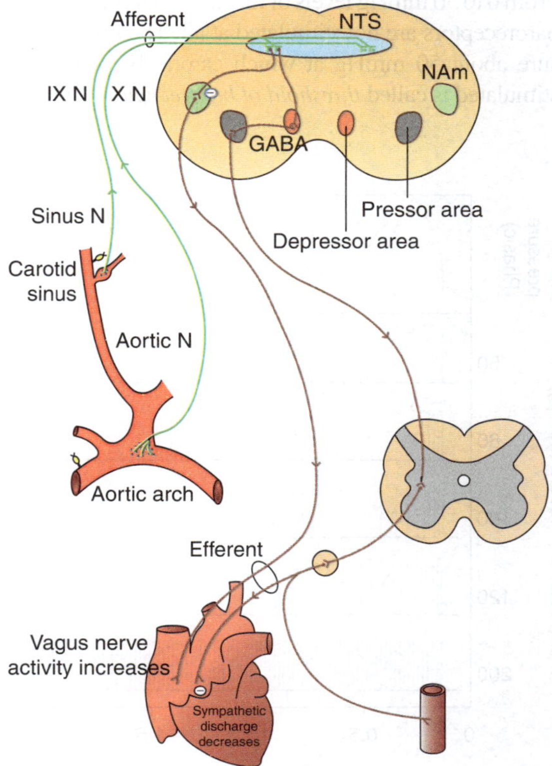

FIGURE 4.5-8 Neural pathway of baroreceptor reflex.

- *Depressor area of VMC (CVLM),* where they stimulate GABA, secreting inhibitory neurons, which produce decrease in the sympathetic activity by inhibiting the tonically discharging impulses from the pressor area of VMC, and *sympathetic preganglionic neurons* of spinal cord and to decrease sympathetic activity, and
- *Cardiac vagal centre* (nucleus ambiguus), after receiving the impulses from NTS, *sends inhibitory* pathway along the vagus nerve to:
- *Heart* through cardiac branches of the vagus nerve to decrease heart rate and force of contraction.

Response of Carotid and Aortic Baroreceptors to Pressure Response from carotid baroreceptors has been studied in detail and that from aortic receptors has not been studied in such great deal. However, there is no reason to believe that responses of aortic receptors differ significantly from those of the carotid receptors. Salient features of these receptor responses to pressure are:

Baroreceptor Response. At normal blood pressure levels, the fibres of the buffer nerves discharge at a low rate which increases when the pressure in the carotid sinus and aortic arch rises, and declines when the pressure falls (Figs 4.5-9 and 4.5-10).

The Effect of Different Arterial Pressure Levels on the Discharge Rate in carotid sinus nerve shown in Figure 4.5-10 depicts that:

- From 0 to 50 mmHg levels of mean arterial pressure, carotid baroreceptors are not stimulated at all. The minimum pressure about 50 mmHg at which carotid baroreceptors are stimulated is called *threshold of baroreceptor reflex.*

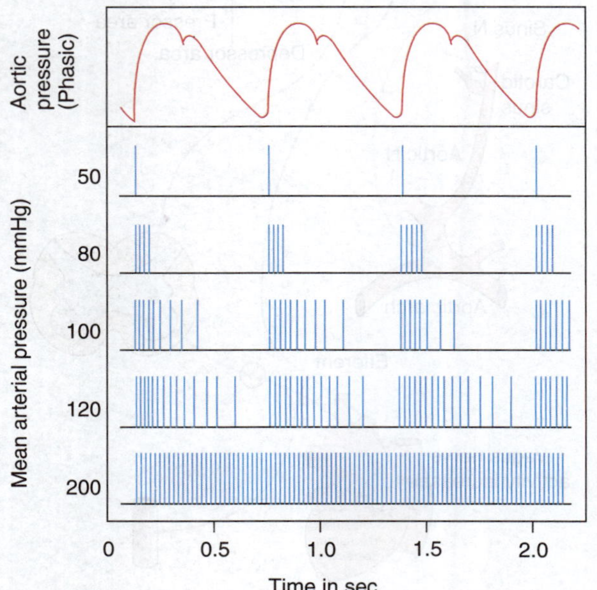

FIGURE 4.5-9 Discharges (vertical lines) in a single afferent nerve fibre from carotid sinus at various levels of mean arterial pressure, plotted against changes in aortic pressure with time.

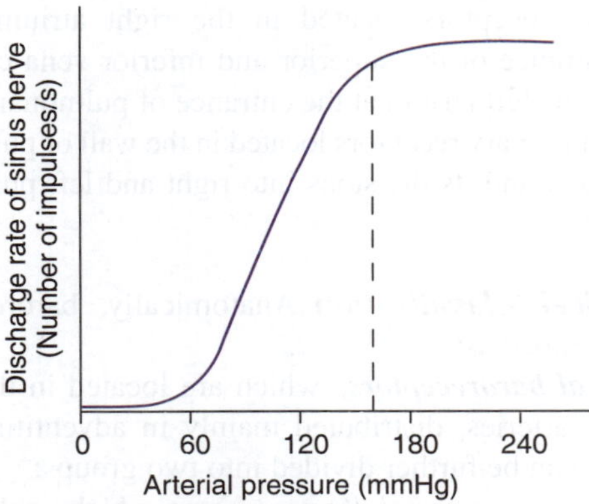

FIGURE 4.5-10 Response of carotid baroreceptors at different levels of arterial pressure.

- Above threshold level the baroreceptors respond progressively more rapidly till the discharge rate reaches a *plateau,* at 180–200mmHg, i.e. there is no further increase in response. Thus, the carotid baroreceptors exhibit a great sensitivity as they respond to pressure that vary from approximately 50–200 mmHg.
- In the normal operating rate at 95–100 mmHg, even a slight change in pressure causes a strong change in the baroreceptor reflex signals to readjust the arterial pressure back towards the normal. Thus, the baroreceptor feedback mechanism functions most effectively in the pressure range where it is most needed.
- When pressure decreases below normal levels the baroreceptor discharge decreases and reflexly brings the pressure to normal. Conversely, when pressure increases above normal the baroreceptor discharge also increases and reflexly brings the pressure to normal. The effect of carotid receptors response to change in arterial pressure can be demonstrated experimentally as:
  - *Bilateral occlusion of common carotid arteries at their origin* reduces the carotid sinus pressure, as a result the carotid baroreceptors become inactive and lose their inhibitory effect on the VMC and the blood pressure is raised. Because aortic and cardiac baroreceptors respond to raised pressure so the occlusion of both carotid arteries cause only a moderate pressure response. When the common carotid occlusion is removed the arterial pressure returns to normal (Fig. 4.5-11).

The Carotid Baroreceptors Respond Both to the Mean Pressure and the Pulse Pressure. Thus, the baroreceptor discharge would increase:

- When the mean pressure rises and the pulse pressure remains unchanged or
- When the pulse pressure rises and the mean pressure remains unchanged.

Carotid Baroreceptors Respond Much More to a Rapidly Changing Pressure than to a stationary pressure, i.e. if the mean arterial pressure is 150 mmHg and at that

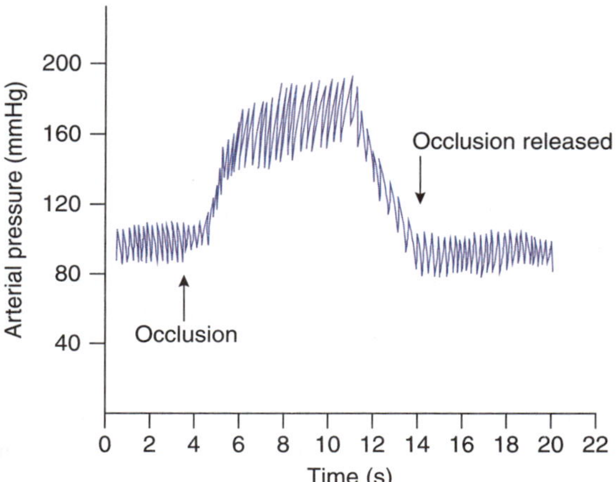

FIGURE 4.5-11 Effect of occlusion of both common carotid arteries on arterial pressure in dog.

moment is rising rapidly, the rate of impulse transmission may be as much as twice than that when the pressure is stationary at 150 mmHg. Conversely, if the pressure is falling, the rate might be as little as one quarter that for the stationary pressure.

Pressure-Buffer System of Baroreceptors. From the above description, it is clear that baroreceptor system opposes both increase as well as decrease in arterial pressure. Therefore, it is called a *pressure-buffer system,* and the nerves from the baroreceptors are called buffer nerves. The role of the pressure-buffer system of baroreceptors can be demonstrated experimentally by bilateral denervation of carotid and aortic baroreceptors.

- The arterial pressure recording for 2 hours from a dog where bilateral buffer nerves have been cut shows extreme variability of the pressure caused by simple routine events such as lying down, standing, excitement, eating and defecation (Fig. 4.5-12B), which are absent in the normal dog with intact innervation (Fig. 4.5-12A).
- The frequency distribution curve of mean arterial pressure recorded for 24 h from a normal dog shows that during most of the day with all routine activities the arterial pressure wave maintained at 95–105 mmHg (Fig. 4.5.13A); while that from a dog where baroreceptors have been denervated shows that the arterial pressure varied extremely from 50 to 160 mmHg (Fig. 4.5-13B).
- From the above experiment it can be confirmed that baroreceptors serve as *pressure-buffer system* and reduce the minute by minute variation in the arterial pressure occurring with daily routine activities.

Baroreceptors Resetting. Baroreceptors posess a property to reset themselves in 1–2 days to whatever pressure they are exposed. Therefore, in chronic hypertension the baroreceptor reflex mechanism resets to maintain an elevated rather than a normal arterial pressure. This fact can be demonstrated by perfusion studies on hypertensive experimental animals

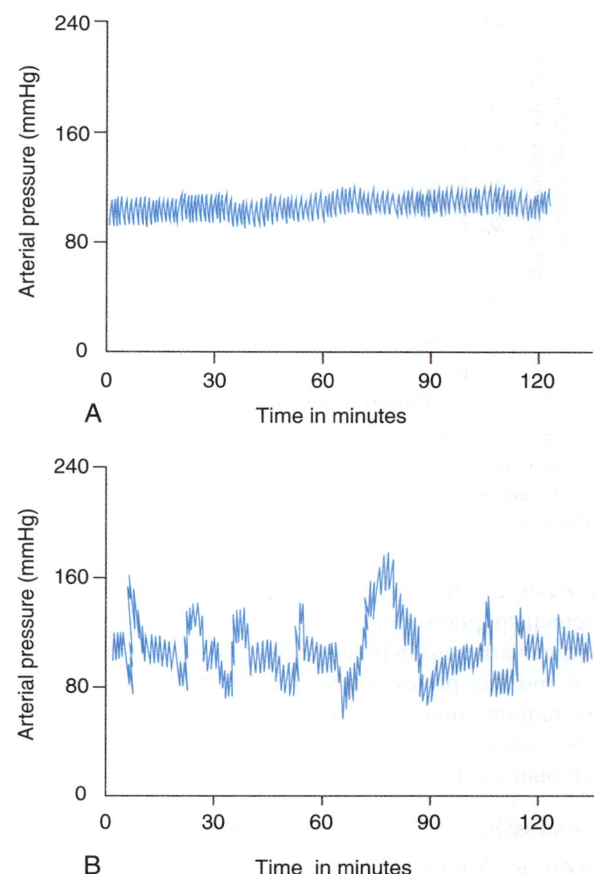

FIGURE 4.5-12 **(A)** Two-hour record of arterial pressure in a normal dog with intact innervation, and **(B)** in same dog after several weeks after denervation of baroreceptors.

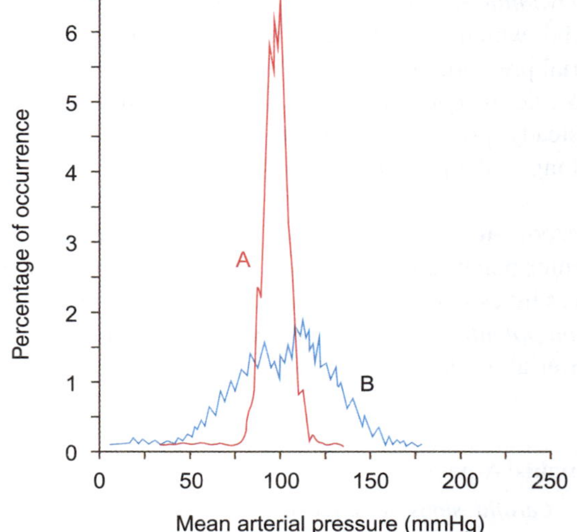

FIGURE 4.5-13 Frequency distribution curve of the arterial pressure for 24-hour period: **(A)** in a normal dog; and **(B)** in the same dog several weeks after denervation of baroreceptors.

(Fig. 4.5-14). Little is known about how and why this occurs, but resetting occurs rapidly in experimental animals. It is also rapidly reversible, both in experimental animals and in clinical situations. Because of this property the *baroreceptor system has no role to play for long-term regulation of*

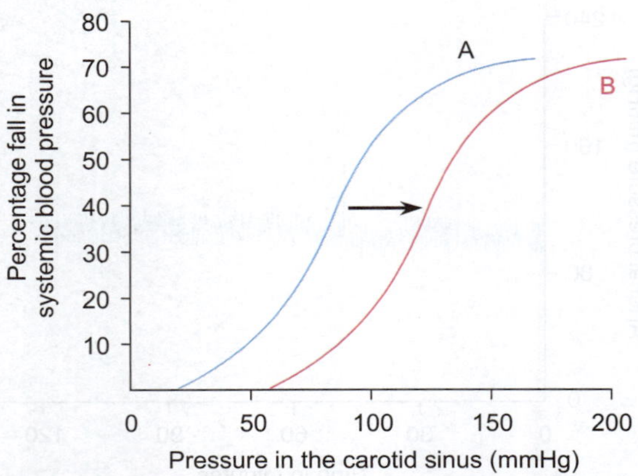

FIGURE 4.5-14 Percentage fall in systemic blood pressure produced by raising the pressure in the isolated carotid sinus: **(A)** in a normal monkey; and **(B)** in a hypertensive monkey. Note the graph obtained is similar (due to resetting of baroreceptors to raised pressure).

the mean arterial pressure. Thus, the baroreceptor reflex mechanism plays important role only in preventing the extreme variations in blood pressure which occur for a short term and that prolonged regulation of mean arterial pressure requires other control system, principally, the *renal-body fluid-pressure control system* along with its associated hormonal mechanisms (see page 330).

Transmission of Baroreceptors Response

Receptor Potential. The systemic arterial baroreceptors generate a receptor potential in response to pressure induced distension of the vascular walls. The receptor potential so generated has two components:

- *Dynamic receptor response* is the initial receptor potential, which is proportional to the rate of change in arterial pressure.
- *Static receptor response* is proportional to the new steady pressure and continues without adaptation as long as the pressure is maintained.

Afferent Action Potentials (APs) are generated by the receptor potentials and are carried over the sinus and aortic nerves in response to increasing arterial blood pressure. The *action potential frequency* is linearly related to the increase in arterial pressure over a wide range.

> **Applied Aspects**
>
> ***Carotid sinus massage*** is used clinically to interrupt paroxysmal atrial tachycardia by inducing a vagally mediated slowing of the heart.
>
> ***Stokes-Adams syndrome*** refers to an increased sensitivity of the carotid sinus seen in some elderly individuals who experience syncope as a result of vagally mediated sinus arrest, which causes a prolonged period of ventricular systole.

Effect of Carotid Clamping and Bilateral Vagotomy

- Bilateral clamping of the carotid arteries proximal to the carotid sinus lowers the pressure in the sinuses which is followed by a decline in dischage rate from the carotid baroreceptors leading to rise in blood pressure and heart rate.
- When along with bilateral occlusion of the common carotid arteries, bilateral vagotomy is also performed, the blood pressure rises to 300/200 mmHg or higher and is unstable.
- Bilateral destruction of nucleus of tractus solitarius (NTS), the site of termination of the baroreceptor afferents, also causes a marked pressure response producing severe hypertension which can be even fatal.
- These forms of experimentally induced hypertension due to neurogenic lesions are called *neurogenic hypertension.*

Cardiac Baroreceptors

Cardiac baroreceptors are located in the walls of heart subendocardially. All cardiac receptors are innervated by vagus nerve. These include:

- Atrial stretch receptors, and
- Ventricular receptors.

Atrial Stretch Receptors Atrial stretch receptors present in the walls of atria are also called *low-pressure receptors.*

Types of atrial stretch receptors. Atrial stretch receptors have been studied in detail by Prof AS Paintal (an Indian Scientist) in 1953. These can be divided into following types:

1. Atrial Stretch Receptors with Large Myelinated Afferent Fibres. These receptors are located at the various *venoatrial junctions* and depending upon their location are named as:

- *Atriocaval receptors,* which are located in the right atrium just at the entrance of superior and inferior vena cavae.
- *Pulmonaryvenoatrial receptors,* which are located in the left atrium just at the entrance of pulmonary vein.

Depending upon the discharge pattern, the atrial stretch receptors with large myelinated afferents fibres are of three types:

i. ***Type A receptors*** discharge during atrial systole only and their impulse activity occurs in the PR interval of the electrocardiogram (Fig. 4.5-15).
ii. ***Type B receptors*** discharge in the later part of atrial diastole when the atria are distended with blood. That is, these receptors discharge just before the onset of atrial contraction and reach peak after T-wave of the electrocardiogram (Fig. 4.5-15). Type B receptor discharge increases when the venous return is increased.

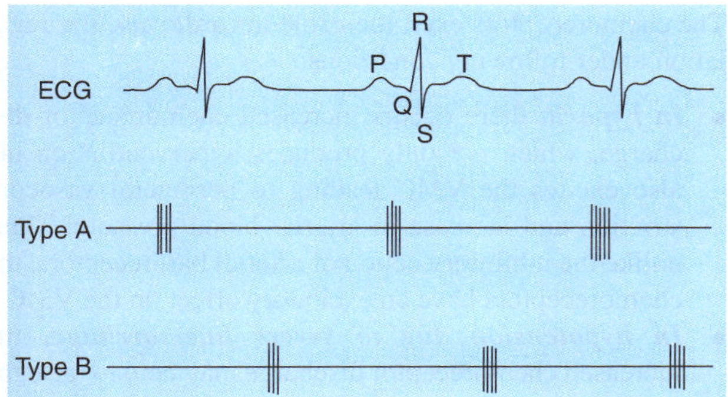

FIGURE 4.5-15 Discharge pattern of type - A, and type- B atrial stretch receptors as recorded from vagus nerve and their correlation with electrocardiogram recording.

iii. ***Intermediate type of receptors*** discharge both during atrial systole as well as diastole. Therefore, there discharge pattern is characterized by type A receptors discharge followed by type B receptors discharge.

2. Atrial Stretch Receptors with Non-myelinated Afferent Fibres. These receptors are scattered throughout the atria and the interatrial septum. Their discharge is sparse (1 impulse/sec) and irregular.

Role of Atrial Stretch Receptors. The atrial stretch receptors have been associated with following roles in the cardiovascular control:

1. As Low-pressure Receptors. the atrial stretch receptors (especially type B receptors) along with pulmonary receptors play an important role to minimize arterial pressure changes in response to change in blood volume. For example, when about 300 ml of blood is suddenly infused into a dog with all the receptors intact, the arterial pressure rises only by about 15 mmHg. With the *systemic arterial baroreceptors* denervated, the pressure rises by about 40 mmHg. If the *low-pressure receptors* are also denervated, the pressure rises by about 100 mmHg. From these observations it is quite clear that even though the low-pressure receptors cannot detect the systemic arterial pressure, they do detect simultaneous increase in pressure in the low-pressure area of circulation caused by increase in volume, and they elicit reflexes parallel to the baroreceptor reflexes to make the total reflex system much more potent for control of arterial pressure. In other words, the atrial stretch receptors provide information about the circulating blood volume, i.e. greater the venous return, greater will be the discharge from the receptor fibres.

2. Atrial Reflex Control of Heart Rate (Bainbridge Reflex). Bainbridge noted that sudden rise in atrial pressure after rapid infusion of saline or blood in anaesthetised animals produced tachycardia, if the initial heart rate was low. This effect is known as Bainbridge reflex. Atrial stretch receptors of both the sides may be responsible for this reflex. The afferent signals from these receptors pass through the vagus nerves to the medulla of brain. The efferent signals are transmitted back through both the vagal and the sympathetic nerves to increase the heart rate and force of contraction. Thus, this reflex helps to prevent damming of blood in the veins, atria and pulmonary circulation. This reflex has a different purpose from that of controlling arterial pressure.

3. Atrial Reflex Control of Blood Volume (Volume Reflex). when there is volume overload the atrial stretch receptors help to return the blood volume back towards normal by following mechanisms, which collectively are called volume reflex:

1. Stretch of the atria causes very significant reflex dilatation of the afferent arterioles in the kidney leading to rise in glomerular capillary pressure, with resultant increase in filtration of fluid into the kidney tubules.
2. *Stretch of the atria also transmits signals to the hypothalamus* to decrease the secretion of antidiuretic hormone (ADH), which diminishes the reabsorption of water from tubules (see page 520).

   The mechanisms (1) and (2) reduce the increased blood volume back toward normal.
3. Stretch of the atria also causes release of a chemical called *atrial natriuretic peptide* (ANP) which causes powerful diuresis and thus adds still further to the loss of fluid in the urine and return of blood volume back to normal. For details see page 535.

The above described mechanisms (1, 2 and 3) which combined constitute volume reflex, act as volume controller and thus indirectly act as *pressure controller* as well. Because excess volume increases the cardiac output and thus the arterial pressure as well.

Ventricular Receptors The ventricular baroreceptors are scattered throughout the left ventricle and interventricular septum. They discharge irregularly. These receptors exhibit following responses:

• ***Response to Increased Left Ventricular Pressure.*** When the left ventricle is distended in experimental animals, there occurs bradycardia and hypotension. The distension required to produce these effects is so high that no physiological significance can be attached to these receptors. However, left ventricular stretch receptors may play a role in the maintenance of the vagal tone that keep the heart rate low at rest.

• ***Bezold-Jarisch Reflex or Coronary Chemoreflex*** refers to reflex apnoea followed by rapid breathing, hypotension and bradycardia which occur following injection of certain drugs like capsaicin, phenylguanide, serotonin, veratidine or nicotine into the coronary arteries supplying the left ventricle (injection into the right coronary artery is ineffective) in experimental animals. This reflex is probably produced by the chemical stimulation of left ventricular stretch receptors. The receptors are probably C fibre endings, and the afferents are vagal. A similar response is produced by stimulation of C fibre endings in the lungs (pulmonary chemoreceptors).The reflex has been named after the person who first reported this response pattern.

- *Physiological significance of* this reflex is uncertain, but it has been speculated that the persistent hypotension in some patients of acute myocardial infarction may be due to stimulation of ventricular receptors by substances released from the necrotic cardiac tissue.
- Defense against chemical toxic pollutants and temperature is also provided by activation of cardiopulmonary reflexes.
- Vasovagal syncope, i.e. syndrome of cardiac slowing and hypertension has also been attributed to activation of this reflex.

Pulmonary Baroreceptors

Pulmonary baroreceptors are located in the walls of pulmonary trunk and its divisions, the right and left pulmonary artery. The pulmonary receptors along with atrial receptors constitute the so-called *low-pressure receptors or cardiopulmonary receptors* and play an important role to minimize arterial pressure changes in response to change in blood volume as discussed above (see page 345).

Role of Chemoreceptor Reflexes in Cardiovascular Control

Chemoreceptors are chemosensitive cells that respond to following changes in blood:

- Oxygen lack (decreased PO_2)
- Carbon dioxide excess (increased pCO_2) and
- hydrogen ion excess (decreased pH).

Location of Chemoreceptor. The peripheral chemoreceptors are present in (Fig. 4.5.7):

1. ***Carotid bodies.*** These are 1–2 mm in size and are located in the bifurcation of each common carotid artery. These are innervated by carotid sinus nerve which is a branch of glossopharygeal nerve.
2. ***Aortic bodies*** are one to three in number located adjacent to arch of aorta. These are innervated by aortic nerve (branch of vagus nerve).

Functions of Chemoreceptors

1. Respiratory Control. Chemoreceptors are primarily concerned with the regulation of pulmonary ventilation and are discussed in much more detail in Chapter 5.6 page 447.

2. Cardiovascular Control. In physiological conditions, i.e. in healthy individuals breathing normal air, there is very little discharge from the chemoreceptors and there is no contribution to the regulation of the cardio-vascular system. The chemoreceptors exert their role in cardiovascular regulation under following conditions:

- ***In hypoxia*** there occurs increased chemoreceptor discharge, which not only produces hyperventilation but also excites the VMC leading to peripheral vasoconstriction and increase in arterial blood pressure. Thus, unlike the inhibitory action of arterial baroreceptors, the chemoreceptors have an excitatory effect on the VMC.
- ***In hypotension due to severe haemorrhage,*** the increased chemoreceptor discharge may help to raise the arterial blood pressure. The role of chemoreceptors in severe hypotension can be demonstrated experimentally. Bilateral section of sinus and aortic nerves in animals which have been bled severely to produce hypotension, causes further fall in blood pressure. Since in such animals the baroreceptor discharge is already absent, the section of sinus and aortic nerves abolishes the chemoreceptor drive as well. Thus, further fall in blood pressure in such animals indicates that chemoreceptors were contributing to some extent to the maintenance of blood pressure.

Chemoreceptor discharge may contribute to *Mayer's waves.* Mayer waves are observed as slow, regular oscillations in arterial pressure recordings at the rate of about one/20–40 s, during hypotension (produced by haemorrhage in experimental animals). Hypoxia under these conditions stimulates chemoreceptors leading to rise in arterial pressure which improves the blood flow to chemoreceptors and therefore, there is an elimination of stimulus to the chemoreceptors. The BP again falls and a new cycle of chemoreceptor stimulation get activated and again rise in pressure.

NOTE. It is important to note that the chemoreceptor reflex is not a powerful arterial pressure controller in the normal arterial pressure range because the chemoreceptors themselves are not stimulated strongly until the arterial pressure falls below 60 mmHg. Therefore, it is at lower pressures that this reflex becomes important and help to prevent still further fall in pressure.

Important Note

Mayer waves should not be confused with Traube-Hering waves, which are fluctuations in blood pressure recordings synchronizing with phases of respiration. In early phase of inspiration inflation of lungs there is vasodilation and fall in blood pressure. This response is mediated via vagal afferents from the lungs that inhibit vasomotor discharge, but in later part of inspiration blood pressure increases due to increase in end diastolic pressure due to decrease in intra thoracic pressure and rise in intraabdominal pressure.

During expiration first there is rise and further fall in blood pressure occurs due to opposite effects.

Direct Effects on Vasomotor Area

The VMC is directly affected by locally produced hypoxia and hypercapnia. Examples of direct effects are central nervous system ischaemic response and Cushing reflex.

1. Central Nervous System Ischaemic Response

- When blood pressure falls below 60 mmHg, the blood flow to the vasomotor area in the brainstem is decreased enough to cause CNS ischaemia.
- As a result of CNS ischaemia, the CO_2/lactic acid are accumulated locally near the VMC and excite the neurons of VMC strongly.
- Excitation of VMC causes strong sympathetic stimulation leading to vasoconstriction. Peripheral vessels become totally occluded at certain areas, e.g. kidney. There occurs immediate increase in the blood pressure. This most powerful response that activates sympathetic vasoconstrictor system strongly is called *CNS ischaemic response.* This acts as an emergency arterial pressure control system. If rise of pressure does not relieve CNS ischaemia, neural cells begin to suffer and within 3–10 min become totally inactive.

2. Cushing Reflex When intracranial pressure is increased and becomes equal to the arterial pressure, it compresses the arteries in the brain and blood supply to the vasomotor area is compromised. The hypoxia and hypercapnia produced locally increase the discharge from VMC. The resultant rise in systemic pressure tends to restore the blood supply to medulla. This effect, which protects the vital centres in the brain is called *Cushing reflex.* The resultant increase in blood pressure also causes reflex bradycardia via baroreceptor response. Thus, bradycardia is an important feature of raised intracranial pressure.

Important Note

A rise in arterial pCO_2 activates RVLM, but direct peripheral effect of hypercapnia is vasodilation. The peripheral and direct effects of hypercapnia cancel each other, therefore there is little change in blood pressure, but exposure to high concentration of CO_2 causes vasodilation of cerebral (the effect is mediated via increase in H^+ concentration in the CSF) and vasoconstriction of splanchnic and cutaneous vessels through activation of peripheral chemoreceptors, hence there is slow rise in blood pressure.

Afferents from Nociceptive Stimuli. Afferents carrying pain sensations also affect VMC and evoke either pressor or depressor reflex effect as:

- *Pressor effect* in the form of increase in the blood pressure and tachycardia is caused due to sympathetic activity by *somatic pain afferents,* i.e. unmyelinated C-fibres which stimulate the pressor area of VMC (RVLM).
- *Depressor effect* in the form of hypotension and bradycardia is produced by *visceral pain afferents,* i.e. thin myelinated fibres which synapse with depressor area of VMC (CVLM) and cause inhibition of sympathetic activity.

Role of Skeletal Nerves and Muscles in Controlling Blood Pressure

Though ANS plays the main role in control of circulation, the skeletal muscles and nerves also contribute as:

1. Abdominal Compression Reflex Whenever VMC is stimulated, e.g. by baroreceptor reflex or chemoreceptor reflex, other areas of reticular formation of brainstem are also stimulated along with. They send simultaneous impulses through skeletal nerves to skeletal muscles of the body especially abdominal muscles. The contraction of abdominal muscles compresses the abdominal venous reservoirs increasing the venous return to heart and thereby the cardiac output. This response as a whole is called abdominal compression reflex.

2. Role of Skeletal Muscles during Exercise During exercise, the skeletal muscles especially that of limbs contract and compress the venous reservoirs. This causes translocation of large quantities of blood from the peripheral vessels into heart and lungs. This increases the cardiac output.

HUMORAL CONTROL MECHANISMS

Humoral regulation of circulation refers to the regulation by substances secreted into or absorbed into body fluids, e.g. hormones, ions, etc. Most important humoral factors affecting circulation are:

1. Circulating vasodilators,
2. Circulating vasoconstrictors and
3. Ions and other chemical factors.

Circulating Vasodilators

The circulating vasodilators include kinins, VIP (see page 578) and ANP (see page 794).

Kinins

Kinins are peptides which cause vasodilation. Two forms of kinins with similar action found are:

- ***Bradykinin*** is nonapeptide found in the plasma and
- ***Lysyl-bradykinin*** or kallidin is a decapeptide found in body tissues.

Synthesis and Secretion

- The kinins are formed from high molecular weight kininogen (HMWK) and low molecular weight kininogen (LMWK) by the action of plasma and tissue kallikreins:

$$\text{HMWK} \xrightarrow{\textit{Plasma kallikrein}} \text{Bradykinin}$$

$$\text{LMWK} \xrightarrow{\textit{Plasma Kallikrein}} \text{Lysyl-bradykinin}$$

- Lysyl-bradykinin can be converted to bradykinin by aminopeptidase.

$$\text{Bradykinin} \xrightarrow{\textit{Aminopeptidase}} \text{Lysyl-bradykinin}$$

- Kinins are metabolized to inactive fragments by the enzymes kininase I and II and angiotensin-converting enzyme (ACE).

$$\text{Kinins} \xrightarrow[\text{ACE}]{\text{Kinase I and II}} \text{Inactive peptides}$$

- Kinin release is inhibited by glucocorticoids.

Note: Kininase II is the same enzyme as angiotensin converting enzyme, which removes histidine and leucine from the terminal carboxyl end of angiotensin I

Functions of Kinins

- They cause *vasodilation* by relaxing vascular smooth muscle (VSM) via NO and increase *capillary permeability.*
- Kinins play role in regulating blood flow especially to skin, salivary glands and GIT glands. Therefore, they are formed during active secretion in sweat glands, salivary glands, and in exocrine portion of pancreas.
- By regulating blood flow to skin, the kinins probably play a role in thermoregulatory vascular adjustments.
- Kinins appear to be responsible for some episodes of vasodilation in patients with carcinoid tumours.
- Kinins are responsible for inflammation because of their following actions:
  - Increase in vascular permeability especially of venules and capillaries leading to escape of plasma proteins into tissues,
  - Excitation of sensory nerve endings and production of pain (which is enhanced by 5HT) and
  - Attraction and migration of leucocytes from blood to tissues.
- Kinins cause contraction of visceral smooth muscles of ileum, uterus and bronchioles (leading to bronchoconstriction in patients with asthma).
  Mechanism of action. The actions of kinins are mainly paracrine and quite similar to histamine. Kinins act through their receptors. Two types of bradykinin receptors have been identified (B_1 and B_2), both types of receptors are coupled with G protein. The B_1 receptors mediate pain producing effect of kinins and the B_2 receptors have homology to histamine (H_2) receptors.

Circulating Vasoconstrictors

The circulating vasoconstrictors include catecholamines, angiotension II and vasopressin.

Catecholamines

Catecholamines are released on sympathetic stimulation and include epinephrine and norepinephrine. The effects of epinephrine and norepinephrine are brought about by action on α and β adrenergic receptors, which are further subdivided into as: $\alpha_1$and α_2 subtypes and β receptors into β_1, β_2 and β_3 subtypes.

Epinephrine. It stimulates both α and β adrenergic receptors:

- *Stimulation of α-receptors* results in vasoconstriction in skin and splanchnic areas.
- *Stimulation of β-receptors* results in dilation of the vessels in skeletal muscles, liver and coronary arteries.
- The β receptor induced vasodilation is more dominant than α receptors induced vasoconstriction. So, the net effect is slight lowering of peripheral resistance producing slight fall in diastolic blood pressure.
- β receptor induced increase in stroke volume and heart rate results in higher cardiac output, a rise in systolic blood pressure and widening of pulse pressure.

Norepinephrine. has a generalized vasoconstrictor action as it has much greater effect on α than on β receptors.

- Therefore, it increases peripheral resistance and raises the diastolic blood pressure.
- Since it has negligible effect on β receptors, so direct cardiac stimulation is insignificant. Rather, there occurs reflex cardiac inhibition due to the rise in diastolic blood pressure.

Renin–Angiotensin System

The renin–angiotensin system has important roles in the regulation of blood pressure and in the regulation of extracellular fluid volume.

Renin Secretion and Angiotensin Formation

- *Renin,* a protease enzyme is secreted by *juxtaglomerular cells* of the kidney into the blood. Its secretion is stimulated by a decrease in the blood pressure.
- Renin catalyzes the conversion of *angiotensinogen* (α_2 – globulin substrate present in the plasma) to angiotensin I.
- *Angiotensin I* is converted into angotensin II by the action of *angiotensin converting enzyme* (ACE) present in the endothelium of blood vessels throughout the body, especially in the lungs and kidneys.
- *Angiotensin II* persists in the blood until it is rapidly inactivated by multiple blood and tissue enzymes collectively called *angiotensinases*

$$\text{Angiotensinogen} \xrightarrow{\text{Renin}} \text{Angiotensin I}$$

$$\text{Angiotensin I} \xrightarrow{\text{ACE}} \text{Angiotensin II}$$

Effects of Angiotensin II Angiotensin II has three principal effects by which it can elevate the arterial pressure:

1. Vasoconstriction. Angiotensin II is the most potent pressor substance being 4 to 8 times more potent than norepinephrine. By producing generalized vasoconstriction of arterioles and veins throughout the body it raises both systolic and diastolic pressure. This effect of angiotensin II is important in intermediate blood pressure control during circumstances such as acute haemorrhage.

2. Decrease in Salt and Water Excretion by Kidney. This action slowly increases extracellular fluid volume, which increases arterial pressure over a period of hours and days. Thus, this effect of angiotensin II plays important role in the long-term control of arterial pressure.

Mechanisms by which angiotensin II causes salt and water retention by the kidneys. Angiotensin II causes salt and water retention by the kidney in two ways:

- *By following direct actions on the kidneys:*
  - Angiotensin II constricts the efferent arterioles which diminishes blood flow through the peritubular capillaries, allowing rapid osmotic reabsorption from the tubules.
  - Angiotension II directly stimulates the epithelial cells of renal tubules to increase reabsorption of sodium and water.
- *By stimulating secretion of aldosterone.* Angiotensin II stimulates the adrenal glands to secrete aldosterone which in turn increases salt and water reabsorption by the epithelial cells of the renal tubules.

3. Stimulation of Thirst. Angiotensin II is a powerful stimulator of thirst. It leads to consumption of large volumes of water, leading to a rise in blood volume. This mechanism also plays some role in long-term control of blood pressure.

Vasopressin

Vasopressin or ADH is a powerful vasoconstrictor, but it is secreted in minute quantities and therefore mainly affects water reabsorption in renal tubules. However, after a severe haemorrhage its concentration rises to a high level and then it has vasoconstrictor effect. Its role in blood pressure regulation is discussed on page 692.

Urotensin II

Urotensin II is a potent vasoconstrictor present in cardiac and vascular tissue. Urotensin II is a polypeptide first isolated from the spinal cord of fish.

Applied In patients with hypertension and heart failure the levels of urotensin II and its receptors have been shown to be elevated, therefore may be the markers of the disease.

Ions and Other Chemical Factors

The increased concentration of many different ions and chemical factors can also alter local blood flow by causing vasodilation or vasoconstriction.

- Calcium ions cause vasoconstriction,
- Potassium ions cause vasodilatation,
- Hydrogen ions (decreased pH) cause vasodilation,
- Carbon dioxide causes vasodilation in most tissues and marked vasodilation in the brain.
- Glucose or other vasoactive substances, when increased in quantities raise the osmolarity of blood and cause vasodilation.

LOCAL CONTROL MECHANISMS

Need of Local Control Mechanisms

Local cardiovascular control mechanisms are primarily concerned with the control of blood flow to the tissues locally. The ability of the tissues to regulate their own blood flow locally serves many *functions,* a few examples are:

1. Local control of blood flow permits the tissues to maintain adequate nutrition and perform necessary functions in maintaining homeostasis. In general, the blood flow to the tissues is related to rate of metabolism of the organ, greater the rate of metabolism, greater is the blood flow.
2. These mechanisms help in temporarily curtailing blood flow to some organs so as to divert more blood to a metabolically active organ.
3. Control of blood flow to skin helps in control of body temperature.
4. Control of blood flow to kidney allows them to rapidly excrete the waste products of the body.

Classification of Local Control Mechanisms

A. Mechanisms involved in acute control of blood flow:
   1. General mechanisms
   2. Special mechanisms
B. Mechanisms involved in long-term blood flow regulation.

Mechanisms Involved in Acute Control of Blood Flow

Acute control occurs within seconds to minutes through constriction or dilation of arterioles, meta-arterioles and precapillary sphincters. The mechanisms involved in acute control of blood flow include:

I. General Mechanisms

These are the mechanisms that are present in most tissues of the body are:

1. Autoregulation, i.e. control of flow during changes in arterial pressure,

2. Role of local vasodilator metabolites and factors,
3. Role of local vasoconstrictors,
4. Role of substances secreted by endothelial cells.

1. Autoregulation (Control of Flow during Changes in Arterial Pressure) Autoregulation is the ability of an organ or tissue to adjust its vascular resistance and maintain a relatively constant blood flow over a wide range of arterial pressure. For details see page 315.

2. Role of Local Vasodilator Metabolites The accumulation of local vasodilator metabolites increase local blood flow. The greater the rate of metabolism in the tissue, the greater the rate of production of tissue metabolites.

Metabolic Changes that Produce Vasodilation Include:

- *Decrease in O_2 tension and pH* causes vasodilation in most tissues. These changes cause relaxation of the arterioles and precapillary sphincters. Decrease in O_2 tension occurs either due to decreased O_2 availability such as high altitude and in pneumonia or due to increased O_2 demand during increased tissue activity.
- A local fall in pO_2 produces a Hypoxia Inducible Factor-1α (HIF-1α) that causes expression of a vasodilatory gene.
- *Increase in pCO_2 and osmolality* also dilates the vessels. The direct dilation action of CO_2 is most pronounced in the skin and brain.
- *Rise in temperature* exerts a direct vasodilator effect, and the temperature rise in active tissues (due to the heat of metabolism) may contribute to vasodilation.
- *Potassium (K^+) and lactate ions* are other substances that accumulate locally and play role in vasodilation especially in skeletal muscles. The vasodilation effect of K^+ is produced by hyperpolarization of VSMs.
- *Histamine* released from damaged cells in injured tissues increases capillary permeability.
- *Adenosine* may play a vasodilator role in cardiac muscles but not in skeletal muscles. It also inhibits the release of norepinephrine.

Active Hyperaemia refers to the vasodilation which occurs when the tissue metabolic rate increases. The dilation of local blood vessels helps the tissues to receive the additional nutrients required to sustain its new level.

Metabolic Theory of Autoregulation states that any vasodilator metabolites which accumulate in the tissues during active metabolism will produce autoregulation. When blood flow decreases, they accumulate and the vessels dilate; when blood flow increases, they are washed away.

Reactive Hyperaemia is a phenomenon by which the local blood flow to the organ is controlled after a period of ischaemia (also see page 315). This phenomenon also appears to be a manifestation of local metabolic blood flow regulation mechanisms. After vascular occlusion, there occurs accumulation of tissue vasodilator metabolites and the development of oxygen deficiency in the tissues. The extra blood flow during reactive hyperaemia lasts long enough to almost exactly repay the tissue oxygen deficiency and to wash out accumulated vasodilator metabolites.

3. Role of Localized Vasoconstrictors

- ***Serotonin*** released from platelets in the injured tissue is responsible in part for the vasconstriction which occurs in haemostasis.
- ***Decrease in tissue temperature*** causes vasoconstriction, and this local response to cold plays a part in temperature regulation (see page 367).

4. Role of Substances Released by Endothelium Vascular endothelial cells make up a large and important organ. These cells secrete many growth factors and vasoactive substances which play important role in the local control of blood flow. The vasoactive substances include:

- Prostaglandins and thromboxane A_2,
- Endothelium-derived relaxing factor (EDRF), and
- Endothelins.

i. Prostaglandins and Thromboxane A_2

- *Prostacyclin* is prostaglandin produced by endothelial cells from arachidonic acid via cyclo-oxygenase pathway. It inhibits platelet aggregation and promotes vasodilation.
- *Thromboxane A_2* is produced by platelets also from arachidonic acid. It promotes platelet aggregation and vasoconstriction.
- *Balance between prostacyclin and thromboxane A_2* fosters localized platelet aggregation and consequent clot formation while preventing excessive extension of clot and maintaining blood flow around it.

Important Note

The prostacyclin-thromboxane A_2 balance can be shifted towards prostacyclin by administering low doses of aspirin. Aspirin produces irreversible inhibition of cyclo-oxygenase. Obviously, this reduces production of both prostacyclin and thromboxane A_2. However, endothelial cells produce new cyclo-oxygenase in a matter of hours whereas platelets cannot manufacture the enzyme, and the level rises only as new platelets enter the circulation. This is slow process because platelets have a half-life of about 4 days. Therefore, administration of small amounts of aspirin for prolonged periods reduces clot formation and has been shown to be of value in preventing myocardial infarction, unstable angina, transient ischaemic attacks and stroke.

ii. Endothelium-derived Relaxing Factor. Endothelial derived relaxing factor (EDRF) is the name given to a substance which is released by vascular endothelial cells and produces vasodilation. Later on it was identified to be *nitric oxide (NO)* in chemical structure.

Synthesis of NO. It is synthesized from arginine (Fig. 4.5.16) in a reaction catalyzed by *nitric oxide synthase (NOS).* NO synthase is a very complex enzyme, employing co factors like: NADPH, FAD, FMN and Tetrahydrobiopetrin. Three isoforms of NOS have been identified:

- NOS-1, is found in the nervous tissue,
- NOS-2, is found in macrophages and other immune cells, and
- NOS-3 is found in endothelial cells.

NOS-1 and NOS-3 are activated by agents that increase intracellular Ca^{2+} concentration, including the vasodilators acetylcholine and bradykinin, while NOS-2 is activated by cytokinase.

Inactivation of NO. NO has a very short life (3-5 sec) as it is highly reactive. It is inactivated by haemoglobin. NO and its products are inactivated through oxidation into nitrite (NO_2^-) and nitrate (NO_3^-) which are excreted in urine. The plasma and urine concentration of NO_3^- and cGMP are useful indicators for NO production rate.

Mechanism of vasodilation by NO. The NO that is synthesized in the endothelium diffuses to smooth muscle cells, where it activates soluble guanylyl cyclase, producing cyclic GMP (Fig. 4.5-16), which in turn mediates the relaxation of VSM by decreasing intracellular Ca^{2+} concentration.

Functions of NO. It has been recognised by direct and indirect evidences that NO performs many functions in the body which include:

1. ***Relaxation of vascular smooth muscle*** produced by NO. Serves various functions in different circumstances:
   - *Flow-induced vasodilation* is thought to occur due to local release of NO. When flow to a tissue is suddenly increased by arteriolar dilation, the large arteries to the tissue also dilate.
     - *Post-stenotic vasodilation* is an example of flow-induced vasodilation. Any narrowing of arterial vessels increases the local blood flow velocity which stimulates NO release and results in post-stenotic vasodilation.
     - *Vasodilation during physical exercise* is also supposed to be flow induced. It is evidenced by an increase in urinary NO_3^- and cyclic GMP excretion rates after submaximal exercise in healthy subjects. Exercise-induced NO release may explain the beneficial effects of endurance training on the cardiovascular system.
   - *Tonic release of NO* under basal physiological conditions is necessary to maintain normal blood pressure. This is evidenced by the observation that when various derivatives of arginine that inhibit NO synthase (NOS) are administered to experimental animals, there is prompt rise in blood pressure. Nitroglycerine and other nitro vasodilators that are of great value in the treatment of angina act by stimulating guanylyl cyclase in the same manner as NO does.
   - *Penile erection* which is consequent to vasodilation and engorgement of corpora cavernosa is also thought to be produced by release of NO. The drug *sildenafil* (Viagra), a selective inhibitor of GMP specific phosphodiesterase, acts by inhibiting the inactivation of NO.
   - *Modulation of effect of vasoconstrictor and vasodilator substances.* Adenosine, ANP, and histamine Via H_2 receptors produce relaxation of VSM that is independent of endothelium. However, acetylcholine, bradykinin, VIP, substance P, and some other polypeptides act via the endothelium. Various vasoconstrictors that act directly on VSM would produce much greater constriction if they did not simultaneously cause the release of NO. Conversely, the vasodilators that have direct actions of VSM produce greater vasodilation by triggering the simultaneous release of NO.

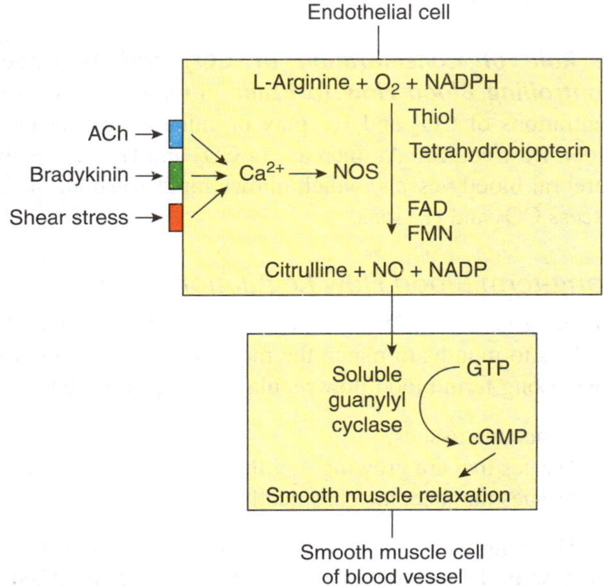

FIGURE 4.5-16 Synthesis and mechanism of action of endothelium-derived relaxing factor (EDRF).

Many of these substances are products of platelet aggregation and cause release of NO, and thus resulting vasodilation helps to keep blood vessels patent with an intact endothelium. This is in contrast to injured blood vessels, where the endothelium is damaged at the site of injury and platelets therefore aggregate and produce vasoconstriction. NO interferes with the secretion and action of endothelin, a potent vasoconstrictor. There seems to be a balance between endothelium derived vasoconstrictor and vasodilators.

2. ***Inhibition of platelet adhesion and aggregation*** caused by NO is somewhat complementary to its vasodilator effect, both of which are extremely important for the maintenance of normal blood flow.
3. ***Anti-atherosclerotic effect.*** NO decreases LDL oxygenation and inhibits superoxide anion (O_2^-) production by

inhibiting NADPH reductase activity. These actions are related to the strong anti-atherosclerotic effect exerted by NO.

4. ***Role of NO in vascular remodelling and angiogenesis*** is also suggested. NO may also be involved in pathogenesis of atherosclerosis. It is interesting in this regard that some patients with heart transplants develop an accelerated form of atherosclerosis in the vessels of the transplant, and there is reason to believe that this is triggered by endothelial damage.
5. ***NO plays role in cytotoxic activity of macrophages,*** including their ability to kill cancer cells.
6. ***NO acts as a mediator of inflammatory*** response, therefore its production is increased in inflammatory disease. NO inhibits leucocyte adhesion and migration.
7. ***In GIT,*** NO produces smooth muscle relaxation.

iii. Endothelins. Endothelins (ET) are family of three similar polypeptides: ET-1, ET-2 and ET-3. Endothelin-1 produced by endothelial cells is one of the most potent vasoconstrictor agents yet isolated. The structure of ET is similar to polypeptide sarefotoxin, found in venom of a type of snake.

Synthesis and secretion. In endothelial cells, the product of endothelin-1 gene is processed to a 39-amino acid prohormone, called *big endothelin-1* which is cleaved to form endothelin-1 by endothelin-converting enzyme. Small amounts of big endothelin-1 and endothelin-1 are secreted into the blood, but most of the endothelin-1 is secreted into the tunica media of the blood vessels and act in a paracrine fashion.

Factors affecting endothelin-1 secretion. *Stimulators* of endothelin-1 secretion are angiotensin II, catecholamines, growth factors, hypoxia, insulin, oxidized LDL, HDL, shear stress and thrombin. *Inhibitors* of endothelin-1 secretion include NO, ANP, PGE and prostacyclin.

Mechanism of action. Endothelin-1 exerts its vasoconstrictor effect through the ET_A receptor which is found predominantly on VSM. ET_B receptor is found on endothelial cells and responds to all the three ET (ET-1, ET-2 and ET-3). When activated ET_B receptor stimulates release of NO and thus favours vasodilation.

Biologic actions of endothelins include the following:

- ***Effect on cardiovascular system.*** Endothelin-1 is primarily a local paracrine regulator of vascular tone. Veins are possibly more sensitive than arteries.
  - ET increase the heart rate and force ofcontraction of myocardium.
  - ET play a role in closing the ductus arteriosus at birth.
- ***Effect on central nervous system.*** In the brain, ET play a role in regulating transport across the blood–brain barrier and across the synapses.
- ***Effect on kidneys.*** In the renal glomerulus endothelin causes contraction of mesangial cells and decreases glomerular filtration rate (GFR), renal blood flow and regulates Na^+ reabsorption.
- ***Effect on endocrines.*** ET increase plasma levels of renin, aldosterone, catecholamines and ANP.
- ***Effect on lungs.*** ET produce bronchospasm.
- ***Effect on GIT.*** ET enhance glucogenesis and regulate gastrointestinal blood flow. Megacolon (Hirschsprung disease) occurs when cells that form myentric plexus fail to migrate to the distal colon, has also been associated with endothelin-1 gene.
- ***Promitogenic effects.*** Stimulate cell growth in numerous cell lines. Carbon monoxide, hydrogen sulphide and nitric oxide are the gaseo transmitters present in cardiovascular tissue also regulate vascular tone, but their relative role yet to be established.

II. Special Mechanisms

In addition to the above-described general mechanisms, there are special mechanisms that control blood flow in special areas. These are discussed in relation to specific organs, but the following two are notable mechanisms:

1. Tubuloglomerular Feedback Mechanism in Kidneys In the kidneys, blood flow control is vested, in part, in a mechanism called *tubuloglomerular feedback*, in which the composition of fluid in the early distal tubule is detected by the macula densa, which is located where the tubule abuts the afferent and efferent arterioles at the juxtaglomerular apparatus. When too much fluid filters from the blood through the glomerulus into the tubular system, feedback signals from the macula densa cause constriction of the afferent arterioles, thereby reducing renal blood flow and GFR back toward normal (see page 487 for further details).

2. Role of Concentration of CO_2 and Hydrogen Controlling Blood Flow to Brain In the brain, the concentrations of CO_2 and H^+ play prominent roles in local blood flow control. An increase in CO_2 and H^+ dilates the cerebral blood vessels, which allows rapid washout of the excess CO_2 and H^+ ions.

Long-term Blood Flow Regulation

The long-term blood flow regulation develops over a period of days to months to match the metabolic needs of the tissues. Long-term blood flow regulation is required by:

- Ischaemic tissues,
- Tissues that are growing rapidly or
- Tissues that become chronically hyperactive.

The long-term blood flow regulation is brought by an increase in the physiological size of the vessels in a tissue, and in certain circumstances even by an increase in the number of blood vessels. One of the major factors that stimulate the increased vascularity of the tissues is a low oxygen concentration. The growth of the new vessels is called angiogenesis.

Angiogenic Factors. These are the substances which are responsible for angiogenesis. Three of the best characterized angiogenic factors which have been isolated from tumours or from other tissues that are rapidly growing or have inadequate blood supply are:

- Vascular endothelial growth factor (VEGF),
- Fibroblast growth factor (FGF), and
- Angiogenin.

Mechanism of Angiogenesis. Essentially all of the angiogenic factors promote new vessel growth by causing the vessels to sprout from small venules or, occasionally from capillaries. The basement membrane of endothelial cells is dissolved, followed by the rapid production of new endothelial cells that stream out of the vessel in extended cords directed towards the source of angiogenic factor. The cells continue to divide and eventually fold over into a tube. The tube then connects with another tube budding from another donor vessel and forms a capillary loop through which blood begins to flow. If the flow is sufficiently great, smooth muscle cells eventually invade the wall so that some of these vessels grow to be small arterioles and venules, or perhaps even larger vessels.

Development of Collateral Blood Vessels. Collateral blood vessels refer to those new vessels which develops around a blocked artery or vein and allow the affected tissue to be at least partially resupplied with blood. An important example is the development of collateral blood vessels after thrombosis of one of the coronary arteries in old people.

Chapter 4.6

Regional Circulation

INTRODUCTION

After discussing the 'dynamics of circulation' and 'cardiovascular regulation mechanisms, it will be worthwhile to know how these basic principles apply to circulation in various regions of the body. This chapter includes:

- Coronary circulation,
- Cerebral circulation,
- Cutaneous circulation,
- Skeletal muscle circulation and
- Splanchnic circulation.

Circulation to other regions, such as pulmonary circulation, renal circulation and fetal circulation have been described in the concerned sections.

CORONARY CIRCULATION

Coronary Blood Vessels

Coronary Arteries

Two Coronary Arteries (right and left) arise from the root of ascending aorta and supply blood to the myocardium.

Right coronary artery (RCA) supplies blood to the right ventricle, right atrium, the posterior part of left ventricle, posterior part of interventricular septum and major portion of the conducting system of heart including SA node.

Left coronary artery (LCA) thus supplies blood mainly to the anterior part of left ventricle, left atrium, anterior part of the interventricular septum and a part of the left branch of bundle of His.

Predominant supply by right coronary artery described above is seen in about 50% individuals. In 20% individuals, the predominant supply to myocardium is by left coronary artery. In 30% individuals it is the balanced supply, i.e. equal supply by the two arteries.

Major Coronary Arteries, (i.e. right coronary artery and its main branch posterior interventricular branch, and left coronary artery and its main branches the circumflex artery and anterior interventricular artery) travel in the epicardium of heart *(superficial vessels)* (Fig. 4.6-1) and subdivide sending *penetrating branches* through the myocardium. The penetrating branches subdivide into arcades that distribute blood to the myocardium.

End Arteries. Normally, the coronary arteries appear to function as *end arteries*. However, the presence of an arterial plaque or occlusion allows the *anastomoses* present between vessels to become functional. These anastomoses are of two types:

- ***Cardiac Anastomoses*** are those which are present between branches of two coronary arteries and between the branches of coronary artery and deep venous system.

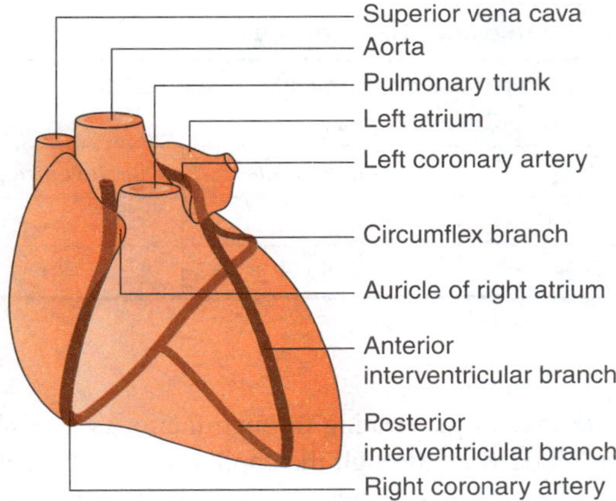

FIGURE 4.6-1 Major coronary arteries and their branches.

- ***Extracardiac Anastomoses*** include those present between the branches of coronary arteries and vessels lying near the heart such as vasa vasora of aorta, vasa vasora of pulmonary arteries, intrathoracic arteries, bronchial arteries and phrenic arteries.

Coronary Veins

Coronary Sinus is a wide vein about 2-cm long, which drains most of the venous blood from the myocardium (mainly left ventricle) into the right atrium. Its tributaries are the *great cardiac vein,* the *small cardiac vein,* the *posterior vein of left ventricle* and the *oblique vein of left ventricle* (Fig. 4.6-2).

Anterior Cardiac Vein draining venous blood mainly from the right ventricle opens directly into the right atrium.

Thebesian Veins and *coronary-luminal vessels* (connections between the coronary vessels and the lumen of heart) constitute the deep venous system. These vessels drain only less than 10% of the venous blood from myocardium directly into the various cardiac chambers, contributing to an *anatomic shunt effect.* The coronary luminal connections carry a larger proportion of the flow in the right ventricle than in the left ventricle.

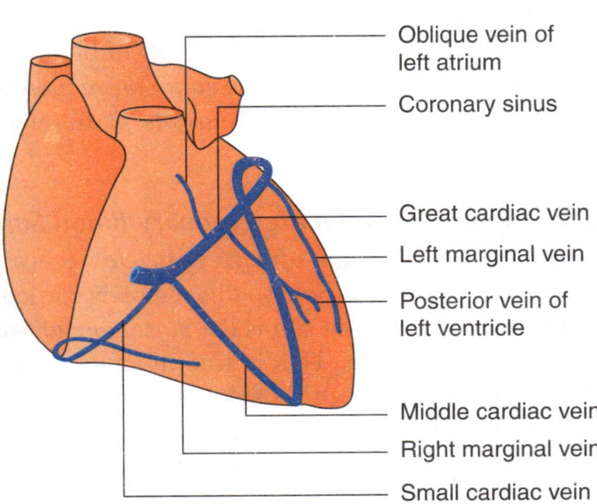

FIGURE 4.6-2 Coronary sinus and its tributaries.

Coronary Blood Flow: Characteristic Features

Normal Coronary Blood Flow and Oxygen Demand

- ***A continuous flow of blood*** to the heart is essential to maintain an adequate supply of O_2 and nutrients.
- ***Normal coronary blood flow*** at rest is about 250 ml (70 ml/100 g tissue/min), i.e. about 5% of the resting cardiac output (5 L). Three- to sixfold increase in the coronary blood flow may occur during exercise. Blood flow to the left ventricle (80 ml/100 g/min) is twice the flow to right ventricle. Atrial blood flow is about one-fourth of the ventricular flow.
- ***Oxygen consumption by the myocardium*** is very high (8 ml/min/100 g at rest). Because of this, even at rest 70–80% of the oxygen is extracted from each unit of the coronary blood compared with the whole body (average of 25%) oxygen extraction at rest. The increased oxygen demand of the myocardium during exercise is met with by almost total (nearly 100%) extraction of oxygen and by manifold increase in the coronary blood flow. Oxygen supply and utilization by myocardium vis-à-vis rest of the body (average) is shown in Table 4.6-1.

Phasic Changes in Coronary Blood Flow

The coronary blood flow shows changes during phases of cardiac cycle. The blood flow is determined by the balance between *pressure head* (i.e. aortic pressure) and the resistance (i.e. extravascular pressure exerted by the myocardium on the coronary vessels) offered to blood flow during various phases of cardiac cycle is shown in Table 4.6-2 and Fig. 4.6-3 and described here:

Blood Flow to Left Ventricle

During Systole, the tension developed in the left ventricle is so high that it has throttling effect on the branches of

TABLE 4.6-1 Oxygen Supply and Consumption by Myocardium vis-à-vis Rest of the Body (Average)

Parameter	Rest of the body (average)	Myocardium
Oxygen content		
– Arterial blood	19 ml%	19 ml%
– Venous blood	14 ml%	06 ml%
A–V O_2 difference	5 ml%	13 ml%
Coefficient of O_2 utilization	5/19 × 100 = 26%	13/19 × 100 = 70%
Oxygen saturation of venous blood	14/19 × 100 = 74% with PO_2 40 mmHg	6/19 × 100 = 32% with PO_2 <20 mmHg

TABLE 4.6-2 Pressure Gradients between Ventricles and Aorta during Systole and Diastole

Phase of cardiac cycle	Pressure (mmHg)		Pressure gradient (mmHg) between aorta and ventricle		
	Right ventricle	*Left ventricle*	*Aorta*	*Right ventricle*	*Left ventricle*
Systole	25	121	120	95	−1
Diastole	0	0	80	80	80

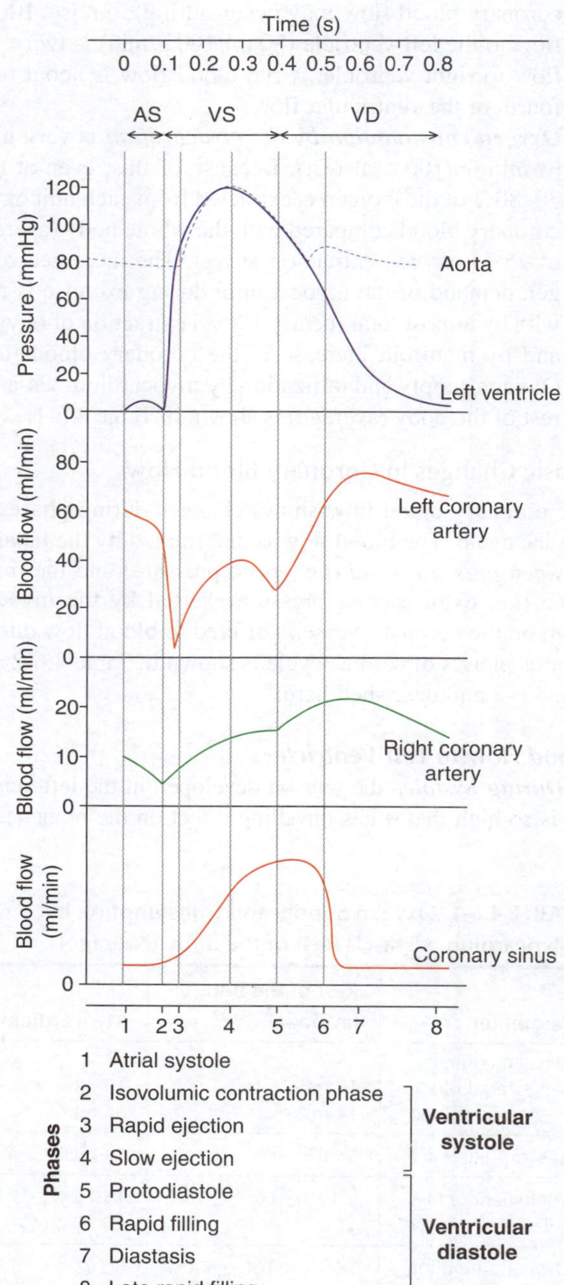

FIGURE 4.6-3 Blood flow in right and left coronary arteries and coronary sinus during different phases of cardiac cycle. AS = atrial systole, VS = ventricular systole and VD = ventricular diastole.

coronary arteries penetrating through them. As a result, the average blood flow through the capillaries of left ventricles falls to the extent that during some moments of the isometric contraction phase the blood flow to the left ventricle practically ceases, i.e. becomes zero. This is particularly true for the subendocardial region of the left ventricle. However, the epicardial parts of the left ventricle do receive some flow of blood during systole as the effect of intraventricular pressure is sufficiently dampened in these parts.

During Diastole, the cardiac muscles relax and blood flow increases. *Maximal flow in the left coronary vessels usually occurs during isovolumic relaxation phase,* while the arterial pressure is still relatively high and the myocardium is relaxed. Thus, most of the coronary blood flow (over 70%) occurs during diastole (Fig. 4.6-3). In severe tachycardia, the duration of diastole is drastically reduced. This tends to reduce the coronary blood flow during diastole as well, but due to local metabolic regulation the blood flow to the myocardium is not seriously affected.

Blood Flow to Right Ventricle and Atria. Blood passing through coronary capillaries of right ventricle also shows phasic changes similar to left ventricle. However, the changes in right ventricular flow are far less because force of contraction of the right ventricle is much less (Table 4.6-2). Thus, the blood flow to the right ventricle and atria occurs both during systole and diastole.

Blood Flow through Coronary Sinus. As shown in Fig. 4.6-3, in the coronary sinus the inflow of blood gradually rises from the *isovolumic ventricular contraction phase* and reaches its peak during *protodiastole phase* and then gradually falls.

Clinical Importance of Phasic Coronary Blood Supply

1. ***Subendocardial region of left ventricle*** receives no blood supply during systole so this region is particularly vulnerable to ischaemia and is the *most common site of myocardial infarction.* This is true in spite of the fact that this region has been provided with following *compensatory (protective) mechanisms:*
   - *Capillary density* in subendocardial region of left ventricle is much higher (1100 capillaries/mm^2) than the epicardial region (750 capillaries/mm^2). Therefore,

during diastole, flow to the subendocardial region of the left ventricle is considerably higher.

- *Minimum diffusion distance* between the capillaries and myocardial cells is 20% shorter in subendocardial region of left ventricle (16.5 μm) compared with epicardial region (20.5 μm).
- *Myoglobin content* (O_2 storage pigment) is higher in the subendocardial region than the epicardial region of the left ventricle.

2. ***In aortic stenosis,*** pressure in the left ventricle is much higher than that in aorta, because the ventricle has to force the blood against a narrow aortic orifice. This leads to severe compression of coronary vessels during systole and thus chances of myocardial infarction are increased in such cases.
3. ***In congestive heart failure (CHF),*** increase in venous pressure decreases aortic diastolic pressure. As a result, the effective coronary perfusion pressure falls and coronary blood flow decreases.

Measurement of Coronary Blood Flow

1. Nitrous Oxide Method (Kety Method)

Principle. Nitrous oxide method is the most common method used for measuring coronary blood flow. It gives almost accurate value and is based on the Fick's principle (see page 285).

Procedure. The individual is made to inhale a mixture of 15% nitrous oxide and air for 10 min..

- During inhalation of gases, serial samples of arterial and coronary sinus venous blood (through a catheter introduced) are taken at fixed intervals for 10 minutes.
- The coronary blood flow (CBF) is then determined from the amount of nitrous oxide taken up per minute (N_2O/min) and the difference of nitrous oxide content of arterial (A) and venous (V) blood, i.e.

$$\text{CBF} = \frac{N_2O \text{ taken up/min}}{(A - V)}$$

2. Radionuclides Utilization Technique

Principle. The radioactive tracers are pumped into cardiac muscle cells by the enzymes Na^+–K^+ ATPase and equilibrate with the intracellular K^+ pool. Distribution of radioactive tracers is directly proportional to myocardial blood flow and this forms the basis of this technique.

Procedure. Radionuclide such as thallium-201 ($^{201}T_1$) is injected intravenously. After 10 min, the amount of $^{201}T_1$ taken up by the myocardial cells is then measured with the help of gamma-scintillation camera over the chest. The amount of coronary blood flow is calculated from these values. Areas of ischaemia are detected by their low uptake. Some radiotracers such as technetium-99m stannous pyrophosphate (^{99m}Tc-PYP) are selectively taken up by the infarcted tissues only by an unknown mechanism. These substances are used to detect areas of myocardial infarcts which stand out as *hot spots* on the scintiscans of the chest.

3. Coronary Angiographic Technique Coronary angiography, when combined with measurement of ^{133}Xe washout using a multiple-crystal scintillation camera, provides detailed analysis of coronary blood flow.

4. Electromagnetic Flowmeter Technique

- This technique is employed in animals to measure the coronary blood flow. The main advantages of this technique are that it tells the phasic flow and the flow per minute.
- In this technique, blood flow through the left ventricle is determined with the help of electromagnetic flowmeter implanted around the main left coronary artery or around its circumflex branch. The arterial and venous (with the help of a catheter passed into coronary sinus) blood samples are analyzed for O_2 content. From the measured flow, and the difference of O_2 content of arterial and venous blood, the myocardial consumption of O_2 is then determined directly.

Regulation of Coronary Blood Flow

I. Local Control Mechanism

1. Autoregulation. Like other vital organs of the body, coronary circulation shows well-developed phenomenon of autoregulation. As described in detail on page 315, autoregulation refers to the ability of an organ/tissue to adjust its vascular resistance and maintain a relatively constant blood flow over a wide range of arterial blood pressure. However, this phenomenon of autoregulation of coronary blood flow fails when blood pressure falls below 70 mmHg and coronary perfusion is seriously compromised.

2. Role of Local Metabolites. Metabolic local factors are the most important factors which regulate the coronary blood flow and therefore, they even override the effect of nervous stimulation.

- It is important to note that under resting state about 50–70% of O_2 is released to the myocardium from the haemoglobin of arterial blood (in contrast, haemoglobin releases about 25% of its O_2 content for the body as a whole). Therefore, not much additional oxygen can be provided to myocardium unless the blood flow increases. Consequently, a direct and almost linear correlation is observed between the coronary blood flow and myocardial O_2 consumption (Fig. 4.6-4). How the O_2 consumption regulates the coronary vascular resistance is not known exactly. Probably following mechanisms are involved:
- ***Role of adenosine*** (Berne's hypothesis). Adenosine is considered the major factor in production of coronary vasodilation during hypoxic states. In myocardial ischaemia, either due to generalized hypoxia or due to increased myocardial metabolism the intracellular myocardial *adenine nucleotides* are degraded to *adenosine*. The adenosine is capable of crossing myocardial cell

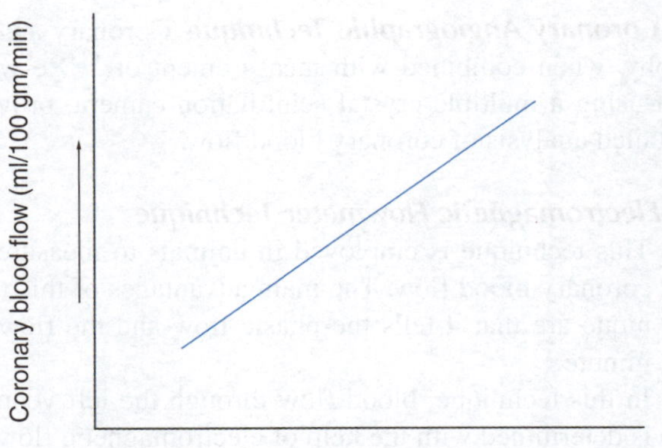

FIGURE 4.6-4 Relation between coronary blood flow and myocardial oxygen consumption.

membrane and thus comes out in the ECF and gains access to the resistance vessels, including the precapillary sphincters of the coronary system producing an extremely strong vasodilator response (Fig. 4.6-5). The adenosine is then reabsorbed back into the cardiac cells to be reused.

- ***Direct effect of O_2.*** It has been proposed that a decrease in the tissue PO_2 could also act directly on the arterioles and cause vasodilation.
- ***Role of other local metabolites.*** Hydrogen ions, bradykinin, CO_2 and prostaglandins are the other suggested vasodilator substances.

3. Role of Endothelial Cells

- Endothelial cells release several *vasodilator* autacoids that contribute to the physiologic regulation of coronary vasomotor tone. These include EDRF, prostacyclin (PGI_2) and endothelium-derived hyperpolarizing factor (EDHF).

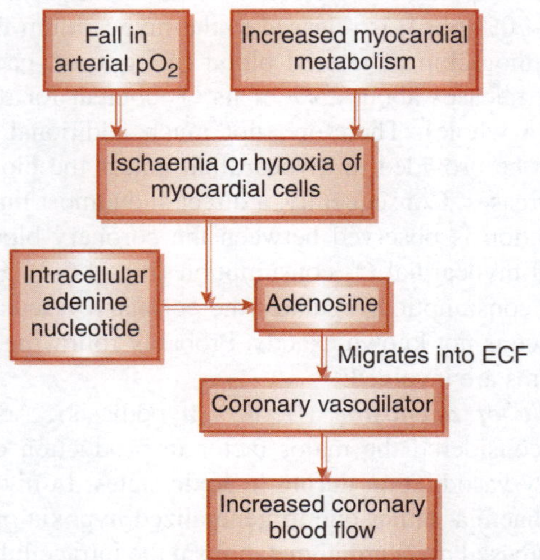

FIGURE 4.6-5 Berne's hypothesis (adenosine mechanism) of increase in coronary blood flow.

- Endothelial cells also release *vasoconstrictor autacoids* that may have a pathologic role, such as endothelin-1 (ET-1), angiotensin II and endothelium-derived contracting factors (EDCF).

II. Nervous Control Mechanism

Autonomic nerves control the coronary blood flow directly as well as indirectly.

1. Direct Nervous Control. Direct nervous control on coronary circulation is exerted through sympathetic and parasympathetic nerve supply to the coronary vessels.

- ***Parasympathetic nerve fibres*** to coronary vessels through vagus are so less that parasympathetic stimulation has very little direct effect, causing vasodilation.
- ***Sympathetic nerve fibres*** extensively innervate the coronary vessels. The transmitters released at their nerve endings are epinephrine and norepinephrine. The coronary vessels contain both $\alpha-$ and β-receptors.
  - Norepinephrine acts on α-receptors and causes vasoconstriction. Epicardial vessels have preponderance of α receptor.
  - Epinephrine acts on β-receptors of coronary vessels, causing vasodilation. Intramuscular arteries have preponderance of β-receptors.
  - The net result of direct effect of sympathetic stimulation is vasoconstriction.

2. Indirect Nervous Control. Indirect control of nervous stimulation on coronary blood flow is through their action on the heart.

- ***Sympathetic stimulation*** causes increase in the heart rate and increase of force of contraction of the heart. Thus, increased activity of heart helps conversion of ATP to ADP which by producing coronary vasodilation increases the coronary blood flow. This indirect effect of sympathetic stimulation overrides the direct effect of sympathetic discharge on coronary vasculature. Thus, the overall effect of sympathetic stimulation is coronary vasodilation and increased coronary blood flow.
- ***Parasympathetic stimulation*** causes decreased heart rate and decreased force of contraction of heart. Thus, indirectly the coronary blood flow is reduced.

3. Neurohumoral Control Factors. In addition to direct and indirect nervous control through sympathetic and parasympathetic neurotransmitters, several nonadrenegic–noncholinergic neurotransmitters also play a modulatory role:

- ATP (purine) which is co-released with norepinephrine from nerve terminals produces vasoconstriction through P_1 receptors and vasodilation through P_2 receptors present on vascular smooth muscles.
- *Neuropeptide Y (NPY)* is released with norepinephrine during sympathetic stimulation and causes severe vasoconstriction.

- *Calcitonin gene-related peptide (CGRP)* and substance P which are also found in cardiac nerves cause release of endothelium-derived relaxing factor (EDRF) and produce maximal dilation of epicardial coronary arteries.

Factors Affecting Coronary Blood Flow

1. Mean Aortic Pressure. This is the force for driving blood into the coronary arteries. Rise in mean aortic pressure increases the blood flow and vice versa. But if pressure remains high for a long time, because of increased work load on the heart, heart will go into congestive heart failure.

2. Muscular Exercise. Normal coronary blood flow (CBF) at rest is about 70 ml/100 g tissue/min. During exercise, CBF increases about 4 times because of sympathetic stimulation by following mechanisms:

- Increased activity of heart,
- Increased cardiac output (≥5-fold) and
- Increase in mean arterial pressure.

3. Emotional Excitement. During emotional excitement states such as fright, auditory and olfactory stimuli, the CBF is increased due to increased sympathetic discharge.

4. Hypotension. There occurs reflex increase in noradrenergic discharge during hypotension, which produces coronary vasodilation to increase CBF. This effect is observed secondary to the metabolic changes in myocardium at a time when there occurs vasoconstriction of splanchnic, renal and cutaneous vessels.

5. Hormones affecting CBF are:

- *Thyroid hormones* increase CBF because of increase in metabolism.
- *Adrenaline and noradrenaline* cause increase in CBF as already explained, indirectly by acting on β-receptors in heart.
- *Acetylcholine* may increase CBF by its action on heart similar to parasympathetic stimulation.
- *Pitressin* is known to decrease CBF by increasing coronary resistance.
- *Nicotine* is reported to increase CBF through the liberation of norepinephrine.

6. Heart Rate. When heart rate is increased, stroke volume decreases; therefore, phasic CBF and O_2 consumption per beat also decreases.

7. Effect of Ions. Potassium ions (K^+) in low concentration causes dilation of coronary vessels increasing CBF, whereas, high K^+ ion concentration causes constriction of coronary vessels decreasing CBF.

8. Metabolic Factors. Increased metabolism of the heart increases O_2 consumption leading to relative hypoxia. Hypoxia causes vasodilation due to direct effect and also due to release of adenosine leading to increased CBF.

9. Temperature. Hyperthermia increases metabolism and so causes increase in CBF while hypothermia decreases metabolic rate and thus decreases CBF as well.

Coronary Artery Disease

Coronary artery disease (CAD) also known as ischaemic heart disease (IHD) results due to insufficient coronary blood flow.

It is a condition associated with development of atherosclerosis in the coronary arteries, which supply the heart muscles (myocardium). With atherosclerosis, the arterial wall is hardened and its lumen becomes narrow due to plaque formation which may consist of calcium deposits, fatty deposits, smooth muscle proliferation and abnormal inflammatory cells.

Risk Factors for CAD Include:

- *Age and sex.* Men over 60 and women over 65 are more prone.
- *Family history* is a predisposing factor.
- *Diseases* like diabetes, hypercholesterolaemia and hypertension are proven risk factors.
- *Smoking* is a big risk factor.
- *Obesity.*
- *Diet* rich in saturated fats and low in antioxidants.
- *Life style.* Sedentary worker with lack of exercise.

Pathophysiology and Manifestations of CAD

Coronary artery atherosclerosis per se or with superadded arterial spasm or thrombus leads to limitation of blood flow to the heart muscle causing ischaemia (cell starvation due to a lack of oxygen) of the myocardial cells. Myocardial ischaemia clinically may manifest as:

1. Stable angina pectoris or
2. Acute coronary syndrome: Unstable angina, myocardial infarction.

Angina Pectoris

Definition. Angina pectoris refers to a transient form of myocardial ischaemia, especially occurring during increased oxygen demand (e.g. during exercise) in patients with coronary artery disease having about 60–70% narrowing of coronary arteries. Superadded thrombus formation causing incomplete coronary occlusion results in an unstable angina.

Characteristic Features. Typically, the angina is described as a feeling of uncomfortable pressure, fullness, squeezing or pain in the substernal region, which may be localized or may be referred to the inner border of left arm, neck or jaw. Pain occurs due to accumulation of anoxic myocardial metabolites and *factor P*, which stimulates pain nerve endings.

Types. Angina is of two types; stable and unstable.

- ***Stable angina***, also known as effort angina, refers to the occurrence of above described features of angina precipitated by some activity (walking, running, exercise, etc.) with minimal or nonexistent symptoms at rest.
- ***Unstable angina*** occurs at rest and usually lasts for more than 10 min. Attacks are frequent.

Diagnosis

1. *Electrocardiography* The characteristic ECG changes observed during angina episode are:
   - ST segment depression, that reverses after disappearance of ischaemia.
   - T-wave flattening/inversion may also occur.

   Stress test/ exercise electrocardiography is most useful for detecting ischemia that is not present at rest but precipitated by exercise (stress). Exercise testing can be done on motorized treadmill or with bicycle ergometer. The speed of treadmill is increased every 3 min until limited by symptoms.
2. *Laboratory testing* include serum lipid levels,

Treatment

- ***Nitroglycerine***—sublingual nitroglycerine is the drug of choice. Nitrates decrease arteriolar and venous tone, reduce preload and after load, and lower the oxygen demand.

  Nitrates also improve myocardial blood flow by dilating collaterals and in the presence of increased vasomotor tone.
- ***Prevention of further angina attacks include:***
  - Aggravating factors like hypertension, strenuous activity, emotional stress and cold temperature should be identified and treated or avoided.
  - Nitroglycerine: use of nitroglycerine sublingually/ translingually by spray or long acting nitrates should be taken before any strenuous activity.
  - Beta blockers prevent angina by reducing myocardial oxygen requirement during exertion or stress. This effect is accomplished by reducing the heart rate, myocardial contractility and blood pressure.
  - Calcium channel-blocking agents like verapamil, diltiazem and dihydropyridine prevent angina by reducing myocardial oxygen requirements.

Myocardial Infarction. Myocardial infarction (MI) or acute myocardial infarction (AMI), commonly known as a 'heart attack' refers to a degree of myocardial ischaemia (due to interruption of blood supply) that causes irreversible changes (necrosis, i.e. cell death or infarction) in the myocardium. Commonly, MI occurs when partially occluded coronary artery is constricted further by vasospasm or plaque (most common cause), which triggers formation of thrombus and occludes coronary artery.

Causes of myocardial infarction include:

- Atherosclerosis of coronary arteries,
- Thrombus formation,
- Embolus coming from other areas and
- Spasm of coronary vessels.

Since atheromatous coronary artery stenosis is the commonest cause, it has become synonymous with CAD.

Signs and Symptoms

- Sudden severe chest pain is a classical symptom of MI. Pain lasts for more than 30 min and typically may radiate to left arm and left side of neck. Pain occurs due to the anoxic metabolites and necrotic tissue products.
- Associated symptoms often complained with pain are shortness of breath, nausea, vomiting, palpitation, sweating and anxiety (often described as a sense of impending doom).

Note. Approximately 25% of all myocardial infarction are 'silent', i.e. without chest pain or other symptoms. Silent MI usually occurs in diabetics with associated autonomic neuropathy in elderly and also in patients with heart transplants.

Diagnosis Diagnosis of MI is made by triad of:

- Typical signs and symptoms associated with
- ECG changes seen on serial tracings and
- Changes in serum levels of certain enzymes and proteins (cardiac biomarkers).

ECG Changes in Myocardial Infarction are very important to diagnose, localize the area of infarction and to know the duration of infarction. Typical ECG changes (hallmark) seen in MI include:

- Elevation of ST segment in the leads overlying the infarct area and
- Depression of ST segments in the reciprocal leads.

For details see page 269.

Measurement of Serum Enzymes and Proteins Related to MI. Certain enzymes and proteins called as cardiobiomarkers leak into the circulation from the damaged myocardial cells. These include:

- ***Troponin-T and troponin-I*** are cardiac specific proteins, released 2–4 h after MI. Peak levels are seen after 12 h and persist up to 7 days. These are the most sensitive and specific for MI
- ***Creatine Kinase (CK-MB)*** levels increase within 4–6 h and lasts for 2–3 days. It is relatively specific when skeletal muscle damage is not present.
- ***Lipoprotein(a) [Lp(a)].*** There is a relation between atherosclerosis and circulating levels of Lp(a). Lp(a) interferes with the fibrinolysis by decreasing plasmin generation.
- ***Lactate dehydrogenase (LDH)*** levels peak within 72 h. LDH is not specific as troponin.
- ***Homocysteine.*** This substance damages endothelial cells of coronary vessels. There is a strong positive correlation of circulating levels of homocysteine I and MI.

Note. Homocysteine is converted into nontoxic substance (methionine) by vitamin B_{12} and folic acid. Therefore, supplements of folate and vitamin B_{12} lower the incidence of MI.

- ***Highly sensitive C-reactive protein*** and other inflammatory markers are correlated with the presence of inflammatory cells in the atherosclerotic lesion. Therefore, estimation of plasma C-reactive protein is also helpful in diagnosis.

- ***Glycogen phosphorylase isoenzyme BB (GPBB)*** is one of the new cardio-biomarkers. A rapid rise in blood levels can be seen in MI and unstable angina within 3 h after process of ischaemia and peak levels are seen within 7 h. It has a high sensitivity and specificity, if estimated early after chest pain.
- ***Serum transaminases (AST/ALT).*** These are nonspecific cardiac biomarkers as they exist in other tissues, namely liver skin, RBC, etc. However, rise and fall with characteristic symptoms and ECG changes, these can be used as a marker.

For localization of the infarct and to decide further management other investigations included are;

- ***Echocardiography*** provides assessment of left ventricular and regional functioning, and can help in diagnosis and management of infraction.
- ***Doppler echocardiography*** is most convenient procedure for diagnosing postinfarction damage.
- ***Scintigraphic studies*** with technetium-99m stannous pyrophosphate and thallium 201 identify the regions of ischemia.
- ***Radionuclide angiography*** demonstrates akinesis in the area of infraction and also measure ejection fraction.

Treatment In myocardial infarction, treatment should be started immediately to avoid irreversible changes. Therefore, main aim is to restore blood flow to the affected area.

A. ***General measures:*** Coronary care unit monitoring should be instituted as early as possible.

B. ***Drug therapy***

1. *Aspirin* (for mechanism of action see page 242)
   Analgesia: To relieve pain, sublingual nitroglycerine should be attempted first, if no relief than intravenous opioids provide effective and rapid analgesia.
2. *Thrombolytic therapy* reduces mortality and limits the infarct size. The greatest benefit occurs if treatment is initiated within first 3 h. Thrombolytic agents commonly used are:
   - Streptokinase, the first thrombolytic agent, it is less clot specific and less effective, cause hypotension and allergic reaction, therefore not generally administered.
   - Anistreplase (anisoylated plasminogen streptokinase activator complex; APSAC) It is injected as a bolus and provides continued thrombolytic activity.
   - Ateplase (recombinant tissue plasminogen activator tPA) is a naturally-occurring thrombolytic agent. Two additional clot-specific agents available are reteplase (closely related to tPA) and tenecteplase (TNK-tPA).
   - Heparin-post-thrombolytic management should be done by anticoagulation therapy with intravenous heparin (60 units/kg bolus followed by 12 units/kg/min to maintain a PTT of 50–75 s).
3. *Beta adrenergic agents* (see page 292)
4. *Angiotensin-converting enzyme (ACE) inhibitors* (see page 333)
5. *Calcium channel blockers* (see page 333)

C. ***Surgical treatment*** includes:

- *Aortic coronary bypass surgery* is performed to remove discrete points of blockage due to atherosclerosis. In this procedure, a section of subcutaneous vein either from arm or leg is removed and then grafting is done from root of aorta to the peripheral artery (beyond the blockage point).
- *Coronary angioplasty.* This procedure is used to open partially blocked coronary vessels. A small balloon-tipped catheter about 1 mm in diameter, is passed under radiographic guidance into the coronary system and pushed through partially occluded vessel till balloon reaches to blocked point. Then, the balloon is inflated under pressure, which stretches the diseased artery. After the procedure, blood flow increases by three- to fourfolds and 75% patients are relieved of ischemic symptoms.
- *Stents* are small stainless steel mesh tubes, which are placed inside the coronary artery (dilated by angioplasty) to keep the artery open and preventing restenosis. The endothelin usually grows over the stents and allows smooth blood flow through the stent. Drug-eluting stents are usually preferred because these slowly release the drugs, which prevent the excessive growth of scar tissue and decrease the incidence of restenosis.
- *Laser beam coronary artery catheterization* is a new procedure alternative to thrombolysis.

Complications. A variety of complications can occur even after when treatment is initiated promptly in MI. These include:

- Postinfarction angina. Approximately 30% of patients will have postinfarction angina.
- Arrhythmia. Abnormalities of rhythm and conduction are common in MI (for details see page 262)
- Myocardial dysfunction. The severity of myocardial dysfunction is proportionate to the extent of myocardial necrosis. Acute left heart failure, hypotension and shock are common myocardial dysfunctions.
- Mechanical defects in the form of partial or complete rupture of papillary muscle or of interventricular septum or myocardial rupture may occur in less than 1% of acute myocardial infarction.
- Left ventricular aneurysm may develop in 10–20% patients surviving acute MI
- Pericarditis and postmyocardial infarction syndrome (Dressler's syndrome) occurs in less than 5% of

patients. This is an autoimmune phenomenon and presents as pericarditis, associated with fever, leucocytosis and pericardial/pleural effusion.
- Mural thrombosis. Mural thrombi are also common, and can be detected by echocardiography or CT scan.

CEREBRAL CIRCULATION

Cerebral Blood Vessels

Arteries of the Brain

- The arteries which supply the brain are derived from two internal carotid arteries and the basilar artery (formed by union of the right and left vertebral arteries). Branches of the internal carotid arteries and of basilar artery anastomose on the inferior surface of the brain to form the circulus arteriosus (Circle of Willis).
- The *Circle of Willis* (Fig. 4.6-6) is thus basically a free anastomoses between the two internal carotid arteries and the two vertebral arteries, which equalize pressure on the arteries of the two sides. In this way, the circulus arteriosus allows blood that enters by either internal carotid or vertebral artery to be distributed to any part of both cerebral hemispheres.
- *Six large arteries,* taking part in formation of Circle of Willis, supply blood by their central and cortical branches to the brain substance.
- *Anatomical peculiarities of cerebral capillaries* and their role in *blood–brain barrier* are discussed on page 994.

Venous Drainage of the Brain The cerebral hemisphere has two sets of veins: the superficial and deep. The veins draining the brain open into the various dural venous sinuses. Ultimately, the blood from all these sinuses reaches the sigmoid sinuses which become continuous with the two internal jugular veins. The venous drainage of individual part of the brain is as follows:

Veins of the Cerebral Hemisphere

- The veins of the cerebral hemisphere consist of two sets: superficial and deep veins.

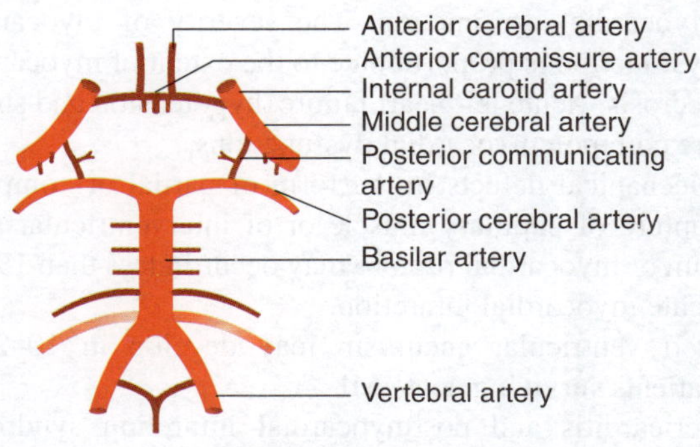

FIGURE 4.6-6 The Circle of Willis.

- *Superficial veins* drain into neighbouring venous sinuses.
- *Deep veins* of the cerebral hemisphere are two internal cerebral veins and two basal veins. The internal cerebral veins join to *great cerebral veins.* Basal veins end in the great cerebral vein which in turn ends in straight sinus.

Cerebral Blood Flow: Characteristic Features

Normal Blood Flow

- Brain relies on a continuous blood flow for adequate function. It is most susceptible to ischaemia. Interruption of blood flow only for 5–10 s causes a loss of consciousness, and circulatory arrest for only 3–4 min results in irreversible brain damage. The vegetative structures in brainstem are more resistant to hypoxia than cerebral cortex.
- Brain has a very rich blood supply. Normal blood flow to brain (which forms <2% of the body weight) represents approximately 15% of the resting cardiac output (75 ml/min), or about 50–55 ml blood/100 g tissue/min. The average weight of brain is 1400 g, therefore blood flow to brain is about 750ml/min.
- When cerebral blood flow falls below 18 ml/100 g tissue/min (*critical flow level*), there occurs unconsciousness.

Normal O_2 Consumption

- Total O_2 consumption of the brain is approximately 50 ml/min (3.3 ml/100 g tissue/min), i.e. 20% of the whole body at rest.
- O_2 consumption of grey matter (GM) is much more (3 ml/100 g tissue/min) than the white matter (WM) which consumes only 0.3 ml/100 g tissue/min. The greater O_2 demand of GM is essential for its functioning and is made possible because of high density of capillary network (4000 capillaries/mm^2 of GM).

Distribution of Blood

- The major cerebral arteries are not end arteries as they anastomose at Circle of Willis. Because of this, blood flows adequately to different parts of the brain. However, under normal circumstances, blood from each carotid artery is distributed largely to the same side of the brain and very little mixing occurs between the two circulations because a pressure gradient is normally not present due to equal blood pressure on the two sides.
- The major cerebral arteries supply the brain tissue through their central and cortical branches.
- The *central branches* of the cerebral arteries are end arteries, i.e. they do not anastomose with each other. Therefore, thrombosis or rupture of any of them invariably causes infarction.
- *Cortical branches* of the anterior, middle and posterior cerebral arteries supplying the surfaces of hemispheres overlap, forming border zones between the areas supplied by these arteries. However, these border zones susceptible to ischaemic damage and under condition of inadequate perfusion develop the so-called *watershed infarcts.*

- *Anterior watershed infarct* results due to inadequate perfusion of the border zone between supply of anterior and middle cerebral arteries and is characterized by development of contralateral hemiparesis of the leg and expressive language or behavioural changes.
- *Posterior watershed infarct* results due to inadequate perfusion of the border zone between supply of middle and posterior cerebral arteries and commonly produces a partial visual loss accompanied by a variety of language problems.

Measurement of Cerebral Blood Flow

1. Kety Method

Principle. It is based on Fick's principle (see page 285).

Procedure. In this method, subject is made to breathe a mixture of 15% nitrous oxide and air for 10 min. During this period, serial samples are taken every minute from the internal jugular vein (representing venous blood from brain) and a peripheral artery. The cerebral blood flow (CBF) then is calculated as:

$$CBF = \frac{N_2O \text{ taken up by brain tissue per min}}{A - V \text{ diff of } N_2O \text{ concentration}}$$

Disadvantages of this technique are:

- It gives an average value but no information about regional differences in the blood flow. For example, a reduction in flow to one part of the brain may be completely compensated by an increase in flow to other part so that total blood flow remains unchanged in spite of the fact that a region may be damaged.
- It measures the blood flow to only perfused areas of brain.
- It can only be used in steady state and not for the measurement of rapidly changing blood flow.

2. By Using Radioactive Substances, i.e. Single Photon Emission Computed Tomography (SPECT)

Principle. In this technique, blood flow to a region of brain is measured from the clearance curve of an inert radioactive tracer.

Procedure. Commonly used radioactive substance in this method is radioactive xenon (^{133}Xe or ^{123}Xe). A known amount of ^{133}Xe gas dissolved in saline is injected within 1–2 s in the internal carotid artery with the help of a thin catheter. The arrival and clearance of the tracers is detected for 10 min by multiple collimated scintillation detector built into a helmet that fits over the cranium. Each detector collimated to scan about 1 cm^2 of brain surface. The output from the detectors is processed in computer and displayed on coloured television screen. The colour is proportional to amount of blood flow. Resolution can be improved by computerized tomographic reconstruction. The mean cerebral blood flow (CBF) in ml/g/min is calculated from the following equation:

$$CBF = \frac{\lambda b(H_{max} - H_{10})}{A_{10}}$$

λb = Brain blood partition coefficient,
H_{max} = Maximal height of clearance,
H_{10} = Clearance height at 10 min and
A_{10} = Area under clearance curve.

Advantage of this technique is that blood flow to different regions of the cerebral cortex can be measured in conscious humans.

3. Positron Emission Tomography (PET)

It can also be employed to measure regional cerebral blood flow. As blood flow is coupled to brain metabolism, therefore, a short half-life radioisotope such as ^{18}F, ^{11}O or ^{15}O is labelled to a compound such as 2-deoxyglucose and compound is injected.

The arrival and clearance of the tracer is detected by scintillation detector placed over the head. The local uptake of 2-deoxyglucose is a good index of blood flow and its concentration in different parts can be easily monitored.

4. Magnetic Resonance Imaging (MRI)

In this technique regional concentration of individual metabolites is measured and changes in local O_2 utilization are mapped from which regional cerebral blood flow is studied.

This technique is based on detecting signals from different tissues in a magnetic field. Functional magnetic resonance imaging (fMRI) measures the amount of blood flow in a tissue area. During activity, the local blood flow and oxygen utilization by the tissue increases; therefore, when neural activity increases there is an increase in discharge activity that changes field potentials. The fMRI detects increase in oxygenated blood.

Advantages of fMRI-As fMRI does not involve the use of radioisotope activity, therefore, fMRI can be used at frequent intervals to detect regional brain blood flow changes in same individual during different types of activity (e.g. awake state, during sleep and involvement in specific activity like solving mathematical problems, etc).

Applied Aspects

Certain brain diseases are associated with regional/general changes in cerebral blood flow, which are detected by fMRI. A few conditions are:

- In epileptic seizure, blood flow to ectopic foci increases, whereas it reduces to other parts of brain.
- In Alzheimer disease, first change noticed is decreased metabolic activity and reduced blood flow to superior parietal cortex than to frontal cortex.
- In Huntington disease, there is reduction in blood flow to caudate nuclei.
- In manic depressive disorder, there is generalized reduction of blood flow.
- In schizophrenia, evidence suggests reduction of blood flow to frontal and temporal lobes, and to basal ganglia.

Regulation of Cerebral Blood Flow

The perfusion pressure which determines cerebral blood flow is the difference between the mean arterial pressure at the head level and the internal jugular pressure (cerebral venous pressure). Therefore, the factors which affect the cerebral blood flow are:

- Arterial blood pressure,
- Intracranial pressure,
- Resistance, i.e. viscosity of the blood and
- Diameter of the cerebral blood vessels.

The cerebral blood flow is regulated by the following mechanisms:

1. Metabolic Regulation Measurement of local cerebral blood flow has revealed that blood flow in individual segments of the brain changes within seconds in response to local neuronal activity. For example, the act of making a fist with the hand causes an immediate increase in blood flow in the motor cortex of the opposite cerebral hemisphere; similarly, the act of reading elevates the blood flow in the occipital cortex and in the language perception area of temporal cortex.

This change in blood flow with the neuronal activity of the particular area of the brain is related to the level of metabolism. The important metabolic factors which play important role are:

i. Carbon Dioxide. Physiologically, pCO_2 is the most potent vasodilator of cerebral blood vessels. With increase in pCO_2 there occurs a linear increase in the cerebral blood flow (Fig. 4.6-7). However, when arterial pCO_2 increases above 80 mmHg, no further increase in cerebral blood flow occurs due to maximal dilation of blood vessels. Similarly, when arterial pCO_2 falls below 20 mmHg, there occurs no further decrease in cerebral blood flow due to cerebral venoconstriction.

It has been observed that a maintained increase of arterial pCO_2 of 1mmHg above its normal range increases cerebral blood flow by 3 ml/100 g/min while a maintained decrease in arterial pCO_2 of 1mmHg below its normal range decreases cerebral blood flow by 1.5 ml/100 g/min. This is an important factor in the production of cerebral symptoms during hyperventilation.

Effect of CO_2 is mediated via change in pH as described: A rise in pCO_2 is associated with a rise in H^+ concentration. Carbon dioxide easily diffuses through the blood–brain barrier and reaches the CSF. In the CSF, CO_2 combines with water to form carbonic acid, which partially dissociates to form H^+ ions. The H^+ ions induce cerebral vasodilation in proportion to their concentration. The H^+ ions, however, do not cross the blood–brain barrier. Therefore, any substance that increase the acidity of brain and, therefore, the H^+ ion concentration will increase cerebral blood flow; such substances include lactic acid, pyruvic acid or other acidic compounds that are formed during the course of metabolism.

ii. pO_2. Slight fall in pO_2 causes vasodilation and produces increase in cerebral blood flow. Any stimuli, which either reduces the O_2 supply to the brain or increases the O_2 need of the brain, results in rapid formation of *adenosine,* which is potent dilator of pial arterioles.

Inhalation of hyperbaric O_2 causes cerebral vasoconstriction and thus cerebral blood flow decreases. High cerebral pO_2 disrupts neuronal metabolism producing convulsions, coma and death.

iii. K^+ ions. An increase in K^+ concentration in the CSF following hypoxia, electrical stimulation of brain and seizures cause rapid increase in cerebral blood flow. However, increase in K^+ is not sustained throughout the period of stimulation. Hence, only the initial increase in cerebral blood flow is attributable to the release of K^+ ions.

2. Autoregulation of Cerebral Blood Flow Like other vital organs of the body, cerebral circulation also shows phenomenon of autoregulation (for details see page 315). Due to autoregulation, cerebral blood flow remains nearly constant between 60 and 140 mmHg of blood pressure (Fig. 4.6-7). When blood pressure falls below 60 mmHg, the cerebral blood flow becomes extremely compromised, and syncope may result. When blood pressure rises above 140 mmHg, there may occur disruption of blood–brain barrier due to stretching and cerebral oedema or cerebral haemorrhage may result.

- ***Mechanism of autoregulation.*** Both metabolic and myogenic theories of autoregulation are considered (see details at page 315). In metabolic theory, main regulating substance of cerebral blood flow appears to be pCO_2.

  Autoregulation is abolished easily by trauma, hypoxia or other noxious stimuli. In such states, the flow and apparently the pressure in micro-circulation increases with an increase in cerebral perfusion pressure.

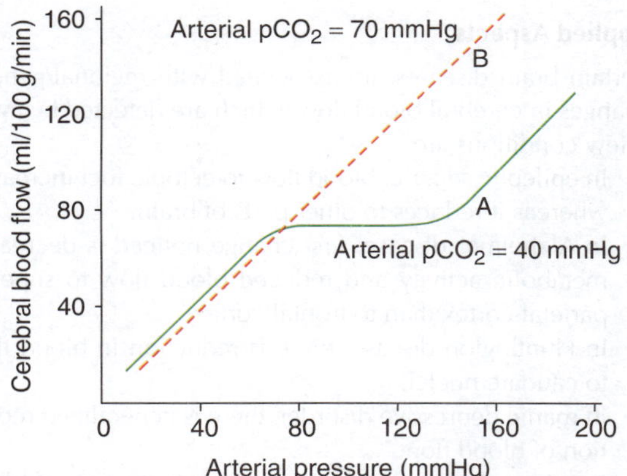

FIGURE 4.6-7 Effect of pCO_2 on cerebral blood flow and autoregulation of cerebral blood flow.

3. Role of Intracranial Pressure in Regulation of Cerebral Blood Flow The intracranial pressure level regulates cerebral blood flow by following two mechanisms:

i. Monro–Kellie Doctrine. According to this doctrine the brain, CSF and blood in the cerebral vessels are three elements enclosed in a rigid cranial cavity; and when any of them increases, it is at the expense of other two. This relationship helps to maintain the cerebral blood flow when changes in the arterial blood pressure occur at the level of head as explained:

- *When the body is accelerated upwards (positive g.),* blood moves towards the feet and the arterial pressure at the level of head decreases, and theoretically the cerebral blood flow should be severely compromised. However, practically it does not occur so because due to gravity the venous pressure and intracranial pressure are also decreased, and so the pressure on the vessels is decreased. Thus, the blood flow is less severely affected.
- *When the body is accelerated downwards (negative g),* the reverse occurs, i.e. the arterial pressure at the level of head increases and theoretically the cerebral vessels could have ruptured. However, practically it does not occur so, because due to negative 'g' intracranial pressure also rises, which supports the vessels and prevents them for rupturing. The Monro–Kellie doctrine also explains the maintenance of normal cerebral blood flow during posture changes, coughing and Valsalva manoeuvre.

ii. Cushing Reflex. When intracranial pressure is increased and becomes equal to the arterial pressure, it compresses the arteries in the brain and blood supply to vasomotor area is compromised. The hypoxia and hypercapnia produced locally increases the discharge from VMC. The resultant rise in systemic pressure tends to restore the cerebral blood flow. The rise in blood pressure is proportionate to rise in intracranial pressure up to a certain limit, beyond which cerebral circulation ceases. This effect which protects the vital centres in brain is called Cushing reflex. The resultant increase in blood pressure also causes reflex bradycardia via baroreceptor response. Thus, bradycardia is an important feature of raised intracranial pressure.

4. Nervous Regulation of Cerebral Blood Flow The cerebral blood vessels are innervated by noradrenergic vasoconstrictor fibres and cholinergic vasodilator fibres. The precise role of these fibres in regulation of cerebral blood flow is still a matter of debate. However, under normal conditions vasomotor nerves do not regulate the cerebral blood flow. These nerves may act indirectly by release of substances from the astrocytes which act paracrinally and regulate vasomotor tone.

- *In severe hypertension,* the noradrenergic sympathetic nerves cause vasoconstriction reducing cerebral blood flow. This prevents cerebral vascular haemorrhage and stroke and also protects the integrity of blood–brain barrier, which gets disrupted at high blood pressure.
- *In severe hypotension,* the cholinergic sympathetic vasodilator nerves play role in maintaining the cerebral blood flow.

Applied Aspects

Syncope

Syncope refers to transient fainting, i.e. transient loss of consciousness due to momentary but significant decrease in cerebral blood flow. Syncope may be cardiogenic or noncardiogenic.

Cardiogenic syncope occurs in the following cardiac conditions:

- *Obstruction to cardiac output,* e.g. in aortic stenosis. It usually occurs due to exertion and is also called effort syncope.
- *Cardiac arrhythmias,* such as sinus arrest, heart blocks and Stokes-Adams syndrome.
- *Myocardial infarction.*

Noncardiogenic syncope occurs in following forms:

- *Vasovagal syncope* occurs due to vasovagal reflex causing sudden hypotension and bradycardia.
- *Postural syncope* results due to inadequate vasomotor response to postural changes in blood pressure.
- *Carotid sinus syncope* or the carotid sinus syndrome results due to excessive sensitivity of the carotid sinus to compression, e.g. as by a tight collar.
- *Valsalva manoeuvre syncope* is associated with increased intrathoracic pressure in following situations:
  - Micturition (micturition syncope),
  - Defecation (defecation syncope) and
  - Coughing (tussive syncope).
- *Metabolic syncope* occurs in following situations:
  - *Hyperventilation* leads to hypocapnia, which causes cerebral vasoconstriction and
  - *Hypoglycaemia* impairs the activity of vasomotor centre.

CUTANEOUS CIRCULATION

Cutaneous Blood Vessels (Fig. 4.6-8)

Cutaneous Arterioles form a dense network just under the dermis layer of the skin.

- *Meta-arterioles,* which arise from the arterioles, are relatively high-resistance conduits present between the arterioles and capillaries.
- *Cutaneous capillaries.* The meta-arterioles subdivide into capillary loops, which provide a large surface area for heat exchange.
- *Venules* form an extensive subpapillary venous plexus, which hold large quantity of blood and lie parallel to the surface of skin and play important role in maintaining the body temperature.

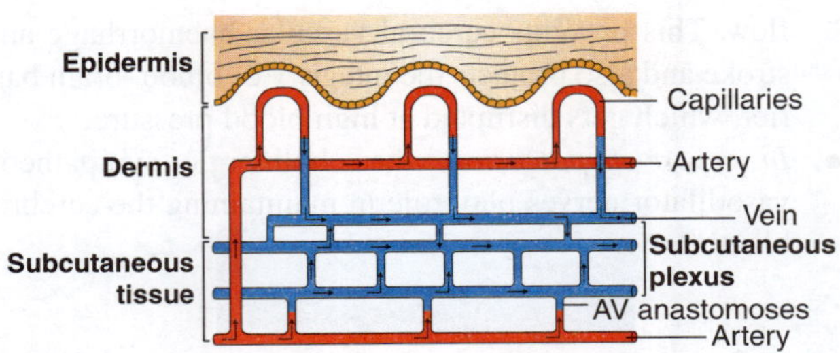

FIGURE 4.6-8 Arrangement of blood vessels in subcutaneous region.

- *Arteriovenous anastomoses* are located in the distal parts of the extremities (hands and feet), the nose, lips and ear lobules. These vessels are wide, low-resistance connections that serve as shunts and allow blood to bypass the superficial capillary loops and play major role during control of body temperature.

Cutaneous Blood Flow: Characteristic Features

- ***Main function of cutaneous circulation*** is to aid in the regulation of body temperature. The metabolic rate of the skin is relatively small so that a minimal amount of blood flow to the skin can supply the nutritive function.
- ***Resting cutaneous blood flow,*** i.e. the flow when a person is at thermal equilibrium with the environment (at approximately 27°C atmospheric temperature), is about 10–15 ml/min/100 g of skin tissue.
- ***During exposure to cold,*** when sweating is minimal, the cutaneous blood flow falls to about 1/10th of resting blood flow, i.e. about 1 ml/min/100 g tissue.
- ***During exposure to heat,*** when sweating is maximum, the cutaneous blood flow may increase 10 times of resting blood flow, i.e. about 150 ml/min/100 g tissue. Maximum cutaneous blood flow that occurs on heat exposure imposes a heavy circulatory load on the heart. That is why persons working under maximal heat loads may simply collapse with circulatory failure unless supervised adequately.
- ***Regional variation in cutaneous blood flow*** exists due to presence of A-V anastomoses in abundance in certain area such as hands, feet, nose and ear lobules. During heat stress, the blood flow to the area with rich A-V anastomoses increases much more (about 75 ml/100 g/min) compared with the rest of the skin (about 25 ml/min/100 g tissue).
- ***Cutaneous blood flow and skin colour.*** The colour of skin is basically determined by the pigment present; however, the amount of blood and degree of oxygenation also affect the skin colour tinge which may be reddish, bluish or some shade in between.

Regulation of Cutaneous Blood Flow

The skin has very little metabolic activity. Consequently, it has little O_2 consumption, i.e. only 0.3 ml/min/100 g compared with 3.3 ml/min/100 g in brain and 9.7 ml/min/100 g in cardiac muscles. Therefore, in contrast to most other tissues, the cutaneous blood flow is predominantly regulated by the nervous control instead of metabolic control.

Nerve Supply of Cutaneous Vessels

- ***Sympathetic vasoconstrictor*** nerves supplying the cutaneous vessels exhibit a sympathetic constrictor discharge under resting condition. The sympathetic tonic discharge is more marked on AV anastomoses vessels than the other vessels.
- ***Parasympathetic vasodilator nerves*** do not supply the cutaneous blood vessels. Vasodilation of cutaneous vessels results due to:
  - Reduction of sympathetic vasoconstrictor effect,
  - Local production of bradykinin (a potent vasodilator polypeptide) in sweat glands and
  - Production of other local vasodilator substances (see page 350).

Neural Control Mechanisms The cutaneous blood flow is regulated by following neural control mechanisms.

1. Hypothalamic Control Mechanism. The reflex increase or decrease in sympathetic discharge to cutaneous vessels during thermoregulation is mediated through the temperature regulation centres of the hypothalamus as:

- ***Under resting conditions,*** i.e. when the person is at thermal equilibrium with the environment (at about 27°C atmospheric temperature), the sympathetic vasoconstrictor fibres have a mild tonic discharge. The tonic sympathetic discharge normally keeps the A-V anastomoses closed.
- ***During exposure to heat stress,*** the tonic sympathetic discharge is reflexly abolished by a hypothalamic mechanism. Thus, the blood flow to skin is increased by following responses in a chronological sequence:
  - First of all, A-V anastomoses of hands, feet, and ear lobules dilate due to reduction in the sympathetic tonic discharge.
  - Secondly, rest of the cutaneous vessels dilate due to progressive withdrawal of sympathetic vasoconstrictor activity.
  - Finally, sweat glands get activated due to cholinergic sympathetic discharge. The *bradykinin* produced by the secretory activity of the sweat glands acts locally as a powerful vasodilator and increases blood flow to skin.

All the above mechanisms combinedly may increase the cutaneous blood flow to as high as 150 ml/min/100 g tissue. Thus, total cutaneous blood flow during heat stress may be over 3 L/min. The increased blood flow carries heat to the surface of the body, where it is dissipated by *radiation, evaporation* and *conduction* to the environment. If the environmental temperature is higher than the body temperature, heat can only be dissipated by means of evaporation of sweat; under these conditions radiation and conduction would cause the body to gain heat.

- ***During exposure to cold stress,*** via hypothalamic mechanism, there occurs widespread cutaneous vasoconstriction due to increased sympathetic discharge. Consequently, cutaneous blood flow is markedly decreased to as low as 1 ml/min/100 g. Thus, total blood flow to skin during exposure to cold stress may be even less than 50 ml/min. In this way, *heat conservation* is accomplished by markedly diminishing the rate of blood flow to skin. Body heat is preserved because less heat is dissipated to the environment. For details of temperature regulation see page 1246.

2. Baroreceptor-mediated Reflex Cutaneous blood vessels participate in baroreceptor-mediated reflexes during conditions of circulatory stress such as exercise and haemorrhage. They exhibit considerable vasoconstriction and act as compensatory mechanism to divert blood from periphery to the central pool.

3. Cortical Control Mechanism The *emotions* affect the cutaneous circulation through corticohypothalamic pathway. The impulses are relayed from the corticohypothalamic centres to the thoracolumbar sympathetic cell bodies and thence to the skin vessels. The effects of emotions on cutaneous circulation manifest in following forms:

- ***Blanching of skin*** during situations of fear (pale with fear) occurs due to vasoconstriction mediated through cortical mechanism.
- ***Phenomenon of blushing,*** i.e. emotional embarrassment, occurs due to vasodilation of vessels. It is supposed to be the result of bradykinin (a potent vasodilator) release, secondary to a brief corticohypothalamically controlled discharge of sympathetic cholinergic fibres to the sweat glands.

Cutaneous Vascular Responses

Certain peculiar cutaneous vascular responses are:

- White reaction,
- Triple response,
- Dermatographia,
- Axon reflex,
- Reactive hyperaemia,
- Cold vasodilation and
- Cold vasoconstriction.

White Reaction White reaction refers to appearance of a pale stroke line when a pointed object is drawn lightly over the skin. This occurs due to the fact that the mechanical stimulus initiates contraction of the precapillary sphincter, and blood drains out of the capillaries and small veins. This response appears in about 15 s.

Triple Response Triple response is three-part response, consisting of the red reaction, wheal and flare, which occurs as a normal reaction to the skin which is more in intensity than that simply causes white reaction. In other words, even when the skin is stroked more firmly with a pointed instrument, instead of white reaction, there occurs triple response.

The Red Reaction refers to the red line which appears at the site of injury in about 10 s.

- It occurs due to dilation of the precapillary sphincters in the injured area.

The dilation of the precapillary sphincters is not mediated by nerves but is produced by histamine and/or some polypeptides such as bradykinin released from the damaged skin.

- Since it is not neurally mediated, local anaesthesia of skin does not prevent the red reaction.

The Flare refers to the diffusely spreading and irregularly outlined redness of the skin surrounding the red line.

- It occurs after a few minutes of the appearance of red line.
- It occurs due to the dilation of the arteriole and precapillary sphincters. An arteriole supplies blood to the capillaries in an irregularly outlined area. This explains the irregular outline of flare.
- The dilation of the arteriole increases local blood flow.
- The dilation of arteriole is mediated by nerves, since it is abolished by the local anaesthetic agents.
- Since the blockade of the concerned afferent nerve fibres away from the site of injury does not abolish the response, it is believed that the flare is mediated by the *axon reflex* in the cutaneous fibres, which does not involve the CNS like a typical reflex. For details of axon reflex see page 339.

Wheal refers to the swelling or localized oedema that develops within the area of flare when the stroke stimulus is strong enough.

- It occurs due to increased capillary permeability with consequent extravasation of fluid.
- The increase in capillary permeability responsible for wheal formation is produced in part by histamine or histamine-like substance released from local mast cells and mediated via H_1 receptors, in part by P substance and calcitonin gene-related peptide, the transmitter released at the central termination of the sensory fibre neurons. Thus, there is histaminergic as well as a peptidergic component of the wheal.

Note. The use of effective nonapeptide antagonist to substance P reduces extravasation of the fluid, thus prevent wheal formation.

Dermatographia Dermatographia refers to striking triple response that occurs as an unusual reaction in some individuals. Thus, in the prone individuals anything drawn on the skin even with a blunt point becomes conspicuous within a few minutes. The exact cause of dermatographia is not known. Possibly, it is due to excessive release of the histamine from the involved skin area.

Reactive Hyperaemia Reactive hyperaemia is a phenomenon by which the vessels control blood flow to the organ after a period of *ischaemia* following occlusion of the artery to an organ or tissue. This response of the blood vessels occurs in many organs but is visible in the skin. Due to this phenomenon, the blood flow exceeds the control level when the occlusion is removed. For example, when the blood supply to a limb is occluded, the cutaneous arterioles below the occlusion dilate. When the circulation is re-established, blood flowing into the dilated vessels makes the skin fiery red. Oxygen diffuses a short distance through the skin, and reactive hyperaemia is prevented if the circulation of the limb is occluded in an atmosphere of 100% O_2. Therefore, it has been proposed that the arteriolar dilation is apparently due to local effect of hypoxia. The magnitude and duration of reactive hyperaemia depends upon the duration of occlusion.

Cold Vasodilation As discussed above, normally during exposure to cold stress, there occurs widespread cutaneous vasoconstriction via hypothalamic mechanism. However, prolonged and severe vasoconstriction may lead to tissue damage known as *frostbite.* This usually occurs when skin temperature falls below 10°C. The tissue injury so produced is painful and associated with the release of histamine and/or some other polypeptide, which excites the sensory terminals and produce *vasodilation* due to *axon reflex* operating particularly on A-V anastomoses. In addition, exposure to severe cold promotes the formation of *plasma kinins,* which also produce vasodilation; cold vasodilation is the cause of ruddy cheeks seen in fair-complexioned individuals on a cold day.

Cold Vasoconstriction Exposure to cold causes vasoconstriction via hypothalamic mechanism. Cutaneous vasoconstriction results in decrease in nutrient supply to the skin and also decreases metabolic rate of the tissue. Due to decreased metabolism, the metabolites accumulation is very slow so, unlike in muscles, the local metabolites of the skin are not able to produce local vasodilation and oppose (escape) the sympathetic vasoconstriction. As a result, the maximal vasoconstrictor discharge to the precapillary resistance vessels of the skin is well sustained. So, prolonged cold-induced vasoconstriction especially in damp conditions results in cutaneous ischaemia-producing lesions such as *trench foot*.

SKELETAL MUSCLE CIRCULATION

Skeletal Muscle Blood Flow: Characteristic Features

At Rest the blood flow to the skeletal muscle is about 2–4 ml/min/100 g of muscle tissue.

- Since the whole body skeletal muscles weight is approximately 30 kg in adults, the total blood flow to the body muscle mass is about 750–800 ml/min.
- At rest, only 20–25% of muscle capillaries have flowing blood.

During Exercise. During strenuous exercise, muscle blood flow can increase up to 20 times, i.e. about 50–80 ml/min/100 g muscle tissue or over 20 L/min to the whole body skeletal mass. This is called exercise hyperaemia.

- The tremendous increase in muscle blood flow mainly occurs due to local metabolite-induced vasodilation (see control of muscle blood flow). During exercise, there occurs dilation of the arterioles and precapillary sphincters, and all the dormant capillaries open up, greatly increasing the surface area and the rate of blood flow to the skeletal muscles.
- During exercise, the blood flow to the muscle is intermittent because during each contraction muscle fibres squeeze the blood vessels passing through them and thus the blood flow decreases or even stops (Fig. 4.6-9). During relaxation period, muscle blood flow increases and myoglobin acts as an O_2 acceptor and it yields its O_2 to the myofibrils during the subsequent muscle contraction.
- Sustained and severe contractions lasting more than 10 s lead to cessation of blood flow, myoglobin supply of O_2 is exhausted and anaerobic metabolites accumulate causing fatigue and ischaemic pain.
- Following heavy phasic exercise, the blood flow does not subside immediately, but falls exponentially from its high level during the exercise to resting values. This is due to the *oxygen debt of exercise* (see page 1208).

Reactive Hyperaemia. When the blood supply to a limb is occluded, the muscular and cutaneous arterioles below the occlusion dilate. When the circulation is re-established, blood flowing into the dilated vessels causes *muscle hyperaemia* (muscle blood flow may increase to 35–40 ml/100 g/min). Reactive hyperaemia seems to be mediated by local hypoxia.

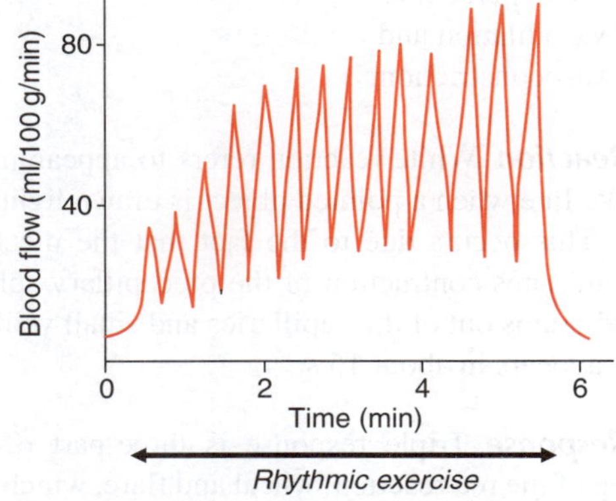

FIGURE 4.6-9 Blood flow through skeletal muscles.

White versus red muscle blood flow. White versus red muscles have been described on page 95. Some of the essential differences related to blood flow are enumerated:

- White muscles constitute 3/4th of the total mass and show rapid phasic contractions. While red muscles constitute 1/4th of total mass and show steady prolonged contraction. These muscles are concerned with maintenance of posture.
- White muscles have a resting blood flow 2–4 ml/min/100 g, which may increase to 50–80 ml/min/100 g, during maximal exercise. While red muscle fibres employ aerobic metabolism and contract all the times. So, their O_2 demand is much higher (30 ml/min/100 g).
- White muscles are prone to O_2 debt, red muscles do not, because of greater surface area of the capillary bed (three times the size of white muscles) and higher resting blood flow the red muscles are unlikely to be exposed to O_2 debt.

Regulation of Muscle Blood Flow

The blood flow to the skeletal muscles is regulated by autoregulation mechanism, metabolic control mechanism and nervous control mechanism. These mechanisms exhibit their role in different situations as described.

1. Autoregulation Mechanism Autoregulation is the ability of an organ or tissue to adjust its vascular resistance and maintain a relative constant blood flow over a range of arterial pressure. Mechanism of autoregulation is well developed in skeletal muscles like that of kidney, heart and brain. The precapillary resistance vessels in the skeletal muscles have a *high basal myogenic tone.* A rise of the transmural pressure excites a stretch-induced contraction of the sphincter smooth muscles, which by raising the precapillary vessel tone protects the capillaries from an undue rise of pressure *(myogenic theory of autoregulation)* also (see page 315). These responses are particularly important in leg muscles, where they reduce the rate of capillary filtration in erect posture and thus prevent pedal oedema under normal circumstances.

2. Metabolic Control Mechanism Local metabolic control mechanism is chiefly responsible for the tremendous increase in skeletal muscle blood flow during exercise (exercise hyperaemia). The muscle contraction increases the metabolic rate of tissue, which in turn reduces *oxygen concentration* in the muscle. The decreased tissue pO_2 leads on to vasodilation. In addition, the exercising skeletal muscle, potassium ions, hydrogen ions, lactic acid, carbon dioxide and further rise of *tissue temperature* due to muscular activity may also contribute to the dilation of arterioles and precapillary sphincter. As a result, there is 10- to 100-fold increase in the number of open capillaries in the skeletal muscles.

Metabolic control also explains the *reactive hyperaemia* that occurs following a period of occlusion of arterial blood supply, as discussed above.

3. Nervous Control Mechanisms Vessels of the skeletal muscles are supplied by both sympathetic vasoconstrictor and sympathetic vasodilator fibres.

Sympathetic Vasoconstrictor Control

- ***Under resting conditions***, the noradrenergic sympathetic nerve fibres discharge at a rate of 1 impulse/s in recumbent position and 2–3 impulses/s in the upright position. This sympathetic discharge contributes relatively small part to the high basal tone of the resistance vessels of the muscles. Most of the basal tone of these vessels is myogenic. Because of this relatively low sympathetic contribution to the total basal tone, blockade or the permanent loss (by surgical removal) of sympathetic vasoconstrictor supply to the skeletal muscles only doubles the blood flow.
- ***During muscular exercise.*** Because of the low sympathetic contribution to total basal tone, it is obvious that *exercise hyperaemia* is independent of sympathetic discharge to muscle vessels and is due to metabolic factors as described above.

  Further, skeletal blood vessels contain both α-adrenergic and β-adrenergic receptors. Alpha receptors are located in close proximity of the terminals of vasoconstrictor sympathetic nerve fibres, and β receptors are independent of any innervation. During strenuous exercise norepinephrine and epinephrine are released into the systemic circulation from adrenal medulla, which tend to produce vasoconstriction and vasodilation by acting on α- and β-receptors, respectively. These two factors tend to counter each other and hence may not contribute significantly to the increased skeletal blood flow during exercise.
- ***During circulatory shock and other type of circulatory stress*** the sympathetic vasoconstrictor mechanism assumes a great physiological importance. Sympathetic vasoconstriction reduces muscle blood flow profoundly. Since the muscle capillary bed is very large, these help in diverting substantial amount of blood from the muscles towards the heart and other vital organs.

Sympathetic Vasodilator Fibres

- Skeletal blood vessels are also supplied by sympathetic vasodilator fibres. In some animals, these fibres release acetylcholine at their nerve endings, but in primates the vasodilator effect is believed to be caused by epinephrine-exciting β-adrenergic receptors in the skeletal muscle vasculature.
- These fibres are activated by *corticohypothalamic reticulospinal* pathways (see page 338), which are quite separate from the *VMC–thoracolumbar pathways.* Therefore, they are not influenced by the baroreceptor and chemoreceptor afferents and do not participate in changes in peripheral resistance by usual cardiovascular reflexes.
- These fibres probably operate during emergencies, i.e. during mental stress and emotions. Since there is stimulation of different areas in hypothalamus in these situations, therefore due to activation of corticohypothalamic reticular pathway there occurs vasodilation in muscle blood vessels also.

- Some experiments suggest that the sympathetic vasodilator system might cause initial vasodilation in skeletal muscles to allow anticipatory increase in blood flow, even before the onset of exercise.
- These fibres play an important role in preventing the sudden rise in systemic blood pressure at the beginning of exercise, i.e. these provide a *safety valve mechanism.* Just before the start of exercise, there occurs a considerable increase in the sympathetic activity. This is brought by the mere thought of exercise. As a result, the increase in stroke volume and heart rate should produce a marked increase in the blood pressure to a dangerous level. However, this does not happen so, because the discharge of sympathetic vasodilator fibres reduces the total peripheral resistance and thus lowers the blood pressure to safety level. Since the sympathetic vasodilator fibres dilate only the arterioles and not the precapillary sphincters, they do not increase the blood flow to the muscles. When exercise commences, the precapillary sphincters are dilated by the local metabolites and blood flow to the muscle is increased tremendously.

SPLANCHNIC CIRCULATION

Splanchnic Vessels

Splanchnic circulation includes the combined vascular beds of the intestines, pancreas, spleen and liver. The main vessels which constitute the splanchnic circulation are:

- ***Arteries*** supplying the blood to intestines, pancreas, spleen and liver (Fig. 4.6-10) include:
  - *Coeliac trunk* is about 1 cm long and after arising from the abdominal aorta it divides into three main branches the *left gastric artery, hepatic artery and splenicartery,*
  - *Superior mesenteric artery* and
  - *Inferior mesenteric artery.*
- ***Hepatic portal system*** is formed by the veins draining blood from the abdominal part of the GIT. The veins comprising the hepatic portal system are shown in Fig. 4.6-11. All these veins end in the *portal vein.* The portal vein supplies the blood collected from GIT to the liver by its right and left branches.
- ***Hepatic veins*** are terminal parts of an elaborate venous tree that permeates the liver. The hepatic veins emerging from the liver tissue end in the inferior vena cava.

Splanchnic Circulation: Characteristic Features

- During rest, the abdominal GIT, viscera and liver receive about 1500 ml blood per minute (about 30% of cardiac output) via coeliac, superior mesenteric and inferior mesenteric arteries (Fig. 4.6-10).
- If the entire GIT becomes simultaneously active, the splanchnic blood flow would have increased to about 4.0 L/min. However, since during digestion and absorption, the GIT is sequentially activated, the maximum circulation is about 3.0 L/min.

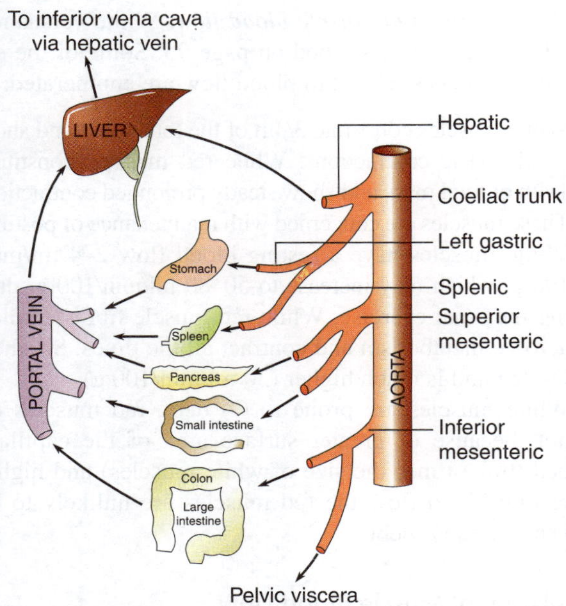

FIGURE 4.6-10 Splanchnic circulation.

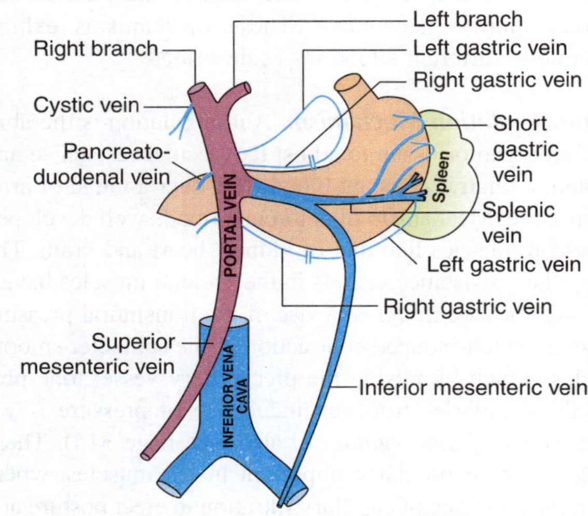

FIGURE 4.6-11 Tributaries of portal vein.

- The unique feature of the splanchnic circulation is that the venous blood from GIT viscera is not directly carried to the heart through systemic veins, but is carried to the liver forming hepatic portal system.

For the purpose of discussion the splanchnic circulation is considered to consist of three parts:

- Intestinal (mesenteric) circulation,
- Splenic circulation and
- Hepatic circulation.

Intestinal Circulation

Intestinal or Mesenteric Circulation is constituted by the blood supplied to the intestines and pancreas (about 100 ml/min) by a series of parallel circulations via the branches of superior and inferior mesenteric arteries.

Extensive Anastomoses between the vessels constituting mesenteric circulation, but blockage of a large intestinal artery still leads to infarction of the below.

The Blood Flow to Intestinal Mucosa is much more (about 5 times) than that of rest of the intestinal wall (Table 4.6-3).

Capillary Filtration Coefficient for mucosal capillaries is about 10 times than that for skeletal muscles, that is why the mucosal vessels have an enormous capillary surface available for absorption and pore bound secretion.

During Metabolic Activity the blood flow to GIT increases (Table 4.6-3) due to vagal activity (in the stomach), humoral activity, the local release of bradykinin from the mucosal glands and metabolites in the intestinal tract itself.

- ***Countercurrent system*** exists in the capillaries and venules in a villus, i.e. the direction of blood flow in the capillaries and venules in a villus is opposite to that in the main arteriole (Fig. 4.6-12). This system has both advantages and disadvantages.
- *Advantages of countercurrent system* of villus blood vessels shows that it slows down the entrance of rapidly absorbed solutes into the blood as explained below:

  The lipid-soluble substances when carried in the *venous descending limb* of vascular hair pin loop pass by diffusion across into the *ascending arterial limb* because of a concentration gradient (Fig. 4.6-12A). In this way, high concentration of absorbed substances reaches in outer parts of the villi and then these substances leave relatively slowly via the venous blood.
- *Disadvantage of countercurrent system* of villus blood vessels is that it decreases pO_2 at the tip of villi as explained.

This system permits diffusion of O_2 from the ascending arterial limb of villi into the descending venous limb (Fig. 4.6-12B). In this way, at low flow rates substantial amount of O_2 from the arterioles is shifted to venules near the base of villi resulting in decrease in O_2 supply to the mucosal cells at the tips of villi. When intestinal blood flow is very low, the transfer of O_2 from arterioles to venules is exaggerated and may cause extensive necrosis of intestinal villi.

TABLE 4.6-3 Blood Flow to Intestines (in ml/100 g/min)

Structure	At rest	During maximum metabolic activity
• Intestinal mucosa	50–60	300–400
• Rest of the intestinal wall	10	40

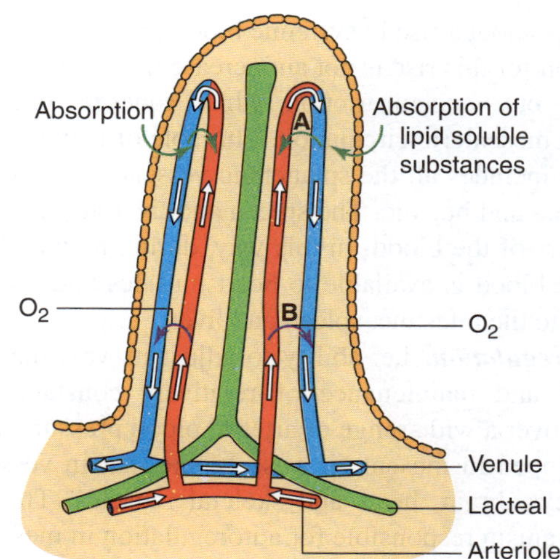

FIGURE 4.6-12 Countercurrent system of villus blood vessels depicting transfer of lipid-soluble substances from venous limb to arterial limb (**A**) and that of O_2 from arterial to venous limb (**B**).

Regulation of Intestinal Circulation

1. ***Local chemical control (functional hyperaemia).*** During increased intestinal activity, i.e. after food ingestion there occurs a marked increase in the intestinal blood flow (*functional hyperaemia).* It is proposed that *gastrin, secretin, bradykinin and cholecystokinin,* which are secreted from mucosal glands during food ingestion, cause local vasodilation and augment the blood flow.

   The absorption of digested food is also associated with increased intestinal blood flow. The principal mediators of mesenteric hyperaemia present in the digested food are glucose and fatty acids.
   - As the digestive and reabsorptive process proceed in different parts of the alimentary canal in a sequential manner the blood flow also increases in the same pattern and so the maximum blood flow during these activities is about 3 L/min.
2. ***Neural regulation.*** The splanchnic vessels are richly innervated by noradrenergic sympathetic nerve fibres. These nerve fibres have mild tonic discharge, which causes a moderate vascular resistance in the splanchnic blood vessels. The direct effect of sympathetic stimulation is intense vasoconstriction of the arterioles leading to decrease blood flow. After few minutes of the vasoconstriction, blood flow returns back to normal by 'autoregulatory escape' phenomenon. Autoregulatory escape is the local metabolic vasodilator mechanism elicited by ischemia that overrides sympathetic vasoconstriction. Therefore, sympathectomy causes only 25% increase in intestinal blood flow.

   The main role of neural regulation of splanchnic vessels is in time of cardiovascular crisis, e.g. sudden hypotension, when more blood is to be transferred from the splanchnic vessels to systemic circulation. Under such situation, the splanchnic vasomotor nerves participate in the baroreceptor-mediated reflexes and their stimulation brings about a rise in systemic blood pressure. The main reason for this rise is not an increase in peripheral resistance but venoconstriction, which squeezes out blood from mesenteric circulation. This role of neural mechanism includes all the splanchnic vessels, viz. intestinal, splenic and hepatic. The spleen and liver are major reservoirs of the blood. In this way, during hours of crisis more blood is available to heart muscles and the brain than to the intestine, spleen and liver.

3. ***Autoregulation,*** i.e. ability to adjust its vascular resistance and maintenance of relatively constant blood flow over a wide range of arterial blood pressure is well developed in mesenteric vessels like that in vessels of kidneys, brain, heart and skeletal muscles. The main mechanism responsible for autoregulation in mesenteric vessels is *metabolic,* though the *myogenic* mechanism may also play some role. The principal metabolic mediator here is *adenosine.* However, potassium ions and altered osmolality may also contribute to autoregulation.

Splenic Circulation

Splenic Artery, which is branch of coeliac trunk, supplies about 200 ml of blood/min to the spleen during rest via its splenic branches, which enter the hilum of the spleen.

Spleen Serves as Reservoir of Blood. In spleen, two structures are involved in storage of blood, namely splenic venous sinuses and splenic pulp. The small arteries and arterioles open directly into the splenic venous sinuses (Fig. 4.6-13). Due to dilation of venous sinuses, a large amount of blood is stored in spleen and the spleen distends. The capillaries of the splenic pulp are highly permeable. So, lot of blood cells pass through the capillary membrane and are stored in the pulp.

The constriction of Splenic Venous Sinuses by sympathetic stimulation causes release of blood into the circulation.

Regulation of Splenic Blood Flow Regulation of splenic blood flow is similar to that of intestinal blood flow. As mentioned earlier, the main role of neural control of splanchnic vessels is to transfer blood to circulation during hours of crisis. The spleen in the dogs and other carnivores contain lot of smooth muscles in its capsule, which contract strongly on sympathetic stimulation and discharge lot of blood into the circulation. This function of spleen is quantitatively not important in human. However, reservoir function of the whole visceral circulation plays a vital role in this mechanism.

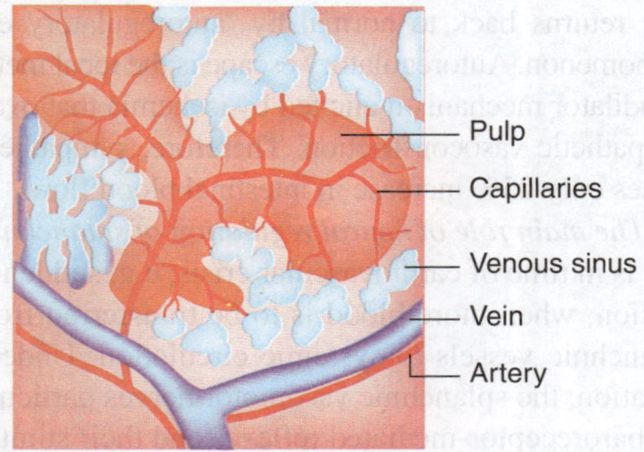

FIGURE 4.6-13 Storage of blood in splenic venous sinuses and splenic pulp.

Hepatic Circulation

Characteristic Features of Hepatic Circulation

- ***Source of Blood.*** Liver receives about 1500 ml blood/min from two sources:
  - ***Hepatic Artery*** which is a branch of coeliac trunk supplies about 20–25% (300–400 ml) of the total blood which caters to the metabolic requirements of the liver tissue.
  - ***Portal Vein*** which collects blood from the mesenteric and splenic vascular bed supplies about 75–80% (1100–1200 ml/min) of the total blood.

  The hepatic and portal blood streams meet in the sinusoids.

Functional Unit of Liver The functional unit of liver is *acinus.* The acini have been likened to grapes or berries, each on a vascular stem. There are about 10000 acini in human liver. Thus, each acinus is at the end of vascular stalk containing terminal branches of portal vein, hepatic arteries and bile ducts (Fig. 4.6-14). Blood flows from these terminal vessels into the sinusoids, which represent the capillary network of the liver. The sinusoids radiate toward the periphery of acinus, where they drain into the terminal branches of hepatic veins. Blood from these terminal hepatic venules drains into progressively larger branches of the hepatic veins, which are tributaries of the inferior vena cava. For details, see page 616.

Zones of Acinus. Each acinus can be considered to have three zones: 1, 2 and 3 based on the pattern of vessels in the acinus described above. The blood supply to different zones of acinus is:

- ***Zone 1*** refers to the central portion of acinus immediately surrounding the terminal hepatic arteriole and terminal portal venule. This zone is *well oxygenated.* Enzymes involved in oxidative metabolism and glucogenesis predominate here.
- ***Zone 2,*** i.e. the intermediate zone which is present in between zone 1 and 3 is *moderately well oxygenated.* It contains a mixed complement of enzymes.

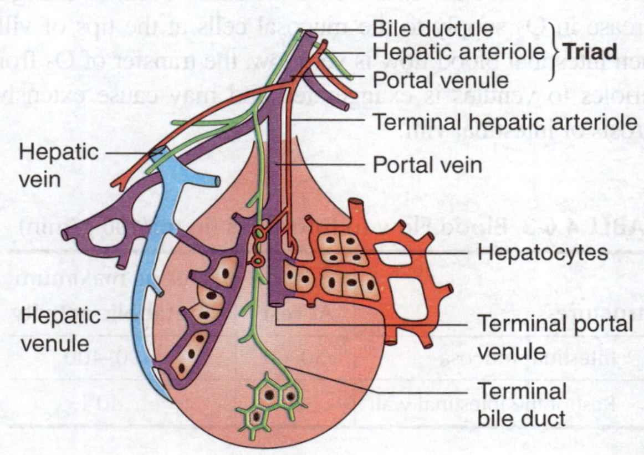

FIGURE 4.6-14 Concept of acinus as functional unit of liver.

- ***Zone 3*** refers to most peripheral part of the acinus. It is least well oxygenated and most susceptible to anoxic injury. It is rich in enzymes involved in glycolysis, lipid and drug metabolism.

Hepatic Artery versus Portal Vein Blood Flow

Pressure gradients and hepatic arterial and venous blood flow. The mean pressure in the hepatic artery branches that converge on the sinusoids is about 90 mmHg and that in the terminal portal venules which converge on the sinusoids is 10 mmHg. The hepatic venous pressure is about 5 mmHg (Fig. 4.6-15). From the above pressures, one would expect that sinusoid pressure to be very high. However, the sinusoidal pressure is only 10 mmHg. This is because of the fact that due to high presinusoidal resistance in hepatic arterial tree there is a marked pressure drop along the hepatic arterioles. The pressure drop in the hepatic arterial tree is adjusted so that there is an *inverse relationship between hepatic arterial and portal venous blood flow.* That is when portal venous blood flow is low the hepatic arterial blood flow increases and when the portal venous blood flow is high the hepatic arterial blood flow decreases. This inverse relationship may be maintained in part by the rate at which adenosine is removed from the region around the arterioles. According to this hypothesis, adenosine is produced by metabolism at a constant rate. When portal flow is reduced, it is washed away more slowly, and local accumulation of adenosine dilates the terminal arterioles increasing the hepatic arterial blood flow and vice versa. Thus, the hepatic arteriolar blood flow has *autoregulation* but the portal vein blood flow system does not have autoregulation.

Important Note

- As portal pressures do not increase linearly with portal blood flow, therefore, is important to prevent fluid loss through highly permeable liver sinusoids. Ascitis in cirrhosis of liver occurs because the parenchymal cells get destroyed and replaced with fibrous tissue that greatly increases resistance to blood flow. High hepatic vascular pressure can cause fluid transudation into the peritoneal cavity from hepatic and portal capillaries (ascitis).

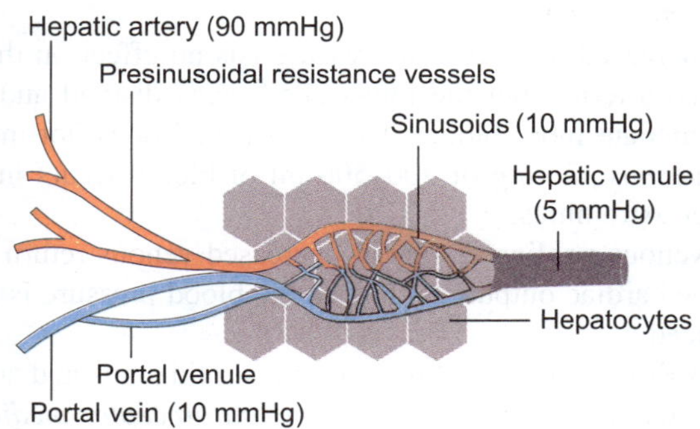

FIGURE 4.6-15 Pressure gradient across the blood vessels of an acinus.

Oxygen supply to liver. The hepatic arterial flow contributes 30% and rest of the 70% of the O_2 used by the liver is contributed by the portal blood flow. This is because of the fact that about 80% of the blood entering the liver is from portal venous system and 20% is from hepatic arterial system. During periods of activity, i.e. ingestion and digestion there is marked increase of portal blood flow (functional hyperaemia) which compensates for the reduced content of O_2 per 100 ml of blood.

Though the rate of O_2 delivery to the liver is varied, it tends to maintain a constant O_2 consumption. This is made possible because of two reasons: firstly the extraction of O_2 from the hepatic blood is very efficient, and secondly liver has the capability to compensate by an appropriate change in the fraction of O_2 extracted from the blood. This extraction is facilitated by the distance between the presinusoidal vessels at the centre of acinus and postsinusoidal vessels at the periphery of acinus. In other words, the substantial distance between these types of vessels prevents a countercurrent exchange of O_2 as seen in intestinal villi.

Filtration across Hepatic Sinusoids The hepatic sinusoids are perforated and show large fenestrations; and therefore, allow a free exchange of macromolecules across their wall compared with capillaries elsewhere in the body. Because of this reason, the liver lymph has very high protein contents (6 g/100 ml), i.e. similar to that of plasma while the lymph from other places has low protein contents (2 g/100 ml).

Regulation of Hepatic Circulation

1. Autoregulation. The hepatic arterial blood flow is autoregulated and the portal blood flow is not autoregulated. As described above, the hepatic arterial blood flow changes reciprocally with portal blood flow and that the adenosine is involved in this adjustment.

2. Functional Hyperaemia of the intestinal tract after meals is associated with increased portal blood flow to liver.

3. Neural Regulation. The hepatic vessels are innervated by the noradrenergic sympathetic nerve fibres via T_3 to T_{11} roots and splanchnic nerves and the vasoconstrictor fibres reach the liver from hepatic plexus. There is no known vasodilator innervation to the liver vasculature. The liver serves as a blood reservoir, storing about 400 ml of blood in its sinusoids. The sympathetic nerves constrict the presinusoidal resistance vessels in the portal venous system and hepatic arterial system. As described in the neural control of intestinal blood flow, the neural effects on capacitance vessels are more important. Sympathetic stimulation causes a marked reduction in the capacitance of the portal system and other splanchnic capacitance vessels, and mobilizes about 1 L of blood towards the heart in less than a minute. In severe shock, hepatic blood flow gets reduced markedly and may produce patchy necrosis of the liver.

Chapter 4.7

Cardiovascular Homeostasis in Health and Disease

CARDIOVASCULAR HOMEOSTASIS IN HEALTH

- Cardiovascular adjustments during gravitational changes
  - Posture change from lying to standing
  - Prolonged quiet standing
  - Postural hypotension
  - Gravity acceleration
  - Gravity deceleration
  - Zero gravity
- Cardiovascular adjustments during intrathoracic pressure changes
  - Valsalva manoeuvre
  - Muller's manoeuvre
- Cardiovascular adjustments during muscular exercise
  - Changes in muscle blood flow
  - Other cardiovascular changes

CARDIOVASCULAR HOMEOSTASIS IN DISEASES

- Circulatory shock
  - Types and causes
  - Stages and clinical features
    - Nonprogressive shock
    - Progressive shock
    - Refractory shock
  - Physiology in treatment of shock
- Heart failure

CARDIOVASCULAR HOMEOSTASIS IN HEALTH

Cardiovascular homeostasis in health refers to the compensatory adjustments of the cardiovascular system (CVS) to challenges faced by the circulation in everyday life. The common situations during which cardiovascular adjustment are required in day to day life include:

- Gravitational changes,
- Intrathoracic pressure changes and
- Exercise.

Cardiovascular Adjustments During Gravitational Changes

Gravitational changes occur under following conditions in life:

- Posture change from lying to standing,
- Prolonged quiet standing,
- Gravity acceleration (positive g), deceleration (negative g) and zero gravity (zero g).

Adjustments During Posture Change From Lying to Standing

When posture is changed from lying (recumbent) to standing (erect) the haemodynamic changes occur as a result of the effect of gravity on the blood column which tends to reduce the cardiac output and blood pressure. However, since in humans the compensatory mechanisms are so well developed that in normal persons no effect is felt on posture changes in day-to-day life. The sequence of events which occurs during change in posture from lying to standing is explained below.

In standing position, due to *hydrostatic (gravitational) effect of blood column*, for every centimetre below or above the heart level, the pressure increases or decreases by 0.77 mmHg, respectively. Therefore, in normal adults, the blood pressure at the level of feet (about 100 cm below heart level) in both arteries and veins is increased approximately by 80 mmHg. Thus, the mean arterial pressure and venous pressure which are 90 and 10 mmHg, respectively, in supine position will change to 170 and 90 mmHg, respectively, on standing.

Increased intraluminal pressure has no effect on thick-walled arteries, but the thin-walled veins distend and accommodate more blood. If the individual does not move, the *venous pooling* of 300–500 ml of blood occurs in the lower extremities.

Venous pooling results in decreased venous return and so the cardiac output and thence the blood pressure is also reduced.

A drop in the blood pressure in carotid sinus and aortic arch within seconds triggers the *baroreceptor-mediated compensatory mechanism* which causes the following changes.

- ***Heart rate*** is increased by 5–10 beats/min.
- ***Force of cardiac contraction*** is increased leading to increase in stroke volume and cardiac output.
- ***Peripheral resistance*** is increased due to arteriolar constriction in the cutaneous, renal and splanchnic circulation. Increase in peripheral resistance increases the diastolic pressure.
- ***Venoconstriction*** in the body transfers blood from the capacitance vessels towards the heart increasing the venous return.
- ***Increased secretion of renin and aldosterone*** also helps in normalization of blood pressure.

In spite of the above mentioned compensatory changes, the stroke volume and cardiac output in standing posture are about 25% less than in supine position. However, due to 25% increase in the total peripheral resistance, the blood pressure becomes almost normal.

The above events are summarized in Fig. 4.7-1.

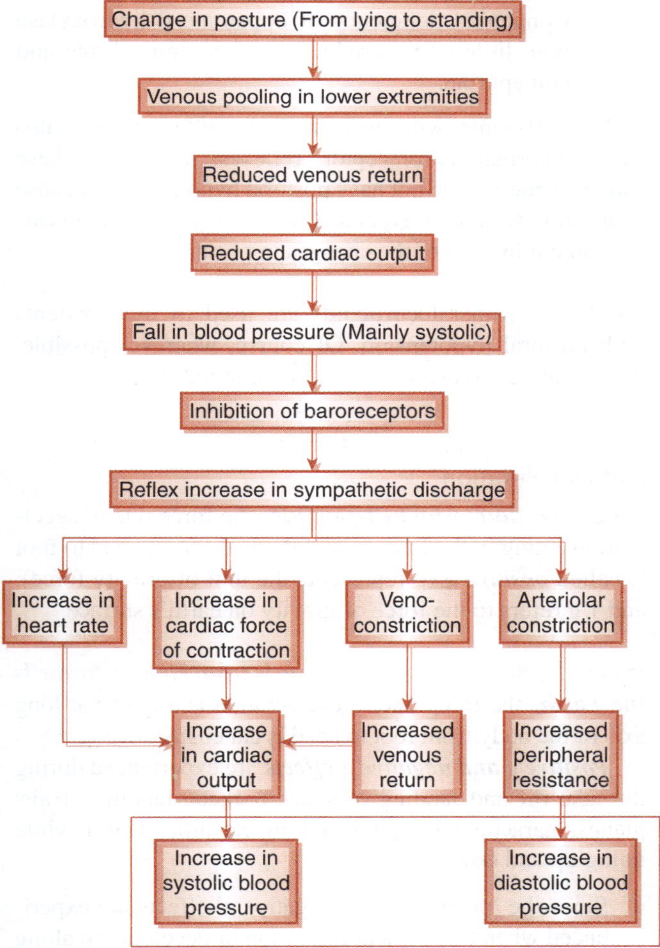

FIGURE 4.7-1 Summary of events maintaining normal blood pressure during change of posture from lying to standing.

Net Effects on CVS of Rising from the Supine to Upright Position Average net effects which occur on the CVS of rising from supine to upright position after the compensatory mechanism are

- *Central venous pressure* is decreased slightly (3 mmHg).
- *Heart rate* is increased by 25%.
- *Abdominal and limb flow* is decreased by 25%.
- *Stroke volume* is decreased by 40%.
- *Cardiac output* is decreased by 25%.
- *Total peripheral resistance* is increased by 25%.
- *Systolic blood pressure* is slightly reduced due to fall in stroke volume.
- *Diastolic blood pressure* is slightly increased due to increased total peripheral resistance.
- *Pulse pressure* (systolic BP – diastolic BP) is reduced.
- *Mean arterial pressure* is nearly unchanged.

Maintenance of Cerebral Blood Flow ***Cerebral blood flow*** in standing position is maintained by certain additional compensatory changes:

- ***Decrease in jugular venous pressure (JVP) to*** 5 mmHg due to gravity compensates for the drop in arterial pressure at head level to 20–40 mmHg by reducing the drop in perfusion pressure (arterial pressure minus venous pressure).
- ***Fall in intracranial pressure*** due to fall in venous pressure reduces cerebral vascular resistance and thus facilitates cerebral blood flow.
- ***Increased*** pCO_2 ***and decreased*** pO_2 ***and decreased pH*** in brain tissues occurring due to decreased cerebral blood flow causes vasodilation, improving the blood flow.

Because of the operation of the above-mentioned *autoregulatory mechanisms*, the cerebral blood flow decreases only 20% on standing. In addition, the amount of *O_2 extracted per unit of blood increases,* and the net effect is that cerebral O_2 consumption is about the same in supine and erect positions.

The above events are summarized in Fig. 4.7-2.

For details see page 380

Changes During Prolonged Quiet Standing

When one changes posture from lying to standing, certain cardiovascular adjustments occur (described above) which maintain the almost normal blood pressure and normal blood flow to various organs of the body.

The prolonged standing presents an additional problem due to increasing interstitial fluid volume in the lower extremities. If the person keeps on moving, the operation of 'muscle pump' (see page 289) keeps the venous pressure below 30 mmHg at the feet level and maintains adequate venous return. However, on prolonged quiet standing (a situation particularly met with military or police personnel, i.e. standing in attention for long periods), along with the

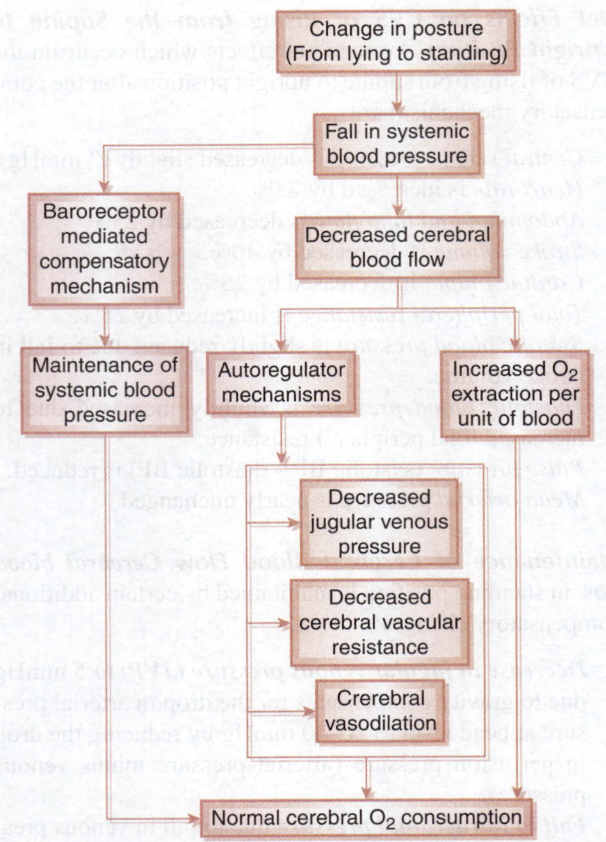

FIGURE 4.7-2 Summary of events maintaining normal cerebral O_2 consumption in standing posture.

venous pooling, the fluid begins to accumulate in the interstitial spaces because of increased hydrostatic pressure in the capillaries. The cardiac output is decreased due to decreased venous return. A stage may come when cerebral blood flow decreases to less than about 60% and symptoms of cerebral ischaemia develop. The individual may faint and fall down.

The fainting, in a sense, is also a homeostatic mechanism, because falling to horizontal position promptly restores venous return, cardiac output and cerebral blood flow to adequate levels.

Postural Hypotension

In postural hypotension or *orthostatic hypotension* there occurs a sudden fall in blood pressure on changing posture from lying to erect, which causes symptoms of cerebral ischaemia. The individual experiences transient blurring of vision, dizziness or even fainting. It is diagnosed by recording blood pressure in lying and standing postures. A decrease in systolic blood pressure by 30 mmHg or more on standing from supine position is diagnostic.

Pathophysiology Postural hypotension develops in individuals in whom the cardiovascular compensatory mechanism (described above) which maintains normal blood pressure and adequate cerebral blood flow is very slow to develop.

Causes of Postural Hypotension

1. Decreased Blood Volume. The effects of gravity on the circulation in humans depend in part upon the blood volume. When the blood volume is low, the compensatory mechanisms are slow to develop and the individual may suffer from postural hypotension.

2. Sympatholytic Drugs. Postural hypotension is common in patients receiving sympatholytic drugs.

3. Dysfunctions of Sympathetic Nervous System are obviously associated with postural hypotension. Dysfunction of sympathetic nervous system may be grouped as

i. Surgical sympathectomy
ii. Autonomic neuropathy occurring in diseases such as diabetes mellitus, syphilis and Parkinson's disease
iii. Primary autonomic failure seen in following conditions:
   - Bradbury–Eggleston syndrome (idiopathic orthostatic hypotension),
   - Shy–Drager syndrome (multiple system atrophy),
   - Riley–Day syndrome (familial dysautonomia),
   - Congenital deficiency of dopamine β-hydroxylase with little or no production of norepinephrine and epinephrine.

Note. Patients with *primary hyperaldosteronism* also have abnormal baroreceptor reflexes. However, these patients generally do not have postural hypotension, because their blood volume is expanded sufficiently to maintain cardiac output in spite of the changes in posture.

Treatment Mineralocorticoids are used to treat patients with postural hypotension. Of course, wherever possible, the causative disease should be ameliorated.

Cardiovascular Effects of Gravity Acceleration and Deceleration

When the Body Moves Upwards, the force due to acceleration acting in the long axis of the body from head to foot is called *positive g* (g represents the unit of gravity force), and 1 g refers to the force of gravity on earth's surface.

When the Body Moves Downwards from Height Towards the Earth, the force due to deceleration acting in the long axis of the body from foot to head is called *negative g*.

Positive g and negative g effects are experienced during the take off and landing of space rockets, landing of airplanes, parachute jumping and in elevators (lifts) while going up and down.

- Since the 'positive g and negative g' effects are experienced when there is a acceleration or deceleration along the long axis of the body, the astronauts avoid these effects by positioning themselves perpendicular to the direction of g, i.e. in a *chest-to-back direction.*

Effect of Positive g The effects of 'positive g' on the CVS are due to throwing down of blood in lower part of the body and similar to those occurring from change of posture from lying to standing, but they are multiplied depending upon the speed of acceleration.

At Acceleration Less than 5 g the compensatory mechanisms (described in effect of posture change) are able to maintain vital cardiovascular status. *Cardiac output* is maintained for a time when blood is drawn from the pulmonary venous reservoir and as the force of cardiac contraction is increased, *cerebral circulation* is protected due to associated fall in the JVP and intracranial pressure.

At Acceleration More than 5 g with body in long axis, the pressure in the veins in the lower limbs rises to over 450 mmHg. The consequent passive dilatation of veins of the lower limbs retains so much blood that the venous return and therefore, cardiac output is markedly reduced. Under such a situation, vision fails (*blackout*) in about 5 s and unconsciousness almost hits immediately thereafter.

Antigravity Suit or the g-suit is used by the astronauts to effectively cushion the effects of gravitational force. The 'g-suit' is a double walled pressure suit containing water or compressed air. When there is 'positive g', there is a tendency of venous pooling and simultaneously the water in the g-suit also rushes to the lower parts. The g-suit is regulated in such a way that it compresses the abdomen and legs with a force proportionate to the positive g. This decreases venous pooling and helps to maintain venous return.

Effect of Negative g The effects of 'negative g' on the CVS are due to the rushing up of blood towards head when the body suddenly moves down. As a result of accumulation of blood in the head and neck, following changes occur:

- *Cardiac output* is increased due to general increase in venous return. Most of the cardiac output, however, moves towards upper parts of the body.
- *Cerebral arterial pressure* is increased markedly. In spite of the great increase in cerebral arterial pressure, the vessels in the brain do not rupture, because there occurs a corresponding *increase in intracranial pressure and their walls are supported.* In other words, the CSF acts like a g-suit.
- Blood vessels of head and neck show intense congestion.
- *Ecchymosis* appears around the eyes.
- *Severe throbbing headache,* pain, and eventually
- *Mental confusion* (red out).

Effect of Zero Gravity The 'zero gravity' situation occurs when the astronauts in a spacecraft go out of the earth's gravitational effect, e.g. during orbital flights to other planets. The absence of gravity leads to:

- Weightlessness,
- Movements of the body become effortless,
- Absence of hydrostatic pressure on the blood column.

A data of 14 months stay in the zero gravity zone are available, which shows the following documental effects.

Effects on the CVS

- ***Transient postural hypotension*** has been present after return to earth from space flights, and full readaptation to normal gravity has been reported to occur in 4 weeks.
- ***Some atrophy of myocardium*** is reported to occur, because of the fact that heart did not have to function for increases in cardiac output required in everyday life as on earth. *More severe disuse atrophy of myocardium* is speculated in prolonged period of weightlessness during future trips to planets.

Other Effects of Zero Gravity

- ***Flaccidity and atrophy of skeletal muscles*** to some extent occurs since, due to zero gravity the muscular effect is much reduced when objects to be moved are weightless and the normal proprioceptive input is decreased. A programme of regular exercises against resistance, e.g. pushing against a wall of spacecraft or stretching a heavy rubber band may decrease the muscle atrophy.
- ***Space motion sickness,*** (the nausea, vomiting and vertigo) develops in astronauts, when they are first exposed to 'zero gravity' and often wears off after a few days of space flight. It can occur with re-entering in the gravity. It occurs due to vestibular apparatus dysfunctioning.
- ***Changes in the blood*** noted are:
  - Loss of plasma volume, probably because of head ward shift of body fluids, with subsequent diuresis,
  - Loss of red cell mass and
  - Alterations in the plasma lymphocytes.
- ***Bone mineral*** is lost steadily with increased Ca^{2+} excretion. A loss of body Ca^{2+} is equivalent to 0.4% of the total body Ca^{2+} per month initially, but later tapers off during prolonged space flight. Further, a high-calcium diet helps to overcome this problem.
- ***Psychological problems*** associated with isolation and monotony of prolonged space flight are also a matter of concern.

Cardiovascular Adjustments During Intrathoracic Pressure Changes

Intrathoracic pressure changes are not uncommon in everyday life. Depending upon the mechanism of intrathoracic pressure changes, the activities responsible for these may be grouped into Valsalva manoeuvre and Muller's manoeuvre.

Valsalva Manoeuvre

Valsalva manoeuvre refers to a forced expiration against a closed glottis. The common everyday activities in which Valsalva manoeuvre effect is seen on the intrathoracic pressure are straining during defecation, initial phase of coughing and straining during parturition.

Intrathoracic Pressure Changes During Valsalva Manoeuvre and Their Effects on CVS The changes exerted on the CVS due to a sudden and sharp rise in intrathoracic pressure occurring due to Valsalva manoeuvre effect can be described in four phases (Fig. 4.7-3).

- ***Phase 1*** is characterized by a transient rise in the arterial pressure. It coincides with compression of the aorta due to sudden increase in the intrathoracic pressure.
- ***Phase 2***, which follows phase 1 is characterized by:
  - A fall in arterial pressure which plateau after few seconds owing to reflex vasoconstriction.
  - Heart rate usually increases slightly.

  Mechanism. The phase 2 changes in CVS are initiated by a decrease in venous return which occurs due to increase in intrathoracic pressure changes. The sequence of events which follow decreased cardiac output is depicted in Fig. 4.7-3.
- ***Phase 3*** is characterized by a transient fall in blood pressure which follows 1–2 s after release of the strain. It coincides with release of pressure compressing the aorta due to decreased intrathoracic pressure. In other words, events in phase 3 are just reverse of the events in phase 1.
- ***Phase 4*** is characterized by:
  - *Increase in arterial blood pressure* above the resting level within 10 s. This overshoot of blood pressure is due to the lingering effect of vasoconstriction induced during phase 2. The blood pressure returns to resting level after about 1.5 min of strain release.

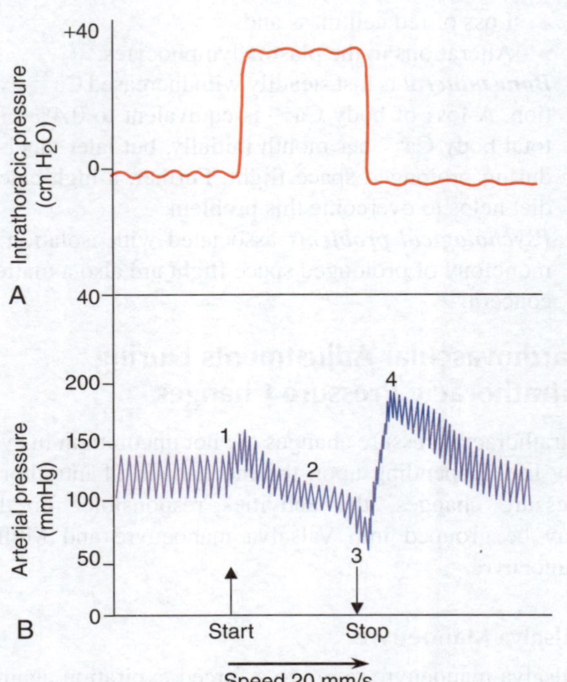

FIGURE 4.7-3 Response to Valsalva manoeuvre in a normal man: **A**, intrathoracic pressure changes; and **B**, arterial pressure changes (in phase 1, 2, 3, 4).

- *Slowing of heart rate* occurs due to baroreceptor-mediated vagal stimulation in response to overshoot of blood pressure.

Clinical Application of Valsalva Manoeuvre In clinical practice, Valsalva manoeuvre is employed for testing of baroreceptor reflexes and also as a test for autonomic insufficiency where the vagal response may be impaired.

- ***Procedure.*** The subject is asked to blow for about 15 s into a mouthpiece which is attached to a sphygmomanometer at a pressure of 40 mmHg. A continuous recording of ECG is made during and after this manoeuvre.
- ***Interpretation of results.*** Results of this test are interpreted in the form of *Valsalva ratio.* Valsalva ratio is the ratio of the longest RR interval (noted within 20 beats of the end of Valsalva manoeuvre) to the shortest RR interval (noted during the Valsalva manoeuvre). The normal Valsalva ratio is >1.5, but in autonomic insufficiency, the Valsalva ratio is less than 1.11.

Muller's Manoeuvre

Muller's manoeuvre refers to forced inspiration against closed glottis. It is just the reverse of the Valsalva manoeuvre, i.e. it reduces the intrathoracic pressure (up to 80 mmHg). Therefore, the cardiovascular changes occurring during Muller's manoeuvre are exactly opposite to those which occur during Valsalva manoeuvre described above.

Cardiovascular Adjustments During Muscular Exercise

Severe muscular exercise is the most stressful physiological condition that the cardiovascular homeostasis mechanisms face in everyday life. In addition to CVS adjustments, respiratory and other adjustments also occur in the body, so they are comprehensively discussed in Chapter 12.1 on 'Physiology of exercise' (see page 1209).

CARDIOVASCULAR HOMEOSTASIS IN DISEASES

Cardiovascular homeostasis mechanism operates in almost all cardiorespiratory and many other multiorgan diseases. The most important conditions which need special description are:

- Circulatory shock and
- Cardiac failure.

Circulatory Shock

Circulatory shock or simply called as shock is a syndrome (collection of different entities that share certain common features) characterized by *serious reduction of tissue perfusion* with a relatively or absolutely inadequate cardiac output. In other words, the shock is a condition characterized by inadequate delivery of oxygen and nutrients to critical organs such as heart, brain, liver, kidneys and gastrointestinal tract.

Types and Causes of Shock

Depending upon the cause of inadequacy of cardiac output (relative or absolute) the circulatory shock may be of the following types:

I. Hypovolaemic shock,
II. Low-resistance or distributive or vasogenic shock,
III. Cardiogenic shock and
IV. Obstructive shock.

I. Hypovolaemic Shock Hypovolaemic shock also known as cold shock is caused by a low blood volume resulting in decreased cardiac output.

Causes. Depending on the causes, the hypovolaemic shock may be of following types:

1. ***Haemorrhagic shock*** occurs as a result of external or internal blood loss caused by ruptured vessels.
2. ***Dehydration shock.*** Fluid loss, when insufficient amount, can dehydrate the body and reduce the circulating blood volume. Fluid loss can occur from
   - Gastrointestinal tract (GIT) in diarrhoea or vomiting.
   - *Kidney* in diabetes mellitus, diabetes insipidus or excessive use of diuretics.
   - *Skin* in burns, exudative lesions and sweating. In burns, large part of the skin gets denuded and large amount of plasma is exuded through the exposed parts. Hypovolaemia due to plasma loss is a common complication of severe burns (burns shock).
3. ***Traumatic shock*** is a special type of hypovolaemic shock in which there is associated neurogenic shock caused by severe pain which inhibits the vasomotor centre (VMC).

II. Low-Resistance or Distributive or Vasogenic Shock Low-resistance or distributive or vasogenic shock occurs when neural reflexes or toxic substances cause excessive vasodilation within the vascular system. Due to vasodilation, the size of capacitance vessels is increased and thus the cardiac output is decreased in spite of normal blood volume. Low-resistance shock is also called *warm shock* because skin is warm and not cold and moist as it is in hypovolaemic shock.

Causes. Depending upon the causes, the low-resistance shock is of the following types:

1. ***Neurogenic shock*** occurs due to two types of nervous effects:
   i. *Marked reduction in sympathetic vasomotor tone* is responsible for most cases of neurogenic shock as seen in:
      - Deep general anaesthesia,
      - Spinal anaesthesia,
      - Brain damage, prolonged ischaemia causes inactivation of VMC (Note: Short periods of medullary ischaemia increase vasomotor activity),
      - Effects of antihypertensive drugs and
      - Postural syncope.
   ii. *Pronounced increased in the vagal tone* of the heart is responsible for neurogenic shock in some cases, as seen in:
      - Vasovagal syncope or emotional fainting.
2. ***Anaphylactic shock.*** Anaphylaxis refers to an acute allergic reaction. Large quantities of histamine and histamine-like substances released in allergic reaction cause widespread and marked *vasodilation* reducing peripheral resistance. Also, there is a marked *increase in capillary permeability* leading to fluid loss and adding hypovolaemic element to the low-resistance shock.
3. ***Septicaemic shock.*** Septicaemia is a condition in which bacteria circulate and multiply in the blood and form toxic products and cause high fever. Septicaemia may occur in conditions like acute peritonitis, perforation of bowel, strangulated bowel, puerperal sepsis, etc. Septicaemic shock develops due to the following effects of bacteria and toxic products:
   - Marked vasodilatation due to peripheral arteriolar paralysis,
   - Sludging of blood, presumably caused by red cell agglutination in response to degenerating tissues and
   - Disseminated intravascular coagulation (DIC).
4. ***Endotoxic shock*** refers to the shock produced by endotoxins released by gram-negative bacteria. Endotoxins produce shock due to their following effects:
   - Marked vasodilation reducing peripheral resistance,
   - Depressing myocardial contractility reducing cardiac output and
   - Increasing capillary permeability and causing hypovolaemia.

III. Cardiogenic Shock Cardiogenic shock occurs due to decreased pumping ability of the heart because of some cardiac abnormality. Severe depression of the systolic cardiac performance is the key factor in causing this type of shock. Since the heart is not able to pump out all the venous return, there occurs congestion of the lungs and viscera and that is why it is also called *congested shock.*

Causes of cardiogenic shock are:

1. ***Myocardial*** infarction involving 40% or more of the left ventricular myocardium is the commonest cause.
2. ***Other causes are:***
   - Cardiac arrhythmias,
   - Congestive heart failure,
   - Toxic states of heart and
   - Severe valvular dysfunctions.

IV. Obstructive Shock Obstructive shock or more precise to be, the extracardiac obstructive shock occurs due to impairment of ventricular filling during diastole due to some external pressure on the heart. Due to decreased ventricular filling, the stroke volume and hence the cardiac output is decreased causing circulatory shock.

Causes of obstructive effusion shock are:

1. Pericardial cardiac tamponade, i.e. bleeding into the pericardium with external pressure on the heart,
2. Tension pneumothorax,
3. Constrictive pericarditis,
4. Pulmonary embolism and
5. Post end-expiratory pressure respiration.

Stages and Clinical Features of Shock

Stages and clinical features of all types of shock are similar with minor differences. However, since the haemorrhagic shock is of more common, the discussion in this section will be centred on it. Depending upon the severity, the circulatory shock can be divided into three stages:

- First stage or nonprogressive shock,
- Second stage or progressive shock and
- Third stage or refractory (irreversible) shock.

I. First Stage of Shock or NonProgressive Shock

Nonprogressive shock also known as *compensated shock* or initial stage of shock occurs when there is a moderate reduction in cardiac output secondary to fluid loss or venous pooling or negative inotropic effect on the heart depending upon the type of shock.

Hypovolaemic shock due to acute blood loss, in other words, the *haemorrhagic shock*, occurs when at least 10% to 15% of total blood volume is lost. Thus, about 10% of the total blood volume may be lost without any significant effect.

Compensatory mechanisms of rapid onset (short-term mechanisms) immediately set into motion following the acute loss of blood and try to maintain the blood flow to vital organs in spite of reduced cardiac output. These mechanisms are effective in immediately controlling the blood pressure in nonprogressive shock and are followed by long-term compensatory mechanisms which restore the circulatory plasma proteins and red cell mass in 4–8 weeks. The compensatory mechanisms are described below in detail.

A. Rapid Compensatory Mechanisms (Neural Mechanism). Rapid or the so-called short-term control mechanisms primarily include the following three nervous reflexes.

1. ***Baroreceptor reflex.*** When the blood pressure is decreased there occurs decrease in the impulse discharge from the arterial baroreceptors (for detail see page 340). Even when the blood pressure has not fallen, the decrease in pulse pressure is sufficient to decrease the impulse discharge from baroreceptors. As a result there is a generalized increase in the sympathetic vasomotor discharge to heart, arterioles and veins. There occurs generalized vasoconstriction (sparing vessels of brain and heart). Vasoconstriction is more marked in the cutaneous, splanchnic, renal and skeletal muscle vessels. This causes shifting of greater amount of blood in circulation. Venoconstriction on account of sympathetic stimulation also causes increased shifting of stored venous blood in circulation leading to increased venous return and cardiac output. In kidneys both afferent and efferent blood vessels constrict, but afferent vessels constrict to a greater extent leading to reduction in GFR. All these mechanisms maintain blood pressure at such a level that the blood flow to the vital organs like heart and brain is not affected. However, blood flow to the vital organs is provided at the cost of other body tissues such as skin, abdominal viscera, kidney, and skeletal muscles.
2. ***Chemoreceptor reflex.*** Acute haemorrhage causes loss of red blood cells leading to reduced O_2 carrying capacity. The resultant anaemia and stagnant hypoxia as well as acidosis stimulate chemoreceptors which also excite VMC to cause the same effects as these caused by baroreceptor reflex. Fall in blood pressure below 60 mmHg usually initiates chemoreceptor reflex.
3. ***CNS ischaemic response.*** When blood pressure falls below 50 mmHg this response is initiated (for details see page 347). It causes more powerful sympathetic stimulation. This effect of central nervous system ischaemic response is called 'Last-ditch stand' of sympathetic reflexes.

The rapid compensatory mechanisms discussed above account for following:

Symptoms and Signs observed in patients with shock:

- ***Pale, cold and moist skin*** occurs due to decreased blood flow to skin and increased sweating (due to increased sympathetic discharge).
- ***Cyanotic tinge of skin*** may sometimes occur because of increased O_2 extraction from the blood.
- ***Tachycardia and fall in pulse pressure*** produce *thin and thready pulse,* the characteristic feature of hypovolaemic shock.
- ***Increased rate and force of respiration*** is due to greater sinoaortic chemoreceptors discharge.
- ***Oliguria,*** another important feature of hypovolaemic shock is due to renal arteriolar constriction.
- ***Restlessness and apprehension*** may occur due to stimulation of brainstem reticular formation by circulating catecholamines, since haemorrhage is a potent stimulator of secretion of these hormones from the adrenal medulla.

B. Intermediate Compensatory Mechanisms.

1. Renin–angiotensin vasoconstrictor mechanism (see page 348),
2. Reverse stress relaxation (see page 329) and
3. Capillary fluid shift mechanism (see page 330).
   - The angiotensin–vasopressin, as well as reverse stress relaxation mechanism require 10 min to 1 h to respond completely and help in raising the arterial pressure or circulatory filling pressure, thereby increases venous return to the heart.
   - Readjustment of blood volume by absorption of fluid from interstitial spaces and intestinal tract, as well as oral ingestion and absorption of additional quantity of water and salt may require 1–48 h.

C. Long-Term Compensatory Mechanisms.

1. ***Restoration of plasma volume and proteins.*** After a moderate haemorrhage, the plasma volume is restored to normal in 12–72 h. However, the improvement in blood volume is merely because of the increase in the amount of plasma water along with electrolyte content. The plasma protein concentration and haematocrit value is actually reduced *(haemodilution)*. There is rapid entry of preformed albumin from extravascular stores. After this initial influx, albumin and rest of the plasma protein loss are restored by hepatic synthesis over a period of 3–4 days.
2. ***Restoration of red cell mass.*** In the mean time, there is excess release of erythropoietin which increases the rate of cell production in the bone marrow within 10 days. Normal cell mass is restored in 4–8 weeks.

Note. Under normal circumstances, the circulatory compensatory mechanisms described above eventually cause full recovery without help of outside therapy during the stage of nonprogressive shock. However, a timely outside therapy may hasten the recovery.

II. Progressive Shock Second stage of the circulatory shock is a progressive stage which occurs after a 15–25% loss of total blood volume. In this stage, the compensatory mechanisms are not able to stop the progression of the shock. In other words, the *intense arteriolar vasoconstriction* seen in this stage is usually not adequate for maintenance of normal blood pressure. In progressive shock, the structures of circulatory system begin to deteriorate and various types of *positive feedback mechanisms* develop. Therefore, timely therapeutic interventions are essential in this stage, otherwise the vicious cycle of positive feedback mechanisms will cause progressive decrease in the cardiac output and ultimately the patient will go into a stage of refractory shock.

Positive Feedback Cycles. Positive feedback cycles responsible for continuous progression of shock, if not interrupted by therapeutic intervention, leading to refractory stage are (Figs 4.7-4, 4.7-5):

1. ***Cardiac failure.*** Due to severe decrease in arterial pressure, particularly diastolic pressure, the coronary blood flow also decreases, and coronary ischaemia occurs. This weakens the myocardium and further decreases cardiac output and blood pressure. This positive feedback causes progressive cardiac deterioration and may ultimately cause complete heart failure.
2. ***Vasomotor failure.*** Blood flow to heart and brain is usually preserved when cardiac output is decreased. However, there occurs very severe fall in blood pressure,

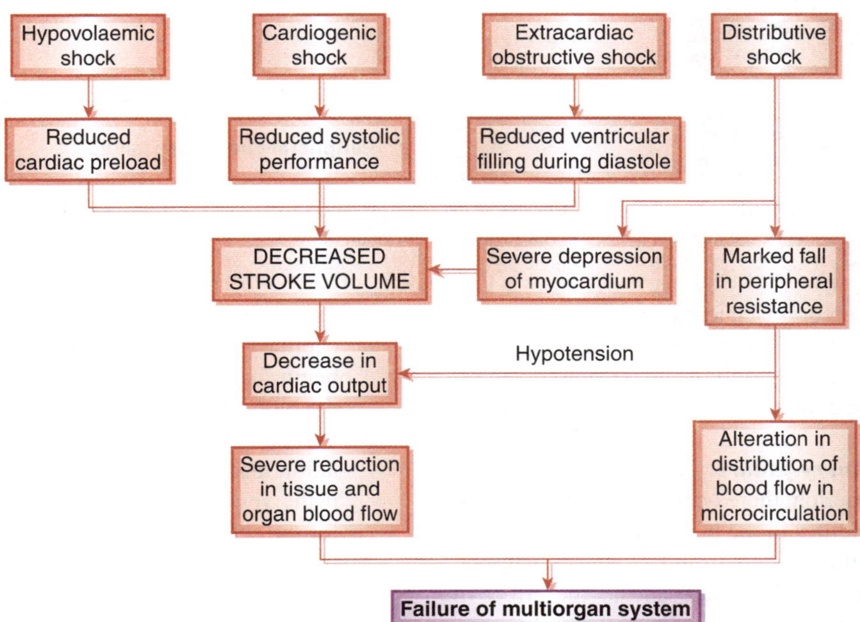

FIGURE 4.7-4 Chain of events that ultimately cause failure of multiple organ system and refractive shock in different types of shocks.

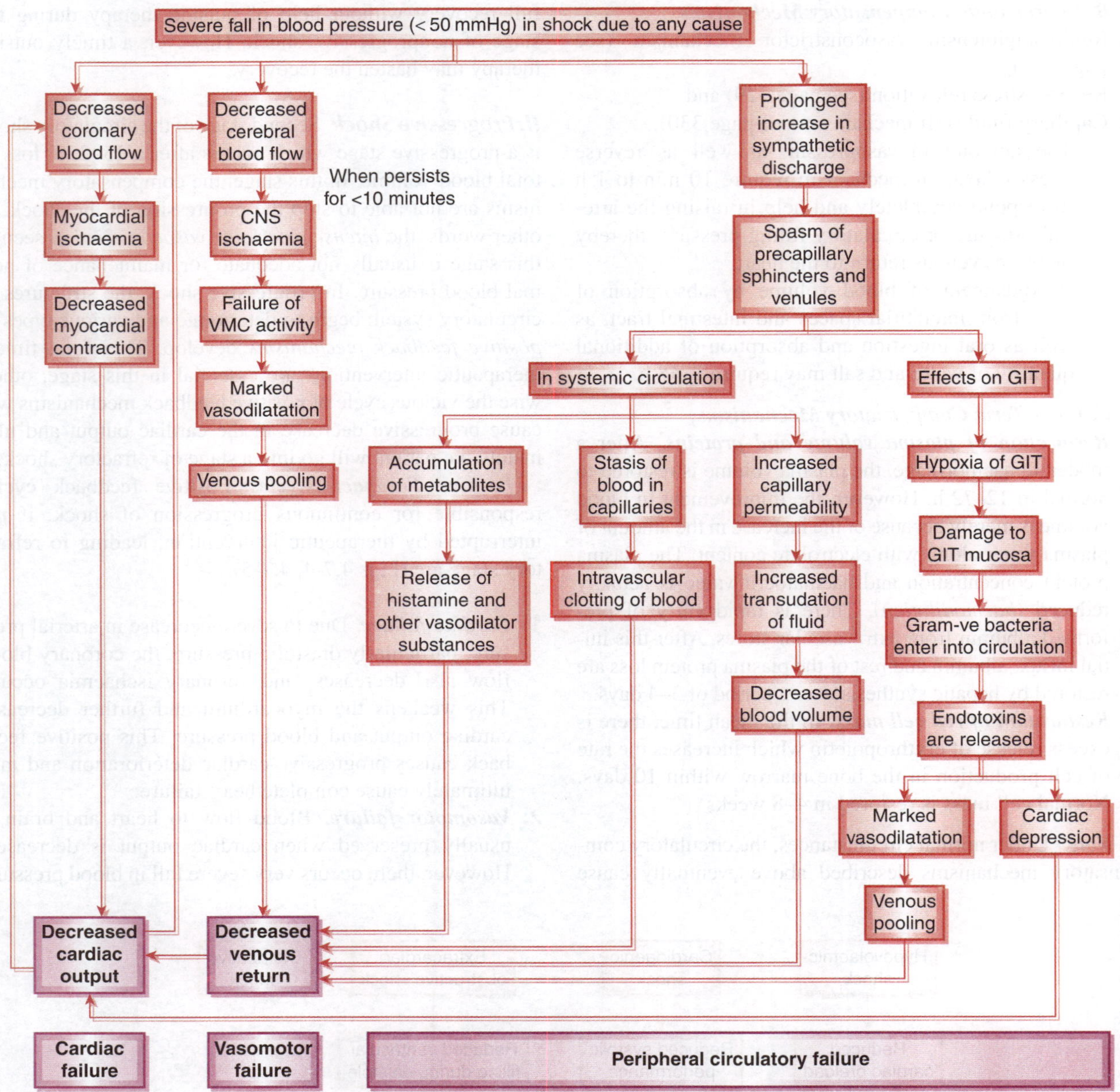

FIGURE 4.7-5 Chain of events of various positive feedback cycles which cause progression of shock to refractory stage. **NOTE**: In severe haemorrhage (blood loss > 40% of blood volume), the refractory shock develops due to these chain of events.

there may occur cerebral ischaemia and failure of medullary VMC. Failure of VMC results in marked vascular dilatation causing venous pooling and decreased venous return. The cardiac output and blood pressure are further decreased.

3. ***Peripheral circulatory failure.*** Due to prolonged and intense vasoconstriction, there occurs hypoxia and accumulation of metabolites in the body tissues. The peripheral circulatory failure results from following changes:
   - Capillaries and venules dilate due to the effect of local metabolites and there occurs peripheral venous pooling.
   - Prolonged capillary hypoxia results in increase in capillary permeability, and large quantity of fluid begin to transudate into the tissues. This decreases the blood volume and increases the shock.
   - The pooling and sluggish blood flow in microcirculation leads to *intravascular clotting of blood.* Even if the vessels do not become plugged, the tendency for the cells to stick to each other makes it more difficult for the blood to flow through microvasculature, giving rise to a condition called *sludged blood.*
4. ***Septicaemia and toxaemia.*** Due to prolonged vasoconstriction of splanchnic vessels there occurs hypoxia of

GIT. The hypoxic damage causes a breakdown of normal protective mucosal barrier in the gut leading to the entry of the intestinal bacteria into the portal circulation. Simultaneous deterioration of hepatic functions permit bacteria and bacterial endotoxins to reach the systemic circulation leading to septicaemia and toxaemia. The endotoxins cause widespread failure of arteriolar and precapillary sphincter functions and cardiac depression. There occurs extensive vasodilatation. At this stage, no amount of treatment can restore the circulatory functions to normal.

Effect on Body Tissues in Progressive Shock. In progressive shock, there occurs *widespread cellular degeneration* in the body tissues. Generalized cellular damage usually occurs first in highly metabolic tissues such as liver, lung and heart. Liver cells are usually the first to be affected because hepatic cells have very high rate of metabolism and also liver is the first organ exposed to toxins from the intestine through the portal vein.

The different damaging cellular effects that are known to occur include:

- Great decrease in active transport of sodium and potassium through cell membrane results in the accumulation of sodium in the cells and loss of potassium from the cells. So, the cell begins to swell.
- Mitochondrial activity in liver cells as well as in cells of many other tissues of the body is decreased.
- Lysosomes begin to split in tissues throughout the body, with release of hydrolases that causes widespread intracellular damage.
- Cellular metabolism of nutrients, such as glucose is eventually greatly depressed in last stages of shock. The activity of some hormones are depressed as well, including a marked suppression of insulin action.
- Poor delivery of oxygen to tissues, greatly diminishes oxidative metabolism and the cells switch to anaerobic glycolysis. This leads to the accumulation of lactic acid in the blood. Moreover the sluggish blood flow through the tissue also results in the accumulation of CO_2 in tissue. The CO_2 dissolves in water to produce H^+ ions causing acidosis. Acidosis causes vasodilation which further aggravates the shock and a vicious cycle starts.

III. Refractory Shock As mentioned above, when the shock is in the progressive stage and is not treated adequately, a vicious cycle of various positive feedback mechanisms (Fig. 4.7-5) set in and patient passes into the third stage of shock, the *refractory shock* (previously known as *irreversible shock).* In this stage, all therapeutic interventions are usually ineffective and eventually the patient dies.

Causes of refractiveness (point of no return) of shock. The main factor responsible for irreversibility of shock is the *depletion of high-energy phosphate compounds.* The high-energy phosphate reserves in the cells of the body, especially liver and heart are greatly diminished in severe degrees of shock. The adenosine triphosphate degraded in the cells to adenosine diphosphate and adenosine monophosphate and finally to adenosine. The adenosine diffuses out of the cell and is converted to uric acid, which cannot reenter the cell. New adenosine is synthesized rather slowly (at a rate of 2% of the total cellular amount per hour), hence once depleted, the high-energy phosphate stores of the body cells are difficult to replenish during shock and this contributes to the final stage of irreversibility.

Tissue damage in refractory shock. Slowly, necrosis of some cells of body sets in especially the cells adjacent to the venous ends of capillaries which receive less nutrition than the cells near the arterial ends of same capillaries. Patchy necrosis first appears in the cells of liver, kidney tubules, lungs and heart.

- In the kidney, there may occur *acute tubular necrosis* leading to acute renal failure and uraemic death.
- Deterioration of the lungs often leads to respiratory distress, the *shock lung syndrome.*

Treatment of Shock with Physiological Basis

The treatment of shock is aimed at correcting the causes and helping physiological compensatory mechanisms.

1. General Measures for Shock treatment are

- ***Room temperature.*** Where the patients of shock are kept should be cold. If exposed to warm, there will be sweating which will cause further hypovolaemia and aggravate the shock. It is important to note that most patients with shock are cold and therefore reflex warming of the body of a shock patient with water bottles or providing warm environment such as covering the patient with blankets, etc. will abolish the sympathetic discharge. So, the compensatory mechanism will be disturbed and shock will be aggravated and patient may even die.
- ***Raising the foot end of the patient's bed*** by 6" to 12" (*Trendelenburg position*) helps in promoting the venous return and thereby increasing the cardiac output. It is especially useful in haemorrhagic and neurogenic shock when the blood pressure is too low.

2. Replacement Therapy is very useful in hypovolaemic shock.

- ***In haemorrhagic shock*** the best therapy is transfusion of whole *blood.* When whole blood is not available the *plasma* may be used. Plasma maintains the colloid osmotic pressure of the blood, but the haematocrit decreases with this therapy. If neither whole blood nor plasma is available, a plasma substitute such as *dextran* may be used. Dextran is a large polysaccharide which does not pass through capillary pores. It therefore promotes osmosis of water from the interstitial fluid to intravascular spaces, thereby increasing the plasma volume.

- *In patients with burns or interstitial obstruction,* plasma infusion is the appropriate therapy. If plasma is not available *dextran* can be used.
- *In hypovolaemic shock due to dehydration* intravenous infusion of *balanced electrolytic solution* (e.g. lactated Ringer's solution is the appropriate therapy.

3. Sympathomimetic Drugs are useful as:

- Sympathomimetic drugs are usually not useful in haemorrhagic shock where the sympathetic system is already very active.
- These are especially useful in *neurogenic shock* and *anaphylactic shock* where the cause of shock is marked vasodilation due to lost neurogenic vascular tone.
- *Dopamine* should be the sympathomimetic drug of choice, because it produces renal vasodilation and at the same time, produces vasoconstriction elsewhere in the body. It also has a positive inotropic effect on heart.
- Epinephrine or norepinephrine drug may also be used when dopamine is not available.

4. Oxygen Therapy. Oxygen therapy may have some beneficial effects. In general, it does not have marked effect since the hypoxia of shock is of the anaemic or stagnant type and not of hypoxic type.

5. Glucocorticoids. Glucocorticoids are useful in shock because of their below-mentioned effects. They are particularly useful in anaphylactic shock:

- They increase the strength of heart in the last stages of shock,
- By stabilizing lysosomal membranes, they prevent release of enzymes of cells and
- They help in metabolism of glucose by the severely damaged cells.

Heart Failure

Heart failure is a pathophysiological state of the heart when cardiac performance is too low to maintain the cardiac output to meet the demands of the metabolizing tissues.

Pathophysiology

Cardiac failure can occur in the following three situations (Fig. 4.7-6):

1. Increase in Preload. According to *Starling law of heart*, an increase in preload (end-diastolic volume) augments cardiac function, but when there is too much increase

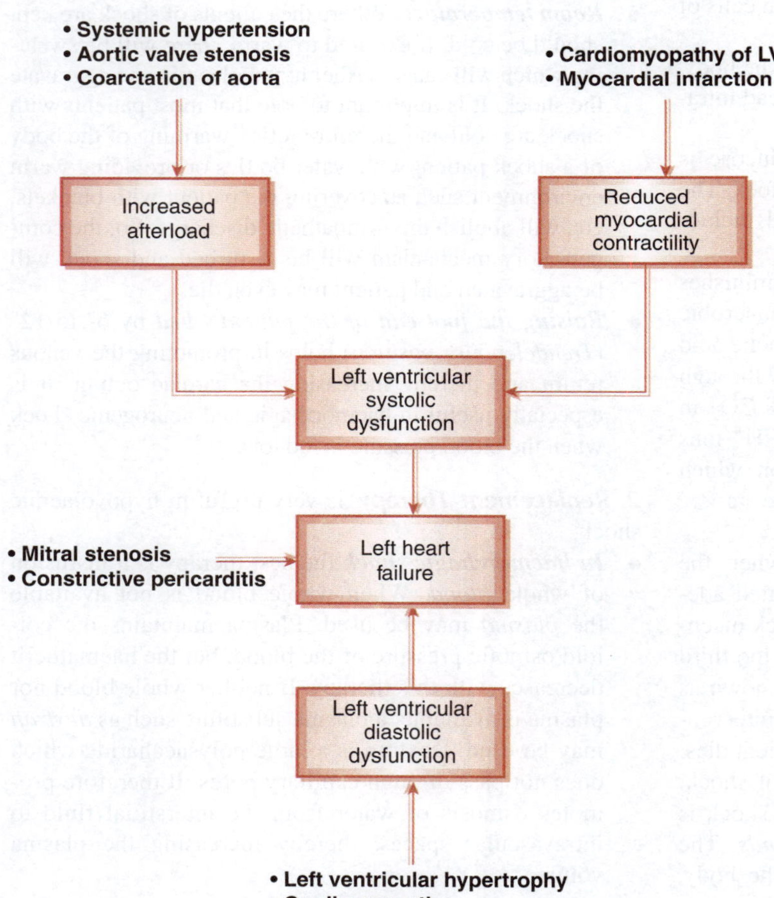

FIGURE 4.7-6 Pathophsiology of heart failure.

in preload then (it operates through descending limb of Starling curve, see page 246) it leads to ventricular dilatation and heart failure.

2. Increase in Afterload (resistance), e.g. in hypertension, there is resistance to outflow of blood from the heart which causes overstretching leading to ventricular dilatation and heart failure.

3. Reduction in Myocardial Contractility, i.e. decrease in pumping ability of the heart decreases the cardiac output.

The interaction of these three variables leads to development of cardiac failure.

Types and Causes of Heart Failure

Heart failures can be classified by various ways.

I. Depending on the Onset

1. Acute Heart Failure develops suddenly as in patient with myocardial infarction.

2. Chronic Heart Failure develops due to gradual deterioration of heart functions, as in patients suffering from valvular diseases.

II. Depending on the Operation of Compensatory Mechanisms

1. Compensated Heart Failure. It means impairment of cardiac performance is being compensated by certain adaptive changes that prevent development of overt heart failure. The adaptive changes are of two types (Fig. 4.7-7):

i. ***Local changes***, which are in the form of:
- Enlargement of chambers of heart,
- Myocardial hypertrophy and
- Increase in heart rate.

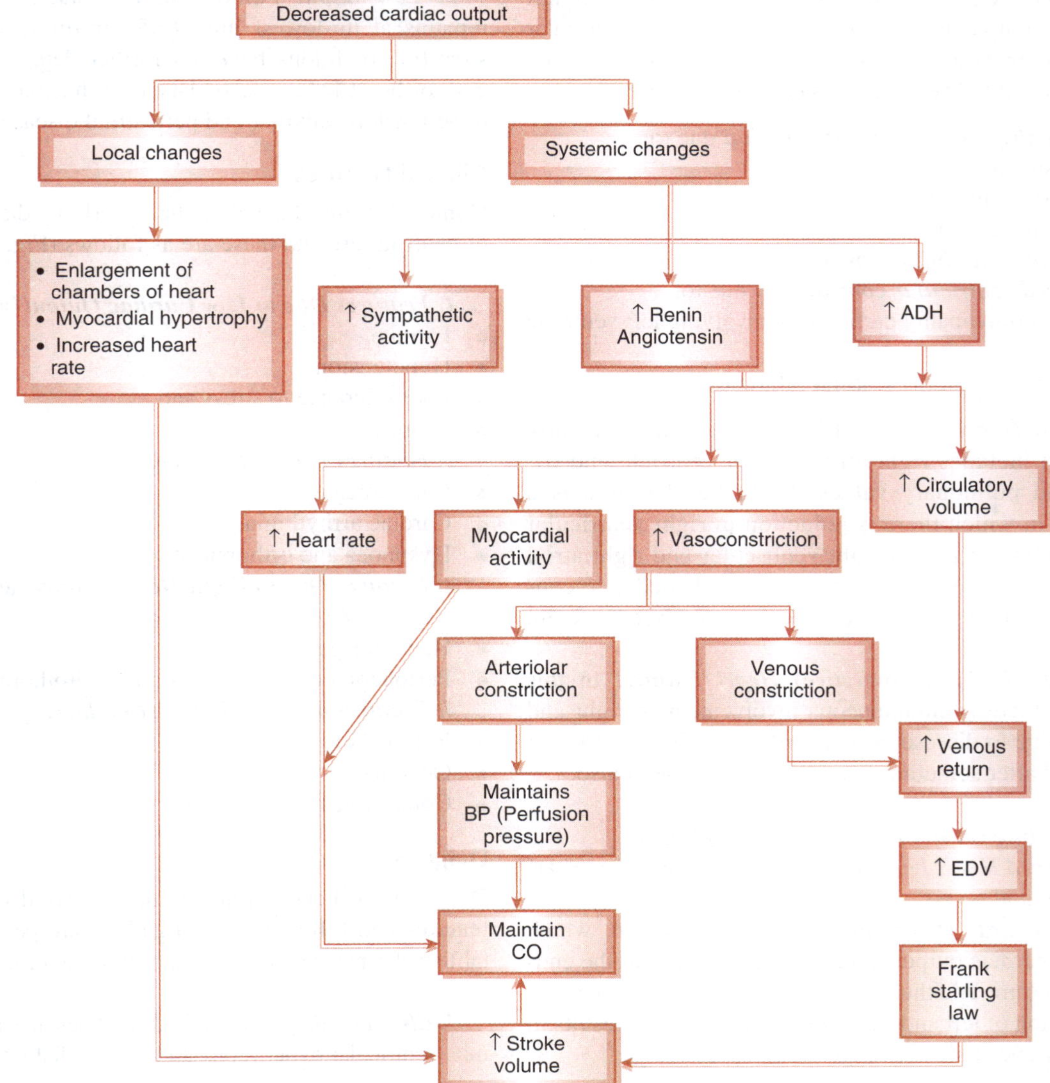

FIGURE 4.7-7 Compensatory/adaptive changes in heart failure.

ii. ***Systemic changes*** are:

- Activation of renin–angiotensin–aldosterone system and sympathetic system and
- Release of antidiuretic hormone and atrial natriuretic peptide.

Initially, compensatory changes improve cardiac performance, but as the disease advances they fail and become counterproductive.

2. Decompensated or Overt Heart Failure. In the presence of certain precipitating factors such as infections, anaemia, pregnancy, thyrotoxicosis, arrhythmia and myocardial infarction or due to failure of compensatory mechanisms, compensated heart failure leads to decompensated heart failure.

III. Depending on the Involvement of Side of Heart

1. Left Heart Failure. Anatomically, left heart comprises left atrium, left ventricle, aortic valve and mitral valve. The left heart failure (LHF), therefore, refers to reduction in left ventricular output leading to elevation of left ventricular volume and pressure and its transmission to left atrium and pulmonary veins. The conditions causing LHF are:

i. ***Left ventricular outflow obstruction*** due to:
- Systemic hypertension
- Aortic valve stenosis
- Coarctation of aorta

ii. ***Left ventricular inflow obstruction*** due to mitralstenosis

iii. ***Reduced ventricular contractility*** due to:
- Cardiomyopathy particularly involving left ventricle and
- Anterior wall myocardial infarction.

2. Right Heart Failure. Like left heart anatomically right heart includes right atrium, right ventricle and tricuspid and pulmonary valves. Right heart failure is a condition in which there is reduction in right ventricular output leading to rise in right ventricular and right atrial pressure, which further causes rise in JVP, oedema, congestive hepatomegaly and congestion of viscera except lungs.

3. Biventricular (Congestive) Heart Failure. In this condition, there is simultaneous involvement of right and left heart due to disease of myocardium, or left ventricular failure and after sometime involves the right heart also.

IV. Depending on Inadequate Cardiac Output

1. Forward Heart Failure results due to inadequate cardiac output and

2. Backward Heart Failure is the one in which decreased cardiac output results in the elevation of the end-diastolic volume and thus increases the ventricular pressure. The elevation of left and right ventricular pressure results in pulmonary and systemic congestion, respectively.

V. Systolic and Diastolic Heart Failure

1. Systolic Heart Failure occurs due to poor myocardial contractility (systolic dysfunction) and

2. Diastolic Heart Failure results due to poor ventricular filling because of defective relaxation.

Both systolic and diastolic heart failures coexist particularly in myocardial infarction.

VI. High-Output and Low-Output Failure

1. High-output Failure is a state in which cardiac output remains high, i.e. at the upper limit of normal cardiac output (3.5 $l/m^2/min$) even though cardiac functions are depressed. Various conditions which result in high output failure are:

- Fever,
- Thyrotoxicosis,
- Anaemia and
- Beriberi.

2. Low-output Failure. In this state, cardiac output remains at its lowest limit (2.5 $l/m^2/min$) at rest and in stressful conditions becomes further depressed, as in the case of heart failure secondary to ischaemic heart disease, hypertension, valvular and pericardial diseases.

Clinical Features

Clinical features depend on the underlying disease and type of heart failure and these are as follows (Fig. 4.7-8):

1. Features Due to Low Cardiac Output are:
- Fatigue,
- Hypotension,
- Poor tolerance to stress and
- Oliguria.

2. Features Due to LHF are:
- Cardiomegaly,
- Cardiac arrhythmia,
- Dyspnoea and orthopnoea.

3. Features Due to Right Heart Failure are:
- Rise in JVP,
- Hepatomegaly,
- Peripheral oedema, ascites and hydrothorax.

4. Features of Chronic Heart Failure:
- Raised JVP,
- Oedema,
- Congestive hepatamegaly.

Diagnosis

Diagnosis of heart failure is mainly based on its clinical features and following investigations are performed to establish the nature, severity, and complications which have occurred.

1. Electrocardiography (ECG) findings may reveal arrhythmia, ventricular hypertrophy and myocardial infarction.

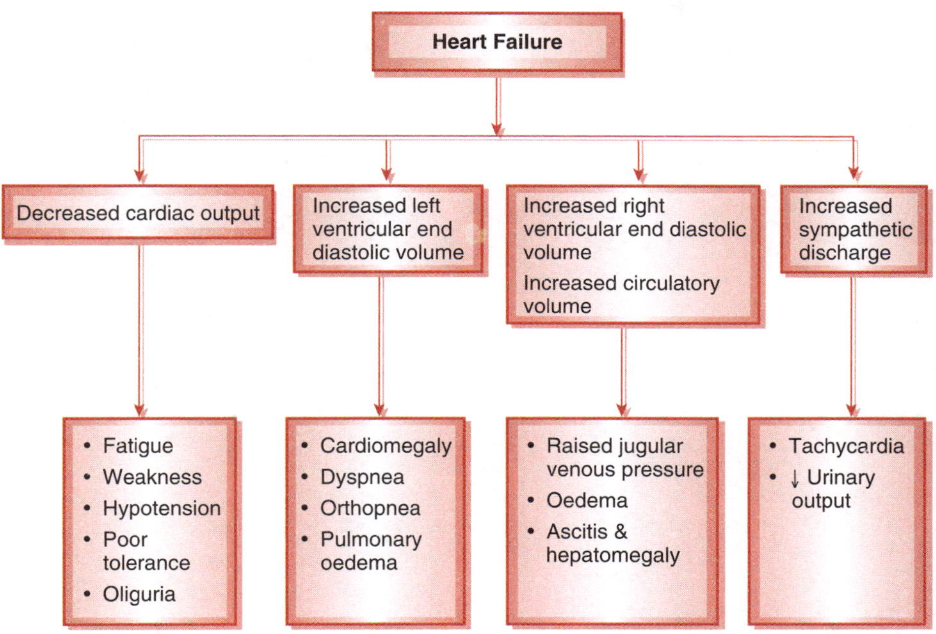

FIGURE 4.7-8 Pathophysiological features leading to sign and symptoms in heart failure.

2. Radiography of Chest may show enlargement of heart, congestion of lungs and certain valvular defects.

3. Biochemical Tests include estimation of blood urea and electrolytes for renal failure, hypokalaemia and hyponatraemia.

Treatment

The basic principles of treatment of heart failure are aimed at to:

- Remove the precipitating factors,
- Correct the underlying cause,
- Control the congestive heart failure state and
- Prevent complications.

In general, following measures are employed as a treatment of cardiac failure.

A. To Reduce Cardiac Work Load

- Complete bed rest is advised or patient is hospitalized for 1–2 weeks,
- Small and light meals are recommended and
- Drugs (like sedatives and antianxiety) are prescribed.

B. To Improve Myocardial Contractility

Drugs like cardiac glycosides (digitalis) and sympathomimetic amines (dopamine) are prescribed.

C. ***To Control Fluid Retention.*** Dietary salt intake is restricted, and diuretics are given.

D. ***To Reduce Afterload,*** use of vasodilator drugs specially angiotensin converting enzyme inhibitors (captopril and enalapril) is recommended.

Section 5

Respiratory System

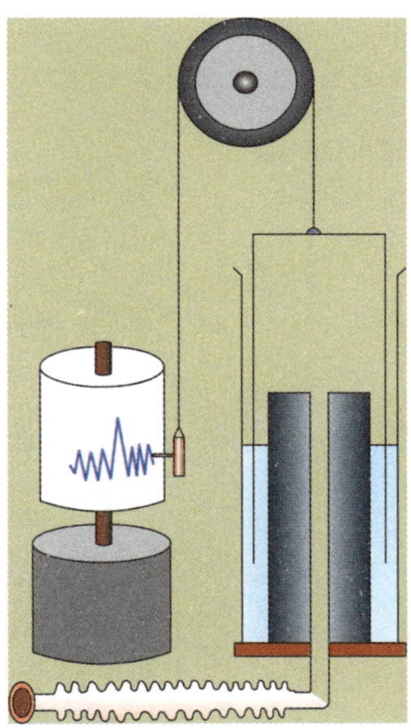

The word respiration has been derived from the Latin word 'respirae' which means to breathe. The primary role of the respiratory system is to provide O_2 to the tissues for metabolic needs and remove the CO_2 formed by them. An adult body consumes about 250 ml of O_2 and produces about 200 ml of CO_2 per minute. Respiration entails two processes: the external respiration and internal respiration.

The *internal respiration* or tissue respiration refers to utilization of O_2 and production of CO_2 by the tissue. It is generally considered the domain of biochemistry.

The *external respiration* includes supply of O_2 to the tissues from the environment and excretion of CO_2 released by the tissues into the atmosphere. The process of external respiration involves three major events:

- *Pulmonary ventilation,* i.e. exchange of gases between the environment and lungs. It includes mechanics of respiration.

- *Pulmonary diffusion* refers to transfer of gases from alveoli to the blood by diffusion across the respiratory membrane. To understand the process of pulmonary diffusion it is essential to understand facts about *pulmonary circulation* and the *properties of gases* and the laws governing diffusion of gases.
- *Transport of gases* from the blood to the body cells and back.

The *respiratory adjustments in health and diseases* are essential for life; and to understand these, knowledge about *regulation of respiration* is must.

The study of respiration without the concepts about functional anatomy of the respiratory system will not be easy, and so has been discussed in the very first chapter of this section.

Chapter 5.1

Respiratory Tract: Structure and Functions

FUNCTIONAL ANATOMY

The chief organs of the respiratory system are right and left *lungs.* The oxygen contained in the atmospheric air reaches the lungs by passing through a series of *respiratory passages* which also serve for removal of CO_2 from the alveoli to the atmosphere. The respiratory system also includes a pump that ventilates the lung. This pump consists of the chest wall and respiratory muscles. Salient points about functional anatomy of respiratory passages and lungs are discussed here. Functional anatomy of chest wall and respiratory muscles is discussed in Chapter 5.2 on 'Pulmonary Ventilation' which includes the mechanics of respiration.

Respiratory Passages

Respiratory passages include the following structures (Fig. 5.1-1):

1. Nasal Cavities. The air enters the body through right and left anterior (external) nares which open into the right and left nasal cavities. Through the posterior (internal) nares, the nasal cavities open into the pharynx. The nasal cavities warm up the air to the body temperature, humidify the air to 100% saturation, clean and filter the air of its particulate content by channeling the air through a tortuous path between the turbinates. The particles are deposited at the bends where they adhere to the mucus layering the nasal cavity.

2. Pharynx. From above downwards the pharynx is divided into nasopharynx, oropharynx and laryngopharynx. Air from nasal cavities enters the nasopharynx and passes down through the oropharynx and laryngopharynx to larynx. From the mouth the air can directly pass to oropharynx.

3. Larynx. It is continuous above with laryngopharynx and below with trachea. The air passes through the glottis (the triangular space between vocal cords) into the trachea. Apart from being a respiratory passage, the larynx also acts as a voice box.

4. Tracheobronchial Tree. The air passages between trachea and alveoli divide 23 times to form the extensive tracheobronchial tree (Fig. 5.1-2). These multiple divisions greatly increase the total cross-sectional area of the airway from 2.5 cm^2 in the trachea to 11,800 cm^2 in the alveoli. Consequently, the velocity of air flow in the small airway declines to very low values. The 23 generation divisions of tracheobronchial tree have been numbered as:

The trachea is designated as generation zero.

The principal bronchi right and left which are two major divisions of trachea constitute the first generation.

- *Lobar bronchi,* which are division of the principal bronchus form the second generation.
- *Segmental bronchi* which are further division of each lobar bronchus forms the third generation. Each segmental bronchus divides into several generations of branches that ultimately end in very small tubes called *bronchioles.*
- *Terminal bronchioles* is the name given to 16th generation of the divisions. Upto this generation of division no exchange of gases is possible.
- *Respiratory bronchiole* is the name given to 17th–22nd generation of divisions. These are labelled as respiratory bronchioles, because some exchange of gases is possible in these tubes.

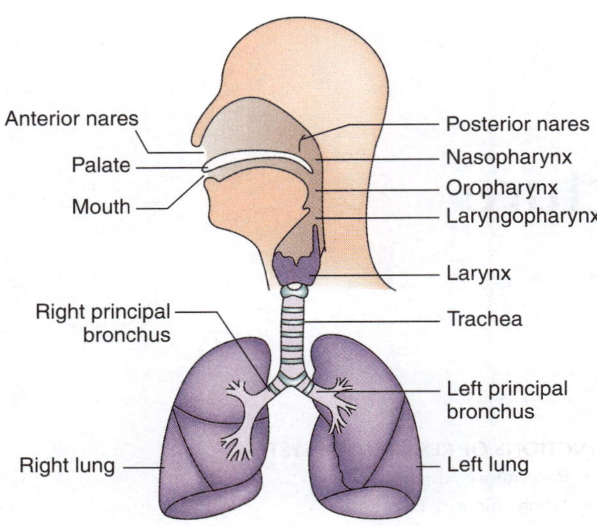

FIGURE 5.1-1 The air passages.

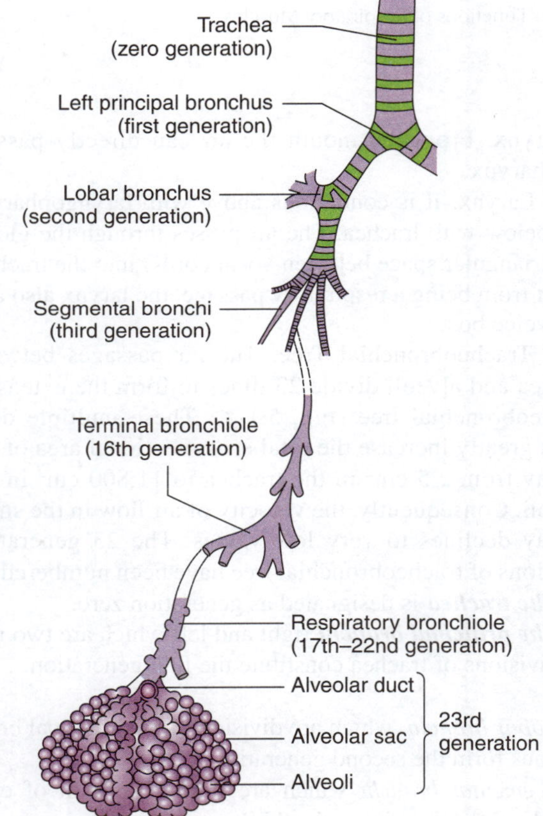

FIGURE 5.1-2 The tracheobronchial tree.

Alveolar ducts and in the alveoli or the alveolar sacs which form the 23rd generation division. It is here that most of the O_2 and CO_2 exchange occurs.

Thus, from the functional point of view the tracheobronchial tree can be divided into two major zones:

i. ***Conducting zone*** of the air passages is formed by the first 16 generations of passages and it only transports gases from and to the exterior. Thus, conducting zone starts from trachea and extends upto terminal bronchioles. Since no exchange of gases is possible here, so starting from nose to the terminal brochioles forms the so-called *dead space* which has a total capacity of approximately 150 ml.
ii. ***Respiratory zone.*** The remaining seven generations of the tracheobronchial tree which includes the respiratory bronchioles, alveolar ducts and alveoli form the respiratory zone, where exchange of gases occurs. Its volume is approximately 4 L.

Histological Features of the Tracheobronchial Tree

1. Cartilaginous Rings are present in trachea and initial bronchi of few generations. These are absent in terminal bronchioles and respiratory bronchioles. The cartilaginous rings of trachea are incomplete on their posterior aspect. This allows some contraction of trachea but tracheal lumen cannot be completely obliterated easily.

2. Smooth Muscles. Ends of cartilagious rings of trachea are approximated by transverse smooth muscle fibres. In bronchi, bands of fibres tend to become circular so that in terminal bronchioles they are present in large amount and form a sphincter. Smooth muscles are not present in alveoli.

3. Epithelial Lining in trachea and large bronchi is columnar and becomes cuboidal in bronchioles and simple squamous in alveoli. The epithelial cells of the tracheobronchial tree are ciliated. Cilia are absent in alveoli. Efficiency of ciliated cells of trachea and bronchi in propelling mucus and waste products is of higher order. Cilia are not influenced by nerve impulses. The mucous secreting goblet cells and deep serous glands are present in trachea and bronchi but are absent in bronchioles and alveoli (Fig. 5.1-3).

Respiratory Parenchyma

Each respiratory unit consists of one respiratory bronchiole which opens into a number of alveolar ducts, and each alveolar duct in turn opens into number of alveoli. The two lungs contain about 300 million alveoli. Each alveolus has a diameter of about 0.2 μm. The alveoli are surrounded by pulmonary capillaries. The total area of the alveolar walls in contact with capillaries in both the lungs is about 70 m^2.

Microscopic Structure of Alveolus (Fig. 5.1-4) Each alveolus is lined by two types of epithelial cells:

- ***Type I cells*** are flat cells with large cytoplasmic extensions and are the primary lining cells.
- ***Type II cells*** (granular pneumocytes) are thicker and contain numerous lamellar inclusion bodies. These cells secrete *surfactant.*

The alveolar wall also contains:

- ***Other special type of epithelial cells,***

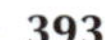

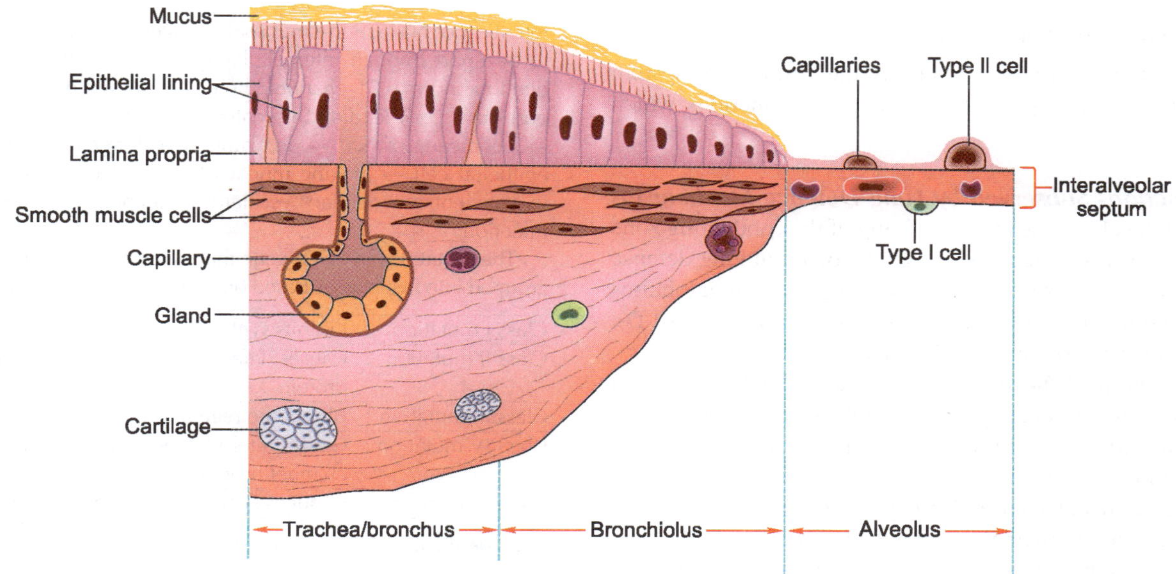

FIGURE 5.1-3 Histological features of epithelial lining of tracheobronchial tree.

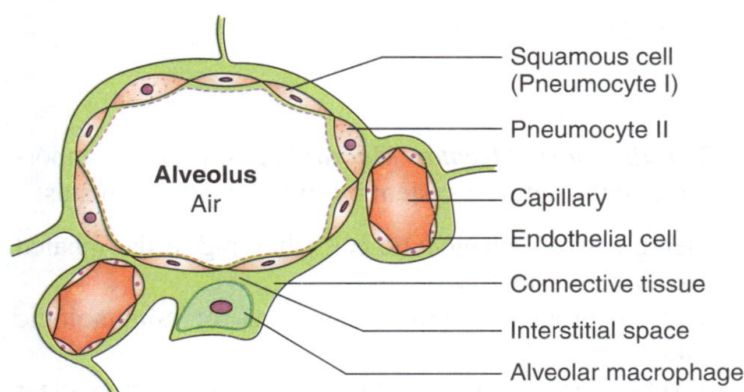

FIGURE 5.1-4 Microscopic structure of alveolus.

- *Pulmonary alveolar macrophages* (PAM) which are active phagocytic cells,
- *Lymphocytes,*
- *Plasma cells* which form and secrete immunoglobulins,
- *Amine precursor uptake and decarboxylation* (APUD) *cells* which store and secrete many biologically active peptidases, e.g. vasoactive intestinal peptide (VIP) and substance P, etc.
- *Mast cells* which contain heparin, various lipids, histamine and various proteases that participate in allergic reactions.

Communication between the two alveoli occurs through small pores, called *pores of Kohn.*

Respiratory Membrane

It is the name given to the tissues which separate the capillary blood from the alveolar air. It is important to understand the structure of a respiratory membrane for better understanding of diffusion of gases between alveoli and capillary blood, so it is described in detail in Chapter 5.4 on Pulmonary Diffusion (page 418).

Blood Supply

Conducting airway is supplied by systemic blood, whereas the respiratory zone of the lung is supplied by deoxygenated (venous) blood coming through pulmonary arteries to lungs. Blood is oxygenated in lungs and is returned to left atrium via pulmonary veins.

Innervation

The walls of bronchi and bronchioles are innervated by the autonomic nervous system.

- *Parasympathetic* fibres innervate through vagus nerve. Their stimulation causes cholinergic discharge producing bronchoconstriction and increased bronchial secretion via muscarinic receptors.
- *Sympathetic nerves* supplying the lungs when stimulated causes bronchodilation and decreased bronchial secretion via adrenergic receptors, predominantly by β_2 receptors while α_1 adrenergic receptors inhibit bronchial secretions.
- *Afferents* from the lungs pass through vagi nerves.

FUNCTIONS OF THE RESPIRATORY SYSTEM

Respiratory Functions

The main function of the respiratory system in general and lung in particular is exchange of gases between atmosphere and blood.

Nonrespiratory Functions

Besides the respiratory functions the respiratory system performs many important nonrespiratory functions which include:

A. Functions Subserved by Lung Defence Mechanisms

Epithelial cells in the mucosal lining of the conducting zone secrete various molecules that are involved in lung defense mechanism. These include secretory immunoglobulins (IgA), collectins, surfactant proteins—(SP-A) and (SP-D), defensins, chemokines, cytokines, etc.

1. Immunoglobulin-A (IgA) is secreted in the bronchial secretion and protects against respiratory infections. *Ciliary escalator action* is an important defence system against airborne infection. The dust particles in the inhaled air are often laden with bacteria. While passing through the repeatedly branched bronchial tree the dust particles and the bacteria are caught in the mucous layer present at the mucosal surface of respiratory passages and are moved up towards pharynx by the rhythmic upward beating action of cilia Fig. 5.1-5 and swallowed. Cigarette smoke disturbs the ciliary function. That explains the higher incidence of respiratory infections in smokers than in nonsmokers.

Applied Aspects

Cystic fibrosis is an autosomal recessive disorder occurs due to abnormal gene (located on long arm of chromosome 7), that encodes cystic fibrosis transmembrane conductance regulator (CFTR). The basic abnormality lies in transport protein for Cl^- on apical membrane of epithelial lining of respiratory, gastrointestinal and genitourinary tracts.

Normally in the airways of epithelial cells , Cl^- channel (transport protein) transports Cl^- out of the cell, resulting in retention of Na^+ on the mucosal surfaces that causes water to transport through intercellular spaces. In cystic fibrosis, due to abnormal Cl^- channel, there is inhibition of Cl^- transport out of cell leading to greater influx of Na^+ in the cell → deficiency of Na^+→ dehydration of luminal border of epithelial cell → making mucous thick and viscid leading to deficient mucocilliary escalator clearance→ leading to infection.

The mutations in CFTR gene that cause cystic fibrosis are grouped into five classes based on their cellular functions as :

Class I mutation :	Inhibits synthesis of Cl^- channel protein
Class II mutation :	Causes defective processing of channel protein
Class III mutation :	Blocks the regulation of channel protein
Class IV mutation :	Causes altered conductance through channel protein
Class V mutation :	Reduces synthesis of channel protein

Therapeutic measures advised in cystic fibrosis include:

- Chest physiotherapy and mucolytic agents should be used to loosen thick mucus.
- Antibiotics— to prevent infection.
- Bronchodilators and anti-inflammatory agents to expand and clear the airways.

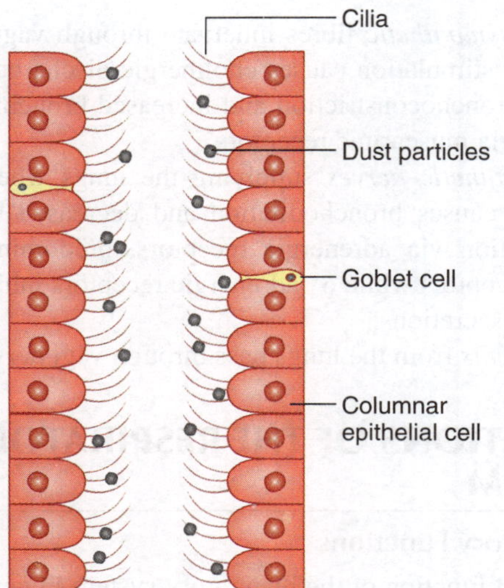

FIGURE 5.1-5 Ciliary escalator action of the respiratory mucosa.

2. Pulmonary Alveolar Macrophages play an important role in the defence system by following mechanisms:

- Being actively phagocytic cells they ingest the inhaled bacteria and small particles.
- Help in processing inhaled antigens for immunologic attack.
- PAMs secrete substances that attract polymorhonuclear cells to the lungs.
- By some secretions they stimulate granulocyte and monocyte formation in the bone marrow.

Note. The deterimental function of PAM is to digest substances inhaled in cigarette smoke or other irritants. During the digestive process they release lysosomal products into the extracellular spaces and cause inflammatory reaction.

3. Cough Reflex. The laryngeal, tracheal and bronchial mucous membranes contain vagal afferent terminals which act as *irritant receptors.* Stimulation of these receptors by chemical or mechanical stimuli (excessive mucus, inadvertently inhaled foodstuff, etc.) produces a bout of coughing which helps in the expulsion of the foreign material.

For details of cough reflex see page 446.

B. Functions Subserved by Pulmonary Circulation

1. Reservoir for Left Ventricle. When left ventricle output becomes transiently greater than systemic venous return, the blood stored in pulmonary circulation helps in maintaining the left ventricular output for few strokes.

2. Pulmonary Circulation Acts as a Filter and filters out particles from the blood, which may include: small fibrin or blood clots, detached cancer cells, fat cells, gas bubbles, agglutinated RBCs, masses of platelets and debris from stored blood.

The filtered particles in the lung are removed by lytic enzyme in capillary endothelium, ingestion by macrophages and penetration into the lymphatic system.

3. Removal of Fluid from Alveoli. Because of low pulmonary hydrostatic pressure, the fluid entering the alveoli is absorbed by the capillaries. This protects the gas exchange function of lungs and opposes transudation of fluid from capillaries to the alveoli.

4. Role in Absorption of Drugs. Certain drugs that rapidly pass through the alveolar capillary barrier by diffusion are administered by inhalation, e.g. anaesthetic gases, aerosol and other bronchodilators.

C. Metabolic Functions of Lungs

1. Surfactant produced in the lungs plays an important role in respiration (for details see page 405).

2. Protein Synthesis for maintenance of the structural framework.

3. Conversion of Angiotensin I to II is performed by the enzyme angiotensin converting enzyme (ACE) present in the pulmonary capillary endothelium.

4. Inactivation Partly or Completely of many vasoactive substances present in the blood is done by capillary endothelial cells as they pass through pulmonary circulation. These substances include bradykinin, serotonin, some prostaglandins, norepinephrine, acetylcholine, etc. Amount of serotonin and norepinephrine reaching the systemic circulation is decreased by lungs. Vasoactive substances that pass through the lungs without being metabolized include epinephrine, dopamine, oxytocin, vasopressin and angiotensin I.

5. Fibrinolytic Mechanism present in the lung lyses clot in the pulmonary vessels.

6. Storage of Hormones and Certain Biologically Active Peptides is done in the APUD cells and nerve fibres present in the alveoli. These substances include VIP, substance P, opioid peptides, cholecystokinin-pancreozymin (CCK-PZ) and somatostatin. These substances are later released into the systemic circulation.

D. Functions Subserved by Respiratory Muscles Respiratory muscles are also used during laughing and singing.

Chapter 5.2

Pulmonary Ventilation

INTRODUCTION

As we know, respiration, to be more precise the *external respiration* (supply of O_2 from atmosphere to body tissues and removal of CO_2 from the body to atmosphere), involves three major processes:

- *Pulmonary ventilation,* i.e. exchange of gases between the environment and lungs,
- *Pulmonary diffusion,* i.e. transfer of gases from the alveoli to capillary blood across the respiratory membrane and
- *Transport of gases* from the blood to tissue cells and back.

In this chapter, following aspects and concepts related to pulmonary ventilation are discussed:

- Mechanics of pulmonary ventilation,
- Lung volumes and capacities,
- Pulmonary elastance and compliance and
- Work of breathing.

MECHANICS OF PULMONARY VENTILATION

Mechanism of Breathing

- *Pulmonary ventilation* is accomplished by two processes: inspiration and expiration.
- *Inspiration* refers to inflow of atmospheric air into the lungs. This obviously occurs when the intrapulmonary pressure falls below the atmospheric air pressure.
- *Expiration* refers to outflow of air from the lungs into the atmosphere. This obviously occurs when the intrapulmonary pressure rises above the atmospheric air pressure.
- *Changes in the intrapulmonary pressure* which govern the respiratory cycle of inspiration and expiration are related to changes in the intrapleural pressure.
- *Changes in the intrapleural pressure* are brought about by changes in the size of the thoracic cavity. Expansion of the thoracic cage leads to fall in intrapleural pressure and decrease in the size of the thoracic cavity leads to rise in the intrapleural pressure.
- *Changes in the size of the thoracic cavity* are brought about by the actions of respiratory muscles:
  - Muscles of normal tidal inspiration are diaphragm and external intercostal muscles.
  - Accessory muscles of inspiration are scaleni, sternomastoid and serratus anterior, and alae nasi.
  - Muscles of expiration are internal intercostal muscles and abdominal muscles (abdominal recti muscles, transverse abdominis muscles and internal oblique muscles).

Mechanism of Tidal Respiration

Inspiration Inspiration is an active process, normally produced by contraction of the *inspiratory muscles* (*negative-pressure breathing*). Use of a respirator to inflate the respiratory system produces positive pressure (*positive-pressure breathing*). During tidal inspiration (quiet breathing), the diaphragm and external intercostal muscles contract and cause an increase in all the three dimensions of the thoracic cavity.

Role of a Diaphragm. In tidal inspiration (quiet breathing), 70–75% of the expansion of chest is caused due to the contraction of diaphragm. The diaphragm is a dome-shaped, musculotendinous partition between the thorax and abdomen. The convexity of this dome is directed towards the thorax. When the diaphragm contracts, the following changes occur:

- The dome becomes flattened, and the level of diaphragm is lowered *increasing the vertical diameter* of the thoracic cavity (Fig. 5.2-1A). During quiet breathing, the descent of diaphragm is about 1.5 cm, and during forced inspiration it increases to 7 cm.
- The descent of diaphragm causes the rise in intra-abdominal pressure which is accommodated by the reciprocal relaxation of the abdominal wall musculature.
- The contraction of diaphragm also lifts the lower ribs causing thoracic expansion laterally and anteriorly (the bucket handle and pump handle effect, respectively) (Figs 5.2-1B and C). The abdominal organs support the diaphragmatic dome and act as a fulcrum, while the diaphragmatic contraction raises the lower ribs.

Role of External Intercostal Muscles. The fibres of external intercostal muscles slope downwards and forwards. They are attached close to the vertebral ends of the upper ribs than the lower ribs (Fig. 5.2-2). From pivot-like joint with the vertebrae, the ribs slope obliquely downwards and forwards. So, when the external intercostal muscles contract (because of the lever effect), the ribs are elevated causing the lateral and anteroposterior enlargement of the thoracic cavity due to the so-called bucket- and pump-handle effects, respectively (Figs. 5.2-1B and C).

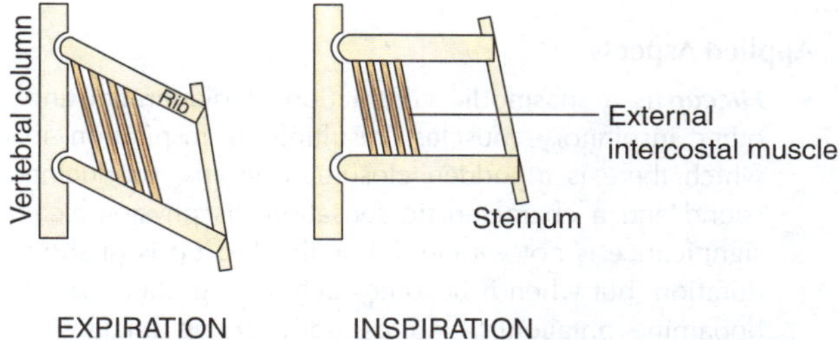

FIGURE 5.2-2 Contraction of external intercostal muscle favours elevation of ribs due to mechanical leverage effect of the attachments of its fibres close to the pivot on the upper ribs as compared to lower ribs.

Role of Laryngeal Muscles. The abductor muscles of the larynx contract during inspiration pulling the vocal cords apart.

Expiration Expiration in quiet breathing is largely a passive phenomenon and is brought about by the following:

- Elastic recoil of the lungs,
- Decrease in the size of the thoracic cavity due to the relaxation of diaphragm and external intercostal muscles,
- An increase in the tone of muscle of the anterior abdominal wall which forces the relaxing diaphragm upwards and
- The serratus posterior inferior muscles that play a minor role in pulling down the ribs.

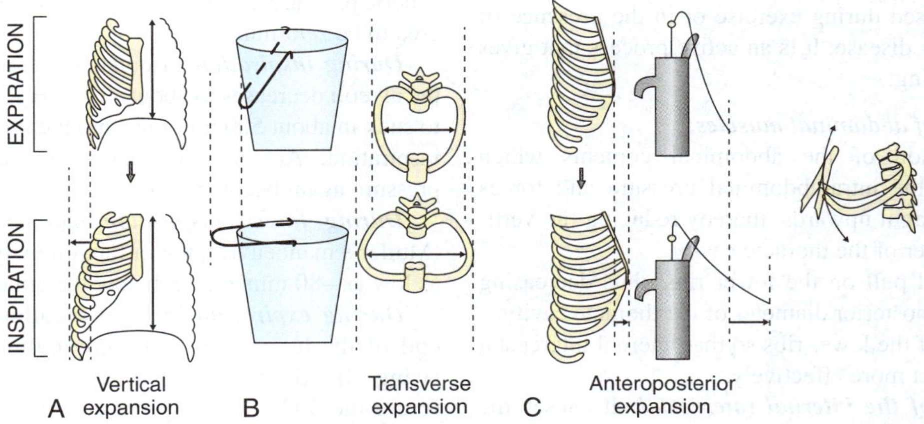

FIGURE 5.2-1 Mechanism of increase in diameter of thoracic cavity: **(A)** increase in vertical diameter (descent of diaphragm); **(B)** increase in transverse diameter (bucket handle effect) and **(C)** increase in anteroposterior diameter (pump handle effect).

Applied Aspects

- ***Hiccup*** is a spasmodic contraction of diaphragm and other inspiratory muscles, resulting in inspiration in which there is a sudden closure of glottis, producing sound and a characteristic sensation. Its physiological significance is not yet clear. Usually, hiccup is of short duration, but when it becomes debilitating, then use of dopamine antagonist and centrally acting analgesics may help.
- In bilateral phrenic nerve palsy, adequate ventilation at rest can be maintained by the external intercostal muscles alone but respiration is somewhat laboured to maintain life.
- Spinal cord transaction above the level of the third cervical segment is fatal without artificial respiration, whereas in transaction below the fifth cervical segment, respiration remains normal as the phrenic nerve (C_3, C_4, C_5) that innervates the diaphragm remains intact.

Mechanism of Forced Respiration

Forced Inspiration Forced inspiration is characterized by:

1. ***Forceful contraction of diaphragm*** leading to the descent of diaphragm by 7–10 cm as compared to 1–1.5 cm during quiet inspiration.
2. ***Forceful contraction of external intercostal muscles*** causing more elevation of ribs leading to more increase in transverse and anteroposterior diameter of the thoracic cavity.
3. ***Contraction of accessory muscles of inspiration*** which causes the following effects:
   - Sternomastoid muscles contract and lift the sternum upwards.
   - Anteriorserrati muscles contract and lift many of the ribs upwards.
   - Scaleni muscles contract and lift the first two ribs.

Forced Expiration Forced expiration is required when respiration is increased during exercise or in the presence of severe respiratory disease. It is an active process that gives rise to the following:

1. ***Contraction of abdominal muscles:***
   - Compression of the abdominal contents which increases the intra-abdominal pressure and forces the diaphragm upwards, thereby reducing the vertical diameter of the thoracic cavity.
   - Downward pull on the lower ribs, thus decreasing the anteroposterior diameter of the thoracic cavity.
   - Fixation of the lower ribs so that internal intercostal muscles act more effectively.
2. ***Contraction of the internal intercostal:*** It causes the effect which is just opposite to that of external intercostal muscles. This is because of the leverage mechanism of the direction of the muscle fibres which slope downwards and backwards, creating a longer force arm for the upper ribs (Fig. 5.2-3). Hence, their contraction tends to pull all the ribs downwards, thereby reducing the anteroposterior diameter (because of the falling of the pump-handle effect) as well as the transverse diameter (because of the action of ribs like the falling of the bucket-handle effect) of the thoracic cavity.

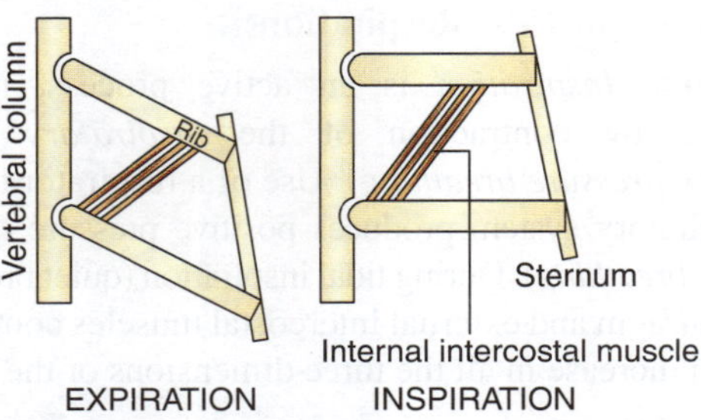

FIGURE 5.2-3 Contraction of internal intercostal muscle pulls the ribs down due to mechanical leverage effect of its fibres close to the pivot on the lower ribs as compared to upper ribs.

Note. Besides their role in deep breathing, the expiratory muscles are also involved in other forced expiratory efforts, e.g. in coughing, vomiting, defaecation and Valsalva manoeuvre, etc.

Pressure and Volume Changes during the Respiratory Cycle

Pressure Changes

***Intrapulmonary Pressure Changes during the Respiratory Cycle** (Fig. 5.2-4).* The movement of air in and out of the lungs depends primarily on the pressure gradient between the alveoli and the atmosphere (i.e. *transairway pressure).* The intrapulmonary or alveolar pressure is the air pressure inside the lung alveoli.

At End-Expiration and End-Inspiration, i.e. when the glottis is open and there is no movement of air, the pressures in all parts of the respiratory tree are equal to the atmospheric pressure, and the intrapulmonary pressure is considered to be *zero* mm of Hg.

During inspiration in quiet breathing, the pressure in the alveoli decreases to about –1 mmHg, which is sufficient to suck in about 500 ml of air into the lungs within 2 sec of inspiration. At the end-inspiration, the intrapulmonary pressure again becomes zero.

During forced inspiration against a closed glottis (Muller's manoeuvre), the intrapulmonary pressure may be as low as –80 mmHg, i.e. below the atmospheric pressure.

During expiration in quiet breathing, the elastic recoil of the lungs causes the intrapulmonary pressure to swing slightly to the positive side (+1 mmHg) which forces the 500 ml of inspired air out of the lungs during 2–3 sec of expiration. At the end-expiration, once again the alveolar pressure regains the atmospheric pressure (zero mm of Hg).

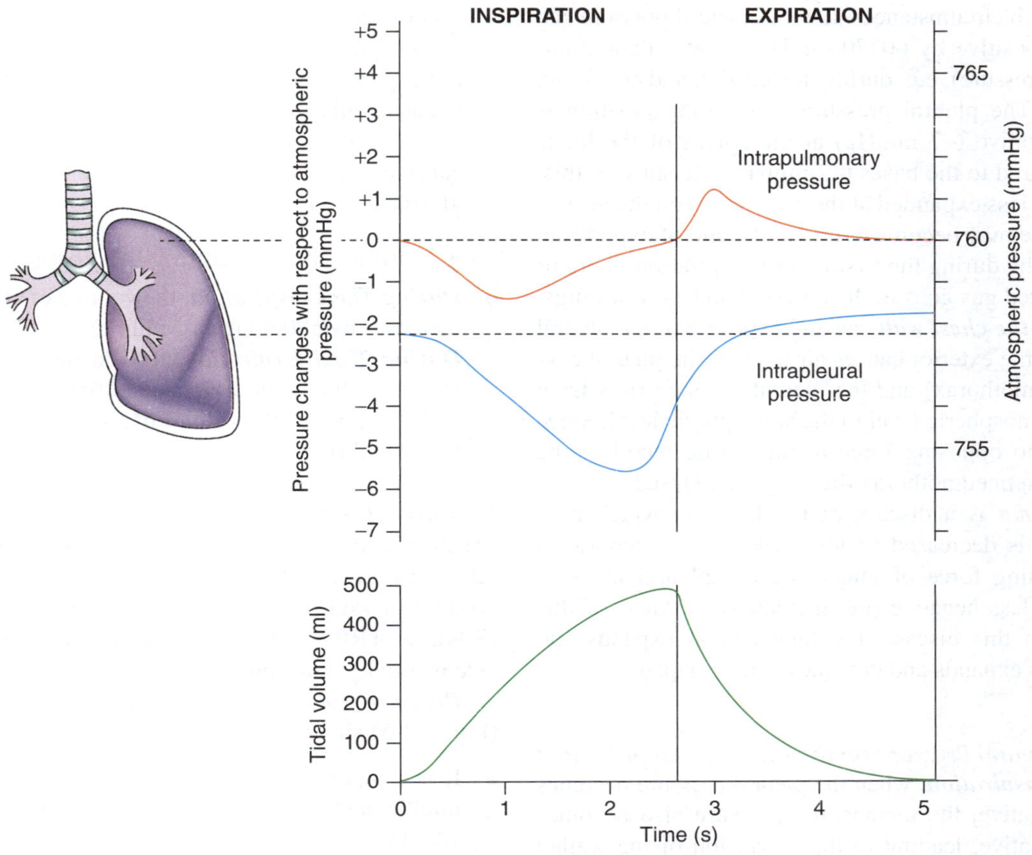

FIGURE 5.2-4 Pressure and volume changes during the respiratory cycle.

Forceful expiration against closed glottis (Valsalva's manoeuvre) may produce the intrapulmonary pressure of as much as 100 mmHg.

Intrapleural (Pleural) Pressure Changes during the Respiratory Cycle *(Fig. 5.2-4)* Pleural pressure is the pressure of fluid in the space between the visceral pleura and parietal pleura.

• ***Normal Pleural Pressure*** when the respiratory muscles are completely relaxed and the airways are open is about –2.5 mmHg.

- The negative pleural pressure (–2.5 mmHg) is the amount of suction required to hold the lungs at their equilibrium volume or the functional residual capacity (FRC). FRC is the lung volume at the end of normal (eupnoeic), relaxed expiration and is about 2–2.5 L of gas.
- The negative pleural pressure (–2.5 mmHg) is the result of balance of two opposite forces: the recoil tendency of the lungs and the recoil tendency of the thoracic cage.
- Recoil tendency of the lungs (continuous tendency to collapse) is caused by:
  - The presence of many elastic fibres in the alveolar walls which are under constant stretch in the inflated lungs and
  - Surface tension of the fluid lining the alveoli due to which the alveoli tend to become progressively smaller and collapse.
- Recoil tendency of the thoracic cage, i.e. a constant tendency to expand (to pop outwards), is because of the fact that the chest wall is an elastic structure which is normally partially pulled inwards. The elastic property of the thoracic cage is because of the elastic nature of ribs, muscles and tendons.
- ***During Inspiration*** due to the expansion of the chest wall, the pleural pressure becomes more negative (–6 mm of Hg) and pulls the surface of lungs with greater force creating negative intrapulmonary pressure.
- ***During Expiration.*** At the end of inspiration, the inspiratory muscles relax and the recoiling force of lungs begins to pull the chest wall back to expiratory position. At end-expiratory position, where the recoil force of the lungs and recoil force of thoracic cage balance, the pleural pressure returns back to –2.5 mmHg.

Factors Affecting Pleural Pressure

1. ***Deep inspirations.*** The pleural pressure may become as low as –30 mmHg during deep inspiration.
2. ***Valsalva manoeuvre*** or when expiratory muscles work against closed glottis, there occurs a marked decrease in the thoracic volume causing deflation of lungs.

Under such circumstances, the intrapleural pressure can become positive by 60–70 mmHg (greater than atmospheric pressure), e.g. during defaecation and coughing.

3. ***Gravity.*** The pleural pressure in standing position is more negative (–7 mmHg) at the apices of the lungs as compared to the bases (–2 mmHg). Because of this, lungs are less expanded at the base and even the airway at the base may become closed at the end of expiration. This is why during the first part of inspiration, more of the inspired gas goes to the apices than bases of lungs.
4. ***Injury to the chest wall*** causing exposure of the pleural cavity to the exterior causes air to enter the pleural cavity (pneumothorax) and the pleural pressure rises from the subatmospheric level to the atmospheric level. Since there is no opposing force to the elastic recoil of the lung, so in pneumothorax the lung is collapsed.
5. ***Emphysema*** is a disease of the lungs in which lung elasticity is decreased or lost. Due to the decrease in the recoiling force of lungs, the intrapleural pressure becomes less negative (i.e. increases). Because of this reason, in this disease, the lung alveoli expands and chest also expands and becomes barrel shaped.

Effects of Pleural Pressure on the Cardiovascular System

1. ***During inspiration,*** when the pleural pressure becomes more negative, the mediastinal pressure also becomes more negative, leading to the expansion of the walled structures in the thorax, especially large veins (superior and inferior vena cavae) and thereby decreasing pressure on them. This causes blood to be sucked into these veins from extrathoracic regions. Thus, there is *increased venous return* to the heart during inspiration due to suction action of the respiratory pump. The descent of diaphragm during inspiration causes a slight rise in intra-abdominal pressure, thereby increasing the pressure gradient between abdomen and thorax further. The increase in the venous return during inspiration *increases the cardiac output.* This respiratory pump action is especially marked during exercise.
2. ***During Valsalva manoeuvre*** or when expiratory muscles are working violently against closed glottis, e.g. while severe bouts of cough, the pleural pressure becomes positive leading to a decrease in the venous return. So the cardiac output is markedly decreased and there may occur cerebral ischaemia, visual blackouts and unconsciousness, especially in old persons.

Measurement of Pleural Pressure

1. ***Manometric measurement*** can be made by inserting a needle into the intrapleural space whose other end is attached to a water manometer with the help of a rubber tubing.
2. ***Intraoesophageal*** pressure can be recorded with the help of an air-containing rubber balloon sealed over a catheter placed in the lower part of thoracic part of oesophagus. Intraoesophageal pressure in the thoracic part is equivalent to the intrapleural pressure because this part of oesophagus becomes a closed cavity due to the closure of its lower end by the cardiac sphincter and upper end by the closure of glottis.

Lung Volume Changes during the Respiratory Cycle

- ***During Tidal Inspiration,*** the volume of air in the lungs increases by 500 ml (tidal volume).
- ***During Tidal Expiration,*** the elastic forces compress the gas in the lungs which starts flowing out and at the end of expiration the volume of air in the lungs decreases by 500 ml (Fig. 5.2-4).

Pressure–Volume Curve of Respiratory System The transrespiratory pressure (TRP) refers to the transmural pressure across the entire respiratory system. It equals alveolar pressure (PA) minus pressure at the body surface (PBs), i.e. TRP = PA – PBs. The pressure at the body surface is usually atmospheric pressure.

Pressure–volume curve of the respiratory system (Fig. 5.2-5) shows that:

- It is a sigmoid-shaped curve which is steepest in the middle and almost flat at both high- and low-lung volumes.
- FRC is determined by the volume at which the transrespiratory pressure (TRP) is zero.
- Residual volume (RV) and total lung capacity (TLC) are limited by the decreased compliance of the system, as indicated by the reduced slope of the curve at both extreme of volumes.

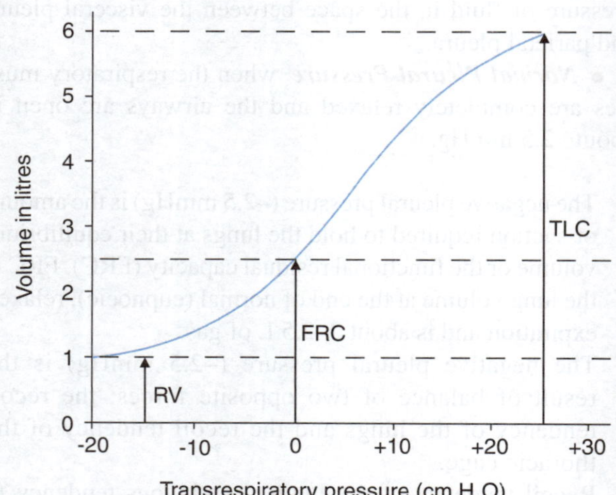

FIGURE 5.2-5 Pressure–volume curve of the respiratory system. RV= residual volume, FRC= functional residual capacity and TLC= total lung capacity.

LUNG VOLUMES AND CAPACITIES

Static Lung Volumes and Capacities

Lung Volumes

The maximum volume to which a lung can be expanded has been divided into four nonoverlaping volumes (Fig. 5.2-6).

1. Tidal Volume (TV). It is the volume of air inspired or expired with each breath during normal quiet breathing. It is approximately 500 ml in a normal adult male.

2. Inspiratory Reserve Volume (IRV). It is the extra volume of air that can be inhaled by a maximum inspiratory effort over and beyond the normal tida l volume. It is about 3000 ml in a normal adult male.

3. Expiratory Reserve Volume (ERV). It is the extra volume of air that can be exhaled by maximum forceful expiration over and beyond the normal tidal volume, (i.e. after the end of normal passive expiration). It is approximately 1100 ml in a normal adult male.

4. Residual Volume (RV). It is the volume of the air that still remains in the lungs after the most forceful expiration. It is about 1200 ml in a normal adult male.

Lung Capacities

Lung capacities are combination of two or more pulmonary volumes and include (Fig. 5.2-6):

1. Inspiratory Capacity (IC). This is the maximum volume of the air that can be inspired after normal tidal expiration. Therefore, it equals the tidal volume plus inspiratory reserve volume (TV + IRV) and is approximately 3500 ml in a normal adult male.

2. Expiratory Capacity. It is the maximum volume of air that can be expired after normal tidal inspiration. It equals tidal volume plus expiratory reserve volume (TV + ERV) and is approximately about 1600 ml in a normal adult male.

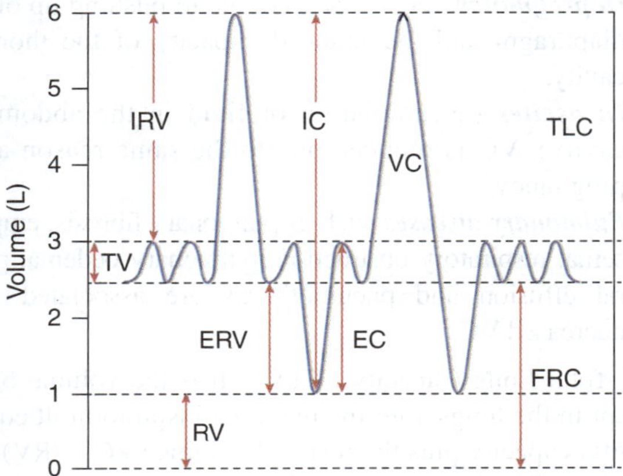

FIGURE 5.2-6 A spirogram showing various lung volumes and capacities: RV = residual volume; TV= tidal volume; IRV= inspiratory reserve volume; ERV = expiratory reserve volume; FRC= functional residual capacity; TLC= total lung capacity; IC= inspiratory capacity; VC= vital capacity and EC = expiratory capacity.

3. Functional Residual Capacity (FRC). It is the volume of the air remaining in the lungs after normal tidal expiration. Therefore, it equals the expiratory reserve volume plus the residual volume (ERV + RV) and is about 2300 ml in a normal adult male.

• ***Significance of FRC.*** The FRC (RV + ERV) of about 2300 ml represents the air that remains in the lungs most of the times. Even after the most forceful expiration about 1200 ml (residual volume) air is always present in the lungs. This has several advantages:

i. ***Continuous exchange of gases*** is possible due to presence of some air always in the lungs, and thereby concentration of O_2 and CO_2 in blood are maintained constant. Without FRC, pO_2 would have risen to 150 mmHg during inspiration, and reduced nearly to zero during expiration, which is maintained at about 100 mm of Hg due to the FRC.

ii. ***Breath holding*** is made possible due to the FRC.

iii. ***Dilution of toxic inhaled gases*** occurs due to the reserve of 2300 ml of air in the lungs (FRC) most of the times.

iv. ***Load on respiratory mechanism and left ventricle would*** have been much more if there was no FRC, since:
   - Without FRC, lungs would have collapsed at the end of each expiration, and re-expansion would have required tremendous breathing effort, and
   - The collapsed lungs would have increased pulmonary vascular resistance and imposed a heavy load on left ventricle.

• ***Factors Affecting FRC.*** Hyperinflation of the lungs seen in following conditions may be associated with increased FRC:

- Old age due to loss of elasticity of lungs,
- Emphysema, and
- Bronchial asthma.

• ***Measurement of FRC.*** Functional residual capacity can be measured by the nitrogen wash-out method or the helium dilution method.

Nitrogen wash-out method for measuring FRC. This method is based on the assumption that the alveolar air has 80% nitrogen. In this method, the subject is made to wash out nitrogen from the lungs completely by inhaling pure O_2 for 5 min and expiring into a large gas bag called the Douglas bag (washed with pure O_2 and, hence, made nitrogen free). The volume of gas collected in the *Douglas bag* and its nitrogen content are measured and the value of FRC is calculated as follows.

- Suppose that the expired gas collected at the end of 5 min is 40 L and its nitrogen concentration is 5%.
- Then the volume of nitrogen (*Vn*) in the expired gas will be

$$\frac{40 \times 5}{100} = 2 \text{ L or } 2000 \text{ ml}$$

- Since the nitrogen content of the expired gas is solely from the subject's lungs where it forms 80% of the gas present in the lungs (FRC); therefore,

$$\text{FRC} = \frac{2000 \times 100}{80} \text{ ml}$$
$$= 2500 \text{ ml or } 2.5 \text{ L}$$

Helium dilution method for FRC estimation. This method is based on the basic principle that the amount (A) of a substance present is equal to its volume (V) multiplied by its concentration (C), i.e.

$$A = V \times C.$$

- In this method, a closed circuit system is prepared with a mixture of helium, oxygen and air. The amount of helium is added in the mixture such as to achieve a helium concentration of 10%.
  - The subject is then made to breathe in the closed system till the concentration of helium in the lungs and the bag becomes equal. The helium concentration is measured at the end of a normal expiration (because the FRC is the volume of air remaining in the lungs at the end of normal expiration).

Since no helium was present in the lungs to start with, The same amount of helium which was added in the mixture in the close circuit system gets distributed between the bag and the lungs (Figs 5.2-7A and B).

- The FRC can be calculated as follows:
  - Suppose that the volume of helium added in the mixture to make its concentration to 10% is 560 ml,
  - Volume of the bag is 5000 ml and
  - Concentration of helium (He) in the bag and lungs after breathing in the close circuit system is 8%.

Then, the

$$\text{volume of He} = \frac{(\text{Volume of lungs} + \text{bag})}{\text{Concentration of helium}} \times \left(\frac{8}{100}\right)$$

i.e. $$560 = (\text{volume of lungs} + 5000) \times \frac{8}{100}$$

or

$$\text{volume of lungs} + 5000 = \frac{500 \times 100}{8}$$

or

$$\text{Volume of lungs} = 7000 - 5000$$
$$\text{Hence,} \quad \text{FRC} = 2000 \text{ ml.}$$

4. Vital Capacity (VC). This is the maximum amount of air a person can expel from the lungs after the deepest possible inspiration. Therefore, it equals the tidal volume plus the inspiratory reserve volume plus the expiratory reserve volume (TV + IRV + ERV) and is about 4600 ml in a normal adult male.

Significance of Vital Capacity

- Estimation of VC allows the assessment of maximum inspiratory and expiratory efforts and, thus, gives useful information about the strength of respiratory muscles.
- VC also provides useful information about other aspects of pulmonary functions through FEV (see page 407).

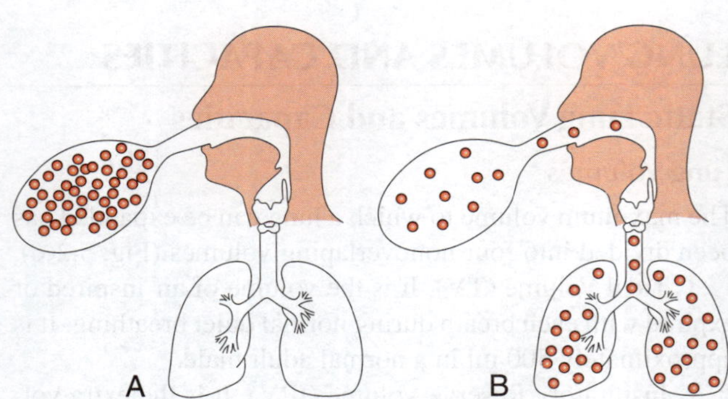

FIGURE 5.2-7 Helium dilution method for estimation of functional residual copacity (FRC): **(A)** in the beginning no helium present in the lungs and **(B)** The helium present in close circuit distributed equally between bag and the lungs.

Factors Affecting Vital Capacity

i. ***Size of the thoracic cavity.*** VC is more in males (2.6 L/m^2 body surface area) because of large chest size and more muscle power than females.

ii. ***Age.*** In old age, VC decreases due to the decrease in the elasticity of the lungs.

iii. ***Strength of respiratory muscles.*** In swimmers and divers, VC is more because of the increased strength of the respiratory muscles.

iv. ***Gravity.*** In standing position, VC is more than in sitting and lying position because of:
   - Increased size of the thoracic cavity in standing (diaphragm moves down), and
   - Reduced pulmonary blood flow due to decreased venous return.

v. ***In pregnancy,*** VC is reduced due to pushing up of the diaphragm and the reduced capacity of the thoracic cavity.

vi. ***In ascites*** (accumulation of fluid in the abdominal cavity), VC is reduced due to the same reason as in pregnancy.

vii. ***Pulmonary diseases*** such as pulmonary fibrosis, emphysema, respiratory obstruction, pulmonary oedema, pleural effusion and pneumothorax are associated with decreased VC.

5. Total Lung Capacity (TLC). It is the volume of air present in the lungs after the maximal inspiration. It equals the vital capacity plus the residual volume (VC + RV) and is about 5800 ml in a normal adult male.

Measurement of Static Lung Volumes and Capacities. All volumes and capacities except residual volume, functional residual capacity and TLC are recorded by a *spirometer*. Functional residual capacity is determined by the nitrogen wash-out method or the helium dilution method, and then residual volume and TLC are calculated.

Recording of lung volumes and capacities are the important lung function tests (for details see page 473).

Dynamic Lung Volumes and Capacities

Timed Vital Capacity (TVC) or Forced Vital Capacities

Forced vital capacity is the volume of the air that can be expired rapidly with a maximum force following a maximum inspiration. The volume of air expired can be timed by recording the vital capacity on a spirograph moving at the known speed.

Components of TVC or FVC (Fig. 5.2-8)

i. Forced Expiratory Volume in 1 sec (FEV_1). It represents the volume expired in the first second of an FVC.

- Estimation of FEV_1 is the most commonly used secreening test for airway diseases.
- The FEV_1 is actually a flow rate: its unit is L/sec.
- FEV_1% is the per cent of FVC expired in 1 sec (i.e. $FEV_1\% = FEV_1/FVC \times 100$); normally, FEV_1% is about 80% of the FVC (Fig. 5.2-9A).

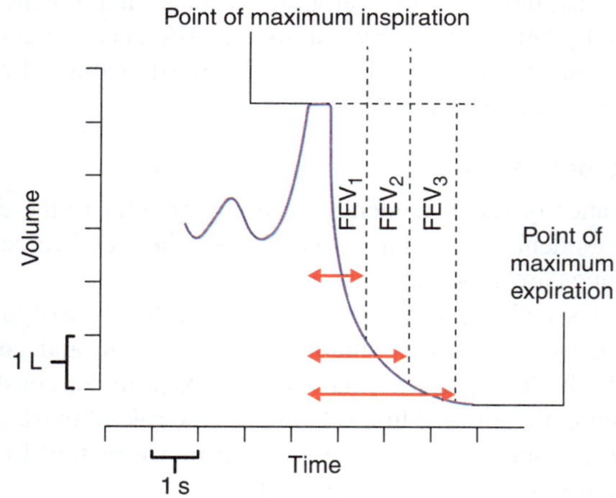

FIGURE 5.2-8 Components of timed vital capacity.

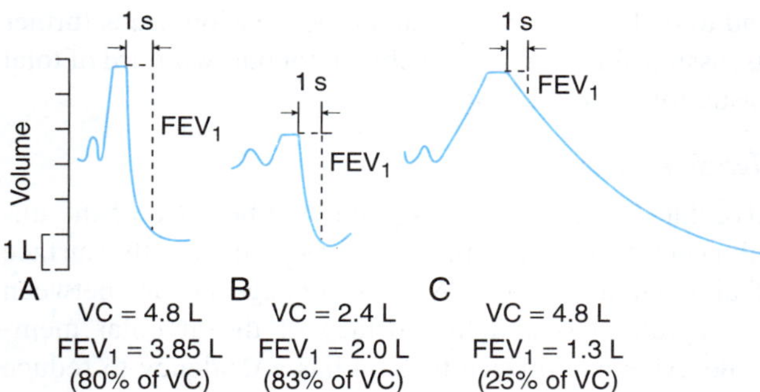

FIGURE 5.2-9 Forced expiratory volume in first second (FEV_1) component of timed vital capacity: **(A)** in normal subject; **(B)** in a patient with restrictive lung disease (RLD); and **(C)** in a patient with obstructive lung disease (OLD).

Clinical application. Useful in distinguishing between restrictive and obstructive lung diseases:

- Patients with *restrictive lung disease* (RLD), e.g. kyphoscoliosis and ankylosing spondylitis, have a reduced FVC; but they are able to achieve relatively high flow rates; therefore, their FEV_1% exceeds 80% (Fig. 5.2-9B).
- Patients with *obstructive lung disease* (OLD), e.g. bronchial asthma, have low flow rates as a result of high airway resistance; therefore, their FEV_1% is abnormally low (Fig. 5.2-9C).

ii. Forced Expiratory Volume in 2 sec (FEV_2). It represents the volume of air expired in the first 2 sec of FVC; FEV_2% is about 90% of FVC under the normal condition.

iii. Forced Expiratory Volume in 3 sec (FEV_3). It represents the volume of air expired in the first 3 sec. Normally FEV_3% is 98%–100% of FVC.

Forced Expiratory Flow during 25%–75% of Expiration (FEF 25%–75%)

- It is the mean expiratory flow rate during middle 50% of FVC (Fig. 5.2-10A).
- Normal FEF 25%–75% is 300 L/min.
- Mid expiratory time (MET) refers to the time taken for FEF 25&–75%. Its normal value is 0.5 sec which is increased in obstructive lung disorders.

Forced Expiratory Flow during 200–1200 ml of Expiration (FEF 200–1200)

- FEF 200–1200 refers to the mean expiratory flow rate between the 200 and 1200 ml segment of FVC (Fig. 5.2-10B).
- Normal values of FEF 200–1200 is 350 L/min.

Minute Ventilation (MV) or Pulmonary Ventilation (PV)

It is the volume of air inspired or expired per minute. It equals the tidal volume multiplied by the respiratory rate (TV × RR). The TV at rest averages 500 ml (0.5 L), and the normal respiratory rate is 12–15 breaths/min; therefore, normal minute volume is 6–7.5 L/min.

Maximum Breathing Capacity (MBC) or Maximum Voluntary Ventilation or Maximum Ventilation Volume (MVV)

- It is the maximum volume of air that can be ventilated on command during a given interval.
- This index of ventilatory function depends upon the complete co-operation of the subject, who is asked to breathe as rapidly and deeply as he/she can for a 15-sec interval. The volume of the air moved is either recorded by a spirometer fitted with a writing point or is collected in a Douglas bag; the result is expressed in L/min.
- A normal adult male can attain anMVV of 80–170 L/min (average 100 L/min).

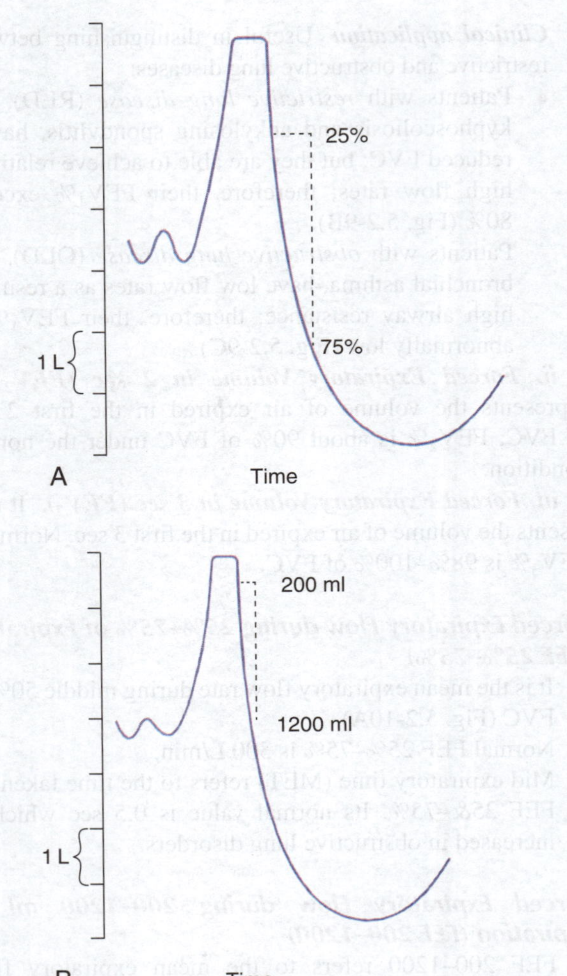

FIGURE 5.2-10 Forced expiratory flow: **(A)** during 25–75% of expiration (FEF 25–75%); and **(B)** during 200–1200 ml of expiration (FEF 200–1200 ml).

- MVV is profoundly reduced in patients with emphysema, airway obstruction and very poor respiratory muscle strength.

Important Note

Hyperventilation causes CO_2 washout which leads to respiratory depression. This may result in fainting; therefore, voluntary hyperventilation should be done for the brief periods (15 sec only).

Pulmonary Reserve or Breathing Reserve

- Pulmonary reserve (PR) refers to the maximum amount of the air above the pulmonary ventilation that can be inspired or expired in 1 min.
- It equals the maximum ventilation volume minus pulmonary ventilation (minute ventilation), i.e.

$$PR = MVV - PV/min.$$

- Pulmonary reserve is usually expressed as the percentage of MVV and is known as the percentage pulmonary reserve or the *dyspnoeic index (DI), i.e.*

$$DI\ \frac{MVV - PV}{MVV} \times 100$$

- Normal values of DI or per cent PR range from 60% to 90% with an average of 75%.
- Dyspnoea is usually present when the value of DI becomes less than 60%.

PULMONARY ELASTANCE AND COMPLIANCE

Pulmonary Elastance

Elastance refers to the *recoil* (retractive) tendency of a structure. Both the thoracic cage and lungs have elastance.

Elastance of Thoracic Cage

Elastance or the recoil tendency of the thoracic cage refers to the constant tendency of the thoracic cage to expand (to pop outward). The elastance of the thoracic cage is because of the fact that the chest wall is an elastic structure which is normally kept partially pulled inward. The elastic property of the thoracic cage is because of the elastic nature of ribs, muscles and tendons.

Elastance of Lungs

Elastance or recoil tendency of the lungs refer to the constant tendency of the lungs to collapse. The recoil forces in the lungs are generated by:

1. Tissue Forces. These are due to the presence of many elastic tissues such as smooth muscle, elastic and collagen in the lung parenchyma which are kept under constant stretch in the inflated lungs. However, the role of these connective tissue fibres in generating elastic (retractile) forces in the lungs is not fully elucidated.

2. Surface Forces. These are generated at the alveolar surface lined by fluid (*alveolar surface tension*) due to which the alveoli tend to become progressively smaller and tend to collapse. The alveolar surface tension needs further discussion since it is responsible for about two-third of total elastic forces in the lungs.

Alveolar Surface Tension

Alveolar surface tension is generated because of the unbalanced attraction of the liquid molecules at the surface of alveolar membrane. A phase change occurs between the alveolar gas and the surface of the alveolar membrane. Alveolar surface tension has a tendency to reduce the size of each alveolus, thus resulting into recoil tendency of the lung, i.e. surface tension increases the tendency of the lungs to deflate. An increased transmural pressure is necessary to counteract the effects of surface tension. According to the *law of Laplace,* in a spherical structure like alveoli the transmural pressure generated equals two times the (surface) tension divided by radius, i.e. P = 2T/r. In other words, the pressure in the alveoli is directly proportionate to the surface tension and inversely proportionate to the radii. Therefore, small alveoli tend to become still smaller whereas large alveoli tend to become still larger (Fig. 5.2-11). Thus, surface tension tends to produce collapse of the alveoli.

Alveolar surface tension playing a major role in generating elastance forces in the lungs can be demonstrated by an experiment (see page 408).

Pulmonary Surfactant

The alveolar surface tension opposes the expansion of the lungs during inspiration. The surface tension of pure water and air interface is so high that every inspiration would require an exhausting muscular effort. However, the presence of pulmonary surfactant in the fluid lining the alveoli reduces the surface tension markedly.

Source. Pulmonary surfactant is secreted by type II alveolar epithelial cells (granular pneumocytes). In the cells, it is stored in lamellar bodies. It comes to the surface of alveoli by the process of exocytosis and mixes with the water molecules present there.

Composition. Pulmonary surfactant is a complex mixture of several phospholipids, proteins and ions. Four unique proteins have been identified in surfactant: SP-A, SP-B, SP-C and SP-D. SP-A and SP-D are hydrophilic proteins, and SP-B and SP-C are strongly hydrophobic proteins. Dipalmitoylphosphatidylcholine (DPPC) along with several other phospholipids is responsible for reducing surface tension.

Mechanism of Action. One portion of each phospholipid molecule is hydrophilic and dissolves in the water lining the alveoli. Lipid hydrophobic portion of the molecule is oriented towards the air. This causes spreading of surfactant molecules over the surface of fluid lining the alveoli. Apoproteins and calcium ions are responsible for uniform and quick spreading of surfactant molecules over the surface. Such a hydrophobic surface exposed to air has one-twelfth to one-half of the surface tension of a pure water surface depending upon the concentrations and orientation of surfactant molecules on the surface.

Surface tension with normal alveolar fluid lining without surfactant is about 50 dynes/cm^2 and with surfactant it varies between 5 and 30 dynes/cm^2, depending upon the concentration of surfactant.

Functions of Pulmonary Surfactant

1. Reduces the Tendency of Alveoli to Collapse. The surface tension in a thin-walled sphere like alveolus tends to make the sphere smaller to collapse. Surfactant, by reducing surface tension decreases the tendency to collapse.

2. Reduces Work of Breathing. According to Laplace's law, due to reduction in the surface tension, the mean alveolar radius is increased. This reduces the transmural pressure required for expanding the alveoli. As alveoli are easily expanded, so work of breathing is reduced. The low surface tension also facilitates the reopening of collapsed airway and alveoli.

3. Prevents Pulmonary Oedema. Surface tension is retracting force which not only pulls alveolar wall to the centre of alveolus but also pulls fluid from capillaries into the interstitial space surrounding the alveoli and into the alveoli leading to pulmonary oedema. Surfactant prevents this phenomenon by lowering the surface tension.

4. Alveolar Stabilization. Surfactant causes stability of alveoli, i.e. it maintains almost uniform size of alveoli. Due to pulmonary surfactant pulling pressure in the alveoli is reduced from 18 cm of H_2O to 4 cm of H_2O. The mechanism of alveolar instability and how the pulmonary surfactant causes alveolar stabilization is explained.

Alveolar instability due to surface tension effect is produced as follows:

- In the two alveoli (with unequal size) connected to each other the amount of pressure generated in each according to Laplace's law will be:

$$\text{Pressure} = \frac{2 \times \text{surface tension}}{\text{radius}}$$

- Thus, when the surface tension is constant, the pressure developed in the smaller alveolus will be more than the larger alveolus. This will cause pushing of air from smaller alveolus (with higher pressure) to large alveolus (with lower pressure). As a result, the smaller alveolar sac will become more smaller and larger alveolar sac will become more larger (Fig. 5.2-11).

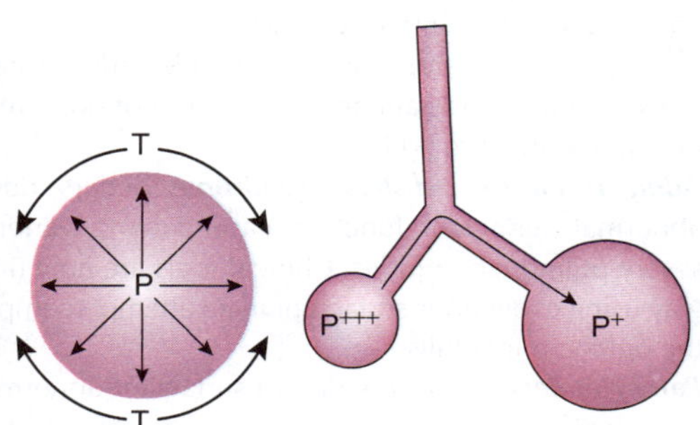

FIGURE 5.2-11 Pressure in the alveoli **(P)** is directly proportionate to the surface tension **(T)** and inversely proportionate to the radii (r). Therefore, small alveoli tend to become still smaller and large alveoli tend to become still larger.

- The above cycle of pushing air from smaller to larger sac will continue till the smaller sac totally collapses leading to large distension of the other sac, thereby producing instability of the alveoli.

Pulmonary surfactant causes alveolar stabilization by following mechanisms:

- In the presence of surfactant, the surface tension developed in the alveoli is inversely proportionate to the concentration of surfactant per unit area.
- In the smaller alveolus, the surfactant molecules form a thick layer, while in a larger alveolus the surfactant molecules are scattered on the larger surface (as number of molecules is limited) (Fig. 5.2-12).
- Thus, in a smaller alveolus the tendency to develop more pressure due to smaller radius will be neutralized by the tendency to develop less pressure due to more concentration of surfactant per unit area; and the reverse will occur in larger alveolus. In this way, there will not be much pressure gradient between the two alveoli helping to maintain the size of alveolar sac constant. Thus, due to the presence of surfactant stability of alveoli is maintained.

Other factors which help in alveolar stabilization along with surfactant are interdependence and fibrous tissue.

- ***Interdependence*** is a mechanical method of alveolar stabilization. The alveolar septa form a continuous network that is under tension because of lung inflation. Alveoli are tethered together by their adjoining walls and cannot change volume independently of the neighbouring lung tissue.
- ***Fibrous tissue.*** The lung is constructed of about 50,000 functional units, each of which contains one or a few alveolar ducts and their associated alveoli. All of these are surrounded by fibrous septa that act as additional splints and stabilize the alveoli.

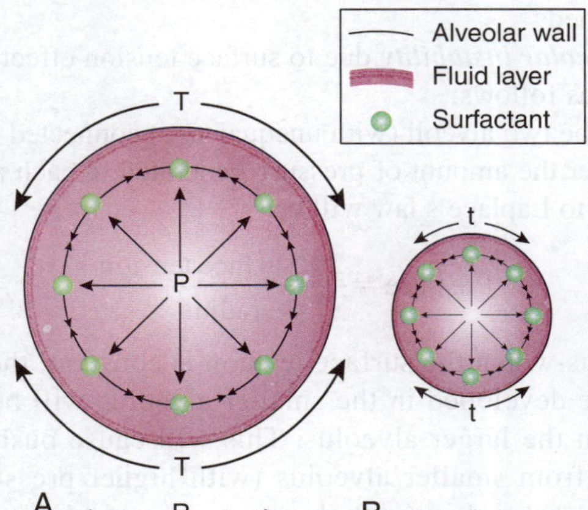

FIGURE 5.2-12 Distribution of surfactant in a **(A)** large and **(B)** small alveoli.

Factors Affecting Pulmonary Surfactant

Factors which Decrease the Pulmonary Surfactant

- Long-term inhalation of 100% O_2,
- Occlusion of main bronchus,
- Occlusion of one pulmonary artery,
- Cigarette smoking, and
- Cutting both the vagii.

Factors which Increase Surfactant Production

- Thyroid hormones increase the secretion of pulmonary surfactant by increasing the size and number of inclusion bodies in type II alveolar lining epithelial cells.
- Glucocorticoids accelerate the maturation of pulmonary surfactant.

Applied Aspects

Clinical Significance of Pulmonary Surfactant

1. ***Respiratory distress syndrome of newborn*** or the *hyaline membrane disease* occurs in the newborn babies (especially premature) due to inadequate formation of surfactant, resulting in an elevated alveolar surface tension. Retention of fluid in the lung is an additional factor in respiratory distress syndrome (RDS). During fetal life pulmonary epithelium secretes Cl^- in the fluid but at birth epithelial cells start absorbing Na^+ through epithelial Na^+ channels (ENaCs) and fluid gets absorbed along with Na^+. Immaturity of EnaCs is responsible for pulmonary oedema in RDS. Under this condition it is extremely difficult to expand the lungs.

   Dysfunction/overproduction of surfactant proteins is the cause of pulmonary alveolar proteinosis and can lead to respiratory distress. Under this condition it is extremely difficult to expand the lungs.

   Sign and symptoms—Respiratory work is greatly increased and there is inadequate exchange of gases due to alveolar instability, pulmonary oedema and collapse of alveoli (atelectasis) in many areas. This results in severe respiratory insufficiency, and the infant may die.

   Diagnosis—Plasma levels of thyroid hormones and cortisol are low in infants with RDS.

   Treatment—Therapy of RDS includes administration of exogenous surfactant and application of positive-end expiratory pressure (PEEP).
2. ***Adult respiratory distress syndrome*** occurs due to abnormal surfactant function caused by a variety of severe pulmonary injuries. Clinical trials are now underway using exogenous surfactant in an attempt to improve the outcome in adults.
3. ***Patchy atelectasis*** occurs due to surfactant abnormality in patients who have undergone cardiac surgery during which a pump oxygenator is used and the pulmonary circulation is interrupted.

Pulmonary Compliance

Definition and Normal Value

- Compliance (C) refers to change in lung volume (ΔV) per unit change in transpulmonary pressure (ΔP), i.e.

$$C = \frac{\Delta V}{\Delta P}$$

Transpulmonary pressure is the difference in the pressure between alveolar pressure and pleural pressure.

- Compliance expresses the distensibility (expansibility) of the lung and chest wall.
- Normal value of compliance for the lungs and chest wall combined is 0.13 L/cm of H_2O and for the lung alone it is 0.22 L/cm of H_2O.

Measurement of Total Compliance

Total respiratory compliance (combined compliance of chest wall and lungs) can be measured by the pressure–volume curve of the respiratory system. The pressure–volume curve of the respiratory system can be obtained in living subjects by using a spirometer as below:

Procedure The subject is connected to the spirometer and asked to breathe air through mouth (with nostrils closed). The manometer attached with the spirometer measures airway pressure (transpulmonary pressure). The subject inhales known volume of air from end-expiratory position, and the valve of the spirometer is than shut off to close the airway. The subject holds the breath and then releases the respiratory muscles and change in the airway pressure is measured. The procedure is repeated with actively inhaling or exhaling different air volumes up to the maximum.

The change in the airway pressure is plotted against each air volume and a curve obtained is called the pressure–volume curve of the respiratory system (Fig. 5.2-13).

Observations and Inferences

1. The pressure–volume curve of the respiratory system is a sigmoid shape curve which is steepest at the middle and almost flat at both ends (i.e. high and low lung volumes).
2. The volume at which air pressure is 0 mmHg (atmospheric pressure) is called *relaxation volume* which is equal to FRC. At relaxation volume, the recoil of chest wall and recoil of lung balance each other.
3. Above relaxation volume, on increasing lung volumes there is increase in the airway pressure and at maximum inspiration pressure rises up to 30 mmHg. On the other hand, decrease in the lung volumes below relaxation volume airway pressure decreases and at maximum expiration point it decreases up to –30 mmHg.
4. The RV and TLC are limited by decrease compliance of the system as indicated by the reduced slop at both extreme volumes.

Factors Affecting Compliance of Lungs and Chest Wall *Downward and right shift* of the pressure–volume curve indicates decreased total respiratory compliance. The causes of decreased compliance are:

- Pulmonary congestion
- Interstitial pulmonary fibrosis
- Pulmonary oedema

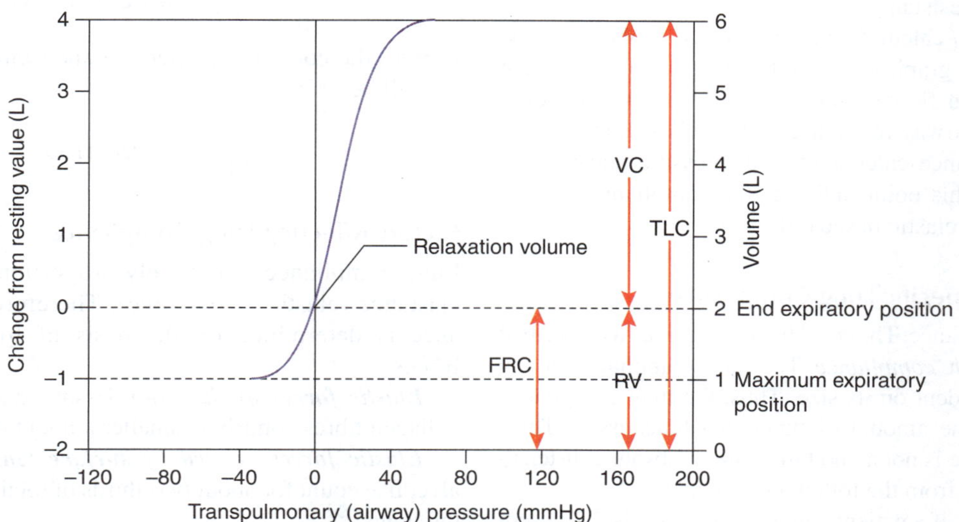

FIGURE 5.2-13 Pressure–volume curve of the respiratory system.

Upward and left shift of the pressure–volume curve indicates increases total respiratory compliance. The causes of increased compliance are:

- Emphysema
- Old age

Measurement of Pulmonary Compliance

- The compliance of lung alone can be measured by measuring the intrapleural pressure at different lung volumes.
- The intrapleural pressure (being similar to intra-oesophageal pressure) is measured with the help of an intraoesophageal balloon connected to a manometer.
- The subject is made to inspire air from a spirometer in steps of 100 ml and each time the intrapleural pressure is recorded.
- The relationship of lung volume to intrapleural pressure is plotted on a graph, which gives the *inspiratory compliance curve* (Fig. 5.2-14).
- Similarly expiration is also done in steps and *expiratory compliance* curve is obtained (Fig. 5.2-14).
- The inspiratory and expiratory compliance curves do not coincide but form a loop called *hysteresis loop.*
- So, Figure 5.2-14 shows that the lung volume at any given pressure is greater during expiration than during inspiration. This is due to difference in the distensibility (stretchability) of the lungs between inspiratory and expiratory phases. The volume midway between the hysteresis loop (dashed linear line (Fig. 5.2-14) gives the average compliance of the lungs. Had the lungs been a perfectly elastic structure like a spring the pressure–volume relation line would have been linear (Hook's law).
- The curved lines obtained during inspiration and expiration are because of two resistances:
  - Viscous resistance due to nonelastic tissues in the lungs, and
  - Airway resistance.
- Therefore, to calculate the compliance of the lung, the point on the graph at the end of inspiration, i.e. when there is no air flow should be considered. At this point, there is no airway resistance and no viscous resistance. The compliance calculated from pressure and volume changes at this point indicates the compliance of lung alone due to elastic tissue only.

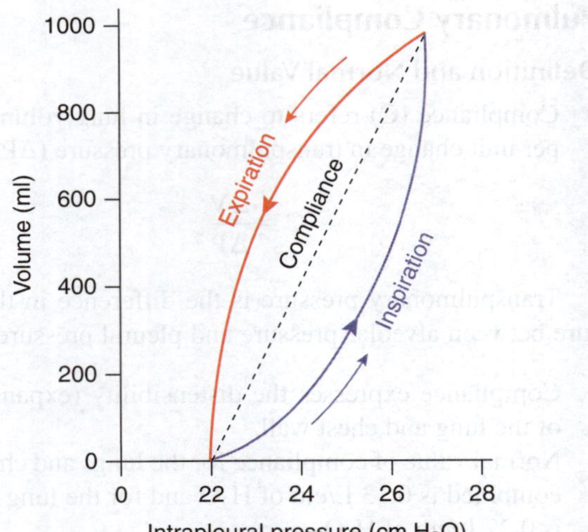

FIGURE 5.2-14 Change in volume per unit change in intrapleural pressure during quiet respiration.The dotted line represents the pulmonary compliance.

Static Versus Specific Lung Compliance

Static Compliance. The compliance measured as described above is the *static compliance*. The static compliance of any system is dependent on its size. Thus, the lung compliance depends upon the amount of functional lung tissue. Thus, static compliance is not a good measure of absolute distensibility, as is clear from the following example:

For example, if a patient's lung compliance is 0.22 L/cm H_2O, then both lungs together are able to expand 0.22 L for each cm H_2O change in pleural pressure. Assuming equal compliance in both lungs, each lung will take up 0.11 L of gas. If the patient undergoes a pneumonectomy, the compliance measured will be only 0.11 L/cm H_2O, in spite of the fact that distensibility of the remaining lung is normal. Therefore, clinically term specific compliance is used.

Specific Compliance is the compliance of the lung at relaxation volume (the point at the end of a tidal expiration), i.e. the functional residual capacity. The specific compliance is expressed per litre of functional residual capacity (FRC). It is a measure of the absolute distensibility of a structure. For instance, in the above cited example if the FRC is 2.2 L then:

- Specific compliance with both intact lungs will be:

$$= \frac{0.22}{2.2} = 0.1 \text{ L /cm } H_2O$$

- Specific compliance after pneumonectomy of one lung will be

$$\frac{11}{11} = 0.1 \text{ L/cm } H_2O.$$

Factors Affecting Lung Compliance

Lung compliance is inversely proportionate to the lung elastance (elastic recoil force). Therefore, lung compliance is determined on the basis of following elastic forces:

Elastic forces of the lung Tissues due to elastic and collagen fibres contribute smaller amount of elasticity.

Elastic forces caused by surface tension within the alveoli account for about two-thirds of total elastic forces in the lungs.

Alveolar surface tension plays a major role in generating elastance forces in the lungs and thus is very important factor affecting lung compliance. It can be demonstrated experimentally by recording the compliance of an isolated lung of an animal by first distending it with air and then with saline. Filling the lungs with saline theoretically eliminates the force of surface tension so that only the elastic forces of the lung tissue produce recoil. Figure 5.2-15 shows the results of such an experiment. Compared with air-filled lungs (Fig. 5.2-15A), the saline-filled lungs (Fig. 5.2-15B) markedly reduce recoil forces, leading to the conclusion that the elastic forces caused by alveolar surface tension play a major role in generating elastance forces in the lungs.

Changes in the Lung Compliance

- ***Decreased Compliance*** of the lungs can be caused by lung diseases, (e.g. tuberculosis, silicosis) that produce scarring or fibrosis of the lungs, destruction of the functional lung tissue or both. Reduced compliance produces a condition termed RLD. Patients with RLD must generate greater than normal forces to expand the lungs.
- ***Increased Compliance*** is produced by the pathologic processes that occur in emphysema as well as from the aging process. Alveolar septa which provide some of the retractive forces in lungs are destroyed under both conditions, but emphysema causes a much more extensive loss of septa than the normal aging process.

WORK OF BREATHING

The contraction of respiratory muscles causes the expansion of the thoracic cage and thereby causes expansion of lungs and fall in intra-alveolar pressure and allows the atmospheric pressure to push air into the lungs during inspiration. Thus, to move the air into the lungs, the respiratory muscles have to do work to overcome the following *resistances*.

Resistance to Breathing

Tissue Resistance. It is the resistance offered by the tissues as they expand or contract. Tissue resistance comprises:

1. ***Elastic resistance.*** It is the sum of forces of elastic recoil exerted by the lung and the chest wall. The elastic recoil of the lungs is due to the presence of elastic fibres in the lungs and due to the alveolar surface tension.
2. ***Viscous resistance*** is the resistance offered by the non-elastic tissues in the lungs.

Airway Resistance. It is the resistance caused by friction of gas molecules between themselves and the walls of the airways. Factors affecting airway resistance are:

1. ***Rate of gas flow.*** Greater the rate of gas flow, greater is the resistance. The rate of gas flow is highest in the intermediate sized bronchi as they have highest cross-sectional area; so the highest resistance to flow occurs in this part of a tracheobronchial tree.
2. ***Airway radius.*** It is the most powerful determinant of resistance. Smaller the radius of airway, greater is the resistance. According to *Poiseuille-Hagen formula* (see page 302),

$$\text{resistance} \; \alpha \frac{1}{r^4}.$$

In other words, if radius decreases by half (keeping the other factors constant), the resistance increases by 16 times.

Airway radius increases when lungs expand (during inspiration) and it decreases when lungs contract (during expiration). Therefore, airway resistance is high during expiration as compared to inspiration. Because of this reason in bronchial asthma patients (where broncho-constriction develops) inspiration is possible but there is extreme difficulty in expiration.

Control of Airway Diameter

- *Sympathetic adrenergic stimulation* to the airway causes bronchodilation. In human, direct sympathetic nerve activation causes only slight bronchodilation. Because these nerves do not actually innervate the bronchial smooth muscles. However, the bronchial smooth muscles contain a large number of β_2 receptors that respond to circulating adrenergic substances such as epinephrine, norepinephrine and isoproterenol.
- *Vagus nerve (cholinergic) stimulation* causes bronchoconstriction and increase in mucous formation.

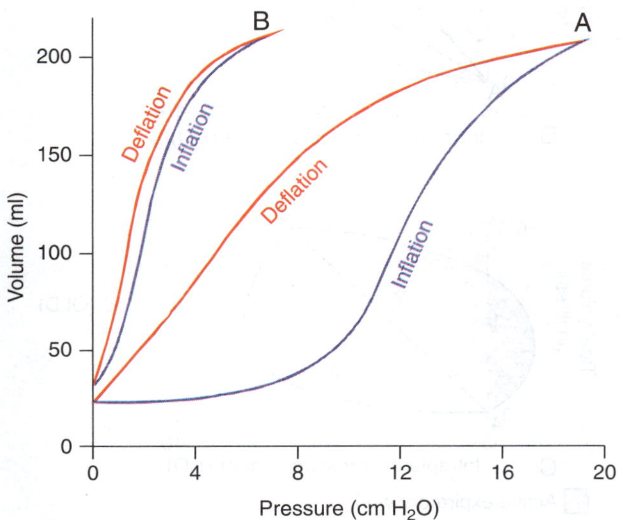

FIGURE 5.2-15 Pressure–volume relationship of an isolated lung filled (A) with air and (B) with saline. The saline filled lung has far greater compliance due to absence of surface tension at water–air interface seen with air filled lung.

Cholinergic activity may be the cause of asthma in some individuals.

- *Nonadrenergic noncholinergic* control of bronchial smooth muscle is exerted through following substances:
  - Noncholinergic excitatory compounds such as substance P and neurokinins A and B cause bronchoconstriction, mucous secretion and increased vascular permeability. These substances may be involved in pathogenesis of asthma in some individuals.
  - Nonadrenergic inhibitory system consists of postganglionic neurons that release vasoactive intestinal polypeptide (VIP) and other mediators that cause smooth muscle relaxation and inhibit mucus production.

3. ***Length of airway.*** It does not change much during respiration or in lung diseases and therefore, is not an important factor.
4. ***Type of air flow.*** The airway resistance is more in turbulent flow (e.g. during rapid respiration) than in laminar flow or streamline flow in quiet breathing.

Components of Work of Breathing

The total work done by the respiratory muscles during quiet breathing may be divided into following components:

- Work done to overcome elastic resistance (65%),
- Work done to overcome viscous resistance (7%) and
- Work done to overcome airway resistance (28%).

Calculation of Work of Breathing

The work of breathing, i.e. the work of inflating the lungs can be calculated by plotting the change in lung volume (ΔV) versus the change in intrapleural pressure (ΔP) (Fig. 5.2-16). The total area represented by $\Delta P \times \Delta V$ in Figure 5.2-16 is proportional to the work that must be performed by the respiratory muscles and to the O_2 utilized by them. The work done by the respiratory muscles can be calculated separately for inspiration and expiration.

Work Done During Inspiration In Figure 5.2-16A, the area AXBC denotes the total work done during normal inspiration. The work of inspiration can be divided into three fractions:

- ***Compliance work*** refers to the work done by respiratory muscles to inflate the lungs against the *elastic resistance* of chest wall and lungs. It is represented by the grey triangular area AYBCA in Figure 5.2-16A. Thus, most of the work done (65%) is used to overcome elastic resistance.
- ***Nonelastic resistance work*** is done to overcome the nonelastic resistance. It includes the work done to overcome:

- Viscous resistance of lungs (7%) and
- Airway resistance (28%).

It is represented by pink area AXBYA in Figure 5.2-16A. Thus, only a small amount (7%) of the work done is used to overcome the viscosity of the lungs and 28% of the work done is utilized to overcome the resistance of air flow through the respiratory passages.

Work Done During Expiration Since in quiet breathing, expiration is a passive process so no work is done during expiration. The grey triangle AYBCA in Figure 5.2-16 A represents the stored elastic energy that is present at the end of inspiration. This stored energy can compress the alveolar gas and create expiratory flow. When the lungs are recoiling back some energy is required to overcome *nonelastic resistance,* i.e. the airway resistance plus viscous tissue resistance. This is represented by the area AYBZA which in normal quiet expiration falls within the triangle AYBCA (stored energy) and so no extra work is required to overcome this resistance.

Work of Breathing Done in Restrictive Lung Disease In the presence of RLD, the patient has to overcome significantly

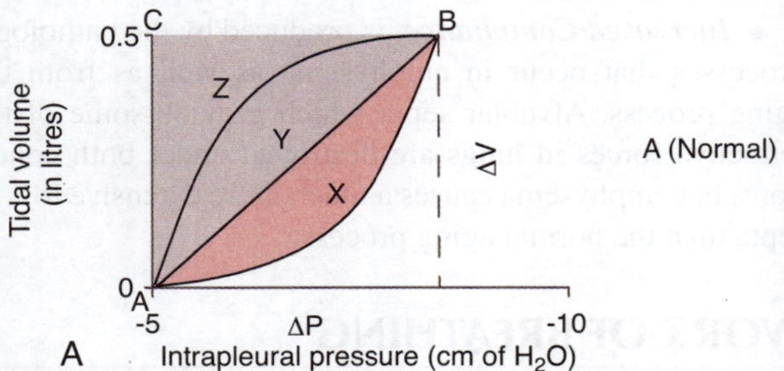

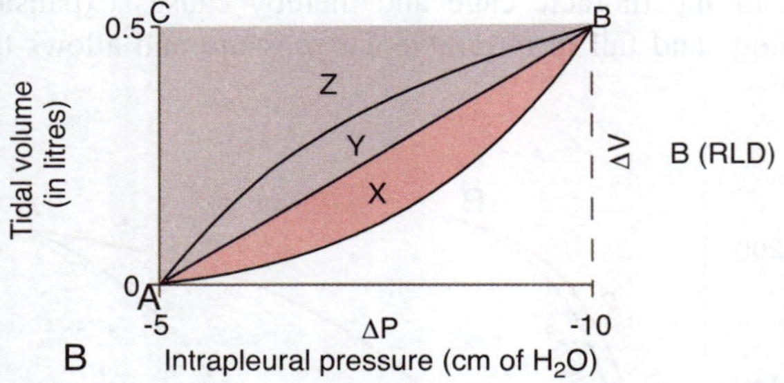

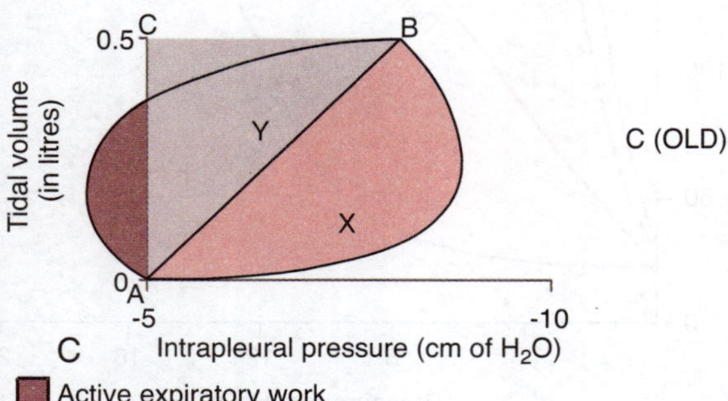

FIGURE 5.2-16 Calculation of work done during breathing by plotting the change in volume (ΔV) against change in intrapleural pressure (ΔP): **(A)** in normal quiet breathing; **(B)** in restrictive lung disease (RLD) and **(C)** in obstructive lung disease (OLD).

higher elastance forces for the normal tidal breathing. So, in RLD more work has to be performed by the respiratory muscles during inspiration to overcome the decreased compliance (Fig. 5.2-16B).

Minimal Work of Breathing is a function of airway resistance and respiratory system compliance (Fig. 5.2-17A). All species of animals use the combination of tidal volume and respiratory rate that requires the minimal work of breathing. The increase in the elastance, work done in patients with RLD can be minimized by breathing rapidly and shallow (Fig. 5.2-17B). The tidal volume is decreased but the increased respiratory rate ensures adequate ventilation of lungs.

Work of Breathing Done in Obstructive Lung Diseases

In patient with OLD, the airway resistance is increased due to narrowing of passages. The patients must generate increased pressure gradients to produce adequate air flow. So, *during inspiration* more work by respiratory muscles is done to overcome the increased nonelastic resistance, as a result the work loop broadens significantly as is evident from the pink area AXBYA in Figure 5.2-16C vis-à-vis 5.2-14A. Under such circumstances when the work loop extends beyond Y-axis active contraction of expiratory muscles is required to accomplish the task of expiration, as the elastic recoil (stored energy represented by grey triangular area) is not sufficient for it. The extra work performed by expiratory muscles is represented by brown area in Figure 5.2-16C.

Compensatory Mechanism. The resistance work can be minimized by breathing more slowly and deeply (see Fig. 5.2-17B). This prolongs the time of expiration, which reduces the pressure gradient necessary to generate gas flow. The increased tidal volume compensates for the decreased respiratory rate so that normal alveolar ventilation is maintained.

Factors Affecting Total Work of Breathing Total work of breathing during quiet respiration under normal circumstances ranges from 0.3 to 0.8 kg mt/min. Normally, the work of breathing represents 2–3% of the resting O_2 consumption.

- If either the respiratory resistance increases or the compliance decreases, the respiratory work will increase and therefore the respiratory muscles will use more O_2 to overcome the added load.
- The work of breathing is also increased markedly during muscular exercise (physiological).

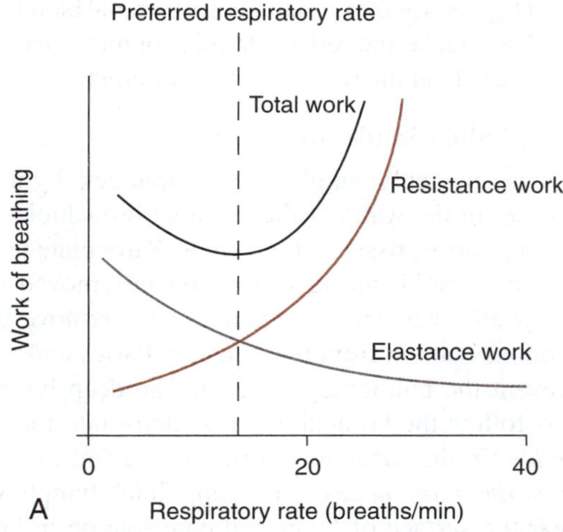

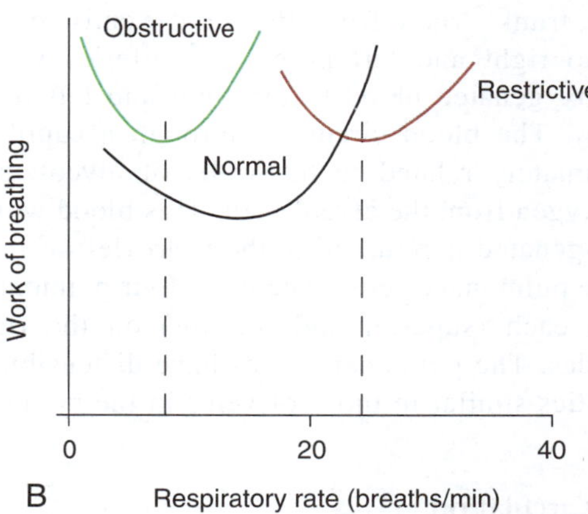

FIGURE 5.2-17 Determinants of an optimal breathing to do minimal work of breathing: **(A)** variations in different components of work of breathing—the preferred respiratory rate to do minimal work of breathing normally is 12–15 breaths/min, with tidal volume 0.5 L and **(B)** total work of breathing curve reflects that the patients with obstructive lung disease (OLD) minimizes their work of breathing by decreasing respiratory rate and increasing tidal volume and those with restrictive lung disease (RLD) do so by decreasing tidal volume and increasing respiratory rate.

Chapter 5.3

Pulmonary Circulation

FUNCTIONAL ANATOMY

The lungs have three circulations—pulmonary, bronchial and lymphatic.

Pulmonary Circulation

Pulmonary trunk arises from the right ventricle and divides into right and left pulmonary arteries which convey deoxygenated blood to the right and left lung, respectively. The blood circulates through a capillary plexus intimately related to the walls of alveoli and receives oxygen from the alveolar air. This blood which is now oxygenated is returned to the heart (left atrium) through the pulmonary veins. There are four pulmonary veins, two each (superior and inferior) on the right and left sides. The pulmonary veins have distensibility characteristics similar to those of veins in the systemic circulation.

Bronchial Circulation

The lungs also receive oxygenated blood like other tissues in the body. This is conveyed through *bronchial arteries* (two left and one right) which are branches of the descending thoracic aorta. Bronchial blood flow amounts to about 1 to 2% of total cardiac output. The oxygenated blood in the bronchial arteries supplies the connective tissues, septa and large and small bronchi of the lungs. Because the bronchial blood empties into the pulmonary veins and bypasses the right heart, the bronchial circulation therefore constitutes a *physiological shunt,* i.e. a channel that bypasses oxygenation in the lungs. The other example of physiological shunt is coronary vessels that drain into the left side of the heart. These physiological shunts have two effects:

- They reduce the O_2 saturation of arterial blood slightly and
- They make the left ventricular output greater by about 1–2% than the right ventricular output.

Lymphatic Circulation

Lungs are richly supplied by lymphatics. Lymphatics are present in the walls of the terminal bronchioles and in all the supportive tissues of the lungs. Particulate matter entering the alveoli during inspiration is removed by way of lymphatic channels. Lymphatics also remove the plasma proteins leaking from the lung capillaries and thus help to prevent the pulmonary oedema. The deep lymphatic vessels follow the bronchi and first drain into the *pulmonary nodes* (in the substance of the lungs) and then into *bronchopulmonary nodes.* The superficial lymph vessels lie near the surface of lungs and converge on to bronchopulmonary nodes. From bronchopulmonary node lymph drains into *tracheobronchial nodes* and from there into the *bronchomediastinal trunk.*

CHARACTERISTIC FEATURES OF PULMONARY CIRCULATION

Introduction

- The pulmonary arteries and their branches are thin walled and distensible, giving the pulmonary arterial tree a large compliance. The distensibility of pulmonary vessels makes the pulmonary circulation a *low pressure, low-resistance* and *high-capacitance system.*

- The thickness of the right ventricle and pulmonary artery is approximately one-third of the thickness of left ventricle and aorta, respectively.
- The pulmonary arterioles have very little smooth muscles in their walls. The pulmonary capillaries are larger in diameter than systemic capillaries and have multiple anastomoses.
- The pulmonary capillaries surround the alveoli and are sandwiched between their walls, as a result each alveolus seems to be enclosed in a basket of capillaries (Fig. 5.3-1).

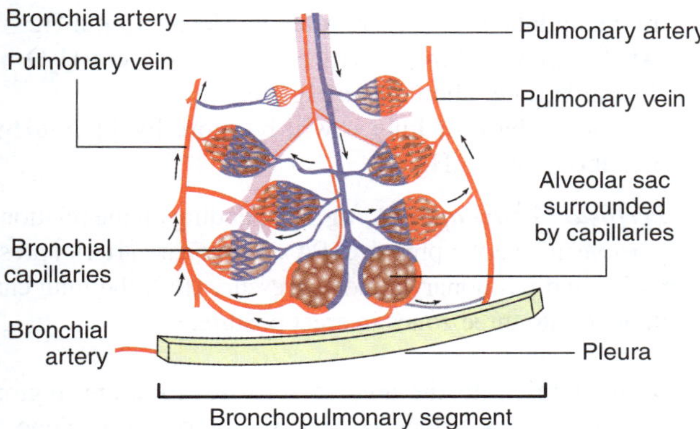

FIGURE 5.3-1 Organization of pulmonary circulation.

Pressures in the Pulmonary System (Fig. 5.3-2)

Right Ventricular Pressure during each cardiac cycle reaches a peak value of 25 mmHg in systole (if 120 mmHg in the left ventricle) and falls to 0–1 mm in diastole (if 5 mmHg in left ventricle).

Pulmonary Artery Pressures vis-à-vis aorta, respectively are:

- Systolic pressure 25 mmHg and 120 mmHg,
- Diastolic pressure 8 mmHg and 80 mmHg,
- Mean arterial pressure 15 mmHg and 100 mmHg, and
- Pulse pressure 17 mmHg and 40 mmHg.

Left Atrial Pressure in major pulmonary veins averages about 5 mmHg in the recumbent human being. Therefore, the pressure gradient in the pulmonary system (mean pulmonary artery pressure–mean pulmonary vein pressure) is 15–5 = 10 mmHg (if 120 mmHg in the systemic circulation).

Pulmonary Capillary Pressure, the mean values estimated through indirect means is about 10 mmHg. Since this pressure is far below the colloid osmotic pressure (25 mmHg), so a net suction force of 15 mmHg tends to draw fluid from alveolar interstitial space into the pulmonary capillaries *which keeps the alveoli dry.* However, if the pulmonary capillary hydrostatic pressure rises above 25-mmHg fluid can escape into the interstitial space leading to *pulmonary oedema.* This can happen during exercise, particularly at high altitude, in left heart failure, mitral stenosis and pulmonary fibrosis. It is

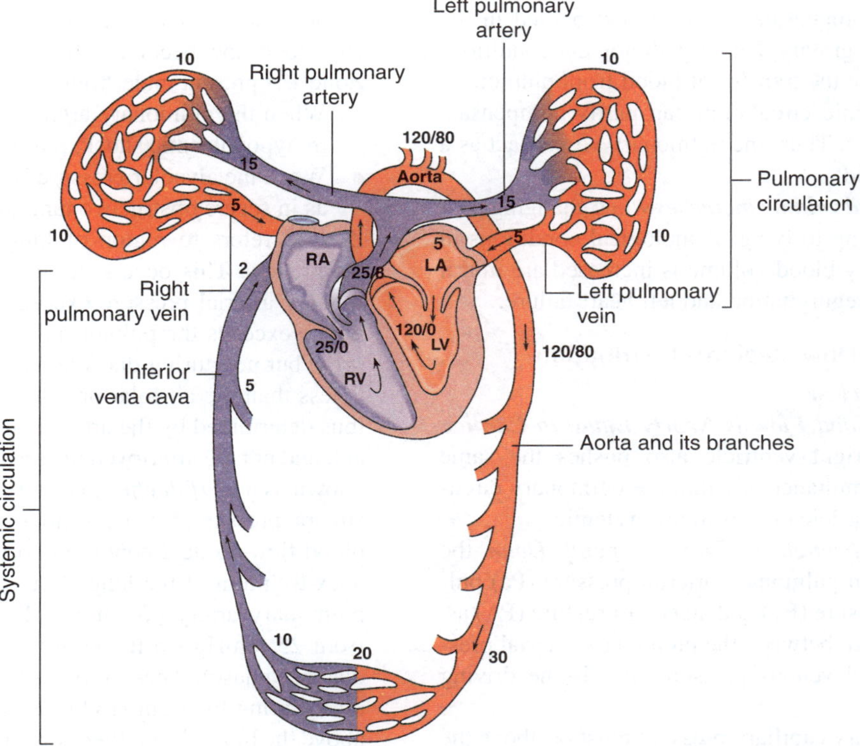

FIGURE 5.3-2 Blood pressure (mmHg) in pulmonary and systemic circulation. RA= right atrium, LA=left atrium, RV=right ventricle and LV=left ventricle

important to know that even a thin layer of interstitial fluid increases the distance between blood in pulmonary capillaries and gases in alveoli. Since the rate of diffusion is inversely proportional to the diffusion distance, increase in the distance would reduce the rate of gas exchange in the lungs. The resultant hypoxia may be fatal.

Pulmonary Wedge Pressure is measured to give an estimate of left atrial pressure. Direct measurement of left atrial pressure is difficult because it requires passing a catheter through left ventricle. Pulmonary wedge pressure is measured by inserting a balloon tipped catheter through the right side of the heart and pulmonary artery until the catheter wedges tightly in a smaller branch of the artery and stops the blood flowing in it. Under such circumstances the ballooned tip of the catheter makes an almost direct connection through the pulmonary capillaries with the blood in pulmonary veins which have the pressure similar to left atrium. The wedge pressure so measured is usually only 2 to 3 mm greater than the left atrial pressure. Clinically, wedge pressure measurements are employed frequently for studying changes in left atrial pressure in patients with congestive heart failure.

Pulmonary Blood Volume

- ***Pulmonary vessels*** *contain* about 600 ml of blood at rest. Since the pulmonary vessels act as capacitance vessels their blood content can vary from 200 ml to 900 ml.
- ***Pulmonary blood volume*** *decreases* under physiological conditions like standing and is shifted to systemic circulation to compensate for the blood pooled in the leg veins due to gravity. Under pathological conditions like haemorrhage the transfer of blood from pulmonary vessels to systemic circulation can partly compensate for the blood loss. Thus, the pulmonary vessels act as a reservoir of blood.
- ***Pulmonary blood volume*** *increases* when changing posture from standing to lying. Pathological conditions in which pulmonary blood volume is increased are mitral stenosis, mitral regurgitation and left heart failure.

Pulmonary Blood Flow: Regional Distribution

Pulmonary Blood Flow

• ***Pulmonary Blood Flow is Nearly Equal to Cardiac Output*** since the right ventricle also pushes the same amount of blood simultaneously into the pulmonary circulation as the left ventricle pushes in the systemic.

• ***Blood Flow Through the Lungs Depends Upon*** the relationship between pulmonary arterial pressure (Pa) pulmonary venous pressure (Pv) and alveolar pressure (PA) as:

- The difference between the pulmonary arterial pressure (Pa) and venous pressure (Pv) is the driving pressure and
- The pulmonary capillary pressure must be above the alveolar pressure for the blood flow to continue.

• ***Effect of Gravity on Regional Pulmonary Blood Flow.*** In normal adults in supine position the mean arterial pressure is same all over the lung and so all regions of the lung are uniformly perfused. However, in erect posture the gravity affects the regional distribution of blood through the lung by altering the pulmonary vasculature pressure due to hydrostatic pressure effect. The hydrostatic pressure adds or subtracts from the pressure levels in supine position if levels are below or above the zero reference plane, respectively. The zero reference plane is at the level of the right atrium, which is approximately in the middle of lung in the region of hilum. Therefore, in standing posture the mean pulmonary arterial pressure in a 30-cm-long lung will be:

- In the middle of lung (zero reference level) 15 mmHg
- At the apex of lung it will be less by 15 cm H_2O or 11 mmHg, i.e. about 4 mmHg, and
- But at the base of lung it will be more by 11 mmHg, i.e. about 26 mmHg.

Perfusion Zones of the Lung. Depending on the relationship between alveolar pressure (PA), pulmonary arterial pressure (Pa) and pulmonary venous pressure (Pv), the lung can be divided into three zones in erect posture:

- ***Zone 1*** refers to the area of zero flow, i.e. any region of the lung that does not receive blood flow. Zone 1 *does not exist in normal lungs.* Zone 1 occurs when the regional pulmonary arterial pressure becomes less than the alveolar pressure (Pa $<$ PA) under these conditions, the pulmonary capillaries collapse (Fig. 5.3-3) and blood flow becomes zero.
  Zone 1 is present under following abnormal conditions:
  - When the pulmonary arterial pressure is too low as in hypovolaemic shock, pulmonary embolism, or
  - When the alveolar pressure is too high to allow flow as in severe obstructive lung disorder.
- ***Zone 2*** refers to region of lung that has intermittent blood flow. This occurs during systole when the pulmonary arterial pressure exceeds the alveolar pressure which exceeds the pulmonary venous pressure Pa$>$PA $>$Pv, but not during diastole when the arterial pressure is less than the alveolar pressure. Zone 2 blood flow is thus determined by the arterial–alveolar pressure gradient, and not the arteriovenous gradient. This condition is known as *waterfall effect,* because changes in the downstream pressure, or the venous pressure do not alter blood flow. Zone 2 condition normally occurs from the apex to hilum of the lung. At the middle of lung mean pulmonary artery pressure is 15 mmHg, but it varies from 25 mmHg (in the systole phase) to 8 mmHg (in diastole phase). These levels of arterial pressure keep on lowering by 1 cm H_2O (0.8 mmHg) for every 1 cm above the hilum level; therefore, at the apex of the lungs the mean arterial pressure becomes about 4 mmHg

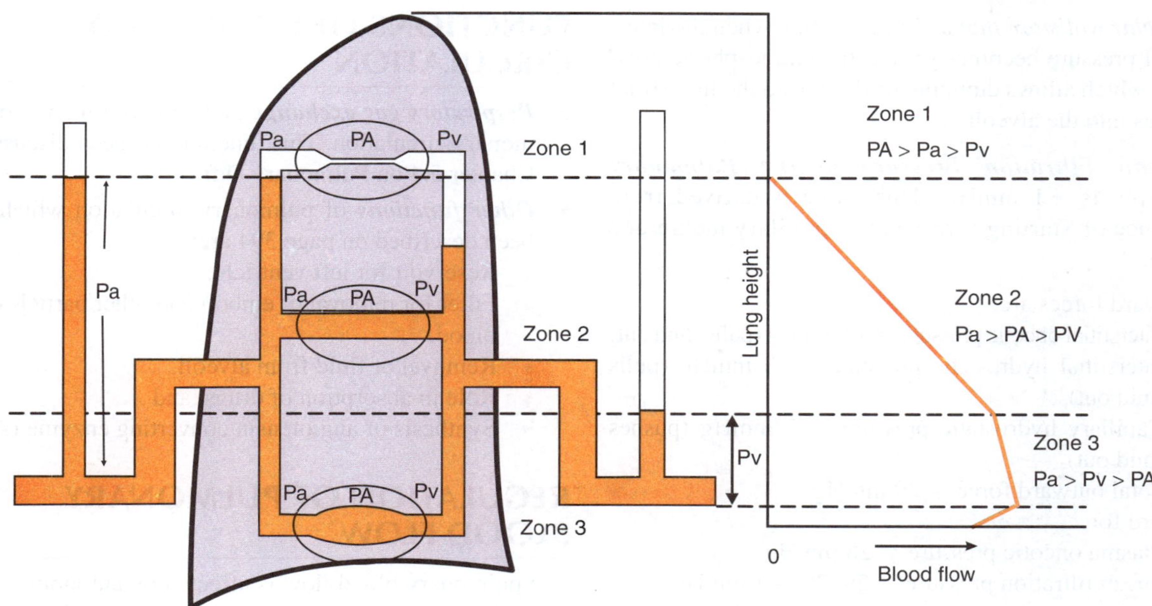

FIGURE 5.3-3 Effect of gravity on regional distribution of pulmonary blood flow in standing posture.

and varies from 14 mmHg in a systole to –3 mmHg in diastole. However, the alveolar pressure remains constant, and thus the blood flow (which depends in arterio-alveolar gradient) increases linearly from the top to the bottom of zone 2 (Fig. 5.3-3).

- ***Zone 3*** refers to region of high continuous blood flow where the capillary pressure remains greater than alveolar pressure during the entire cardiac cycle. So, Zone 3 occurs when the pulmonary artery pressure exceeds the pulmonary venous pressure which exceeds the alveolar pressure (Pa>Pv>PA). This condition occurs near the bottom of the lung. Since the pulmonary vascular pressure increases as we go down from the middle of the lung to its bottom, so the blood flow increases down Zone 3 (Fig. 5.3-3).

Effect of Exercise on Regional Pulmonary Blood Flow. During exercise, the blood flow increases in all the regions of the lungs. During heavy exercise pulmonary blood flow increases 4 to 7 times. Near the base of the lung blood flow increases by 2 to 3 times, while in the upper regions it can increase to 8 times. Thus, the entire lung becomes equivalent to zone 3 during exercise. The marked increase in pulmonary blood flow occurs due to two effects:

- *Recruitment of capillaries,* i.e. increasing the number of open capillaries, and
- *Distension of the capillaries* increasing the rate of flow.

Both distension and recruitment of capillaries decrease the resistance to blood flow so much so that even during exercise the pulmonary artery pressure rises very little. This ability of the lungs to accommodate markedly increased flow during exercise has two advantages:

- Conserves the energy of right side of heart, and
- Prevents development of pulmonary oedema during the increased cardiac output.

Pulmonary Capillary Dynamics

Pulmonary Transit Time The mean transit time in the pulmonary circulation from pulmonary valves to the left atrium is about 4 seconds. A red cell traverses the pulmonary capillary in approximately 0.8 seconds at rest (capillary transit time); and 0.3 seconds during exercise. Even in this brief duration, adequate gaseous exchange between red cells and the alveolar air can occur.

Capillary Exchange of Fluid in the Lung, and Pulmonary Interstitial Fluid Dynamics

- ***Dynamics of Fluid Exchange Through Pulmonary Capillaries*** are qualitatively the same except for following quantitative differences from the peripheral tissues in systemic circulation:

- *Pulmonary capillary pressure* is low about 7 mmHg (c.f. 17 mmHg in peripheral tissues).
- *Interstitial fluid pressure* is slightly more negative (–5 to –8 mmHg) than in the peripheral subcutaneous tissue.
- *Capillary permeability* is high, so more proteins leak in the interstitial fluid; consequently the interstitial oncotic pressure is also high, averaging about 14 mmHg (c.f. 7 mmHg in peripheral tissues).

- *Alveolar walls are thin* and may rupture when the interstitial pressure becomes greater than atmospheric pressure, which allows dumping of fluid from the interstitial spaces into the alveoli.

• ***Mean Filtration Pressure at the Pulmonary Capillaries*** is +1 mmHg. This value is derived from the balance of Starling forces at the capillary membrane as given:

- Outward forces are:
  - Interstitial oncotic pressure = 14 mmHg (pulls fluid out)
  - Interstitial hydrostatic pressure = –8 mmHg (pulls fluid out),
  - Capillary hydrostatic pressure = 7 mmHg (pushes fluid out)
  - Total outward force = 29 mmHg
- Inward force
  - Plasma oncotic pressure = 28 mmHg
- Net mean filtration pressure = 29–28 = 1 mmHg

• ***Filtration of Fluid*** from the pulmonary capillaries into the interstitial space caused by the net filtration pressure of +1 mmHg is very small in amount. Except for a meagre amount that evaporates in the alveoli, most of this fluid is pumped back to the circulation through the pulmonary lymphatic system. So practically a negligible amount of fluid is present in the interstitial space.

Pulmonary Oedema

- Theoretically, pulmonary oedema can occur due to change in any of the four Starling forces resulting in increased capillary filtration in the same way as peripheral oedema can occur.
- *Increase in the capillary hydrostatic pressure* is by far the most common factor responsible for pulmonary oedema in conditions leading to left heart failure or mitral valvular disease. The pulmonary capillary pressure normally must rise equal to the plasma colloid osmotic pressure, i.e. above 28 mmHg. Thus, there is safety factor against pulmonary oedema of about 21 mmHg.
- *Increase in capillary permeability* due to damage to capillary membrane caused by infections or breathing of irritating gases produces rapid leakage of both plasma proteins and fluid out of the capillaries (exudation).
- *In acute left heart failure,* when capillary pressure rises above the safety level, lethal pulmonary oedema can occur within minutes to hours. When capillary pressure rises to 50 mmHg, death frequently ensures within less than 30 minutes from acute pulmonary oedema.
- *In chronic cases of pulmonary oedema,* there occurs a compensatory increase in the lymphatic drainage as much as tenfold which prevents pulmonary oedema even at higher capillary pressure. In a patient with chronic mitral stenosis, pulmonary capillary pressure of 40 to 50 mmHg has been measured without the development of significant pulmonary oedema.

FUNCTIONS OF PULMONARY CIRCULATION

- ***Respiratory gas exchange*** is the major function of pulmonary circulation. This function has been discussed in Chapter 5.4 on Pulmonary Diffusion.
- ***Other functions*** of pulmonary circulation which have been described on page 394 are:
  - Reservoir for left ventricle,
  - Filter for removal of emboli and other particles from blood,
  - Removal of fluid from alveoli,
  - Role in absorption of drugs, and
  - Synthesis of angiotensin converting enzyme (ACE).

REGULATION OF PULMONARY BLOOD FLOW

The pulmonary blood flow is affected by autonomic innervation and large number of circulating humoral factors.

Neural Control

Efferent Sympathetic Vasoconstrictor Nerves richly innervate the pulmonary blood vessels. But these nerves have *no resting discharge and tone,* which means they can only show an increase in activity when stimulated. These participate in the vasomotor reflexes, e.g.

- *Baroreceptor stimulation* produces reflex dilatation of pulmonary vessels, while
- *Chemoreceptor stimulation* causes pulmonary vasoconstriction.

However, the effect of vasodilatation and vasoconstriction is more on the capacity rather than the resistance of pulmonary vessels. The vasoconstriction produced in the lungs due to sympathetic discharge is considerable and results in transfer of pulmonary blood in systemic circulation, e.g. during acute haemorrhage.

Afferent Control Through Vagus is Mediated Through Following Receptors:

- ***Pulmonary baroreceptors*** are present in the tunica adventitia of pulmonary trunk and its two major branches. These vagal mechanoreceptors detect rise in pressure in pulmonary artery and produce reflex bradycardia and hypotension.
- ***Pulmonary volume receptors*** are the vagal mechanoreceptors present at the junction of pulmonary vein with left atrium. Stimulation of these receptors produces tachycardia and diuresis which help in regulating blood volume. These vagal receptors could be afferent limb of the Bainbridge reflex.
- ***J receptors*** (juxtapulmonary receptors) are present adjacent to pulmonary capillaries in the alveolar interstitial

space. These are stimulated by multiple microemboli in the small pulmonary vessels and also by the fluid entrapped in interstitial space specially after exercise and at high altitude. Stimulation of J receptors leads to *reflex tachypnoea* (increases in rate of breathing) and reduction of skeletal muscle tone. A.S. Paintal, an Indian physiologist who discovered J receptors postulated that stimulation of these receptors induces dyspnoea, which together with reduction of muscle tone would discourage exercise, thereby taking away the trigger for pulmonary congestion.

Conclusion. On the whole the neural control on the pulmonary circulation is not very strong, since all the cardiac output has to pass through the pulmonary circulation. Mostly pulmonary vessels act as passive distensible tubes that enlarge with increasing luminal pressure and become narrow with the decrease in pressure.

Chemical Control

1. Local Hypoxia is responsible for most significant alterations in pulmonary blood flow by producing *vasoconstriction.* This is a local and direct action, since it can be demonstrated in isolated (denervated) perfused lungs. This is exactly opposite to what happens in systemic circulation where low pO_2 produces vasodilatation. Both of these opposite responses are very useful for the body:

- *In systemic circulation, low pO_2* in tissues indicates that oxygen supply is insufficient for the demands of the tissues. Therefore, low pO_2 induced vasodilation increases the blood flow and corrects the deficiency.
- *In lungs low pO_2* in a region means that the alveoli in that region are not well ventilated. Therefore blood flow through that region is waste. Since it will not get adequately oxygenated, thus, the local low pO_2 induced vasoconstriction in the lungs is a phenomenon that diverts pulmonary blood flow from the alveoli that are poorly ventilated to better ventilated regions so that blood can be properly oxygenated.

Mechanism. The smooth muscles of pulmonary arteries contain O_2 sensitive K^+ channels, which mediate the vasoconstriction caused by hypoxia. This is in contrast to systemic arteries, which contain adenosine triphosphate (ATP) dependent K^+ channels that permit more K^+ efflux with hypoxia and causes vasodilation rather than vasoconstriction.

2. Hypercapnia and Acidosis also produce vasoconstriction. The effects of pCO_2 and acidosis on pulmonary vessels are just opposite to those in the systemic vessels where these stimuli produce vasodilation. The functional significance of this response is same as in the case of local hypoxia.

3. Chronic Hypoxia, as occurs in high altitude dwellers, is associated with a marked increase in pulmonary arterial pressure *(pulmonary hypertension),* which imposes a heavy afterload on the right ventricle that results in right ventricular hypertrophy, right heart failure and pulmonary oedema. This is the reason that:

- Thick pulmonary precapillary vessels develop in high altitude dwellers and
- Children born and raised at high altitude show pulmonary hypertension.

Humoral Control

The pulmonary vessels respond to circulating agents through their receptors located on smooth muscles of the vasculature (Table 5.3-1).

TABLE 5.3-1 Receptors on Smooth Muscles of Pulmonary Vasculature and Their Effects

Receptor	Subtype	Response
Adrenergic	α_1	Contraction
	α_2	Relaxation
	β_2	Relaxation
Adenosine	A_1	Contraction
	A_2	Relaxation
Angiotensin	A_{T1}	Contraction
ANP	ANP_A	Relaxation
Bradykinin	ANP_B	Relaxation
	B_2	Relaxation
Cholinergic (muscarinic)	M_3	Relaxation
C GRP		Relaxation
Endothelin	ET_A	Contraction
	ET_B	Relaxation
5-HT	$5HT_1$	Contraction
	$5HT_{1C}$	Relaxation
Histamine	H_1	Relaxation
	H_2	Relaxation
Purinergic	P_{2X}	Contraction
	P_{2Y}	Relaxation
Tachykinin	NK_1	Relaxation
	NK_2	Contraction
Thromboxane	T_P	Contraction
Vasopressin	V_1	Relaxation
VIP		Relaxation

Chapter 5.4

Pulmonary Diffusion

INTRODUCTION
- Physics of gas diffusion and gas partial pressures
  - Gas pressure
    - Boyle's law
    - Charles' law
  - Partial pressure
    - Dalton's law
  - Partial pressure of gas in water and tissues
    - Henry's law
  - Water vapour pressure

ALVEOLAR VENTILATION
- Physiological significance
- Dead space air
- Measurement of dead space
- Effect of gravity on alveolar ventilation

ALVEOLAR VENTILATION–PERFUSION RATIO (VA/Q)
- Effect of gravity
- Causes of alterations in VA/Q
- Effects of alterations in VA/Q
  - Normal VA/Q
  - Increased VA/Q
  - Decreased VA/Q

ALVEOLAR AIR
- Composition of alveolar air
- Composition of expired air
- Alveolar gas equation

DIFFUSION OF GASES THROUGH RESPIRATORY MEMBRANE
- Respiratory unit and respiratory membrane
- Factors affecting diffusion across respiratory membrane
- Diffusion and equilibration of gases through respiratory membrane
- Perfusion-limited versus diffusion-limited gas exchange
- Effect of VA/Q ratio on pulmonary gas exchange
- Diffusion capacity of lungs

INTRODUCTION

As discussed earlier, the external respiration (supply of O_2 from atmosphere to body tissues and removal of CO_2 from the body tissues to atmosphere) is accomplished by three major processes:

- *Pulmonary ventilation,* i.e. exchange of gases between the environment and lungs,
- *Pulmonary diffusion,* i.e. transfer of gases from alveoli to capillary blood across the respiratory membrane, and
- *Transport of gases* from the blood to the tissue cells and back.

To understand the *intricacies* of diffusion of gases across the respiratory membrane it is essential to have knowledge about the following related aspects and concepts, most of which form the contents of this chapter:

- *Pulmonary perfusion,* i.e. *pulmonary blood flow.* Special problems related to pulmonary haemodynamics have important implications for gas exchange in the lungs. Most of these have been discussed in Chapter 5.3.
- *Physics of gas diffusion and gas partial pressures.* The rate at which the respiratory gases diffuse across the respiratory membrane is a much more complicated problem, requiring a deeper understanding of the physics of diffusion and gas exchange.
- *Alveolar ventilation,* i.e. the rate at which new air reaches the gas exchange area of the lungs. Alveolar ventilation governs the process of pulmonary diffusion in its own way.
- *Alveolar ventilation–perfusion ratio.* It is the ratio of alveolar ventilation and pulmonary blood flow. This is highly quantitative concept which was developed to help in understanding respiratory exchange when there is imbalance between alveolar ventilation and alveolar blood flow.
- *Diffusion of gases through the respiratory membrane* is the main process which transfers gases from the alveoli into the capillaries. Various important aspects of this process have also been discussed in this chapter.

PHYSICS OF GAS DIFFUSION AND GAS PARTIAL PRESSURES

It is worthwhile to recapitulate some of the basic principles and laws governing the behaviour of gases, for a better understanding of the process of diffusion between alveolar air and pulmonary capillary blood. Consequently, the present discussion is on some of the important aspects concerning physics of gas diffusion and gas partial pressures.

Gas Pressure

The gas molecules have a kinetic energy so they are in a continuous random motion. These molecules bounce against each other and/or against the walls of container and exert a pressure. The gas pressure (P) exerted depends upon following factors:

Concentration of Molecules (n). It is obvious that greater the concentration of the molecules of gas, the greater would be the force exerted by the molecules against the container walls at any given time. Therefore, the pressure of a gas is directly proportional to its concentration, i.e.

$$P \alpha n \qquad \text{(i)}$$

Volume (V). Unlike liquids, gases expand to fill the volume available to them. Therefore, it is obvious that the pressure exerted by a constant number of gas molecules will be more if the volume is less and vice versa. Therefore, at a constant temperature, the pressure (P) of a given mass of gas is inversely proportional to its volume (V), i.e.

$$p \alpha \frac{1}{v} \qquad \text{(ii)}$$

This is called *Boyle's law* of gases.

Absolute Temperature (T). According to *Charles' law,* at a constant pressure the volume of gas is directly proportional to its absolute temperature, i.e. V α T, and as mentioned above according to Boyle's law

$$P \alpha \frac{1}{v}.$$

Therefore, it can be derived that:

$$P \alpha T \qquad \text{(iii)}$$

From equation (i), (ii) and (iii) it can be derived that:

$$P = \frac{nRT}{V} \text{ where}$$

P = Pressure of gas,
n = Number of molecules of gas,
T = Absolute temperature,
V = Volume of gas and
R = Gas constant.

Partial Pressure

According to *Dalton's law* of partial pressure, the total pressure exerted by a mixture of gases is equal to the sum of the partial pressure of all gases present in the mixture. Thus, the partial pressure (p) refers to the pressure exerted by any one gas present in a mixture of gases. It is equal to the total pressure exerted by the mixture of gases times the fraction of the total amount of mixture of gases it represents. Hence, the partial pressure (p) of a gas can be calculated by multiplying its fractional concentration by the total pressure. For example, environmental air (which has atmospheric pressure (at sea level) of about 760 mmHg) is a mixture of 21% oxygen (O_2) and 79% nitrogen (N_2). Therefore, the partial pressure (p) of O_2 and N_2 respectively will be:

$$pO_2 = 760 \times \frac{21}{100} = 160 \text{ mmHg, and}$$

$$pN_2 = 760 \times \frac{79}{100} = 600 \text{ mmHg.}$$

Partial Pressure of Gases in Water and Tissues

It is important to have knowledge about the partial pressure of gases in water and tissues, because the respiratory gases to cross the respiratory membrane must first dissolve in the tissues and then diffuse into the plasma of pulmonary capillaries. The pressure (p) of a gas in a solution is determined not only by its concentration but also by its solubility coefficient. According to *Henry's law,* when temperature is kept constant, the content of gas (n) dissolved in any solution is directly proportional to the partial pressure of a gas, i.e.

n = p.c., where
n = concentration (amount) of a gas in a solution,
p = partial pressure of gas, and
c = solubility coefficient of the gas.

Gas Content, Partial Pressure and Solubility need further clarification. When a gas under pressure comes in contact with a liquid, some of the gas molecules get dissolved in it. As more and more molecules become dissolved, they diffuse all over the liquid medium and some of them start bouncing out of the liquid phase into the gas phase. Ultimately, an *equilibrium* is reached when the number of gas molecules entering the liquid phase equals the number of molecules leaving it.

Partial Pressure of a gas in a liquid represents the pressure it would exert in the gas phase. *At equilibrium,* the partial pressure in the liquid phase equals the partial pressure in the gas phase. *In the absence of equilibrium,* the partial pressure of a gas in liquid phase is less than in the gas phase.

Gas Content represents the volume of the gas per unit volume of liquid that is present. The units of gas content are volume of gas/volume of solvent (e.g. ml/L, ml, dl and so on).

Solubility of a gas is a major determinant of the number of molecules present. A higher solubility increases the rate of diffusion, because this indicates the presence of an increased number of molecules.

Solubility Coefficient is a constant for each gas that equates gas content and partial pressure. Solubility coefficient of gases (important to respiratory physiology) is given in

Table 5.4-1. Increasing the temperature reduces the solubility coefficient of gases (Table 5.4-1). It is important to note that *solubility coefficient of carbon dioxide (CO_2) is about 24 times more and that of nitrogen (N_2) is one half that of oxygen (O_2).*

Water Vapour Pressure

The atmospheric air entering the respiratory passages during inspiration is humidified by the water vapours from the conducting passages. By the time, the atmospheric air reaches the alveoli it is saturated with water vapours. Thus, in the alveolar air, besides O_2 and N_2, water vapours also exert its partial pressure. Vapour pressure of water is dependent upon its temperature. At body temperature (37°C) the vapour pressure of water in alveolar air is 47 mmHg.

ALVEOLAR VENTILATION

Alveolar ventilation is the volume of the fresh air which reaches the gas exchange area of the lung each minute. During inspiration some of the air inhaled never reaches the gas exchange areas but instead fills the non-gas exchange areas (conducting zone) of the respiratory tract called the *dead space,* which is equal to about 150 ml. Thus, alveolar ventilation is not equal to pulmonary ventilation (PV) or the so-called minute respiratory volume (MV), which equals tidal volume (500 ml in quiet respiration) multiplied by the respiratory rate (12 breaths/min), i.e. about 6 L/min.

During expiration out of 500 ml of tidal volume 150 ml of the alveolar expired air remains in the conducting passages. Therefore, of 500 ml air entering the lungs only 350 ml/breath is the fresh air which contributes to alveolar ventilation. Thus, alveolar ventilation can be calculated as:

Alveolar ventilation (VA) = Respiratory rate × (tidal volume – Dead space volume), with a normal tidal volume of 500 ml, a normal dead space of 150 ml, and a respiratory rate of 12 breaths per minute, alveolar ventilation equals 12 × (500 – 350), or 4200 ml/min.

TABLE 5.4-1 Solubility Coefficient Coefficient of Important Gases to Respiratory Physiology

Temperature (°C)	Solubility coefficient (ml gas/ ml saline/ mmHg gas tension)			
	O_2	N_2	CO_2	CO
0	0.049	0.024	1.71	0.035
20	0.032	0.016	0.90	0.023
37	0.024	0.012	0.58	0.019

Physiological Significance of Alveolar Ventilation

The physiological significance of alveolar ventilation can be understood by comparing the alveolar ventilation of two subjects with following parameters:

- ***Subject A,*** having normal breathing with TV of 500 ml and respiratory rate (RR) of 12 breaths/min will have:
  - Pulmonary ventilation = 12 × 500 = 6 L/min, and
  - Alveolar ventilation = 12 × 500 – 150 =4.2 L/min.
- ***Subject B,*** having rapid shallow breathing with tidal volume of 200 ml and respiratory rate 30/min will have:
  - Pulmonary ventilation = 30 × 200 = 6L/min and
  - Alveolar ventilation = 30 × (200–150) = 1.5 L/min.
- ***On Comparison,*** we see that both the subjects A and B have similar amounts of pulmonary ventilation (6 L/min), but the subject B has the alveolar ventilation (1.5 L/min) which is much less than that of subject A (4.2 L/min). Consequently, the subject B is likely to suffer from hypoxia and hypercapnia.

Dead Space Air

Dead space air is the portion of minute ventilation that does not take part in exchange of gases. There are three types of dead spaces (Fig. 5.4-1):

1. Anatomical Dead Space refers the volume of air present in the conducting zone of the respiratory passage, i.e. from nose to terminal bronchioles. The anatomical dead space ventilation (V_D) is a function of the anatonical dead space and respiratory rate. As mentioned earlier, the anatomical dead space contains approximately 150 ml of air, therefore, at a normal respiratory rate of 12 breaths/min, the anatomical dead space ventilation will be 150 × 12, i.e. 1.8 L/min.

2. Alveolar Dead Spaceair refers to the volume of air present in those alveoli which do not take part in gas exchange. Normally, all the alveoli take part in gas

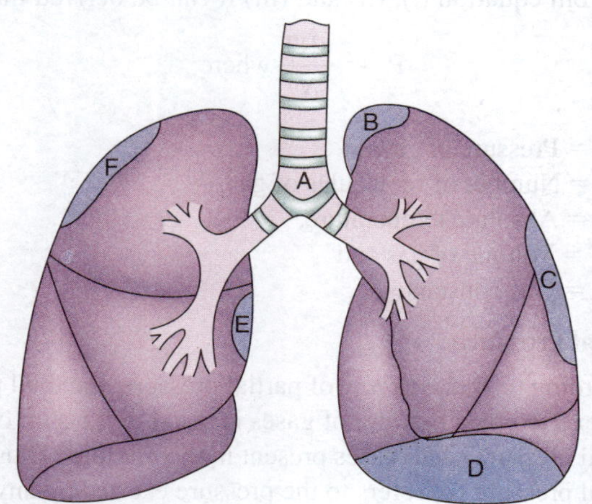

FIGURE 5.4-1 Dead space: (A)Anatomical, (B+C+D+E+F) Alveolar and (A+B+C+D+E+F) Physiological.

exchange, but in some lung diseases, some alveoli do not take part in gas exchange because of following reasons:

- ***When alveoli have zero blood flow*** (Zone 1 condition), the volume of air ventilating such alveoli does not take part in gas exchange,
- ***When alveoli are over ventilated,*** some of the air which is in excess of the volume required to equilibrate with the blood is not able to take part in gas exchange. These alveoli form the alveolar dead space and the air present in them is called the alveolar dead space air.

3. Physiological Dead Space refers to the total dead space which includes both the anatomical and alveolar dead spaces. In a normal healthy person, physiological dead space nearly equals the anatomical dead space. However, in certain respiratory disorders with many nonfunctioning alveoli the physiological dead space may be as much as 10 times the anatomical dead space; obviously, such patients would have very little effective alveolar ventilation which results in respiratory distress. Some of such common respiratory disorders include advanced stages of:

- Emphysema,
- Bronchiectasis and
- Pulmonary embolism.

Measurement of Anatomical Dead Space

Single Breath, Oxygen Technique. This technique is also called Single breath Nitrogen washout test. In this test, nitrogen contents in the expired air are used as an indicator for determining the dead space.

Procedure. The subject is asked to take a deep breath of pure oxygen (100% O_2). Then steadily exhales into the nitrometer, which continuously measures N_2 contents in the expired air. The anatomical dead space can be measured by the analysis of single breath nitrogen curve (Fig. 5.4-2). The curve has four phases labelled by roman letters (I, II, III and IV).

- During inspiration, N_2 contents are nil (zero %) as subject has inspired pure O_2.
- During initial phase of expiration (Phase I), N_2 contents are nill (zero %) as the expired air is from the dead space (which is filled with pure O_2).
- Subsequently (Phase II), there is rise in N_2 contents in expired air because exhaled air contains mixture of dead space air and alveolar air.
- In phase III, the N_2 contents reach to a plateau (60%) and phase III of single breath nitrogen curve ends at closing volume (CV) and followed by the phase IV. The CV is the lung volume at which the airways in lower (basal) part of the lung begin to close because of lesser transmural pressure in these regions. The CV is always above residual volume.
- Phase IV. In this phase N_2 contents of the expired air are further increase, because the upper parts of the lung are

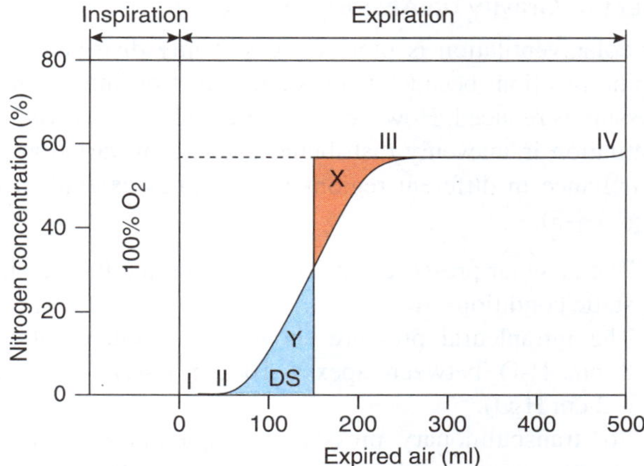

FIGURE 5.4-2 Single breath curve for measuring dead space air. The changes in N_2 concentration of expired air during expiration are indicated by various phases (I-IV). (DS = dead space)

more distended at the beginning of inspiration, therefore N_2 in these regions get less diluted with oxygen.

- The volume of the anatomical dead space is measured by placing a vertical line on the record from mid-poriton of phase II of expiration (red area X = blue area Y).

Measurement of Physiological Dead Space

Bohr's Equation is used to measure the physiological (total) dead space by determining CO_2 tensions in the expired and alveolar gas. Bohr's equation is based on the fact that inspired air contains negligible quantity of CO_2 (almost zero). Therefore, all the CO_2 in expired air is derived from the functional alveoli. The equation is:

(VT – VD) × $pACO_2$ + (VD × pCO_2 in inspired air, i.e. zero) = VT × $pECO_2$

$$\text{or } VT - VD = \frac{VT \times pECO_2}{pACO_2}$$

$$\text{or } VD = \frac{VT - VT \times pECO_2}{pACO_2}$$

$$\text{or } VD = VT \times (1 - pECO_2),$$

where

VD = Physiological (total) dead space air,

VT = Tidal volume,

$pECO_2$ = Carbon dioxide tension in mixed expired air and is represented by average pCO_2 and of the total expired air.

$pACO_2$ = Carbon dioxide tension in alveolar air and is theoretically represented by the pCO_2 of end-tidal samples of expired gases.

For example, if

$$pECO_2 = 28 \text{ mmHg}$$
$$pACO_2 = 40 \text{ mmHg}$$
$$VT = 500 \text{ ml}$$

then, $VD = 150$ ml

Effect of Gravity on Alveolar Ventilation

Alveolar ventilation is more or less evenly distributed in supine position, because hydrostatic effect on intrapleural pressure is reduced. However, in a vertical lung the alveolar ventilation is unevenly distributed because of variation in compliance in different regions of the lungs as explained (Fig. 5.4-3):

- The alveolar pressure is zero throughout the lung under static conditions.
- The intrapleural pressure shows a gradient of about 8 cm H_2O between apex (–10 cm H_2O) and base (–2 cm H_2O).
- So, transpulmonary pressure (intrapleural pressure – alveolar pressure) also varies from –10 cm H_2O at apex to –2cm H_2O at the base.
- Consequently, the lung compliance (change in lung volume per unit change in transpulmonary pressure) also shows corresponding gradient between apex and base.
- Because of more negative intrapleural pressure at apex (–10 cm H_2O) the apical alveoli are larger but poorly ventilated. While the basal alveoli because of less negative (–2 cm H_2O) intrapleural pressure is smaller but better ventilated.
- There is a linear reduction in regional alveolar ventilation from base to apex in erect position (Fig. 5.4-4).

Clinical Significance of Effect of Gravity on Alveolar Ventilation. Arterial oxygenation can be improved in patients with unilateral lung disease by making them lie on their sides so that the good lung is in the dependent position. Somehow, the situation is opposite in infants, who do better with the diseased lung in dependent position.

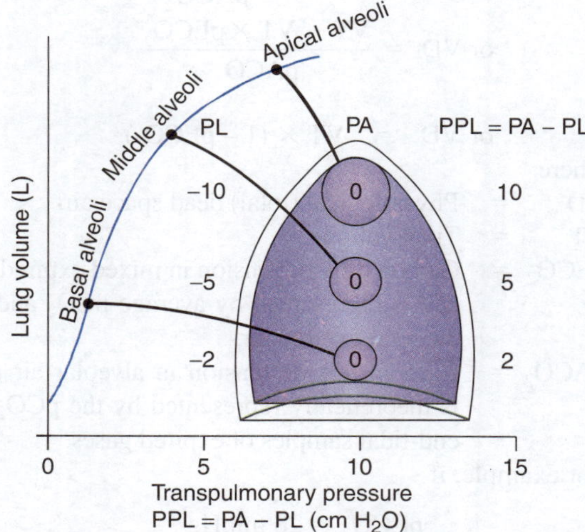

FIGURE 5.4-3 Correlation of transpulmonary pressure (PPL = PA – PL) and lung inflation in different regions during erect posture. PA = alveolar pressure, PL= intrapleural pressure, and PPL = transpulmonary pressure.

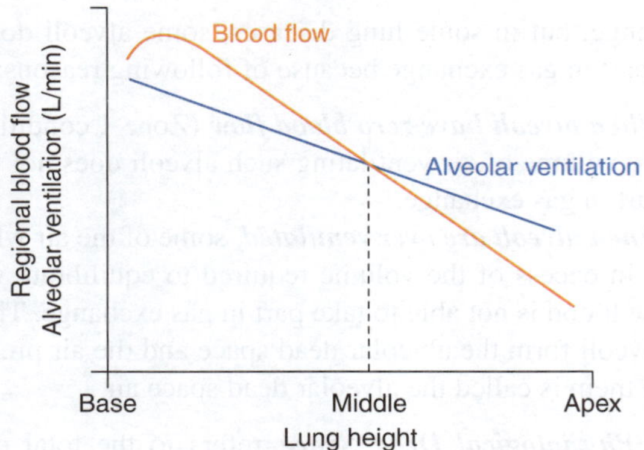

FIGURE 5.4-4 Distribution of alveolar ventilation and pulmonary blood flow in different regions of lung during standing.

ALVEOLAR VENTILATION–PERFUSION RATIO

Alveolar ventilation–perfusion ratio (VA/Q) is the ratio of alveolar ventilation per minute to quantity of blood flow to alveoli per minute. Normally, alveolar ventilation (VA) is 4.2–5.0 L/min, and the pulmonary blood flow (equal to cardiac output) is approximately 5 L/min. So, the normal VA/Q is about 0.84 to 0.9. At this ratio maximum oxygenation occurs.

Effect of Gravity on VA/Q

- Because of the effect of gravity the basal alveoli are over perfused and apical alveoli are under perfused (see details on page 414). There is almost of a linear reduction in the blood flow from base to apex (Fig. 5.4-4).
- The alveolar ventilation also reduces linearly from the base to apex (Fig. 5.4-4), and thus the basal alveoli are over ventilated and apical alveoli are under ventilated (For detailed mechanism see page 400).
- However, gravity affects perfusion much more than it affects ventilation. Hence, as shown in Fig. 5.4-4, the apical alveoli are more under perfused than under ventilated. Because of this relationship the VA/Q is more than 1. In the middle of lung the alveolar ventilation equilibrates the perfusion. As we go up from middle of the lung to apex the VA/Q ratio goes on increasing and is about 3 at the apices. Conversely, at the bases the alveoli are more over perfused than over ventilated, as a result the VA/Q is always less than normal. As we move down from the middle of the lungs to the bases, the VA/Q ratio goes on decreasing, at the bases it is about 0.6.

Applied Aspects

- Because of high VA/Q ratio, the apical alveolar air has low pCO_2 and high pO_2. Since high alveolar pO_2 provides favourable environment for the growth of *Mycobacterium tuberculosis* so the apices of lungs are more predisposed to tuberculosis.

Causes of Alteration in the VA/Q Ratio Obviously, the factors altering alveolar ventilation or/and pulmonary perfusion will alter the VA/Q ratio.

Causes of Uneven Alveolar Ventilation include:

- Bronchial asthma,
- Emphysema,
- Pulmonary fibrosis,
- Pneumothorax, and
- Congestive heart failure.

Causes of Uneven Pulmonary Perfusion are:

- Anatomical shunts, e.g. Fallot's tetralogy,
- Pulmonary embolism,
- Regional decrease in pulmonary vascular bed in emphysema, and
- Increased pulmonary resistance in conditions like pulmonary fibrosis, pneumothorax and congestive heart failure.

Effects of Alterations in the VA/Q Ratio

1. Normal VA/Q Ratio implies that there is both normal alveolar ventilation and normal alveolar perfusion. The exchange of gases is optimal and the alveolar pO_2 is about 104 mmHg and pCO_2 is about 40 mmHg.

2. Increased VA/Q Ratio means that alveolar ventilation is more than the perfusion. As a result the whole of the alveolar air is not utilized for gaseous exchange. The extra air in the alveoli which goes waste forms the so-called *alveolar dead space air.* There will also be change in the composition of alveolar air (Fig. 5.4-5).

When VA/Q ratio increases to infinity, i.e. when alveolar perfusion becomes zero, no exchange of gases can occur. Under such circumstances the composition of alveolar air becomes equal to the humidified inspired air, which has a pO_2 of 149 mmHg and a pCO_2 of 0 mmHg (Fig. 5.4-5).

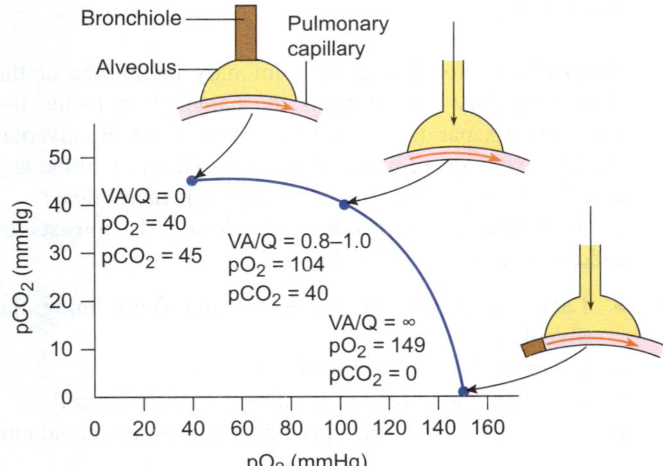

FIGURE 5.4-5 Relationship of alveolar ventilation–perfusion ratio (VA/Q) with alveolar air pO_2 and pCO_2.

Thus, the *effects of increased VA/Q are*:

- Decreased exchange of gases at respiratory membrane,
- Alveolar dead space formation, leading to increase in physiological (total) dead space, and
- Change in alveolar air composition.

3. Decreased VA/Q Ratio occurs when the rate of blood *flow is more than the rate* of alveolar ventilation. Since the alveolar ventilation is not enough to provide oxygen, a fraction of venous blood passes through the pulmonary capillaries without becoming oxygenated. This fraction is called *shunted blood.* This shunted blood along with additional deoxygenated blood from bronchial veins to pulmonary vein (about 2% of cardiac output) forms the so-called *physiological shunt.* The greater the physiological shunt, the greater is the amount of blood that fails to be oxygenated as it passes through the lungs.

When VA/Q becomes zero, there is no alveolar ventilation, so that the air in the alveolus comes to equilibrium with O_2 and CO_2 in the venous blood flowing through the pulmonary capillaries. So, alveolar air will have a pO_2 of 40 mmHg and pCO_2 of 45 mmHg.

Thus, the *effects of decreased VA/Q ratio are*:

- Decreased exchange of gases at the respiratory membrane,
- Shunting of part of venous blood, and
- Change in alveolar air composition (Fig. 5.4-5), under such circumstances an *anatomical shunt* is said to exist. The presence of an anatomical shunt means that true venous blood is mixing with oxygenated blood. The anatomical shunt may be intra-or extrapulmonary. An extrapulmonary anatomical shunt may result from congenital cardiac malformations suchas atrial or ventricular septal defect with right to left blood flow.

ALVEOLAR AIR

Volume of air which is available for exchange of gases in the alveoli per breath is called alveolar air, which is equivalent to tidal volumeminus dead space, i.e. (500–150) or 350 ml.

Composition of Alveolar Air

Composition of alveolar air can be studied by *alveolar air sampling* that involves analysis of the last few millilitres of air that issues from the lungs during expiration. Alveolar air composition is considerably different than that of atmospheric air (Table 5.4-2) because of the following reasons:

1. Water Vapours Dilute the other Gases in the Inspired Air. As shown in Table 5.4-2, the atmospheric air is composed mostly of nitrogen (79%) and oxygen (21%). It contains almost no carbon dioxide or water vapour. The dry atmospheric air becomes totally humidified as it passes through the respiratory passages. Water vapour pressure rises to 47 mmHg at body temperature. As total pressure

TABLE 5.4-2 Composition and Partial Pressure of Gases in Atmospheric Air, Humidified Air, Alveolar Air and Expired Air

	Partial pressure (mmHg) and concentration (percentage) of various gases			
Gas	*Atmospheric air*	*Humidified air*	*Alveolar air*	*Expired air*
N_2	597.0 (78.62%)	563.4 (74.09%)	569.0 (74.9%)	566.0 (74.5%)
O_2	159.0 (20.84%)	149.3 (19.67%)	104.0 (13.6%)	120.0 (15.7%)
CO_2	0.3 (0.04%)	0.3 (0.04%)	40.0 (5.3%)	27.0 (3.6%)
H_2O	3.7 (0.5%)	47 (6.20%)	47.0 (6.2%)	47.0 (6.2%)
Total	760.0 100%	760 100%	760 100%	100%

remains the same, so pO_2 decreasesfrom 159 mmHg in atmospheric air to 149 mmHg in humidified air, and

- pN_2 decreases from 597 mmHg in atmospheric pressure to 563 mmHg in the humidified air.

2. Alveolar Air is Renewed Very Slowly by Atmospheric Air. Since with each breath only 1/7th of the alveolar air is replaced by fresh air, so the composition of the two is different. This slow replacement of alveolar air prevents sudden changes in gas concentrations in the blood.

3. Oxygen is Constantly Being Absorbed from the Alveolar Air so its pO_2 is reduced to 104 mmHg. The alveolar O_2 concentration is controlled by a dynamic equilibrium between the rate of O_2 absorption into the blood and the rate of entry of new O_2 into the lungs.

4. Carbon Dioxide is Constantly Diffusing from the Pulmonary Blood to Alveoli so the pCO_2 of alveolar air become 40 mmHg which is almost negligible in the atmospheric air.

Composition of Expired Air

As shown in Table 5.4-2, the composition of expired air is different than that of alveolar air. This is because of the fact that the expired air is a combination of dead space air and alveolar air. The expired air can be split into three portions:

- ***First portion*** of the expired air represents the dead space air and its composition is similar to typical humidified air.
- ***Middle portion*** of the expired air is a mixture of more and more alveolar air with the dead space air until the dead space air is washed out.
- ***Last portion*** of the expired air represents the alveolar air and so is used to study the alveolar air composition (*alveolar air sampling*).

For alveolar air sampling last 10 ml of expired air, during quite breathing can be collected using modern apparatus with suitable automatic valve.

Alveolar Gas Equation

The alveolar pO_2 and pCO_2 are interrelated to each other, since both are related to alveolar ventilation and alveolar perfusion. The alveolar gas equation which gives the relationship between alveolar pO_2 and pCO_2 is as follows:

$$pAO_2 = pIO_2 - pACO_2 \times \left(FIO_2 + \frac{1 - FIO_2}{RQ} \right), \text{ where}$$

- pAO_2 = Alveolar air pO_2 (normally 104 mmHg)
- pIO_2 = Inspired air, i.e. atmospheric pO_2 (normally 159 mmHg)
- $pACO_2$ = Alveolar air pCO_2 (normally 40 mmHg)
- FIO_2 = Fraction of O_2 in dry air (normally 0.2)
- RQ = Respiratory quotient, i.e. the ratio of CO_2 output and O_2 intake by tissues per minute (normally 0.8).

The gas analysis for composition of gas mixture or in body fluids is done by the use of O_2 and CO_2 electrodes. These are small probes sensitive to O_2 and CO_2 are inserted into the airway, or into blood vessels or tissues, and partial pressure of O_2 and CO_2 (pO_2& pCO_2) can be recorded continuously.

DIFFUSION OF GASES THROUGH THE RESPIRATORY MEMBRANE

Respiratory Unit and Respiratory Membrane

Each Respiratory Unit is composed of a respiratory bronchiole, alveolar ducts, atria and alveoli. There are about 300 million respiratory units in the two lungs. Gas exchange occurs through the membranes of all the structures forming a respiratory unit, not merely in the alveoli themselves.

Respiratory Membrane or pulmonary membrane or the alveolocapillary membrane is the name given to the tissues which separate the capillary blood from the alveolar air. The exchange of gases between the capillary blood and alveolar air requires diffusion through this membrane.

Structure of Respiratory Membrane. It consists of following layers (Fig. 5.4-6):

- Layer of pulmonary surfactant and fluid lining the alveolus,
- Layer of alveolar epithelial cells,
- Basement membrane of the alveolar epithelial cells,
- A very thin interstitial space between the epithelial and endothelial cells,
- Basement membrane of capillary endothelial cells, and
- Layer of capillary endothelial cells.

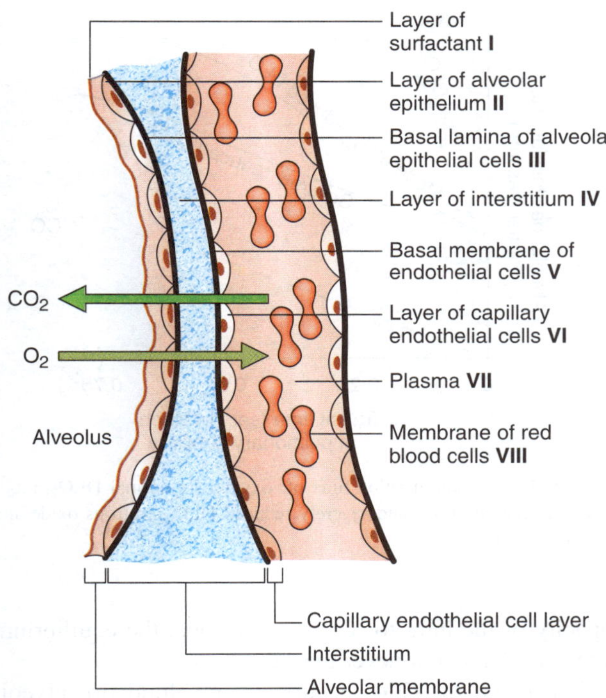

FIGURE 5.4-6 Layers of respiratory membrane.

Characteristic Features of respiratory membrane which optimize for the gas exchange are:

- *Thickness* of the respiratory membrane, despite the large number of layers forming it averages about 0.6 μm.
- *Surface area* of the total respiratory membrane is about 70 square metres in the normal adult.

Factors Affecting Diffusion across Respiratory Membrane

The diffusion of gases across the respiratory membrane is affected by following factors:

1. Thickness of Respiratory Membrane. As mentioned above the thickness of respiratory membrane (about 0.6 μm) has been optimized for gas exchange. The rate of diffusion through the membrane is inversely proportional to the membrane thickness (diffusion distance, denoted by d), i.e.

$$\text{Vgas (volume of gas diffused)} \ \alpha \ 1/d \qquad \text{(i)}$$

Any factor which increases thickness will therefore significantly decrease the gaseous exchange. Examples are:

- Pulmonary oedema, i.e. collection of fluid in the interstitial space and alveoli,
- Pulmonary fibrosis occurring in certain lung diseases increases the thickness of respiratory membrane.

2. Surface Area of Respiratory Membrane. Normally, the total surface area of the respiratory membrane is about 70 square metres. Rate of diffusion is directly proportional to the surface area (A), i.e. with the decrease in total surface area, the rate of diffusion of gases decreases, i.e.

$$\text{Vgas} \ \alpha \ A \qquad \text{(ii)}$$

Some causes of decrease in surface area are:

- Pulmonectomy, i.e. removal of one complete diseased lung reduces surface area to half the normal.
- In emphysema, many of the alveoli coalesce, with dissolution of alveolar walls; this often causes the total surface to decrease by as much as five fold.

3. Diffusion Coefficient. The rate of diffusion is directly proportional to the diffusion coefficient (D) of the gas, i.e.

$$\text{Vgas} \ \alpha \ D \qquad \text{(iii)}$$

- The diffusion coefficient of CO_2 is about 20 times that of O_2 through water (and therefore through fluid of respiratory membrane). Therefore, CO_2 diffuses much more easily through the respiratory membrane.
- The diffusion coefficient of a gas is a function of molecular weight (diffusion is inversely related to the square root of the molecular weight), solubility in a particular solvent, and absolute temperature (310 K, normal body temperture), i.e.

$$D = \frac{\text{Solubility of the gas}}{\sqrt{\text{Molecular weight of the gas}}}$$

4. Pressure Gradient across Respiratory Membrane. The rate of diffusion across the respiratory membrane is directly proportional to the pressure difference between the partial pressure of a gas in alveoli (PA) and in pulmonary capillary (Pc), i.e.

$$\text{Vgas} \ \alpha \ (\text{Pc} - \text{PA}) \qquad \text{(iv)}$$

Further details about pressure gradient during diffusion of gases is discussed later.

From the equations (i), (ii), (iii) and (iv) it can be derived that:

$$\text{Vgas} = (\text{PC} - \text{PA}) \frac{\text{D.A.}}{\text{d}}$$

This is called *Fick's law of diffusion*. Thus, it can be concluded that the rate of pulmonary gas diffusion, i.e. the volume of gas that crosses the respiratory membrane per minute is determined by several factors as defined by Fick's law of diffusion.

Diffusion and Equilibration of Gases Across the Respiratory Membrane

Diffusion of O_2. The normal alveolar pO_2 is 104 mmHg, whereas the blood entering the pulmonary capillary normally has a pO_2 of 40 mmHg. Pressure gradient therefore is 64 mmHg in the beginning. After dissolving in the respiratory membrane, the O_2 molecules diffuse into the blood. As O_2 diffuses from alveoli to blood the pO_2 of blood becomes the same as in alveolar air (104 mmHg), the gradient becomes zero, and no diffusion occurs (Fig. 5.4-7). By the time blood passes to one-third of distance in capillary the pO_2 of blood equals that of alveoli. This means the pressure gradient is there only for one-third of blood flow in capillary. As stated above, the pressure gradient which is 64 mmHg in the beginning becomes lesser and lesser with diffusion of O_2 into the blood. Average pressure gradient is therefore calculated considering the pressure gradients at various sites and the time for which particular pressure gradient was present. This time integrated average pressure gradient is about 11 mmHg.

Equilibration Time. The blood remains for about 0.75 seconds in the capillary (*transit time*). As mentioned above, normally, enough O_2 diffuses across the respiratory membrane so that blood pO_2 and alveolar pO_2 equalize in one-third of the transit time, i.e. about 0.25 seconds (Fig. 5.4-8); then no further gas transfer normally takes place for the rest 0.50 seconds of transit time. This time provides a *safety margin* that ensures adequate O_2 uptake during periods of stress (e.g. exercise, exposure to high altitude) or impaired diffusion. When the normal diffusing capacity of the lung for O_2 is diminished, the equilibrium time is prolonged or never reached.

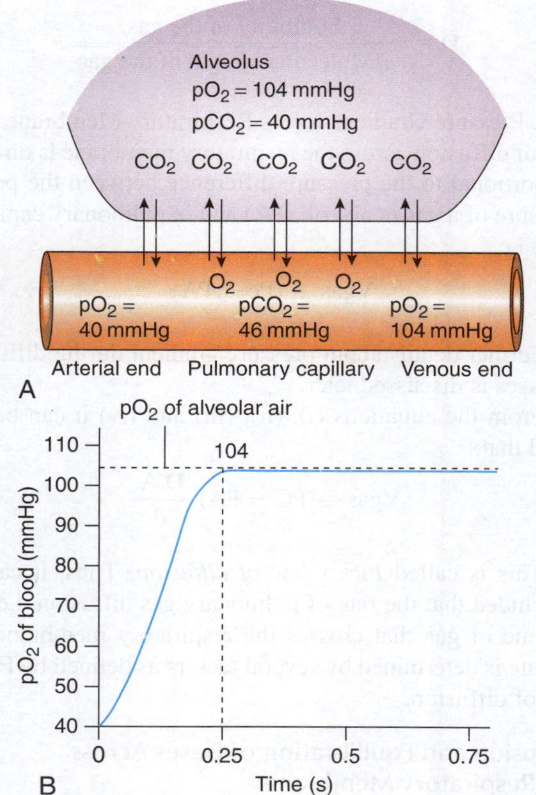

FIGURE 5.4-7 (A) Diffusion of oxygen across respiratory membrane (B) leading to progressive increase in capillary blood pO_2.

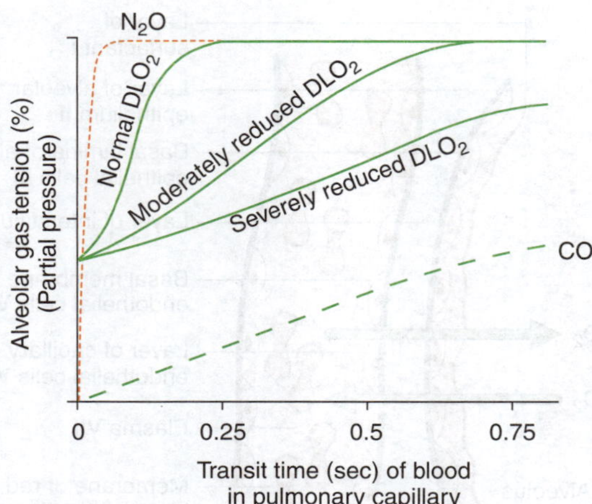

FIGURE 5.4-8 Equilibration time of: oxygen (in normal DLO_2, moderately decreased DLO_2 and severely reduced DLO_2), nitrous oxide and carbon monoxide.

Diffusion of CO_2 occurs from blood to alveoli because pCO_2 is higher in blood than in alveolar air. The average pCO_2 in the pulmonary capillary blood is 46 mmHg, as opposed to 40 mmHg in the alveoli. Therefore, pressure gradient in the beginning is 6 mmHg and time integrated pressure gradient calculated for CO_2 (in a manner similar to O_2) across the respiratory membrane is only 1 mmHg. Although the pressure gradient for CO_2 is only one-tenth of the O_2 diffusion gradient, CO_2 diffuses almost 20 times more rapidly than O_2 because of higher diffusion coefficient.

Equilibration Time. It is estimated that the time required for the blood pCO_2 and alveolar air pCO_2 to equalize is also approximately 0.25 second.

Perfusion-Limited versus Diffusion Limited Gas Exchange

Pulmonary gas exchange is determined by either perfusion or diffusion properties of the system (Fig. 5.4-9):

- ***Perfusion-Limited Gas Exchange*** occurs when equilibration takes place between the alveolar gas and the pulmonary capillary blood. Normally, O_2 and CO_2 are transferred by perfusion-limited gas exchange as they equilibrate in about 0.25 second (while transit time in 0.75 sec). Therefore, when pulmonary blood flow increases, the diffusion of O_2 and CO_2 across the respiratory membrane also increases.

  Nitrous oxide (N_2O) an anesthetic gas reaches at equilibrium in about 0.1 second, therefore, N_2O taken up is not diffusion limited, but by the amount of blood flowing through pulmonary capillaries (i.e perfusion limited).

- ***Diffusion-Limited Gas Exchange*** occurs whenever equilibration does not take place between the alveolar and pulmonary gas tensions.

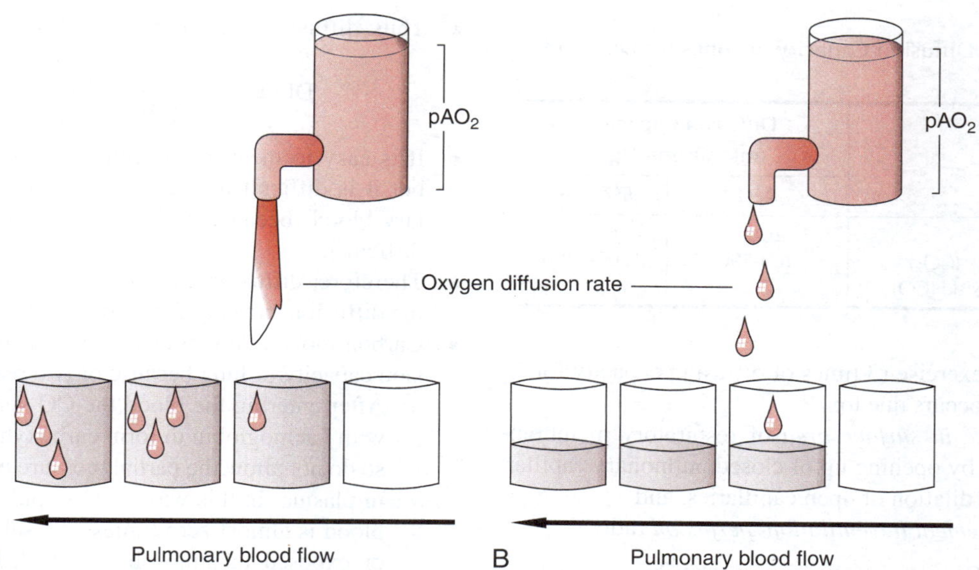

FIGURE 5.4-9 (A) In perfusion-limited gas exchange, the blood is equilibrated (as symbolized by full beakers), so that the only method of increasing gas uptake is to increase pulmonary blood flow (by moving more beakers through the system). (B) In diffusion-limited gas exchange the blood is not equilibrated (symbolized by partially filled beakers), so that diffusion rate must be increased to improve the exchange (so that available beaker in the above symbolization may become full). The diffusion rate can be increased by raising partial pressure of the alveolar air (pAO_2) and increasing the driving force for diffusion.

- Carbon monoxide (CO) which does not reach equilibrium in 0.75 second (transit time of blood in pulmonary capillary) has a diffusion limited transport, i.e. its transport across the respiratory membrane will increase only if the rate of diffusion increases. Increase in blood flow will not increase the transport of carbon monoxide.
- Since, CO exchange is diffusion limited, so measuring the diffusion capacity of CO is an effective means of evaluating the diffusion properties of respiratory system.
- In certain systemic diseases and at a significant increase in altitude pO_2 of alveolar air is reduced, which in turn reduces the diffusion rate. Raising the fraction of inspired O_2 (FIO_2) is one way to treat diffusion-limited gas exchange.

Effect of Alveolar Ventilation–Perfusion Ratio on Pulmonary Gas Exchange

- Optimum gas exchange across the respiratory membrane occurs when the alveolar ventilation–perfusion ratio (VA/Q) is normal, i.e. between 0.8 and 1.
- Both, a decrease as well as an increase in VA/Q ratio reduces the gas exchange. For details see page 423.

Diffusion Capacity of Lung

Diffusion capacity (DL) of the lung is quantitative expression of the ability of the respiratory membrane to exchange a gas between the alveoli and the pulmonary blood. It is defined as the volume of gas (V gas) that diffuses through the respiratory membrane of lung each minute for a pressure gradient of 1 mmHg.

Factors Affecting Diffusion Capacity All the factors discussed in detail that affect the rate of diffusion through the respiratory membrane (see page 425) will obviously affect the diffusing capacity of lung. To summarize once again the diffusion capacity of lung (DL) is

- Inversely proportional to thickness of the respiratory membrane, i.e. diffusion distance (d),
- Directly proportional to the surface area (A) of respiratory membrane,
- Directly proportional to the diffusion coefficient (D) of the particular gas. Diffusion coefficient in turn is directly proportional to the solubility (S) of the gas in respiratory membrane and inversely proportional to the square root of molecular weight (MW) of the gas.
- Directly proportional to the pressure gradient between the partial pressure of gas in alveolar air (pA) and capillary blood (pC), i.e. pA–pC.

Diffusion Capacity of Lung for Different Gases Depending upon the above factors, the diffusion of lungs is bound to be different for different gases. Diffusion capacity of the lungs for common gases is (Table 5.4-3):

Diffusion Capacity of Lungs for O_2

- ***At rest*** the diffusing capacity of lungs for O_2 is about 20–25 ml/min/mmHg. As the mean oxygen pressure gradient across the respiratory membrane is about 11 mmHg, so at rest about 250 ml of O_2 diffuses through the lungs per minute.
- ***During exercise*** the diffusing capacity of lungs for O_2 is increased. It may reach upto 65ml/min/mmHg during

TABLE 5.4-3 Diffusion Capacity of Lungs for Different Gases

Gas	Diffusion Capacity (ml/min/mmHg)	
	Rest	Exercise
Oxygen (O_2)	20-25	65
Carbon-dioxide (CO_2)	400-500	1200-1300
Carbon monoxide (CO)	17	

strenuous exercise (3 times of diffusing capacity for O_2 at rest). It occurs due to:

- *Increase in surface area* of respiratory membrane caused by opening up of closed pulmonary capillaries and dilation of open capillaries, and
- *Improvement in ventilation–perfusion* ratio.

Diffusion Capacity of Lungs for CO_2 has never been measured because of technical difficulties. Carbon dioxide diffuses across the respiratory membrane so rapidly that the difference between the average pCO_2 of the capillary blood and pCO_2 of alveolar air is only 1 mmHg. Such a small difference cannot be detected by any available technique. However, from the available knowledge about diffusion coefficient of CO_2, the diffusion capacity of lungs for CO_2 is estimated.

- ***At rest*** the diffusing capacity of lungs for CO_2 is about 20 times that for O_2, i.e. about 400 ml to 500 ml/min/mmHg.
- ***During strenuous exercise*** the diffusing capacity for CO_2 is increased to 1200 ml to 1300 ml/min/mmHg.

Clinical significance of higher diffusion capacity of CO_2. When diffusing capacity of respiratory membrane is markedly decreased due to certain diseases, one expects retention of CO_2 and lack of O_2. But due to vast difference in the diffusing capacities for O_2 and CO_2, a serious impairment of diffusion of O_2 causes significant lack of O_2 with little signs of CO_2 retention.

Measurement of Diffusion Capacity of Lungs Diffusion capacity of lungs for different gases can be measured using *Fick's law,* according to which diffusion capacity is given by:

$$DL = \frac{V}{(pA - pC)}, \text{ where}$$

DL = Diffusion capacity of lungs for a given gas,
V = Volume of the gas uptake in one minute, and (increase in the gas content of blood in one minute),
pA–pC = Pressure gradient between alveolar air and pulmonary capillary blood.

- Thus, diffusion capacity for O_2 (DLO_2) is:

$$DLO_2 = \frac{O_2 \text{ consumption/min}}{pAO_2 - pO_2)}$$

- It is easy to measure O_2 consumption/min and pAO_2, but it is difficult to measure pO_2 in pulmonary capillary blood (because collection of sample is extremely difficult).
- Therefore, diffusion capacity for O_2 is measured from the diffusion capacity for carbon monoxide.
- Carbon monoxide is preferred for measuring the diffusion capacity of lung because of two reasons:
  - After entering the blood the CO very rapidly reacts with haemoglobin to form carboxyhaemoglobin and so do not allow the partial pressure of CO to build up in plasma. In this way, pCO in pulmonary capillary blood is almost zero (unless the subject is a smoker or exposed to atmospheric CO levels). Therefore, problem of collecting of CO in the pulmonary capillary blood is avoided.
  - Diffusion of CO across respiratory membrane is diffusion limited. Therefore, the amount of CO transferred to blood is correct estimate of the diffusion capacity. Since diffusion of O_2 across the respiratory membrane is flow limited, so measuring the amount of O_2 transferred to blood will underestimate the true diffusion capacity.

Procedure of Single-Breath Carbon Monoxide Technique of Measuring Diffusion Capacity of Lung

- The subject is made to take a single breath of gas mixture containing dilute concentration (0.01%) of carbon monoxide (CO). He is asked to hold the breath for 10 seconds to allow the diffusion.
- The CO uptake/min is calculated from the difference between the inspired air and expired air CO concentration, and FRC. The pCO of alveolar air is estimated from the end-expiratory sample. The pCO of pulmonary capillary blood is considered zero and so the diffusion capacity for CO (DL CO) is calculated as:

$$DL\ CO = \frac{\text{CO uptake/min}}{\text{pCO in alveolar in}}$$

- The diffusion capacity measured for CO at rest is about 17 ml/min/mmHg
- Diffusion capacity for O_2 is determined by multiplying the diffusion capacity for CO by 1.27, because diffusion coefficient of O_2 is about 1.2 times that of CO: $DLO_2 = 17 \times 1.2$, or about 20 ml/min/mmHg.

Chapter 5.5

Transport of Gases

INTRODUCTION

It is being repeated, probably, for the fourth time in this section, but is essential as an introductory remark that *external respiration* refers to supply of O_2 from atmosphere to tissues and removal of CO_2 from the tissues into the atmosphere. It is accomplished by three major processes:

- *Pulmonary ventilation,* i.e. exchange of gases between the environment and lungs (discussed in Chapter 5.2),
- *Pulmonary diffusion,* i.e. transfer of gases from alveoli to capillary blood across the respiratory membrane (discussed in Chapter 5.4) and
- *Transport of gases* from blood to the tissue cells and back.

TRANSPORT OF OXYGEN

Transport of oxygen from the lungs to tissues occurs due to constant *circulation of blood,* and *diffusion* of O_2 that occurs at various sites in the direction of concentration gradient which is represented by O_2 tension (pO_2) differences given:

- Alveolar air pO_2 : 104 mmHg
- Arterial blood pO_2 : 95 mmHg
- Venous blood pO_2 : 40 mmHg
- Tissue interstitial fluid pO_2 : 40 mmHg

From the above, it is clear that:

- Oxygen from the alveolar air is taken up by the pulmonary capillary blood along a pressure gradient of 104-40, or 64 mmHg, and
- Oxygen from the arterial blood is released into the tissues by a pressure gradient of 95–40, or 55 mmHg.

Transport of oxygen from the lungs to the tissues can be described as under:

A. Uptake of oxygen in the lungs by pulmonary blood,
B. Transport of oxygen in arterial blood, and
C. Release (diffusion) of oxygen from blood to the interstitial fluid in tissues.

Uptake of Oxygen by Pulmonary Blood

- As mentioned above, pO_2 of pulmonary arterial blood is about 40 mmHg and that of alveolar air is 104 mmHg. Therefore, due to this great concentration gradient, oxygen readily diffuses from the alveoli into the blood.
- The process of diffusion across the respiratory membrane has been described in Chapter 5.4
- It is important to note that this process is very rapid and even if the stay of blood in lungs is reduced (as occurs during strenuous exercise due to increased cardiac output) there occurs complete oxygenation.

Transport of Oxygen in Arterial Blood

PO_2 in pulmonary venous blood is 104 mmHg, however, by the time blood reaches the aorta pO_2 falls to about 100 mmHg. This happens due to ***venous admixture***, i.e. mixing of venous blood to arterial blood. The venous blood which mixes with arterial blood is:

- Blood present in bronchial veins (which forms about 2% of cardiac output) mixes with the pulmonary capillary blood at the repiratory bronchioles which are supplied by systemic as well as pulmonary capillaries.
- Part of the coronary venous blood flows into the chambers of left side of heart through thebesian veins.

Arterial blood contains about 20 ml and venous blood about 15 ml of O_2 per 100 ml. Thus, about 5 ml of O_2 is transported per 100 ml of blood from lungs to the tissue cells.

Oxygen is transported in the blood in two forms: as dissolved form and in combination with haemoglobin.

Oxygen Transport in Dissolved Form

- The solubility of O_2 in water (plasma) is so little that at pO_2 value of 100 mmHg, out of the 20 ml of O_2 present in 100 ml of blood, only 0.3 ml is in dissolved form and rest is combined with haemoglobin (as oxyhaemoglobin).
- The dissolved oxygen obeys Henry's law, i.e. amount dissolved is proportional to the pO_2. Thus, there is no limit to the amount of O_2 that can be carried in dissolved form provided the pO_2 is sufficiently high. This is a distinct advantage over O_2 transport as oxyhaemoglobin which cannot exceed a certain limit.
- Therefore, dissolved O_2 at high pO_2 (hyperbaric oxygen) is utilized in clinical practice for the oxygenation of tissues when the haemoglobin gets denatured in certain types of poisoning, e.g. carbon monoxide poisoning.

Oxygen Transport in Combination with Haemoglobin

Oxygenation of Haemoglobin After entering the blood from the alveolar air, most of the oxygen combines with haemoglobin to form a *loose and reversible* combination. The iron present in heme molecule stays in the ferrous form; therefore, this process is called *oxygenation* (not oxidation) and converts deoxyhaemoglobin into oxyhaemoglobin. The reaction is very rapid requiring < 0.01 second. The driving force for this reaction is O_2 tension in the pulmonary capillaries.

One molecule of oxygen combines with one iron ion of the heme molecule. The O_2 molecule occupies the sixth *co-ordination* position of the iron atom. Since haemoglobin contains four molecules of heme, so each molecule of haemoglobin can combine with as many as *four* O_2 molecules. The reaction proceeds in four steps:

$$Hb_4 + O_2 \rightarrow Hb_4O_2,$$
$$Hb_4O_2 + O_2 \rightarrow Hb_4\,O_4,$$
$$Hb_4O_4 + O_2 \rightarrow Hb_4O_6, \text{ and}$$
$$Hb_4O_6 + O_2 \rightarrow Hb_4O_8$$

After the first step, affinity of haemoglobin for O_2 increases with each next step because in deoxyhemoglobin, the globin units are tightly bound (that is intense configuration), which reduces affinity for O_2. This happens so, because the insertion of O_2 molecule ruptures all the salt links and changes the quaternary structure of haemoglobin from the tense or *T-configuration* to relaxed or *R-configuration* which exposes more O_2 binding sites, which favours O_2 binding. Subsequent molecules of oxygen, therefore, find it easier to bind to haem moieties and there is 500 fold increase in O_2 affinity. This phenomenon is termed as *co-operative binding kinetics*. This is the reason for the sigmoid nature of oxygen haemoglobin association or dissociation curve. In tissues the reactions are reversed resulting in O_2 release.

Oxygen Carrying Capacity of Haemoglobin One gram of haemoglobin can bind with maximum of 1.34 ml of O_2. Thus, 100 ml of blood with haemoglobin level of 15 gm% can carry 1.34×15, or 20.1 ml of oxygen. However, due to the presence of various physiological shunts (venous admixture) only 97% of the haemoglobin is available for carrying the oxygen. Therefore, practically, 100 ml of the arterial blood carries about 19.8 ml of oxygen out of which about 19.5 ml as oxyhaemoglobin and 0.3 ml as dissolved form in plasma.

Thus, under normal circumstances, the haemoglobin carries most of the bulk of oxygen present in the blood. The only *disadvantage* is that there is a ceiling on the amount of oxygen that can be carried by the haemoglobin (depending upon the concentration of haemoglobin in the blood). The limit can never be surpassed.

Haemoglobin saturation is the percentage of haemoglobin that is combined with oxygen. When all the four sites on haemoglobin are occupied by O_2 (1.34 ml), then that molecule of haemoglobin is 100% saturated. When one gram of haemoglobin is combined with 0.67 ml of O_2, it is said to be 50% saturated. The *percentage saturation* is the average saturation of the entire haemoglobin molecules in the blood and is calculated as:

$$\text{percentage saturation} = \frac{O_2 \text{ content of blood/100 ml}}{O_2 \text{ carrying capacity of blood}} \times 100$$

Oxygen–haemoglobin Dissociation Curve

The Oxygen–haemoglobin Curve refers to the curve obtained when the relation between the pO_2 and the percentage of haemoglobin saturation is plotted (Fig. 5.5-1).

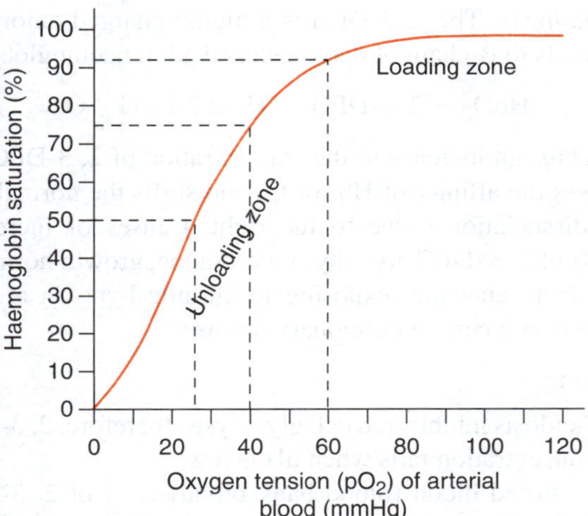

FIGURE 5.5-1 Normal oxygen–haemoglobin dissociation curve.

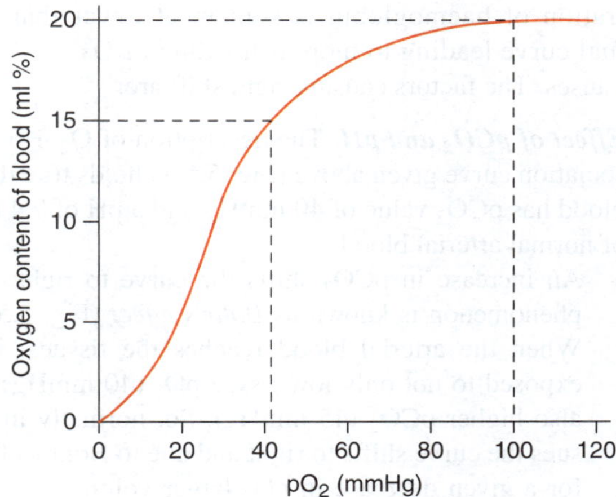

FIGURE 5.5-2 The relationship between pO_2 and oxygen contents of the blood.

The O_2–Hb dissociation curve shows that the percentage saturation of haemoglobin increases with the increase in pO_2 of arterial blood. However the relation is not linear but *sigmoid or S-shaped* (because of the reason explained above), but it has several physiological advantages (vide infra).

Two distinct zones of the O_2–Hb dissociation curve are recognized:

- ***Loading (Association) Zone*** refers to upper flat part (plateau) of the curve, which is related to the process of O_2 uptake in the lungs. The curve shows that at pO_2 values of 100 mmHg or above, the haemoglobin is 100% saturated. More important to note is the fact that even if pO_2 falls to 60 mmHg, the Hb saturation is still 90%. Thus, the loading zone provides a margin of safety, because it ensures fairly high uptake of O_2 by pulmonary blood even when alveolar pO_2 is moderately decreased in situations like:

- Climbing mountains to moderate altitude, and
- Pulmonary diseases.

- ***Unloading (Dissociation) Zone*** of the O_2–Hb dissociation curve refers to the *steep portion* of the curve that occurs at pO_2 below 60 mmHg. The steep part of the curve is concerned with O_2 delivery in the tissues and shows that large amounts of oxygen can be liberated from the blood with relatively minor fall of O_2 tension. This property keeps the O_2 tension in the capillary blood relatively high so that the diffusion gradient for O_2 is maintained. At pO_2 value of 40 mmHg, Hb is 75% saturated with O_2 (Fig. 5.5-1). Thus, each 100 ml of blood can hold only 15ml of O_2 as compared to 20 ml at pO_2 of 100 mmHg (Fig. 5.5-2). Thus, 5 ml of O_2 is extracted by the tissues at rest. At values of pO_2 lower than 40 mmHg still larger volume of O_2 would be offloaded and become available to the tissue (e.g. during exercise). The greater release of O_2 with slight decrease in tissue pO_2 (due to increased O_2 consumption) minimizes decrease of tissue pO_2 that would otherwise take place. Thus, it will regulate tissue pO_2 (buffering effect).

Physiological Advantages of S-shaped O_2–Hb Dissociation Curve, which can be summarized from the above discussion are:

- It allows greater uptake of O_2 at lungs despite great variation in alveolar air pO_2,
- Tissues are supplied with O_2 according to their needs and
- Haemoglobin acts as a buffer and maintains tissue pO_2 at about 40 mmHg.

Shifts in O_2–Hb Dissociation Curve Several factors affect the affinity for haemoglobin for O_2 and thus shift the O_2–Hb dissociation curve to either right or left.

Shift to Right Shift to the right of O_2–Hb dissociation curve signifies decreased affinity of haemoglobin for O_2 (Fig. 5.5-3). Thus at every level of pO_2, the oxygen

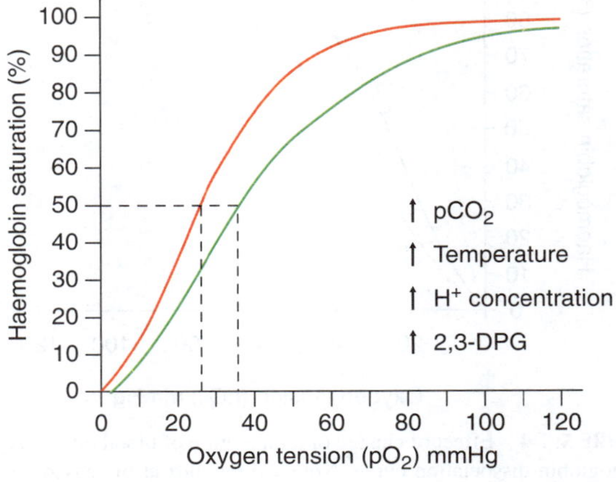

FIGURE 5.5-3 Right shift of oxygen–haemoglobin dissociation curve which occurs due to increase in pCO_2, H^+ concentration, temperature or 2, 3-DPG. Note P_{50} is increased.

saturation of haemoglobin is somewhat lower than the normal curve leading to more offloading of O_2.

Causes. The factors causing right shift are:

1. ***Effect of pCO_2 and pH.*** The description of O_2–Hb dissociation curve given above (Fig. 5.5-1) holds true if the blood has pCO_2 value of 40 mmHg and a pH of 7.4 (pH of normal arterial blood).
   - An increase in pCO_2 shifts the curve to right; this phenomenon is known as *Bohr's effect* (Fig. 5.5-3). When the arterial blood reaches the tissues, it is exposed to not only low tissue pO_2 (40 mmHg) but also higher pCO_2 (45 mmHg). So, normally in tissues the curve shifts to right and due to Bohr's effect for a given decrease in pO_2 larger volume of O_2 is shed off (about 2% more).
   - A decrease in pH of blood, as occurs in the tissues, also shifts the O_2Hb dissociation curve to the right.
2. ***Effect of temperature.*** An increase in the temperature of blood shifts the curve to right (Fig. 5.5-4). During *exercise* the demand of O_2 is increased in skeletal muscles. The factors which facilitate the delivery of the required larger amounts of O_2 (by causing right shift in the curve) are:
   - Increased temperature in skeletal muscles due to more heat production,
   - Increased pCO_2 due to accumulation of CO_2 resulting from rapid metabolism,
   - Decreased pO_2 due to rapid consumption, and
   - Decreased pH due to accumulation of lactic acid produced in muscular exercise.
3. ***Effect of diphosphoglycerate or biphosphoglycerate.*** The red blood cells are rich in 2, 3 - diphosphoglycerate (2, 3-DPG) which is formed from 3-phosphoglyceraldehyde produced during glycolysis via *Embden-Meyerhof pathway*. The 2, 3-DPG is a highly charged anion that binds to β-chain of deoxygenated adult haemoglobin.

$$HbO_2 + 2,3\text{-DPG} \rightarrow Hb\ 2,3\text{-DPG} + O_2$$

Thus, an increase in the concentration of 2, 3-DPG decreases the affinity of Hb for O_2 and shifts the normal O_2–Hb dissociation curve to the right. Causes of increased levels of 2, 3 -DPG are : thyroid hormone, growth hormone, androgen, anaemia, exposure to chronic hypoxia at high altitude and certain pulmonary diseases.

Note:

- Acidosis inhibits red cell glycolysis, therefore, 2, 3-DPG concentration falls when pH is low.
- In stored blood (blood bank blood) level of 2, 3-DPG falls and ability to release oxygen in the tissues is reduced; therefore transfusion of stored blood especially in hypoxic patients has limited benefit.

Advantages versus disadvantages of right shift:

- Right shift is advantageous in the tissues where greater O_2 is released from haemoglobin (at the same pO_2).
- However, right shift is disadvantageous in the lungs because (at the same pO_2) blood takes up less oxygen.

Shift to Left. Shift to left of O_2–Hb dissociation curve signifies increased affinity of haemoglobin for O_2 (Fig. 5.5-5). Thus, at every pO_2 level the oxygen saturation of haemoglobin is somewhat greater than in a normal curve.

Causes for left shift of the curve are:

- Decreased pCO_2 of blood,
- Increased pH of blood,
- Decreased temperature, and
- Fetal haemoglobin.

Advantages versus disadvantages of left shift. Left shift of the curve has limited advantage because though it

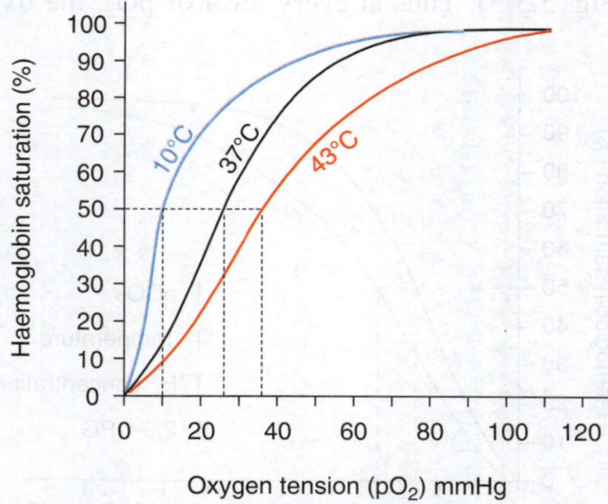

FIGURE 5.5-4 Effect of change of temperature of blood on the oxygen–haemoglobin dissociation curve. Note a right shift at increased temperature (43°C) and left shift at decreased temperature (10°C) as compared to the normal curve (37°C).

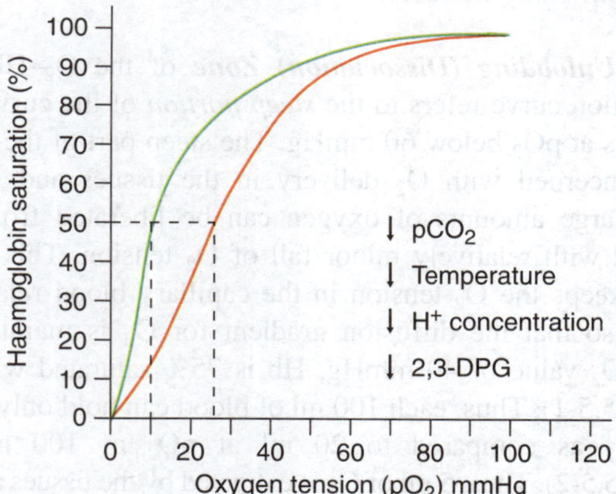

FIGURE 5.5-5 Left shift of oxygen–haemoglobin dissociation curve which occurs due to dercrease in pCO_2, H^+ concentration, temperature and 2,3-DPG. Note—p_{50} value is decreased.

allows greater uptake of O_2 at lungs (at same pO_2) but it decreases release of O_2 to the tissues (at same pO_2).

Concept of p_{50} and Its Significance

p_{50} refers to the partial pressure of O_2 that produces a 50% saturation of the haemoglobin with O_2; Normal p_{50} for arterial blood in an adult at 37°C body temperature and at pCO_2 of blood 40 mmHg is 25–27 mmHg (Fig. 5.5-1).

Haemoglobin affinity for O_2 is inversely related to the p_{50} value, therefore:

- Decreased p_{50} (Hb gets 50% saturated at lower pO_2) indicates increased affinity of haemoglobin for O_2. Thus, decreased p_{50} is equivalent to shift of Hb–O_2 dissociation curve to left (Fig. 5.5-5). A decreased p_{50} is an obvious benefit in the lungs because it enhances the haemoglobin saturation with O_2. Fetal haemoglobin and myoglobin have lower p50 value than adult haemoglobin.
- Increased p_{50} (Hb gets 50% saturated at higher pO_2) indicates decreased affinity of haemoglobin for O_2. Thus, increased p_{50} is equivalent to right shift of O_2–Hb dissociation curve (Fig. 5.5-3). Increase in pCO_2, H^+ concentration, temperature and 2, 3-DPG causes increased p_{50}.

O_2–Hb Dissociation Curve of Fetal Haemoglobin

- As shown in Figure 5.5-6, the O2–Hb dissociation curve of fetal haemoglobin (HbF) is shifted to the left in comparison with O_2–Hb dissociation curve of adult haemoglobin (HbA).
- The O_2–Hb dissociation curve of HbF is shifted to left because its affinity for 2, 3-DPG is considerably less than that of HbA. This is because two gamma (γ) chains present in HbF have very little affinity for 2, 3-DPG as compared to the beta (β) chains of HbA.
- Thus, affinity of HbF to combine with O_2 is more than that of HbA. This property of HbF helps it to take up normal volumes of O_2 in spite of the fact that fetal blood is exposed to rather low pO_2 values of the maternal blood in placenta. As shown in Figure 5.5-6 at pO_2 20 mmHg where HbA is only 35% saturated the HbF is 70% saturated, that is why HbF can store more O_2.

Effect of Carbon Monoxide on O_2 Transport

- Carbon monoxide (CO) interferes with O_2 transport because it has about 200 times the affinity (of oxygen) for haemoglobin.
- CO combines with Hb at the same site on its molecule as O_2 and forms the carboxyhaemoglobin, and thus decreases the functional haemoglobin concentration.
- Because of the extreme affinity of CO for haemoglobin the carboxyhaemoglobin curve lies along the Y-axis and a CO tension of only 0.5 mmHg inactivates about 50% of the haemoglobin, i.e. p50 for CO is only 0.5 mmHg (Fig. 5.5-7).

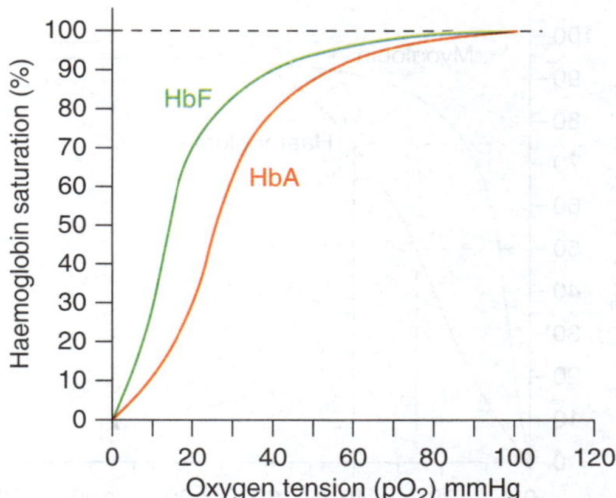

FIGURE 5.5-6 Oxygen haemoglobin dissociation curves of adult haemoglobin (HbA) and fetal haemoglobin (HbF).

- CO lowers the tissue O_2 tension by decreasing the O_2 content and the p50 for O_2.

Oxygen Dissociation Curve for Myoglobin Myoglobin is present in higher quantities in the muscles specialized for sustained contraction, e.g. muscles of legs and heart. The characteristic features of O_2 dissociation curve of myoglobin vis-à-vis haemoglobin are (Fig. 5.5-8):

- Dissociation curve of myoglobin is rectangular hyperbola rather than sigmoid in shape, because it takes up O_2 at low pressure much readily, i.e. rate of association of myoglobin with O_2 is very fast.
- Myoglobin does not show Bohr's effect.
- At pO_2 40 mmHg the myoglobin is 95% saturated while haemoglobin is 75% saturated. Even at pO_2 5mmHg myoglobin is saturated by slightly less than 60%. Thus, it acts as a temporary store house for O_2 in the muscles.

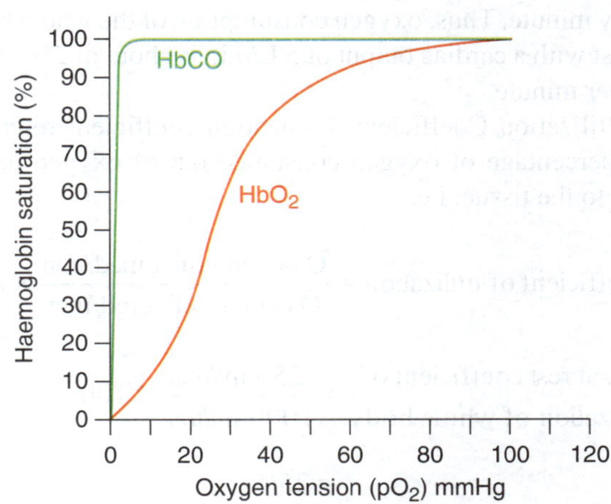

FIGURE 5.5-7 Haemoglobin saturation curves for both O_2 (HbO_2) and carbon monoxide (HbCO). Note that HbCO curve lies along the Y axis which indicates extreme high affinity of haemoglobin for carbon monoxide. Note the p_{50} for CO is only 0.5 mmHg.

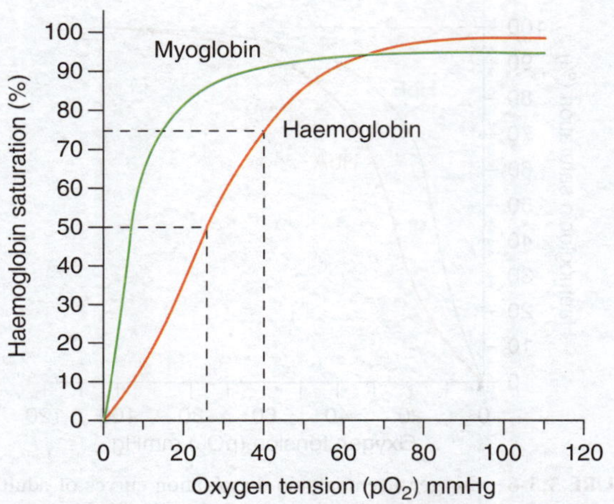

FIGURE 5.5-8 Oxygen dissociation curve of myoglobin versus haemoglobin.

Release of Oxygen in Tissues

Oxygen Release at Rest

Oxygen Delivery. represents the amount of O_2 that is presented to body cells per minute and is equal to the arterial O_2 content multiplied by cardiac output. Since 100 ml of arterial blood at pO_2 of about 100 mmHg contains about 20 ml of oxygen, thus with a cardiac output of about 5 L/min, the normal oxygen delivery to the entire body is about 1L/min. The oxygen delivery to the tissues decreases with either decrease in arterial O_2 content or decrease in cardiac output.

Oxygen Consumption. When the arterial blood with approximate pO_2 100 mmHg reaches the tissues with tissue fluid pO_2 40 mmHg; because of pressure gradient, about 5 ml of O_2 diffuses from the tissue capillaries to the interstitial fluid out of 100 ml of blood (containing ~ 19 ml O_2) every minute. Thus, oxygen consumption of the whole body at rest with a cardiac output of 5 L/min is about or 250 ml of O_2 per minute.

Utilization Coefficient. Utilization coefficient refers to the percentage of oxygen consumed out of oxygen delivered to the tissue, i.e.

$$\text{Coefficient of utilization} = \frac{\text{Oxygen consumed/min}}{\text{Oxygen delivered/min}} \times 100$$

$$\text{So, at rest coefficient of utilization of whole body} = \frac{250 \text{ ml/min}}{1000 \text{ ml/min}} \times 100 = 25\%$$

Oxygen Release during Exercise

Oxygen release during exercise or activity depending upon the severity of exercise the O_2 consumption is increased per min. The oxygen demand of the tissues is met with following changes:

Delivery of Oxygen to the Tissues is *increased* by:

- Increase in blood flow to the tissues occurs due to:
  - Increase in cardiac output,
  - Local arteriolar dilatation, and
  - Increase in the number of open capillaries.
- *Increase in RBC count* due to splenic contraction.

Release of Oxygen in the Tissue is increased by:

- Right shift of oxygen dissociation curve occurs due to increase in pCO_2, H^+ concentration, temperature and 2, 3-DPG. As a result more O_2 is released to the tissues at the same pO_2. This can increase the oxygen uptake of tissues to 750 ml/min, i.e. 3 times the resting level.
- Fall in PO_2 of interstitial fluid. Depending upon the degree of activity, the O_2 tension in the interstitial fluid may fall to even zero. This leads to a very steep pressure gradient between blood and tissues increasing release of O_2.

All the above factors combined can increase the oxygen released in the tissues by 15 times the resting levels.

Vehicles for Transport of Oxygen: A Comparison of Plasma, Haemoglobin and Whole Blood

The oxygen dissociation curves of plasma, haemoglobin solution and whole blood (Fig. 5.5-9) and the amount of oxygen that can be loaded and unloaded by different transport vehicles reveal that:

From the Lungs at pO_2 of about 100 mmHg, the amount of O_2 loaded by 100 ml of transport vehicle is:

- Whole blood : 19.8 ml
- Haemoglobin solution : 19.5 ml
- Plasma solution : 0.3 ml only

In the Tissue at pO_2 of 40 mmHg, the amount of oxygen released by 100 ml of transport vehicle is:

- Whole blood : 5 ml,
- Haemoglobin solution : 1.5 ml and
- Plasma : 0.18 ml

At Maximum Haemoglobin Saturation the whole blood can release:

- 5 ml of O_2 at rest when tissue pO_2 is about 40 mmHg,
- 13 ml of O_2 during moderate exercise when tissue pO_2 is about 25 mmHg, and
- 15–16 ml of O_2 during severe exercise, when tissue pO_2 is about 15 mmHg.

From the above, it is quite clear that whole blood is an ideal vehicle for transport of O_2, to load itself in lungs with O_2 and to release O_2 in tissues as per requirement.

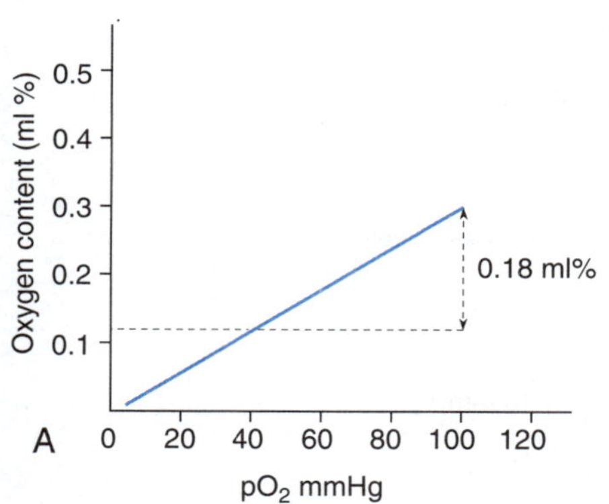

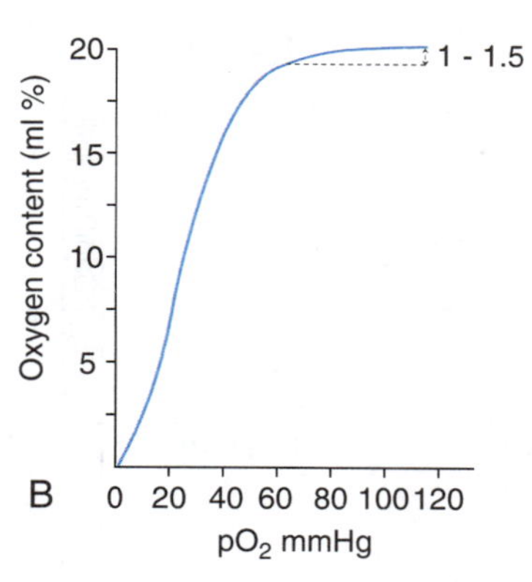

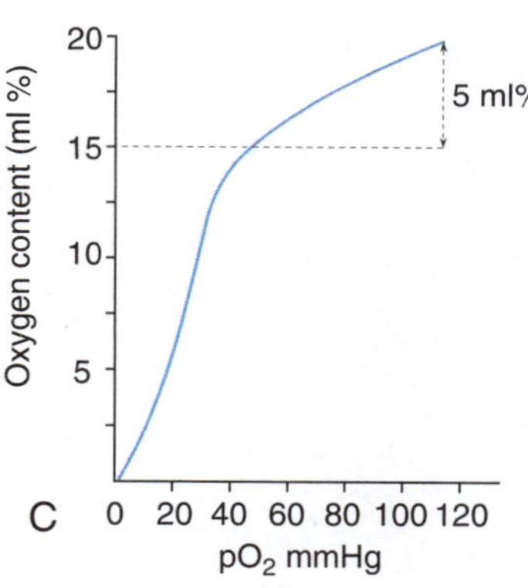

FIGURE 5.5-9 Oxygen dissociation curves: **(A)** for plasma; **(B)** for haemoglobin solution and **(C)** for whole blood.

TRANSPORT OF CARBON DIOXIDE

Transport of carbon dioxide from tissue cells to the lungs occurs due to *constant circulation* of blood and diffusion of CO_2 that occurs at various sites in the direction of concentration gradient which is represented by CO_2 tension differences as given:

- Intracellular pCO_2 : 46 mmHg,
- Interstitial fluid pCO_2 : 45 mmHg
- Arterial blood pCO_2 (in tissue capillaries) : 40 mmHg
- Venous blood pCO_2 : 45 mmHg
- Alveolar air pCO_2 : 40 mmHg

From the above pCO_2 levels, it is clear that:

- CO_2 from the cells diffuses into the interstitial fluid against a tension gradient of 1 mmHg,
- From the interstitial fluid the CO_2 diffuses into the capillaries at a tension gradient of 5 mmHg, and
- From the venous blood that is supplied to pulmonary capillaries the CO_2 diffuses across the respiratory membrane into the alveoli against a tension gradient of 5 mmHg.

Transport of carbon dioxide from the tissue cells to the lungs can be described as under:

A. Diffusion of CO_2 in the blood,
B. Transport of CO_2 in the blood and
C. Release of CO_2 in the lungs.

Diffusion of CO_2 in the Blood

Tissue cells constantly form CO_2 inside the cells due to metabolism. As mentioned above intracellular pCO_2 is 46 mmHg and that of interstitial fluid surrounding the cells is 45 mmHg. Though the cells are continuously forming CO_2 but still the CO_2 tension gradient between inside and outside of the cells is only 1 mmHg. This is owing to the rapid diffusion of CO_2 (20 times that of O_2) out of the cells into the interstitial fluid. Since pCO_2 of the arterial blood flowing in tissue capillaries is lower (40 mmHg) than that of interstitial fluid, so CO_2 diffuses inside the capillary blood which flows in the systemic venous system.

Transport of CO_2 in Blood

Venous blood contains about 52 ml and arterial blood about 48 ml of CO_2 per 100 ml. Thus, 4 ml of CO_2 is transported per 100 ml of blood from tissue cells to the lungs. Thus, total CO_2 transported from the whole body tissue cells at rest with a cardiac output of 5 L/min is about 4 × 5000/100, or 200 ml/min.

Carbon dioxide is transported in the blood in three forms (Fig. 5.5-10):

- In dissolved state (7%)
- In bicarbonate form (70%), and
- In carbamino compound form (23%).

Carbon Dioxide Transport in Dissolved Form

- The venous blood, with pCO_2 45 mmHg contains about 2.7 ml/100 ml of CO_2 in the dissolved state.
- The arterial blood with pCO_2 40 mmHg contains about 2.4 ml/100 ml of CO_2 in the dissolved state.
- Thus only 0.3 ml of CO_2 is transported in dissolved state per 100 ml of blood from tissues to the lungs. This represents about 7% of all CO_2 that is transported.

Carbon Dioxide Transport in Bicarbonate Form

Approximately 70% of the carbon dioxide is transported in the form of *plasma bicarbonate ions.* However, these bicarbonate ions are formed in the RBCs and then diffuse into plasma as explained:

- After entering the blood, most of the CO_2 enters the RBCs, wherein the presence of carbonic anhydrase, it rapidly reacts with water to form carbonic acid (H_2CO_3).
- Carbonic acid (H_2CO_3) dissociates into bicarbonate ions (HCO_3^-) and hydrogen ions (H^+).
- The bicarbonate ions diffuse out of the RBCs into plasma and are transported as sodium bicarbonate

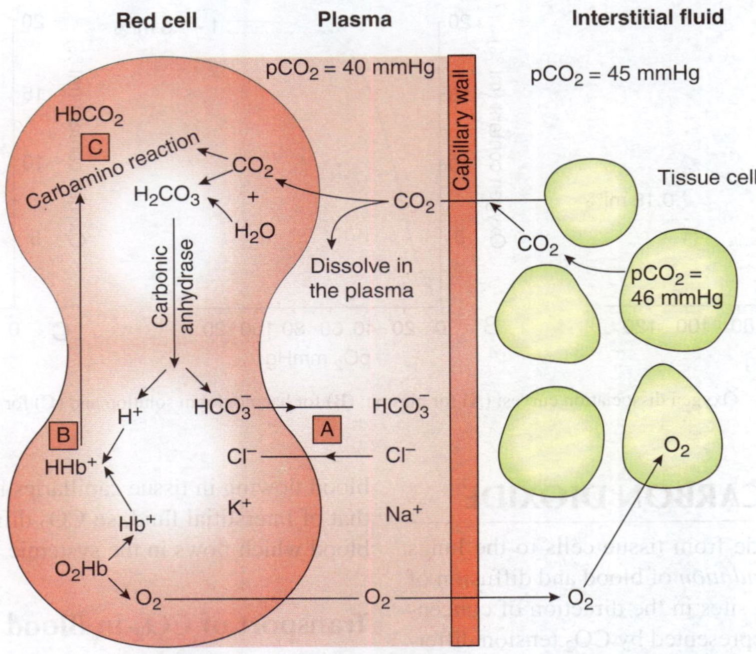

FIGURE 5.5-10 **(A)** Transport of carbon dioxide (CO_2) in blood demonstrating formation of HCO_3^- and chloride shift phenomenon; **(B)** H^+ buffering by haemoglobin; and **(C)** formation of carbaminohaemoglobin.

(alkali reserve of blood). Thus, although HCO_3^- is formed within the RBCs, most of the CO_2 is carried in the plasma as HCO_3^- and some in the RBCs as well.

- The H^+ are buffered by deoxygenated haemoglobin, which is a weaker acid than oxyhaemoglobin. This enables the reaction to proceed unabated in the forward direction.
- Chloride shift *(Hamburger phenomenon)* the HCO_3^- diffuses out of the RBCs into the plasma, the inside of the cells become less negatively charged. Because the RBC membrane is relatively impermeable to cations, so in order to neutralize this effect, negatively charged chloride ions (Cl^-) diffuse from the plasma into the RBCs to replace the HCO_3^-. The movement of chloride ions into the RBCs is called chloride shift or Hamburger phenomenon. This process is mediated by Band 3, a major ion exchange membrane protein also called Anion Exchange-I (AE-I). The chloride shift occurs very rapidly and essentially completed within 1 second.
- As a result of chloride shift, the total number of ions inside the RBCs increase, so the osmotic pressure inside the RBCs becomes higher than that of plasma. This causes osmotic absorption of fluid into the RBCs. Thus, venous RBCs contain the greater quantity of fluid as compared to the arterial blood RBCs. Because of this:
  - Packed cell volume (PCV) of venous blood is slightly higher (~3%) than that of arterial blood, and
  - Venous RBCs are more fragile than the arterial RBCs.

Transport of Carbon Dioxide in Carbamino Form

Approximately 23% of the total CO_2 is transported in the blood in the form of carbamino compounds. After entering the blood, some of the CO_2 combines with the amino group ($-NH_2$) of proteins to form carbamino compounds:

• ***In the Plasma,*** CO_2 combines with amino group of plasma proteins to ($Pr\ NH_2$) form carbamino proteins:

$$CO_2 + PrNH_2 \rightarrow Pr.\ NH.\ COOH$$

- This reaction is much less significant because quantity of these proteins is one-fourth that of haemoglobin.

• ***In the RBCs,*** CO_2 combines with amino group of haemoglobin ($HbNH_2$) to form a compound called carbamino haemoglobin.

$$CO_2 + HbNH_2 \rightarrow Hb.\ NH.\ COOH$$

- This combination of CO_2 with haemoglobin is a reversible reaction that occurs with a loose bond, so that the CO_2 is easily released into the alveoli where pCO_2 is lower than that in the tissue capillaries.
- This reaction of CO_2 with Hb is much slower than the reaction of CO_2 with water in RBCs. This is because, more CO_2 (70%) is transported as bicarbonates and less as carbamino compounds (23%).
- This reaction of CO_2 with Hb is further decreased to a great extent when 2, 3-DPG concentration is more, because both 2, 3-DPG and CO_2 compete for the same sites on Hb.

Carbon Dioxide Dissociation Curve

- Carbon dioxide dissociation curve is obtained by plotting the relationship between pCO_2 and total CO_2 content of the blood (Fig. 5.5-11).
- The graph shows that relationship between the two is nearly linear over wider range of pCO_2 (if compared with O_2–Hb, dissociation curve, which is sigmoid shaped).
- It is important to note that practically in the body the pCO_2 value of arterial and venous blood varies within a narrow range of 40 to 45 mmHg (in contrast the corresponding values of pO_2 vary from 100 to 40 mmHg). Therefore, the full range of CO_2 dissociation curve shown in Figure 5.5-11 is an experimental theoretical phenomenon and does not operate in the body practically. Physiologically the curve operates only within A-V range (Fig. 5.5-11).

Factors Affecting CO_2 Dissociation Curve

1. Oxygen. Deoxyhaemoglobin present in the tissue capillaries is capable of loading more CO_2 than the oxyhaemoglobin. And also the oxygenation of haemoglobin in the lungs increases the CO_2 unloading. This effect is called *Haldane's effect.* Haldane's effect on the transport of CO_2 depicts that:

- Blood with pCO_2 40 mmHg reaching the tissues is capable of drawing CO_2 from the tissues more at pO_2 40 mmHg (point A) than at pO_2 of 100 mmHg (point B). Thus, because of Haldane's effect, the CO_2 dissociation curve shifts to the left when blood flows to the tissues.
- Blood with pCO_2 45 mmHg reaching the lungs is capable of retaining less or in other words releasing more CO_2 in the lungs at pO_2 100 mmHg (point C) than at $pO_2$40 (point D). Thus, because of Haldane's effect, the CO_2 dissociation curve shifts to the right when blood flows in the pulmonary capillaries.

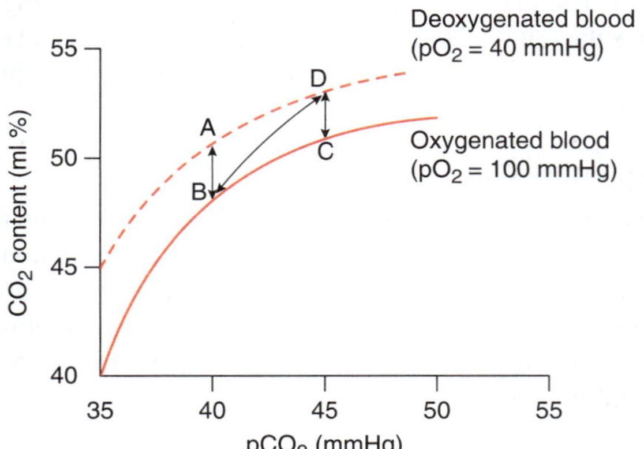

FIGURE 5.5-11 Carbon dioxide dissociation curve for oxygenated (solid line) and for deoxygenated blood (dotted line) to demonstrate Haldane's effect.

- Figure 5.5-11 also depicts that Haldane's effect is beneficial because it almost doubles the quantity of CO2 to be carried from the tissues to lungs and also doubles the amount of CO2 to be excreted by the lungs.

2. 2,3-DPG. decreases the formation of carbamino haemoglobin because it competes with CO_2 for the same sites on Hb especially in case of reduced Hb. Thus, 2, 3-DPG shifts the CO_2 dissociation curve to the right meaning thereby that CO_2 carrying capacity is decreased.

3. Increase in Body Temperature. causes release of O_2 from Hb, this causes left shift of the CO_2 dissociation curve, i.e. larger amount of CO_2 can be taken of at given pCO_2.

Release of CO_2 in the Lungs

When the venous blood with pCO_2 of 45 mmHg, CO_2 content of 52 ml per 100 ml, and pO_2 of 40 mmHg reaches the pulmonary capillaries, it is separated by the respiratory membrane from the alveolar air having pCO_2 40 mmHg. CO_2 content of 48 ml/100 ml and pO_2 104 mmHg. Then following changes occur which lead to diffusion of 4 ml of CO_2 100 ml of blood/min in the alveoli (Fig. 5.5-12):

Release of CO_2 from Carbamino Haemoglobin into Plasma (Fig. 5.5-12A)

- O_2 diffuses into the capillary blood with a concentration gradient of 104 mmHg – 40 mmHg or 64 mmHg.
- The O_2 enters the RBCs and converts the deoxyhaemoglobin into oxyhaemoglobin which has very low affinity for CO_2. In this CO_2 is released from the carbamino haemoglobin which diffuses into the plasma.

Release of CO_2 from Carbonate into Plasma (Fig. 5.5-12B)

- The oxyhaemoglobin so formed is a strong acid. Increased acidity of the blood results in increased H^+ concentration. To neutralize it the bicarbonate (HCO_3^-) ions diffuse into the RBCs where H^+ and HCO_3^-react to form H_2CO_3 (carbonic acid) which dissociates to form H_2O and CO_2. This whole reaction occurs in the presence of enzyme carbonic anhydrase. CO_2 so released diffuses into the plasma.
- With the movement of HCO_3^-inside the RBCs, inside of the cell becomes more negative. To neutralize them, either the positive charged cations should move in or –ve charge anions should flow out of the cell. Since RBC membrane is relatively impermeable to cations, so the Cl^- anions return in the plasma from the RBC. This whole reaction catalysed by carbonic anhydrase inhibitor is called *reversal of chloride shift.*

Diffusion of CO_2 from Plasma to Alveoli The CO_2 dissolved in plasma plus that released from the carbamino

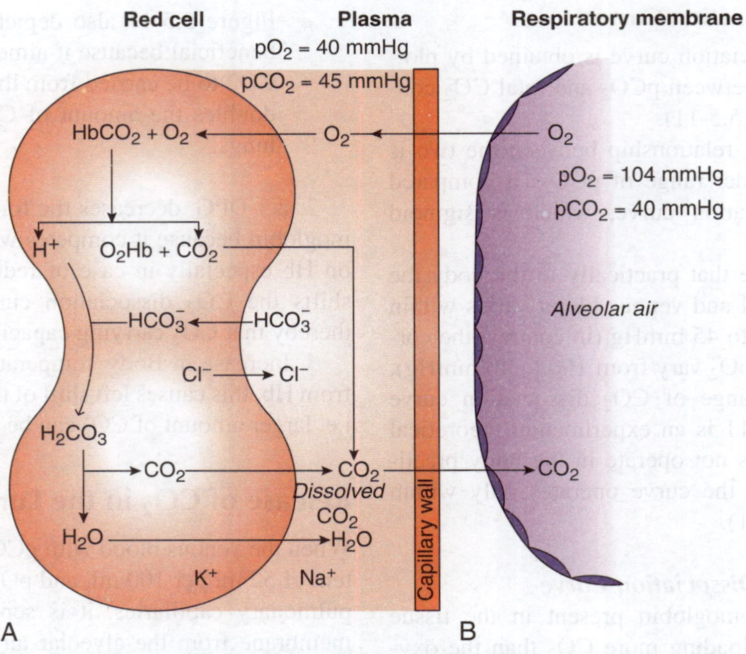

FIGURE 5.5-12 (A) Release of carbon dioxide in the plasma from carbaminohaemoglobin and from bicarbonate ionsand (B) diffusion of CO_2 from plasma into the alveoli through respiratory membrane.

haemoglobin and bicarbonates combinedly exerts pCO_2 of 45 mmHg. Since the pCO_2 of alveolar air is 40 mmHg, so because of pressure gradient CO_2 diffuses from blood to alveoli. Due to constant ventilation CO_2 from alveoli is transported to atmosphere.

Other Facts about CO_2 Transport

Comparison of Different Vehicles for CO_2 Transport

The carbon dioxide dissociation curve of plasma, bicarbonate solution and whole blood (Fig. 5.5-13 and the amount of CO_2 that can be loaded and unloaded by different transport vehicles from the tissues at pCO_2 45 mmHg (Table 5.5-1) reveal that:

- *Plasma* is not a good transport vehicle as very small amount of CO_2 (only 0.2 ml) can be taken from tissues/100 ml of blood/min.
- *Bicarbonate solution* is also not a good transport vehicle because beyond pO_2 40 mmHg there is no further transport of CO2.
- *Whole blood* is an ideal vehicle for transport of CO_2, to load itself in tissues with CO_2 and to release CO_2 in the lung.

Rate of Total CO_2 Transport

In Resting Conditions, each 100 ml of blood transports about 4 ml of CO_2 from the tissues to the lungs. Thus, with an average cardiac output of 5L/min, a total of (4 × 5000)/100 or 200 ml of CO_2 is transported per min.

During Exercise the amount of CO_2 transported increases depending upon the severity of exercise. In severe exercise, as much as 4 L of CO_2 may be transported per minute. Because of greater solubility and transport in different forms, the transport of such a large amounts of CO_2 occurs without any difficulty. The conversion of most of CO_2 into bicarbonate ions prevents any significant change in the pH of blood even when such a large volume of CO_2 enters the circulation.

Changes in Blood pH during Transport of CO_2

Normally, the pH of arterial blood is 7.4. As it passes through the tissues, it acquires CO_2 and the pH of blood falls due to formation of carbonic acid (H_2CO_3) in venous blood. The pH may fall by about 0.4. However, during exercise the fall in pH may become to the tune of 0.5 and even more. Nevertheless most of it is neutralized by the blood buffers.

Respiratory Quotient

Definition. Respiratory quotient (RQ) refers to the ratio of the rate of CO_2 excretion and rate of O_2 consumption per minute. It is also called the *respiratory exchange ratio.*

Normal Value. Normally, the rate of CO_2 excretion is 4 ml/100ml/min, and rate of O_2 consumption is 5 ml/100 ml/min. So, RQ = 4/5, or 0.8.

The RQ Depends Upon the Type of Fuel Consumed

- In a person who is utilizing carbohydrates as the entire source of energy for the body metabolism, value of

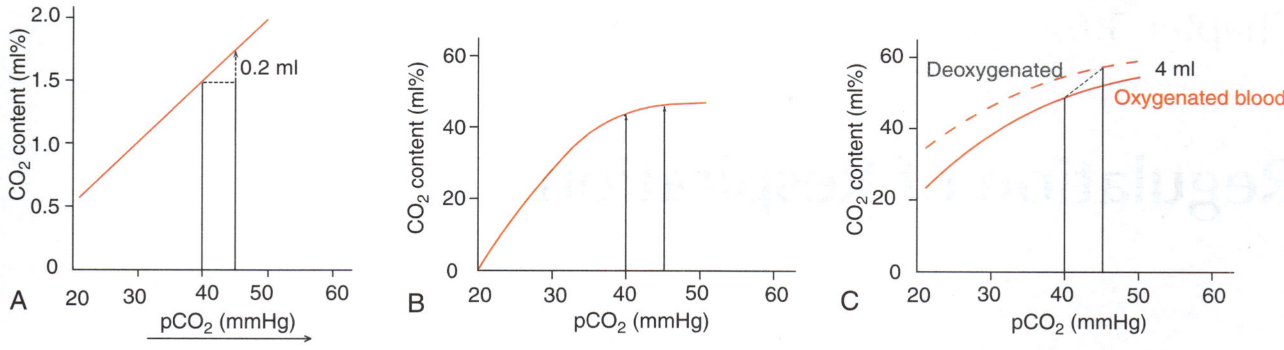

FIGURE 5.5-13 Carbon dioxide dissociation curve: **(A)** for plasma; **(B)** for bicarbonate solution and **(C)** for whole blood.

RQ is 1, because in metabolism of carbohydrates, one molecule of CO_2 is formed for each molecule of O_2 consumed.

- The RQ is <1.0 for proteins and fats. When only fats are metabolized, the value of RQ falls to 0.7, because 0.7 molecules of CO_2 are formed, for each molecule of O_2 consumed in the metabolism of fat.
- A lower RQ, thus suggests that a greater than usual proportion of proteins and fats are being catabolized in the body.
- RQ can be easily estimated by knowing the amount of O_2 removed from inspired air and the amount of CO_2 added to the expired air per minute.

TABLE 5.5-1 Amount of CO_2 That can be Loaded and Unloaded by Different Transport Vehicles

Vehicle	Content of CO_2/100 ml/min		
	In venous blood at pCO_2 45 mmHg	*In arterial blood at pCO_2 40 mmHg*	*Loaded by the blood*
Plasma	1.8 ml	1.6 ml	0.2 ml
Bicarbonate solution	48 ml	48 ml	Nil
Whole blood	52 ml	48 ml	4 ml

Chapter 5.6

Regulation of Respiration

INTRODUCTION

Respiration is regulated by a complex integration of neural control mechanisms which are modified by certain respiratory reflexes and chemical control mechanisms.

Neural control mechanisms include:

- *A system for automatic control* of respiration as an involuntary function. The involuntary control system of respiration is located in the medullary and pontine centres of the brain stem.
- *A system for voluntary control* of respiration is located in the cerebral cortex.

Thus, respiration enjoys the distinction of being an involuntary function which can be influenced voluntarily. This *dual control* has great functional significance, i.e.

- Involuntary control which allows human to breathe without conscious efforts under all circumstances including sleep and is thus essential for life.
- The voluntary control system facilitates acts like talking, singing, swimming, breath holding and voluntary hyperventilation.

Respiratory reflexes which modify the effects of neural mechanisms are those initiated by stimulation of stretch receptors, irritant receptors, J-receptors and chest wall receptors.

Chemical control mechanisms are influenced by alterations in arterial pO_2, pCO_2 and H^+ concentration. The chemical control mechanisms are initiated by stimulation of the chemoreceptors (central and peripheral).

Functions of respiratory regulatory mechanisms include:

- *Genesis of normal respiratory spontaneous rhythm.* This is the function of medullary and pontinecentres of neural mechanism.
- *Control of rate and depth of respiration,* i.e. adjustment of total ventilation to match metabolic needs of the body so that arterial oxygen tension (pO_2), carbon dioxide tension (pCO_2) and H^+ concentration (pH) are almost maintained constant whether it be during quiet breathing, sleep or muscular exercise. This function is accomplished by all the respiratory control mechanisms acting in unison (Fig. 5.6-1):
  - *Sensors,* i.e. chemoreceptors and other receptors (e.g. stretch, irritant, chest wall and J receptors) perceive the respiratory needs of the body and convey via afferent nerves to the central controller.
  - *Central controller*, i.e. medullary, pontine and other parts of the brain adjust the efferent outputs as per the body needs and convey to the effectors.

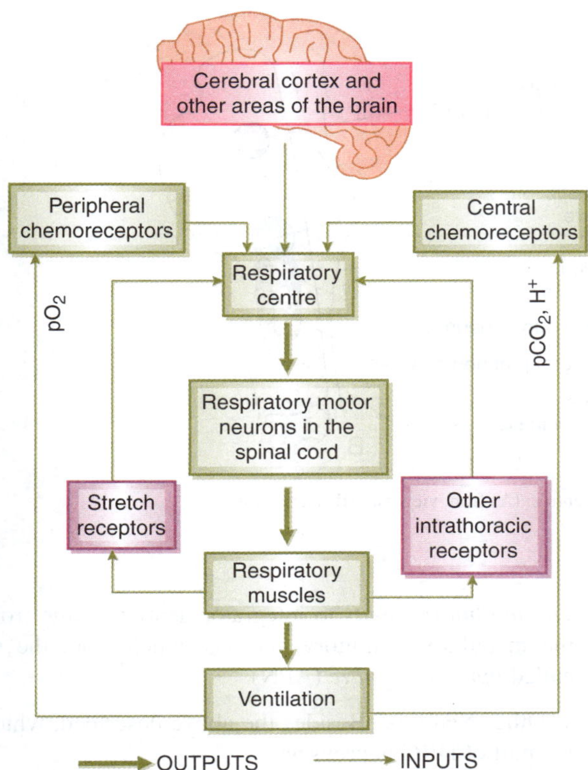

FIGURE 5.6-1 Diagrammatic representation of the inputs to respiratory centre that generate the output to the respiratory muscles.

- *Effectors* are the respiratory muscles which perform their activity as per the neural discharges received.

NEURAL REGULATION OF RESPIRATION

The neural mechanisms regulating respiration can be described under two headings:

- Automatic control system, and
- Afferent impulses to respiratory centres.

Automatic Control System

Neural Genesis of Respiratory Rhythm

The involuntary neural control system regulates respiration by several groups of neurons situated bilaterally in medulla and pons which include medullary respiratory centres, pontine respiratory centres and reticular activating system (RAS).

I. Medullary Respiratory Centres

The medullary respiratory centres include two groups of neurons: the dorsal respiratory group (DRG), and ventral respiratory group (VRG) which generate the basic respiratory rhythm.

The Respiratory Control Pattern Generator. The respiratory control pattern generator, which is responsible for automatic respiration, is located in the medulla. A group of neurons called pacemaker cells from the pre-Botzinger complex, which are situated between nucleus ambiguus and lateral reticular nucleus. The rhythmic activity is initiated by these synaptically coupled neurons. These neurons discharge rhythmically and generate rhythmic motor activity in phrenic nerve, hypoglossal nerve and intercostal nerves.

Important Note

On the neurons of pre-Botzinger complex the receptors for substance P, Tachykinin (NK_1), $5HT_4$ and μ- opioid are present. Opioids are used as analgesic, but at the same time it causes respiratory depression as a side effect. However, it is now known that $5HT_4$ receptor agonists block the inhibitory effect of opioids on respiration without inhibiting analgesic effect.

1. Dorsal Respiratory Group Neurons Most of the neurons are located within the nucleus of tractus solitaries (NTS) and some in the adjacent reticular substance (Fig. 5.6-2). The neurons of DRG are of three types:

i. Inspiratory Neurons. The DRG mainly contains inspiratory cells called *I-neurons* that discharge during inspiration only. The axons of I-neurons cross the mid-line and descend on the contralateral side of spinal cord to make contact with the spinal motor neurons of inspiratory muscles, namely, the diaphragm (supplied by the phrenic nerve arising from C_3 to C_5 spinal segments) and the external intercostal muscles (supplied by the intercostal nerves). In other words, the neurons in the DRG are the upper motor neurons of respiratory muscles.

From I-neurons, nerve signals pass to the muscles of inspiration. The signal is not instantaneous but is a ramp signal, i.e. it is weak in the beginning and it steadily increases in a ramp manner for about 2 seconds and is thus called *inspiratory ramp*. This leads to a steady increase in the lung volume during inspiration rather than the respiratory gasps (abrupt distension). Ramp signal then abruptly ceases for approximately next 3 seconds.

ii. Inspiratory Off-switch (IOS) Neurons. IOS neurons refer to a group of neurons that are responsible for terminating the activity of I-neurons and causes turning off of excitation of muscles of inspiration (diaphragm and external intercostal muscles). These muscles, therefore relax allowing elastic recoil of the chest wall and the lungs to cause expiration. After expiration again there is a signal for starting another cycle.

iii. Integrator Neurons. Integrator neurons are other type of neurons of DRG present near the I-neurons and are stimulated by them. They subserve following integrating functions:

- The integrator neurons when depolarize to a critical level lead to firing of the so-called IOS neurons which are responsible for terminating the inspiratory ramp.

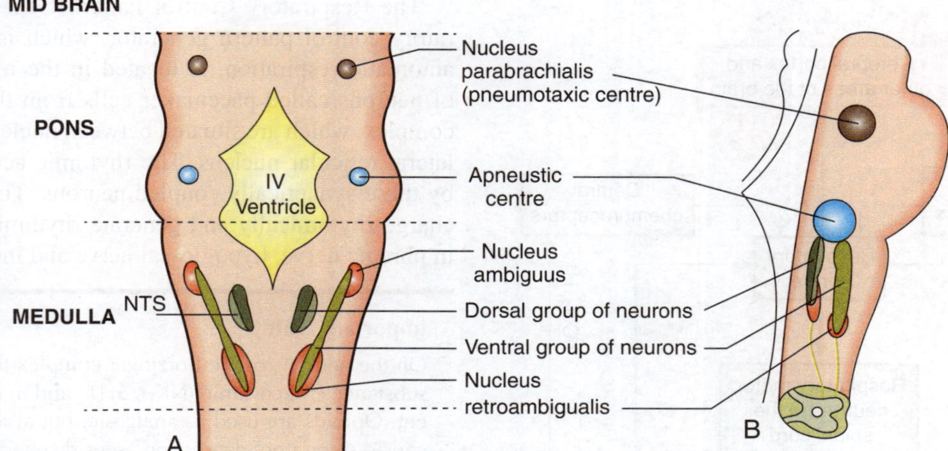

FIGURE 5.6-2 Medullary and pontine respiratory centres: (**A**) front view and (**B**) lateral view.

The *I-neurons* trigger the IOS neurons indirectly through integrators and thereby bring about the termination of their own discharge. This forms the basic circuity of an automatic respiratory rhythm (Fig. 5.6-3). In this way, the cycle of inspiration/expiration goes on continuously to cause tidal respiration.

- The *integrator neurons* receive both excitatory and inhibitory inputs (Fig. 5.6-3) and thus integrate the activity of *I-neurons* and IOS neurons accordingly.
- *The excitatory inputs* to integrator neurons come from:
  - Cerebral cortex
  - Pneumotaxic centre (PNC)
  - Vagal afferents from stretch receptors

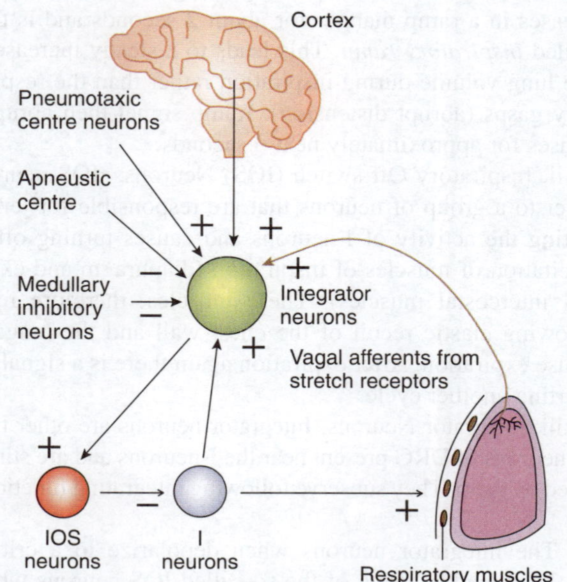

FIGURE 5.6-3 Basic circuity for generation of respiratory rhythm.

- *The inhibitory inputs* to integrator neurons come from the medullary inhibitory neurons which from the so called *apneustic centre* (APN).

iv. Other Neurons. Besides the above described, which form a part of DRG neurons are:

- *P-neurons or pump cells* are the second order pulmonary stretch receptor sensory neurons. These do not receive other respiratory inputs.
- *Propriobulbar inspiratory ramp interneurons, early inspiratory or early-burst neurons, late onset inspiratory neurons* and *post inspiration* (PI)-related neurons are other inspiratory neurons of the DRG.

Detailed functioning of these other neurons of the DRG is beyond the scope of this book.

2. Ventral Respiratory Group Neurons VRG neurons contain both inspiratory cells called I neurons and expiratory cells called E-neurons (c.f. DRG which contain only I-neurons).

Parts of VRG Neurons. The VRG neurons can be subdivided into three main parts (Fig. 5.6-2):

i. ***Caudal part or nucleus retroambigualis (NRA)*** contains mainly E-neurons which constitute the bulbospinal premotor neurons. Their axons cross the midline and descend on the contralateral side to make contact with the motor neuron pool for the muscles of expiration, i.e. internal intercostal muscles and abdominal muscles. In other words, these neurons in the VRG seem to form the *upper motor neurons of expiratory muscles.*

ii. ***Intermediate part*** of VRG neurons denote *nucleus parambigualis* because it parallels the ambiguus nucleus. This part mainly contains I-neurons called the bulbospinal inspiratory premotor neurons. These control the activity of inspiratory upper motor neurons.

iii. ***Most rostral part of VRG*** coincides with nucleus retrofacialis (NRF). It contains several types of E-neurons which form a complex called *Botzinger complex.* Some of these neurons control the pharyngeal and laryngeal musculature which must relax during expiration.

Interaction of I and E Neurons. The I and E neurons have inhibitory connections to each other, i.e. there exists *reciprocal innervation* between the two. Therefore, the motor neurons to the expiratory muscles are inhibited when those supplying the inspiratory muscles are active and vice versa. This reciprocal innervation is mediated via collaterals from excitatory pathway that synapse on inhibitory interneurons. Thus, an impulse that stimulates the one will inhibit the other and vice versa (Fig. 5.6-4):

Role of VRG Neurons. The VRG neurons, normally remain totally inactive during quiet breathing. The VRG neurons become active during inspiration (role of I-neurons) as well as expiration (role of E-neurons) during forceful respiration. This area is especially important in providing powerful expiratory signals to expiratory muscles. Thus, VRG operates when high levels of pulmonary ventilation is required, for example, during exercise.

II. Pontine Respiratory Centres

The pontine centres include the apneustic (APN) and pneumotaxic (PNC), both of which modify the activity of medullary respiratory centres.

1. Apneustic Centre APN refers to a group of inhibitory neurons located bilaterally in the lower part of pons (Fig. 5.6-2). It sends signals to integrator neurons of DRG that affects the inspiratory off switch (IOS) neurons and prevent the switch-off of the inspiratory activity (Fig. 5.6-3).

$$\text{I-neurons} \overset{(-)}{\underset{(-)}{\Longleftrightarrow}} \text{E-neurons}$$

FIGURE 5.6-4 Reciprocal innervation of I and E-neurons.

This increases the tidal volume and duration of inspiration, resulting in a deeper and more prolonged inspiratory effort termed as *apneusis.* However, normally the APN is inhibited by impulses carried by the vagus nerves and also by the activity of PNC. Either of these two influences, penumotaxic centre or the vagii, seems to be adequate to keep apneusis in check. The above-described facts are based on the experimental observations made in dogs and cats under general anaesthesia. The situation in conscious animals may be different. The existence and functions of APN are based on following experimental observations (Fig. 5.6-5):

- Sectioning of brain between the medulla and pons (level 1 in Fig. 5.6-5) leaves the basic rhythm intact indicating thereby that medullary respiratory centres are working normally.
- Sectioning the brain at mid-pontine level, i.e. between PNC and APN, (i.e. at level 2 in Figure 5.6-5) along with bilateral vagotomy leads to prolonged periods of inspiration, i.e. apneusis or apneustic breathing. This indicates that removal of two inhibitor influences (PNC and vagii) on the APN allows APN to exert its influence on medullary centres producing apneusis.
- Sectioning the brain rostral to the pons (level 3 in Fig. 5.6-5) leaves the respiratory rhythm intact even if combined with bilateral vagotomy. This indicates that mere presence of check by PNC is sufficient to control the apneustic effect of APN on medullary centres.

2. Pneumotaxic Centre The PNCs are located bilaterally in *nucleus parabrachialis* of the upper pons.

Functions. As described above, the PNC inhibits the APN. Therefore, stimulation of PNC shortens inspiration, leading to shallow and more rapid respiratory pattern. In other words the PNC by inhibiting activity of APN indirectly controls the switch-off point of inspiratory ramp, thus controlling the duration of inspiration.

- Strong PNC discharge because of rapid switching-off of ramp signals may cut down the inspiratory phase to

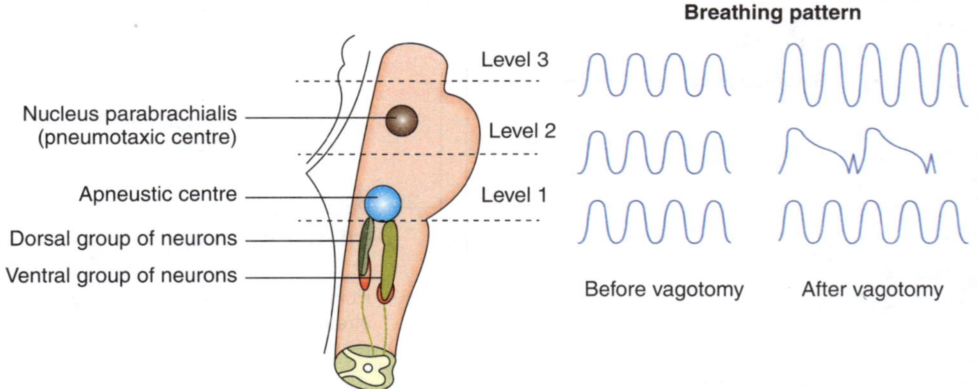

FIGURE 5.6-5 Sectioning of brain at different levels to demonstrate the activity of different respiratory centres.

- 0.5 second only; and as a result the rate of inspiration increases to 30–40 breaths per minute.
- Weak PNC discharge increases the duration of ramp signals and may reduce the rate of respiration to only a few breaths per minute.

Thus, though rhythm of respiration resides in DRG neurons in medulla, PNC and APN control these neurons to regulate the depth and rate of respiration.

III. Reticular Activating System

The RAS stimulates the respiratory centres to increase respiratory drive. During sleep, RAS activity diminishes, decreasing respiratory drive, which diminishes alveolar ventilation and results in a slight elevation of arterial CO_2 tension.

AFFERENT IMPULSES TO RESPIRATORY CENTRES

The respiratory centres generate the respiratory rhythm and execute their effects through the efferent nerves supplying the respiratory muscles. The activity of respiratory centres in turn is influenced by the afferent impulses from the lungs and various other parts of the body. These afferent impulses guide the respiratory centres to regulate their activity so as to serve a number of purposes in the body such as:

- To cope up with the O_2 demand of the body and get rid of CO_2 from the body,
- To help to regulate the H^+ concentration of body,
- To maintain the appropriate O_2 tension of blood in certain conditions of anoxia or hypoxia.
- To help to maintain the normal body temperature, and so on.

Various afferent impulses to the respiratory centres can be grouped as (Fig. 5.6-6):

- Afferent impulses from higher centres,
- Afferent impulses from non-chemical receptors, which may constitute *non-chemical regulation of respiration* and
- Afferent impulses from the chemical receptors, which constitute the 'chemical regulation of respiration' and hence has been described separately.

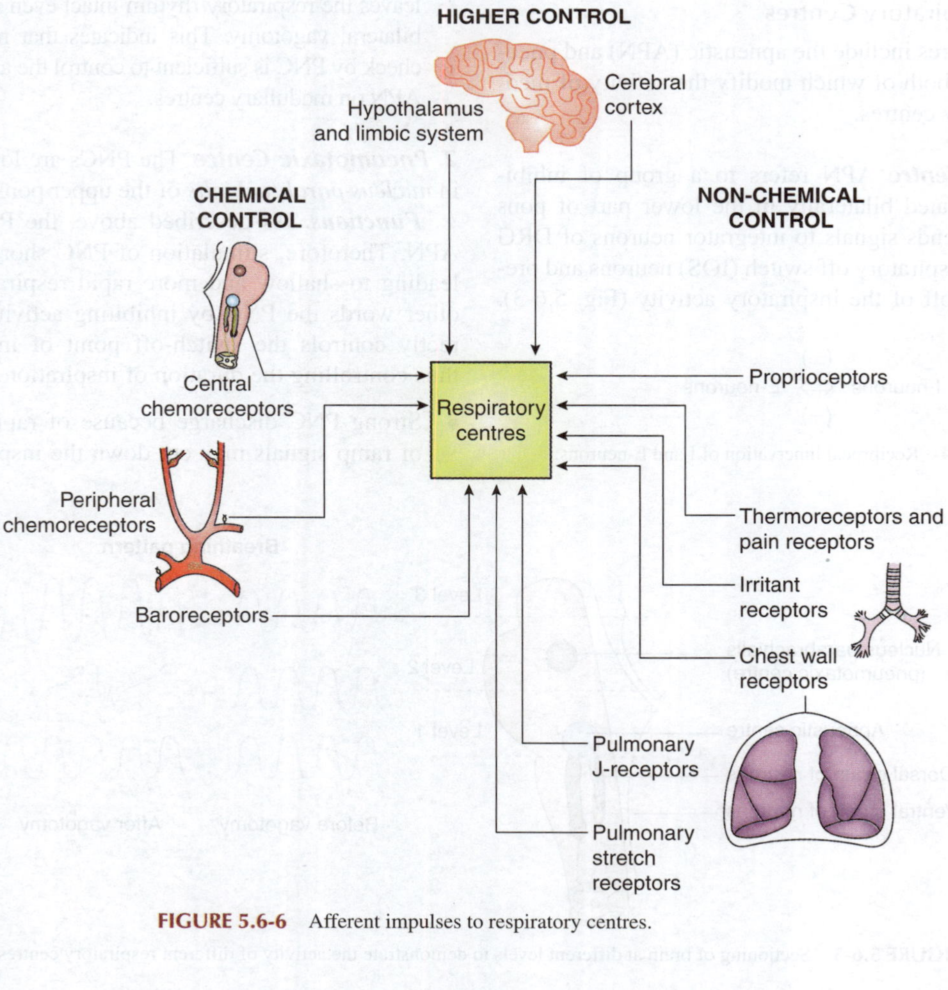

FIGURE 5.6-6 Afferent impulses to respiratory centres.

Afferent Impulses from Higher Centres

The afferent impulses from higher centres which influence the involuntary activity of respiratory centres mainly include voluntary control system and limbic control system.

1. Voluntary Control System As described above, normally, breathing is an involuntary effort and goes on automatically. However, the respiratory muscles are typical skeletal muscle and can also be controlled voluntarily. The voluntary control of respiration is mediated by a pathway which originates from the neocortex, bypasses the medullary respiratory centres to project directly on the spinal respiratory neurons. The voluntary control of breathing is exercised during: *activities like* talking, singing, and swimming; and breath holding.

Breath Holding or Voluntary Apnea. Breathing can be stopped voluntarily for about 50–60 seconds (breath-holding time). But, after this time the chemical drive overrides the voluntary inhibition and the person has uncontrollable desire to breathe and ultimately breathing is resumed involuntarily. That is why it is impossible to commit suicide by holding the breath voluntarily. The decrease in arterial pO_2 and increase in arterial pCO_2 seem to be the chief causes for the end of breath-holding. Breath-holding can be prolonged by 15–20 seconds by an initial hyperventilation which lowers the arterial pCO_2. As a result it takes longer duration of breath-holding to increase the arterial pCO_2 to the critical level. Breath-holding may also be increased by prior inhalation of pure O_2. Some mechanical or reflex factors originating from the chest wall also seem to be involved in limiting the duration of breath-holding.

Voluntary Hyperventilation, i.e. voluntary overbreathing can be done for some time only similar to breath-holding. Effects of hyperventilation are discussed in chemical control of respiration (see page 452)

2. Limbic Control System Pain and emotional stimuli influence the rate and depth of breathing. It indicates the presence of afferents from limbic system to the pontomedullary respiratory neurons. Experimentally also marked changes in respiration are observed on electrical stimulation of various regions of hypothalamus. The influence of hypothalamus and the other parts of limbic system on respiration is only to be expected in view of respiratory changes being a part of emotional expression.

Important Note

Changes in the breathing pattern are the basis for part of polygraph test used as a lie detector.

Applied Aspects

As respiration has two separate controls, coluntary and automatic, sometimes automatic control is disrupted whereas voluntary control remains intact. Clinically, this condition is known as *Ondine curse*. In this state person would stay alive only if he is awake and remembers to breathe. Ondine was a water nymph cursed by the king and all his automatic functions were withdrawn. Due to exhaustion he fell asleep and died because of stoppage of breathing. This condition usually occurs in the patients suffering with bulbar poliomyelitis or conditions which compress the medulla.

Afferent Impulses from Nonchemical Receptors

Afferent impulses from the receptors other than the chemoreceptors, i.e. from nonchemical receptors include the following:

1. Afferent Impulses from Pulmonary Stretch Receptors (Hering–Breuer Reflex) *Hering–Breuer reflex* is one of the first examples of negative feedback. In 1868, Hering and Breuer found that lung inflation inhibits output of the phrenic motor neurons, thereby protecting lung from over-inflation.

The Hering–Breuer inspiratory inhibitory reflex is initiated when the stretch receptors located in the smooth muscles of the bronchi and bronchioles are stimulated by inflation of the lungs. The impulses are then sent through *vagii nerves* to pontomedullary respiratory centres to inhibit respiration. This reflex has an important role in controlling tidal volume during eupnea in human infants. In adults this reflex, therefore, does not play any regulatory role in tidal respiration. This reflex is initiated only when the tidal volume is more than 1–1.5 L. Thus, the reflex tends to limit the tidal volume.

2. Afferent Impulses from J-receptors Afferent impulses from J-receptors constitute the J-reflex. The J-receptors were discovered by an Indian Physiologist AS Paintal in 1954. The name J-receptors (juxtapulmonary capillary receptors) was given to them because of their location very close to the pulmonary capillaries (Fig. 5.6-7). Important features of J-receptors are:

- J-receptors are basically un-myelinated vagal afferent nerve endings (type C fibres).
- These receptors are primarily sensitive to increase in the content of interstitial fluid between the capillary endothelium and alveolar epithelium, therefore they are stimulated in conditions like pulmonary congestion, pulmonary oedema, pneumonia, hyperinflation of lungs and microembolism in pulmonary capillaries.

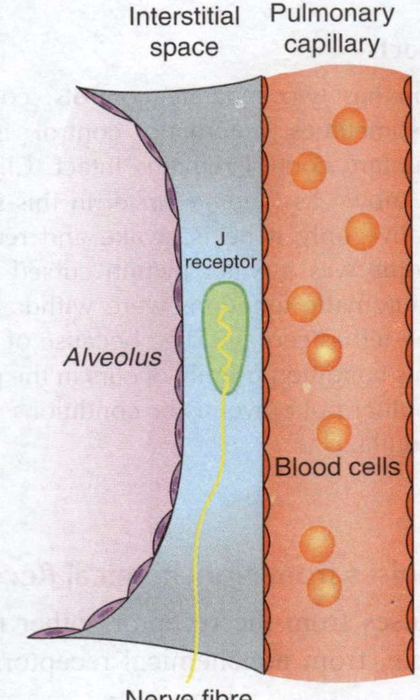

FIGURE 5.6-7 Location of J-receptors.

- J-receptors are also stimulated by some chemical substances like phenyl diguanide, capsaicin, halothane and bradykinin.
- The J-reflex response produced on stimulation of J-receptors is characterized by apnoea followed by hyperventilation, bradycardia, hypotension and weakness of skeletal muscles.
- Physiological role of J-receptors has been postulated by the discoverer Mr Paintal. He states that after exercise especially at high altitude some fluid is entrapped in the alveolar interstitial space which stimulates the J-receptors producing dyspnoea and reduction of skeletal muscle tone. Their combined effect would discourage exercise, thereby taking away the trigger for pulmonary congestion.

3. Afferent Impulses from Irritant Receptors in the Respiratory Tract Irritant receptors are located below the mucosa of whole respiratory tract. These are stimulated by smoke, noxious gases, particulate matter in the inspired air and in a number of other conditions. These receptors initiate a large number of reflexes some of which are:

i. Cough Reflex. This is a protective reflex caused by stimulation of irritant receptors in the pharynx, larynx, trachea and bronchi (conducting zone of respiratory tract). Cough begins with a deep inspiration followed by forced expiration with closed glottis. So, intrapleural pressure rises above 100 mmHg. The glottis is then suddenly opened producing an explosive outflow of air. The velocity of the air flow may reach 960 km per hour. By this endeavour the irritants may be expelled out of the respiratory tract.

ii. Sneezing Reflex is also a protective reflex produced on stimulation of irritant receptors of nasal mucosa. The sneezing begins with deep inspiration, followed by forceful expiration with opened glottis (in cough reflex where glottis is closed).

iii. Hering–Breuer Deflation Reflex is produced on stimulation of irritant receptors located in bronchial epithelium due to distortion of bronchial epithelium caused by large deflations of the lungs as seen in pneumothorax and lung collapses (atelectasis). This reflex may also be responsible for the *sighs* or *yawning* in response to the increase in compliance that occurs periodically due to the collapse of smaller alveoli. The reflex helps in opening up the collapsed alveoli again.

- Yawning is a peculiar respiratory act. Its physiological basis is uncertain. However, one view suggests that deep inspiration and stretching help in opening up of alveoli and prevent them from collapsing. However, experimentally atelectasis preventing effect of yawning could not be demonstrated.
- Yawning increases venous return to the heart.
- In groups of certain animal (monkeys) yawning is used as signal for communication.

iv. Reflex Tachypnoea and Bronchoconstriction is produced on stimulation of irritant receptors present in the respiratory zone of the respiratory tract. Rapid shallow breathing results from reflex stimulation of inspiratory motor neurons. Bronchoconstriction is produced by release of histamine and other chemical substances in the lungs, thereby preventing the irritants to reach the gas exchanging surface. For receptors see page 445.

v. Deglutition Reflex refers to temporary apnoea produced during pharyngeal phase of swallowing of food. It is a protective reflex which prevents the entry of food particles into the respiratory tract. The afferents travel in the glossopharyngeal nerve and produce *deglutition apnoea* by temporary inhibition of respiratory centres.

In the case of vomiting, the chest is fixed so that contraction of intra-abdominal muscle increases intra-abdominal pressure. See page 603.

4. Afferent Impulses from Proprioceptors Proprioceptors are the receptors present in the muscles, tendons and joints and are stimulated during change in the position of different parts of the body. Afferent impulses from proprioceptors stimulate the inspiratory neurons to increase the rate and depth of respiration.

Important Note

This reflex helps in increasing ventilation during exercise. The paediatricians employ this reflex for initiating first breath in the newborn by slapping it.

5. Afferent Impulses from Chest Wall Stretch Receptors Chest wall stretch receptors are nothing but the *muscle spindles* present in the intercostal muscles. Stretching of the intercostal muscles produce a stretch reflex due to stimulation of muscle spindles that is characterized by contraction of intercostal muscles. The muscle spindles present in respiratory muscles help to co-ordinate breathing during change in posture or during speech. They play *a* special role in maintaining normal tidal volume when breathing is impeded by an increase in airway resistance or a decrease in pulmonary compliance.

When the mechanical load on the respiratory system is increased, intercostal muscles are stretched and their muscle spindles are stimulated leading to increased strength of contraction of intercostal muscle. It has been observed that increase in intercostal nerve afferent activity leads to contraction of neighbouring intercostal muscles. This reflex has been termed the *intercostal-to-intercostal reflex*.

Although diaphragm contains very few muscle spindles, but it also shows reflex contraction. This has been attributed to reflex contraction of diaphragm in response to afferent nerve impulses originating in lower intercostal nerves. This reflex has been termed the *intercostal-to-phrenic reflex*.

6. Afferent Impulses from Baroreceptors Baroreceptors or pressure receptors located in the carotid sinus and aortic arch (see details on page 340) are stimulated by increase in the arterial blood pressure. Though they play primary role in regulation of blood pressure, but the impulses do travel to respiratory centres (via vagus from aortic arch and via glossopharyngeal nerve from carotid sinus) and cause inhibition of respiration, in physiological conditions the baroreceptors play an insignificant role in regulation of respiration. The *adrenaline apnoea* observed on injection of high doses of adrenaline has been explained due to the fact that the adrenaline causes a large rise in arterial pressure which in turn inhibits respiration by afferent impulses from the baroreceptors to respiratory centres. However, in small doses, adrenaline stimulates respiration by stimulating the peripheral chemoreceptors.

7. Afferent Impulses from Thermoreceptors Thermoreceptors are those receptors which are stimulated by a change in the body temperature. Thermoreceptors are of two types: the cold receptors and the warmth receptors. When warm receptors are stimulated the impulses are conveyed to cerebral cortex via somatic afferent nerves. Cerebral cortex in turn stimulates the respiratory centres to produce hyperventilation.

Respiration helps to maintain body temperature, as some amount of heat is lost in the expired air. In dogs panting is one of the major mechanisms of thermoregulation.

CHEMICAL REGULATION OF RESPIRATION

The chemical factors regulating respiration are pCO_2, pO_2 and pH of blood. These factors influence respiration in such a way that their own blood levels are maintained constant. The chemical mechanism of regulation operates through chemoreceptors.

Chemoreceptors

Chemoreceptors are the sensory nerve endings, which are highly sensitive to changes in pCO_2, pO_2 and pH of blood. These are of three types:

- Peripheral chemoreceptors,
- Central chemoreceptors, and
- Pulmonary and myocardial chemoreceptors.

Peripheral Chemoreceptors

Location. Peripheral chemoreceptors include the carotid and aortic bodies (Fig. 5.6-8).

- *Carotid body* is located on either side near the bifurcation of common carotid artery.
- *Aortic bodies,* two or more in number, are located near the arch of aorta.

Structure. Each carotid and aortic body consists of:

Capsule surrounding each carotid and aortic body is very thin.

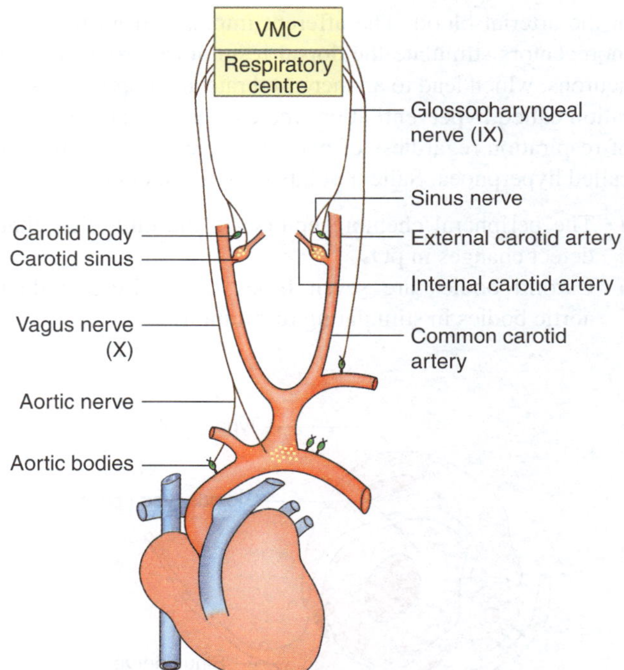

FIGURE 5.6-8 Location of carotid and aortic bodies (peripheral chemoreceptors).

Sinusoidal large capillaries present below the capsule surround the main mass of each body.

Epithelial Cells. The main mass of the body consists of islands of epithelial cells which are of two types: type I and type II (Fig. 5.6-9):

• ***Type I or Glomus Cells*** are similar to chromaffin cells of the adrenal glands. These cells have densecore granules containing catecholamines (probably dopamine). Unmyelinated nerve endings are closely applied to these cells, these nerve endings are cup shaped and have dopamine receptors (D_2) on them. When exposed to hypoxia, the type 1 cells release catecholamine which stimulates the D_2 receptors.

• ***Type II Cells*** which are probably glial cells are also closely applied to the type 1 cells.

• ***Nerve Fibres.*** Outside the capsule of each body, the nerve fibres acquire myelin sheath, they are only 2–5 μm in diameter and conduct at relatively low rate of 7–12 m/s. Afferent fibres from the carotid body join the sinus nerve, a branch of glossopharyngeal (IX) nerve and ultimately ascendes to medulla. Those from the aortic body join the aortic nerve branch of vagus (Xth cranial) nerve and ascend to medulla.

Blood Flow to each carotid and aortic body is highest in the body (2000 ml/100 gm/min). Therefore, the O_2 needs of these cells can be met largely by dissolved O_2 only.

Functions. The peripheral chemoreceptors respond to lowered pO_2 increased pCO_2 and increased H^+ concentration in the arterial blood. The afferent impulses from the chemoreceptors stimulate the dorsal respiratory group (DRG) neurons, which lead to an increased rate and depth of respiration called hyperventilation. Increase in the rate or depth of respiration regardless of patients subjective sensation is called hyperpnoea. Salient points of their functions are:

- The peripheral chemoreceptors are the only sites that detect changes in pO_2.
- Carotid bodies are seven times more effective than aortic bodies in stimulating respiration.

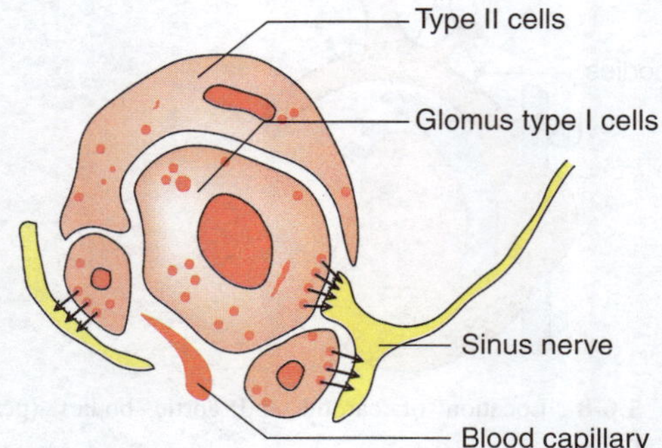

FIGURE 5.6-9 Histological structure of carotid body.

- Carotid bodies increase both rate and depth of respiration, while aortic bodies increase only the frequency of respiration with small increase in ventilation.

Mechanism of Chemoreceptors Stimulation by Hypoxia and Oxygen Transduction in Glomus Cells. The peripheral chemoreceptors are stimulated by the release of neurotransmitter by glomus cells. Oxygen transduction is the process by which changes in the arterial pO_2 results in proportionate changes in the frequency of action potential discharge. The sequence of events is:

- Hypoxia leads to decrease in activity of oxygen-sensitive K^+ channels present in the cell membrane of glomus cells leading to decrease in the K^+ efflux depending upon the level of pO_2.
- Thus, the glomus cells get depolarized in proportion to the fall in arterial pO_2.
- Depolarization of the glomus cells opens up the L-type Ca^{2+} channels in the glomus cell membrane leading to increase in Ca^{2+} influx.
- The Ca^{2+} influx triggers the release of neurotransmitter which stimulates the afferent nerve endings.

Factors Affecting Peripheral Chemoreceptors Stimulation

i. O_2 Tension Versus O_2 Content. The peripheral chemoreceptors monitor the dissolved O_2, i.e. pO_2, rather than its total content. They are stimulated when pO_2 falls below 60 mmHg. Therefore, they respond to various types of hypoxia differently as:

- *Hypoxic hypoxia* in which arterial pO_2 is reduced stimulates peripheral chemoreceptors.
- *Histotoxic hypoxia* in which there is reduced utilization of O_2 by the tissue cells including glomus cells also stimulates chemoreceptors.
- *Anaemic hypoxia,* methaemoglobinemia or carbon monoxide poisoning do not stimulate the peripheral chemoreceptors, because under these conditions, though the total content of O_2 may be low, but the O_2 tension, which is determined by the amount of dissolved O_2, remains normal.
- *Vascular stasis,* in which the amount of O_2 delivered to receptors per unit of time is decreased, which leads to chemoreceptor stimulation.
- *Drugs* such as cyanide, nicotine and lobeline, prevent O_2 utilization at the tissue level, stimulate peripheral chemoreceptors.

ii. Elevated pCO_2. Elevated pCO_2 (by 10 mmHg) also stimulates the peripheral chemoreceptors, but the major effect of CO_2 is on the central chemoreceptors.

iii. H^+ Concentration when increased in the blood (decreased pH by 0.1 unit) stimulates the peripheral chemoreceptors.

iv. Increase in Plasma K^+ Levels may stimulate the peripheral chemoreceptors even in the absence of hypoxia. Increase in plasma K^+ levels during exercise contributes to exercise induced hyperventilation.

v. Asphyxia, i.e. combination of O_2 lack plus CO_2 excess in blood stimulate peripheral chemoreceptors.

Effects of Stimulation of Peripheral Chemoreceptors

- They regulate the respiration from breath to breath and their stimulation increases the rate and depth of respiration.
- They also cause increase in blood pressure and tachycardia.
- About 15–20% of resting respiratory drive is due to stimulatory effect of CO_2 on peripheral chemoreceptors.

Central Chemoreceptors

Location. Central chemoreceptors are the cells (neurons) that lie just beneath the ventral surface of the medulla oblongata and are therefore also called medullary receptors (Fig. 5.6-10).

Innervation. Nerves from the neurons forming central chemoreceptors project directly over to the respiratory centres which are located slightly deeper to central chemoreceptors.

Stimulation Characteristics of central chemoreceptors are:

- They respond to H^+ concentration in the surrounding interstitial fluid and CSF.
- The magnitude of stimulation is directly proportional to the local H^+ concentration, which in turn parallels arterial pCO_2.
- *Mechanism by which increase in CO_2 concentration affects central chemoreceptors.* CO_2 readily crosses the blood–brain barrier, because it is a small, very soluble, uncharged molecule. In the CSF, CO_2 combines with water to form H_2CO_3 which dissociates into H^+ and HCO^-_3 ions. The increase in H^+ concentration of CSF and interstitial fluid stimulates the central chemo-receptors, whereas a decrease in the H^+ concentration inhibits respiration. It is important to note that the blood–brain barrier does not allow the charged ions (e.g. H^+, HCO_3^- etc.) to cross through readily. Because of this reason if the arterial pCO_2 is kept constant experimentally a decrease in arterial pH (raised H^+ concentration) fails to stimulate central chemoreceptors.
- *Increase in pCO_2 of CSF is more effective in stimulating central chemoreceptors than increased pCO_2 in interstitial fluid of brain.* As mentioned above actual stimulus for central chemoreceptors is the increased H^+ concentration. In CSF, there are no buffers (proteins) to buffer the H^+ ions formed from H_2CO_3. The interstitial fluid is surrounded by cells having proteins to act as buffers. Therefore, for the same change in CO_2 concentration, H^+ concentration of CSF is more than that of interstitial fluid; thus increased pCO_2 of CSF is more important stimulus.
- Central chemoreceptors are not stimulated by hypoxia, rather like any other cell, they are depressed by hypoxia.
- Central chemoreceptors are also inhibited by anaesthesia, cyanide and during sleep.

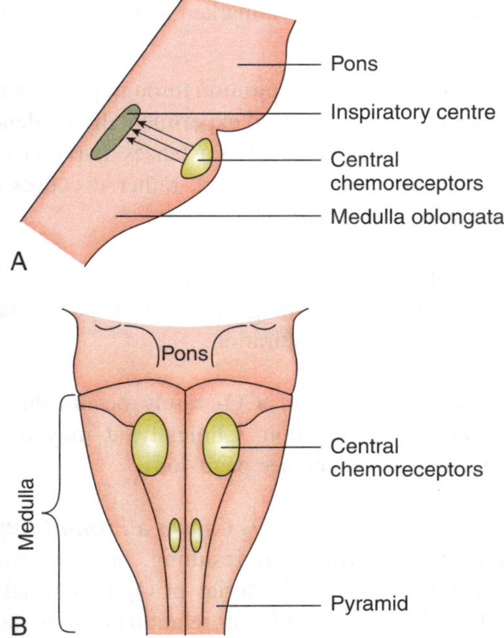

FIGURE 5.6-10 Location of central chemoreceptors in medulla: **(A)** lateral view and **(B)** front view.

Effects of Stimulation of central chemoreceptors are:

- The central chemoreceptors regulate the respiration from minute to minute. Their stimulation leads to increase in the rate and depth of respiration.
- It is important to note that about 80–85% of the resting respiratory drive is due to stimulatory effect of CO_2 on the central chemoreceptors. While peripheral chemoreceptors provide only 15–20% of initial drive to increase respiration.

Pulmonary and Myocardial Chemoreceptors

Location. Pulmonary and myocardial chemoreceptors are located in the pulmonary and coronary blood vessels, respectively.

Innervation. These are innervated by the vagus (Xth cranial) nerve.

Stimulation Characteristics and Effects of these receptors are:

- ***Pulmonary Chemoreceptors*** are stimulated by injection of veratridine or nicotine into pulmonary circulation and produce the so-called *pulmonary chemoreceptor reflex,* which is characterized by bradycardia, hypotension and apnoea followed by tachypnoea (rapid shallow breathing). Physiological role of this reflex is not established. It occurs in pathological states like pulmonary congestion or embolism.

• ***Myocardial Chemoreceptors*** are similarly stimulated when these agents are injected into coronaries supplying the left ventricle and produce the so-called *coronary chemoreflex* or *Bezold-Jarisch reflex* having features similar to pulmonary chemoreflex. *Physiological role* of this reflex is not established. It is known to occur after myocardial infarction (see page 345).

Effect of pO_2, pCO_2 and H^+ Concentration on Respiration

- The pO_2, pCO_2 and H^+ concentration influence the respiration by their effects on chemoreceptors.
- The peripheral and central chemoreceptors work in unison to bring about increased ventilation in response to a rise in pCO_2, rise in H^+ concentration or a fall in arterial pO_2. Of the three, hypercapnia provides the strongest respiratory drive.
- Chemical regulation of breathing ensures that the arterial pCO_2 is kept constant at normal value of 40 mmHg, arterial pO_2 is not allowed to fall below 60 mmHg and changes in blood pH are opposed.
- Denervation or removal of carotid chemoreceptors produces about 40% decrease in response to hypercapnia as well as H^+ concentration and complete abolition of response to drop in pO_2. The predominant effect of hypoxia after denervation of the carotid bodies is a direct depression of the respiratory centre.

With these introductory remarks, effect of each chemical factor on respiration will be discussed followed by the interaction of chemical factors in regulation of respiration.

Effect of Hypoxia on Respiration

The Normal Arterial pO_2 is 100 mmHg, which may fall in many conditions (see page 459), producing the so-called hypoxic hypoxia.

A Decrease in Arterial pO_2 is the most potent stimulus for the peripheral chemoreceptors; consequently, the rate of discharge in the peripheral chemoreceptors begins to increase.

When the Arterial pO_2 Levels Falls between 100 and 60 mmHg not much effect is produced on ventilation. However, a marked increase in pulmonary ventilation occurs when the pO_2 falls below 60 mmHg (Fig. 5.6-11). This can be explained as:

At pO_2 Levels from 100 to 60 mmHg, though there is significant increase in the afferent nerve discharge from the peripheral chemoreceptors, however, pulmonary ventilation does not increase significantly because of following two reasons:

• ***Breaking Effect of CO_2*** When decrease in pO_2 of arterial blood stimulates ventilation, increased ventilation causes washing out of CO_2. This leads to decrease in pCO_2 of blood which inhibits the respiration through its effect on central chemoreceptors. It opposes and neutralizes the effect of decreased pO_2 and thus there is no marked effect on ventilation. This phenomenon is called breaking effect of CO_2.

This fact can be confirmed experimentally by holding the pCO_2 constant at 40 mmHg and decreasing arterial pO_2 simultaneously. Under these conditions hyperventilation is observed even pO_2 between 100 and 60 mmHg.

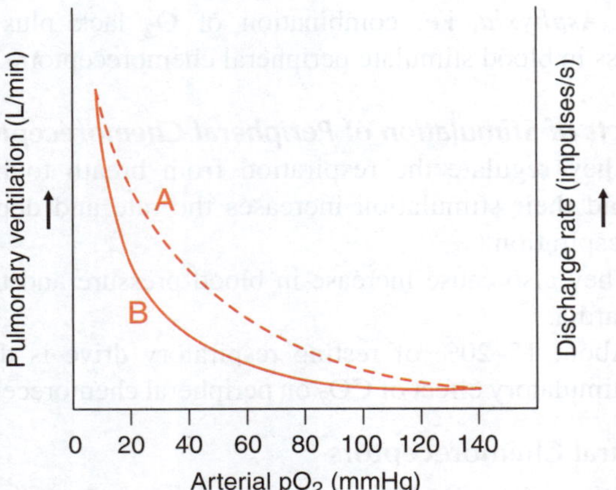

FIGURE 5.6-11 Relationship of pO_2 with sinus nerve discharge rate (A) and pulmonary ventilation (B).

- Due to hypoxia, the amount of deoxyhaemoglobin is increased which is a weaker acid as compared to oxyhaemoglobin. This results in mild decrease in H^+ concentration of blood which tends to nullify the hypoxic drive on pulmonary ventilation.

At pO_2 Levels Below 60 mmHg, the stimulation of peripheral chemoreceptors is so strong that it overrides the inhibitory effects of decreased arterial pCO_2 and decreased H^+ concentration and produces a marked increase in pulmonary ventilation.

- Hypoxia stimulating respiration through peripheral chemoreceptors can be proved experimentally by denervating them. Under such circumstances hypoxia cannot increase pulmonary ventilation, rather it causes direct depression of the respiratory centre.

Effect of Hypercapnia on Respiration

Normal pCO_2 is 40 mmHg, which is kept constant by chemical regulation of respiration.

Hypercapnia, i.e. rise in pCO_2 rarely occurs due to an increase in CO_2 production. Clinically, it may occur in restrictive lung disorders (see page 468).

An Increase in Arterial pCO_2 Causes a Prompt Increase in Pulmonary Ventilation resulting in CO_2 washout and a near restoration of arterial pCO_2 to normal level (40 mmHg). There exists a linear relation between increase in arterial pCO_2 and increase in pulmonary ventilation. This can be demonstrated experimentally by breathing from a bag of air with different concentration of CO_2, varying from 4 to 7% (Fig. 5.6-12).

CO_2 Increases Pulmonary Ventilation Mainly by Stimulating the Central Chemoreceptors. This can be demonstrated experimentally by removing the peripheral chemoreceptors and then making the person to breathe from a bag of air with different concentration of CO_2. The same effect is obtained as above (Fig. 5.6-12).

CO_2 is Capable of Increasing the Pulmonary Ventilation by Stimulating the Peripheral Chemoreceptors as Well. When central chemoreceptors are depressed by anaesthesia, CO_2 increases respiration through stimulation of peripheral chemoreceptors.

CO_2 Acts as a Main Regulator of Respiration because of following facts:

- It has a direct effect on respiratory centre through the central chemoreceptors.
- It can cross the blood–brain or blood–CSF barrier easily; therefore, CO_2 concentration in CSF and in interstitial fluid of brain increases soon after the increase in concentration of CO_2 in the blood.
- CO_2 has a very strong breaking effect on the action of either decreased pO_2 or pH,
- pO_2 or pH does not have very strong breaking effect on the action of increased CO_2 on ventilation (Fig. 5.6-12).

Carbon Dioxide Narcosis. It develops when arterial pCO_2 increases above 50 mmHg. Accumulation of such a large amount of CO_2 (hypercapnia) in the body depresses the CNS, including respiratory centres producing headache, confusion, convulsions and finally coma and death may occur.

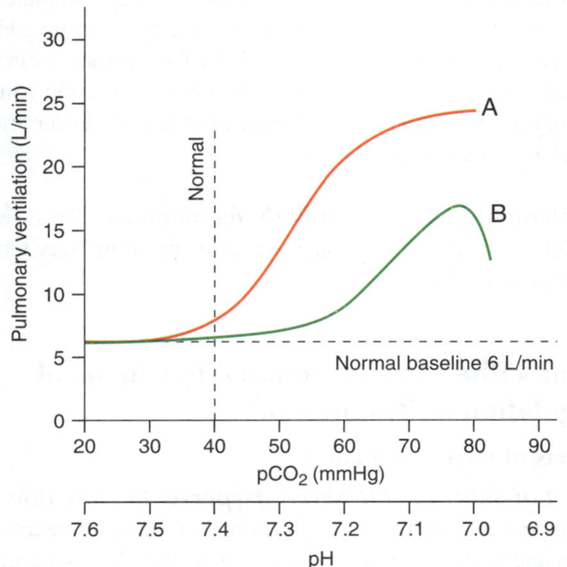

FIGURE 5.6-12 Effect of increase in **(A)** arterial pCO_2 and **(B)** decreased pH on pulmonary ventilation.

Causes. Carbon dioxide narcosis may occur in patients with prolonged severe emphysema or due to accidental inhalation of CO_2 (in breweries, refrigeration plants, etc). Experimentally, it can be produced by making the person to inhale the air containing more than 7% CO_2. When the inspired air pCO_2 approaches close to the alveolar pCO_2, as a result elimination of CO_2 becomes difficult which causes alveolar and arterial pCO_2 to rise abruptly in spite of the hyperventilation.

Important Note

Clinical significance. Whenever CO_2 is to be used to stimulate respiration in a comatose patient with respiratory depressions it is always advisable to estimate the CO_2 content of blood, to avoid occurrence of death from carbon dioxide narcosis.

Effect of Arterial pH on Respiration

i. Increased H^+ Concentration (metabolic acidosis) produces prolonged respiratory centre stimulation via peripheral chemoreceptors, leading to a decrease in the arterial pCO_2 by elimination of larger amounts of CO_2, producing compensatory fall in blood H^+ concentration. The related aspects of renal correction of acid–base balance are discussed in Chapter 12.3 page 1227.

Causes of metabolic acidosis, i.e. decrease in HCO^-_3 concentration in blood secondary to increase in H^+ concentration of blood are:

- Diabetic ketoacidosis (hyperventilation occurring in this condition is called *Kussmaul breathing).*
- Renal failure (when kidney fails to excrete their normal quota of H^+).
- Due to accumulation of lactic acid in severe muscular exercise.
- Ketoacidosis in starvation and
- Infantile diarrhoea associated with loss of $NaHCO_3$.

ii. Decreased H^+ concentration (metabolic alkalosis) depresses respiratory centre via peripheral chemoreceptors, leading to retention of CO_2 and an increase in arterial pCO_2. The secondary changes in arterial pCO_2 compensate for the primary metabolic defects and help to restore H^+ concentration of blood.

Common Causes of metabolic alkalosis, i.e. increase in HCO^-_3 concentration in blood secondary to decreased H^+ concentration in blood: excessive vomiting with loss of HCl from the body.

Respiratory acidosis and alkalosis. It may be added here that primary changes in the pulmonary ventilation also effect the pH of blood causing respiratory acidosis or alkalosis.

iii. Primary Pulmonary Hypoventilation may lead to elevation of arterial pCO_2 (hypercapnia) producing the so-called *respiratory acidosis.*

Causes of hypercapnia responsible for respiratory acidosis are:

- Respiratory depression due to narcotic poisoning or cerebral diseases.
- Neuromuscular disorders with impaired breathing.
- Chronic obstructive pulmonary disease such as emphysema in which effective alveolar ventilation is decreased due to ventilation–perfusion mismatch.

Compensatory Mechanism through chemoreceptors produces hyperventilation, washes out CO_2 and tries to restore arterial pCO_2.

iv. Primary Pulmonary Hyperventilation may cause a decrease in the arterial pCO_2 producing the so-called *respiratory alkalosis.*

Causes of respiratory alkalosis are:

- Voluntary hyperventilation,
- Excessive artificial respiration,
- Compulsive hyperventilation in hysteric patients and
- Chronic O_2 lack (hypoxia) producing CO_2 wash due to hyperventilation, e.g. as seen in high altitude hypoxia.

Signs and Symptoms

- *Hypocapnia* produced causes faintness and paraesthesias due to reduction of cerebral blood flow.
- *Respiratory alkalosis* produced causes lowering of ionized Ca^{2+} in plasma and the appearance of symptoms of tetany, e.g. carpopedal spasm.

Compensatory mechanism through chemoreceptors slows down the respiration, leading to retention of CO_2, which in turn restores H^+ concentration of blood towards normal.

Interaction of pO_2, pCO_2 and pH in Regulation of Respiration

In the above discussion, we have seen that each of hypoxia, increased pCO_2 and acidosis individually cause an increase in the respiration. In many physiological or clinical situations more than one factor may be present. Their interaction is summarized here:

1. Interaction of pCO_2 and pO_2 ***Hypoxia*** sensitizes the respiratory mechanism to excess of CO_2 or H^+ concentration, therefore increased pCO_2 and H^+ concentration produce a much greater effect (Fig. 5.6-13.).

When pCO_2 is held constant at a level 2–3 mm of Hg above normal (i.e. in the presence of hypercapnic drive) there is an inverse relationship between ventilation and alveolar pO_2, even in the 90–110 mmHg range (Fig. 5.6-14). ***When pCO_2 is held constant at a level 2–3 mmHg below normal,*** (i.e. in the absence of CO_2 related drive), a fall in pO_2 level between 110 and 60 mmHg does not produce any effect on ventilation. However, a marked increase in pulmonary ventilation occurs when pO_2 falls below 60 mmHg (Fig. 5.6-14).

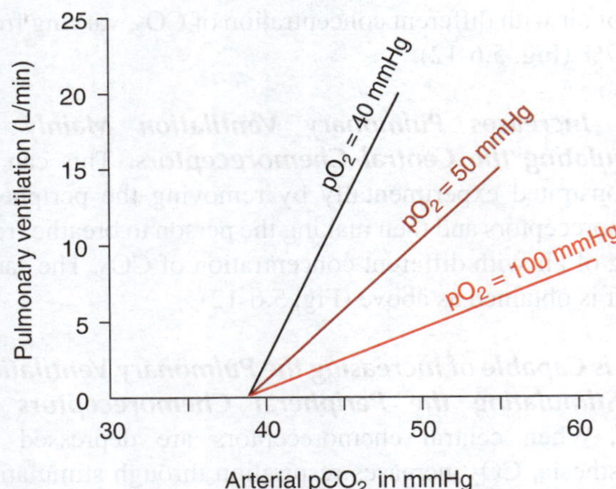

FIGURE 5.6-13 Interaction of arterial pO_2 and pCO_2 depicting effect of pCO_2 on pulmonary ventilation at different levels of pO_2.

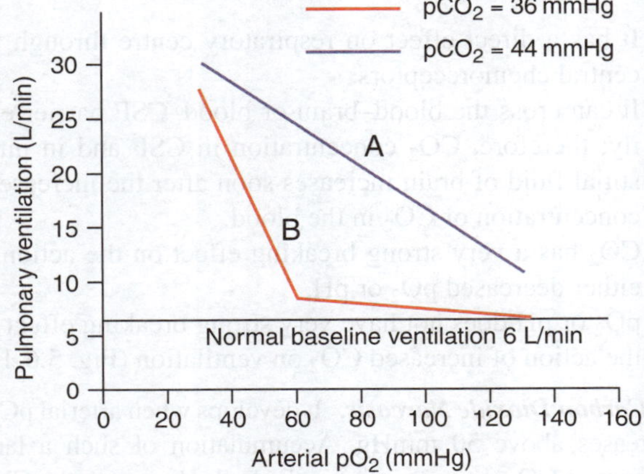

FIGURE 5.6-14 Effect of hypoxia (pO_2) on pulmonary ventilation with arterial pCO_2 being kept (**A**) 2–3 mm above normal and (**B**) 2–3 mm below normal.

2. Interaction of pH and CO_2 Response The stimulatory effects of H+ concentration and CO_2 on respiration are additive, i.e. a fall in pH (acidosis) shifts the CO_2 response curve to left without change in slope. In other words, the same amount of respiratory stimulation is produced by lower arterial pCO_2 levels (Fig. 5.6-15).

3. Interaction of CO_2 and Body Temperature The effect of CO_2 on respiration increases with increase in body temperature (Fig. 5.6-16).

Some Other Aspects Related to Chemical Regulation of Respiration

Effects of Hyperventilation

Effect of Short Lasting Severe Hyperventilation Effects of hyperventilation on respiration can be demonstrated experimentally by making a person to breathe as rapidly and as deeply as possible for him for one to two minutes and

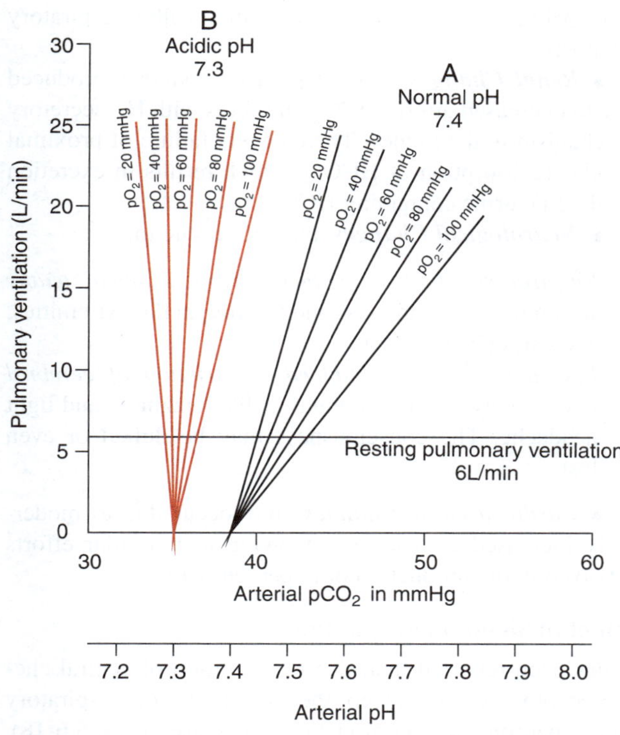

FIGURE 5.6-15 Effect on CO_2 response curve of varying amount of hypoxia and pH.

FIGURE 5.6-16 Effect of temperature on CO_2 response curve.

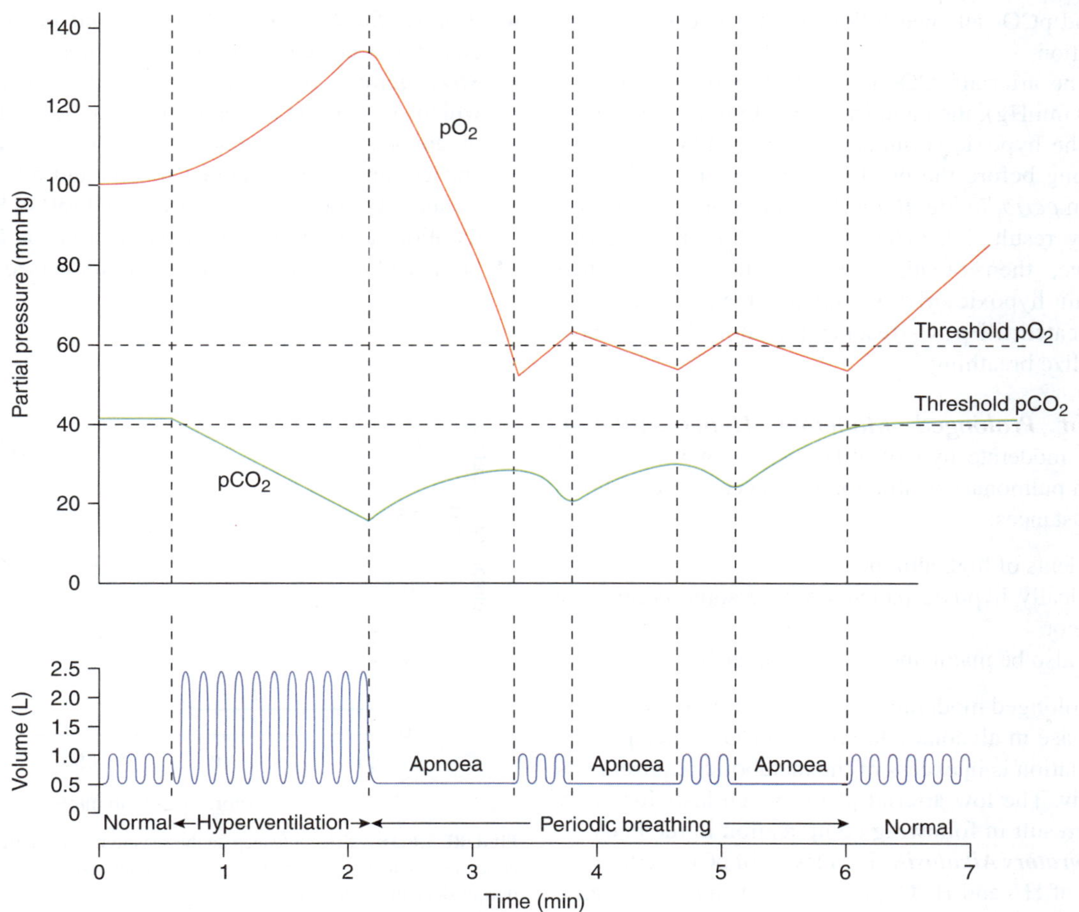

FIGURE 5.6-17 Effect of hyperventilation on arterial pO_2, pCO_2 and respiration.Note correlation between pCO_2, pO_2 and periods of hyperventilation, apnoea and periodic breathing and normal breathing.

then stop. The voluntary hyperventilation may show following effects (Fig. 5.6-17):

i. Effects on Respiration. After a period of hyperventilation, any of the following pattern of respiration may be seen for a small period before normal respiration is restored:

- *Hypoventilation* for a prolonged period is seen in most of the individuals.
- *Apnoea,* i.e. complete cessation of breathing for 1–2 minutes may occur in some individuals.
- *Periodic breathing (Cheyne-Stokes breathing),* i.e. alternate phases of apnoea and breathing may occur for sometime in a few individuals.

ii. Effects on Arterial pCO_2 and pO_2 and Their Correlation with Effect on Respiration (Fig. 5.6-17)

- Arterial pO_2 may go as high as 150 mmHg and pCO_2 as low as 15 mmHg after a period of voluntary hyperventilation.
- Apnoea occurring in some individuals at the end of hyperventilation seems to be related to lack of CO_2, because it does not occur if the person hyperventilates a gas mixture containing 5% CO_2 and 20% oxygen.
- During phase of apnoea, due to metabolism of body, there occurs a decline in arterial pO_2 and an increase in pCO_2. Depending upon the interaction between levels of pO_2 and pCO_2 attained following effects can occur on respiration.
  - If the arterial pCO_2 is reached at threshold level (40 mmHg), then a normal breathing is resumed,
  - If the hypoxic stimulus (decreased pO_2) becomes strong before the pCO_2 reaches a threshold level, then *periodic breathing* (Cheyne-Stokes breathing) may result, i.e. a few breaths eliminate hypoxic drive, then breathing stops and restarts when again hypoxic drive stimulates it. Such cycles are repeated till pCO_2 reaches threshold level to normalize breathing.

Effects of Prolonged Moderate Hyperventilation

Prolonged moderate hyperventilation, i.e. two to fivefold increase in pulmonary ventilation may occur under following circumstances:

- In residents of high altitude,
- In clinically hypoxic patients due to some pulmonary disease or
- It may also be maintained even voluntarily.

The prolonged moderate hyperventilation is associated with decrease in alveolar and arterial pCO_2, since pulmonary ventilation is in excess of the metabolic requirements of the body. The low arterial pCO_2 which lasts for many days may result in following complication in the body:

• ***Respiratory Alkalosis.*** Low levels of pCO_2 reduce the formation of H^+ and HCO^-_3 in the blood causing increase in its pH to 7.55 or even 7.6, a condition called respiratory alkalosis.

• ***Renal Changes.*** The respiratory alkalosis produced due to decreased arterial pCO_2 interferes with H^+ secretory mechanism in the kidney. There occurs failure of proximal tubular reabsorption of HCO^-_3, which results in excretion of alkaline urine containing HCO^-_3.

• ***Neurological Changes*** may occur due to:

- *Respiratory alkalosis induced hypocalcaemic tetany* which include numbness and tingling in the extremities, and carpopedal spasm.
- *Low arterial pCO_2 induced constriction of cerebral vessels* may produce symptoms like dizziness and light headache. The consciousness may be dulled or even lost.

• ***Cardiovascular Changes*** may occur due to moderately increased cardiac output owing to muscular efforts involved in the production of hyperventilation.

Effect of Sleep on Respiration

It has been reported that, due to inhibition of central chemoreceptors during sleep the sensitivity of respiratory centre neurons to arterial pCO_2 is decreased (Fig. 5.6-18). It may cause following effects:

- ***Apnoea for brief period (10 second duration)*** is of common occurrence during sleep in normal individuals.
- ***Sleep apnoea syndrome*** is a serious clinical problem which may occur in some individuals. Such episodes of apnoea are more common in obese male snorers and children with enlarged tonsils and adenoids. The frequent episodes of more prolonged (30 to 90 seconds duration) apnoea many produce hypoxic damage to the brain leading to intellectual deterioration (see page 457).

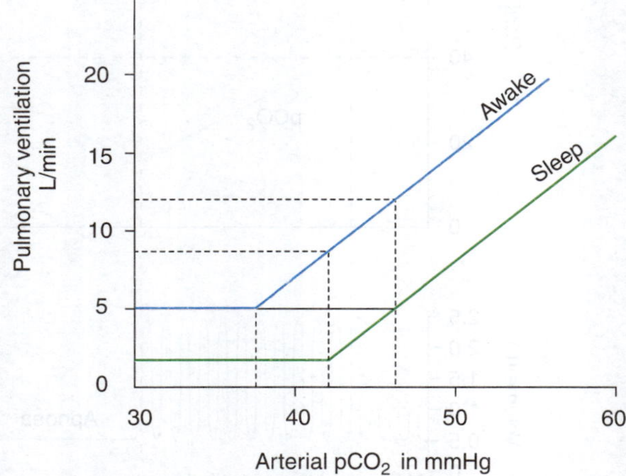

FIGURE 5.6-18 Effect of sleep on the sensitivity of respiratory neurons. Note the amount of pulmonary ventilation of the same level of pCO_2 is less during sleep than during awakening.

Chapter 5.7

Respiration: Applied Aspects

INTRODUCTION

Applied respiratory physiology forms a link between the basics of respiration and clinical manifestations of respiratory diseases. The pulmonary function tests performed to diagnose respiratory disorders require an understanding of basic physiological principles of respiration and gas exchange. In fact, respiratory diseases cannot be managed satisfactorily without a proper understanding of the basic and applied aspects of respiratory physiology. This chapter is concerned with some of the important applied aspects of respiration which include:

- Respiratory adjustments to stresses in health,
- Disturbances of respiration,
- Artificial respiration,
- Pulmonary function tests.

RESPIRATORY ADJUSTMENTS TO STRESSES IN HEALTH

Respiratory adjustments to stresses in health illustrate the integrated operation of the respiratory regulatory mechanisms. The stresses faced by respiration requiring adjustments in day-to-day life include:

1. Respiratory Adjustments during Exercise. Exercise is the most frequently faced stress in day-to-day life. Since during exercise, many complex adjustments of muscular blood flow, metabolism, respiration, circulation and temperature are required, so they have been comprehensively discussed in Chapter on 'Physiology of Exercise' (page 1207).

2. Respiratory Adjustments at High Altitude. At high altitude barometric pressure is low and so the partial pressure of O_2 is also low, however, the amount of O_2 in the atmosphere is same as it is at the sea level. When a person is exposed to high altitude particularly by rapid ascent, the different systems of the body cannot cope with the lowered O_2 tension and the effects of hypoxia start. Respiratory adjustments are thus a part of changes in the body at high attitude, so these have been discussed comprehensively under the title '*Physiology of high altitude*' (see page 1219).

3. Respiratory Adjustments to High Atmospheric Pressure. form a part of physiological problems faced by

the body while going under the sea and have been discussed comprehensively under the title *Deep sea physiology* (see page 1223).

4. Respiratory Adjustments on Exposure to Cold and Heat. have been discussed under the title *Effects of exposure to heat and cold on the body* (see page 1246).

5. Respiratory Adjustments at Birth. Birth is the most traumatic event that the respiratory system must withstand during the entire life span of an individual. These form a part of *Fetal physiology* and that have been discussed in the concerned chapter at page 1254.

Note. Students are advised to go through the respiratory changes occurring during the above-mentioned situations along with the study of respiratory system for better understanding.

DISTURBANCES OF RESPIRATION

From the physiological viewpoint, disturbances of respiration can be discussed under following headings:

- Abnormal respiratory patterns,
- Disturbances related to respiratory gases and
- Pulmonary diseases: pathophysiological aspects.

Abnormal Respiratory Patterns

Eupnoea refers to normal respiratory pattern, which implies a normal rate, rhythm and depth of respiration. Various abnormal respiratory patterns (Fig. 5.7-1) can be produced by changes in the environment or diseases affecting the respiratory system, cardiovascular system, or brain. The terms used for the altered pattern of respiration are:

- *Tachypnoea* refers to increase in the rate of respiration
- *Bradypnoea* means decrease in the rate of respiration.
- *Polypnoea* is used to denote the rapid but shallow breathing resembling panting in dogs. In this, the rate of respiration is increased but the force does not change significantly.
- *Apnoea* refers to temporary cessation of breathing.
- *Hypoventilation* term is used to describe a decrease in rate and force of respiration.
- *Hyperventilation* refers to increase in rate as well as force of respiration.
- *Hyperpnoea* signifies a marked increase in pulmonary ventilation due to increase in rate and/or force of respiration.
- *Dyspnoea.* When hyperpnoea involves 4–5 fold increase in pulmonary ventilation, an unpleasant sensation or discomfort is felt. This type of respiration is called dyspnoea.
- *Periodic breathing* refers to a respiratory pattern characterized by alternate periods of respiratory activity and apnoea. Some of the abnormal respiratory patterns are discussed in detail.

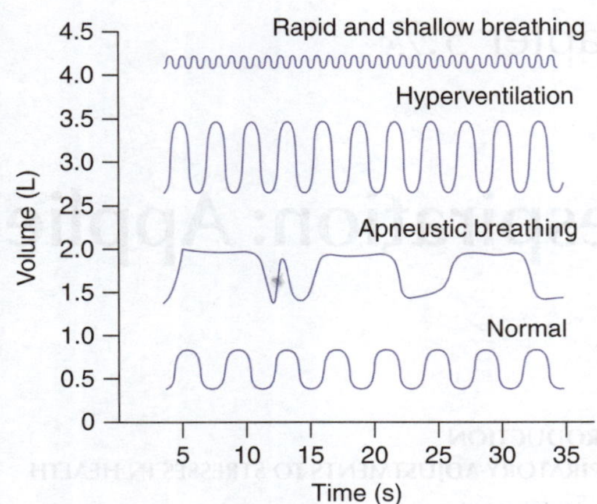

FIGURE 5.7-1 Various abnormal respiratory patterns.

Apnoea

Apnoea refers to temporary cessation of breathing. Depending upon the cause, apnoea may be of following types:

1. Voluntary Apnoea refers to temporary arrest of breathing due to voluntary control of respiration. It is also called breath-holding. The breath-holding time or apnoea time during which breathing can be witheld voluntarily is about 40–60 seconds in a normal person, after a deep inspiration (for details see page 445).

Breaking point is the point at which breathing can no longer be voluntarily inhibited. At this point, chemical regulation overcomes the neural regulation. The breaking point is due to an increased arterial pCO_2 and a decreased pO_2.

2. Apnoea after Hyperventilation occurs due to reduced stimulation of respiratory centre owing to CO_2 wash caused by hyperventilation (for details see page 454).

3. Deglutition Apnoea occurs reflexly during swallowing (about 0.5 second). During the pharyngeal stage of swallowing, the fluid or food stimulates the sensory nerve endings (5th, 9th and 10th cranial nerves) around the pharynx. Nerve impulses from these irritant receptors, via the swallowing centres specifically inhibit the respiratory centre, stopping the breathing at any point of the cycle (deglutition apnoea). Simultaneously, there is closure of glottis (the opening between vocal cords). Both these effects prevent aspiration of fluid or food into the lungs (also see page 585).

4. Breath-Holding Attacks are attacks of brief period of apnoea which occur in infants and young children, and are generally precipitated by emotional distress, such as fright, frustration, pain or anxiety. The child starts to cry, and then suddenly holds his/her breath, becomes limp or stiff, and may become blue and lose consciousness. The attacks last briefly and recovery is rapid and complete. In some cases, there may be a rigid phase followed by tonic and clonic convulsions. These attacks are harmless and stop by the age of three years; they are not considered epileptic in origin.

5. Vagal Apnoea can be produced experimentally in animals by stimulation of vagus nerve. Stimulation of vagus nerve produces apnoea by inhibiting the inspiratory centre.

6. Adrenaline Apnoea occurs after injection of high doses of adrenaline (see page 447).

7. Sleep Apnoea refers to cessation of breathing for a brief period (10 second) during sleep in normal individuals. It has been related to reduced sensitivity of respiratory centre neurons to arterial pCO_2 owing to inhibition of central chemoreceptors.

Sleep Apnoea Syndrome has been recognized as a serious clinical problem or disorders of respiratory control that affects middle-aged and elderly men. It may occur in two forms:

- ***Obstructive sleep apnoea*** occurs when inspiration is prevented by transient blockage of the airway due to collapse of hypopharynx as a result of loss of tone of pharyngeal muscles which prevent airflow though strong contractions of inspiratory muscles occur (Fig. 5.7-2). Partial airway obstruction causes snoring. The association of sleep apnoea with extreme obesity is referred to as the *pickwickian syndrome*.
- ***Nonobstructive (central) sleep apnoea*** refers to complete stoppage of rhythmic activity from respiratory centres. Obviously, during apnoea there is no respiratory muscle contraction (Fig. 5.7-2). It is supposed to result from decreased chemoreceptor sensitivity to O_2 and CO_2. Central sleep apnoea has been proposed as one of the many possible causes of *sudden infant death syndrome*.

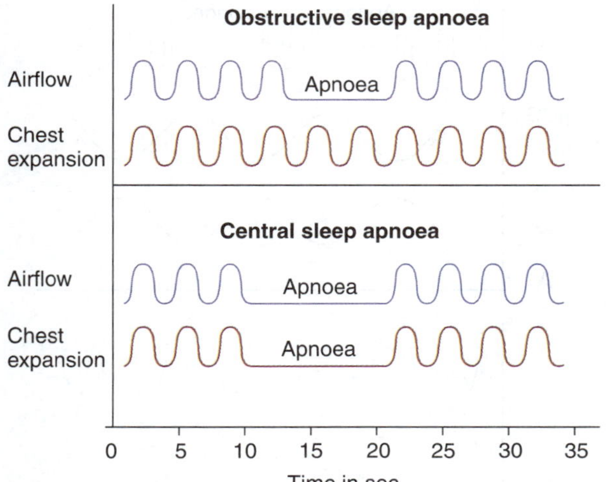

FIGURE 5.7-2 Record of air flow and chest movements in patients with obstructive and central sleep apnoea.

Hypoventilation

Hypoventilation is used to describe a decrease in rate and force of respiration. Thus, in hypoventilation the amount of air moving in and out of lungs is reduced.

Causes of hypoventilation are:

- Depression of respiratory centres by some drugs
- Partial paralysis of respiratory muscles.

Effects. Hypoventilation leads on to hypoxia and hypercapnia which result in increase in rate and force of respiration and patient may develop dyspnoea.

Hyperventilation

Hyperventilation refers to increase in rate as well as force of respiration. Thus, in hyperventilation the amount of air moving in and out of lungs is increased; that is why it is also called increased pulmonary ventilation or overventilation.

Causes of hyperventilation are:

- During exercise due to stimulation of respiratory centres by increased pCO_2
- Voluntary hyperventilation
- Secondary to hypoxia.

Effects of hyperventilation on respiration and other systems of the body are described on page 452.

Dyspnoea

Dyspnoea literally means distressed breathing. Increased respiration without discomfort is called *hyperpnoea.* One is not aware of one's respiration till resting pulmonary ventilation becomes more than double. When hyperpnoea involves four-Fivefold increase in pulmonary ventilation, an unpleasant sensation or discomfort is felt. This type of respiration is called dyspnoea. The word 'air-hunger' is used as synonym to dyspnoea in general language. Thus, desire for air or mental anguish associated with inability to ventilate enough to satisfy the air demand is the essence of dyspnoea.

Dyspnoea point refers to the height of hyperpnoea at which dyspnoea appears.

Predisposing factors for dyspnoea include:

1. *Low vital capacity.* People with low vital capacity are more predisposed to get dyspnoea than those with normal or high vital capacity.
2. *Maximum ventilatory volume* (MVV). Patients with reduced MVV (maximum volume of air that can be taken in or given out per minute, normal value is 120 L/min) are more predisposed to get dyspnoea.
3. *Breathing reserve* (BR) is the difference between MVV and respiratory minute volume (RMV). RMV is the volume of air that is taken in or given out per minute (Normal $500 \times 12 = 6$L/min). Individuals with

increased RMV (also called pulmonary ventilation) by 4–5 times get dyspnoea. Individuals with less breathing reserve are more prone to get dyspnoea.

$$BR = MVV - RMV = 114 \text{ L/min}$$

Dyspnoeic index (DI) refers to breathing reserve percentage of MVV, i.e.

$$DI = \frac{BR \times 100}{MVV} = \frac{110 \times 100}{120} = 95\%$$

- Normal value of DI range from 70–95%
- Dyspnoea occurs when DI is <60%.

Causes of dyspnoea are:

- *Physiologically dyspnoea occurs* in severe muscular exercise
- *Pathalogical causes* include:
  - *Respiratory disorders* such as bronchial asthma, emphysema, pneumonia, pulmonary oedema and penumothorax.
  - *Cardiac failure:* It causes dyspnoea by the mechanism explained in Figure 5.7-3).

Important Note

It is important to note that patients with cardiac failure prefer to sit rather than lie down, because in lying position pulmonary congestion is increased which causes dyspnoea. Dyspnoea occurring in lying down position is called *orthopnoea.*

- *Metabolic disorders* causing dyspnoea are diabetic acidosis, uraemia, increased H^+ concentration. Metabolic acidosis causes dyspnoea by increasing pulmonary ventilation.

Periodic Breathing

Periodic breathing is characterized by alternate periods of respiratory activity and apnoea. It is of two types:

- Cheyne-Stokes respiration and
- Biot's breathing.

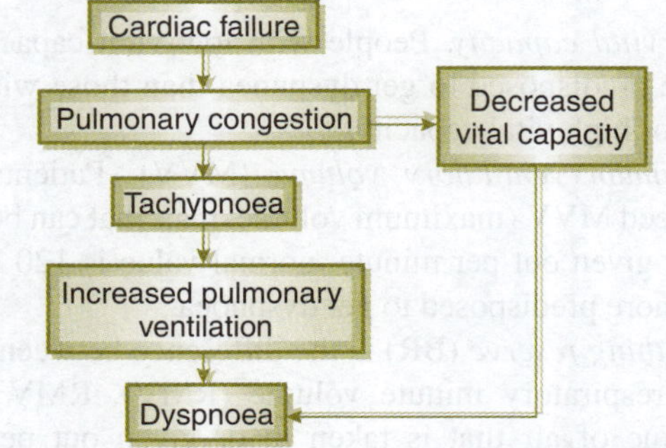

FIGURE 5.7-3 Cardiac failure causing dyspnoea: mechanism.

Cheyne-Stokes Respiration Cheyne-Stokes respiration is periodic type of breathing in which the alternate periods of respiratory activity and apnoea occur at regular intervals; and during the period of respiratory activity there is waxing and waning of tidal volume. The duration of one cycle is about one minute. The arterial pO_2 and pCO_2 fluctuate during each cycle. The pO_2 is lowest and the pCO_2 is highest at the end of apnoea (Fig. 5.7-4A).

Causes of Cheyne-Stokes respiration are:

1. ***Physiological causes*** include:
   - Voluntary hyperventilation,
   - High altitude and
   - During sleep in some normal individuals especially infants.
2. ***Pathological causes*** are:
   - Chronic heart failure, due to increased circulation time from lungs to brain,
   - Brain damage due to increased negative feedback gain in the respiratory centre,
   - Uraemia and
   - Poisoning by narcotics.

Mechanism of Development of Cheyne-Stokes Respiration in Three Most Important Conditions is Described

Voluntary Hyperventilation. Mechanism of development of Cheyne-Stokes breathing in hyperventilation has been described on page 454.

Heart Failure. Mechanism of development of Cheyne-Stokes breathing is summarized as:

- Left ventricular failure → Pulmonary congestion → Hypoxia → Stimulation of respiratory centres → Increased ventilation → Increased alveolar pO_2 and decreased pCO_2 → Decreased arterial pCO_2.

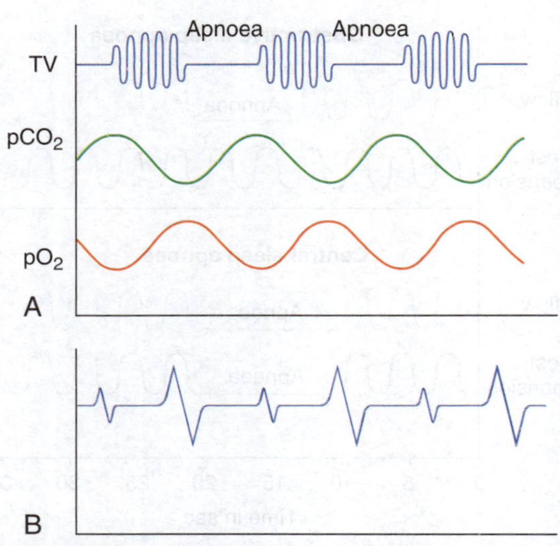

FIGURE 5.7-4 Periodic breathing: **(A)** Cheyne-Stokes breathing; and **(B)** Biot's breathing.

- As in heart failure *circulation time* is prolonged, so it takes longer than normal time for the blood with low pCO_2 to reach the brain and cause apnoea by inhibiting respiratory centre.
- Since in heart failure the pulmonary congestion continuously present, so hypoxia is maintained and the above-described cycle of apnoea followed respiratory activity keeps on repeating till the heart failure is treated or alveolar pCO_2 comes back to normal.

Brain Damage. In brain damage, when supramedullary inhibitory pathway is damaged the medullary (central) chemoreceptors become more sensitive to the action of CO_2 and produces Cheyne-Stokes breathing as:

- Increased sensitivity of central chemoreceptors to CO_2 → Hyperventilation → CO_2 washout → Apnoea → Accumulation of CO_2 → Increased pCO_2 → Hyperventilation → Cycle of respiratory activity and apnoea continues.

Biot's Breathing Biot's breathing also known as *ataxic breathing* is a type of periodic breathing showing alternate periods of respiratory activity and apnoea (Fig. 5.7-4B). It differs from Cheyne-Stokes breathing in following aspects:

- It occurs at irregular intervals,
- There is no waxing and waning of tidal volume during the period of respiratory activity and
- It can never occur physiologically.

Causes. Biot's breathing indicates a disruption of the normal medullary rhythmicity of respiration. It may occur when medulla is involved in disorders such as meningitis, head injury, medullary compressions like pontine haematomas or cerebellopontine herniation. *Central medullary lesions* are the most common cause of Biot's breathing. So, it is rare in cerebral ischaemia, which has to be bilateral to infarct the central medulla.

Disturbances Related to Respiratory Gases

Respiratory disturbances related to respiratory gases include:

- Hypoxia,
- Hypercapnia,
- Hypocapnia,
- Asphyxia and
- Carbon monoxide poisoning.

Hypoxia

The term hypoxia is used to denote deficiency of oxygen supply at the tissue level. It has almost replaced the term anoxia (complete absence of oxygen), which rarely occurs practically.

Causes and Types

Causes. Hypoxia can occur because of any one or more of the following defects:

- Decreased oxygen tension (pO_2) of the arterial blood,
- Decreased oxygen carrying capacity of the blood,
- Decreased rate of blood flow to the tissue or
- Decreased utilization of oxygen by tissue cells.

Types. Depending upon the mechanism of occurrence there are four types of hypoxia:

- Hypoxic hypoxia,
- Anaemic hypoxia,
- Stagnant hypoxia and
- Histotoxic hypoxia.

1. **Hypoxic Hypoxia**

Hypoxic hypoxia occurs due to decreased oxygen tension (pO_2) of the arterial blood, hence also called *arterial hypoxia*. Therefore, in this condition O_2 carrying capacity of blood, rate of blood flow to tissue and utilization of O_2 by tissues is normal.

Causes of hypoxic hypoxia are:

1. ***Low oxygen tension (pO_2) in inspired air,*** e.g.
   - High altitude, where person is exposed to low atmospheric pO_2,
   - Breathing artificial gas mixture with low pO_2 and
   - Breathing in a closed space.
2. ***Hypoventilation*** due to any causes, e.g.
   - Obstruction in respiratory passages as in asthma,
   - Decreased lung compliance as in pneumothorax,
   - Paresis or paralysis of respiratory muscles, as in poliomyelitis,
   - Pump failure due to fatigue of respiratory muscles and
   - Damage to respiratory centres by drugs like morphine (that causes depression of respiratory neurons in the medulla)or brain tumours.

   Hypoventilation decreases alveolar pO_2 and hence arterial pO_2.
3. ***Reduced diffusion of oxygen across respiratory membrane*** occurs due to:
   - Marked reduction in area of respiratory membrane as in emphysema,
   - Increased thickness of respiratory membrane as in pulmonary oedema and
   - Nonfunctioning respiratory membrane as in fibrosis.
4. ***Physiological shunt*** formation due to abnormalities of ventilation–perfusion (VA/Q) ratio.
5. ***Anatomical shunts,*** i.e. when venous blood mixes with arterial blood lowering its pO_2, as occurs in:
   - Congenital heart diseases such as Fallot's tetralogy.

Characteristic features of hypoxic hypoxia are:

- *Low*—Arterial pO_2, arterial O_2 content, percentage saturation of haemoglobin and low A-V pO_2 difference.
- *Normal* – O_2 carrying capacity of blood, blood flow to tissues and utilization of O_2 by tissue cells.

2. Anaemic Hypoxia

Anaemic hypoxia occurs due to the decreased O_2 carrying capacity of blood.

Causes of anaemic hypoxia are:

1. *Decreased RBC count* as occurs in:
   - Bone marrow depression and
   - Haemorrhage.
2. *Decreased haemoglobin content* of blood as occurs in:
   - Anaemias of all types.
3. *Altered haemoglobin* which is not capable of carrying O_2, e.g.
   - Methaemoglobin, in which iron is present in ferric (Fe^{3+}) form instead of ferrous (Fe^{2+}) form
   - Carboxyhaemoglobin, in which carbon monoxide combines with haemoglobin due to its 200 times more affinity than O_2.

Characteristic features of anaemic hypoxia are:

- Arterial pO_2 is normal (95–100 mmHg),
- Oxygen carrying capacity of blood is reduced due to anaemia or altered haemoglobin,
- Percentage saturation of haemoglobin is decreased,
- A–V pO_2 difference is normal (95–40 = 55 mmHg).

Pathophysiology of low O_2 supply to tissues in anaemic hypoxia

- Mild to moderate anaemia usually does not produce hypoxia at rest because there is compensatory increase in 2,3-DPG amount in the RBCs which combines with oxyhaemoglobin and results in increased liberation of O_2,

$$HbO_2 + 2,3-DPG \rightarrow Hb\ 2,3-DPG + O_2$$

- However, during exercise the increased demand of O_2 by tissues is not met with and hence symptoms of hypoxia appear.
- Anaemic hypoxia in carbon monoxide poisoning is severe and needs emergency treatment. CO produces severe hypoxia by:
  - Preventing the Hb to combine with O_2 and
  - Shifting O_2-Hb dissociation curve to left (Fig. 5.7-5) thereby decreasing the amount of O_2 that can be released.

3. Stagnant Hypoxia

Stagnant hypoxia occurs due to decreased blood flow to the tissues so that in spite of normal pO_2 and haemoglobin, adequate O_2 is not delivered to the tissues.

Causes. Stagnant or ischaemic hypoxia may be generalized or localized.

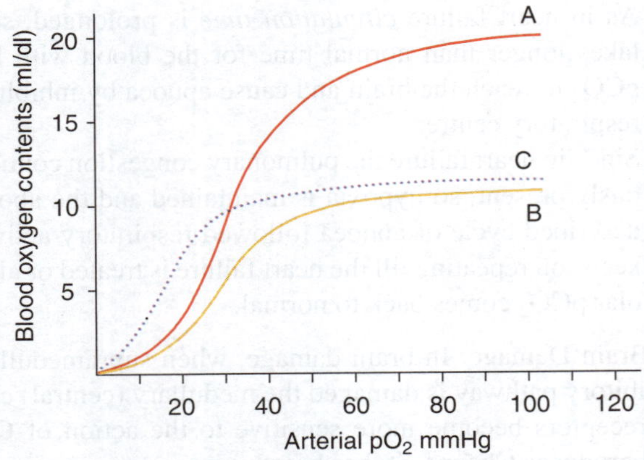

FIGURE 5.7-5 Oxygen–haemoglobin dissociation curves: **(A)** normal curve (when haemoglobin concentration is 15 gm/dl); **(B)** anaemic curve (when haemoglobin concentration is 7 gm/dl); and **(C)** carbon monoxide poisoning curve (when 50% carboxyhaemoglobin) shifted to left of the anaemic curve.

Generalized stagnant hypoxia occurs in:

- ***Shock*** due to circulatory failure and haemorrhage. In this condition via baroreceptors there occurs reflex vasoconstriction and thus blood flow to the tissues is decreased. Worst affected are kidneys and heart which have very high O_2 demand.
- ***Congestive heart failure*** is associated with decreased venous return and hence decreased blood flow to the tissues causing hypoxia. Liver and brain are worst affected by venous congestion. Further, the associated pulmonary congestion produces defect in oxygenation and thus the patients also suffer from hypoxic hypoxia in addition to stagnant hypoxia.
- ***Localized stagnant hypoxia*** is caused by abnormalities in regional vessels such as:
  - Atherosclerosis,
  - Thrombosis and
  - Embolism.

Characteristic features of stagnant hypoxia are:

- Normal arterial pO_2,
- Normal arterial O_2 content,
- Normal arterial percentage oxygen saturation of haemoglobin,
- A-V pO_2 difference is more than normal because resting O_2 uptake of tissues increases from 5 ml % to 10 ml % or the blood stays in the tissue for longer period. Thus in venous blood:
  - pO_2 is reduced from ~ 40 mmHg to ~ 25 mmHg.
  - O_2 content is reduced from 14 to 9 ml % and
  - O_2 saturation of Hb is reduced from 75% to 45%.

4. Histotoxic Hypoxia

Histotoxic hypoxia occurs due to decreased ability of the tissues themselves to utilize the oxygen. So, strictly speaking, it is not a true hypoxia, because O_2 supply to the tissues is adequate.

Causes. Histotoxic hypoxia is caused by certain poisonous substances which destroy the cellular oxidative enzymes and completely paralyse the cytochrome oxidative system of the cells. These include:

- Cyanide poisoning and
- Sulphide poisoning.

Characteristic features. Since O_2 supply is adequate and the tissue cells are not able to utilize the O_2, so histotoxic hypoxia is characterized by:

- Normal arterial pO_2
- Normal arterial % O_2 saturation of haemoglobin
- No difference in the O_2 content of arterial and venous blood and
- A-V pO_2 difference is practically nil.

Characterstic features of four types of hypoxia are summarized in Table 5.7-1.

Symptoms of Hypoxia Symptoms of hypoxia depend upon:

- Rapidity of development of hypoxia,
- Severity of hypoxia and
- Effectiveness of the body's compensatory mechanisms.

Based on the above the hypoxia may be fulminant, acute or chronic.

1. Fulminant Hypoxia refers to severe hypoxia developing very fast, i.e. which occurs within seconds after exposure to an arterial O_2 tension of less than 20 mmHg. Such a situation may occur if an aircraft loses cabin pressure (becomes impressurized) above 20,000 feet and no supplemental O_2 is available. It results in:

- *Unconsciousness* within 15 to 20 second due to lack of O_2 supply to brain and
- *Brain death* may follow in 4–5 minutes.

2. Acute Hypoxia is produced by exposure to arterial O_2 tensions of 25–40 mmHg (e.g. as would occur at altitudes of 18,000–25,000 feet). Symptoms of acute hypoxia are very similar to the effects of ethyl alcohol and include:

- Lack of co-ordination,
- Slowed reflexes,
- Slurring of speech,
- Overconfidence and eventually,
- Unconsciousness,
- Coma and death can occur in minutes to hours if the compensatory mechanisms of the body are inadequate.

3. Chronic Hypoxia. It occurs due to exposure to low pO_2(40–60 mmHg) for long periods (e.g. as would

TABLE 5.7-1 Characteristic Features of Different Types of Hypaxia

Features	Hypoxic hypoxia	Anaemic hypoxia	Stagnant hypoxia	Histotoxic hypoxia
Pathophysiology	Occurs due to decreased O_2 tension (decreased arterial pO_2)	Occurs due to low O_2 carrying capacity of blood	Occurs due to decreased blood flow to tissue	Occurs due to decreased ability of the tissue to utilise O_2
Causes	• Low O_2 tension (low pO_2 in inspired air) • Hypoventilation • ↓ Diffusion of O_2 across respiratory membrane • Physiological shunt • Anatomical shunt	• ↓ RBC count • ↓ Hb content of blood • Altered Hb	• Shock • Circulatory failure	• Cyanide poisoning
Arterial p O_2	Decreased	Normal	Normal	Normal
Arterial O_2 contents	Decreased	Markedly Decreased	Normal	Normal
Arterial Hb contents	Normal	Reduced	Normal	Normal
% O_2 saturation (in arterial blood)	Decreased	Decreased	Normal	Normal
O_2 carrying capacity of arterial blood	Normal	Decreased	Normal	Normal
A-V (arterial—venous) pO_2 difference	Decreased	Normal	More than normal	Less than normal (nil)
Cyanosis	Present	Absent	Present	Absent
Peripheral chemoreceptor stimulation	Present (because dissolved oxygen in plasma is reduced)	Absent (because dissolved oxygen in plasma is sufficient)	Present (because arterial pCO_2 increases and pO_2 decreases)	Present (cyanide decreases oxygen utilisation at tissue level)
Tachypnoea	Present	Absent	Present	Present

occur after stay for extended period of time at altitudes of approximately 10,000–18,000 feet). Most of the clinical cases of hypoxia are of this category. Patients with chronic hypoxia may be bedridden or limited to chair because respiratory and cardiac disease prevents them from increasing O_2 supply to tissues. Symptoms of chronic hypoxia are:

- Severe fatigue,
- Dyspnoea,
- Shortness of breath,
- Respiratory arrhythmias (e.g. Cheyne-Stokes breathing) can occur in patients with chronic hypoxia, especially during sleep, which can contribute to the hypoxic state.

Signs of Hypoxia

1. Cyanosis is the bluish discolouration of skin and mucous membrane caused by presence of more than 5 gm of deoxyhaemoglobin/100 ml of the capillary blood. There are two types of cyanosis:

Peripheral cyanosis is seen in the nailbeds and is suggestive of *stagnant hypoxia*. This is because perfusion in these distally located areas are worst affected in hypotensive states. Large amount of O_2 is extracted from haemoglobin and the concentration of deoxyhaemoglobin rises to produce cyanosis.

Central cyanosis is seen in the earlobes where skin is thin and in the mucous membrane of lips and tongue. These areas receive a good blood supply and become cyanotic only if the O_2 saturation of blood is low, as occurs in *hypoxic hypoxia*.

Cyanosis is not a reliable sign of hypoxia because:

- Anaemic paients may never develop cyanosis, even though they are extremely hypoxic because of an inadequate haemoglobin concentration,
- Cyanosis does not occur in histotoxic hypoxia either, because the O_2 saturation of haemoglobin is normal and
- In contrast, patients with polycythemia may be cyanotic as a result of high concentration of haemoglobin, even though their tissues are adequately oxygenated and further
- Methaemoglobin, with its slate-grey colour, can also impart a bluish colour to tissues.

2. Tachycardia. It occurs as a peripheral chemoreceptor reflex response to the low arterial oxygen tension.

3. Tachypnoea, (i.e. rapid breathing and *hyperpnoea* (i.e. deep breathing) are also reflex responses to hypoxia that are activated by arterial chemoreceptors. Therefore, tachypnoea and hyperpnoea are:

- Present in hypoxic hypoxia where arterial pO_2 is low and are
- Absent in both anaemic hypoxia and stagnant hypoxia in which the arterial pO_2 is normal.

Physiological Compensatory Responses to Chronic Hypoxia Two types of physiologic compensatory responses known to occur in hypoxia are *accommodation and acclimatization.*

I. Accommodation. Accommodation, refers to immediate reflex adjustments of the respiratory and cardiovascular systems to hypoxia. These include:

- ***Hyperventilation.*** As mentioned above, hyperventilation occurs secondary to stimulation of peripheral chemoreceptors by low O_2 tension in the arterial blood. The increased ventilation is compensated by:
  - Increasing pO_2 and reducing pCO_2,
  - Reduced pCO_2 causes a respiratory alkalosis, which in turn, lowers the respiratory drive. The respiratory drive continues to increase during this time as the alkalosis is corrected.
- ***Tachycardia,*** as mentioned above, also occurs as a peripheral chemoreceptor response to the low arterial oxygen tension. It increases O_2 delivery to the tissues by increasing cardiac output. In the individuals who go to high altitudes, the cardiac output returns to normal after several weeks.
- ***Increase in 2,3-diphosphoglycerate (2,3-DPG) concentration*** in RBCs occurs in response to hypoxia and alkalosis. The increased 2,3-DPG concentration raises p_{50} of haemoglobin, which helps to maintain the tissue O_2 tension at slightly higher level than it would be otherwise.

II. Acclimatization. Acclimatization refers to the changes in body tissues in response to long-term exposure to hypoxia, such as when a person living at sea level goes and stays at high altitude for a long time. With longer stay, the person gradually gets acclimatized to low pO_2 by following changes in the body tissues:

- ***Increase in red blood cell count*** or the polycythaemia secondary to tissue hypoxia results from the release of *renal erythropoietic factor,* which acts on a plasma globulin to form erythropoietin. Erythropoietin stimulates the production of RBCs by the bone marrow. This leads to:
  - Increase in haemoglobin concentration from 15 gm% to about 20 gm%,
  - Increase in haematocrit from normal value of 40–45% to 60% after full acclimatization and
  - Increase in blood volume by 20–30% leading to total increase in circulating haemoglobin by 50%.

  These changes allow each unit of blood to carry additional O_2, which compensates for the decreased O_2 tension. Increase in haemoglobin and blood volume starts after 2 weeks, reaches half development in a month and is fully developed only after many months.
- ***Increase in pulmonary ventilation.*** When an individual stays at high altitude for many days, there is gradual

increase in ventilation to an average of about five times the normal. This is because of loss of breaking effect of CO_2 due to renal correction of alkalosis, leading to decreased HCO^-_3 ion concentration in CSF and brain tissues.

- ***Cardiovascular changes*** in the form of increased heart rate, force of contraction and increased cardiac output which occur in the initial accommodation period, later on decrease back to normal once the O_2 supply to tissues becomes normal due to changes in blood.
- ***Pulmonary hypertension.*** It occurs secondary to the generalized hypoxic pulmonary vasoconstriction. The increased pulmonary artery pressure causes a more even distribution of pulmonary blood flow, which can improve gas exchange. However, the elevated pulmonary artery pressure can induce cor pulmonale if the hypoxia is sufficiently severe.
- ***Increase in total lung capacity and diffusing capacity of the lung*** occur in high altitude natives as compared to their sea-level counterparts. The increase in total lung capacity is evidenced by the enlarged chest that high altitude natives develop.

  Diffusing capacity of lungs increases due to increase in surface area of respiratory membrane. The greatly increased pulmonary capillary blood volume expands the capillaries thereby increasing surface area. Hypoxia increases pulmonary ventilation leading to increase in lung volume which expands surface area of alveolar membrane. Pulmonary hypertension forces blood into greater number of alveolar capillaries than normally, especially in upper parts of lungs which are poorly perfused.
- ***Cellular and tissue acclimatization*** occurs after a long stay at high altitude. These include:
  - *Increase in oxidative enzyme concentrations* within the mitochondria of many tissues, which allows more rapid generation of ATP via oxidative phosphorylation.
  - *Increase in mitochondrial density* within the cells, which reduces the diffusion distance and provides more sites for O_2 utilization.
  - *Increase in capillary density* in skeletal and cardiac muscles, which reduces the diffusion distance from the blood into the cells.
- ***Decreased respiratory drive*** is caused by lifelong exposure to hypoxia, i.e. for very prolonged periods. The reduced respiratory drive leads to higher CO_2 tension and lower O_2 tension, but it diminishes the work of respiration, which reserves more O_2 for use by other skeletal muscles.

Oxygen Therapy

Physiological Basis of Oxygen Therapy in Hypoxia

Oxygen therapy is of great value in certain types of hypoxia and at the same time of almost no value in other types. With the basic knowledge of physiological principles of different types of hypoxia, one can readily decide when oxygen therapy will be of value and, if so how valuable.

In general, simple O_2 therapy is not of much help in treatment of hypoxia because diffusion across respiratory membrane depends upon partial pressure of gases, therefore, alveolar pO_2 can be increased by:

- Inhalation of 100% pure oxygen, or
- Inhalation of 100% pure oxygen at high barometric pressure, called hyperbaric oxygen therapy.

Oxygen Therapy with 100% Pure Oxygen at Atmospheric Pressure, i.e. at 760 mmHg.

1. Oxygen Therapy is Useful in most types of hypoxic hypoxia. The way the oxygen therapy is useful in different causes of hypoxic hypoxia are highlighted:

- *In atmospheric hypoxia,* oxygen therapy can correct the depressed oxygen level in the inspired gases and therefore provide 100 per cent effective therapy.
- *In hypoventilation hypoxia*, a person breathing 100 per cent oxygen can move five times as much oxygen into the alveoli with each breath as when breathing normal air. Again, here oxygen therapy can be extremely beneficial.
- *In hypoxia due to impaired respiratory membrane diffusion,* oxygen therapy can increase the pO_2 in the lungs from a normal value of about 100 mmHg to as high as 160 mmHg thus raising the oxygen diffusion gradient.

2. Oxygen Therapy is of Limited Value in anaemic hypoxia, stagnant hypoxia and hypoxic hypoxia caused by physiological or anatomical shunts; because in all these conditions oxygen is already available in the alveoli. However, in these conditions some extra oxygen can be transported in dissolved state in the blood when alveolar oxygen is increased to the maximum level; and this extra oxygen may some times be the difference between life and death.

Therefore, hyperbaric O_2 therapy is more useful in such conditions than O_2 therapy at atmospheric pressure.

3. Oxygen Therapy is of No Use in histotoxic hypoxia, because in this type of hypoxia, the tissue metabolic enzyme system is simply incapable of utilizing the oxygen that is delivered.

4. Caution is Required While Giving Oxygen Therapy to patients with severe pulmonary failure associated with hypercapnia (increased pCO_2), as it may cause death. The central chemoreceptors in these patients are inhibited following excessive overdrive by the pCO_2. In such a situation, whatever respiration is there, it is due to hypoxic stimulation of peripheral chemoreceptors. So, O_2 therapy at such a juncture may produce apnoea by taking away this hypoxic drive and soon death may occur due to direct depression of respiratory centre by severe hypoxia and hypercapnia.

Hyperbaric Oxygen Therapy (Inhalation of 100% Pure Oxygen at High Barometric Pressure)

Advantage of Hyperbaric O_2 therapy over O_2 therapy at atmospheric pressure is that the former increases the amount of dissolved O_2 in plasma, and is therefore unaffected by the haemoglobin concentration.

Amount of O_2 Dissolved in Plasma depends upon its partial pressures:

- Normally, plasma can have 0.3 ml of dissolved oxygen per 100 ml per 100 mmHg pO_2, or 0.003 ml per 100 ml per mmHg pO_2.
- *At 1 atmospheric pressure (760 mmHg).* inhalation of 100% O_2 (in a patient with normal pCO_2 40 mmHg and pH_2O 47 mmHg) can raise the arterial pO_2 to a maximum of 760 – (40 1 47), or 673 mmHg.
- Therefore, the maximum amount of O_2 that can be dissolved in plasma will be:
  - At 1 atmospheric pressure: 673 × 0.003, or 2 ml/100 ml.
  - At 2 atmospheric pressure: 673 × 0.003 3 2, or 4 ml/100 ml and
  - At 3 atmospheric pressure: 673 × 0.003 3 3, or 6 ml/100 ml.
- The normal demand of the body tissues (5 ml/100ml/min), thus can be met only by dissolved O_2 in plasma, if administered at atmospheric pressure of 2.5 or more.

Indications of Hyperbaric O_2 Therapy, thus include those types of hypoxias in which normal Hb is not available to carry the O_2 to the tissues, and so the main dependence is on dissolved O_2 in plasma. These conditions include:

- Carbon monoxide poisoning
- Anaemic hypoxia (due to severe anaemia)
- Decompression sickness and air embolism
- Wounds with poor blood supply
- Stagnant hypoxia (very limited value).

Caution. For therapeutic use, the hyperbaric 100% O_2 should not be used with pressures beyond 2–3 times atmospheric and should not be used more than five hours; because of high chances of developing O_2 toxicity.

Side Effects of 100% O_2 (O_2 Toxicity)

- ***Mechanism of side effects.*** Inhalation of 100% O_2 produces side effects (harmful effects) due to conversion of molecular oxygen into active oxygen, i.e. superoxide anion ($O^-{}_2$), which is free radical and H_2O.
- ***Side effects noted by inhalation of 100% O_2*** include:
  - *Irritation of airways* in the form of nasal congestion, sore throat, substernal discomfort, sneezing and coughing and bronchoconstriction may occur after about 8 hours of inhalation.
  - *Bronchopneumomia* may be initiated when O_2 therapy is continued for more than 24 hours because of:
    - Inhibition of ability of lung macrophages to kill bacteria and
    - Decreased production of surfactant.
  - *Complications in newborn infants* are very common, as they are very sensitive to get O_2 toxicity. Therefore, special care is needed while treating newborns in incubators with O_2 therapy. It is cautioned that infants should never be given more than 40% O_2. Special dangers of O_2 therapy in premature infants are occurrence of:
    - *Retinopathy of prematurity* (old name retrolental fibroplasia), which is characterized by retinal neovascularization and proliferation of fibrovascular tissue ultimately forming an opaque retrolental mass, leading to bilateral permanent blindness. Normally, the retinal receptors get matured from central part towards the peripheral part of the retina, and at the same time vascularization also occurs in an orderly manner (centre towards periphery). A large amount of oxygen is being utilized in the process of maturation, therefore, if premature babies are treated with 100% oxygen, the normal pattern of maturation fails and consequently there is proliferation of fibrovascular tissue resulting in formation of opaque reterolental mass.
    - *Bronchopulmonary dysplasia* is characterized by formation of lung cysts and opacities.
  - *Nervous system complications,* i.e. derangement of cerebral activity is especially known to occur with administration of *hyperbaric O_2* therapy. At high pressures of O_2, dissolved O_2 in plasma is greatly increased, which in turn causes rise in tissue pO_2. As mentioned above, oxygen toxicity is caused by production of free oxygen radicals which oxidize polyunsaturated fatty acids (essential compounds of cells membrane) and also oxidize cellular enzymes (damaging cellular metabolic systems). Nervous tissues are especially susceptible because of their high lipid content. Nervous symptoms include muscular twitching, tinnitus (ringing of bells in ears), convulsions, coma and even death.

Hypercapnia

Hypercapnia refers to increase in arterial pCO_2 (normal value 40 mmHg). When hypercapnia is the primary problem, it is associated with respiratory acidosis (see page 451) since an increase in CO_2 promptly generates excess H^+ through following reaction:

$$H_2O + CO_2 \xrightarrow{\text{Carbonic anhydrase}} H_2CO_3 \rightarrow H^+ + HCO^-{}_3$$

Causes of Hypercapnia Hypercapnia rarely occurs due to increased production of CO_2, because an increase in arterial pCO_2 causes a prompt increase in pulmonary ventilation through stimulation of central chemoreceptors, resulting in CO_2 washout and a near restoration of arterial pCO_2 to normal levels of about 40 mmHg.

There exists a linear relationship between increase in arterial pCO_2 and increase in pulmonary ventilation (see page 451). Increased production of CO_2 without hypercapnia occurs in fever, following excess consumption of carbohydrate and in metabolic acidosis with respiratory compensation.

Hypercapnia occurs due to:

1. *Defective elimination of CO_2* as occurs in:
   - Reduced pulmonary ventilation due to restrictive lung disorder, or
   - Reduced effective alveolar ventilation due to ventilation-perfusion mismatch as seen in chronic obstructive pulmonary disease (COPD).
2. *Accidental inhalation of CO_2* in persons working in breweries and refrigeration plants.

Signs and Symptoms of Hypercapnia

1. ***Hyperpnoea*** occurs due to stimulation of respiratory centre through central chemoreceptors. Since, most of the times, clinically hypercapnia occurs due to restrictive lung disorders, so hyperpnoea fails to improve pulmonary ventilation.
2. ***Carbon dioxide narcosis*** develops when arterial pCO_2 increases above 50 mmHg. Retention of large amount of CO_2 causes depression of central nervous system leading to confusion, diminution of sensory acuity and eventually coma and death.

These patients present with severe respiratory acidosis, therefore, as a compensation for acidosis, large amount of HCO_3^- are excreted in urine (for details see page 451).

Hypocapnia

Hypocapnia, i.e. reduced pCO_2 is usually associated with *respiratory alkalosis,* since decrease in CO_2 promptly drives the following reaction in backward direction, resulting in a decrease in H^+ concentration.

$$H_2O + CO_2 \xleftarrow{\text{Carbonic anhydrase}} H_2CO_3 \leftarrow H^+ + HCO^-_3$$

Causes. Hypocapnia occurs due to hyperventilation (see page 452). The effects of hypocapnia are-

- Vasoconstriction due to direct effect on cerebral blood vessels causes reduction in cerebral blood flow by 30%. The resulting ischemia causes headache, dizziness and parasthesia.
- Due to alkalosis pH increases to 7.5–7.6, and low plasma HCO_3^- level, the renal compensation results in absorption of HCO_3^- due to inhibition of acid secretion.
- Plasma ionic calcium level (Ca^{2+}) falls, therefore, hypocapnic patient develops signs of tetany i.e *carpopedal spasm* and a *positive Chevostek's sign.*

Asphyxia

Asphyxia refers to a condition in which hypoxia (decreased pO_2) is associated with hypercapnia (increased pCO_2).

Causes. Asphyxia can be general or local.

- *Local asphyxia* occurs following complete obstruction or ligation of blood vessel.
- *General asphyxia* can be chronic or acute.
- *Chronic asphyxia* may occur in patient with cor pulmonale, i.e. right ventricular failure due to lung diseases, and
- *Acute asphyxia* occurs due to sudden blockage in airways. Common causes are:
  - Strangulation,
  - Drowning,
  - Acute tracheal obstruction (due to entry of food or due to choking),
  - Paralysis of diaphragm, as in acute poliomyelitis.

Clinical Stages of Acute Asphyxia. There are three stages of acute asphyxia:

Stage 1: Stage of Hyperpnoea. This stage lasts for one minute and is characterized by:

- Increase in rate and depth of respiration, with more pronounced expiratory effort,
- Dyspnoea, cyanosis and sudden prominence of eyeballs.
- This stage occurs due to sudden and powerful stimulation of respiratory centres by acutely occurring rise in pCO_2. O_2 lack is not yet enough to stimulate ventilation.

Stage II: Stage of Central Excitation. This stage occurs due to excess CO_2 stimulating the centres directly, and lack of O_2 stimulating the centres reflexly. It lasts for about 1 minute and is characterized by all signs of central excitation, such as:

- Expiration becomes more *violent*,
- Heart rate is increased,
- Systemic blood pressure rises due to widespread vasoconstriction,
- Pupils are constricted,
- All the reflexes are exaggerated,
- Convulsions occur due to excess of pCO_2 and
- Consciousness is lost.

Stage III: Stage of Central Depression. This stage occurs due to direct effect of O_2 lack on vital centres causing their inhibition. It lasts for 2–3 minutes and its characteristic features are:

- Convulsions disappear,
- Respiration becomes slow and finally it becomes gasping (shallow and with low frequency),
- Heart rate is decreased,
- Blood pressure falls,
- Pupils are dilated,
- All the reflexes are abolished,

- The whole body lies still,
- Duration between the gasps is gradually increased and
- Finally the death occurs.

Drowning There are two main mechanisms by which effects of drowning, ultimately causing death:

1. Asphyxia is the cause of death in only 10% cases of drowning. Asphyxia occurs initially due to *breath-holding,* and after the breaking in effect due to the severe *laryngospasm* induced by first gasp of water. The laryngospasm prevents entry of water into the lungs, but soon produces death due to asphyxia. Thus, the lungs remain dry in asphyxial deaths due to drowning.

2. Flooding of Lungs with Water occurs in 90 per cent cases of drowning. The muscles of glottis relax and allow entry of water into the lungs. Further events depend upon the type of water:

- *Fresh water drowning* is associated with rapid absorption of water (since it is hypotonic) into the circulation, which causes plasma dilution and intravascular haemolysis.
- *Sea water drowning* is associated with hypovolaemia due to draining of water from the circulation into the lungs (since the sea water is hypertonic).

Note. When the patients with drowning are timely rescued and resuscitated with artificial respiration, the above described circulatory effects must be taken care of depending upon the type of water.

Carbon Monoxide Poisoning

Carbon monoxide (CO) is a dangerous gas present in exhaust of gasoline engines, coal mines, gases from deep wells and underground drainage systems.

Toxic Effects. Carbon monoxide produces anaemic hypoxia and derangement of cellular metabolic system.

1. Anaemic Hypoxia. When CO inhaled accidently from the abovementioned sources, carbon monoxide having 200 times more affinity than O_2 for haemoglobin combines with it to form *carboxyhaemoglobin.* The carboxyhaemoglobin produces severe anaemic hypoxia by following mechanisms:

- It does not allow the haemoglobin to take up oxygen from alveolar air and
- The presence of carboxyhaemoglobin decreases the release of oxygen from haemoglobin, i.e. the oxygenhaemoglobin dissociation curve shifts to the left (Fig. 5.5-7) see page 433.

2. Derangement of Cellular Metabolic System. Carbonmonoxide causes toxic effects on cytochrome system of the cells causing derangement of the cellular metabolic system but the amount of CO required for producing cytochrome toxic effects is 1000 times (the lethal dose).

Sign and Symptoms of CO Poisoning depending upon its concentration in the inspired air are:

- *When the inspired air contains 1% CO,* saturation of haemoglobin with CO becomes 15 to 20%. Patients get headache and nausea within one hour of inhalation.
- *When the inspired air contains more than 1% CO,* the haemoglobin saturation becomes 30–40 %. This causes loss of consciousness.
- *When haemoglobin saturation with CO* becomes 50% death occurs.
- The symptoms of CO poisoning are of hypoxia, but there is no stimulation of respiration because arterial blood pO_2 remains normal.
- The cherry red color of COHb is visible on the skin, nail bed and mucous membrane.

Treatment of CO Poisoning. When diagnosed timely, following measures should be taken promptly:

- Immediate termination of exposure to carbon monoxide,
- Immediate hyperbaric 100% O_2 therapy,
- Administration of air with few per cent of CO_2 to stimulate respiratory centres.

Pulmonary Diseases: Physiological Peculiarities

Physiological peculiarities of some of the common pulmonary diseases are described to understand the pathophysiology of respiratory insufficiency occurring in these diseases.

From the physiological point of view the pulmonary diseases can be divided into two groups:

- Obstructive lung diseases and
- Restrictive lung diseases.

Obstructive Lung Diseases The chronic obstructive lung diseases include asthma, chronic bronchitis and emphysema. The obstructive lung diseases are characterized by increased resistance to airflow.

The airway resistance mainly depends on the radius of the airway and on type of air flow. Resistance is low when air flow is laminar and high when air flow is turbulent. Upper airway resistance usually does not increase, except in conditions like nasal congestion, deviated nasal septum or enlarged adenoids. Mouth breathing is common in these conditions.

Lower Airway Resistance chiefly lies in the medium sized bronchi (2-4 mm diameter). Smooth muscle contraction mainly increases airway resistance by reducing airway's radius. The diameter of these bronchi is altered by following factors:

- ***Bronchomotor tone*** is chiefly regulated by autonomic neural discharge (see page 393) and also by local chemical mediators like prostaglandins, leukotrienes, kinins etc.
- ***Radial traction by lung parenchyma-*** Bronchi and bronchioles are surrounded by lung parenchyma. The constant

pull of lung parenchyma helps in maintaining patency of the airway. This supportive action is known as radial traction. During expiration small airways (bronchioles) collapse.

- ***Transmural pressure-*** In quite breathing, during inspiration, pressure is negative (because of negative intra pleural pressure with respect to intra-pulmonary pressure). Therefore, the airways remain patent. Same situation prevails during tidal expiration, however in forced expiration transmural pressure becomes positive, which tends to collapse the small airways. The condition worsened in emphysema due to loss of radial traction.
- ***Mucous secretion.*** Presence of mucous or any other material in airways also increases airway resistance.

Mechanisms of Airway Obstruction in the obstructive lung diseases include:

- ***The airway lumen,*** may be partially obstructed by excessive secretions (chronic bronchitis), oedema fluid, or aspiration of food or fluids.
- ***The airway wall smooth muscles*** may be contracted (asthma) or thickened because of inflammation and oedema (asthma, bronchitis), or mucous glands may be hypertrophied (chronic bronchitis).
- ***Outside the airway,*** the destruction of lung parenchyma may decrease radial traction, causing the airways to be narrowed (emhysema).

1. Asthma

Asthma is considered an inflammatory disease of the bronchioles caused by the hypersensitivity of the bronchioles to foreign substances in the air. Asthma is a chronic life-long disease with periods of remissions and *exacerbation.*

Aetiopathogenesis. Functional abnormality in asthma is airway narrowing produced by following effects of allergic reactions:

- *Spasm of bronchial smooth muscle,* which is triggered by exposure to provoking agents such as allergen or exercise,
- *Inflammation of bronchial wall (*predominantly eosinophilic/producing mucosal oedema) and
- *Secretion of thick mucus* into the lumen of bronchioles.

Symptoms. The above changes increase the airway resistance; thus asthma is an obstructive lung disease. The asthmatic person can usually inspire adequately but has great difficulty during expiration. During attack of asthma patient may have:

- Dyspnoea, or air hunger,
- Cough,
- With repeated acute attacks patient may get progressive fatigue and even eventual respiratory arrest.
- *Pulmonary function abnormalities* may occur in patients over the years. During asthmatic attack because of difficulty in expiring air there occurs:
- Reduced maximum expiratory rate,
- Increase in FRC and in RV.
- There is a reduction in TV), VC and forced expiratory volume-one (FEV_1).

Gas Exchange Abnormalities. There is no decrease in diffusion capacity in asthma. Alveolar ventilation is uneven and decreased causing *mild hypoxia.* However, with increasing severity of attack pO_2 decreases in direct proportion to the drop in FEV_1. Hyperventilation in response to hypoxia leads to decreased pCO_2. When the attack is prolonged patient may get acidosis, dyspnoea and cyanosis. A normal or increased pCO_2 in asthma along with increasing hypoxaemia is an ominous sign of impending respiratory arrest.

Treatment Therapeutically the drugs used are:

- β adrenergic agonists are used to treat mild to moderate asthmatic attack.
- Steroids both as inhaler or systemically may be used to reduce inflammation.
- Agents that block synthesis of leukotrienes or their receptors are also useful in certain cases.

2. Chronic Bronchitis and Emphysema

Chronic Bronchitis, i.e. inflammation of the bronchial tree occurs due to cigarette smoking, exposure to oxidant gases, dust and irritants. Mucosal inflammation is exacerbated by superadded infection. It is characterized by an increase in volume of submucosal glands and increase in number of goblet cells in the surface epithelium.

- Chronic cough and hypersecretion of mucus are the hallmark of chronic bronchitis.
- Increased air flow resistance occurs due to chronic inflammation of the small airways and the condition is termed *small airway disease.*

Pulmonary Emphysema literally means excess air in the lung. Chronic pulmonary emphysema, however, signifies a complex obstructive and destructive process of the lungs and is usually a consequence of long-term smoking.

Development of Emphysema involves two main events:

- ***Airway obstruction*** is caused by changes of chronic bronchitis (as described above) which include chronic infection, excess mucus and inflammatory oedema of the bronchial epithelium. Furthermore, the smaller peripheral bronchi are thickened and distorted by the scar tissue and at the segmental level there may be loss of bronchial cartilage. All these changes are termed as *small airway disease.*
- ***Destruction of alveolar walls.*** The obstruction of the airway makes it especially difficult to expire, causing entrapment of air in the alveoli and overstretching of the alveoli. This combined with lung infection causes marked destruction of alveolar cells. Usually there is loss of some elastic tissues because of the proteolytic enzyme called elastase.

3. Chronic Obstructive Pulmonary Disease

Chronic obstructive pulmonary disease (COP) is the term used to denote the clinical entity having combined effects of chronic bronchitis and chronic pulmonary emphysema. Genetic factors also predispose to COPD by producing deficiency of anti trypsin activity. In the lungs normally action of elastase and other proteolytic enzymes (produced by leucocytes) is antagonized by anti trypsin activity. It is characterized by following respiratory physiological changes:

Increased Airway Resistance occurs due to chronic bronchial obstruction. So, the movement of air through the respiratory passages become difficult. Expiration is especially difficult because the force on the outside of the lung compresses the bronchioles, which further increases their resistance.

Decreased Diffusing Capacity of the lungs results from destruction of alveolar membrane. So, ability of the lungs to oxygenate the blood and to remove the carbon dioxide is reduced.

Abnormal Ventilation–Perfusion Ratio (VA/Q) occurs as:

- ***Very low VA/Q ratio*** occurs in the areas of lungs with bronchiolar obstruction. In these areas alveolar ventilation (VA) is much less than the blood supply (perfusion), resulting in poor aeration of blood (*physiological shunt formation).*
- ***Very high VA/Q ratio*** occurs in the areas of lungs having marked loss of alveolar walls. In such areas, VA is much more as compared to perfusion, resulting in wasted ventilation (*physiological dead space formation*).

Increased Pulmonary Resistance may occur due to decrease in number of capillaries owing to the destruction of lung parenchyma. The increased pulmonary vascular resistance may in turn cause pulmonary hypertension.

Pulmonary Function Tests in patients with moderate to severe COPD may reveal following abnormalities:

- *Decreased forced expiratory flow* occurs due to: loss of lung elasticity, increase in airway resistance upstream from equal pressure point and an increase in compliance of the airway downstream from equal pressure points.
- *Forced vital capacity (FVC)* may be normal or decreased (reflecting increased residual volume).
- Forced expiratory volume in first second (FEV_1) is reduced as is the ratio of FEV_1/FVC.
- RV and FRC are increased. TLC may also be increased in some cases.

Restrictive Lung Diseases

The restrictive lung diseases include pulmonary fibrosis, silicosis, asbestosis, tuberculosis, pneumothorax, pleural effusion and paresis of respiratory muscles (e.g. in poliomyelitis and myasthenia gravis).

Characteristic Features. Restrictive lung diseases are characterized by low lung volumes. Patients with restrictive lung disease find it easier to breath at low lung volumes because it is difficult to expand the lungs.

Mechanisms of Restriction of Lung Expansion include:

- *Abnormalities of lung parenchyma.* Diseases in which excessive pulmonary fibrosis decreases lung elasticity as occur in pulmonary fibrosis, pneumonia, silicosis, asbestosis and tuberculosis.
- *Abnormalities of pleura* as occur in pneumothorax and pleural effusion.
- *Paresis of respiratory muscles* as occurs in poliomyelitis and myasthenia gravis.

I. Lung Parenchymal Diseases

1. Pneumonia. The term pneumonia includes an inflammatory condition of the lung in which alveoli are filled with fluid and inflammatory cells. It is characterized by clinical and radiological consolidation of the involved parts of lung parenchyma.

Causes. The pneumonia is usually an infective process caused by bacterial (commonly pneumococcal or viruses) but can also result from noninfective causes such as chemical or radiation injury to the lungs.

Functional Abnormalities which occur in patients with pneumonia are:

- *Restrictive pulmonary function defect* as occurs due to total replacement of alveolar gases by the inflammatory exudates in the involved part of lung.
- *VA/Q* is decreased because in the involved areas of lung, perfusion is normal but alveolar ventilation is markedly decreased, resulting in *physiological shunt formation.*
- *Hypoxia* may develop depending upon the extent of involvement of lung parenchyma.

Clinically patient may develop:

- *Fever which* occurs in response to infection
- *Compression of chest* and feeling of chest pain.
- *Respiratory efforts may be increased* due to stimulation by hypoxia and associated fever, leading to hypocapnia and respiratory alkalosis.
- *Heart rate* may be increased in response to hypoxia.
- *Retention of CO_2* occurs only in later stages in severe disease when patient gets exhausted and respiratory effort is failing.
- *Cerebral hypoxia* may develop in severe cases causing delirium which is characterized by confused mental state, illusion, hallucination, disorientation, hyperexcitability and loss of memory.

2. Pulmonary Tuberculosis

- Pulmonary tuberculosis is a chronic infection of the lung parenchyma caused by the acid-fast bacteria called *Mycobacterium tuberculosis* or tubercle bacilli.

- The invasion of lung parenchyma by tubercle bacilli causes infiltration of the infected area by macrophages and walling off of the lesion by fibrous tissue to form the so-called tubercle.
- Tuberculosis in its late stages causes many areas of fibrosis and reduces the total amount of lung tissue.
- Initially the alveoli in the affected part become nonfunctioning due to thickness of respiratory membrane. When a large part of the lung is involved, the diffusing capacity is very much reduced.

3. Atelectasis. Atelectasis refers to the collapse of alveoli with absence of air in the involved parts.

Causes. Atelectasis may develop due to:

- ***Obstruction of bronchus or a bronchiole.*** Air trapped distal to the bronchial obstruction is absorbed causing collapse of the alveoli attached to the bronchus or bronchiole.
- ***Lack of surfactant*** increases the surface tension of alveolar fluid and causes collapse of the alveoli. Marked lack of surfactant is seen in a disease called hyaline membrane disease or the so-called respiratory distress syndrome.
- ***Pressure from the pleural cavity*** caused by presence of air (pneumothorax), fluid (hydrothorax) or blood (haemothorax) in the pleural cavity may cause collapse of the lung, depending upon their amount present.

Functional Abnormality. When a large portion of the lung is collapsed, the partial pressure of oxygen is reduced in blood leading to respiratory disturbances. Marked collapse is a common cause of dyspnoea.

4. Pulmonary Oedema. Pulmonary oedema refers to collection of serous fluid in the alveoli and the interstitial spaces of the lung tissue.

Causes of pulmonary oedema are:

- *Increased pulmonary capillary pressure* as occurs in left ventricular failure or mitral valve disease.
- *Pneumonia*
- Effect of harmful chemicals like chlorine or sulphur dioxide.

Functional Abnormalities produced by pulmonary oedema are:

- *Diffusion capacity of the lung* is decreased due to increased thickness of respiratory membrane. So the ability of the lungs to oxygenate the blood and to remove the carbon dioxide is reduced.
- *Marked alveolar oedema* is fatal and causes sudden death due to suffocation.

II. Diseases of Pleura

The disease of pleura includes:

1. Pleural Effusion. Pleural effusion refers to accumulation of large amount of fluid in the pleural cavity. Normally, there is very little pleural fluid because the fluid which is produced by a pressure gradient pushing fluid from parietal capillaries to pleural space is promptly absorbed by a net force driving pleural fluid from pleural space to visceral capillaries and lymphatics.

Causes of pleural effusion include:

- ***Excessive transudation*** of fluid from the pulmonary capillaries due to:
  - Increased hydrostatic pressure as occurs in left ventricular failure or
  - Decreased oncotic pressure as occurs in hypoproteinaemia.
- ***Exudation in inflammatory conditions*** of pleura (pleuritis or pleurisy) results due to damage of capillary membranes, allowing leakage of fluid and plasma proteins into the pleural cavity. The high-protein content of pleural fluid increases its osmotic pressure which pulls more fluid.
- ***Obstruction to lymphatics*** in inflammatory and neoplastic conditions also leads to collection of fluid in the pleural cavity.

Functional Abnormalities produced in pleural effusion depend on the size of effusion and the rate at which fluid accumulates.

- Pleural effusion essentially produces a *restrictive abnormality* with decrease in FVC, FRC, TLC and RV.
- When large pleural effusion develops quickly, it causes atelectasis which is associated with dyspnoea and *hypoxia* producing hyperventilation and hypocapnia.
- Moderate to massive effusion causes shift of the mediastinal structures to the opposite side. When this occurs rapidly, this may compromise cardiac output and hypotension.

2. Pneumothorax. Pneumothorax refers to presence of air in the pleural cavity. Normally, there is a negative pressure in the pleural space (about –0.66 kPa), which becomes positive in pneumothorax.

Causes. Pneumothorax occurs due to entry of air into the pleural cavity either due to a hole in the chest wall and parietal pleura or a hole in the lung parenchyma and visceral pleura as may occur in accidents, bullet injuries or stab injuries.

Types of Pneumothorax and Functional Abnormalities produced in them are:

i. ***Open pneumothorax*** refers to the condition in which an open communication is developed between the pleural cavity and the atmosphere. So the air is present in the pleural cavity at atmospheric pressure which reduces all lung volumes. Thus, there occurs a restrictive ventilatory impairment leading to reduction in FVC, FRC and TLC in proportion to the volume of pneumothorax. Depending upon the degree of lung collapse produced there occurs proportionate hypoxia, hypocapnia, dyspnoea and cyanosis.
ii. ***Closed pneumothorax*** develops when after the entry of air into the pleural cavity the hole in the pleura is

sealed. As normally, the partial pressure of gases in the capillaries in the pleura are about 5.3 to 6 kPa less than atmospheric pressure, so there is a significant gradient for absorption of gases from pleural space to capillaries. Thus, the air entrapped in the pleural cavity is slowly absorbed; and so not much functional abnormalities are produced.

iii. ***Tension pneumothorax*** occurs when the hole produced in pleura is valvular which allows entry of air into the pleural cavity during inspiration but prevents the exit of air during expiration. As a result the intrapleural pressure keeps on rising progressively leading to collapse of ipsilateral lung and pushing the mediastinum and contralateral lung.
- Squeezing of both lungs leads to marked hypoxaemia.
- Displacement of mediastinal structures leads to progressive fall in cardiac output.
- Decreased cardiac output and hypoxia combined produce loss of consciousness and hypotension, and ultimately may prove fatal soon.

Tension pneumothorax requires treatment as a medical emergency.

III. Pulmonary Vascular Disorders

Pulmonary vascular disorders include: pulmonary hypertension and pulmonary embolism.

1. Pulmonary Hypertension. The mechanisms responsible for genesis of pulmonary hypertension are:

- *Increased pulmonary resistance*. The most common cause of pulmonary hypertension occurs due to:
  - Pulmonary vasoconstriction because of alveolar hypoxia (see page 417)
  - Obstruction of pulmonary vessels e.g thromboembolism
  - Pulmonary capillaries obliteration e.g in emphysema
- *Increase in left atrial pressure*-for details see page 467
- *Increased pulmonary blood flow* due to congenital heart diseases like ASD, VSD or patent ductus arteriosus, the high blood flow is accommodated by recruitment and distension of pulmonary blood vessels. However, sustained high blood flow results in structural changes in smaller vessels leading to rise in pulmonary arterial pressure and ultimately shunt in the heart is reversed (i.e instead of left to right, become right to left).

2. Pulmonary Embolism. Occlusion of pulmonary vessels by an embolus results in following effects:

A. ***When a large embolus gets lodged in a major branch of the pulmonary artery,*** it results in reduction in cardiac output and cor- pulmonale.Whereas, when small segmental arteries get blocked by medium sized emboli, then pulmonary infarction, cyanosis, tachypnea and pleural pain occurs. In nut shell there is high VA/Q ratio due to increase in physiological dead space and hypoxia, and pulmonary hypertension occurs.

B. ***The substances released from the thrombo-emboli*** (e.g Histamine, serotonin and prostaglandins) cause constriction in pulmonary vasculature and bronchoconstriction.

C. ***Surfactant synthesis*** also get reduced due to compromised blood flow, and results in collapse of alveoli and exudation of fluid (pulmonary oedema).

The above-mentioned effects are responsible for dyspnoea and syncope may occur in massive embolism.

ARTIFICIAL RESPIRATION AND CARDIOPULMONARY RESUSCITATION

Artificial Respiration

Artificial respiration (AR) alone is required as an emergency life saving procedure:

I. *When there is sudden stoppage of breathing* as seen in:
- Drowning,
- Electrocution,
- Anaesthetic accidents,
- Carbon monoxide poisoning,
- Strangulation and
- Accidents.

II. *AR may also be needed when breathing is expected to stop gradually* as in paralysis of muscles in:
- Poliomyelitis,
- Diphtheria and
- Ascending paralysis.

It is important to note that the tissues of brain, particularly cerebral cortex, develop irreversible damage if oxygen supply is stopped for 5 minutes. So, the resuscitation must be started quickly without any delay, before the development of cardiac failure.

Methods of Artificial Respiration

Presently, AR can be given by two types of methods:

- Manual methods, e.g. mouth-to-mouth breathing method.
- Mechanical methods.

Mouth-to-Mouth Breathing Method Various manual methods of AR have been described in past and discarded. Presently, the only manual method employed is mouth-to-mouth breathing (exhaled air ventilation) because:

- It can be applied quickly without waiting for the availability of any aid.
- It is simple and effective measure of resuscitation.
- It can be applied in all age groups.
- It is the only technique capable of producing adequate ventilation.
- It also works by expanding the lungs.

Procedure

- The procedure should be performed swifty and alertly.
- The procedure is performed after placing the patient in supine position.
- It is essential to provide and maintain a clear airway for the procedure to be effective. Therefore, any foreign material present in the mouth cavity must be removed with fingers, e.g. grass, straw, etc. (in case of drowning patients), artificial denture if any: mucus, saliva and blood clot. The tongue must be drawn forward and it must be prevented from falling posteriorly causing airway obstruction. The clothes around the neck and chest region must be loosen. If the mouth is full of blood, mouth-to-nose respiration should be given.
- To begin with patient's neck is extended by placing one hand under the neck and lifting it and pressing the forehead with the other hand (Fig. 5.7-6A). This prevents the flaccid tongue from falling back into the pharynx.
- Then the patient's nostrils are closed by the thumb and index finger of the hand (Fig. 5.7-6B).
- The resuscitator then takes a deep breath and exhales air into the patient's airway after tightly placing his mouth over patient's mouth and noting the expansion of the chest at the same time. The volume of the air exhaled must be twice the normal tidal volume. This expands the patient's lungs.
- Then, the resuscitator removes his mouth from that of the patient, allowing expiration to occur passively due to the elastic recoil of the lungs and chest (Fig. 5.7-6C).
- Some of the air is likely to enter the stomach through the oesophagus. It can be easily expelled by pressure on the epigastrium.
- The above procedure is repeated 12 to 16 times per minute till spontaneous breathing returns, or till the patient is shifted to a hospital.
- It is important to remember that:
  - Mouth-to-mouth method is the most effective manual method, because the CO_2 present in the expired air by the resuscitator can also directly stimulate the respiratory centres and facilitate the onset of respiration.
  - The expired air by the resuscitator contains 16% oxygen which is sufficient to revive the patient.

Mechanical Methods of AR The mechanical respirators are employed when AR has to be continued for long periods. The mechanical respirators are of two types:

- Tank respirators and
- Ventilators.

1. Tank Respirators or the so-called iron lung chambers as the name indicates consist of an airtight chamber made of iron or steel. There are various types of mechanical respirators. A commonly used respirator is the Drinker respirator. In this respirator, the patient is kept inside the tank by placing the head outside the chamber. In the Drinker method, alternate positive and negative pressure breathing machines produce periodic inflation and deflation of the lungs.

2. Ventilators are the AR mechines by which air or oxygen is pumped into the lungs with pressure intermittently through a rubber tube introduced into the patient's trachea. Inflation occurs when air is pumped and expiration occurs by elastic recoil of chest and lungs, when it is stopped. Presently two types of ventilators are available:

- ***Volume ventilator pumps*** a constant volume of air into the patient's lungs intermittently with minimum pressure.
- ***Pressure ventilator pumps*** the air with a constant high pressure into the patient's lungs.

Cardiopulmonary Resuscitation

Cardiopulmonary resuscitation (CPR) is required in some patients when heart and respiration both stop. Breathing

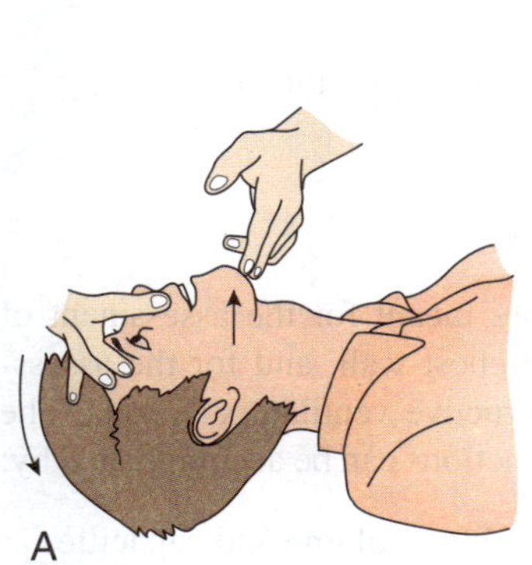

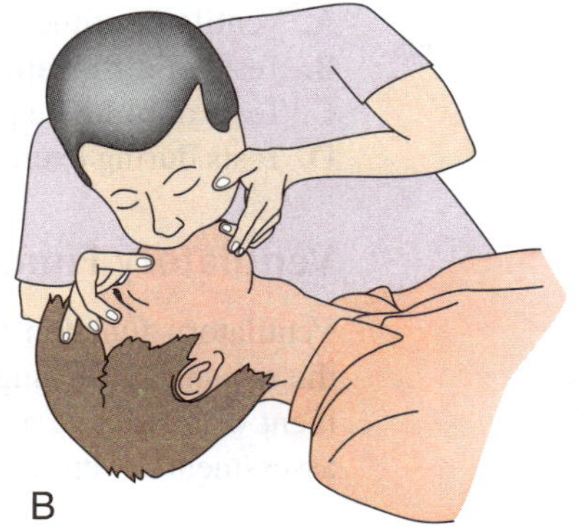

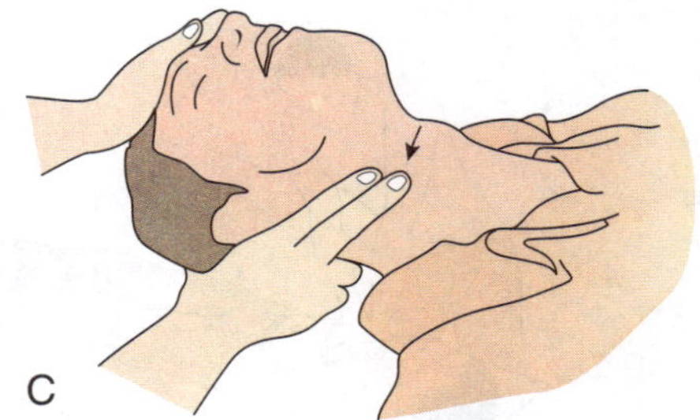

FIGURE 5.7-6 Mouth-to-mouth breathing: (**A**) the neck is extended by placing one hand under the neck and pressing the forehead with other hand; (**B**) nostrils are closed with thumb and index finger and resuscitator exhales into the patient's airway by tightly placing his mouth over the patients mouth; and (**C**) allows the patient to exhale passively by unsealing nose and mouth.

usually stops before the heart stops, so AR should be started immediately. The CPR may be required in patients with:

- Ventricular fibrillation following a heart attack,
- Victim of electrocution,
- Drowning.

Emergency Plan of CPR The following plan called ABC of CPR has proved useful in reviving such patients:

A: Airway Care is required in unconscious patients. Immediately, tilt head back with a hand under the neck to maintain an open airway (Fig. 5.7-6A).

B: Breathing by the AR method is required when the patient is not breathing. Mouth-to-mouth respiration should be immediately started (see page 480). Feel carotid pulse, if present continue AR only.

C: Cardiac Massage is required when carotid pulse cannot be felt. During external cardiac massage (procedure described below) sternum should be depressed by 4–5 cm at a rate of 80 to 90 times per minute. The cardiac compression should be alternated with mouth-to-mouth respiration at a rate of one ventilation to five chest compression (1:5).

Procedure of External Cardiac Massage. Effective cardiac massage can be carried out without opening the chest. The person conducting external cardiac massage places the heel of one hand on the lower sternum above the xiphoid process and the heel of the other hand on top of the first (Fig. 5.7-7). Pressure is applied straight down, depressing the sternum 4 or 5 cm toward the spine. This procedure is repeated 80–90 times per minute. Manually squeezing the ventricles is also effective, if the chest is already open, but emergency thoracotomies should not be performed.

Precautions to be taken during CPR are:

- CPR must be started at the earliest, because a delay of more than 4–5 minutes may cause irreversible damage to the brain.
- The patient should not be made to sit or stand. No pillow should be put under his head, because it will bend the head and occlude trachea.
- Nothing orally should be given to an unconscious person.

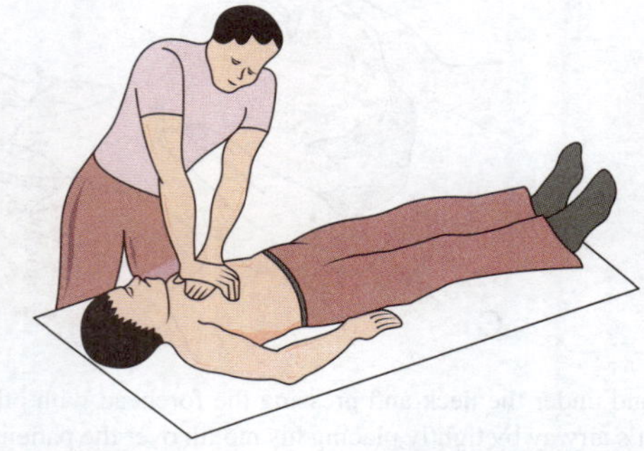

FIGURE 5.7-7 Procedure showing external cardiac massage.

- The feet and legs should be raised with a pillow under the hip to improve cerebral blood flow.
- While giving cardiac massage, the pressure should not be applied over the ribs as they are likely to fracture.

PULMONARY FUNCTION TESTS

Role of Pulmonary Function Tests in Clinical Practice

The evaluation of pulmonary function begins with a careful history taking meticulous clinical examination and radiographs of chest. In addition, various pulmonary function tests are employed to help the clinician to make a physiological assessment of lung function rather than to make a pathological diagnosis. The roles of pulmonary function tests in clinical practice are:

1. In diagnosis of pulmonary diseases, pulmonary function tests may be employed:
    - For early diagnosis of a disease, e.g. decreased diffusing capacity is the earliest change seen in interstitial lung disease,
    - For confirmation of clinical diagnosis and
    - For exclusion of a diagnosis.
2. To follow the progress of disease and its response to treatment.
3. To objectively assess the severity of disease.
4. To assess respiratory status before anaesthesia and also to assess the capacity of the individual to tolerate the risk of surgery especially cardiothoracic surgery involving removal of a lung or its part.
5. To assess physical fitness for certain jobs such as those involving strenuous physical exercise, flying at high altitude, etc.
6. To obtain medicolegal information in certain situation.

Classification

Pulmonary function tests can be classified into following groups:

A. Ventilatory function tests,
B. Tests of diffusion,
C. Tests of ultimate purpose of respiration and
D. Tests during exercise.

Ventilatory Function Tests

Ventilatory function tests are meant for the assessment of the expansion of lungs and chest wall, and for the assessment of restrictive and obstructive ventilatory defects. The assessment of ventilatory functions can be accomplished by:

I. Measurement of various lung volume and capacities,
II. Measurement of dead space,
III. Measurement of compliance and
IV. Measurement of airway resistance.

I. Measurement of Various Lung Volumes and Capacities

Various lung volumes and capacities have been described on page 401. Most of the lung volumes and capacities except residual volume, functional residual capacity and total lung capacity can be measured by spirometry. Functional residual capacity is determined by nitrogen wash-out method or helium dilution method, and then residual volume and total lung capacity are calculated.

Spirometry Spirometry refers to recording of volume changes during various clearly defined breathing manoeuvres. It can be performed using a simple spirometer, a modified spirometer called respirometer or computerized spirometer.

• ***Simple Spirometer*** (Fig. 5.7-8) is made of metal. It consists of following parts:

- *Outer chamber* or container which is filled with water.
- *Floating drum* or a gas bell with 6-litre capacity, floats in the water in an inverted manner. It is attached to a chain which passes over a pulley bearing a balancing weight and a writing needle (pen). The needle (pen) moves with the movement of the floating drum. The floating drum is thus counterpoised and has very little inertia and friction.
- *Inner chamber* is open at the top end which lies above the water level in outer chamber and is connected to a tube at the bottom end. At the end of tube, a mouthpiece is attached through which the subject is made to respire.

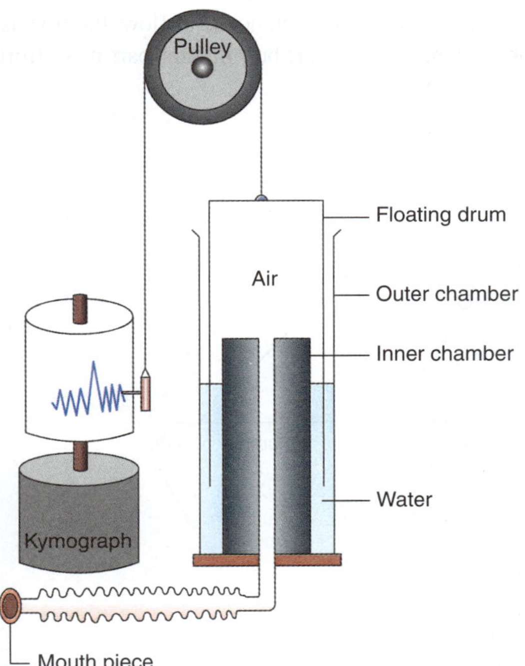

FIGURE 5.7-8 Simple spirometer.

- *Kymograph* is a recording drum on which the movements of the needle are recorded.

• ***Procedure.*** The whole procedure is explained to the subject thoroughly and then he is made to breathe through the mouthpiece of the spirometer. As explained above and shown in Figure 5.7-8, the arrangement in spirometer is such that when the subject expires the floating drum (gas bell) moves up and the counterweight along with writing needle (pen) moves down, and thus the expiration is recorded as downward deflection on the kymograph. Conversely, when the subject inspires, the floating drum moves down and the counterweight with writing pen moves up; and thus the inspiration is recorded as an upward deflection on the kymograph. The record of various lung volume and capacities so obtained on the kymograph is called spirogram.

To measure the various lung volumes and capacities the subject is instructed to expire or inspire as described:

- First, he is asked to breath normally (tidal respiration) for a few times,
- Then he is asked to inspire as deeply and fully as possible and
- Thus, while keeping the nostrils closed with his thumb and index finger, he is asked to expire with a maximum effort. It is preferable to take three recordings, at intervals of 5 minutes, for each determination. The maximum volume of the three readings should be considered the reporting value. The various lung volumes and capacities are then calculated from the record (spirogram so obtained) (see page 401 Fig. 5.2-6) which in general give information about the ventilatory functions.

Of the various static and dynamic lung volumes and capacities which serve as more useful pulmonary function tests are:

1. Vital Capacity

Measurement of vital capacity under different conditions is the most commonly performed pulmonary function test.

Slow Vital Capacity Slow vital capacity is the volume of air expired (after maximum inspiration) during a slowly performed maximum expiratory effort. It is used to evaluate the size of the lungs (see Fig. 5.2-6). The vital capacity can be decreased by either decrease in TLC as seen in restrictive lung disease or by increase in reserve volume ie seen in obstructive lung disease.

Forced Vital Capacity FVC or TVC is the volume of air that can be expired rapidly with a maximal expiratory effort after a maximal inspiration.

FVC is reduced in:

- *Conditions producing restrictive defect,* such as kyphoscoliosis, pleural effusion, pneumonia, etc. and

- *Condition producing trapping of air* due to collapse of distal air during a forced expiratory manoeuvre.

Components of FVC The volume of air expired can be timed by recording the forced vital capacity on a spirograph moving at the known speed. From the graph so obtained (Fig. 5.2-7), the FVC can be divided into following components:

i. Forced Expiratory Volume During First Second (FEV_1)

- FEV_1 is the volume of air expired during the first second of FVC.
- It is the most commonly used screening test for airway diseases.
- The FEV_1 is actually a flow rate,its unit are L/sec.
- FEV_1% is the percentage of VC expired in one second, i.e. $FEV_1\% = FEV1/FVC \times 100$) normally FEV_1% or about 80% of the FVC (Fig. 5.2-8A).

Clinical application. Useful in distinguishing between restrictive and obstructive lung disease:

- Patients with *restrictive lung disease* (e.g. kyphoscoliosis and ankylosing spondylitis) have a reduced FVC but are able to achieve relatively high flow rates; therefore, their FEV_1% exceeds 80% (Fig. 5.2-8B).
- Patients with *obstructive lung disease* (e.g. bronchial asthma) have low flow rates as a result of high airway resistance therefore their FEV_1% is abnormally low (Fig. 5.2-8C).

ii. Forced Expiratory Volume in 2 sec (FEV_2). It represents the volume of air expired in first 2 second of an FVC, FEV_2% is about 90% of FVC under normal condition.

iii. Forced Expiratory Volume in 3 sec (FEV_3). It represents the volume of air expired in first 3 second. Normally FEV_3% is 98–100% of FVC.

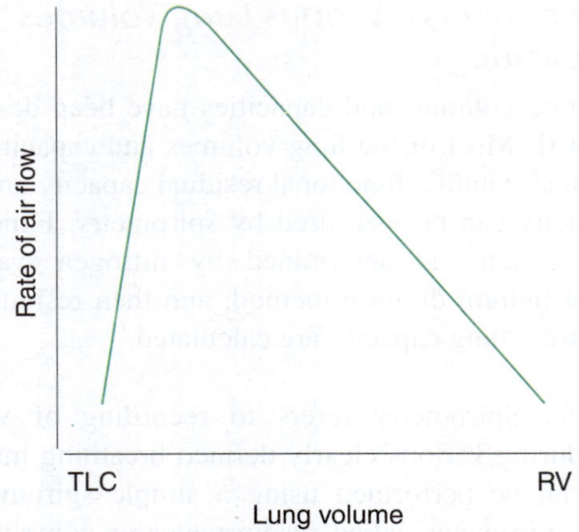

FIGURE 5.7-9 Flow–volume curve during maximum expiration.

Flow–Volume Curve The rate of air flow noted during maximum expiration can be plotted versus volume change to give a flow–volume curve (Fig. 5.7-9). This curve may be altered dramatically in obstructive and restrictive diseases. However, due to technical problems, flow-volume curve is not routinely plotted in clinical respiratory laboratories.

Flow Volume Loop Flow Volume loop is a relationship between volume and flow during maximum inspiratory and expiratory effort, which can be recorded with recent computerized recorders for ventilatory function. The normal pattern of pressure volume loop is a 'triangle sitting on a semi circle'. (Fig 5.7-10).

Clinical significance of Flow Volume loop is as under:

During expiration depending on the mechanical properties of the lung and resistance to airflow; the flow is effort dependent in early part but, in later part it is effort independent. Therefore,

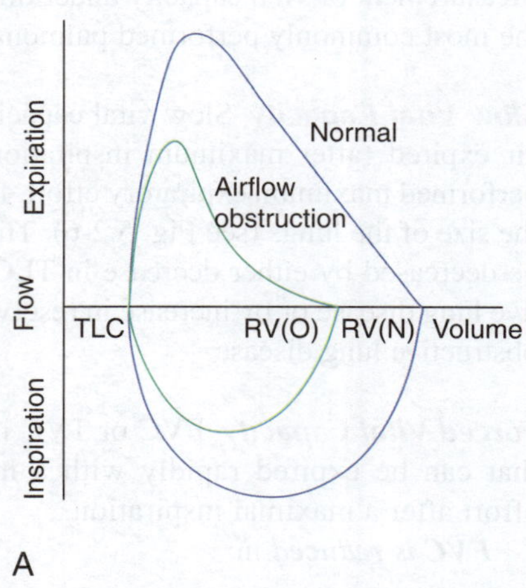

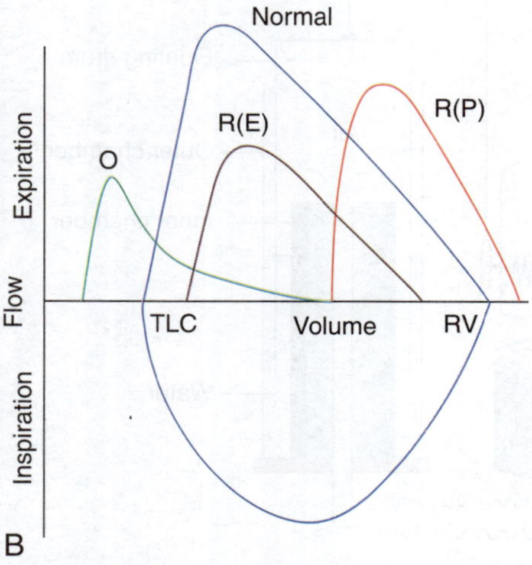

FIGURE 5.7-10 Flow–volume loops in a normal individual and a patient with airflow obstruction - **A;** and in different conditions - **B;** R(E) - extraparenchymal restrictive disease; O = obstructive disease. R(P) Parenchymal restrictive disease

- In case of air flow obstruction, the flow rate at any given volume is decreased, particularly in later part of expiration and scooped out appearance to the expiratory curve (Fig 5.7-10B). Therefore, in obstructive lung disease an abnormal flow-volume loop may appear before any abnormality is appreciated in FEV_1/FEV or $FFF_{25-75\%}$

2. Forced Expiratory Flow Rate during 25–75% of Expiration ($FEF_{25-75\%}$)

- It is the mean expiratory flow rate during middle 50% of FVC (Fig. 5.2-9A), and so is also called the mid-expiratory flow rate.
- This measurement can be done from the same record as FEV_1. The total expired volume is divided into four equal parts. The flow rate is calculated for the middle two parts (25 to 75%), i.e. the middle half.
- Mid expiratory time (MET) refers to the time taken for FEF 25-75%. Its normal value is 0.5 sec which is increased in obstructive lung disorders. It may be the only abnormality indicating early disease in smokers with COPD.

3. Peak Expiratory Flow Rate

Park expiratory flow rate (PEFR) refers to the maximum rate of air flow observed during a sudden forced expiration, from the position of full inspiration. It can be measured by a simple device known as peak flow meter (Fig. 5.7.11) which can be used by the patients even at home. The best of three efforts should be noted as the value of PEFR. It is a good and reproducible measure of degree of airflow obstruction.

4. Maximum Breathing Capacity (MBC) or Maximum Voluntary Ventilation (MVV)

For details see page 403.

5. Spirometric Response to Inhaled Bronchodilators

In this test forced expirogram is recorded before and 10–20 mins after inhalation of two puffs of Salbutamol inhaler (separated by 30–60 seconds interval). Each puff delivers 100 μg of bronchodilator. Test is used for finding out:

- Whether the air flow obstruction is reversible or not, specially in suspected asthma patients and also
- To know the degree of reversiblility in severe cases of asthma.

6. Functional Residual Capacity

FRC is the volume of the air remaining in the lungs after normal tidal expiration. For details see page 401.

Functional residual capacity can be measured by nitrogen wash-out method or helium dilution method.

For details see page 401

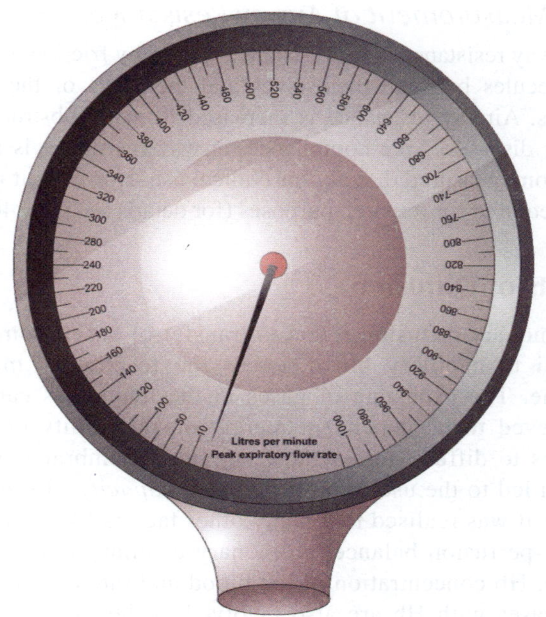

FIGURE 5.7-11 Peak flow meter.

Common Abnormal Patterns of TLC, FRC and RV

- *Normal TLC with increased FRC, RV and RV/TLC ratio* is seen in patients with severe airway obstruction with air trapping. Since FVC is reduced in such patients so FRC and RV are increased.
- *Reduced TLC, RV and FRC* is seen in patients with restrictive lung disorders like interstitial lung disease. On spirometry, FVC is also reduced in such patients.
- *Reduced TLC with increased RV and FRC* may be seen in patients with mixed obstructive and restrictive lung disorders.

II. Measurement of Dead Space

Dead space air is the portion of minute ventilation that does not take part in exchange of gases. Normally, it is constituted by the air present in the conducting zone of respiratory passages *(anatomical dead space),* but in some diseases may additionally include also poorly perfused alveoli (physiological dead space). For details see page 421.

III. Measurement of Compliance

Compliance (C) expresses the distensibility (expansibility) of the lungs and chest wall. Reduced compliance produces a condition called RLD. In clinical testing, the restrictive lung diseases are evaluated indirectly by measurement of various lung volumes and capacities as described above. Thus, direct measurement of compliance in the respiratory system is rarely done for clinical use; however it may be required for research purposes. For details see page 408.

IV. Measurement of Airway Resistance

Airway resistance is the resistance caused by friction of gas molecules between themselves and the walls of the airways. Airway resistance is increased in many obstructive lung diseases. Like compliance, airway resistance is also seldom measured directly for clinical use. However, it may be required for research purposes (for details see page 409).

Tests of Diffusion

Pulmonary diffusion refers to transfer of gases from alveoli to capillary blood across the respiratory membrane. The exchange of gases in the lungs was earlier believed to be dependent merely on the ability of the gases to diffuse across the respiratory membrane. This term led to the use of term *diffusion capacity.* However, later it was realised that many other factors like ventilation–perfusion balance, pulmonary capillary blood volume, Hb concentration of the blood and rate of reaction of gases with Hb are also involved in the exchange of gases. Therefore, nowadays, the term *transfer factor,* rather than diffusion capacity is used.

For estimation of transfer factor (diffusion capacity) of O_2 see page 428.

Tests of Ultimate Purpose of Respiration

Since the ultimate purpose of respiration is to supply O_2 from atmosphere to tissues and removal of CO_2 from the tissues into the atmosphere; so, the estimation of arterial blood pO_2, pCO_2 and pH (blood gas analysis) are most fundamental of all the pulmonary function tests.

Estimation of Arterial pO_2, pCO_2 and pH For blood gas analysis, arterial blood sample is usually taken from the radial artery or femoral artery. The estimation of pO_2, pCO_2 and pH can be done within a minute or so using a very small sample of blood with the help of miniaturised glass electrodes.

Arterial pO_2 levels in young healthy adult vary from 85 to 105 mmHg with a mean of 95 mmHg. The value may drop by upto 15% in healthy elderly subjects due to an increase in ventilation-perfusion inequality.

Causes of decreased arterial pO_2 are:

- Alveolar hypoventilation, i.e. inadequate intake of air.
- Diffusion defect, i.e. inadequate transport of O_2 across the respiratory membrane.
- Arteriovenous admixture, i.e. right to left vascular shunt and
- Decreased ventilation-perfusion ratio, i.e. physiological shunt as seen in patients with emphysema.

Arterial pCO_2 and pH level in normal adult are about 40 mmHg and 7.4, respectively and are basically determined by the volume of alveolar ventilation:

- *Hypoventilation* causes increased pCO_2 and reduction in arterial pH (respiratory acidosis),
- *Hyperventilation* produces decreased pCO_2 and increase in arterial pH (respiratory alkalosis).

Tests during Exercise

Because of enormous physiological reserves, both the cardiac and pulmonary functions may be normal at rest in early stages of the disease. Exercise testing provides information about the total cardiopulmonary performance of the individual and unmasks the abnormality not detected by the function tests performed at rest. The exercise may be performed on a treadmill or a cycle ergometer. Measurement of pulse rate, minute ventilation, O_2 uptake and arterial blood gas tension during graded exercise are extremely useful specially when the cause of dyspnoea is obscure.

Section 6

Excretory System

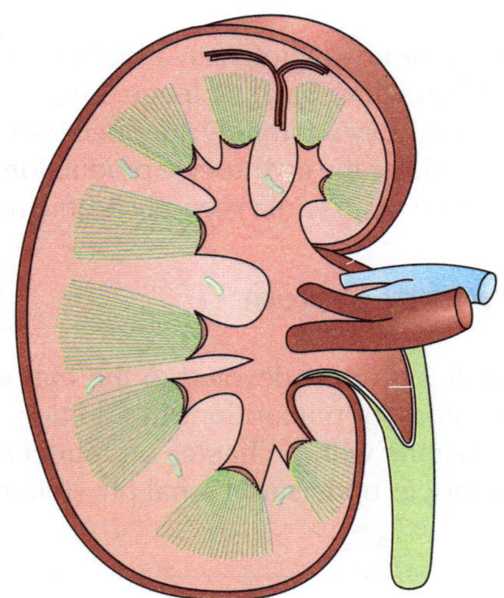

Concept of excretory system: *Excretion*. Literally, the word excretion means elimination of any matter from the body of an organism. The organs that are involved in the process of excretion include:

- *Kidneys,* which excrete water and water-soluble waste products,
- *Lungs,* which excrete carbon dioxide, water vapour and other volatile substances such as acetone,
- *Skin,* which excretes water and salts mainly in the form of sweat and
- *Gastrointestinal tract,* which excretes faeces (excreta).

However, *sensu stricto,* the term excretion refers to elimination of principal products of metabolism except carbon dioxide. The principal products of metabolism, other than carbon dioxide, are ammonia, urea, uric acid, creatinine, various pigments and inorganic salts. Of these, carbon dioxide is a universal metabolic waste which is discharged by the respiratory organs. The remaining excretory substances, in bulk, are excreted by the kidneys. Small quantities of some of the excretory substances are also eliminated by the skin.

Excretory organs. Thus, in the strictest sense, kidneys are the excretory organs. Together with a pair of ureters and a urinary bladder, kidneys constitute the excretory system. Most excretory substances are in solution in water. Water itself is not considered a waste product, but any excess of it is eliminated along with the excretory substances dissolved in it. The final product is called urine. That is why, the kidneys may also be called as urinary organs and the excretory system as urinary system.

Functions of Excretory Organs

Excretory organs, i.e. the kidneys, serve several major functions:

1. *Excretory function*. As mentioned above, the kidneys excrete a number of end products of metabolism in urine. Thus, formation of urine is the major function of the kidneys. The kidneys eliminate these substances from the body at a rate that matches their production. Thus, they regulate their concentration within the body fluids. In addition to the metabolic wastes, they also excrete foreign substances from the body, such as drugs, pesticides and other chemical ingested in food.
2. *Regulation of water and inorganic ion balance*. Control of volume of body fluids and their inorganic ion balance is an important homeostatic role of kidneys. The kidneys accomplish this task by working in concert with components of cardiovascular system, endocrine and central nervous system. Therefore, it has been discussed in chapter on 'Regulation of Body Fluid, Osmolality, Composition and Volume' on page 529.
3. *Regulation of acid–base balance*. Kidneys, in co-ordination with lungs, liver and buffers in the body play a role in regulation of the acid–base balance. This co-ordinated function has been discussed in a separate chapter on 'Physiology of Acid–Base Balance', in Section 12 on 'Specialized Integrative Physiology' (page 1227).
4. *Hormonal function*. As an endocrine gland, the kidneys produce and secrete renin, calcitriol and erythropoietin.
   - *Renin* activates the renin–angiotensin–aldosterone system that influences the blood pressure and sodium and potassium balance (page 534).
   - *Calcitriol* (1,25-dihydroxy vitamin D_3) influences calcium balance (page 727).
   - *Erythropoietin* stimulates the erythrocyte production by the bone marrow. Decreased erythrocyte production is a cause of anaemia seen in chronic renal failure (page 545).

Overview of Excretory System

This section on excretory system is devoted to the major function of excretory system—the formation of urine and physiology of micturition. In addition, important applied aspects have also been included. This section begins with a chapter on 'Functional Anatomy of Kidneys and Renal Blood Flow', which is mandatory to understand renal physiology.

Chapter 6.1

Kidneys: Functional Anatomy and Blood Flow

FUNCTIONAL ANATOMY OF KIDNEYS

Gross Anatomy

External Features Gross anatomical features of a human kidney, illustrated in Fig. 6.1-1A, are:

Location. The kidneys are bean-shaped organs that lie retroperitoneally on the posterior abdominal wall, one on each side of the vertebral column at the level of T_{12} to L_1 vertebrae. The right kidney lies slightly inferior to the left kidney.

Size and Shape. During life, the kidneys are reddish-brown in colour. Each kidney in an adult human weighs about 150 g and measures approximately 10 cm in length, 5 cm in width and 2.5 cm in thickness.

Surface, Borders and Poles. Each kidney has anterior and posterior surfaces, medial and lateral margins, and superior and inferior poles. The lateral margin is convex and the medial margin is concave, where the renal sinus and renal pelvis are located.

Renal Hilum and Sinus. The renal hilum is a vertical cleft present on the concave medial margin. It is the entrance to space within the kidney—the renal sinus. Through the renal hilum the renal artery enters, and the renal vein and renal pelvis leave the renal sinus. The *renal sinus* is thus occupied by the renal pelvis, calyces, vessels, nerves and a variable amount of fat.

Renal Pelvis and Calyces. The renal pelvis is the flattened, funnel-shaped expansion of the superior end of ureter. Within the renal sinus, the pelvis divides into two (or three) parts called *major calyces*. Each major calyx divides into a number of *minor calyces*. The end of each minor calyx is shaped like a cup into which fits a projection of kidney tissue called renal papilla (the apex of renal pyramid).

Gross Internal Structure Gross internal structure of the kidney, as seen in coronal section through the organ, exhibits that kidney tissue consists of an outer region called the cortex and an inner region called the medulla (Fig. 6.1-1B).

Medulla. It is made up of triangular areas of renal tissue that are called the renal pyramids. Pyramids are 4–14 in number and separated from each other by cortical columns of Bertin. Each pyramid has a base directed towards the cortex, and an apex (or renal papilla) which is directed towards the renal pelvis and fits into the minor calyx. Pyramids show striations that pass radially towards the apex. These striations are due to straight portion of the nephron and extend some distance upwards into the cortex where they are called medullary rays. The medulla can be subdivided into two parts:

- ***Outer medulla*** that is further subdivided into the outer stripe, and the inner stripe.
- ***Inner medulla*** is also called papillary zone.

Cortex. The renal cortex can be divided into two parts which are continuous with each other:

- ***Cortical arches*** or cortical lobules refer to the tissue lying between the bases of pyramids and surface of the kidney.
- ***Renal columns refer*** to the cortical tissue that lies in between the pyramids.

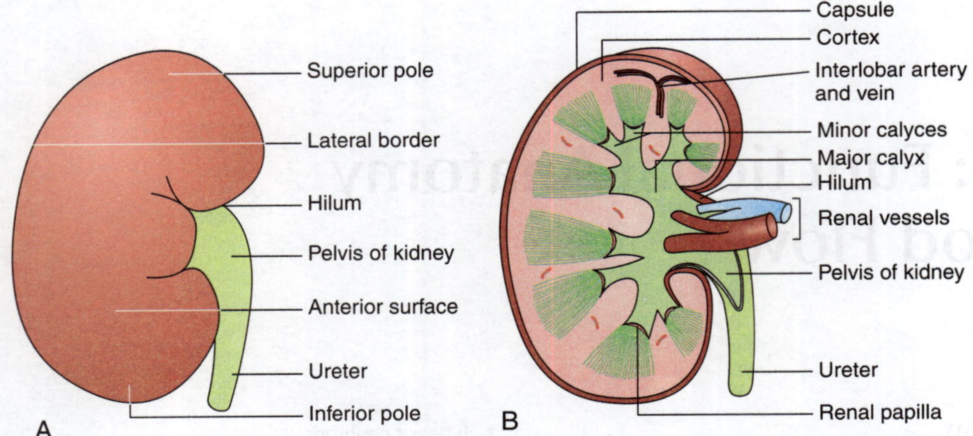

FIGURE 6.1-1 Gross anatomical features (**A**) and coronal section through human kidney (**B**).

- ***Lobe of kidney***. *Each* pyramid, surrounded by a shell of cortex, constitutes a lobe of the kidney. This lobulation is obvious in the fetal kidney.

Microscopic Structure of Kidney

Microscopically, the cortex and medulla of the kidney are composed of nephrons, blood vessels, lymphatics and nerves.

Nephron is a structural and functional unit of the kidney. Each kidney contains approximately 1.2 million nephrons. Each nephron is capable of forming urine.

Structure of the Nephron A nephron consists of two major parts (Fig. 6.1-2):

- Renal corpuscle, and
- Renal tubule.

Renal Corpuscle. Renal corpuscle or Malpighian corpuscle is a rounded structure comprising glomerulus surrounded by glomerular capsule (Fig. 6.1-3A).

Glomerulus. Glomerulus refers to a rounded tuft of anastomosing capillaries about 200 μm in diameter. Blood enters the glomerulus through an *afferent arteriole* and leaves it through an *efferent arteriole* (note that the efferent vessel

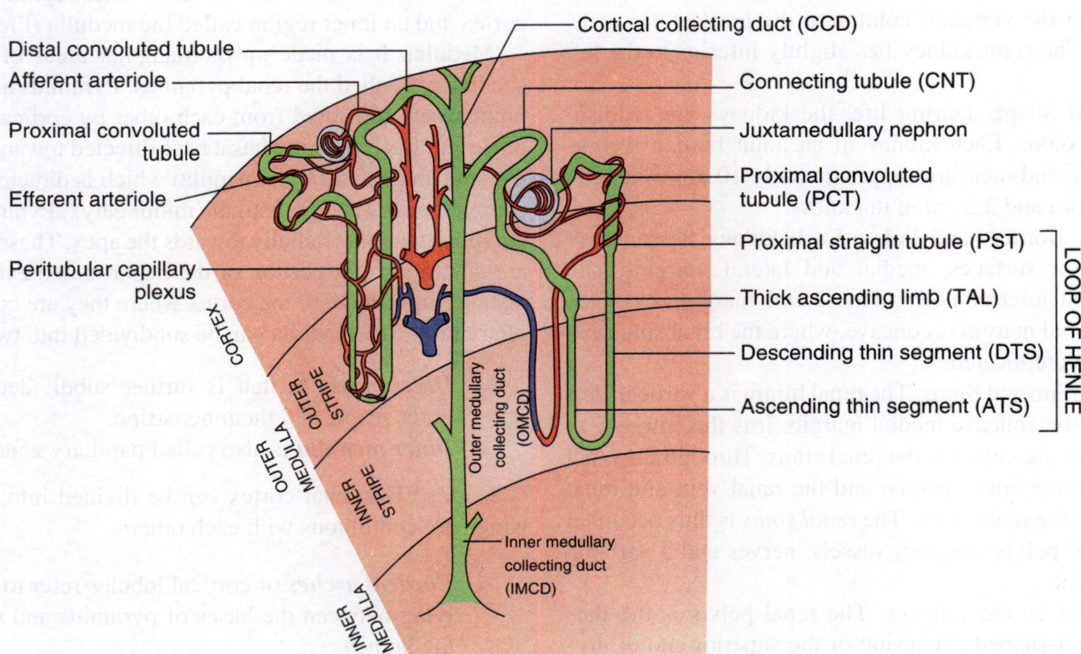

FIGURE 6.1-2 Part of a typical nephron. Organization of cortical and juxtamedullary nephrons showing different parts. Note differences between two types of nephrons.

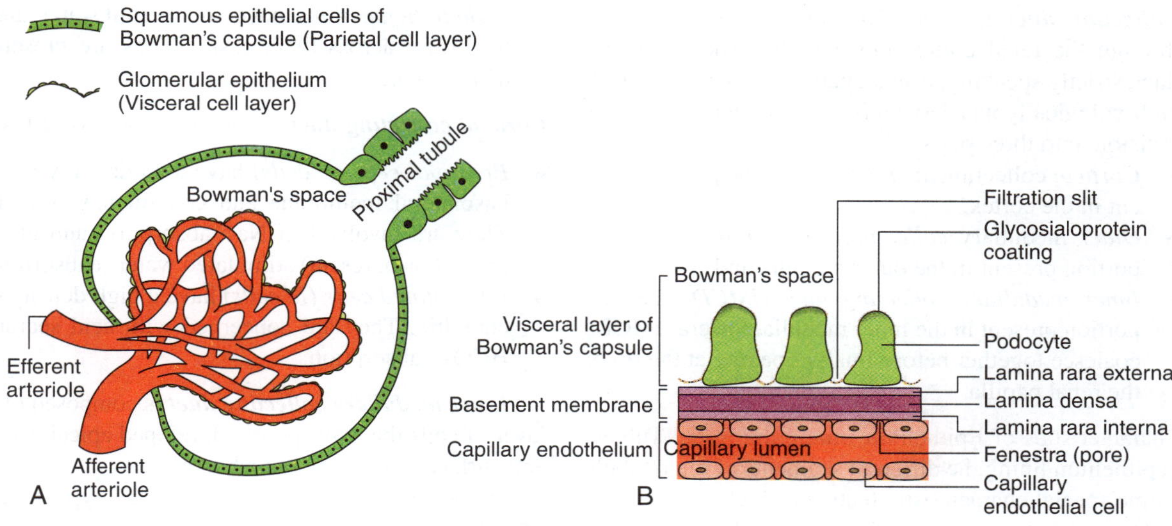

FIGURE 6.1-3 Structure of a glomerulus (**A**) and glomerular membrane (**B**).

is an arteriole and not a venule). The afferent and efferent arterioles lie close together at a point that is referred to as the *vascular* pole of the renal corpuscle.

Glomerular Capsule. Glomerular capsule, also known as Bowman's capsule, encloses the glomerulus and is formed of two layers: the inner layer covering the glomerular capillaries is called *visceral layer*, and the outer layer is called *parietal layer*. In fact, the Bowman's capsule represents the cup-shaped blind beginning of the renal tubule. The space between the visceral and parietal layer of the capsule (called Bowman's space or urinary space) is continuous with the lumen of the renal tubule.

Ultrastructure of Glomerular Membrane. Glomerular membrane refers to the membrane that separates blood of glomerular capillaries from the fluid present in the Bowman's space. It is also called *filtration barrier* and consists of three major layers (Fig. 6.1.3B):

1. ***Capillary endothelium***. It is fenestrated (i.e. it contains pores with diameter 70–90 nm) and is freely permeable to water, small solutes and even to small proteins.
2. ***Basement membrane***. It consists of a matrix of glycoproteins and mucopolysaccharides. Compared with typical membranes, the glomerular basement membrane is very thick. It comprises three layers:
   - Lamina rara externa or outer cement layer,
   - Lamina densa and
   - Lamina rara interna.

   No pores have been demonstrated in the basement membrane; however, its permeability corresponds to pore size (of about 8 nm).
3. ***Bowman's visceral epithelium*** or the inner layer of Bowman's capsule, which forms the third layer of glomerular membrane, is formed by special cells called *podocytes*. Podocytes have finger-like processes that encircle the outer surface of capillaries. The processes of podocytes interdigitate to cover the basement membrane and are separated by gaps called the *filtration slits* (~25 nm diameter). Each filtration slit is covered by a layer of fine filaments that constitute the diaphragm.

Mesangium is an important component of renal corpuscle; it consists of mesangium cells that are present between the capillary endothelial cells and the basement membrane, especially where the basement membrane encloses more than one capillary. These cells provide structural support for the glomerular capillaries, secrete the extracellular matrix and exhibit phagocytic activity.

Renal Tubule. Renal tubule is a long complicated tubule, which is divisible into the following main parts (Fig. 6.1-2), is about 15 mm long and 55 μm in diameter:

1. ***Proximal tubule***. The proximal tubule initially forms several coils, *proximal convoluted tubule (PCT)*, followed by a straight segment, *proximal straight tubule (PST)* or *pars recta* that descends towards the medulla.
2. ***Intermediate tubule or loop of Henle*** that consists of:
   - Descending thin segment (DTS),
   - Ascending thin segment (ATS) and
   - Thick ascending limb (TAL).

   In *juxtamedullary nephrons,* the DTS joins ATS to form the hair pin band (loop). The ATS reaches up to the junction of outer and inner medulla. In *cortical nephrons,* there is no ATS; the DTS is continuous at the bend of loop with the thick ascending limb (TAL). Near the end of thick ascending limb (TAL), the nephron passes between its afferent and efferent arteriole. This short segment of the thick ascending limb is called the *macula densa*.
3. ***Distal convoluted tubule (DCT)*** is about 5 mm long. It begins a short distance beyond the macula densa and extends to a point in the cortex where the connecting tubules (CNT) of two or more nephrons join to form the cortical collecting ducts.

4. ***Collecting duct*** is about 20 mm long which passes through the renal cortex and medulla. The collecting duct, strictly speaking, is not a part of the nephron, since embryologically it is derived from the ureteric buds. It is divisible into three parts:
   - *Cortical* collecting *duct (CCD),* i.e. the portion present in the cortex,
   - *Outer* medullary *collecting duct (OMCD),* i.e. the portion present in the outer medulla and
   - *Inner medullary collecting duct (IMCD),* i.e. the portion present in the inner medulla. Several IMCDs coalesce together before finally opening at the tip of the renal papilla.

Characteristics of Epithelium Lining the Renal Tubule. The epithelium lining the different segments of renal tubule has some special characteristic features which are suited to perform specific transport functions (Figs 6.1-2, 6.1-4).

Type of cells. The cells lining the renal tubule are mostly cuboidal, except in the thin segment where these are flat or squamous type.

Apical surface of cuboidal cells bear a few microvilli in general, which are numerous, dense and amplified in proximal tubule cells to form the so-called brush border.

Basolateral membrane of the proximal convoluted tubule cells, thick ascending segment cells and distal convoluted tubule cells is highly invaginated and contains many mitochondria. These infoldings create basal spaces. In contrast, the cells of descending thin limb and ascending thin limb of loop of Henle have poorly developed basolateral surfaces and contain a few mitochondria.

Lateral surfaces of the cells of renal tubules bear the lateral cell process which interdigitate with lateral processes of the adjacent cells. *Lateral intercellular* spaces are present in between the interdigitations. Lateral intercellular spaces do not communicate with the basal spaces. The lateral surfaces of cells form two types of tight junctions:

- *Leaky tight junctions* that permit water and solutes to diffuse across them. These are present in the *proximal tubule.*

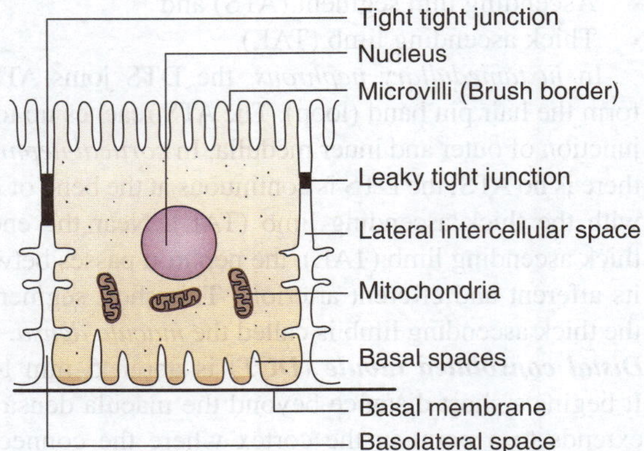

FIGURE 6.1-4 Ultrastructure of an epithelial cell lining the proximal convoluted tubule.

- *Tight tight junctions* that do not permit water and solutes to diffuse across them easily. They are present in the *distal tubule.*

Cortical collecting duct is composed of two cell types:

- *Principal cells (P cells)* have a moderately invaginated basolateral membrane and contain few mitochondria. They are involved in Na^+ absorption and also antidiuretic (vasopressin) stimulated water reabsorption.
- *Intercalated cells (Ic cells)* have a high density of mitochondria. They are concerned with acid secretion and HCO_3^- absorption.

Inner medullary collecting duct is composed of a single layer of cells that have poorly developed apical and basolateral surfaces and a few mitochondria.

In the interstitial tissue of medulla, type I medullary interstitial cells are present, which contain lipid droplets and also secrete prostaglandins (predominantly PGE_2).

Types of Nephrons There are two types of nephrons: cortical (superficial) and juxtamedullary. Differences between the cortical and juxtamedullary nephrons are depicted in Fig. 6.1-2 and Table 6.1-1.

Juxtaglomerular Apparatus Juxtaglomerular apparatus as the name indicates (juxta—near) refers to collection of specialized cells located very near to the glomerulus. It forms the major component of renin–angiotensin–aldosterone system The juxtaglomerular apparatus comprises three types of cells (Fig. 6.1-5):

- Juxtaglomerular cells,
- Macula densa cells and
- Mesangial cells.

1. Juxtaglomerular Cells. Juxtaglomerular (JG) cells are specialized *myoepithelial* (modified vascular smooth muscle) cells located in the media of the *afferent arteriole* in the region of juxtaglomerular apparatus.

Characteristic features of juxtaglomerular cells are:

- They have well-developed Golgi apparatus and endoplasmic reticulum, abundant mitochondria and ribosomes.
- They synthesize, store and release an enzyme called *renin.* Renin is stored in the secretory granules of JG cells and, therefore, these are also called *granular cells.*
- They act as *baroreceptors* (tension receptors) and respond to changes in the transmural pressure gradient between the afferent arterioles and the interstitium.
- They are densely innervated by *sympathetic nerve* fibres and release their renin content in response to sympathetic discharge.
- As these cells act as vascular volume receptors, they monitor renal perfusion pressure and are stimulated

TABLE 6.1-1 Differences between Cortical and Juxtamedullary Nephron

Feature	Cortical nephron	Juxtamedullary nephron
Location of glomerulus	Upper region of cortex	Near junction of cortex and medulla
Percentage of total nephron	85%	15%
Size of glomeruli	Small	Larger
Size of loop of Henle	Small, extends up to outer layer of medulla	Large, extends deep into the medulla
Descending limb of loop of Henle comprises	Thin segment	Thin segment
Ascending limb of loop of Henle comprises	Thick segment	Thin segment
Efferent arterioles	Have large diameter and break up into peritubular capillaries	Have small diameter and continue as vasa recta
Rate of filtration	Slow	High
Major function	Excretion of waste products in urine	Concentration of urine by countercurrent system

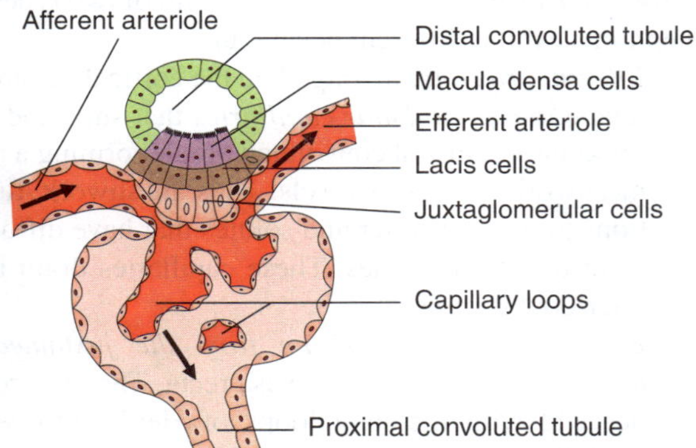

FIGURE 6.1-5 Juxtaglomerular apparatus.

by hypovolaemia or decreased renal perfusion pressure. The granulation of these cells increases when there is sustained hypotension in afferent arteriole, in sodium deficiency.

2. Macula Densa Cells. Macula densa cells refer to the specialized renal tubular epithelial cells of a short segment of the thick ascending limb of loop of Henle which passes between the afferent and efferent arterioles supplying its glomerulus of origin.

Characteristic features of macula densa cells are:

- They are not well adapted for reabsorption.
- They are not innervated.
- They have prominent nuclei, and their Golgi complex is usually located between the nucleus and the cell base (i.e. towards the afferent arteriole), while in other tubular cells the Golgi complex is located near the apical membrane. These characteristics suggest that these cells may be secreting a substance towards the arteriole.
- These cells are in direct contact with the mesangial cells and in close contact with the juxtaglomerular cells.
- They act as chemoreceptors and are stimulated by decreased NaCl concentration and causing increased renin release.

3. Mesangial Cells. Mesangial cells or *lacis* cells are the interstitial cells of the juxtaglomerular apparatus.

Characteristic features of these cells are:

- They are in contact with both the macula densa cells (on one side) and juxtaglomerular cells (on the other side).
- Structurally, these cells act as supporting cells and plugging device at the glomerular entrance.
- Functionally, these cells possibly relay the signals from macula densa to granular cells after modulating the signals. In this way, a decreased intraluminal Na^+ load, Cl^-load or both in the region of macula densa stimulates the juxtaglomerular cells to secrete renin.
- They also show granulation to secrete renin in conditions of extreme hyperactivity.
- They also secrete various substances and take up immune complexes.

Innervation of Kidney Renal vessels are innervated by sympathetic and parasympathetic fibres.

Parasympathetic Innervation is by vagus nerve, but its function is uncertain.

Sympathetic Innervation. Preganglionic sympathetic fibres arise from the neurons of lower thoracic and upper lumbar (T_{10}–L_2) intermediolateral segments of spinal cord. The cell bodies of the postganglionic neurons are located in the ganglia of sympathetic chain and superior mesenteric ganglion. The fibres from these neurons are carried by the renal nerves, which travel along the renal blood vessels as they enter the kidney. The efferent fibres are mainly distributed to afferent and efferent arterioles, cells of renal tubule and also to JG cells.

Afferents from the kidney (afferents of renorenal reflex and pain fibres) run along with the efferent fibres and enter in the spinal cord through the thoracic and upper lumbar dorsal roots.

Note. *Renorenal reflex.* An increase in uteteral pressure of one kidney reflexly reduces efferent nerve activity of contralateral kidney and causes increased excretion of sodium and water, known as renorenal reflex.

RENAL BLOOD FLOW

Renal Blood Vessels

Arrangement of Arterial Vessels (Renal Artery and Its Branches) in the Kidney (Fig. 6.1-6)

- ***Renal artery*** (one for each kidney), a major branch from the aorta, divides into a number of lobular arteries at the hilum of kidney.
- ***Lobular artery*** (one for each pyramid) divides into two or more interlobar arteries.

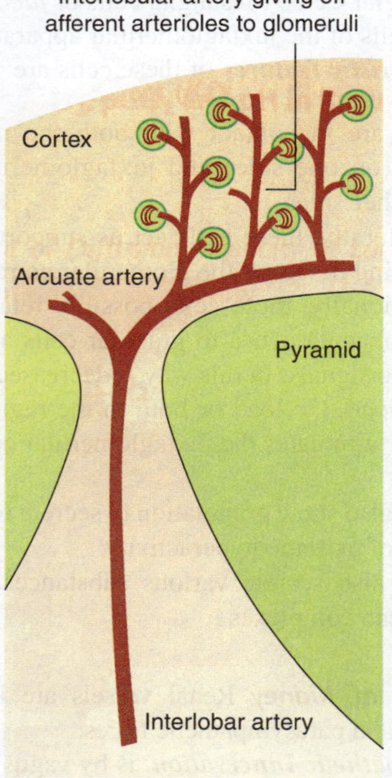

FIGURE 6.1-6 Scheme to show arrangement of arteries within the kidney.

- ***Interlobar arteries*** enter the tissue of the renal columns and run towards the surface of kidney. Reaching the level of the bases of the pyramids, the interlobar arteries divide into arcuate arteries.
- ***Arcuate arteries*** run at right angles to the parent interlobar arteries. They lie parallel to the renal surface at the junction of pyramid and cortex. They give a series of interlobular arteries.
- ***Interlobular arteries*** run through the cortex at right angles to the renal surface to end in a subcapsular plexus. It has been held that interlobular arteries divide the renal cortex into small lobules. Each interlobular artery gives off a series of afferent arterioles.
- ***Afferent arterioles***. Each afferent arteriole enters the Bowman's capsule and divides into a rounded tuft of anastomosing capillaries called *glomerulus*. As mentioned earlier, this capillary network has special features owing to which it works as a sieve allowing plasma filtration with retention of plasma proteins and blood cells. The glomerular capillaries join to form the efferent arteriole.
- ***Efferent arterioles*** leaving the glomeruli of two types of nephrons exhibit different behaviour:
  - *Efferent arterioles* arising from the cortical nephrons divide into *peritubular capillaries* that surround the proximal and distal convoluted tubule forming a rich meshwork of microvessels. This meshwork functions to remove water and solutes that have diffused from the renal tubules. These capillaries drain into interlobular veins.
  - *Efferent arterioles arising from the juxtamedullary nephrons* give rise to vasa recta. The vasa recta descend with the long loops of Henle into renal medulla and return to the area of the glomerulus, and drain into interlobular or arcuate vein.

Side branches arising from the vasa recti form capillary network at different levels along the loop of Henle (Fig. 6.1.7).

Arrangement of Venous Vessels (Renal Veins) The pattern of renal venous system is similar to that found in the end arterial system, except for the presence of multiple anastomoses between veins at all levels of the venous circulation. The corresponding veins which run parallel to the arterial vessels are the interlobular veins, the arcuate veins, the interlobar veins and the renal veins which exit the kidney at the hilus.

Characteristics of Renal Blood Flow

Amount and Rate of Blood Flow

- *Rate of renal blood flow* under basal conditions, approximately 1200 ml/min (400 ml/100 g tissue/min), is very high compared to other tissues, e.g.
  - Coronary blood flow: 80 ml/100 g/min,

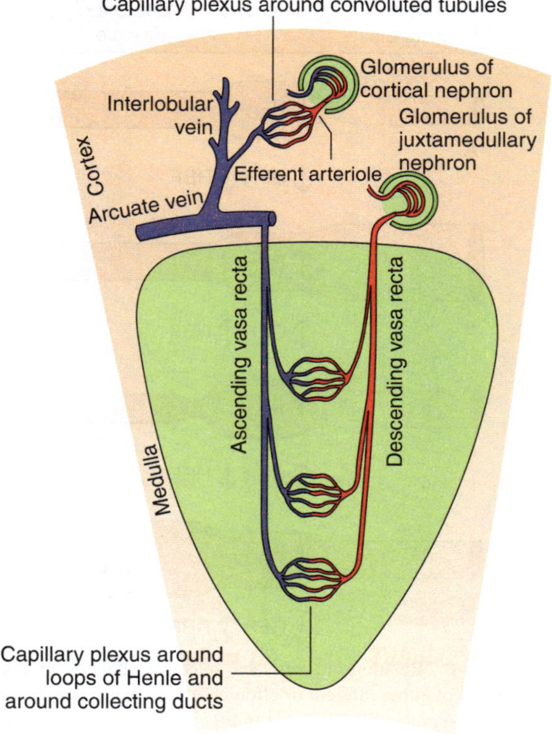

FIGURE 6.1-7 Scheme to show behaviour of efferent arterioles arising from the glomeruli of cortical and juxtamedullary nephrons.

- Brain blood flow: 55 ml/100 g/min and
- Skeletal muscle blood flow: 4 ml/100 g/min.

- *Total renal blood flow* is approximately 20% of resting cardiac output, while the two kidneys make <0.5% of total body weight.
- *Range of blood flow* to kidney is rather narrow. It allows only a 25% increase (300 ml) over the basal renal blood flow of 1200 ml/min. This reserve is much higher in other organs.
- *Higher blood flow* to kidneys is related to its excretory function rather than its metabolic requirement.
- Blood flow to the kidneys is directly proportional to the pressure difference between the renal artery and renal vein, and is inversely proportional to the resistance of the renal vasculature. Because the afferent arteriole, the efferent arteriole and the intralobular artery are the major resistance vessels in the kidneys, they determine renal vascular resistance.
- *In face of blood pressure changes,* the renal blood flow shows remarkable constancy due to autoregulation.
- *During exercise,* sympathetic tone to renal vessels increases and shunts renal blood flow to the skeletal muscles.

Renal Blood Flow and Oxygen Consumption

- *Renal O_2 consumption* (approximately 6 ml/100 g tissue/min) is very high being only second to the heart (i.e. 8 ml/100 g tissue/min) in the body.
- *Arteriovenous O_2* difference (approximately 1.5 ml/dL) of blood is smallest of the major organ system (Table 6.1-2).
- *Oxygen consumption* (VO_2) in kidneys is directly proportional to the renal blood flow, and arteriovenous O_2 difference does not change in spite of massive alteration in blood flow. This is a unique feature of kidneys, because in most body organs, the (A-V) O_2 difference is inversely proportional to their blood flow. Thus, unlike other organs, where the blood flow is related to O_2 requirements of the organ, in the kidneys, the O_2 consumption is a function of blood flow.
- *Renal oxygen consumption correlates* best with the active reabsorption of Na^+, but a significant fraction is also required for H+ secretion via the H^+–ATPase pumps.
- Some basic differences in the determinants of blood flow in the kidney vis-à-vis other organs, notably the muscular vascular bed, are summarized in Table 6.1-3.

Intrarenal Distribution of Renal Blood Flow Of the total renal blood flow, approximately 90% perfuses the cortex, while only 10% perfuses the medulla (9% outer medulla and 1% inner medulla). As the main function of the renal cortex is filtration, therefore renal cortical blood flow is relatively greater. Low blood flow to the medulla is due to

TABLE 6.1-2 Arteriovenous O_2 Difference in Major Organ Systems of the Body

Organ	Arterial O_2 content (ml%)	Venous O_2 content (ml%)	A-V O_2 difference (ml%)
Kidneys	19	17.5	1.5
Heart	19	8	11
Brain	19	12	07
Whole body	19	14	05

TABLE 6.1-3 Basic Differences in the Determinants of Renal Blood Flow vis-à-vis Muscular Blood Flow

Muscle blood flow (MBF)	Renal blood flow (RBF)
MBF increases or decreases to maintain a constant O_2. MBF changes according to O_2 demands	RBF is regulated to maintain a constant GFR. O_2 consumption changes with GFR, which in turn changes with RBF
When O_2 consumption increases, the blood flow increases in excess of the requirement. Hence, the (A-V) O_2 difference falls	O_2 consumption parallels the change in RBF; hence, (A-V) O_2 difference remains constant despite marked changes in RBF

relatively high vascular resistance in vasa recta because of the following three reasons:

- *Long length* (40 mm) of vasa recta (vascular resistance is proportional to the length of the vessel),
- *Increased viscosity of blood* near the hair pin bend of loop of Henle (resistance is proportional to the viscosity of blood). Sudden increase in the viscosity of blood in the region of inner medulla occurs due to loss of large amounts of water, as the osmotic pressure of interstitium in this region is very high (2000 mOsm/L) and
- *Low hydrostatic pressure head,* because the diameter of efferent arterioles arising from the juxtamedullary nephrons is small.

Physiological significance of low perfusion of medulla. Low medullary blood flow plays an important role in the urinary concentration mechanism (page 518).

Hydrostatic Pressure in Renal Vessels and Their Physiological Significance

- ***Glomerular capillaries*** have relatively high hydrostatic pressure (45 mmHg), which is an important factor in the formation of glomerular filtrate.
- ***Peritubular capillaries*** have very low hydrostatic pressure (8 mmHg only) due to drop in the pressure in efferent arterioles. This low hydrostatic pressure in peritubular capillaries facilitates the reabsorptive function of the proximal and distal *convoluted* tubules.
- Renal veins have hydrostatic pressure of only 4 mmHg.

Renal Portal Circulation. It has been mentioned above that the afferent arterioles arise from the interlobular arteries and each breaks up into a bunch of capillaries, called the glomerulus. The glomerular capillaries drain into efferent arterioles which again break up into peritubular capillary network which ultimately drains into an interlobular vein.

Vein. In this way, two sets of capillaries are formed and thus renal circulation becomes a sort of portal circulation.

Regulation of Renal Blood Flow

The regulatory mechanisms affect the renal blood flow (RBF) and glomerular filtration rate (GFR) by changing the arteriolar resistance. Therefore, before discussing the various regulatory mechanisms, it will be worthwhile to understand the ***relationship between selective changes in the resistance of afferent and/or efferent arterioles and RBF and GFR*** (Fig. 6.1-8):

- Constriction of afferent arteriole decreases both RBF and GFR, without change in filtration fraction (FF) (Fig. 6.1-8A).
- Dilatation of the afferent arteriole increases both RBF and GFR, without change in FF (Fig. 6.1-8B).
- *Constriction of the efferent arteriole* decreases the RBF and increases GFR, and FF (Fig. 6.1-8C).

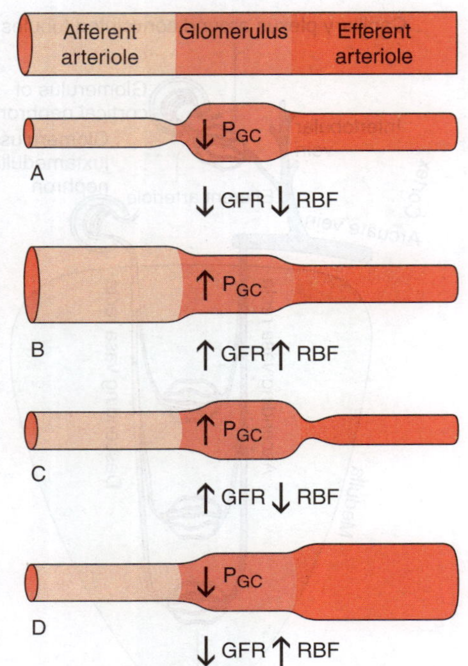

FIGURE 6.1-8 Relationship between selective changes in arteriolar resistance and of either afferent or efferent arteriole and renal blood flow (RBF) and glomerular filtration rate (GFR). P_{GC}: hydrostatic pressure in glomerular capillaries.

- *Dilatation of the efferent arteriole* increases the RBF and decreases the GFR, and FF (Fig. 6.1-8D).

Regulatory mechanisms of renal blood flow include:

- Autoregulation,
- Hormonal regulation and
- Nervous regulation.

Autoregulation of Renal Blood Flow Renal blood flow (RBF) and thus the glomerular filtration rate (GFR) remain constant over a wide range of renal arterial pressures (80–200 mmHg) (Fig. 6.1-9). This occurs due to an intrarenal mechanism known as autoregulation (also see

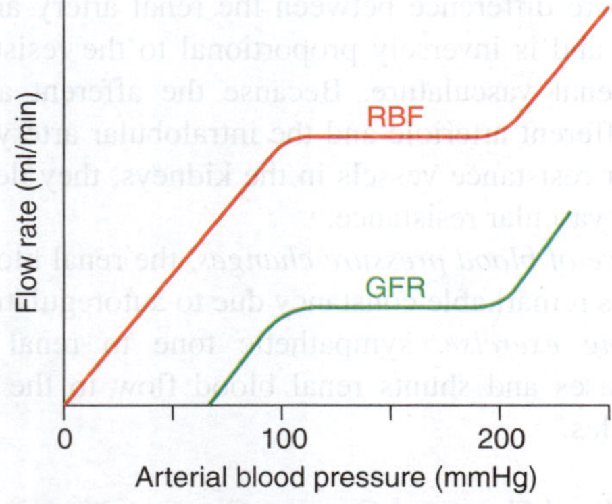

FIGURE 6.1-9 Autoregulation maintains renal blood flow (RBF) and glomerular filtration rate (GFR) constant over a wide range of arterial pressure (80–200 mmHg).

page 315). Autoregulation of RBF is accomplished by changing renal vascular resistance. When arterial pressure changes (between 80–200 mmHg), a proportionate change occurs in the renal vascular resistance which maintains a constant RBF.

Mechanisms of Autoregulation. Autoregulation has been observed to persist after renal denervation, in the isolated perfused kidney, in the transplanted kidney, after adrenal demedullation, and even the absence of erythrocytes; thus ruling out the role of all these factors.

Two mechanisms are considered responsible for autoregulation of RBF and GFR: one mechanism that responds to changes in arterial pressure, and another that responds to changes in NaCl concentration of tubular fluid.

1. ***Myogenic mechanism.*** It is related to an intrinsic property of vascular smooth muscle: the tendency to contract when it is stretched. Thus, when renal arterial pressure is raised, the afferent arterioles are stretched, which contract and increase the vascular resistance. The increased vascular resistance offsets the effect of increased arterial pressure and thereby maintains a constant RBF and GFR (Fig. 6.1-9).
2. ***Tubuloglomerular feedback mechanism.*** Tubuloglomerular feedback (TGF) mechanism is based on the NaCl concentration of tubular fluid. It involves a feedback loop which operates as (Fig. 6.1-10):
   - Changes in the GFR cause changes in NaCl concentration of fluid in the loop of Henle.
   - Changes in the NaCl concentration are sensed by the macula densa cells and converted into a signal.
   - The signal from the macula densa cells changes the vascular resistance in afferent arterioles.
   - Signals obtained due to increased concentration of NaCl produce vasoconstriction; conversely signals obtained due to decreased NaCl cause vasodilatation of afferent arterioles.
   - The effector mechanism responsible for vasoconstriction and vasodilatation is not exactly known. Perhaps, adenosine triphosphate (ATP), which selectively constricts the afferent arterioles and metabolites of arachidonic acid, may contribute to TGF mechanism.

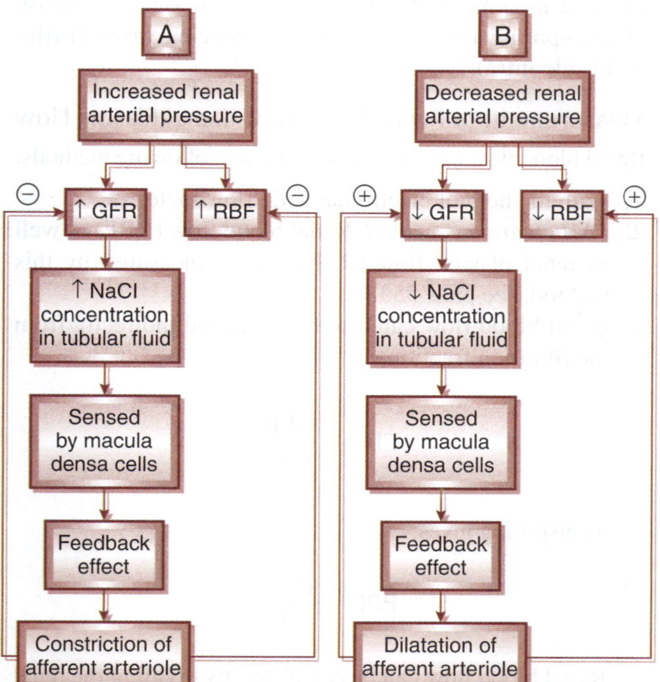

FIGURE 6.1-10 Tubuloglomerular feedback mechanism which maintains a constant RBF and GFR when renal arterial pressure increases (**A**) or decreases (**B**).

Physiological Significance and Certain Important Facts about Autoregulation

Physiological significance. A small change in GFR has great effect on urinary output and therefore on loss of solutes and water. If RBF and GFR were to change suddenly in proportion to change in blood pressure, urinary excretion of fluid and solute would also change suddenly. Such changes in water and solute excretion, without comparable alterations in intake, would prove disastrous due to alterations in fluid and electrolyte balance. Thus, autoregulation of RBF and GFR is an effective mechanism for uncoupling renal function from fluctuations in arterial pressure and maintain fluid and electrolyte balance.

Certain important facts about autoregulations to be noted are:

- Autoregulation of RBF and GFR is virtually absent at the mean arterial blood pressure below 80 mmHg,
- Autoregulation is not a perfect mechanism, i.e. RBF and GFR do change slightly with variation in arterial blood pressure and
- Several hormones and other factors can change RBF and GFR, despite autoregulation mechanisms.

Hormonal Regulation As mentioned above, despite autoregulation, several hormones and other factors have a major effect on RBF and GFR by affecting afferent and/or efferent arteriolar resistance (Table 6.1-4).

1. Hormones that Cause Vasoconstriction, and thereby decrease RBF and GFR include:

- ***Norepinephrine*** causes an intense vasoconstriction of both afferent and efferent arterioles.
- ***Angiotensin II,*** in low concentrations, causes a predominant constriction of the efferent arterioles. However, at higher concentrations, it causes constriction of both afferent as well as efferent arterioles.
- ***Endothelin*** causes profound vasoconstriction of the afferent and efferent arterioles. It is secreted by endothelial cells of renal vessels, mesangial cells and distal tubular cells. Its production is elevated in a number of glomerular diseases.

TABLE 6.1-4 Hormones Influencing the RBF and GFRs

Hormone	Stimulus	Effect on GFR	Effect on RBF
Vasoconstrictors			
• Norepinephrine	↓ ECV	↓	↓
• Angiotensin II	↓ ECV	↓	↓
• Endothelin	↑ Stretch, ↓ ECV, Angiotension II, bradykinin, epinephrine	↓	↓
Vasodilators			
• Prostaglandins (PGI_2 and PGE_2)	↓ ECV, Stretch, Angiotensin II	NC	↑
• Nitric oxide (NO)	↑ Stretch, ACh, Histamine, bradykinin, ATP	↑	↑
• Bradykinin	Prostaglandin, ↓ ACE	↑	↑
• ANP	↑ ECV	↑	↑
• Glucocorticoids	Administration in therapeutic dose	↑	↑
• Dopamine	–	NC	↑
• Histamine	Inflammation, injury	NC	↑

ECV: effective circulatory volume; NC: no change; ACE: angiotensin-converting enzyme.

2. *Hormones that Cause Vasodilatation,* and thereby increase RBF and GFR include:

- ***Prostaglandins*** (PGE_2 and PGI_2) are produced locally within the kidneys in conditions such as haemorrhage and increase RBF by dampening the vasoconstrictor effects of sympathetic nerves and angiotensin II.
- ***Nitric oxide (NO)*** causes vasodilatation of both afferent and efferent arterioles. In addition, it also decreases total peripheral resistance.
- ***Bradykinin*** is a vasodilator that acts by stimulating the release of NO and prostaglandins.
- ***Atrial natriuretic peptide (ANP).*** Its secretion by the heart rises with hypertension and expansion of extracellular fluid volume. It causes vasodilatation of the afferent arterioles and vasoconstriction of efferent arterioles. The net effect of ANP is therefore to produce a modest increase in GFR with little change in RBF.
- ***Glucocorticoids,*** when administered in therapeutic doses, increase RBF and GFR.
- ***Dopamine.*** The proximal tubule produces the vasodilator hormone dopamine which increases RBF and inhibits renin secretion.
- Histamine increases RBF without elevating GFR, by decreasing the resistance of afferent and efferent arterioles.

Nervous Regulation The afferent and efferent arterioles are innervated by sympathetic nerve fibres from T_{10} to L_2 intermediolateral grey segments of spinal cord through the splanchnic nerves. The sympathetic cell bodies are located in the superior mesenteric ganglion.

- ***Under normal circulatory conditions,*** sympathetic tone is minimum.
- ***Mild to moderate stimulation*** of sympathetic nerves usually has mild effects on RBF because of autoregulation mechanism.
- ***Strong acute stimulation*** of sympathetic nerves may produce marked fall in RBF (even to 10–30% of normal) temporarily due to constriction of both afferent and efferent arterioles. This effect is mediated mainly by α_1-adrenergic receptors and to a lesser extent by post-synaptic α_2-adrenergic receptors.

Note. This system works to preserve arterial pressure at the expense of maintaining normal RBF in conditions of acute hypotension due to severe haemorrhage. Further, an increase in sympathetic activity also increases the release of epinephrine and angiotensin-II, enhancing vasoconstriction (vide infra).

Measurement of Renal Blood Flow/Renal Plasma Flow

Renal blood flow can be measured by the following methods:

1. With the help of electromagnetic flow meter.
2. *PAH clearance method*. Renal blood flow (RBF) as well as renal plasma flow (RPF) can be measured by this method, see page 553.
3. Renal blood flow can also be measured indirectly from the filtration fractions:

$$FF = \frac{GFR}{RPF}$$

Transposing gives:

$$RPF = \frac{GFR}{FF}$$

Renal blood flow can be calculated by dividing the renal plasma flow by 1 − haematocrit (see page 133).

Chapter 6.2

Mechanism of Urine Formation: Glomerular Filtration and Tubular Transport

INTRODUCTION

The main function of the kidneys is to clear waste products from blood and excrete them in the urine. In addition to the metabolic wastes, the kidneys also excrete foreign substances from the body such as drugs, pesticides and other chemicals ingested in food. The kidneys accomplish their excretory function by formation of urine.

Processes Concerned with Urine Formation. Three processes are involved in urine formation (Fig. 6.2-1):

- *Glomerular filtration,* i.e. filtration of plasma from the glomerular capillaries into the renal tubules is the first step in the formation of urine.
- *Tubular reabsorption,* i.e. the return of needed solutes and water from the tubules into the blood, is the second step in the process of urine formation. It changes the composition of glomerular filtrate and reduces its volume markedly.
- *Tubular secretion* involves net movement of water and unwanted solutes (that could not be filtered) from the blood into the tubules.

Thus, the excretion of each substance in the urine involves a specific combination of filtration, reabsorption and secretion as expressed by the following relationship: Urinary excretion = Filtration − Reabsorption + Secretion (Fig. 6.2-1).

GLOMERULAR FILTRATION

Glomerular filtration refers to the process of ultrafiltration of plasma from the glomerular capillaries into the Bowman's capsule. The understanding of the process of glomerular filtration involves a review of:

- Characteristics of filtration membrane,
- Composition of glomerular filtrate,
- Dynamics of glomerular filtration,
- Glomerular filtration rate,
- Filtration fraction,
- Factors affecting glomerular filtration,
- Regulation of glomerular filtration and
- Measurement of glomerular filtration.

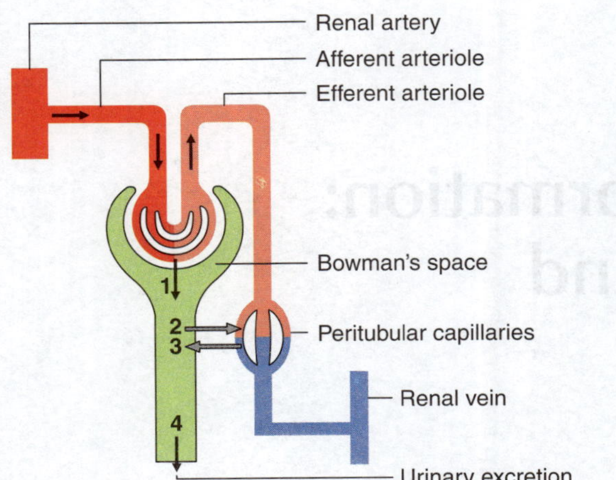

FIGURE 6.2-1 Steps involved in the formation of urine: 1, filtration; 2, reabsorption; 3, secretion; and 4, excretion.

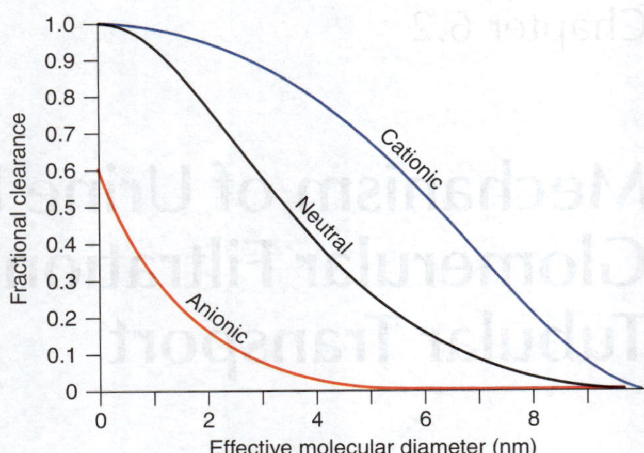

FIGURE 6.2-2 Effect of electrical charge and effective molecular diameter on filterability of dextran molecule through glomerular filtration membrane. A value of one indicates that it is filtered freely, whereas a value of zero indicates that it is not filtered.

Characteristics of Filtration Membrane

As described on page 481 (Fig. 6.1-3B), the filtration membrane consists of three layers: capillary endothelium, glomerular basement membrane (GBM) and Bowman's visceral epithelium (podocytes). Glomerular filtration occurs across this membrane.

Characteristic features of the filtration membrane are:

High Permeability. The glomerular membrane is highly permeable to water and 100% dissolved substances because of its porous nature.

Permeability Selectivity. The filtration membrane exhibits a high degree of permeability selectivity based on two factors:

- *Pore size*. The capillary endothelial cells have pores that are 70–90 nm in diameter, the glomerular basement membrane (GBM) has no pores but its permeability corresponds to pore size of 8 nm, and the podocytes form filtration slits which are approximately 25 nm wide. From this it is clear that the glomerular filtration barrier for solutes resides at the level of GBM. The permeability of the membrane to various neutral solutes depending on their effective molecular diameter is (Fig. 6.2-2):
  - Molecules less than 4 nm in size are freely filtered.
  - Molecules with diameter more than 8 nm are not filtered at all (i.e. zero permeability).
  - Filtration of molecules having diameter between 4–8 nm is inversely proportional to their diameter.
- *Electrical charge*. It may however, be realized that permeability of the filtration membrane is not simply related to molecular size but also to its shape and electrical charge. The pores in the filtration membrane are negatively charged due to presence of glycoproteins rich in sialic acid. Thus, with the same molecular size, compared to anionic particles, there is, in order, increasing permeability for neutral and cationic particles (Fig. 6.2-2). This explains why albumin (with a molecular diameter of 7 nm but a negative charge) is not filtered.

Composition of Glomerular Filtrate

The unique characteristic features of the glomerular filtration membrane determine the composition of glomerular filtrate, in that it is like that of plasma except for the absence of proteins (colloids) and cells. Capillary permeability alterations in disease do not alter rate of filtration of diffusible molecules. Thus, transfer of such substances into glomerular filtrate depends only on GFR. Filtration membrane permeability alteration in diseases, however, may alter diffusibility of colloids and cells. For example, in a number of glomerular diseases, the negative charge on the filtration membrane is reduced because of immunological damage and inflammation. As a result filtration of proteins is increased, and albumin appears in the urine in significant amounts (albuminuria or proteinuria). It is important to note that normally the amount of proteins in the urine is less than 100 mg/dL, and most of this is not filtered but comes from the sheded tubular cells.

Dynamics of Glomerular Filtration

The forces which determine the bulk flow or ultrafiltration of protein free plasma across the glomerular membrane are the same which determine formation of tissue fluid, i.e. fluid exchange across capillaries in the rest of the body. Thus, the driving force for glomerular filtration is the net ultrafiltration pressure across the glomerular capillaries. Filtration is always favoured in the glomerular capillaries because the net ultrafiltration pressure always favours the movement of fluid out of the capillaries.

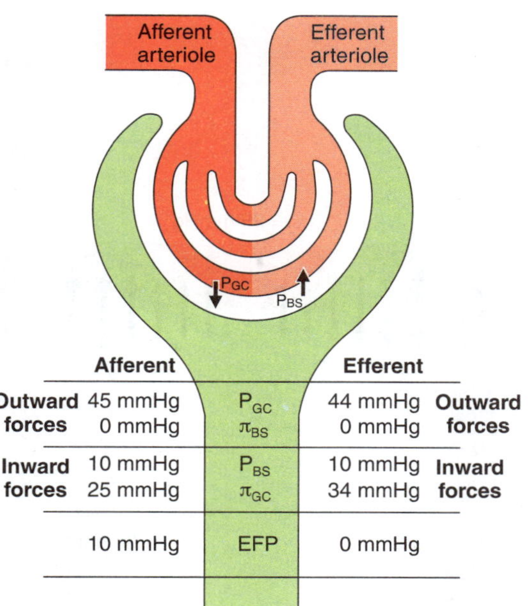

FIGURE 6.2-3 Depiction of Starling forces across the glomerular filtration membrane: P_{GC}: glomerular capillary hydrostatic pressure, P_{BS}: Bowman's space hydrostatic pressure, π_{GC}: glomerular capillary oncotic pressure, π_{BS}: Bowman space oncotic pressure.

The glomerular filtration rate (GFR) will depend upon the balance of Starling forces (Fig. 6.2-3). For detailed information about Starling forces see page 318. According to Starling hypothesis, the GFR can be expressed as:

$$\text{GFR} = \text{Kf}\left[\left(P_{GC} - P_{BS}\right) = \left(\pi_{GC} - \pi_{BS}\right)\right]$$

where:

GFR is the filtration across the glomerular membrane.

Kf or the filtration coefficient of the glomerular membrane.

- It is the product of glomerular membrane hydraulic permeability and the effective filtration surface area.
- The filtration coefficient (Kf) normally equals 12.5 m^2/min/mmHg.

P_{GC} is glomerular capillary hydrostatic pressure

- It tends to force the fluid out through the glomerular membrane.
- It depends upon the arterial blood pressure, and pre- and postglomerular capillary resistance.
- Its normal value is about 45 mmHg.

P_{BS} *or Bowman's space hydrostatic pressure*

- It is analogous to P_i (hydrostatic interstitial pressure) in systemic circulation.
- It tends to force fluid inwards through the glomerular membrane.
- Its normal value is about 10 mmHg.

π_{GC} *or glomerular capillary oncotic pressure*

- It results from the osmotic pressure of plasma proteins.
- It tends to pull fluid inward through the glomerular membrane.
- Its normal value is 25 mmHg.

π_{BS} *or Bowman's space oncotic pressure*

- It is the oncotic pressure of the fluid in Bowman's space.
- Its normal value is zero, because glomerular filtrate contains no proteins.

Effective filtration pressure (EFP) is the net outward force and is calculated as the difference between the outwardly (i.e. P_{GC} and π_{BS}) and inwardly (P_{BS} and π_{GC}) directed forces (Fig. 6.2-3).

Thus, under normal circumstances,

$$\text{GFR} = 12.5(45 - 10) - (25 - 0) = 125 \text{ ml/min}$$

Normal Glomerular Filtration Rate

As calculated above, the normal glomerular filtration rate (GFR) in an average-sized man is about 125 ml/min (range 90–140 ml/min).Its magnitude correlates fairly well with surface area, but values in women are 10% lower than those in men even after correction for surface area. Thus, in a 24 h period, as much as 180 L/day of plasma is filtered at the glomerulus. In other words, in one day kidneys filter an amount of fluid equal to 4 times the total body water, 15 times the ECF and 60 times the plasma volume. Of the 180 L/day of glomerular filtrate which passes through the remaining part of the nephron, 99% or more is reabsorbed and only 1% or less is excreted as urine.

After age of 30 years, GFR declines with age. However, this decline in GFR usually does not adversely affect the kidney's excretory function, or their ability to maintain fluid, electrolyte and acid–base balance.

Filtration Fraction

The filtration fraction (FF) is the ratio of GFR to the renal plasma flow (RPF).

At normal values of GFR 125 ml/min and RPF 650 ml/min; the filtration fraction is approximately 0.2% (125/650). In other words, normally only about 20% of the renal plasma flow is actually filtered per minute.

Glomerular Versus Systemic Filtration

Total Filtration Approximately 180 L of fluid is filtered from the glomerular capillaries; in contrast, only 20 L of fluid is filtered out per day in the rest of the systemic capillaries of the body. These figures demonstrate the massive scale at which glomerular filtration occurs.

Filtration Coefficient (Kf). The considerable greater rate of filtration in glomerular capillaries than systemic capillaries is mainly because the Kf is approximately 100 times higher in glomerular capillaries.

Hydrostatic Pressure within the glomerular capillaries is approximately twice as high in systemic capillaries. It also contributes to greater glomerular filtration.

Total Capillary Exchange Area. The total glomerular capillary exchange area is estimated to be 1.6 m^2, of which 2–3% is available for filtration. Thus, the glomerular filtration surface area measures between 500–810 cm^2. In contrast, the total exchange area of the systemic capillary bed is estimated to be 1000 m^2, of which only 25% is open at any time at rest. Thus, the systemic filtration area at rest measures about 250 m^2.

Balance of Starling Forces. In the systemic capillary, the oncotic pressure does not vary over the length of capillary, as the filtration of fluid is small. The hydrostatic pressure at the arteriolar end exceeds the oncotic pressure of plasma proteins and favours filtration. However, over the length of the capillary, the hydrostatic pressure gradually declines and the net filtration pressure (NFP) becomes zero near the middle of the capillary. From here, the inward forces become dominant and the reabsorption process starts to reach its maximum at the venular end (Fig. 6.2-4A).

In the Glomerular Capillary, the hydrostatic pressure does not decline over the length, because of the efferent arteriolar resistance. But, because of massive filtration of fluid, the oncotic pressure in the glomerular capillary increases over the length and becomes equal to hydrostatic pressure at the efferent end. Thus, there is no filtration of fluid in distal 25% of glomerular capillary (Fig. 6.2-4B).

However, if the rate of renal blood flow is increased, the equilibrium between the hydrostatic pressure (P_{GC}) and oncotic pressure (π_{GC}) would be reached more slowly, i.e. filtration would continue over a larger length of the glomerular capillary. From this it can be concluded, that besides Starling forces, the rate of renal blood flow is also an important factor determining the GFR.

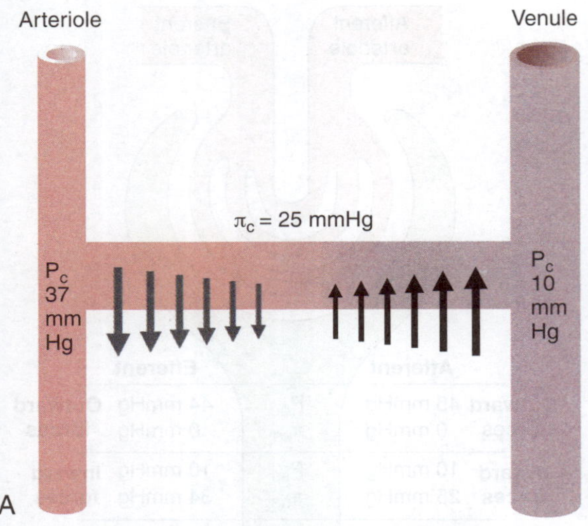

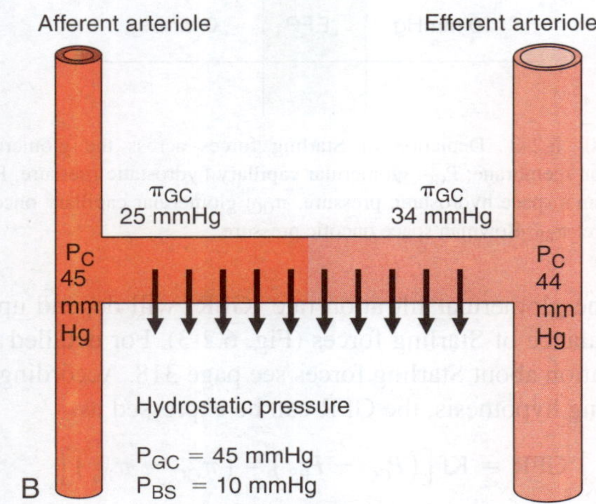

FIGURE 6.2-4 Balance of Starling forces: systemic capillary (**A**) versus glomerular capillary (**B**).

Factors Affecting Glomerular Filtration Rate

1. Filtration Coefficient (Kf). Increased Kf raises GFR and decreased Kf reduces GFR. As mentioned earlier, Kf is the product of permeability and filtration area of the glomerular capillary membrane.

   i. ***Permeability of the glomerular capillaries is increased*** in abnormal conditions like hypoxia and presence of toxic agents. In such conditions GFR is increased, because plasma proteins are also filtered to a variable degree. This causes increase in colloid osmotic pressure of Bowman's space fluid (normally this is zero because proteins are not filtered), which in turn increases GFR.
      - *Decreased capillary permeability* occurs due to thickening of capillary membrane in some diseases leading to decreased GFR.

   ii. ***Alteration in GFR filtration area of glomerular capillaries*** can alter the Kf. *Mesangial cells* contraction or relaxation is associated with alteration in coefficient of filtration.
      - *Contraction of mesangial cells* leading to decreased Kf is caused by vasoconstrictors like angiotensin II, endothelin, norepinephrine, thromboxane A_2, leukotrienes C_4 and D_4 and histamine. *Relaxation of mesangial cells* leading to increased Kf is caused by vasodilators like dopamine, cAMP, ANP, nitric oxide (NO) and prostaglandins (PGE).

2. Hydrostatic Pressure in Bowman's Space Fluid (P_{BS}) opposes filtration, and therefore GFR is inversely related to it. It is increased in acute obstruction of urinary tract (e.g. a ureteric obstruction by stone).

3. Glomerular Capillary Hydrostatic Pressure (P_{GC}). GFR is directly related to P_{GC}. Changes in P_{GC} serve as a primary means for physiological regulation of GFR. P_{GC} is mainly dependent on arterial pressure, renal blood flow, afferent arteriolar resistance and efferent arteriolar resistance.

   i. ***Arterial pressure.*** GFR is autoregulated between arterial pressure of 80–200 mmHg. Increased arterial pressure above 200 mmHg may raise GFR and decreased arterial pressure below 70 mmHg may lower GFR.

ii. ***Renal blood flow.*** GFR is directly proportional to the renal blood flow (as described above page 484). However, renal blood flow is controlled by autoregulatory mechanisms.

iii. ***Afferent and efferent arteriolar resistance.*** Relation of afferent and efferent arteriolar resistance with GFR is described on page 486).

Note. In *acute renal failure*, GFR declines because of fall in P_{GC}.

4. Glomerular Capillary Oncotic Pressure (π_{GC}). GFR is inversely proportional to π_{GC}. In hyperproteinaemia and in haemoconcentration ratio, the π_{GC} is raised leading to decrease in GFR. Conversely, in hypoproteinaemia and haemodilution the π_{GC} is reduced leading to increased GFR.

5. Sympathetic Stimulation. See page 488.

Regulation of GFR

Regulation of GFR, like that of renal blood flow includes:

- Autoregulation,
- Nervous regulation and
- Hormonal regulation.

For details see page 486.

Measurement of Glomerular Filtration

Glomerular filtration rate can be measured by renal clearance of inulin, urea and creatinine. For details see page 551.

TUBULAR REABSORPTION AND SECRETION

Of the 180 L glomerular filtrate formed per day, about 1.5 L (i.e. <1%) per day is excreted as urine. The different segments of the renal tubule viz. proximal tubule, loop of Henle, distal tubule and collecting duct determine the composition and volume of the urine by process of *selective reabsorption* of solutes and water and *selective secretion* of solutes. Consequently, the tubules precisely control the volume, osmolality, composition and pH of intracellular and extracellular fluid compartments. For conceptual understanding, this section on renal tubular reabsorption and secretion can be considered in the following subsections:

- *General Principles of Renal Tubular Transport*
  - Transport mechanisms across cell membranes,
  - Transepithelial transport pathways,
  - Tubular mechanisms and patterns of renal handling of a substance and concept of renal clearance and
  - Parameters of renal active transport.
- *Transport across different segments of renal tubule*
  - Transport across proximal tubule,
  - Transport across Henle's loop,
  - Transport across distal tubule and
  - Transport across collecting duct.
- *Tubular transport of common solutes and water*
  - Tubular transport of Na^+,
  - Tubular transport of Cl^-,
  - Tubular transport of K^+,
  - Tubular transport of glucose and
  - Tubular transport of water.

General Principles of Renal Tubular Transport

Transport Mechanisms across Cell Membrane The water moves across the cell membrane of renal tubular cells passively, while the solute movement occurs by both passive and active mechanisms.

- ***Passive transport*** does not need energy and occurs spontaneously, down an electrochemical gradient by the following mechanisms:
  - Diffusion,
  - Facilitated diffusion (channels, uniport, coupled transport, uniport or symport) and
  - Solvent drag.
- ***Active transport*** requires direct input of energy and is abolished if cell metabolism is inhibited. Active transport can occur against an electrochemical gradient, but it does not mean that it only occurs against such gradients in the body. Most of the active transports are carrier mediated. Endocytosis is also a type of active transport and it will prove prudent to revise the various transport mechanisms described in Chapter 1.3 page 26, before proceeding further.

Transepithelial Transport Pathways In the renal tubule, a substance can be reabsorbed or secreted by two pathways:

- ***Paracellular pathway*** refers to transport between the cells (Fig. 6.2-5A). Examples of paracellular pathway include:
  - Reabsorption of Ca^{2+} and K^+ across the proximal tubule,
  - Some of the water reabsorbed across the proximal tubule crosses the paracellular pathway and
  - Some solutes dissolved in this water (in particular Ca^{2+}, and K^+) are carried along with the reabsorbed fluid across the paracellular pathway by the process of solvent drag.
- ***Transcellular pathway*** refers to transport through the cells. Its example includes transcellular Na^+ reabsorption by the proximal tubule, which is a two-step process (Fig. 6.2-5B):
  - *Movement of Na^+ into the cell* across the apical membrane occurs down an electrochemical gradient established by Na^+–K^+–ATPase.
  - *Movement of Na^+ into the ECF* across the basolateral membrane occurs against an electrochemical gradient via Na^+–K^+–ATPase.

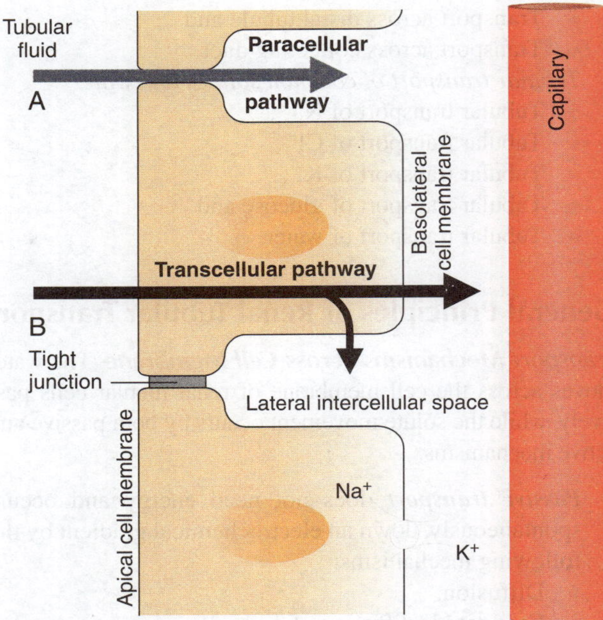

FIGURE 6.2-5 Pathways of transepithelial transport: **A,** paracellular pathway; and **B,** transcellular pathway.

Tubular Mechanisms, Patterns of Renal Handling of Substances and Concept of Renal Clearance

Tubular Mechanisms. As mentioned earlier, the two main tubular mechanisms involved in renal handling of a substance are tubular reabsorption and tubular secretion.

- ***Tubular reabsorption*** denotes the active transport of solutes and passive movement of water from the tubular lumen into peritubular capillaries. In other words, reabsorption is the removal of substances of nutritive value such as glucose, amino acids, electrolytes (Na^+, K^+, Cl^-, HCO_3^-) and vitamins from the glomerular filtrate. Small proteins and peptide hormones are reabsorbed in the proximal tubules by endocytosis.
- ***Tubular secretion*** refers to the transport of solutes from the peritubular capillaries into the tubular lumen, i.e. it is the addition of a substance to the glomerular filtrate.

Active secretion of substances occurs into the tubular fluid with the help of certain nonselective carriers. The carrier which secretes para-aminohippuric (PAH) acid can also secrete uric acid, bile acids, oxalic acid, penicillin, probenecid, cephalothin and furosemide. It is because of the common carrier that probenecid can block secretion of penicillin and maintain its plasma concentration for a longer time. For bases there is another carrier, which is also nonselectively involved in secretion of substances like acetylcholine, creatinine, dopamine, histamine, 5HT, thiamine, quinine, procaine, morphine and other bases.

Important Notes

The ensuing discussion includes the list and mechanism of the substances reabsorbed and/or secreted in different segments of renal tubule (page 496).

- Only two natural constituents of plasma (K^+ and H^+) are secreted by the distal tubules.
- Proximal tubular cells may secrete uric acid, and many drugs.
- Uric acid is the only organic substance that can be both reabsorbed and secreted.
- K^+ is the only inorganic substance which can be both reabsorbed and secreted.

Patterns of Renal Handling of a Substance and Concept of Renal Clearance.

Different Patterns of Renal Handling of a Substance Include:

1. ***Glomerular filtration only,*** i.e. the substances are freely filtered, but neither reabsorbed nor secreted (e.g. inulin) (Fig. 6.2-6A). Such substances are called glomerular markers and are said to have renal clearance equal to GFR.
2. ***Glomerular filtration followed by partial reabsorption*** (Fig. 6.2-6B). Such substances have renal clearance less than GFR.
3. ***Glomerular filtration followed by complete tubular reabsorption*** (Fig. 6.2-6C). Such substances have lowest renal clearance, e.g. Na^+, glucose, amino acids, HCO_3^- and Cl^-. The substances that are not filtered at all (e.g. protein), also have the lowest renal clearance.
4. ***Glomerular filtration followed by tubular secretion*** (Fig. 6.2-6D). Such substances that are both filtered across the glomerular capillaries and secreted from the peritubular capillaries into urine have the highest renal clearances (e.g. PAH).
5. ***Glomerular filtration followed by partial reabsorption and secretion*** (Fig. 6.2-6E). In such circumstances, depending upon which of the two process is dominant, there may be net reabsorption or net secretion of the substance.Net absorption is said to occur if the amount of substance excreted in urine is less than GFR in the same time. Similarly, net secretion is said to occur when the amount excreted is more than GFR in the same time.
6. ***No glomerular filtration, no absorption, only secretion*** (Fig. 6.2-6F). Many organic compounds are bound to plasma proteins and are therefore unavailable for ultrafiltration. Secretion is thus their major route of excretion in urine.

Renal Clearance. From the above, the renal clearance can be defined as the volume of plasma that is cleared of a substance in 1 min by excretion of the substance in the urine. Further, from the above description and examples, the relative clearances of the common substances are:

PAH $>$ K^+(high K^+ diet) $>$ inulin $>$ urea $>$ Na^+ $>$ glucose, amino acids and HCO_3^-.

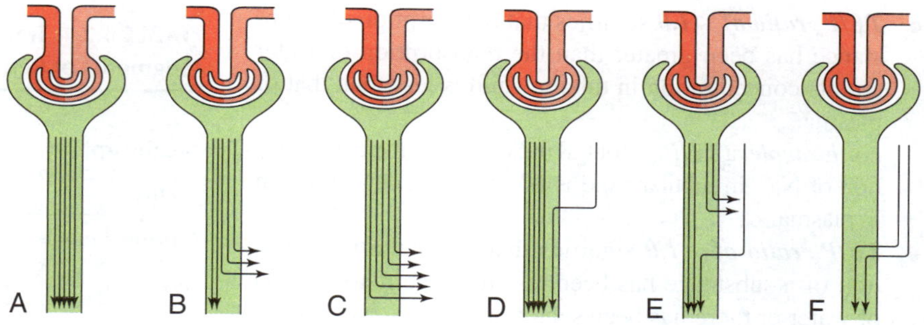

FIGURE 6.2-6 Different patterns of tubular handling of substances (for details see text).

Quantification of Renal Tubular Transport The parameters used for quantitative analysis of renal tubular transport are denoted by the capital letters with dots above them and include:

- Filtered load (F^o),
- Excretion rate (E^o),
- Reabsorption rate (R^o),
- Secretion rate (S^o),
- Renal tubular transport maximum (T_m) and
- Tubular fluid (TF) concentration and plasma concentration (P) ratio.

Filtered Load. It is the amount of a substance entering the renal tubule by glomerular filtration per unit time.

- Filtered load (F^o) is calculated by multiplying the glomerular filtration rate (GFR) with plasma concentration of the substance (P_x), i.e. $F^o = \text{GFR} \times P_x$ mg/min. As described on page 551, the GFR is equal to the clearance of inulin (C_{in}), therefore, $F^o = C_{in} \times P_x$.

Excretion Rate. It is the amount of substance that appears in the urine per unit time. The excretion rate (E^o) can be calculated by multiplying urine flow rate (V) *and the urinary concentration of the substance* (U_x).

That is, $$E^o = V \times U_x \text{ mg/min.}$$

Reabsorption Rate (R^o). Reabsorption of a substance is said to occur when the filtered load exceeds the excretion rate. The reabsorption rate of a substance is calculated by subtracting excretion rate from the filtered load, that is:

$$R^o = F^o - E^o$$

Secretion Rate (S^o). The net secretion of a substance is said to occur when the excretion rate is more than the filtered load. Under such circumstances, the secretion rate is calculated by subtracting filtered load from the excretion rate, that is:

$$S^o = E^o - F^o$$

Renal Tubular Transport Maximum (T_m). Renal tubular transport maximum T_m refers to the maximal amount of a solute that can be actively transported (reabsorbed or secreted) per minute by the renal tubules. In other words, the point at which carriers are saturated is the T_m. Therefore, it is important to note that T_m pertains to solutes that are actively transported only and the substances that are passively transported (e.g. urea) do not exhibit T_m.

Maximum tubular secretory capacity (T_s) is the highest attainable rate of secretion. All substances secreted by the kidney do not have T_m.

- Secreted substances that have T_m include para-aminohippuric acid (PAH), penicillin, certain diuretics, salicylate and thiamine (vitamin B_1).
- Secreted substances that do not have T_m are secretion of K^+ by the distal tubules.

Maximal tubular reabsorptive capacity (T_r) is the highest attainable rate of reabsorption. All substances reabsorbed by an active carrier-mediated mechanism do not have T_m.

- Substances that have T_m are phosphate ion, sulphate, glucose, many amino acids, uric acid and albumin, acetoacetate, β-hydroxybutyrate and α-ketoglutarate.
- Substances that do not have T_m include reabsorption of Na^+ along the nephron and HCO_3^-.

Threshold concentration is defined as the plasma concentration at which a substance first appears in the urine.

Tubular Fluid Concentration (TF)/Plasma Concentration (P_x) Ratio The TF/P_x ratio compares the concentration of a substance in tubular fluid at any point along the nephron with its concentration in plasma. The tubular fluid, for such studies, is collected by micropuncture technique. A micropipette is inserted into the Bowman's space and different portions of the tubules of the living kidney in experimental animals and the composition of aspirated tubular fluid is determined by the use of microchemical techniques.

Significance of TF/P_x Ratio. The TF/P_x ratio may be 1, <1 or >1.

- ***TF/Px ratio of 1.0*** signifies that either there has been no reabsorption, or reabsorption of the substance has been exactly proportional to the reabsorption of water.
  For example, a TF/P_x of 1.0, indicates that concentration of Na^+ in tubular fluid and plasma is identical. For any freely filterable substance, TF/P_x ratio is 1.0 in Bowman's space (before any reabsorption or secretion has taken place to modify the tubular fluid).

- ***TF/P$_x$* ratio of <1.0** signifies that reabsorption of a substance has been greater than the reabsorption of water and its concentration in tubular fluid is less than that of plasma.
  For example, a TF/P_{Na+} of 0.8 indicates that the concentration of Na^+ in tubular fluid is 80% of Na^+ concentration in plasma.
- ***TF/P$_x$* ratio of >1.0** signifies that either the reabsorption of a substance has been less than the reabsorption of water or there has been secretion of the substance.

Tubular Fluid Concentration (TF)/Plasma Concentration of Inulin (P_{inulin}) The substance inulin is freely filtered by glomerular capillaries but is neither reabsorbed nor secreted into the tubules. Thus, its concentration in tubular fluid is determined solely by how much water remains in the tubular fluid. So, TF/P inulin is used as a marker for water reabsorption along the nephron. Its value increases as water is reabsorbed. From the value of TF/P inulin, the *fraction of the filtered water that has been reabsorbed* can be calculated by following equation:

- Fraction of filtered H_2O reabsorbed = $1/TF/P_{inulin}$
- When TF/P_{inulin} is 2, then FF of H_2O reabsorbed is $1 - ½ = 0.5 = 5\%$
- Similarly, when TF/P_{inulin} is 3, then FF of H_2O reabsorbed is $1 - 1/3 = 0.67 = 67\%$.

$[TF/P_x]/[TF/P_{inulin}]$ Ratio
The double ratio corrects the TF/P_x ratio for water reabsorption and gives the fraction of the filtered load remaining at any point along the nephron.

For example, a $[TF/P_K]/[TF/P_{inulin}]$ ratio of 0.3 at the end of proximal tubule indicates that 30% of filtered K^+ remains in the tubular fluid and 70% has been reabsorbed into the blood.

Transport across Different Segments of Renal Tubule

The substances transported across the different segments of renal tubules are described below and enlisted in Table 6.2-1.

Transport across Proximal Tubule

The proximal tubule reabsorbs:

- Approximately 67% of the filtered water, Na^+, Cl^-, K^+ and other solutes and
- Almost all the glucose and amino acids filtered by the glomerulus.
  The proximal tubule does not reabsorb inulin, creatinine sucrose and mannitol.
  The proximal tubule secretes H^+, PAH, urate, penicillin, sulphonamides and creatinine.

TABLE 6.2-1 **Transport of Substances across Different Segments of Renal Tubule**

Reabsorption		Non-reabsorption	Secretion
Active	*Passive*		
Proximal tubule			
Na^+	Cl^-	Inulin	H^+
K^+	HCO_3^-	Creatinine	Water
Ca^{2+}	HPO_4^-	Sucrose	Penicillin
Mg^{2+}	Water	Mannitol	Sulphonamide
HPO_4^{2-}	Urea		Creatinine
SO_4^{2-}			
NO_3^-			
Glucose			
Amino acids			
Protein			
Urate			
Vitamins			
Acetoacetate			
β-hydroxybutyrate			
Henle's loop			
Na^+	Cl^-		
K^+	HCO_3^-		
Ca^{2+}	Water		
Distal tubule and collecting duct			
Na^+	Cl^-		K^+
Ca^{2+}	HCO_3^-		H^+
Mg^{2+}	Water		
Water			

Reabsorption

Characteristics of Proximal Tubule Cells. As shown in Fig. 6.1-3, the proximal tubular cells are characterized by the presence of brush border on their luminal surfaces. The brush is composed of thousands of villi which increase the absorptive surface area of each cell 20-fold. The substances absorbed are transferred to the peritubular capillaries from the basolateral membrane of the cells.

Key element in the proximal tubular reabsorption is $Na^+–K^+–ATPase$ in the basolateral membrane. The reabsorption of every substance including water is linked in some way to the operation of $Na^+–K^+–ATPase$.

Sodium Reabsorption The process of sodium reabsorption in proximal tubule is *isosmotic*, i.e. the reabsorption of sodium and water are exactly proportional. Therefore, both TF/P_{Na+} and TF/P_{osm} are 1.0.

Mechanisms of Na^+ Reabsorption. Mechanism of Na^+ reabsorption in the early proximal tubule and late proximal tubule is different.

In early proximal tubule, Na^+ is reabsorbed by *cotransport with H^+ or organic solutes (glucose, amino acids, phosphate and lactate)*. The Na^+ absorption is a two-step process (Fig. 6.2-7):

- *Across the basolateral membrane*, Na^+ moves against an electrochemical gradient via Na^+–K^+–ATPase pump, which pumps Na^+ into the paracellular spaces and lowers the intracellular Na^+ concentration.
- *Across the apical membrane*, the sodium moves down an electrochemical gradient as above. The entry of Na^+ is mediated by specific antiporter and symporter proteins, and not by diffusion through channels:
  - *Na^+–H^+–antiporter* is the main determinant of Na^+ and H_2O reabsorption in the proximal tubule. Na^+–H^+ exchange is linked directly to the reabsorption of HCO_3^-.

    Note: Carbonic anhydrase inhibitors (e.g. acetazolamide) are diuretics that act in the early proximal tubule by inhibiting the reabsorption of filteredHCO_3^-.
  - *Na^+–glucose (and other organic solutes) symporter* mechanisms are also involved in the entry of Na^+ in the proximal cells. The glucose, amino acids, phosphate and lactate are almost completely absorbed along with Na^+ (Fig. 6.2-8) by the symporter (carrier) proteins which are different for different molecules.

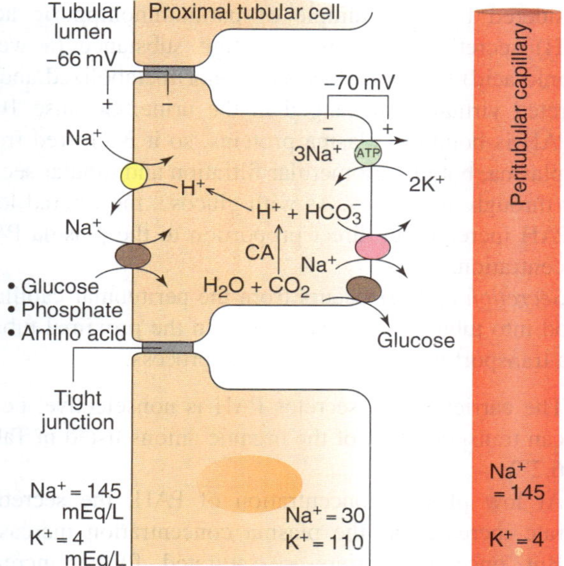

FIGURE 6.2-7 Mechanism of reabsorption of sodium and other solutes across early proximal tubule.

The carrier for glucose in proximal tubule is called sodium-dependent–glucose transporter-I (SGLT-1). The glucose and other organic solutes that enter the cell with Na^+ leave the cell across the basolateral membrane by passive transport mechanism.

Note. The reabsorption of Na^+–HCO_3^- and Na^+-organic solutes across the proximal tubule establishes a transtubular osmotic gradient that provides the driving force for the passive absorption of water by osmosis. Because more water than Cl^- is reabsorbed in the early segment of proximal tubule, the Cl^- concentration in tubular fluid rises along the length of the early proximal tubule (Fig. 6.2-8).

In the late proximal tubule the Na^+ is reabsorbed primarily by *chloride-driven sodium transport mechanism* across both the transcellular and paracellular pathways.

- *Reabsorption via paracellular pathway*. The filtered glucose, amino acids and HCO_3^- have already been almost completely removed from the tubular fluid by reabsorption in the early proximal tubule. So the fluid entering the late proximal tubule contains very little of these substances but contains a high concentration of Cl^- (140 mEq/L) compared with that in the early proximal tubule (105 mEq/L). This high Cl^- (140 mEq/L) concentration in the lumen of late proximal tubule and comparatively low concentration (105 mEq/L) in the interstitium creates a concentration gradient which favours the diffusion of Cl^- from the tubular lumen across the tight junctions into lateral intercellular space. Movement of negatively charged Cl^- causes the tubular

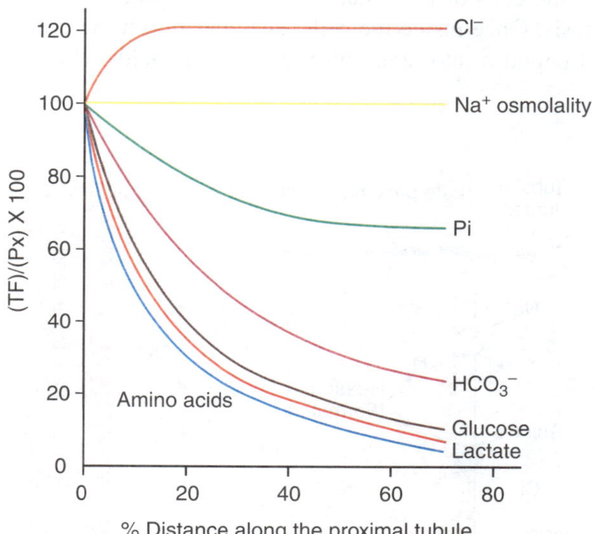

FIGURE 6.2-8 Concentration of solutes in tubular fluid as a function of length along the proximal tubule. TF is the concentration of substance in the tubular fluid, and P_x is the concentration of substance in the plasma. Values above 100 indicate that relatively less of substance than water was absorbed; and values below 100 indicate that relatively more of substance than water was reabsorbed.

fluid to become positively charged relative to the blood. This causes the diffusion of Na^+ across the tight junctions into the blood.

- *Transcellular Na^+ reabsorption* across the luminal membrane of late proximal tubule cells occurs due to parallel operation of Na^+–H^+ and one or more Cl^- anion (formate) antiporters (Fig. 6.2-9).
- *Across the basolateral membrane*, the Na^+ leaves the cell by the action of Na^+–K^+–ATPase pump, and Cl^- leaves by K^+–Cl^- cotransporter (Fig. 6.2-9).

Water Reabsorption Approximately 67% of the filtered water is absorbed in the proximal tubule by osmosis in response to a transtubular osmotic gradient established by the solute reabsorption (i.e. Na^+–Cl^-, Na^+–glucose and so forth).

- Two-thirds of H_2O reabsorption occurs through the transcellular pathway and one-third through the tight junction's paracellular pathway (Fig. 6.2-10).
- The osmotic water flowing across the proximal tubule also causes some reabsorption of K^+ and Ca^{2+} by the process of *solvent drag*.
- The osmotic water absorption is termed as *obligatory water absorption* as it cannot be changed according to the needs of the body.

Protein Reabsorption Normally, only a small amount of proteins is filtered by the glomerulus (40 mg/L). However, because of high GFR (180 L/day) the total amount of protein filtered per day is significant (180 L/day × 40 mg/L = 7.2 g/day). Normally, the proteins are completely taken into the cells of proximal tubules by the process of endocytosis. Once inside the cells, enzymes digest the proteins and peptides into their constituent amino acids which exit across the basolateral membrane and return to the blood in the peritubular capillaries.

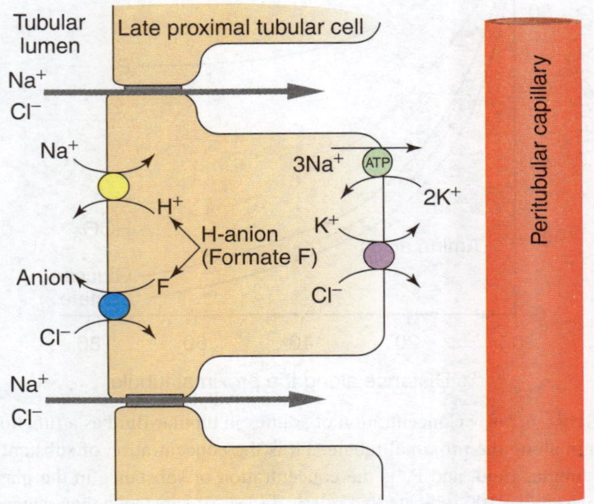

FIGURE 6.2-9 Mechanism of reabsorption of sodium and other solutes across late proximal tubule (for understanding see text).

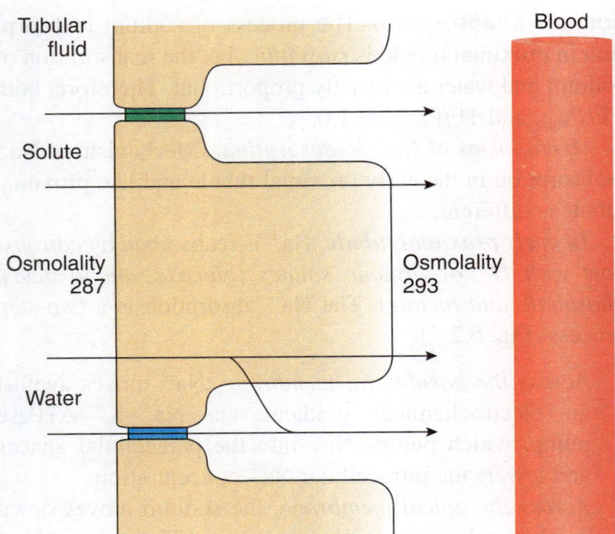

FIGURE 6.2-10 Routes of water and solute reabsorption across the proximal tubule (for understanding see text).

When the amount of filtered proteins increases (due to disruption of glomerular filtration barrier in kidney diseases), the reabsorbing mechanisms saturate and the proteins may appear in the urine (*proteinuria*).

Secretion in Proximal Tubule. The cells of proximal tubule, in addition to reabsorbing solutes and water, also secrete organic anions and organic cations, which include some end products of metabolism circulating in plasma, exogenous organic compounds and certain drugs (Table 6.2-2).

Mechanism of Secretion of Organic Anions can be considered by the example of para-aminohippuric acid (PAH) secretion. PAH is a foreign substance (a weak organic acid) that is neither stored nor metabolized and is excreted virtually unchanged in the urine. Because 10% of PAH is bound to plasma proteins, so it is cleared from the plasma, both by glomerular filtration and tubular secretion through the kidney. As with glucose, the filtered load of PAH increases in direct proportion to the plasma PAH concentration.

Secretion of PAH occurs from the peritubular capillary blood into tubular fluid via carriers in the proximal tubule by a transport maximum T_m limited process.

- The carrier which secretes PAH is nonselective, i.e. it can transport most of the organic anions listed in Table 6.2-2.
- At low plasma concentration of PAH, the secretion rate increases as the plasma concentration increases. But, once the carriers are saturated, further increase in plasma PAH concentration does not cause further increase in secretion rate T_m (Fig. 6.2-11).

TABLE 6.2-2 Some Organic Anions, Cations, Organic Compounds and Drugs Secreted by Proximal Tubule Cells

Anions Secreted by Proximal Tubule	
Endogenous anion	**Drugs**
PAH	Acetazolamide
cAMP	Furosemide
Bile salts	Penicillin
Oxalate	Probenecid
Prostaglandins	Salicylate (aspirin)
Water	NSAIDs
Cations Secreted by Proximal Tubule	
Endogenous cation	**Drugs**
Creatinine	Atropine
Dopamine	Cimetidine
Epinephrine	Morphine
Norepinephrine	Quinine
	Procainamide
	Verapamil

- The PAH is taken into the cell across the basolateral membrane against its chemical gradient, in exchange for α-ketoglutarate (αKG) via a PAH–αKG *antiport mechanism.* The resultant high intracellular concentration of PAH provides the driving force for PAH exit across the luminal membrane into the tubular fluid via a PAH–anion (A^-) antiporter and possibly a voltage-driven PAH transporter (Fig. 6.2-11).

Note. PAH clearance can be used to measure renal plasma flow (see page 553).

Mechanism of Secretion of Organic Cations

- *Across the basolateral membrane,* the organic cations enter the cell by facilitated diffusion. This mechanism is driven by the magnitude of the voltage difference (negative potential) across the basolateral membrane.
- *Across the luminal membrane,* the organic cations enter into the tubular fluid by an OC^+– H^+ antiport (Fig. 6.2-12).
- The carrier which secretes organic cation into the tubular fluid is nonselective, i.e. it can transport most of the organic cations listed in Table 6.2-2.

Transport across Loop of Henle About 20% of filtered Na^+ and Cl^-, 15% of filtered water and cations such as K^+, Ca^{2+} and Mg^{2+} are reabsorbed in the loop of Henle.

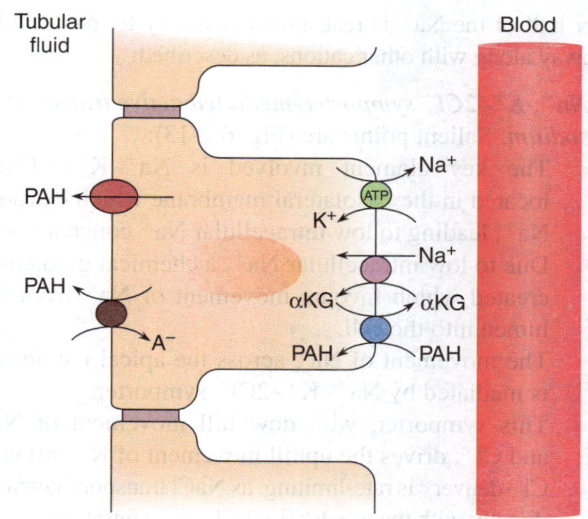

FIGURE 6.2-11 Mechanism of secretion of organic anion (e.g. PAH) across the proximal tubule.

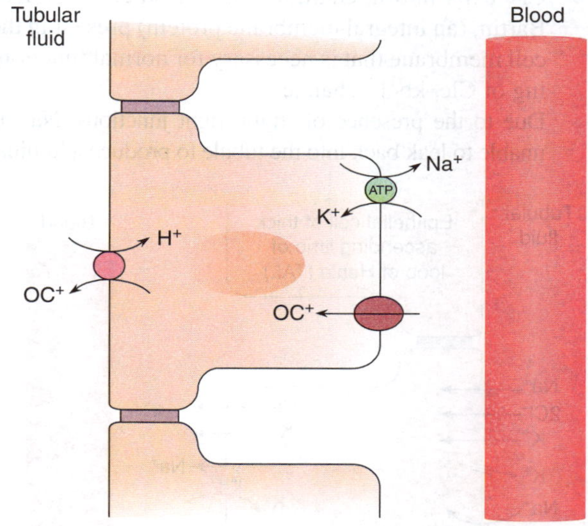

FIGURE 6.2-12 Mechanism of secretion of organic cations (OC^+) across the proximal tubule (for understanding see text).

Reabsorption occurring in different parts of the loop of Henle is:

Thin Descending Limb of Loop of Henle. *Water absorption* occurs passively (because of hypertonic interstitial fluid) exclusively in this part of loop of Henle. It is accompanied by diffusion of sodium ions from interstitial fluid into tubular lumen.

Thin Ascending Limb of Loop of Henle. Limited passive reabsorption of Na^+ and Cl^- occurs in this water-impermeable limb. Because of impermeability to water, the fluid leaving this limb is hypotonic relative to plasma.

Thick Ascending Limb of Loop of Henle. This limb is impermeable to water but is involved in the reabsorption of 20% of the filtered Na^+, Cl^- and other cations. About half of the Na^+ is reabsorbed actively and transcellularly, while the other half of the Na^+ is reabsorbed passively by paracellular pathway along with other cations, as described:

- ***Na^+, K^+–$2Cl^-$ symporter-mediated active transport of sodium.*** Salient points are (Fig. 6.2-13):
  - The key element involved is Na^+–K^+–ATPase located in the basolateral membrane which extrudes Na^+, leading to low intracellular Na^+ concentration.
  - Due to low intracellular Na^+, a chemical gradient is created which favours movement of Na^+ from the lumen into the cell.
  - The movement of Na^+ across the apical membrane is mediated by Na^+–K^+–$2Cl^-$ symporter.
  - This symporter, with downhill movement of Na^+ and Cl^-, drives the uphill movement of K^+ influx.
  - Cl^- delivery is rate-limiting, as NaCl transport increases directly with the tubular fluid Cl^- concentration.
  - Na^+ leaves the cell across the basolateral membrane by the action of Na^+–K^+–ATPase.
  - Cl^- exits into interstitium via Clc–kbcl$^-$ channels. Bartin, (an integral membrane protein) present in the cell membrane that is necessary for normal functioning of Clc–kbcl$^-$ channel.
  - Due to the presence of 'tight' tight junctions, Na^+ is unable to leak back into the tubule to produce a luminal potential, however, some of the K^+ which enters the cell leaks back across the apical membrane into the tubular lumen, and into the interstitium by ROMK and other K^+ channels, generating a lumen-positive transepithelial potential difference of +6–+10 mV.

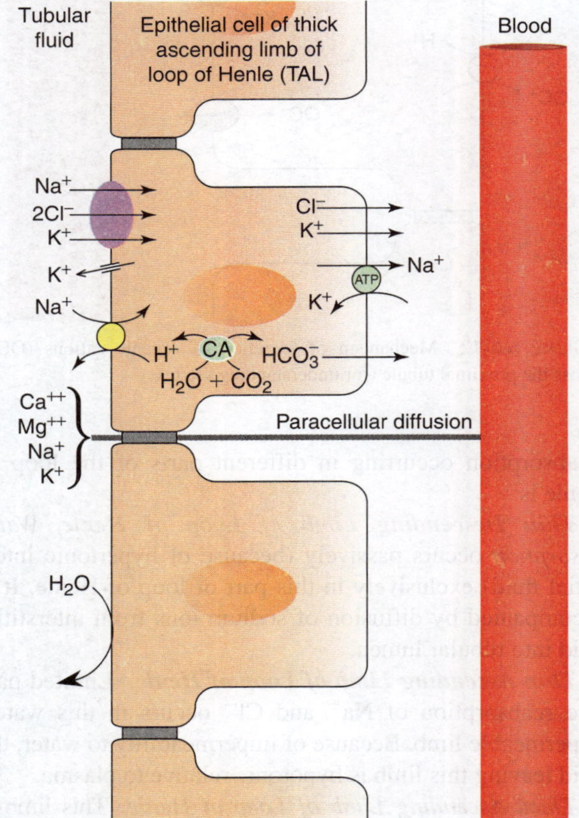

FIGURE 6.2-13 The active (transcellular) and passive (paracellular) transport mechanism operating across the tubular cells in thick ascending limb (TAL) of loop of Henle.

Note. Thick ascending limb is the site of action of the loop diuretics (e.g. furosemide, ethacrynic acid), which inhibit Na^+–K^+–$2Cl^-$ transporter.

- ***Dent disease.*** Some of Cl^- absorption in thick ascending loop of Henle occurs with Na^+, K^+ and Ca^{2+}. In kidneys, a type of Cl^- channel has been identified which is linked with Ca^{2+}. Gene mutation of this channel is associated with Ca^{2+} containing renal stones and hypercalciuria, is known as Dent disease.
- ***Na^+–H^+ antiporter-mediated active reabsorption*** of sodium also occurs transcellularly leading to H^+ secretion (HCO_3^- reabsorption) (Fig. 6.2-13).
- ***Paracellular passive reabsorption of Na^+, K^+, Ca^{2+} and Mg^{2+}*** is the function of voltage across the thick ascending limb. Because of the unique location of transport proteins in the apical and basolateral membranes, the tubular fluid is positively charged relative to the blood. The increased salt reabsorption by the thick ascending limb increases the magnitude of positive charge in the lumen which plays a major role in driving the passive paracellular reabsorption of cations (Fig. 6.2-13)

Note. Thick ascending limb is *impermeable* to water. Thus, NaCl and other solutes are reabsorbed without water. As a result, tubular fluid Na^+ and tubular fluid osmolarity decreases to less than their concentration in plasma (i.e. $TF/P_{osm} < 1.0$). This segment is therefore called the *diluting segment*. Further, Na^+ reabsorbed from this segment is the main driving force behind the countercurrent multiplier system which concentrates Na^+ and urea in medullary interstitium.

Applied Aspects

Bartter's syndrome: Bartter's syndrome is a rare disease that most often presents in neonatal period or early childhood with polyuria, polydipsia, salt craving and growth retardation. Blood pressure remains normal or low. It may result due to mutation affecting any of the ion transport proteins in TAL: Na^+–K^+–$2Cl^-$ symporter, the ROMK K^+ channel, Clc–kbcl channel or bartin. The TAL transporters function in an integrated manner to maintain electrical potential difference and Na^+ gradient between the tubular lumen and cell.

- Loss of lumen positive electric transport potential, (that normally derives paracellular absorption of Na^+, Ca^{2+} and Mg^{2+}) causes NaCl wasting, hypercalciuria and hypomagnesium.
- Bartter's syndrome due to mutation of bartin is also associated with deafness, because striavascularis in the inner ear is responsible for maintaining high K^+ concentration in scala media.

Transport Across Distal Tubules and Collecting Duct

Approximately 7% of the filtered NaCl and about 8–17% of water is reabsorbed and K^+ and H^+ are secreted in these segments.

Early distal tubule (initial segment of distal tubule) reabsorbs Na^+, Cl^- and Ca^{2+}, and is impermeable to water.

- *Na^+–Cl^- symporter* mechanism is involved in the transport of Na^+–Cl^- across the apical membrane. Across the basolateral membrane, Na^+ leaves the cell via the action of Na^+–K^+–ATPase, and Cl^-leaves the cell by diffusion via channels (Fig. 6.2-14).
- Because of *impermeability to water,* the reabsorption of NaCl in this segment occurs without water leading to dilution of tubular fluid. This is why it is also called cortical diluting segment.
- *Thiazide diuretics* reduce NaCl reabsorption by inhibiting Na^+–Cl^- cotransport.

Late distal tubule and collecting duct have two cell types (principal cells and intercalated cells) which perform both reabsorption and secretory functions:

Principal cells reabsorb Na^+, Cl^- and H_2O and secrete K^+ (Fig. 6.2-15):

- *Na^+ reabsorption.* Na^+ is actively transported using Na^+–K^+–ATPase across the basolateral membrane. Across the apical membrane, Na^+ diffuses passively due to chemical gradient.
- *Cl^- reabsorption* occurs passively through paracellular pathway. Cl^- is driven by the lumen negative charge generated by the diffusional influx of sodium.
- *H_2O absorption* occurs in response to the effect of antidiuretic hormone (ADH) on the principal cells. ADH increases H_2O permeability by directing the insertion of H_2O channels in the luminal membrane. In the absence of ADH, the principal cells are virtually impermeable to water.

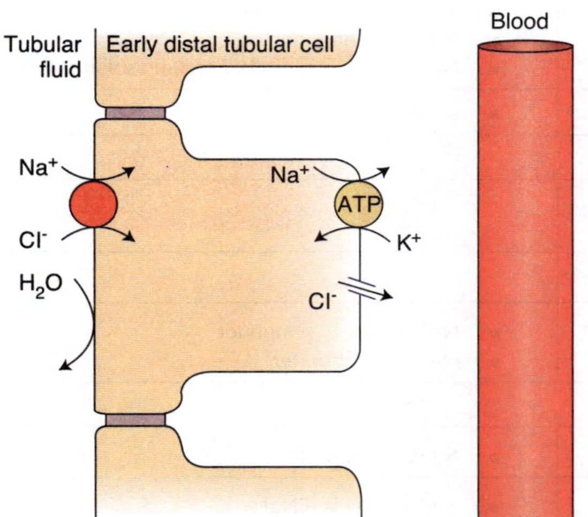

FIGURE 6.2-14 Mechanism of reabsorption of Na^+ and Cl^- in the early distal tubule. This segment is impermeable to water (see text for details).

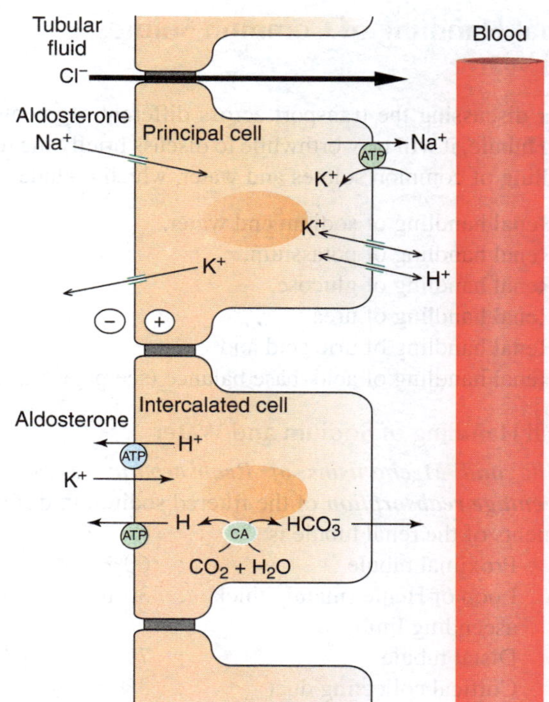

FIGURE 6.2-15 Mechanism of transport in principal cells and intercalated cells of the late distal tubule and collecting duct (see text for details). CA = carbonic anhydrase.

- *K^+ secretion.* K^+ uptake across the basolateral membrane occurs via the action of Na^+–K^+–ATPase followed by diffusion down its electrochemical gradient across the apical cell membrane into the tubular fluid.

Role of aldosterone on principal cell functions. Aldosterone increases Na^+ reabsorption and increases K^+ secretion. Like other steroid hormones, the action of aldosterone takes several hours to develop because new protein synthesis is required. About 2% of overall Na^+ absorption is affected by aldosterone.

Effect of amiloride. Amiloride is a diuretic that inhibits Na^+ reabsorption by distal tubule and collecting duct by directly inhibiting Na^+ channels in the luminal cell membrane. Thus, indirectly, by reducing the negative charge in lumen, the amiloride also inhibits Cl^- reabsorption and K^+ secretion. As the K^+ excretion in urine is decreased, it is called *potassium sparing diuretic*. Other potassium sparing diuretics are spironolactone and triamterene.

Intercalated cells reabsorb K^+ and secrete H^+

- *K^+ reabsorption*, occurs probably by a H^+–K^+–ATPase located in the apical cell membrane.
- *H^+ secretion* (HCO_3^- reabsorption) or HCO_3^- secretion (H^+ reabsorption) can occur by H^+–ATPase. This function is important for acid–base balance (see page 523).
- *Aldosterone* increases H^+ secretion by intercalated cells by stimulating the H^+–ATPase (in addition to its actions on the principal cells).

Renal Handling of Common Solutes and Water

After discussing the transport across different segments of renal tubule, it will be worthwhile to discuss briefly the renal handling of common solutes and water, which include:

- Renal handling of sodium and water,
- Renal handling of potassium,
- Renal handling of glucose,
- Renal handling of urea,
- Renal handling of uric acid and
- Renal handling of acid–base balance (see page 523).

Renal Handling of Sodium and Water

Site and Mechanisms of Reabsorption of Sodium. ***Percentage reabsorption*** of the filtered sodium in different segments of the renal tubule is:

- Proximal tubule : 60%
- Loop of Henle (mainly thick ascending limb) : 30%
- Distal tubule : 7%
- Cortical collecting duct : 3%

Mechanisms of reabsorption, as described in detail above in the subsection on transport across different segments of renal tubule are summarized in Table 6.2-3.

Sodium recycling. The sodium which is actively pumped out from the thick ascending limb (TAL) into the outer medullary interstitium mostly enters the outer medullary descending thin segment (DTS). This results in recycling of Na^+ in the long loops of the juxtamedullary nephrons. The recycling causes accumulation of Na^+ in the interstitium of the renal medulla.

Reabsorption of Water

Site and Mechanism of Reabsorption. Water is absorbed passively by osmosis in response to a transtubular osmotic gradient. Rapid diffusion of water across the cell membrane occurs through water channels made up of proteins called *Aquaporins*. Different types of aquaporins are aquaporin-1, 2, 5 and 9. Mostly, these aquaporins are present in the kidney. The other sites include are: leucocytes, liver, lung and lacrimal gland. In the collecting ducts, reabsorption of water is controlled by antidiuretic hormone (ADH). Renal handling of water by different segments of renal tubule is as:

Proximal tubule: Passively reabsorbed (67%).

Loop of Henle

- Descending thin segment (DTS) : Passively reabsorbed (15%)
- Ascending thin segment (ATS) : Impermeable
- Thick ascending limb (TAL) : Impermeable

TABLE 6.2-3 Summary of Mechanism of Na^+ Absorption across Different Segments of Renal Tubule

Segment of the tubule	Absorption active/ passive/impermeable	Mediated by
Proximal tubule		
• Early proximal tubule	Active	• Na^+–K^+ antiporter and • Na^+–H^+ antiporter • Na^+–glucose (and other organic solutes) symport
• Late proximal tubule	Active	• Cl^--driven Na^+ transport
Loop of Henle		
• Descending thin segment (DTS)	Passively secreted in interstitium	
• Ascending thin segment (ATS)	Passive	
• Thick ascending limb (TAL)	Active (transcellular)	• Na^+–K^+–$2Cl^-$ symporter • Na^+–H^+ antiporter
Distal tubule and collecting duct		
• Early distal tubule	Active	• Na^+Cl^- symporter
• Late distal tubule and collecting duct (principal cell)	Active	• Na^+ channels (ENa) • Regulated by aldosterone

Distal tubule and collecting duct (8–17%)

- Distal convoluted tubule (DCT) : Impermeable
- Connecting tubule (CNT) : Impermeable
- Cortical collecting duct (CCD) : Reabsorbed (ADH)
- Outer medullary duct collecting (OMCD) : Reabsorbed (ADH)
- Inner medullary duct collecting (IMCD) : Reabsorbed (ADH)

Obligatory and Facultative Reabsorption of Water

Obligatory Reabsorption. About 85% of the filtered water is always reabsorbed, irrespective of the body water balance. This reabsorption occurs by osmosis in response to a transtubular osmotic gradient and is called obligatory (must occur) reabsorption.

- About 67% of obligatory reabsorption occurs in the proximal tubules and
- About 15–18% of obligatory reabsorption occurs in the descending thin segment of loop of Henle.

Facultative Reasborption. The remaining 15–18% of the water may or may not be absorbed depending upon the body water balance. It is called facultative (optional) reabsorption.

Facultative reabsorption of water occurs from the collecting tubule and is under the control of ADH.

Regulation of NaCl and Water Absorption

1. ***Hormonal regulation.*** Various hormones including angiotensin II, aldosterone, ADH, ANP, urodilatin epinephrine and norepinephrine (released from sympathetic nerves) and dopamine regulate NaCl reabsorption. ADH is the only major hormone that directly regulates the amount of water excreted by kidney. Table 6.2-4 summarizes for each hormone, the major stimulus for secretion, the nephron site of action and the effect on transport.
2. ***Role of Starling forces.*** Although Na^+ reabsorption is an active process, it is affected by the passive Starling forces operating between the intercellular spaces and the peritubular capillaries in the proximal tubule.
   - *Starling forces that favour* the movement of reabsorbed substances into the capillaries are capillary oncotic pressure (π_C) and the hydrostatic pressure in the intercellular spaces (P_i).
   - *Opposing Starling forces* are the interstitial oncotic pressure (π_i) and the capillary hydrostatic pressure (P_C).
   - Starling forces do not affect transport by the loop of Henle, distal tubule and collecting duct because these segments are less permeable to water than the proximal tubule.

TABLE 6.2-4 Hormonal Regulation of NaCl and Water Reabsorption

Hormone	Major stimulus for secretion	Nephron (site of action)	Effect on transport
Angiotensin II	↑ Renin	PT	↑ Na^+, $Cl^-$and H_2O reabsorption
Aldosterone	↑ Angiotensin and ↑ $[K^+]_P$	TAL, DT CD	↑ NaCl and H_2O reabsorption
Atria natriuretic peptide	↑ ECV	CD	↓ NaCl and H_2O reabsorption
Urodilatin	↑ ECV	CD	↓ NaCl and H_2O reabsorption
Sympathetic nerves	↓ ECV	PT, TAL, DT/CD	↑ NaCl and H_2O reabsorption
Dopamine	↑ ECV	PT	↓ NaCl and H_2O reabsorption
ADH	↑ Posm	DT/CD	↑ H_2O reabsorption

PT, proximal tubule; TAL, thick ascending limb; DT/CD, distal tubule and collecting duct; ECV, effective circulatory volume; $[K^+]_P$, plasma K^+ concentration; and P_{osm}, plasma osmolarity.

- Starling forces across the peritubular capillaries around the proximal tubule are changed by:
  - Dilatation of efferent arteriole (↑es P_C)
  - Constriction of efferent arteriole (↓es P_C).

3. ***Role of glomerulotubular balance in the proximal tubule.*** Glomerulotubular balance (GTB) in the proximal tubule maintains reabsorption at a constant fraction (2/3 or 67% of the filtered Na^+ and H_2O). For example, if GFR spontaneously increases, the filtered load of Na^+ also increases. Without a change in reabsorption, this situation would lead to increased Na^+ excretion. However, GTB functions such as Na^+ reabsorption will also increase, ensuring that a constant fraction is reabsorbed.

   Mechanism of GTB is based on Starling forces in the peritubular capillaries, which alter the reabsorption of Na^+ and H_2O in the proximal tubule (Fig. 6.2-16):
   - *Route of isosmotic fluid reabsorption* is from the lumen, to the proximal tubule cell, to the lateral intercellular space and then to the peritubular capillary blood.
   - *Starling forces in the peritubular capillary blood* govern how much of this isosmotic fluid will be reabsorbed.
   - *Fluid reabsorption* is increased by increase in oncotic pressure of the peritubular capillaries blood (π_C) and decreased by decrease in π_C.

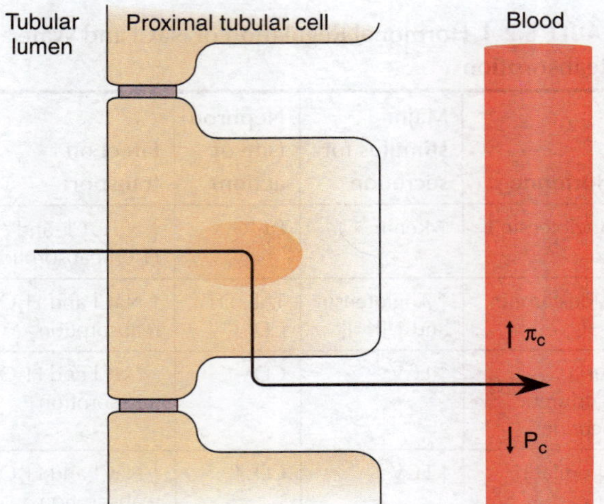

FIGURE 6.2-16 Mechanism of glomerulotubular balance (isosmotic reabsorption).

- *Increase in GFR and filtration fraction* causes the protein concentration and π_C of peritubular capillary blood to increase. This increase, in turn, produces an increase in fluid reabsorption. Thus, there is matching of filtration and reabsorption, i.e. GTB.

4. ***Effects of ECF volume on proximal tubular reabsorption***
   - *ECF volume contraction increases reabsorption.* ECF volume contraction increases peritubular capillary protein concentration and oncotic pressure (π_C) and decreases peritubular capillary hydrostatic pressure (P_C). Together, these changes in Starling forces in peritubular capillary blood cause an increase in proximal tubular reabsorption.
   - *ECF volume expansion decreases reabsorption.* ECF volume expansion decreases peritubular capillary protein concentration and oncotic pressure (π_C) and increases peritubular capillary hydrostatic pressure (P_C). Together, these changes in Starling forces in peritubular capillary blood cause a decrease in proximal tubular reabsorption.

Renal Handling of Potassium and Potassium Homeostasis

General Considerations

Functions of K^+ Potassium (K^+) is one of the most abundant cations in the body. It is the *principal intracellular cation*, and is equally important in the extracellular fluid for specific functions. Potassium is required for following biochemical functions:

- Maintenance of intracellular osmotic pressure,
- Optimal activity of enzyme pyruvate kinase (of glycolysis),
- Proper synthesis of DNA and proteins by ribosomes,
- Optimal cell growth,
- Transmission of nerve impulse,
- Generation of cell membrane potential and muscle contraction,
- Extracellular K^+ influences cardiac muscle activity and
- Regulation of acid–base balance and water balance in the cells.

Daily Requirement and Sources

- ***Daily requirement*** of K^+ is about 3–4 g/day.
- ***Sources*** of K^+ are bananas, oranges, pineapples, potatoes, beans, chicken, liver and tender coconut water.

Potassium Homeostasis

Distribution of K^+

- *Total body K^+* constitutes about 50 mEq/kg of body weight, or 3500 mEq for a 70 kg individual.
- *Intracellular K^+*. K^+ is predominantly an intracellular cation. Ninety-eight per cent of the K^+ in the body is located within cells, where its average concentration is 150 mEq/L.
- *Extracellular fluid* (ECF) contains only 2% of the total body K^+, where its normal concentration is approximately 4 mEq/L.

Shifts of K^+ between ICF and ECF Hyperkalaemia, i.e. ECF K^+ concentration $>$ 5.0 mEq/L, occurs when K^+ is shifted out of cells in following conditions:

- Insulin deficiency,
- β-adrenergic antagonists,
- Acidosis (exchange of extracellular H^+ for intracellular K^+),
- Hyperosmolarity (H_2O flows out of the cells, K^+ diffuses out with H_2O),
- Inhibition of Na^+–K^+ pump (e.g. digitalis), as when pump is blocked, K^+ is not taken up into cells,
- Exercise and
- Cell lysis (therefore, care should be taken to avoid haemolysis of RBCs for the estimation of serum K^+).

Hypokalaemia, i.e. ECF K^+ concentration $<$ 3.5 mEq/L, occurs when K^+ is shifted into the cells, as is caused by:

- Insulin,
- β-adrenergic agonists,
- Alkalosis (exchange of intracellular H^+ for extracellular K^+) and
- Hypoosmolarity (H_2O flows into the cell, K^+ diffuses in with H_2O).

External versus Internal K^+ Balance Despite wide fluctuations in dietary K^+ intake, its concentration in ICF and ECF remains constant. Two sets of regulatory mechanisms safeguard K^+ homeostasis: one type of mechanism maintains external K^+ balance and the second set of mechanism maintains the internal K^+ balance.

External K^+ balance refers to maintenance of constant amount of K^+ in the body. It is accomplished by adjusting renal K^+ excretion to match the dietary K^+ intake. Normally, all the K^+ absorbed by GIT is excreted by the kidneys. However, it is a slow process and at least takes 6 h. This arrangement ensures a long-term, chronic constancy of K^+ content. However, rapid loses of large amount of K^+ can cause serious hypokalaemia. Conversely, hyperkalaemia can occur when K^+ is absorbed from GIT or infused intravenously much faster than the kidney can excrete it.

Internal K^+ balance refers to the constancy of K^+ distribution in ICF and ECF. Rapid changes in ECF are not uncommon. After a meal, the K^+ absorbed by the GIT enters the ECF within minutes and as mentioned above, the kidney takes at least 6 h to excrete it. Therefore, certain mechanisms are required to keep a balance between ECF and ICF, otherwise even after normal meals the plasma K^+ levels will rise to fatal levels. The internal K^+ balance is maintained by various hormones which allow a rapid to and fro shift between ECF and ICF (Fig. 6.2-17).

Maintenance of Internal K^+ Balance The internal K^+ balance is maintained by rapid redistribution of K^+ between ICF and ECF. Factors involved in it are summarized in Fig. 6.2-17. Before discussing the role played by each factor, it will be worthwhile to understand the mechanism involved in the regulatory process.

Mechanism of Control of K^+ Entry into the Cells. The primary mechanisms which affect the movement of K^+ into and out of the cells are:

1. ***Na^+–K^+–ATPase activity*** is the main factor controlling entry of K^+ into the cells. All the major hormones involved in maintaining internal K^+ balance (i.e. epinephrine, insulin and aldosterone), increase K^+ uptake of cells (particularly of skeletal muscle, liver, bone and red blood cells) by stimulating activity of the Na^+–K^+–ATPase pump. The activity of Na^+–K^+–ATPase is increased.
   - *Rapidly* (within minutes) by increased turnover rate of existing Na^+–K–ATPase to handle the acute changes in plasma K^+ levels.
   - *Slowly* (within hour to day) by an increase in the number of Na^+–K^+–ATPase units in the membrane. The slow increase in Na^+–K^+–ATPase activity is required to produce a chronic increase in K^+ uptake by the cells.

   For example, an increase in plasma K^+ levels that follows K^+ absorption by GIT, stimulates insulin secretion from the pancreas, aldosterone release from the adrenal cortex and epinephrine secretion from the adrenal medulla to stimulate Na^+–K^+–ATPase activity for handling the raised K^+ plasma levels. In contrast, a decrease in plasma K^+ levels inhibits the release of these hormones. It is important to note that insulin and epinephrine act within a few minutes, while aldosterone requires about 1 h to stimulate K^+ uptake into the cells.
2. ***Potassium permeability***. Increase in K^+ permeability will result in loss of intracellular K^+ to ECF and vice versa. K^+ permeability increases in a condition called hypokalaemic periodic paralysis.
3. ***Intracellular anions***, e.g. organic phosphates, DNA and RNA serve to counterbalance the positive charge of K^+. Loss of these anions is associated with loss of K^+ from the cells.

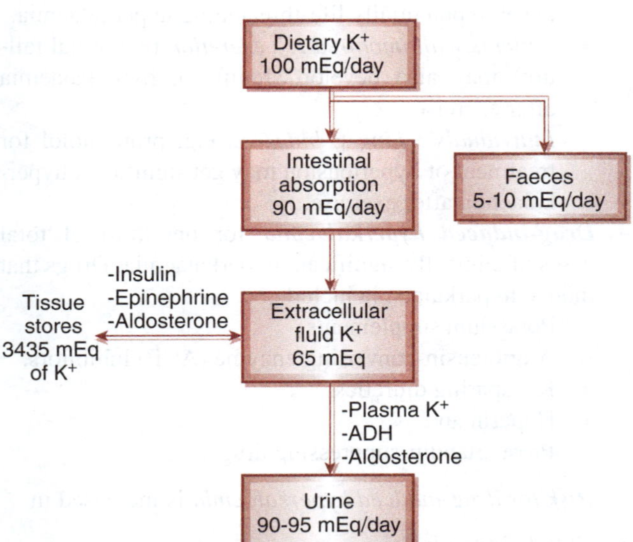

FIGURE 6.2-17 An overview of potassium homeostasis (for explanation see text).

Shift of K^+ between ECF and ICF Common causes of shift of K^+ from ECF to ICF and from ICF to ECF are depicted in Fig. 6.2-18.

Role of Hormones in Maintaining Internal k^+ Balance

1. ***Epinephrine***. It influences the K^+ distribution across the cell by activating α and β_2 receptors.
   - Stimulation of α-receptors releases K^+ from cells, especially in the liver. This mechanism is important in producing local hyperkalaemia in the muscle, which subserves two beneficial functions: vasodilatation and activation of glycogenolysis. Both activities support vigorous exercise.
   - Stimulation of β_2 receptors causes K^+ uptake by cells. This mechanism lowers plasma K^+ during acute stress, e.g. myocardial ischaemia.
2. ***Insulin***. It is the most important hormone that shifts K^+ into cells after ingestion of K^+ in a meal by stimulating Na^+–K^+–ATPase. The role of insulin explains:
   - Greater rise in plasma K^+ after a K^+ rich meal in an individual with diabetes mellitus (insulin deficiency) as compared to a normal person.
   - Role of insulin infusion (with glucose to prevent insulin-induced hypoglycaemia) in correcting hyperkalaemia.

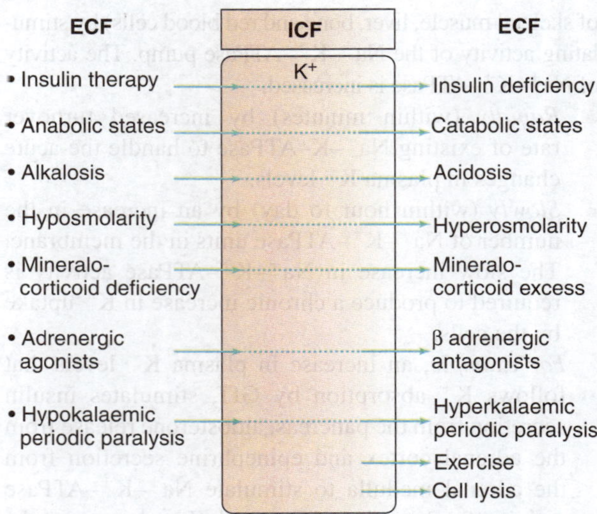

FIGURE 6.2-18 Causes of shift of K^+ between ECF and ICF.

3. ***Aldosterone***. It promotes K^+ uptake into the cells by activating Na^+–K^+–ATPase; therefore:
   - *Hypokalaemia* occurs when aldosterone levels are increased (e.g. in primary aldosteronism) and
   - *Hyperkalaemia* occurs when aldosterone level falls (e.g. in Addison's disease).

The aldosterone also stimulates urinary K^+ excretion (discussed later in this chapter).

Effect of Other Factors on Internal K^+ Balance. Certain factors which do not contribute to K^+ homeostasis, but do affect the internal K^+ balance are described below. The extent to which these factors are able to alter plasma K^+ depends upon the integrity of homeostatic mechanisms that regulate plasma K^+ (e.g. secretion of epinephrine, insulin and aldosterone).

1. ***Acid–base balance*** influences the internal K^+ balance in following ways:
   - *Metabolic acidosis produced by inorganic acids* (e.g. HCl and H_2SO_4) is associated with entry of H^+ into the cells and movement of K^+ into the ECF, producing hyperkalaemia.
   - *Metabolic acidosis produced by organic acids* (e.g. lactic acid, acetic acid and keto acids) usually does not produce hyperkalaemia. It is because in such circumstances, the anions enter the cell along with H^+, and thereby eliminate the need for K^+/H^+ exchange across the cell membrane. Further, organic anions may stimulate insulin secretion which moves K^+ into the cells. This movement may counteract the direct effect of acidosis, which moves K^+ out of the cell.
   - *Respiratory acidosis* has very little effect on plasma K^+ levels, because the resting membrane potential does not change when CO_2 enters the cells, or when it reacts with water to form H^+ and HCO_3^-.
   - *Metabolic alkalosis* decreases plasma K^+ because K^+ enters the cells in exchange of H^+.
2. ***Plasma osmolarity*** influences the internal K^+ balance as:
   - *Hyperosmolarity*. In this condition, water moves out of the cells because of the osmotic gradient across the cell membrane until the intracellular osmolarity equals that of ECF. The loss of water shrinks cells and causes K^+ to rise. The rise in intracellular K^+ leads to diffusion of K^+ into the ECF, producing hyperkalaemia.
   - *Hypoosmolarity*, results in hypokalaemia because of movement of K^+ into the cells by the effect just opposite to that seen in hyperosmolarity.
3. ***Exercise***. During exercise, more K^+ is released from the skeletal muscle cells than during rest. This is because during the depolarization that accompanies muscle contraction, K^+ exits from the muscle cells. However, most of the K^+ released enter the T tubules, from which K^+ is rapidly taken back into the cell on repolarization, but a little K^+ does enter the interstitial fluid and plasma. Therefore, the ensuing hyperkalaemia depends on the degree of exercise. After slow walking, plasma K^+ level increases by 0.3 mEq/L, but with more vigorous exercise the K^+ levels may increase upto 2.0 mEq/L above normal. However, exercise-induced hyperkalaemia usually does not produce symptoms and is reversed after several minutes of rest. Exercise-induced hyperkalaemia is unusual under the following circumstances:
   - *Patients with disturbed T tubule architecture of muscles*. Such patients may develop hyperkalaemia with minimal exercise. For example, even fist clenching may be associated with significant hyperkalaemia.
   - *Patients with certain endocrine disorders* that effect release of insulin, epinephrine or aldosterone may develop potentially life-threatening hyperkalaemia.
   - *Patients with impaired K^+ excretion* (e.g. renal failure) may also develop significant hyperkalaemia after exercise.
   - *Individuals taking β-blockers*, e.g. propranolol for treatment of hypertension may get significant hyperkalaemia after exercise.
4. ***Drug-induced hyperkalaemia*** for one-third of total cases of clinically significant hyperkalaemia. Drugs that induce hyperkalaemia include:
   - Potassium supplements,
   - Angiotensin-converting enzyme (ACE) inhibitors,
   - K^+-sparing diuretics,
   - Heparin and
   - Prostaglandin-suppressing drugs.

Risk for drug-induced hyperkalaemia is increased in:

- Elderly individuals,
- Patients with diabetes mellitus and
- Patients with renal insufficiency.

Maintenance of External Potassium Balance As mentioned earlier, external potassium balance refers to maintenance of constant body potassium, i.e. renal excretion matches dietary intake.

Intestinal Absorption versus Renal Excretion ***Absorption.*** The average diet contains approximately 100 mEq/day (~5 g/day) of potassium. Normally, 90% of the dietary K^+ is absorbed and about 10% is lost through faeces and sweats (Fig. 6.2-17). This amount (90%) of absorption is essentially constant, and not physiologically regulated and therefore, play little role in maintenance of the external potassium balance.

Excretion. Normally, kidneys excrete 90–95% of K^+ ingested in the diet (Fig. 6.2-17) and thus play a major role in maintaining external potassium balance. Excretion equals intake, even when intake increases by as much as 10-fold. Therefore, the K^+ excretion can vary widely from 1 to 110% of the filtered load, depending upon the dietary intake, aldosterone levels and acid–base balance. The transport pattern of K^+ by the major nephron, i.e. renal handling of the K^+ is described. It will be noted that the *main event that regulates external potassium balance is K^+ secretion* from the blood into the tubular fluid by the cells of the distal tubule and collecting duct system, and not the reabsorption in the proximal tubule which is load dependent.

Transport of Potassium across Major Nephron

Glomerular Filtration. Filtration occurs freely across the glomerular capillaries and potassium is not bound to plasma proteins. Therefore, TF/Pk^+ in Bowman's space is 1.00.

Tubular Reabsorption and Secretion. As shown in Fig. 6.2-19, 67% of the filtered K^+ is reabsorbed in the proximal tubule, 20% in loop of Henle and approximately 10% is delivered to the early distal tubule. In contrast to proximal tubule and loop of Henle, which are capable of only reabsorbing K^+, the distal tubule (DT) and collecting duct (CD) are able to either reabsorb or secrete K^+. The role of reabsorption or secretion by DT and CD depends on a variety of hormones and factors.

Reabsorption of K^+ by Proximal Tubule. In proximal tubule, potassium reabsorption is load dependent like that of Na^+. Two mechanisms involved in K^+ reabsorption are:

1. ***Beek flow*** or solvent drag. By this mechanism, approximately 7% of the filtered K^+ is reabsorbed passively in proportion to the H_2O reabsorption.
2. ***Paracellular transport***. About 60% of the filtered K^+ is reabsorbed actively by a unique paracellular transport, which has the following steps (Fig. 6.2-20):
   - *Concentration gradient* is created between the paracellular space and tubules fluid by active K^+ uptake via Na^+–K^+–ATPase located in the lateral cell membrane facing the lateral intercellular spaces.
   - *Diffusion of K^+ along the concentration gradient* occurs from the tubular lumen into the lateral intercellular spaces. In this way, luminal fluid equilibrates with low K^+ concentration in the intercellular space.
   - *Exit from basolateral membrane* of most of the K^+ that enters the cell actively from lateral surface (as described above), occurs by three pathways (Fig. 6.2-20):
     - The conductive K^+ channel,
     - The K^+–Cl^- cotransporter and
     - The Na^+–K^+–ATPase pump.

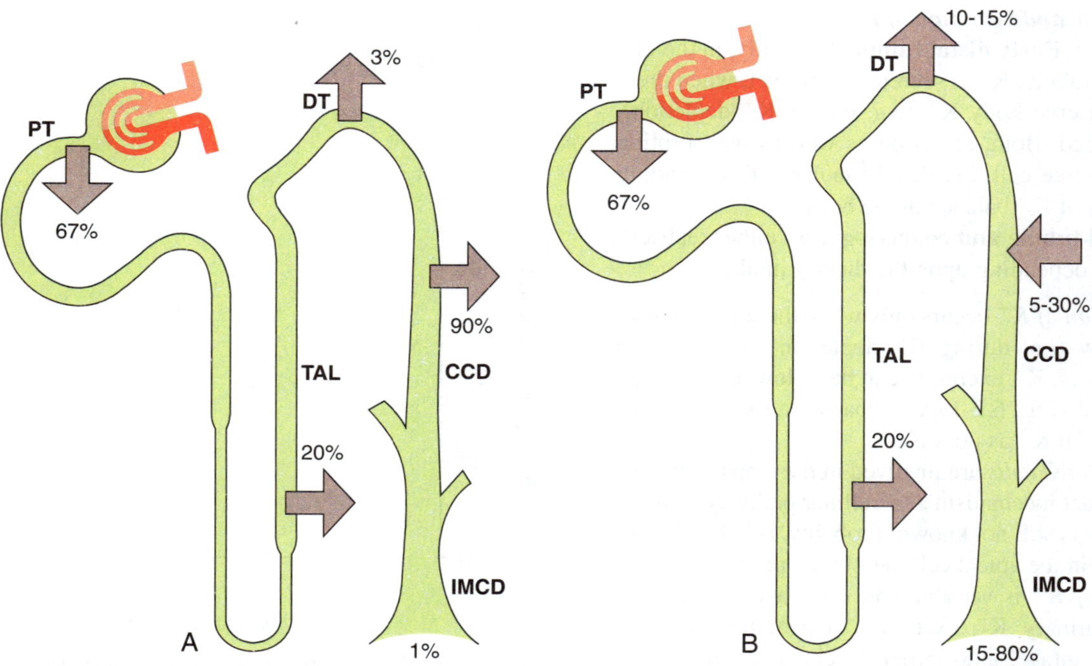

FIGURE 6.2-19 Potassium transport along the nephron: **A,** during dietary potassium depletion; and **B,** during normal and increased dietary intake.

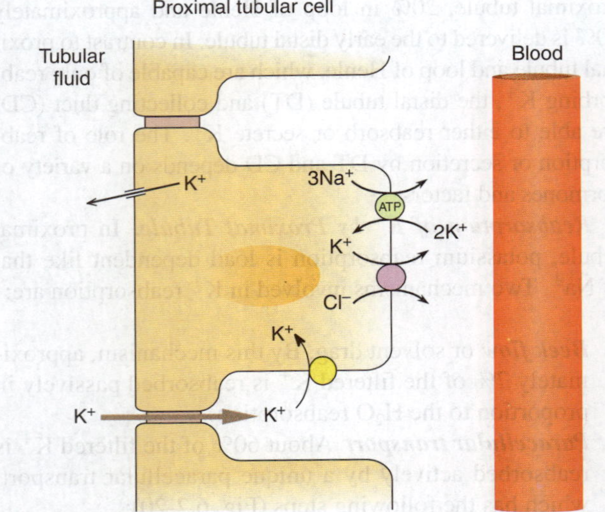

FIGURE 6.2-20 Mechanism of K^+ reabsorption in proximal tubule cells.

The K^+ that exits from the basolateral membrane is immediately absorbed in the peritubular capillaries.

Reabsorption of K^+ by Loop of Henle. Twenty per cent of the filtered K^+ is reabsorbed in the thick ascending limb (TAL) of loop of Henle, along with Na^+ reabsorption by two mechanisms:

1. *Na^+–K^+–$2Cl^-$ active transport mechanism.* Salient points of this mechanism are described on page 500 and depicted in Fig. 6.2-13.
2. *Paracellular passive reabsorption* occurs as a function of voltage gradient across the thick ascending limb. For details see page 493 and Fig. 6.2-13.

Reabsorption and Secretion of K^+ by Distal Tubule and Collecting Duct **Early distal tubule.** Normally, in the distal convoluted tubule, K^+ is secreted. However, when there is need to conserve body K^+ (e.g. during K^+ depletion), K^+ is reabsorbed. Both, secretion as well as reabsorption occurs in the same cell, i.e. distal tubular cell, depending upon the status of K^+ balance in the body.

Late distal tubule and collecting duct either reabsorb or secrete K^+, depending upon the dietary intake.

- ***Reabsorption of K^+*** occurs only when the dietary intake is very low (i.e. during K^+ depletion). Under these circumstances, K^+ excretion can be as low as 1% of the filtered load (Fig. 6.2-19A), because the kidneys conserve as much K^+ as possible.
  - *Intercalated cells* are involved in the reabsorption of K^+. Exact mechanism and cellular pathway of reabsorption is still not known. Probably, H^+–K–ATPase located in the apical cell membrane plays a role.
- ***Secretion of K^+*** is variable and accounts for the wide range of urinary K^+ excretion, depending upon the dietary K^+ intake, aldosterone levels, acid–base status and urine rate of flow.
  - *Principal cells* are involved in the K^+ secretion.
  - *Mechanism of K^+* secretion is as follows (Fig. 6.2-15):
    - At the basolateral membrane, K^+ is actively transported into the cell by Na^+–K^+–ATPase. As in all cells, this mechanism maintains a high intracellular K^+ concentration.
    - At the apical membrane, K^+ is passively secreted into the lumen through K^+ channels, down its electrical and chemical gradient.
    - *Regulation of K^+ secretions.* See regulation of urinary K^+ excretion.

Hormones and Factors that Regulate Urinary K^+ Excretion As mentioned earlier, regulation of urinary K^+ excretion is achieved mainly by alterations in K^+ secretion by principal cells of the distal tubule and collecting ducts. In a nutshell, K^+ secretion by the principal cells is increased when the electrochemical driving force for K^+ across the apical membrane is increased and vice versa. Hormones and other factors involved in regulation of K^+ tubular secretion and thus of urinary K^+ excretion, include:

- Plasma K^+ level,
- Aldosterone,
- Glucocorticoids,
- Antidiuretic hormone,
- Acid–base balance,
- Flow of tubular fluid and
- Luminal anions.

1. ***Plasma K^+ level,*** which mainly depends on
   - *Dietary intake* of K^+, is an important determinant of K^+ secretion by principal cells (Fig. 6.2-21). Hyperkalaemia, resulting from a high K^+ diet or any other factor (e.g. rhabdomyolysis), stimulates K^+ secretion within minutes.

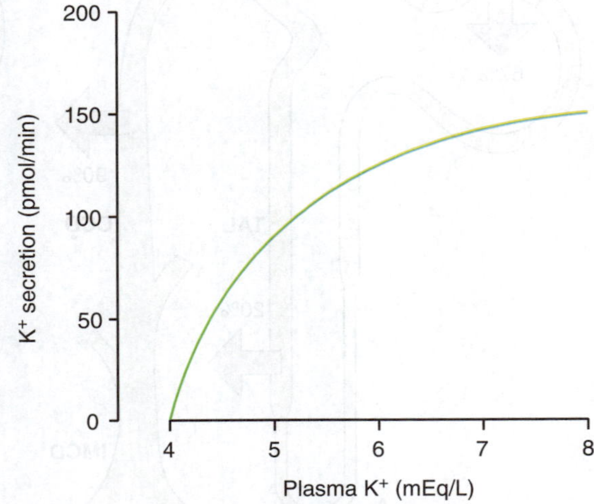

FIGURE 6.2-21 Relationship between plasma K^+ level and K^+ secretion by principal cells.

- *Mechanisms* involved in high secretion of K^+ in hyperkalaemia are:
  - *Stimulation of Na^+–K^+–ATPase*, caused by hyperkalaemia, increases K^+ uptake across the basolateral membrane. Increased levels of intracellular K^+ increase the electrochemical gradient across the apical membrane.
  - *Permeability of apical membrane* to K^+ is increased by hyperkalaemia.
  - *Aldosterone secretion* is increased by hyperkalaemia, which (as discussed below), acts synergistically with plasma K^+ levels to stimulate K^+ secretion.
  - *Flow rate of tubular fluid* is increased by hyperkalaemia, which (as discussed below) stimulates K^+ secretion by principal cells.
- *Hypokalaemia*, resulting from a low K^+ diet or other factors (e.g. diarrhoea) decreases K^+ secretion by mechanisms opposite to those described for hyperkalaemia. In addition, hypokalaemia also *stimulates α-intercalated cells* to reabsorb K^+ by the H^+–K^+–ATPase.

2. ***Aldosterone***. Salient points on the role of aldosterone in regulating K^+ secretion by principal cells are:
   - *Aldosterone secretion is increased* by hyperkalaemia and angiotensin II (after activation of renin–angiotensin system).
   - *Aldosterone secretion is decreased by* hypokalaemia and atrial natriuretic peptide (ANP).

   Acute increase in aldosterone does not increase K^+ secretion. This is because of the fact that due to acute increase in Na^+ and water reabsorption caused by aldosterone the tubular flow is decreased, which in turn decreases K^+ secretion (as discussed below in detail).
   - *Chronic rise in aldosterone level increases* K^+ secretion by the principal cells via following mechanisms:
     - **i.** *By increasing Na^+–K^+–ATPase activity*. Aldosterone increases the amount of Na^+–K^+–ATPase in principal cells. This leads to increased pumping of Na^+ out of the cell in the basolateral membrane and increased Na^+ entry into the cells across the luminal membrane. Stimulation of Na^+–K^+–ATPase simultaneously increases K^+ uptake into the principal cells, increasing the intracellular K^+ concentration and the driving force for K^+ secretion. It is important to note that chronic stimulation of Na^+ reabsorption results in volume expansion and thereby returns tubular flow to normal and thus does not affect the K^+ secreting action of aldosterone. Further, like other steroid hormones, the action of aldosterone takes hours to develop because new protein synthesis is required.
     - **ii.** *By making the transepithelial potential difference (TEPD) more lumen negative*. By increasing the Na^+ reabsorption from lumen, the aldosterone makes the TEPD more lumen negative which in turn favours K^+ secretion;
     - **iii.** *By increasing the permeability* of apical membrane to K^+, aldosterone increases K^+ secretion.
3. ***Glucocorticoids*** indirectly increase K^+ excretion by increasing GFR, which increases tubular flow. Increased tubular flow increases K^+ secretion (as discussed below).
4. ***Antidiuretic hormone***. ADH increases Na^+ and water reabsorption and decreases the tubular flow, which in turn decreases K^+ secretion (as discussed below). However, the ADH-induced increased Na^+ uptake across the luminal membrane of the principal cells creates an electrochemical gradient which increases K^+ secretion into the lumen. In this way, the inhibitory effect (through decreasing tubular flow) and stimulatory effect (through increasing electrochemical driving force for K^+) of ADH on K^+ secretion enable urinary K^+ excretion to be maintained constant, despite wide fluctuations in water excretion.
5. ***Flow of tubular fluid***. Salient points of effect of flow of tubular fluid on K^+ secretion are:
   - *Tubular flow rate* is increased by ECF volume expansion and with diuretic therapy; while it is decreased in volume contraction caused by severe haemorrhage, or vomiting or diarrhoea.

   Increase in tubular fluid flow increases K^+ secretion rapidly, while decrease in tubular fluid flow decreases the secretion of K^+ by distal tubule and collecting ducts by following two mechanisms:
     - *Change in the electrochemical driving force for K^+ across the apical membrane*. K^+ secretion in the tubular fluid leads to increased K^+ levels in the fluid and thus reduces the electrochemical driving force for K^+ exit across the apical membrane. The increased tubular fluid flow rate prevents the rise in K^+ concentration as the secreted K^+ is immediately washed down the stream.
     - *Stimulation of K^+ uptake across basolateral membrane*. Increased tubular flow rate increases the amount of Na^+ reabsorbed across the apical membrane of principal cells. The increased Na^+ reabsorption in turn increases the K^+ uptake across the basolateral membrane by increasing the Na^+–K^+–ATPase activity.

     Note 1. The increase in K^+ secretion with the increase in tubular fluid flow rate is directly proportional to the dietary intake of K^+ (Fig. 6.2-22).

     Note 2. Thiazide and loop diuretic increase the K^+ secretion by increasing the tubular fluid flow through the distal tubule and collecting ducts.
6. ***Acid–base balance*** effects the K^+ secretion by distal tubule and collecting ducts in the following manner:
   - *Acute acidosis* reduces K^+ secretion by two mechanisms:
     - *By decreasing Na^+–K^+–ATPase activity* across the basolateral membrane, it reduces the intracellular

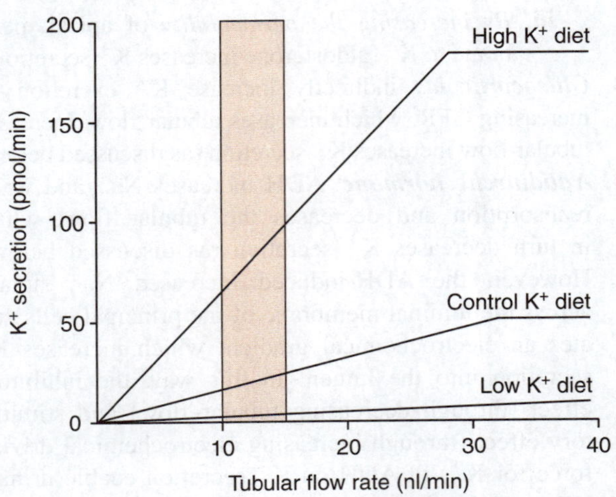

FIGURE 6.2-22 Effect of dietary intake of K^+ on the relationship between tubular flow rate and K^+ secretion by the distal tubule and collecting duct.

K^+ concentration and thus reduces the electrochemical driving force for K^+ exit across the apical membrane.

- *By reducing the permeability of apical membrane K^+*, it decreases K^+ secretion and also tends to increase intracellular K^+ concentration.

  So, as a net result of the above two mechanisms, K^+ secretion by the principal cells decreased while their K^+ content remained unchanged.

- *Acute alkalosis* has exactly the opposite effect to acute acidosis and thus as a net result increases K^+ secretion by the principal cells.
- *Chronic acidosis,* i.e. when metabolic acidosis lasts for several days, there occurs an increase in K^+ secretion by the mechanisms: depicted in Fig. 6.2-23.

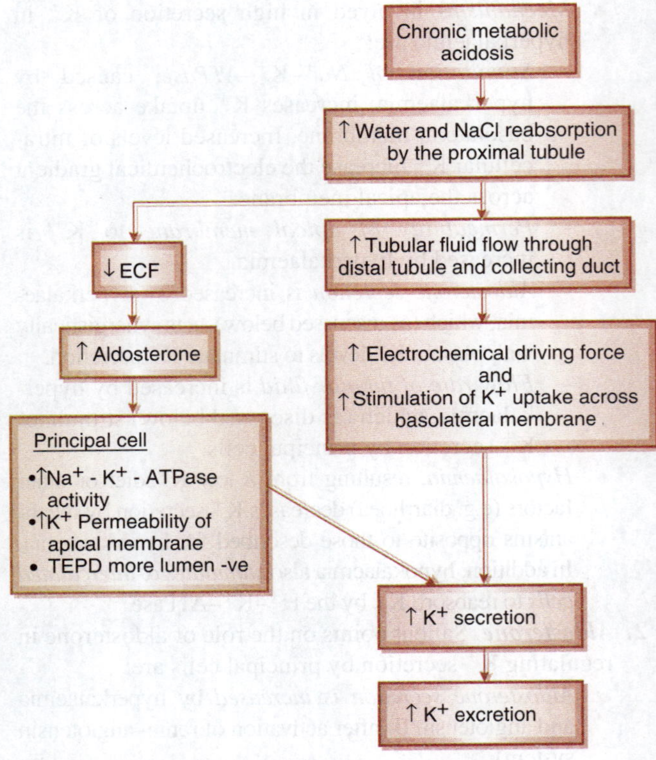

FIGURE 6.2-23 Mechanism of increase in K^+ secretion in patients with chronic metabolic acidosis.

Renal Handling of Organic Substances

Renal Handling of Glucose

Glomerular Filtration Glucose is freely filtered into the glomerular filtrate. Filtration load of glucose increases in direct proportion to the plasma glucose concentration (P glucose). Filtered load of glucose = GFR × P glucose P_G.

Mechanism of Tubular Reabsorption. All the filtered glucose is completely reabsorbed into the proximal tubule by an active transport mechanism (Fig. 6.2-24):

- ***Carrier-mediated Na^+–glucose cotransport.*** Carrier protein located at the apical membrane in the proximal tubule reabsorbs glucose from tubular fluid into the blood.
  - The carrier protein for glucose in early and late proximal tubule is called SGLT-2 and SGLT-1, respectively (SGLT = sodium-dependent glucose transporter).
  - The carrier is driven by the Na^+ concentration gradient which exists between the high tubular (Na^+) concentration and the low intracellular (Na^+) gradient produced by the pumping out of Na^+ through the basolateral surface.
  - Phlorhizin, (a plant glucoside) inhibits glucose transport in kidney by binding with carrier protein $SGLT_2$.
- ***Facilitated diffusion*** moves the glucose out of the cell through the basolateral membrane. The carrier for facilitated diffusion across the basolateral membrane in early and late proximal tubule is called GLUT-2 and GLUT-1, respectively (GLUT = glucose transporter).

Characteristics of Glucose Transport and Glucose Excretion. Glucose is reabsorbed by a transport maximum process, i.e. there is a limited number of Na^+-glucose carriers. The characteristics of glucose transport and glucose excretion can be elicited from the glucose titration curve which is constructed by plotting the following pairs of variables:

- The filtered load against plasma glucose concentration,
- The excretion rate against plasma glucose concentration and
- The difference between the filtered load and excretion rate (i.e. maximum tubular reabsorption capacity, T_r) against plasma concentration.

Glucose titration curve (Fig. 6.2-25) depicts that:

Filtered load increases with the plasma glucose concentration (P_G).

Renal threshold, i.e. the plasma glucose concentration at which glucose first appears in the urine (glycosuria) is about 180–200 mg%. At plasma levels below the renal threshold, the reabsorption of glucose is complete (100%), i.e. all of the filtered glucose can be reabsorbed because plenty of carriers are available and hence no glucose is excreted in urine. In this region, the line of reabsorption is the same as that of filtration.

Transport maximum (T_m) refers to the plasma concentration at which carriers are fully saturated. As shown in Fig. 6.2-25, beyond plasma glucose concentration of 350 mg% (T_{mG}), the reabsorption rate does not increase, i.e. becomes constant and is independent of P_G. Thus, beyond T_{mG} levels, all the additional filtered glucose is excreted in the urine. Therefore, as the T_{mG} is reached, the urinary excretion rate increases linearly with increase in plasma glucose concentration (Fig. 6.2-25).

Splay refers to the region of the glucose curve between threshold and T_{mG}, i.e. between P_G 180 and 350 mg%. It represents the excretion of glucose in urine before the T_{mG} is fully achieved. Note in the region of splay, the reabsorption curve is rounded, indicating that though the reabsorption rate is increasing with increase in P_G, the reabsorption is less than filtration. Similarly, the excretion curve is also rounded in the region of splay, indicating that though the urinary excretion is increasing with increase in P_G, there is no linear relation.

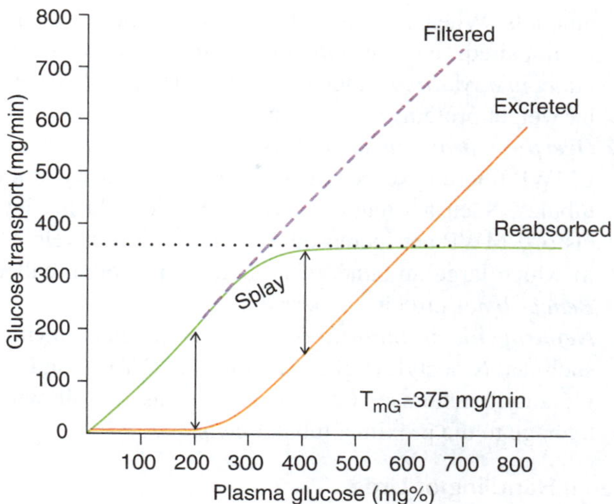

FIGURE 6.2-25 Glucose titration curve (for details see text).

Causes of splay are:

- *Heterogenicity in glomerular size*, proximal tubular length and number of carrier proteins for glucose reabsorption. For example, a nephron with a large glomerulus (i.e. a high filtered load), or a short proximal tubule (i.e. low reabsorptive capacity) will spill glucose into the urine at a lower P_G than predicted from the T_{mG} for the whole kidney.
- *Variability in T_{mG} of the nephron.* For example, there is variability in the number of glucose carriers, the transport rate of the carriers and the binding affinity of the Na^+–glucose carriers.

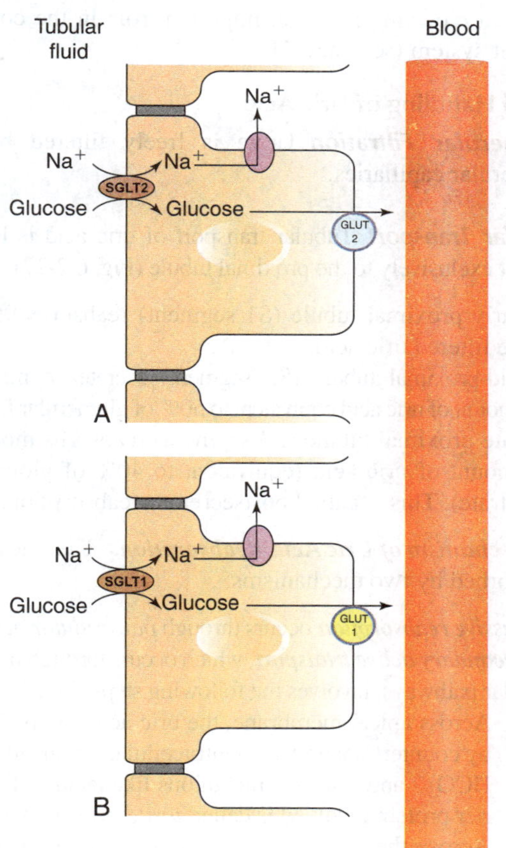

FIGURE 6.2-24 Mechanism of glucose reabsorption in: **A,** early proximal tubule; and **B,** late proximal tubule.

Renal Handling of Proteins, Peptides and Amino Acids

Normally, a small amount of protein is filtered by the glomerulus and almost all is absorbed in the proximal tubule (see page 497). Normally, upto 150 mg of proteins are excreted daily in urine and of this only 15 mg is albumin and the rest are low molecular weight proteins (LMWP). About 25 mg of LMWP are the *Tamm–Horsfall* proteins derived from the cells of thick ascending limb (TAL). The rest are derived from plasma proteins and include microproteins, lysozymes and light chains of immunoglobulins.

Proteinuria Proteinuria is labelled when excretion of proteins in urine is more than 150 mg/day. It may be of the following types:

1. ***Glomerular proteinuria*** occurs when the glomerular permeability increases and allows albumin and other large proteins to be filtered.
2. ***Tubular proteinuria.*** Normally, low molecular weight proteins enter the glomerular filtrate in fairly large

amounts. When tubular reabsorption for these proteins is impaired, e.g. in *tubulointerstitial disorders and Fanconi's syndrome*, then large amounts of low molecular weight proteins are excreted in urine.

3. ***Overflow proteinuria*** occurs when the amount of LMWP filtered exceeds the reabsorptive capacity of the tubules. Such a situation may arise when plasma levels of LMWP are increased, e.g. in multiple myeloma, in which large amounts of an abnormal protein called *Bence–Jones* proteins appear in the plasma.
4. ***Nephrogenic proteinuria*** occurs when tubular enzymes such as N-acetyl β-glucosaminidase (NAG) and γ-glutamyltransferase (γ-GT) are released following damage to the proximal tubular cells.

Renal Handling of Urea

Glomerular Filtration Urea is freely filtered into the glomerular filtrate. The amount of urea filtered by glomerular capillaries varies with the protein intake. A high protein diet increases the amount of urea filtered, which in turn increases the ability of kidney to concentrate the urine and low protein diet reduces filtration and thus the ability to concentrate the urine.

Tubular Transport

- ***Proximal tubules*** reabsorb 5% of the filtered urea passively.
- ***Proximal straight tubule*** (PST), *descending thin segment* (DTS) and *ascending thin segment* (ATS) of the nephron receive urea by diffusion (*tubular secretion*) from the interstitium of renal medulla, in which urea is present in high concentration.
- ***Thick ascending limb*** (TAL), DCT, CNT, CCD and OMCD are all impermeable to urea.
- ***Inner medullary collecting duct*** (IMCD) reabsorbs large amounts of urea employing a specialized *urea transport protein* (UT-A). There are at least four isoforms of transport protein UT-A in the kidneys (UT-A1–UT-A4), (UT-B is found in erythrocytes). This protein is stimulated by ADH which consequently increases urea permeability of the IMCD.

Urea recycling. Urea recycling involves following steps (Fig. 6.2-26):

1. ***Concentration of urea in collecting duct*** (CCD and OMCD), as mentioned above, the nephron segment distal to ATS (i.e. TAL, DCT, CNT, CCD and OMCD) are all impermeable to urea. Therefore, as water is reabsorbed from the CCD, OMCD and the initial part of IMCD, urea gets more and more concentrated within the collecting duct.
2. ***Rapid and massive reabsorption of urea by IMCD***, as described above, increases the concentration of urea in medullary interstitium. Urea transport in collecting duct is mediated by $UT\text{-}A_1$.
3. ***Carriage of urea by vasa recta to renal cortex interstitium***. From the medullary interstitium, most of the urea enters the vasa recta and is carried upwards towards the renal cortex by the ascending vasa recta.

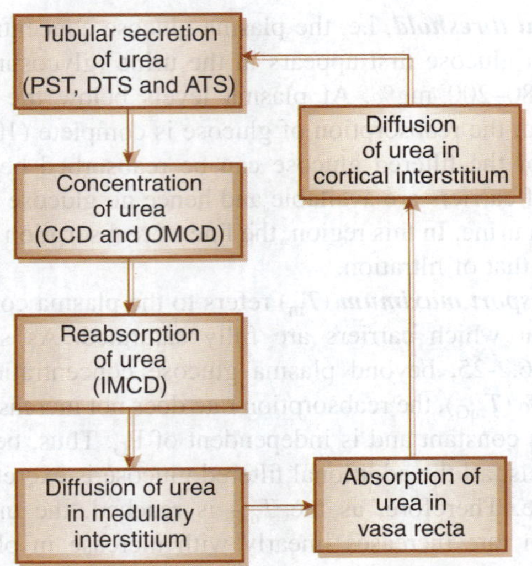

FIGURE 6.2-26 Steps involved in urea recycling.

4. ***Tubular secretion of urea*** from the renal cortical interstitium occurs into the PST of cortical nephrons. Some of the urea also enters the thin segment of the long loops of the juxtamedullary nephrons. In this way, the urea is again carried back to the IMCD from where it diffuses out again resulting in a constant recycling.

Urea recycling plays an important role in the countercurrent system (see page 517).

Renal Handling of Uric Acid

Glomerular Filtration Urate is freely filtered by the glomerular capillaries.

Tubular Transport Tubular transport of uric acid is limited almost exclusively to the proximal tubule (Fig. 6.2-27):

- Early proximal tubule (S1 segment) reabsorbs 95% of the filtered uric acid.
- Mid-proximal tubule (S2 segment) secretes a moderate amount of uric acid equivalent to 50% of glomerular filtrate).
- Late proximal tubule (S3 segment) reabsorbs moderate amount of uric acid (equivalent to 40% of glomerular filtrate). This is called postsecretory reabsorption.

Mechanism of Uric Acid Reabsorption. The uric acid is reabsorbed by two mechanisms:

- ***Passive reabsorption*** occurs through *paracellular* pathway.
- ***Secondary active transport***, which occurs through transcellular pathways, involves the following steps (Fig. 6.2-28).
  - Across apical membrane, the uric acid enters the cell by countertransport with intracellular anions like Cl^-, HCO_3^- and also organic anions like lactate. The carrier protein involved is called *urate transport protein*.
  - Across the basolateral membrane, the urate moves out using another anion-exchanger. The same anion-exchangers are employed for urate secretion also.

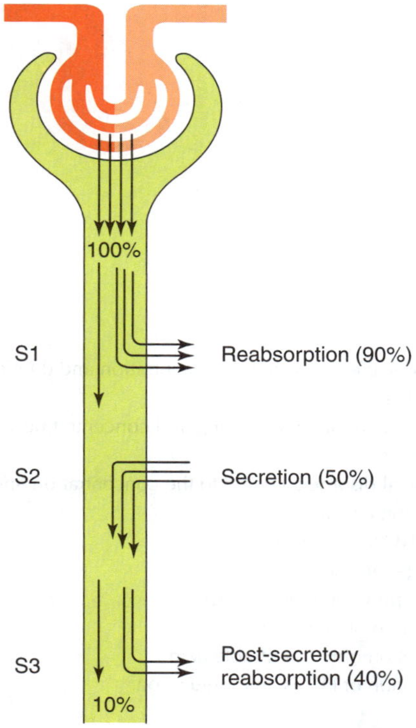

100%

S1 Reabsorption (90%)

S2 Secretion (50%)

S3 Post-secretory reabsorption (40%)

10%

FIGURE 6.2-27 Tubular transport of uric acid: reabsorption, secretion and postsecretory reabsorption.

Summary of Effects of Renal Handling of Common Solutes and Water

Effects of renal handling (glomerular filtration and tubular transport) of common solutes and water are summarized in Table 6.2-5.

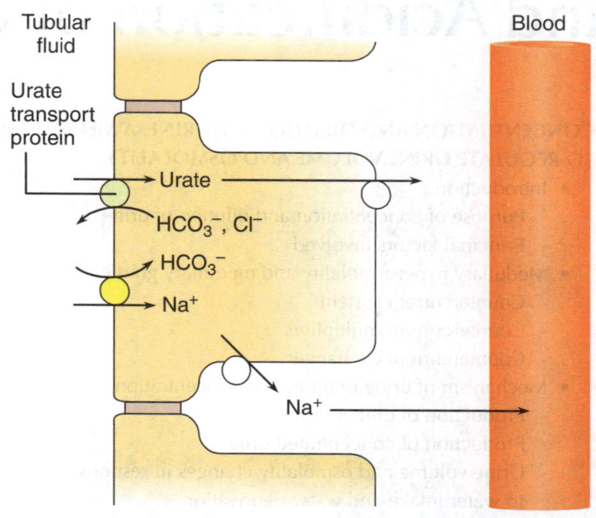

FIGURE 6.2-28 Mechanism of urate reabsorption in proximal tubule cell.

TABLE 6.2-5 Effects of Glomerular and Tubular Function on Water, Electrolytes and Solutes in a Normal Human Adult on an Average Diet

Substance	Measure	Filtered	Reabsorbed	Secreted	Excreted	Percentage reabsorption	Location
Na^+	mEq	26,000	25,850		150	99.4	P, L, D, C
K^+	mEq	720	620		100	86.1	P, L, D, C
Cl^-	mEq	18,000	17,850	–	150	99.2	P, L, D, C
HCO_3^-	mEq	4900	4900	–	0	100	P, D
Ca^{2+}	mEq	540	530	–	10	98.2	P, L, D, C
Glucose	mmol	800	800	–	0	100	P
Urea	mmol	870	435	–	435	50	P, L, D, C
Creatinine	mmol	12	1	1	12	–	–
Uric acid	mmol	50	49	4	5	98	P
Total solutes	mosm	54,000	53,400	100	700	98.9	P, L, D, C
Water	L	180	178.5	–	1.5	99.2	P, L, D,C

P, proximal tubule; L, loop of Henle; D, distal tubule; and C, collecting duct.

Chapter 6.3

Concentration, Dilution and Acidification of Urine

CONCENTRATION AND DILUTION OF URINE: A MECHANISM TO REGULATE URINE VOLUME AND OSMOLALITY

Introduction

The kidneys possess a unique property of regulating the volume and osmolality of the urine formed by the mechanism of concentrating and diluting the urine as per the need of the body.

Purpose of concentration and dilution of urine. The main purpose is to maintain the osmolality and volume of the body fluids within a narrow range, which is accomplished by kidneys in concert with other systems by regulating the excretion of water and NaCl, respectively. The present discussion pertains to urine concentration and dilution, the mechanism which controls the amount of water excreted relative to the amount of solute excreted and thus regulates the plasma osmolality by varying urine osmolality.

The kidney can produce urine with osmolality as low as 30 mOsm/kg H_2O to as high as 1400 mOsm/kg H_2O by changing the water excretion as high as 23.3 L/day to as low as 0.5 L/day, respectively (Table 6.3-1). From the figures shown in Table 6.3-1, two important facts which need to be noted are:

- First, at least 87% of the filtered water is reabsorbed even when urine volume is 23.3 L/day; and
- Second, that the reabsorption of the remainder of the filtered water be varied without affecting the total solute excretion, i.e. when the urine is concentrated, water is retained in excess of solutes, and when it is dilute, water is lost from the body in excess of solutes.

Principal Factors. Principal factors responsible for mechanism of concentration and dilution of urine are:

- Antidiuretic hormone and
- Hyperosmolality and osmolality gradient in medullary interstitium of kidneys.

The details about antidiuretic hormone (ADH) are described on page 691. It will be useful to go through these pages before proceeding further. After an overview of hyperosmolality and osmolality gradient of medullary interstitium, the role of these two principal factors is concentration and dilution of the urine, which is discussed separately.

Medullary Hyperosmolality and Medullary Gradient

Interstitial fluid of the medulla is critically important in concentrating the urine, because the osmotic pressure of this fluid provides the driving force for reabsorbing water from both the descending thin segment (DTS) and the collecting duct.

Normal osmolality of plasma and other body fluids is about 300 mOsm/kg H_2O. The interstitial fluid of the renal cortex has the same osmolality as that of

TABLE 6.3-1 Effects of Concentration and Dilution Mechanism on Volume and Osmolality of Urine. In Each Case, the Osmotic Load Excreted is Same (700 *mOsm* /Day)

Character of urine formed	GFR (ml/min)	Percentage of filtered water reabsorbed	Urine volume (L/day)	Urine concentration (mOsm/kg H_2O)	Gain or loss of urine formed of water in excess of solute (L/day)
Urine isotonic to plasma	125	98.7	2.4	290	–
Concentrated urine (vasopressin : maximal antidiuresis)	125	99.7	0.5	1400	1.9 gain
Diluted urine (no vasopressin: complete diuresis diabetes insipidus)	125	87.1	23.3	30	20.9 loss

plasma, i.e. 300 mOsm/kg H_2O with virtually all osmoles attributable to NaCl. The osmolality of the renal medulla is higher than the plasma (i.e. *hyperosmolar*) and that it goes on increasing progressively from about 300 mOsm/kg H_2O at corticomedullary junction to about 1200 mOsm/kg H_2O at papilla (medullary gradient) where a maximally concentrated urine is excreted (Fig. 6.3-1). This hyperosmolality and medullary gradient is generated and maintained by the so-called countercurrent system.

Counter Current System

A countercurrent system refers to a system in which the inflow runs parallel to, counter to, and in close proximity to the outflow for some distance. The countercurrent flow system is formed by U-shaped tubules. The effect of countercurrent system can be best understood by studying the effect of a heater on a straight water pipe and a pipe bent in U shape (Fig. 6.3-2). Let us suppose, the heater raises the temperature of flowing fluid through the straight tube at a constant flow rate by 10°C from 30 to 40°C (Fig. 6.3-2A). Now, if the pipe is bent in a U shape and the two limbs are brought in close proximity, the temperature at the outlet is again 40°C, but a gradient of temperature is set up along the pipe in such a way that at the bend of the pipe the temperature is not raised from 30 to 40°C but from 30 to 100°C (Fig. 6.3-2B). This is because the outgoing fluid warms the incoming fluid and sets up the countercurrent system.

In the kidney, the structures which form the countercurrent system are loop of Henle and the vasa recta. In both, the direction of flow of fluid in the descending limb is just the opposite to that of the ascending limb. Thus, the countercurrent system of the kidney consists of two components:

- *Countercurrent multiplier,* which is formed by the operation of loop of Henle and is responsible for the production of hyperosmolality and a gradient in renal medulla and
- *Countercurrent exchanger,* which is formed by the operation of vasa recta and is responsible for maintenance of the medullary gradient and hyperosmolality.

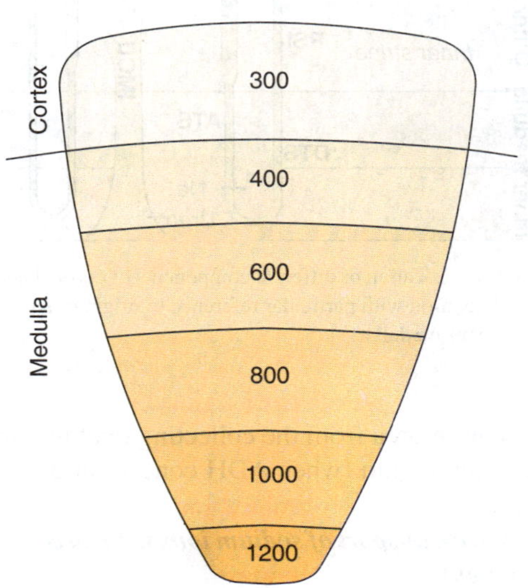

FIGURE 6.3-1 Osmolality gradient of renal medullary interstitium (values are in mOsm/kg H_2O).

Counter Current Multipliers

The working of countercurrent multiplier, that operates in the loop of Henle and generates hyperosmolarity and medullary gradient, can be best understood by describing it as two processes:

- Origin of single effect and
- Multiplication of the single effect.

Origin of Single Effect. The single effect is the main driving force behind the countercurrent multiplier. It is the name given to the osmotic gradient of approximately 200 mOsm

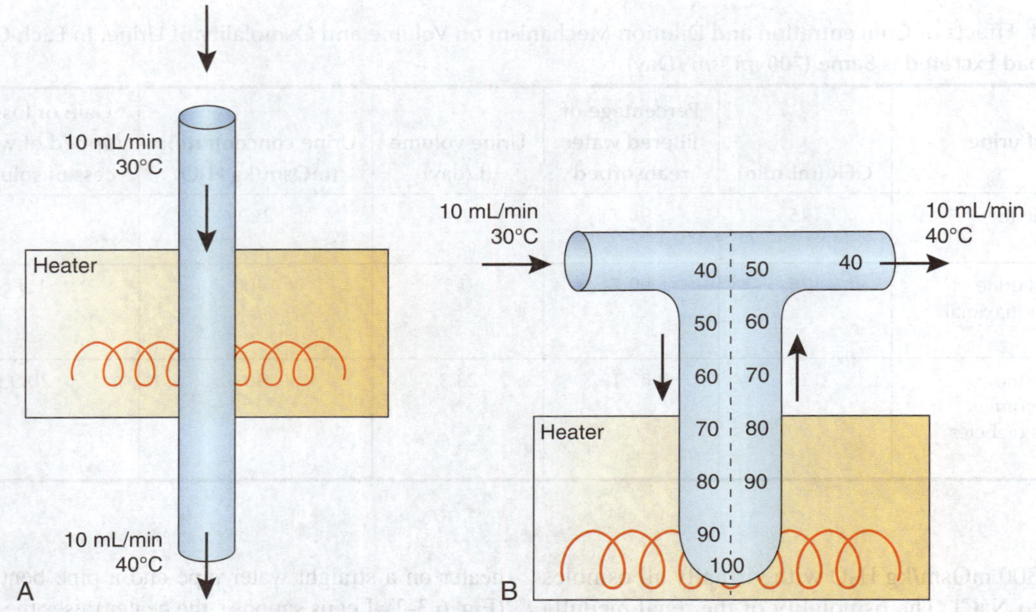

FIGURE 6.3-2 Understanding the principle of countercurrent system. Effect of heating on water flowing at a constant rate: **A,** from a straight pipe; and **B,** from a U-shaped bent pipe (countercurrent effect).

that exists between the ascending limb of loop of Henle and the surrounding interstitial fluid. These are the juxtamedullary nephrons which are more important for the production of medullary hyperosmolarity. The cortical nephrons contribute to production of hyperosmolarity in the outer medulla mainly. The mechanism of origin of single effect in outer medulla is different from that of the inner medulla.

Mechanism of Origin of Single Effect in Outer Medulla. As shown in Fig. 6.3-3, the thick ascending limb (TAL) of loop of Henle is located in the outer medulla, and not in the inner medulla. TAL is impermeable to water. So NaCl and other solutes are actively absorbed in this segment without water, as a result, the tubular fluid osmolality decreases to less than plasma. This is why; this segment is called the diluting segment. The NaCl reabsorbed in this segment raises the osmolality of outer medullary interstitium by about 200 mOsm. This separation of solute and water by the TAL leading to osmolality difference between that tubular fluid and interstitial fluid is called single effect and is the main driving force behind the countercurrent multiplier.

Origin of Single Effect in Inner Medulla. Three different mechanisms contribute to the origin of single effect (and thus, ultimately to the development of medullary gradient and hyperosmolality after multiplication) in the inner medullary interstitium. These include:

- Passive transport of sodium ions from ascending thin segment into the interstitium,
- Active transport of sodium from the inner medullary collecting duct and

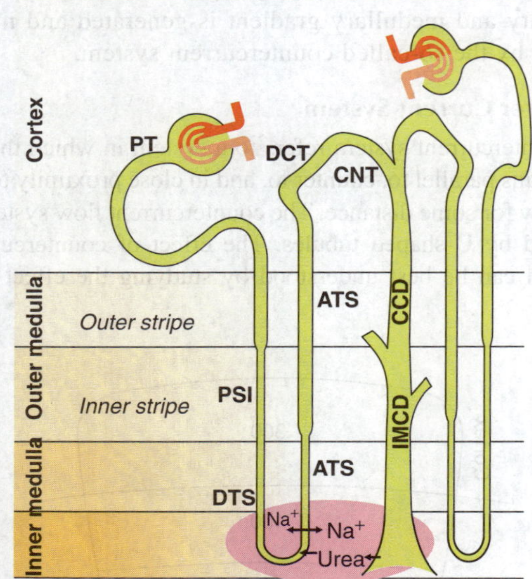

FIGURE 6.3-3 Location of different components of cortical nephron and juxta cortical nephron with particular reference to origin of single effect in outer versus inner medulla.

- Diffusion of urea from the collecting duct into the medullary interstitium (when ADH concentration is high in blood).

1. ***Passive transport of sodium ions from ascending thin segment***

   As shown in Fig. 6.1-2, the inner medulla contains ascending thin segment (ATS) of loop of Henle of juxtamedullary nephrons, which is impermeable to water and does not have the property to actively absorb solutes (c.f. TAL). The single effect is, therefore, produced by the passive diffusion of solutes, which occurs because of difference in the composition of tubular fluid and that of interstitium. The tubular fluid in the ATS is relatively rich in NaCl and but has less urea in it compared with the interstitium. Consequently, NaCl moves out from the ATS into the interstitium and urea moves into the ATS from the interstitium. However, the rate at which NaCl diffuses out far exceeds the rate at which urea diffuses into the lumen of ATS. Thus, as a net result, more solute diffuses out in the interstitium, raising the inner medullary osmolality (single effect).

2. ***Reabsorption of sodium ions from medullary part of collecting duct***
   In addition to the passive diffusion of Na^+ from ascending thin segment (ATS), smaller quantities of ions are also transported from medullary part of the collecting duct into the medullary interstitium, particularly in the inner part of medulla near renal sinus. As described on page 501, Na^+ is actively transported by the principal cells of the collecting duct, which is followed by electrogenic passive absorption of chloride ions.
3. ***Role of urea***
   Urea plays an important role in the development of medullary osmotic gradient, especially when concentration of ADH is high in the blood. Under such circumstances, inner medullary collecting duct (IMCD) absorbs large amount of urea employing a specialized urea transport protein (UT-A) (see page 512). Further, there occurs urea recycling (see page 512), which plays an important role in the countercurrent system.

Multiplication of the Single Effect. The hyperosmolality and medullary gradient is in fact generated by the multiplication of the single effect by the countercurrent multiplier. The main characteristics of the components of countercurrent multiplier which play role in multiplication of single effect are (Table 6.3-2):

- High permeability of a descending thin segment to water.
- Impermeability to water but high permeability to NaCl.
- Impermeability to water and ability to actively absorb solutes by thick ascending limb (TAL).
- In renal medulla, all other tubular structures (except ascending limb) are in osmotic equilibrium. The descending limb, therefore, acquires the increased osmolality of the surrounding fluid. The effect is multiplied as new iso-osmolar filtrate arrives at the descending limb and forces the concentrated tubular contents towards the tip of loop of Henle (hair pin band).

The process of multiplication of single effect can be best understood by dividing the whole process in hypothetical steps, leading to normal equilibrium condition. These steps are summarized (Fig. 6.3-4):

- *Initially*, let us assume the osmolality of fluid in the descending limb and the ascending limb of loop of Henle and medullary interstitium is 300 mOsm/kg H_2O (Fig. 6.3-4A).

TABLE 6.3-2 Permeability and Transport in Various Segments of the Nephron

Segment of nephron	Permeability and transport of			
	H_2O	*Urea*	*NaCl*	*Na^+*
Loop of Henle	4+	+	±	0
• Thin descending limb	0	+	4+	0
• Thin ascending limb	0	±	±	4+
• Thick ascending limb	±	±	±	3+
Distal convoluted tubule	±	±	±	3+
Collecting duct				
• Cortical collecting duct (CCD)	*3+	0	±	2+
• Outer medullary collecting duct (OMCD)	*3+	0	±	1+
• Inner medullary collecting duct (IMCD)	*3+	3+	±	1+

*These values are in the presence of ADH. In the absence of ADH, these values are positive.

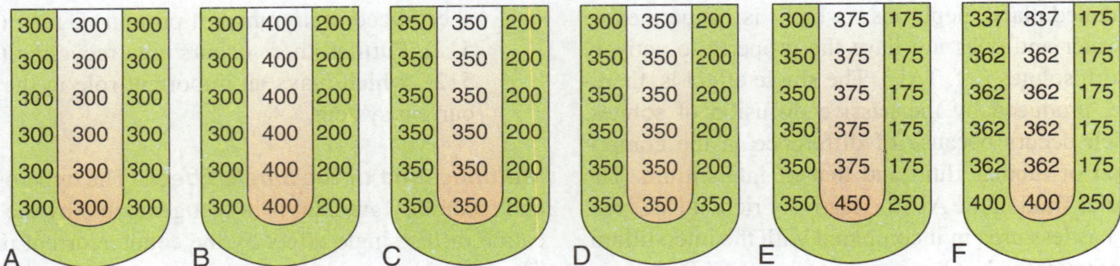

FIGURE 6.3-4 Operation of loop of Henle as countercurrent multiplier producing a gradient of hyperosmolality in the medullary interstitium **A, B, C, D. E** and **F** are hypothetical steps involved in the process of generation of the gradient (see text for details).

- Further, let us assume that the thick ascending limb (TAL) actively pumps out 100 mOsm/kg H_2O of NaCl into the medullary interstitium. Since the TAL is impermeable to water, this effect will lower the osmolality of fluid in TAL to 200 mOsm/kg H_2O and raise the osmolality of the adjacent interstitium to 400 mOsm/kg H_2O (Fig. 6.3-4B). Establishment of this osmotic gradient of 200 mOsm/kg H_2O, as described earlier, is called single effect.
- The portion of descending thin segment (DTS) which is located in the outer medulla is moderately permeable to Na^+ and highly permeable to water.
- Due to osmotic gradient created, the water moves out and Na^+ from the interstitium (osmolality 400 mOsm/kg H_2O) moves into the DTS (osmolality 300 mOsm/kg H_2O) till equilibrium is reached with osmolality of 350 mOsm/kg H_2O (Fig. 6.3-4C).
- The fresh iso-osmolar filtrate at 300 mOsm/kg H_2O trickles down into the descending loop and pushes some of the hyperosmolar fluid (350 mOsm/kg H_2O) into the ascending limb (Fig. 6.3-4D).
- In the meanwhile, hypotonic fluid flows into the distal tubule, and isotonic and subsequently hypertonic fluid (Fig. 6.3-4 E, F) flow into the ascending thick limb.
- As the process with above steps keeps repeating, the final result is a gradient of osmolality from top to bottom of the loop and surrounding interstitium.

Counter Current Exchanger

Vasa Recta (the Countercurrent Exchanger). If the vasa recta would have been a straight blood vessel, the osmotic gradient in the medullary pyramid would not last long, as the Na^+ and urea in the interstitial spaces would have been removed by the circulation (Fig. 6.3-5A). However, because of the hair pin (U-shaped) anatomical arrangement, the vasa recta operates as countercurrent exchanger and retains these solutes in the medullary interstitium (Fig. 6.3-5B). Thus, the countercurrent exchanger formed

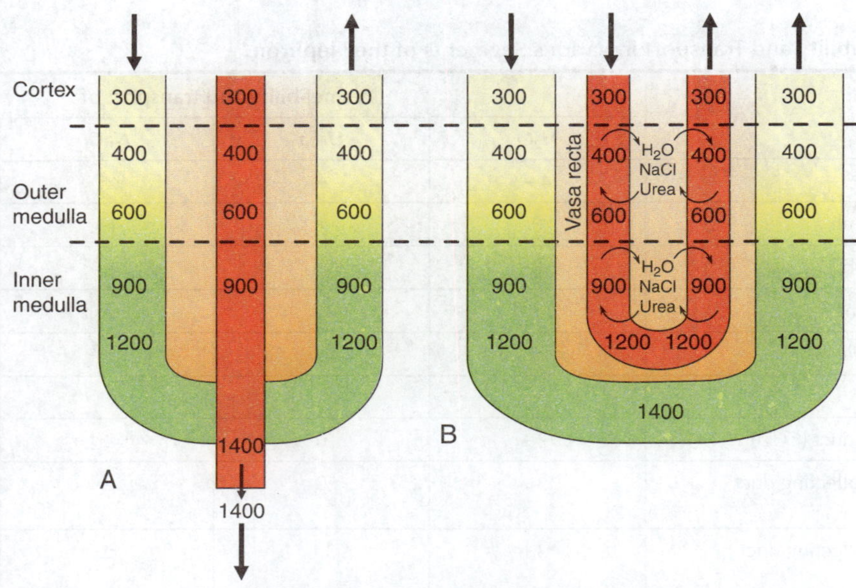

FIGURE 6.3-5 Operation of vasa recta as countercurrent exchangers in the kidney: **A,** effect on medullary osmolality if vasa recta would be a straight vessel without hairpin arrangement; and **B,** as it is a U-shaped vessel.

by the vasa recta is responsible for the maintenance of the hyperosmolality medullary gradient generated by the countercurrent multiplier.

Operation of Countercurrent Exchanger. The vasa recta, the capillary network supplying blood to the medulla, is highly permeable to the solute and water. So, in addition to bringing nutrients and oxygen to tubules within the medulla, these capillaries more importantly remove excess water and solutes, which are continuously added to the medullary interstitium by the nephron segments in this region.

- ***Operation at the level of descending vasa recta.*** As shown in Fig. 6.3-5B, when the descending vasa recta dips down in the medulla having a progressively increasing osmolality (from 300 to 1200 mOsm/kg H_2O), the solutes diffuse into its lumen and water diffuses out so that the blood flowing in it (with osmolality 300 mOsm/kg H_2O) equilibrates with the medullary interstitium and thus its osmolality also increases progressively.
- ***Operation at the level of ascending vasa recta.*** The vasa recta then loops around and ascends towards the cortex (Fig. 6.3-5B). As at the beginning of the ascending vasa recta, its blood has attained an osmolality of 1200 mOsm/kg H_2O and when it passes through an interstitium where osmolality is progressively decreasing from 1200 to 300 mOsm/kg H_2O, the solutes move out and water diffuses in, and thus the blood in it once again equilibrates with the interstitium around it.
- ***Effect of operation of countercurrent exchanger on the medullary interstitium.*** By the above-described operations, the solutes tend to recirculate in the medulla and water tends to bypass it, so that hypertonicity of the medulla is maintained. Since solutes (sodium and urea) are exchanged for water between the ascending and descending limbs of vasa recta, this system has been named countercurrent exchanger.

Another factor which ensures retention of sodium in the medullary interstitium is very slow rate of blood flow through the medullary parenchyma. Some important facts about working of countercurrent exchanger which need elaboration are:

- *The ability of the vasa recta to maintain the medullary interstitial gradient is flow dependent.* A substantial increase in blood flow through the vasa recta will ultimately dissipate the medullary gradient, i.e. wash out the medullary gradient. Alternatively, if blood flow is reduced, the nephron segments within the medulla will receive inadequate oxygen. Under such conditions, the tubular transport, especially by the thick ascending limb (TAL) is impaired. As a result, the medullary interstitial osmotic gradient cannot be maintained.
- Countercurrent exchanger is a passive process, as it depends upon the diffusion of water and solutes in both directions across the permeable walls of the vasa recta. Therefore, it could not maintain the osmotic gradient along the medullary pyramids if the process of countercurrent multiplier were to cease.

Mechanism of Urine Dilution and Concentration

Production of Diluted Urine

Conditions in which Dilute Urine is Formed Dilute urine is called hypo-osmotic urine, in which urine osmolality is less than blood osmolality. It is produced under the following circumstances:

- When the circulating levels of ADH are low (e.g. after water drinking), central diabetes insipidus (see page 696) or
- When ADH is ineffective (e.g. nephrogenic diabetes insipidus (see page 696).

Principal Factors Governing Formation of Dilute Urine As mentioned earlier, the principal factors governing formation of dilute and concentrated urine are hyperosmolality medullary gradient and the presence or absence of ADH. The renal medullary osmotic gradient is smaller in the absence of ADH. This is because ADH stimulates both countercurrent multiplication and urea cycling.

Segmental Changes in Tubular Fluid during Formation of Dilute Urine Segmental changes occurring in tubular fluid during the formation of dilute urine are summarized (Fig. 6.3-6A):

- ***Proximal Tubule.*** The osmolality of glomerular filtrate entering the proximal tubule is identical to that of plasma (300 mOsm/L). About 60–70% of the H_2O is reabsorbed isosmotically (with Na^+, Cl^-, HCO_3^-, glucose, amino acids and so forth). As H_2O is reabsorbed isosmotically, the TF/Posm = 1.0 throughout the proximal tubule.
- ***Descending Thin Segment of Loop of Henle*** receives isosmotic fluid (i.e. osmolarity 300 mOsm/L) from the proximal tubule, because this segment is highly permeable to water but much less to solutes (Table 6.3-2). As thin segment descends deeper in the renal medulla, water is reabsorbed owing to the osmotic gradient set up by the progressive increasing hyperosmolality of the medulla. At the bend of loop of Henle, though the osmolality of tubular fluid and interstitium is equal, but their composition differs. The NaCl concentration is higher and that of urea is lower in the tubular fluid compared with the interstitial fluid.
- ***Ascending Thin Segment of Loop of Henle*** is impermeable to water but permeable to NaCl and urea (Table 6.3-2). As the tubular fluid moves up in this segment, NaCl moves out and urea moves in. As a net result, the volume remains

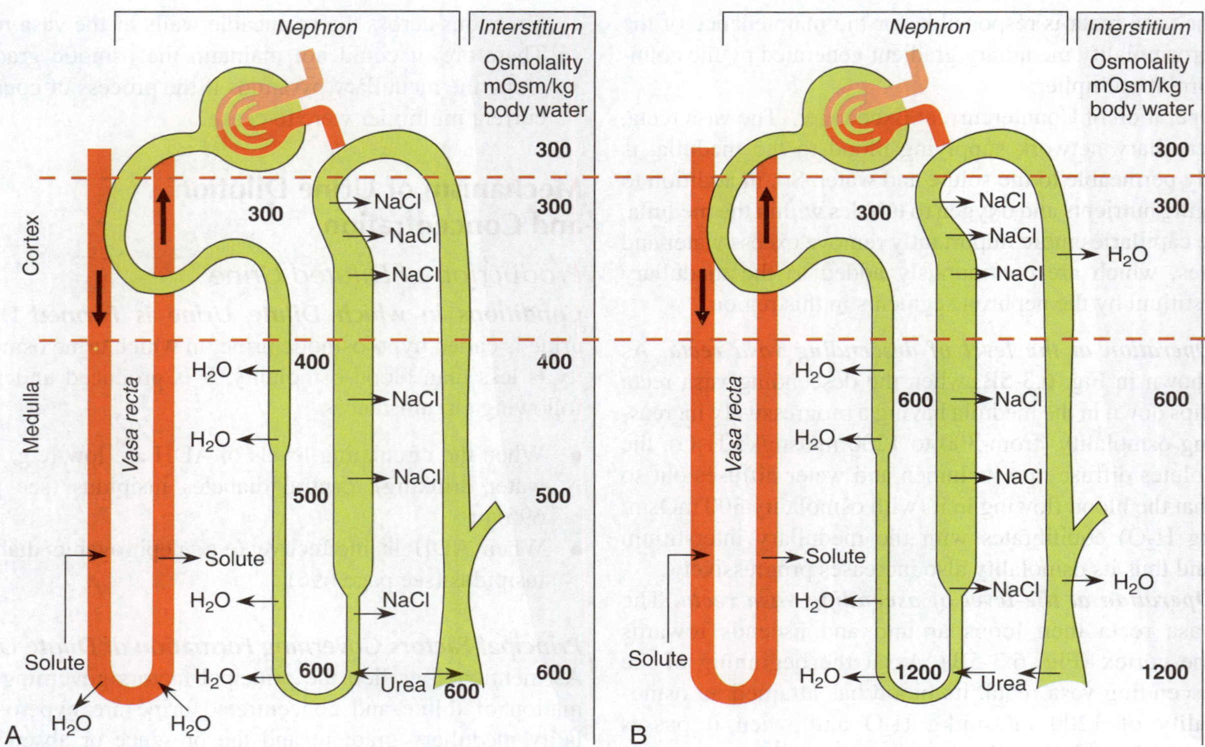

FIGURE 6.3-6 Mechanism of producing: A, dilute urine in the absence of ADH; and B, concentrated urine in the presence of ADH.

the same, osmolarity decreases and the concentration of NaCl decreases, but that of urea increases in the tubular fluid.

- ***Thick Ascending Limb (TAL)*** of loop of Henle is impermeable to water and urea. Because of active absorption of NaCl without water, the tubular fluid becomes dilute (although not quite as dilute as in the presence of ADH). In this diluting segment, urine becomes hypo-osmolar for the first time, and the only time. The minimum possible osmolarity of the tubular fluid is 100 mOsm/L (i.e. 200 mOsm less than the surrounding interstitium).
- ***Early distal tubule*** behaves like TAL and the tubular fluid is further diluted.
- ***Late distal tubule and cortical collecting ducts.*** Cells of these segments actively reabsorb NaCl but are impermeable to urea. In the absence of ADH, the cells of these segments are impermeable to water. So, due to reabsorption of NaCl without the water, the osmolality of the tubular fluid is further reduced.
- ***Medullary collecting duct*** actively reabsorbs NaCl. Even in the absence of ADH, this segment is slightly permeable to H_2O and urea. So, some urea enters the collecting duct from the interstitium and about 2% of H_2O is reabsorbed. So, in the absence of ADH, the urine will have an osmolality between 30 and 50 mOsm/L and will contain low NaCl and urea (TF/Posm < 1.0). The volume of urine excreted can be about 18 L/day or approximately 10% of glomerular filtrate: however, in extreme conditions, it may reach to 23–32 L/day (Table 6.3-2).

Production of Concentrated Urine

Conditions in which Concentrated Urine is Formed Concentrated urine is also called *hyperosmotic urine,* in which urine osmolality is more than that of blood. It is produced when circulating ADH levels are high, e.g.

- Water deprivation,
- Haemorrhage and
- Syndrome of inappropriate antidiuretic hormone, i.e. SIADH (see page 695).

Principal Factors Governing Formation of Concentrated Urine The high level of ADH is the main factor governing the formation of concentrated urine, because it:

- Increases the size of hypersomolality medullary gradient and
- Augments the urea cycling from the inner medullary collecting ducts into the medullary interstitial fluid.

Segmental Changes in the Tubular Fluid during Formation of Concentrated Urine Segmental changes occurring in the tubular fluid during the formation of concentrated urine are summarized (Fig. 6.3-6B):

- ***From proximal tubule to ascending thick limb and even early distal tubule,*** the changes occurring in the tubular fluid are the same as during the formation of dilute urine. Only point to be noted here is that the ADH stimulates NaCl reabsorption in the thick ascending limb and therefore increases the size of medullary gradient by *countercurrent multiplier,* which is important for formation of concentrated urine.

- ***Late distal tubule***. The tubular fluid entering the late distal tubule is *hypo-osmolar* (osmolality about 150 mOsm/L). In the presence of ADH, H_2O permeability of the principal cells is increased and consequently H_2O is reabsorbed until the osmolality of distal tubular fluid equals that of the surrounding cortical interstitium (300 mOsm/L) (Fig. 6.3-6B). So, at the end of the distal tubule, TF/Posm = 1.0, because osmotic equilibrium occurs in the presence of ADH. It is important to note that though the osmolality of the fluid in this segment is similar to that of the fluid, which entered the descending thin segment from the proximal tubule, its composition has altered dramatically. Because of NaCl reabsorption by the preceding nephron segments (NaCl accounts for a much smaller portion of the total tubular fluid osmolality), urea, filtered and that added in descending thin and ascending thin limb of loop of Henle, mainly accounts for the osmolality at this juncture.

  Note. ADH increases the H_2O permeability of the principal cells of late distal tubule and collecting duct through aquaporin-2 (For details about mechanism of action see page 602).

- ***Collecting ducts***. ADH markedly increases the permeability of the principal cells (see page 602). As the tubular fluid flows through the collecting ducts, it passes through the corticopapillary gradient (regions of increasingly higher osmolality, from 300 to 1200 mOsm/L), which was previously established by countercurrent multiplication (see page 518) and urea cycling (see page 512). Consequently, H_2O is reabsorbed from the collecting ducts until the osmolality of tubular fluid equals that of the surrounding interstitial fluid. Because initial portion of the collecting duct is impermeable to urea, it remains in the tubular fluid, and its concentration in the tubular fluid increases. In the presence of ADH, the urea permeability of the last portion of the medullary collecting duct is increased, and so some urea diffuses out into the medullary interstitium.

  The final osmolality of urine is about 1200 mOsm/L, and it contains high concentration of urea and other nonreabsorbed solutes. The TF/Posm > 1.0, because osmotic equilibrium occurs with the medullary gradient in the presence of ADH. In humans, the osmolality of urine may even reach 1400 mOsm/L, almost five times the osmolality of plasma, with a total of 95.7% or more of the filtered water being reabsorbed; and urine under this condition can be as low as 0.5 L/day (Table 6.3-1). In other species, the ability to concentrate urine is even greater. Maximal urine osmolality is about 2500 mOsm/kg H_2O in dogs, about 3200 mOsm/kg H_2O in laboratory rats and as high as 5000 mOsm/kg in certain desert rodents. In fact, the ability to concentrate urine depends upon the number of long-looped juxtamedullary nephrons, which form about 15% of total nephrons in human.

Note. It is important to note that the tubular response to ADH is not an all-or-none phenomenon, but a graded response. Therefore, varying grades of plasma ADH concentrations can produce proportionate increase in permeability of collecting ducts to H_2O. Consequently, depending on the status of body water and plasma osmolality, considerable variations in the rate of urine flow and urinary osmolality normally occur in different parts of the day. After an overnight fast, the morning urine samples tend to be relatively more concentrated.

Urine Volume and Osmolality Changes in Response to Water Intake and Water Deprivation

Water Diuresis versus Osmotic Diuresis

Water Diuresis. Water diuresis refers to increased urinary output following excessive intake of water or hypotonic solution.

Pathophysiology. It occurs due to the absence of ADH in the plasma. Steps involved in its occurrence are summarized in Fig. 6.3-7. Due to the absence of ADH, the distal tubule and collecting ducts become impermeable to water leading to marked decrease in reabsorption. However, water reabsorption in the proximal tubule and loop of Henle is not affected.

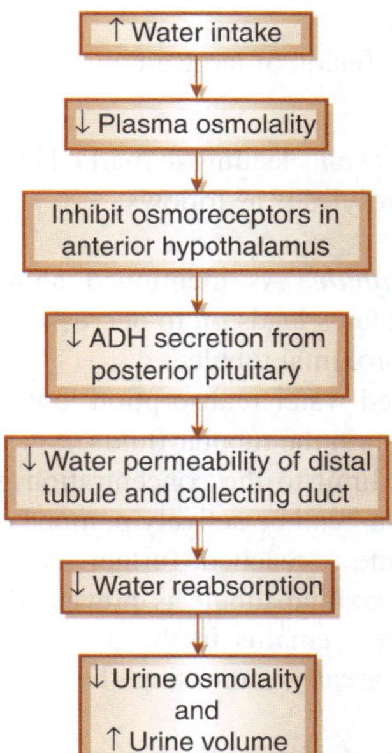

FIGURE 6.3-7 Steps involved in urine osmolality changes in response to increased water intake.

Characteristic Features

- Water diuresis begins about 15 min after ingestion of water and reaches its maximum in 40 min.
- Urine output may be increased to 20 L/day.
- Urine formed is diluted, osmolality is low (50 mOsm/kg H_2O).
- Specific gravity of urine is always below 1.010.

Water intoxication. During water diuresis, the maximum urine flow that can be produced is 16 ml/min. When water ingestion exceeds this limit of water excretion, there occurs water stasis, leading to a marked increase in ECF. Similar situation may also occur when water intake is not reduced after administration of exogenous vasopressin or secretion of endogenous vasopressin in response to nonosmotic stimuli such as surgical trauma. Consequently, the body cells are swollen because of uptake of water by the cells from increased hypotonic ECF. Symptoms of water intoxication occur rarely when swelling of the brain cells may cause convulsions, coma and eventually death.

Osmotic Diuresis. Osmotic diuresis refers to increased urine output because of an osmotic effect.

Pathophysiology. Presence of large quantities of unreabsorbed solutes in the proximal tubules exerts an appreciable osmotic effect. Osmotic diuresis may occur under the following circumstances:

- When the filtered load of naturally occurring substances such as Na+, glucose (e.g. in diabetes mellitus), urea, etc. exceeds the maximum capacity of the tubules to reabsorb (T_m).
- Following administration of compounds such as mannitol and related polysaccharides that are filtered but not reabsorbed.
- Following infusion of large amounts of sodium chloride and urea.

Sequence of events leading to marked loss of Na^+ water and other electrolytes is as follows:

- ***Proximal tubule.*** As mentioned above, presence of excessive solutes leads on to decreased water reabsorption in the proximal tubule.
  - Decreased water reabsorption lowers the Na^+ concentration in the tubular fluid.
  - When a limit to the concentration gradient against which Na^+ can be actively pumped out of the proximal tubule is reached, further reabsorption of Na^+ in the proximal tubule is prevented. Consequently, more Na^+ remains in the tubule, and water stays with it, greatly increasing the volume of isotonic fluid.
- ***In the loop of Henle.*** Reabsorption of Na^+, K^+ and Cl^- in the ascending limb of loop of Henle is decreased because the limiting concentration gradient for Na^+ reabsorption is reached. This leads to decreased medullary gradient, which in turn further decreases the reabsorption of water and Na^+.
- ***Collecting ducts*** thus receive a large volume of fluid but can reabsorb very less amount of water because of decreased medullary gradient. Consequently, the urine output and excretion of Na^+ and other electrolytes increased.

Characteristic Features

- Urine output may be >20 L/day, in spite of maximal ADH secretion.
- Urine osmolality is higher than 300 mOsm/kg H_2O.
- Urine specific gravity is over 1.010.

Water Deprivation

Water deprivation is followed by a sequence of changes which consume water for the body needs. As a consequence, urine volume is decreased but urine osmolality is increased (Fig. 6.3-8).

Factors Affecting Urinary Concentration and Dilution Mechanisms

1. Functioning of Thick Ascending Limb (Tal) of Loop of Henle. The active reabsorption of NaCl in TAL is the most important event for the generation of medullary hyperosmolality by the countercurrent system. If this

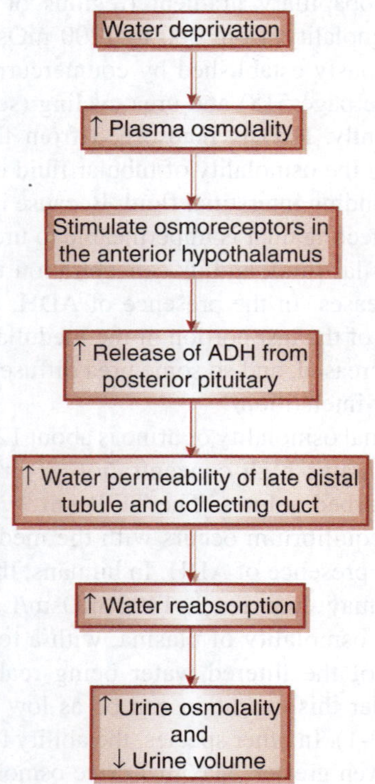

FIGURE 6.3-8 Steps involved in urine osmolality changes in response to water deprivation.

event is blocked (e.g. by loop diuretics), the entire medullary gradient of hyperosmolality disappears within minutes. As a result, urine can neither be concentrated nor diluted.

2. Length of Loop of Henle. In the human kidney, long-looped juxtamedullary nephrons, which are mainly responsible for the development of hyperosmolality gradient, constitute 15% of the total nephrons. Consequently, human kidney can produce urine with a maximum osmolality of 1400 mOsm/kg H_2O. Animals with a large number of long-looped nephrons (e.g. cat, dog) can produce more concentrated urine (with osmolality of 2500 mOsm/kg H_2O).

3. Availability of Urea. Development of single effect in the inner medulla (and subsequently development of hyperosmolality) requires the presence of high concentration of urea in the medullary interstitium (see page 517). Therefore, factors which affect the availability of urea will affect urine-concentrating mechanism. For example:

- Individuals who genetically lack the urea transport protein (UT) have lesser urine-concentrating ability.
- Low-protein diet makes lesser quantity of urea available and thus decreases urine-concentrating ability. The reverse occurs in high-protein diet.

4. Effect of Tubular Fluid Flow Rate. Increased tubular fluid flow is associated with reduced medullary hyperosmolality because of the following reasons:

- Greater reabsorption of water from the thin descending limb dilutes the solutes in the medullary interstitium.
- Active transport of Na^+ is not able to dilute the tubular fluid in TAL, and the single effect is reduced in magnitude.
- The reabsorption of water from the collecting tubule is not able to sufficiently concentrate urea in the IMCD.

Causes of increased tubular flow rate are:

- Increased GFR
- Osmotic diuretics (like mannitol or excessive glucose) when present in the proximal convoluted tubules interfere with reabsorption of NaCl and water. Therefore, intratubular flow rate is increased throughout the nephron leading to impairment of urinary concentration ability.

Conversely, a decrease in tubular flow rate (e.g. due to decreased GFR) tends to cause increased urinary concentration even in the absence of ADH.

5. Blood Flow Through Vasa Recta. It affects the ability of countercurrent exchanger to maintain medullary gradient (see page 518).

6. Effect of Prostaglandins. Certain prostaglandins impair the urinary concentration ability by:

- Increasing blood flow through vasa recta, or
- Inhibiting active transport of NaCl in the thick ascending limb of Henle loop (TAL) or
- Inhibiting the enzyme adenylyl cyclase which is involved in the genesis of cAMP (required for ADH action).

Assessment of Renal Diluting and Concentrating Ability

Assessment of renal dilution and concentration process can be made by performing the following tests:

- Measurement of urine osmolality,
- Measurement of urine specific gravity,
- The urine concentration test,
- The urine dilution test and
- Estimation of free water clearance (CH_2O).

All these tests are described in detail in the subsection on "Kidney function test", see page 549.

Clinical Disorders Related to the Concentration and Dilution of Urine Common clinical disorders related to the concentration and dilution of urine include:

- Primary psychogenic polydypsia (compulsive water drinking),
- Diabetes insipidus, which may be:
  - Central diabetes insipidus and
  - Nephrogenic diabetes insipidus
- Water deprivation and
- Syndrome of inappropriate hypersecretion of antidiuretic hormone (SIADH).

Most of these have been described in detail on page 695, and for a ready reference are summarized in Table 6.3-3.

ACIDIFICATION OF URINE

The pH of urine is variable depending upon the concentration of H^+ ions. Under normal circumstances, the pH of urine is acidic (~ 6.0). This clearly indicates that kidneys have contributed to the *acidification of urine,* when it is formed from the plasma (pH 7.4). In other words, H^+ ions generated in the body in the normal circumstances are eliminated by acidified urine. Thus, the role of kidneys in the maintenance of acid–base balance of the body (blood pH) is highly significant, as the renal mechanism tries to provide a permanent solution to the acid–base disturbances. This is in contrast to the temporary buffering systems of the blood and short-term respiratory mechanisms described in the chapter on 'Physiology of Acid–base Balance' (see page 1227).

The kidneys regulate the blood pH by three main mechanisms:

- Reabsorption of the filtered HCO_3^-,
- Generation of $NaHCO_3^-$ of the alkali reserve of the body and

TABLE 6.3-3 Summary of Clinical Disorders Related to the Concentration and Dilution of Urine

Clinical disorder	Serum ADH	Serum osmolality/ serum Na^+	Urine osmolality	Urine flow rate	Free water clearance (C_{H_2O})
Primary polydypsia	Decreased	Decreased	Hyposmotic	High	Positive
Central diabetes insipidus	Decreased	Increased (because of excretion of too much water)	Hyposmotic	High	Positive
Nephrogenic diabetes insipidus	Increased (because of increased plasma osmolality)	Increased (because of excretion of too much water)	Hyposmotic	High	Positive
Water deprivation	Increased	High/normal	Hyperosmotic	Low	Negative
SIADH	Markedly increased	Decreased (because of reabsorption of water)	Hyperosmotic	Low	Negative

- Excretion of acid in the form of titrable acid and ammonium ions.

All these mechanisms are accomplished through the process of H^+ secretion by the nephron.

Hydrogen Ion Secretion

The tubular cells of proximal tubule, distal tubule and collecting ducts are capable of secreting H^+. The kidney is the only organ which can eliminate the fixed acids by active secretion of H^+.

Mechanism of H^+ Secretion by Proximal Tubule. Steps involved are (Fig. 6.3-9):

- *Formation of carbonic acid.* Carbonic acid (H_2CO_3) is first formed in the cells of proximal tubules from CO_2 and H_2O by a reaction that is catalysed by the intracellular *carbonic anhydrase*. Therefore, the carbonic anhydrase inhibitors depress the secretion of acid by proximal tubule.
- *Dissociation of carbonic acid* (H_2CO_3) then occurs in H^+ and HCO_3^-.
- Secretion of H^+ into the lumen occurs via *Na^+–H^+* exchange mechanism in the luminal membrane. This is an example of secondary active transport, in which first Na^+ is extruded actively from the cell into the interstitium by Na^+–K^+-ATPase, and intracellular Na^+ is lowered. This is followed by the entry of Na^+ into the cell from the lumen coupled with H^+ secretion into the lumen by *Na^+–H^+* antiporter (Fig. 6.3-9).
- The secreted H^+, in the lumen, combines with the filtered HCO_3^- and helps its reabsorption (as described below). Therefore, this process does not result in net secretion of H^+.
- *HCO_3^- formed in the cell* (from the dissociation of H_2CO_3) diffuses into the interstitial fluid. Thus, for each H^+ secreted, one Na^+ ion and one HCO_3^- ion enter the interstitial fluid. The later adds up to the alkali reserve of the body.

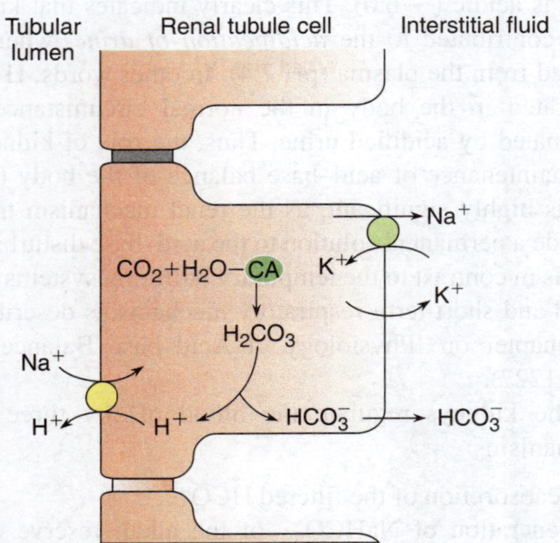

FIGURE 6.3-9 Cellular mechanism for secretion of H+ by proximal tubular cell in the kidney (for details see text).

Mechanism of H^+ Secretion by Distal Tubules and Collecting Ducts. In the distal tubule and collecting ducts, H^+ secretion occurs independent of Na^+. Two mechanisms involved in secretion of H^+ by the intercalated cells in these parts of tubules are (Fig. 6.3-10):

- ATP-driven proton pump is mainly responsible for the secretion of H^+ in the distal tubules and collecting ducts. It can increase the H^+ concentration of the luminal fluid 1000 times the plasma concentration. Aldosterone acts on this pump to increase distal H^+ secretion.
- H^+, K^+–ATPase is also responsible for secretion of some of the H^+ coupled with reabsorption of K^+ in these parts of renal tubules.

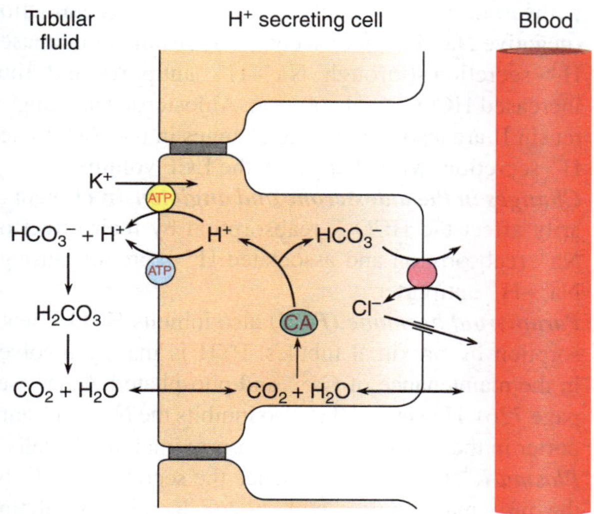

FIGURE 6.3-10 Cellular mechanism for secretion of H^+ and reabsorption of HCO_{32} by intercalated cells of the late distal tubule and collecting ducts (for details see text).

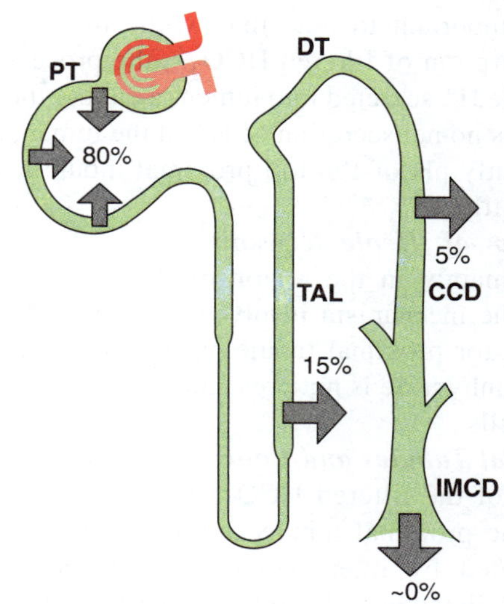

FIGURE 6.3-11 Reabsorption of filtered HCO_3^- load along various segments of nephron.

Fate of H^+ Secreted in the Renal Tubule. The secretion of H^+ in the renal tubule can continue only if the H^+ is immediately buffered in the luminal fluid. The tubular cells can secrete H^+, up to a luminal fluid pH of about 4.5, i.e. an H^+ concentration in the urine that is 1000 times the concentration in plasma. In the absence of buffering of H^+ in the lumen, this pH would be reached rapidly, stopping further H^+ secretion. The pH 4.5 is thus the *limiting pH*. However, the free H^+ secreted in the renal tubules is immediately buffered (permitting more acid to be secreted):

- In proximal tubule, the secreted H^+ ions are buffered by the filtered HCO_3^- (i.e. consumed in reabsorption of filtered HCO_3^-, vide infra) and
- In distal tubule and connecting ducts, the secreted H^+ ions are buffered by Na_2HPO_4 and NH_3 and are excreted as titrable acid and ammonium ion (NH_4^+), (vide infra).

Reabsorption of Filtered HCO_3^-

The concentration of HCO_3^- in plasma, and consequently in the glomerular filtrate, is about 24 mEq/L. Thus, glomerular filtration delivers about 4320 mEq of HCO_3^- (180 L × 24 mEq/L) per day to the nephron. The reabsorption of the filtered HCO_3^- is critically important for the prevention of its loss in the urine and thus for the maintenance of acid–base balance in the body. Under normal circumstances, virtually all the filtered HCO_3^- is reabsorbed by different segments of nephron (Fig. 6.3-11) and none appears in the urine. The mechanisms involved in reabsorption of filtered HCO_3^- in different segments are summarized.

• ***Proximal Tubule*** reabsorbs approximately 80% of the filtered HCO_3^-. Steps of cellular mechanism involved are:

- H^+ secreted in the lumen of proximal tubule (as described above (Fig. 6.3-9) combines with the filtered HCO_3^- to form carbonic acid (H_2CO_3) (Fig. 6.3-12).
- The H_2CO_3 is rapidly converted to CO_2 and H_2O. This reaction is catalysed by the brush border carbonic anhydrase.
- The CO_2 diffuses into the tubular cell along the concentration gradient. In the tubular cell, the CO_2 again combines with H_2O to form H_2CO_3, which then dissociates into H^+ and HCO_3^-, followed by secretion of H^+ in tubule and diffusion of HCO_3^- in the interstitial fluid as described above (Figs 6.3-9, 6.3-12). Thus, for each mole of HCO_3^- reabsorbed from the lumen, one mole of HCO_3^- diffuses from the tubular cell into the blood, even though it is not the same mole that disappeared from the tubular fluid. Further,

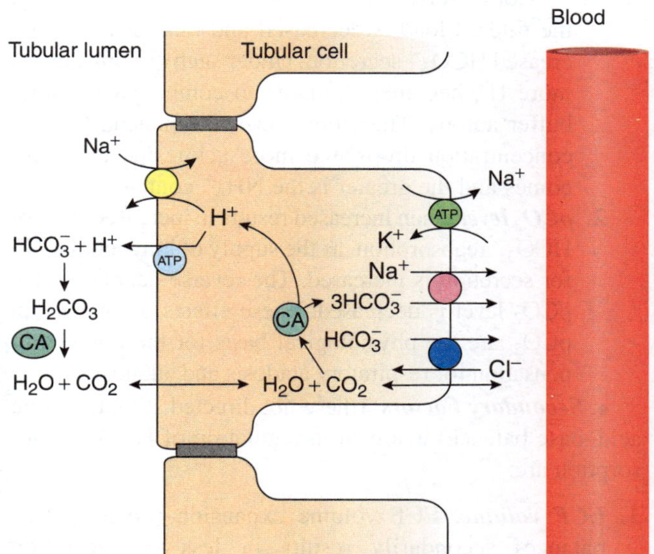

FIGURE 6.3-12 Cellular mechanism involved in reabsorption of filtered HCO_3^- in proximal tubular cell.

it is important to note that, while there occurs net reabsorption of filtered HCO_3^-, the process neutralizes the H^+ secreted into lumen, meaning thereby that there is no net secretion of H^+ in the lumen, and consequently pH of fluid in proximal tubule is changed very little.

• ***Loop of Henle*** reabsorbs 15% of the filtered HCO_3^-, mainly in the region of thick ascending limb (TAL). The mechanism involved is exactly the same as described for proximal tubule, except that brush border carbonic anhydrase is not present in the apical membrane of TAL cells.

• ***Distal Tubules and Convoluted Tubules*** reabsorb only 5% of the filtered HCO_3^- which escapes absorption in the proximal tubule and TAL. So, some of the H^+ secreted by intercalated cells of these parts of tubule is utilized in reabsorption of HCO_3^- (Fig. 6.3-10), while most of the H^+ secreted in these segments is excreted with non-HCO_3^- urinary buffers (described in later discussion).

Regulation of HCO_3^- Reabsorption Various factors that regulate HCO_3^- reabsorption (i.e. H^+ secretion) can be divided into two groups of primary and secondary factors.

• ***Primary Factors*** (those directed at maintaining acid-base balance) involved in regulation of HCO_3^- reabsorption include:

1. ***Plasma HCO_3^- level.*** An increase in the plasma HCO_3, increases the filtered load of HCO_3, resulting in increased HCO_3^- reabsorption. However, if the plasma concentration becomes very high (above 28 mEq/L, e.g. metabolic alkalosis), the filtered load will exceed the reabsorptive capacity (the renal threshold for HCO_3^-), the HCO_3^- appears in the urine and urine becomes alkaline.

   Conversely, with the decrease in plasma HCO_3, the filtered load is decreased and this results in decreased HCO_3^- secretion. Under such circumstances, more H^+ becomes available to combine with other buffer anions. Therefore, lower the plasma HCO_3^- concentration drops, the more acidic the urine becomes and the greater is the NH_4^+ content.
2. ***pCO_2 level*** when increased results in increased rates of HCO_3^- reabsorption, as the supply of intracellular H^+ for secretion is increased. The reverse happens when pCO_2 level is decreased. These effects of changes in pCO_2, are the physiological basis for the renal compensation for respiratory acidosis and alkalosis.

• ***Secondary Factors*** (these not directed at maintaining acid–base balance) involved in regulation of HCO_3^- reabsorption are:

1. ***ECF volume.*** ECF volume expansion (positive Na^+ balance) secondarily results in less H^+ secretion (through Na^+–H^+ antiport) and thus decreased HCO_3^- reabsorption. Conversely, ECF volume contraction (negative Na^+ balance) secondarily results in increased H^+ secretion (through Na^+–H^+ antiport) and thus increased HCO_3^- reabsorption. Aldosterone and angiotensin II are also involved in changes in the Na^+-linked H^+ secretion, with changes in the ECF volume.
2. ***Changes in the aldosterone and angiotensin II*** secondarily affect the HCO_3^- reabsorption by their effect on Na^+ reabsorption and associated H^+ secretion through Na^+–H^+ antiporter.
3. ***Parathyroid hormone (PTH)*** also inhibits HCO_3^- reabsorption by proximal tubules. PTH is mainly involved in the maintenance of Ca^{2+} and phosphate balance (see page 726). However, PTH also inhibits the Na^+–H^+ antiporter in the apical membrane of proximal tubule cells.
4. ***Plasma K^+*** levels also influence the secretion of H^+ by the proximal tubules, with hypokalaemia stimulating and hyperkalaemia inhibiting secretion.

Generation of New HCO_3^-

As discussed above, the kidneys play an important role in the maintenance of acid–base balance of the body by completely reabsorbing the filtered HCO_3^-. However, in reality, HCO_3^- reabsorption alone does not replenish the HCO_3^- lost during the titration of nonvolatile acids which are daily added to the plasma, from the diet and produced by metabolism. Therefore, to maintain acid–base balance, the kidneys replace this lost HCO_3^- with new HCO_3^- by the following processes:

- Excretion of H^+ as titrable acid and
- Excretion of H^+ as NH_4.

As discussed below, by these processes, the kidneys not only synthesize new HCO_3^- but also result in net secretion of H^+.

Excretion of H^+ as Titrable Acid Excretion of H^+ as titrable acid (as explained below) refers to the excretion of secreted H^+ along with the primary urinary buffer, the dibasic phosphate (HPO_4^{2-}). This reaction occurs in the distal tubules and collecting ducts, because it is here that the phosphate which escapes proximal reabsorption is greatly concentrated by the reabsorption of water. The cellular mechanism involved in the synthesis of new HCO_3^- and net excretion of H^+ with dibasic phosphate urinary buffer are (Fig. 6.3-13):

- H^+ and HCO_3^- are produced in the cell from CO_2 and H_2O.
- The new HCO_3^- is reabsorbed into the blood.
- H^+ secreted into the lumen (mainly of by H^+-ATPase) combines with filtered HPO_4^{2-} to form $H_2PO_4^-$, which is excreted as titrable acid. The amount of H^+ excreted as titrable acid is determined by the amount of urinary buffer and the pK of the buffer.

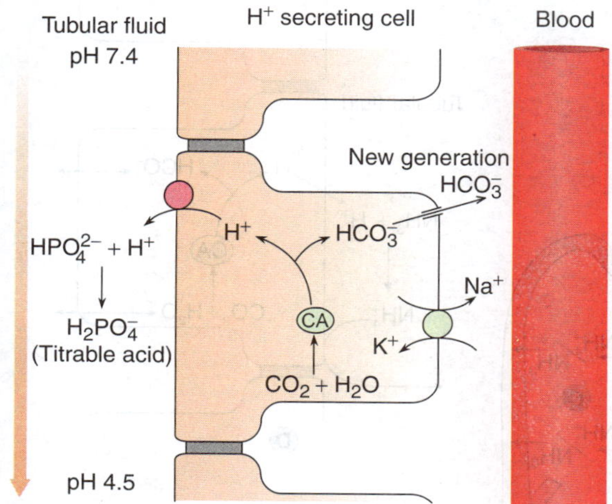

FIGURE 6.3-13 Mechanism for excretion of H^+ as titrable acid and synthesis of new HCO_3^-.

As a result of H^+ excretion in the form of titrable acid, the pH of urine is progressively decreased (from 7.4, that of blood). The *acidification of the urine* may lower its pH to a minimum of 4.5, i.e. H^+ concentration of urine is approximately 1000 times the concentration of H^+ in the plasma. Thus, titrable acidity is a measure of acid excreted in the urine by the kidney. This can be estimated by titrating urine back to normal pH of blood (7.4). In quantitative terms, titrable acidity refers to the number of millilitres of N/10 NaOH required to titrate 1 L of urine to pH 7.4. However, the titrable acidity obviously measures only a fraction of the acid secreted, since it does not account for the H_2CO_3 that has been converted to H_2O and CO_2.

In addition, the pK of ammonia system is 9.0, and the ammonia system is titrable only from the pH of urine to pH 7.4, so it contributes very little to titrable acidity.

Further, as mentioned earlier, although nearly 4000 mEq of H^+ are secreted into the proximal tubule, the pH of the fluid does not change because almost all the H^+ secreted into proximal tubule is neutralized during the process of reabsorption of filtered HCO_3^-. Practically, there is no buffering of H^+ by the $NHPO_4^{2-}$ in proximal tubules.

Excretion of H^+ as Ammonium Ion Excretion of H^+ as NH_4^+ is another mechanism of excretion of secreted H^+ and formation of new HCO_3^-. However, it is important to note that new HCO_3^- formation by this process depends on the kidney's ability to excrete the NH_4^+ in the urine. If NH_4^+ is not excreted in the urine, but instead enters the systemic circulation, it will titrate the plasma HCO_3^-, thus negating the process of generating new HCO_3^-. The amount of H^+ excreted as NH_4^+ depends upon both the amount of NH_3 synthesized by renal cells and the urine pH. The process by which the kidneys excrete NH_4^+ is complex and can be described to have four stages (for the purpose of understanding only) (Fig. 6.3-14):

- A: Synthesis of NH_4^+ and new HCO_3^- in proximal tubule,
- B: Reabsorption of NH_4^+ across thick ascending limb,
- C: Accumulation of NH_4^+ in medullary interstitium and
- D: Anionic diffusion and diffusion trapping in collecting ducts.

A. Synthesis of NH_4^+ and New HCO_3^- in Proximal Tubule. Ammonium ions (NH_4^+) are produced in the cells of proximal tubules from the metabolism of *glutamine*. Each molecule of glutamine is metabolized into two molecules each of NH_4^+ and HCO_3^-.

- HCO_3^- diffuses across the basolateral membrane into the peritubular blood as new HCO_3^-.
- NH_4^+ is secreted into the lumen via Na^+–H^+ antiporter, with NH_4^+ substituting for H^+. Some NH_4^+ is converted into NH_3^+ and H^+. NH_3^+ diffuses into the lumen where it combines with the secreted H^+ to form NH_4^+.

B. Reabsorption of NH_4^+ across Thick Ascending Limb. NH_4^+ then moves along the tubular fluid. In the thick ascending limb (TAL) of loop of Henle, a significant amount of NH_4^+ is reabsorbed via two mechanisms:

- *Transcellularly*, via $1Na^+$–$1K^+$–$2Cl^-$ symporter with NH_4^+ substituting for K^+ and
- *Paracellularly* driven by the lumen positive transepithelial voltage in this segment.

C. Accumulation of NH_4^+ in Medullary Interstitium. The NH_4 reabsorbed across the TAL accumulates in the medullary interstitium, where it exists in chemical equilibrium with NH_3^+.

D. Anionic Diffusion and Diffusion Trapping in Collecting Ducts. The cells of collecting duct are not permeable to NH_4^+, but permeable to NH_3^+. From the medullary interstitium, NH_3^+ diffuses into the lumen of collecting ducts by a process called nonionic diffusion and is protonated to NH_4^+ by combining with H^+ secreted by the cells of collecting duct. Since the cells of collecting ducts are impermeable to NH_4^+, NH_4^+ is trapped in the lumen of collecting duct (*diffusion trapping*) and is excreted in the urine. Thus, for every NH_4^+ excreted in the urine, a new HCO_3^- is returned to the systemic circulation. Therefore, excretion of NH_4^+ can be used as a marker of proximal tubule glutamine metabolism, which in turn determines new HCO_3^- formation.

Certain Important Points to Note about NH_4^+

- *NH_4^+* is a major urine acid. It is estimated that about half to two-third of body acid load is eliminated in the form of NH_4^+ ions. For this reason, renal regulation via NH_4^+ excretion is very effective to eliminate large quantities of acids produced in the body.

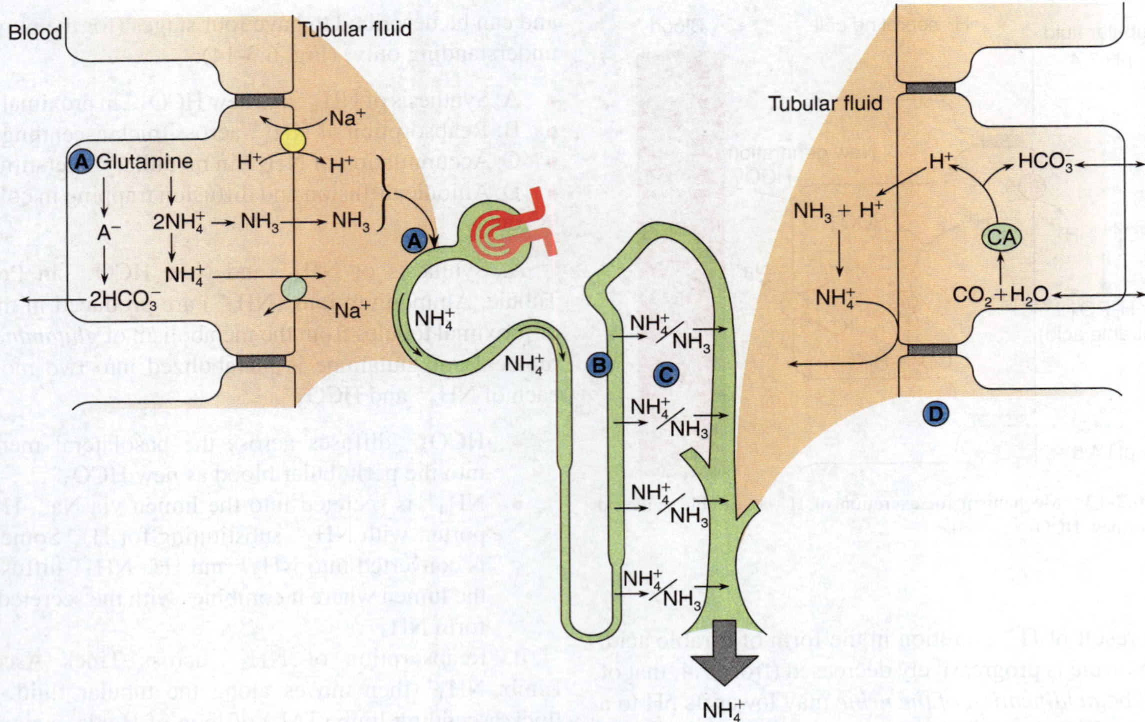

FIGURE 6.3-14 Excretion of H^+ as NH_4^+ and generation of new HCO_3^- can be considered in four stages: **A,** synthesis of NH_4^+ and HCO_3^- from glutamine in proximal tubule; **B,** reabsorption of NH_4^+ across thick ascending limb; **C,** accumulation of NH_4^+ in medullary interstitium in equilibrium with NH_3^+; and **D,** anionic diffusion and diffusion trapping in collecting ducts.

- The ammonium content of urine is negligible until the urinary pH falls below 6. Below this urinary pH, the ammonium secretion increases linearly with the fall in pH.
- Unlike phosphate buffer, the capacity of ammonia buffer is not limited by the amount filtered in the glomerular filtrate. In states of chronic acidosis (e.g. diabetic ketoacidosis, respiratory acidosis), the amount of H^+ excreted as NH_4^+ may increase to 10-fold, due to an *adaptative increase in NH_3* synthesis.
- Since the pK value of this buffer system is 9, H^+ excreted as NH_4^+ does not contribute to titrable acidity of the urine.

Chapter 6.4

Regulation of Body Fluid Osmolality, Composition and Volume

INTRODUCTION

The control of body fluid osmolality, composition and volume, and thus the water and electrolyte balance in the body, is concerted function of the kidneys, blood, skin, lungs, digestive system, certain hormones and neural mechanisms. However, the kidneys play a major role in these homeostatic mechanisms. For the ease of understanding, this chapter has been divided into following sections:

- The body fluid compartments,
- Control of body fluid osmolality,
- Regulation of extracellular fluid volume and composition,
- Defence of specific ions composition and
- Water and electrolyte disturbances.

BODY FLUID COMPARTMENTS

Volumes and Composition of Body Fluid Compartments

The total body water (TBW) and the body fluid compartments have been described in Chapter 1.1 (see page 6). The salient features are summarized here:

- Total body water (TBW), intracellular fluid (ICF) and extracellular fluid (ECF) form 60, 40 and 20% of the total body weight, respectively (60-40-20 rule).
- Percentage of TBW is the highest in newborns and adult males, and lowest in adult females and in adults with a large amount of adipose tissue.
- The major cation of ECF is Na^+, while that of ICF is K^+.
- The major anions of ECF are Cl^- and HCO_3^-, while that of ICF are protein and organic phosphates [adenosine

triphosphate (ATP), adenosine diphosphate (ADP) and adenosine monophosphate (AMP)].

Fluid Exchange between Body Fluid Compartments

Basic Principles Basic principles of fluid exchange which are also useful for analysis of fluid shifts between ICF and ECF are:

- ***Osmolality of ECF and ICF*** are equal at steady state. Because the plasma membranes of cells are highly permeable to water, a change in the osmolality of either ECF or ICF results in the rapid movement of water between these compartments to achieve the equality in osmolality.
- ***Movement of water across plasma membrane*** between ECF and ICF is determined mainly by the osmotic difference between the two compartments. Whereas, fluid exchange between plasma and interstitial fluid across the capillary wall is determined by Starling forces (see page 318).
- ***Movement of ions across the cell membrane*** is variable and depends on the presence of specific membrane transporters. However, for the sake of simplification in analysing fluid shifts between compartments, it can be assumed that equilibration between ECF and ICF occurs only by the movement of water and that solutes like NaCl and mannitol do not cross cell membranes and are confined to the ECF.
- ***Exchanges of solutes and water with external environment*** occur through the ECF (e.g. intravenous administration, oral intake or loss via GIT and urinary tract, etc.). Changes in ICF are secondary to changes in ECF, and occur only if perturbation of the ECF alters its osmolality.
- ***Gross estimation of volume of various fluid compartments*** in the normal adult can be made from their standard ratio:
  - Total body water (TBW) = 0.6 × body weight,
  - Intracellular fluid (ICF) = 0.4 × body weight,
  - Extracellular fluid (ECF) = 0.2 × body weight,
  - Interstitial fluid = 0.75 × ECF and
  - Plasma volume = 0.25 × ECF.

CONTROL OF BODY FLUID OSMOLALITY

At steady state, the major fluid compartments of the body, i.e. ECF and ICF are in osmotic equilibrium and thus have the same osmolality. This equilibrium is maintained by free water shifts between the ECF and ICF compartments. Therefore, a measurement of plasma osmolality provides a measure of both ECF and ICF osmolality. It is important to note that though the osmolality of ECF and ICF osmolality is similar, there is marked difference in the concentration of electrolytes (cations and anions) between the ECF and ICF. As described in body electrolytes (Chapter 1.1, page 9), Na^+ is the principal cation of ECF, while in the ICF, the principal cation is K^+. This difference in the concentration is essential for the cell survival, and is maintained by Na^+–K^+ pump.

Normal plasma osmolality ranges from approximately 280 to 295 mOsm/kg H_2O. Table 6.4-1 shows the distribution of constituents in plasma osmolality. Sodium and its associated anions make the largest contribution (~90%) to plasma osmolality.

Computation of plasma osmolality, for practical purposes, can be done from the concentration (mmol/L) of Na^+, K^+, urea and glucose:

$$\text{Plasma osmolality} = 2\,(Na^+) + 2\,(K^+) + \text{urea} + \text{glucose}.$$

The factor of 2 is used for Na^+ and K^+ ions to account for the associated anion concentration. Since plasma Na^+ is the most predominant contributor to osmolality, the above calculation can be simplified (provided plasma glucose and urea are in the normal range) as follows:

$$\text{Plasma osmolality (mmol/kg)} = 2 \times \text{plasma } Na^+ \text{ (mmol/L)}.$$

Plasma (Na^+) and ECF. It is important to realize that Na^+ and its associated anions (mainly Cl^-) are mainly confined to ECF. Therefore, the retention of water in the ECF is directly related to the osmotic effect of these ions. Thus, the amount of Na^+ in the ECF ultimately determines its volume. When evaluating abnormal plasma (Na^+) in an individual, it is tempting to suspect a problem in Na^+ balance. However, the problem most often relates to water balance not with Na^+, alterations in the volume of ECF, and neither its osmolality.

Determinants of body fluid osmolality. The total body osmolality is directly proportionate to the total body sodium plus the total body potassium divided by the total body water. Therefore, changes in the body fluid occur when there is disproportion between the amounts of these electrolytes and the amount of water ingested or

TABLE 6.4-1 Distribution of Constituents in Plasma Osmolality

Constituent (solute)	Osmolality (mOsm/kg H_2O)
Sodium	135
Associated anions	135
Potassium	3.5
Associated anions	3.5
Calcium	1.5
Associated anions	1.5
Magnesium	1.0
Associated anions	1.0
Urea	5.0
Glucose	5.0
Protein	1.0
Total	293

lost from the body. In other words, water balance in the body is the most important determinant of the body fluid osmolality.

Water Balance in the Body

The kidneys possess tremendous capacity to regulate the body water balance. In a healthy individual, this is achieved by balancing the daily water input and output.

Water Input Water is added to the body fluids by:

1. Ingestion of Water in the form of fluid and as constituent of foodstuffs (Table 6.4-2). The water intake is highly variable, which may range from 0.5 to 20 L/day depending upon the social and personal habits and environmental conditions. In general, people living in hot climate drink more water. Ingestion of water is mainly controlled by the thirst centre. Increase in the plasma osmolality stimulates thirst centre and promotes water ingestion.

2. Endogenous Production of Water during oxidation of foodstuffs adds about 300 ml of water to the body fluids per day (Table 6.4-2).

Water Output A variable amount of water is lost from the body in urine, faeces, sweat and as insensible loss (Table 6.4-2).

1. Insensible Loss of Water (about which the individual is unaware) occurs by evaporation from the cells of skin and respiratory passages.

2. Water Loss in Sweat. Water loss by the production of sweat from skin can vary from 100 ml/day in routine at room temperature of 23°C to 1400 ml in hot weather, to 5000 ml following prolonged exercise (Table 6.4-3).

3. Water Loss in Faeces. Most of the water entering the GIT is reabsorbed by the intestine. About 200 ml/day is lost through faeces in a healthy individual (Table 6.4-2).

TABLE 6.4-2 Water Balance in the Body Represented by Daily Water Input and Output in Adults at Room Temperature (23°C)

Water intake (ml/day)		Water output (ml/day)	
Source	*Volume*	*Route*	*Volume*
Ingested water	1200*	Insensible	700
In food	1000	Sweat	100
Metabolic water	300	Faeces	200
		Urine	1500**
Total	2500		2500

*Fluid ingestion varies from 1000 to 2000 ml/day; obligatory water ingestion is 400 ml/day.

**Urine flow varies depending upon the water ingested; obligatory urine volume is 500 ml/day.

TABLE 6.4-3 Effect of Environmental Temperature and Exercise on Water Loss and Intake in Adults

Route of water loss	Volume (ml/day)		
	Normal temperature	*Hot weather*	*Prolonged heavy exercise*
• Insensible loss			
Skin	350	350	350
Lungs	350	250	650
• Sweat	100	1400	5000
• Faeces	200	200	200
• Urine	1500	1200	500
• Total loss	2500	3400	6700
• Water intake to maintain balance	2500	3400	6700

Faecal loss of water is tremendously increased in diarrhoea. GIT water losses can also occur with vomiting.

4. Water Loss in Urine. About 1500 ml of water is eliminated from the body in urine. Water losses through kidney are highly variable.

It is important to note that water loss in sweat, faeces and evaporation from the lungs and skin is *not regulated.* However, the renal loss, though variable, is well regulated to maintain the water balance. For water balance, the water output is precisely matched with water intake by the kidneys:

- The kidneys produce small amount of concentrated urine (hyperosmotic with respect of plasma), when the intake is low or losses are more, and conversely,
- The kidneys produce large amount of dilute urine (hypo-osmotic with respect to plasma), when the water intake is high.

Thus, in a normal individual, depending primarily on the ADH concentration, the urine osmolality may vary from 50 to 1200 mOsm/kg H_2O with a corresponding urine volume of 18 to 0.5 L/day.

Disorders of Water Balance alter body fluid osmolality. Changes in body fluid osmolality are manifested by a change in plasma (Na^+):

- *Positive water balance* (intake > excretion) results in decrease in body fluid osmolality and hyponatraemia.
- *Negative water balance* (intake < excretion) results in an increase in body fluid osmolality and hypernatraemia.

Factors Controlling Water Balance The input of water (i.e. thirst) and output of water (i.e. urinary excretion) are both controlled by plasma osmolality and blood volume.

1. Plasma Osmolality controls water balance by stimulating thirst centre and ADH secretion through the osmoreceptors as mentioned below. Significant changes in ADH secretion occur by a small (2%) change in the plasma osmolality.

2. Blood Volume. Under normal circumstances, the water balance of the body is mainly regulated through osmoreceptors. However, a significant (more than 10%) decrease in blood volume also stimulates thirst and ADH secretion from the posterior pituitary. If blood volume is markedly decreased, ADH release is stimulated even if plasma osmolality is low. Whenever there is conflict between plasma osmolality and blood volume, the latter is maintained at the cost of plasma osmolality. Decreased blood volume is sensed by low-pressure receptors in the atria and pulmonary vessels.

For further details see pages 345 and 346.

Mechanisms Controlling Body Fluid Osmolality

The control of body fluid osmolality, i.e. defence of the tonicity of the ECF, is primarily the function of the vasopressin secretion and thirst mechanisms:

When the Effective Osmotic Pressure of Plasma rises, the *osmoreceptors* located in the anterior hypothalamus are stimulated. The stimulation of receptors results from their shrinkage caused by cellular dehydration. Cellular dehydration may occur because of:

- Deficiency of total body water or
- Excessive intake of NaCl, which causes the water to shift from ICF to ECF.

The *stimulated osmoreceptors* in turn cause (Fig. 6.4-1):

- Increase in thirst, which regulates water intake and
- Increase in vasopressin release, which regulates water excretion by the kidneys.

When the Effective Osmotic Pressure of Plasma decreases, i.e. when plasma becomes hypotonic, the vasopressin secretion is decreased (increasing water excretion in excess of solute) and thirst is decreased (decreasing water intake).

Thus, the main mechanisms which are related with regulation of body fluid osmolality are:

- Role of antidiuretic hormone (see page 692),
- Role of thirst mechanism and
- Renal mechanisms for dilution and concentration of urine (see page 514).

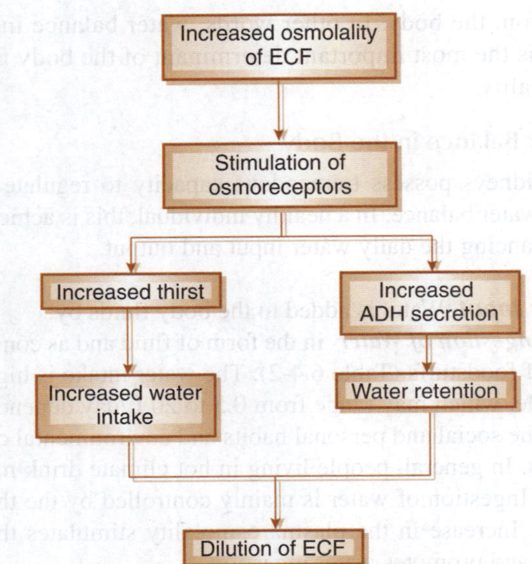

FIGURE 6.4-1 Mechanisms regulating body fluid osmolality.

REGULATION OF EXTRACELLULAR FLUID VOLUME AND COMPOSITION

The regulation of extracellular fluid (ECF) volume is primarily mediated through the regulation of the amount of osmotically active solute in it. The major solutes of the ECF are the salts of Na^+; of these, NaCl is the most abundant. Since the kidneys are major route of NaCl excretion from the body, they play an important role in the regulation of ECF. The kidneys get signals from the volume-sensing system to make appropriate adjustment in NaCl excretion. The volume sensors generate signals in response to changes in the effective circulatory volume (ECV). The volume sensor signals then control the volume of ECF by controlling the renal excretion of NaCl and water. Therefore, the process of regulation of ECF volume can be described in following subsections:

- Concept of effective circulating volume and volume-sensing system,
- Volume sensor signals neural and hormonal control of NaCl excretion and
- Sodium balance.

Effective Circulatory Volume and Volume Sensors

Concept of Effective Circulating Volume

Effective Circulatory Volume (ECV) is not a measurable and distinct body fluid compartment. In physiologically conceptual term, the ECV refers to the portion of extracellular fluid (ECF) volume that is present in the arterial system under particular pressure and is effectively perfusing the tissues. Thus, ECV cannot be simply regulated with the volume of fluid in the vascular tree. In a 70-kg man with 42 L of total body water (60% of body weight), the ECF volume is about 14 L (20% of body weight), out of which interstitial fluid volume is 10.5 L (75% of ECF) and plasma volume (vascular volume) is 3.5 L (25% of ECF). Only about 0.7 L of vascular volume (i.e. 20% of plasma, or 5% of ECF or 1.7% of TBW or 1% of the body weight) forms the ECV. The ECV is regulated by the volume sensors which are located entirely within the vascular tree. Sensation of ECV is related to 'fullness', i.e. 'volume and pressure' in the vascular tree.

In the Normal State, variations in ECV are reflected as parallel variations in ECF volume and also in vascular volume arterial blood pressure and cardiac output. In other words, a decrease in ECF, vascular volume, arterial pressure or cardiac output will be sensed in the body as decrease in effective circulatory volume (ECV).

Maintenance of ECV and regulation of Na^+ balance are closely related. Therefore, Na^+ loading produces expansion of ECV and Na^+ loss leads to depletion of ECV. In other words, when ECV is decreased, the renal NaCl excretion is reduced. This adaptive response restores the ECV to normal and thereby maintains adequate tissue perfusion. Conversely, an increase in ECV results in an enhanced renal NaCl excretion termed the *natriuresis*. Again, this is an adaptive response to restore the ECV to its normal point.

In Pathological Conditions such as congestive heart failure and hepatic cirrhosis, the ECV may be independent of ECF volume, i.e. ECV is reduced though ECF volume is markedly increased. Since the kidneys regulate the excretion of NaCl in response to changes in ECV rather than in ECF volume, there occurs renal retention of Na^+ and H_2O, despite the increased content of total body Na^+ and H_2O, which is a paradoxical renal response. The increase in ECF and retention of Na^+ in such patients manifests as accumulation of fluid in the lungs (*pulmonary oedema*) and peripheral tissues (*generalized oedema*).

ECV Sensors (Volume-Sensing System)

The ECV sensors, commonly known as volume sensors or volume receptors, refer to the receptors which are located in the vascular system and respond to the degree of stretch of the vessel wall and not to the volume of the vessel (hence, also called as baroreceptors). Various volume sensors known are:

I. *Vascular volume receptors*
  - **a.** Low-pressure volume receptors are located in:
    - Cardiac atria and
    - Pulmonary vasculature
  - **b.** High-pressure volume receptors include:
    - Carotid sinus,
    - Aortic arch and
    - Juxtaglomerular apparatus of kidney

II. *Hepatic volume receptors* and

III. *Central nervous system* Na^+ sensors.

The sensors within the liver and central nervous system (CNS) are less well understood, and do not seem to be as important as the vascular sensors in monitoring the effective circulating volume. The vascular receptors are described in detail in Chapter 4.5 (see page 344); only salient points are mentioned here.

Vascular Low-pressure Volume Receptors, located within the walls of cardiac atria and large pulmonary vessels, respond to fullness of vascular tree. Afferents from these receptors travel to the solitary tract nucleus of the medulla oblongata via vagus nerve and reflexly modulate:

- Sympathetic discharge,
- ADH secretion and
- ANP secretion (only by cardiac atrial receptors).

Vascular High-pressure Volume Receptors. *The sino-aortic baroreceptors* respond primarily to the arterial blood pressure. Afferents from these receptors travel to the solitary tract nucleus of the medulla via glossopharyngeal and vagus nerves and reflexly regulate:

- Sympathetic discharge to heart and resistance vessels including the renal arterioles and
- ADH secretion.

  Juxtaglomerular apparatus of the kidneys (see page 482), particularly the afferent arterioles, respond directly to change in the pressure and modulate the renin–angiotensin mechanism.

Hepatic Sensors, though not as important as vascular volume receptors, but do play a role in regulating renal NaCl excretion by reflexly regulating renal sympathetic discharge. The hepatic sensors also appear to be involved in the regulation of gastrointestinal Na^+ absorption. For example, when the Na^+ concentration of the portal vein blood is increased, there is reflex reduction in jejunal NaCl absorption.

CNS Na^+ Receptors, like the hepatic sensors, play only a little role in regulating renal NaCl excretion. Probably, these are located in the hypothalamus and respond to Na^+ concentration in carotid blood or CSF, and regulate renal sympathetic nerve activity.

Neural and Hormonal Regulation of Renal Sodium Chloride Excretion

Both neural and hormonal volume sensor signals arise in response to afferents from the above described volume sensors and regulate the renal excretion of NaCl (Table 6.4-4):

Neural Regulation

As described in Chapter 6.1 (page 484), the sympathetic nerve fibres innervate the afferent and efferent arterioles of the glomerulus as well as nephron cells.

TABLE 6.4-4 Summary of Neural and Hormonal Control of Renal NaCl and Water Excretion

Neural Control
↑ **Sympathetic activity decreases NaCl excretion by:**
• ↓ Glomerular filtration rate
• ↑ Renin secretion
• ↑ Tubular NaCl reabsorption
Hormonal Control
↑ **Renin–angiotensin–aldosterone secretion decreases NaCl excretion by:**
• ↑ Proximal tubule absorption and
• ↑ ADH secretion by angiotensinogen-II
• ↑ Tubular reabsorption by aldosterone
↑ **ANP secretion increases NaCl excretion by:**
• ↑ Glomerular filtration rate
• ↓ Renin secretion
• ↓ Aldosterone secretion
• ↓ NaCl and water reabsorption by the collecting duct
• ↓ ADH secretion and action of ADH on the collecting duct
↑ **ADH secretion decreases H_2O excretion by:**
• ↑ H_2O absorption by the collecting duct

Renal Sympathetic Stimulation, which is induced by vascular low- and high-volume sensors, in conditions of negative Na^+ balance (i.e. decreased ECV), leads to decrease in NaCl excretion by the following mechanisms:

1. Reduction in GFR occurs due to vasoconstriction of afferent arterioles induced by sympathetic stimulation. Reduced GFR leads to a decrease in the filtered load (filtered load = GFR × plasma Na^+ concentration). Reduction in filtered load does help in Na^+ conservation; however, changes in filtered load of Na^+ are not reflected in parallel changes in the urinary Na^+ excretion because of the following effects:

- Glomerular tubular balance (see page 503) and
- Tubuloglomerular feedback (see page 487).

2. Increased Na^+ Reabsorption, along the nephron is directly produced by stimulation of a-adrenergic receptors. Proximal tubule is the most important segment influenced by sympathetic nerve stimulation.

3. Stimulation of Renin Secretion from the cells of afferent arterioles is produced by the activation of β-adrenergic receptors. As described below, it results in increased plasma concentration of angiotensin II and aldosterone.

Renal Sympathetic Inhibition, which is induced by vascular low- and high-pressure volume receptors in conditions of positive Na^+ balance (i.e. increased ECV), leads to increased NaCl excretion by the reverse effect of the above-described mechanisms.

Hormonal Regulation

1. Renin–angiotensin–aldosterone System. Renin–angiotensin–aldosterone system when stimulated with volume depletion results in decreased NaCl excretion; conversely, when suppressed with volume expansion enhances NaCl excretion.

Renin is secreted by smooth muscles of afferent arterioles of kidney in response to:

- Reduced perfusion pressure,
- Increased renal sympathetic discharge (as mentioned above) and
- Decreased delivery of NaCl to the macula densa cells (tubuloglomerular feedback mechanism) (see page 487).

Renin converts angiotensinogen (produced by liver) into angiotensin I, which is converted to angiotensin II by angiotensin-converting enzyme (ACE) (Fig. 6.4-2).

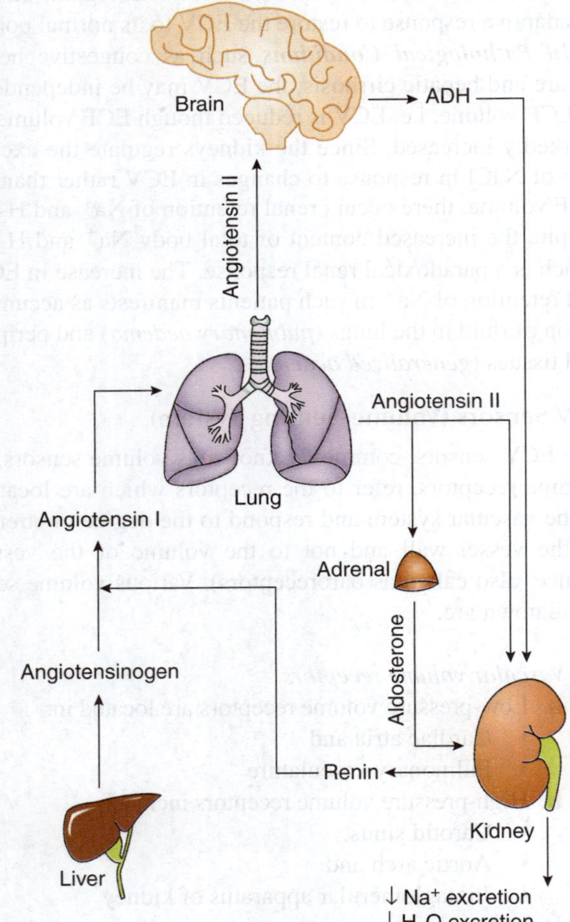

FIGURE 6.4-2 Mechanism of decreased Na^+ excretion by the renin–angiotensin–aldosterone system (for explanation see text).

Angiotensinogen II subserves the following physiological functions:

- Stimulates aldosterone secretion by the adrenal cortex,
- Increases blood pressure by arteriolar vasoconstriction,
- Stimulates ADH secretion and thirst and
- Enhances NaCl reabsorption by proximal tubules.

Aldosterone enhances NaCl reabsorption from the thick ascending limb (TAL) of loop of Henle by stimulating Na^+–K^+–$2Cl^-$ symporter at apical membrane and Na^+–K^+–ATPase at the basolateral membrane.

2. Atrial Natriuretic Peptide (ANP) is released from the atrial myocytes by the atrial stretch caused by volume expansion (increased ECV). Its actions are opposite to that of renin–angiotensin–aldosterone system and result in increased urinary excretion of NaCl by the following mechanisms:

- *Increased GFR* by vasodilation of afferent and vasoconstriction of efferent arterioles.
- *Inhibition of renin secretion* by the afferent arterioles.
- *Inhibition of aldosterone secretion* by inhibiting renin secretion and also by its direct effect on the adrenal cortex cells.
- *Inhibition of ADH secretion* by posterior pituitary and inhibition of ADH action on the collecting duct.
- *Inhibition of NaCl reabsorption* by the collecting duct by inhibiting aldosterone secretion, by inhibiting ADH secretion, and also by its direct effect on the collecting duct cells.

3. Antidiuretic Hormone (ADH) secretion by the posterior pituitary is increased with volume depletion (decreased ECV) leading to retention of water by the kidneys and thus re-establishing euvolaemia. Reverse occurs in volume expansion (see pages 693 and 694).

Sodium Balance Sodium is actively pumped out of the cells by Na^+–K^+–ATPase pump. As a result, 85–90% of all Na^+ is extracellular, and the ECF volume is reflection of total body Na^+ content. Normal volume regulatory mechanisms ensure that Na^+ loss balances Na^+ gain. If this does not occur, conditions of Na^+ excess or deficit ensure and manifest as oedematous or hypovolaemic states, respectively.

Sodium Intake An individual consumes about 150 mmol of NaCl daily. This normally exceeds basal requirements. Since Na^+ is the principal extracellular cation, the dietary intake of Na^+ results in ECF volume expansion. This, in turn promotes enhanced renal Na^+ excretion to maintain steady state Na^+ balance.

Sodium Excretion The neural and hormonal regulation of the Na^+ excretion, as described above, is multifactorial and is the major determinant of Na^+ balance. Therefore, further discussion is devoted to:

- Characteristics and mechanisms of responses to varying salt intake,
- Regulation of Na^+ excretion during euvolaemia,
- Regulation of Na^+ excretion with volume expansion and
- Regulation of Na^+ excretion with volume contraction.

Characteristics and Mechanisms of Responses to Varying Salt Intake

Wide Range of Na^+ Excretion. The kidneys can maintain normal ECF volume and normal ECV by varying the amount of NaCl excretion over a wide range depending upon the circumstances. Consequently, under conditions of salt restriction (e.g. low-NaCl diet), the kidneys conserve all the Na^+, and virtually no Na^+ appears in the urine. Conversely, with large quantities of intake, renal excretion can exceed 1000 mEqL/day.

Response to variation in salt intake takes a few days and during the transition period, excretion does not match intake as explained below:

1. ***When NaCl intake is suddenly increased,*** the individual remains in a positive balance (intake > excretion) for 2–3 days. With positive balance, water retention occurs, which manifests as an increase in the body weight. After a period of adaptation (that depends upon the magnitude of change in NaCl intake), the daily urinary excretion of NaCl matches the amount ingested (Fig. 6.4-3).

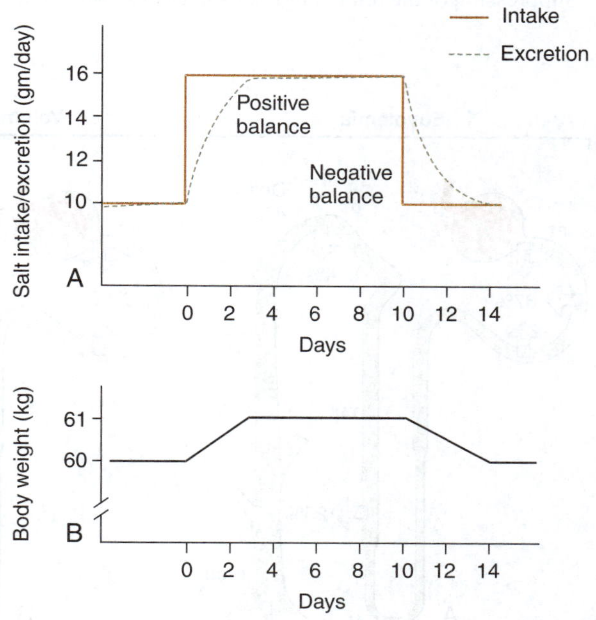

FIGURE 6.4-3 Effect of sudden increase and decrease in dietary salt intake on sodium and water balance: **A,** showing the positive and negative during adaptive period; and **B,** showing corresponding increase and decrease in body weight.

2. ***When the salt intake is abruptly decreased,*** the individual remains in a negative balance (intake < excretion) for 2–3 days. With negative balance, there occurs loss of water, which manifests as decrease in the body weight. After a period of adaptation, the daily urinary excretion of NaCl matches the amount ingested (Fig. 6.4-3).

Mechanism. The role of different regulatory mechanisms (described above) in controlling Na^+ excretion in different situations is described.

Regulation of Na^+ Excretion during Euvolaemia During euvolaemia, the kidneys match Na^+ excretion with intake simply by adjusting the reabsorption in the collecting duct. A change of about 2% in fractional excretion of Na^+ can produce more than 3 L of change in the volume of ECF. *Aldosterone* is the primary regulator of collecting duct Na^+ reabsorption.

As long as variations in dietary intake of NaCl are minor, this mechanism can regulate renal Na^+ excretion appropriately, and thereby maintain euvolaemia (Fig. 6.4-4 A, Table 6.4-5).

Regulation of Na^+ Excretion with Volume Expansion Volume expansion, i.e. a large increase in ECF volume and ECV, may occur following excessive salt intake or excessive administration of intravenous saline.

An increase in ECV (volume expansion), as detected by the vascular volume receptors, initiates a response that ultimately leads to increased sodium excretion by the following mechanisms (Fig. 6.4-5):

- Decreased renal sympathetic discharge,
- Suppression of the renin–angiotensin–aldosterone system,
- Increased ANP secretion from the atrial myocytes and
- Suppression of ADH release.

Renal response to the above signals, which results in increased Na^+ excretion, consists of (Fig. 6.4-4 B, Table 6.4-5):

- Increased glomerular filtration rate,
- Reduced Na^+ reabsorption in the proximal tubule (thus, glomerulotubular balance, as described on page 503, does not occur under this condition),
- Increased delivery of NaCl to the beginning of collecting duct (i.e. about 8%) and
- Decreased Na^+ reabsorption in the collecting duct.

In *summary,* the important difference between a situation of euvolaemia and volume expansion is that the renal response in the later involves the entire nephron and is not limited to the collecting duct as in the former.

Regulation of the Na^+ Excretion with Volume Contraction Volume contraction, i.e. a large decrease in ECF and ECV, may occur due to severe extra renal loss of NaCl, e.g. due to heavy sweating or diarrhoea. A decrease in ECV as detected by vascular volume sensors initiates a response that ultimately leads to decreased excretion by the following mechanisms, and the reverse effects to these are shown in Fig. 6.4-5:

- Increased renal sympathetic discharge,
- Stimulation of renin–angiotensin–aldosterone mechanism,
- Decreased ANP secretion from the atrial myocytes and
- Stimulation of ADH release.

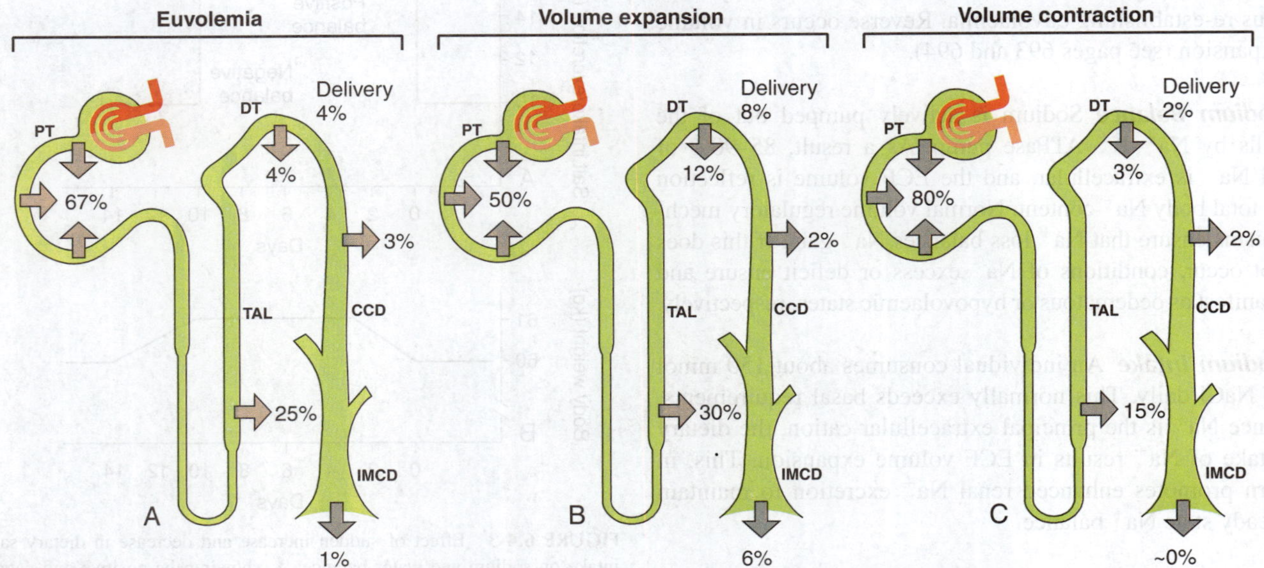

FIGURE 6.4-4 Segmental Na^+ reabsorption during: **A,** euvolaemia; **B,** volume expansion; and **C,** volume contraction. Note that the delivery of Na^+ to collecting duct in euvolaemia, volume expansion and volume contraction is 4, 8 and 2%, and Na^+ excretion, i.e. 1, 6 and 0%, respectively.

TABLE 6.4-5 Neural and Hormonal Signals Producing Different Renal Response in Euvolaemia, Volume Expansion and Volume Contraction

Signals	Euvolaemia	Volume expansion	Volume contraction
Neural signal			
• Renal sympathetic activity	N	↓	↑
Hormonal signal			
• Renin–angiotensin–aldosterone system activity	N	↓	↑
• ANP secretion	N	↑	↓
• ADH secretion	N	↓	↑
Renal response			
• GFR	N	↑	↓
• Na^+ reabsorption in proximal tubule	N (67%)	↓ (50%)	↑ (80%)
• Delivery of Na^+ to collecting duct	(4%)	↑ (8%)	↓ (2%)
• Na^+ excretion	(1%)	↑ (6%)	↓ (0)

N, normal; ↑ increased; and ↓ decreased.

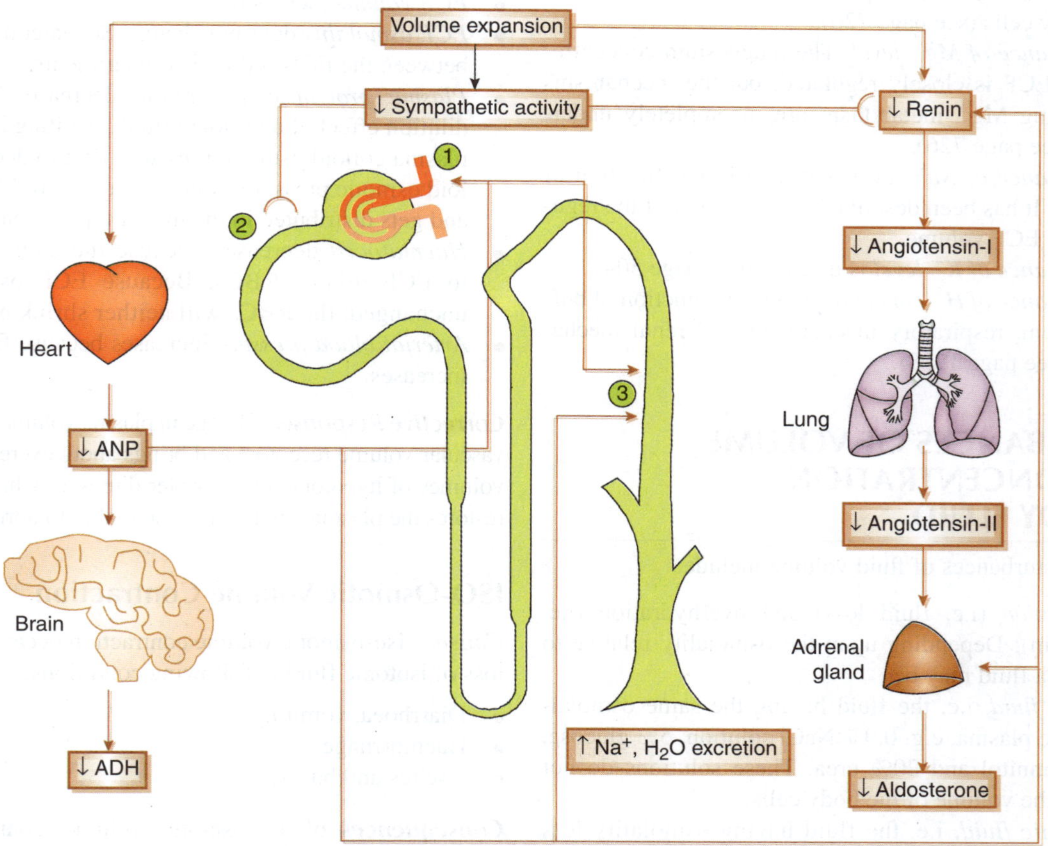

FIGURE 6.4-5 An integrated neural and humoral response to volume expansion: increased glomerular filtration rate (1); decreased sodium reabsorption in proximal tubule (2); and decreased sodium absorption in collecting duct (3). Note a response just reverse of the above occurs in response of volume contraction.

Renal response to the above signals, which results in decreased Na^+ excretion, consists of (Fig. 6.4-4 C and Table 6.4-5):

- Decreased glomerular filtration rate,
- Increased Na^+ reabsorption in the proximal tubule (Thus, G–T balance, as described on page 503 does not occur under this condition).
- Decreased delivery of NaCl to the beginning of collecting duct (i.e. about 2%), and increased Na^+ reabsorption in the collecting duct.

In *summary,* the important difference between a situation of euvolaemia and volume contraction is that the renal response in the later involves the entire nephron and is not limited to the collecting duct as in the former.

DEFENCE OF SPECIFIC ION COMPOSITION

The regulation of ion composition of extracellular fluid is the function of special regulatory mechanisms that maintain the level of these ions as:

- *Maintenance of ionized Ca^{2+} level* is governed by the feedback of Ca^{2+} on the parathyroids and the calcitonin secretory cells (see page 726).
- *Maintenance of Mg^+ level.* The magnesium concentration of ECF is closely regulated, but the mechanisms controlling Mg^+ metabolism are incompletely understood (see page 726).
- *Maintenance of Na^+ level* is primarily the function of kidneys. It has been described above as part of the regulation of ECF volume.
- *Maintenance of K^+ level* is discussed on page 504.
- *Maintenance of H^+ concentration* is the function of buffer system, respiratory mechanisms and renal mechanisms (see page 1228).

DISTURBANCES OF VOLUME AND CONCENTRATION OF BODY FLUID

Broadly, disturbances of fluid volume include:

- *Dehydration* (i.e. fluid loss) and overhydration (i.e. fluid gain): Depending upon the osmolality relative to plasma, a fluid may be:
- *Isotonic fluid,* i.e. the fluid having the same osmolality as the plasma, e.g. 0.9% NaCl solution, 5% glucose, 10% mannitol and 20% urea. These solutions do not change the volume of the body cells.
- *Hypotonic fluid,* i.e. the fluid having osmolality less than that of plasma, such solutions cause the cells to swell and if sufficiently dilute, to burst (lyse).
- *Hypertonic fluid,* i.e. the fluid having osmolality more than that of plasma, such solutions cause cells to shrink (i.e. to undergo crenation).

Disturbances of fluid volume and concentration can be classified as:

- Iso-osmotic volume expansion,
- Iso-osmotic volume contraction,
- Hyperosmotic volume expansion,
- Hyperosmotic volume contraction,
- Hypo-osmotic volume expansion and
- Hypo-osmotic volume contraction.

The causes, consequences and corrective responses of disturbances of volume and concentration in dehydration and over hydration are summarized in Table 6.4-6.

ISO-Osmotic Volume Expansion

Causes of iso-osmotic volume expansion include:

- Infusion of isotonic fluids, e.g. 0.9% NaCl solution.

Consequences of iso-osmotic volume expansion are (Fig. 6.4-6A):

- *ECF volume* increases.
- *ECF osmolality* does not change. So water does not shift between the ECF and ICF compartments.
- *Plasma protein* concentration decreases because of dilution effect of additional fluid, resulting in decreased plasma colloid osmotic pressure. Due to decreased colloid osmotic pressure, water moves out of blood vessels and gets distributed in the interstitial compartment.
- *Haematocrit* decreases because the addition of fluid to ECF dilutes RBCs. Because ECF osmolality is unchanged, the RBCs will neither shrink nor swell.
- *Arterial blood pressure* increases because ECF volume increases.

Corrective Response. Change in plasma volume is sensed by vascular volume receptors and brings about excretion of large volumes of hypotonic urine (water diuresis), which gradually restores the plasma volume and osmolality to normal.

ISO-Osmotic Volume Contraction

Causes. Iso-osmotic volume contraction occurs because of loss of isotonic fluid in following conditions:

- Diarrhoea, vomiting,
- Haemorrhage,
- Ascites and burns.

Consequences of iso-osmotic volume contraction are (Fig. 6.4-6B):

- *ECF volume* is decreased,

TABLE 6.4-6 Summary of Disturbances of Volume and Concentration of Body Fluids

Type of disturbance	Volume (L)		Osmolality (mOsm/L)		Causes	Consequences	Corrective response
	ICF	*ECF*	*ICF*	*ECF*			
Dehydration							
Iso-osmotic contraction	—	↓	— (Fig. 6.4-6B)	—	• Water loss due to: • Diarrhoea, • Vomiting, • Haemorrhage, • Burns and • Ascites	• Plasma protein concentration *increases* • Haematocrit increases • Arterial BP falls	Decrease plasma volume → inhibition of volume sensors → reflexly **restoration of plasma volume** due to decrease excretion of Na^+ and water ***Note.*** Thirst sensation is quenched by drinking isotonic salt solution
Hyperosmotic contraction	↓	↓	↑ (Fig. 6.4-6D)	↑	• Water loss due to: • Decreased water intake • Excessive sweating • Diabetes (mellitus and insipidus) • Alcoholism • Tracheostomy patients (if loss > 500 ml)	• Increase plasma protein concentration due to decreased ECF volume • Haematocrit increases	↑ ECF osmolality → stimulates osmoreceptors → decreased plasma volume → **restoration of plasma volume and osmolality** → inhibit volume receptors
Hypo-osmotic contraction	↑	↓	↓ (Fig. 6.4-6F)	↓	• Loss of NaCl or hypertonic fluid from body, e.g. vomiting • Adrenocortical insufficiency (Addison's disease)	• Increase plasma protein concentration causes increase oncotic pressure therefore, shift of fluid from plasma to interstitial fluid. • However in grave salt depletion plasma volume decreases. • Thirst is inhibited because thirst cells swell up • Haematocrit increases due to decreased ECF • Arterial BP decreases	• The ECF volume decreased but thirst is absent • Salt craving or salt appetite stimulates person to consume more NaCl → ECF osmolality restoration → shift of water from ICF to ECF → shrinkage of thirst centre cells → thirst stimulation → drinking of water → **normalization of plasma volume and osmolality**
Overhydration							
Iso-osmotic expansion	—	↑	— (Fig. 6.4-6A)	—	• Infusion of isotonic fluids (0.9% NaCl)	• Plasma protein concentration decreases • Haematocrit decreases • Arterial pressure increases (due to increase in ECF volume)	• Change in plasma volume sensed by volume receptors → excretion of large volume of hypotonic urine (water diuresis) → **normalisation of ECF volume**

Continued

TABLE 6.4-6 Summary of Disturbances of Volume and Concentration of Body Fluids—cont'd

Type of disturbance	Volume (L)		Osmolality (mOsm/L)		Causes	Consequences	Corrective response
	ICF	*ECF*	*ICF*	*ECF*			
Hyperosmotic expansion	↓ (Due to fluid shift from ICF to ECF)	↑	↑ (equalization with ECF) (Fig. 6.4-6C)	↑	• Administration of excessive amount of hypertonic saline	• Plasma protein concentration decreases • Haematocrit decreases • Arterial pressure increases (due to increase in ECF volume)	• Increase plasma osmolality promotes water retention • Increase in plasma volume • Thirst and ADH secretion is suppressed (increase *plasma volume oversides osmolality)* → excretion of excessive hypotonic urine → **plasma volume normalized** • ANP secretion increases → promote Na excretion → **osmolality normalized**
Hypo-osmotic expansion	↑ (shift of water from ECF to ICF)	↑ due to water retention)	↓ (Fig. 6.4-6E)	↓	• SIADH (syndrome of inappropriate ADH secretion) and • Ingestion of large volume of water	• Water shifts from ECF to ICF → decreased ICF osmolality • Plasma protein concentration decreases • Haematocrit remains unchanged (because water shifts from plasma into RBCs)	Vascular volume receptor sand osmoreceptors sense volume changes → excretion of large amount of hypotonic urine → **volume and osmolality normalized**

ICF = intracellular fluid; ECF = extracellular fluid; = increased; ¯ = decreased; — = no change.

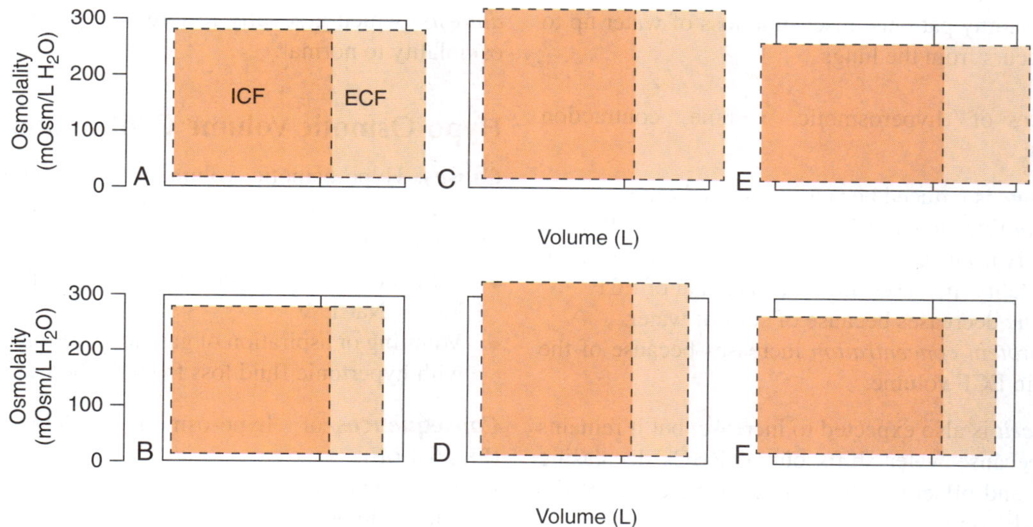

FIGURE 6.4-6 Showing volume and osmolality of ECF and ICF and shift of water between two compartments during disturbances of fluid volume; **A,** iso-osmotic volume expansion; **B,** iso-osmotic volume contraction; **C,** hyperosmotic volume expansion; **D,** hyperosmotic volume contraction; **E,** hypo-osmotic volume expansion; and **F,** hypo-osmotic volume contraction. Volume and osmolality of normal ECF and ICF are indicated by solid lines. Changes in volume and osmolality as consequences of various situations are indicated by dashed lines.

- *ECF osmolality* does not change. So, water does not shift between the ECF and ICF compartments.
- *Plasma protein* concentration is increased because loss of ECF concentrates the protein. Due to presence of plasma protein (which hold fluids), the plasma volume is less reduced compared with interstitial fluid.
- *Haematocrit* is increased because loss of ECF concentrates the RBCs. Because ECF osmolality is unchanged, the RBCs will neither shrink nor swell.
- *Arterial blood pressure* is decreased because of decrease in ECF volume.

Corrective Response. Decreased plasma volume inhibits the vascular volume sensors and reflexly restores the plasma volume by decreasing Na^+ and water excretion. It is important to note that the thirst produced by volume receptors is quenched with isotonic salt solution, instead of plain water.

Hyperosmotic Volume Expansion

Causes. Hyperosmotic volume expansion results when excessive amount of hypertonic saline is administered.

Consequences of hyperosmotic volume expansion (Fig. 6.4-6C):

- ECF osmolality is increased, because osmoles (NaCl) have been added to ECF.
- *Water shifts from ICF to ECF*. As a result of this shift, ICF osmolality increases until it equals that of ECF.
- *ECF volume* increases because of addition of fluid as well as shift of fluid from ICF to ECF (volume expansion).
- *ICF volume* is decreased due to fluid shift.
- *Plasma protein* concentration decreases because of the increase in ECF volume.
- *Haematocrit* decreases because of increase in ECF volume. RBCs shrink and ECF osmolality is increased.
- *Arterial blood pressure* is increased because of increase in ECF volume.

Corrective Response. Increased plasma osmolality promotes water retention, while an increase in plasma volume inhibits the same. Under such circumstances, volume oversides tonicity. Therefore, the increased plasma volume would suppress thirst and ADH, leading to excretion of large volume of hypotonic urine, which brings down the plasma volume. The natriuretic hormones, which are secreted only in response to osmolality and not to volume changes, promote Na^+ excretion and correct osmolality.

Hyperosmotic Volume Contraction

Causes. Hyperosmotic volume contraction occurs due to loss of water in following conditions:

- Decreased water intake,
- Diabetes mellitus,
- Diabetes insipidus,
- Excessive sweating in a desert,
- Alcoholism and

- In tracheostomy patients, insensible loss of water up to 500 ml occurs from the lungs.

Consequences of hyperosmotic volume contraction (Fig. 6.4-6D):

- *ECF volume* is reduced because of loss of water.
- *ECF osmolality* increases because more water is lost.
- *Water shifts from ICF to ECF*. As a result of this shift, ICF osmolality increases until it equals that of ECF.
- *ICF volume* decreases because of shift of water.
- *Plasma protein concentration* increases because of the decrease in ECF volume.

Haematocrit is also expected to increase, but it remains unchanged because water shifts out of RBCs decreasing their volume and offsetting the concentrating effect of the decreased ECF volume.

Corrective Response. Increased ECF osmolality stimulates the osmoreceptors, while reduced plasma volume inhibits the volume receptors. Either of them would reflexly restore the plasma volume and plasma osmolality to normal level.

Hypo-Osmotic Volume Expansion

Causes. Hypo-osmotic volume expansion occurs due to gain of water in the following conditions:

- Syndrome of inappropriate ADH (SIADH) secretion,
- Ingestion of large volume of water and
- Recto-colonic washouts with plain water.

Consequences (Fig. 6.4-6E)

- *ECF osmolality* decreases because of the excess water retention.
- *ECF volume* increases because of excess water retention.
- *Water shifts from ECF to ICF* increasing the volume of ICF.
- *ICF osmolality* decreases until it equals ECF osmolality.
- *Plasma protein concentration* decreases because of the increase in the ECF volume.
- *Haematocrit* might be expected to decrease, actually remains unchanged because water shifts into the RBCs, increasing their volume and offsetting the diluting effect of the gains of ECF volume.

Corrective Response. The vascular volume receptors and osmoreceptors sense the changes in plasma volume and osmolality, respectively. The signals from either of them lead to excretion of large amount of hypotonic urine (*water diuresis*) which gradually restores the plasma volume and osmolality to normal.

Hypo-Osmotic Volume Contraction

Causes. Hypo-osmotic volume contraction results from loss of NaCl or hypotonic fluid from the body in the following conditions:

- Adrenocortical insufficiency is associated with renal loss of NaCl
- Vomiting or aspiration of gastric secretions is associated with hypertonic fluid loss from the body.

Consequences of hypo-osmotic volume contraction (Fig. 6.4-6F):

- *ECF osmolality* is decreased because of loss of NaCl or other solutes
- *Water shifts from ECF to ICF*, increasing the volume of ICF and decreasing the ECF volume.
- *ICF osmolality* decreases until it equals ECF osmolality.
- *Plasma volume* and osmolality changes tend to parallel those of ECF. However, a decrease in plasma volume raises *plasma protein* concentration. Due to the raised colloid oncotic pressure, the shift of fluid from the plasma to interstitial fluid is decreased. Because of this, plasma volume is better preserved than is the volume of interstitial fluid. However, in severe cases (*grave salt deficiency syndrome*), the plasma volume reduces sufficiently to produce a shock-like state with signs of renal failure. But, unlike in shock there is no sensation of thirst, as explained:
  - *Cells of thirst centre* swell up due to shift of water from ECF to ICF. The thirst centre interprets this as the presence of excess water in the body. Consequently, thirst is inhibited.
  - *Haematocrit* increases because of the decrease in ECF volume and because the RBCs swell as a result of water entry.
  - *Arterial blood pressure* decreases because of the decrease in ECF volume.

Corrective Response. The ECF volume is decreased but thirst is absent; this seems to be nature's defence mechanism, since any water ingested would promptly leave the ECF and expand the ICF further. Therefore, salt craving or salt appetite which stimulates the individual to consume a large amount of NaCl is useful in restoring ECF osmolality. Normalization of ECF osmolality shifts water from ICF to ECF, leading to partial restoration of ECF volume shift of fluid from ICF to ECF which shrinks the cells of thirst centre and restores the thirst. Consequently, drinking of water restores the remaining deficit in ECF volume.

Chapter 6.5

Applied Renal Physiology Including Renal Function Tests

PATHOPHYSIOLOGY OF COMMON RENAL DISORDERS

The applied aspects of common renal disorders which need some elaboration are:

- Common urinary symptoms,
- Renal failure and
- Nephrotic syndrome.

Common Urinary Symptoms

Polyuria, Nocturia and Urinary Frequency. Normal urine output per day is 800–2500 ml. Therefore, a reasonable criterion to satisfy the definition of polyuria is excretion of 3.0 L of urine daily provided the patient is not on high fluid diet.

Nocturia means excessive amount of urine passed at night.

Urinary frequency means the increase in the number of times the patient goes for urination. Polyuria is differentiated from increased frequency by measuring the 24 h urine output.

Common causes of polyuria are:

I. *Physiological* (primary polydypsia or excessive water drinking), which can be
   - Psychogenic or
   - Drug-induced (chlorpromazine, anticholinergics).

II. *Pathological* (defective water conservation by the kidney):
   - Diabetes insipidus.
   - Solute diuresis, as in chronic renal failure, diabetes mellitus and mannitol infusion.
   - Natriuresis as occurs in salt losing nephropathy and effects of diuretics.

Dysuria and Urgency of Micturition. *Dysuria* refers to pain or burning during micturition. *Urgency of micturition* is the exaggerated sense or urge to micturate. It is due to either irritative or inflammatory disorders of the urinary bladder. This is often associated with increased frequency of urination.

Incontinence. This refers to inability to retain urine in the bladder. It results from neurological or mechanical disorders of the complicated system that controls normal micturition (see page 562).

Common causes of incontinence are:

- Neurogenic incontinence due to disturbances of neural control of micturition (see page 564),
- Stress incontinence, e.g. in postmenopausal parous women,
- Mechanical incontinence, e.g. damage to urethral sphincters following transurethral resection of prostate (TURP),
- Overflow incontinence, e.g. in obstruction due to benign prostatic enlargement,
- Psychogenic incontinence, as in anxious children and
- Functional incontinence is seen in very old persons who have mental derangement.

Enuresis refers to the involuntary passage of urine at night or during sleep. It is also called night bedwetting or nocturnal enuresis. It is normal in children up to 2–3 years of age. In some children it continues for long.

Oliguria refers to urine output less than 500 ml/day in an average adult. It invariably occurs in acute on chronic renal failure or acute renal failure.

Anuria is said to occur when the patient does not pass any urine or passes less than 50 ml of urine/day. In a physiological sense, the term anuria means less formation or absence of formation of urine by the kidney.

Common causes of anuria are:

- Complete urinary tract obstruction,
- Total bilateral renal arterial or venous occlusion,
- Bilateral renal cortical necrosis and
- Rapidly progressive acute glomerulonephritis.

Renal Failure

Renal failure refers to the deterioration of renal functions resulting in a decline in glomerular filtration rate (GFR) and rise in urea and non-nitrogenous substances in the blood. It is of two types:

- Acute renal failure and
- Chronic renal failure.

Acute Renal Failure Acute renal failure (ARF) refers to the sudden decline in GFR over a period of days or weeks associated with a rapid rise in blood urea.

Pathophysiology of Acute Renal Failure. Common causes of acute renal failure (ARF) can be grouped as:

1. *Prerenal causes* include:
   - Reduced blood supply to the kidneys. Normally, kidneys receive about 20–25% of the cardiac output (1100 ml/min). Decreased renal blood flow is usually accompanied by decreased GFR and reduced urinary output. When blood flow is reduced below the basal requirements (i.e. 20–25% less than normal renal blood flow), renal ischemia occurs causing damage to renal cells, particularly tubular epithelial cells. The common causes of reduced blood flow to kidney are severe haemorrhage, shock, severe burns, hypovolaemia, septicaemia, cardiac failure and so on.
2. *Intrarenal causes* include: acute glomerulonephritis and acute tubular necrosis
   - Acute glomerulonephritis is usually caused by an abnormal immune reaction, which causes damage to the glomeruli. In 95% of cases of glomerulonephritis, streptococcal infection involving other parts of body (tonsillitis or skin infection). The antibodies develop against the streptococcal antigen (within few weeks), react and form insoluble antigen–antibody complexes, which get deposited in the glomeruli and evoke an inflammatory reaction. The glomeruli get blocked and those which are not blocked, their permeability increases and allow leak of proteins and red cells from the glomerular capillaries into the glomerular filtrate. In severe cases, there is renal shutdown and this results in acute renal failure.
   - Acute tubular necrosis means destruction of tubular epithelial cells. Tubular necrosis occurs due to diminution of oxygen and nutrition to epithelial cells. Toxins, poisons and certain drugs also damage the tubular epithelium resulting in acute renal failure due to toxins or ischaemia.
3. *Obstructive causes* include urinary tract obstruction at any site.

Postrenal or obstructive renal failure occurs due to abnormalities of lower urinary tract which partially or completely blocks urinary flow (though renal blood flow is normal). If the urine output of only one kidney is blocked, no major changes occur in body fluids composition because the contralateral kidney undergoes compensation. The causes of postrenal acute renal failure include:

- Bilateral obstruction of ureters, or of renal pelvis, by large stones or blood clots and
- Bladder or urethral obstruction

Physiological effects of acute renal failure include:

i. Retention of salt and water, waste metabolites and electrolytes (rise in creatinine and urea) in blood and extracellular fluid can lead to oedema and hypertension.
ii. Excessive retention of potassium (hyperkalaemia) is a serious threat to a patient with acute renal failure.
iii. Kidneys are unable to excrete hydrogen ions resulting in metabolic acidosis and that itself is a fatal condition and also aggravates hyperkalaemia.
iv. In severe cases of acute renal failure, oliguria or complete anuria occurs and the patient may die unless kidney functions are restored.

Characteristic features of ARF include:

- No history of pre-existing renal disease,
- Presence of oliguria or anuria,
- Rapid rise in blood urea and creatinine levels and
- High urine osmolality (>400 mOsm/kg H_2O).

Management during the oliguria phase is directed with the sole aim of keeping the patient alive with appropriate measures till diuretic phase sets in:

1. *Medical management* consists of:
   - Maintenance of adequate water and electrolyte balance,
   - Control of infection,
   - Control of blood pressure,
   - Control of metabolic acidosis by I/V use of sodium bicarbonate, so that the bicarbonate levels are maintained around 18 mmol/dL.
   - Control of diet—protein, Na^+, K^+, Mg^+ and water. About 20–40 g of protein should be given per day to prevent endogenous breakdown of proteins.
2. *Dialysis* is frequently needed in cases with oliguria, hyperkalaemia, or acidosis or fluid overload (for details see page 556).

Chronic Renal Failure Chronic renal failure (CRF) refers to a slow, insidious, irreversible deterioration of renal functions resulting in the development of clinical syndrome of *uraemia*, manifested by excretory, metabolic, neurological, haematological and endocrinal abnormalities.

Common Causes which lead on to slow, progressive nephron loss and ultimately chronic renal failure can be grouped as under:

1. ***Congenital disorders,*** e.g. polycystic kidney.
2. ***Vascular diseases of kidney,*** renal hypertension. Injury to renal vasculature can lead to renal ischemia. The most common cause of renal vascular injury is atherosclerosis. Atherosclerosis of the larger renal arteries leads to hypertension and involvement of smaller arteries (interlobular arteries and efferent arterioles) results in thickening of vessel walls due to deposits of fibrinoid tissue (nephrosclerosis), eventually leading to constriction (ischemic injury).
3. ***Glomerular diseases,*** e.g. proliferative glomerulonephritis and diabetic nephropathy. Chronic glomerulonephritis: injury to glomeruli can be caused by several diseases. In most cases, it begins with accumulation of antigen–antibody complexes in the glomerular membrane and ultimately glomeruli are replaced by fibrous tissue, therefore unable to filter the fluid. Therefore, glomerular capillary filtration coefficient gets markedly reduced.
4. ***Tubulointerstitial disease,*** e.g. chronic pyelonephritis and analgesic nephropathy. These diseases are referred to as interstitial nephritis. Injury to renal interstitium can be caused by bacterial infection (called as pyelonephritis) or as a result of vascular, glomerular and tubular damage by poison and toxic drugs.
5. ***Obstructive renal diseases,*** e.g. benign enlargement of prostate, renal calculi and ureteral constriction.

Pathophysiology of Chronic Renal Failure. Chronic renal failure, like acute renal failure, also occurs in a wide variety of diseases, but the end result is reduction of functional nephrons and deterioration of the kidney function to the point, where the patient must be placed on dialysis treatment or transplanted with a functional kidney for survival. This condition is referred as *end-stage renal disease (ESRD).*

The exact mechanism of this stage is not well understood, but a slowly progressing vicious cycle due to renal adaptive changes may be responsible (Fig. 6.5-1).

Acute versus chronic renal failure. Differentiating features of acute and chronic renal failure are summarized in Table 6.5-1.

Treatment

I. *Medical management* consists of:
   a. Treat, if the cause is reversible, e.g. hypertension, urinary tract obstruction, etc.
   b. Nephrotoxic drugs to be avoided.
   c. Measures to limit the adverse effects of uraemia and to prevent further progression include:
      - Control of infection,
      - Control of hypertension,
      - Control of diet as regards proteins, Na^+, K^+, water and Mg^+ content,
      - Control of anaemia,
      - Control of metabolic acidosis and
      - Maintenance of electrolyte and water balance.

II. *Dialysis* and *renal transplantation* is frequently needed (see page 556).

Nephrotic Syndrome

Nephrotic syndrome refers to massive proteinuria (more than 3.5 g/day), mainly albuminuria and its associated consequences which include:

- Hypoalbuminaemia,
- Oedema,
- Hyperlipidaemia,

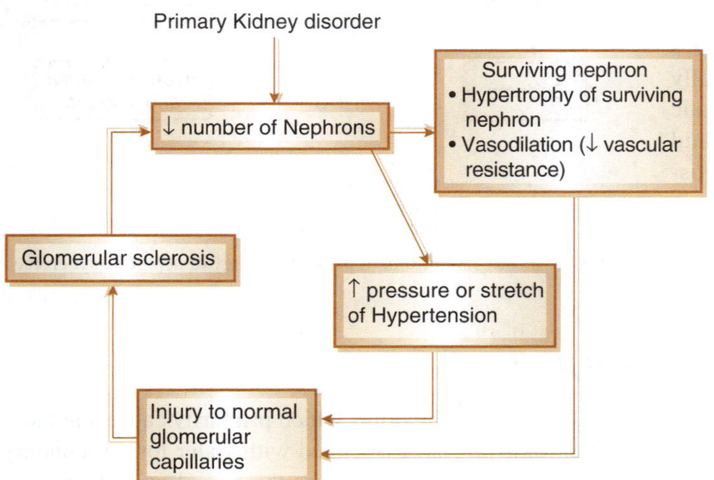

FIGURE 6.5-1 Flow diagram depicting sequence of event in pathophysiology of chronic renal failure.

TABLE 6.5-1 Distinguishing Features of Acute and Chronic Renal Failure

Feature	Acute renal failure	Chronic renal failure
Onset	Sudden over days or to weeks	Gradual, over months or years
Reversibility	Invariably reversible	Usually irreversible
Causes	May be prerenal	Mostly renal or postrenal but may be extrarenal
Urinary volume	Oliguria and anuria	Polyuria and nocturia
Signs and symptoms of uraemia	Of recent onset	Of more than 3 months duration
Characteristic features	Of acute reduction in GFR, e.g. oedema, hypertension, salt and water retention	Of chronicity, i.e. uraemic symptoms of long duration, small-sized kidneys, anaemia, hypertension and so on
Renal failure casts (broad casts) in urine	Absent	Present
Specific gravity of urine	High	Low and fixed
Past history of renal disease	Absent	Present
Dialysis	Required for short period	Repeated chronic maintenance dialysis required
Renal transplantation	Usually not required	Usually is the final answer

- Lipiduria and
- Hypercoagulability.

Pathophysiology. A wide variety of disease processes including immunological disorders, toxic injuries, metabolic abnormalities, biochemical defects and vascular disorders involving glomeruli contribute to development of the nephrotic syndrome. The sequence of events involved in pathophysiology of the nephrotic syndrome is summarized in Fig. 6.5-2.

Minimal change nephrotic syndrome is a condition in which there is no abnormality of the glomerular capillary membrane. Minimal change nephropathy is associated with loss of normal negative charges from the basement of the glomerular membrane resulting in easy passage of albumin. Normally, negative charges in the basement membrane repel negatively charged plasma protein molecules. Incidence of minimal change nephropathy in children between ages 2–6 years is more. Plasma protein concentration usually falls below 2 g/L, leading to a decrease in colloidal osmotic pressure (<10 mmHg). Therefore, a large amount of fluid leaks out from the capillaries all over the body into the tissue, causing oedema

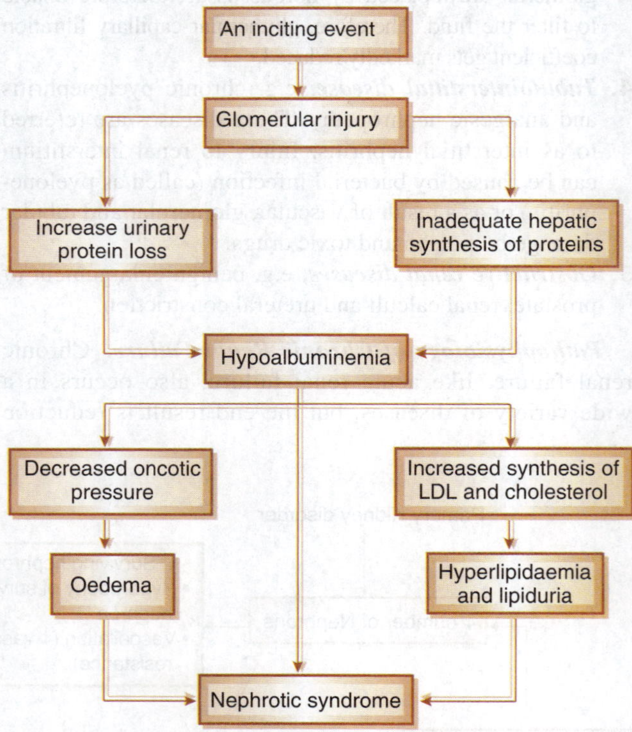

FIGURE 6.5-2 Algorithm of pathophysiology of nephrotic syndrome.

Specific Tubular Disorders

There are many tubular disorders due to abnormal transport of individual or groups of substances through the tubular epithelial membrane. These disorders mainly occur due to an absence of enzyme, deficient or mutations of genes encoding carrier proteins required for transport. The specific tubular disorders are summarized in Table 6.5-2.

DIURETICS

The diuretics are the drugs which primarily cause a net loss of Na^+ (*natriuresis*) associated with water loss (secondary to natriuresis) and thus increase the rate of urine flow.

TABLE 6.5-2 Specific Tubular Disorders, Their Causes and Effects

Tubular disorder	Cause	Effect
1. Renal glycosuria	Tubular transport mechanism of glucose is limited or absent	• Blood–glucose level: normal • Renal excretion of glucose: greatly increases
2. Amino acid uria	Rare condition, occurs due to deficiency of specific carrier proteins for cystine, glycine and beta-amino-isobutyric acid	• Essential cystinuria → cystine stone (renal stone) due to crystallization • βeta amino-isobutyricaciduria and • Glycinuria
3. Renal phosphatemia	Failure to absorb phosphate	• Long-standing low level of phosphate leads to reduced calcification of bones resulting in rickets • Rickets is refractory to vitamin D therapy
4. Renal tubular acidosis	Hereditary disorder, failure to secrete H^+	• Loss of $NaHCO_3^-$ in the urine leading to continued state of metabolic acidosis
5. Nephrogenic diabetes insipidus	Deficiency of vasopressin receptors or renal tubules do not respond to ADH	• Water diuresis leading to • Dehydration
6. Fanconi syndrome	A generalized reabsorptive defect	In severe cases leads to: • ↓ Excretion of all amino acids • ↓ Absorption of HCO_3^- leading to metabolic acidosis • ↑ Excretion of potassium and calcium • Nephrogenic diabetes insipidus
7. Bartter's syndrome	Autosomal recessive disorder, occurs due to defect in: • 1sodium–2chloride–1potassium cotransporter or • K^+ channels on luminal surface or • Cl^- channels on basolateral membrane of thick ascending loop of Henle	• ↑ Urinary excretion of Na^+ and water ↓ Water depletion leads to activation of renin–angiotensin–aldosterone system ↓ Stimulate K^+ and H^+ secretion in collecting duct ↓ Hypokalaemia and metabolic alkalosis
8. Gitelman's syndrome	An autosomal recessive disorder due to thiazide-sensitive sodium chloride cotransporter	• Effects are same as of Bartter's syndrome
9. Liddle's syndrome	An autosomal dominant disorder due to mutations in amiloride sensitive epithelial sodium channel (ENaC) in distal and collecting tubule	• Excessive activity of ENaC causing ↑ reabsorption of Na^+ and H_2O leading to hypertension and metabolic alkalosis

Classification Depending upon their efficacy, the diuretic drugs can be classified as:

1. ***High efficacy diuretics*** (inhibitors of Na^+–K^+–$2Cl^-$ transport), also called loop diuretics, e.g.
   - Furosemide,
   - Bumetanide and
   - Ethacrynic acid.
2. ***Medium efficacy diuretics*** (inhibitors of Na^+–Cl^- symport)
   - Thiazide diuretics, e.g. chlorothiazide, hydrochlorothiazide and benzthiazide and
   - Thiazide-like, e.g. metolazone.
3. ***Weak or adjunctive diuretics***
   - Carbonic anhydrase inhibitors, e.g. acetazolamide,
   - Potassium sparing diuretics, e.g. spironolactone, triamterene and amiloride,
   - Osmotic diuretics, e.g. mannitol, isosorbide and glycerol and
   - Xanthines, e.g. theophylline.

Site of Action, Mechanism of Action and Major Effects

Site of Action. The different sites of a nephron, where the diuretics act are (Table 6.5-3):

1. ***Proximal tubule.*** Diuretics acting on proximal tubules have limited efficacy since the thick ascending loop (TAL), which has a great reabsorptive property compensates for any decrease in Na^+ and H_2O reabsorption that might occur in proximal tubule.
2. ***Thick ascending loop (TAL).*** Diuretics acting on TAL are called loop diuretics. They abolish the urine

TABLE 6.5-3 Site of Action, Mechanism of Action and Major Effects of Various Classes of Diuretics

Class of diuretic	Site of action	Mechanism of action	Major effects	Other effects	K^+ depletion	Acidosis/ alkalosis
High efficacy diuretics Loop diuretics, e.g. • Furosemide • Bumetanide • Ethacrynic acid	TAL	Inhibition of Na^+–K^+–$2Cl^-$	↑ NaCl excretion ↑ K^+ excretion ↑ Ca^{2+} excretion ↓ Ability to concentrate urine ↓ Ability to dilute urine	↑ Venous capacitance by venodilatation	Yes	Alkalosis
Medium efficacy diuretics Thiazide diuretics, e.g. • Chlorothiazide • Hydrochlorothiazide	Early distal tubule	Inhibition of Na^+–Cl^- symport	↑ NaCl excretion ↑ K^+ excretion ↓ Ca^{2+} excretion ↓ Ability to dilute urine	Antihypertensive	Yes	Alkalosis
Weak or adjunctive diuretics						
i. Carbonic anhydrase inhibitor, e.g. • Acetazolamide	Proximal tubule	Inhibition of carbonic anhydrase	↑ HCO_3^- excretion	↓ Formation of aqueous humour (antiglaucoma drug)	Yes	Acidosis
ii. Potassium sparing diuretics, e.g. • Spironolactone • Triamterene • Amiloride	Late distal tubule and collecting duct	Inhibition of Na^+ reabsorption, inhibition of K^+ secretion	↑ Na^+ excretion ↓ K^+ excretion ↓ H^+ excretion	–	No	Acidosis
iii. Osmotic diuretics, e.g. • Mannitol • Isosorbide	Proximal tubule	Retain water iso-osmotically and inhibits NaCl reabsorption	↑ Na^+ excretion ↑ K^+ excretion ↑ Cl^- excretion	–	Yes	Acidosis

concentrating ability of the nephron and, therefore, are also classified as high efficacy diuretics.

3. ***Early distal convoluted tubule.*** Thiazide diuretics act on this cortical diluting segment and have medium efficacy, because only a small part of the filtered solute load reaches this part of the tubule.
4. ***Late distal convoluted tubule and collecting duct.*** Various K^+ sparing diuretics act on this site. These diuretics have weak efficacy.

Mechanism of Action and Major Effects of the diuretics are summarized in Table 6.5-3.

(i) Osmotic Diuretics such as urea, mannitol and sucrose are not easily absorbed by the renal tubules. The increased concentration of osmotically active molecules cause an increase in osmotic pressure resulting in reduced water reabsorption. Therefore, a large amount of tubular fluid is excreted. In diabetes mellitus, polyuria is an example of osmotic diuresis. (see page 522)

(ii) Loop Diuretics (such as furosemide, ethacrynic acid and bumetanide) decrease the active transport of sodium–chloride–potassium reabsorption by blocking 1 sodium–2 chloride–1 potassium cotransporter at luminal surface of epithelial cells of thick ascending limb of loop of Henle

(iii) Thiazide Diuretics include thiazide derivatives such as chlorothiazide and hydrochlorothiazide. They inhibit sodium-chloride reabsorption by blocking sodium–chloride cotransporter in luminal membrane of early distal tubular cells.

(iv) Carbonic Anhydrase Inhibitors, e.g. acetazolamide inhibits sodium bicarbonate reabsorption in the proximal tubule (mainly) and collecting duct by inhibiting the action of the enzyme carbonic anhydrase. As H^+ secretion and HCO_3^- reabsorption is coupled to sodium reabsorption through sodium–hydrogen ion counter transport (see page 497). Increased concentration of sodium and bicarbonate in tubular fluids acts as osmotic diuresis. The carbonic anhydrase inhibitors cause some degree of acidosis due to loss of $HCO^-{}_3$ in the urine.

(v) Potassium Sparing Diuretics, e.g. spironolactone and eplerenone are mineralocorticoid receptor antagonists, which act as competitive inhibitors of aldosterone for receptors present on the epithelial cells in cortical collecting ducts and can decrease reabsorption of sodium and secretion of potassium. Therefore, sodium remains in tubules causing osmotic diuresis.

(vi) Sodium Channel Blockers like amiloride and triamterene inhibit sodium reabsorption and potassium secretion by blocking sodium channels present on the luminal membrane of epithelial cells of the collecting duct.

Other Substances which Act as Diuretics. In addition to the above described drugs, following other substances also act as diuretics, e.g.

- *Water*. It acts by inhibiting ADH secretion.
- *Alcohol*. It also acts by inhibiting ADH secretion.
- *Glucose* (e.g. in diabetes mellitus). It acts as osmotic diuretic.
- *Caffeine*. It increases GFR and probably decreases renal tubular Na^+ reabsorption.

RENAL FUNCTION TESTS

Renal function tests are carried out to assess the functional capacity of the kidneys. The main aim of these tests in clinical medicine is the detection of renal impairment as early as possible in its course and the quantitative measure of change in function with time. However, it must be remembered that about two-thirds of renal tissue must be functionally damaged to show any abnormality by these tests. Renal function tests can be divided into the following groups:

- Analysis of urine,
- Analysis of blood,
- Renal clearance tests,
- Radiology and renal imaging and
- Renal biopsy.

Analysis of Urine

Analysis of urine helps, of course, to a limited degree, to assess kidney functioning. In patients with suspected renal disorder, the urine analysis should be performed for volume, specific gravity, osmolality, pH, abnormal constituents, microscopic examination and bacteriological finding.

1. Volume. Normal urine output per day is 800–2500 ml. Abnormalities of urine volume include polyuria, oliguria and anuria (see page 544).

2. Colour. The normal light yellow colour of the urine is due to the presence of urochrome pigment (a compound of urobilin and urobilinogen with peptide). On standing, the colour deepens due to oxidation of uribilinogen into urobilin. Abnormalities of urine colour include:

- *Brownish-yellow,* due to presence of conjugated bilirubin in patients with hepatic and posthepatic jaundice.
- *Cloudy appearance* is seen in strongly alkaline urine due to precipitation of calcium phosphate and due to precipitation of urates.
- *Frothy appearance* is indicative of proteinuria.
- *Red–dark brown* tinge of urine is seen in porphyria.

3. Osmolality and Specific Gravity. Normal urinary osmolality varies from 50 to 1200 mOsm/kg and specific gravity from 1.003 to 1.030, depending upon the state of hydration of the body. If the early morning urine sample after an overnight fast has an osmolality of >600 mOsm/kg H_2O (and specific gravity > 1.018), then the patient has a normal urine concentrating ability. Certain abnormalities are:

- Fixed urinary osmolality of 300 mOsm/kg H_2O (specific gravity 1.010) is an evidence of fairly advanced urinary failure.
- Persistently low urinary osmolality (<100 mOsm/kg H_2O) even after 8 h of fluid deprivation is diagnostic of diabetes insipidus.

4. Urine pH. Normal pH of urine varies from 4.5 to 8.0. Urine is normally slightly acidic, except for a short postprandial alkaline tide. Intake of high protein nonvegetarian diet shifts the urinary pH towards the acidic side, while vegetarian diet shifts it towards the alkaline side.

Causes of abnormal pH include:

- Infection with urea-splitting organisms raises the pH and
- Impairment of tubular acidification.

5. Chemical Analysis for Abnormal Urinary Constituents may reveal:

i. Proteinuria. Normally, up to 150 mg of proteins are excreted daily in urine (see page 498). Excretion of >150 mg/day of protein is called proteinuria. Depending upon the cause, proteinuria may be of following types:

- ***Mild transient proteinuria*** occurs in congestive heart failure, high fever and severe anaemia.
- ***Orthostatic proteinuria*** occurs after prolonged walking or standing, in some otherwise healthy individuals.
- ***Glomerular proteinuria*** occurs in diseases in which permeability of glomerular membrane is increased. Massive glomerular proteinuria is seen in nephrotic syndrome. Other causes of glomerular proteinuria are acute glomerulonephritis, pyelonephritis and toxaemia of pregnancy.
- ***Tubular proteinuria*** occurs in conditions in which tubular reabsorption of low molecular weight proteins (which are normally filtered by glomeruli) is impaired, e.g. tubulointerstitial disorders and Fanconi's syndrome.

ii. Glycosuria refers to presence of glucose in the urine. Glycosuria may be due to diabetes mellitus, renal disorders (renal glycosuria) or GIT disorder (alimentary glycosuria). Other sugars like galactose and fructose may also be present in urine in certain inborn errors of metabolism.

iii. Ketonuria refers to presence of ketone bodies (acetoacetic acid, β hydroxybutyric acid and acetone) in the urine. Ketonuria occurs in patients suffering from ketosis due to severe diabetes mellitus or prolonged starvation.

iv. Bilirubinuria refers to appearance of bilirubin in the urine in patients with elevated conjugated bilirubin levels, in hepatic or posthepatic jaundice. Normally, 1–3.5 mg of urobilinogen is excreted daily in the urine. Its excessive excretion in the urine is one of the characteristic features of haemolytic jaundice.

v. Haemoglobinuria, i.e. presence of haemoglobin in the urine, indicates intravascular haemolysis, as seen in blackwater fever, due to falciparum malarial infection.

vi. Porphobilinogen appears in urine in acute intermittent porphyria. This is not detected in fresh voided urine but gives a red–brown colour (Burgundy wine) to urine on standing for some time.

vii. Haematuria, i.e. presence of blood in the urine is seen in acute glomerulonephritis, renal stone disease and in malignancy of the urinary tract. Urine becomes reddish in colour in gross haematuria.

viii. Aminoaciduria occurs in a variety of congenital tubular disorders.

6. Microscopic Examination. Examination of centrifuged sediment of urine may show casts, cells and crystals.

i. Casts are proteinaceous plugs formed by coagulation of Tamm–Horsfall protein within the renal tubules and washed out by the flow of tubular fluid. They have cylindrical shapes, broken ends and various shapes corresponding to the tubule in which the formed casts may be cellular or noncellular.

In cellular casts, certain cells are coagulated with the protein material. Cellular casts include:

- ***Red cell casts*** are typically seen in acute glomerulonephritis.
- ***Leucocytic casts*** are a feature of acute bacterial pyelonephritis.
- ***Epithelial casts*** made of tubular epithelial cells are present in acute tubular necrosis (ATN).
- ***Fatty casts*** containing epithelial cells laden with fat drops are seen in nephrotic syndrome.
- ***Noncellular casts*** are hyaline and granular casts.

ii. Crystals are usually present in normal urine and thus have no pathological significance. Commonly seen are crystals of calcium oxalate, calcium phosphate, calcium ammonium–magnesium phosphate (triple phosphate) or uric acid. Uric acid crystals and cysteine crystals, when present in large amounts have some diagnostic significance.

iii. Cells found on microscopic examination may be RBCs, leucocytes, tubular epithelial cells and squamous epithelial cells.

7. Bacteriological Examination of Urine. The midstream sample of urine is examined for pus cells and bacteria. Bacteriuria and pyuria indicate urinary tract infection.

Analysis of Blood

Estimation of blood levels of the substances that are excreted by the kidneys throws some light on the functional status of kidney, although these tests are less sensitive than clearance tests.

1. Blood Urea level (normal 20–40 mg%) is an index of glomerular function. The blood urea levels begin to rise after about 50% glomerular damage has occurred.

2. Plasma Creatinine Concentration (normal 0.6–1.5 mg%) is more reliable than blood urea, as the latter is subjected to variations by dietary proteins, hydration and tissue breakdown. The relationship between GFR and serum creatinine levels depicts that GFR must fall to about 50% of its normal value before a significant increase in serum creatinine occurs (Fig. 6.5-3). Therefore, a normal serum creatinine level does not necessarily mean that all is well with the kidney.

> ***Note.*** Cystatin C, a member of the superfamily of cysteine protease inhibitors, is produced by nucleated cells. The production of cystatin C is not affected by diet or nutrition status. Hence, it is a more sensitive marker of renal function than creatinine. Even minor changes in GFR in the early stages of chronic renal diseases are associated with increased cystatin C (normal range is 0.8–1.2 mcg/dL).

3. Serum Proteins Levels. (Normal: total protein 6.7–8 g%; albumin 3–5 g%; globulins 2–3 g% and A/G ratio 1.7:1) are reduced if there is significant proteinuria with renal failure. In nephrotic syndrome, the albumin levels decrease and globulin levels increase, leading to reversal of A/G ratio.

4. Serum Cholesterol Levels (normal 150–200 mg%) are increased in nephrotic syndrome.

5. Serum Electrolyte levels (normal: Na^+, 152 mEq/L; K^+, 5 mEq/L; Ca^{2+}, 9–11 mg%; PO_4^{3-}, 3–4.5 mg%;

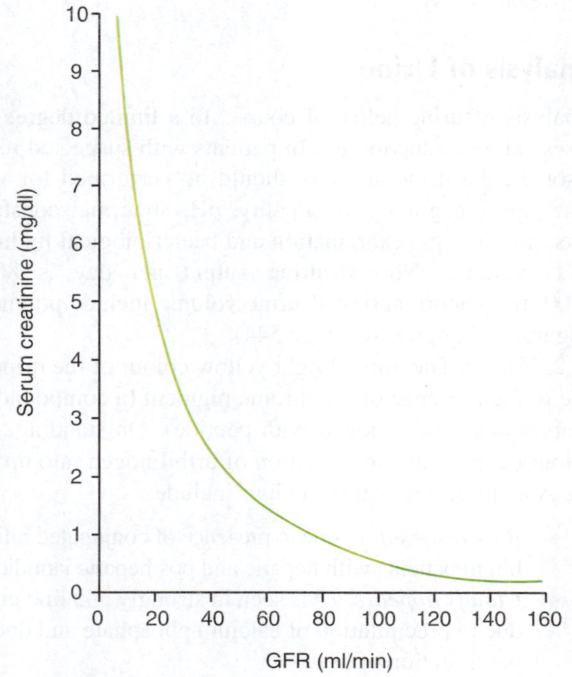

FIGURE 6.5-3 Relationship between plasma creatinine concentration and glomerular filtration rate.

SO_4^{2-}, 0.5–1.5 mEq/L; and Mg^{2+}, 1.5–2.5 mEq/L) are of value in a variety of renal disorders. For example, chronic renal failure is mostly accompanied by high potassium and phosphate but low sodium and calcium levels in blood.

Renal Clearance Tests

The term 'renal clearance' is related to the ability of the kidneys to clear out the plasma of various substances. The concept of renal clearance can be applied to any substance that is present in the blood and is excreted in the urine. *The renal clearance can be defined as the volume of plasma that is cleared of a substance in 1 min by excretion of the substance in the urine.* It is a 'virtual volume'. The unit of renal clearance (*C*) is ml/min, and is calculated from the following formula:

$$C = \frac{UV}{P}, \text{ where}$$

C = renal clearance, U = urine concentration of the substance, V = rate of flow of urine and P = plasma concentration of the substance.

Principles Governing Renal Clearance of a substance, described on page 494, are summarized briefly:

- Substances that are freely filtered, but neither reabsorbed nor secreted (e.g. *inulin*), have renal clearance rate equal to GFR, and hence are called glomerular markers.
- Substances that are freely filtered, but are partially reabsorbed in the tubules have renal clearance rate less than GFR.
- Substances that are freely filtered, but are completely reabsorbed (e.g. Na^+, glucose, amino acids, Cl^- and HCO_3^-) have the lowest renal clearance rate.
- Substances that are filtered and also secreted by the tubules but not reabsorbed (e.g. *PAH* and Diotrast) have the highest renal clearance rate. Such substances are thus entirely excreted by a single passage of blood through kidneys. Clearance of such substances represents the range of blood flow.

Renal Clearance as Kidney Function Test. Renal clearance of a substance is correlated more directly with the status of kidney function. It shows a deviation from normal (earlier) in the course of renal damage.

Renal clearance tests, therefore, can be employed to assess the different functions of a nephron, e.g.

- To assess glomerular filtration,
- To assess tubular secretory capacity,
- To assess renal plasma flow (RPF) and renal blood flow (RBF) and
- To assess 'osmotic' and 'free water' clearance ability.

Renal Clearance Tests to Measure GFR

Glomerular filtration rate can be accurately measured by renal clearance of inulin, urea and creatinine. In practice, however, measurement of clearance for the substances already present in the blood is preferred. Further, the renal clearance tests are not commonly employed in the clinical practice. The plasma levels of urea and creatinine are used as indicators of glomerular function.

1. Inulin Clearance Test Inulin is a dye (chemically a fructopolysaccharide) with molecular weight 5200 that does not exist naturally in the body. It is found in roots of certain plants. Inulin clearance (C_{in}) is a measure of GFR because the volume of plasma completely cleared of inulin per unit time equals the volume of plasma filtered per unit time. Inulin clearance gives the measure of GFR because of its following characteristics:

- It is freely filtered by the glomeruli and neither reabsorbed nor secreted by the tubules,
- It is biologically inert and nontoxic,
- It is neither metabolized nor stored in the kidney and
- Its concentration can be easily estimated in the laboratory.

Method. To perform this test, a single bolus dose of inulin is injected intravenously, which is followed by a continuous intravenous infusion at a rate which compensates for its loss in urine. This endurance is important to achieve a fairly constant level of the plasma concentration of inulin. The inulin clearance (C_{in}) and thus, the GFR is then calculated from the values of urine concentration of inulin (U_{in}) 35 mg/ml, urine flow rate (V) is 0.9 ml/min and plasma concentration of inulin (P_{in}) 0.25 mg/ml, as:

$$C_{inulin} \text{ (or GFR)} = \frac{U_{in}V}{P_{in}}$$

$$GFR = 35 \times 0.9/0.25 = 126 \text{ ml/min}$$

Clinical Applications (Significance) of Inulin Clearance. In addition to its use as a measure of GFR, the inulin clearance rate is also used as ***an indicator of plasma clearance mechanisms***. A comparison of the clearance of a given substance (C_x) with the clearance of inulin (C_{in}) provides information about the renal transport processes used to remove the substance from the plasma (Fig. 6.5-4):

i. ***When C_x equals C_{in}***, i.e. when clearance ratio is one [ratio of clearance of ~ given substance (C_x) and clearance of inulin (C_{in})], such a substance has characteristics similar to the inulin, i.e. it is only filtered by glomeruli and neither reabsorbed nor secreted by the tubules. Further, the mass of such a substance excreted in the urine per unit time ($U_x.V$) equals the mass of the substance filtered during the same time (GFR P_x), i.e.

$$U_x.V = C_{in}.P_x \text{ (or GFR)} = C_{in}$$

Examples of substances with clearance ratio close to 1 are: mannitol, sorbitol, ferricyanide, Vitamin B_{12} and sucrose. Although inulin is used most commonly,

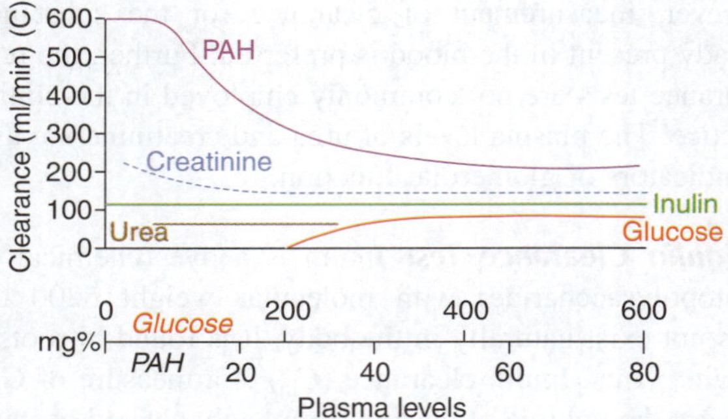

FIGURE 6.5-4 Clearance of various substances plotted against their plasma concentration.

however, these substances can also be used to measure GFR.

ii. ***When C_x is less than C_{in}***, i.e. clearance ratio (C_x/C_{in}) is less than 1. Such substances with clearance below that for inulin (Fig. 6.5-4), are filtered and reabsorbed, i.e. excretion is by filtration and reabsorption. *Examples* of substances with clearance ratio <1 are glucose, xylose and fructose.

iii. ***When C_x is greater than C_{in}***, i.e. when clearance ratio (C_x/C_{in}) is more than 1. Such substances with clearance above that of inulin (Fig. 6.5-4) are filtered and secreted, i.e. excretion is by filtration and secretion. Examples of substances with clearance ratio more than 1 are para-aminohippuric acid (PAH) and phenol red.

2. Creatinine Clearance Test Though the creatinine clearance test is less accurate than the inulin clearance test for measurement of GFR, in clinical practice the former is preferred over the latter because the latter is more cumbersome as it requires a continuous intravenous infusion. Creatinine is an endogenous substance (a by-product of muscle metabolism) having a fairly constant plasma value (P) of about 0.6–1.5 mg/dL. It is filtered by the glomeruli and only marginally secreted by the tubules. The value of creatinine clearance is close to GFR; hence its measurement is a fairly good method of measuring GFR.

Method. In the traditional method, creatinine content of 24 h urine collection and the plasma concentration in a sample collected at midpoint of the urinary collection period are estimated. The creatinine clearance (C) is then calculated by the usual formula:

$$C_{cr} = \frac{U_{cr}V}{P_{cr}}$$

Normal Value of creatinine clearance ranges from 80–110 ml/min in an adult and declines with age in healthy individuals. Because creatinine clearance is an index of GFR, it reflects the normal decline in GFR with age, although plasma creatinine concentration remains constant because of decreased muscle mass.

Sometimes, it is difficult to collect urine for measuring creatinine clearance. In such cases, the approximate GFR changes can be obtained by plasma concentration of creatinine, which is inversely proportional to GFR

$GFR = C_{cr} = U_{cr} \times V/P_{cr}$ where

C_{cr} = Creatinine clearance,

U_{cr} = Urine concentration of creatinine and

P_{cr} = Plasma concentration of creatinine.

Creatinine Clearance as Kidney Function Test in Disease. As shown in Fig. 6.5-3, the plasma creatinine concentration varies inversely with GFR and the product of GFR and plasma creatinine concentration is constant. Thus, a fall in GFR may be the earliest clinical sign of renal disease (i.e. a decline in functional renal mass).

3. Urea Clearance Test Urea is the end product of protein metabolism. After being filtered by the glomeruli, it is partly reabsorbed by the renal tubules. Hence, urea clearance is less than the GFR, and further, it is influenced by the protein content of the diet. For these reasons, urea clearance is not as sensitive as creatinine clearance for assessing renal function. Despite this fact, several laboratories traditionally use this test.

Method. At the beginning of the test, the patient is asked to completely empty the bladder by voiding the urine and the exact time is recorded. Exactly after 1 h, the patient is asked to void again and the quantity of urine is exactly measured. The levels of urea are estimated in the urine and the blood sample collected at the midpoint of the test. Since the urea clearance drastically changes when the volume of urine is less than 2 ml/min, so two empirical indices have been developed to calculate the urea clearance, which are called the maximal urea clearance and standard urea clearance.

i. *Maximal urea clearance* ($C_{urea(m)}$) is calculated from the usual formula. This is applicable when the urine output is more than 2 ml/min.

$$\text{Maximum urea clearance} = \frac{U \times V}{P}, \text{ where}$$

U = Urea concentration in urine (mg/ml),
V = Volume of urine excreted (ml/min) and
P = Urea concentration in plasma (mg/ml).

ii. *Standard urea clearance* ($C_{urea(s)}$). When the volume of urine is less than 2 ml/min, the standard urea clearance ($C_{urea(s)}$) is calculated by a modified formula:

$$C_{urea(s)} = \frac{U \times \sqrt{V}}{P}$$

Normal values of maximal urea clearance is 75 ml/min, while that of standard urea clearance is 54 ml/min.

Diagnostic importance. A urea clearance value below 75% of the normal is viewed seriously. Since it is an indicator of renal damage, blood urea level as such is found to increase only when the clearance falls below 50% normal.

Calculation of GFR from urea clearance. Since the proportion of urea reabsorbed by the renal tubules remains relatively constant at about 40% of the filtered, the urea clearance test can serve as a measure of GFR. The urea clearance expressed as a percentage of normal multiplied by 1.2 is a rough clinical estimation of GFR. As already mentioned, creatinine clearance test is a better indicator of GFR compared with urea clearance.

Renal Clearance Tests to Assess Tubular Secretory Capacity

The tubular secretory capacity can be assessed by the renal clearance of substances that are actively secreted by the tubular cells. As described on page 495, secretion of PAH (para-aminohippuric acid) occurs into the tubular fluid via carriers in the proximal tubule by a transport maximum (T_m) limited process. Once T_m of PAH is reached, the clearance of PAH (C_{PAH}) becomes progressively more a function of glomerular filtration and hence the C_{PAH} approaches C_{in}, and the constant amount of PAH secreted becomes a smaller fraction of the total amount excreted. Because the T_m (PAH) is nearly constant, it is used clinically to estimate tubular secretory capacity (T_s).

Renal Clearance Test to Assess Renal Plasma Flow

The renal plasma flow (RPF) can be calculated by applying *Fick's principle* to the kidneys. According to this principle, the amount of a substance excreted by the kidney per unit time (UV) is equal to the renal plasma flow (RPF) multiplied by the arteriovenous difference in its plasma concentration:

$$UV = \text{RPF}\,(P_a - P_v)$$

$$\text{RPF} = \frac{UV}{P_a - P_v}$$

P_a = Concentration of the substance in renal arterial plasma (mg/ml),
P_v = Concentration of the substance in renal venous plasma (mg/ml),
U = Concentration of the substance in urine (mg/ml) and
V = Volume of urine excreted (ml/min).

PAH Clearance is Used to Measure RPF Method. PAH is continuously infused at low doses, so as to keep its plasma concentration constant. The RPF is calculated as

$$\frac{U_{PAH}V}{P_{a(PAH)} - P_{v(PAH)}}$$

- At low plasma concentration of PAH, all the PAH is excreted into the urine and none is returned to the circulation via the renal vein. As a result, the PAH concentration in the renal vein is zero and can be eliminated. The equation now becomes

$$\text{RPF} = \frac{U_{PAH}V}{P_{a(PAH)}}$$

- Since $\frac{U_{PAH}V}{P_{PAH}}$ is equal to clearance of PAH (CPAH), so the equation can be written as

$$\text{RPF} = C_{PAH}$$

- About 10% of total renal plasma flow perfuses the nonexcretory portions of the kidney. Therefore, RPF calculated from the clearance of PAH is referred to as the effective RPF (ERPF) because only 90% of the plasma PAH is extracted. Therefore, the equation can be written as

$$\text{ERPF} = C_{PAH}$$

- Normally concentration of PAH in urine (U_{PAH}): 14 mg/ml
  - Urine flow (V): 0.9 ml/min.
  - Concentration of PAH in plasma (P_{PAH}): 0–02 mg/ml.
  - Therefore, ERPF = 14 × 0.9/0.02 = 630 ml/min.
- To obtain true RPF, it is necessary to divide C_{PAH} by 0.9

$$\text{True PF} = \frac{C_{PAH}}{0.9}$$

Therefore, actual RPF = 630/0.9 = 700 ml/min.
- From the value of true RPF, the value of RBF can be easily determined, if haematocrit value (Hct) is known as:

$$\text{RBF} = \text{RPF} \times \frac{1}{1-\text{Hct}}$$

Normally, Hct is 45%; therefore,
RBF = 700 × 1/1−0.45
= 700 × 1/0.55 = 1273 ml/min.
- Normal values of ERPF are 650 ml/min/1.73 m^2 body surface area (BSA) in males and 600 ml/min/1.73 m^2 BSA in females. Accordingly, renal blood flow is approximately 1200 ml/min.

Renal Clearance Test to Assess 'Osmotic' and 'Free Water' Clearance

1. Osmotic Clearance (C_{osm}) Osmotic clearance (C_{osm}) is the amount of plasma (in ml) completely cleared of osmotically active solutes that appear in the urine each minute. It measures the rate at which plasma is cleared of osmotic particles and is calculated by the usual renal clearance formula of $C = \frac{U \times V}{P}$, which can be written as:

$$C_{osm} = \frac{U_{osm}.V}{P_{osm}}, \text{ where}$$

U_{osm} = urinary osmolality,
V = rate of urine flow ml/min and
P_{osm} = Plasma osmolality.

Normal value of C_{osm} is about 3 ml/min. It is increased in osmotic diuresis and decreased in fasting or diet deficient in proteins.

2. Free Water Clearance (CH_2O) The quantitative measure of the kidney's ability to excrete water is termed *free water clearance* (CH_2O). Free water clearance (CH_2O) denotes the volume of pure (i.e. solute free) water that must be removed from, or added to, the flow of urine (in ml/min) to make it iso-osmotic with plasma. In other words, it is a measure of the ability of the kidneys to generate solute-free water. It is not a true clearance, because no osmotically free water exists in plasma.

Free water, or solute-free water, is generated in the diluting segments of the kidney (i.e. thick ascending limb and early distal tubule), where NaCl is reabsorbed and free water is left in the tubular fluid.

In the absence of ADH, this solute-free water is excreted and CH_2O is positive.

In the presence of ADH, this solute-free water is not excreted but is reabsorbed by the late distal tubule and collecting ducts and CH_2O is negative.

Calculation of CH_2O

$CH_2O = V - C_{osm}$ where:
CH_2O = Free water clearance (ml/min),
V = Urine flow rate (ml/min),

$$C_{osm} = \text{Osmolal clearance } \frac{U_{osm}V}{P_{osm}} \text{ (ml/min).}$$

Example. If the urine flow rate (V) is 10 ml/min, urine osmolality (U_{osm}) is 100 mOsm/kg H_2O and when plasma osmolality is 300 mOsm/kg H_2O, then the CH_2O can be calculated as:

$$CH_2O = V - C_{osm}$$

$$= 10\text{ ml/min} - \frac{100\text{ mOsm/kgH}_2\text{O} \times 10\text{ ml/min}}{300\text{ mOsm/kgH}_2\text{O}}$$

$$= 10\text{ ml/min} - 3.33\text{ ml/min}$$
$$= +6.7\text{ ml/min.}$$

Relationship between Free Water Clearance, Urine Volume and Osmolal Clearance

1. ***With iso-osmotic urine*** (Fig. 6.5-5 A), neither excretion nor reabsorption of solute-free water occurs, i.e.
   - Solute-free water clearance (CH_2O) = 0 and
   - Urine flow (V) is equal to osmolal clearance (C_{osm}).

   Clinical situation when zero CH_2O can occur in treatment with a loop diuretic. Treatment with loop diuretic inhibits NaCl reabsorption in the thick ascending limb (TAL), inhibiting both dilution in TAL and production of the corticopapillary osmotic gradient. Therefore, the urine cannot be diluted during water drinking (because a diluting segment is inhibited) or concentrated during water deprivation (because the corticopapillary gradient has been abolished).
2. ***With hypo-osmotic urine*** (Fig. 6.5-5 B), the urine is divided into two virtual volumes; one that contains solutes that is iso-osmotic to plasma (C_{osm}) and a volume that is solute-free water (CH_2O). Thus:
   - Osmolal clearance (C_{osm}) is equal to solute-free water clearance (CH_2O), i.e. $C_{osm} = CH_2O$,
   - Urine flow rate (V) is equal to the sum of osmolal clearance (C_{osm}) and free water clearance, i.e. $V = C_{osm} + CH_2O$, and
   - CH_2O is positive.

   Clinical situations in which a positive CH_2O occurs include:
   - Excessive water intake (in which ADH release from the posterior pituitary is suppressed),
   - Central diabetes insipidus (in which pituitary ADH is insufficient) or
   - Nephrogenic diabetes insipidus (in which the collecting ducts are unresponsive to ADH).
3. ***With hyperosmotic urine***, TCH_2O ($-CH_2O$) represents the volume of free water that would have to be added to the urine to make it iso-osmotic to plasma (Fig. 6.5-5 C), i.e.
   - Urine volume (V) is equal to the difference between osmolal clearance (C_{osm}) and free water reabsorption.
   - The osmolal clearance (C_{osm}) is equal to the sum of urine volume (V) and free water reabsorption (TCH_2O) and
   - CH_2O is thus negative.

   Clinical situations in which negative CH_2O or positive free water reabsorption (TCH_2O) occurs include:
   - Water deprivation (ADH release from the pituitary is stimulated) and
   - SIADH.

Tests for Tubular Functions

The reabsorptive and secretory functions of renal tubules can be tested by the following tests:

1. Urine Concentration Test. The ability of tubules to concentrate the urine is assessed by measuring the specific gravity of urine either after 12 h of water deprivation or 12 h after injection of vasopressin (ADH). In either case, if the specific gravity of urine is above 1.020, the tubular function is considered to be normal.

2. Urine Dilution Test. In this test, the patient is asked to drink 1 L of water and the urine sample is collected every hour for the next 4 h. Normally, at least 750 ml (75%) of urine should be excreted during this period and at least one

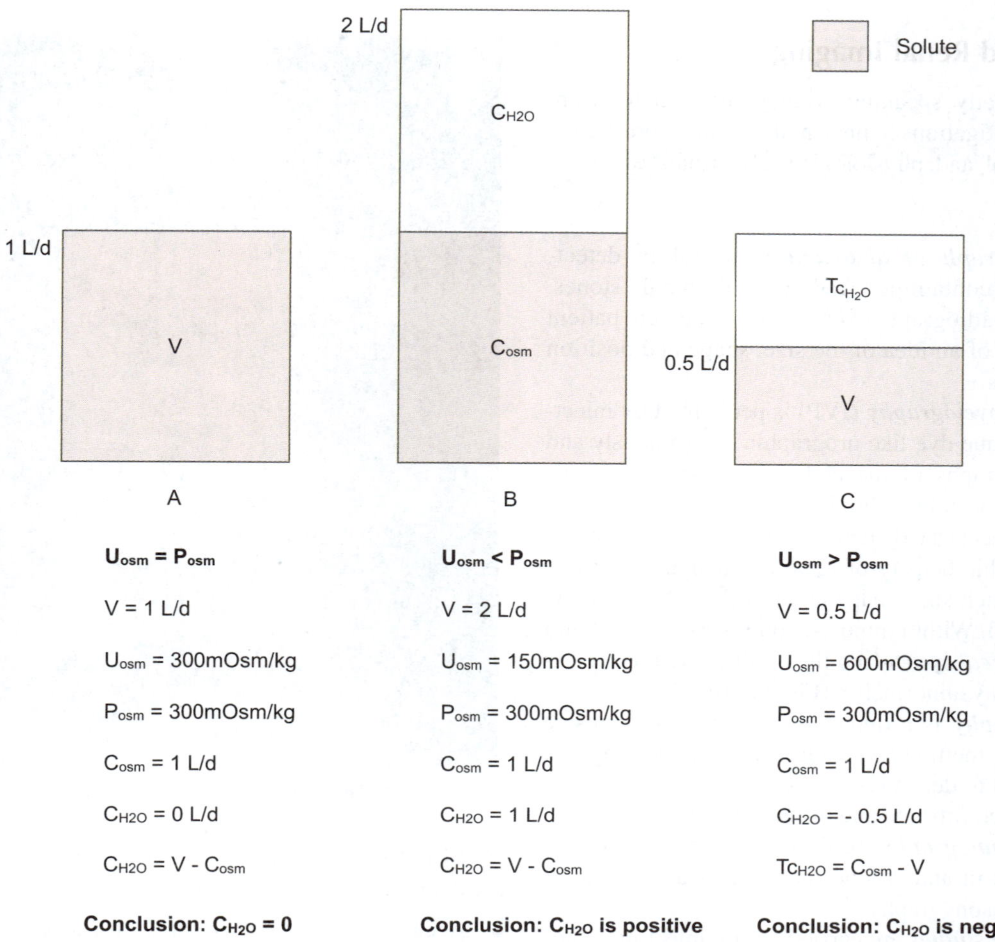

FIGURE 6.5-5 Relationship between free water clearance (CH_2O), urine volume (V) and osmolal clearance ($Cosm$): **A**, with iso-osmotic urine; **B**, with hypo-osmotic urine; and C, with hyperosmotic urine.

of the samples should have osmolality less than 100 mOsm/kg H_2O (or specific gravity below 1.004).

3. Urine Acidification Test. In this test, the patient is given ammonium chloride (NH_4Cl) orally in the dose of 0.1 g/kg BW and pH of the urine is tested in a sample collected after 6 h. Normally, urine pH should be below 5.3 because after metabolism in the liver, the NH_4Cl yields HCl:

$$NH_4Cl \rightarrow NH_3 + HCl$$

NH_3 is metabolized to urea and HCl is excreted by the kidney leading to a fall in urinary pH. Urine pH above 5.3 indicates inability of the tubules to excrete the acid (H^+).

4. Tubular Secretory Capacity. is also tested by:

i. *PAH clearance test* (see page 553)

ii. *Urea clearance test* (see page 552)

iii. *Phenolsulphonephthalein Px* (PSP) excretion test. In this test, the dye PSP is injected intravenously and the time of its first appearance in the urine and the quantity eliminated within a definite period are taken as a measure of the functional capacity of the kidney. In the normal individual, 25% or more of the dye is excreted during the first 15 min and not less than 70% will be excreted during a 2-h period. The status of nephron function is graded as:

Status of nephron function	Excretion of dye
• Normal	70% or above
• Slight impairment	59–40%
• Moderate impairment	39–25%
• Marked impairment	24–11%

5. Other Methods of Study of the Tubular Function, usually employed in research laboratory, include:

i. *Micropuncture technique* to analyse the tubular fluid at various levels.

ii. *Microcryoscopic studies* of renal tissue slices at different depths.

iii. *Microelectrode studies* to measure the membrane potential of the tubular cells.

Radiology and Renal Imaging

Though, not strictly speaking, kidney function tests are quite useful investigations in present day clinical practice to assess anatomical and physiological abnormalities of the kidneys.

1. ***Plain radiograph of abdomen*** is useful in detecting calcium-containing (radiopaque) renal stones. However, a radiograph from a well-prepared patient gives enough of an idea of the size, shape and position of the kidneys.
2. ***Intravenous pyelography*** (IVP) is performed by injecting a radiopaque dye like urographin intravenously and taking radiographs of the abdomen at short intervals (1, 5, 10 and 30 min). The dye is filtered by the glomeruli and concentrated in the renal tubules increasing the radiographic density of renal parenchyma (*nephrogram*), by which size, shape and position of the kidney can be studied. Within minutes, contrast is excreted into the *pelvicalyceal system* and the outlines are made clear to study for any abnormality (Fig. 6.5-6).
3. ***Ultrasonography*** is a quick, noninvasive, inexpensive and harmless method to evaluate size, shape, position of kidney and to detect tumour, stones, cysts, etc. of the kidneys, ureter, prostate and urinary bladder.
4. ***Computed tomography (CT)*** is performed to detect abnormalities in and around the kidneys as mentioned above in ultrasonography.
5. ***Radionuclide studies*** are carried out by injecting radioactive compounds which are concentrated and excreted by the kidneys. Radioactivity of the kidneys is recorded by a gamma camera.

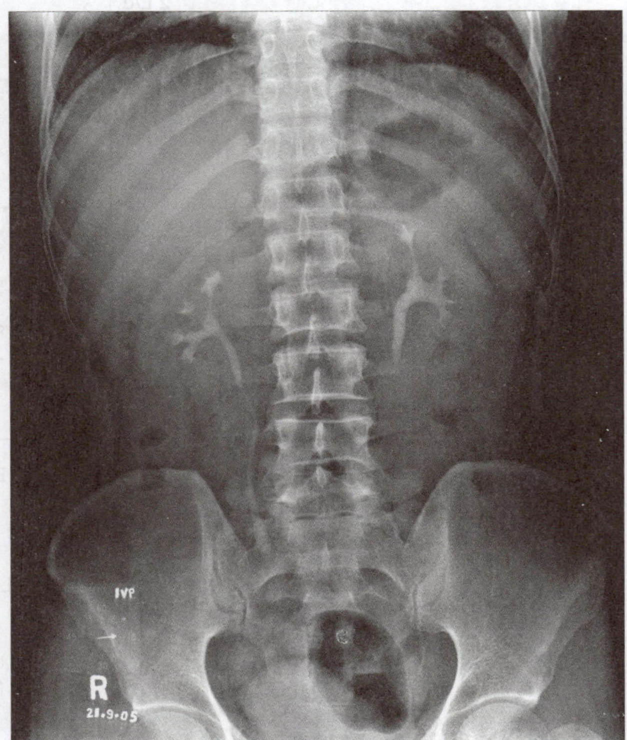

FIGURE 6.5-6 Intravenous pyelogram.

Renal Biopsy

Renal biopsy is performed percutaneously with the help of *Vim–Silverman* needle. This is useful in diagnosis of patients with proteinuria of unknown origin, an unexplained renal failure with normal sized kidneys or in systemic diseases associated with abnormal urinary constituents. The biopsy specimen is subjected to light, electron and immunofluorescence microscopic studies. This technique has increased knowledge and a better understanding of glomerular and tubular diseases.

DIALYSIS AND RENAL TRANSPLANTATION

Dialysis

The term dialysis in physiological sense refers to the diffusion of solutes from an area of higher concentration to an area of lower concentration through a semipermeable membrane. This principle has been used to dialyze the blood of patients with renal failure, especially those developing uraemia.

Uraemia develops when more than 75% of nephrons are damaged and is characterized by:

- Accumulation of nitrogenous waste products in the blood,
- Metabolic acidosis and
- Hyperkalaemia.

Uraemic coma is the terminal event in chronic renal failure. It has been attributed chiefly to acidosis and hyperkalaemia. Accumulation of nitrogenous waste products contributes relatively less to the loss of consciousness in uraemic coma.

Types of dialysis. By dialysis, the dissolved crystalloids of the plasma pass through a semipermeable membrane so that their levels are brought down to lower levels. Two types of dialysis procedures are available:

- Haemodialysis or artificial kidney and
- Peritoneal dialysis.

Haemodialysis or Artificial Kidney

Haemodialysis can save a life in many types of *acute renal failure* produced by reversible pathological processes, specially circulatory shock or mercury poisoning. The intermittent haemodialysis may prolong the life of many patients with chronic renal failure, which may lead to an active life for many years.

The dialysis can partially replace the excretory function of the kidneys but does not replace endocrine and metabolic functions.

Procedure. The haemodialysis machine is also called as artificial kidney. Haemodialysis is done in a hospitalized patient through an intravenous line for 3–5 h. During haemodialysis, the patient's radial artery is connected to the haemodialysis machine. Inside the haemodialysis machine, the blood is passed through a long and coiled cellophane tube immersed in a dialysis fluid (Fig. 6.5-7). Heparin is used as an anticoagulant while passing the blood through the machine.

Dialyzing Fluid. The composition of dialyzing fluid is similar to that of plasma, except it is free of waste products like urea, uric acid, etc. The fluid contains less amounts of sodium, potassium and chloride ions than in uraemic blood. But the quantity of glucose, bicarbonate and calcium ions are more in the dialyzing fluid than in the uraemic blood (Table 6.5-4).

During Haemolysis, the semipermeable cellophane membrane permits the free diffusion of the constituents of plasma, except proteins. In this way, the dialysis of patient's blood removes the toxic waste products and restores normal electrolyte concentration in the plasma. The dialyzed blood is returned back to the patient's body through a peripheral vein (Fig. 6.5-7). At a time, about 500 ml is passed through the artificial kidney. Haemodialysis is done usually thrice a week in severe uraemia.

Peritoneal Dialysis

In this type of dialysis, the peritoneum is used as a semipermeable membrane. Continuous ambulatory peritoneal dialysis is a form of long-term dialysis done by the patients at home or at work.

Procedure. Two litres of dialyzing fluid is introduced through a permanent intraperitoneal catheter. It is then kept in the peritoneal cavity for exchange to take place for a period of 15–20 min, called dwell time. Fluid is then drained out and measured. A strict input and output chart is maintained. The whole procedure constitutes one cycle. It is done at 6-h intervals (four cycles per day), even when the patient is ambulatory or mobile. There is no need for hospitalization and it is useful for young children and old patients with cardiovascular disorders. It prolongs survival in patients with chronic renal failure for many years.

Peritoneal dialysis versus haemodialysis

Table 6.5-5 compares and contrasts the peritoneal dialysis versus haemodialysis.

Renal Transplantation

The haemodialysis is an expensive procedure and needs to be repeated almost every week. Therefore, it cannot be regarded as a remedy in individuals with irreversible terminal renal failure (*end stage renal disease*). Renal transplantation is the final answer to all the problems in cases with chronic renal failure. It reverses metabolic and excretory abnormalities. The graft is taken from a cadaver donor or from a sibling or a parent. Usually the left kidney of the donor is transplanted to the right iliac fossa of the recipient. Long-term immune suppression with prednisolone and cyclosporine is needed. It offers complete rehabilitation and is the most cost-effective option.

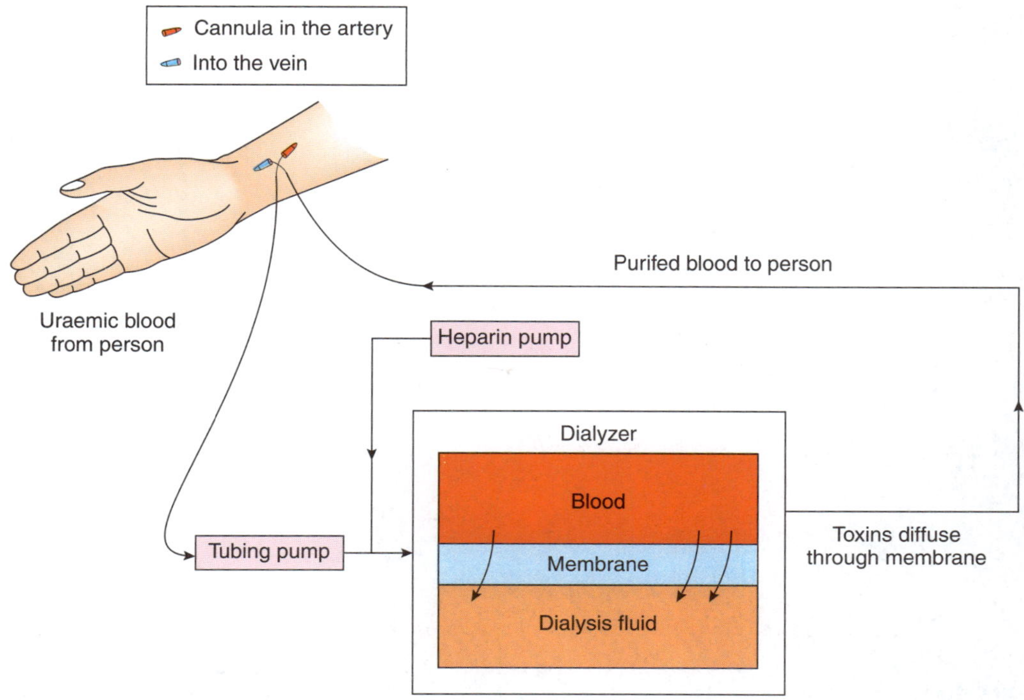

FIGURE 6.5-7 Basic principle of haemodialysis.

TABLE 6.5-4 Composition of Dialyzing Fluid as Compared to That of a Typical Uraemic Patient

Constituent	Uraemic plasma	Dialyzing fluid
Electrolytes (mEq/L)		
Na^+	142	142
K^+	7	4
Ca^{2+}	2	3
Mg^{2+}	1.5	1.5
Cl^-	103	107
HCO_3^-	14	27
Lactate	1.2	1.2
HPO_4	9	0
Urate	2	0
SO_4^{2-}	3	0
Nonelectrolytes (mg%)		
Glucose	100	125
Urea	200	0
Creatinine	6	0

TABLE 6.5-5 Peritoneal Dialysis versus Haemodialysis

Peritoneal dialysis	Haemodialysis
Costly machine not required	Costly machine required
Less effective	More effective
Takes nearly 24 h to bring down urea level from 200 mg/dL to 100 mg/dL	Takes 6 h to bring down urea level from 200 to l50 mg/dL
May be uncomfortable	Usually not uncomfortable
Haemodynamic disturbances are less	Haemodynamic disturbances are more
Suitable to patients with coagulopathy	May have haemorrhagic problems following heparinization
May be done in patients with low blood pressure	Difficult in patients with hypotension
Not very suitable for drug poisoning cases	Very helpful in drug poisoning with toxic kidney
Not very effective in patients with gross fluid overload.	Very effective in patients with gross fluid overload and water can be filtered out very fast by haemofiltration

Chapter 6.6

Physiology of Micturition

URINARY BLADDER AND URETHRA

Gross Anatomy

External Features. The urinary bladder, a hollow muscular viscus, is a temporary reservoir for urine. The main body of empty bladder is pyramidal, having an apex, a base, and a superior and two inferolateral surfaces. The lowest part of the bladder is called neck, which is the most fixed part of the bladder. The neck continues as posterior urethra.

Interior of the Bladder. In an empty bladder, the greater part of the mucosa shows irregular folds due to its loose attachments to the muscular coat. The interior of the base (posterior surface) of the bladder presents a triangular area, the trigone where the mucosa is smooth due to its firm attachment.

Internal urethral orifice is located at the apex (inferior angle) of the trigone. The ureters open into the bladder at superior angles of the trigone (Fig. 6.6-1). The ureters pierce the bladder wall obliquely, and this provides a valve-like action, which prevents a reverse flow of urine towards the kidneys as the bladder fills.

Structure of the Bladder. The wall of the urinary bladder consists of three layers: an outer serous layer, a thick coat of smooth muscle and the inner mucous membrane.

Mucous membrane is lined by transitional epithelium. Its characteristic features are:

- It stretches when the bladder distends.
- It forms a complete barrier to the passage of fluid and electrolytes. Therefore, urine stored in the bladder remains unchanged in chemical composition.
- It secretes a glycosaminoglycan barrier that prevents bacterial adherence.

Muscular layer is formed by smooth muscle fibres which constitute the detrusor muscle. The detrusor muscle is arranged in interlacing longitudinal, circular and spiral bundles. Contraction of this muscle coat is responsible for emptying of the bladder.

Urethra and Its Sphincters

Male urethra, about 20 cm in length, is divided into three parts: prostatic urethra (3 cm), membranous urethra (1.25 cm) and penile urethra (15.75 cm). Membranous urethra is surrounded by the external sphincter.

Female urethra is about 3.8 cm long. It extends from the neck of the bladder to the external meatus. It traverses the external sphincter and lies immediately in front of the vagina.

Sphincters of the Urethra

1. Internal Sphincter. The circular smooth muscle fibres in the area of the neck of bladder are thickened to form the internal sphincter (sphincter vesicae). The natural tone of the internal sphincter prevents emptying of the bladder until the pressure in the body of bladder rises above a threshold level.

2. External Sphincter. Beyond the bladder neck, as the urethra passes through the urogenital diaphragm, it is encircled by a ring of voluntary (skeletal type) muscle known as external sphincter of the bladder. The external sphincter

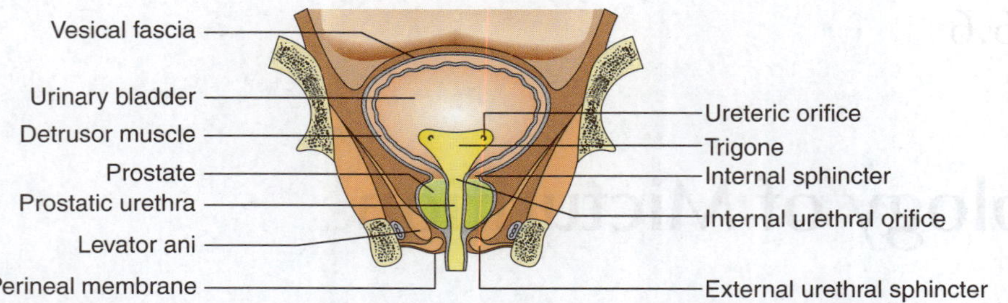

FIGURE 6.6-1 Coronal section through the bladder and prostate to show the interior of the bladder, internal urethral sphincter and external urethral sphincter.

provides voluntary control over micturition. In males, its stronger action can stop micturition midstream even after it has been reflexly initiated.

Innervation of the Urinary Bladder (Fig. 6.6-2)

Motor Innervation

Parasympathetic Innervation. The parasympathetic efferent fibres (nervi erigentes) are derived from the second, third and fourth sacral segments (mainly S_2 and S_3). These fibres carry motor impulses to the urinary bladder causing contraction of detrusor muscle and emptying of the bladder. These fibres are inhibitory to the internal sphincter. If these fibres are destroyed, normal micturition is not possible.

Sympathetic Innervation. These nerves arise in the 11th thoracic to the second lumbar segments (T_{11}–L_2). These fibres are said to be inhibitory to detrusor muscle and motor to the sphincter vesicae. Many workers regard them to be chiefly vasomotor.

Sympathetic activity is not involved in micturition. Increased sympathetic discharge to the bladder occurs during ejaculation and helps to prevent the reflux of sperms from the prostatic urethra into the bladder.

Somatic Motor Innervation. The somatic pudendal nerve (S_2, S_3 and S_4) supplies the external sphincter which is voluntary.

Sensory Innervation

Sensation of Bladder Distension. Afferents from the detrusor stretch receptors travel to the spinal cord via the pelvic splanchnic nerve (nervierigentes). From the region of the bladder neck and trigone, the afferents travel via the hypogastric plexus to spinal cord segments T_{11}–L_2.

In the spinal cord, the fibres of awareness of bladder distension run in the posterior column (fasciculus gracilis)

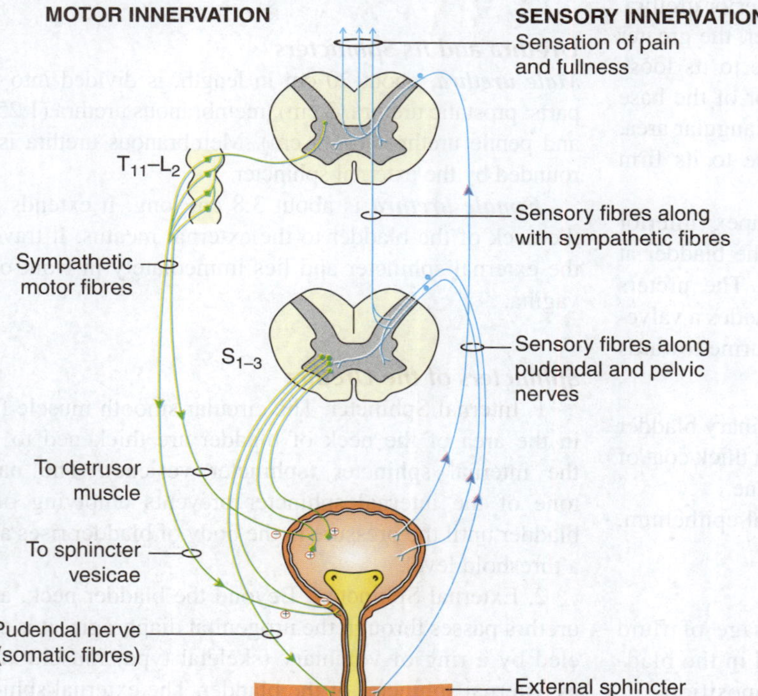

FIGURE 6.6-2 Innervation of urinary bladder.

to reach the spinal, pontine and suprapontine micturition centres.

Sensation of Bladder Pain. The pain fibres are stimulated by excessive distension or spasm of the bladder wall, or by stone, inflammation or malignant disease irritating the bladder. The pain fibres run predominantly in the hypogastric plexus but are also present in the nervi erigentes.

In the spinal cord, the fibres carrying pain sensation run in the lateral spinothalamic tract. Bilateral anterolateral cordotomy, therefore, selectively abolishes pain without affecting the awareness of bladder distension and the desire to micturate (which runs in the posterior column),

Urethral Sensations, including sensation of imminent voiding associated with maximal bladder filling, reach the spinal cord via the pudendal nerve.

In the spinal cord, fibres carrying urethral sensations travel in the dorsal column.

PHYSIOLOGY OF MICTURITION

Micturition is the process by which urinary bladder empties when filled. Micturition begins in the fifth month of intrauterine life with the onset of urinary secretion. It remains purely a reflex act until approximately 2–2.5 years of age, at which time it begins to come under voluntary control. The main physiological events in the process of micturition are:

- Filling of urinary bladder, and
- Emptying of urinary bladder.

Filling of Urinary Bladder

Transport of Urine into Urinary Bladder through Ureters As urine collects in the renal pelvis, the pressure in the pelvis increases and initiates a peristaltic contraction beginning in the pelvis and spreading along the ureter to force urine towards the bladder. This peristaltic wave, travelling at a velocity of about 3 cm/s, occurs from once every second to once every 2–3 min. The peristaltic wave can move urine against an obstruction with a pressure as high as 25–50 mmHg

Capacity of the Bladder

- ***Physiological capacity*** of the bladder varies with age, being 20–50 ml at birth, about 200 ml at 1 year and can be as high as 600 ml in young adult males. In all cases, the physiological capacity is about twice that at which the first desire to void is felt.
- ***Anatomical capacity*** refers to the capacity of the bladder beyond which rupture occurs. It is about 1 L or more, and is never approached under physiological conditions.

Volume and Pressure Changes in Bladder during Filling

The normal bladder is completely empty at the end of micturition and the intravesical pressure is equal to the intra-abdominal pressure. As the bladder is filled up, it adjusts its tone and a fairly large volume of urine can be accommodated with minimal alterations in the intravesical pressure. This is possible because of phenomenon of adaptation. The *adaptation* occurs because of the inherent property of *plasticity,* the smooth muscles of detrusor and *because of law of Laplace*. According to Laplace's law, pressure in a hollow organ is inversely proportional to its radius; the tone remaining constant. That is, if tone remains constant, an increase in radius decreases the pressure and vice versa:

$P = T/R$, where P = pressure, T = tension, and R = radius.

In the bladder, as volume of fluid rises, the radius increases due to relaxation of detrusor and therefore the pressure rise is almost nil. It is important to note that adaptation is independent of nervous mechanism and it, therefore, presents in the denervated bladder, but not after birth.

Cystometry. This refers to the process of studying the relationship between the intravesical volume and pressure; the cystometrogram refers to graphical record of this relationship.

Method of Recording Cystometrogram. A double-lumen catheter is introduced into the bladder. The fluid is introduced through one lumen and pressure changes are recorded by connecting the other lumen to the pressure transducer of a polygraph (Fig. 6.6-3). The bladder is filled with 50 ml increments of water and at each volume, the intravesical pressure is recorded.

Normal Cystometrogram shows three phases of filling (Fig. 6.6-4):

- ***Phase Ia.*** It is the initial phase of filling in which pressure rises from 0 to 10 cm of H_2O, when about 50 ml of fluid is collected in the bladder.
- ***Phase Ib.*** It is the phase of plateau which lasts till the bladder volume is 400 ml. During this phase, the pressure in the bladder does not change much and remains approximately at 10 cm H_2O. This is because of adaptation of urinary bladder by relaxation, as described above.
- ***Phase II.*** This phase starts beyond 400 ml volume when the pressure begins to rise markedly, triggering the micturition reflex. Normally, the voiding contraction raises the intravesical pressure by about 20–40 cm of H_2O. If voiding is avoided (not initiated), the pressure rises from 10 cm of H_2O onward, as shown by dotted lines beyond the phase II in Fig. 6.6-4. Beyond 600 ml, the urge to void urine becomes almost unbearable.

Emptying of the Bladder

Micturition is the process by which urinary bladder empties when it becomes filled. Emptying of the bladder is basically a reflex action called the micturition reflex, which is controlled

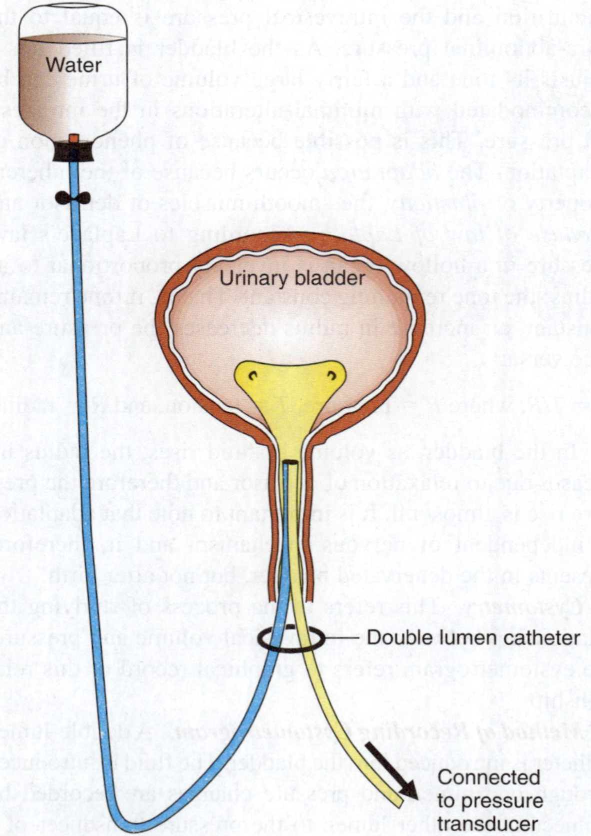

FIGURE 6.6-3 Procedure of cystometry to demonstrate pressure–volume relationship in urinary bladder.

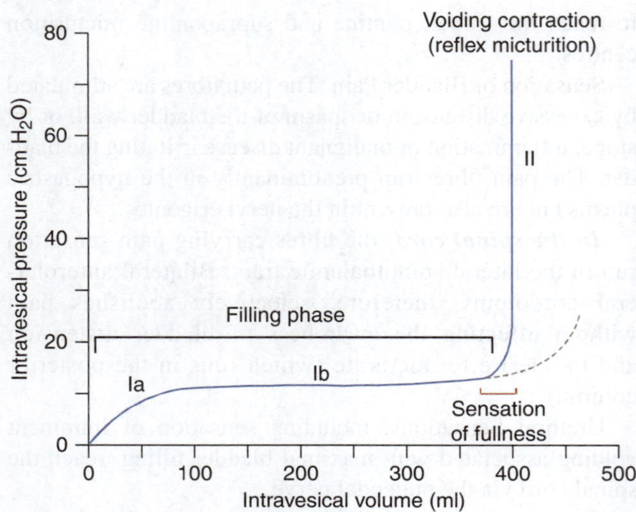

FIGURE 6.6-4 Normal cystometrogram.

by supraspinal centres and is assisted by contraction of perineal and abdominal muscles. Therefore, discussion on emptying of the urinary bladder focuses on:

- Micturition reflex,
- Voluntary control of micturition and
- Role of perineal and abdominal muscles in micturition.

Micturition Reflex

Initiation. Micturition reflex is initiated by stimulation of the stretch receptors located in the wall of urinary bladder.

Stimulus. Filling of bladder by 300–400 ml of urine in adults constitutes the adequate stimulus for the micturition reflex to occur. Though, under natural circumstances, the first urge to empty the bladder occurs at approximately 150 ml of urinary volume but it can be easily suppressed.

Afferents. Micturition reflex is a spinal reflex. The afferents from the stretch receptors in the detrusor muscle and urethra travel along the pelvic splanchnic nerves and enter the spinal cord through dorsal roots to S_2, S_3 and S_4 segments to reach the sacral micturition centre (Fig. 6.6-5).

Sacral Micturition Centre is formed by the sacral detrusor nucleus and sacral pudendal nucleus.

- ***Sacral detrusor nucleus*** is a cluster of preganglionic parasympathetic neurons located in the intermediolateral grey matter of S_2, S_3 and S_4 segments. Afferents of micturition reflex excite the neurons of this nucleus.
- ***Sacral pudendal nucleus*** refers to a cluster of neurons found in the ventral horn primarily of the S_2 and to a lesser degree of S_3 and S_4 segments. The afferents from the stretch receptors in the bladder wall inhibit this nucleus thereby exciting the external sphincter of urethra.

Efferents. Efferents arising from the sacral detrusor nucleus are the preganglionic parasympathetic fibres which relay in the ganglia near or within bladder and urethra (Fig. 6.6-5). The postganglionic parasympathetic fibres are excitatory to the detrusor muscle and inhibitory to the internal sphincter.

Response. Once micturition reflex is initiated, it is self-regenerative, i.e. initial contraction of the bladder wall further activates the receptors to increase sensory impulses (afferents) from the bladder and urethra which cause further increase in reflex contraction of detrusor muscle of the bladder. The cycle thus keeps on repeating itself again and again until the bladder has reached a strong degree of contraction. After a few seconds, reflex fatigues and regenerative cycle cease. Once a micturition reflex has occurred but not succeeded in emptying the bladder, the nervous elements of the reflex usually remain in an inhibited state for at least a few minutes to an hour before another micturition reflex occurs.

Once the micturition reflex becomes powerful enough, this causes another reflex which passes through pudendal nerves to external sphincter to cause its inhibition. If this

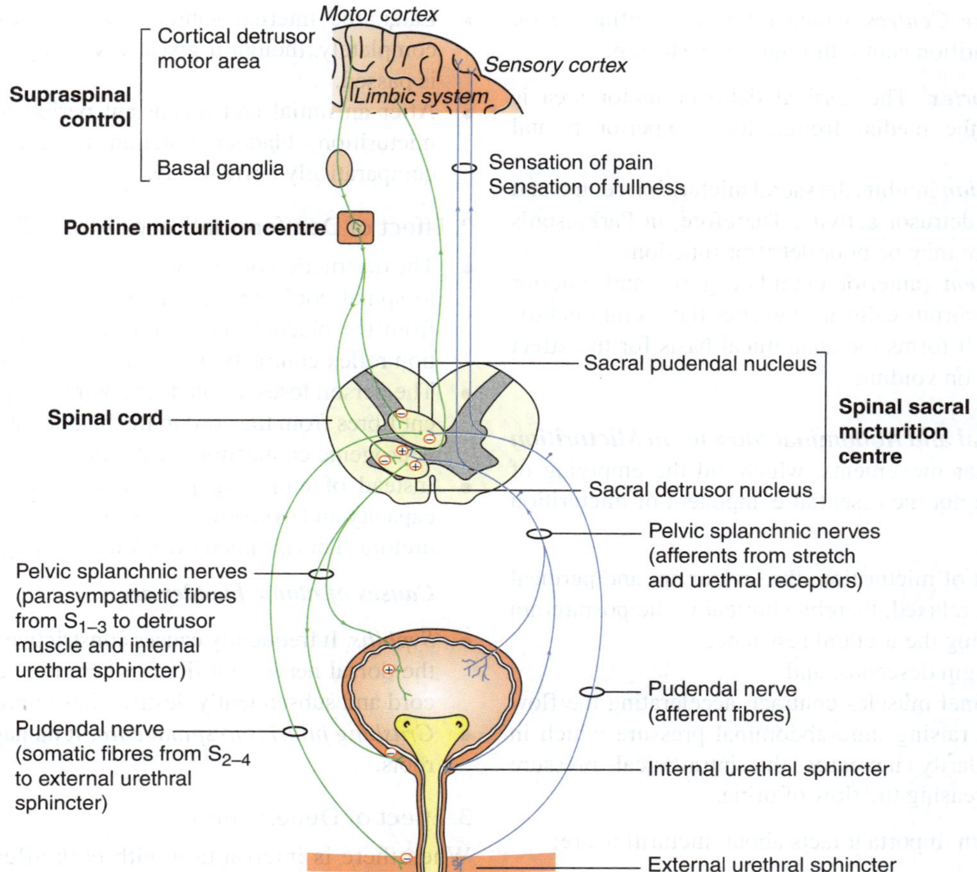

FIGURE 6.6-5 Pathway and supraspinal control of micturition reflex.

inhibition is more potent than the voluntary constrictor signals from brain, then urination will not occur. If not so, urination will not occur unless the bladder fills still more and micturition reflex becomes more powerful.

Voluntary Control of Micturition

Role of Supraspinal Centres. The micturition reflex is fundamentally a *spinal reflex* facilitated and inhibited by higher brain centres (*supraspinal centres*) and, like defaecation, is subjected to voxluntary facilitation and inhibition. In infants and young children, micturition is purely a reflex action. *Voluntary control* is gradually acquired as a learned ability of the toilet training. Once voluntary control is acquired, the supraspinal control centres exert final control of micturition by the following means:

- The higher centres keep the micturition reflex partially inhibited all the time except when it is desired to micturate.
- Even if the micturition reflex occurs, still the higher centres can prevent micturition by continual tonic contraction of external urinary sphincter until a convenient time presents.
- When the convenient time to urinate presents, the higher centres facilitate the sacral micturition centre (SMC) to initiate a micturition reflex and inhibit the external urinary sphincter so that urination can occur.

Supraspinal control centres which control the micturition reflex (a completely automatic cord reflex) include the pontine micturition centre (PMC) and suprapontine centres.

Pontine Micturition Centre (PMC), also called Barrington centre, corresponds to the locus ceruleus of the rostral pons. Neurons from PMC descend in the reticulospinal tract and exert control over the sacral micturition centre (SMC) and thoracolumbar sympathetics. Functions of PMC are:

- ***Co-ordination of detrusor contraction and sphincter relaxation,*** which is important for proper micturition. Therefore, in the absence of control from PMC, there occurs loss of co-ordination between the bladder and external sphincter mechanism (*detrusor–sphincter dyssynergia*).
- ***To relay inputs from the suprapontine centres,*** therefore, in the lesions of PMC due to disruption of suprapontine influences, there occurs decreased storage and incomplete voiding.

Suprapontine Centres which relay their influence on the sacral micturition centre through the PMC are:

- ***Cerebral cortex.*** The cortical detrusor motor area is located in the medial frontal lobe (superior frontal gyrus).
- ***Basal ganglion*** inhibits the sacral micturition centre, and thereby the detrusor activity. Therefore, in Parkinson's disease, there may be poor detrusor function.
- ***Limbic system*** (anterior cingulate gyrus and anterior genu of the corpus callosum) excites the sacral micturition centre. It forms the anatomical basis for the effect of emotions on voiding.

Role of Perineal and Abdominal Muscles in Micturition

Certain muscular movements, which aid the emptying of bladder, but are not the essential component of micturition process are:

- At the onset of micturition, the levator ani and perineal muscles are relaxed, thereby shortening the posturethra and decreasing the urethral resistance.
- The diaphragm descends, and
- The abdominal muscles contract, accelerating the flow of urine by raising intra-abdominal pressure which in turn secondarily increases the intravesical pressure thereby increasing the flow of urine.

Note. Certain important facts about micturition are:

- A voiding contraction, once initiated, is normally maintained until all the urine has been discharged from the urinary bladder. This is a function of facilitating impulses from the higher centres. However, if required so, the micturition can be voluntarily stopped in between by inhibitory impulses from the higher centres.
- The bladder contracts in all directions like a toy balloon deflating from its neck.
- After urination, the female urethra empties by gravity, whereas the urine remaining in the urethra of male is expelled by several contractions of bulbospongiosus muscle.

ABNORMALITIES OF MICTURITION

Effect of Interference with Nervous Control of Bladder

1. Transection of Sympathetic Supply

Following effects are produced:

- In man, the immediate effect would be relaxation of: ureteric reflexes, trigone and internal sphincter.
- After complete denervation, ejaculation no longer can take place, though physical orgasm and erection occur; therefore, sterility takes place.
- Later, the internal sphincter may recover and closes completely, though it gives way easily when a catheter is passed.
- After an initial and inconstant period of frequency of micturition, bladder function is re-established in a comparatively normal way.

2. Effect of Deafferentation or Atonic Bladder

- The destruction of sensory nerve fibres from the bladder to spinal cord prevents transmission of stretch signals from the bladder and therefore, also prevents micturition reflex contractions. In this condition:
- The person loses all bladder control despite intact efferent fibres from the cord to the bladder and despite intact neurogenic connections with brain.
- Instead of emptying periodically, the bladder fills to capacity and overflows a few drops at a time through the urethra. This is called *overflow dribbling*.

Causes of atonic bladder are:

- *Syphilis.* It frequently causes constrictive fibrosis around the dorsal nerve root fibres where they enter the spinal cord and subsequently destroy these fibres.
- *Crushing injuries to spinal cord.* It damages the sensory roots.

3. Effect of Denervation

When there is interruption with both afferent and efferent nerves of bladder, the following consequences are observed:

- The bladder is flaccid and distended for a while,
- Gradually, however, the muscle of *decentralized bladder* becomes active, with many contraction waves that expel dribbles of urine out of the urethra and
- The bladder becomes shrunken and the bladder wall hypertrophies.

The reason for the difference between the *small, hypertrophic bladder* seen in this condition and the *distended, hypotonic bladder* seen only when afferent nerves are interrupted is not known. The hyperactive stage in the former condition suggests the development of denervation hypersensitization even though the neurons interrupted are preganglionic rather than postganglionic.

Conditions—e.g. tumours of the cauda equina.

4. Effect of Spinal Cord Transection

During Spinal Shock

- Voluntary micturition is completely abolished. The activity of detrusor muscle remains in abeyance for a long period, but sphincter now returns very soon. At this stage, bladder responds to filling in the same manner as the dead organ or an elastic bag. Retention of urine is

therefore complete from an early stage. If no catheter is passed, the bladder becomes increasingly overstretched. The sphincter is finally forced open by a high intravesical pressure and small quantities of urine escape at frequent intervals—a condition of *retention with overflow*.
- The capacity is reduced and its walls become hypertrophied. This type of bladder is sometimes called *spastic neurogenic bladder*.
- Owing to excessive stretching of bladder wall, its nutrition suffers and it becomes very prone to infection. *Cystitis* may occur, and death results from the usual complications of *ascending urinary infection*.

After Spinal Shock has Passed, the voiding reflex returns, although there is no voluntary control. Some paraplegic patients train themselves to initiate voiding by pinching or stroking their thighs, provoking a mild mass reflex.

Effects of Obstruction

Conditions causing obstruction to the outflow of urine from the bladder may be:

- *Anatomical obstacles,* e.g. enlarged prostatic or urethral stricture.
- *Functional derangements,* e.g. atonic sphincter with a relatively weak detrusor.

Effects

- Retention of urine consequently tends to occur, and the intravesical pressure rises till it causes expulsion of urine.
- When the obstruction is mechanical, the stretching of bladder wall acts at first as a growth stimulus resulting in hypertrophy of its fibres and increase in their expulsive power which for a time enables the obstacle to overcome. But when, finally, the bladder wall is overstretched, it becomes paralyzed and normal evacuation no longer takes place.

Section 7

Gastrointestinal System

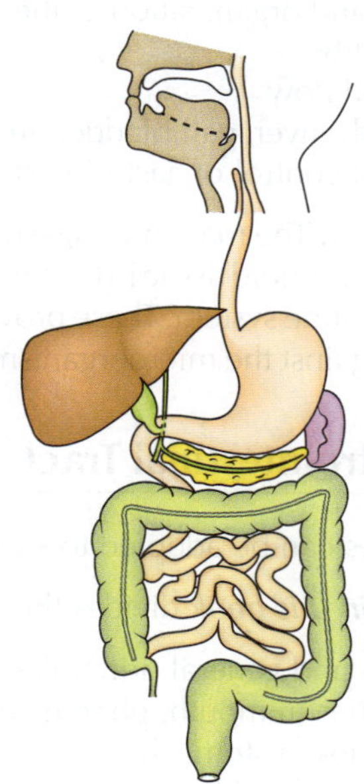

To sustain life, the body needs a continual supply of water, electrolytes and nutrients. This function is served by the gastrointestinal or the so-called digestive system.

Gastrointestinal system comprises alimentary canal and other associated organs such as liver, gall bladder and pancreas. Alimentary canal is a long tube starting at the mouth, passing through the pharynx, oesophagus, stomach, small intestine, large intestine, rectum and ending at anus.

Functions of Gastrointestinal System

I. Digestive functions. The major function of the gastrointestinal system is to transfer nutrients, minerals and water from external environment to the circulating body fluids for distribution to all the body tissues. This function is accomplished by the following processes:

1. ***Ingestion of food.*** It involves:
   - Placing the food into the mouth. Most of the foodstuffs are taken into mouth as large particles, mainly made of carbohydrates, proteins and fats.
   - Chewing the food into smaller pieces is carried out with the help of teeth and jaw muscles. This process is called mastication.
   - Lubrication and moistening of the food is done by the saliva.
   - Swallowing the food (deglutition). It refers to pushing the bolus of food from mouth into the stomach. It is accomplished in three phases: oral phase, pharyngeal phase and oesophageal phase.
2. ***Digestion of food.*** It refers to conversion of complex insoluble large organic molecules (food) into soluble, smaller and simpler molecules which can be easily absorbed. Digestion of food is accomplished with the help of hydrochloric acid and digestive juices containing various enzymes.
3. ***Absorption of digested food.*** Absorption of food refers to movement of digested molecules from the lumen of alimentary canal across its epithelial lining to the blood or lymph. The absorbed water, electrolytes and nutrients are carried away to the various tissues by the circulating blood.
4. ***Egestion,*** i.e. excretion of unwanted undigested food by the alimentary canal in the form of faeces is called defaecation.

To understand the digestive function of gastrointestinal system, it is imperative to have knowledge about:

- Functional anatomy and organization of the gastrointestinal system,
- Gastrointestinal motility,
- Gastrointestinal blood flow
- Role of salivary glands, liver, gall bladder and pancreas and
- Neural and hormonal control of gastrointestinal functions.

II. Nondigestive functions. The main nondigestive function of the gastrointestinal system is its role as immune system. The lymphoid tissue in the tonsils, adenoids and Peyer's patches constitute an important part of body's immune system. These provide both the humoral and cellular immunity which is especially effective against the microorganisms trying to enter the body from the alimentary canal.

Physiology of Gastrointestinal Tract

Two different approaches can be adopted to study the physiology of the gastrointestinal tract (GIT).

The approach adopted in this book divides the subject matter into the following chapters:

7.1 Functional anatomy and general principles of functions of gastrointestinal system
7.2 Physiological activities in mouth, pharynx and oesophagus
7.3 Physiological activities in stomach
7.4 Pancreas, liver and gall bladder
7.5 Physiological activities in small intestine
7.6 Physiological activities in large intestine
7.7 Digestion and absorption

The alternative approach which can be adopted to study physiology of GIT is summarized with reference page numbers given in parenthesis:

1. Functional anatomy of GIT (page 571)
2. Motility of the GIT
   - Chewing (page 579)
   - Deglutition (page 584)

- Gastric motility (page 597)
- Motility of small intestine (page 631)
- Motility of large intestine (page 638)
- Defaecation (page 639)

3. Gastrointestinal secretions
   - Salivary secretion (page 581)
   - Gastric secretion (page 590)
   - Pancreatic secretion (page 608)
   - Bile secretion (page 619)
   - Secretions of the small intestine (page 630)
   - Secretion of the large intestine (page 637)
4. Gastrointestinal hormones

   Gastrin family of hormones
   - Gastrin (page 593)
   - Cholecystokinin (page 612)

   Secretin family of hormones
   - Secretin (page 612)
   - GIP, i.e. gastric inhibitory polypeptide (page 594)
   - VIP, i.e. vasoactive intestinal peptide (page 578)
   - Glucagon (page 780)

   GLI, i.e. glucagon-like immune reactivity (page 780)

   Other GIT hormones
   - Motilin (page 577)
   - Neurotensin (page 578)
   - Substance P (page 338)
   - GRP, i.e. gastrin-releasing peptides (page 594)
   - Somatostatin (page 594)
5. Digestion and absorption in GIT (page 645)
6. Gastrointestinal function tests
   - Gastric function tests (page 605)
   - Pancreatic function tests (page 614)
   - Liver function tests (page 625)
   - Tests of intestinal absorption (page 659)
7. Physiology of gastrointestinal disorders
   - Disorders of swallowing (page 587)
   - Disorders of stomach (page 602)
   - Disorders of pancreas (page 613)
   - Disorders of small intestine (page 635)
   - Disorders of liver and gallbladder (page 624)
   - Disorders of large intestine (page 643)
   - Disorders of absorption (page 658).

Chapter 7.1

Functional Anatomy and General Principles of Functions of Gastrointestinal System

FUNCTIONAL ANATOMY

Functional Organization

The digestive system comprises gastrointestinal tract (GIT) and accessory organs of digestion like teeth, tongue, salivary glands, liver and exocrine part of pancreas.

Gastrointestinal Tract, also known as alimentary canal, is basically a muscular tube extending from the mouth to the anus (Fig. 7.1-1). At either end, the lumen is continuous with external environment. It measures about 10 m (30 feet) and comprises following parts:

Mouth. Mouth is a loosely used term to denote the external opening and for the cavity it leads to. Strictly speaking, the term mouth should be applied only for the external opening which is also called oral fissure. The cavity containing anterior two-third of tongue and teeth is the *mouth cavity* or *oral cavity* or *buccal cavity* (Fig. 7.1-2). The oral cavity extends from the lips to the oropharyngeal isthmus, i.e. junction of the mouth with the pharynx. The oral cavity is subdivided into two parts: the vestibule and oral cavity proper (Fig. 7.1-2).

- *Vestibule* lies between the lips and cheeks externally, and the gums and teeth internally.
  - *Oral cavity proper* lies within the alveolar arches, gums and teeth.

Tongue, in the digestive system, plays two important roles:

- Tells the taste of food and
- Helps in chewing and swallowing of the food.

Teeth. Functions of different types of teeth in chewing are:

- *Incisors* provide strong cutting action.
- *Canines* are responsible for tearing action.
- *Premolars and molars* have grinding action.

Pharynx. The pharynx is a median passage that is common to the gastrointestinal and respiratory systems. It is divisible, from above downwards, into three parts:

- *Nasal part* or *nasopharynx* into which nasal cavities open,
- *Oral part* or *oropharynx* which is continuous with the posterior end of oral cavity and
- *Laryngeal part* or *laryngopharynx* which is continuous in front with larynx, and below with oesophagus.

Oesophagus. It is a fibromuscular tube about 25 cm long. At its junction to the pharynx, upper oesophageal sphincter is present and at its junction with the stomach, lower oesophageal sphincter is present. During swallowing, the upper oesophageal sphincter opens and food passes into the

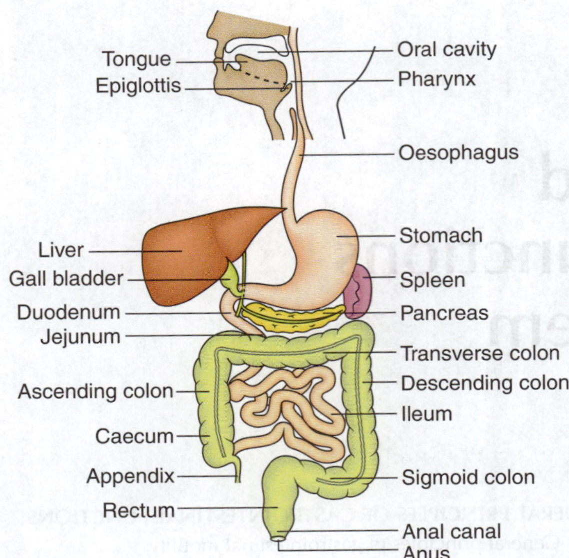

FIGURE 7.1-1 The gastrointestinal system.

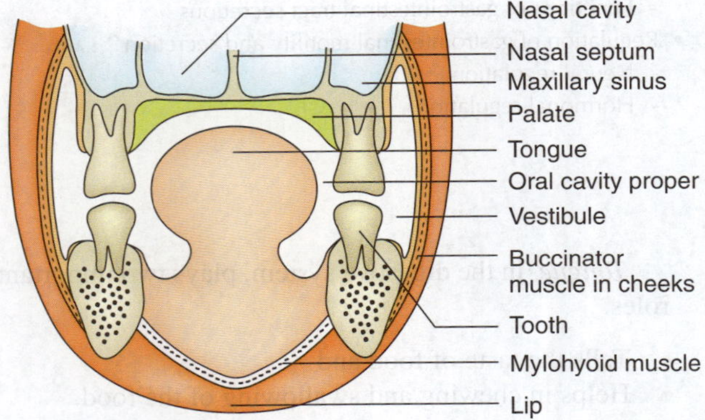

FIGURE 7.1-2 Schematic coronal section through oral cavity.

oesophagus. The peristaltic movements of the oesophagus propel the food into stomach.

Stomach. It is a hollow muscular bag connected to the oesophagus at its upper end and to the duodenum at the lower end. It serves the following motor functions:

- Storage of food till it can be accommodated in the duodenum,
- Mixing of food with gastric secretions to form a semiliquid mixture called chyme and
- Slow emptying of food into the small intestine.

Small Intestine. It is a long tubular structure which can be divided into three parts:

- *Duodenum* is the first part of small intestine. It is C shaped and measures about 25 cm in length.
- *Jejunum,* the middle part of the small intestine is about 25 m long and
- *Ileum,* the last part of small intestine, is about 3.5 m long.

Gastric chyme enters the duodenum where it meets with pancreatic juice, bile and secretions of the small intestine (succus entericus). The partially digested foodstuffs in the gastric chyme are digested further and the final products of digestion are absorbed by the villi of small intestine. The movements of small intestine help in mixing, digestion and absorption of the food. The peristaltic activity of small intestine also helps in moving the undigested and unabsorbed food material to the large intestine.

Large Intestine. It arches around and encloses the coils of the small intestine and tends to be more fixed than the small intestine. It is divided into following parts (Fig. 7.1-1):

- *Caecum* is a blind-ended sac into which opens the lower end of ileum. The ileocaecal junction is guarded by the ileocaecal valve which allows on flow but prevents backflow of intestinal contents.
- *Appendix* is a worm-shaped tube that arises from the medial side of caecum which in humans is a vestigial organ.
- *Ascending colon* extends upward from the caecum along the right side of the abdomen up to the liver. On reaching the liver, it bends to the left, forming the *right hepatic flexure.*
- *Transverse colon* extends from the right hepatic flexure to the *left splenic flexure.* It forms a wide U-shaped curve.
- *Descending colon* extends from the left splenic flexure to the pelvic inlet below.
- *Sigmoid colon* begins at the pelvic inlet as continuation down of the descending colon and joins the rectum in front of the sacrum.
- *Rectum* descends in front of the sacrum to leave the pelvis by piercing the pelvic floor. Here it becomes continuous with the anal canal in the perineum.
- *Anal canal* opens to the exterior through the anus, the opening which is guarded by two sphincters.

In large intestine, there occurs absorption of water and electrolytes from the intestinal contents. The remaining material is called *faecal matter.* The mucus secreted from the wall of large intestine lubricates the faecal matter. The faecal matter is stored in the sigmoid colon (pelvic colon) till expelled by the process of defaecation which is assisted by the movements of large intestine, activity of anal canal and anal sphincters.

Structural Characteristics of GIT Wall

Different parts of the gastrointestinal tract are specialized for carrying out different functions, particularly digestion and absorption, but the basic structural characteristics of the wall of whole gastrointestinal tract are similar. The intestinal wall from inside to outwards consists of following layers (Fig. 7.1-3):

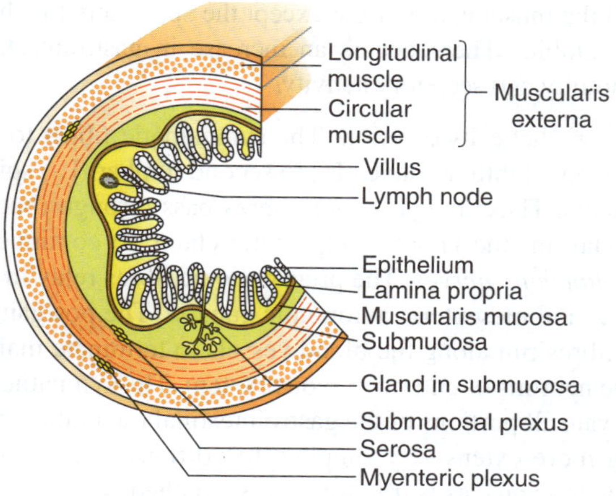

FIGURE 7.1-3 Cross-section of the alimentary canal depicting structural characteristics of its wall.

1. Mucosa (mucous layer). It is innermost coat consisting of three layers:

- *Surface epithelium* lining the luminal surface consists of epithelial cells which vary in type from simple squamous to tall columnar depending upon the function of the part of GIT.
- *Lamina propria* is composed of loose connective tissue which contains numerous glands, small blood vessels, lymphatics and nerve fibres.
- *Muscularis mucosa* is composed of two thin layers of smooth muscle fibres which help in localized movements of the mucosa.

2. Submucosa. This refers to the layer of connective tissue present outside the mucosa. It contains blood vessels, lymphatics and a network of nerve fibres and nerve cells called submucosal nerve plexus (Meissner's plexus).

3. Muscle Coat. It is formed by a thick layer of smooth muscle fibres surrounding the submucosa. The smooth muscle fibres are arranged in two layers:

- *Circular muscle fibres* form the inner layer and
- *Longitudinal muscle fibres* form the outer layer.

In between the circular and longitudinal muscle fibres is present an extensive network of nerve cells and fibres named *Auerbach's plexus* (myenteric plexus).

4. Serosa (serous layer). This is the outermost layer consisting of a layer of connective tissue. This layer helps in the attachment of gut to the surrounding structures.

Innervation of the GIT

The innervation of the gastrointestinal tract includes intrinsic and extrinsic system (Fig. 7.1-4).

1. Intrinsic Innervation. The intrinsic nervous system, also called as *enteric nervous system,* consists of nerve cells and fibres which originate and are located in the intestinal wall itself. This system supplies the smooth muscles of gastrointestinal tract (i.e. musculature of GIT except upper oesophagus and external anal sphincter which contain striated muscle). This system controls most of the gastrointestinal functions like secretion and

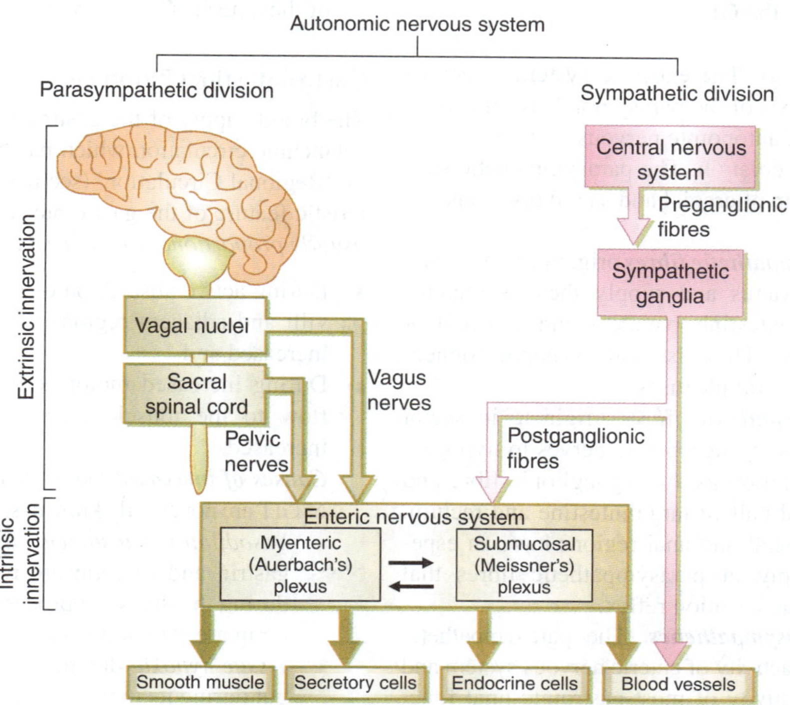

FIGURE 7.1-4 Schematic illustration of the innervation of gut.

motility. The enteric nervous system is composed mainly of two plexuses:

Myenteric Plexus or Auerbach's plexus is present in between the circular and longitudinal muscle fibres of muscular coat of the GIT. Stimulation of myenteric plexus causes increase in tone of the gut wall, intensity of rhythmical contractions of gut wall, rate of contraction and velocity of contraction.

Functions of myenteric plexus include:

- *Control of motility of gut* is the main function of this plexus.
- *Inhibition of pyloric sphincter,* which controls the emptying of stomach and
- *Inhibition of the ileocaecal valve,* which controls the emptying of the small intestine into the caecum.

Meissner's Plexus or submucosal plexus is present in the submucosal layer. It *controls the secretory activity* and blood flow to the gut. In contrast to the myenteric plexus, it is mainly concerned with controlling function within the inner wall of each minute segment of the intestine. By receiving sensory signals from the mucosal epithelium and from stretch receptors in the wall of alimentary canal, it helps to control local intestinal secretion, local absorption and local contraction of the submucosal muscle.

The Auerbach's and Meissner's plexuses are interconnected with each other and are under the control of parasympathetic and sympathetic components of the extrinsic nervous system. In both the plexuses, the axons branch profusely, so that stimulation of one region produces a widespread response in the GIT.

2. Extrinsic Innervation. The extrinsic system of nerves supplying the gut consists of the parasympathetic and sympathetic components of autonomic nervous system.

Parasympathetic Innervation. The parasympathetic supply to the gut is made up of cranial and sacral divisions:

- ***Cranial parasympathetic fibres*** originate in medulla, come through vagus and supply the oesophagus, stomach, small intestine, pancreas and first half of the large intestine. They also make synaptic connections with intramural plexuses.
- ***Sacral parasympathetic fibres*** originate in sacral spinal cord, pass through pelvic nerves to hypogastric (pelvic) ganglion as a postganglionic fibre and supply the distal half of large intestine and rectum. The sigmoid, rectal and anal regions have an especially rich supply of parasympathetic fibres that function in the defaecation reflex.

Functions of parasympathetics. The parasympathetic nerves increase the activity of enteric nervous system and thus enhance the activity of most gastrointestinal functions. Parasympathetic stimulation causes excitation of all the musculature of gut except the sphincters to which it inhibits. There occurs an increase in gastrointestinal motility and secretory activity.

Sympathetic Innervation. The sympathetic fibres to gut arise from eighth thoracic (T_8) to second lumbar (L_2) spinal segments. These preganglionic fibres pass through (but do not relay in) the lateral sympathetic chain, to continue as the *splanchnic nerves.* The preganglionic fibres relay in the coeliac and mesenteric autonomic ganglia. The postganglionic fibres run along the blood vessels to terminate mainly on the neurons of enteric nervous system. The sympathetics innervate all portions of the gastrointestinal tract rather than being more extensively supplied to portions near the oral cavity and anus, as is true for parasympathetics.

Functions of sympathetic innervation. Sympathetic stimulation causes:

- Vasoconstriction,
- Excitation of ileocaecal and internal anal sphincters and smooth muscles of muscularis mucosa throughout (to increase number of folds) and
- Inhibition of motility in the gut.

Thus, most of the effects of sympathetic stimulation are opposite to that of parasympathetic stimulation.

Mechanism of action. The sympathetic nerve endings secrete norepinephrine, which exerts its effects in two ways:

- To slight extent by a *direct action* that inhibits smooth muscle and
- To a major extent by an inhibitory effect on the neurons of the enteric nervous system.

Gastrointestinal Blood Flow

The blood supply of the gastrointestinal tract forms part of splanchnic circulation which has been described in chapter on 'Regional Circulation' (see page 370). The main characteristic feature of the gastrointestinal blood flow is that it is *usually proportional to the level of local activity.* Therefore:

- During active absorption of nutrients, blood flow in the villi and adjacent regions of the submucosa is greatly increased and
- During increased motor activity of the gut, the blood flow to the muscle layers of the intestinal wall is increased.

Causes of increased blood flow during increased activity of GIT are not exactly known; some of the known facts are:

- *Vasodilator substances* such as cholecystokinin, gastrin and secretin are released from the mucosa during the digestive process, and kallidin and bradykinin are released from the gastrointestinal glands.
- *Tissue hypoxia* due to decreased oxygenation of the gut during its increased activity causes marked vasodilation and increased blood flow by at least 50%.

Nervous Control of Gastrointestinal Blood Flow

- *Parasympathetic stimulation* increases glandular secretion and local blood flow in the gut.
- *Sympathetic stimulation* causes vasoconstriction and decrease in blood flow. This phenomenon is especially useful when blood is to be shifted from the splanchnic circulation to the heart in conditions like heavy exercise and circulatory shock.

GENERAL PRINCIPLES OF GASTROINTESTINAL FUNCTIONS

The main activities involved in the functioning of gastrointestinal tract are gastrointestinal tract motility and gastrointestinal tract secretion. The general principles governing these activities are discussed here.

General Principles of Gastrointestinal Motility

Characteristics of Gastrointestinal Smooth Muscle Functioning

The motor functions of the gut are performed by different layers of smooth muscles in its wall. The *gastrointestinal smooth muscle functions as a syncytium,* i.e. when an action potential is elicited within the muscle mass, it travels in all directions in the muscle and it contracts as a whole mass. The distances that it travels depend on the excitability of the muscle. This occurs because of the fact that the smooth muscle fibres in the longitudinal and circular muscle layers are electrically connected through the gap junctions that allow the ions to move from one cell to the next.

Electrical Activity of Gastrointestinal Smooth Muscle

Resting Membrane Potential (RMP) of gut smooth muscle fluctuates between −50 and −60 mV and thus shows undulating changes in the form of slow waves. The cause of these waves is not exactly known; it probably might be due to slow undulation of the activity of sodium–potassium pump. These waves determine the rhythm of most gastrointestinal contractions.

Factors affecting RMP of gastrointestinal smooth muscles. The basic level of RMP of gastrointestinal smooth muscle can be increased or decreased.

Factors that depolarize the membrane include:

- Stretching of the muscle,
- Stimulation by acetylcholine,
- Stimulation by parasympathetic nerves that secrete acetylcholine at their endings and
- Stimulation by gastrointestinal hormones.

Factors that hyperpolarize the membrane are:

- Effect of norepinephrine or epinephrine on the muscle membrane and
- Stimulation by sympathetic nerves that secrete norepinephrine at their endings.

Action potentials that cause muscle contraction occur in the form of spike potentials. They occur when the RMP becomes more positive than about −40 mV. The channels responsible for the action potentials are called *calcium–sodium channels.* These channels allow particularly large number of calcium ions to enter along with smaller number of sodium ions.

Functional Types of Gastrointestinal Movements

Peristalsis refers to the movement of gut. Functionally, two types of peristalsis are recognized: propulsive movements and mixing movements.

1. Propulsive Movements. The propulsion of food in the gut towards anus is accomplished by peristalsis:

- *Contraction ring* around a segment of intestine appears when it is distended, which moves forward propelling the food a few centimetres before ending.
- *Receptive relaxation* of the gut several centimetres towards the anus occurs along with appearance of contraction ring. This allows the food to be propelled more easily towards the anus.

The propulsive movements comprising appearance of contraction rings and receptive relaxation do not occur in the absence of myenteric plexus; therefore, it is also called *myenteric reflex* or *peristaltic reflex.* The peristaltic reflex plus the direction of movement toward the anus is called *law of the gut.*

2. Mixing Movements. The mixing of food in the gut is accomplished by peristalsis and local constrictive contractions:

- *Peristaltic contractions* cause most of the mixing of food. The churning is made possible more effectively when forward propulsion of intestinal contents is blocked by a sphincter.
- *Local constrictive contractions* which occur every few centimetres in the gut cause mixing of intestinal contents by their chopping action.

General Principles of Gastrointestinal Tract Secretion

Functions of Gastrointestinal Tract Secretions The secretions of gastrointestinal tract subserve three primary functions:

1. Lubrication of Food is carried by the mucus present in the secretion. Lubrication helps in propulsion of the intestinal contents.

2. Protection of Mucosa of alimentary tract is also done by the mucus present in the secretion.

3. Digestion of Food. Digestive enzymes present in the secretions degrade the food into usable nutrients. For example:

- *Starches* are degraded by amylases into monosaccharides.

- *Proteins* are degraded by a variety of enzymes (e.g. pepsin and trypsin) into dipeptides and amino acids.
- *Fats* are digested by lipases and esterases into monoglycerides and free fatty acids.

Stimulation of Alimentary Tract Secretion The alimentary tract secretion is initiated by direct mechanical stimulation of glandular cells by food. The stimulated local glands secrete digestive juices.

Regulation of Gastrointestinal Motility and Secretion

Regulation of gastrointestinal motility and secretion provides optimal conditions for digestion and absorption of the foodstuffs. The regulation reflexes are initiated by stimulation of receptors located in the walls of the intestinal tract, especially in the mucosa. *Receptors* located in the gut wall include:

- Mechanoreceptors,
- Chemoreceptors and
- Osmoreceptors.

Stimulation of above receptors activates the enteric nervous system of the gut wall. The types of stimuli that do this are:

- Distension of the gut wall by luminal contents,
- Tactile stimulation by the foodstuff,
- Chemical stimulation by acidity of the chyme,
- Stimulation of osmoreceptors by the osmolality of the chyme and
- Chemical stimulation by products of protein, fat and carbohydrate digestion, e.g. peptides, fatty acids, etc.

The regulation of gastrointestinal motility and secretion is mediated through neural and hormonal mechanisms:

Neural Regulation

Neural Innervation involved in the regulation of gastrointestinal function is described on page 573.

Characteristics of Neural Regulation are:

- *Enteric nervous system* is responsible for basic gut motility and secretions.
- *Stimulation of receptors* present in the gut mucosa modifies the activity of enteric nervous system.
- *Sensory signals* arising from one part of the gut may modify the secretory activity of another part of the gut, e.g. low pH of chyme in the duodenum decreases the acid secretion in the stomach.
- *Extrinsic nervous system* is involved in the regulation of gut motility and secretion in response to changes in the environment, e.g. effect of emotions, smell or taste on the gastric secretion and motility. This system is also involved in the long-loop reflexes in the gut, e.g. gastroileal reflex.

Gastrointestinal Reflexes that essentially control the gut motility and secretion can be grouped as:

Reflexes that Occur Entirely within the Enteric Nervous System of Gut. These reflexes control the gastrointestinal secretion, peristalsis, mixing contractions and local inhibitory effects.

Reflexes Involving Sympathetic Innervation. Such reflexes transmit signals for long distances (long-loop reflexes). These include:

- *Gastrocolic reflex* involves the signals from stomach to cause evacuation of the colon.
- *Enterogastric reflex* involves the signals from the small and large intestine that inhibit gastric motility and secretion.
- *Colo-ileal reflex* involves the signals from the colon which inhibit emptying of ileal contents into the colon.

Reflexes Involving Central Nervous System, Spinal Cord or Brainstem. These include:

- Reflexes that control motor and secretory activity of stomach through the vagus nerve.
- *Pain reflexes* that cause general inhibition of the entire gastrointestinal tract.
- *Defaecation reflexes* that travel to the spinal cord and back again to produce the powerful colonic, rectal and abdominal contraction required for defaecation.

Autonomic Control of Gastrointestinal Tract can be summarized as:

Motility of the Gut exhibits the following effects:

- ***Parasympathetic stimulation*** produces increase in motility and tone of the gut wall but causes relaxation of sphincters.
- ***Sympathetic stimulation*** produces decrease in motility and tone of the gut wall but causes contraction of sphincters.

Secretions of the Gut exhibit the following effects:

- ***Parasympathetic stimulation*** increases the secretions. This is especially true of salivary glands, oesophageal glands, gastric glands, the pancreas, Brunner's glands in the duodenum and the glands of distal portion of the large intestine. Secretions in the remaining of small intestine and in the first two thirds of large intestine occur mainly in response to local neural and hormonal stimuli.
- ***Sympathetic stimulation*** can have a dual effect on glandular secretion, i.e. may increase or decrease, depending on the existing secretory activity of the gland. This dual effect is highlighted:
  - *Sympathetic stimulation alone* usually slightly increases secretions.
  - *When secretion is already increased,* superimposed sympathetic stimulation usually inhibits the secretion by reducing blood flow to the gland.

Hormonal Regulation

Gastrointestinal Hormones: An Overview

- Gastrointestinal hormones regulate the secretions and even to some extent the motility of gastrointestinal tract.
- The *glandular cells* secreting gastrointestinal hormones are individually scattered in the epithelium of the stomach and small intestine and not in the form of clusters of cells as in the endocrine glands.
- The luminal surface of glandular cells when stimulated by various chemicals present in the chyme releases hormone from the opposite surface into blood capillaries of portal circulation.
- Through portal circulation, the released hormone reaches the target tissue situated in the nearby region of GIT and exhibits physiological actions on the target cells with specific receptors for the hormone. For example, the hormone gastrin released by G cells present in mucosa of pyloric part of the stomach in response to presence of peptides in chyme reaches the body of stomach via portal circulation and increases the acid secretion as well as motility of the stomach.
- The effects of gastrointestinal hormones persist even after nervous connections between the site of release and the site of action have been severed.
- Gastrointestinal hormones are characterized by two specific features:
  - Each hormone (even at physiological concentration) may affect more than one target tissue. For instance, the secretin increases the secretion of not only pancreatic juice but also of bile).
  - Each target tissue usually responds to more than one gastrointestinal hormone. For example, acid-secreting cells of gastric glands are stimulated by gastrin but inhibited by secretin.

Classification of Gastrointestinal Hormones The gastrointestinal hormones, based on their physio-anatomical similarities, can be broadly classified into three types:

1. *Gastrin family of hormones* includes:
   - Gastrin (for details see page 593) and
   - Cholecystokinin PZ or CCK-PZ
2. *Secretin family of hormones* includes:
   - Secretin (for details see page 612),
   - Gastric inhibitory polypeptide or GIP (for details see page 594),
   - Vasoactive intestinal peptide or VIP (for details see page 1016),
   - Glucagon (for details see page 780) and
   - Glucagon-like immune reactivity or GLI or glycentin (see page 780).
3. *Other gastrointestinal hormones* include:
   - Motilin,
   - Neurotensin,
   - Substance P,
   - Gastrin-releasing peptide or GRP (see page 594) and
   - Somatostatin (see page 594).

Actions of Gastrointestinal Hormones The details about the action of various gastrointestinal hormones are described somewhere else (see pages given in parentheses above). However, the outlines of the action of each gastrointestinal hormone as well as the stimulus for secretion and site of secretion are depicted in Table 7.1-1.

TABLE 7.1-1 Stimuli for Secretion, Site of Action and Actions of Gastrointestinal Hormones

Hormone	Stimuli for secretion	Site of secretion	Actions						
			Gastric secretion	*Gastric motility*	*Pancreatic secretion*	*Bile secretion*	*Gall bladder contraction*	*Small intestine secretion*	*Small intestine motility*
• Gastrin	Small peptides, amino acids, gastric disten- tion, vagal stimulation	G cells of gastric antrum	+	+	+	0	0	0	0
• Cholecystokinin (CCK)	Small peptides, amino acids, fatty acids	Type I cells of duodenum and jejunum	0	–	+	0	+	0	+
• Secretin	Acid Fatty acids	S cells of duodenum	–	0	+	+	0	0	0

Continued

TABLE 7.1-1 Stimuli for Secretion, Site of Action and Actions of Gastrointestinal Hormones—cont'd

Hormone	Stimuli for secretion	Site of secretion	Actions						
			Gastric secretion	*Gastric motility*	*Pancreatic secretion*	*Bile secretion*	*Gall bladder contraction*	*Small intestine secretion*	*Small intestine motility*
• Gastric inhibitory polypeptide (GIP)	Fatty acids, amino acids and oral glucose	Duodenum and jejunum	–	–	0	0	0	+	–
• Vasoactive Intestinal Polypeptide (VIP)	Fatty acids	Jejunum	–	–	0	0	0	0	0
• Somatostatin	Acid in stomach	D cells of islets of Langerhans	–	–	–	0	–	0	0

0 = no effect, + = stimulatory effect, – = inhibitory effect.

Immunology of the Gastrointestinal Tract

The gastrointestinal tract helps in replenishment of nutrient supply that comes from the external environment, and also is equipped with defence mechanisms.

Architecture. The immunological architecture of gut comprises:

- ***Epithelium:*** The mucosal epithelium overlying the Peyer's patches in small intestine has specialized microfold cells (M cells) for absorption of antigenic substances.
- ***Peyer's Patches*** are dense aggregates of lymphoid tissue having a collection of T and B lymphocytes.
- ***Lamina Propria:*** In the lamina propria of small intestine, large number of lymphocytes and plasma cells are scattered. The antigens absorbed by M cells get processed in these lymphocytes and get converted into lymphoblasts that ultimately form plasma cells.
- ***The Plasma Cells*** are responsible for secretion of IgA antibodies which provide secretory immunity against infested antigens.

Physiological Role of Immune Mechanism of the GIT

- These mechanisms prevent the absorption of intestinal-derived antigens such as food antigens and micro-organism origin antigens (bacteria and viruses). IgA antibodies present in the intestinal lumen prevent their access to the epithelial lining. The mechanism is known as *immune exclusion.*
- Luminal IgAs check bacterial colonization in the gut by preventing adherence of bacteria to the mucous membrane.
- IgAs play some role in bacteriolysis in presence of complement system.
- IgAs neutralize the adverse effect of viral toxins by inactivation of viruses.

The lymphocytes interspread in the epithelial lining mount an antigen-specific cell-mediated immune response that is especially useful in viral infection and tumour surveillance.

Chapter 7.2

Physiological Activities in Mouth, Pharynx and Oesophagus

INTRODUCTION

The digestive system is responsible for breaking down food and supplying the body with water, nutrients and electrolytes needed to sustain life. The functioning of the digestive system starts from the mouth (oral cavity) and ends at the anus.

INGESTION of food involves following processes:

- Placing of food into the mouth,
- Mastication, i.e. chewing the food into smaller pieces,
- Lubrication of the food with saliva and
- Swallowing, i.e. deglutition.

The aforementioned physiological activities which take place in the mouth, pharynx and oesophagus are discussed in this chapter.

MASTICATION

Mastication or chewing refers to the process by which the food placed in the mouth is cut and ground into smaller pieces. It involves:

- Movements of the jaws,
- Action of teeth—the incisors provide a strong cutting action, whereas the molars have a grinding action and
- Co-ordinated movements of the tongue and muscles of the oral cavity.

Chewing Reflex Mastication or chewing, though a voluntary act, is co-ordinated by a chewing reflex that facilitates the opening and closing of the jaw. The chewing reflex operates as:

- When the mouth is opened to place the food inside it, the muscles of jaw are stretched which leads to their contraction due to stretch reflex, thereby raising the jaw to cause closure of the mouth.
- When the mouth is closed, the food comes into contact with buccal receptors which cause reflex inhibition of the muscles of mastication and also initiate a reflex contraction of the digastric and lateral pterygoid muscles, causing the mouth to open.
- When the jaw drops, again there occurs contraction of jaw muscles due to stretch reflex and causes the entire cycle to be repeated. Again and again repetition of the cycle of opening and closing the jaw leads to mastication. The tongue contributes to the grinding process by positioning the food between the upper and lower teeth.
- Jaw muscles working together are capable of exerting a force of about 11–25 kg for incisiors and about 29–30 kg

for molars. As the force is exerted over a small area, therefore, the pressure exerted is hundreds of kg/cm2.

Muscles of Mastication

- *Masseter* raises the mandible, *clenches* the teeth and helps to protract the mandible.
- Temporalis raises the mandible and helps to retract the mandible after protraction.
- *Internal and external pterygoids* protrude the mandible, depress the chin and, therefore, help in opening the mouth. Grinding movements are produced by these when right and left muscles are acting alternatively.
- *Buccinator* is an accessory muscle of mastication which prevents accumulation of food between the cheek and teeth.

Functions of Mastication

1. Breaking of food into smaller pieces increases the total surface area. As the digestive enzymes act mainly on the surface of food particles, so the digestion rate is increased.
2. Undigestive cellulose membrane present around the nutrition portion of most fruits and raw vegetable is broken, making it easier for them to be digested.
3. Mixing of food with saliva initiates the process of starch digestion by salivary amylase, and lipid digestion by lingual lipase.
4. Swallowing becomes easy because of breaking of food into smaller pieces, and lubrication and softening of the food bolus by saliva.
5. Chewing brings food into contact with taste receptors and releases odour that stimulates the olfactory receptors. Stimulation of taste receptors and olfactory receptors increase the pleasure of eating and stimulate gastric secretions.

Net Effect of Mastication. The bolus of food becomes a homogenized mixture of small food particles, saliva and mucus, which is easy to swallow and digest.

LUBRICATION OF FOOD BY SALIVA

Salivary Glands

In addition to the chewing, another important physiological activity which takes place in the mouth is lubrication of food by saliva. Saliva is secreted by three pairs of major salivary glands:

1. Parotid Glands

Location. Parotid glands are the largest salivary glands (each weighing 20–30 g), located near the angles of jaw.

Acini. The parotid glands are purely serous glands (Fig. 7.2-1) which secrete watery saliva containing more than 90% water. Parotid glands secrete 25% of the total salivary secretion (which is about 1500 ml/day).

Ducts. Ducts of the parotid glands open on the inner side of the right and left cheek and pour their secretions in the vestibule.

2. Sublingual Glands

Location. The sublingual gland is the smallest of the three main salivary glands. It lies just below the mucosa on the floor of mouth. Each gland raises a ridge of mucosa which starts at the sublingual papilla and runs laterally and backwards. The ridge is called the sublingual fold.

Acini. The sublingual gland contains both serous and mucous acini (Fig. 7.2-1), the latter predominating.

Ducts of sublingual gland are 8–20 in number. Most open into the mouth on the summit of sublingual fold but a few may open into the submandibular duct.

3. Submandibular Glands

Location. The submandibular glands are large salivary glands which lie (one on each side) partly under cover of the body of the mandible. Each gland is made up of a large superficial part and a small deep part.

Acini. The submandibular gland is composed of a mixture of serous and mucous acini, the former predominating (Fig. 7.2.1).

Ducts. S-shaped duct of each submandibular gland opens on the sublingual papilla located just lateral to the frenulum lingua.

Note. The sublingual and submandibular glands secrete a fluid that contains a higher concentration of proteins and so is more viscous compared with the watery secretion of parotid glands.

Smaller Salivary Glands In addition to the three pairs of salivary glands described above, several smaller glands are located throughout the oral cavity. Those in the tongue secrete lingual lipase.

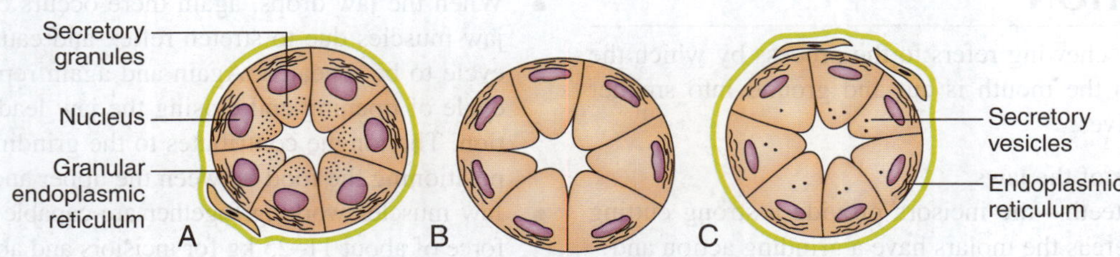

FIGURE 7.2-1 Different types of acini in salivary glands: **A**, serous; **B**, mucous; and **C**, seromucous.

Saliva

Secretion and Composition

The composition of salivary secretion depends on its source and rate of secretion. Serous secretion is watery and mainly contains electrolytes and amylase, whereas mucous secretion is viscous in nature, and it contains electrolytes and mucin.

Amount. Under normal circumstances, the salivary glands secrete about 500–1500 ml of saliva every day. pH of saliva varies from 6 to 7.4.

Composition. Saliva is composed of:

Water: 99%, and

Solids: 1%, which include:

- Organic substances such as L-amylase (ptyalin), lingual lipase, kallikrein, lysozyme, small amounts of urea, uric acid, cholesterol and mucin.
- Inorganic substances are Na^+, Cl^-, K^+ and HCO^-_3.

Note. Composition of saliva varies with the salivary flow rate.

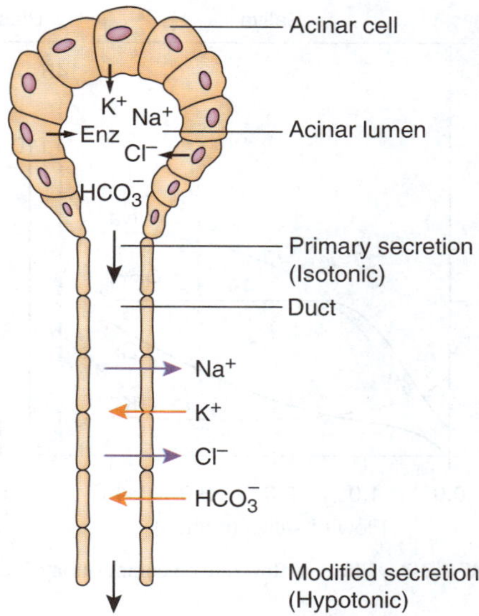

FIGURE 7.2-2 Mechanism of formation of saliva.

Mechanism of Formation of Saliva Mechanism of formation of saliva involves two processes:

1. Primary Secretion of Saliva. The acinar cells of salivary glands secrete the initial saliva into the salivary ducts. The initial saliva is formed by transudation (pressure filtration) of plasma and therefore is isotonic, i.e. has the same Na^+, Cl^-, K^+ and HCO^-_3 concentrations as plasma (Fig. 7.2-2). However, the initial saliva is soon modified by the salivary ducts.

2. Modification of Saliva. The ductal cells that line the tubular portions of the salivary ducts change the composition of initial saliva by the following processes (Fig. 7.2-2).

- ***Reabsorption of Na^+ and Cl^-*** occurs in the ductal cells; therefore, the concentration of these ions is lower than their plasma concentration.
- ***Secretion of K^+ and HCO^-_3*** is caused by the ductal cells; therefore, the concentration of these ions is higher than their plasma concentrations.
- ***Modified saliva becomes hypotonic*** in the ducts because the ducts are relatively impermeable to water. Because more solutes than water are reabsorbed by the ducts, the saliva becomes dilute relative to plasma.

Note. Aldosterone acts on the ductal cells to increase the reabsorption of Na^+ and Cl^- from salivary ducts (analogous to its actions on renal tubule). Thus a high Na^+/Cl^- ratio is seen when aldosterone is deficient in Addison's disease (see page 757). Conversely, in presence of excess aldosterone, the greatly increased sodium chloride concentration of saliva falls almost to zero and increases K^+ concentration equal to or higher than that of plasma.

Effects of Flow Rate on the Composition of Saliva Effects of flow rate on the composition of saliva occur due to changes in the contact time available for reabsorption and secretion processes to occur in the ducts.

1. At High Flow Rates, there is less time for reabsorption and secretion, and therefore the saliva is most likely the initial secretion by the acinar cells. Thus, with the increase in flow rate, the concentration of ions changes (Fig. 7.2-3):

- *Sodium ion (Na^+)* concentration increases progressively to a plateau value of 80–90 mEq/L.
- *Chloride ions (Cl^-)* concentration increases to about 50 mEq/L.

Note. Na^+ and Cl^- concentrations of saliva are always lower than that in the plasma.

- Potassium ion (K^+) concentration decreases to 15–20 mEq/L.
- Bicarbonate ion (HCO^-_3) concentration increases when salivary flow rate increases, because HCO^-_3 secretion is increased when salivary glands are stimulated by the parasympathetic nervous system. HCO^-_3 concentration then increases in saliva than that of plasma at high flow rates (up to 50–70 mEq/L).

2. At Low Flow Rates, there is more time for reabsorption and secretion; therefore, the modified saliva under resting conditions contains:

- Low concentration of Na^+ (about 15–20 mEq/L),
- Low concentration of Cl^- (15–20 mEq/L),
- Low concentration of HCO^-_3 (10–15 mEq/L) and
- High concentration of K^+ (25–30 mEq/L).

Phases of Salivary Secretion

1. ***Cephalic phase*** refers to secretion of saliva before entering of food into the mouth. It is caused by a conditioned reflex initiated by the mere sight or smell of food.
2. ***Buccal phase*** refers to secretion of saliva caused by stimulation of buccal receptors by the presence of food

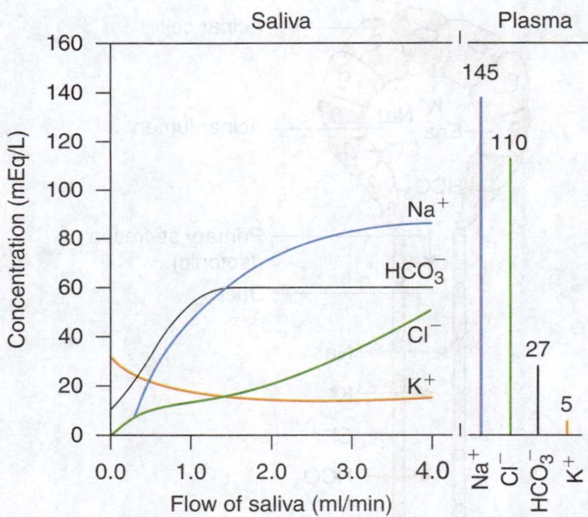

FIGURE 7.2-3 Effect of flow rate on composition of saliva.

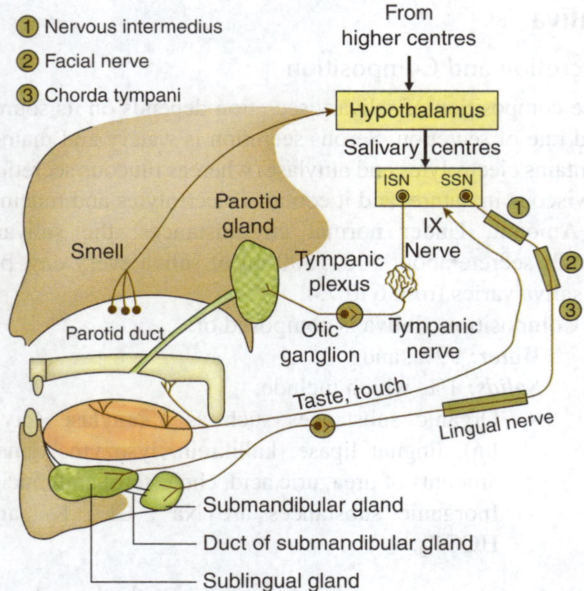

FIGURE 7.2-4 Parasympathetic nerve supply to salivary glands.

in the mouth. It is an unconditioned reflex, partially regulated by the appetite area of the brain.

3. ***Oesophageal phase*** occurs due to stimulation of salivary glands to a slight degree by the food passing through oesophagus.
4. ***Gastric phase*** refers to secretion of saliva by the presence of food in the stomach. It specially occurs when irritant food is present in the stomach (e.g. increased salivation before vomiting).
5. ***Intestinal phase*** refers to salivary secretion caused by presence of irritant food in the upper intestine.

Control of Salivary Secretion

- Salivary secretion is controlled entirely by autonomic nervous system (ANS) reflexes.
- Unlike other gastrointestinal glands, there is no hormonal regulation of salivary secretion.
- Salivary secretion production is unique in that it is increased by both parasympathetic and sympathetic activity; however, the activity of former is more important.

I. Parasympathetic Control

Parasympathetic Nerve Supply (Fig. 7.2-4)

Parotid glands are supplied by parasympathetic fibres (preganglionic) which arise from the inferior salivary nucleus (dorsal nucleus of IXth nerve) of medulla.

- Preganglionic fibres run via tympanic nerve and small superficial petrosal nerve to otic ganglion.
- Postganglionic fibres from the otic ganglion join auriculotemporal nerve to reach parotid gland where fibres are supplied along with blood vessels of gland.

Submandibular and sublingual glands are supplied by the parasympathetic fibres originating from superior salivary nucleus (dorsal nucleus of VIIth nerve).

- Preganglionic fibres run in nervous intermedius (sensory division of VII nerve), join the facial nerve and leave by its chorda tympani branch to join the lingual nerve. They synapse in the ganglia present near the glands.
- Postganglionic fibres arising from the ganglia present near the glands are supplied to the glands along with the blood vessels.

Parasympathetic Reflexes. Parasympathetic nerves are secretomotor to the salivary glands and control their secretion via following reflexes:

1. Conditioned Reflexes. Sight, smell or even thought of palatable food increase the salivary secretion by conditioned reflexes. In conditioned reflexes, the parasympathetics supplying the salivary glands are stimulated by impulses coming from higher centres of brain.

2. Unconditioned Reflexes are initiated by stimulation of receptors in the buccal cavity. Receptors and afferents, and efferents of unconditioned reflexes are:

- ***Receptors and afferents***
  - *Mechanoreceptors* which are excited by tactile stimulation from the tongue, mouth and pharynx. The tactile stimuli occur due to the presence of food in the buccal cavity, chewing movements and irritation of buccal mucosa.
  - *Afferent path* of tactile stimulation reflexes run in trigeminal nerve branches (such as lingual, buccal and palatine nerves), pharyngeal branches of vagus and glossopharyngeal nerve.
  - *Chemoreceptors*, i.e. taste buds are stimulated by sensation of taste and chemicals in the food. Afferents for taste sensation from:
    - *Posterior* 1/3rd of tongue pass via glossopharyngeal nerve to end in inferior salivary nucleus (dorsal nucleus of IXth nerve), and

- From anterior 2/3rd of tongue pass via nervous intermedius (branch of VIIth nerve) to end in superior salivary nucleus (dorsal nucleus of VIIth nerve).
- *Salivary centre* is thus constituted by superior and inferior salivary nuclei.
- *Efferents* from superior salivary nucleus stimulate the submandibular and sublingual salivary glands, while those from the inferior salivary nucleus stimulate the parotid glands.

Effects of Parasympathetic Stimulation Parasympathetic nerve stimulation causes the salivary gland cells to secrete a large volume of watery fluid that is high in electrolytes but low in proteins. Parasympathetic stimulation (cranial nerves VII and IX) increases saliva production by the following mechanisms (Fig. 7.2-5).

Stimulation of parasympathetic nerves liberates a proteolytic enzyme kallikrein from the gland cells which acts on α_2-globulin in interstitial fluid to form bradykinin. It also causes local release of VIP (vasoactive intestinal peptide). These increase the saliva production by:

- Increasing transport processes in the acinar and ductal cells, and
- Causing vasodilatation of blood vessels of salivary gland.

It is important to note that:

- Cholinergic receptors on acinar and ductal cells are muscarinic.
- The second messenger is inositol 1,4,5-triphosphate (IP3) and increased in transcellular calcium (Ca^{2+}) (Fig. 7.2-5).

- Anticholinergic drugs (e.g. atropine) inhibit the production of saliva and cause dry mouth.

II. Sympathetic Control

Sympathetic Nerve Supply

- Preganglionic fibres originate from the lateral horn cells of T_1 and T_2 segments of spinal cord and enter paravertebral sympathetic chain via ventral roots to synapse with the cells in *superior cervical ganglion*.
- *Postganglionic fibres* run along the carotid artery branches and are supplied to the three pairs of salivary glands along with their blood supply.

Effects of Sympathetic Stimulation Stimulation of sympathetic fibres causes vasoconstriction in the salivary glands, and transient secretion of a very small amount of thick viscid saliva rich in mucus and other organic constituents. Sympathetic stimulation causes salivary secretion if the gland is already activated by parasympathetic activity. However, in humans, the role of sympathetic nerves in physiological stimulation of salivary secretion is doubtful.

Receptors on acinar and ductal cells are ß-adrenergic and the second messenger is cyclic adenosine monophosphate—cAMP (Fig. 7.2-5).

Paralytic Secretion Claude Bernard observed that cutting the chorda tympani nerve (parasympathetic) in dog or cat produces scanty secretion of thin turbid saliva, which increases to peak on 7th day and diminishes in 3 weeks. He called it as paralytic secretion because it was caused by cutting the nerve supply. However, later on, it was shown that the increased secretion is due to increased sensitivity of the gland to adrenaline after cutting the chorda tympani nerve.

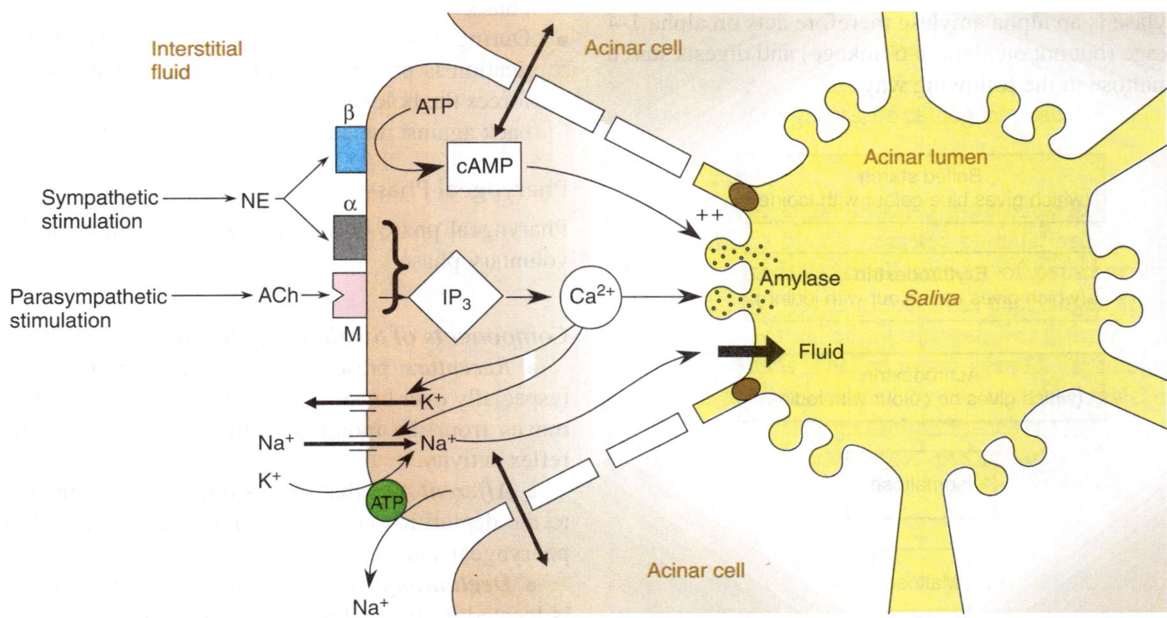

FIGURE 7.2-5 Mechanism of salivary regulation by parasympathetic and sympathetic nerves.

Functions of Saliva

1. Protective Function

- *Dilutes hot and irritant* food substances thus preventing injury to the buccal mucosa.
- *Washes away food particles* that remain in the oral cavity at the end of meal and thus cleans the oral cavity, i.e. helps in maintaining oral hygiene. In this way, growth of several harmful bacteria in the oral cavity is prevented.
- *Destroys harmful bacteria* in the mouth and thus minimizes risk of buccal infection and dental caries because of its following constituents:
  - *Lysozymes* which have bactericidal action,
  - *IgA* which provides immunological defence against bacteria and viruses and
  - *Lactoferrin* which has bacteriostatic action, i.e. prevents multiplication of bacteria.
- *Thiocyanate:* Saliva also contains thiocyanate ions (which are bactericidal) and an enzyme that facilitates the entry of thiocyanate ions into the bacteria.
- *Dilutes any hydrochloric acid (HCl) and bile* which regurgitate into oesophagus and mouth.

2. Role in Mastication and Deglutition

- Salivary mucus lubricates the food and buccal mucosa and thus aids in mastication and swallowing.
- Helps bolus formation by acting as a glue.

3. Digestive Functions

- *Initial starch digestion* starts by α-amylase (ptyalin) present in the saliva. However, the role of salivary amylase in the digestion of polysaccharides is limited by the short duration of salivary action. When the bolus of food reaches the stomach and mixes with the gastric juice, the gastric acidity (pH 1) stops the action of salivary amylase (which acts at an optimum pH of 6.5–7). Salivary amylase is an alpha amylase therefore acts on alpha 1-4 linkage (but not on alpha 1-6 linkage) and digests starch to maltose in the following way:

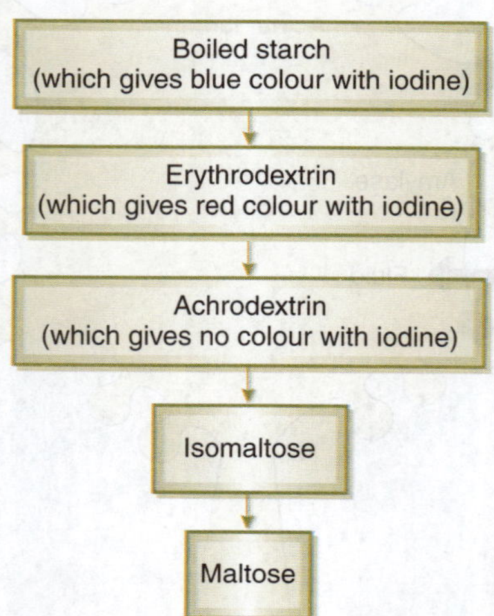

- *Initial triglyceride digestion* is caused by lingual lipase present in the saliva.

4. Role in Taste Sensation Saliva acts as a solvent for various foodstuffs, and is therefore necessary for taste. As taste is a chemical sense, the taste receptors respond only to dissolved substances.

5. Role in Speech Salivary mucus lubricates the oral mucosa and thus aids speech by facilitating movements of lips and tongue.

6. Excretory Function Saliva acts as a vehicle for excretion of certain heavy metals, thiocyanate ions, alcohol and morphine.

7. Role in Temperature Regulation

- During state of dehydration, the salivary secretion is reduced which induces thirst.
- Panting mechanism. In dogs, saliva is evaporated from the surface of tongue to cause evaporative heat loss.

DEGLUTITION (SWALLOWING)

Phases of Swallowing

Deglutition or swallowing refers to passage of food from the oral cavity into the stomach. It comprises three phases:

- Oral phase (voluntary),
- Pharyngeal phase (reflex or involuntary) and
- Oesophageal phase (reflex or involuntary).

Oral Phase

- Oral phase or the first stage of swallowing is a voluntary phase.
- During this phase. the bolus of food formed after mastication is put over the dorsum of tongue. The tongue forces the bolus into the oropharynx by pushing up and back against the hard palate (Fig. 7.2-6A).

Pharyngeal Phase

Pharyngeal phase or second stage of swallowing is an involuntary phase.

Components of Swallowing Reflex *(Fig. 7.2-7)*

- ***Receptors*** present around the opening of pharynx (especially over tonsillar pillars) are stimulated when bolus moves from the mouth into the pharynx and initiate the reflex activity.
- ***Afferent Arc*** that carries impulses from the receptors to the deglutition centre comprises the trigeminal, glossopharyngeal and vagus nerves.
- ***Deglutitioncentre*** co-ordinating the reflex activity is located in the medulla oblongata and lower pons (i.e. in

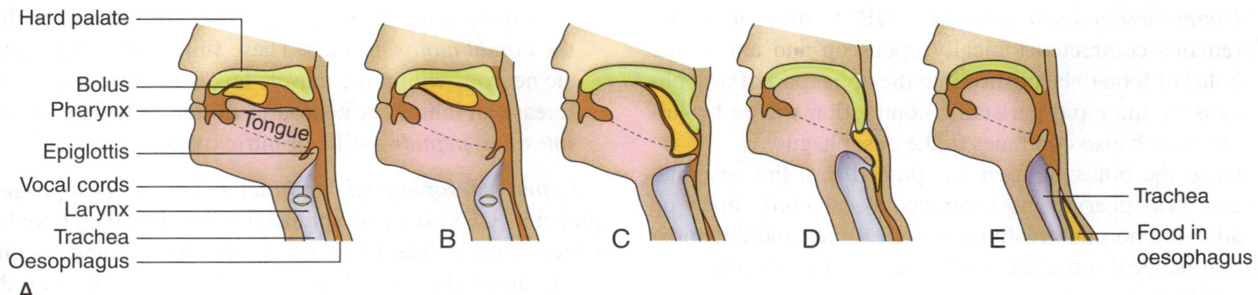

FIGURE 7.2-6 Phases of swallowing: **A,** oral phase; **B, C, D,** early, middle and late pharyngeal phase; and **E,** oesophageal phase.

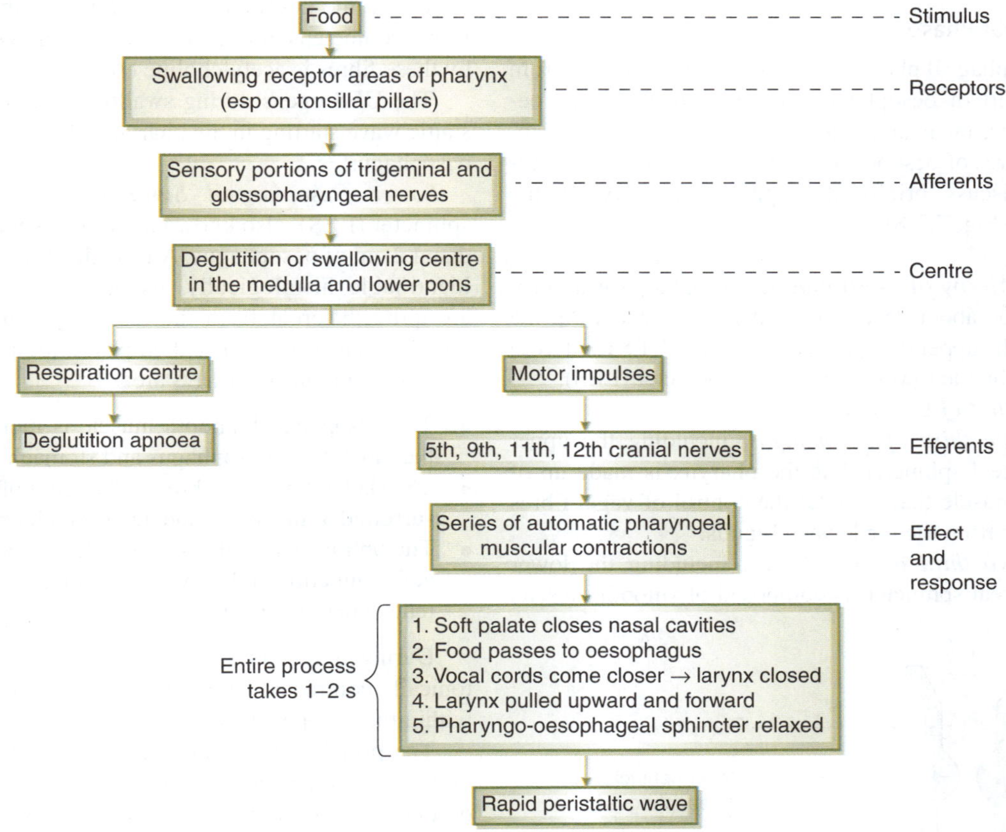

FIGURE 7.2-7 Summary of swallowing reflex.

the nucleus of the tractussolitarius (NTS) and the nucleus ambiguus).

- ***Efferent Arc*** which initiates a series of muscular contraction reaches the pharyngeal musculature and tongue through the 5th, 9th, 10th and 12th cranial nerves.

Events during Pharyngeal Phase Events which take place during movement of bolus from the pharynx into the oesophagus occur in the following sequence (Figs 7.2-6B, C and D).

- *Oral cavity is shut off* from the pharynx by the approximation of posterior pillars of the fauces.
- *Nasopharynx is closed* by the upward movement of soft palate, preventing regurgitation of food into the nasal cavities.
- *Palatopharyngeal folds are pulled medially*, to make a slit-like opening for food, allowing only properly masticated food to pass through (selective action).
- *Vocal cords* strongly approximate stopping the breathing temporarily (*deglutition apnoea*), *larynx* is pulled upward and anteriorly by neck muscles enlarging the opening of oesophagus which is normally a slit and *epiglottis* swings backwards to close the laryngeal opening. All this guides the food towards the oesophagus and prevent its entry into the trachea.

- *Upper oesophageal sphincter* (UES) which normally remains contracted tonically opens up and allows the bolus of food to be pushed into the upper part of oesophagus by the rapid peristaltic contraction wave of pharynx which also continues in the oesophagus.
- Once the bolus of food has passed into the oesophagus, cricopharyngeus contracts, vocal cords open up allowing normal breathing to be resumed and the upper oesophageal sphincter (UES) once again goes into tonic contraction.

The entire process of pharyngeal phase is completed in 1–2 s.

Oesophageal Phase

During oesophageal phase, the food bolus is propelled from the upper part of oesophagus to the stomach by the oesophageal peristalsis and aided by gravity. Before describing the features of oesophageal peristalsis, it will be worthwhile to discuss briefly the applied anatomy of the oesophagus (Fig. 7.2-8).

Applied Anatomy of Oesophagus Oesophagus is a fibromuscular tube about 25 cm long. It is separated from the pharynx by the upper oesophageal sphincter (UES) and from the stomach by the lower oesophageal sphincter (LES).

Musculature of Oesophagus

- *Upper one third of oesophagus,* including the upper oesophageal sphincter, like the pharynx is made up of striated muscle that is under the control of vagal fibres emerging from the nucleus ambiguus.
- *Lower two third of oesophagus,* including the lower oesophageal sphincter, is composed of smooth muscle.

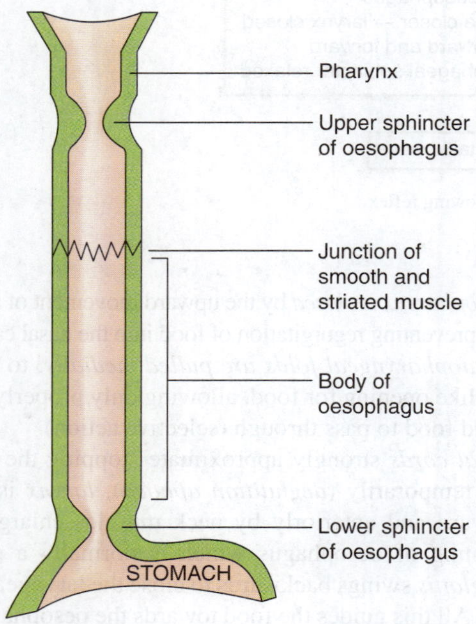

FIGURE 7.2-8 Schematic structure of oesophagus.

Its activity is regulated by vagal fibres originating within the *dorsal motor nucleus*. These fibres innervate intrinsic neurons within the muscle layers of oesophagus that release an inhibitory neurotransmitter (either vasoactive *intestinal peptide*—VIP, or nitric oxide).

Upper Oesophageal Sphincter Upper oesophageal sphincter (UES) is a true sphincter formed by the cricopharyngeal muscle. The UES is a striated muscle and is completely under the control of vagal fibres that innervate the upper one third of oesophagus. The UES is normally contracted tonically and serves to prevent the entry of air into the oesophagus during normal respiration. Its tone is maintained by the continual firing of vagal fibres originating from the nucleus ambiguus. The neurotransmitter released by these fibres is acetylcholine (ACh).

The UES opens during swallowing when a rapid peristaltic wave starting in the pharyngeal muscles passes on to oesophagus.

Lower Oesophageal Sphincter Lower oesophageal sphincter (LES), also known as cardiac sphincter, refers to distal 2 cm of oesophagus. Although LES is not separately identifiable histologically, its contractile characteristics are quite different from the rest of oesophageal smooth muscle (that is why it is called physiological sphincter).

The components of LES are:

- The oesophageal smooth muscle is more prominent at the junction of oesophagus and stomach.
- The skeletal muscle fibres of the crura of the diaphragm surround at this point and act as pinch cock.
- The oblique sling fibres of gastric wall act as flap valve at this junction and prevent regurgitation of gastric contents when there is increase in intragastric pressure.

During quiescent (nonperistaltic) periods, the LES is tonically contracted while the remainder of smooth muscle within the oesophagus is relaxed.

The principal function of LES is to prevent regurgitation of gastric contents (food, gastric juice and air) into the oesophagus; when the intragastric pressure is markedly raised (e.g. after a heavy meal or ingestion of carbonated drinks), the resistance of LES is overcome and air escapes into the mouth (belching). The local hormone, gastrin, increases the tone of LES and helps to keep the sphincter more tightly closed during digestion.

Oesophageal Peristalsis

- The oesophageal phase of deglutition (Fig. 7.2-6E) is completed by two types of oesophageal peristalsis, primary and secondary.

Primary Oesophageal Peristalsis

- Primary oesophageal peristalsis is initiated by swallowing, i.e. it is a part of swallowing and is thus coordinated by vagal fibres emerging from the swallowing centre.

- As soon as the food bolus enters the oesophagus from pharynx, the UES contracts to prevent regurgitation of food into the mouth, and primary oesophageal peristalsis begins which propels the food downwards.
- The peristaltic wave travels rather slowly (3–4 cm/s), taking about 8 s to push the food into the stomach. In the upright position, the force of gravity causes the liquids and semisolid to pass through the oesophagus at a much faster rate.
- The lower oesophageal sphincter (LES) (which normally remains tonically contracted) relaxes as the peristaltic wave approaches the sphincter and allows the bolus of food to enter the stomach without causing any resistance.

Secondary Oesophageal Peristalsis

- When the primary oesophageal peristalsis is not able to push a bolus of solid food all the way down the oesophagus, the food remaining in the oesophagus stretches mechanical receptors and initiates another peristaltic wave called the secondary oesophageal peristalsis.
- Secondary oesophageal peristalsis is co-ordinated by the *intrinsic nervous* system of the oesophagus. Afferent fibres innervate stretch receptors within the wall of the oesophagus and thereby activate the appropriate fibres in the intrinsic nervous system. Therefore, vagotomy would have little or no effect on secondary oesophageal peristalsis.
- Thus, the secondary oesophageal peristalsis is initiated by the presence of food within the oesophagus and the waves continue until all the swallowed food is removed from the oesophagus.

Note. After the food enters the stomach, the LES contracts to prevent regurgitation of food into the oesophagus. With this the oesophageal phase of deglutition is completed.

Disorders of Swallowing

1. Abolition of Deglutition Reflex Abolition of deglutition reflex causes regurgitation of food into the nose or aspiration into the larynx and trachea. It may occur:

- When IX or X nerve is paralyzed in lesions of medulla, and
- When pharynx is anaesthetized with cocaine (deglutition reflex is abolished temporarily).

2. Aerophagia

- Aerophagia refers to unavoidable swallowing of air along with the swallowing of food bolus and liquids.
- It usually occurs in nervous individuals having low tone of the upper oesophageal sphincter (UES).
- Some of the gases present in the air swallowed are absorbed, partly the air is regurgitated into the oral cavity and out in the atmosphere (belching), and majority of it passes on the colon and is then expelled as flatus through the anus.

3. Cardiac Achalasia

- Cardiac achalasia is a neuromuscular disorder of the lower two thirds of oesophagus, characterized by absence of oesophageal peristalsis and failure of the lower oesophageal sphincter (LES) to relax during swallowing.
- Because of this, food transmission to stomach is impeded. In severe cases, oesophagus fails to empty the swallowed food into stomach for several hours.
- Over months and years, oesophagus becomes enlarged and infected due to long-standing stasis of food.

  Causes: The myenteric plexus of the oesophagus is usually deficient in the region of LES; therefore, the release of VIP and NO is also defective leading to increased resting tone of LES and incomplete relaxation during swallowing.

  Treatment: Cardiac achalasia can be treated by the following procedures:

  - Pneumatic dilatation of the LES.
  - Incision of oesophageal smooth muscle (myotomy).
  - Injection of botulinum toxin into LES to prevent release of acetylcholine. This treatment is effective for about several months.

4. Gastroesophageal Reflux Disease Gastroesophageal reflux disease (GRD) refers to a condition in which incompetence of lower oesophageal sphincter (LES) causes reflux of acidic gastric contents into oesophagus. Reflux of stomach acid causes oesophageal pain (heartburn) and may lead to irritation of oesophagus or bronchioles (due to aspiration).

Conditions Associated with Gastroesophageal Reflux Disease include:

- Conditions in which emptying of the stomach is not normal (e.g. as in pyloric sphincter disease).
- When the gastric contents are pushed up against the oesophagus (e.g. when the patient is lying down).
- When the LES is forced through the diaphragm into the thoracic cavity (e.g. hiatal hernia).
- During pregnancy, the growing fetus may push the top of the stomach into the thorax. The low intrathoracic pressure (compared with the higher intra-abdominal pressure) causes the LES to expand, allowing reflux to occur.
- Conditions in which LES fails to contract between swallows.

5. Dysphagia Dysphagia is a term used to denote difficulty in swallowing due to any cause.

Chapter 7.3

Physiological Activities in Stomach

FUNCTIONAL ANATOMY
- Gross anatomy
- Structural characteristics
- Innervation of stomach

PHYSIOLOGY OF GASTRIC SECRETION
- Gastric juice
  - Composition
  - Secretion
- Regulation of gastric secretions
  - Regulatory mechanisms
  - Phases and regulation of gastric secretion
  - Experimental demonstration of regulation of gastric secretion

PHYSIOLOGY OF GASTRIC MOTILITY
- General considerations
- Initiation of gastric motility
- Motility of empty stomach
  - Migratory motor complexes
  - Hunger contractions
- Gastric motility related to meals
  - Receptive relaxation
  - Mixing peristaltic waves
  - Gastric emptying

FUNCTIONS OF STOMACH
- Mechanical functions
- Digestive functions
- Absorptive functions
- Excretory functions
- Stimulating functions
- Reflex functions
- Antiseptic functions

APPLIED ASPECTS
- Gastric mucosal barrier and pathophysiology of peptic ulcer
- Physiology of vomiting
- Total gastrectomy
- Gastric function tests

FUNCTIONAL ANATOMY

Gross Anatomy

General Features

- Stomach is a J-shaped hollow muscular bag connected to the oesophagus at its upper end and to the duodenum at the lower end.
- Gastric contents are isolated from the rest of the gastrointestinal tract proximally by the lower oesophageal sphincter (LES) and distally by the pyloric sphincter.
- The *volume* of stomach is 1200–1500 ml, but its *capacity* is greater than 3000 ml.
- The stomach has two curvatures. The concavity of the right inner curve is called *lesser curvature* and the convexity of the left outer curve is the *greater curvature*. An angle along the lesser curvature, the *incisura angularis* marks the approximate point at which the stomach narrows before its junction with the duodenum.

Parts of Stomach The stomach can be divided into five anatomic regions (Fig. 7.3-1):

- *Cardia* is the narrow conical portion of the stomach immediately distal to the gastroesophageal junction.
- *Fundus* is the dome-shaped proximal portion of the stomach.
- *Body or corpus* is the main part of the stomach that extends up to the incisura angularis.
- *Pyloric antrum* extends from the incisura angularis to the pyloric canal.
- *Pyloric canal or pylorus* is the distal-most 1-inch-long tubular part of stomach.

Note. Anatomically, the antrum and pylorus are continuous and respond to the nervous control as a unit. Functionally, the first part of the duodenum is associated with the pyloric part of the stomach.

Structural Characteristics

As elsewhere in the gut (page 572), the gastric wall consists of mucosa, submucosa, muscular coat and serosa (serous layer). The mucosa and muscular coats of the stomach need to be described in detail to understand the physiology of the stomach.

Gastric Mucosa

Gross Features

- The inner surface of the stomach exhibits coarse *rugae.* These infoldings of mucosa and submucosa extend

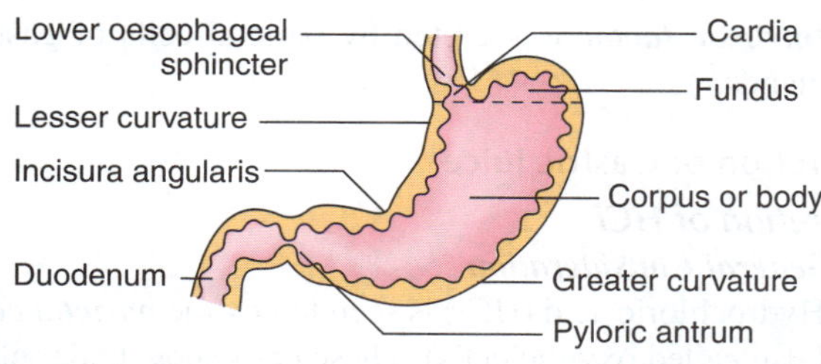

FIGURE 7.3-1 Gross anatomy of stomach.

longitudinally and are most prominent in the proximal stomach.

- A finger mosaic-like pattern is delineated by small furrows in the mucosa.
- The delicate texture of the mucosa is punctured by millions of gastric *foveolae* or pits, leading to the mucosal glands.

Histological Features. Gastric mucosa comprises (Fig. 7.3-2):

- ***Surface foveolar cells*** are tall columnar mucin-secreting cells which line the entire gastric mucosa, as well as the gastric pits. These cells have basal nuclei and mucin-containing granules in the supranuclear region.
- ***Mucous neck cells*** are present deeper in the gastric pits. These cells have a lower content of mucin granules and are thought to be the progenitors of both, the surface epithelium and the cells of gastric glands.
- ***Glandular cells*** form the gastric glands. There are three types of gastric glands, main gastric glands, cardiac tubular glands and pyloric (antral) glands.

1. ***Main gastric glands,*** found in the body and fundus of stomach, are much more in number than in the other gastric glands. These are simple tubular glands (Fig. 7.3-2). The alveoli of main gastric glands contain two types of cells:
   - *Chief cells*, also known as peptic or zymogen cells are basophilic. These cells are concentrated at the base of the main gastric glands. These cells secrete proteolytic proenzymes and pepsinogen I and II.
   - *Parietal cells*, also known as oxyntic cells are acidophilic. These cells predominantly line the upper half of the glands and have an extensive intracellular canalicular system. These secrete *hydrochloric acid* (HCl) and the *intrinsic factor*.
2. ***Cardiac tubular glands*** are found in the mucosa of cardia (a small conical part of the stomach), just around the distal end of the oesophagus. These secrete *soluble mucus*.
3. ***Pyloric (antral) glands*** are found in the antrum and pylorus region of the stomach. These glands contain two types of cells:
   - *Mucus cells*, which secrete *soluble mucus* and
   - *G-cells*, which are responsible for release of the hormone gastrin.

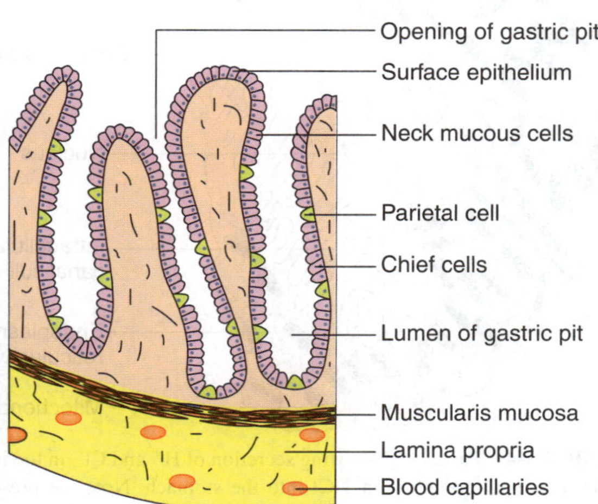

FIGURE 7.3-2 Histological features of gastric mucosa.

Musculature of Stomach Characteristic features of gastric musculature are:

- The muscle coat of the stomach has three layers, an outer longitudinal, middle circular and an inner oblique (Fig. 7.3-3).
- As elsewhere in the gut, each muscle layer in the stomach forms a *functional syncytium* and, therefore, acts as a unit. In the fundus, where the layers are relatively thin, the strength of contraction is weak; in the antrum, where the muscle layers are thick, the strength of contraction is greater.
- The stomach and duodenum are divided by a thickened, circular smooth muscle layer called the *pyloric sphincter*.

Innervation of Stomach

Innervation of stomach, as elsewhere in the gut (page 573), includes an intrinsic and an extrinsic system.

1. Intrinsic Innervation comprises two interconnected plexuses:

- *Myenteric (Auerbach's) plexus*, located between the layers of circular and longitudinal muscles of the stomach and
- *Submucosal (Meissner's) plexus*, located in the submucosal layer.

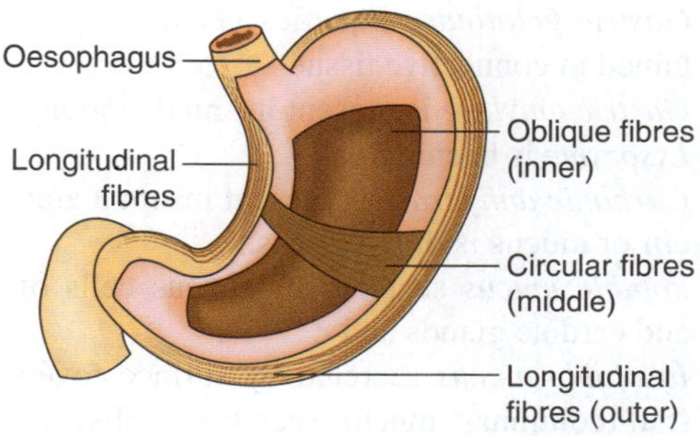

FIGURE 7.3-3 Three layers of gastric mucosa.

The intrinsic innervation is directly responsible for peristalsis and other contractions. Because this system is continuous between the stomach and duodenum, peristalsis in the antrum influences the duodenal bulb.

2. Extrinsic Innervation modifies the co-ordinated motor activity that arises independently in the intrinsic nervous system. It consists of the two components of the autonomic nervous system:

- *Sympathetic innervation* comes via coeliac plexus and *inhibits motility* and
- *Parasympathetic innervation* comes via the vagus nerve and *stimulates motility*.

PHYSIOLOGY OF GASTRIC SECRETION

The gastric secretions include:

- *Exocrine secretions,* i.e. gastric juice and
- *Endocrine secretions*, i.e. gastrin hormone (see regulation of gastric secretion, page 593).

Gastric Juice

Composition

Gastric glands secrete about 2–2.5 L of gastric juice in the lumen of stomach per day. It is acidic with a pH varying from 1 to 2. Important constituents of gastric juice are:

- ***Water*** 99.45%
- ***Solids*** 0.55%, which include:
- ***Electrolytes*** such as Na^+, K^+, Mg^{2+}, Cl^-, HCO_3^-, HPO_4^{-2} and SO_4^{-2}. The electrolyte content of gastric juice varies with the rate of secretions. At low secretory rates, Na^+ concentration is high and H^+ concentration is low, but as acid secretion increases Na^+ concentration falls.
- ***Enzymes*** present in the gastric juice are:
  - *Pepsin* is a proteolytic enzyme which is secreted by chief cells of gastric glands in an inactive form pepsinogen. Pepsinogen is activated to pepsin in the presence of HCl at an optimal pH of about 2.
  - *Gastric lipase* is a weak fat-splitting enzyme. It is of little importance in fat digestion except in pancreatic insufficiency.
  - *Gastric gelatinase* liquefies gelatin, a protein contained in connective tissue.
  - *Gastric amylase* is present in small amounts.
  - *Lysozyme* is bactericidal.
  - *Carbonic anhydrase* is present in small amounts.
- ***Mucin*** or mucus is of two types:
  - *Soluble mucus* secreted by mucus cells of pyloric and cardiac glands and
  - *Insoluble mucus* secreted by surface foveolar cells (tall columnar mucin secreting cells) lining the entire gastric mucosa.
- ***Intrinsic factor*** is secreted by parietal cells of gastric glands.

Secretion of Gastric Juice

Secretion of HCl

General Consideration

- Hydrochloric acid (HCl) is secreted by the *parietal cells* (also called oxyntic cells). These cells show under electron microscope, as a complex network of *intracellular canaliculi* (Fig. 7.3-4) into which HCl is secreted
- Gastric glands secrete about 2.5 L of HCl in a day. The HCl secreted by gastric glands is concentrated having a pH of approximately 1.0.
- The gastric HCl dissociates completely into H^+ and Cl^-. The concentration of H^+ in the gastric juice increases with the increase in the rate of its secretion. At high rates of secretion H^+ concentration maybe as high as 155 mEq/L, i.e. about three million times greater than its concentration in the blood.

Mechanism of HCl Secretion. Various theories have been put forward to explain the origin of H^+ of HCl (e.g. Davenport and Fisher theory, Davies theory and Hollander hypothesis). However, it is still not known exactly. The hypothesis more widely accepted is shown in Fig. 7.3-5. Hydrochloric acid is made up of hydrogen (H^+) and chloride ions (Cl^-) and, therefore, its secretion can be described in two steps, i.e. secretion of H^+ and secretion of Cl^-.

Secretion of H^+

- The H^+ ions are believed to be generated inside the parietal cell from metabolic CO_2 and H_2O present in the cell. The enzyme carbonic anhydrase present in abundance in

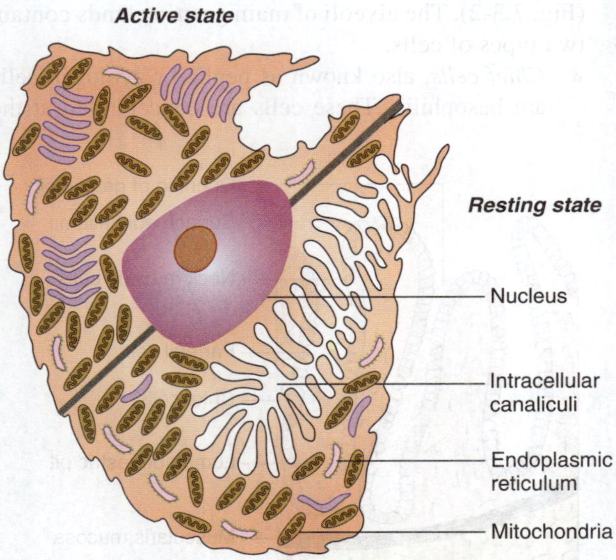

FIGURE 7.3-4 Partial cell showing secretion of H^+ and Cl^- in the intracellular canaliculi which pour HCl into the stomach. Note the presence of numerous mitochondria which provide energy for the active transport process.

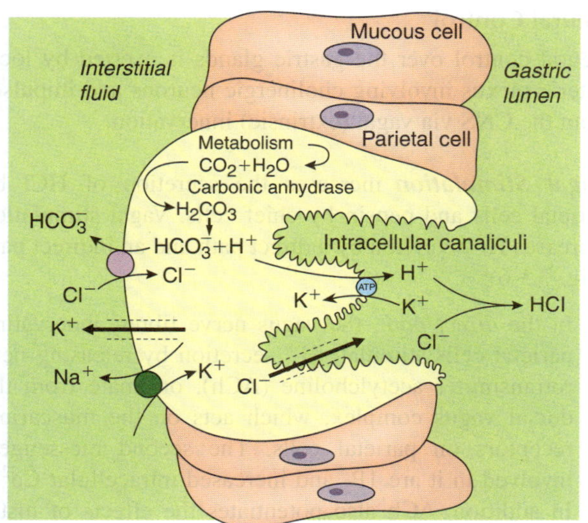

FIGURE 7.3-5 Mechanism of HCl secretion in the parietal cells of the stomach.

the parietal cells is essential for the secretion. It accelerates the formation of H_2CO_3 which dissociates to release H^+ and HCO^-_3 as:

$$CO_2 + H_2O \xrightarrow[\text{anhydrase}]{\text{Carbonic}} H_2CO_3 \rightarrow H^+ + HCO_3^-$$

- The H^+ ions generated by the above reaction are then secreted into the lumen of the canaliculi in exchange for K^+ by a primary active transport mediated by H^+–K^+–ATPase pump or proton pump (Fig. 7.3-5). This H^+–K^+ exchange is obviously electroneutral.

Note. The drug omeprazole, used to decrease HCl formation, inhibits the H^+–K^+–ATPase and blocks H^+ secretion.

- In resting condition, the proton pumps are sequestered as tubulovesicles within the parietal cell membrane. In active stage, these proton pumps get fused with the canaliculi present on the apical membrane, thereby positioning of proton pumps on the membrane helps in acid secretion.
- The K^+ channels present on the apical membrane supply K^+ for exchange of H^+ secretion.
- The HCO^-_3 ions produced in the parietal cell are transported by an antiport in the serosal (basolateral) membrane into the blood in exchange of Cl^- by an active transport via Cl^-/HCO^-_3 exchange. The HCO^-_3–Cl^- exchange is again electroneutral.

The HCO_3^- released into the blood is responsible for the postprandial alkaline tide associated with increased gastric acid secretion after meals, which is characterized by: alkaline urine, slightly depressed breathing and raised alveolar pCO_2.

Note. Eventually, this HCO_3^- from the blood will be secreted in pancreatic secretion to neutralize H^+ in the small intestine. If vomiting occurs, gastric H^+ never arrives in the small intestine, there is no stimulus for pancreatic HCO_3^- secretion and the arterial blood becomes alkaline (metabolic alkalosis).

Secretion of Cl^-. Because of the high intracellular negativity, the Cl^- present in the parietal cell is forced out into the lumen of gland through the Cl^- channels located on the apical membrane of the cell. These Cl^- channels are activated by cAMP. The high intracellular negativity is the result of the following (Fig. 7.3-5):

- The Na^+–K^+ pump located on the basolateral membrane of parietal cells pumps out 3 Na^+ for every 2 K^+ pumped in, thereby creating intracellular negativity.
- The K^+ pumped in diffuses out through the K^+ channels present on the basolateral as well as apical membranes. This diffusion further increases intracellular negativity of parietal cells.

Note. It is important to note that the active transport processes involved in the generation of HCl require a large amount of adenosine triphosphate (ATP). The ATP generated by mitochondria is found in very high concentration (40% of cell volume) within the parietal cell (Fig. 7.3-4).

Factors Affecting HCl Secretion

- ***Factors stimulating HCl secretion are:***
  - Vagal stimulation,
  - Gastrin and
  - Histamine.
- ***Factors that inhibit HCl secretion are:***
  - Low pH in stomach (<3) by negative feedback mechanism,
  - Intestinal influences,
  - Somatostatin and
  - Prostaglandins (PGE and PGI), epidermal growth factor (EGF) and transforming growth factor (TGF)

(For details see page 800)

Functions of HCl

- HCl participates in the breakdown of protein,
- It provides an optimal pH for the action of pepsin and
- It hinders the growth of pathogenic bacteria.

Pepsinogen Secretion

- ***Pepsinogen is an inactive precursor*** (proenzyme) of pepsin. It is mainly secreted by *chief cells* of the main gastric glands. A small amount of pepsinogen is also secreted by pyloric glands. The pepsinogen secreted by chief cells is called *pepsinogen I* and that secreted by pyloric glands is called *pepsinogen II*. Pepsinogen I and II can be differentiated by the immunological method but their physiological significance is not known.
- ***Pepsinogen is synthesized and stored*** as zymogen granules in the apical region of chief cells.
- ***Pepsinogen secretion is stimulated by*** vagal stimulation, gastrin and histamine.
- ***Pepsinogen is converted to pepsin*** (the active form) by the action of HCl or preformed pepsin.

$$\text{Pepsinogen} \xrightarrow{\text{HCl}} \text{Pepsin}$$
$$\text{Pepsinogen} \xrightarrow{\text{Pepsin}} \text{Pepsin}$$

Function of Pepsinogen. Pepsin, the active form of pepsinogen, is a proteolytic enzyme that begins the process of protein digestion. It splits protein into proteoses, peptones and polypeptides. It is important to note that the optimum pH for the action of pepsin is 2.0; therefore, acid secretion by the stomach is as essential as pepsinogen secretion for the digestion of proteins.

Secretion of Mucus Mucus is of two types, insoluble and soluble.

Insoluble mucus is secreted by the mucous-secreting cells lining the entire gastric mucosa. The insoluble mucus is such a viscid that it forms a gel-like coat over the mucosa. These cells also secrete bicarbonate ions which make the mucus with alkaline pH of 7 that forms an extremely important protective layer saving the stomach from the destruction of HCl and substances known as trefoil peptides that stabilize the mucus bicarbonate layer.

Soluble mucus is secreted by mucus cells of pylorus and cardiac glands.

Mucus secretion is increased by direct stimulation of mucosa by the rough food. Neural or hormonal control over secretion of mucus, if any, is not known.

Secretion of Intrinsic Factor

Secretion. Intrinsic factor (IF), a glycoprotein, is secreted by the parietal cells of gastric mucosa, chiefly by those in the fundus. The secretion of intrinsic factor by the parietal cells is linked to the action of histamine through cAMP mechanism.

Functions. The intrinsic factor is essential for the absorption of vitamin B_{12}. It forms a complex with B_{12}, which is carried to the terminal ileum where the vitamin is absorbed.

Deficiency of intrinsic factor in some patients with idiopathic atrophy of gastric mucosa may cause a serious disorder called pernicious anaemia (see page 162).

Regulation of Gastric Secretion

Regulation of gastric secretion can be discussed under three subheads:

- Regulatory mechanisms,
- Phases of gastric secretion and their regulation and
- Experimental demonstration of the role of regulatory mechanisms.

Regulatory Mechanisms

Mechanisms regulating the gastric secretion include neural control and chemical control.

Neural Control

Neural control over the gastric glands is exerted by local enteric plexus involving cholinergic neurons and impulses from the CNS via vagal (extrinsic) innervation.

Vagal Stimulation increases the secretion of HCl by parietal cells and pepsin by chief cells. Vagal stimulation increases H^+ secretion by a direct path and an indirect path (Fig. 7.3-6):

- In the *direct path,* the vagus nerve fibres, innervating parietal cells stimulate H^+ secretion by releasing neurotransmitter acetylcholine (ACh), originate from the dorsal vagus complex, which acts on the muscarinic receptors on parietal cells. The second messengers involved in it are IP_3 and increased intracellular Ca^{2+}. In addition, ACh also potentiates the effects of histamine on H_2 receptors of parietal cells.
- In the *indirect path,* the vagus nerve innervates G-cells and stimulates the release of gastrin into circulation through gastrin-releasing peptide (GRP). GRP is a

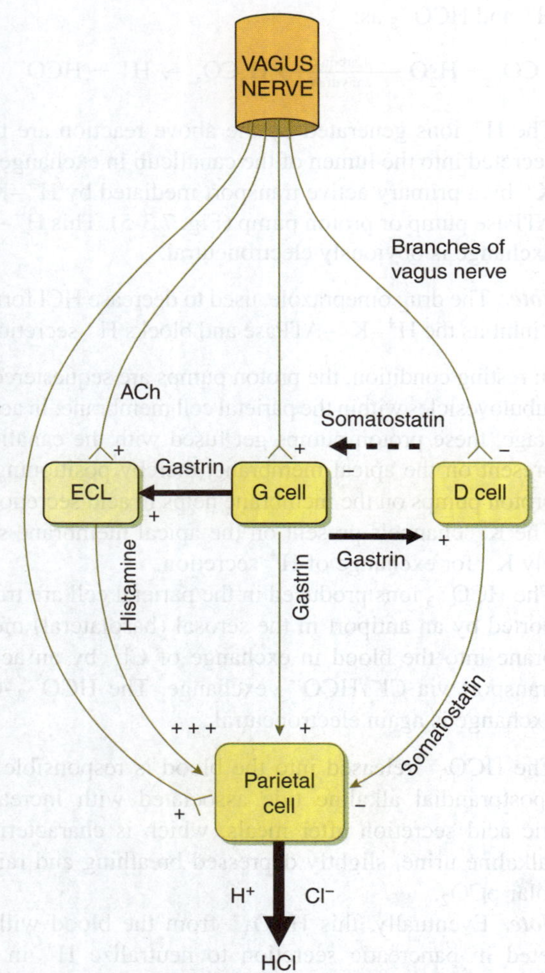

FIGURE 7.3-6 Mechanisms by which vagal stimulation increase H^+ secretion in parietal cells.

neurotransmitter released from enteric plexus nerve endings. The gastrin, in turn, stimulates H^+ secretion by the mechanism, described a bit later:

- Further, vagal stimulation also inhibits the release of *somatostatin* and thus indirectly stimulates H^+ secretion by removing the inhibitory effect of somatostatin on the parietal cells.
- ACh released on vagal stimulation also acts on the enterochromaffin-like cells (ECL), which release histamine. Histamine increases H^+ secretion by acting on H_2 receptors on the parietal cells.

Chemical Control

Chemical control on gastric glands is exerted mainly through:

- *Gastrin*, a hormone secreted by G-cells,
- *Histamine*, a paracrine agent released from the mast cells of gastric mucosa,
- *Somatostatin*, secreted by D-cells,
- *Low pH* (<3.0) in stomach acts in a negative feedback mechanism and
- *Local hormones* released in the duodenum inhibit the gastric secretion, in addition to promoting the secretion of pancreatic juice and bile.

1. Role of Gastrin Gastrin, a hormone, is secreted by the G-cells into the blood circulation (and not into gastric juice). It reaches the stomach through the arterial circulation and stimulates secretory activity of the parietal cells and chief cells.

G-cells or the gastrin-secreting cells are located at the base of the gastric glands and are especially abundant in the *pyloric glands*. The G-cells are also called APUD cells, as these are also responsible for amine precursor uptake and decarboxylation. G-cells are flask-shaped with a broad base and contain many gastrin granules near the base. The gastrin granules disappear after feeding, leaving the empty vacuoles.

Types of Gastrin. The precursor for gastrin is preprogastrin gastrin and is secreted in an inactive form, *progastrin,* which gets converted to active form (gastrin) by HCl or products of digestion. There are three types of gastrin, namely G-34, G-17 and G-14 (depending upon the number of amino acids). G-17, containing 17 amino acids, is the principal product concerned with gastric acid secretion. It has a half-life of 2–3 min in the circulation and is inactivated mainly in the kidney and small intestine.

Other forms of gastrin are:

- Large form with 45 amino acid residues and
- Sulphated form.

Depending on the activity, there are differences in activity of different forms of gastrin.

Functions of Gastrin

- *Stimulates HCl secretion* by binding with CCK-β/gastrin receptors on the parietal cell. It acts to open Ca^{2+} channels and to release Ca^{2+} from intracellular stores in order to increase cytosolic-free Ca^{2+} concentration. The Ca^{2+}, along with cyclic AMP act via protein kinase to increase the transport of H^+ into the gastric lumen by H^+–K^+–ATPase (Fig. 7.3-7) interacting with unidentified receptors on the parietal cell. The second messenger for the gastrin on the parietal cell has not been identified, but is clearly different from those for ACh and histamine because their actions are additive with those of gastrin.

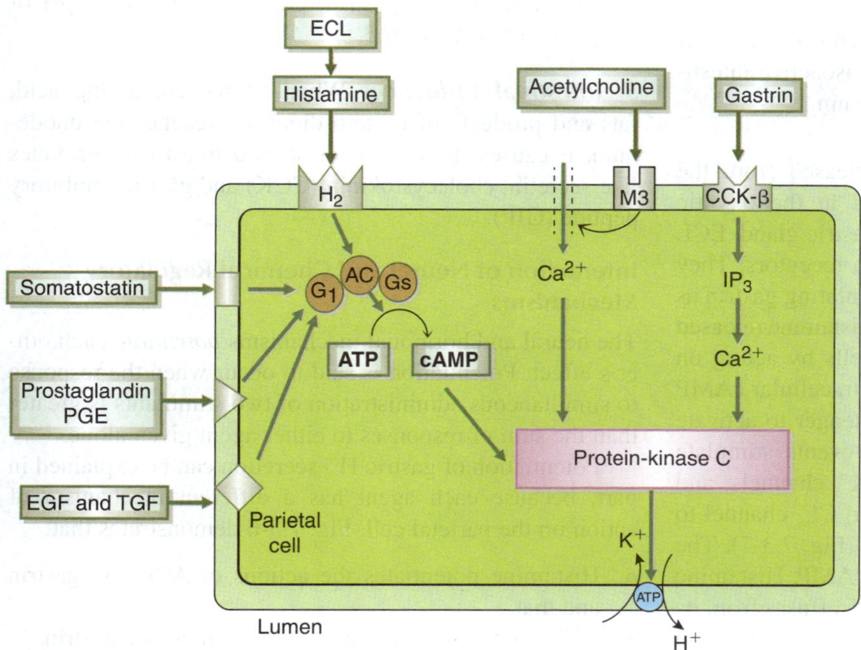

FIGURE 7.3-7 Control of HCl secretion at the parietal cell level. Acetylcholine (ACh), histamine and gastrin act agonists of HCl secretion by distinct mechanism (for details see text). Somatostatin, prostaglandins (PGE), epidermal growth factor (EGF) and transforming growth factor (TGF) act as endogenous antagonists of HCl secretion by inhibiting adenylyl cyclase.

Gastrin also increases the HCl secretion by stimulating secretion of histamine from the *enterochromaffin-like cells* (ECL) present in the body of stomach.

- *Increases gastric and intestinal motility*. It also causes contraction of lower oesophageal sphincter (LES) and it has a feeble influence on gall bladder contraction.
- *Increases pancreatic secretion* of insulin and glucagon, but only after a protein meal.
- *Trophic action*, i.e. it is necessary for the proper growth of gastrointestinal mucosa.

Factors Affecting Gastrin Secretion

Factors that stimulate gastrin secretion:

- *Vagal stimulation*. Vagal stimulation increases gastrin release through gastrin-releasing peptide (GRP) and not through release of neurotransmitter ACh. Because of this, atropine (which blocks muscarinic receptors) does not affect release of gastrin from G-cells.
- *Distension of the pyloric antrum* increases gastrin secretion through the intrinsic innervation. This fact can be proved experimentally by Heidenhain pouch (see page 597).
- *Products of protein digestion* (e.g. peptides and amino acids), alcohol and coffee also increase gastrin secretion.
- *Calcium and epinephrine* are also reported to increase gastrin secretion.

Factors that inhibit gastrin secretion:

- *Low pH of gastric juice* (<3) inhibits gastrin secretion and forms the basis of negative feedback mechanism controlling HCl release (see page 594).
- *Somatostatin*, released by D cells (located adjacent to G-cells or parietal cells in gastric mucosa) inhibit gastrin secretion by G-cells.
- *Other substances* that inhibit gastrin secretion are secretin, gastric inhibitory peptide (GIP), vasoactive intestinal peptide (VIP), glucagon and calcitonin.

2. *Role of Histamine* Histamine is released from the enterochromaffin-like (ECL) cells found in the oxyntic region of the stomach in the base of the gastric gland. ECL cells bear both gastrin receptors and ACh receptors. They release histamine in response to both, circulating gastrin as well as ACh released by vagal fibres. The histamine released stimulates *HCl secretion* from parietal cells by acting on H_2 receptors. The H_2 receptors increase intracellular cAMP via Gs. The cAMP acts as a second messenger to activate cAMP-dependent protein kinase. These events stimulate HCl secretion by activating basolateral K^+ channels; and also cause H^+–K^+–ATPase molecules and Cl^- channel to be inserted into apical plasma membrane (Fig. 7.3-7). The second messenger for histamine is cyclic AMP. Histamine is classified as a paracrine agent because it diffuses from its release site to the parietal cells (rather than travelling within the circulation, as does a hormone). H_2 receptor-blocking drugs, such as cimetidine and ranitidine, inhibit H^+ secretion by blocking the stimulatory effect of histamine.

3. *Role of Somatostatin* Somatostatin, a growth-inhibiting hormone is released from D cells in gastrointestinal mucosa and of pancreatic islets. There are two types of somatostatins, i.e. somatostatin 14 and 28.

- Somatostatin is secreted by D-cells located adjacent to G cells or the parietal cells in the gastric glands.
- Somatostatin secretion by D-cells is stimulated by secretin, enteroglucagon, GIP and VIP.
- Somatostatin inhibits HCl secretion in two ways:
  - Directly by its action on parietal cells and
  - Indirectly by inhibiting gastrin secretion by G-cells.
- Somatostatin, prostaglandins, epidermal growth factor and transforming growth factor act on parietal cells to inhibit HCl secretion by inhibiting adenylyl cyclase (Fig. 7.3-7).

4. *Role of Low pH (<3) in Stomach* Low pH (<3) in the stomach inhibits the secretion of H^+ by parietal cells by a negative feedback mechanism:

- After a meal is ingested, H^+ secretion is stimulated by cephalic and gastric influences.
- After the meal is digested and the stomach emptied, further H^+ secretion decreases the pH of stomach contents.
- When the pH of stomach contents is <3.0, *gastric secretion is inhibited*, which in turn inhibits H^+ secretion. This forms the so-called *negative feedback mechanism*.
- On the other hand, if the pH of gastric contents rises above 3.5 (due to buffering action of food), the release of gastrin is stimulated. In this way, the negative feedback control over gastrin release maintains the pH of gastric contents near 3.

5. *Intestinal Influences* When chyme containing acid, fats and products of protein digestion reaches the duodenum, it causes the release of several intestinal hormones like secretin, cholecystokinin (CCK) and gastric inhibitory peptide (GIP).

Interaction of Neural and Chemical Regulatory Mechanisms

The neural and hormonal mechanisms *potentiate* each other's effect. Potentiation is said to occur when the response to simultaneous administration of two stimulants is greater than the sum of responses to either agent given alone.

Potentiation of gastric H^+ secretion can be explained in part, because each agent has a different mechanism of action on the parietal cell. Fig. 7.3-6 demonstrates that:

- Histamine potentiates the actions of ACh and gastrin and that
- ACh potentiates the actions of histamine and gastrin.

Phases of Gastric Secretion and Their Regulation

Meal-related gastric secretion can be divided into three phases:

- Cephalic phase,
- Gastric phase and
- Intestinal phase.

1. Cephalic Phase

- Cephalic phase of gastric secretion occurs before the entry of food into the stomach.
- Rate of gastric juice secretion during this phase is high, about 500 ml/h, but this phase lasts for a short time and accounts for about 45% of total gastric juice secretion during a meal.
- Cephalic phase of gastric secretion is *initiated* by the thought, sight, smell or taste of food. Neurogenic signals originate in the cerebral cortex and appetite centres of amygdala or hypothalamus. The impulses are transmitted to dorsal vagal nuclei and from there through the vagi to the stomach (Fig. 7.3-8). The vagal efferent fibres stimulate secretion of hydrochloric acid (HCl) from parietal cells, gastrin from G-cells and pepsinogen from peptic (chief) cells.

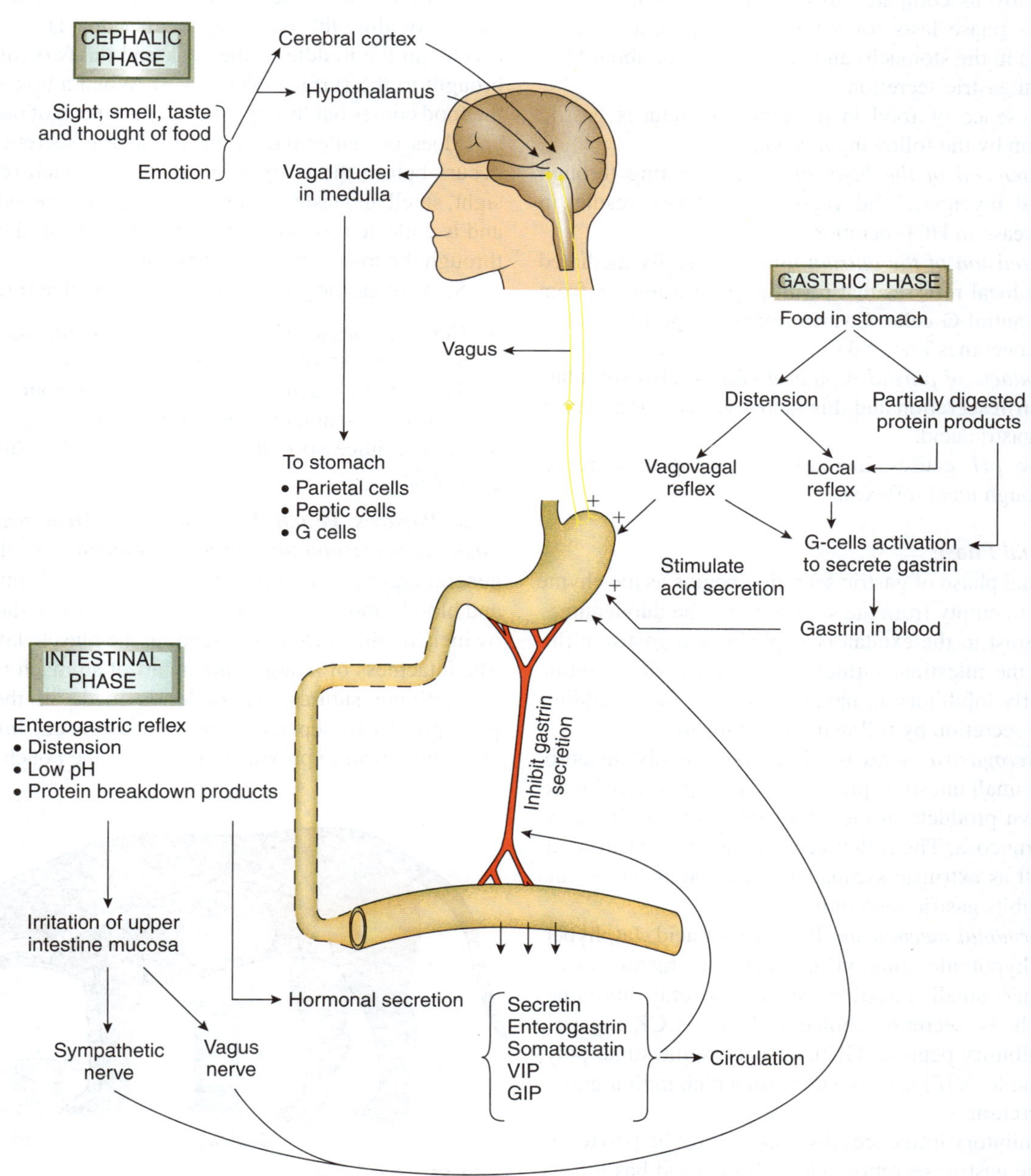

FIGURE 7.3-8 Phases and regulation of gastric secretion.

- Emotions also influence this vagally mediated gastric secretion. *Anger and hostility* are associated with increased gastric secretion and motility. *Fear and depression* decrease the gastric secretion and motility. In high-stung and aggressive individuals, increased vagal discharge produces gastric secretion even during non-digestive periods, leading to hyperacidity or even peptic ulceration.

2. Gastric Phase

- Gastric phase of gastric secretion occurs when food enters the stomach.
- Rate of gastric juice secretion during this phase is less (200 ml/h) as compared to that in the cephalic phase. But this phase lasts for a long time (as long as food remains in the stomach) and so accounts for about 50% the total gastric secretion.
- The presence of food in the stomach induces gastric secretion by the following *mechanisms:*
  - *Distension of the body of stomach* acting through local myenteric and vagovagal reflexes, results in increase in HCl secretion.
  - *Distension of the antrum* initiates vagally mediated and local reflexes that result in gastrin release from the antral G-cells. Gastrin release is inhibited when pH becomes low (<3).
  - *Products of partial protein digestion* also stimulate gastrin secretion and this increases secretion mainly of gastric acid.
  - *Low pH* causes increased pepsinogen secretion through local reflexes.

3. Intestinal Phase

- Intestinal phase of gastric secretion begins as the chyme begins to empty from the stomach into the duodenum.
- In contrast to the excitatory cephalic and gastric influences, the intestinal influence on the gastric secretion is chiefly inhibitory in nature. Intestinal factor inhibits gastric secretion by following mechanisms:
  - *Enterogastric reflex* is initiated by the distension of the small intestine, presence of acid or protein breakdown products in the upper intestine and irritation of mucosa. The reflex activity involves intrinsic, as well as extrinsic sympathetic and vagus nerves and inhibits gastric secretion.
  - *Hormonal mechanism*. Presence of acid, fat, hyper- or hypotonic solution and irritating factors in the upper small intestine release several hormones such as secretin, cholecystokinin (CCK), gastric inhibitory peptide (GIP), vasoactive intestinal polypeptide (VIP) and somatostatin which inhibit gastric secretion.
- The inhibitory influences discussed above help to terminate the gastric secretion when all the food has left the stomach.
- Products of protein digestion, however, have a slight stimulatory effect on gastric acid secretion and account for 50% or 5% of the total gastric acid secretion that occurs following a meal.

Experimental Demonstration of Regulation of Gastric Secretion

Phases and regulation of gastric secretion has been studied by certain experiments which are described briefly.

1. Sham Feeding: an Experiment to Demonstrate Cephalic Phase of Gastric Secretion. Cephalic phase of gastric secretion, i.e. secretion of gastric juice before the entry of food can be demonstrated by sham feeding experiment. For this, the oesophagus of a dog is exposed and divided in the middle of the neck and the two cut ends are brought to the surface (Fig. 7.3-9). When a dog swallows, the food comes out through the upper cut end of oesophagus and does not enter the stomach. Gastric secretion, which occurs before the entry of food into stomach (caused by sight, smell and taste of food) represents the *cephalic phase* and is collected for study by passing a tube in the stomach through the lower cut end of oesophagus.

Study of gastric juice so collected shows that (Fig. 7.3-10):

- Cephalic phase of the so-called appetite juice begins after a latency of 5–7 min,
- The volume reaches the peak within an hour,
- Gastric secretion continues for 3 h and
- Gastric juice so collected is highly acidic and rich in pepsin.

2. Pavlov's Pouch Experiment to Demonstrate that Vagus is Secretomotor Nerve to Stomach. For this, under general anaesthesia, a pouch of stomach with intact nerve and blood supply is separated from the body of the stomach by incising the mucosa and keeping the muscle layer intact. The intactness of a larger, main part of stomach is restored by applying sutures. An outlet is made in the smaller part (pouch) so separated and is brought out through the abdominal wall to provide drainage for the pouch secretion

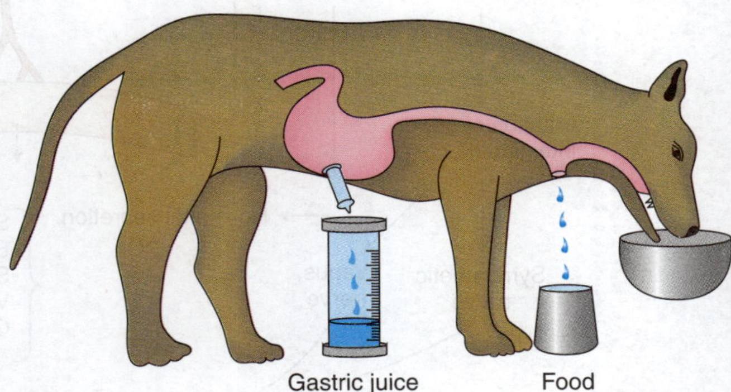

FIGURE 7.3-9 Sham feeding experiment to demonstrate initiation of cephalic phase of gastric secretion.

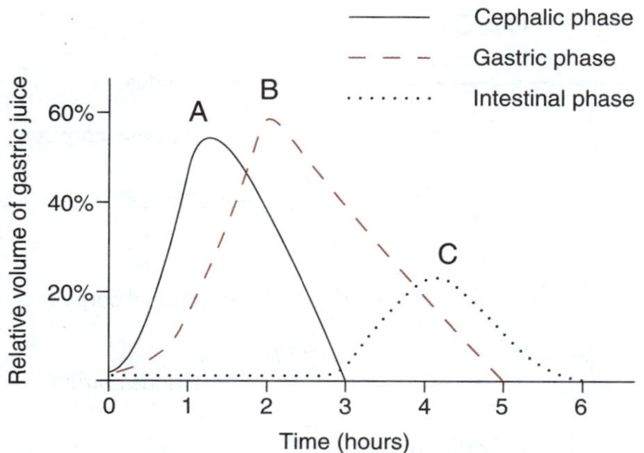

FIGURE 7.3-10 Volume and time curve of different phases of gastric secretion: A, cephalic phase; B, gastric phase; and C, intestinal phase.

(Fig. 7.3-11). The vagus nerve is exposed and divided in the neck and the animal is allowed to recover.

After some days, the peripheral cut end of the vagus is stimulated in the unanaesthetized dog. Flow of gastric juice rich in HCl and pepsin after a short latent period demonstrates that the vagus nerve is the secretomotor to the stomach.

3. Heidenhain's Pouch Experiment to Demonstrate Existence of Some Blood-borne Mechanism Regulating Gastric Secretion.

- Heidenhain's pouch is a modified Pavlov's pouch, which is separated in such a way from the antral part of stomach that it is denervated but with intact blood supply (Fig. 7.3-12).
- Distension of the denervated pouch (with intact blood supply) induces gastric secretion. Occurrence of gastric secretion in a denervated pouch of stomach demonstrates that there exists some blood-borne mechanism which also regulates gastric secretion.
- Intravenous injection of gastrin is followed after 5 min by secretion of gastric juice from the denervated Heidenhain's pouch. This demonstrates that the blood-borne mechanism is mediated by the gastrin hormone released from the antral mucosa.

Note. Bickel's, Farrell's and Ivy's pouches are other examples of completely denervated pouches, which have been used to study the gastric secretion.

PHYSIOLOGY OF GASTRIC MOTILITY

General Considerations

- Gastric motility is the function of gastric musculature, which consists of three layers of oblique layer.
- As elsewhere in the gut, each muscle layer in the stomach forms a *functional syncytium* and therefore, acts as a single unit. In the fundus, where the layers are relatively thin, the strength of contraction is weak; and in the antrum, where the muscle layers are thick the strength of contraction is greater.
- From the viewpoint of gastric contractions, the stomach can be divided into two regions:
  - *Oral region* of the stomach includes the fundus and proximal body. This region is responsible for receiving the ingested food.
  - *Caudal region* of the stomach includes the antrum and the distal part of the body of the stomach. This region is responsible for the contractions that mix food and propel it into the duodenum.

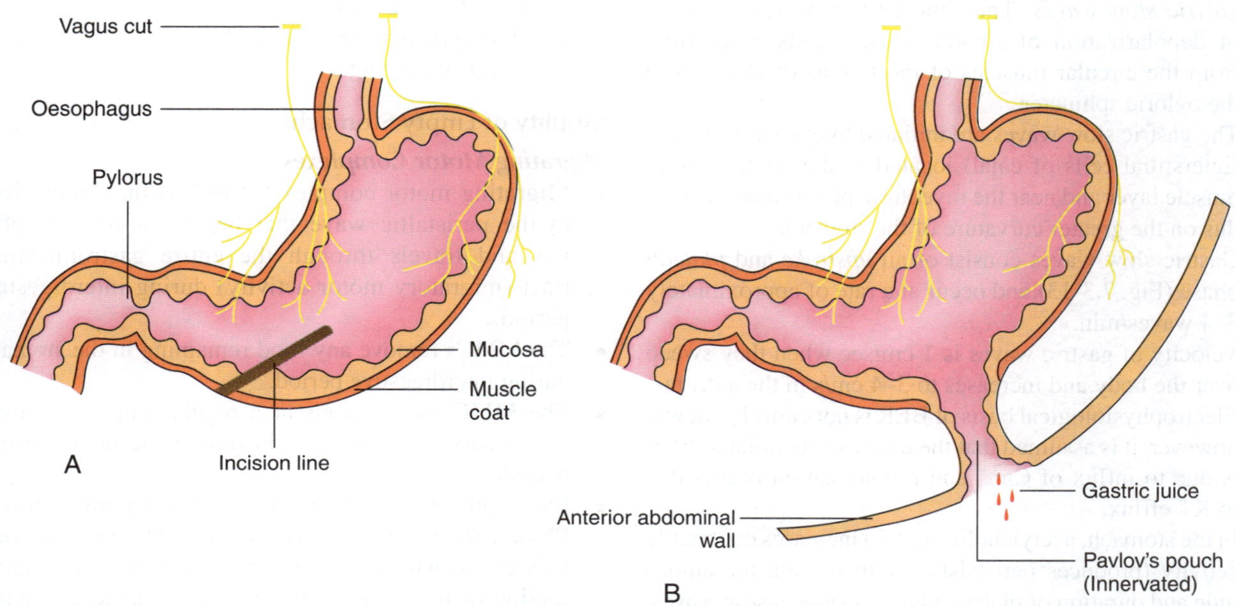

FIGURE 7.3-11 Preparation of Pavlov's pouch: **A,** showing the site of incision; and **B,** Pavlov's pouch opening outside through anterior abdominal wall.

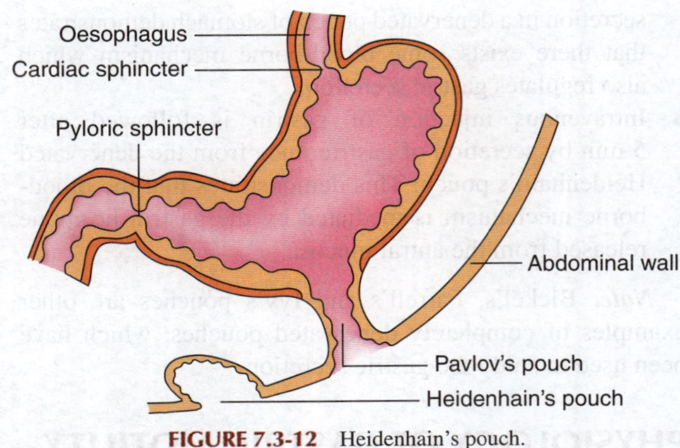

FIGURE 7.3-12 Heidenhain's pouch.

Motor Functions of Stomach observed by gastric motility are:

- *Storage of food*. It is accomplished by a special gesture of gastric musculature of the oral region called the receptive relaxation.
- *Mixing of food* with gastric juice to form semisolid paste (chyme). It is accomplished by enhanced contractile activity (combination of peristalsis and retropulsion) in the caudal region.
- *Slow emptying of food* into the small intestine. It is carried out by contractions in the caudal region of the stomach.

Initiation of Gastric Motility

Basal Electrical Rhythm

- The musculature of the stomach, being a single-unit smooth muscle has its only rhythmic contractile myogenic tone called the *basic electrical rhythm* (BER) or *gastric slow waves*. Thus, the BER represents a wave of depolarization of smooth muscle cells proceeding from the circular muscles of the fundus of stomach to the pyloric sphincter.
- The gastric slow waves are initiated by *pacemaker cells* (interstitial cells of cajal) located in the outer circular muscle layer and near the myenteric plexus near the fundus on the greater curvature of the stomach.
- Gastric slow waves consist of an *upstroke* and *plateau* phase (Fig. 7.3-13) and occur at a rate of approximately 3–4 waves/min.
- Velocity of gastric waves is 1 cm/sec when they sweep over the body and increases to 3–4 cm/s in the antrum.
- Electrophysiological basis of BER is not entirely known, however, it is assumed that the upstroke (depolarization) is due to influx of Ca^{2+} and repolarization occurs due to K^+ efflux.
- In the stomach, acetylcholine (ACh) increases contractile activity (produces peristalsis) by increasing the amplitude and duration of plateau phase of slow gastric waves. Other agents that initiate contraction of smooth muscles of the stomach are gastrin, histamine, nicotine, barium and K^+. Agents that inhibit the activity are enterogastrone, epinephrine, norepinephrine, atropine and Ca^{2+}.

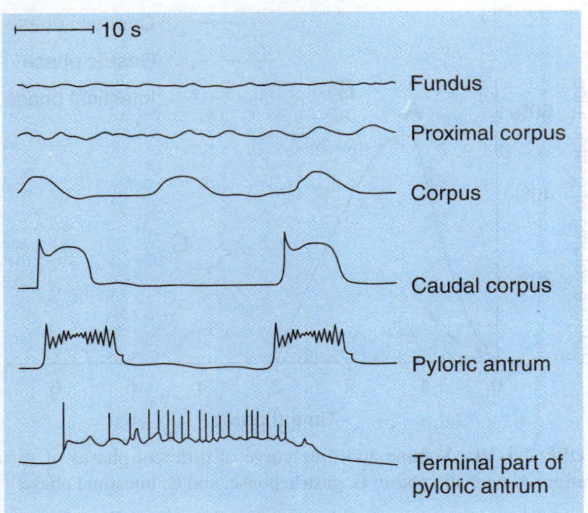

FIGURE 7.3-13 Basic electrical rhythm (BER) recorded from different parts of the stomach.

Types of Gastric Motility

The peristaltic activity of the gastric musculature has been given various names depending upon its features and motor function subserved by it. Gastric motility can be described as:

- Motility of the empty stomach, which includes:
  - Migrating motor complex and
  - Hunger contractions.
- Gastric motility related to meal, includes:
  - Receptive relaxation,
  - Mixing peristaltic waves and
  - Gastric emptying.

Motility of Empty Stomach

Migrating Motor Complexes

- Migrating motor complex (MMC) is the name given to the peristaltic wave that begins in the oesophagus and travels through the entire gastrointestinal tract (migratory motor activity) during interdigestive period.
- The MMCs remove any food remaining in the stomach during interdigestive period.
- The MMC wave travels at a regular rate (5 cm/min) and occurs every 60–90 min during the interdigestive period.
- Each cycle of migrating motor complex has three phases: Phase I (quiescent period), each migrating motor complex begins with quiescent period, continues to phase II (period of irregular electrical and mechanical activity) and ends with a burst of regular activity (Phase III).

- There is a close correlation of the basal electrical rhythm (BER) and migratory motor complexes (MMCs). When there are no MMCs, the BER consists of rhythmic oscillation of the RMP between about −65 and −45 mV. During the MMC, the electrical oscillations are superimposed with spikes (Fig. 7.3-14).
- Each MMC is associated with increase in gastric secretion, bile flow and pancreatic secretion.
- As the MMC clears the stomach and small intestine of luminal contents in preparation for the next meal, they have been called the *interdigestive housekeepers*.
- The hormone motilin, which is released from the endocrine cells within the epithelium of small intestine, increases the strength of MMC.
- The MMCs are abolished immediately after the entry of food in the stomach.

Hunger Contractions Mild peristaltic contractions occur in the empty stomach, which over a period of hours increase in intensity and are called hunger contractions. MMCs are probably responsible for hunger contractions. When they become extremely strong, they fuse to cause *tetanic* contraction lasting for 2–3 min which can be felt and may even be painful. These are associated with the sensation of hunger.

Gastric Motility Related to Meals

Receptive Relaxation and Accommodation

- Storage function of stomach is accomplished by receptive relaxation and accommodation.
- The empty stomach has a volume of about 50 ml only and the diameter of its lumen is only slightly more than that of the small intestine.
- As stated earlier, as soon as the food enters the stomach the MMCs are abolished and the fundus and upper part of the body of stomach, i.e. the *oral region* relaxes to accommodate the ingested food without any increase in intramural pressure. This phenomenon is called *receptive relaxation* (Fig. 7.3-15).
- The passage of each bolus of food stimulates the stretch *receptors of oral region* and produces further relaxation. By the end of the meal, the smooth muscles of the oral region of the stomach relax to such an extent that 1–2 L of food can be accommodated.

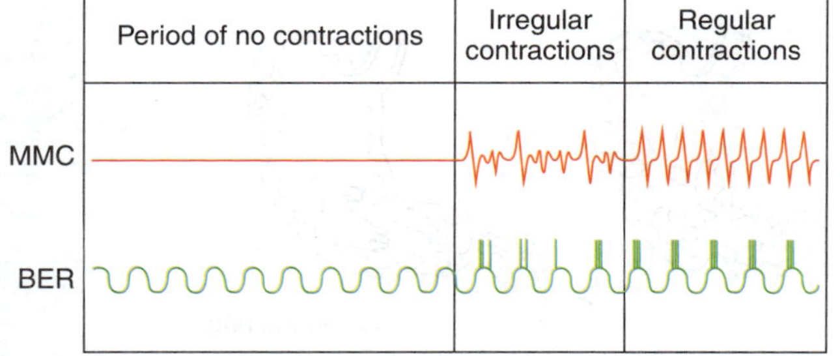

FIGURE 7.3-14 Relation of basic electrical rhythm (BER) with migratory motor complexes (MMCs).

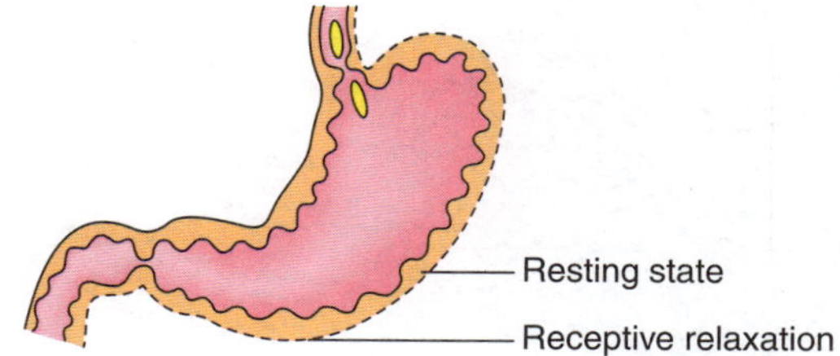

FIGURE 7.3-15 Receptive relaxation of stomach.

- Receptive relaxation is a *vagovagal reflex* initiated by distension of stomach and is synchronized with the primary peristaltic waves in the oesophagus.
- CCK participates in receptive relaxation by increasing the distensibility of the oral stomach.
- The inhibitory neurotransmitter responsible for receptive relaxation and accommodation is either VIP or NO.
- Vagotomy abolishes receptive relaxation.

Mixing Peristaltic Waves The presence of food in the caudal region (distal body and antral part) of stomach increases the contractile activity of this part of the stomach. This enhanced contractile activity (a combination of peristalsis and retropulsion) is called mixing waves which mix the food with stomach acid and enzymes and break it into smaller and smaller pieces. When the food is mixed into a pasty consistency it is called *chyme*.

Initiation and Production of Peristalsis

Peristalsis is the co-ordinated pattern of smooth muscle contraction and relaxation where a wave of relaxation precedes the wave of contraction. Peristaltic contractions are produced by periodic changes in membrane potential (basal electrical rhythm, described earlier). The rhythmicity of gastric peristalsis is determined by the BER which has a frequency of 3–4/min (slow waves). Certain neurotransmitters like acetylcholine or hormone gastrin cause generation of depolarizing spikes at the peak of BER cycles resulting in mechanical contraction (peristalsis). The number of spikes fired in a slow wave determines the force of each peristaltic contraction (Fig. 7.3-16).

Regulation of Force of Peristalsis From the above, it is clear that frequency of peristalsis is determined by BER, and thus, does not vary. However, the force of peristaltic contractions is under neural and hormonal control.

- Distension of the stomach or increased gastrin secretion increases the force of gastric peristalsis.
- Gastric contractions are increased by vagal stimulation and decreased by sympathetic stimulation.
- Acetylcholine and gastrin increase the size of slow wave plateau potential, which increases the amount of Ca^{2+} entering the cell from the extracellular fluid (ECF) and

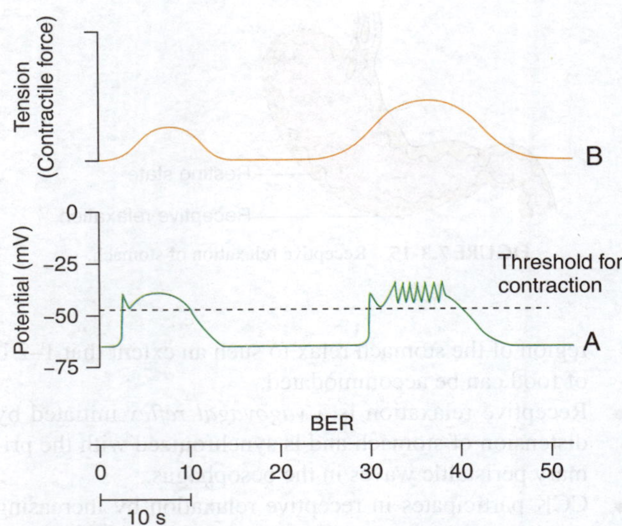

FIGURE 7.3-16 Membrane potentials of smooth muscle of stomach (A) and their relation to mechanical response (B).

activate second messengers that release Ca^{2+} from the sarcoplasmic reticulum. The amount of Ca^{2+} present in the smooth muscle cell determines the force of contraction.

Mixing Mechanism of Peristalsis and Retropulsion

- Peristaltic contractions begin in the mid-stomach (Fig. 7.3-17A) and proceed caudally. As the wave proceeds towards the pylorus, it deepens. Thus, the peristaltic waves are most marked in the distal half of the stomach (called antral systole).
- The food particles also move towards the pylorus (Fig. 7.3-17B), along with the deep wave of contraction, but the wave of contraction reaches pyloric sphincter and causes its contraction before the food reaches there.
- When the food reaches the pylorus, it strikes against the closed pyloric sphincter with a force. As a result, most of the antral contents are forced back into the body of stomach and only a small amount of chyme passes into the duodenum (Fig. 7.3-17C). The backward movement of the food is called *retropulsion*.
- The forward and backward movements (caused by forceful propulsion and retropulsion) of the gastric contents helps to break the food particles into smaller pieces and mixes it with gastric secretion, converting it into a semiliquid paste called chyme.

Gastric Emptying

- Gastric emptying results from a progressive wave of forceful contraction, which sequentially involves antrum, pylorus (pyloric sphincter) and proximal duodenum, thus all the three function as a unit. It is the force of gastric peristalsis which determines emptying and not the variations in tone of pyloric sphincter. The forceful gastric emptying waves spread over the antrum as a strong peristaltic ring-like contraction creating pressure of 50–70 cm of H_2O (six times as powerful as that produced by mixing waves).
- Gastric emptying occurs when the chyme is decomposed into enough small pieces (typically <1 mm^3) to fit through the pyloric sphincter.
- Each time the chyme is pushed against the pyloric sphincter, contraction ahead of advancing gastric contents prevent bigger food particles from entering the duodenum. Therefore, chyme is pumped in a bit (2–7 ml) at a time into the small intestine.
- The peristaltic waves which provide this pumping action are known as *pyloric pump*.
- Regurgitation from duodenum, normally does not occur, because the contraction of the pyloric segment tends to persist slightly longer than that of the duodenum. The prevention of regurgitation may also be due to the stimulating action of CCK and secretin on the pyloric sphincter.

Factors Regulating the Gastric Emptying. After a normal meal, the emptying time is 2–3 h. The gastric emptying is regulated by various factors:

1. Fluidity of the Chyme. The rate of gastric emptying of solids depends on the rate at which the chyme is broken down into smaller particles. Liquids empty much faster than

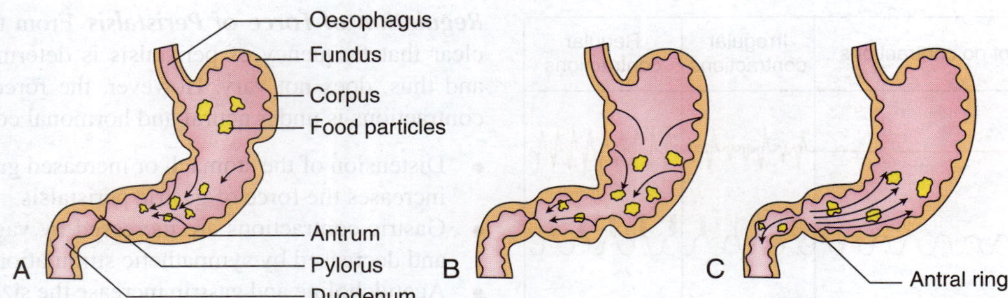

FIGURE 7.3-17 Mixing peristaltic waves of stomach: **A,** peristaltic contractions begin in the mid-stomach and pushes the food towards pylorus; **B,** when food reaches the pylorus it strikes against closed pyloric sphincter; and **C,** antral contents forced back (retropulsion).

solids. The rate at which liquids empty is proportional to the pressure within the oral stomach, which increases slowly during the digestive period.

2. Gastric Factors which affect emptying are:

- *Volume of food in the stomach.* Greater the volume of food in the stomach, greater is the stretching of the stomach wall. Distension of the stomach triggers long (vagally mediated) and short (intrinsic neural plexus mediated) reflexes leading to strong peristalsis waves and increased rate of gastric emptying.
- *Gastrin hormone.* Presence of certain types of food (e.g. meat) causes release of gastrin from antral mucosa. Gastrin enhances the activity of pyloric pump and therefore promotes gastric emptying.
- *Type of food ingested* (present in the stomach) affects the gastric emptying as:
  - Carbohydrate-rich food causes rapid gastric emptying,
  - Protein-rich food causes slow gastric emptying and
  - Fat-rich food causes the slowest gastric emptying. Because of this reason, some people consume fats before a cocktail party. The fat keeps the alcohol in the stomach longer, slowing the absorption and reducing the chances of intoxication.

3. Duodenal Factors, which inhibit gastric emptying are:

- *Enterogastric reflex.* It is a neural-mediated reflex. It is initiated by stimulation of receptors in the duodenal mucosa. The important stimuli are: distension of duodenum, acidity of the contents (pH <4), high or low osmolarity of chyme, presence of fat and protein digestion products in the chyme.

  The enterogastric reflex is initiated in the duodenum and passes to stomach through the myenteric plexus and also extrinsic nerves to inhibit or even stop emptying by inhibiting antral propulsive contractions and increasing slightly the tone of the pyloric sphincter.
- *Enterogastric hormones.* A variety of intestinal hormones, collectively called enterogastrones inhibit gastric contractions. Some of the hormones, which have been identified are:
- *Cholecystokinin (CCK).* It is released from the duodenum in response to fat or protein digestion product. CCK probably acts by blocking the excitatory effects of gastrin on gastric smooth muscles.
- *Secretin.* It is released from the duodenum in response to presence of acid. Secretin most likely has a direct inhibitory effect on smooth muscle.
- *Gastric inhibitory peptide (GIP).* It is released from the upper small intestine in response to fat in chyme and reduces gastric motility under some conditions.

Purpose of duodenal inhibitory effect on gastric emptying. The duodenal inhibitory effects (exerted through enterogastric reflex and enterogastrones) prevent the flow of chyme from exceeding the ability of intestine to handle it (especially longer time is required for fat digestion). It does not allow disturbance in electrolyte balance even if hypo- or hypertonic solutions are drunk.

4. Other factors affecting gastric emptying:

- *Emotions* have a strong effect on gastric motility. Anger and aggression increase gastric motility, whereas depression and fear decrease it.
- *Vagotomy* decreases the magnitude and co-ordination of stomach contractions and thus slows emptying.

FUNCTIONS OF STOMACH

After studying the physiological activities of the stomach, its functions can be summarized as:

1. Mechanical or Motor Functions include:

- ***Storage of food.*** Stomach serves as a reservoir for the food ingested. Stomach can store about 1–L of food. Food remains in the stomach for several hours.
- ***Mixing of food*** with gastric juice is performed by gastric motility until it forms a semisolid paste known as chyme.
- ***Slow emptying of food*** into duodenum occurs to provide proper time for digestion and absorption by small intestine.

2. Digestive Functions. Only small amounts of foods are digested in the stomach as:

- ***Carbohydrate digestion*** in the stomach depends on the action of salivary amylase, which remains active until halted by the low pH of stomach.
- ***Protein digestion.*** About 10% of ingested protein is broken down completely in the stomach. *Gastric pepsin* facilitates later digestion of protein by breaking protein into peptone.
- ***Fat digestion*** in stomach is minimal due to the restriction of gastric lipase activity to triglycerides containing short chain (<10 carbon) fatty acids. Acid and pepsin break emulsions so that fats coalesce into droplets, which float and empty last.

3. Absorptive Function. Stomach contributes little in the absorption function.

- ***Absorption of nutrients.*** Very little absorption of nutrients takes place in the stomach. The only substances absorbed to any appreciable extent are highly lipid-soluble substances (e.g. the nonionized triglycerides of acetic, propionic and butyric acids). *Aspirin* at gastric pH is nonionized and fat soluble and after absorption it ionizes intracellularly, damaging mucosal cells and ultimately producing bleeding.
- ***Ethanol*** is absorbed rapidly in proportion to its concentration.
- ***Water absorption.*** Water moves in both directions across the gastric mucosa. It does not, however, follow

osmotic gradients. Water soluble substances, including Na^+, K^+, glucose and amino acids, are absorbed in insignificant amounts.

- ***Intrinsic factor*** released from gastric glands helps in absorption of vitamin B_{12} from the small intestine.

4. Excretory Function. Stomach excretes following substances:

- Certain toxins, as in case of uraemia and
- Certain alkaloids, such as morphine.

5. Stimulating Functions. Stomach performs stimulatory function for release of:

- Gastrin,
- Enterogastrin and
- Intrinsic factor of Castle.

6. Reflex Functions. Various reflexes initiated from the stomach are:

- Gastro–salivary reflex,
- Gastro–ileal reflex,
- Gastro–colic reflex and
- Presence of food in the stomach reflexly stimulates secretion of pancreatic juice and expulsion of bile.

7. Antiseptic Action. HCl present in the gastric juice kills the bacteria and other harmful substances.

APPLIED ASPECTS

Important applied aspects of stomach which need special attention are:

- Gastric mucosal barrier and pathophysiology of peptic ulcer,
- Physiology of vomiting,
- Gastrectomy and
- Gastric function tests.

Gastric Mucosal Barrier and Pathophysiology of Peptic Ulcer

Gastric Mucosal Barrier

The gastric mucosal barrier protects the gastric mucosa from damage by intraluminal HCl, i.e. autodigestion. Indeed, it is a physiologic marvel, or gastric walls would suffer the same fate as a piece of swallowed meat. It is created by the following:

- ***Mucin secretion.*** The thin layer of surface mucus in the stomach and duodenum exhibits a diffusion coefficient for H^+ that is one-fourth that of water. Acid- and pepsin-containing fluid exits the gastric glands as jets passing through the surface mucus layer, entering the lumen directly without contacting surface epithelial cells.
- ***Bicarbonate secretion.*** Surface epithelial cells, in both the stomach and the duodenum secrete bicarbonate into the boundary zone of adherent mucus, creating an essentially pH neutral microenvironment immediately adjacent to the cell surface.
- ***Epithelial barrier.*** Intercellular tight junctions provide a barrier to the back-diffusion of H^+. Any damaged cells are quickly replaced, as the turnover rate of gastric mucosa is very high. Approximately, 5×10^5 mucosal cells are shed each minute, replacing the entire mucosa in 1–3 days.
- ***High mucosal blood flow.*** It rapidly carries away any acid that penetrates the cellular lining. The rich mucosal blood supply also provides oxygen, bicarbonate and nutrients to epithelial cells.
- ***Prostaglandins,*** are responsible for maintaining the gastric mucosal barrier.

Pathophysiology of Peptic Ulcer

Peptic ulcer refers to excavation of mucosa of duodenum or pyloric part of stomach caused by the digestive action of gastric juice. Peptic ulcer can be caused by either of two ways:

1. Diminished Ability of the Gastroduodenal Mucosal Barrier to protect against the digestive properties of the acid–pepsin complex. Factors that disturb the mucosal barrier include:

- ***Bacterial Infection by Helicobacter Pylori,*** breakdown the gastroduodenal mucosal barrier. At least 75% patients with peptic ulcer have recently been found to have chronic infection by *H. pylori*. The sequence of events in the pathology of the peptic ulcer by *H. pylori* infection is as follows:
  - *H. pylori* is a gram negative bacterium, with multiple flagella at one end which makes it highly motile. The bacterium burrows the mucus layer and lives deep adherent to the epithelial surface.
  - *H. pylori* uses an adhesion molecule (Bab A) to bind itself to the antigen called *Lewis b* antigen present on the epithelial cells. The surface pH nearly remains neutral because if there occurs any acidity, it gets buffered by production of urease (an enzyme produced by the bacteria), which produces ammonia from urea that raises the pH (Fig. 7.3-18). The bacterium stimulates gastritis by local inflammatory reaction in the underlying epithelium that depends on expression of gene, i.e.:
    - Cytotoxin-associated gene A (Cag A), which interacts with various cell signalling pathways involved in cell replication
    - Vaculating cytotoxin gene A (Vac A) is a pore forming Adhesin (Bab A)
    - Cytokine interleukin-1β (IL-1β) associated with gastric atrophy

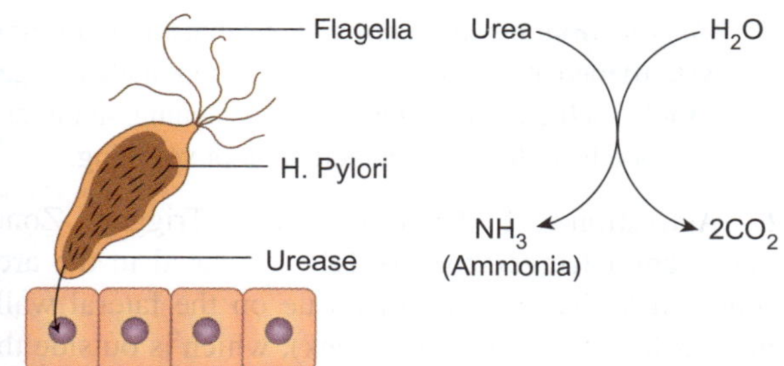

FIGURE 7.3-18 Buffer action of *H. pylori* by production of urease enzyme.

- *H. pylori* causes gastritis due to depletion of somatostatin from D cells and increased gastrin release from G-cells (Fig. 7.3-19).

  The bacterium releases digestive enzymes that liquefy the barrier, which allows gastric secretion to digest the epithelial cells leading to peptic ulceration.

- ***Nonsteroidal Anti-inflammatory Drugs*** (NSAIDs), such as aspirin, ibuprofen and diclofenac sodium.
  - NSAIDs act through inhibition of prostaglandin H synthase and cyclooxygenase (COX) enzyme. NSAID damage the gastric mucosal barrier by reducing prostaglandin synthesis.
- ***Other Factors*** which can disrupt the mucosal barrier are ethyl alcohol, vinegar, bile salts and cigarette smoking.

2. Excessive Secretion of Gastric Acid Hyperacidity leads to ulcer formation in the duodenum and pyloric part of the stomach. Hyperacidity may occur due to:

- Increased parietal cell mass,
- Increased sensitivity for secretory stimuli,
- Increased basal acid secretory drive and

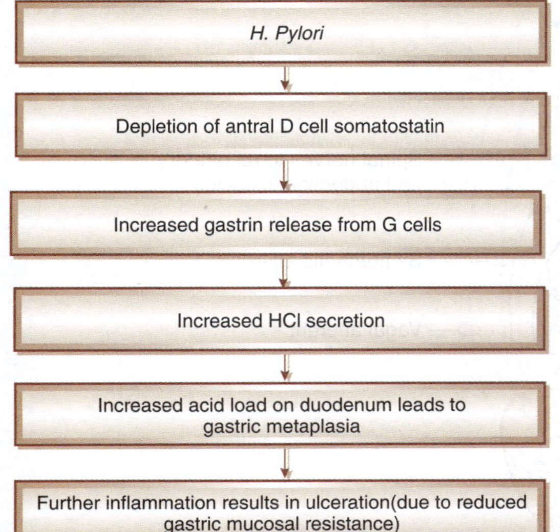

FIGURE 7.3-19 Sequence of events of pathophysiology of peptic ulcer by *H. pylori*.

- Excess gastric secretion, as seen in Zollinger–Ellison syndrome, in which patients have *gastrinomas* (tumours that secrete gastrin).

Investigations

1. *Endoscopy* is the procedure by which microscopic details can be observed with the help of an endoscope. It is used for both diagnostic and therapeutic purpose.
2. The tests for diagnosis of *H. pylori* infection include both non invasive and invasive tests.

The noninvasive tests are; serology, C urea breath test for higher sensitivity and faecal antigen test (a specific test).

Invasive tests include biopsy for histology, microbiological culture and rapid urease test.

Physiologic Basis of Management of Peptic Ulcer. The aims of peptic ulcer management are to:

- Reduce symptoms,
- Induce healing and
- Prevent recurrence.

Commonly employed measures for treatment of peptic ulcer, along with their physiological bases are:

- ***Antacids.*** These form a gel that coats the mucosa and neutralizes the acid. Most of the antacids contain aluminium hydroxide, magnesium hydroxide or calcium bicarbonate.
- ***H_2-receptor blocking drugs*** such as cimetidine, ranitidine and nizatidine, decrease HCl secretion by blocking the effect of histamine on H_2-receptors of parietal cells.
- ***M_1 muscarinic receptor blocking drugs*** such as atropine and pirenzepine decrease H^+ secretion by blocking the effect of ACh on M_1-muscarinic receptors of parietal cells.
- *Gastric H^+–K^+–ATPase* inhibiting drugs such as omeprazole, obviously decrease H^+ secretion by blocking the action of gastric H^+–K^+–ATPase in the parietal cell.
- ***H. pylori eradication:*** All proven cases of acute or chronic gastric ulcer with *H. pylori* should be given eradication as primary therapy.
- ***Bilateral vagotomy combined with resection of gastrin producing pyloric part of stomach,*** is performed in very severe cases of duodenal and pyloric ulcers. This surgical treatment abolishes the effects of both ACh and gastrin, and thus markedly reduces HCl production.

Physiology of Vomiting

Vomiting refers to forceful expulsion of contents from the stomach and intestine. Vomiting is a complex reflex involving both autonomic and somatic pathways.

Initiation of Vomiting Vomiting may be initiated by either activation of vomiting centre or by activation of the chemoreceptor trigger zone.

1. Activation of Vomiting Centre. Vomiting centre is situated in the reticular formation of medulla oblongata near the vagal nucleus. It may be activated directly or through afferents:

i. ***Direct activation of the vomiting centre*** occurs due to initiation caused by injury to the area or by raised intracranial pressure, and causes projectile vomiting—a rapid, forceful emesis not accompanied by nausea.

ii. ***Afferent impulses*** activating vomiting centre include (Fig. 7.3-20):

- *Visceral afferent pathway* in the sympathetic and vagi relay impulses arising due to irritation of mucosa of upper GIT. There are 5HT receptors in the stomach and small intestine, and 5HT (serotonin) released from the enterochromaffin cells appears to initiate impulses in afferents that trigger nausea and vomiting. These receptors are stimulated by local irritants such as: drugs, viruses, radiations, bacteria, $CuSO_4$ and cytotoxic agents.
- *Afferent impulses from the vestibular nuclei* mediate nausea and vomiting of motion sickness.
- *Afferents from higher centres* (diencephalon and limbic system) mediate emetic response to emotionally charged stimuli such as nauseating smell, sickening sights and memory, fear, dread and anticipation of vomiting.

2. Activation of Chemoreceptor Trigger Zone. Chemoreceptor trigger zone (CTZ) is located in the area *postrema* (a V-shaped band of tissue on the lateral walls of the fourth ventricle near the obex), which is outside the blood–brain barrier and is thus more permeable to many substances than the underlying medulla (Fig. 7.3-20). Chemoreceptor cells present in CTZ contain dopamine (D_2) receptors and $5HT_3$ receptors and initiate vomiting when they are stimulated by:

- Circulating emetic substances in patients with uraemia and radiation sickness,
- Drugs: such as NSAIDs, opioids, glycoside (digoxin) antibiotics and cytokines,
- Infections: viral and bacterial infections, hepatitis, gastroenteritis and urinary tract infection and
- Emetic agents such as apomorphine and emetin, digitalis and glucosides.

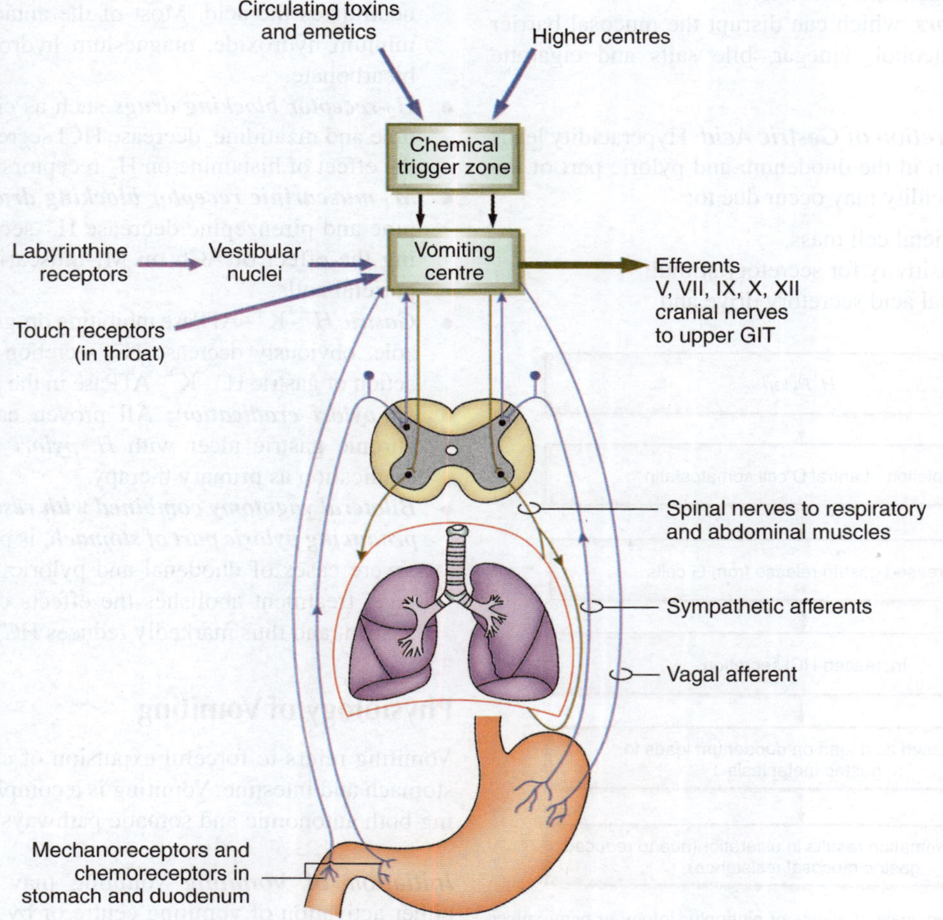

FIGURE 7.3-20 Pathway for vomiting reflex.

Note: $5HT_3$ antagonists such as ondansetron and D_2 antagonists such as chlorpromazine and haloperidol, cannabinoids, corticosteroids and benzodiazepines are effective antiemetic agents.

Efferent Impulses from Vomiting Centre and CTZ. Efferent impulses from the vomiting centre and CTZ, which give effect to act of vomiting, are transmitted via V, VII, IX, X and XII cranial nerves to upper GIT and through spinal nerves to the muscles of respiration.

Sequence of Mechanical Events of Vomiting Vomiting is a complex process and consists of following phases:

1. ***Pre-ejection phase***. During this phase there occurs gastric relaxation and retroperistalsis. It is characterized by a feeling of nausea, excessive salivation, deep, rapid and irregular breathing.
2. ***Retching phase*** may precede in many cases. It is characterized by:
   - *Closure of glottis,* which remains so till the end of the act of vomiting. It increases intrapulmonary pressure causing compression of the oesophagus. It also prevents aspiration of vomitus in trachea.
   - *Rhythmic action of respiratory muscles* preceding vomiting and consisting of contraction of abdominal, intercostal and diaphragmatic muscles against a closed glottis.
3. ***Ejection phase,*** during which the GIT contents are actually expelled out, consists of events which occur in the following sequence:
   - Closure of glottis is continued.
   - Pyloric part of stomach contracts firmly and its contents are transferred to flaccid body of stomach.
   - Simultaneous intense contraction of abdominal muscles and the descent of the diaphragm raise the intra-abdominal pressure to such an extent, that all the contents are squeezed out of the stomach into the oesophagus as a reflex relaxation of its cardiac sphincter, which also occurs at this moment.
   - From the oesophagus the contents are expelled into the mouth due to the effect of positive intrapulmonary pressure and antiperistaltic waves in the oesophagus. At this juncture, a soft palate is raised and it shuts-off the nasal cavity from the throat.
   - Towards the end of the act of vomiting, the diaphragm relaxes (i.e. ascends) and the expiratory muscles and abdominal wall contract.

Total Gastrectomy

The patients who undergo a surgical removal of the stomach or gastric bypass surgery (in which the stomach is stapled), the loss of reservoir function of the stomach may produce the following effects:

Nutritional Disturbances after Gastrectomy

1. Effect on Carbohydrate Metabolism. The carbohydrates directly enter the duodenum and are digested and absorbed rapidly resulting in *hyperglycaemia.* As a result of *hyperglycaemia,* there occurs an abrupt rise in insulin secretion, which leads to hypoglycaemia after about 2 h of meals. Thus, there occur sharp oscillations between hypoglycaemia and hyperglycaemia.
2. Effect on Protein Metabolism. The stomach plays an important role in the digestion of protein, but the near-normal digestion of protein can occur in the absence of pepsin and nutrition can be maintained.
3. Effect on Fat Digestion. Almost no effect on fat digestion is seen except on butter fat, for which gastric juice has an enzyme tributarase.
4. Effect on Absorption of Vitamin B_{12}. Due to deficiency of intrinsic factor, absorption of vitamin B_{12} is affected markedly and there may occur *pernicious anaemia*.
5. Effect on Iron Absorption. Conversion of iron from ferric (Fe^{3+}) to ferrous (Fe^{2+}) form requires HCl. Therefore, iron absorption, which occurs in ferrous form, is affected, predisposing the individual to iron deficiency anaemia. However, only traces of iron are absorbed in the stomach.

Dumping Syndrome Dumping syndrome refers to a condition characterized by development of weakness, dizziness and sweating after meals. This is seen in the cases of partial or total gastrectomy, where the oesophagus is directly anastomosed with duodenum.

Causes of Symptoms of Dumping Syndrome

1. Main cause of symptoms in dumping syndrome is sharp oscillations between hyperglycaemia and hypoglycaemia, as described above.
2. Another cause of symptoms is the rapid entry of hypertonic meals into the intestine. It provokes the movement of so much water into the gut that the resultant reduction of plasma volume is great enough leading to a significant decrease in cardiac output.

Treatment

- Avoid large meal,
- Meals should be small in bulk and dry,
- Milk and carbohydrate meals should be avoided and meals should have some dietary fibres and
- Daily and regular supplement of iron and Vitamin B complex is necessary to prevent development of anaemia.

Gastric Function Tests

Gastric function tests are employed to establish the presence of *hyperchlorhydria* (associated with peptic ulcer) or achlorhydria (complete absence of acid secretion) associated with pernicious anaemia. Gastric function tests include:

1. Fractional Test Meal Test Fractional test meal (FTM) test, previously used to be employed commonly for analysis of gastric juice. Presently, it is no more used because of its relative insensitivity and inconvenience.

Procedure, in brief, is described:

- After an overnight fast, the gastric fluid present in the stomach is aspirated with the help of Ryles' tube passed into the stomach through the nose or throat.
- A test meal is then given to stimulate the gastric juice. Any one of the standard test meals can be given: 300 ml of oatmeal gruel or dry toast and cup of tea or wheat biscuits and 300 ml of water.
- After 15 min of giving test meal, a sample of gastric content (10 ml of fluid) is aspirated. The procedure is repeated every 15 min for 3 h. Thus, including the fasting sample, a total of 13 samples are collected in separate containers.
- Each sample is analysed for free acidity, combined acidity (Fig. 7.3-21) starch and sugar, bile, total chlorides, blood lactic acid and mucus.

2. Histamine Test Histamine test is a comparatively more sensitive test than the fractional test meal test for studying the gastric acid secretion. It is because:

- Firstly, the histamine is a powerful stimulator of acid secretion and
- Secondly, due to histamine injection, acid level increases very rapidly and therefore there is no time for neutralization of acid.

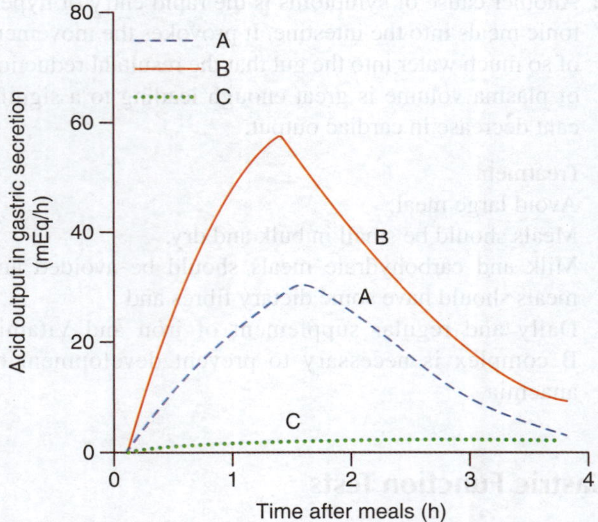

FIGURE 7.3-21 Human gastric acid secretion in response to fractional test meal: **A,** normal response; **B,** hyperchlorhydria in duodenal ulcer; and **C,** hyposecretion or achlorhydria.

Procedure. After overnight fast, in the morning the stomach is aspirated and washed with distilled water. Then, 0.5 mg histamine is injected subcutaneously and the gastric samples are aspirated and analysed as described in FTM test.

If there is no free acid present in any of the samples, then it is called true achlorhydria or histamine fast achlorhydria.

3. Augmented Histamine Test

- This test is performed with progressively increasing doses of histamine in a stepwise manner till a maximal secretory response is obtained.
- The maximal secretory response correlates well with the total number of parietal cells in the gastric mucosa.

4. Pentagastrin Test This test is also performed to assess the gastric acid status. It is performed similar to the histamine test except that in this, instead of histamine, 6 mg of pentagastrin (a synthetic gastrin) is given as subcutaneous injection.

5. Insulin Test

- This test is based on the fact that hypoglycaemia (blood sugar below 45 mg%) produces vagal stimulation through hypothalamus and that vagal stimulation causes secretion of acid from the stomach.
- In this test, 7 units of insulin are given intravenously and the gastric samples are tested for presence of free acid, as done in histamine test.
- Acid secretion occurs after insulin injection (positive test) only if vagus is intact. Therefore, insulin test performed after vagotomy operation (for gastric ulcer) to know whether all the fibres of nerves supplying stomach are cut or not. If vagotomy is done properly, insulin test is negative.

6. Barium Meal Study Barium meal study is a radiographic evaluation of the status of mucosa and lumen of the upper intestinal tract. In this test, the patient swallows a suspension of radiopaque barium sulphate, while its passage through the GIT is observed by radiograph on a fluorescent screen and films are taken to provide a permanent record. Diagnosis of gastric ulcer, duodenal ulcer or other abnormalities in the lumen of GIT is made from the typical finding.

7. Endoscopic Examination and Biopsy Nowadays, the condition of the oesophagus, gastric and duodenal mucosa can be directly visualized by endoscopic examination. This is a more reliable method than the conventional barium meal studies. The endoscopes carry a channel through which biopsy forceps or a brush can be introduced to obtain specimens for histological and cytological examination.

Chapter 7.4

Pancreas, Liver and Gallbladder

Pancreas, liver and gallbladder are accessory organs of the digestive system. After studying the physiological events occurring in the stomach and before considering the physiological activities of the small intestine, it will be worthwhile to know about the physiological role of the pancreas, liver and gallbladder in the digestive system, because secretions of these organs affect the activities of the small intestine.

PANCREAS

Functional Anatomy

General Considerations

- The pancreas—an elongated, accessory digestive gland—lies retroperitoneally and transversely across the posterior abdominal wall, posterior to the stomach between the duodenum on the right and the spleen on the left (Fig. 7.4-1).
- *Anatomically,* for the purpose of description, the pancreas is divided into four parts: head, neck, body and tail.
- *Physiologically,* on the basis of functions performed, the pancreas consists of two parts:
  - *Exocrine part*, which produces a secretion called pancreatic juice that contains enzymes capable of hydrolysing proteins, fats and carbohydrates.
  - *Endocrine part* of the pancreas, the islets of Langerhans, produces the hormones insulin and glucagon, which play a key role in the carbohydrate metabolism. The endocrine part is discussed in Section 8 (page 768).

Structural Characteristics of Exocrine Part of Pancreas

The exocrine part of the pancreas is in the form of a serous, compound tubuloalveolar gland, very similar to the parotid gland in the general structure (Fig. 7.4-2).

Acinar cells lining the alveoli appear triangular in section. Numerous secretory (or zymogen) granules can be demonstrated in the cytoplasm, especially in the apical part of the cells. These granules are eosinophilic and decrease considerably after the cells have poured out their secretions.

The acinar cells produce a thick secretion containing numerous enzymes (listed in composition of pancreatic juice).

Centroacinar cells. In addition to the secretory acinar cells, the alveoli of exocrine pancreas contain centroacinar cells that are so-called because they appear to be located near the centre of the acinus (alveolus). These cells really belong to the intercalated ducts which are invaginated into the acinus (Fig. 7.4-2).

Ductal cells lining the ductal system of the pancreas produce a watery secretion rich in bicarbonate ions

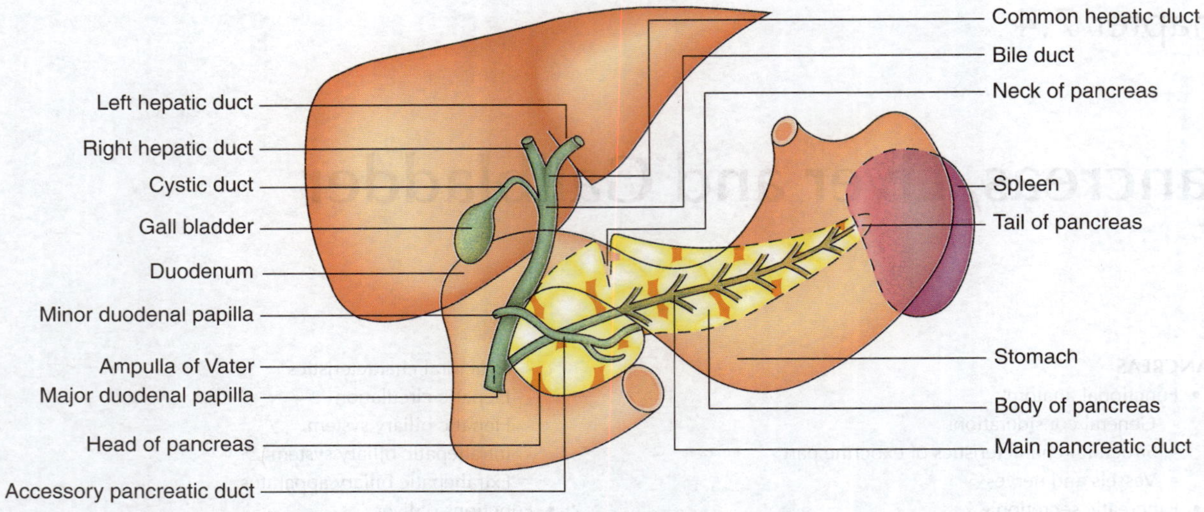

Common hepatic duct
Bile duct
Neck of pancreas
Left hepatic duct
Right hepatic duct
Cystic duct
Spleen
Gall bladder
Tail of pancreas
Duodenum
Minor duodenal papilla
Stomach
Ampulla of Vater
Major duodenal papilla
Body of pancreas
Head of pancreas
Main pancreatic duct
Accessory pancreatic duct

FIGURE 7.4-1 Anatomical relations of pancreas, pancreatic duct and extrahepatic biliary system.

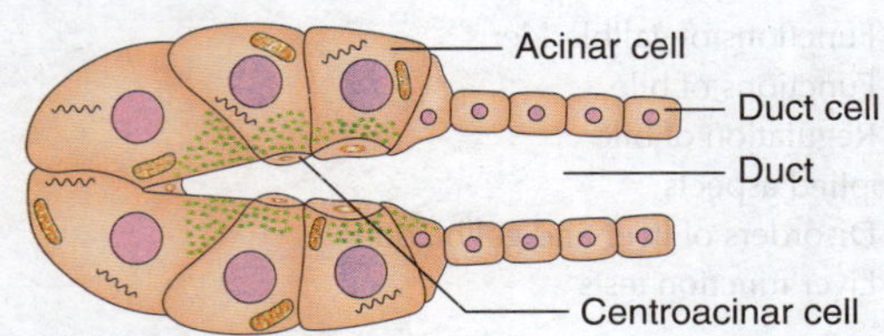

FIGURE 7.4-2 Histology of functional unit of pancreas.

(HCO_3^-), which mixes with the thick secretion produced by acinar cells to constitute the pancreatic juice.

Pancreatic Ducts

The intercalated ducts, which receive secretions produced by acini, pass it on to interlobular ducts. Ultimately, the pancreatic secretion passes into the duodenum through the main pancreatic duct and the accessory pancreatic duct.

Main pancreatic duct, also known as duct of Wirsung, begins in the tail and runs the length of the gland, receiving numerous tributaries on the way. It joins the common bile duct to form the ampulla of Vater, which opens into the second part of the duodenum at about its middle on the major duodenal papilla (Fig. 7.4-1). Ampulla of Vater is guarded by the sphincter of Oddi.

Accessory pancreatic duct, also called the duct of Santorini, when present, drains the upper part of the head and then opens into the duodenum about 2 mm above the main duct on the minor duodenal papilla. The accessory duct frequently communicates with the main duct.

Vessels and Nerves of Pancreas

- ***Arterial supply*** to the pancreas comes from the splenic and superior as well as inferior pancreatico–duodenal arteries.
- ***Veins***, corresponding to arteries, drain into the portal system.
- ***Lymphatics*** drain into the lymph nodes situated along the arteries that supply the gland. The efferent vessels ultimately drain into the coeliac and superior mesenteric lymph nodes.
- ***Nerve supply*** comes from both sympathetic and parasympathetic (vagi) nerves. Preganglionic vagal fibres synapse with ganglionic cells embedded in the pancreatic tissue; the postganglionic fibres innervate both the acinar cells and smooth muscles of the ducts. Vagal stimulation increases pancreatic juice secretion.

Pancreatic Juice

Properties

- Pancreatic juice is a transparent, colourless fluid isotonic with plasma.
- About 1200–1500 ml of pancreatic juice is secreted per day.
- Its specific gravity varies from 1.010 to 1.018.
- Pancreatic juice is markedly alkaline (pH 7.8–8.4), due to very high concentration of HCO_3^- (113 mEq/L about 4–5 times that of plasma).

Composition

Pancreatic juice is composed of 99.5% water and 0.5% solids, which include organic and inorganic substances.

Organic Constituents of pancreatic juice are certain enzymes and other substances.

- ***Enzymes.*** The pancreas secretes four major types of enzymes: amylase, lipase, protease and trypsin inhibitor.
- ***Other organic substances*** present in traces are albumin and globulin.

Inorganic Substances present in the pancreatic juice are cations like Na^+, K^+, Ca^{2+}, Mg^{2+} and Zn^{2+}; and anions such as HCO_3^-, Cl^- and traces of SO_4^{2-} and HPO_4^{2-}. Electrolyte composition varies with rate of secretion (see page 611).

Pancreatic Enzymes Pancreatic acini secrete four major types of enzymes: amylase, lipase, protease and trypsin inhibitor.

1. Pancreatic ∝ Amylase. It is secreted in its active form. It is the only amylytic enzyme present with pancreatic juice. Its action on the carbohydrates is like that of salivary amylase. It hydrolyses glycogen, starch and most other complex carbohydrates, except cellulose, to form disaccharides.

2. Pancreatic Lipases or lipolytic enzymes include pancreatic lipase, cholesterol ester hydrolase and phospholipase A_2.

- ***Pancreatic lipase.*** It is a powerful lipolytic enzyme. It hydrolyses neutral fats to glycerol esters and fatty acids. Its activity is accelerated in the presence of bile salts.
- ***Cholesterol ester hydrolase*** converts cholesterol esters to cholesterol.
- ***Phospholipase A_2.*** It is secreted in an inactive form pro-phospholipase A_2 and gets converted to active form phospholipase A_2 by the action of trypsin. Phospholipase A_2 splits fatty acid phoshatidylcholine (PC) forming Lyso-PC. Lyso-PC damages the cell membrane.

Important Note

It is *important to note* that in acute pancreatitis, phospholipase A_2 gets activated in the pancreatic ducts causing disruption of pancreatic tissue and necrosis of surrounding fat, which may be fatal. Acute pancreatitis is invariably associated with high serum amylase level.

---

3. Pancreatic Proteases or proteolytic enzymes include three endopeptidases (trypsin, chymotrypsin and elastase) and two exopeptidases (carboxypeptidase A and B). Endopeptidases break the peptides somewhere in the middle. Exopeptidases break the peptide chain near its end, releasing single amino acid.

- ***Trypsin.*** It is the most powerful proteolytic enzyme of the pancreatic juice. It is secreted in an inactive form of trypsinogen, which is activated by the enzyme enterokinase (enteropeptidase) secreted by the duodenal mucosa. Once formed, trypsin also activates trypsinogen—an autocatalytic reaction.

$$\text{Trypsinogen} \xrightarrow{\text{Enterokinase}} \text{Trypsin}$$

$$\text{Trypsinogen} \xrightarrow{\text{Trypsin}} \text{Trypsin}$$

  - Trypsin hydrolyses proteins into proteoses and to polypeptides.
  - It activates trypsinogen and other pancreatic enzymes.
- ***Chymotrypsin.*** It is also secreted in an inactive form chymotrypsinogen and is activated by trypsin. It hydrolyses the proteins into small polypeptides.
- ***Elastase.*** It is secreted as proelastase, which is activated by trypsin. It digests elastin.
- ***Carboxypeptidase A and B.*** These are secreted as procarboxypeptidase A and B and are activated by enterokinase and trypsin.
  - Carboxypeptidase A cleaves the carboxyl-terminal amino acid that has aromatic or branched aliphatic side chains.
  - Carboxypeptidase B cleaves the carboxyl-terminal amino acids that have basic side chains.
- ***Nucleases*** (ribonuclease and deoxyribonuclease). They split nucleic acids of ribose and deoxyribose type into nucleotides.
- ***Collagenase.*** It is also activated by trypsin and digests collagen.

4. Trypsin Inhibitor. If even a small amount of trypsin is released into the pancreas, the resulting chain reaction would produce active enzymes that could digest the pancreas. It is therefore, not surprising that the pancreas normally contains a trypsin inhibitor, which is secreted by the same cells and at the same time as the pancreatic proenzymes. The trypsin inhibitor protects the pancreas from autodigestion.

Functions of Pancreatic Juice

1. Digestive Functions. The pancreatic juice is the major source of digestive enzymes that digest all components of the food—proteins, carbohydrates, fats and nucleic acid. For details see page 646.

2. Neutralizing Function. Pancreatic juice is highly alkaline due to high concentration of HCO_3^- and neutralizes the gastric HCl in the chyme that enters the duodenum.

Mechanism of Pancreatic Secretion

Secretion of Pancreatic Enzymes

- The acinar cells of the exocrine part of the pancreas produce the pancreatic enzymes which are synthesized in the ribosomes of the rough endoplasmic reticulum. The raw material for the synthesis of enzymes is amino acids-derived from the blood.
- After synthesis in the rough endoplasmic reticulum, the enzymes pass to the Golgi complex where they are surrounded by membranes and then released into the cytoplasm as *secretory (zymogen) granules*.
- The zymogen granules move to the luminal surface of the cells. When stimulated, the acinar cells pour the enzymes in the lumen of acini by *exocytosis*. After passing through the intercalated and interlobar ducts, ultimately the

pancreatic juice containing these enzymes is poured into the duodenum through the main and accessory pancreatic ducts.

- Within the cells, these enzymes are stored in inactive form (proenzymes). They become active only after mixing with duodenal contents. Activation is initiated by the brush border enzyme enteropeptidase (enterokinase) present in the epithelial cells lining the duodenum.

Formation of Aqueous Component of Pancreatic Secretion The aqueous component of the pancreatic juice is produced principally by the columnar epithelial cells which line the pancreatic ducts. However, acinar cells, which are primarily responsible for secreting pancreatic enzymes, also have some contribution towards aqueous component. The characteristics of the aqueous component of pancreatic juice secreted by acinar cells are intralobular ductal cells and extralobular ductal cells (Fig. 7.4-3) are as:

Secretion by Acinar Cells. The acinar fluid is isotonic and resembles plasma in its concentrations of Na^+, K^+, Cl^- and HCO_3^-. The secretion of acinar fluid and the proteins it contains is stimulated by cholecystokinin and acetylcholine.

Secretion by Intralobular Ductal Cells. The spontaneous secretion that is produced by intralobular ductal cell has a higher concentration of K^+ and HCO_3^- than does plasma.

Secretion by Extralobular Ductal Cells is stimulated by the hormone secretin. The secretin stimulated secretion by the extralobular ductal cells is still richer in HCO_3^- than the spontaneous secretion.

Cellular Mechanism for Secretion of HCO_3^- Rich Fluid by the Ductal Epithelial Cells. Bicarbonate in the blood, perfusing the pancreatic duct, rather than HCO_3^- that is produced by the ductal epithelial cells, is the major source of the HCO_3^- that is secreted into the lumen of the extralobular duct. The steps involved in the secretion rate of HCO_3^- are (Fig. 7.4-4):

- Blood perfusing the ducts is acidified by Na^+–H^+ exchangers and H^+–K^+–ATPase in the basolateral membrane resulting in the formation of CO_2 from blood HCO_3^-.
- CO_2 diffuses into the ductal cells, where it combines with water (H_2O) to form carbonic acid (H_2CO_3) in the presence of enzyme carbonic anhydrase (CA).
- Dissociation of H_2CO_3 to H^+ and HCO_3^-, together with extrusion of H^+ across the basolateral membrane, produces a high intracellular HCO_3^-.
- HCO_3^- flows down its electrochemical potential gradient across the luminal membrane via the Cl^-, HCO_3^- exchanger.
- Cl^- is recycled back into the lumen by the electrogenic Cl^- channels in the luminal membrane.
- Na^+ enters the luminal fluid by flowing through the tight junctions in response to the negative electrical potential in the lumen that is produced by electrogenic Cl^- transport.
- Efflux of K^+ through basolateral K^+ channels maintains the intracellular electronegativity that is part of the driving force for the transport of Cl^- and HCO_3^- across the luminal membrane.

Modification in the Main Collecting Ducts. As the secretion flows through the main ducts, water moves into the duct across the epithelium (because the pancreatic duct cells are permeable to water), and makes the pancreatic juice isotonic to plasma. In addition, some HCO_3^- move out of the ducts in exchange for Cl^- (Fig. 7.4-3).

Effect of Flow Rate on Composition of Aqueous Component of Pancreatic Juice. The electrolyte composition of pancreatic juice varies with the secretion rate (Fig. 7.4-5).

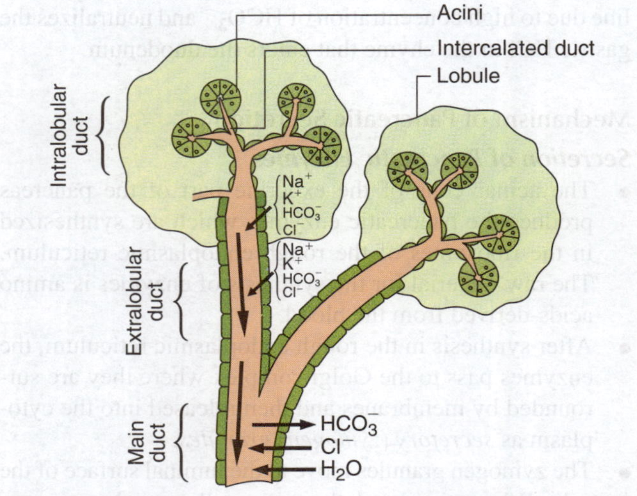

FIGURE 7.4-3 Formation of the aqueous component of pancreatic juice at the level of acinar cell, intralobular ductal cells and extralobular ductal cells; and modification at the level of the main collecting duct.

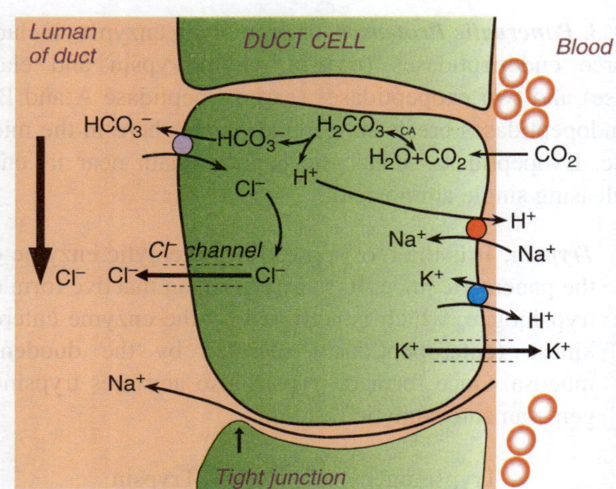

FIGURE 7.4-4 Mechanism of secretion of HCO_3^- by the ductal epithelial cells.

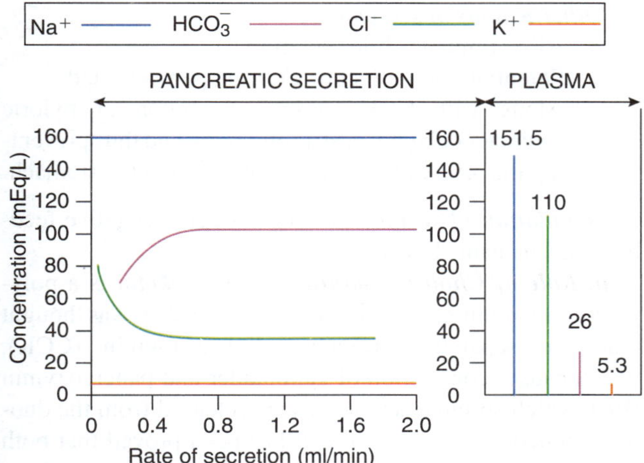

FIGURE 7.4-5 Effect of rate of secretion of pancreatic juice on its electrolyte composition.

- *Bicarbonate ion (HCO_3^-)* concentration of pancreatic juice at low secretory rate is as high as 80 mEq/L (much more than that of plasma, 26 mEq/L) and increases up to 120 mEq/L at high flow rates.
- *Chloride ion (Cl^-)* concentration decreases, as the flow rate of pancreatic juice increases, in other words, the HCO_3^- concentration rises. Thus, the total concentration of HCO_3^- and Cl^- remains constant and there exists a reciprocal relationship between their concentrations (Fig. 7.4-5).
- *Sodium (Na^+)* and potassium (K^+) concentrations in the pancreatic juice, unlike the saliva, are similar to those in the plasma and do not vary with the rate of secretion.
- *Tonicity of pancreatic juice*. From the above, it is clear that regardless of the flow rate, pancreatic secretions are *isotonic*. *At low flow rates,* the pancreas secretes an isotonic fluid that is composed mainly of Na^+ and Cl^-, as at low flow rates, equal volume of pancreatic juice comes from acinar and ductal cells. At high flow rates, the pancreas secretes an isotonic fluid that is composed mainly of Na^+ and HCO_3^-, as at high flow rates the proportion of the pancreatic juice secreted by the ductal cells, which have a high concentration of HCO_3^- increases.

Regulation of Pancreatic Secretion

Both, neural and hormonal mechanisms are involved in the regulation of pancreatic secretion, with the latter playing the predominant role. *Neural regulation* is through vagal efferents supplying the exocrine gland of pancreas and hormonal regulation is through secretin, cholecystokinin (CCK), gastrin and somatostatin. The exact role of these regulatory mechanisms in regulating the different phases of pancreatic secretion viz. cephalic phase, gastric phase and intestinal phase is summarized in Table 7.4-1.

TABLE 7.4-1 Summary of Regulation of Cephalic, Gastric and Intestinal Phases of Pancreatic Secretion

Phase	Stimulus	Mediator	Pancreatic response
Cephalic	Conditioned reflex initiated by: • Taste, • Smell and • Thought of food Unconditioned re-flex initiated by taste of food in mouth.	Vagus	Little secretion of pancreatic enzymes and HCO_3^-
Gastric	• Distension of stomach by food	Vagus	Low volume of pancreatic HCO_3^- and enzymes
	• Amino acids and peptides	Gastrin	Low volume high enzyme secretion
Intestinal	• Low pH of chyme in duodenum	Secretin	Large amount of aqueous secretion with high HCO_3^- concentration
	• Amino acids and peptides in chyme in duodenum	CCK	Pancreatic juice rich in enzymes
	• Food in small intes-tine	Vagus through - Secretin - CCK	Pancreatic juice rich in enzymes and HCO_3^-

1. Regulation of Cephalic Phase *Cephalic phase* of pancreatic secretion like that of gastric secretion occurs before the entry of food into the stomach. This phase is characterized by very little flow of secretions from pancreatic ducts into the duodenum because of the secretion of small quantities of enzymes and aqueous components of the pancreatic juice.

Regulation of this phase is mainly through the *reflex vagal stimulation,* which occurs:

- **By conditioned reflexes,** initiated by sight, smell and thought of food and
- **Unconditioned reflexes,** initiated by stimulation of taste buds by the food in the mouth cavity, the act of chewing and swallowing.

Afferent impulses, from the cerebral cortex (during conditioned reflexes) and from the mouth (during unconditioned reflexes) reach the dorsal nucleus of vagus. Stimulation of efferents in vagus nerve supplying the exocrine part of pancreas enhances secretion from both, acinar as well as ductal cells:

- *Enzyme secretion* from acinar cells is enhanced due to stimulation of enteric neurons, which release acetylcholine. Acetylcholine exerts its effect on the acinar cells by activating *phospholipase*.
- *Bicarbonate secretion* from the ductal cells is enhanced by stimulation of enteric neurons which release noradrenergic transmitters.

2. Regulation of Gastric Phase Gastric phase of pancreatic secretion occurs when the stomach is distended by the food. This phase is regulated by *neural control* exerted through the vagus and *hormonal control* executed through the hormone gastrin:

- ***Vagus stimulation*** (vagovagal reflex), which occurs due to distension of the body of the stomach by the food results in secretion of low volumes of pancreatic juice containing HCO_3^- and enzymes. Acetylcholine is the transmitter.
- ***Gastrin hormone*** is released from antral G-cells by the food breakdown products (primarily amino acids and peptides). Gastrin released into the blood, while reaching the pancreas, stimulates the acinar cells and produces a low-volume, high-enzyme pancreatic secretion.

3. Regulation of Intestinal Phase The intestinal phase of pancreatic secretion begins when the chyme enters the duodenum and jejunum. It is characterized by a marked increase in the secretion of both enzymes and aqueous component of pancreatic juice. This phase is regulated by the hormones secretin and cholecystokinin (CCK).

i. Role of Secretin Secretin was the first hormone ever discovered by Bayliss and Starling in 1902. It is a polypeptide with 27 amino acids.

Source of secretin is endocrinal S-cells located among the epithelial cells of the mucous membrane of duodenum and jejunum.

Stimulant for release of secretin is *low pH* (<4.5) of chyme caused by presence of gastric HCl.

Actions. Secretin is released in an inactive form—*prosecretin,* which is converted into secretin by the gastric HCl and salts of fatty acids present in the chyme. Secretin enters the blood circulation and after reaching the pancreas it *acts on the duct* cells via cyclic AMP (second messenger) and produces large amounts of watery juice with a high concentration of HCO_3^-. The alkaline pancreatic juice with high concentration of HCO_3^- subserves the following functions:

- *Neutralizes the HCl* present in the chyme and thus protects the intestinal mucosa from the acid and
- *Provides a required pH* (7–9) for the activation of pancreatic enzymes.

Other actions of secretin are:

- Also stimulates bile secretion,
- Potentiates the effect of CCK on pancreas and
- Along with CCK causes contraction of pyloric sphincter delaying gastric emptying and thus preventing the reflux of duodenal contents into the stomach.

Regulation of secretin occurs through a negative feedback mechanism shown below Fig. 7.4-6.

ii. Role of Cholecystokinin *Cholecystokinin* is a polypeptide containing 33 amino acids. Previously it was thought that two separate hormones—cholecystokinin (CCK), which causes contraction of gallbladder and pancreozymin (PZ), which stimulates pancreas are released from the duodenal mucosa. However, now it has been proved that both the actions (on gallbladder and pancreas) are brought about by a single hormone which is called cholecystokinin-pancreozymin (CCK-PZ) or simply cholecystokinin (CCK).

Source of secretion of CCK is the *endocrinal I-cells* located among the epithelial cells of the mucosa of duodenum and jejunum. CCK, is produced from the precursor prepro-CCK, contains 58 amino acid residues (CCK-58) processed into many fragments. Different forms of CCK are: CCK-39, CCK-12, CCK-8 and CCK-4. Like gastrin, all these forms of CCK have five amino acids same at the carboxyl-terminal. The half-life of CCK is 5 min, about its metabolism, very little is known.

Stimulants for release of CCK are amino acids (primarily phenylalanine), fatty acids, and monoglycerides present in the chyme.

Actions. CCK passes via blood to pancreas and causes *secretion of pancreatic juice rich in enzymes* by causing discharge of zymogen granules from the pancreatic acinar cells via second messenger inosine triphosphate (IP_3) and increased intracellular Ca^{2+}.

Other actions of CCK are:

- Contraction of gallbladder to release bile,
- Potentiates the effect of secretin to produce more alkaline pancreatic juice,
- Increases the secretion of enterokinase (enteropeptidase) from the duodenum,

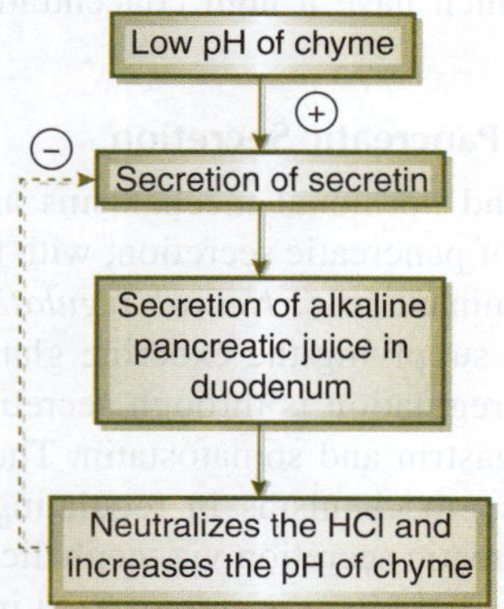

FIGURE 7.4-6 Regulation of secretin secretion.

- Inhibits the gastric motility and gastric emptying,
- Increases the motility of small and large gut,
- Increases the pancreatic growth (trophic effect) and
- It is also found in neurons in the brain (especially in the cerebral cortex) where it is involved in the regulation of food intake and is related to the production of anxiety and analgesia.

Mechanism of action. CCK act through its receptors. Two types of CCK receptors have been identified. CCK-A receptors are located primarily in the periphery whereas both CCK-A and CCK-B receptors are found in the brain. Both types of receptors cause activation of phospholipase-C, causing increase production of IP_3 and diacylglycerol (DAG).

Regulation of CCK secretion occurs through a positive feedback mechanism (Fig. 7.4-7).

The secretion of CCK is increased by contact of intestinal mucosa with product of digestion (particularly peptides of amino acid and fatty acid containing more than 10 carbon atoms).Two releasing factors that activate CCK secretion have been identified, which are CCK-releasing peptide (from intestinal mucosa)and monitor peptide (from pancreas).

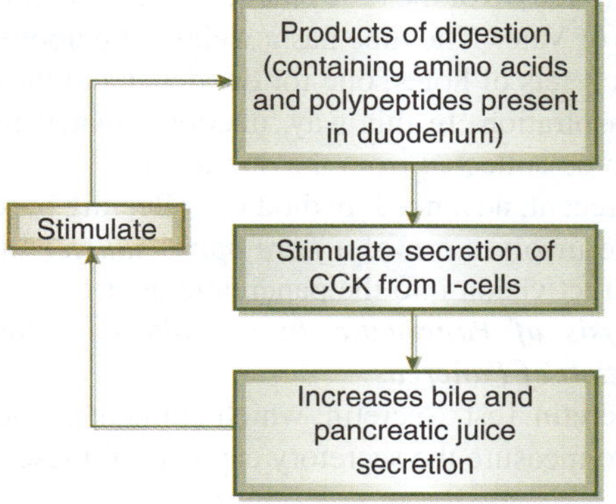

FIGURE 7.4-7 Regulation of cholecystokinin secretion.

Potentiation of effect of secretin and CCK

- Secretin potentiates the effect of CCK. By itself, secretin has no effect on enzyme secretion.
- CCK potentiates the effect of secretin. By itself, CCK has no effect on HCO_3^- secretion.
- Because they are potentiators of each other's action, small concentrations of CCK and secretin together can produce significant amounts of pancreatic HCO_3^- and enzyme secretions.

Interaction of nervous and humoral regulation

- A vagovagal reflex is initiated during intestinal phase of digestion, which greatly potentiates the effects of secretin and CCK through the acetylcholine. Thus, vagus stimulation is much more potent in stimulating pancreatic secretions when CCK and secretin are present in the plasma.

Applied Aspects

Disorders of Pancreas

Common disorders of pancreas are:

1. Acute Pancreatitis. It is an acute inflammatory disease of the pancreas, thought to result from autodigestion of pancreatic tissue by the proteolytic enzymes which leak out of the acini and are activated within the pancreas. Recently, it has been hypothesized that the proteolytic enzymes become activated by lysosomal hydrolases within the pancreatic acini itself. Patient usually presents with acute pain in upper abdomen, nausea and vomiting. It is a serious disease and

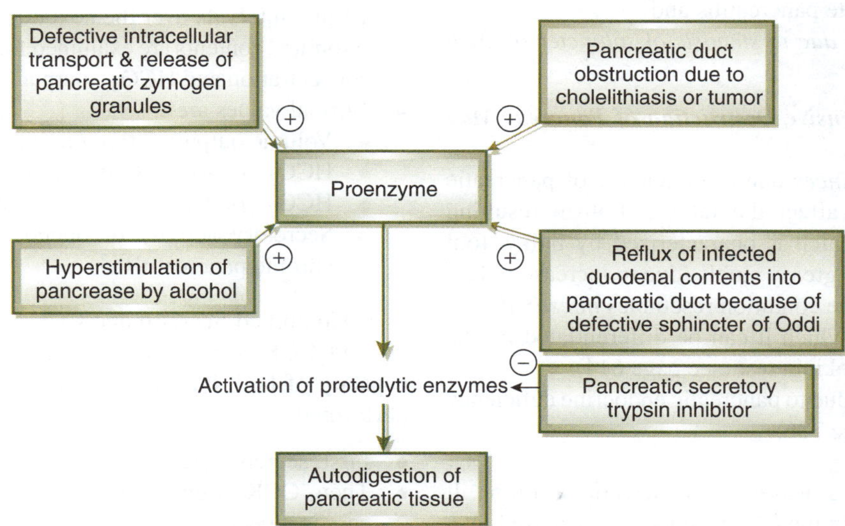

FIGURE 7.4-8 Pathophysiology of acute pancreatitis.

may be fatal sometimes. Marked elevation of serum amylase (threefold rise) usually *clinches* the diagnosis.

Pathophysiology of acute pancreatitis. Acute pancreatitis occurs as a consequence of premature activation of zymogen granules, releasing proteases which digest the pancreatic epithelium and surrounding tissue. The severity of the condition depends on the balance between the activity of released proteolytic enzymes and antiproteolytic factors such as intracellular pancreatic trypsin inhibitor protein, circulating β_2-macroglobulin, α_1-antitrypsin and Cl-esterase inhibitor. The conditions that can cause acute pancreatitis have been given in Fig. 7.4-8.

Diagnosis of acute pancreatitis is made by signs, symptoms and investigations.

Management. Acute pancreatitis is often self-limiting. The management comprises of several steps:

- Proper diagnosis and its severity to be established.
- Early treatment depending on the severity of the disease, i.e. management of analgesia by:
  - Analgesic such as pethidine.
  - Correction of hypovolemia using normal saline/colloids.
- Detection and treatment of complications.
- Treatment of underlying cause, specially gallstones.

2. Chronic Pancreatitis is a chronic inflammation of pancreas which results in slow destruction of the tissue resulting in the deficiency of pancreatic secretions.

The Causative Factors are:

- *Toxic* metabolic factors include: alcohol, smoking and hypercalcaemia,
- *Chronic* renal failure,
- *Genetic factors.* Hereditary pancreatitis occurs due to trypsinogen mutation, SPINK-1 mutation and cystic fibrosis,
- *Autoimmunity.* It may be isolated or involve multiple organs,
- *Recurrence* of acute pancreatitis and
- *Obstructive cause due to stenosis of sphincter of Oddi or tumours.*

Patients with Extensive Destruction of Pancreas May Develop:

- *Digestive disturbances* due to deficiency of pancreatic enzymes, mainly affect the fat metabolism resulting in *steatorrhoea* which is characterized by bulky, foul smelling, pale and greasy stools (due to increase in faecal fat content). The condition resembles *intestinal malabsorption*, from which it can be differentiated by the secretin cholecystokinin test (see page 614).
- *Diabetes mellitus* due to pancreatic endocrine deficiency of insulin (see page 786).

3. Cystic Fibrosis is a disorder of pancreatic secretion. It results from a defect in the Cl^- channel that is caused by a mutation in the cystic fibrosis transmembrane conductance regulator (CFTR) gene. It is associated with a deficiency of pancreatic enzymes resulting in steatorrhoea (features described above).

4. Pancreatectomy, i.e. surgical removal of pancreas is usually performed in carcinoma of the pancreas. It results in deficiency of pancreatic enzymes characterized by the same features as described in chronic pancreatitis.

Pancreatic Function Tests

Pancreatic function tests are performed to evaluate the normal functioning of the pancreas and to detect abnormality, if any. The function tests to evaluate the functioning of the exocrine part of the pancreas can be divided as follows:

- Analysis of pancreatic juice,
- Analysis of products of digestion and
- Estimation of serum amylase levels.

I. Analysis of Pancreatic Juice

Collection of Pancreatic Juice. *A double lumen radiopaque* tube (D veiling tube) is inserted through the nose or mouth, till the tip of the tube reaches the duodenum near the ampulla of Vater. The tube has a weighted bulbous end and contains 2 sets of holes, one for duodenal and the other for gastric aspiration. In this way, uncontaminated pancreatic juice can be collected from the duodenum.

The recent, advanced method of collecting pure pancreatic juice involves use of a *fibre optic catheter* introduced under direct vision into the pancreatic duct.

Analysis of Pancreatic Juice Collected after Direct Stimulation of Pancreas

1. Secretin Test. Secretin, which stimulates ductal cells, is used to measure the secretory capacity of these cells:

- After overnight fasting, duodenal and gastric contents are aspirated in the morning.
- Intravenous infusion of secretin (12.5 units/kg body weight) is given, and duodenal aspirate is collected at 10-min intervals over the next 80 min.
- Aspirated contents are examined for volume, pH, HCO_3^- concentration and HCO_3^- output.
- Normal values are:
  - Volume output: .2.0 ml/kg in 80 min.
  - HCO_3^- concentration: .80 mEq/L.
  - HCO_3^- output: .10 mEq/L in 30 min.
  - Secretory activity of ductal cells is decreased in chronic pancreatitis.

2. Combined Secretin and CCK Test. Combined secretin and CCK test is employed to evaluate the secretory capacity of both ductal cells and acinar cells. The test is performed as:

- First, secretin test is performed as described above.
- Then, CCK is given intravenously and the whole process is repeated.

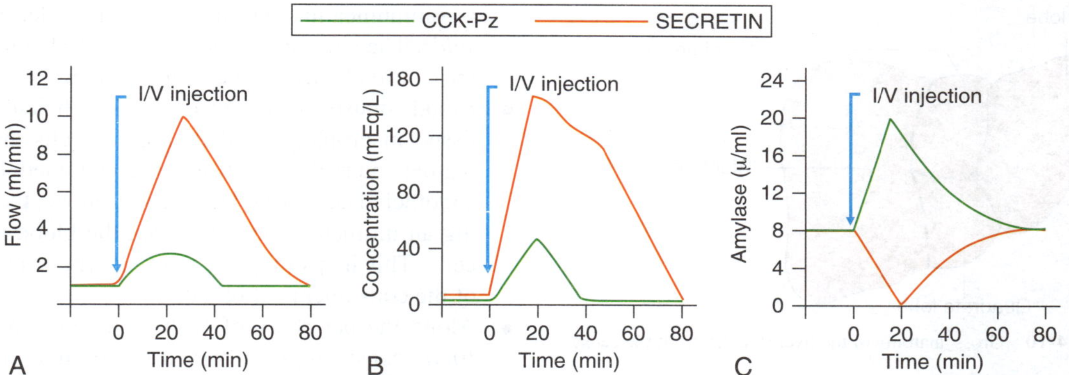

FIGURE 7.4-9 Normal curves for combined secretin–cholecystokinin test: A, volume of pancreatic juice; B, HCO_3^- concentration of pancreatic juice; and C, enzyme (amylase) level of pancreatic juice.

- Curves for normal values of volume of pancreatic juice, HCO_3^- concentration and enzyme levels obtained by this test are shown in Fig. 7.4-9.
- Abnormalities can be detected from the results. With mild pancreatic damage, there is dissociation between the bicarbonate and enzyme output, i.e. only the former is affected, though with advanced damage, both are affected.
- This test helps to differentiate patients with steatorrhoea due to intestinal malabsorption (in which the test will be normal) from that, due to chronic pancreatitis (in which there will be decreased secretion of enzymes).

Analysis of Pancreatic Juice Collected after Indirect Stimulation of Pancreas

1. Lundh Test. In this test, pancreas is stimulated indirectly, by ingestion of a test meal (containing fats, proteins and carbohydrates) and assessment of trypsin activity is made from the pancreatic juice collected. The mean trypsin activity of <6 IU/L indicates presence of pancreatic exocrine insufficiency.

II. Analysis of Products of Digestion

1. Faecal Fat Excretion Test. For this test, subject is placed on a diet containing 100 g of fat per day. The stools are collected over 3–5 days and tested for fat content by Van de Kramer method and results are interpreted as:

- Normally fats are digested by lipase (mainly from pancreas) and about 5–6 g/day are excreted in stools.
- In patients with exocrine pancreatic insufficiency it may increase to 40–50 g/day.

2. Faecal Nitrogen Excretion Test. Normally, about 7 g of nitrogen is excreted in the stools per day. In patients with exocrine pancreatic insufficiency due to deficiency of proteolytic enzymes, the nitrogen excretion in stools is increased.

3. Tripeptide Hydrolysis Test. In this test, patient is given a synthetic peptide B_2–T_4–PABA. Normally, B_2–T_4–PABA is cleaved by the chymotrypsin into B_2–T_4 and PABA. PABA is rapidly absorbed and excreted in urine. In exocrine pancreatic insufficiency cleavage of B_2–T_4–PABA is decreased leading to decreased excretion of PABA in the urine. Thus, from the values of PABA in urine, activity of pancreatic chymotrypsin can be studied.

4. Dual Label Schilling Test. In this test, ability of the gut to absorb vitamin B_{12} is studied. It is based on the fact that pancreatic proteases (trypsin) play an important role in the absorption mechanism of vitamin B_{12} and that in pancreatic insufficiency the absorption of vitamin B_{12} is abnormal.

III. Estimation of Serum Amylase Levels This test is particularly useful in ruling out acute pancreatitis in patients presenting with acute pain in upper abdomen. Normal values of serum amylase are 50–120 units/L. The levels of serum amylase are markedly raised in patients with acute pancreatitis.

LIVER AND GALLBLADDER

Liver: Physiological Anatomy

General Considerations

- Liver, the largest gland in the body, weighs approximately 1500 g and accounts for approximately 1/40th of adult body weight.
- Traditionally, the liver has been divided into *right and left lobes*. Right lobe is much larger and includes the caudate and quadrate lobes. The left lobe is much smaller and consists of 1/6th of total weight of liver.
- In current terminology, the liver consists of right and left functionally independent parts called the *portal lobes*, that are approximately equal in size. Thus, functionally the left part of the liver includes the caudate lobe and most of the quadrate lobe (Fig. 7.4-10).
- The right and left functional parts of the liver have their own blood supply from the hepatic artery and portal vein and their own venous and biliary drainage.

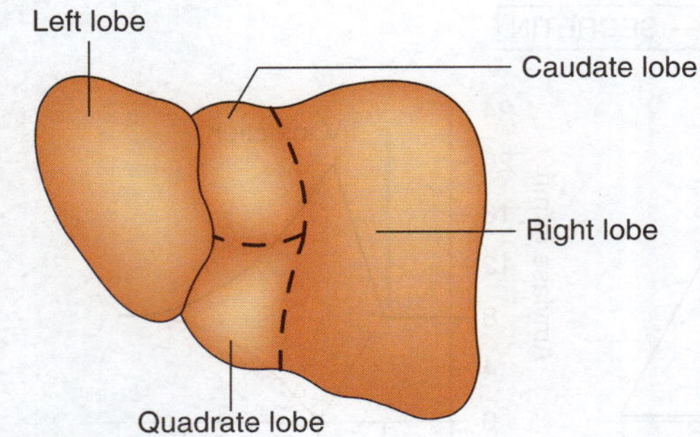

FIGURE 7.4-10 Gross anatomy of the liver (viewed from the back).

- The liver has got considerable physiological reserve. Even after removal of 80% of liver tissues, all *physiological* functions of the liver can be accomplished normally. Furthermore, even if 90% of bile ducts are ligated, the volume of bile secreted remains normal.
- The liver possesses considerable *regeneration power*. Original liver mass is restored within 6–8 weeks of removal of up to 3/4ths of liver. This occurs due to active mitotic division of the cells.

Structural Characteristics

- The liver tissue comprises about one lakh hexagonal areas that constitute the *hepatic lobules* (Fig. 7.4-11A).
- Each hepatic lobule is made-up of ramifying columns of hepatic cells (*hepatocytes*) that are arranged in the form of one cell thick plates. In between the cells are present bile canaliculi. These hepatic cell plates are tunnelled by a communicating system of lacunae called *blood sinusoids*. The sinusoids open into a central vein present in the centre of each lobule (Fig. 7.4-11B).
- Blood sinusoids are lined by endothelial cells. Few tissue macrophages called *Kupffer* cells are found at regular intervals in between the endothelial cells. The endothelial cells have large fenestrations, thereby forming an intimate contact between the blood and hepatic cells. This helps the liver to transform or modify many of the constituents of blood.
- Along the periphery of each lobule are present *portal triads* consisting of a branch of portal vein, branch of hepatic artery and an interlobular bile duct. Blood from the branch of the portal vein and hepatic artery enters the sinusoids which drain into the central vein.
- *Concept of portal lobule*, instead of hepatic lobule has been suggested by some workers. It has been described to consist of adjoining parts of three hepatic lobules centred on a portal triad.
- Presently acinus is considered the functional unit of the liver. Each acinus is considered to have three zones: 1, 2 and 3.
  - *Zone 1* refers to the central portion of the acinus immediately surrounding the terminal hepatic arteriole and terminal portal venule. This zone is well oxygenated. Enzymes involved in oxidative metabolism and glucogenesis predominate here.
  - *Zone 3* refers to most peripheral part of the acinus. It is the least oxygenated and most susceptible to anoxic injury. It is rich in enzymes involved in glycolysis, lipid and drug metabolism.
  - *Zone 2,* i.e. the intermediate zone, which is present in between zones 1 and 3 is moderately well oxygenated. It contains a mixed complement of enzymes.

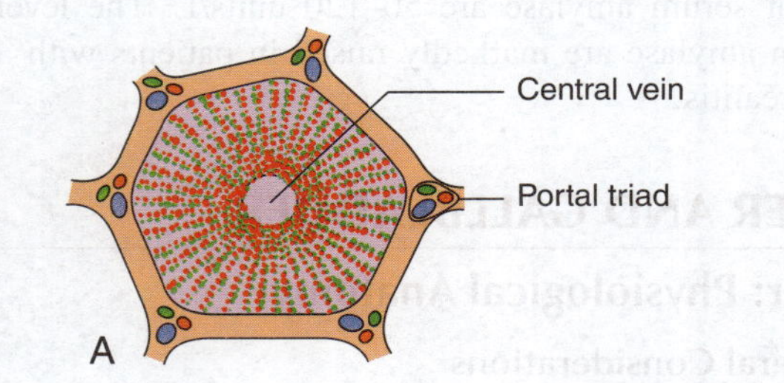

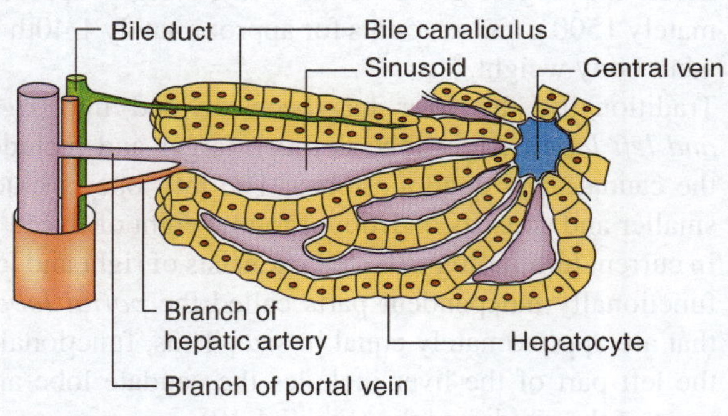

FIGURE 7.4-11 Histological characteristics of the liver: A, hexagonal lobule with portal triad; and B, hepatocyte, sinusoid and biliary canaliculi seen under high magnification.

Hepatic Circulation

Liver receives about 1500 ml blood/min from two sources:

Hepatic Artery, which is a branch of the coeliac trunk supplies about 20–25% (300–400 ml/min) of total blood which caters to the metabolic requirement of the liver tissue.

Portal vein, which collects blood from the mesenteric and splenic vascular bed, supplies about 75–80% (1100–1200 ml/min) of the total blood.

Hepatic vein. The hepatic and portal streams of blood meet in the sinusoids. The various substances produced by liver cells, the waste products and CO_2 are discharged into the sinusoids. The sinusoids drain into the central vein of the lobule. The central veins from different lobules unite to form bigger veins. These veins ultimately form the right and left hepatic veins which open into the inferior vena cava.

For details about the hepatic circulation and oxygen consumption see page 372.

Hepatic Biliary System

Intrahepatic Biliary System

The bile is secreted by liver cells into bile canaliculi. These canaliculi have no walls of their own. In fact, the bile canaliculi are the spaces bounded by canalicular surfaces of adjacent hepatic cells. On either side of the canaliculus, the two cell membranes are united by junctional complexes. These canaliculi form a hexagonal network around the liver cells. At the periphery of a lobule, the canaliculi become continuous with delicate *intralobular ductules,* which in turn become continuous with larger interlobular ductules of portal triads. The *interlobular ductules* are lined by cuboidal epithelium. Some smooth muscle is present in the wall of larger ducts. Ultimately, the larger ducts join to form the *right and left hepatic ducts* which leave the right and left parts of the liver and form part of the extrahepatic biliary system.

Extrahepatic Biliary Apparatus

The extrahepatic biliary apparatus consists of the gallbladder and the extrahepatic bile ducts (Fig. 7.4-1).

Gallbladder The gallbladder is a pear-shaped sac lying on the undersurface of the liver. It has a capacity of about 30–50 ml and stores bile, which it concentrates by absorbing water.

For descriptive purposes, the gallbladder is divided into fundus, body and neck. The neck becomes continuous with the *cystic duct.*

Extrahepatic Ducts

Hepatic Ducts. The right and left hepatic ducts emerge from the right and left lobes of the liver and after a short course join to form the *common hepatic duct* which is about 4 cm long.

Cystic Duct. It is also about 4 cm long and connects the neck of the gallbladder to the common hepatic duct to form the common bile duct.

Common Bile Duct (CBD) is about 8 cm long. It joins the pancreatic duct to form the common hepato-pancreatic duct which is otherwise called the ampulla of Vater. Ampulla of Vater opens into the duodenum at major duodenal papilla. The terminal parts of bile ducts and ampulla of Vater are surrounded by circular muscle fibres known as sphincter of Oddi, which play an important role in the storage and release of bile from the gallbladder.

Functions of Liver

The fact that mitochondria are maximally present in the liver emphasizes that the liver is involved in many biochemical functions. Although details of the various functions performed by the liver are discussed under their respective places, they are summarized here briefly.

I. Secretory Functions Liver cells act as exocrine glands and continuously secrete bile which is important for digestion and absorption of fats. Various aspects of the bile juice are discussed in this chapter.

II. Metabolic Functions Liver is the key organ and the principal site where the metabolism of carbohydrates, lipids and proteins takes place. Liver is also involved in the metabolism of vitamins and minerals to a certain extent.

1. Role in Carbohydrate Metabolism Includes:

- Liver acts as a glucostat in three ways:
  - *Glycogenesis,* i.e. glycogen is formed from glucose and stored in liver,
  - *Glycogenolysis,* i.e. breaking down of liver glycogen to glucose and
  - *Glucogenesis,* i.e. formation of glucose from non-carbohydrate sources such as non-nitrogenous residues of amino acids.

  The liver plays an important role in maintaining blood glucose level. In postprandial period, the liver removes excess of glucose from blood and returns it back when needed. Therefore, this action is called as *glucose buffer function.*
- Liver is the main site of alcohol metabolism for which liver cells contain the enzyme *alcohol dehydrogenase*.
- The interconversion of three monosaccharides, as glucose, galactose and fructose, also occurs in the liver.

2. Role in Fat Metabolism. Both, degradation and synthesis of fats take place in liver.

- *Degradation of fat.* Liver contains the enzyme lipoprotein lipase which hydrolyses triglycerides, cholesterol and phospholipids into fatty acids.
  - ß-oxidation, i.e. a process which oxidizes the fatty acids into acetoacetic acid occurs within the mitochondria.
- *Synthesis of fat* also takes place in liver.
  - Liver synthesizes triglycerides from carbohydrates.
  - Cholesterol and phospholipids are synthesized from unused free fatty acids.
  - Saturated fatty acids are synthesized from the active acetate via Krebs' cycle within the mitochondria.
  - Lipoproteins such as HDL, LDL, VLDL and chylomicrons are also synthesized in liver.

  Liver maintains cholesterol homeostasis by synthesizing it. During excess, the cholesterol is converted into bile acids.

3. Role in Protein Metabolism. In man, the protein turnover involves breakdown and resynthesis of 80–100 g of tissue protein per day, and its 50% part (i.e. 40–50 g) occurs in the liver. Important activities are:

- Liver brings about *deamination* of amino acids and this is essential for energy production, and their conversion into carbohydrates or fats.
- Liver is the main site of *urea formation.*

- Liver is the main site for formation of all nonessential amino acids by transamination of ketoacids.
- Albumin is solely resynthesized in liver and also to some extent α- and ß-globulins.

III. Detoxicating and Protective Functions

- Kupffer cells efficiently remove bacteria and other foreign bodies from portal circulation. This is the blood cleansing action of the liver.
- The biochemical detoxifying action of liver is brought about by a large number of cytochrome P_{450} enzymes from hepatocytes. These enzymes convert xenobiotics and other toxins into their inactive form. The detoxification reactions can be divided into two phases:

  Phase I reactions, e.g. oxidation, hydroxylation and others are mediated by P_{450} enzymes and

  Phase II reactions include esterification.
- Liver detoxifies certain drugs by either oxidation, or hydrolysis, or reduction or conjugation and excretes out through bile.

IV. Storage Functions Liver stores glucose (in the form of glycogen), vitamin B_{12} and vitamin A.

- Liver acts as a blood iron buffer and iron storage medium. It stores 60% of excess of iron mainly in the form of ferritin and partly as haemosiderin.

V. Excretory Functions

Ammonium Excretion. The liver is the only site where circulating ammonia is converted into urea and then excreted by the kidney into the urine.

- In the circulating blood, ammonium is derived from colon, kidney, breakdown of red blood cells and metabolism in the muscles.
- In the liver, ammonium is taken up by the hepatocytes. In the mitochondria of the hepatocyte it is converted into carbonyl phosphate, which reacts with ornithine to generate citrullin, and by series of cytoplasmic reactions produces arginine, which can be dehydrated to form urea and ornithine (Fig. 7.4-12A).

  The ornithine taken back into the mitochondria begins another urea cycle whereas, urea diffuses back into sinusoidal circulation and gets excreted by the kidney into the urine (Fig. 7.4-12B). Certain exogenous dyes like bromsulphthalein (BSP) and rose Bengal dye are exclusively excreted through liver cells.
- Cholesterol, alkaline phosphate and bilirubin are excreted in the bile.
- A number of drugs, adrenocortical and other steroid hormones are excreted in the bile.
- Ammonia is critically handled by the liver, as it is freely permeable across the blood–brain barrier; therefore, it is toxic to CNS tissue.

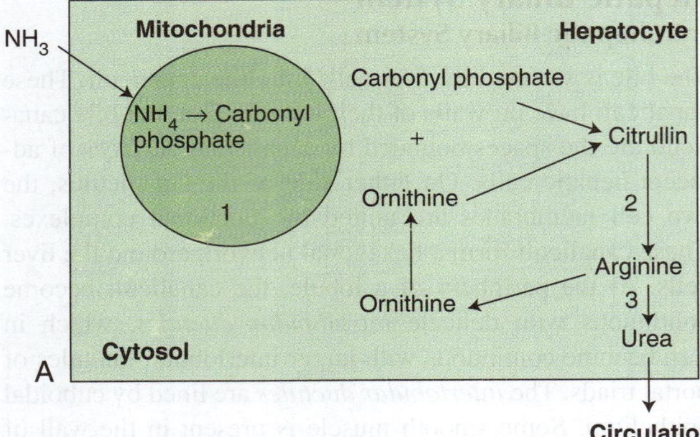

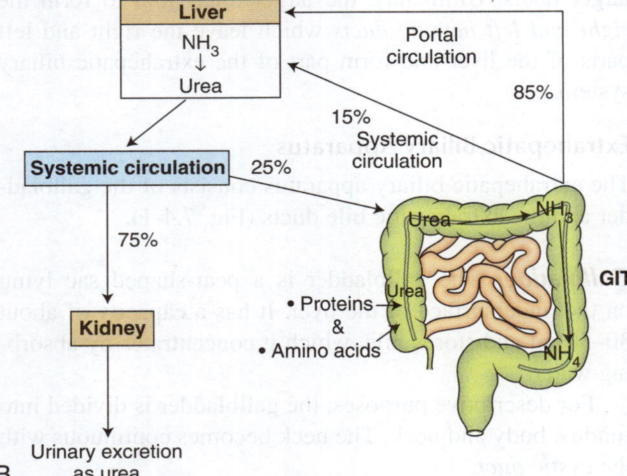

FIGURE 7.4-12 A. Urea cycle. B. Ammonia excretion as urea by the kidney.

VI. Synthesis Function Liver is the site for synthesis of:

- ***Plasma proteins,*** especially albumin and to some extent α- and β-globulins.
- ***Some blood coagulation factors.*** Liver cells are responsible for conversion of preprothrombin (inactive) to active prothrombin in the presence of vitamin K. It also produces other clotting factors such as fibrinogen factor (I), factors V, VII, IX and X.
- ***Enzymes,*** such as alkaline phosphatase, serum glutamic oxaloacetic transaminase (SGOT), serum glutamic pyruvic transaminase (SGPT) and serum isocitrate dehydrogenase (SICD).
- ***Urea.*** Liver removes ammonia from the body to synthesize urea.
- ***Cholesterol.*** It is synthesized from the active acetate.

VII. Miscellaneous Functions

- ***Reservoir of blood.*** Liver acts as a reservoir of blood and it stores about 650 ml of blood. It also helps in regulation of blood volume.

- ***Erythropoiesis.*** Liver is an important site of erythropoiesis in fetal life.
- ***Hormone metabolism.*** Liver causes:
  - *Inactivation* of some hormones such as insulin, glucagon and vasopressin.
  - *Reduction and conjugation* of adrenal and gonadal steroid hormones such as cortisol, aldosterone, oestrogen and testosterone.
  - *Conversion of thyroid hormone,* i.e. tetraiodothyronine (T_4) into tri-iodothyronine (T_3).
- ***Destruction of RBCs,*** also occurs in liver.
- ***Thermal regulation.*** Liver also helps in thermoregulation, as it produces large amount of heat.

Bile and Gallbladder

General Considerations

- Bile is a digestive juice, formed continuously in the liver by the hepatic cells (hepatocytes), and by epithelial cells lining the bile ducts (ductal cells).
- It is poured into the bile canaliculi from where it ultimately goes to the common hepatic duct which join with cystic duct to form the common bile duct. During interdigestive period when the sphincter of Oddi is closed, the bile is directed via the cystic duct to the gallbladder, where it is stored and concentrated.
- During meals, the sphincter of Oddi is relaxed, and when food reaches the duodenum, there occurs release of CCK which causes contraction of the gallbladder. Then the bile is released into the duodenum along with the pancreatic juice through the common opening ampulla of Vater.

Formation and Composition of Bile

The bile is formed by the hepatocytes and ductal cells lining the hepatic ducts. The hepatocytes, one surface of which is adjacent to the blood sinusoids and other to the biliary canaliculi, pick up some constituents of bile from the blood (e.g. *bile pigments*), synthesize some constituents (e.g. *bile salts*) and secrete a mixture into the biliary canaliculi. Ductular cells contribute HCO_3^- and Cl^- to the mixture giving rise to *hepatic bile* (Fig. 7.4-13). The substances that are actively secreted into the bile are bile acids, cholesterol, bilirubin, phosphatidylcholine and xenobiotics. There are specific canalicular transporters for their excretion. The canalicular bile is transiently hypertonic, because a number of substances such as glucose, glutathione, water, calcium and urea passively diffuse from plasma through tight junctions. In the bile ductules and ducts it undergoes modifications. The tight junctions of epithelial cells of ductules (cholangiocytes) are less permeable than that of hepatocytes, but freely, permeable to water, making the bile isotonic. The bile so formed is an alkaline juice comprising:

- Water and solids,
- Solids include organic and inorganic substances,

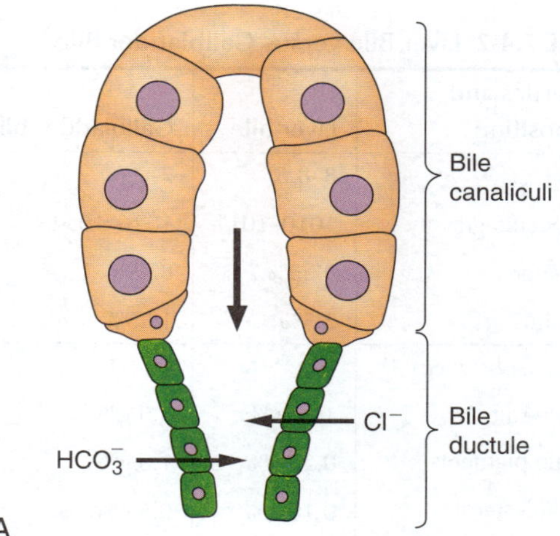

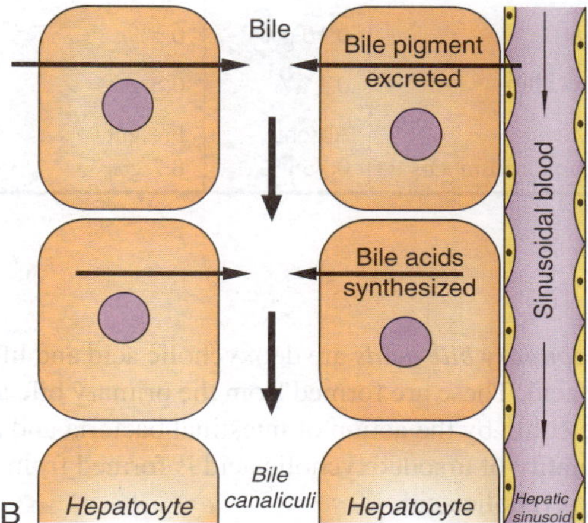

FIGURE 7.4-13 Mechanism of bile formation: **A,** secretion by hepatocytes and ductal cells; and **B,** bile pigments picked up from blood sinusoids are excreted while bile salts are synthesized and secreted by hepatocytes.

- Organic substances are bile salts, bile pigments, cholesterol, lecithin, fatty acids lipid soluble end products of fat metabolism and xenobiotics, phosphatidylcholine, glucose, glutathione, amino acid, urea and enzyme alkaline phosphatase and
- Inorganic substances are Na^+, K^+, Ca^{2+}, HCO_3^- and Cl^-.

Since the bile is concentrated in the gallbladder, so the concentration of its ingredients in the liver bile and gallbladder bile are bound to differ as shown in Table 7.4-2.

Salient features of the some of the ingredients of bile are described here:

1. Bile Salts

Formation of Bile Salts. Bile salts are sodium and potassium salts of bile acids conjugated with either taurine or glycine. Bile acids are of two types: primary and secondary. Steps in the formation of bile salts (Fig. 7.4-14) are:

- ***Primary bile acids*** are cholic acid and chenodeoxycholic acid. These are synthesized by hepatocytes from cholesterol.

TABLE 7.4-2 Liver Bile versus Gallbladder Bile

Properties and composition	Liver bile	Gallbladder bile
• pH	8–8.6	7–7.6
• Specific grav-ity	1010–1011	1026–1032
• Water	97.5%	87.5%
• Solids	2.5%	12.5%
Organic substances		
• Bile salts	1.10 g%	8.0 g%
• Bile pigments	0.20 g%	1.0 g%
• Cholesterol	0.10 g%	0.5 g%
• Fatty acid	0.15 g%	0.5 g%
• Fat	0.10 g%	0 g%
• Lecithin	0.1 g%	0.8 g%
• Mucin	Absent	Present
Inorganic substances	0.75 g%	8.7 g%

- ***Secondary bile acids*** are deoxycholic acid and lithocholic acid. These are formed from the primary bile acids in the colon by the action of intestinal bacteria and a small quantity of ursodeoxycholic acid is formed from chenodeoxycholic acid.
- ***The conjugation of bile acids.*** In the liver, the bile acids are conjugated with either glycine (an amino acid) or taurine (an amino acid derivative) forming the conjugated bile acids.
- The conjugated bile acids namely glycocholic acid and taurocholic acid form bile salts in combination with sodium or potassium.

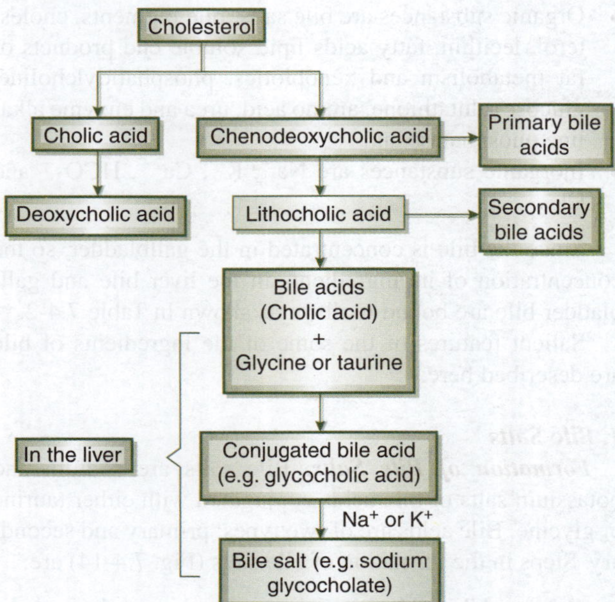

FIGURE 7.4-14 Formation of bile salts from the bile acids.

Functions of Bile Salts Bile salts help in digestion as well as absorption of fat by their following actions:

- ***Emulsification of fat,*** i.e. breaking of large fat drops into smaller droplets and their stabilization is caused by the bile salts because of their power of lowering surface tension. The emulsification is a prerequisite for action of pancreatic lipase, which is water soluble and acts only on the surface of a lipid droplet.
- ***Acceleration of action of pancreatic lipase*** occurs in the presence of bile salts due to binding of colipase for the lipase.
- ***Micelle formation.*** The bile salts combine with the products of hydrolysis of triglycerides to form *small water*=soluble cylindrical disc-shaped particles called micelles, which are transported to the brush border of the epithelial cells for absorption.
- ***Absorption of fat soluble vitamins*** (A, D, E and K) is aided by the bile salts by forming complexes more soluble in water (hydrotropic action).
- ***Choleretic action,*** i.e. they stimulate liver to secrete bile (as long as bile salts are absorbed) and then make more bile salts available for fat digestion.
- ***Cholesterol is kept in soluble form*** in the gallbladder bile by the bile salts. This property of bile salts prevents formation of gall stone.
- ***Intestinal motility*** is stimulated by bile salts. This action of bile salts help in defaecation (laxative action).

Enterohepatic Circulation of Bile Salts Enterohepatic circulation is the recirculation of bile salts from the liver to small intestine and back again. This circulation is necessary because of the *limited pool of bile salts available* to help breakdown and to absorb fat.

Path of Circulation (Fig. 7.4-15). Bile salts travel from the liver to duodenum via the common bile duct.

- When the bile salts reach *terminal ileum,* 90–95% of bile salts are reabsorbed into the portal circulation. It is important to note that no absorption of bile salts occurs in the duodenum and jejunum. The liver then extracts the bile salts from the portal blood and secretes them once again into the bile.
- The remaining 5–10% of bile salts are excreted into the faeces.

Circulating pool. The total circulating pool of bile salts (consisting of salts of primary and secondary bile acids) is approximately 3.6 g. About 4–8 g of bile salts are required (more if the meal is high in fat) for digestion of fats during each meal; thus of the total content of bile salts in the body

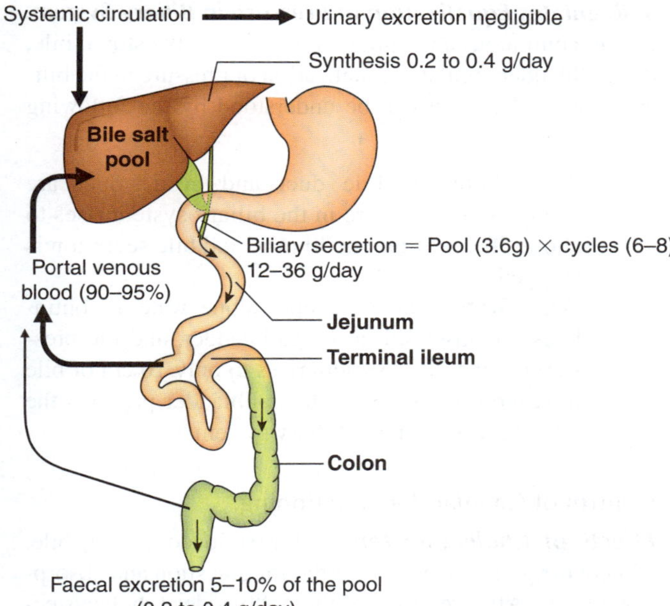

FIGURE 7.4-15 Enterohepatic circulation of bile salts.

(3.6 g), most circulate twice during the digestion of each meal. Consequently, the bile salts usually circulate 6–8 times daily.

Bile salt synthesis and replacement. The rate of bile salt synthesis is determined by the rate of return to liver by enterohepatic circulation. Usually only 0.2–0.4 g (5–10% of 3.6 g) of bile salts are lost in the faeces, which are replaced by synthesis. The maximal synthesis rate can go up to 3–6 g/day. If faecal losses exceed this rate, the total pool size decreases.

Clinical implications of enterohepatic circulation. As bile salts are required for proper digestion and absorption of fats, therefore any condition that disrupts enterohepatic circulation (e.g. ileal resection or small intestinal diseases such as sprue or Crohn's disease) leads to decreased bile salt pool and malabsorption of fat and fat-soluble vitamins. The clinical manifestations of such conditions are:

- Steatorrhoea, i.e. increased fat content in the stools,
- Nutritional deficiency due to malabsorption and
- Watery diarrhoea because the bile salts which inhibit water and sodium absorption from the colon are decreased due to excessive loss in stools.

2. Bile Pigments

- The two principal bile pigments, *bilirubin* and *biliverdin,* are the other major constituents of bile which have no digestive function.
- Bile pigments are metabolites of haemoglobin formed in the liver.
- The hepatic cells extract bilirubin and biliverdin from the blood, conjugate them with glucuronic acid and transfer them into the bile canaliculi by an active transport mechanism (Fig. 7.4-16). They are responsible for the golden yellow colour of bile.
- Intestinal bacteria metabolize bilirubin further to urobilinogen, which is responsible for the brown colour of stools.
- Hepatocellular dysfunction leading to failure of bilirubin passages causes accumulation of bile pigments in the blood producing hepatic or posthepatic jaundice, respectively.

Formation and circulation of bile pigments and jaundice are described on page 153.

3. Phospholipids

- The phospholipids (primarily lecithins) are, after bile salts, the most abundant organic compound in the bile.
- Phospholipids, which are normally insoluble in water, are solubilized by the bile salt micelles.
- Micelles are able to solubilize other lipids more effectively when they are composed of bile salts and phospholipids than when they are composed of bile salts alone.

4. Cholesterol

- Cholesterol is another important constituent of bile that does not have a digestive function. Its presence in the bile seems to be a by-product of bile salt synthesis in the hepatic cells. Normal biliary content of cholesterol is about 100 mg% (60–170 mg%) as compared to 150–240 mg% in blood.

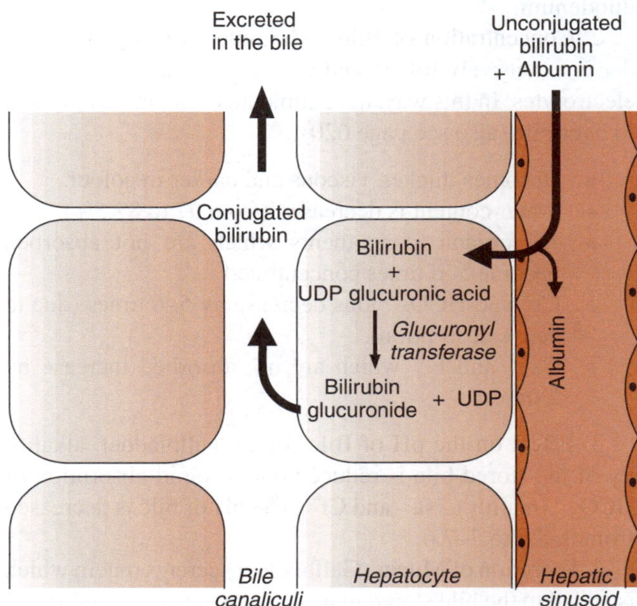

FIGURE 7.4-16 Bile pigment metabolism in the hepatocyte.

- Cholesterol is essentially insoluble in water and thus must be solubilized by bile salt micelles before it can be secreted in the bile.
- Biliary secretion of cholesterol is important because it is one of the few ways in which cholesterol stores can be regulated.
- Biliary cholesterol forms an important component of gallstones (large sand-like particles) found in the gallbladder of some patients.

5. Electrolytes

- Biliary content of inorganic substances is about 0.75 g%.
- The cations Na^+, K^+, and Ca^{2+} are all present in concentration about 20% greater than in the plasma.
- Two major anions are Cl^- and HCO_3^-. Cl^- is present in concentrations lesser than in plasma while HCO_3^- is far greater than in plasma, which makes the bile juice considerably alkaline. Further, HCO_3^- concentration increases with an increased rate of bile secretion. Intravenous administration of acetazolamide (in high doses), decreases HCO_3^- concentration of bile, thereby decreases pH from 8.6 to 7.4.

Functions of Gallbladder

Gallbladder is a thin walled sac-like structure with a storage capacity of about 50 ml. It is not essential for life. Removal of gallbladder (cholecystectomy) in patients suffering from dysfunction of gallbladder does not result in any major disadvantages. Functions of gallbladder are:

1. Storage of Bile. The bile secreted during interdigestive period is stored in the gallbladder. The gallbladder typically stores 30–50 ml of bile. During meals, the gallbladder contracts and releases its contents into the duodenum.

2. Concentration of Bile. The mucosa of the gallbladder is extensively folded and can actively absorb fluid and electrolytes. In this way, the gallbladder bile, in comparison to liver bile (also see page 620).

- Becomes thicker, viscous and darker in colour.
- Water content is decreased (from 97 to 87.5%).
- All organic constituents which are not absorbed become 5–6 times concentrated.
- Cl^- and HCO_3^- ions decrease by 5–6 times (due to active absorption).
- Ca^{2+} and K^+ which are not absorbed increase by 2 times.

3. Effect on the pH of Bile. In the gallbladder, alkalinity of the stored bile is reduced due to rapid absorption of HCO_3^- (mainly), Na^+ and Cl^-. The pH of bile is decreased from 8–8.6 to 7–7.6.

4. Secretion of Mucus. Gallbladder secretes mucin which is added to the bile stored in it. The mucin acts as a lubricant in the intestine for the chyme.

5. Regulates Equalization of Pressure in Biliary System. Due to continuous absorption of water from the stored bile, the gallbladder regulates equalization of pressure in the biliary system. This fact can be understood by the following observations:

- When both the bile duct and cystic duct are clamped, the pressure in the biliary system rises to above 30 cm of bile in 30 min, and bile secretion is stopped.
- When the bile duct is clamped alone, water is continuously reabsorbed in the gallbladder, and the pressure in the biliary system rises to only 10 cm of bile in several hours. Thus, the gallbladder prevents the rise of pressure in the biliary system.

Control of Gallbladder Functioning.

Effects of Cholecystectomy As mentioned earlier, bile, and not the gallbladder is essential for digestion and absorption of fats. After removal of the gallbladder (cholecystectomy), the bile empties slowly but continuously into the intestine, allowing digestion of fats sufficient to maintain good health and nutrition. Only high-fat meals need to be avoided.

- Bile ducts become dilated to accommodate some of the bile which is continuously secreted by liver.

Functions of Bile

Functions subserved by the bile poured into the duodenum are because of its constituents (mainly bile salts), which have already been discussed. However, they are compiled and summarized once again:

1. ***Digestive function.*** Bile salts help in digestion of fats by *emulsifying fat drops* (see page 620).
2. ***Absorptive functions.*** Bile salts help in absorption of fats (by micelle formation) and fat soluble vitamins (see page 620).
3. ***Excretory function.*** Bile pigments are the major excretory products of the bile. The other substances excreted in bile are, heavy metals (e.g. copper and iron), some toxins, some bacteria (e.g. typhoid bacteria), cholesterol, lecithin and alkaline phosphatase.
4. ***Laxative action.*** Bile salts increase the gastrointestinal motility and act as a laxative.
5. ***Protective action.*** Bile is a natural detergent. So, it inhibits the growth of certain bacteria in the lumen of intestine.
6. ***Choleretic action,*** i.e. bile salts stimulate the liver to secrete bile.
7. ***Maintenance of pH of GIT.*** Being highly alkaline the bile juice neutralizes the gastric HCI present in the chyme entering the small intestine. Thus, an optimum pH is maintained for the action of digestive enzymes.

8. ***Prevention of gall stone formation.*** Bile salts keep the cholesterol and lecithin in solution and thus prevent the formation of gallstones. In the absence of bile salts, the cholesterol precipitates along with lecithin and may form gallstones.
9. ***Lubricating function.*** The mucin secreted by gallbladder mucosa into the bile lubricates the chyme in the intestine.
10. ***Cholagogue function.*** Cholagogue is an agent, which increases the release of bile from gallbladder into the intestine. The bile salts perform this function indirectly. The bile salts stimulate the secretion of hormone CCK, which has got the cholagogue action.

Regulation of Bile

The regulation of bile juice released into the duodenum after the meals is performed at two levels:

- Regulation of biliary secretion and
- Regulation of release of bile from the gallbladder.

A. Regulation of Biliary Secretion The secretion of aqueous component (water and electrolytes) and the bile (containing bile salts and other organic substances), though occurring together, are controlled separately by the following mechanisms (Fig. 7.4-17A):

- Regulation of bile-independent fraction of biliary secretion and
- Regulation of bile-dependent fraction of biliary secretion.

1. Regulation of Bile-independent Fraction of Biliary Secretion. The bile-independent fraction of biliary secretion refers to the amount of *fluid containing water and electrolytes*. Secretion of this fraction of the bile juice is (similar to the fluid secreted by ductal cells of pancreas) controlled by secretin and vagal stimulation.

- *Secretin* is a hormone secreted by S-cells of duodenum and jejunum in response to stimulation of acidic chyme (for details see page 612). It acts on the ductal cells of hepatic ducts (Fig. 7.4-17A) via cyclic AMP, second messenger and produces large amounts of watery fluid with high concentration of HCO_3^-.
- *Vagovagal reflex* initiated during intestinal phase of digestion also affects the ductal secretion by potentiating the effects of secretion through the acetylcholine.

Note. The agents (e.g. secretin and acetylcholine), which cause secretion of bile from liver with more amount of water and less amount of solids, are called hydrocholeretics.

2. Regulation of Bile-dependent Fraction of Biliary Secretion. The bile-dependent fraction of biliary secretion refers to the quantity of bile salts secreted by the liver. It depends upon the following factors (Fig. 7.4-17):

- The amount of bile salts secreted by the hepatocytes is directly proportional to the *amount of bile salts*

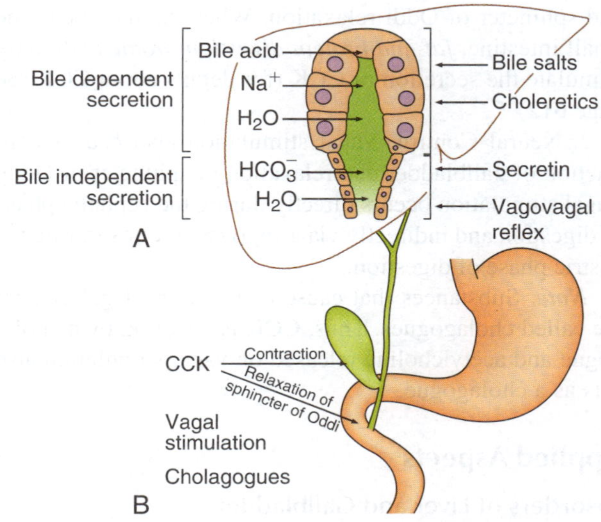

FIGURE 7.4-17 Regulation of bile secretion (A) and release from gallbladder (B).

reabsorbed by them from portal circulation. As the bile salts are recycled in the enterohepatic circulation, they maintain a high level of bile secretion during the digestive period. The secretion of bile increases about 1 h after a meal (when the gastric emptying starts). The maximum rate of bile secretion is achieved 3–5 h after intake of food.
- Synthesis of bile salts in hepatocytes occurs to a limited amount. Bile salts and bile acids are the major agents which enhance synthesis of bile salts. Substances that enhance the secretion of bile salts by the hepatocytes are called choleretics.

Note. Synthesis of bile salts by liver is not controlled by any hormonal or nervous factor.

B. Regulation of Release of Bile Juice from Gallbladder

- ***Filling of gallbladder*** by the bile is simply controlled by a pressure gradient. During the interdigestive period, the sphincter of Oddi remains closed. As bile is secreted continuously, it gets accumulated in the common bile duct (CBD). When pressure of bile in the CBD rises, it forces its way through the cystic duct into the gallbladder. During the interdigestive period, the pressure in the CBD and gallbladder reaches to 7 cm of water.
- ***Emptying of gallbladder.*** When the chyme enters the duodenum, the gallbladder is contracted along with relaxation of sphincter of Oddi, raising the pressure to about 20 cm of water. Because of the increase in pressure, the bile from the gall bladder enters the duodenum. The contraction of gallbladder and relaxation of sphincter of Oddi is regulated by the following factors (Fig. 7.4-17B):

1. Hormonal Control. The hormone *cholecystokinin* (CCK) is the major stimulus for gallbladder contraction

and sphincter of Oddi relaxation. When chyme enters the small intestine, *fat and protein digestion products* directly stimulate the secretion of CCK (for details about CCK see page 612).

2. Neural Control. Vagal stimulation also causes contraction of gallbladder and relaxation of sphincter of Oddi. Vagal stimulation occurs directly during the cephalic phase of digestion and indirectly via a vagovagal reflex during the gastric phase of digestion.

Note. Substances that cause contraction of gallbladder are called cholagogues. Thus, CCK is a well-known cholagogue and acetylcholine released on vagal stimulation also acts as a cholagogue.

Applied Aspects

Disorders of Liver and Gallbladder

Some of the important disorders of gallbladder and liver which need emphasis are mentioned here.

Jaundice or Icterus Jaundice or icterus refers to yellow discolouration of skin and mucous membrane due to raised levels of bilirubin in the blood.

- *Normal values* of serum bilirubin range between 0.3 and 1 mg%,
- *Latent jaundice,* which cannot be detected clinically, occurs when serum bilirubin level is between 1–2 mg%.
- *Jaundice* manifests when serum bilirubin becomes more than 2 mg%.

Types of Jaundice. Jaundice is of three types:

- ***Haemolytic jaundice*** also called as prehepatic jaundice, and occurs due to overproduction of unconjugated bilirubin due to excessive destruction of RBCs owing to any reason.
- ***Hepatocellular jaundice*** occurs due to damage to hepatocytes, as seen in viral hepatitis, cirrhosis and drug-induced hepatitis. In this condition, bilirubin is conjugated but cannot be excreted into the bile by the hepatocytes. So, the conjugated bilirubin returns to the blood, producing jaundice.
- ***Obstructive jaundice,*** also called posthepatic jaundice, occurs due to blockage in bile duct either due to a stone or any growth (e.g. in carcinoma of head of pancreas). The bile cannot be poured into the intestine, so due to back pressure, the biliary ducts and canaliculi are dilated and the bile salts and bile pigment enter the blood producing jaundice.

For further details and differences in the three types of jaundice see page 155.

Cirrhosis of Liver Cirrhosis of liver refers to an irreversible chronic damage to liver with extensive fibrosis and regenerative nodule formation.

Causes. Depending upon the cause, the cirrhosis of liver may be alcoholic, postviral, postnecrotic, biliary, cardiac, metabolic and cirrhosis due to miscellaneous causes.

Clinical features. Loss of functioning of liver tissue may lead to jaundice, oedema, a variety of metabolic disorders, portal hypertension (due to fibrosis and disordered vasculature). Ascites and hepatic encephalopathy result from both hepatocellular insufficiency and portal hypertension.

Viral Hepatitis

Aetiology. Viral hepatitis (inflammation of liver) is caused by hepatitis virus A, B, C, D or E.

Hepatitis A is caused by the hepatitis A virus and spread by faecal-oral route. The infected individual excretes the virus in faecal matter for about 2-3 weeks.

Hepatitis B is more common, and is caused by hepatitis B virus. The sources of hepatitis B infection are: by horizontal (blood) transmission, i.e.

- Injection of unscreened blood products,
- Tattoo/acupuncture needle or
- Sexual.

Clinical features. Patients usually present with history of anorexia, fever, and malaise, followed by yellow discolouration of urine, eyes and skin. Liver may be enlarged, and the patient may have some discomfort in the upper abdomen.

Investigation:

- In *hepatitis A,* presence of antibodies against hepatitis A virus (anti-HAV) is of IgM type. Detection of anti-HAV can be used as a marker for previous HAV infection.
- In *hepatitis B,* presence of Hepatitis B surface antigen is detected on serology. Vertical transmission occurs in 90% of cases, i.e. from hepatitis B surface antigen (HBsAg)-positive mother to child.

Treatment is usually strict bed rest and ingestion of high-carbohydrate diet.

***Hepatitis B** vaccine* prevents occurrence of hepatitis B.

Liver Failure Any cause of liver damage can produce liver failure. Liver failure, though uncommon, is a serious syndrome. Hepatic encephalopathy is the cardinal presentation of acute liver failure. The mental changes start as confusion, but extend to stupor and coma.

- ***Hepatic encephalopathy*** in liver failure occurs due to an increased ammonia level due to defective hepatic ammonia metabolism.

Treatment The treatment of liver failure is primarily to reduce the ammonia load on the liver:

- By increasing amounts of nonabsorbable carbohydrates such as lactulose, which is converted into short-chain fatty acids in the colon, can trap ammonia in its ionized form.
- In severe disease, the only effective treatment is liver transplantation.

Cholecystitis Cholecystitis refers to the inflammation of gallbladder. It is not uncommon, though more common in fatty, fertile females in their forties (4Fs). It is of two types:

- ***Acute cholecystitis.*** Patient usually presents with acute pain in upper abdomen (biliary colic). The triad of symptoms: sudden onset of tenderness in right upper quadrant of abdomen, fever and leucocytosis is highly suggestive of acute cholecystitis.
- ***Chronic cholecystitis*** is almost always associated with gallstones. Patient gets repeated attacks of pain in the abdomen and vomiting.

  Cholecystectomy, i.e. surgical removal of the gallbladder is indicated in patients with continued and recurrent discomfort.

Gallstones (Cholelithiasis)

Gallstone formation is not an uncommon problem.

Two types of gallstones are known:

- ***Cholesterol stones*** account for 80–85% of the cases. These are formed due to precipitation of cholesterol. Normally, cholesterol is present in soluble form due to a proper ratio of cholesterol and bile salts (1:20–1:30). When this ratio falls below 1:13, the cholesterol is precipitated forming many small crystals. This stimulates further formation of crystals, so that the crystals grow larger and larger. In these crystals, bile pigments and calcium also get inspirated forming gallstones. These stones are *radiolucent*, i.e. cannot be visualized on radiograph.
- ***Pigment stones,*** also called *calcium bilirubinate stones* account for 15–20 cases of gallstones. These stones are formed when the conjugated bilirubin in the bile is disconjugated by the action of β-glucuronidase found in certain bacteria. The free bilirubin combines with calcium to form calcium bilirubinate, which is highly insoluble in bile. These stones are radiopaque.

Symptoms. Gallstones may be asymptomatic or may produce symptoms either due to inflammation (biliary colic) or obstruction (obstructive jaundice) following their migration into the cystic or common bile duct. The most specific and characteristic symptom of gallstones is biliary colic.

Treatment of gallstones, when required, is surgical removal of the gallbladder (cholecystectomy).

Liver Function Tests

The liver function tests (LFTs) are the investigations to assess the capacity of the liver to carry out any of the functions it performs. Thus, LFTs help in:

- Assessing the extent of functional damage to the liver,
- Diagnosing the cause of hepatic insufficiency and
- Assessing the progress/regress of the disease.

The major LFTs may be classified as:

I. Tests to assess secretory functions,
II. Tests to assess metabolic functions,
III. Tests to assess synthesis functions,
IV. Tests to assess detoxicating functions,
V. Tests to assess hepatic cellular integrity and
VI. Miscellaneous tests.

I. Tests to Assess Secretory Functions of Liver

1. Serum bilirubin. The normal values are:

- Total serum bilirubin: 0.3–1.0 mg%,
- Conjugated bilirubin: 0.1–0.3 mg% and
- Unconjugated bilirubin: 0.2–0.7 mg%.

Van den Bergh test is specific to identifying the increase in serum bilirubin (above reference level). For procedure, see page 154. The results of the test are interpreted as:

- Normal serum: Negative reaction,
- Haemolytic jaundice: Indirect positive reaction,
- Obstructive jaundice: Direct positive reaction and
- Hepatic jaundice: Biphasic reaction.

2. Urine Bilirubin and Bile Salts. Normally, urine does not contain bilirubin and bile salts. In liver insufficiency, when the serum bilirubin levels increase above 2 mg%, the bilirubin is excreted in the urine (*bilirubinuria*).

3. Urine Urobilinogen. In normal individuals with urine flow of about 1 ml/min, less than 4 mg of urobilinogen is excreted in the urine. In liver insufficiency, initially there occurs a mild increase in the daily excretion of urine urobilinogen. However, in the later stages urobilinogen is absent in the urine. This occurs because of the fact that the swollen liver cells block the bile canaliculi and prevent excretion of conjugated bilirubin in the bile.

4. Faecal Stercobilinogen.

- Normal levels 20–25 mg%.
- Increased initially in liver insufficiency producing dark brown stools.
- Decreased in later stages of liver insufficiency producing pale coloured stools.

5. Faecal Fat Levels.

- Normally, 5–6% of total fat intake per day in excreted in the faeces.
- In liver insufficiency, fat excretion in faeces increases up to 40–50% of total intake (steatorrhoea). This is because of the fact that due to deficiency of bile salts, emulsification and absorption of fat is inadequate in the intestine.

II. Tests to Assess Metabolic Functions of Liver

1. Galactose Tolerance Test. This test is based on the principle that galactose after absorption from the gut gets converted into glycogen in the liver. Therefore, in liver insufficiency its level in the blood rises.

Procedure. In a fasting individual, 40 g galactose is administered orally and blood samples are collected at 30 min intervals for 2 h. From the blood galactose levels in these samples, the galactose index (GI) is calculated. Galactose index (GI) is the sum of the four values of blood galactose levels in mg%. Its normal value is 68–160 mg%. In hepatic insufficiency, GI value is markedly increased.

2. Blood Glucose Level. The normal fasting blood glucose level is 70–90 mg%. In hepatic insufficiency its level decreases.

3. Blood and Urine Amino Acids Levels. Blood and urine amino acids levels are estimated to assess protein metabolism. In liver damage, blood amino acid levels (normal 30–65 mg%) and urine amino acid levels are increased.

4. Lipid Profile. In hepatic insufficiency lipid profile is affected as:

- Plasma NEFA and FFA : Increase (normal 10–30 mg%)
- Serum cholesterol : Decrease (normal 150–240 mg%)
- Serum triglycerides : Decrease (normal 30–150 mg%)
- Serum phospholipids : Decrease (normal 150–300 mg%)
- Total lipids : Decrease (normal 350–800 mg%)
- Ketone bodies : Increase (normal 7–15 mg%)

Abnormalities of serum lipid levels are sensitive but nonspecific indicators.

III. Tests to Assess Synthesis Functions of Liver

1. Estimation of Plasma Proteins

- *Albumin.* Liver cell damage causes hypoalbuminaemia (normal 6.4–8.3 g%).
- *Globulins.* Hyperglobulinaemia is usually associated with hypoalbuminaemia.
- *A:G ratio.* In liver disorder, there occurs reversal of A:G ratio (normal 1.7:1).

2. Serum Levels of Liver Enzymes.

- *Transaminases.* The activity of transaminases like SGPT and SGOT increases in hepatic insufficiency. Serum SGPT levels are increased by 10–1000 times in acute phase (normal value < 40 IU%). Raised levels of SGPT are more specific as it is primarily present in the liver, whereas SGOT is also present in other cells like, red blood cells, skeletal muscle, GIT, brain and kidney.
- *Alkaline phosphatase.* Alkaline phosphatase is not a liver specific enzyme because it arises from bone, intestine and also from the liver and is secreted into the bile. In obstructive jaundice its level is markedly increased (>30 KA units).
- *Gamma glutamyl transferase* is a microsomal enzyme. Raised level of GT is a sensitive index of liver damage.

3. Blood Urea. Liver is the main site for urea formation from ammonia. Decreased levels of blood urea (normal 20–40 mg%) and raised blood ammonia level (normal 20–80 mg%) occur in liver insufficiency.

4. Blood Ammonia. Raised blood ammonia level indicates severe liver disease (hepatic encephalopathy).

5. Urine Ammonia level also increases (normal 350–1200 mg/day).

6. Coagulation Factors. Factors II, V, VII, IX and X and vitamin K needed to activate these factors are synthesized by the liver. The integrity and activity of these factors is determined by prothrombin time test (PTT) (for prothrombin test see page 223). Prolonged prothrombin time (PT) (normal 10–16 s) indicates severe liver disease.

- *Prothrombin time index (PTI).* It is calculated as:

$$\text{PTI} = \frac{\text{Normal prothrombin time (PT)}}{\text{Prothrombin time of patient}} \times 100$$

Normal PTI is 100%. Its value less than 70% is indicative of severe liver damage.

IV. Tests to Assess Detoxication Functions of Liver

1. Bromsulphthalein (BSP) Excretion Test. BSP is taken up by the liver cells from the blood and detoxified and excreted in the bile. The rate of removal of BSP from the blood depends upon the functional efficiency of liver and rate of hepatic blood flow.

Procedure. BSP is injected intravenously (dose 5 mg/kg body weight) and its concentration in blood samples (collected at an interval of 5 and 45 min) is measured.

Assuming BSP concentration as 100% at the beginning, normally its concentration should fall to 85% in the blood sample collected after 5 min and 5% only in the blood sample collected after 45 min. A concentration of > 10% indicates liver insufficiency. Nowadays, this test is used only for diagnosis of Dubin–Johnson syndrome (congenital hyperbilirubinaemia).

2. Hippuric Acid Excretion Test. Sodium benzoate when ingested orally gets conjugated with glycine in the liver and excreted as hippuric acid in the urine.

Normally, when 6 mg of sodium benzoate is ingested orally, about 2.7–3.5 g is excreted in the urine as hippuric acid within 4 h, provided the kidneys are functioning normally. Decreased excretion of hippuric acid occurs in liver damage.

V. Tests to Assess Hepatic Cellular Integrity

1. Ultrasonography is done to detect diffuse disease of parenchyma of the liver (cirrhosis liver, fatty liver), abscess,

cysts, tumours, gallstones and dilatation of biliary system proximal to site of obstruction.

2. Computed Tomography (CT). CT scan has the same diagnostic significance as ultrasonography except that it can also detect even smaller lesions.

3. Radionucleotide Imaging. Technetium (^{99m}Tc) is a sulphur colloid, which is easily taken up by the liver cells monocyte macrophage system (Kupffer cells) and emits γ-rays. Gamma camera picks up these rays and is used to find out the size of the liver and the lesions of the liver (such as filling defect, diffuse liver disease and portal hypertension).

4. Liver Biopsy. This is performed by a special needle passed through intercostal space under local anaesthesia to obtain tissue for histopathological examination.

5. Fine Needle Aspiration (FNA). A very fine needle is usually guided by ultrasound and material is aspirated for cytological, histopathological and bacteriological examination.

6. Cholecystography is done to assess the functions and diseases of the gallbladder. Iodinated compounds given orally are concentrated in the gallbladder and excreted in bile. The gallbladder gets opacified on cholecystography. Therefore, conditions like gallstones and nonfunctioning gallbladder fail to produce opacification. Nowadays, this test is less commonly performed than ultrasonography.

7. Other Elaborate Tests include:

- Percutaneous cholangiography (PTC),
- Portal venography and
- Endoscopic retrograde cholangiography (ERCP).

VI. Miscellaneous Tests

Serological tests to detect hepatitis viruses, antigens and antibodies.

Chapter 7.5

Physiological Activities in Small Intestine

FUNCTIONAL ANATOMY
- Gross anatomical considerations
- Structural characteristics of intestinal wall

SMALL INTESTINAL SECRETIONS
- Composition and formation
- Regulation
- Functions

MOTILITY OF SMALL INTESTINE
- Segmentation contractions
- Peristaltic contractions
- Motility reflexes

FUNCTIONS OF SMALL INTESTINE

APPLIED ASPECTS
- Paralytic ileus
- Intestinal obstruction

FUNCTIONAL ANATOMY

Gross Anatomical Considerations

The small intestine is a convoluted tube that extends from the pylorus to the ileocaecal valve, where it joins with caecum, the first part of large intestine. It is about 6–7 m in length, and its diameter gradually diminishes from its commencement to its termination. It is divided into three parts: the duodenum, the jejunum and the ileum (see Fig. 7.1-1.).

Duodenum. The first and *shortest* part (25 cm long) of the small intestine is also the *widest* and most fixed part. It is C shaped, and for descriptive purposes is divided into four parts: superior (1st) part, descending (2nd) part, horizontal (3rd) part and ascending (4th part). Superior part of duodenum is also called *duodenal cap* or bulb. It is the region which is struck by acidic gastric contents when they pass through pylorus and is a *common site for the peptic ulcer*. The bile and pancreatic ducts open by a common hepatopancreatic ampulla of Vater on the posteromedial wall of descending (2nd) part of duodenum. Ligament of Treitz demarcates the continuation of duodenum with jejunum.

Jejunum and ileum. Jejunum and ileum form respectively, the proximal 2/5th and distal 3/5th of the remaining part of small intestine. There is no sharp demarcation between jejunum and ileum. The inner mucosal surfaces of jejunum and ileum, however, can be differentiated from each other.

Structural Characteristics of Small Intestine

Histologically, the wall of small intestine is made up of four layers, which from within to outwards consist of mucosa, submucosa, muscle coat and serosa (for details see page 572).

Characteristic Features of Mucous Membrane of Small Intestine Characteristic features of mucous membrane of small intestine need special emphasis.

Although the small intestine is about 6 m long, it has an absorptive area of over 250 m^2. This larger surface is created by:

- Numerous folds of the intestinal mucosa *plicae circulars* (Fig. 7.5-1),
- Densely packed villi, which line the entire mucosal surface,
- *Microvilli,* which protrude from the surface of intestinal cells and
- The presence of numerous depressions (crypts of Lieberkuhn) that invade the lamina propria.

Plica Circulares. The mucosal surface shows numerous circular folds (*plicae circulars* or valvulae conniventes), which are absent in the first 2 inches of duodenum but are larger, more numerous and closely set in rest of the duodenum and jejunum, whereas in the upper part of ileum, they are smaller and more widely separated and in the lower part they are absent (Fig. 7.5-1). Unlike the folds in stomach, the plicae circulares are permanent and do not obliterate when intestine is distended. Each fold is made up of all layers of the mucosa (lining epithelium, lamina propria and muscularis mucosa). The submucosa also extends into the fold. The circular folds serve the following functions:

- They increase the surface area for absorption, and also slow down the passage of contents through small intestine, which facilitate absorption.

Villi Villi are finger-like projections of mucous membrane seen throughout the length of small intestine (Fig. 7.5-2).

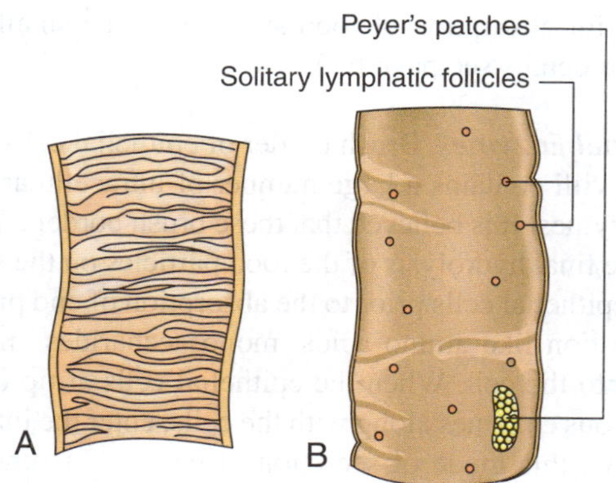

FIGURE 7.5-1 The mucosal surface of jejunum (**A**) and ileum (**B**).

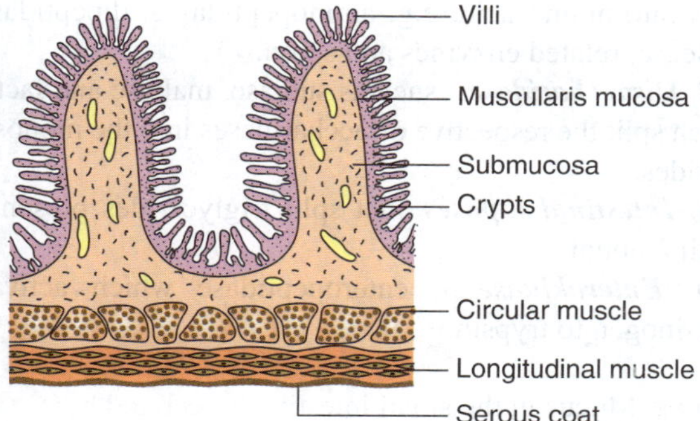

FIGURE 7.5-2 Longitudinal section of small intestine showing plica circulares and villi.

Total number of villi is about 5 million and they are distributed about 20–40 villi per square mm. Each villus is about 0.5–1 mm long.

Structure. Each villus is covered by a single layer of columnar epithelial cells called enterocytes. The core of each villus contains (Fig. 7.5-3):

- An arteriole and venule with their communicating capillary plexus; the venules of the villi, which carry absorbed nutrients that ultimately drain into the portal vein. Blind-ended lymphatic vessel called lacteal which carry the absorbed fats to the thoracic duct, few smooth muscle fibres extending from the muscularis mucosa and
- A fine network of nerves, which has connections with submucosal and myenteric plexus.

Activity. During digestion and absorption, the villi contract quickly with an irregular rhythm and relax slowly. Their muscular fibres serve to pump the lymph from core of villi towards the submucosal lacteals.

The Crypts of Lieberkuhn. The crypts of Lieberkuhn are single tubular intestinal glands that invaginate deep into the lamina propria and are present between the villi throughout the length of small intestine (Fig. 7.5-3). These glands are lined by undifferentiated columnar cells, and also contain goblet cells, argentaffin cells and Paneth cells.

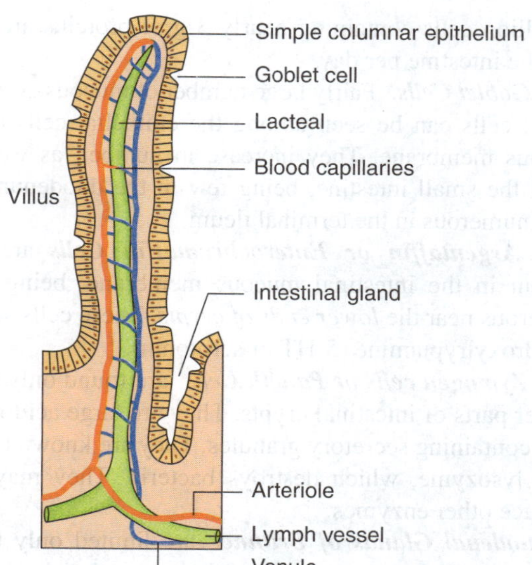

FIGURE 7.5-3 Structure of an intestinal villus, an enterocyte and crypts of Lieberkuhn.

Epithelial Cells of the Mucous Membrane of the Small Intestine and Intestinal Glands The mucous membrane of small intestine is made up of following types of epithelial cells:

1. Absorptive Columnar Cells or the so-called enterocytes are the cells of epithelium which cover the villi, and the areas of the mucosal surface intervening between them. These cells are specialized for absorptive function. The luminal surface of each enterocyte shows small multiple projections of the cell membrane called the *microvilli* or the *brush border* (Fig. 7.5-3), which increase the surface area to some 30-fold. Each enterocyte has about 1000 microvilli. Whole of the system of folds, villi and microvilli combinedly increase the surface area about 600 times as follows: folds (3 times) × villi (10 times) × microvilli (20 times) = 600 times. The surface of each microvillus is covered by a layer of fine fibrils and mucus (glycocalyx).

The lateral surfaces of adjacent enterocytes are joined by *tight junctions.* Enzymes *capable of breaking down* small peptides and disaccharides are associated with microvilli of the absorptive columnar epithelial cells.

2. Undifferentiated Columnar Cells line the crypts of Lieberkuhn. They are similar to absorptive cells, but their microvilli are not as developed and their cytoplasm contains secretory granules. The cells of the lower parts of the crypts *proliferate actively* by mitosis. The newly formed cells migrate upwards from the crypt to reach the walls of villi. Here they differentiate into typical absorptive cells, or into goblet cells. These cells migrate towards the tips of villi, from where they are *shed off in the lumen* of the intestine. Thus, the epithelial lining of the small intestine is being replaced constantly. The *total cycle of cell migration,* from the bases of crypts to the tips of villi and then shedding off, takes about up to 5 days only. In this way, about

17 billion cells containing nearly 3 g of proteins are shed into the intestine per day.

3. Goblet Cells. Fairly large number of mucous-secreting goblet cells can be seen among the epithelial cells of the mucous membrane. They increase in number, as we pass down the small intestine, being few in the duodenum and most numerous in the terminal ileum.

4. Argentaffin or Enterochromaffin Cells are also present in the intestinal mucous membrane, being most numerous near the *lower ends of crypts*. These cells secrete 5-hydroxytryptamine (5-HT or serotonin).

5. Zymogen cells or Paneth Cells are found only in the deeper parts of intestinal crypts. They are large acidophilic cells containing secretory granules. They are known to produce lysozyme, which destroys bacteria. They may also produce other enzymes.

Duodenal Glands of Brunner are limited only to the duodenum. These are compound tubulo-alveolar glands present in submucosa of duodenum. Their ducts pass through the muscularis mucosa to open into the crypts of Lieberkuhn. They are situated mostly near the pylorus; beyond pylorus their number greatly diminishes and they disappear at the junction of duodenum and jejunum. Secretions of these glands contain *mucus and* HCO_3^-, which neutralizes gastric acid entering the duodenum and thus protects its mucosa.

SMALL INTESTINAL SECRETIONS

Composition and Formation

The intestinal juice, also called succus entericus, comprises the intestinal secretions which include:

- Aqueous component (water and electrolytes),
- Intestinal enzymes and
- Mucus.

Aqueous Component of Intestinal Juice Aqueous component of intestinal juice primarily refers to water and electrolytes secreted by the epithelial cells of small intestine, especially those present in the crypts of Lieberkuhn. About 2 L of secretion is produced per day by these cells, whose chemical composition is almost similar to the extracellular fluid, except that it is slightly more alkaline (pH 7.5–8.6). This fluid is colourless; however, it becomes slightly cloudy due to admixture of mucus, shed epithelial cells and cholesterol.

Mechanism of formation. There is an active secretion of chloride and bicarbonate ions into the crypts, which causes electrical force leading to diffusion of sodium ions. All these ions cause osmotic movement of water. Thus, there is marked secretion of watery fluid without enzymes.

Functions. The watery secretion provides a solvent into which the products of digestion are dissolved. This fluid is rapidly reabsorbed by the intestinal villi. Thus, circulation of this fluid from the crypts to the villi supplies a watery vehicle for absorption of food stuffs from the small intestine. For details see page 645.

Intestinal Enzymes Brush border of epithelial cells covering the villi contains a large number of intracellular digestive enzymes. It is believed that these brush border enzymes produce final hydrolysis of the food particles on the surface of the epithelial cells prior to the absorption of end products of digestion like amino acids, monosaccharides and fatty acids into the cell. When the epithelial cells at tip of villi, the various enzymes along with the cells, enter the intestinal secretion, this mode of secretion of enzymes is known as *holocrine mode of secretion*. The enzymes which have been identified in the brush border are:

1. Peptidases (proteolytic enzymes) which digest peptides into amino acid, e.g. aminopeptidases, dipeptidases, nuclease, related enzymes and so on.

2. Disaccharidases such as sucrase, maltase and lactase which split the respective disaccharidases into the monosaccharides.

3. Intestinal Lipases that split triglycerides present in small amount.

4. Enterokinase or enteropeptidase which activates trypsinogen to trypsin.

Mucus Mucus in the small intestine is secreted by:

1. Brunner's Glands, which are located in the duodenum, secrete thick, alkaline mucoid secretion that serves a protective role, preventing HCl and chyme from damaging the duodenal mucosa.

2. Goblet Cells, located along the length of the intestinal epithelium and in the intestinal crypts of Lieberkuhn, secrete lot of mucus which protects the intestinal mucosa and lubricates the chyme.

Regulation of Small Intestinal Secretions

1. Local Stimuli. Local mechanical and chemical stimuli to the intestinal mucosa form the most important means of regulation of intestinal secretions. Mechanical distension of intestinal mucosa by the food or irritation by chemicals, via local myenteric reflexes, increases the volume and total enzyme output of the small intestine; that is why, the greater is the chyme, greater is the secretion of intestinal secretion.

2. Role of Vasoactive Intestinal Polypeptide (VIP). Though the secretion of the crypts of Lieberkuhn is mainly regulated by the local stimuli, but the local hormone VIP is also reported to increase its secretion.

3. Secretion of Brunner's Gland is increased by:

- Vagus stimulation,
- Direct tactile stimulation or irritation of the duodenal mucosa and
- Secretin.

Functions of Intestinal Juice

See functions of small intestine (page 635).

MOTILITY OF SMALL INTESTINE

Motility of small intestine can be described as:

A. *Motility of the small intestine during interdigestive period*, which includes:
- Migrating motor complexes (MMC),

B. *Motility of the small intestine during digestive period* (related to meals), which includes:
- Mixing movements such as segmentation contractions and pendular movements,
- Propulsive movements such as peristaltic contractions and peristaltic rush and
- Movements of villi.

C. *Motility reflexes*, which include:
- Peristaltic reflex,
- Gastroileal reflex and
- Intestino-intestinal reflex.

Motility of Small Intestine during Interdigestive Period

Migrating Motor Complexes

- The migrating motor complex (MMC) is the name given to the peristaltic wave that begins in the oesophagus and travels through the entire gastrointestinal tract during the interdigestive period.
- The MMCs sweep out the chyme remaining in the small intestine.
- The MMCs occur every 60–90 min and last for about 10 min.
- For further details about MMCs, see page 598.

Motility of Small Intestine during Digestive Period

1. Mixing Movements The mixing movements of small intestine are responsible for proper mixing of chyme with digestive juices like pancreatic juice, bile juice and intestinal juice. The mixing movements of small intestine include:

- Segmentation contractions and
- Pendular movements.

i. Segmentation Contractions Features:

- Segmentation is the most common type of intestinal contractions, which occurs throughout the digestive period in a rhythmic fashion, and hence also called *rhythmic segmentation contractions*.
- During segmentation contraction, a section of the small intestine (about 2–5 cm) contracts, sending the intestinal contents (chyme) in both oral and caudal directions. That section of the small intestine then relaxes, and the contents move back into the segment. At the same time, the adjoining segment which was relaxed, now contracts (Fig. 7.5-4A).
- The alternate contracted and relaxed segments give a ring-like appearance resembling the chain of sausages (Fig. 7.5-4B).

Function. These back-and-forth movements of chyme, produced by segmentation contractions, cause thorough mixing without any net forward movement of chyme (Fig. 7.5-4A).

- The segmentation contractions slow down the transit time in the small intestine and thus increase the contact time with the absorption surfaces of the intestinal mucosa.
- The higher frequency of segmentation in the proximal intestine (duodenum) than in the distal intestine (ileum) also propels the chyme slowly towards the colon.

Rate and duration. Segmentation contractions occur about 12 times/min in the duodenum and 8 times/min in the ileum. The contractions last for 5–6 s.

Types. Two types of segmentation contractions have been described:

- ***Eccentric contractions.*** They consist of contractions located in a localized segment less than 2 cm in length, and are eccentric in appearance. They are mainly due to contraction of outer longitudinal smooth muscle layer.

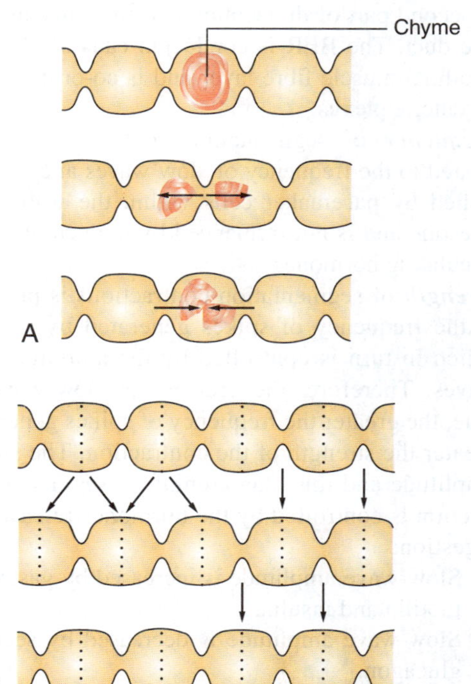

FIGURE 7.5-4 Segmentation contraction of small intestine: **A,** steps of segmentation are shown to reveal back and forth movements of chyme; **B,** the alternate contracted and relaxed segments give a ring-like appearance resembling the chain of sausages.

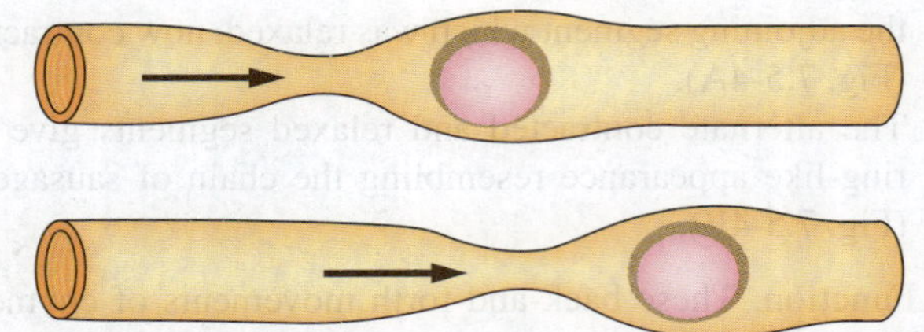

FIGURE 7.5-5 Peristaltic contraction moves the food through intestine by pushing bolus ahead of muscle contraction.

- ***Concentric contractions.*** The segments are usually longer than 2 cm and are of relatively uniform circumference. They are mainly due to contraction of inner circular smooth muscle layer.
- ***Tonic contractions*** are variants of segmentation contractions, which last somewhat longer, isolating one segment of the intestine from another for quite some time.

Control

- ***Initiation.*** Segmentation contractions can occur only if the slow waves (basal electrical rhythm, i.e. BER) produce spikes, or action potentials. Spikes appear on the slow waves when the membrane potential is sufficiently depolarized. The slow waves (BER) are initiated by the pacemaker cells (interstitial cells of Cajal) which are stellate mesenchymal cells having long branched processes reaching up to intestinal smooth muscles located in second part of duodenum near the entry of common bile duct. The BER is conducted caudally by the longitudinal muscle fibre layer and is co-ordinated by the myenteric plexus.
- ***Frequency*** of segmentation contractions is directly related to the frequency of slow waves and is thus controlled by pacemaker cells within the walls of small intestine and is not influenced by the neural activity or circulating hormones.
- ***Strength*** of segmentation contractions is proportional to the frequency of spikes generated by slow waves which in turn is controlled by the amplitude of slow waves. Therefore, the greater the slow-wave amplitude, the greater the frequency of spikes generated, the greater the strength of the contraction. The slow-wave amplitude and thus the strength of segmentation contraction is controlled by the hormones released during digestion:
  - Slow-wave amplitude is increased by gastrin, CCK, motilin and insulin.
  - Slow-wave amplitude is decreased by secretin and glucagon.

ii. Pendular Movements. These are small constrictive waves which sweep forward and backward or upward and downward in pendular fashion. These mixing movements can be noticed only by close observation.

2. Propulsive Movements The propulsive movements of small intestine are involved in pushing the chyme towards the aboral end of intestine. These include:

- Peristaltic contractions and
- Peristaltic rush.

i. Peristaltic Contractions.

Characteristic Features. Peristalsis refers to a wave of contraction preceded by wave of relaxation. Ideally, in the small intestine, peristalsis is superimposed over the segmentation contractions after digestion and absorption have taken place.

- The peristaltic contractions are highly coordinated, and typically, a peristaltic contraction involves contraction of a segment behind the bolus, and simultaneous relaxation of the segment in front of the bolus, causing the chyme to be propelled caudally (Fig. 7.5-5).
- A peristaltic contraction consists of deep circular ring of contraction, which passes down the intestine at a rate of 0.5–2 cm/s. Each contraction travels for a variable but short distance and then dies out. A new contraction is then initiated from a site little distal to the site of origin of the previous contraction. In this way, a continuous peristaltic wave is set up in the intestine. Several of these wave-like contractions occur simultaneously along the length of the intestine, resulting in vermiform movements (worm-like movements). That is why they are called vermicular or peristaltic movements.
- Along with the peristaltic movements, the chyme moves at a rate of about 1 cm/min. Thus, the net movement of chyme in anal direction is very slow and it takes about 3–5 h for the chyme to move from the pylorus to the ileocaecal valve.

Law of Intestine. As a matter of fact, the peristaltic contraction travels from the point of stimulation in both directions. But under normal conditions, the progress of contraction in an oral direction is inhibited quickly and the contraction disappears. Only the contraction that travels in the aboral direction persists. In this way, the peristaltic waves always travel from the oral end towards the aboral end of the intestine. This phenomenon has been labelled as the *Law of the intestine*, by Starling in 1901. The other names which have been given to this phenomenon are: 'Polarity of intestine' 'Polar conduction of intestine', 'Electrical activity of intestine', 'Law of gut' and 'Theory of receptive relaxation'.

- ***Proof.*** The law of intestine can be proved experimentally. When a piece of gut is resected, and the resected segments are resutured in the same position, the peristaltic wave passes easily over the resected segment (Fig. 7.5-6B). But if the resected segment is resutured in the reverse position, the peristalsis stops at the beginning of the reversely sutured segment, proving the law of intestine.

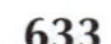

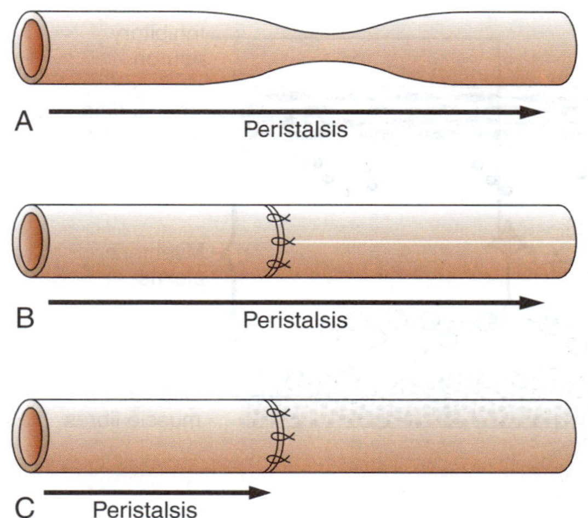

FIGURE 7.5-6 Experiment to prove 'Law of intestine': **A,** normal peristaltic movements of a segment of small intestine; **B,** normal peristalsis continues when a part of small intestine is cut and sutured in the same position; and **C,** when the resected segment is sutured in reverse position the peristalsis stops at proximal sutured end.

- ***Explanation.*** The law of intestine has been attributed to the *descending* rate of rhythmicity of BER from duodenum (12/min) towards ileum (9/min).

Functions. subserved by peristaltic waves are:

- Help to propel the intestinal contents aborally.
- Also help in digestion and absorption of the food particles, because different types of nutrients are digested and absorbed in different segments of the small intestine.

Control of Peristaltic Contractions. *Initiation*. The coordinated peristaltic activity is dependent on the integrity of enteric nerve plexus. The usual stimulus for peristalsis is distension. When the wall of intestine is stretched, the wave of peristalsis is initiated which passes along the intestine towards the rectum at a rate of 2–2.5 cm/s. This response to stretch is called *myenteric reflex*. The local stretch releases serotonin, which activates sensory neurons that stimulate the myenteric plexus. Activity of the myenteric plexus from a stimulus point travels in either direction to activate neurons that release (Fig. 7.5-7):

- *Acetylcholine and substance P* above the point of stimulus, producing a circular constriction and
- *Nitric oxide, VIP and ATP* below the point of stimulus producing receptive relaxation.

a. *Neural control.* Though the peristaltic contractions can occur in the absence of extrinsic innervation, but their magnitude is affected by neural influences (Fig. 7.5-8).
  - *Parasympathetic stimulation* increases intestinal motility through vagus as seen during strong emotions.
  - *Sympathetic stimulation* decreases intestinal movements as seen during anger and pain.

b. *Hormonal control.* Certain hormones also affect the magnitude of peristaltic contraction:
  - Intestinal motility is enhanced by gastrin, CCK, 5-HT, thyroxine and insulin.
  - Intestinal motility is decreased by secretin and glucagon.

ii. Peristaltic Rush

- Peristaltic rush refers to a very powerful peristaltic contraction which occurs when intestinal mucosa is irritated intensely as in some infectious processes.
- It is partly initiated by extrinsic nervous reflex and partly by myenteric reflex.
- This type of powerful contraction begins in duodenum and passes through the entire length of small intestine, and finally reaches the ileocaecal valve within few minutes. Thus, they sweep the contents of the intestine into the colon, thereby relieving the small intestine of irritant or excessive distension, as it occurs in cases of diarrhoea.

3. Movements of Villi

As the smooth muscle fibres of the intestinal wall extend into the villi, movements of villi also occur during the movements of small intestine.

Features. Movements of villi consist of alternate shortening and elongation of the villi caused by contraction and relaxation of the muscle.

Functions. Movements of villi help in emptying lymph from the central lacteal into the lymphatic system. The surface area of villi is increased during elongation. This helps in the absorption of digested foodstuffs from the lumen of intestine.

Initiation. Local nervous reflexes, which occur in response to the presence of chyme in small intestine, initiate the movements of villi. *Villikinin,* a hormone secreted from small intestinal mucosa, is also believed to play an important role in increasing the movements of villi.

Motility Reflexes

1. Gastroileal Reflex

- Gastroileal reflex refers to a marked increase in the peristaltic contractions of ileum associated with relaxation of ileocaecal sphincter which occur immediately after the meals. As a result, the intestinal contents are delivered to the large intestine.
- This reflex is initiated by the distension of stomach by the food.
- The peristaltic contractions are caused by reflex stimulation of vagus and the relaxation of ileocaecal sphincter seems to be produced by the hormone gastrin.

2. Intestino-Intestinal Reflex Intestino-intestinal reflex refers to relaxation of smooth muscles of rest of the small intestine in response to overdistension of one segment of the intestine.

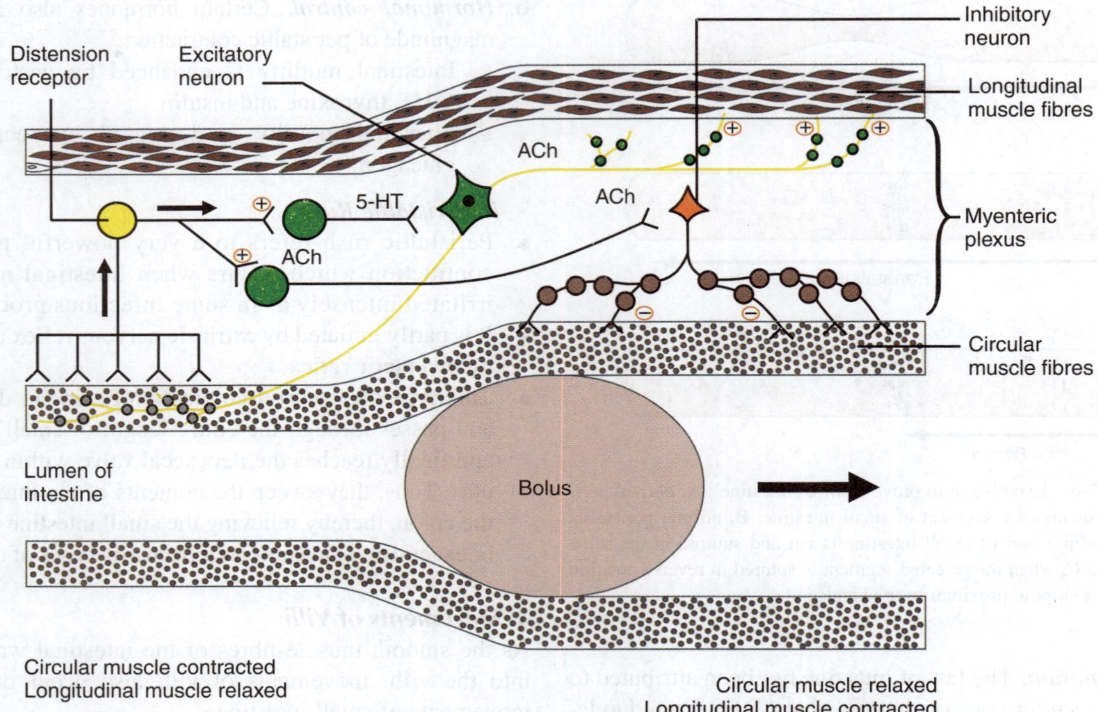

FIGURE 7.5-7 The postulated connection in the myenteric plexus to co-ordinate the peristaltic contraction. (+) indicates an excitatory synapse, (−) an inhibitory synapse; ACh = acetylcholine; 5-HT = 5-hydroxytryptamine.

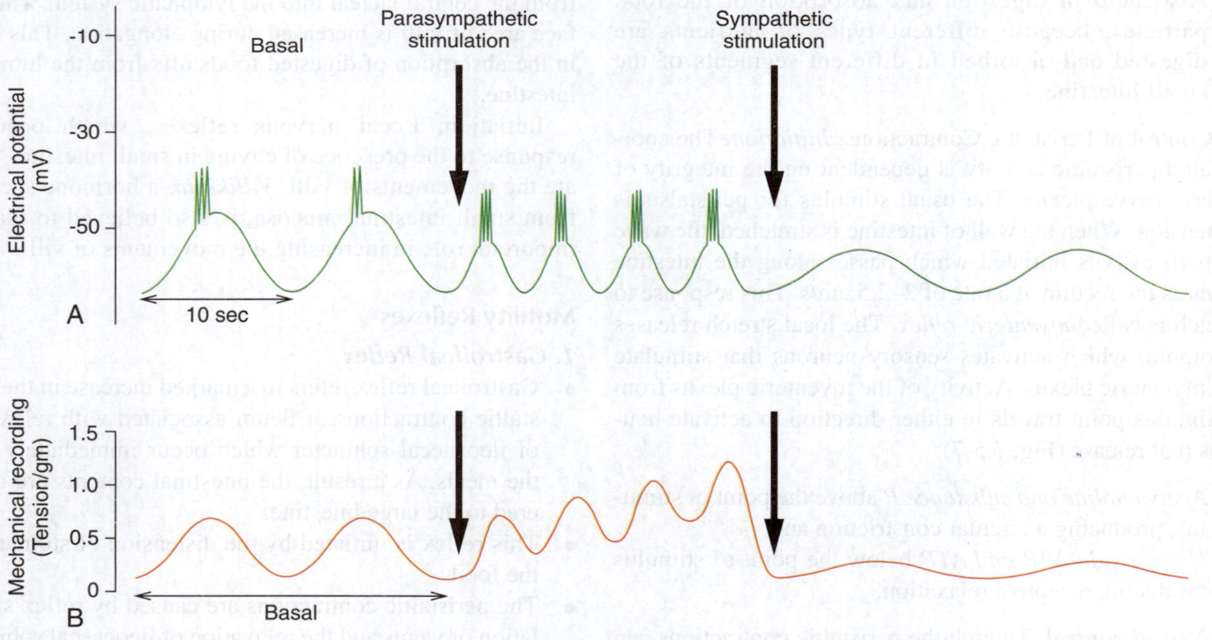

FIGURE 7.5-8 Effect of parasympathetic stimulation and sympathetic stimulation on membrane potential (A) and mechanical activity (B) of small intestine.

FUNCTIONS OF SMALL INTESTINE

After going through the physiology of intestinal secretion and intestinal motility, the functions of small intestine can be summarized as:

1. Mechanical Functions. The mixing and propulsive movements of the small intestine help in thorough mixing of chyme with the digestive juices (pancreatic juice, bile juice and succus entericus), and propel it towards the large intestine.

2. Digestive Functions of small intestine are carried out by the digestive enzymes present in the succus entericus (see page 630), pancreatic enzymes (see page 609) and bile (see page 619).

3. Absorptive Function is accomplished by the huge surface area created by the presence of plicae circulares, villi and microvilli. The end products of digestion of carbohydrates, proteins and fats are absorbed through portal system or through the lymph. For details of absorption, see page 645.

4. Hormonal Functions. The small intestine secretes certain hormones that exert their effect on the secretions and motility of gastrointestinal tract. These hormones include *enterogastrone, secretin* (page 612) and *cholecystokinin* (page 612).

5. Activator Function. The enzyme enterokinase secreted by small intestine activates trypsinogen into trypsin, which in turn activates other enzymes.

6. Protective Function. The mucus secreted into the succus entericus protects the intestinal wall from the gastric acid chyme.

7. Hydrolytic Function. The aqueous component of the succus entericus provides water, and thus helps in all the hydrolytic processes of enzymatic reactions of digestion of various food particles.

APPLIED ASPECTS

Paralytic Ileus Paralytic ileus or the adynamic ileus refers to a condition in which the intestinal motility is markedly decreased leading to retention of its contents (because the contents cannot be propelled into the colon). This produces irregular distension of the small intestine by pockets of gas and fluid.

Causes. Paralytic ileus may occur due to:

1. *Direct inhibition of smooth muscles of small intestine* due to handling of intestine:
   - During intra-abdominal operations and
   - During trauma.
2. *Reflex inhibition of smooth muscles of small intestine* due to increased discharge of noradrenergic fibres in splanchnic nerves, as seen in irritation of peritoneum (in patients with peritonitis and injury to peritoneum).

Treatment. Paralytic ileus can be treated by aspiration of fluid and gas by introducing a tube through nares up to the small intestine.

- The occurrence of paralytic ileus can be reduced by using laproscopic surgery.
- Postsurgical, early ambulation also enhances intestinal motility.
- Use of specific opioid antagonists is also helpful in relieving this condition.

Intestinal Obstruction

Causes. Obstruction of the lumen of small intestine may occur due to many causes, such as tumours, strictures and fibrotic bands in the abdomen.

Features. The intestinal obstruction is characterized by:

- ***Intestinal colic,*** i.e. severe abdominal pain. Pain is caused by peristaltic rush (intense peristaltic wave initiated due to irritation of intestinal mucosa at the site of obstruction).
- ***Distension of small intestine*** with pockets of fluid and gas occur proximal to the site of obstruction.
- ***Local ischaemia*** of intestinal wall may occur due to increased intraluminal pressure.
- ***Stimulation of visceral afferent*** nerves by the increased intraluminal pressure may cause sweating, hypotension and severe vomiting.
- ***When the obstruction is in the upper half of small intestine,*** the antiperistaltic reflux causes intestinal juices to flow into the stomach, and these juices are vomited along with the secretions of stomach. The person becomes severely dehydrated, but the loss of acids and bases may be approximately equal, so that little change occurs in acid–base balance.
- ***When the obstruction is near the lower end of the small intestine,*** it is possible to vomit more basic than acidic substances; in this case, acidosis may result. In addition, after a few days of obstruction, the vomitus becomes faecal in character.

Chapter 7.6

Physiological Activities in Large Intestine

FUNCTIONAL ANATOMY

Gross Anatomical Considerations

Functional Organization The large intestine is a tube about 6 cm in diameter and 100 cm in length. It normally arches around and encloses the coils of small intestine and tends to be more fixed than the small intestine. It is divided into the following parts (Fig. 7.6-1):

- ***Caecum*** is a blind-ended sac into which opens the lower end of ileum. The ileocaecal junction is guarded by the ileocaecal valve which allows inflow but prevents backflow of intestinal contents.
- ***Appendix*** is worm-shaped tube that arises from the medial side of caecum which in humans is a vestigial organ.
- ***Ascending colon*** extends upward from the caecum along the right side of abdomen up to the liver. On reaching the liver, it bends to the left, forming the right hepatic flexure.
- ***Transverse colon*** extends from the right hepatic flexure to the left splenic flexure. It forms a wide U-shaped curve.
- ***Descending colon*** extends from the left splenic flexure to the pelvic inlet below.
- ***Sigmoid colon*** begins at the pelvic inlet as continuation of the descending colon and joins the rectum in front of the sacrum.
- ***Rectum*** descends in front of the sacrum to leave the pelvis by piercing the pelvic floor. Here it becomes continuous with anal canal in the perineum.
- ***Anal canal*** opens to the exterior through the anus, the opening which is guarded by two sphincters.

Ileocaecal Valve

Structure. Ileocaecal valve functioning occurs due to invagination of ileum into the caecum at the ileocaecal junction and a very small ileal opening (only 2–3 mm in diameter).

Functions. The principal function of the ileocaecal valve is to prevent back flow of the faecal matter from the caecum into ileum. The valvular mechanism works in such a way that when the caecal pressure is increased, the ileocaecal opening is closed.

Role of Ileocaecal Sphincter. Ileocaecal sphincter refers to thickened band of circular muscle coat of the terminal part of ileum just above the ileocaecal junction. The rhythmic contractions of ileocaecal sphincter leading to rhythmic opening and closing occur after every 30 s after a meal. During every rhythmic opening, a small jet of ileal fluid (approximately 15 ml) escapes into the caecum. The ileocaecal sphincter slows down the emptying of ileal contents into the caecum and thus helps in completion of the absorption of nutrients in the ileum.

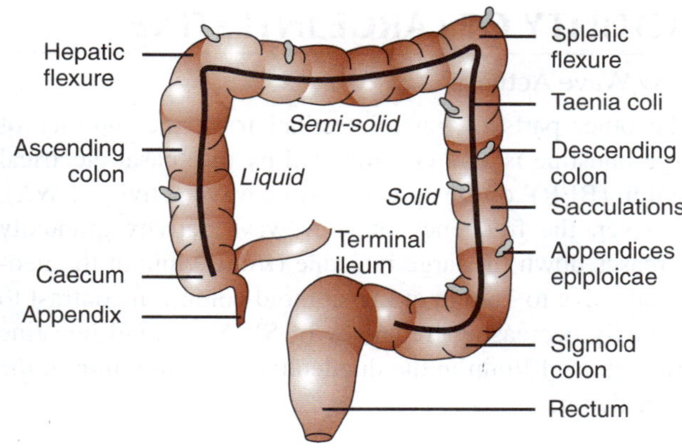

FIGURE 7.6-1 Functional organization of the large intestine and consistency of faecal contents in its different segments.

Control. Gastrin produces relaxation and secretin causes contraction of ileocaecal sphincter. It is important to note that these hormones show opposite effects on cardiac sphincter.

Structural Characteristics

Histological structure of large intestines is similar to that described in general (see page 572) with the following special characteristics. Mucosa of large intestine is characterized by:

- Absence of plica circulares and villi (seen in small intestine).
- It is thrown into folds opposite to the contractions seen in wall of large intestine which produce sacculations.
- A large number of simple tubular glands (crypts of Lieberkuhn) lined by simple columnar epithelial cells with large number of goblet cells which secrete mucus are the histological characteristics of mucosa of large intestine (Fig. 7.6-2). Epithelial cells contain no enzyme.

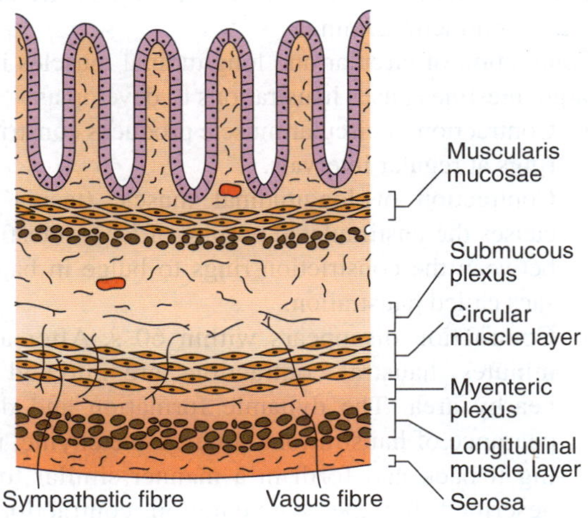

FIGURE 7.6-2 Histological structure of the colon.

- The epithelium overlying solitary lymphatic follicles (in ascending colon, caecum and appendix) contains M-cells similar to those seen in small intestine.

Longitudinal Layer of Muscle Coat of colon is Unusual

- Most of the fibres in it are collected to form three thick bands, the *Taenia coli* which can be seen through the serous layer (Fig. 7.6-1). A thin layer of longitudinal fibres is present in the intestines between the taenia.
- The taenia coli are shorter in length than other layers of the wall of colon. This results in the production of *sacculations* (also called *haustrations*) on the wall of colon.

Serous layer is missing over the posterior aspect of the ascending and descending colon. At places, small peritoneal bags of fat, called *appendices epiploicae,* project from the colonic serosa.

LARGE INTESTINAL SECRETIONS AND BACTERIAL ACTIVITY

Large Intestinal Secretions

- The large intestinal secretions mainly comprise mucus secreted by the goblet cells which are in abundance among the epithelial cells of mucosa and some water, and lot of HCO_3^- are secreted by glands of Lieberkuhn.
- The mucus lubricates the faecal matter and also protects the mucous membrane of large intestine by preventing the damage caused by mechanical injury or chemical substances.
- The alkaline nature (pH 8.0) of the mucoid secretions of the large intestine is due to the presence of HCO_3^-. It serves to neutralize the acids formed by bacterial action on the faecal matter.
- Large quantities of water and electrolytes are secreted by mucosa of large intestine only when it is intensely irritated.

Intestinal Bacterial Activity

Bacterial Flora. At birth, the colon is sterile, but the colonic bacterial flora becomes established early in life and includes:

- *Harmless bacteria* such as *Escherichia coli* and *Enterobacter aerogenes*; and
- *Potentially dangerous bacteria* such as *Bacteroides fragilis*, various types of cocci and gas gangrene bacilli. These bacteria can cause serious disease in tissues outside the colon.

Intestinal Bacterial Activities can be grouped as:

- Beneficial bacterial activities,
- Indifferent bacterial activities and
- Detrimental bacterial activities.

Beneficial bacterial activities include:

- *Synthesis of vitamins* such as vitamin C, a number of B-complex vitamins and folic acid.
- *Trophic effects on colonic mucosa*. Unabsorbed carbohydrates are converted to short-chain fatty acids by colonic bacteria. Some of the short-chain fatty acids produced have a trophic effect on colonic mucosa.
- *Play a role in cholesterol metabolism* by decreasing plasma cholesterol and LDL levels.

Indifferent bacterial activities include:

- *Production of intestinal gases*. The colonic bacteria produce gas in large volumes up to 7–10 L/day, which contribute towards flatus. The gas is produced chiefly through breakdown of undigested nutrients that reach the colon. The gases produced by colonic bacteria include carbon dioxide (CO_2), hydrogen sulphide (H_2S), hydrogen (H_2) and methane (CH_4) which contribute to flatus. Nitrogen gas (N_2) derived from the swallowed air accounts for most of the flatus passed through rectum, or other gases diffuse readily through the intestinal mucosa. Therefore, the volume of flatus expelled is reduced to about 600 ml/day.
- *Organic acids* formed by the colonic bacteria from the carbohydrates are responsible for the slight acidic reaction of the stools (pH 5–7).
- *Substances responsible for odour of the faeces* such as indole, skatole and mercaptans are synthesized by colonic bacteria.
- *Potentially toxic amines* like histamine and tyramine are synthesized by some colonic bacteria. These substances were earlier thought to produce 'auto-intoxication' in constipated patients, but are now known to be harmless.
- *Pigments formed* by the colonic bacteria from the bile pigments are responsible for the known colour of stools.

Detrimental bacterial activities include:

- *Consumption of nutrients* like vitamin C, vitamin B_{12} and choline by some bacteria may lead to deficiency symptoms, unless these are supplemented in adequate amounts in the diet.
- *Production of ammonia*. Colonic bacteria also produce ammonia, which is absorbed by blood and is normally detoxified quickly by the liver. However, in liver dysfunction, hyperammonaemia results, producing neurological symptoms (hepatic encephalopathy); osmotic cathartic such as lactulose is useful in the treatment of such a condition, by its following actions:
  - Reduces the colonic load of ammonia-forming proteins, and also
  - Acidifies the colonic contents and promotes the growth of bacteria that form ammonia.

MOTILITY OF LARGE INTESTINE

Slow Wave Activity

Like other parts of gastrointestinal tract, the motility of large intestine is also co-ordinated by the 'basal electrical rhythm (BER)' or the so-called slow wave activity (SWA). However, the frequency of slow wave activity gradually increases down the large intestine (from 9/min at the ileo-caecal valve to 16/min at the sigmoid colon), in contrast to gradually decreasing frequency of SWA in small intestine (from about 12/min in the duodenum to about 9/min in the lower ileum).

Movements of Large Intestine

Functions The principal functions of colon are absorption of water and electrolytes from the chyme and storage of faecal matter until it can be expelled. The proximal half of the colon is concerned principally with absorption, and the distal half is concerned with storage. The contractile activity of the large intestine serves two main functions:

- It increases the efficiency of colon for water and electrolyte absorption, and
- Promotes the excretion of the faecal matter remaining in the colon.

Types of Movements The movements of colon have been studied by different methods and have been differently classified. The different types of movements (most accepted nomenclature) of colon are:

1. Haustral Shuttling

- The haustral shuttling or haustral contractions are similar to the segmentation contractions of small intestine, which vigorously mix the contents of colon by exposing more of the contents to mucosa (facilitate absorption). During haustral contractions, the pressure rises to about 10–16 mmHg in distal colon, and their frequency is 2–3 contractions/min.
- Contraction of circular and longitudinal muscles in the large intestine causes haustrations to develop as:
  - Contraction of circular muscle produces constriction rings at regular intervals.
  - Contraction of longitudinal muscle (taenia coli) causes the unstimulated portion of large intestine in between the constriction rings to bulge in bag-like sacs called haustration.
  - Contraction disappears within 60 s. After a few minutes, haustral contractions are initiated in a nearby area. The dynamic formation and disappearance of haustrations squeeze the chyme, moving it back and forth in a manner similar to that described for the segmentation contractions in small intestine.

Functions. The haustral contractions perform two main functions:

- *Mixing*. Haustral contractions dig into and roll over the faecal material in the large intestine. In this way, all the faecal material is gradually exposed to the surface of the large intestine, and fluid and dissolved substances are progressively absorbed.
- *Propulsion*. Haustral contractions at times move slowly towards the anus during the period of contraction and thereby provide forward propulsion of the colonic contents.

2. Peristalsis. Peristalsis is a progressive contractile wave preceded by a wave of relaxation. In the colon, the peristaltic waves are very small pressure waves of prolonged duration.

Function. They propel the contents towards the rectum very slowly (5 cm/h). It can take up to 48 h for the chyme to traverse the colon.

3. Mass Movements

- The mass movements are special type of peristaltic contractions which are observed in the colon only.
- These occur 3–4 times a day, generally after meals and each contraction lasts for about 3 min.
- A mass movement is characterized by appearance of a constriction ring at a distended or irritated point in the colon followed by a simultaneous contraction of the smooth muscle as a unit over large confluent areas distal to the constriction.
- The mass movements force the faecal material rapidly in mass down the colon. These powerful peristaltic movements empty about <20 cm segment of the colon. They also move material into the rectum, and rectal distension initiates the defaecation reflex.
- A mass movement can be initiated by:
  - Gastrocolic or duodenocolic reflexes,
  - Intense stimulation of the parasympathetic nerves or
  - Overdistension of a segment of colon.

Gastrocolic Reflex Gastrocolic reflex refers to contraction of colon induced by entry of food into the stomach. This reflex results in an urge to defaecate after a meal. Because of this, defaecation after meals is a rule in children. However in adults, the bowel training suppresses this reflex.

Initiation. It has been reported that perhaps this reflex consists of two phases:

- ***The early or rapid phase*** (which occurs within 10 min of meals) is initiated by distension of stomach and is conducted through the extrinsic nerves of autonomic nervous system. It can be abolished by anticholinergic drugs.
- ***The late or slow phase*** is considered to be mediated by gastrointestinal hormones like gastrin and cholecystokinin (CCK) which are secreted into the bloodstream in significant amounts shortly after a meal.

Transit Time in the Gut The transit time in various parts of the gut studied after a test meal is:

- Up to *caecum* – 4 h,
- Up to *hepatic flexure* – 6 h,
- Up to *splenic flexure* – 8 or 9 h,
- Up to *pelvic colon* – 12 h,
- From *pelvic colon to anus,* transport is made slower, and as much as a quarter (25%) of the residue of a test meal may still be in the rectum for up to 3 days.
- Complete expulsion of the meal in stool takes more than a week. It has been observed that when beads of three different colours are consumed on three consecutive days (e.g. red on first day, green on 2nd day and blue on 3rd day), beads of all the three colours are found in the stool from the 4th day onward and complete expulsion occurs after a week of the consumption. It indicates that there is a pool probably in the caecum and sigmoid colon, where residues get mixed.
- It has been observed that a high residue diet passes more rapidly through the entire gut. This is mainly because of its effect on the colonic movements, as addition of fibres to the diet is actually reported to decrease the rate of flow through the jejunum.

Note. Recent advances have made it possible to study the transit time, pressure fluctuations and changes in pH in the gastrointestinal tract by monitoring the progress of a small pill that contains sensors and a miniature radio transmitter.

DEFAECATION

Functional Anatomy

A brief description of functional anatomy of the anal sphincters which play most important role in the process of defaecation needs special emphasis.

1. Internal or Involuntary Anal Sphincter consists of thickened circular smooth muscles at the pelvic–rectal flexure. This sphincter relaxes reflexly in response to stimulation of stretch receptors when the rectum is distended.

Innervation of internal anal sphincter is by:

- *Parasympathetic* pelvic splanchnic nerves which are inhibitory, and
- *Sympathetic nerves* which are excitatory.

2. External or Voluntary anal Sphincter consists of somatic skeletal muscle fibres innervated by the pudendal nerves. *Characteristic features* are:

- It is maintained in a state of tonic contraction.
- Mild to moderate distension of the rectum increases its force of contraction.
- Moderately severe distension of rectum initiates a reflex which inhibits the discharge of somatic pudendal nerves

(which cause tonic contraction) and thus relaxes the internal anal sphincter.

- The external anal sphincter can be voluntarily relaxed, the action which aids the reflex emptying of the distended rectum.

The Act of Defaecation

Defaecation, the process of excretion of faecal material, involves both voluntary and reflex activity:

- Reflex contraction of smooth muscles of the distal colon and rectum which propel the faecal matter in anal canal.
- Reflex relaxation of internal anal sphincter.
- Reflex relaxation with voluntary control of external anal sphincter and voluntary contraction of abdominal muscles. The events associated with process of defaecation proceed as follows:

Distension of Rectum. Usually the rectum is empty. This is because the frequency of contractions is greater in the rectum than in the sigmoid colon, which causes retrograde movement of faecal material (because of this movement, material placed into the rectum, such as suppository, is pushed up into the colon).

Usually, once or twice a day, the gastrocolic reflex drives the faeces into the rectum which increases the intrarectal pressure passively (Fig. 7.6-3AI, II).

Defaecation Reflexes. As the rectum starts filling, the resultant rise in the intrarectal pressure stimulates the stretch receptors, sets up defaecation reflexes and produces an urge to defaecate (when intrarectal pressure increases to about 18 mmHg). The voluntary external anal sphincter which normally remains tonically contracted further contracts when there is moderate rise in the rectal pressure (Fig. 7.6-3CI–III).

Intrinsic Reflex. It is mediated by intrinsic nerve plexus. Distension of rectum with faeces initiates afferent signals that spread through the myenteric plexus:

- Initiates peristaltic waves in the descending colon, sigmoid colon and rectum causing the active contraction of smooth muscles and further raising intrarectal pressure thus forcing the faeces towards the anus (Fig. 7.6-3AIII, IV).
- Relaxation of internal anal sphincter occurs by inhibitory signals from the myenteric plexus, when the peristaltic wave approaches the anus (Fig. 7.6-3B).

The intrinsic defaecation reflex functioning by itself is relatively weak. To be effective in causing defaecation, this reflex usually must be fortified by a spinal cord reflex.

Spinal Cord Reflex. Distension of rectum by faeces causes transmission of afferent impulses through the pelvic nerves to sacral segments of spinal cord. This induces reflex parasympathetic discharge in nerviergentis (mainly from S_2–S_4) and the pelvic splanchnic nerves (Fig. 7.6-4) to cause:

- Intensification of colonic peristaltic contraction further raising the intra-rectal pressure (Fig. 7.6-3AV),
- When the rectal pressure reaches to about 55 mmHg, there occurs further relaxation of internal anal sphincter (Fig. 7.6-3BV) and external sphincter as well (Fig. 7.6-3CV).

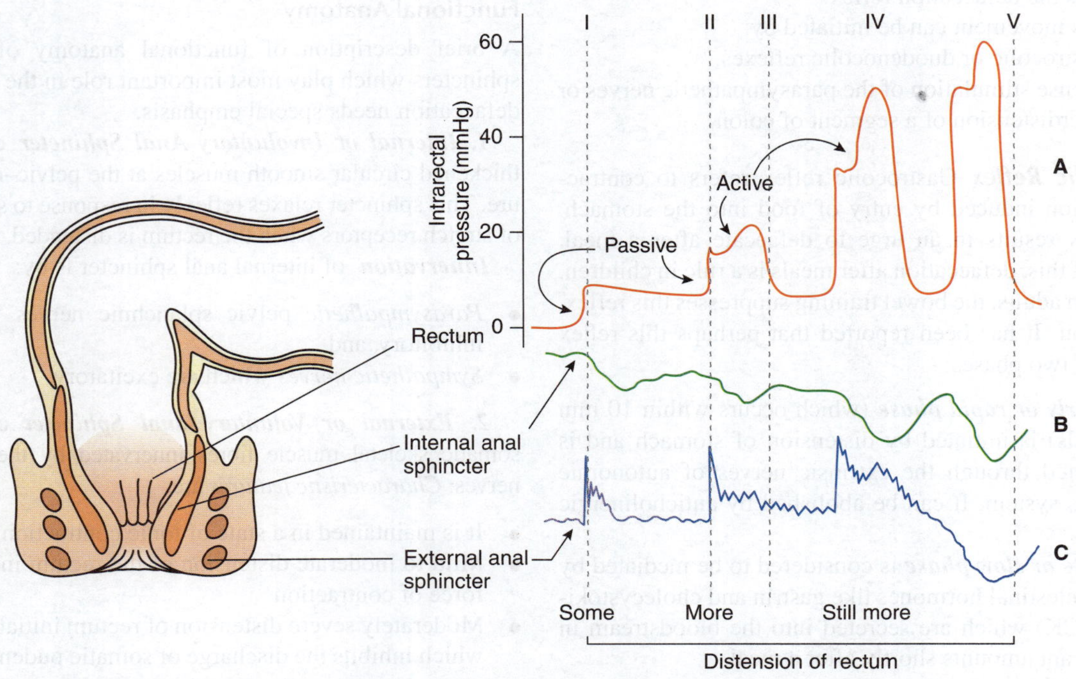

FIGURE 7.6-3 Changes in: A, intrarectal pressure; B, tone of internal anal sphincter; and C, tone of external anal sphincter during distension of rectum by the faeces.

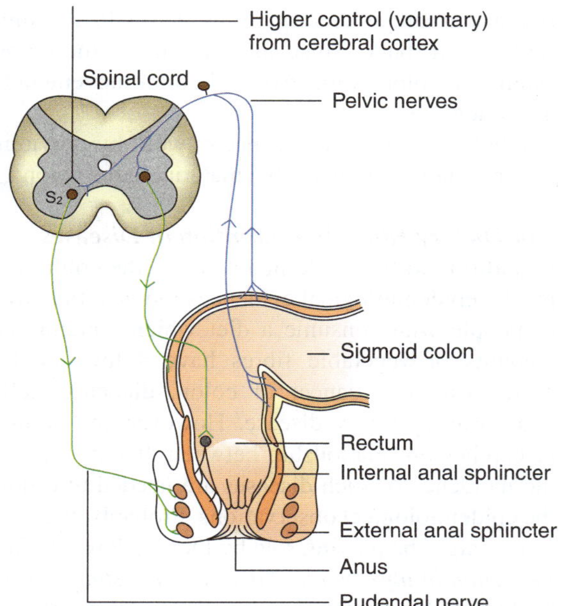

FIGURE 7.6-4 Pathway of spinal defaecation reflex and its voluntary control.

Role of Voluntary Control on Defaecation. Once the above described reflex effects are obtained, the voluntary control mechanism depending upon the convenience may or may not allow the act of defaecation to occur:

When Defaecation is Not Allowed, the voluntary control mechanism maintains the contraction of external anal sphincter, which is composed of skeletal muscle innervated by the pudendal nerves (also see page 639). Soon, the internal anal sphincter also closes, and the rectum relaxes to accommodate the faecal matter within it. Once the defaecation reflex dies out, it recurs after some hours.

When it is Convenient to Defaecate:

- The external anal sphincter is relaxed voluntarily. Thus, both internal and external sphincters are relaxed.
- The intra-abdominal pressure is increased by contraction of abdominal and diaphragmatic muscles (a process of expiring against closed glottis, i.e. Valsalva manoeuvre).
- Normally, the defecation is inhibited because of a 90° angle between rectum and anus (anorectal angle) and contraction of puborectalis muscle. Straining causes contraction of abdominal muscles and lowers the pelvic floor by 1–3 cm, and relaxation of puborectalis. The anorectal angle is also reduced to 15° or less. The combined effect of straining and relaxation of internal and external anal sphincters causes defecation.
- The smooth muscles of the distal colon and rectum contract forcibly, propelling the faecal matter out of the body through the anal canal.

Voluntary Initiation of Defaecation. As per convenience, before the pressure that relaxes the external anal sphincter is reached (i.e. below 55 mmHg but above 18 mmHg), the defaecation can be voluntarily initiated. This is done by voluntarily relaxing the external sphincter and contracting the abdominal muscles (straining), thus aiding the reflex emptying of distended rectum.

Applied Aspects of Defaecation

Defaecation in Infants. In infants, defaecation reflex causes automatic emptying of lower bowel without normal voluntary control on external anal sphincter. The voluntary control of the reflex by higher centres is attained by social training as the child grows.

Defaecation in Individuals with Spinal Cord Injury, Transection. In individuals with spinal cord transection, initially there occurs retention of faeces. But defaecation reflex returns quickly. However, reflex evacuation occurs automatically, without voluntary control, when the rectal pressure increases to about 55 mmHg.

When spinal cord injury occurs between conusmedullaris and brain (lower spinal cord injury), the defecation reflex remains intact, but voluntary control is blocked. In these patients, enema is usually given in the morning shortly after meals to excite defecation reflex.

Role of Dietary Fibres. Dietary fibres increase bulk of faeces, this plays a role in defaecation reflex by distending the rectum (for details see page 640).

Faeces

Composition. Faeces or the faecal matter is derived mainly from the intestinal secretion and partly from the undigested material. If vegetables and coarsely ground cereals are excluded from the diet, faeces have a fairly uniform composition. The faecal matter consists of *water,* forms the main bulk of faeces (75%), and *solids,* contribute 25% to total faecal matter weight. These include inorganic material, mostly calcium and phosphate, undigested plant fibres, epithelial cells, dead bacteria, constituents of intestinal secretions including bile pigments, fats and proteins. It is important to note that:

- *Proteins* in the stools are not of dietary origin but come from bacteria and cellular debris.
- Some of the *fats* in the stools come from the dietary intake but most of them are also derived from desquamated epithelial cells and from bacterial synthesis. On an average, for a fat intake of 100 g/day, 5–6 g/day is normally lost in faeces. Stool fat content is increased in steatorrhoea.
- Since a large fraction of the faecal matter is of nondietary origin, faeces during starvation though decreased in bulk but differ little in composition from those of normally fed persons.

pH of Stools is slightly acidic (5–7) due to the organic acids formed from carbohydrates by colonic bacteria.

Brown Colour of stools is due to the pigment *urobilin* which is formed from oxidation of urobilinogen which is colourless. Urobilinogen is formed from bile pigments by the intestinal bacteria. Oxidation of residual urobilinogen in the stools accounts for the darkening of faeces which occurs upon standing in the air. When the bile fails to enter the intestine, stools become white (*acholic stools*), as seen in obstructive jaundice.

Odour of Stools is due to the presence of substances like indole, skatole, mercaptans and hydrogen sulphide. These substances are formed by the action of colonic bacteria on the food.

FUNCTIONS OF LARGE INTESTINE

After going through the physiology of large intestine secretion and motility, the functions of large intestine can be summarized as:

1. Secretory Functions. The large intestinal secretion mainly comprises mucin which helps to lubricate the faecal matter. The alkaline nature (pH 8) of the secretion serves to neutralize the acids formed by bacterial action on the faecal matter.

2. Synthesis Functions. The bacterial flora of the large intestine synthesizes folic acid, vitamin B_{12} and vitamin K.

3. Absorptive Functions. Absorption of water and electrolytes is the chief function of proximal part of the colon. Organic substances like glucose, alcohol and some drugs like anaesthetic agents, sedatives and steroids can also be absorbed in large intestine. Vitamin K and a number of B complex vitamins which are synthesized in colon by bacterial flora are also absorbed in the large intestine.

4. Excretory Functions. Heavy metals like mercury, lead, bismuth and arsenic are excreted by large intestine through the faeces.

5. Storage Function. After the absorption of nutrients, water and other substances, the unwanted substances form faeces. The faeces are stored in pelvic colon until they can be expelled by the process of defaecation.

APPLIED ASPECTS

Role of Dietary Fibres

Physiological Role of Dietary Fibres on Intestinal Food Transit. Dietary fibres constitute the cellulose, hemicellulose and lignin components of the vegetable products in diet.

- In humans, there is no appreciable digestion of the dietary fibres at all. The ingested dietary fibres reach the large intestine in an essentially unchanged state and thus add bulk to the faeces and play a role in defaecation reflex by distending the rectum.
- If the amount of dietary fibres is small, the diet is said to lack bulk. Since the material in the colon is small, the colon is inactive and colon movements are infrequent.
- The bulk laxatives such as pectin work by providing a larger volume of indigestible material to the colon.

Role of Dietary Fibres in Prevention of Diseases

- In addition to their role in activating the colon movements, epidemiological evidences indicate that groups of people who consume a diet which contains large amounts of vegetable fibres have a low incidence of diverticulitis, cancer of colon, diabetes mellitus and coronary artery disease. However, the definitive researches on relationship between dietary fibres and the incidence of such diseases are needed to establish the epidemiological observations. Probably, the dietary fibres might be playing role by their following effects:
- *Reduction in absorption of digested foodstuffs* is caused by dietary fibres by forming a mechanical barrier between the nutrients and absorptive surface. Due to this effect, the dietary fibres reduce chances of postprandial hyperglycaemia and are thus especially useful in diabetics.
- *Reduction in blood cholesterol level* by dietary fibres is caused by increasing excretion of bile salts in faeces as summarized:

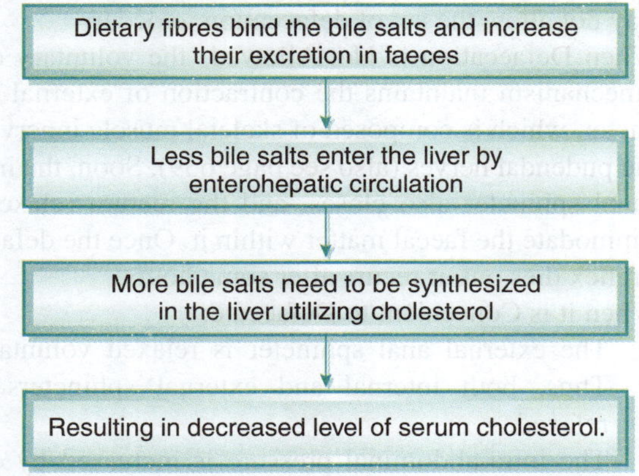

Dietary fibres bind the bile salts and increase their excretion in faeces
Less bile salts enter the liver by enterohepatic circulation
More bile salts need to be synthesized in the liver utilizing cholesterol
Resulting in decreased level of serum cholesterol.

Therefore, dietary fibres are especially useful in patients with atherosclerosis, obesity, hypercholesterolaemia and diabetes mellitus.

- *Prevention of colonic cancers* by dietary fibres is caused by their following effects:
  - Dilution of carcinogens by the water held in them.
  - Reduction of duration of contact between carcinogens and mucous membrane of colon, as they decrease the intestinal transit time.
  - Excretion of carcinogen which get bound to dietary fibres.

Therapeutic Role of Dietary Fibres. The daily recommended intake of dietary fibres is about 25–35 g/day.

High-fibre supplements have therapeutic role in following conditions:

- ***In constipation,*** the dietary fibres work as bulk laxatives by providing a larger volume of indigestible material to the colon. *Plantagolanata* or isabgol-rich in hemicellulose is being used since ages as ancient Indian medicine for constipation.
- ***In spastic colon and diverticular disease,*** the dietary fibres are useful by making the stools softer and thus lowering the intraluminal pressure.
- ***In diabetes and high cholesterol levels,*** the role of dietary fibres have already been discussed.
- ***In diarrhoea, complete avoidance of dietary fibres*** is useful by increasing the transit time, decreasing the frequency and volume of stools.

Precautions for Consuming Fibre Supplements

- ***Should be taken at least 2 h before meals,*** to avoid impairment in absorption of iron and calcium from the diet.
- ***Should not be taken at bed time,*** to avoid the risk of reflux and aspiration.
- ***Should be avoided in disorder of oesophageal motility*** as the smaller dietary fibres can make a solid mass inside the oesophagus called bezoar.

Disorders of Large Intestine Motility

1. Hirschsprung's Disease Hirschsprung's disease, or the aganglionic megacolon, occurs due to congenital absence of the ganglion cells in the myentric as well as submucous plexus (as a result of failure of migration of neural crest cells during development). For normal migration of neural crest cells, endothelins which act on B endothelin receptors are necessary. Recently, it has been postulated that mutation of gene expressing B endothelin receptor is responsible for this disease.

This disease leads to blockage of both the peristalsis and mass contractions at the aganglionic segment. Therefore, the faeces pass the aganglionic segment with difficulty and accumulate in the large intestine leading to dilatation of the colon (megacolon). The affected neonate presents as an emergency and needs to be treated surgically by cutting the aganglionic portion of pelvic–rectal junction and anastomosing the cut ends.

2. Constipation Constipation refers to failure of voiding of faeces which produces discomfort. It results from infrequent mass movement in the colon. As a result, the faecal matter remains in the colon for longer time, so large amount of fluid is absorbed and the faeces become hard and dry.

Aetiopathogenesis. Constipation, most of the time, results from irregular bowel habit. If the sensation of fullness of rectum (i.e. urge to defaecate) is repeatedly ignored voluntarily, over the time there occurs adaptation. Progressively, increasing weakness of the defaecation reflex results in problematic constipation, which is a fairly common problem.

Constipation also occurs due to imbalance between secretion and absorption in the colon.

Symptoms. Persons suffering from constipation may develop anorexia, nausea and abdominal distension and discomfort. Patients may have headache, restlessness and irritability. Symptoms of constipation are not due to absorption of any toxic substances from the colon, as they are quickly relieved with evacuation of rectum.

Treatment. Addition of dietary fibres (which are neither digested nor absorbed) in the meals, adds to the bulk of faeces which helps in initiating the colonic peristalsis by distending the colon. Bulk laxatives may be used. In severe cases, even finger evacuation of the rectum may be needed.

Lubiprostone is used to relieve constipation. It acts by enhancing chloride secretion and water into the colon, resulting in increased fluidity of colonic contents.

3. Diarrhoea Diarrhoea is a condition which is characterized by increased frequency of defaecation with increased water content of the faeces. It may develop in number of bacterial, protozoal and viral infections of the intestinal tract, food poisoning, ulcerative colitis, etc.

Enteritis (inflammation of intestinal tract) is usually caused by viral or bacterial infection. The mucosa gets irritated resulting in increased rate of secretions. At the same time, there is several fold increase in motility of the gut.

Cholera is a severe secretory diarrhoea caused by cholera bacillus which usually occurs in epidemics.

- ***Pathogenesis:*** Cholera bacillus stays in the gut lumen but produces a toxin that binds to receptors (GM-1 ganglioside receptors) present on the apical membrane of enterocytes, leading to entry of toxins into the enterocytes. The cholera toxin increases cyclic AMP concentration by activation of adenyl cyclase which stimulates excessive secretion of electrolytes and reduces NaCl absorption by reducing mucosal transport for Na^+.

  Thus, increase in intestinal water and electrolyte contents causes diarrhoea leading to about 20 L stool volume/day.
- ***Treatment:*** The main physiological basis is replacement therapy to prevent dehydration by infusing fluid intravenously.

  In cholera, however, Na^+–K^+ ATPase and Na^+–glucose transporter are unaffected; therefore, oral administration of solution containing NaCl and glucose is useful in diarrhoea. Oral rehydration solution (prepacked mixture of sugar, salt) dissolved in water is effective to reduce mortality in epidemic of cholera.

Ulcerative Colitis. In this condition, there is inflammation of large intestine leading to ulcerations. The exact cause of ulcerative colitis is not known, but may be allergic or immune response. The irritation of the ulcerative colitis causes increased motility which is so great that mass movements occur and colon secretions are greatly increased.

Psychogenic Diarrhoea accompanies nervous tension and anxiety (such as during examination). This type of diarrhoea, also called psychogenic diarrhoea, occurs due to excessive stimulation of parasympathetic system causing increased motility and mucous secretion in distal colon.

Complications. Severe diarrhoea may cause dehydration, hypovolaemia and electrolyte imbalance due to marked loss of water, Na^+, K^+, HCO_3^- in the stools. There may occur shock, cardiovascular collapse and even death (especially in infants).

Treatment. Treatment consists of maintenance of water and electrolyte balance by oral rehydration therapy (ORT), which is life-saving. In very serious cases, intravenous administration of fluids is required.

Chapter 7.7

Digestion and Absorption

DIGESTION AND ABSORPTION OF CARBOHYDRATES

Dietary Carbohydrates

Dietary intake of carbohydrates is 250–850 g/day, which represents 50–60% of the diet. Major carbohydrates in the human diet are present in the following forms:

1. Polysaccharides. Polysaccharides are made up of many monosaccharides, may be up to a million. These may be present in the following forms:

- *Starch* is the carbohydrate reserve of plants. It consists of two polysaccharide components:
  - Amylose (15–20%). It is a water-soluble straight-chain polysaccharide and
  - Amylopectin (80–85%). It is a water insoluble branched-chain polysaccharide.
- *Glycogen*. It is available in nonvegetarian diet and so often referred to as animal starch. In it, glucose molecules are mostly long chains (1:4 α-linkages and 1:6 αlinkages) at branching points.
- *Cellulose* is another plant polysaccharide, which is present in diet in large amounts. But, there is no enzyme in the human GIT to digest it, so it is excreted.

2. Oligosaccharides. Undigested oligosaccharide contains 2–10 monosaccharide molecules which are liberated on hydrolysis. Based on the number of monosaccharide units present, oligosaccharides are further subdivided into di-, tri-, tetra- and pentasaccharide.

Disaccharides include:

- Sucrose (glucose + fructose) is also known as table sugar (cane or beet sugar).
- Lactose (glucose + galactose) is also called milk sugar.
- Maltose (glucose + glucose). It is a product of starch hydrolysis. It is present in germinating seeds.

3. Monosaccharides. Monosaccharides consumed mostly in human diet are *hexoses* such as:

- Glucose (in fruits, vegetables and honey) and
- Fructose in fruits.

Pentoses do not occur in free form, but are found in nucleic acid and in certain polysaccharides such as pentosans of fruits and gums.

Other carbohydrates that may be present in the human diet are alcohol, lactic acid, pyruvic acid, pectin, dextrin and minor quantities of carbohydrate derivatives in the meat.

Digestion of Carbohydrates

The digestion of carbohydrates begins in mouth, continues in stomach but occurs mainly (almost all) in the small intestine.

Digestion of Carbohydrates in the Mouth. Initial starch digestion starts in the mouth by the enzyme α-amylase (ptyalin) present in the saliva. However, the role of salivary amylase in the digestion of carbohydrates is limited by the short duration of stay of the food in the mouth.

α-*Amylase* present in the saliva acts on the 1-4 linkages (but not on 1-6 linkages). It digests cooked starch to maltose (see page 584):

Digestion of Carbohydrates in the Stomach In the stomach, there occurs minimal carbohydrates digestive activity:

α-Amylase (which enters the stomach with food) activity continues in the stomach for 20–30 min till the highly acidic gastric juice mixes with the food and makes it inactive. The optimum pH for the action of salivary amylase is 6–7, and its activity in the stomach completely stops when pH falls below 4.

The HCl of the gastric juice may hydrolyse some sucrose.

Digestion of Carbohydrates in the Small Intestine In the small intestine, the carbohydrates are digested by the amylolytic enzymes present in the pancreatic juice and brush border enzymes of small intestine.

Pancreatic α-amylase is present in the pancreatic juice which is poured into the duodenum. Its actions on the carbohydrates are similar to that of salivary amylase, but it is much powerful and so it acts on boiled as well as unboiled starch and variety of other carbohydrates except cellulose. It hydrolyses almost all the starch within 15–30 min of the entry of chyme into the duodenum. Its action occurs before the chyme passes beyond the duodenum or upper jejunum.

Pancreatic amylase acts in an alkaline medium and its digestive activity is increased by the presence of bile salts. It converts the starch (polysaccharides) into oligosaccharides such as maltose, maltotriose and dextrin (Fig. 7.7-1).

$$\underset{\text{(e.g. starch and glycogen)}}{\text{Polysaccharides}} \xrightarrow{\text{Pancreatic amylase}} \underset{\text{(e.g. maltose, dextrin etc.)}}{\text{Oligosaccharides}}$$

Brush Border Enzymes of Small Intestine. The carbohydrate-splitting brush border enzymes of small intestine include *dextrinase, maltase, sucrase* and *lactase*. It is believed that these brush border enzymes digest the oligosaccharides into monosaccharides on the surface of epithelial cells of villi as below:

- ***α-Limiting dextrinase.*** It is the only enzyme in GIT which attacks 1,6 α−glycoside linkage, at the branching points of α-limit dextrins. It also attacks 1,4 α-glycoside linkages, resulting in sequential removal of glucose monomers from the dextrins (the breakdown products of starch by the enzyme amylase).

$$\text{Dextrin} \xrightarrow{\alpha\text{-limiting dextrinase}} \text{Glucose}$$

- ***Maltase, sucrase and lactase*** hydrolyse the corresponding disaccharides into monosaccharides as given below:

$$\text{Maltose} \xrightarrow{\text{Maltase}} \text{Glucose}$$
$$\text{Sucrose} \xrightarrow{\text{Sucrose}} \text{Glucose} + \text{Fructose}$$
$$\text{Lactose} \xrightarrow{\text{Lactase}} \text{Glucose} + \text{Galactose}$$

End Products of Carbohydrate Digestion

- The carbohydrate digestion is completed in the small intestine (mainly in jejunum and proximal ileum).
- The end products of carbohydrates are monosaccharides such as glucose, fructose and galactose. Glucose represents 80% and galactose and fructose combinedly represent only 20% of the end products.
- A little amount of other monosaccharide called pentoses are the end products of digestion of nucleic acids and partial digestion of pentosans.

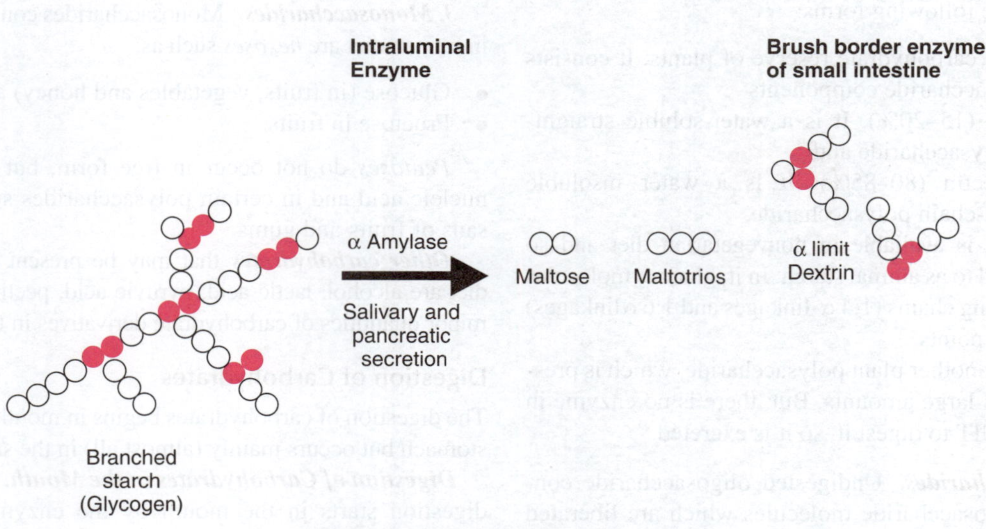

FIGURE 7.7-1 Digestion of carbohydrates.

Absorption of Carbohydrates

Carbohydrates are absorbed from the GIT in the form of monosaccharides. The monosaccharides include those formed at the brush border (described above) and also those ingested as such (e.g. glucose and fructose in fruits).

Site of Absorption Most of the monosaccharides are absorbed from the mucosal surface of jejunum and upper ileum. The absorption is almost completed before the remains of a meal reach the terminal ileum. Negligible absorption also occurs in stomach and colon.

Mechanism of Absorption Various monosaccharides are absorbed by following mechanisms:

- *Glucose* and *galactose* are absorbed by a common Na^+-dependent active transport system.
- *Fructose* is absorbed by *facilitated diffusion*. Fructose absorption occurs readily, because most of the fructose is rapidly converted into glucose and lactic acid within the epithelial cells, thus maintaining a high-concentration gradient for diffusion.
- *Pentoses* are absorbed by simple diffusion.

Absorption of Glucose and Galactose. Glucose and galactose are absorbed into the epithelial cells (enterocytes) lining the mucous membrane of small intestine from their brush border surface (luminal surface) by an *active transport mechanism*—the *sodium cotransport* mechanism. ***Salient points of glucose absorption are*** (Fig. 7.7-2):

Binding of Glucose and Na^+ to Carrier Protein. The carrier protein (present in the cell membrane) has two binding sites, one for sodium and another for glucose. It is called *sodium-dependent glucose transporter-1 (SGLT-1)*. The conformational change in the carrier protein occurs only when the binding sites are occupied by the sodium and glucose present in the gut lumen forming the sodium–glucose–carrier complex.

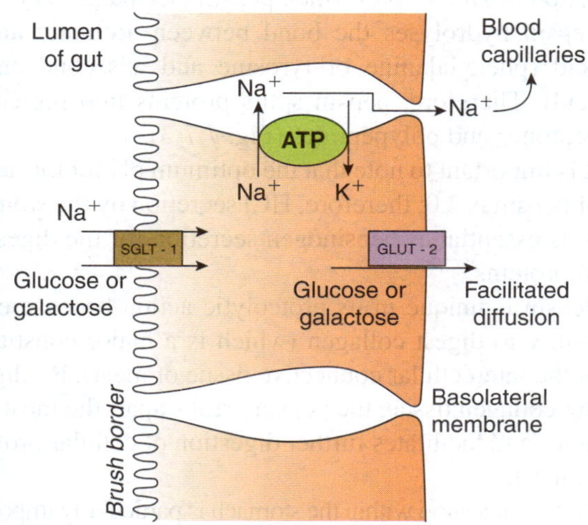

FIGURE 7.7-2 Mechanism of glucose absorption across intestinal epithelial cell.

Creation of Electrochemical Gradient across the Epithelial Cell. The active transport of sodium by Na^+–K^+–ATPase pump through the basolateral membrane into the paracellular spaces lowers the intracellular Na^+ concentration. This creates an electrochemical gradient.

Movement of Sodium and Glucose Inside the Cell. Because of the electrochemical gradient created, sodium moves into the cell (downhill transport). The flow of sodium ions down the gradient is so forceful that the glucose (or galactose) molecule attached to the carrier protein also enters the cell, even against concentration gradient for glucose (uphill movement). Because two Na^+ are transported down their electrochemical gradient, a large amount of energy is available for transport. Thus, almost all of the glucose and galactose present in the intestine can be absorbed (against the concentration gradient). The energy so released is required for Na^+–K^+ pump activity to maintain the sodium gradient.

Transport of Glucose into Blood Capillaries. From the epithelial cell, the glucose is transported into the interstitial space and thence to blood capillaries of portal system, through *facilitated diffusion* by *glucose transporter-2 (GLUT-2)*.

Note: Fructose absorption is independent of Na^+ transport. It is absorbed from intestinal lumen into the enterocyte by GLUT-5, and from enterocyte to interstitium by GLUT-2.

Factors Affecting Glucose Absorption

1. ***Presence of Na^+*** in the intestinal lumen. Due to common carrier protein, the entry of glucose/galactose into the epithelial cells is favoured by the presence of Na^+ in the intestinal lumen (similarly, the presence of glucose and galactose in the lumen favours the absorption of Na^+).
2. ***State of mucous membrane.*** Absorption of glucose is decreased in abnormal states of mucous membrane such as in enteritis and coeliac disease.
3. ***Duration of time during which the carbohydrate remains in contact with mucous membrane.*** Absorption of glucose is decreased because of intestinal hurry in conditions like diarrhoea, excision of small intestine and gastrocolic fistula.
4. ***Role of endocrines*** in glucose absorption is as below:
   - ***Thyroid.*** Thyroxine increases the glucose absorption by directly acting on the mucosa. Therefore, in thyrotoxicosis, glucose absorption is increased and in myxoedema it is decreased.
   - ***Anterior pituitary*** affects the glucose absorption by its effects on the thyroid gland. Hyperpituitarism causes hyperthyroidism and thus increases the glucose absorption and vice versa.
   - ***Adrenal cortex deficiency*** decreases glucose absorption by decreasing the Na^+ concentration.

Note

Regulation of absorption of monosaccharides does not exist, i.e. absorption of monosaccharides is *not regulated.* The intestines can absorb over 5 kg of sucrose per day. Therefore, after ingestion of a high carbohydrate diet, glycosuria can occur, i.e. glucose appears in the urine. This condition is called *alimentary glycosuria.*

Rate of absorption of monosaccharides is variable, being:

- Fastest with glucose and galactose,
- Intermediate with fructose and
- Slowest with mannose or pentoses.

Fate of Glucose in the Body

1. Storage as Glycogen. About 5% of the total glucose absorbed is stored as glycogen in the liver and muscles.

2. Catabolism to Produce Energy. About 50–60% of the glucose absorbed is catabolized in the body tissues to produce energy. A total of 1 g of glucose produces about 4 kcal of energy, when it is completely oxidized to CO_2 and H_2O. Amino acids are formed on transamination of some intermediary products of glucose breakdown.

3. Conversion into Fat. About 30–40% of glucose is converted into fat and is stored in the fat depot.

Abnormalities of Carbohydrate Digestion and Absorption

Lactose Intolerance

Congenital lactose intolerance refers to a condition in which lactose (milk sugar) cannot be digested due to congenital deficiency of enzyme lactase.

- The undigested lactose acts as osmotic particles and draws excessive fluids into the intestine resulting in *diarrhoea.*
- In the colon, the undigested lactose is metabolized by bacteria producing variety of gases (e.g. hydrogen, methane and CO_2) and variety of intestinal irritants, which increase the colonic motility.
- The diarrhoea so produced can lead to life-threatening dehydration and electrolyte imbalance.
- Avoidance of milk and milk products prevents the symptoms from developing if the infant can be fed by synthetic milk containing sucrose instead of lactose.

Secondary lactase deficiency occurring in adults is very common. It produces intestinal distension, diarrhoea and flatulence. For adults, it is usually not a problem, as they can easily avoid milk and milk products.

DIGESTION AND ABSORPTION OF PROTEINS

Sources of Proteins

The proteins that are digested and absorbed in the GIT come from two sources: exogenous and endogenous.

1. Exogenous (Dietary) Proteins

- *Daily requirement* of dietary proteins for adults is 0.5–0.7 g/kg body weight and for children (1–3 years), it is 4 g/kg.
- *Quantity of dietary proteins* varies with the socioeconomic status of the individuals; a balanced diet contains about 95–100 g/day.
- *Sources of dietary proteins* with high biological value are meat, fish, eggs, cheese and other milk products. Soyabeans, wheat and various types of pulses are also rich source of proteins.
- *Proteins of important dietary items* are:
  - Wheat : Glutenin, glycinin and gliadin.
  - Milk : Casein, lactalbumin, albumin and myosin.
  - Egg : Albumin and vitelline.
  - Meat : Collagen, albumin and myosin.
- *Structure of dietary proteins.* Dietary proteins are made of long chains of amino acids bound together by peptide linkages.

2. Endogenous Proteins. Endogenous proteins, totaling 30–50 g/day, are the proteins which reach the intestine through various gastrointestinal secretions and those which are present in the desquamated epithelial cells of the gut.

Digestion of Proteins

Proteins are digested by the proteolytic enzymes to amino acids and small polypeptides, before they are absorbed. Digestion of proteins does not occur in the mouth, as there are no proteolytic enzymes in the saliva. Digestion of proteins thus begins in the stomach and is completed in the small intestine.

Digestion of Proteins in the Stomach

Pepsin, secreted by chief cells of the main gastric glands in an inactive form (pepsinogen), is responsible for digesting about 10–15% proteins entering the gastrointestinal tract.

- Pepsinogen is converted into pepsin (active form) by the action of HCl or preformed pepsin (see page 591).
- Pepsin hydrolyses the bond between aromatic amino acid (phenylalanine or tyrosine and a second amino acid). Therefore, pepsin splits proteins into proteoses, peptones and polypeptides (Fig. 7.7-3).
- It is important to note that the optimum pH for the action of pepsin is 2.0; therefore, HCl secretion by the stomach is as essential as pepsinogen secretion for the digestion of proteins.
- Pepsin is unique in its proteolytic action because of its ability to digest collagen (which is a major constituent of the intercellular connective tissue of meat). By digesting collagen tissue, the pepsin breaks apart the meat particles and facilitates further digestion of cellular proteins of meat.
- Protein digestion within the stomach is particularly important because the protein digestion products act as *secretagogues,* i.e. stimulate secretion of proteolytic enzymes of pancreas.

Digestion of Proteins in the Small Intestine In the small intestine, proteins are digested by the pancreatic proteases, brush border peptidases and intracellular peptidases.

Pancreatic Proteases or proteolytic enzymes of pancreas play a major role in protein digestion. These can digest all the proteins, even if gastric pepsin is absent.

- *Various types of proteases* along with their functions are described on page 609.
- *Pancreatic proteases* digest the proteins and split them into dipeptides, tripeptides and small polypeptides, which are further digested by brush border peptidases (Fig. 7.7-3).
- Some of the dipeptides and tripeptides are absorbed directly into the epithelial cells of mucosa of small intestine, and are further digested by intracellular enzymes into amino acids.

Brush Border Peptidases are the proteolytic enzymes which form an integral constituent of the epithelial cell membrane with active sites projecting into the lumen.

- Brush border peptidases include aminopeptidases, dipeptidases, tripeptidases, nuclease and related enzymes.
- These enzymes continue the digestive process initiated by the pancreatic proteases, eventually converting the proteins to small polypeptides and amino acids (Fig. 7.7-3).

Intracellular Peptidases are the proteolytic enzymes present in the cytosol of epithelial cells of small intestine. The multiple peptidases present in the enterocytes are specific for linkages between the various amino acids. Within minutes, these digest the last dipeptides and tripeptides into amino acids which then enter the blood.

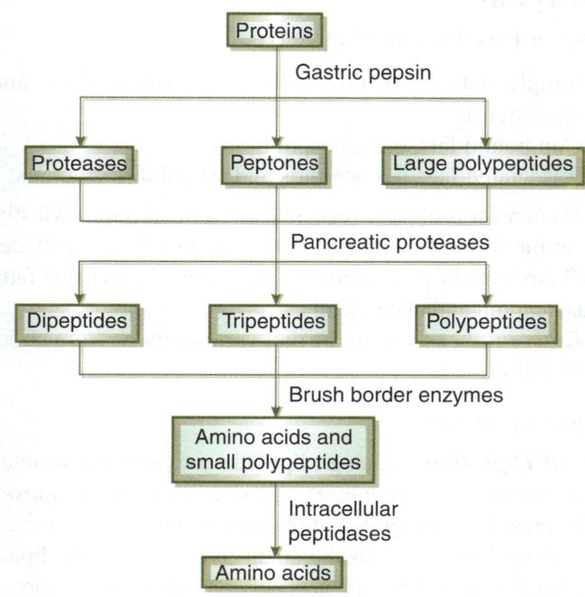

FIGURE 7.7-3 Digestion of proteins.

Digestion of Nucleic Acid and Nucleoproteins

Nucleic Acid and Nucleoproteins are Found in abundance in the foodstuffs, which are rich in nuclei such as liver, kidney, pancreas, yeast, etc.

In the Stomach, HCl hydrolyses the nucleoproteins, removing proteins which are digested together with other proteins as described above.

$$\text{Nucleoproteins} \xrightarrow{\text{HCl}} \begin{matrix}\text{Proteins}\\ + \\ \text{Free nucleic acid}\end{matrix}$$

In the small intestine, the free nucleic acids are digested by the pancreatic enzymes and brush border enzymes.

- *Pancreatic enzymes,* such as ribonuclease and deoxyribonuclease in the duodenum, digest free nucleic acids into nucleotides and nucleosides

$$\begin{matrix}\text{Freen ucleic acids}\\ \text{(RNA and DNA)}\end{matrix} \xrightarrow[\text{Deoxyribonuclease}]{\text{Ribonuclease}} \begin{matrix}\text{Nucleotides}\\ \text{and}\\ \text{nucleosides}\end{matrix}$$

- Brush border enzymes such as nucleases, nucleotidases and nucleosidases convert nucleotides and nucleosides into pentoses (purine and pyrimidine).

$$\begin{matrix}\text{Nucleotides and}\\ \text{Nucleosides}\end{matrix} \xrightarrow[\text{Nucleosidases}]{\text{Nucleases Nucleotidase}} \begin{matrix}\text{Pentoses (purine and}\\ \text{pyrimidine)}\end{matrix}$$

End Products of Protein Digestion. Protein digestion, which starts in the stomach, is completed in the enterocyte of small intestine. The end products of protein digestion are amino acids.

Absorption of Proteins

Mechanisms of Absorption into the Intestinal Epithelial Cells The end products of protein digestion (amino acids, dipeptides and tripeptides) are absorbed through the luminal membrane of the epithelial cells of small intestine. Absorption of amino acids is faster in duodenum and jejunum and slower in ileum. Following mechanisms of absorption are known:

1. Transport Systems: There are seven different transport systems existing for amino acid transport from intestinal lumen into the enterocytes. Five of them require Na^+ (Na^+-dependent cotransport), and out of these, two also require Cl^-, while other two are Na^+-independent transporters.

(i) *Na^+-dependent active transport mechanism.* The levo amino acids, dipeptides and tripeptides are absorbed by a Na^+-dependent active transport mechanism.

- Separate transporters (carriers) are present for the absorption of basic, acidic and neutral amino acids. At least two different polypeptide transporters exist.

- Steps of active transport mechanism are similar to those described for glucose absorption (see page 649). These include (Fig. 7.7-4):
  - Binding of amino acid and Na^+ to carrier protein,
  - Creation of electrochemical gradient across the epithelial cells and
  - Movement of Na^+ and amino acids inside the cell.

(ii) ***Na^+-independent active transport mechanism.*** The carrier is known as Pep T_1 (peptide transporter-1) that requires H^+ instead of Na^+ for transport of di- and tripeptides.

2. Simple Diffusion. The dextro amino acids are absorbed solely by passive diffusion.

3. Endocytosis. Larger polypeptides cannot be absorbed into the epithelial cells. Occasionally, small amounts of larger polypeptides are absorbed by endocytosis. Proteins absorbed by endocytosis usually excite immunological/allergic reaction. In newborn infants, immunoglobulins present in the colostrum are absorbed in the intestinal mucosa by endocytosis and impart passive immunity to child.

Further Digestion in the Epithelial Cells Once amino acids and polypeptides are absorbed into the intestinal epithelial cells, the intracellular peptidases break the remaining linkages of tripeptides and dipeptides causing release of amino acids.

Transport of Amino Acids into Blood Capillaries From inside the epithelial cells, the amino acids are transported into the interstitial space across the basolateral membrane of the cells by a series of basolateral transport proteins. From the interstitium, the amino acids enter the capillaries of villus by simple diffusion, and then via the portal vein, they reach the liver and general circulation. Therefore, after ingestion of a high-protein meal, there occurs a sharp transient rise in the free amino acid content of the portal blood, which provides the whole body requirements of proteins.

Note It is important to note that almost all proteins ingested are absorbed. About 2–5% of proteins that escape digestion and absorption in the small intestine enter the colon and are finally digested by bacterial digestion. Therefore, the proteins that appear in the stool are not of dietary origin, but are derived from the bacterial and cellular debris.

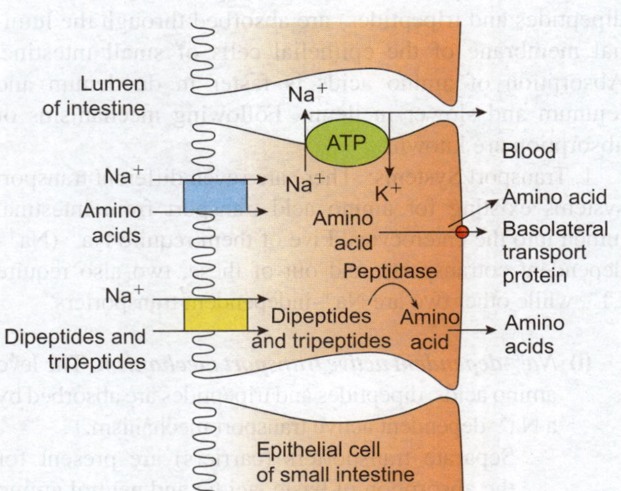

FIGURE 7.7-4 Mechanism of absorption of amino acids, dipeptides and tripeptides by intestinal epithelial cells.

Abnormalities of Protein Digestion and Absorption

1. Inadequate Absorption of Proteins, due to lack of trypsin, is a common consequence of pancreatic diseases.

2. Malabsorption of Amino Acids due to lack of transporters is relatively rare. For example, in *Hartnup disease,* there occurs malabsorption of neutral amino acids due to lack of specific carrier protein, and congenital defect in the transport for basic amino acids causing cysteinuria.

Important Note

The absorption of protein antigens (particularly of bacterial and viral) occurs in the large microfold cells (M cells), specialized epithelial cells overlying the Peyer's patches (aggregates of lymphoid tissue). These cells pass the antigen to lymphoid cells and activate lymphocytes. The activated lymphocytes enter the circulation and return back to intestinal epithelium and other epithelial cells, and secrete IgA antibodies in response to subsequent exposure to same antigen—an important defence mechanism by secretory immunity.

DIGESTION AND ABSORPTION OF FATS

Dietary Fats

Types of Fats. Fats are of three types:

- Simple fats or neutral fats, e.g. triglycerides and cholesterol.
- Compound fats, e.g. phospholipids.
- Associated fats, e.g. steroids and fat-soluble vitamins.

Dietary fat is of both vegetable and animal origin. Mostly, it is in the form of neutral fat (triglycerides). It also includes small amounts of phospholipids, cholesterol, some free fatty acids, lecithin and cholesterol esters.

Daily intake of fats in the diet varies widely, from about 25 to 160 g.

Digestion of Fats

Site of Digestion Although lipolytic enzymes are secreted in the mouth (*lingual lipase*) and stomach (*gastric lipase*), their action is so insignificant that practically digestion of all the dietary fats occurs in the small intestine. Gastric lipase which initiates fat digestion acts only on butter. Under normal conditions, gastric lipase is soon inactivated by gastric juice (pH 1–2), as it is inactivated at pH 2.5 and acts at an optimum pH of 4.5. Some fat digestion in stomach may occur under the following exceptional circumstances:

- Achlorhydria (i.e. gastric juice cannot inactivate gastric lipase),
- Regurgitation of pancreatic lipase from the duodenum into the stomach and
- In young suckling animals which ingest large quantities of milk, the fat of milk is present in an emulsified form and digested, and this inhibits the secretion of gastric juice.

Mechanism of Digestion of Fats The digestion of fat includes three steps:

- Emulsification of fat by bile salts,
- Hydrolysis of fat by pancreatic and intestinal lipolytic enzymes and
- Acceleration of fat digestion by micelle formation.

1. Emulsification of Fat by Bile Salts

- Emulsification, i.e. breaking of large fat drops into smaller droplets, is a prerequisite for action of pancreatic lipase. It is so because the pancreatic lipase being water soluble acts only on the oil–water interface of fat. The surface area available for the action of lipase is increased many thousand times by the emulsification of fats.
- Emulsification of fat is caused by bile salts because of their property of lowering the surface tension (detergent-like action). With the lowered surface tension of the fats, the segmentation movements of small intestine break up large fat globules into fine droplets (1 μm in diameter). Lecithin (a component of bile), which has a stabilization action on the emulsions, greatly enhances the emulsifying action of bile salts. The bile salts surround the fine fat droplets in such a way that their lipophilic nonpolar ends are towards the fat and their hydrophilic polar ends separate the fat droplets from the aqueous phase (Fig. 7.7-5).

2. Hydrolysis of Fat Droplets by Pancreatic and Intestinal Lipolytic Enzymes. Pancreatic juice is markedly alkaline (pH 7.8–8.4). When it mixes with the acidic chyme (pH 6.0) coming from stomach into the duodenum, the pH of chyme is adjusted to about 7 (which is optimal pH for the action of pancreatic lipases).

Pancreatic Lipolytic Enzymes. Pancreatic juice contains three types of lipolytic enzymes. Their hydrolysing effects on fats are given:

i. ***Pancreatic lipase***. Pancreatic lipase is a very powerful lipolytic enzyme. Fat digestion by it occurs very rapidly after emulsification because of the large-surface-to-volume ratio of the small globules. Colipase, a protein present in the pancreatic juice, displaces the bile salts from the fat droplet and allows the action of lipase. Pancreatic lipase hydrolyses almost all the triglycerides (neutral fat) of the food to produce two fatty acids and a 2-monoglycerides.

   Note. Colipase is secreted in an inactive form and is activated by trypsin in the intestinal lumen. When activated, colipase binds to –COOH terminal domain of pancreatic lipase; the activity of this enzyme is facilitated by opening of lid (helix-like structure) that covers its active site.

ii. ***Cholesterol ester hydrolase.*** Most of the dietary cholesterol is in the form of cholesterol esters, which are hydrolysed to cholesterol and fatty acid by the cholesterol ester hydrolase.

   The cholesterol esterase is activated by the bile salts. Cholesterol esterase represents about 4% of the total protein contents of pancreatic juice. The bile salt-activated pancreatic lipase hydrolyses cholesterol esters, esters of fat-soluble vitamins, phospholipids and triglycerides. A similar type of lipase is also present in the human milk.

iii. ***Phospholipase A_2***. It is secreted in an inactive form prophospholipase A_2, and gets converted to active form. It hydrolyses phospholipids and separates fatty acid from them.

Intestinal lipolytic enzymes. Brush border of epithelial cells covering the intestinal villi contains small amount of lipase and cholesterol esterase. Their effects, though minor, but are similar to that of pancreatic lipase.

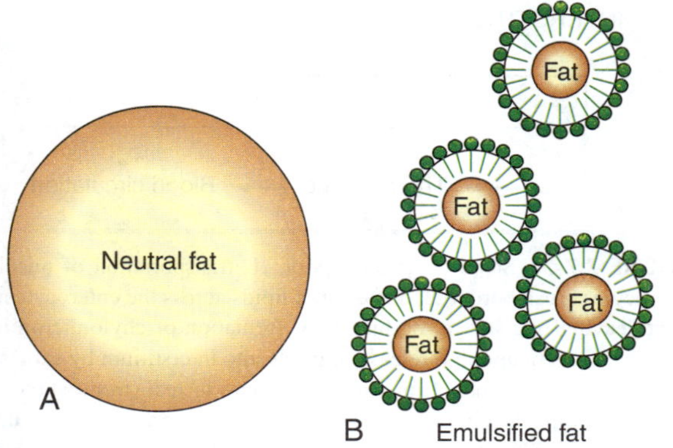

FIGURE 7.7-5 Emulsification of fats by bile salts: **A,** a large fat particle; and **B,** small fat particles surrounded by bile salts.

3. Acceleration of Fat Digestion by Micelle Formation. The hydrolysis of triglycerides is highly reversible; therefore, accumulation of monoglycerides and free fatty acids in the vicinity of digesting fats quickly blocks further digestion. This problem is solved by the property of bile salts to form micelle. ***Micelle formation*** depends on critical micelle concentration of bile salts in the aqueous solution. At a critical micelle concentration, all the bile salts in a solution form micelles. The lipids get collected in the centre of micelle.

Structure

Micelles are small, water-soluble, cylindrical disc-shaped particles. Each micelle is composed of a central fat globule surrounded by about 30 molecules of bile salts in such a way that their lipid-soluble nonpolar ends are in the central fat globule and water-soluble polar ends fan out to form the outer covering of micelle. Monoglycerides and free fatty acids released from the digestion of fat are quickly incorporated into the central fatty portion of the micelles forming, what are known as, the *mixed micelles* (Fig. 7.7-6). In this way, bile salts accelerate the fat digestion by allowing the lipolytic action to continue.

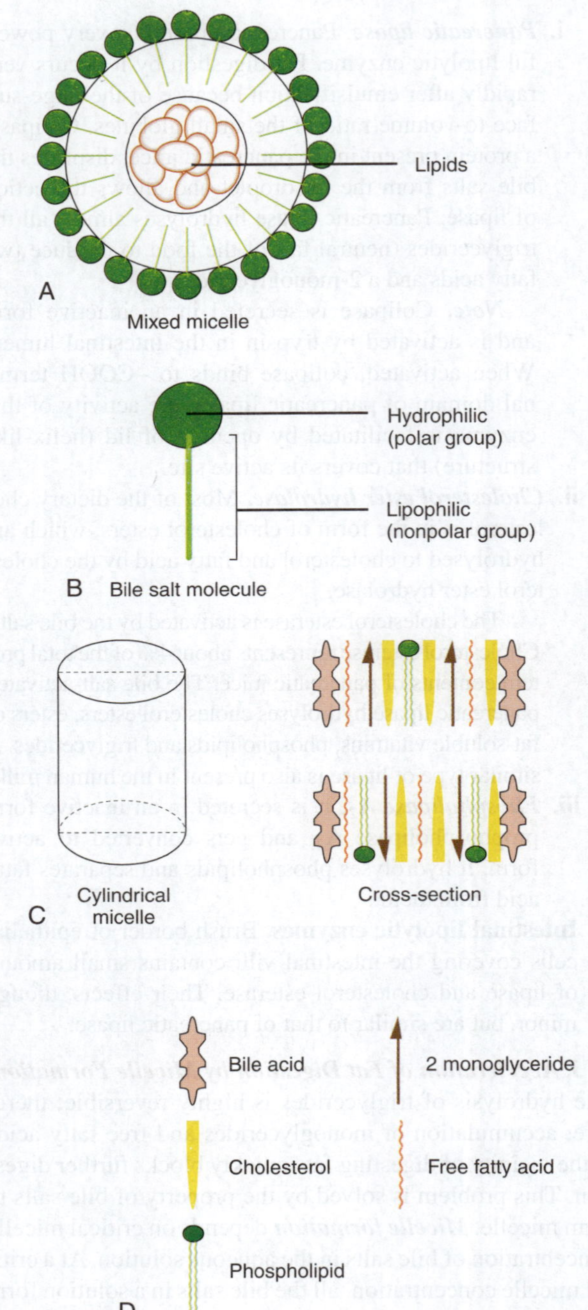

FIGURE 7.7-6 Structure of micelle: **A,** a mixed micelle composed of lipids (monoglycerides, fatty acids and cholesterol) in the centre surrounded by bile salts; **B,** bile salt molecule showing globular (hydrophilic or polar) end and lipophilic (nonpolar) end; **C,** a model of the structure of mixed (bile salt and lipid) micelle and its cross-section showing arrangement of various lipid molecules; and **D,** diagrammatic structure of different lipid molecules.

Absorption of Fats

Most of the fat absorption occurs in the duodenum; almost all the digested lipids are totally absorbed by the time the chyme reaches the mid-jejunum. Absorption of fats is accomplished by the following steps (Fig. 7.7-7):

1. Transportation as Micelles to the Brush Border Membrane. The micelles so formed (as described above) not only accelerate the fat digestion, but are also essential for the fat absorption as explained.

The insolubility of fat globules prevents their diffusion through the aqueous medium of the intestinal lumen to reach the brush border. This problem is solved by the bile salts by forming the micelle. As described above (Fig. 7.7-6), the outer surface of micelle is formed by water-soluble polar ends of bile salts, which help the micelle to diffuse through the aqueous medium to reach the brush border membrane.

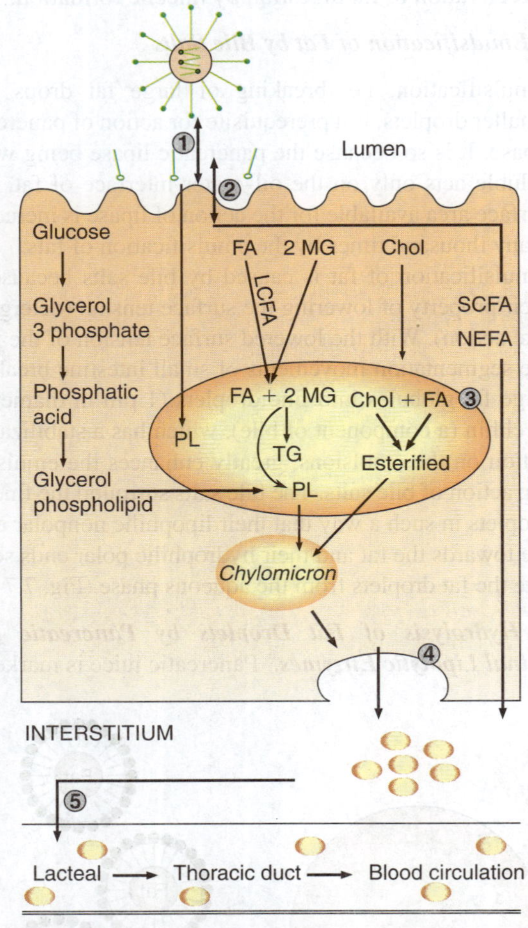

FIGURE 7.7-7 Steps of fat absorption: 1, transportation of micelle to enterocytes brush border; 2, diffusion of lipids across the enterocyte membrane leaving bile salt in the lumen; 3, formation of chylomicron in the endoplasmic reticulum; 4, release of lipids into interstitium by exocytosis; and 5, diffusion of lipids from interstitium into lacteal (from where lipids enter into lymphatic circulation) and through thoracic duct into circulation. FA: fatty acid, MG: monoglycerides, chol: cholesterol, TG: triglycerides, LCFA: long-chain fatty acid, SCFA: short-chain fatty acids, NEFA: non-esterified fatty acids and PL: phospholipid.

Thus, the bile salt micelle acts as a transport vehicle for the products of fat digestion.

2. Diffusion of Lipids across the Enterocyte Cell Membrane. Once the micelle comes in contact with the cell membrane, the monoglycerides, free fatty acids, cholesterol and fat-soluble vitamins (being soluble in the cell membrane) *diffuse passively* at a rapid speed through the enterocyte cell membrane to the interior of the cell, leaving bile salts in the intestinal lumen. Thus, the *rate-limiting* step in lipid absorption is the formation and migration of the micelles from the intestinal chyme to the microvilli surface. It is important to note that the bile salts must be present in certain minimum concentration called *critical micellar concentration,* before micelles are formed.

The bile salts released from micelle after diffusion of their associated lipids are absorbed in the terminal ileum by a Na^+-dependent active transport process.

3. Transport of Lipids from Inside the Enterocytes to the Interstitial Space. Once inside the cell, the end products of fat digestion enter the interstitium by two mechanisms:

i. ***Diffusion across the basal border of enterocyte.*** Small-chain fatty acids (SCFA) with less than 10–12 carbon atoms are water soluble and are able to diffuse across the basal border of enterocytes to enter the interstitium and are actively transported in the portal blood and circulate in unestrified form.

ii. ***Formation and excretion of chylomicrons from enterocytes by exocytosis.*** Large-chain fatty acids, which more than 12 carbon atom, cholesterol and lysophosphatides enter the smooth endoplasmic reticulum, where they are reconstituted:
   - 2-Monoglycerides are combined with fatty acids to produce triglycerides. Some of the triglycerides are also formed from glycerophosphate (a product of glucose catabolism). Glycerophosphate is also converted into glycerophospholipids and participate in chylomicron formation.
   - Lysophosphatides are combined with fatty acids to form phospholipids and
   - Cholesterol is re-esterified.

The reformed lipids coalesce to form a small lipid droplets (about 1 nm in diameter) called chylomicrons, which are lined by the synthesized β-lipoproteins. The chylomicrons are then excreted into the interstitium by exocytosis from the basolateral membrane of enterocyte. Covering of β-lipoproteins is essential for the exocytosis to occur. Therefore, in the absence of β-lipoprotein, exocytosis will not occur, and the enterocytes become engorged with lipids.

4. Transport of Lipids into Circulation. After exiting the enterocytes (i.e. in the interstitium), the chylomicrons merge into larger droplets that vary in size from 50 to 500 nm, depending on the amount of lipid being absorbed. From the interstitium, the lipids diffuse into the *lacteals*, from where they enter the lymphatic circulation, and via thoracic duct gain access into the blood circulation. In an adult, more than 95% of the fat gets absorbed on moderate intake.

Note.

- The process involved in fat absorption at birth is not fully matured; thus, infants are more susceptible to ill effects of disease that reduces fat absorption.

Fate of short-chain fatty acids in the colon

The short-chain fatty acids (SCFA) (2–5 carbon atoms) are weak acids produced by the action of colonic bacteria on unabsorbed complex carbohydrates, resistant starches and components of dietary fibers. They are absorbed from the colon by specific transporter.

Functions:

- SCFA provide significant calories.
- They have trophic effect on colonic epithelium and play an important role during inflammation.
- Help in maintaining acid–base balance.

The principal digestive enzymes, their source and functions are summarized in Table 7.7-1.

Applied Aspects

Lipid Malabsorption

- Lipid malabsorption is much more common than carbohydrate and protein malabsorption.
- Causes of lipid malabsorption include:
  - Deficiency of pancreatic lipase in certain pancreatic diseases and
  - Bile deficiency in disorders of liver and gall bladder.
- Steatorrhoea, i.e. increased amount of fat in the stools, is a common manifestation of fat malabsorption.

Serum Lipid Profile

Lipids are present as lipoprotein complexes. Depending upon the density, the lipoproteins are of following types:

i. Very low-density lipoproteins (VLDL). Density is < 1.060.
ii. Low-density lipoproteins (LDL).
iii. High-density lipoproteins (HDL). Density is 1.060–1.200.

Normal Values:

- Serum triglycerides: 30–150 mg%,
- Serum cholesterol: 150–240 mg%,
- Serum phospholipids: 150–300 mg% and
- Serum free fatty acids (FFA or NEFA = 10–30 mg%).

ABSORPTION OF WATER, ELECTROLYTES, MINERALS AND VITAMINS

Water Absorption

Water Balance in the GIT

- The gastrointestinal tract receives about 9 L of water per day, which includes about 2 L of ingested water and

TABLE 7.7-1 Principal Digestive Enzymes

Substrate	Enzyme	Source	Activator	Function and product
A. Carbohydrate				
Starch (polysaccharide) *Disaccharides*	• Salivary α-amylase • Pancreatic amylase	Salivary gland Exocrine pancreas	Cl^- Cl^-	Hydrolyses 1:4 α-linkages, producing α-limit dextrin, maltotriose, and maltose-same as-
Maltose	• Maltriose • Maltase • α-Dextrins	Intestinal mucosa	–	Glucose
Lactose	• Lactase	Do-	–	Galactose and glucose
Sucrose	• Sucrase	Do-	–	Fructose and glucose
α-Dextrins, maltriose and maltose	• α-Dextrinase	Do-	–	Glucose
Trehlose	• Trehalase	Do-	–	Glucose
B. Nucleic acid	• Nuclease and related enzymes	Do-		Pentoses, purines and pyrimidines
RNA	• Ribonucleasse	Exocrine pancreas	–	Nucleotides
DNA	• Deoxyribonuclease	Do-	–	Nucleotides
C. Proteins and polypeptides	• Pepsinogen (pepsin)	Gastric glands	HCl	Cleave peptide bonds adjacent to aromatic amino acids
	• Trypsinogen (trypsin)	Exocrine pancreace	Enteropeptidase	Cleave peptide bonds on carboxyl side of basic amino acids (arginine and lysine)
	• Chymotrypsin	Do-	Trypsin	Cleave peptide bonds on carboxyl side of aromatic amino acids
Elastin and some other proteins	Proelastase (elastase)	Do-	Trypsin	Cleave peptide bonds on carboxyl side of aliphatic amino acids
	Exopeptidase procarboxypeptidase A (carboxypeptidase)	Do-	Do-	Cleave carboxyl terminal aromatic amino acids having branched aliphatic side chains.
	Carboxypeptidase-B (carboxypeptidase B)	Do-	Do-	Cleave carboxyl terminal amino acid having basic amino acids side chains
Polypeptides	Endopeptidase	Brush border of intestinal mucosa	–	Cleave amino terminal amino acid from peptide
	Carboxypeptidase	Do-	–	Cleave carboxyl terminal amino acid from peptide
	endopeptidase	Do-	–	Cleave between residue of mid-portion of peptide
Dipeptides	Dipeptidase	Do-	–	Two amino acids
Di, tri and tetrapeptides	Various peptidases	Cytoplasm of mucosal cells	–	Amino acids

TABLE 7.7-1 Principal Digestive Enzymes—cont'd

Substrate	Enzyme	Source	Activator	Function and product
4. Fats (lipids) triglycerides	lingual lipase	Lingual gland	–	1,2 Diacylglycerol and fatty acids
	Gastric lipase	Stomach	–	Fatty acids and glycerol
	Colipase	Exocrine pancrease	Trypsin	Facilitate exposure of active site of fancreatic lipase
	Pancreatic lipase	Do-	–	Monoglycerides and fatty acids
Cholesterol esters	Bile salt acid lipase	Do-	–	Cholesterol
	Cholesterol ester hydrolase	Do-	–	Cholesterol

about 7 L contained in salivary, gastric, biliary, pancreatic and intestinal secretions (Table 7.7-2).

- The gastrointestinal tract absorbs about 8.8 L of water (about 95% of total water received) per day. About 60% of absorption occurs in jejunum, 20–25% in ileum and 10–15% in colon (Table 7.7-2).
- The gastrointestinal tract excretes about 0.2 L of water in the faeces per day.

Mechanism of Water Absorption

- In general, water is absorbed passively and iso-osmotically across the gastrointestinal mucosa, following the osmotic gradient created by the active absorption of electrolytes and nutrients.
- Because osmotic equilibrium is rapidly achieved, the fluid in the intestine is always isotonic to plasma.
- Only a small amount of water moves across the gastric mucosa, but water moves in both directions across the mucosa of small intestine and colon in response to the osmotic gradient.
- In the duodenum, the osmotic pressure created by the entering chyme causes water to flow into it.

TABLE 7.7-2 Daily Water Balance in GIT

Input (L)		Absorption (L)		Faecal excretion (L)
Water ingested	: 2	Jejunum (60%)	: 5.5	0.2
Water in GIT	: 7	Ileum (25%)	: 2.0	
Secretions • Saliva: 1.5 • Gastric juice: 2.5 • Bile: 0.75 • Pancreatic juice: 0.75 • Intestinal juice: 1.5		Colon (10–15%)	: 1.3	
TOTAL	9		8.8	0.2

- In the jejunum and ileum, reabsorption of sodium chloride (NaCl) creates an osmotic gradient favouring the reabsorption of water.

Absorption of Sodium

Sodium Balance in GIT. Gastrointestinal tract receives about 40 g of sodium per day, out of which about 10 g is ingested with food and about 30 g is contained in the gastrointestinal secretions. All of it is reabsorbed.

Site of Absorption. Though sodium can be reabsorbed in the entire length of the intestine, but maximum absorption occurs in the jejunum.

Mechanisms of Absorption. Absorption of sodium is a two-step process:

1. ***Transport of sodium from the lumen into the enterocyte*** occurs by following mechanisms (Fig. 7.7-8):
   - Na^+ glucose, Na^+–amino acids and Na^+–di- or tri-peptide cotransport system account for 30% of Na^+ transport into the cell.
   - Neutral Na^+–Cl^- cotransport system also transports about 30% of Na^+.
   - Na^+–H^+ exchange and
   - Passive diffusion (through Na^+ channels) down an electrochemical gradient is responsible for transport of remainder 40% of Na^+.

In the Small Intestine, Na^+–glucose cotransport, Na^+–amino acid cotransport and Na^+–H^+ exchange mechanisms are most important (these cotransport and exchange mechanisms are similar to those in renal proximal tubule) (see page 497). Thus, the presence of glucose in the intestinal lumen facilitates the reabsorpiton for Na^+. Because of this reason, in the treatment of Na^+ and water loss in diarrhoea, glucose is added to the orally administered NaCl solution. Cereals containing carbohydrates are also useful in the treatment of diarrhoea.

In the Colon, passive diffusion via Na^+ channels is most important. These channels of the colon are similar to those in the renal distal tubules, and are stimulated by aldosterone

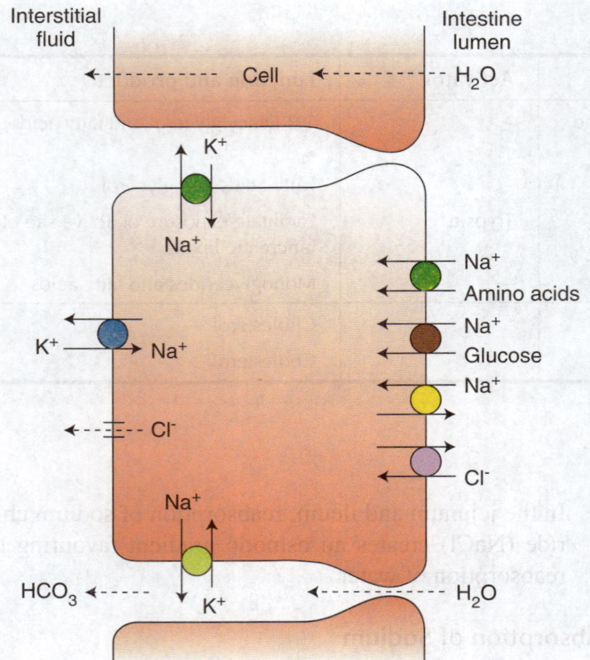

FIGURE 7.7-8 Absorption of sodium, chloride, glucose and amino acids through the intestinal epithelium. The absorption of water 'follows' sodium through the epithelial membrane.

(which greatly enhances sodium absorption). This mechanism is especially useful in dehydration, which leads to aldosterone secretion by the adrenal medulla.

2. ***Transport of Na^+ out of the enterocytes into the interstitium*** occurs against its electrochemical gradient across the basolateral membrane by Na^+–K^+–ATPase active transport system.

Absorption of Chloride

In the jejunum and proximal ileum, most of the Cl^- is absorbed passively through the enterocytes down the electrochemical gradient established by the active transport of Na^+. The mechanisms involved in the transport of Cl^- are:

- Passive diffusion by a paracellular route through the leaky (permeable) junction between the enterocytes and
- Neutral Na^+–Cl^- cotransport system.

In the distal ileum and large intestine, the Cl^- is absorbed by an active Cl^-–HCO_3^- exchange mechanism. In this mechanism, Cl^- is absorbed from the lumen in exchange of HCO_3^-, which is secreted into the lumen. Bicarbonate (HCO_3^-) secreted into the lumen helps to neutralize the acidity produced by the action of colonic bacteria on the food.

Absorption of Bicarbonate

To neutralize acidic chyme in the duodenum and acidic pH in colon (due to bacterial activity), large amount of bicarbonate ions are secreted into pancreatic secretion and bile is poured into the duodenum. At the same time, epithelial cells on the surface of villi in ileum and large intestine also secrete bicarbonate ions in exchange for chloride ion absorption.

- The bicarbonate ion is absorbed indirectly as:
  - During sodium ion absorption, moderate amount of hydrogen ions get secreted into the lumen of gut in exchange to Na^+. These H^+ combine with bicarbonate to form carbonic acid (H_2CO_3), which then dissociates to form water and carbon dioxide.
  - The water remains in the intestine; however, CO_2 is readily absorbed into the blood and ultimately eliminated during expiration through lungs.

Absorption of Potassium

- Passive diffusion via paracellular route down its electrochemical gradient is the mechanism involved in the absorption of dietary K^+ from the small intestine.
- Net movement of K^+ across the intestinal mucosa is directly proportional to the potential difference between the blood and intestinal lumen. The magnitude of which is:
  - Jejunum: 5mV,
  - Ileum: 25 mV and
  - Colon: 50 mV.

Because of this reason, the concentration of K^+ is approximately 6 mEq/L in jejunum, 13 mEq/L in ileum and 30 mEq/L in colon. This accounts for hypokalaemia occurring due to ileal and colonic fluid loss in chronic diarrhoea.

Absorption of Calcium

Body Calcium. Calcium is the most abundant among the minerals in the body. The total content of calcium in an adult man is about 1–1.5 kg of which about 99% is present in the bones and teeth. A small amount (10%) found outside the skeletal tissue performs a wide variety of functions.

Dietary Calcium. Best sources of dietary calcium are milk and milk products. Good sources of calcium are beans, leafy vegetables, fish, cabbage and egg yolk.

Dietary requirements of calcium are:

- Infants (<1 year): 300–500 mg/day,
- Children (1–18 years): 800–1200 mg/day,
- Adult men and women: 800 mg/day and
- Women during pregnancy, lactation and postmenopause: 1500 mg/day.

Site of absorption. Most of the ingested calcium is absorbed in the upper small intestine (duodenum and jejunum).

Mechanism of absorption. Normally, about 75–80% of the daily intake (about 1000 mg) of calcium is absorbed from the upper small intestine. Most of the calcium is absorbed by an active transport mechanism in following two steps:

- *Entry of calcium inside the enterocyte* across its luminal border occurs by the active transport mechanism involving a membrane-bound carrier that is activated by vitamin D.

- Transport of calcium out of the cell into the interstitium, from where it is absorbed into the blood capillaries, occurs by a Ca^{2+}–ATPase active transport system and by a Na^+–Ca^{2+} exchange system.

Regulation of Calcium Absorption Calcium absorption from the small intestine is well regulated to maintain the plasma calcium (*homeostasis of calcium*) levels within a narrow range (9–11 mg%). Vitamin D and parathyroid hormone (PTH) play main role in the regulation of calcium absorption as:

- *Vitamin D_3* is converted to 25-hydroxy vitamin D_3 by the liver.
- *25-Hydroxy vitamin D_3* is converted to 1,25-dihydroxy vitamin D_3 [also known as 1,25-diydroxycholecalciferol (1,25 DHCC) or calciferol] in the kidneys by a process that is regulated by the parathyroid hormone (PTH).
- *1,25-Dihydroxy vitamin D_3* (which is the physiologically active form of vitamin D, acting as hormone) enters the enterocyte and activates the formation of 'calcium-carrier protein' that inserts in the luminal surface of the enterocyte.
- *Calcium-carrier protein* is responsible for carrier-bound transport of calcium inside the cell.

Factors Promoting Calcium Absorption Include:

- *Vitamin D* (through its active form calciferol) promotes calcium absorption by inducing synthesis of calcium-binding protein (as described above).
- *Parathyroid hormone* enhances Ca^{2+} absorption by influencing synthesis of calciferol (as described above).
- *Low pH* is more favourable for Ca^{2+} absorption.
- *Lactose promotes* Ca^{2+} intake by the intestinal cells.
- *Amino acids* (lysine and arginine) facilitate Ca^{2+} absorption.

Factors Inhibiting Calcium Absorption are:

- *Phytates and oxalates* inhibit Ca^{2+} absorption by forming insoluble salts with Ca^{2+} in the intestine.
- *High content of dietary phosphate* also prevents Ca^{2+} absorption by forming insoluble calcium phosphate. The dietary ratio of Ca^{2+} and P between 1:2 and 2:1 is ideal for optimum Ca^{2+} absorption.
- *Free fatty acids* inhibit Ca^{2+} absorption by forming insoluble calcium soaps. It occurs particularly when the fat absorption is impaired.
- *High pH* (alkaline conditions) is unfavourable for Ca^{2+} absorption.
- *Dietary fibres* in high content interfere with calcium absorption.

Importance of Ca:P Ratio. The ratio of Ca:P is important for calcification of bones. The product of Ca × P (in mg/dl) in children is about 50 and in adults it is around 40. This product is less than 30 in rickets.

Excretion of calcium occurs mainly in faeces and partly in urine.

- *Excretion of Ca^{2+} into the faeces* is a continuous process and this is increased in vitamin D deficiency.
- *Excretion of Ca^{2+} into the urine* occurs when the serum Ca^{2+} goes beyond 10 mg/dL. Ingestion of excess proteins causes increased Ca^{2+} excretion in the urine. This is mainly due to an increase in the acidity of urine.

For details of calcium balance, see page 713.

Absorption of Iron

Absorption of iron is discussed in Chapter 3.2, at page 158.

Absorption of Vitamins

Absorption of Fat-soluble Vitamins

- Fat-soluble vitamins (A, D, E and K) become part of micelle formed by bile salts, and are absorbed along with other lipids in the upper part of small intestine (for details see page 652).
- The absorption of fat-soluble vitamins is deficient if fat absorption is depressed because of lack of pancreatic enzymes or if bile is excluded from the intestine by the obstruction of bile duct.

Absorption of Water-soluble Vitamins

- Absorption of water–soluble vitamins is rapid compared with fat-soluble vitamins.
- Most vitamins are absorbed in the upper part of small intestine (jejunum) except vitamins B_{12}, which is absorbed in the ileum.
- Most water-soluble vitamins, e.g. vitamin C and the vitamins B, (biotin, folic acid, nicotinic acid, B_8, i.e. pyridoxine, B_2, i.e. riboflavin and B_1, i.e. thiamine), are absorbed by facilitated transport or by Na^+-dependent active transport system in the proximal small intestine.
- Vitamin B_{12} absorption is most complex than that of other water-soluble vitamins and needs separate description.

Absorption of Vitamin B_{12} involves the following steps:

- ***In the stomach,*** vitamin B_{12} is exposed to specific binding protein R and vitamin B_{12}-binding protein called intrinsic factor (IF). As the affinity of R proteins for vitamin B_{12} is much more than that of IF, so most of the vitamin B_{12} gets bound to R protein in the stomach.
- ***In the lumen of intestine,*** the pancreatic proteases cleave vitamin B_{12} from the R protein. Then, vitamin B_{12} binds to IF to form a complex.
- ***On the brush border of enterocyte,*** IF–B_{12} complex becomes bound to the specific receptors. Following this, the vitamin B_{12} is transported into the cytosol of enterocyte by endocytosis, leaving behind IF at the brush border. It is important to note that absorption of vitamin

B_{12} from the IF–B_{12} complex can occur only after the complex binds to the receptors. In the absence of intrinsic factor, vitamin B_{12} absorption is markedly decreased and the patient may develop pernicious anaemia (see page 162).

- ***From the basolateral border of enterocyte.*** Vitamin B_{12} enters the portal circulation after binding with plasma globulin called transcobalamine-11.
- ***In the liver,*** vitamin B_{12} is stored in large amounts after binding with another globulin called *transcobalamin-1*. The storage of water-soluble vitamin is unique to vitamin B_{12}. Liver may store up to 3 years of supply. Vitamin B_{12} is also stored in the muscles for some extent. Whenever required, it is transported from the liver to the bone marrow.

APPLIED ASPECTS

Malabsorption Syndrome

Malabsorption syndrome is not a simple disease but a group of disorders in which multiple nutritional deficiency states are produced.

Pathophysiology: Malabsorption occurs due to abnormalities of three processes, which are important for normal digestion and absorption.

i. *Intraluminal maldigestion:* When there is deficiency of pancreatic enzymes and bile which results in inadequate solubilization and hydrolyses of nutrients leading to fat and protein malabsorption.
ii. *Mucosal malabsorption* results when there is damage of small intestinal epithelium, thereby diminishing the surface area for absorption and depleting brush border enzyme activity.
iii. *Postmucosal lymphatic obstruction* prevents the uptake and transport of absorbed lipids into lymphatic vessels. Increased pressure in these vessels results in leakage into intestinal lumen leading to protein loosing enteropathy.

General Features of Malabsorption are:

- Deficient absorption of amino acids, fats and carbohydrates result in general weakness.
- Malabsorption of vitamins may produce anaemia and signs of hypovitaminosis.
- Malabsorption of iron results in iron deficiency anaemia.
- Malabsorption of fats produces steatorrhoea (see page 653).
- Water and electrolyte depletion may result in dehydration.

Common Conditions which can produce malabsorption are:

- Coeliac disease
- Sprue
- Lactose intolerance (see page 648)
- Crohn's disease
- Resection of small intestine
- Malabsorption after gastric surgery (see page 605)
- Blind loop syndrome
- Chronic pancreatitis (see page 614)
- Obstruction of common bile duct (see page 624).

Coeliac Disease

Aetiopathogenesis. It occurs due to deficiency of the enzyme gluten hydrolase. As a result, gluten, the principal protein of wheat, rye, barley and oats, is not properly hydrolysed. Consequently, gliadine, a toxic polypeptide, is formed, which produces an inflammatory response in the intestinal mucosa leading to destruction of microvilli.

Clinical features of gluten-induced enteropathy are those of generalized malabsorption. It may occur as:

- Congenital disease manifesting usually within first 3 years of life and
- Acquired disease in adults due to unknown aetiology.

Treatment consists of withdrawal of wheat and other sources of gluten in the diet.

Sprue Sprue or the tropical sprue is a disorder of malabsorption, which is particularly characterized by features of failure of absorption of folate, with or without associated malabsorption of vitamin B_{12}. So, general features of malabsorption with megaloblastic anaemia, which is conspicuous, occur.

Crohn's Disease

Aetiopathogenesis. It is an inflammatory bowel disease (IBD) characterized by idiopathic, nonspecific granulomatous inflammation of the bowel.

Clinical features vary depending upon the part and extent of bowel involved. Common clinical features are: off and on fever, chronic diarrhoea, abdominal discomfort and pain and weight loss is frequent, and many patients have moderate anaemia and other features of malabsorption. Ultimately, the patient may develop narrowing and obstruction of intestinal lumen, fistula formation or intestinal perforation.

Radiological examination (barium meal study) shows pathognomonic features in the form of *string sign,* due to marked narrowing of the lumen and *skip lesions* due to patchy involvement.

Treatment. It is a chronic disease with remissions and relapses over many years. Although there is no specific cure, but *corticosteroids* may induce remission in patients with active disease.

Resection of Small Intestine

Removal of short segment from the jejunum or ileum generally does not produce any severe symptoms. Because there occurs compensatory hypertrophy and hyperplasia of remaining mucosa (*intestinal adaptation*), the capacity of the jejunum to adapt is less than that of ileum.

Removal of ileum produces greater degree of malabsorption compared with removal of jejunum. Because ileal resection prevents absorption of bile salts causing decreased fat absorption, the entry of unabsorbed bile salts in the colon inhibits Na^+ and water reabsorption producing diarrhoea.

Removal of large segment of ileum leaving behind, duodenum, jejunum and a very small length of ileum produce malabsorption which is characterized by:

- *Normal carbohydrate absorption* (99% of ingested carbohydrates are absorbed).
- *Adequate protein absorption* (70% of ingested proteins are absorbed).
- *Markedly decreased fat absorption* which may produce:
  - Steatorrhoea, i.e. increase in faecal fat (see page 621),
  - Deficiency symptoms of fat-soluble vitamins (A, D, E and K),
  - Fatty infiltration of liver and cirrhosis,
- Markedly decreased calcium absorption due to the formation of insoluble calcium salts. Decreased serum calcium (hypocalcaemia) may produce tetany.

Gastrocolic Fistula In this condition, chyme enters directly into transverse colon from the stomach. It is characterized by the following additional features, over and above the features of large segment resection of ileum described above:

- *Pernicious anaemia,* due to the failure of absorption of vitamin B_{12}.
- *Hypovitaminosis* due to both water-soluble as well as fat-soluble vitamins.
- *Amino acid malabsorption,* which produces hypoproteinaemia (causing generalized oedema) and marked muscular weakness with wasting.

Blind Loop Syndrome Blind loop syndrome is characterized by formation of the areas of the intestine where bacteria can proliferate without being subjected to movement down the intestine.

Causes of blind loop formation are multiple diverticula in the small intestine, afferent loop after partial gastrectomy, areas of disordered peristalsis in small intestine and fistula from the upper small intestine to the colon.

Features. Colonization of small bowel by bacteria in blind loop syndrome may produce:

- *Malabsorption of fat* (steatorrhoea). It occurs due to deconjugation of bile salts by bacteria.
- *Megaloblastic anaemia,* due to vitamin B_{12} deficiency (which is taken up by bacteria).
- *Amino acid deficiency* (due to consumption by the bacteria) resulting in weakness and hypoproteinaemia.
- *Diarrhoea* and other nutritional deficiencies.

Diagnosis is confirmed by radiological demonstration of blind loop areas.

Treatment consists of broad-spectrum antibiotics and dietary and vitamin supplements. Occasionally, it may be necessary to correct a structural abnormality by surgical means.

Investigations are performed to confirm the malabsorption and its cause. These include:

i. *Routine blood tests.* If streatorrhea is suspected, these include urea, electrolyte, immunoglobulins, Ca^{2+}, Mg^{2+}, blood counts, clotting tests, albumin, folate and coelic antibodies.
ii. *To investigate small intestine,* the tests include duodenal biopsy, barium studies and sugar absorption test.
iii. *To investigate pancrease*, the tests include pancreatic function test, ultrasonography/CT scan.
iv. *To investigate bile salt malabsorption:*
   - Se HCAT scan and
   - Serum 7 α-hydroxycholestenon.

Tests of Intestinal Absorption

General Principle General principle of the commonly performed tests of intestinal absorption is to give a fixed quantity of nutrient, and measure its blood level, urinary excretion or faecal excretion (Fig. 7.7-9). The nutrient used for the test will depend upon the region to be tested (Fig. 7.7-10).

Carbohydrate Absorption Tests

1. ***D-xylose test.*** D-xylose is a pentose sugar that is completely absorbed from the small intestine as such but is neither metabolized nor stored in the body. The test is conducted in the fasting state, by giving 25 g D-xylose orally with 3–4 glasses of water and measuring its urinary excretion over the next 5 h.
   - Absorption is considered normal if more than 4 g of xylose appears in the urine over the 5-h period.
   - Lesser excretion in urine indicates malabsorption.
   - The diagnostic value of this test is compromised if the patient's kidney function is subnormal.
2. ***Lactose tolerance test***. After overnight fasting, blood glucose level and hydrogen concentration in the end-expiratory air is estimated. The subject is made to ingest 50 g of lactose. Results are interpreted as:
   - Absorption is considered normal if the rise in blood glucose is more than 50 mg/100 ml.
   - Lack of diarrhoea, abdominal discomfort and flatulence also point to adequate absorption.
   - Hydrogen concentration in the end-expiratory air, 90 min after ingestion of lactose, is a fairly reliable indicator of lactose tolerance. Normally, H_2 concentration is less than 15 ppm; a concentration greater than 20 ppm indicates lactose intolerance (in lactose intolerance, the unabsorbed lactose enters the

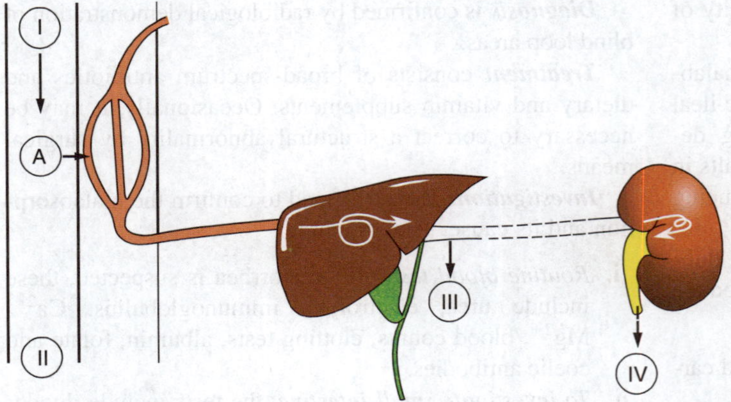

FIGURE 7.7-9 General principle of commonly performed tests of intestinal absorption. The intake is known (I), the quantity absorbed (A) may be estimated from the values of faecal loss (II) and/or blood levels (III) and urinary excretion (IV) of the substance.

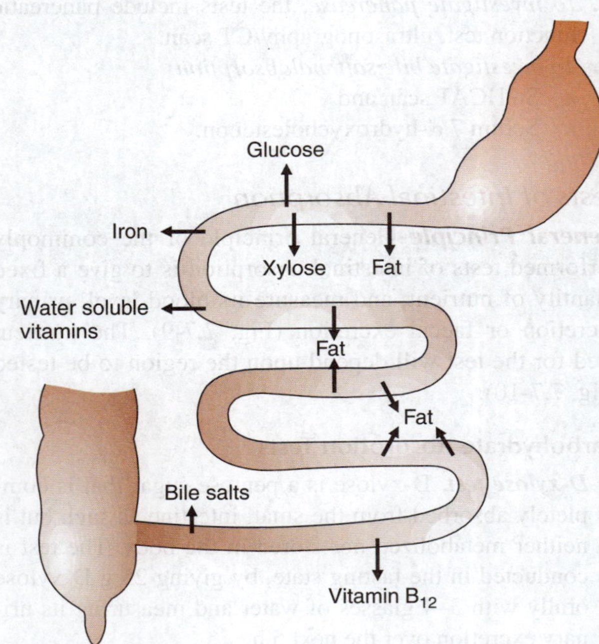

FIGURE 7.7-10 Predominant sites of absorption of nutrients. It helps to decide the nutrient to be used for any particular absorption test.

colon, where it generates H_2 after fermentation. The H_2 is absorbed in bloodstream and eliminated by the lungs).

Tests for Absorption of Fats and Related Substances

1. ***Faecal fat*** (see page 615).
2. ***^{131}I-triolein test.*** A measured quantity of radioactive triolein (a triglyceride) is given orally. The fraction excreted in the stool is assessed by radioactivity.
3. ***Absorption of fat-soluble vitamins*** can also be used as an index of fat absorption.
4. ***^{14}C-glycine–bile acid test*** is performed to test the absorption of bile acids.

Protein Absorption Tests

1. ***Faecal nitrogen excretion test*** (see page 615).
2. ***Serum protein estimation.*** Serum protein concentration is a fair indicator of protein absorption provided:
   - Protein intake is normal,
   - Liver is manufacturing adequate albumin,
   - There is no loss of proteins in urine and
   - There is no protein losing enteropathy.
3. ***Tests for protein losing enteropathy (PLE).*** In PLE, the absorption of proteins is normal but loss from the bowels is abnormally fast, leading to high protein content in stools. It can be tested by tagging the albumin with ^{51}Cr and then radioactive chromium is followed in the blood and stool.

Tests for Absorption of Water-soluble Vitamin

Schilling test (see page 615).

In practice, usually few screening procedures are sufficient to differentiate between the common causes of malabsorption (Table 7.7-3). Coelic disease is an example of generalized malabsorption, Crohn's disease is a localized disease of distal ileum and colon and chronic pancreatitis is an example of exocrine pancreatic insufficiency.

TABLE 7.7-3 Common Causes of Malabsorption and Tests for Differential Diagnosis

Test	Coeliac disease	Crohn's disease	Pancreatic insufficiency
1. Faecal fat contents	Increased	Increased	Increased
2. D-xylose absorption test	Impaired	Normal	Normal
3. Schilling test	Normal	Abnormal	Normal
4. Radiological examination of intestines	Abnormal	Abnormal	Normal

Section 8

Endocrinal System

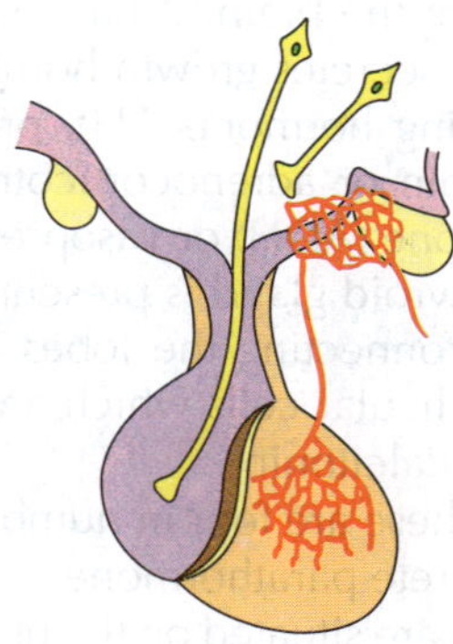

The biological functions of the multicellular living organisms are very well co-ordinated. This co-ordination is achieved by two main control systems, nervous system and the endocrinal system.

Nervous system is principally related with functions of the body in an external and internal environment. The nervous system co-ordinates the body functions through transmission of electrochemical impulses via nerve fibres.

Endocrinal system is mainly concerned with different metabolic functions of the body, especially the chemical reactions and transport of various substances. The endocrinal functions are accomplished through a wide range of chemical messengers, the hormones.

Relationship Between Endocrine and Neural Physiology

In a conceptual sense, the nervous system and the endocrine system have important functional similarities. Each is basically a system for signalling. In fact, the nervous system and the endocrine system often respond together to incoming stimuli so as to integrate the organism's response to changes in its external and internal environment. The co-ordinated function of these systems is well illustrated by the following example.

A significant decrease in the circulating blood volume is sensed by baroreceptors, the cardiac atria, the kidney and the brain. The sympathetic nervous system, a neurohormone from the posterior pituitary gland and hormones from the cardiac atria and ventricles, the adrenal medulla, the adrenal cortex and the kidneys act on target cells in blood vessels and kidneys to restore blood volume. Further, this *close relationship between the nervous and endocrine systems is illustrated by the following common characteristics*:

- Nervous and endocrine cells can both secrete substances into the bloodstream.
- Some endocrine cells and neurons generate electrical potentials and can be depolarized.
- Peptides originally discovered as products of endocrine cells have neurotransmitter function as well. Likewise, molecules normally considered to be neurotransmitters can act as hormones.
- Both biogenic amine neurotransmitters and peptide hormone molecules can be produced by a single cell.
- Certain factors such as neurogenin and nerve growth factor play a role in the development of both endocrine cells as well as nervous system.
- Structural similarities exist between the receptors for hormones and neurotransmitters.

Organization of Endocrine System

The endocrinal system consists of various endocrine glands and neurosecretory cells located in the hypothalamus. The neurosecretory cells of hypothalamus secrete certain neurohormones called releasing and inhibitory factors which influence the secretion of hormones from other endocrine glands. Certain other substances act as neurotransmitters in the brain and influence the secretion of neurosecretory cells of hypothalamus. The environmental factors through these neurotransmitters influence the whole endocrine system. The various endocrine glands present in the body are:

1. ***Pituitary gland (hypophysis).*** Pituitary gland is also known as hypophysis, which in Greek means undergrowth of the brain. It has two main parts: adenohypophysis and neurohypophysis. *Adenohypophysis* secretes growth hormone (GH) or somatotropins, follicle-stimulating hormone (FSH), luteinizing hormone (LH), prolactin, thyrotropin or thyroid-stimulating hormone (TSH) and corticotropin or adrenocorticotropic hormone (ACTH). The *neurohypophysis* stores the antidiuretic hormone (ADH) or vasopressin and oxytocin synthesized by the hypothalamus.
2. ***Thyroid gland***. The thyroid gland is present in the neck in front of trachea. It has two lobes and an isthmus (bridge) connecting the lobes. It secretes thyroxine ($\mathbf{T}_4$) and triiodothyronine ($\mathbf{T}_3$). The C cells or parafollicular cells which are scattered in the spaces between the follicles of the thyroid gland secrete calcitonin.
3. ***Parathyroid glands***. These are four in number; very small glands situated behind the lobes of the thyroid gland and secrete parathormone.
4. ***Adrenal glands***. These are situated on the upper poles of the two kidneys, hence also called suprarenal glands. The outer cortex region of the adrenal glands secretes cortisol, aldosterone and sex steroids, and the inner medullary region secretes catecholamines (adrenaline and noradrenaline).
5. ***Pancreatic islets (islets of Langerhans)***. These are small groups of cells which secrete insulin, glucagon and somatostatin.
6. ***Gonads.*** These include ovaries in females and testes in males. The ovaries secrete oestrogens and progesterone (female sex steroids), and testes secrete male sex hormone (testosterone).
7. ***Pineal gland***. It is a small gland present in the roof of third ventricle in the brain. It secretes melatonin and other biogenic amines.
8. ***Placenta***. During pregnancy, the placenta secretes various hormones like human chorionic gonadotropin (HCG), oestrogen, progesterone, somatotropins and relaxin.
9. ***Gastrointestinal mucosa*** also secretes various hormones collectively known as gastrointestinal (GIT) hormones, e.g. gastrin, secretin, cholecystokinin-pancreozymin (CCK-PZ), etc.
10. ***Kidneys***. In addition to their renal functions, the kidneys secrete erythropoietin, prostaglandins and 1,25-dihydroxycholecalciferol, and also help in activation of angiotensin production.
11. ***Atrial muscle cells***. These secrete atrial natriuretic peptides (ANP) and many other peptides.
12. ***Skin***. This is also considered to act as an endocrine structure by producing vitamin D, which is now considered to be a hormone.

Chapter 8.1

General Principles of Endocrinal System

HORMONES: DEFINITION AND CLASSIFICATION

Definition

The word hormone is derived from the Greek word *hormaein,* which means to execute or to arouse. In the classic definition, hormones are secretory products of the ductless glands which are released in catalytic amounts into bloodstream and transported to specific target cells (or organs), where they elicit physiologic, morphologic and biochemical responses. In reality, the requirement that hormones be secreted into the bloodstream is too restrictive, because they can also act locally. Therefore, the chemical messengers that perform hormonal functions are defined as (Fig. 8.1-1):

1. Endocrine Hormones. These include the chemical messengers whose function is the transmission of a molecular signal from a classic endocrinal cell through the bloodstream to a distant target cell (Fig. 8.1-1A).

2. Neurocrine Hormones. Nervous communication involves the release of chemical messengers from nerve terminals, which may reach their target cells via one of three routes:

- ***Neurotransmitters*** can be released directly into the intercellular space, cross the synaptic junction and inhibit or activate the postsynaptic cell, e.g. acetylcholine and norepinephrine.
- ***Neural signals can be transferred via gap junction,*** which is a membrane stabilization between the nerve cells, between nerve terminals and endocrine cells and between endocrine cells.
- ***Neurohormones*** or peptides are released from a neurosecretory neuron into the bloodstream and then carried to a distant target cells (Fig. 8.1-1B). Example of such neurocrine substances are oxytocin and antidiuretic hormone (ADH). The effector sites of neurohormones are not always endocrine cells.

3. Paracrine Hormones. These chemical messengers, which after getting secreted by a cell, are carried over short distance by diffusion through the interstitial spaces (extracellular fluid) to act on the neighbouring different cell types as or a regulatory substance (Fig. 8.1-1C). For example, in islets of Langerhans, somatostatin secreted by the delta cells acts on the alpha and beta cells.

4. Autocrine Hormones. These refer to those chemical messengers which regulate the activity of neighbouring similar type of cells (Fig. 8.1-1D). Examples of autocrine hormones are prostaglandins.

Note. It is important to note that according to the route by which it is transmitted, the same chemical messenger may act as endocrinal hormone (bloodstream conveyance), or as a paracrine, or as an autocrine hormone (local conveyance),

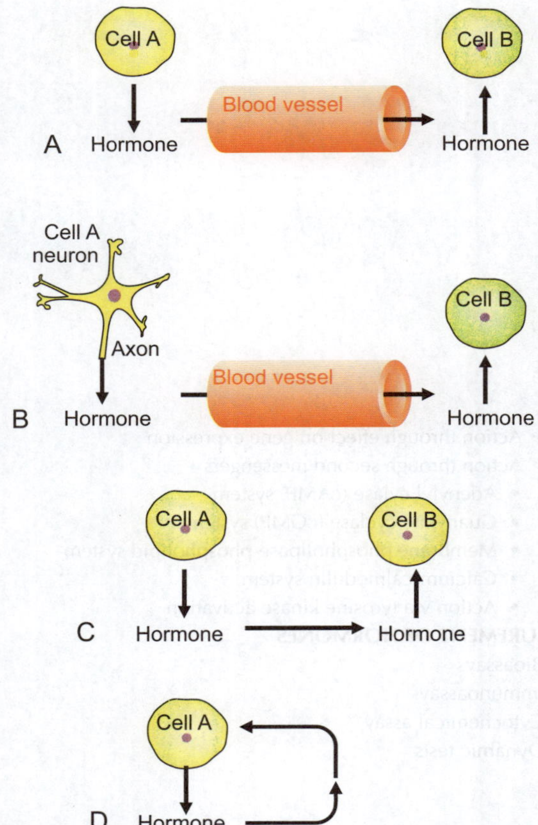

FIGURE 8.1-1 Different types of hormones (by their mechanism of action) are: **A,** endocrine hormone; **B,** neurocrine hormone; **C,** paracrine hormone; and **D,** autocrine hormone.

e.g. insulin secreted by beta cells in the pancreatic islets may act as:

- *Endocrine hormone.* When released into bloodstream, insulin acts on the adipose tissue, muscle, liver and brain to regulate energy stores, carbohydrate, fat and protein metabolism.
- *Paracrine hormone.* Insulin, when released into the islets interstitial fluid, inhibits the neighbouring alpha cells of the islets.
- *Autocrine hormone.* The insulin released in the islets interstitial fluid can regulate growth and function of beta cells themselves as they possess insulin receptors.

Classification of Hormones

A. Depending upon the Chemical Nature

1. ***Amines or amino acid derivatives,*** e.g.

- Catecholamines (epinephrine and norepinephrine),
- Thyroxine (T_4) and triiodothyronine (T_3)

2. ***Proteins and polypeptides***

i. Short-chain polypeptides include:
- Posterior pituitary hormones
- Antidiuretic hormone (ADH) and
- Oxytocin.

ii. Long-chain polypeptides include:
- Insulin,
- Glucagon,
- Parathormone and
- Other anterior pituitary hormones.

3. ***Steroid hormones:*** These include:

- Glucocorticoids,
- Mineralocorticoids,
- Sex steroids and
- Vitamin D.

B. Depending Upon the Mechanism of Action

- ***Group I hormones.*** These act by binding to intracellular receptor and mediate their actions via formation of a hormone receptor complex. These include steroid, retinoid and thyroid hormones.
- ***Group II hormones.*** These involve second messenger to mediate their effect. Depending upon the chemical nature of the second messengers, group II hormones are further divided into four subgroups A, B, C and D (Table 8.1-1).

HORMONES: GENERAL CONSIDERATIONS

Hormone Chemistry, Synthesis, Storage and Release

1. Amines or Amino Acid Derivatives

Synthesis. These hormones include catecholamines, thyroid hormone and calciferol, which are derived from the amino acid tyrosine. Thyroid hormones are derived from two iodinated tyrosine residues. Thyroid hormones are the only substances in the body that contain iodine. These are synthesized in the cell cytoplasm.

Storage and Release

- *Catecholamines* are stored in secretory granules inside the cytoplasm of chromaffin cells. Secretion occurs when the membrane of granule fuses with the plasma membrane, causing the granular contents to be extruded into the circulation.
- *Thyroid hormones* are stored outside the follicular cells in the form of thyroglobulin. Following endocytosis and proteolysis of thyroglobulin, thyroid hormones are secreted into the bloodstream by simple diffusion.
- *Calciferol* (1,25-dihydroxy-vitamin D_3) is stored as a precursor in the form of 7-dehydrocholesterol or cholecalciferol (vitamin D_3) in the skin.

2. Protein and Polypeptide Hormones

Synthesis. The peptide and protein hormones are composed of chains of amino acids linked by peptide bonds. These are synthesized in the granular endoplasmic reticulum of glandular cells in the same manner as other proteins:

- The amino acid sequence is determined by specific deoxyribonucleic acid (DNA) molecules through the messenger ribonucleic acid (mRNA).

TABLE 8.1-1 Types of Group II Hormones Based on the Chemical Nature of Second Messenger Involved in their Mechanism of Action

Group	Second messenger	Hormones
Group II-A	Cyclic AMP (cAMP)	Adrenocorticotropic hormone (ACTH) Antidiuretic hormone (ADH) Angiotensin II Calcitonin Corticotropic hormones (CRH) Catecholamine (α_2 adrenergic) Follicle-stimulating hormone (FSH) Glucagon Luteinizing hormone (LH) Parathormone (PTH) Somatostatin Thyroid-stimulating hormone (TSH)
Group II-B	Cyclic GMP (cGMP)	Atrial natriuretic factor (ANF) and nitric oxide
Group II-C	Calcium/or phosphatidyl inositol or both	Acetylcholine (ACh), catecholamines (α_1 adrenergic), gastrin, oxytocin, thyrotropin releasing hormone (TRH), gonadotropin-releasing hormone (GnRH), platelet-derived growth factor (PDGF) and substances
Group II-D	Kinase or phosphatase cascade	Human chorionic somatotropin (HCS), erythropoietin, growth hormone, insulin and insulin-like growth factors (IGF-I and IGF-II), nerve growth factor (NGF), prolactin and other growth factors

- First the precursor hormone (prohormone, or preprohormone) is synthesized in the rough endoplasmic reticulum.
- Then the precursor hormone is converted into proper hormone within the Golgi complex by post-translational cleavage.

Storage and Release. Protein and polypeptide hormones are stored exclusively in subcellular membrane-bound secretory granules within the cytoplasm of endocrine cell until a release signal is received. On receiving the release signal, these hormones are released into the blood by exocytosis.

3. Steroid Hormones

Synthesis. Steroids are hydrophobic lipid-soluble substances. These are synthesized from cholesterol.

Storage and Release. There is little storage of steroids. Instead, different precursors of cholesterol and intermediate compounds are present in the cells. These serve as precursors and when the necessity of hormone arises, the enzymatic action converts them into steroids which are released in the circulation by simple diffusion.

Hormone Transport, Plasma Concentration and Half-Life

Hormone Transport After secretion into bloodstream, the hormones may circulate in two forms:

Unbound Form. Some hormones circulate as free molecule, e.g. catecholamines and most peptide and protein hormones circulate unbound.

Bound form. Some hormones, such as steroids, thyroid hormones and vitamin D, circulate bound to specific globulins that are synthesized in the liver. The binding of hormones to proteins is advantageous as it:

- Protects the hormone against clearance by the kidney,
- Slows down the rate of degradation by the liver and
- Provides circulating reserve of the hormone.

Some hormones are carried in the blood as inactive forms with proteins. They become active at the target site only. Only unbound hormones pass through capillaries to produce their effects or to degrade.

Plasma Concentration Hormones are usually secreted into the circulation in extremely low concentrations:

- *Peptide hormone concentration is between* 10^{-12} and 10^{-10} mol/L.
- *Epinephrine and norepinephrine concentrations are* 2 $\times 10^{-10}$ and 13 $\times 10^{-10}$ mol/L, respectively.
- *Steroid and thyroid hormone concentrations are* 10^{-9} *and* 10^{-6} *mol/L, respectively.*

Half-Life Most hormones are metabolized rapidly after secretion. In general:

- Peptide hormones have short half-life.
- Steroids and thyroid hormones have significantly longer half-life because they are bound to plasma proteins. Table 8.1-2 depicts half-life of some of the hormones.

TABLE 8.1-2 Half-Life of Some of the Important Hormones

Class of hormone	Hormone	Half-life
Protein and peptide hormones	ADH	<1 min
	Oxytocin	<1 min
	Insulin	5 min
	Prolactin	12 s
	Growth hormone	<30 min
	ACTH	15–25 s
	LH	15–45 min
	FSH	180 min
Amines	Epinephrine	10 s
	Norepinephrine	15 s
	Thyroxine (T_4)	5–7 days
	Triiodothyronine (T_3)	1–3 days
Steroid hormones	Aldosterone	30 min
	Cortisol	90–100 min
	1,25-Dihydroxycholecalciferol	15 h
	25-Hydroxycholecalciferol	15 days

Functions of Hormones

Hormones regulate existing fundamental processes but do not initiate reactions de novo.

1. Regulation of Biochemical Reactions. Hormones regulate the metabolic functions in a variety of ways:

- They stimulate or inhibit the rate and magnitude of biochemical reactions by controlling enzymes and thereby cause morphologic, biochemical and functional changes in target tissues.
- They modulate energy-producing processes and regulate the circulating levels of energy-yielding substances (e.g. glucose, fatty acids). However, they are not used as energy sources in biochemical reactions.

2. Regulation of bodily processes. Hormones regulate different bodily processes such as growth, maturation, differentiation, regeneration, reproduction and behaviour. Thus, the main function of endocrine glands is to maintain homeostasis in an internal environment. For these functions, the hormones do not act directly on the intracellular machinery.

Hormone Disposal

Mechanisms of Hormone Disposal The circulating hormones are disposed off by the following mechanisms:

- Target cell uptake and intracellular degradation,
- Metabolic degradation/inactivation and
- Urinary or biliary secretion.

1. Target cell Uptake and Intracellular Degradation. The interaction of hormones with their target cells is followed by intracellular degradation.

- *Degradation of protein and amine hormones* occurs after binding to membrane receptors, and then internalization of hormone receptor complex.
- *Degradation of thyroid and steroid* hormones occurs after binding the hormone receptor complex to the chromatin.

2. Metabolic Degradation/Inactivation. Only a small fraction of the circulating hormone is removed by target tissue cells; most of the hormone extraction and degradation occurs in the liver and kidneys. Metabolic degradation occurs by enzymatic processes that include proteolysis, oxidation, reduction, hydroxylation, decarboxylation and methylation. Virtually all the hormones are extracted from the plasma and degraded to some extent by the liver. In addition, glucuronization and sulfaction of hormones or their metabolites may be carried out, and the conjugates are subsequently excreted in the bile or urine.

3. Urinary and Biliary Excretion. Renal clearance of hormones is reduced greatly by protein binding in the plasma, e.g. less than 10% of secreted cortisol appears unchanged in the urine, because only the small, free fraction of plasma cortisol is filtered by the glomerulus. On the other hand, about 30% of cortisol metabolites are excreted in urine, because they are generally unbound or only loosely bound to protein. Peptide and smaller protein hormones are filtered to some degree by the glomerulus. However, they may subsequently undergo tubular reabsorption and degradation within the kidney, so that only a small fraction appears in the final urine. Further, as mentioned above, the conjugated hormones are excreted in the bile or urine.

Metabolic Clearance Rate. Metabolic clearance rate (MCR) refers to the sum of all the removal processes, i.e. target cell uptake and degradation, metabolic degradation and urinary or biliary excretion. In a steady rate, MCR is defined as the volume of plasma cleared/unit time, which equals mass removed/unit time divided by circulating mass/unit volume, that is,

$$\text{MCR} = \frac{\text{mg/minute removed}}{\text{mg/ml of plasma}} = \frac{\text{ml cleared}}{\text{minute}}$$

MCR is inversely correlated with plasma half-life.

Functional Turnover Rate (k). Functional turnover rate (k) refers to the ratio of MCR to the volume of distribution of a hormone. The plasma half-life, which is inversely related to k, is a *wider* but more conveniently determined index of hormone disappearance.

Regulation of Hormone Secretion

The quantity of hormones secreted is regulated in accordance with their requirement. General mechanisms that govern the secretion of hormone include:

- Feedback control,
- Neural control and
- Chronotropic control.

1. Feedback Control Regulation of a hormone in terms of requirement is best accomplished through feedback from the blood concentration of the hormone concerned (hormone–hormone) or some result of action of the hormone (substrate–hormone). Feedback control is of two types:

- Negative feedback control and
- Positive feedback control.

Negative Feedback Control. Generally, the influence of blood concentration of the hormone concerned or its effect is to inhibit further secretion of the hormone and is called negative feedback control (Fig. 8.1-2A).

Positive Feedback Control. This is less common and acts to amplify the initial biological effects of the hormone (Fig. 8.1-2B).

Depending upon the product involved, the feedback mechanism may be:

- Hormone–hormone feedback,
- Substrate–hormone feedback and
- Mineral–hormone feedback.

i. Hormone–Hormone Feedback Control. The best example of hormone–hormone negative feedback control is regulation of hormone secretions by hypothalamus and pituitary, which involves three loops (Fig. 8.1-3):

- ***Long-loop feedback*** (Fig. 8.1-3A). The peripheral gland hormone (e.g. thyroid, adrenocortical and gonads) can exert long-loop negative feedback control on both the hypothalamus and the anterior lobe of pituitary.
- ***Short-loop feedback*** (Fig. 8.1-3B). The pituitary trophic hormones decrease the secretion of hypophysiotrophic hormone (e.g. GHRH, GHIH, TRH, GnRH, etc.) by short-loop feedback.
- ***Ultrashort-loop feedback*** (Fig. 8.1-3C). The hypophysiotrophic hormones may inhibit their own synthesis and secretion via an ultrashort-loop feedback mechanism.

ii. Substrate–Hormone Feedback Control. The best example of substrate–hormone feedback control is regulation of insulin secretion from pancreatic beta cells of islets of Langerhans and glucagon secretion from alpha

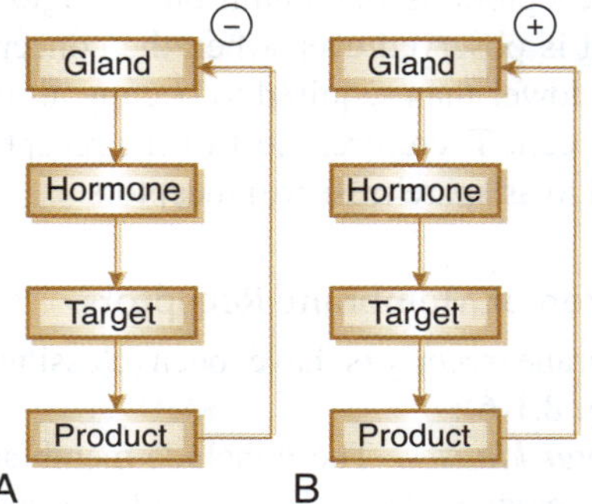

FIGURE 8.1-2 Hormonal regulation by feedback control mechanism: **A,** negative feedback; and **B,** positive feedback.

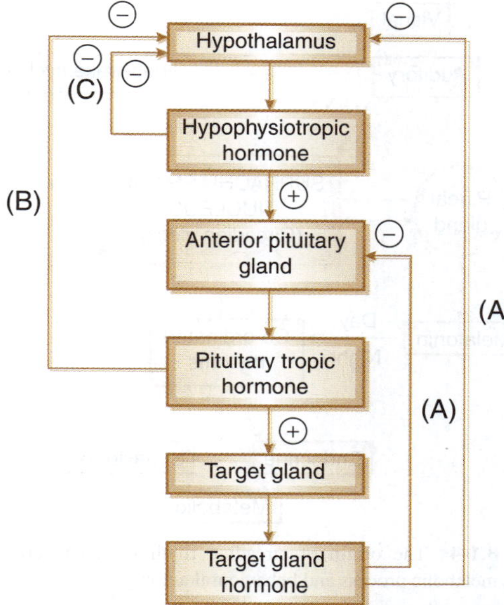

FIGURE 8.1-3 Hormone–hormone negative feedback control by hypothalamus and pituitary: A, long loop feedback; B, short loop feedback; and C, ultrashort loop feedback.

cells by blood glucose levels. A rise in blood glucose level promotes the secretion of insulin, while a fall in blood glucose promotes secretion of glucagon. These responses keep the blood glucose level within narrow limits in spite of variation in carbohydrate intake in diet.

iii. Mineral–Hormone Feedback

2. Neural Control Neural control acts to evoke or suppress hormone secretion in response to both external and internal stimuli.

External stimuli which can modulate hormone release through neural mechanisms may be visual, auditory, olfactory, gustatory and tactile.

Internal stimuli which influence hormonal release through neural mechanism include pain, emotion, sexual excitement, fright, stress and changes in blood volume.

Neural control depending upon the type of nerve fibres involved may be:

- Adrenergic,
- Cholinergic,
- Dopaminergic,
- Serotoninergic and
- Gabaergic.

Examples of neural control of hormones are:

- *Release of oxytocin,* which fills the milk ducts in response to the stimulus of suckling,
- *Release of aldosterone,* which augments the circulatory volume in response to upright posture and
- *Release of melatonin* in response to darkness.

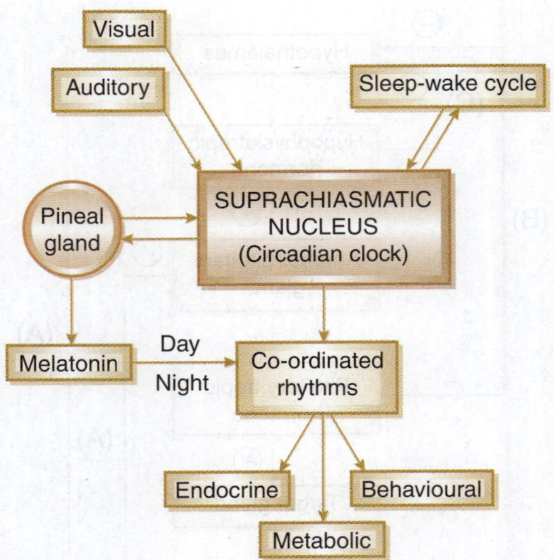

FIGURE 8.1-4 The origin of circadian rhythms in endocrine gland secretion, metabolic process and behavioural activity.

3. Chronotropic Control Chronotropic control of hormone secretion accounts for:

- Oscillating and pulsatile release of certain hormones,
- Diurnal variation in hormonal levels,
- Menstrual rhythm,
- Seasonal rhythm and
- Developmental rhythm.

The source of regular oscillatory cycles is a pulse generator(s) located in the suprachiasmatic nucleus (SCN) of the hypothalamus (Fig. 8.1-4).

The intrinsic circadian clock is also located in the SCN, which is responsible for endocrinal, metabolic and behavioural co-ordinated rhythms.

HORMONE: RECEPTORS AND MECHANISM OF ACTION

Hormone Receptors

All hormones act through specific receptors. Almost all hormone receptors are large proteins present in hormone-sensitive target cells.

Characteristics of Hormone Receptors

Receptor Specificity. There are specific receptors for each hormone. This is the reason that all hormones circulate to all parts of the body, yet each hormone has a specific target tissue for its action (Fig. 8.1-5).

Receptor Location. Depending upon the location, receptors are of two types:

i. *Internal receptors* are located inside the cells, e.g. receptors for steroid hormones and thyroid hormones are localized within the nucleus of target cells.

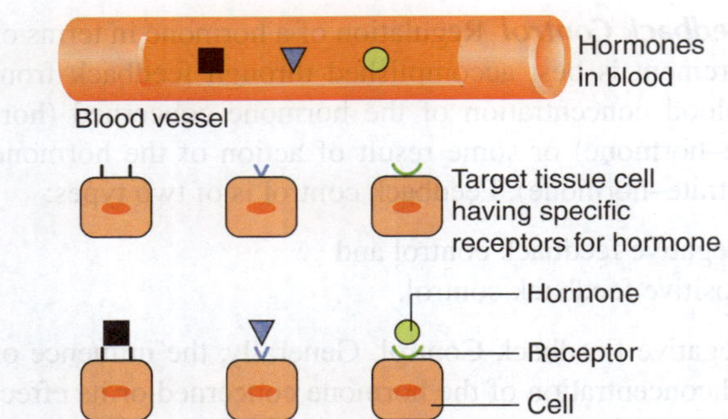

FIGURE 8.1-5 Specificity of hormone action is because of specific receptors.

ii. *External receptors* are located on the plasma membrane of target cells, e.g. peptide and protein hormones, amines and prostaglandins are interspersed within the phospholipid bilayer of the plasma membranes.

Receptor affinity refers to the degree of attraction between the hormone and receptor and is measured from the speed of hormone binding by the receptor.

Receptor capacity refers to the quantity of hormone binding.

Receptor density. Approximately 10^4–10^5 receptors exist on the surface of a polypeptide hormone target cell, and about 3×10^3–3×10^4 intracellular receptors exist per steroid target cell.

Change in Receptor Number. Number of receptors of a cell vary depending upon the situation. It is regulated by two mechanisms: downregulation and upregulation.

i. ***Downregulation*** refers to decrease in the number of active receptors. It occurs to regulate the hormone sensitivity when it is present in excess. For example, elevated ambient insulin concentration causes a loss or inactivation of insulin receptors in liver cells, fat cells and white blood cells (WBCs).

ii. ***Upregulation*** refers to increase in the number of active receptors on a cell. It occurs to regulate the hormone action when its concentration is less. This phenomenon tends to reduce the effect of hormone deficiency.

Spare Receptors. A maximum physiologic response of a target cell is observed even when the concentration of a hormone is lower than required to occupy all of the receptors on that cell. Therefore, most of the receptors (~97%) are referred to as spare (reserve) receptors.

Classification of Membrane Receptors

Cell membrane receptors have been classified into four classes (Fig. 8.1-6):

1. Receptor kinases. These include membrane receptors that contain enzyme activity. For example, receptors for insulin hormone contain tyrosine or serine kinase as an intrinsic part of structure.

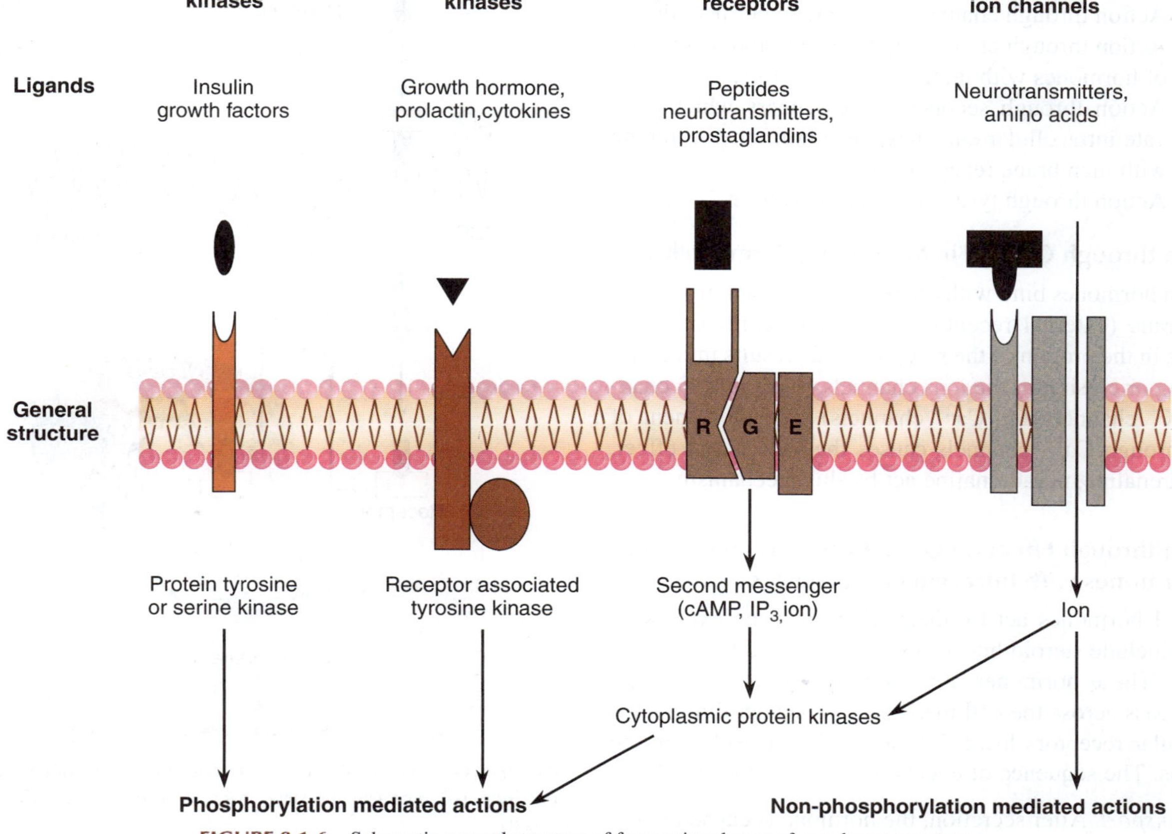

FIGURE 8.1-6 Schematic general structure of four major classes of membrane receptors.

2. ***Receptor-linked Kinases.*** These have no intrinsic enzyme activity, e.g. receptors for growth hormone, prolactin and cytokines.

3. ***G-protein-coupled Receptors.*** Examples are: receptors for pituitary tropic hormones, glucagon, epinephrine norepinephrine, parathyroid hormone and prostaglandins.

4. ***Ligand-gated Ion Channels.*** These act as receptors for neurotransmitters such as acetylcholine (ACh), γ-aminobutyric acid (GABA) and glycine.

Structure of a Receptor

The receptors in general have two parts or domains: a recognition domain (R), and a coupling domain (C) (Fig. 8.1-7).

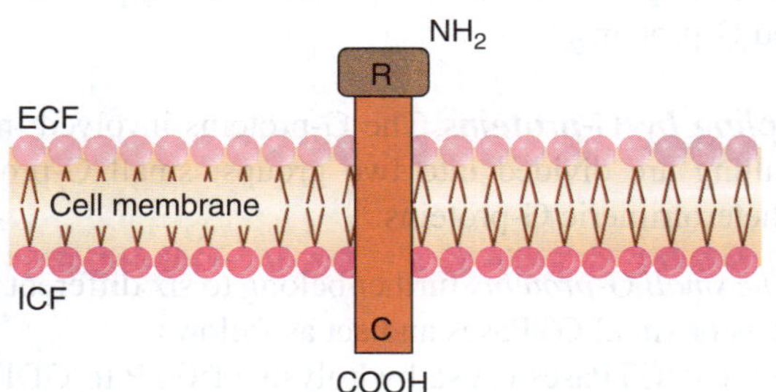

FIGURE 8.1-7 General structure of a hormonal receptor.

Recognition domain (R). It is that part of the receptor where the hormone binds. It is formed by extracellular N-terminus portion of the receptor (extracellularly projected NH_2 group).

Coupling domain (C). It is that part of receptor which initiates signals for intracellular activities after the recognition. It is formed by the intracellular C-terminus tail of the receptor (intracellularly projected carboxyl, i.e. COOH). The membrane receptors wind in and out of the plasma membrane by means of seven transmembrane segments.

Mechanism of Action of Hormones

As mentioned previously, all hormones act through specific receptors, and depending upon the mechanism of action hormones they have been divided into group I and group II (Table 8.1-1).

Group I hormones act by affecting gene expression at cellular level, and

Group II hormones act through intermediary molecules called second messenger, and depending upon the chemical nature of second messenger, the group II hormones have been further divided into subgroups A, B, C and D (Table 8.1-1).

The main mechanisms of hormone actions are:

- Action through change in membrane permeability,
- Action through effect on gene expression by binding of hormones with intracellular receptors,
- Action through secondary messengers which activate intracellular enzymes when hormones combine with membrane receptors and
- Action through tyrosine kinase activation.

Action through Change in Membrane Permeability

Certain hormones bind with the receptors present in the cell membrane (external receptors) and cause conformational change in the protein of the receptors, this results into either opening or closing of the ions channels (such as Na^+ channels, K^+ channels and Ca^{2+} channels). The movement of ions through Ca^{2+} channels causes the subsequent effect, e.g. adrenaline, noradrenaline act by this mechanism.

Action through Effect on Gene Expression by Binding of Hormones with Intracellular Receptors

Group I hormones act by their effect on gene expression which include steroid hormones, retinoids and thyroid hormones. These hormones are lipophilic in nature and can easily pass across the cell membrane. They act through intracellular receptors located either in the cytosol or in the nucleus. The sequence of events involved is (Fig. 8.1-8):

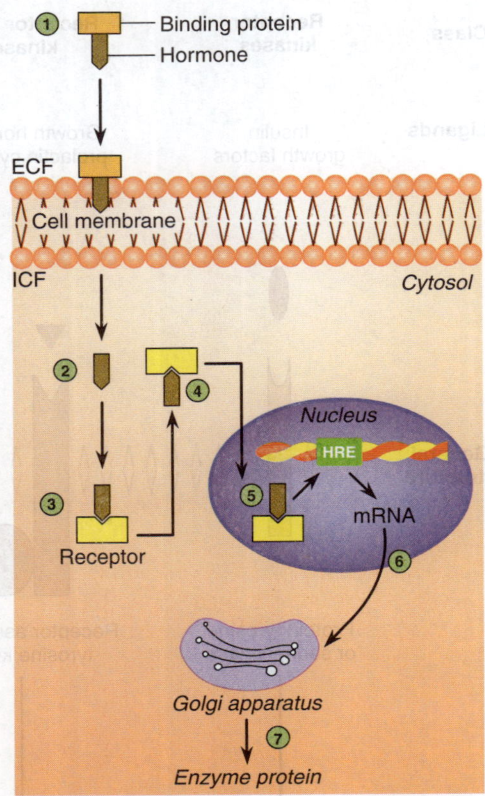

FIGURE 8.1-8 Action of hormones through their effect of gene expression. Note 1–7 represent the steps involved in the process (for details see text).

1. *Transport.* After secretion, the hormone is carried to the target tissue on serum-binding protein.
2. *Internalization.* Being lipophilic, the hormone easily diffuses through the plasma membrane.
3. *Receptor–hormone complex* is formed by binding of hormone to the specific receptor inside the cell. There are three distinct pathways by which primary messenger alter transcription and gene expression as under:
   - Primary messenger (in case of steroid and thyroid hormone) directly binds to nuclear receptor and directly interacts with DNA to alter gene expression.
   - By activation of cytoplasmic receptor protein (kinase) that moves into the nucleus and activates latent transcription factor causing phosphorylation, e.g. *mitogen-activated protein kinase (MAP).*
   - The third pathway is the activation of latent transcription factor present in the cytosol. This pathway is shared by nuclear factor kappa B (NF_KB) and signal transducers of activated transcription (STATs).
4. *Conformational change* occurs in receptor proteins leading to activation of receptors.
5. The activated receptor–hormone complex then diffuses into the nucleus and binds on the specific region on the DNA known as hormone responsive element (HRE), which initiates gene transcription.
6. *Binding of the receptor–hormone complex to DNA* alters the rate of transcription of messenger RNA (mRNA).
7. *The mRNA diffuses in the cytoplasm,* where it promotes the translation process at the ribosomes. In this way, new proteins are formed which result in specific responses. Some of the new proteins synthesized are enzymes.

Note. The hormonal action mediated through intracellular receptors is comparatively slower due to the time (45 min to several hours) involved in the processes described above. Therefore, glucocorticoids may take hours to few days to achieve the therapeutic effect.

Action through Second Messengers

The peptides and biogenic amines are two principal classes of hormones which act through second messengers and are classified as group II hormones (Table 8.1-1). Such hormones are also called first messengers. The release of second messenger is mediated by GTP-binding proteins also called G-proteins.

Coupling by G-proteins The G-proteins involved in cell signalling are divided into two groups: small G-proteins and heterotrimeric G-proteins.

(i) *The small G-proteins* further belong to six different families or small GTPases and act as follows:

- The GTPases cause hydrolysis of GTP to GDP and tend to inactivate small G-proteins.

- Guanine exchange factors (GEFs), present on the active site, activate G-protein by encouraging exchange of GDP for GTP.
- Some small G-proteins lead to lipid modification and thus help to anchor them to the membrane.
- Some small G-proteins are free to diffuse into the cytosol.

Functions:

- The Rab family members of small G-proteins regulate vesicular movement between endoplasmic reticulum, the Golgi apparatus, lysosomes and cell membrane.
- The Rho/Rac family small G-proteins mediate interaction between cytoskeleton and cell membrane.
- Ras family small G-proteins are responsible for regulation of growth by transmission of signals from the cell membrane to the nucleus.

(ii) *Heterotrimeric G-proteins* are large G-proteins that couple the receptors to catalytic units on the cell surface and catalyse the formation of intracellular second messenger. The heterotrimeric G-proteins are made up of three subunits (α, β and γ). The α and γ subunits help in anchoring of G-protein to the cell surface (Fig. 8.1-8). The α subunit is bound to GDP. When hormone or ligand binds to G-protein-coupled receptor the GDP is exchanged with GTP and α subunit separates from the β and γ subunits and is responsible for various biological activities. The intrinsic GTPase activity of separated α subunit converts GTP into GDP and leads to reassociation of α subunit with β and γ subunits.

- The regulators of G-protein signalling (RGS) accelerate α subunit GTPase activity.
- The heterotrimeric G-protein involved in relaying signals for more than 1000 G-protein receptors

  G-protein-coupled receptors structurally (GPCRs) are barrel like.
- The G-protein-coupled receptors (GPCR) are seven helix or serpentine receptors and span the cell membrane seven times.

  Mechanism of action: When a ligand binds the GPCR, a conformational change occurs, which activates heterotrimeteric G-protein-associated cytoplasm, i.e. leaf of plasma membrane which in turn activates many G-proteins, thus leading to amplification of the effect. A large number of ligands act through G-protein-coupled proteins. These include: (Table 8.1-3).
- ***Events involved in coupling by G-protein which lead onto changes in the cellular concentration*** of the second messengers are summarized (Fig. 8.1-9):
  - Group II hormones are water soluble and bind to the plasma membrane of the target cell via cell surface receptors.
  - The hormone-bearing receptor then interacts with a G-protein and activates it by binding GTP. There are two classes of G-proteins: stimulatory G-protein (Gs) and inhibitory G-protein (Gi).

TABLE 8.1-3 The Ligands Act via G-Protein-Coupled Receptors.

Type of ligands	Examples
Neurotransmitters	Epinephrine, norepinephrine, dopamine, 5-HT, acetylcholine, opiods and adenosine
Tachykinins	Substance P, neuropeptide-K and neurokinin
Hormones	Vasopressin, angiotensin II, oxytocin, VIP, GRP, parathyroid, TRH, TSH, FSH, LH, HCG
Arachidonic acid derivatives	Thromboxane A_2
Other	Endothelins, odorants and tastants, platelet-activating factor, cannabinoid and light

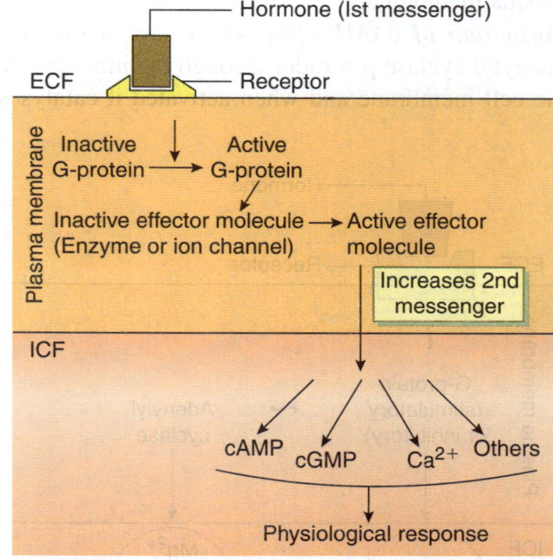

FIGURE 8.1-9 Schematic mechanism of coupling by G-protein leading to increase in second messenger which mediates hormone's physiological response.

- In its activated ("on") state, the G-protein interacts with one or more of the effector protein (most of which are enzymes or ion channels such as adenylyl cyclase, Ca^{2+} or K^+ channels or phospholipase C, A_2 or D) to activate or inhibit them.
- The changed effector molecules in turn generate second messenger that mediates the hormone's intracellular action.

Second Messenger Systems The second messenger systems that are activated through coupling of hormone receptor complexes by G-protein include:

- Adenylyl cyclase–cAMP system,
- Guanylyl cyclase–cGMP system,

- Membrane phospholipase–phospholipid system and
- Calcium–calmodulin system.

1. Adenylyl Cyclase–cAMP System. The adenylyl cyclase–cAMP system was the first to be described by Sutherland in 1961 that initiated the concept of second messenger. The hormones which act through this system constitute the group IIA hormones (Table 8.1-1). The steps involved in the hormone action via adenylyl cyclase–cAMP system are summarized below (Fig. 8.1-10):

i. ***Binding of hormone*** *(Step 1)* to a specific receptor in the cell membrane.

ii. ***Activation of G-protein*** *(Step 2)*. After formation of hormone–receptor complex, the GDP is released from the G-protein and is replaced by GTP, i.e. G-protein is activated.

iii. ***Activation of enzyme adenylyl cyclase*** *(Step 3)*. The hormone–receptor complex via activated G-protein (stimulatory or inhibitory) either stimulates or inhibits the enzyme adenylyl cyclase which is also located in the plasma membrane.

iv. ***Formation of cAMP*** *(Step 4)*. A part of the enzyme adenylyl cyclase protrudes through the inner surface of the cell membrane and when activated it catalyses the formation of cAMP from cytoplasmic ATP with Mg^{2+} as cofactor. A stimulatory G-protein (Gs) therefore increases intracellular cAMP levels, whereas an inhibitory G-protein (Gi) decreases cAMP levels.

v. ***Action of cAMP.*** The cAMP once formed stimulates a cascade of enzyme activation. One molecule of cAMP may stimulate many enzymes. Therefore, even the slightest amount of hormone acting on the cell surface can initiate a very powerful response. The cyclic AMP so formed initiates response by different mechanisms in eukaryotic and prokaryotic cells.

In eukaryotic cells, the cAMP activates protein kinase A *(Step 5)* which phosphorylates the specific proteins, producing highly specific physiological actions *(Step 6):*

- Increase in cell permeability (e.g. ion transport and secretion),
- Increase in synthesis of enzyme system (enzyme induction),
- Activation of enzymes present in the cell.
- Release of hormones from storage pack cells and steroidogenesis,
- Gene regulation and so on.

In prokaryotic cells, in contrast to eukaryotic cells, the cAMP acts directly at the gene level. It binds to a specific protein called *catabolic regulatory protein (CRP).* In association with CRP, it binds to DNA and influences gene expression or transcription. Therefore, cAMP in prokaryotic cells acts just like steroid hormones.

vi. ***Inactivation of cAMP.*** The cAMP is degraded to 5'-AMP (inactive form) by enzyme phosphodiesterase. Hence, the effect of cAMP is short lived if the hormone stimulating adenylyl cyclase is removed. Phosphodiesterase inhibitors such as caffeine and theophylline would be expected to augment the physiologic action of cAMP.

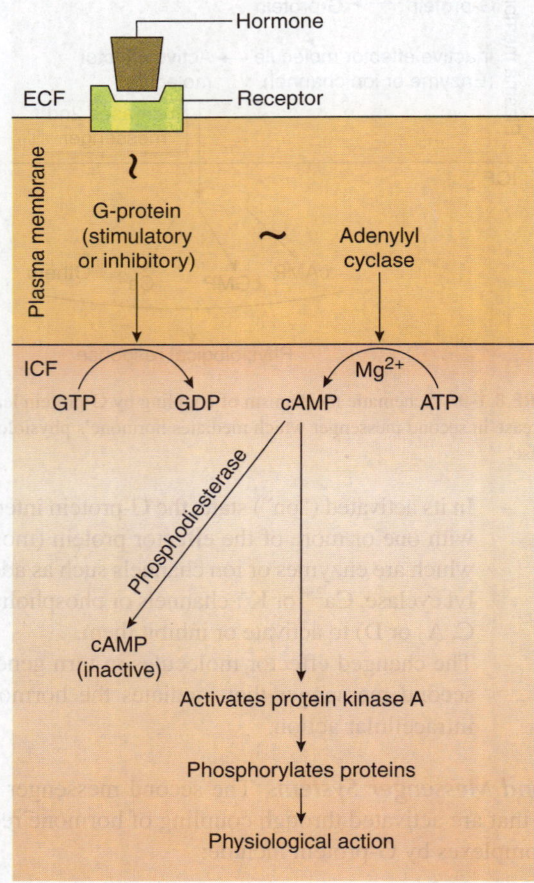

FIGURE 8.1-10 Mechanism of action of hormone through adenylyl cyclase (cAMP) system as second messenger.

Important Note

The bacterial toxins (cholera and pertussis) exert an important effect on adenylyl cyclase.

- *Cholera toxin* catalyses the transfer of ADP ribose on arginine residue of α subunit of G_s protein, which inhibits its GTPase activity thus resulting in prolongation of its stimulation activity.
- *Pertussis toxin* inhibits G-protein activity. This toxin acts by catalysing ADP ribosylation of cystein residue near the carboxyl terminal of α subunit of G_i, thus inhibit its function.

2. Guanylate Cyclase–cGMP System. Group II-B hormones which act via second messenger cGMP include atrial natriuretic factor (ANF) and nitric oxide (NO).

i. ***Synthesis of cyclic GMP*** is analogous to the formation of cAMP. Enzyme guanylate cyclase produces cGMP from GTP.

ii. ***cGMP exerts its biochemical response*** through an enzyme protein kinase G, which when activated initiates a cascade of subsequent enzyme activations that is characteristic of this signalling system.

Note: Cyclic GMP is important in vision. Both rod and cone cells contain ion channels which are regulated by cGMP.

3. Membrane Phospholipase–Phospholipid System or Inositol Triphosphate IP_3 Mechanism. Hormones which exert their response through this system constitute the so-called group II-C hormones (Table 8.1-1). Steps involved in this system are (Fig. 8.1-11):

- Hormone binds to a receptor in the plasma membrane.
- The hormone–receptor complex via a G-protein activates the membrane enzyme phospholipase C present on the inner surface of the membrane.
- Activated phospholipase C (PLC) then releases diacylglycerol and inositol triphosphate (IP_3) from membrane phospholipid.
- Inositol triphosphate (1,4,5 triphosphate) or (IP_3) then mobilizes Ca^{2+} from the endoplasmic reticulum.
- Calcium ions (Ca^{2+}) and diacylglycerol together activate protein kinase C.
- Activated protein kinase C phosphorylates proteins and causes specific physiological action.
- Diacylglycerol also yields arachidonic acid which serves as a substrate for rapid synthesis of prostaglandins that modulate cell response.

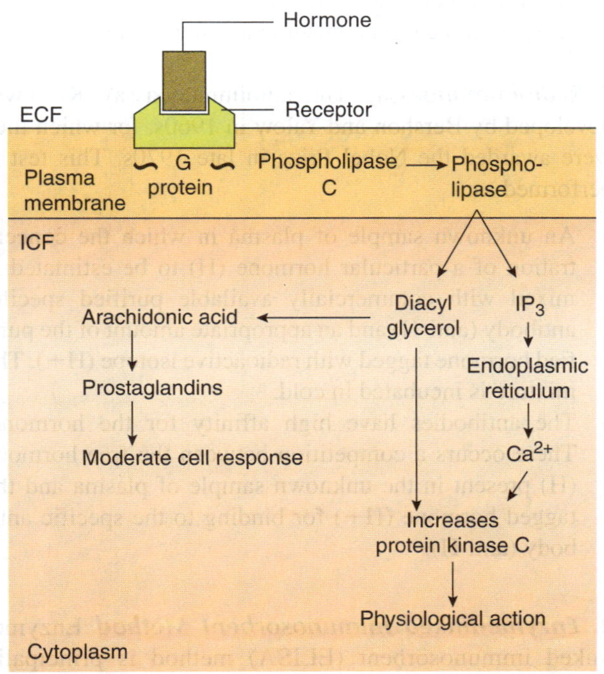

FIGURE 8.1-11 Mechanism of action of hormone via membrane phospholipase–phospholipid system or IP_3 mechanism.

4. Calcium–Calmodulin System. Hormones that act through this system as second messenger are also included in the so-called group-II C hormones (Table 8.1-1). Steps involved in this system are (Fig. 8.1-12):

- Hormone binds to a specific receptor in the plasma membrane.
- Then the hormone–receptor complex, via G-protein opens the Ca^{2+} channels on the cell membrane and also activates mobilization of Ca^{2+} bound to the endoplasmic reticulum.
- Ca^{2+} binds to a specific binding protein, calmodulin, in various proportions.
- The different calcium–calmodulin complexes activate or deactivate various calcium-dependent enzymes producing different physiologic actions.

Mechanism of Action of Hormone via Tyrosine Kinase Activation

Certain hormones act by activating tyrosine kinase system and have been classified as group-II D hormones (Table 8.1-1). This mechanism of signal generation from plasma membrane receptors does not require G-protein intermediaries. These receptors have an extracellular hormone-binding portion, a single transmembrane portion and an intracytoplasmic C-terminal portion.

The activation of tyrosine kinase occurs by two mechanisms:

1. ***Hormone receptors possessing intrinsic tyrosine activity,*** e.g. those for insulin and epidermal growth factor (EGF) involve the following steps (Fig. 8.1-13A):
   - Binding of hormone to the receptor changes its conformation and exposes sites on its intracellular

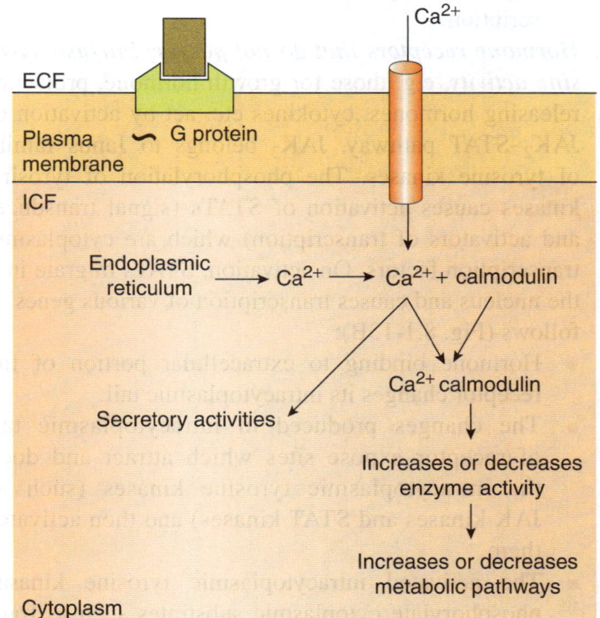

FIGURE 8.1-12 Mechanism of action of hormone via calcium–calmodulin system.

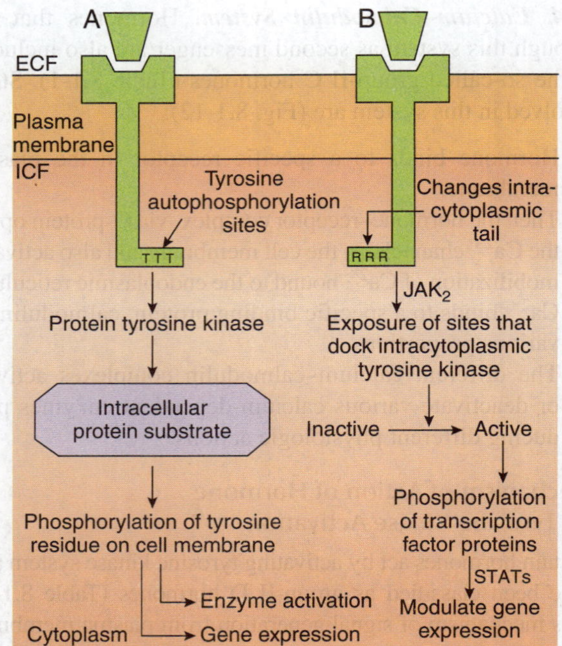

FIGURE 8.1-13 Mechanism of action of hormone via tyrosine kinase activity: **A,** by receptors that possess intrinsic tyrosine activity; and **B,** by receptors that act by activation of JAK_2–STATs pathway.

portion that are capable of receptor autophosphorylation at specific tyrosine sites.

- As a result, the receptor itself becomes a tyrosine kinase that phosphorylates tyrosine residue on intracellular protein substrates.
- This latter activity sets into motion a cascade of events leading to enzyme activation and gene transcription.

2. ***Hormone receptors that do not possess intrinsic tyrosine activity,*** e.g. those for growth hormone, prolactin-releasing hormones, cytokines etc. act by activation of JAK_2–STAT pathway. JAK_2 belongs to Janus family of tyrosine kinases. The phosphorylation of tyrosine kinases causes activation of STATs (signal transducer and activators of transcription) which are cytoplasmic transcription factors. On activation, STATs migrate into the nucleus and causes transcription of various genes as follows (Fig. 8.1-13B):
   - Hormone binding to extracellular portion of the receptor changes its intracytoplasmic tail.
   - The changes produced in intracytoplasmic tail of receptor expose sites which attract and dock the intracytoplasmic tyrosine kinases (such as JAK kinases and STAT kinases) and then activates them.
   - The activated intracytoplasmic tyrosine kinases phosphorylate cytoplasmic substrates such as transcription factor proteins and ultimately modulate gene expression.

MEASUREMENT OF HORMONES

Measurement of blood level of hormones is essential to confirm the endocrinal disorders associated with either deficiency or excess of a hormone. Since hormones exist in the blood at very low concentrations, the conventional methods of estimation, such as colorimetry, are not of much use. Therefore, they are measured by hormone assays and some special techniques which include:

- Bioassay,
- Immunoassay,
- Cytochemical assay and
- Dynamic tests.

Bioassay

Biological assay that was frequently used earlier to measure the level of a hormone in the plasma is now an obsolete technique. In this method, hormone levels were assessed by injecting the unknown sample of plasma in experimental animals and observing quantitatively the specific biological effect. The effect chosen was a characteristic action of the hormone for which a clear dose–response relationship existed. For example, one unit of insulin was defined as one third of the amount of insulin that will lower the blood sugar of a rabbit weighing 2 kg to conclusive levels in 3 h.

Immunoassay

The immunoassay methods, frequently employed for estimation of hormone levels, include:

- Radio immunoassay (RIA) and
- Enzyme-linked immunosorbent assay (ELISA).

1. Radioimmunoassay The radioimmunoassay (RIA) was developed by Bershon and Yalow in 1960s, for which they were awarded the Nobel Prize in late 1970s. This test is performed as:

- An unknown sample of plasma in which the concentration of a particular hormone (H) to be estimated is mixed with commercially available purified specific antibody (anti-H) and an appropriate amount of the purified hormone tagged with radioactive isotope (H+). The mixture is incubated in cold.
- The antibodies have high affinity for the hormone. There occurs a competition between the free hormone (H) present in the unknown sample of plasma and the tagged hormone (H+) for binding to the specific antibody (anti-H).

2. Enzyme-linked Immunosorbent Method Enzyme-linked immunosorbent (ELISA) method is principally similar to RIA, i.e. it is also based on the principle of antigen–antibody reaction. Any antigen that is protein can be measured by this technique. In this method, radioactivity is not measured; instead specific antibody hormone (antigen) complex is stained with suitable dye, e.g. diammonium 2-2' azinobis (3-ethylbenzothiazolene 6 sulphate), also called ABTS, and the intensity of colour is measured by spectrophotometer. This technique is useful in estimating peptide and steroid hormones.

Cytochemical Assay

This test is much more sensitive than the immunoassay, but is cumbersome and time consuming and so rarely used. In this technique, genesis of hormone can be detected in slices cut out of the endocrine gland by incubating them in an ascorbate-enriched culture medium. This test is very useful in measuring the minute basal levels of hormone secretion.

Dynamic Tests

Dynamic tests are needed in certain situations when simple blood hormone level estimation is not enough. Two types of dynamic tests are:

Suppression type of dynamic tests are useful in certain conditions, e.g. to know whether a lung cancer is secreting ACTH.

Stimulation type of dynamic tests are useful in certain other conditions, e.g. metyrapone test is performed to know whether the corticotrophs of the pituitary (which secrete ACTH) are normally functioning or not. For details see page 756.

Chapter 8.2

Endocrinal Functions of Hypothalamus and Pituitary Gland

INTRODUCTION AND FUNCTIONAL ANATOMY

The hypothalamic–pituitary unit forms a unique component of the entire endocrine system that regulates growth, lactation, fluid homeostasis and the functions of the thyroid gland, adrenal glands and gonads.

To appreciate the functional relationship between the hypothalamus and pituitary gland, it is necessary to have knowledge of the functional anatomy and embryological development of the pituitary gland.

Gross Anatomy and Development of Pituitary Gland

Gross Anatomy

Pituitary gland, also called *hypophysis cerebri,* is a small gland, weighs about 0.5 g and is approximately 1 cm in diameter. It is situated in the hypophyseal fossa (sella turcica) of the sphenoid bone. A reflection of the dura mater called the *diaphragm sellae,* extends across the top of sella and separates the pituitary gland from the brain. The diaphragma sellae is perforated in the middle through which passes the *pituitary stalk* that connects the pituitary gland with the hypothalamus.

Physiologically, the pituitary gland consists of three distinct parts or lobes (Fig. 8.2-1):

- Anterior lobe or adenohypophysis,
- Posterior lobe or neurohypophysis and
- Intermediate lobe or pars intermedia.

Development of Pituitary Gland

Anterior pituitary is ectodermal in origin. It develops from *Rathke's pouch,* which is an embryonic upward outpouching from the roof of the primitive oral cavity. This pouch eventually gets separated from the oral cavity by the sphenoid bone of the skull and its lumen is reduced to a small cleft (residual cleft).

Posterior pituitary or neurohypophysis develops from a lowered outpouching of neuroectodermal tissue from the central areas of the hypothalamus (tuber cinereum and median eminence). The lumen of this pouch is obliterated inferiorly and the median eminence continues as infundibular stem and ends as infundibular processes of the posterior pituitary. Superiorly, the lumen remains contiguous with and forms a recess in the adult third ventricle.

From the above, it is quite clear that the anterior and posterior pituitaries develop independently from widely different origins and it is only a coincidence that when fully formed, they happen to lie so close together that they are considered parts of the same organ.

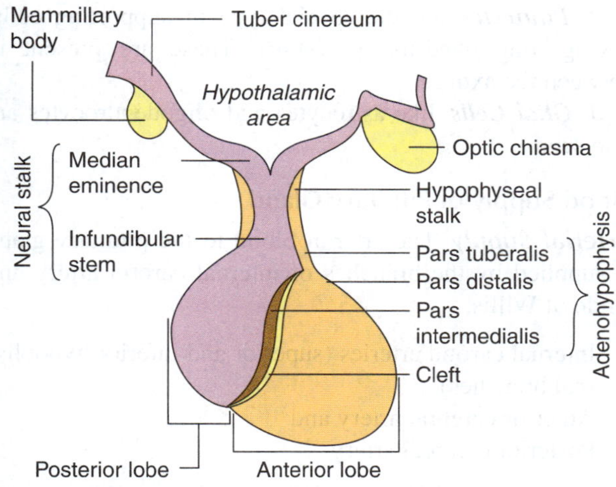

FIGURE 8.2-1 Anatomical subdivisions of pituitary gland.

Parts of Pituitary Gland

Adenohypophysis. The glandular anterior lobe of the pituitary gland is called adenohypophysis. It constitutes about 80% of the pituitary gland. It can be further divided into three parts (Fig. 8.2-1):

- ***Pars distalis.*** It forms the main bulk of the anterior lobe and is a highly vascular area.
- ***Pars intermedia.*** It is an avascular zone that lies between pars distalis and neurohypophysis. In humans, this area is rudimentary, but in lower animals it forms the intermediate lobe of the pituitary.
- ***Pars tuberalis.*** It is the most vascular zone and contains many secretory cells. Superficially it is surrounded by the pituitary stalk.

Neurohypophysis. The posterior lobe of the pituitary is a neural structure and hence called neurohypophysis. It consists of three parts (Fig. 8.2-1):

- ***Pars posterior.*** It is also called pars nervosa or neural lobe or infundibular process and forms the main bulk of neurohypophysis.
- ***Infundibular stem.*** It is the funnel-shaped extension arising from the median eminence at the floor of the third ventricle.
- ***Median eminence.*** It is a small protrusion from the base of the hypothalamus (tuber cinereum). It is situated just beneath the third ventricle and is highly vascular.

Pituitary Stalk. The median eminence and infundibulum constitute the neural stalk. The posterior pituitary maintains its neural connection with the hypothalamus by this neural stalk. The neural stalk surrounded by pars tuberalis of adenohypophysis constitutes the pituitary stalk.

Intermediate lobe of pituitary gland is rudimentary in humans as well as in a few other mammalian species and thus does not secrete melanocyte-stimulating hormone (MSH). In certain lower animals, this lobe secretes MSH in response to changes in exposure to light and other environmental factors. This hormone, in fish, reptiles and amphibia controls the change of the colour of their skin (during thermoregulation, camouflage and behavioural display) by controlling the dispersal and aggregation of pigment granules in the melanophores.

In humans, there are no melanophores-containing pigment granules that disperse and aggregate, but there are *melanocytes,* which have multiple processes containing melanin granules. The ACTH (having sequence of first 13 of the amino acids same as that of MSH) has a weak MSH-like activity. It binds to melanotropin-1 receptors present on the melanocytes. This may probably be the reason why patients with hypersecretion of ACTH develop hyperpigmentation of the skin (e.g. in Addison's disease), and those with hypopituitarism develop abnormal pallor.

Histological Structure of Pituitary Gland

Adenohypophysis

Pars distalis consists of cords of cells separated by fenestrated sinusoids. The cells can be divided into two main types: the chromophobes and chromophils. In addition, folliculostellate cells are also present.

1. Chromophobes. These are agranular cells and contain very few granules in their cytoplasm. It is considered that the chromophils are derived from the chromophobes.
2. Chromophils. These are granular cells, which constitute 50% of the cells of anterior pituitary. Chromophils are further classified as: acidophils (35%) and basophils (15%).
   - **i.** ***Acidophilic cells (α cells).*** The granules of acidophilic cells stain with acidic dyes (like eosin or orange G). The size of granules varies from 200–700 nm. Depending on the size and nature of granules, the acidophils are further divided into following subtypes:
     - *Somatotrophs.* These cells are located mainly in the lateral part of the anterior lobe and constitute 20–40% of acidophilic series of cells and secrete growth hormone (GH) or somatotropin (STH).
     - *Mammotrophs or lactotrophs.* These are scattered throughout the anterior lobe and produce mammotropic hormones, prolactin (PRL) or lactogenic hormone (LTH).
   - **ii.** ***Basophilic cells (β cells).*** The granules of basophilic cells are stained with basic dyes (like haematoxylin) and contain abundant dense core vesicles. The basophils are also further divided into functional subtypes:
     - *Corticotrophs.* The staining characteristics of these cells are intermediate between those of acidophilic and basophilic cells. The granules in these cells contain complex molecules of pro-opiomelano-corticotropin. These secrete ACTH and β-lipoproteins.

- *Thyrotrophs.* These cells produce thyrotropic hormone (thyrotropin or TSH), which stimulates the activity of the thyroid gland.
- *Gonadotrophs (delta* (δ) cells). These basophilic cells are present all along the anterior lobe. They produce two types of hormones: follicular-stimulating hormone (FSH) and luteinizing hormone (LH). Gonadotrophs subserve different actions in males and females.

3. Folliculostellate Cells. These cells send processes between established secretory cells. Recently, it has been demonstrated that these contain and secrete the cytokine 1L-6. Though their physiological role is still not clear, they may act paracrineally to regulate growth and functions of secretory cells.

Capillary network. In addition to the above cells, the anterior pituitary also contains an extensive network of capillaries. The endothelium of the capillaries is fenestrated like that in other endocrine organs. The secretory cells outpour secretory granules by exocytosis. These granules presumably breakdown in the pericapillary space and the hormones released enter the capillaries.

Pars tuberalis. It mainly consists of undifferentiated cells with few acidophils and basophils.

Pars intermedia. It contains β cells, few secretory cells and chromophobe cells.

Neurohypophysis Histologically, posterior pituitary contains following structures;

1. Unmyelinated Nerve Fibres. These are the axons of the neurons located in the supraoptic and paraventricular nuclei of hypothalamus. These carry precursor of posterior pituitary hormones and end as closed terminals near the blood capillaries (Fig. 8.2-2).

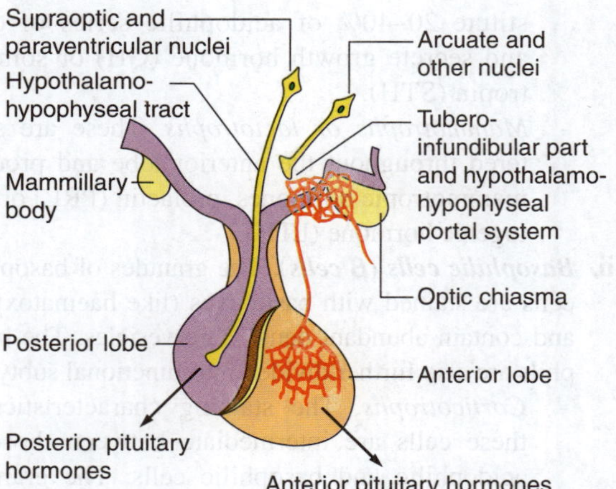

FIGURE 8.2-2 Anatomical and functional relationship between hypothalamus and pituitary gland through hypothalamo–hypophyseal tract and hypothalamo–hypophyseal portal system.

2. Pituicytes are the special type of supporting cells, having long dendritic processes. These are present in between the axons.

3. Glial Cells like astrocytes and oligodendrocytes are also seen.

Blood Supply of Pituitary Gland

Arterial Supply The arterial blood to the pituitary gland is supplied by the branches of internal carotid artery and circle of Willis:

- Internal carotid arteries (superior and inferior hypophyseal branches),
- Anterior cerebral artery and
- Posterior cerebral artery.

Hypothalamo–Hypophyseal Portal System (Figs 8.2-2, 8.2-3)

- The branches from the superior hypophyseal artery form a ring around the upper part of the pituitary stalk and further branch to form a *capillary network* called primary plexus on the ventral surface of the hypothalamus.
- The blood from this capillary network is drained by *long portal veins* in the infundibulum.
- Then, in the anterior lobe, these long portal veins break up into another set of capillary network and are represented as *sinusoids of pars anterior*. This arrangement is called *hypothalamo–hypophyseal portal system.*
- The inferior hypophyseal (branch of internal carotid artery) branches to form a capillary network at the lower end of infundibulum stem called secondary capillary plexus.
- The short portal vessels arise from this capillary network and supply blood mainly to the posterior pituitary and some parts of the anterior pituitary.
- The short portal vessels provide a link between the anterior and posterior pituitary.

Venous Drainage The blood from anterior pituitary is drained to cavernous sinus and then into the jugular vein.

Some Important Points Regarding Circulation of Hypophysis

- The whole of neurohypophysis (median eminence to pars posterior) is permeated by a continuous network of capillaries, in which blood flows in either direction.
- The anterior pituitary lies outside the blood–brain barrier; hence, it is accessible to influences from general circulation (hormones and neurotransmitter by the brain and hormones secreted in general circulation).

Hypothalamic–Pituitary Relationship

The influences from the hypothalamus are conveyed to the pituitary gland by two different tracts:

1. Hypothalamo–hypophyseal Tract. It is composed of axons of the large neurosecretory cells of the supraoptic and

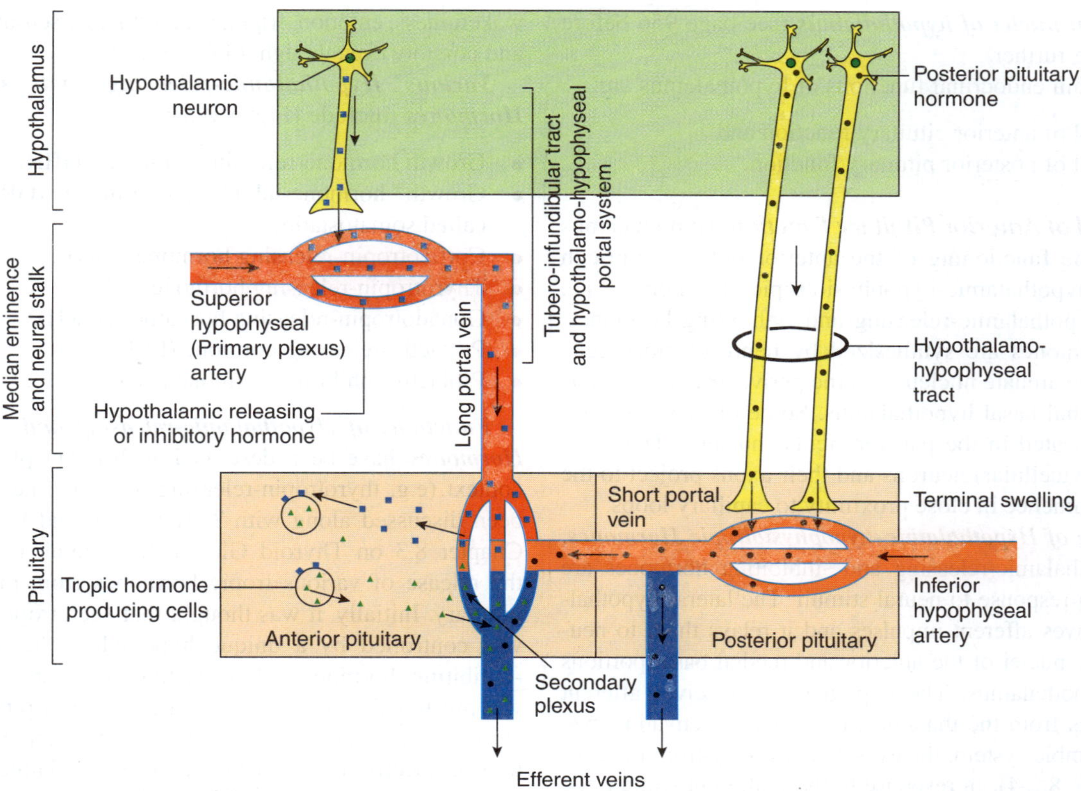

FIGURE 8.2-3 Schematic diagram to explain anatomical and functional relationship between hypothalamus and pituitary gland.

paraventricular nuclei of the hypothalamus. These fibres pass to neurohypophysis through the infundibular stem and form a series of dilated terminals known as *Herring bodies* (Fig. 8.2-2). The neurosecretory cells of supraoptic and paraventricular nuclei secrete peptide hormones (vasopressin and oxytocin), which travel down their axons in neurosecretory granules to be stored in the nerve terminals lying in the neurohypophysis. Upon stimulation of the cell bodies, the granules are released from the axonal terminals by exocytosis. The peptide hormones then enter the peripheral circulation via the capillary plexuses of inferior hypophyseal artery (Fig. 8.2-3). Thus, a single neural cell performs the entire process of hormone synthesis, storage and release.

2. Tuberoinfundibular Tract and Hypothalamo–hypophyseal Portal System. It consists of fibres arising from the arcuate nuclei of the tuberal region of the hypothalamus and extends to the median eminence (Fig. 8.2-2). The cell bodies of these hypothalamic neurons synthesize certain releasing and inhibiting hormones which are conveyed as membrane-bound vesicles by the tuberoinfundibular tract to the median eminence region where they are stored in the nerve terminals. After these hypothalamic neurons are stimulated by nerve impulses, the releasing or inhibiting hormones are discharged into the median eminence and enter the capillary plexus of the superior hypophyseal artery. From here they are transported down the portal vessels (long portal veins) and then exit from the secondary capillary plexus to reach the specific endocrine target cells in the adenohypophysis where they regulate the secretion of tropic hormones of anterior pituitary (Fig. 8.2-3). The tropic hormones released from the secretory cells of adenohypophysis enter the same secondary capillary plexus through which they ultimately reach the peripheral circulation (Fig. 8.2-3).

ENDOCRINAL ASPECTS OF HYPOTHALAMUS

Functional Anatomy

Hypothalamus is a specialized centre in the brain that functions as a master co-ordinator of hormonal action. It is a part of the brain situated below the thalamus and is very closely connected to the pituitary gland, as described above. Thus, the hypothalamus provides an important link between the endocrine system and the nervous system. Before proceeding further, see *details of functional anatomy of hypothalamus* at page 953.

Endocrinal Functions of Hypothalamus

The functions of hypothalamus, in general, are described on page 956. The hypothalamus serves its endocrinal functions through the neurosecretory cells which are arranged in ***different nuclei of hypothalamus*** (see page 956 before proceeding further).

The main endocrinal functions of hypothalamus are:

- Control of anterior pituitary function and
- Control of posterior pituitary function.

1. Control of Anterior Pituitary Function Hypothalamus controls the functioning of the anterior pituitary through various hypothalamic-hypophysiotropic hormones, i.e. various hypothalamic-releasing and -inhibiting hormones. These hormones are synthesized by neurosecretory cells forming the arcuate nucleus and the periventricular nucleus of the medial basal hypothalamus. Some of these neurons are also located in the paraventricular nucleus. These are small (parvicellular) neurons and their axons project to the median eminence in close proximity to capillary loops.

Release of Hypothalamic–hypophysiotropic Hormones. The hypothalamic-releasing and -inhibiting hormones are released in response to neural stimuli. The lateral hypothalamus receives afferent impulses and it relays them to neurosecretory nuclei of the anterior and medial basal portions of the hypothalamus. The hypothalamus receives afferent nerve tracts from the thalamus, the reticular-activating system, the limbic system, the eyes and remotely from the neocortex (Fig. 8.2-4). In response to these afferent stimuli, the hypothalamic-hypophysiotropic hormones are released in the regions of median eminence and reach the anterior pituitary (to control its function) through the hypothalamic–hypophyseal portal vessels as described above and shown in Figs 8.2-2 and 8.2-3. Through these inputs (Fig. 8.2-4), the pituitary functions can be influenced by pain, sleep, wakefulness, emotion, fright, rage, olfactory sensations, light and possibly even thought (Table 8.2-1).

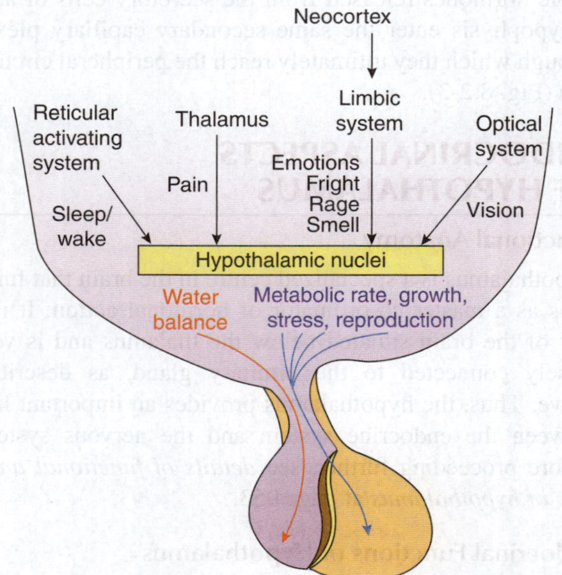

FIGURE 8.2-4 Afferent impulses to different hypothalamic nuclei leading to release of hypothalamic-releasing or -inhibiting hormones controlling pituitary gland.

Various Hypothalamic-releasing and -Inhibiting Hormones include (Fig. 8.2-5):

- Growth hormone-releasing hormone (GHRH),
- Growth hormone-inhibiting hormone (GRIH), also called somatostatin,
- Corticotropin-releasing hormone (CRH),
- Thyrotropin-releasing hormone (TRH),
- Gonadotropin-releasing hormone (GnRH),
- Prolactin-releasing hormone (PRH) and
- Prolactin-inhibiting hormone (PIH).

Functions of Hypothalamic-releasing and -Inhibiting Hormones have been described at different places in the context (e.g. thyrotropin-releasing hormone, i.e. TRH, has been discussed along with TSH and thyroid hormones in Chapter 8.3 on Thyroid Gland). In general, they control the release of various tropic hormones from the anterior pituitary. Initially, it was thought that each tropic hormone was controlled by a unique hypothalamic-releasing and -inhibiting hormone. Also, each hypothalamic hormone was presumed to have only one target anterior pituitary cell. However, now it is known that besides regulating the secretion of specific tropic hormone, a hypothalamic hormone may also influence the secretion of another anterior pituitary hormone. For example:

- TRH, besides promoting secretion of TSH, also stimulates the secretion of prolactin.
- Somatostatin, discovered as a growth hormone-inhibiting hormone (GHIH), also inhibits the secretion of TSH.
- Growth hormone-releasing hormone (GHRH) also stimulates the secretion of ACTH and prolactin.
- GnRH promotes the release of both LH and FSH.

Mechanism of action of Hypothalamic-hypophysiotropic Hormones. The hypothalamic-releasing and -inhibiting peptides are secreted in pulses, and they induce effects via cAMP, Ca^{2+} and phosphatidyl inositol products as second messengers. They stimulate or inhibit transcription, modulate translation and stimulate or inhibit secretion of the target anterior pituitary hormones.

2. Control of Posterior Pituitary Function The large (magnocellular) neurosecretory cells forming the supraoptic and paraventricular nuclei of hypothalamus are responsible for synthesis of the two posterior pituitary peptide hormones (oxytocin and ADH). These hormones reach the posterior pituitary through the hypothalamic–hypophyseal tract described above (Figs 8.2-2, 8.2-3).

ANTERIOR PITUITARY HORMONES

Anterior pituitary is truly the master endocrine organ. It secretes various hormones that influence either directly or

TABLE 8.2-1 Neuroendocrinal Control by Hypothalamus

Hormone	Factor	Afferents (stimuli) from receptors	Integrated area of hypothalamus
Growth hormone	Somatostatin and growth hormone-releasing hormone		Periventricular and arcuate nuclei
Gonadotropins: • Follicular-stimulating hormone (FSH) • Luteinizing hormone (LH)	Gonadotropin-releasing hormone (GnRH)	• Hypothalamic cells sensitive to oestrogen • Touch receptors in skin and genitalia (in reflexly ovulating animals) • Eyes	Preoptic and other areas
Adrenocorticotropic hormone (ACTH) and β lipotropin	Corticotropic-releasing hormone (CRH)	• Emotional stimuli via limbic system • Systemic stimuli via reticular activating system • Hypothalamic and anterior pituitary cells sensitive to circulating cortisol level • Diurnal variations via suprachiasmatic nuclei	Paraventricular nuclei
Thyroid-stimulating hormone (TSH)	Thyrotropin hormone (TRH)	Temperature receptors in infants and others	Paraventricular nuclei and neighbouring areas
Antidiuretic hormone (ADH) or vasopressin		• Osmoreceptors • Volume receptors • Others	• Supraoptic and paraventricular nuclei
Oxytocin	–	• Touch receptors present in breast, uterus and genitalia	• Supraoptic and paraventricular nuclei
Catecholamines	–	Limbic area related to emotions	• Dorsal and posterior hypothalamus

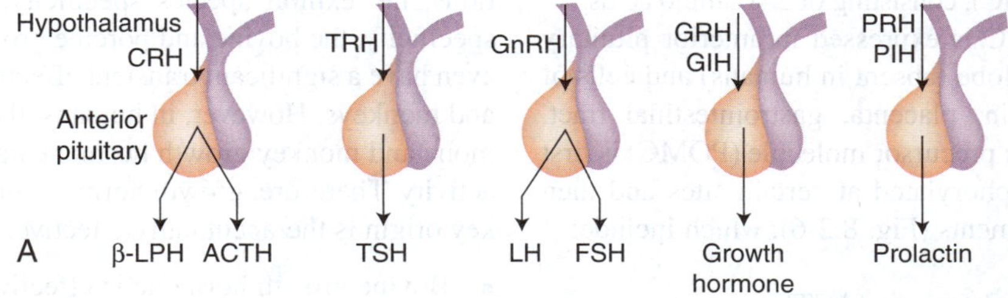

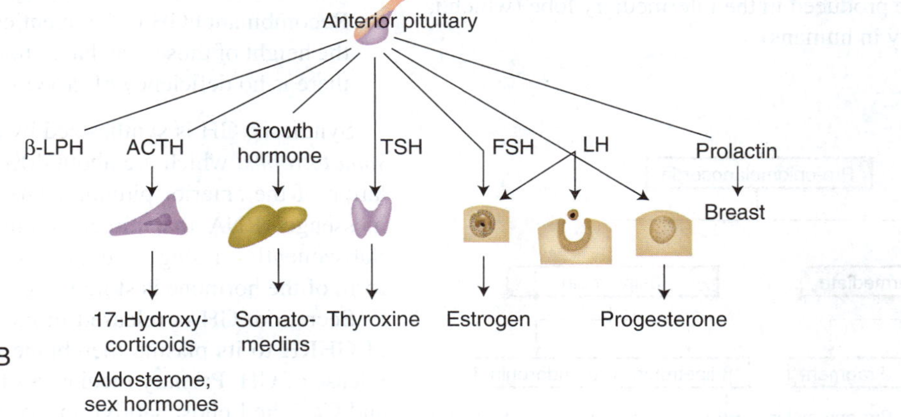

FIGURE 8.2-5 Effect of hypophysiotropic hormones on anterior pituitary **A**; and their effects **B**.

indirectly many biochemical processes in the body. The hormones of adenohypophysis are broadly classified into three categories:

- Growth hormone (prolactin group),
- Glycoprotein hormones and
- Pro-opiomelanocortin (POMC) peptides.

I. Hormones of Growth Hormone Family. Growth hormone (GH), prolactin (PRL) and human chorionic somatomammotropin (HCS) belong to this family and have been thought to have arisen from the same ancestral gene. There is 85% homology between GH and HCS. These hormones have primary regulatory actions of their own.

II. Glycoprotein Hormone Family. The hormones of glycoprotein family secreted by anterior pituitary include:

- Thyroid stimulating hormone (TSH),
- Luteinizing hormone (LH) and
- Follicular stimulating hormone (FSH).

These hormones contain an α and a β subunit. The α subunits of all the hormones are identical. The β subunit of each hormone is different and is responsible for the unique biological activity of each hormone. Each subunit is a product of a separate gene. Hence, synthesis of the whole hormone requires the co-ordinated expression of the α and β subunit genes. The α and β subunits are non-covalently linked and the three-dimensional structures are determined by intramolecular S—S bonds.

III. Pro-opiomelanocortin Peptides. The hormones of this group are derived from a single precursor, the pro-opiomelanocortin (POMC), consisting of 241 amino acids.

The gene for POMC is expressed in anterior pituitary cells, the intermediate lobe (absent in humans) and cells of other tissues like brain, placenta, gastrointestinal tract, lungs and platelets. The precursor molecule (POMC) is first glycosylated and phosphorylated at certain sites and then cleaved into three fragments (Fig. 8.2-6), which include:

- Adrenocorticotropic hormone (ACTH),
- Melanocyte-stimulating hormone (MSH), α-MSH and β-MSH are produced in the intermediary lobe (which is rudimentary in humans),
- β-lipotropin (BLPH) and
- β-endorphin.

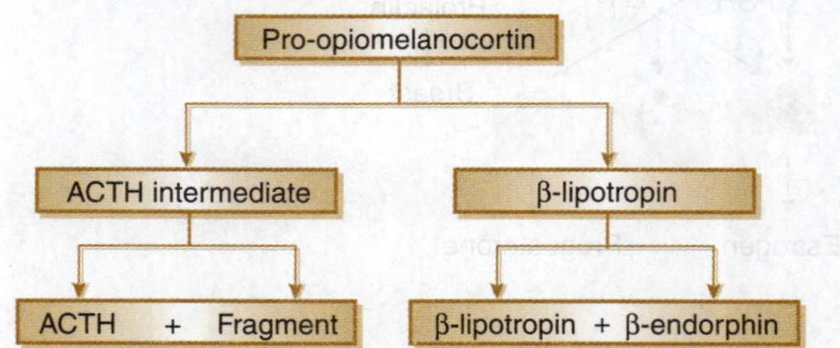

FIGURE 8.2-6 Pro-opiomelanocortin is the precursor of ACTH, β-lipotropin and β-endorphin.

Physiological aspects of the growth hormone are discussed in detail in this chapter. Other hormones are discussed in different chapters (e.g. TSH with thyroid hormone and ACTH with adrenal gland).

Growth Hormone

Growth hormone (GH), also called *somatotropin,* is the most important hormone for postnatal growth and development to adult size. It also helps to maintain lean body mass and bone mass in adults.

Structure, Synthesis and Secretion

Structure. GH consists of a single unbranched chain containing 191 amino acids and two disulphate bondages. Its molecular weight is 2000. It is a member of the large family of 'helix bundle proteins'.

The genes, that code human GH are present on the long arm of the chromosome and are in cluster form. There are five genes for growth hormone.

First two genes encode growth hormone:

- hGH-N—normal human GH (hGH) and
- hGH-V—variant form of GH.

Two other genes encode HCS and fifth gene is hCS pseudogene.

Species Specificity. Growth hormones obtained from different species show chemical and immunological variations, i.e. exhibit species specificity. Because of species specificity, the bovine and porcine growth hormones do not even have a significant transient effect on growth in humans and monkeys. However, in humans, the human growth hormone and monkey growth hormone have similar biological activity. Therefore, growth hormone preparation from monkey origin is therapeutically effective.

- Bovine growth hormone is effectively used for increasing milk production in diary animals and also used as a growth hormone supplement by body builders.
- Recombinant hGH is therapeutically used for increasing the height of those who have short stature, but otherwise there is no deficiency of growth hormone.

Synthesis. GH is synthesized by acidophilic cells called *somatotrophs,* which are about 40% of the total cell population of the anterior pituitary. The GH gene transcribes a messenger RNA that directs synthesis of a prehormone. Subsequently, a single peptide is removed and the final form of the hormone is stored in granules.

Secretion. GH is released in *pulsatile* fashion. Binding of GHRH to its plasma membrane receptor stimulates the release of GH. Primary mediators of GH release are cAMP and Ca^{2+} and phosphatidylinositol products are secondary mediators of GHRH action.

- ***Secretion is increased*** by the stimuli, which are categorized into three parts:
  - **(i)** The conditions which decrease the substrate for energy production in the cell, such as: hypoglycaemia, fasting and exercise,
  - **(ii)** The conditions in which the amount of certain amino acids are increased in the plasma, e.g. protein meal, infusion of arginine and other amino acids and
  - **(iii)** Stressful stimuli, such as fever, psychological stress-sleep, hormones related to puberty, starvation, exercise and hypoglycaemia.
- ***Secretion of GH is decreased*** by somatostatin, somatomedins, obesity, hyperglycaemia, cortisol, free fatty acids and pregnancy.

Regulation of GH Secretion

1. Hypothalamic Control Hypothalamus controls GH secretion by releasing two hormones, growth hormone-releasing hormone (GHRH) and growth hormone release-inhibiting hormone (GRIH) (Fig. 8.2-7).

Growth Hormone-releasing Hormone (GHRH). It is a polypeptide with 44 amino acids that stimulates the secretion of GH from the anterior pituitary.

Mechanism of action. GHRH acts through guanylate cyclase, which releases cyclic GMP, which in turn, stimulates the release of GH from the anterior pituitary. Influx of Ca^{2+} into pituitary cells is an essential event associated with the GHRH-stimulated release of GH.

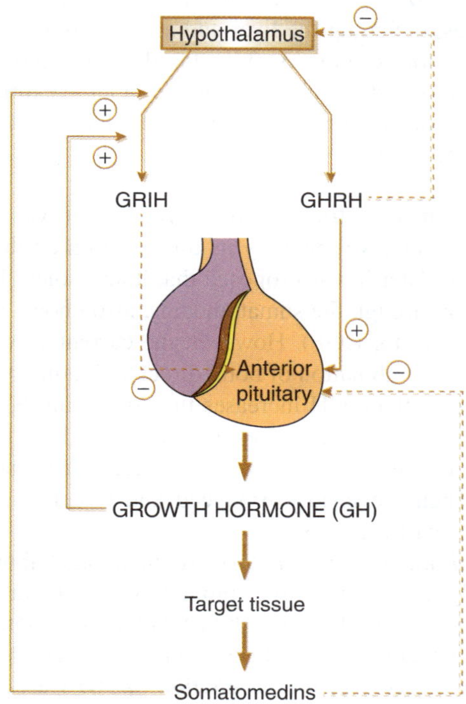

FIGURE 8.2-7 Control of growth hormone secretion GHRH (growth hormone-releasing hormone), and GRIH (growth hormone release-inhibiting hormone).

Factors stimulating GHRH secretion and thus increasing GH release are:

- *Hypoglycaemia* increases GHRH secretion through glucoreceptor cells in the ventromedial nucleus of the hypothalamus. Neurotransmitter involved is epinephrine.
- *Emotions, exercise and physical stress* (pain, trauma, cold, surgery, inflammation, etc.) stimulate GHRH release through nervous pathways (therefore, the effect is seen within a couple of minutes).
- *Slow-wave phase of sleep* is associated with increase in GHRH. The neurotransmitter involved is serotonin.
- *Increase in plasma levels of certain amino acids* such as arginine (after protein meal or infusion of amino acids) increase GHRH secretion by α-adrenergic stimulation of the receptors in neurons that release GHRH.
- *Growth hormone-releasing peptide* (GHRP) also called 'ghrelin' increases GHRH secretion. GHRP is synthesized by the oxyntic glands of the stomach. It increases GH release by its direct action on the anterior pituitary.

Growth Hormone Release-inhibiting Hormone (GRIH), also called somatostatin, is a polypeptide with 14 amino acids. It inhibits the release of GH from the anterior pituitary.

Mechanism of action. GRIH blocks GHRH stimulation in a noncompetitive manner. It acts through its own plasma membrane receptor in part, by decreasing intracellular cAMP and calcium levels.

Factors stimulating GRIH secretion and thus decreasing GH secretion are:

- Hyperglycaemia and
- High plasma FFA concentration.

2. Negative Feedback Control of GH Secretion The negative feedback control mechanism for GH involves the role of somatomedins, GH and GHRH (Fig. 8.2-7).

i. Negative Feedback Control by Somatomedins. Somatomedins are insulin-like growth factor-1 (IGF-1) that are produced when the growth hormone acts on target tissues. Somatomedins inhibit the secretion of GH through two mechanisms:

- By direct inhibitory effect on anterior pituitary and
- By stimulating the secretion of somatostatin from the hypothalamus.

ii. Negative Feedback Control by GH. Growth hormone also inhibits its own secretion by stimulating the secretion of somatostatin from the hypothalamus.

iii. Negative Feedback Control by GHRH. GHRH inhibits its own secretion from the hypothalamus. This mechanism is called *ultrashort feedback loop* and occurs by transport of GHRH via pituitary tanycytes to the cerebrospinal fluid and then back to hypothalamus.

3. Other Factors Controlling GH Secretion Other factors which control GH secretion are:

- ***Thyroxine and cortisol*** at their basal levels synergistically stimulate GH gene expression; while an excess of either hormone decreases the GH responses to GHRH by enhancing somatostatin release.
- ***Insulin*** represses GH gene expression.
- ***Placental GH and placental lactogen*** are responsible for decreased GH secretion noted during later part of pregnancy.
- ***Obesity*** is associated with dampened GH responses to all stimuli including GHRH itself.
- ***Neurotransmitters*** dopamine, norepinephrine, acetylcholine, serotonin, GABA and histamine all increase GH secretion by stimulating the release of GHRH or by blocking the release of somatostatin.
- ***Oestradiol*** increases GH secretion and explains the greater secretion of GH in premenopausal women than in men.

Plasma Levels, Binding and Metabolism

Plasma Levels

Basal plasma GH level varies from 2–4 ng/ml. Its concentration graph shows fluctuations, i.e. after every 1–2 h interval, there is a rise in plasma GH level, i.e. GH is released in 10–20 pulses per day. This pulsatility arises from some combination of the pulsatile release of GHRH and of GRIH into the portal blood.

Diurnal variation in plasma levels of GH is noted. The nocturnal peak occurs 1–2 h after deep sleep (which corresponds to stage three or stage four of slow-wave sleep). This supports the adage, 'If you don't sleep, you won't grow'.

The nocturnal sleep bursts account for nearly 70% of the daily GH secretion. These secretory bursts are greater in children and decrease with age.

Variation in plasma GH levels with age (Fig. 8.2-8).

- *From birth to early childhood* plasma GH levels increase progressively.
- *Children versus adults.* In general, children have only slightly higher plasma GH levels than adults. So, it should not be assumed that plasma GH levels would be very high during childhood and low in adults.
- *Puberty* is associated with peak period of plasma GH levels (Fig. 8.2-8).
- *Senescence* is associated with a reduction in GH secretion in response to GHRH and other stimuli. This decline in GH secretion is partly responsible for the decline in lean body mass, physical fitness, protein synthesis and metabolic rate, as well as the increase in adipose mass that characterizes elderly humans.

Circulation, Half-Life and Metabolism

Circulation. Circulating GH is bound to a plasma protein that is a large fragment of the extracellular domain of the growth hormone receptor. This GH-binding protein appears to arise by cleavage of the receptor at the cell's surface. One molecule of GH binds two of the circulating binding protein molecules.

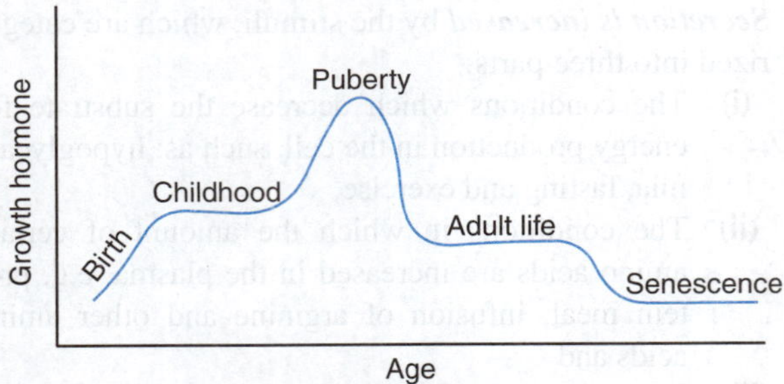

FIGURE 8.2-8 Variations in plasma growth hormone levels with age.

Half-life of circulating GH in humans is 6–20 min and the daily GH output has been calculated to be 0.2–1.0 mg/day in adults.

Metabolism. Growth hormone is rapidly metabolized, probably at least in part in the liver. Metabolic clearance rate is 350 L/day. Although only a trivial portion of secreted GH is excreted unchanged by the kidneys, daily urinary GH excretion correlates well with the integrated 24 h plasma GH profile.

Growth Hormone Receptors and Mechanism of Action of GH

Growth Hormone Receptors Growth hormone receptors of various sizes are present on the cell membrane in target tissues, including the liver and adipose tissue. The GH receptor belongs to the cytokine family of receptors and is a 620 amino acid protein. It comprises a large extracellular portion, a transmembrane domain and a large intracellular cytoplasmic portion.

Mechanism of Action of GH Originally, it was thought that GH promotes growth by its direct action on the target tissues; but later it was proposed that it acts solely by indirect action through the somatomedins, also known as insulin growth factor (IGF). However, the current view is that it acts by a combination of both, direct and indirect effects. By indirect effect, GH increases the circulating IGF-I. By direct effect on the cartilages, GH produces IGF-1 locally and also converts stem cells into the cells that respond to IGF-1. Then the locally produced and circulating IGF-1 makes the cartilage grow.

Insulin-like Growth Factors. As mentioned above, IGF ultimately exerts its growth promoting effect via peptide mediators [(insulin-like growth factors (IGFs) or somatomedins)] that are produced in the liver and many GH target cells.

Steps involved in the production of IGFs are summarized (Fig. 8.2-9):

- Growth hormone has two binding sites for receptors. Binding of two GH receptor molecules at different sites on one molecule of GH produces a homodimer (Fig. 8.2-9, step 1). This process of dimerization activates the receptors.

- The activated receptor dimer then initiates GH actions. The intracytoplasmic portions of the receptors attract, dock and activate *Janus kinases* (JAK-1) (Fig. 8.2-9, step 2). These phosphorylate the signal transducer and activator of transcription factors (STAT) (Fig. 8.2-9 step 3) and induce or repress expression of GH target genes such as IGF genes (Fig. 8.2-9, step 4).
- GH-stimulated expression of IGF genes leads to production of IGFs, primarily, but not solely in the liver. IGFs circulate, bound to at least six carrier proteins known as insulin growth factor-binding proteins (IGFBP 1–6). About 95% of IGF binding is related to IGF-binding protein-3 (IGFBP-3). The characteristic feature of IGF-1 and IGF-2 are depicted in Table 8.2-2.

Structure, Types and Properties of Somatomedins

Structure. IGFs are closely related to insulin except that their C chains are not separated and they have an extension of A chain called D domain.

Types. In humans, two types of IGF are known, IGF-1 and IGF-II. Variants of IGF-1 and IGF-II are also known. The mRNAs for IGF-1 and IGF-II are found in the liver, in cartilage and in many other tissues, indicating that they are synthesized in these tissues.

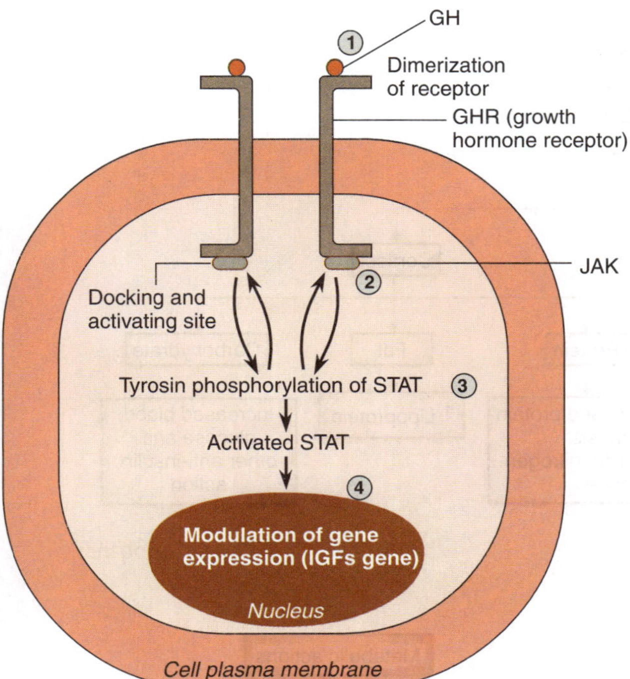

FIGURE 8.2-9 Steps involved in the GH stimulated expression of the IGF genes. For description of steps 1 to 4, see text.

- *IGF-I,* also known as somatomedin-C, is primarily involved in skeletal and cartilage growth. Secretion of IGF-I, before birth is independent of GH, but after birth it is stimulated by GH and its plasma concentration like that of GH (Fig. 8.2-8) rises during childhood, peaks at the time of puberty and then declines to low levels in old age. The IGF-I receptor is very similar to the insulin receptor and probably uses much of the same intracellular machinery.
- *IGF-II,* also known as multiplication-stimulating activity (MSA) is independent of GH. It plays a role in growth during fetal development. Its over expression in the fetus leads to disproportionate growth of organs, especially the tongue, other muscles, kidneys, heart and liver. The *IGF-II receptor* is mannose-6-phosphate receptor, which is involved in the intracellular targeting of acid hydrolases and other proteins to intracellular organelles.

The characteristic feature of IGF-1 and II are depicted in Table 8.2-1.

Actions of Growth Hormone

Growth hormone promotes growth and also influences the normal metabolism, therefore, besides acting on one specific organ, its actions are generalized (Fig. 8.2-10).

1. Growth-Promoting Actions of GH Growth hormone promotes linear growth of an individual by its effects on the bone, cartilage and other connective tissues.

Effects on Cartilage. GH stimulates the proliferation of chondrocytes (cartilage cells) present in the epiphyseal end plates of long bones and thus increases the thickness of the epiphyseal cartilage by depositing new cartilage.

TABLE 8.2-2 Character of Insulin-Like Growth Factors

IGF-I	IGF-II
1. IGF-I is also called somatomedin-C	IGF-II is known multiplication stimulating activity (MSA).
2. Secretion	
Before birth, IGF-I secretion is independent of GH and after birth, its secretion is stimulated by GH and its plasma concentration is correlated with GH (i.e. during childhood, reaches to peak at puberty and declines with increasing age).	Secretion of IGF-II is independent of GH and its level remains constant.
3. Receptors of IGF-I are similar to the insulin receptors.	Receptors of IGF-II are mannose-6 phosphate receptors.
4. Its major role is in the skeletal and cartilage growth.	IGF-II plays a major role in fetal growth.

Effects on Bone. GH stimulates osteoblastic activity which converts cartilage into bone. This process continues up to adolescence till there is fusion of epiphyseal end plate with shaft of the bone. The bone mass also increases during this period.

Mode of Action. As described above, the effects of GH on growth is mediated by somatomedins also called insulin-like growth factors (IGFs).

This action of GH is independent of adrenal glands; probably these electrolytes are diverted from kidney to the growing tissue.

Excretion of amino acid 4-hydroxyproline increases during growth and reflects the stimulation of synthesis of collagen by the GH.

2. Metabolic Actions of GH The actions of GH on protein metabolism resemble that of insulin, while actions on fat and carbohydrate metabolism are antagonistic to insulin and synergistic with cortisol. It appears that influence of GH on carbohydrate and fat metabolism is produced directly and is not mediated through IGF-1.

i. Effects on Protein Metabolism. Growth hormone has an anabolic effect on protein metabolism. It promotes the protein deposition in the tissues by the following effects:

- Increases the rate of amino acid uptake into the cells,
- Increases protein synthesis in ribosomes and
- Stimulates transcription (RNA synthesis from DNA).

The overall effect of GH on protein metabolism is positive nitrogen balance that leads to increase in body weight. In addition, GH also decreases protein breakdown, as well as the rate of amino acid degradation for energy purposes.

ii. Effects on Fat Metabolism. GH promotes lipolysis in adipose tissue (catabolic effect) and then increases fat utilization for energy. Administration of GH is associated with:

- Increased levels of circulating FFA. The plasma FFAs provide a ready source of energy for the tissues during hypoglycaemia, fasting and stressful stimuli.
- Increased hepatic oxidation of FFA produces ketone bodies (ketogenic effect).

iii. Effects on Carbohydrate Metabolism. GH is antagonistic to insulin and produces hyperglycaemia by the following effects on carbohydrate metabolism:

- Increases gluconeogenesis, i.e. increases hepatic glucose output,
- Decreases the uptake as well as utilization of glucose by the tissues for energy production and
- Inhibits glycolysis, and thus glycogen stores tend to increase. This occurs as a consequence of increased mobilization and use of FFA for energy production.

As a consequence of hyperglycaemia (produced by above effects), insulin secretion increases. This is an additional way growth hormone promotes growth, since insulin has a protein anabolic effect.

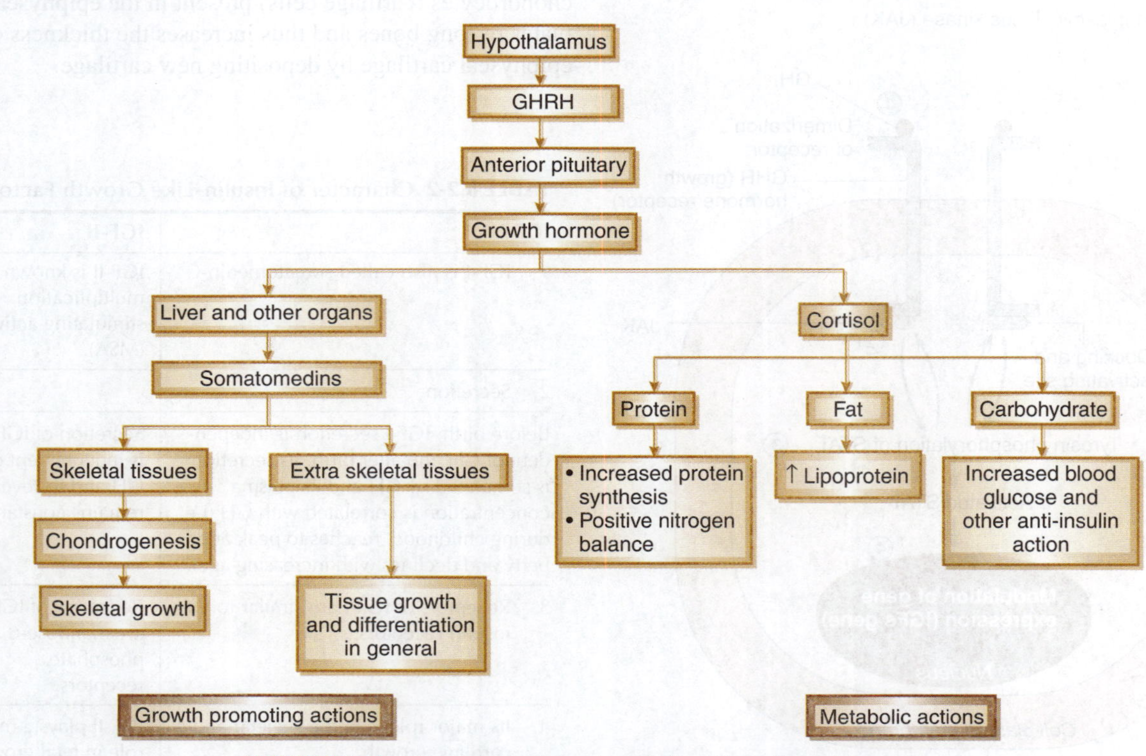

FIGURE 8.2-10 Growth promoting and metabolic actions of growth hormone.

iv. Effects on Mineral Metabolism. Growth hormone promotes bone mineralization in growing children. This effect of growth hormone is probably mediated through insulin-like growth factors (IGF-1), which causes positive balance of calcium, phosphate and magnesium. It promotes renal absorption of Ca^{2+}, phosphate and Na^{+}. It also promotes the retention of Na^{+}, K^{+} and Cl^{-} in the body.

3. Effect on Lactation Growth hormone enhances milk production in lactating animals. Growth hormone acts like prolactin; therefore, this action is referred to as prolactin-like effect of growth hormone.

Applied Aspects: Abnormalities of Anterior Pituitary Hormones

The abnormalities related to pituitary hormones occur either due to excess or deficiency of the hormones secreted. The most common causes of pituitary hormone disturbances are pituitary tumours which may cause symptoms of excess of one or more hormones and simultaneous deficiency of other hormones; hence a mixed picture may evolve. The various hormones of pituitary, their site of action and disease produced by them are given in Table 8.2-3.

Pituitary disorders seen in clinical practice are:

- Hypopituitarism,
- Abnormalities of growth hormone,
- Prolactin deficiency (see page 882) and
- Cushing's syndrome (see page 755).

Hypopituitarism

Hypopituitarism is a clinical condition of hyposecretion of one or more pituitary hormones.

Causes Hypopituitarism can be due to hypothalamic causes or pituitary causes.

A. *Hypothalamic causes of hypopituitarism:*

1. *Congenital conditions*
   - Gonadotropin-releasing hormone (GnRH) deficiency, i.e. Kallmann's syndrome and
   - Isolated growth hormone deficiency.
2. *Acquired conditions* involving hypothalamus include:
   - Tumours such as craniopharyngioma,
   - Radiation,
   - Head injury,
   - Tuberculosis,
   - Sarcoidosis and
   - Histiocytosis 'X'.

B. *Pituitary causes of hypopituitarism:*

- Tumours of anterior pituitary,
- Supracellar cysts,
- Remnants of Rathke's pouch that enlarge and compress the pituitary,
- Surgery,
- Radiotherapy,
- Head injury,
- Postpartum necrosis in females (Sheehan's syndrome),
- Autoimmune and
- Pituitary infarction as occurs in haemorrhagic fever.

TABLE 8.2-3 Pituitary Hormones: Site of Action and Diseases Associated with Their Deficiency and Excess

Hormone	Site of action	Diseases	
		Excess	*Deficiency*
Anterior pituitary			
Growth hormone (GH)	All somatic cells	Gigantism in adolescents	Dwarfism
Adrenocorticotropic hormone (ACTH)	Adrenal cortex	ACTH-dependent Cushing's syndrome	Hypoadrenalism (rare)
Thyroid-stimulating hormone (TSH)	Thyroid	Hyperthyroidism	Hypothyroidism
Prolactin	Breast	Hyperprolactinaemia	–
Gonadotropins	Gonads	Hypergonadism	Hypogonadism
Melanocytic-stimulating hormone (MSH)	Skin	Hyperpigmentation	–
Posterior pituitary			
Antidiuretic hormone	Kidneys	–	Diabetes insipidus

Effects of Hypopituitarism Since anterior pituitary has a large reserve, the endocrine abnormalities are produced only when the large part of pituitary is destroyed. The effects of hypopituitarism are:

1. GH Deficiency. This appears, first of all, with progressive loss of pituitary tissue. Effects of hyposecretion of GH are described on page 690.

2. Gonadotropin Secretion. This is decreased when 70–90% of anterior pituitary is destroyed. It leads to gonadal atrophy decreasing sex hormone levels, which causes:

- In males loss of spermatogenesis, loss of libido, impotency and gynaecomastia.
- In females, abolition of ovulation and stoppage of menstrual cycle results in sterility.
- Some of the secondary sex characteristics disappear, (specially loss of axillary and pubic hair in both the sexes).
- Urinary gonadotropin excretion stops within 2 weeks to 2 months.

3. Thyrotropic Hormone (TSH) Secretion. This is decreased leading to impairment of thyroid function when 90–95% of anterior pituitary is destroyed. Clinical features of hypothyroidism due to hypopituitarism are less marked. Tolerance to cold *is rare*. Frank's myxoedema is not seen.

4. Adrenocorticotropic Hormone (ACTH) Deficiency. This leads to atrophy of adrenal cortex and adrenal insufficiency occurs when almost the whole of the anterior pituitary is destroyed. ACTH-dependent Addison's disease is produced. For details see page 757. In brief, there occurs:

- Pallor of the skin due to decreased ACTH,
- Sensitivity to stress is increased due to decreased glucocorticoids and
- Mineralocorticoid deficiency does not occur, as secretion of aldosterone is controlled by renin secreted from juxtaglomerular apparatus (JGA). So, salt loss and hypovolaemic shock does not occur.

5. Effect on Water Metabolism. Though deficiency of ADH, the posterior pituitary hormone, produces diabetes insipidus, but removal of both anterior and posterior pituitary usually cause no more than a transient polyuria. This occurs because of the following effects:

- Fewer osmotically active products of catabolism are filtered (because ACTH deficiency decreases rate of protein catabolism and TSH deficiency decreases metabolic rate).
- GH deficiency also contributes to the depression of the glomerular filtration rate.

As a consequence of the above, the urine volume decreases even in the absence of ADH. The diuretic activity of anterior pituitary thus can be explained in terms of effects of decreased ACTH, TSH and GH levels.

6. Effect on Insulin Sensitivity. Sensitivity to insulin is markedly increased in hypophysectomized animals. It occurs because of two reasons:

- Due to deficiency of adrenocortical hormones and
- Due to lack of anti-insulin effect of GH.

Abnormalities of Growth Hormone Secretion

The abnormalities of growth hormone secretion include:

- Hypersecretion of GH and
- Hyposecretion of GH.

Hypersecretion of GH Hypersecretion of GH occurs in tumours of acidophilic cells (particularly of somatotrophs) of anterior pituitary. Hypersecretion of GH is also associated with hypersecretion of prolactin. Depending upon the age of an individual, excess of GH may cause:

- Gigantism,
- Acromegaly or
- Acromegalic gigantism (mixed disorder).

*1. **Gigantism.*** It is a clinical condition resulting from hypersecretion of GH in growing children before the closure of epiphysis of long bones.

Clinical features of gigantism include those caused by excess of GH and those produced by compressive and other effects of pituitary tumours.

Features due to excess of GH include gigantism and acromegaly (Figs 8.2.11 and 8.2.12).

Features due to tumour mass include:

- Headache,
- Visual field defects,
- Cranial nerve palsies,
- Enlargement of pituitary fossa with destruction of clinoid processes may be detected on radiograph of skull and
- Hypopituitarism may ultimately result due to compression of other cells of pituitary gland by the tumour.

2. Acromegaly It is a clinical condition that occurs due to excess of GH in adults (after epiphyseal closure of long bones has occurred) and causes excessive growth in those areas where cartilage persists.

Clinical features of acromegaly include those caused by excess of GH and those produced by compressive and other effects of tumour mass.

Features due to excessive GH include:

- *Acromegalic face,* which is characterized by thick lips, macroglossia, broad and thick nose, prominent eyebrows, thickened skin and coarse facial features.
- *Prognathism,* i.e. protrusion of the lower jaw due to elongation and widening of mandible associated with increased spacing of the teeth.

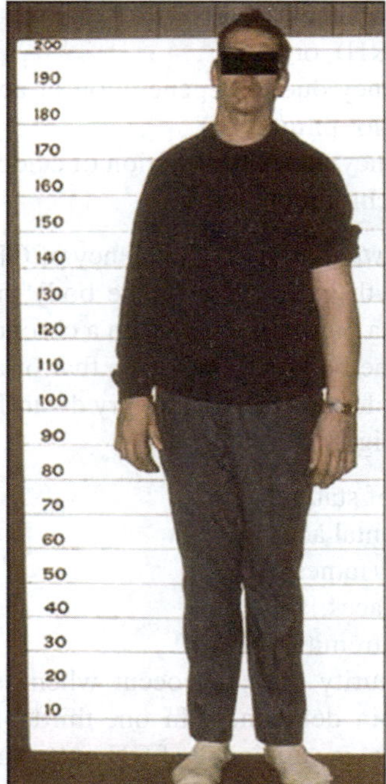

FIGURE 8.2-11 Photograph showing tall stature in a patient with gigantism.

- *Acral part abnormalities* include large spade-like hands, thick wide fingers, increase in head pad and large feet with increase in size of the shoes. Height is normal, build is stout and stocky.
- *Kyphosis* may occur due to improper vertebral growth.
- *Excessive growth of internal organs*, i.e. cardiomegaly, hepatomegaly, splenomegaly and renomegaly may be associated.
- *Increased sympathetic activity* may cause increased sweating and hypertension.
- *Poor gonadal functions* due to hyperprolactinaemia or due to lactogenic effects of GH.
- *Biochemical features* include:
  - Poor glucose tolerance and even occurrence of diabetes in 15% cases,
  - Hypertriglyceridaemia,

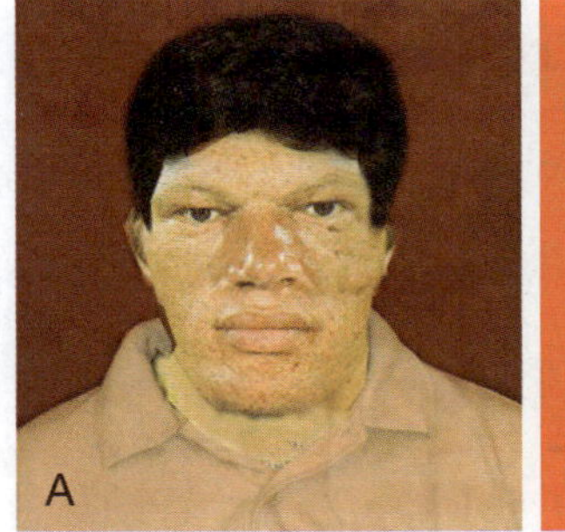

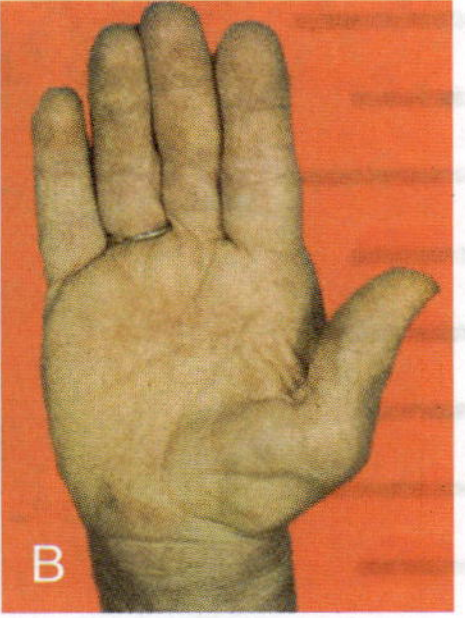

FIGURE 8.2-12 Clinical features of acromegaly. **A,** note coarse facial features, broad thick nose, prognathism, prominent eye brows and thickened skin. **B,** large spade-like hand with short, thick wide fingers.

  - Reduced hepatic and lipoprotein lipase activities and
  - Hypercalcaemia and hyperphosphataemia due to their increased intestinal absorption.

Features due to tumour mass are similar to those seen in gigantism as described above.

3. Acromegalic Gigantism. Acromegalic gigantism, i.e. a mixed picture of acromegaly and gigantism is evolved when the excess of GH occurring in adolescence continues during adult life.

Function Tests for GH In patients with acromegaly and gigantism, following tests are performed:

1. *Basal plasma GH:* level is high.
2. *Plasma prolactin level:* is high in 30% cases.
3. *Glucose tolerance suppression test:* 0.5 μg/L (~2 mU/L) 75 g of glucose is given orally and GH and blood glucose levels are estimated every 2 h.
   - In normal persons hyperglycaemia suppresses GH secretion.
   - In acromegaly or gigantism, there is either no suppression or paradoxical rise in GH (Fig. 8.2-13).
4. *Radiography of skull for pituitary fossa* may show enlargement of pituitary fossa with destruction of clinoid processes.
5. *Visual fields* may be normal or bitemporal, hemianopia or scotoma may be seen due to pressure of pituitary adenoma on the optic chiasma.
6. *CT scan of skull* may show a small or large hypodense microadenoma.

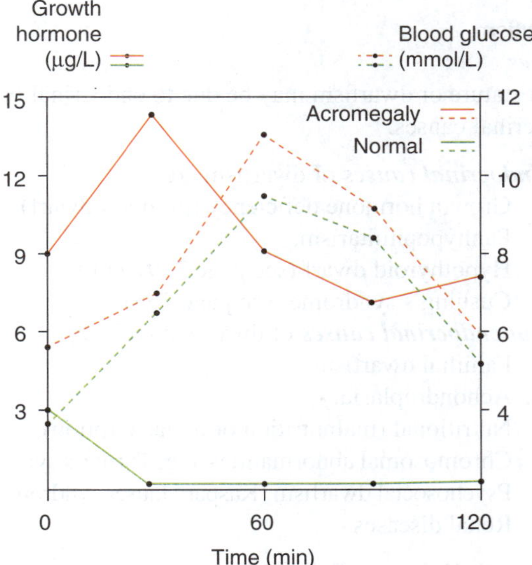

FIGURE 8.2-13 Oral glucose tolerance tests in a normal subject and a patient with acromegaly with measurement of blood glucose and plasma growth hormone. Note the suppression of growth hormone secretion to <0.5 μg/L in the normal subject, and failure to suppress (sometimes accompanied by paradoxical elevation) in acromegaly. Glucose tolerance may also be impaired in acromegaly. (To convert GH in μg/L to mU/L multiply by 3. To convert glucose in mmol/L to mg/dL multiply by 18.)

Treatment may be surgical or medical.

Surgical treatment consists of careful removal of pituitary tumour (adenoma) without damaging other functions.

Radiotherapy. If acromegaly persists even after surgery, then radiotherapy is second line of treatment to stop tumour growth.

Medical treatment includes medical therapy is usually employed to lower GH level to < 1.5 μg/L and to normalize IGF-1 concentration by use of somatostatin analogues:

- *Octreotide* (a somatostatin analogue) is effective in the treatment of long-term acromegaly, but its use is associated with increased chances of gallstone formation.
- *Bromocriptine,* which is a stimulator of GH secretion in normal individuals, is effective in suppressing GH levels in most acromegalic patients.
- *Dopamine agonists* may be helpful if GH hypersecretion is also associated with prolactin excess.
- *Pegvisomant as GH-receptor antagonist* may be indicated, when GH and IGF-1 concentration fails to lower with somatostatin analogue therapy.

Hyposecretion of GH

Deficiency of GH in childhood leads to stunted growth or *dwarfism.*

Deficiency of GH in adulthood results in *mild anaemia* which is refractory to usual treatment with haematinics like iron.

- Reduction in muscle mass and
- Hypoglycaemia may also occur.

Dwarfism

Causes

Short stature or dwarfism may be due to endocrinal or nonendocrinal causes.

- ***Endocrinal causes*** of dwarfism are:
  - Growth hormone deficiency (pituitary dwarf),
  - Panhypopituitarism,
  - Hypothyroid dwarf (see page 709) and
  - Cushing's syndrome (see page 755).
- ***Nonendocrinal causes*** of dwarfism include:
  - Familial dwarfism,
  - Achondroplasia,
  - Nutritional (malnutrition or malabsorption),
  - Chromosomal abnormalities, e.g. Turner's syndrome,
  - Psychosocial dwarfism (Kaspar Hauser syndrome) and
  - Renal diseases.

Growth Hormone-Related Dwarfism

1. Pituitary dwarfism occurs due to deficiency of GH in early childhood. Deficiency of GH may be:

- A part due to the overall lack of anterior pituitary hormones (*panhypopituitarism*),
- An isolated genetic deficiency, or
- Due to deficiency of growth hormone-releasing hormone (GHRH), or
- GH deficiency due to degeneration of acidophilic cells in the anterior pituitary or
- GH deficiency due to destruction of acidophilic cells by tumour of chromophobes.

Characteristic features. Deficiency of GH causes retardation of growth in all parts of the body proportionately. Consequently, a pituitary dwarf with a chronological age of 20 years has the body structure like that of a normal child of 7–10 years of age. Thus, a pituitary dwarf has the following features (Fig. 8.2-14):

- Shortness of stature,
- Normal mental activity,
- Plumpness (fatness),
- Immature faces,
- Delicate extremities and
- Sexual maturity does not occur when associated with gonadotropin deficiency. In one-third of the pituitary dwarfs, there is deficiency of GH only. Such individuals do mature occasionally but do not reproduce.

Functional tests include:

i. *Plasma levels of GH* are low. Since GH levels are undetectable normally in any sample taken during day time, therefore, sample for GH should be taken either:
   - Postexercise; or

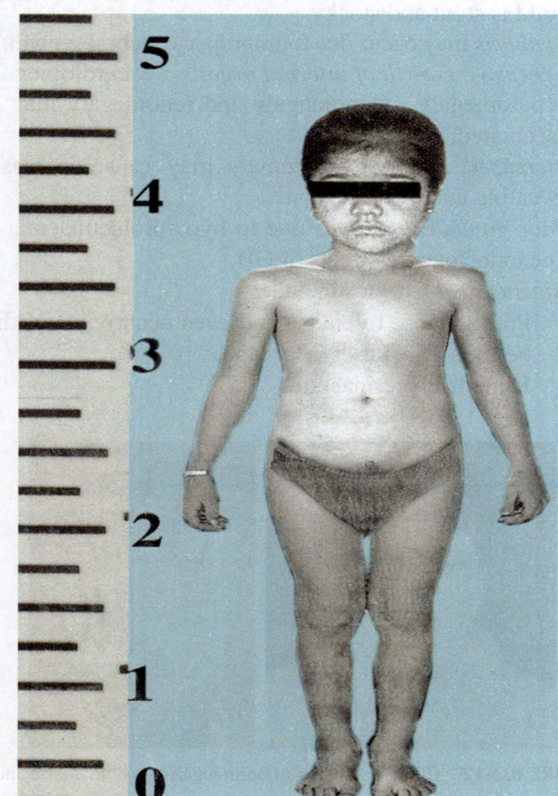

FIGURE 8.2-14 Clinical features of pituitary dwarf.

- One to two hours after going to sleep (at this time there is physiological increase in GH); or
- Frequent samples at night.

ii. *Stimulation test.* Stimulation of GH secretion by insulin-induced hypoglycaemia is a golden standard to confirm or exclude the diagnosis. This test is performed by giving 0.15 U/kg of soluble insulin intravenously to produce hypoglycaemia (blood sugar <40 mg%). The samples are collected at 0, 30, 60, 90 and 120 min for blood glucose and GH. In normal individuals, hypoglycaemia raises GH levels above 20 ng/ml. But in patients with deficiency of GH, the hormone level remains below 7 ng/ml.

Treatment. In children with documented GH deficiency, replacement therapy with GH is useful.

2. African pygmies. In this condition, short stature is due to lack of GH receptors in the tissues, though both GH and somatomedin levels are normal. In addition, their plasma IGF-I levels fail to increase at the time of puberty.

3. Laron dwarfism. In this condition, there is congenital abnormality of the GH receptors, so it is also called *growth hormone insensitivity syndrome*. The plasma concentration of GH-binding protein decreases and IGF-I is not secreted in sufficient amount.

POSTERIOR PITUITARY HORMONES

The two important hormones released from posterior pituitary are:

- Antidiuretic hormone and
- Oxytocin (see page 878).

Antidiuretic Hormone

Antidiuretic hormone (ADH), as the name indicates, prevents diuresis and is chiefly concerned with conservation of body water. Since it also causes vasoconstriction, it is also called vasopressin or more precisely arginine vasopressin (AVP).

Structure, Synthesis, Storage, Release, Transport and Metabolism

Structure, synthesis, storage and release of ADH and oxytocin (OTC) being similar is discussed together.

Structure. ADH and OTC both are homologous neurohormones, polypeptide in nature, containing nine amino acids each, but the amino acids in position 3 and 8 differ in the two hormones.

Synthesis. ADH, as well as OTC, is nonapeptide synthesized in the cell bodies of magnocellular neurons of both paraventricular and supraoptic nuclei of hypothalamus. However, supraoptic nucleus predominately contains ADH-forming neurons while paraventricular nucleus contains mainly the OTC-synthesizing neurons.

- Like all other peptides, they are formed on rough endoplasmic reticulum.
- The ADH and OTC are synthesized as large molecules, the prohormones known as *prepropressophysin* and *preprooxyphysin*, respectively.
- In prepropressophysin, the ADH molecules is associated with neurophysin II and in preprooxyphysin, the oxytocin molecule is associated with neurophysin-I. The neurophysins were originally thought to be binding polypeptides, but it now appears that they are simply parts of the precursor molecules.
- The precursor molecules have their leader molecules removed in the endoplasmic reticulum and are packaged into secretory granules in the Golgi apparatus.

Storage. The axons of ADH and OTC synthesizing neurons end in the posterior pituitary gland as terminal swelling. The secretory granules containing hormone precursors, known as Herring bodies, are transported down the axons by axoplasmic flow to the nerve endings in the posterior pituitary. Cleavage of the precursor molecules occur as they are being transported, and thus the storage granules in the endings contain free ADH or OTC and the corresponding neurophysin. In the case of ADH, a glycopeptide is also present.

Secretion. ADH and OTC are released when a nerve impulse is transmitted from the cell body in the hypothalamus down the axon, where it depolarizes the neurosecretory vesicles. An influx of calcium into the neurosecretory granule then by exocytosis results in secretion of hormones, neurophysins and glycopeptides. Thus, the factors which increase the discharge activity of these neurons cause increased release of hormones and vice versa. All these products are secreted but the functions of the components other than ADH and OTC are not known.

Transport. The hormone and other secreted products separately enter the closely adjacent capillary. Subsequent transport of the hormone into the bloodstream is accomplished by endocytosis into the endothelial cells and then by diffusion through pores in the fenestrated capillary endothelium. The hormone then reaches the target cells and by circulatory interconnections, also to the anterior pituitary.

Evidence to support that ADH and OTC are synthesized in hypothalamus and only stored in posterior pituitary include:

- Herring bodies (coarse large granules) containing ADH and OTC can be visualized in hypothalamus and posterior pituitary by special staining techniques. After sectioning of the hypothalamo–hypophyseal tract, Herring bodies disappear below the section and fill up proximal to the point of section, suggesting that the granules are coming from the hypothalamus.

- Destruction of supraoptic nucleus causes disappearance of Herring bodies with symptoms of ADH deficiency, confirming that the neurons of supraoptic nucleus synthesize ADH.
- Newly synthesized hormone can be released into the circulation from the hypothalamus even in the absence of posterior pituitary depicting that this is not the site of hormone synthesis.

Other Sources of ADH and OTC. In addition to the above-described magnocellular neurons of hypothalamus, the ADH and OTC are also present in the:

- Endings of neurons which project on to brainstem and spinal cord,
- Gonads,
- Adrenal cortex and
- Thymus.

Biological half-life of ADH is 16–20 min after its release into the circulation.

Metabolism. The circulating vasopressin is rapidly inactivated in the liver and kidney.

Vasopressin Receptors

Three types of vasopressin receptors are recognized:

- V_1-A *receptors.* These act through phosphatidylinositol hydrolysis to increase the intracellular Ca^{2+} concentration. These are involved in the vasoconstrictor effect of ADH.
- V_1-B *receptors*. These also act by a mechanism similar to that of V_1-A and are involved in the action of ADH on anterior pituitary.
- V_2 *receptors.* These act through Gs to increase cAMP levels and are involved in the action of ADH on the kidney.

Actions of ADH

1. Action on Kidney. The main role of ADH is regulation of water balance in the body by acting on the kidney, where it decreases the excretion of free water (i.e. antidiuretic and concentrating effect on kidney).

Site of Action. ADH acts on the basolateral membrane of the renal cells that are responsible for reabsorbing free (i.e. osmotically unencumbered) water from the glomerular filtrate. These ADH responsive cells line the distal convoluted tubules and collecting ducts of the renal nephron. ADH increases the permeability of these cells to water. The ADH also acts on the ascending limb of the loop of Henle to enhance sodium transport into the medullary interstitium. The resultant increase in the osmolality of the interstitium helps to create the osmotic gradient for water reabsorption. In this way, ADH increases the osmolality of urine to a maximum that is fourfold greater than that of glomerular filtrate.

Mechanism of Action. The ADH exerts its antidiuretic effect by binding to a specific plasma membrane receptor (known as V_2 receptor) on the capillary (basal) side of the cell, where it activates adenylyl cyclase. The increase in intracellular cAMP activates a protein (kinase) on the opposite (luminal apical) side of the cell. The activated protein kinase leads to rapid insertion of protein water channels (known as aquaporins) in the plasma membranes of the principal cells of the collecting ducts. Through these protein water channels (i.e. aquaporin), water rapidly moves from the tubular lumen into the collecting duct cells.

- *Aquaporins* are of different types: aquaporin-1, -2, and -3 are found in the kidneys; aquaporin-4 is found in the brain and aquaporin-5 is found in the salivary and lacrimal glands and in respiratory tract.
- ADH responsive aquaporin-2 is stored in the endosomes inside the cells and is translocated by the ADH into the luminal membrane of the principal cells of collecting ducts. Through these protein water channels (i.e. aquaporin-2), water rapidly moves from the tubular lumen into the cells of collecting ducts.
- From inside the cells, the water moves into ECF through aquaporin-3 and -4, which are inserted into the basolateral membrane of the cells.

2. Vasoconstrictor Effect. ADH in large doses referred to as supraphysiological or pharmacological doses, cause vasoconstriction and leads to rise in blood pressure. Haemorrhage is a potent stimulus to ADH secretion, and it has been reported that ADH plays an important role in blood pressure homeostasis by causing constriction of splanchnic vascular bed. This effect has been exploited therapeutically in controlling serious gastrointestinal bleeding.

Mechanism of Action. The ADH exerts its vasoconstrictor effect by binding to the V_1-A receptors on the arterial smooth muscles and causes it to constrict. This action is mediated by Ca^{2+} and phospholipase C-generated second messengers.

- Vasopressin also acts as a neurotransmitter on the brain through the V_1-A receptor to decrease cardiac output. The site for this action is area postrema (also known as circumventricular organs) having fenestrated capillaries (out of blood–brain barrier). Therefore, vasopressin plays an important role in blood pressure homeostasis.

3. Action on Anterior Pituitary. ADH travels to the anterior pituitary via the portal veins and combines with the V_1-B receptors (also called V_3 receptors) which appear to be unique to the anterior pituitary. The binding of ADH to V_1-B receptor generates phospholipase C-released second messengers, which cause increased ACTH secretion from the corticotrophs.

4. Action on the Liver. In the liver, ADH causes *glycogenolysis* by combining with the V_1-A receptor.

5. Action on the Brain. V_1-A receptors are also found in brain, where ADH acts as neurotransmitter and is involved in memory, regulation of temperature, regulation of blood pressure, circadian rhythms and brain development.

Synthetic Agonists and Antagonists of ADH

Synthetic agonists of ADH that have selective actions and are more active than naturally occurring ADH have been produced by altering the amino acid residues. For example, 1-deamino-8-D-arginine vasopressin (DDAVP), also called *desmopressin* has very high antidiuretic activity with little pressure activity, making it valuable in the treatment of ADH deficiency.

Synthetic antagonists that selectively block the pressure or antidiuretic activity of ADH have also been synthesized.

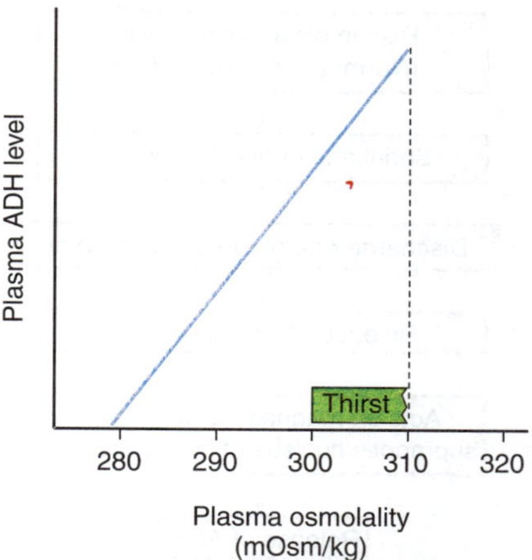

FIGURE 8.2-15 Correlation between plasma osmolality, ADH secretion and onset of thirst in healthy human in whom the plasma osmolality was increased by infusing hypertonic sodium chloride.

Regulation of ADH Secretion

The main factors which regulate the ADH secretion are: effective osmotic pressure of the plasma and changes in blood volume. In addition, some other factors also effect ADH secretion.

1. Effective Osmotic Pressure of Plasma or Plasma Osmolality Plasma osmolality in normal individuals is maintained very close to 285 mOsm/L by ADH. In other words, change in plasma osmolality is a very potent regulator of ADH secretion. A significant change in ADH secretion occurs when plasma osmolality is changed as little as 1%. Thus, water deprivation (which increases plasma osmolality) stimulates ADH secretion, and it thereby decreases free-water clearance and enhances water conservation. On the other hand, a water load (which decreases plasma osmolality) decreases ADH secretion, and thus increases free-water clearance and the efficiency of water excretion.

Thus, ADH and water form a negative feedback loop. When plasma osmolality is increased by infusing hypertonic sodium chloride, ADH secretion is stimulated, and plasma ADH rises over a linear concentration range (Fig. 8.2-15). It is important to note that this response of ADH to hyperosmolality just precedes the response of thirst (Fig. 8.2-15). Both, ADH release and thirst lead to increase in body water that limits further increments in the osmolality of plasma.

Mechanism of Action. Changes in plasma osmolality affect the osmoreceptors.

- ***Osmoreceptors*** refer to the group of neurons located in the anterior hypothalamus in the region of circumventricular organs and organumvasculosum of lamina terminalis (this region is outside the blood–brain barrier). These cells are distinct from the cells which produce ADH.
- ***Osmoreceptors are very sensitive to osmolality of the plasma.*** As mentioned earlier, the normal plasma osmolality is 285 mOsm/L. The rise in plasma osmolality even by 1–2% results in shrinkage of osmoreceptors causing increased rate of discharge and reflexly increased ADH secretion and thus maintained plasma osmolality (Fig. 8.2-16).
- ***Solutes which stimulate osmoreceptors.*** The osmoreceptors are stimulated by those solutes to which the cells are relatively impermeable and cross the blood–brain barrier slowly. Therefore, substances like Na^+, mannitol and sucrose are potent stimulators for ADH secretion.
  - *Na^+* is a very important stimulator of ADH because 95% of effective plasma osmotic pressure is due to plasma Na^+ only.
  - *Glucose and urea.* The hyperglycaemia and uraemia are comparatively less potent stimulators for ADH releases, but in uncontrolled diabetes mellitus (hyperglycaemia associated with insulin deficiency), glucose acts as an effective stimulus for ADH release.

2. Changes in Blood Volume Changes in circulating blood volume, central blood volume, cardiac output and blood pressure (Fig. 8.2-17) affect the secretion of ADH. ADH secretion is increased when ECF volume is low and decreased when ECF volume is high. Quite standing, tilting, or positive-pressure breathing also reduce central blood volume; and therefore, increase ADH secretion, particularly when blood pressure falls. On the other hand, administration of blood or isotonic saline solution, which increases total circulating blood volume, or immersion of body up to the neck in water, which increases central blood volume and decreases ADH release.

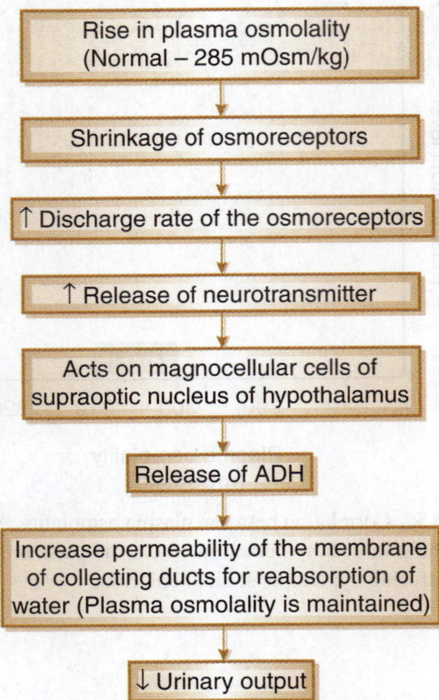

FIGURE 8.2-16 Mechanism of regulation of ADH by plasma osmolality.

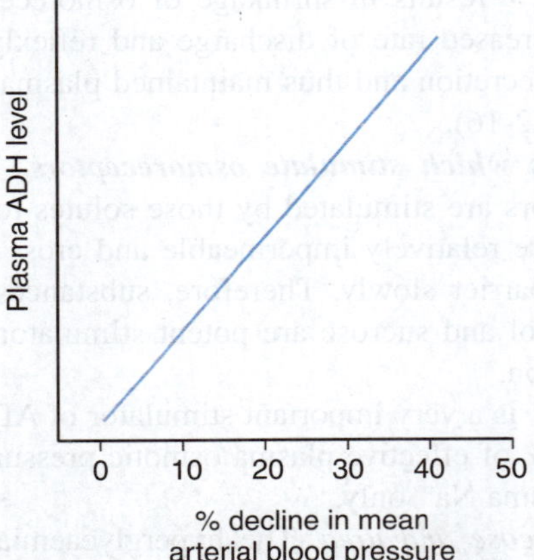

FIGURE 8.2-17 Correlation between declining blood pressure and plasma ADH levels in healthy adult human in whom a progressive decline in blood pressure was induced by infusing trimethaphan (a sympathetic blocking agent).

Mechanism of Action. The changes in blood volume regulate ADH secretion by following mechanisms:

i. ***Pressure receptor mechanism.*** Variations in the discharge from pressure receptors in the circulatory system are inversely related to the rate of ADH secretion. There are two types of pressure receptors in the circulatory system: the low and high pressure receptors.

- *Low pressure receptors* are located in the great veins, right and left atria and pulmonary vessels. They monitor the fullness of vascular system, and thus mainly respond to volume changes (hence also called volume receptors).
- *High pressure receptors* are located in the carotid sinuses and aortic arch (i.e. high pressure portion of the vascular system) and are reported to respond to pressure changes and so are also called baroreceptors.
- *Afferent impulses* from these receptors are carried by the ninth and tenth cranial nerves to their respective nuclei in the medulla. From the medulla the impulses are carried by way of the midbrain via adrenergic neurotransmitters to the supraoptic nuclei of the hypothalamus. Normally, the pressure receptors tonically inhibit ADH secretion by modulating an inhibitory flow of adrenergic impulses from the medulla to the hypothalamus. A decrease in pressure increases ADH secretion by reducing the flow of neural impulses from the pressure receptors to the brainstem. The reduced neural input from these receptors relieves the source of tonic inhibition on the hypothalamic cells that secrete ADH.

ii. ***Renin–angiotensin mechanism.*** Hypovolaemia also stimulates the generation of renin and angiotensin directly within the brain. This renin–angiotensin mechanism reinforces the release of ADH in response to hypovolaemia and hypotension by acting on the circumventricular organs.

iii. ***Atrial natriuretic peptide (ANP) mechanism*** also reinforces the release of ADH in response to hypovolaemia. When circulating volume is increased, ANP is released by cardiac myocytes which acts on the hypothalamus to inhibit ADH release.

Interaction of hypovolaemia and plasma osmolality. The two major stimuli of ADH secretion, i.e. hypovolaemia and plasma osmolality interact with each other.

The hypovolaemia sensitizes the ADH response to hyperosmolality. However, if hypovolaemia is severe (e.g. after severe haemorrhage) baroregulation overrides osmotic regulation, and ADH secretion is stimulated, even though plasma osmolality may be below 270 mOsm/L.

3. Other Factors Affecting ADH Secretion Factors, other than the two major stimuli (i.e. hypovolaemia and plasma osmolality), which affect ADH secretions are:

- ***Stress*** of pain, chronic emotional stress and surgical procedures cause increase in ADH secretion leading to reduction in urine formation under these conditions.
- ***Adrenaline*** decreases the ADH. Hence, one experiences increased frequency of micturition during such acute emotional stresses such as interviews or examinations.
- ***Alcohol*** reduces ADH secretion and thus leads to diuresis.
- ***Sex.*** The size of ADH neurons, the rate of ADH secretion and the plasma level of ADH are all greater in men than women.
- ***Age.*** Elderly individuals secrete more ADH than do younger individuals, probably in compensation for

a diminished ability of their kidneys to concentrate urine.

- ***Cortisol and thyroid hormones*** restrain ADH release. Therefore, in their absence ADH may be secreted, even though plasma osmolality is low.
- ***Some other factors*** that increase ADH secretion include nausea, vomiting, standing posture and drugs like clofibrate, carbamazepine and cytokines.

Summary of factors regulating ADH secretion is given in Fig. 8.2-18.

Abnormalities of ADH Secretion

Abnormalities of ADH secretion include:

- Syndrome of inappropriate hypersecretion of ADH and
- Diabetes insipidus.

Syndrome of Inappropriate Hypersecretion of ADH

Syndrome of inappropriate hypersecretion of antidiuretic hormone (SIADH) refers to a condition in which ADH secretion is increased despite the presence of hypo-osmolality. Excessive ADH secretion leads to water intoxication, i.e. overhydration and because of this SIADH is also called *dilution syndrome*.

Causes

I. Excessive Secretion of ADH from Posterior Pituitary may occur during surgical stress, because of pain and hypovolaemia.

II. Excessive Secretion of ADH from Some Ectopic Source, e.g.

- In cerebral disease (cerebral salt wasting) and
- In pulmonary diseases (pulmonary salt wasting) such as bronchogenic carcinoma.

III. Excess of ADH Due to its Decreased Metabolic Degradation may occur in patients with liver cirrhosis and cardiac failure. In such cases, half-life of ADH is prolonged.

Characteristic Features

1. Water Retention. Excessive ADH leads to water retention causing expansion of blood volume and extracellular fluid (ECF) volume.

2. Hypernatriuria. The expansion in ECF volume reduces aldosterone secretion causing hypernatriuria, i.e. excessive urinary excretion of Na^+.

3. Hyponatraemia, i.e. decrease in plasma Na^+ level (<135 mmol/L) is caused by ADH by its dilatational effect (water retention) as well as by causing hypernatriuria.

4. Oedema. Water retention and excessive urinary excretion of Na^+ causes hypo-osmolality of blood (since ADH secretion is increased despite hypo-osmolality of blood, which is why the condition is called syndrome of inappropriate hypersecretion of ADH). The low plasma osmolality causes shift of water from plasma into the interstitial spaces producing the so-called oedema. The decreased osmolality of fluid in interstitial spaces, i.e. ECF causes shift of water from ECF into the cells.

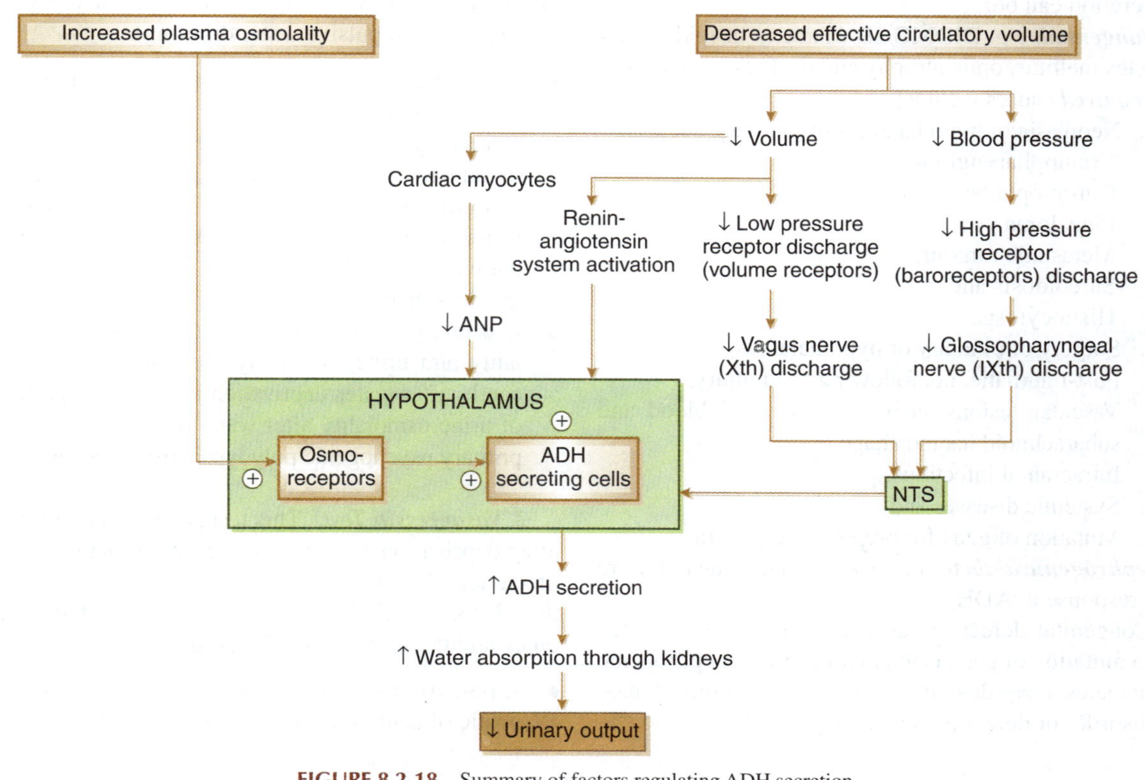

FIGURE 8.2-18 Summary of factors regulating ADH secretion.

5. Increased Urinary Osmolality occurs due to decreased urinary excretion of water and continued excretion of Na^+. The urinary osmolality exceeds plasma osmolality and urinary Na^+ excretion may be more than 20 mEq/L.

Important Note

In this situation, if water intake is restricted then water retention does not occur and ADH secretion has no effect on plasma Na^+ and oedema does not occur. This is because reduced water intake does not cause an increase in ECF volume, and thus aldosterone secretion is not suppressed and hence there is no excessive urinary excretion of Na^+.

- In animals (rats), studies have demonstrated that a prolonged exposure to high vasopressin levels can lead to:
  - Decreased production of aquaporin-2 channels resulting in sudden increase in urinary output and
  - Fall in plasma osmolality.

Treatment. SIADH can be treated with drugs like *demeclocycline,* which blocks the effect of ADH on kidneys.

Diabetes Insipidus

Diabetes insipidus refers to a clinical condition of polyuria that occurs, either due to deficiency of ADH (vasopressin) release or failure of renal response to ADH.

Causes Depending upon the cause, diabetes insipidus is of two types:

A. Central (Cranial) or Neurogenic Diabetes Insipidus results from failure of ADH secretion. Causes of failure of ADH secretion can be:

I. ***Congenital,*** e.g. DIDMOAD (diabetes insipidus, diabetes mellitus, optic atrophy and deafness syndrome.

II. ***Acquired*** causes include:

1. Neoplasia of hypothalamus or pituitary, such as:
   - Craniopharyngioma,
   - Chromophobe adenoma,
   - Pinealoma,
   - Metastatic tumour,
   - Sarcoidosis and
   - Histiocytosis.
2. Surgery of pituitary or hypothalamus,
3. Post-traumatic, i.e. following head injury,
4. Vascular lesions such as intracranial blood and subarachnoid haemorrhage,
5. Intracranial infections,
6. Systemic diseases and
7. Mutation of gene for prepropressophysin.

B. Nephrogenic diabetes insipidus occurs due to failure of renal response to ADH.

- Congenital defect in vasopressin receptor (V_2) due to mutation of gene is the main cause of nephrogenic diabetes insipidus. It is an X chromosome-linked disorder or defect in gene aquaporin-2.
- Other causes of nephrogenic diabetes insipidus are hypokalaemia and hyperkaliuria.

Characteristic Features Diabetes insipidus is characterized by decreased renal absorption of water leading to following features:

- Polyuria,
- Polydypsia and
- Dehydration.

1. Polyurea, i.e. passage of large amounts of urine, is the most important single feature of diabetes insipidus. Patient passes up to 3–20 L of urine of pale colour and of low specific gravity per day. Patient goes for urination after every ½–1 h. In nephrogenic diabetes insipidus, urine output is directly related to the volume of water delivered to collecting ducts.

2. Polydypsia, Polyuria is followed by obligatory polydypsia (drinking of large amount of water). It occurs due to stimulation of thirst mechanism. In fact, polydypsia is an important mechanism which helps to maintain water balance with near normal plasma Na^+ level in patients with diabetes insipidus.

3. Dehydration may occur in severe cases. Its signs and symptoms include dry tongue and dry mouth. Fall of blood pressure and loss of consciousness may be seen in acute severe cases.

Tests for Diagnosis

1. Water Deprivation Test. This test is performed to differentiate diabetes insipidus from primary psychogenic polydypsia (compulsive water drinking).

- Normally, after 8 h of (overnight) water deprivation, plasma osmolality rises and it also raises the urine osmolality, which may reach even up to 800 mOsm/kg.
- In diabetes insipidus, initially, plasma osmolality is high and urine osmolality rises due to ADH deficiency. After water deprivation test, blood osmolality rises further but there is negligible rise in urine osmolality, which is usually less than 300 mOsm/kg.
- In primary psychogenic polydypsia, initial plasma osmolality and urine osmolality are low, which rise significantly after water deprivation test. Thus, significant rise of urine osmolality after water deprivation differentiates primary psychogenic polydypsia from diabetes insipidus.

2. Vasopressin Test. This test is performed immediately after deprivation test and may even form the second part of the test. It helps to differentiate central diabetes insipidus. A total of 5 IU of vasopressin is injected subcutaneously and the response is observed.

- A positive response, i.e. rise in urine osmolality is diagnostic of central diabetes insipidus while

- A negative response, i.e. no rise in urine osmolality even after administration of vasopressin is diagnostic of nephrogenic diabetes insipidus.

3. Other Tests to find out the cause of diabetes insipidus are:

For central diabetes insipidus

- Radiograph of skull may show pituitary fossa enlargement
- Visual field test may be defective
- CT scan and MRI may reveal tumours or other lesions of pituitary or hypothalamus.

For nephrogenic diabetes insipidus

- Serum potassium,
- Serum calcium,
- Radiology of urinary tract and
- Renal function tests.

Treatment

1. ***Central or neurogenic diabetes insipidus*** can be treated by:
   - Hormonal therapy, i.e. ADH or desmopressin administration, and
   - Nonhormonal therapy, i.e. via drugs which increased ADH secretion, such as
   - Chlorpropamide (an oral hypoglycaemic agent), thiazides (diuretics), clofibrate and carbamazepine.
2. ***Nephrogenic diabetes insipidus*** is treated by diuretics, e.g. hydrochlorothiazide. These inhibit Na^+ reabsorption in thick segment of loop of Henle and so urine osmolality does not fall below 300 mOsm/kg.

Chapter 8.3

Thyroid Gland

FUNCTIONAL ANATOMY
- Gross anatomy
- Histological structure

THYROID HORMONES
- Introduction
- Biosynthesis and storage
- Secretion, transport and metabolism
- Regulation of secretion
- Mechanism of action
- Actions

APPLIED ASPECTS OF THYROID HORMONES
- Abnormalities of thyroid gland
  - Hyperthyroidism
  - Hypothyroidism
  - Goitre
- Thyroid function tests

FUNCTIONAL ANATOMY

Gross Anatomy

The thyroid gland has two distinctions: (1) it was the first endocrine gland to be recognized as such on the basis of symptoms associated with excess or deficient functions, and (2) it is the largest endocrine gland in the body (weighing about 15–25 g in adults). It consists of two lobes joined together by a narrow isthmus and is located on either side of the trachea, just below the larynx. It receives high blood supply with its rate of blood flow, 400–600 ml/100 g/min, which is higher than even the myocardium or kidneys.

Histological Structure (Fig. 8.3-1)

Histologically, each *lobe* of the thyroid gland is divided into various *lobules* by fibrous tissue septa. Each lobule is made up of an aggregation of several *follicles*. Follicle (acinus) is the functional unit of the thyroid gland. Each follicle is lined by *follicular cells* that rest on a basement membrane. The reabsorption lacunae are the areas where the colloid is being actively absorbed into the thyrocytes by endocytosis. The follicle is surrounded by a rich capillary plexus.

Follicular Cells. These vary in shape with the degree of glandular activity. Normally (at an average level of activity), the cells are *cuboidal* and the colloid in the follicles is moderate in amount. During high degree of activity, the cells become columnar and flat when inactive (Fig. 8.3-1B). These cells secrete thyroid hormones.

Parafollicular Cells. In addition to follicular cells, the thyroid gland contains parafollicular cells or *C cells*. These do not border on the follicular lumen but are scattered between the follicular cells and basement membrane (Fig. 8.3-1A). They may also lie in the intervals between the follicle cells. These cells secrete calcitonin, which is described in Chapter 8.4.

Colloid. This is a homogeneous material that fills the cavity of each follicle. When stimulated, the follicles are depleted of colloid; and when unstimulated, the follicles accumulate colloid. The major constituent of the colloid is thyroglobulin, a glycoprotein with a molecular weight of 660,000.

THYROID HORMONES

Introduction

The two principal thyroid hormones include thyroxine (T_4) and tri-iodothyronine (T_3). Both T_4 and T_3 consist of iodine-containing amino acids.

- *Thyroxine* or T_4 (3,5,3´,5´-tetraiodothyronine) constitutes 90% of thyroid output.
- *Tri-iodothyronine* or T_3 (3,5,3´-tri-iodothyronine) constitutes 10% of thyroid output; however, it is responsible for most of the tissue actions of thyroid hormone.
- *Reverse tri-iodothyronine* (3,3´,5´-tri-iodothyronine) or reverse T_3 or RT_3, is a biologically inactive thyronine, which forms less than 1% of thyroid output.
- *Calcitonin*, is a hormone secreted by the parafollicular cells of the thyroid gland. It is concerned with calcium homeostasis and is discussed in Chapter 8.4.

Thyroid hormones, for all practical purposes refer to thyroxine (T_4) and tri-iodothyronine (T_3).

- *Molar activity ratio* of T_3 to T_4 is 10:1 in most systems.
- *Storage ratio* of T_4 to T_3 bound to thyroglobulin is 10:1.
- *Secretory ratio of T_4 to T_3* is 10:1.
- *Plasma concentration ratio* of free T_4 to free T_3 is 2:1.

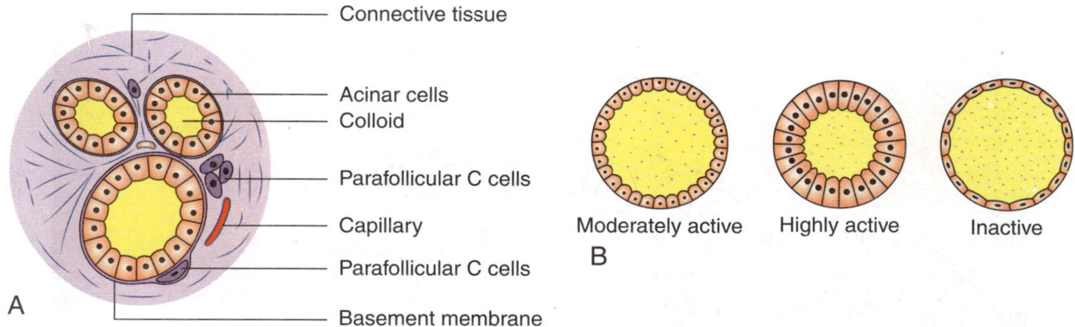

FIGURE 8.3-1 Histological structure of thyroid gland **(A)** and variations in follicular cell size with activity **(B)**.

Iodine Metabolism

Dietary Intake. Iodine is essential for the synthesis of thyroid hormones. It is ingested in the form of iodides. Sources of iodine are sea fish (richest), bread, milk and vegetables. Iodine is added to table salt to prevent iodine deficiency.

- Daily average intake of iodine is 500 μg.
- Daily requirement of iodine is 100–200 μg.
- Minimum intake required to prevent goitre is 75 μg/day.
- Neonatal iodine requirement is 40 μg/day.
- During pregnancy iodine requirement is 200 μg/day.

Fate of Dietary Iodide. Most of (i.e. 400 μg/day) the iodides absorbed from the gastrointestinal tract are rapidly excreted through kidneys, but 100 μg/day is selectively removed from circulation by cells of the thyroid gland. Thyroid uses it for synthesis of the thyroid hormone. Thyroid secretes about 80 μg/day in the form of T_4 and T_3, whereas 40 μg/day diffuses back into the ECF. The circulating T_4 and T_3 are metabolized in the liver and other tissues, with release of 60 μg/day iodine into the ECF and some derivatives excreted into the bile. Some of the iodine is then absorbed by enterohepatic circulation, while about 20 μg/day iodine is lost in the stools.

Plasma iodide level is 0.15–0.3 μg%.

Thyroid iodide. Thyroid gland contains 5–8 mg of iodide, i.e. about 95% of total iodine content of the body. Thus, the thyroid serves as a store for iodine which is sufficient to maintain a euthyroid state for 3 months without hormone synthesis. Of the total thyroid iodide, only 5% is present within the cells of the follicular epithelium. The remaining 95% is present in the follicular lumen, and stored in the colloid as thyroglobulin. In the colloid, two-thirds of the total iodine is present in the form of biologically inactive iodotyrosines and one-third is in the form of biologically active thyronine (T_4 and T_3).

Biosynthesis and Storage of Thyroid Hormones

Thyroxine (T_4) and tri-iodothyronine (T_3) are synthesized from tyrosine and iodide by the enzyme complex, peroxidase. The steps involved in the synthesis of thyroid hormones are (Fig. 8.3-2):

1. **Iodine Trapping.** The first step in the synthesis of thyroid hormones is *uptake of iodide* by the thyroid gland which occurs against the chemical (about 30:1) and electrical gradients by a Na^+-I^- cotransport/symport (NIS) system that is located in the basal membrane of the thyroid epithelial cells. It is an energy requiring process and is linked to the ATPase-dependent Na^+–K^+ pump.

- *TSH controls* the iodide uptake. The thyroid:plasma-free iodide ratio, which is normally maintained at 30, may exceed 100 when the gland is maximally activated by TSH.
- *Antithyroid agents* such as thiocyanate and perchlorate inhibit iodide transport.

2. **Synthesis and Secretion of Thyroglobulin.** Thyroglobulin is a large glycoprotein that is synthesized on the rough endoplasmic reticulum of thyroid epithelial cells as peptide units of molecular weight 330,000 (the primary translation product of its messenger RNA). These units combine into a dimer, after which carbohydrate moieties are added as the molecule moves to the Golgi apparatus. The completed glycoprotein is contained in small vesicles, which move to the apical plasma membrane and release into the lumen of the follicle (Fig. 8.3-2).

- Each molecule of thyroglobulin contains about 140 tyrosine residues which can serve as substrate for iodine for the formation of thyroid hormones. It is also the storage site of the two hormones within the thyroid gland.

3. **Oxidation of Iodide.** Once within the gland, iodide rapidly moves to the apical surface of the epithelial cells. From these, it is transported into the lumen of the follicles by a sodium-independent iodide/chloride transporter called *pendrin*. The iodide (1) is then immediately oxidized to iodine (1°) by the enzyme *peroxidase* present near the apical border of the epithelial cells. The immediate oxidant (electron acceptor) for this reaction is H_2O_2, which is supplied by an NADPH-dependent system (Fig. 8.3-3).

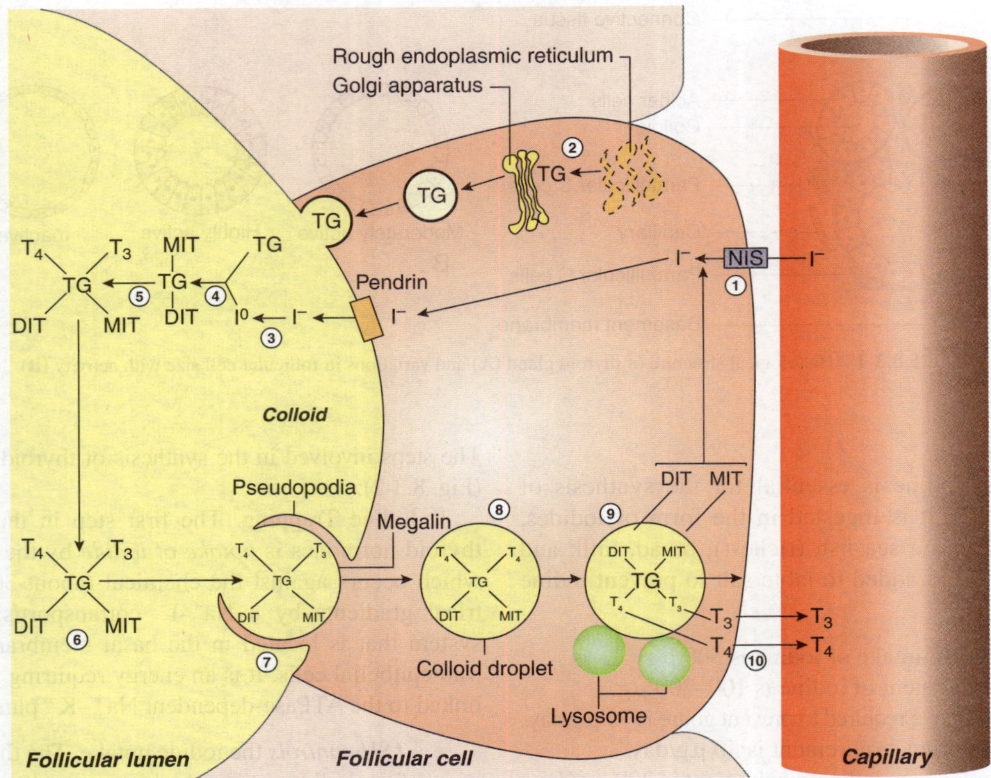

FIGURE 8.3-2 Steps in synthesis and release of thyroid hormones: 1, iodine trapping; 2, synthesis of thyroglobulin; 3, oxidation of iodine; 4, organification of thyroglobulin; 5, coupling reaction; 6, storage of thyroid hormone in colloid; 7, take up of colloid by epithelial cell by endocytosis; 8, colloid vesicle; 9, release of T_3 and T_4 after proteolysis; and 10, diffusion of T_3 and T_4 into the capillary.

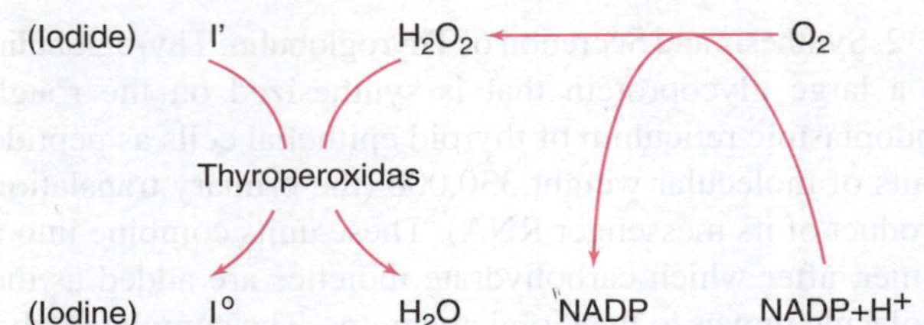

FIGURE 8.3-3 Oxidation of iodide by the enzyme thyroperoxidase.

Thyroid is the only tissue that can oxidize iodide to iodine. TSH promotes this reaction while antithyroid drugs (thiourea, thiouracil, methimazole) inhibit.

Note. Pendrin is an ion exchanger protein in nature, first identified in patients suffering with Pendred syndrome with thyroid dysfunction.

4. **Organification of Thyroglobulin** refers to iodination of tyrosine residues present in the thyroglobulin molecule. This reaction occurs at the apical membrane of the cell as soon as thyroglobulin molecule is released by the secretory granules by exocytosis and requires thyroid peroxidase. Tyrosine (of thyroglobulin) is first iodinated at position 3 to form monoiodotyrosine (MIT) and then at position 5 to form di-iodotyrosine (DIT).

5. **Coupling Reaction.** The process of iodination of tyrosine residues is followed by a coupling reaction, which lasts for the next few minutes to an hour. Two molecules of DIT couple to form thyroxine (T_4). One molecule of MIT, when coupled with one molecule of DIT, tri-iodothyronine (T_3) is produced (Fig. 8.3-4). The mechanism of coupling is not well understood. The enzyme peroxidase is required during coupling as well as for iodination. There are two theories regarding the coupling reaction:

As the process of iodination and coupling is completed, each molecule of thyroglobulin contains about 7 molecules of MIT, 6 molecules of DIT, 2 molecules of T_4 and 0.2 molecules of T_3. Thus, the ratio of T_4 to T_3 in a molecule of thyroglobulin is 10:1.

6. **Storage.** Once thyroglobulin has been iodinated, it is stored in the lumen of the follicle as colloid for several months. It is estimated that the stored thyroid hormones can meet the body requirement for 1–3 months.

Secretion, Transport and Metabolism of Thyroid Hormones

Hormone Secretion Secretion of the thyroid hormone from the colloid stored in the lumen of follicle involves the following steps (Fig. 8.3-2):

Endocytosis. The colloid containing iodinated thyroglobulin is retrieved from the lumen of the follicle by the epithelial cells through endocytosis. This process is facilitated by

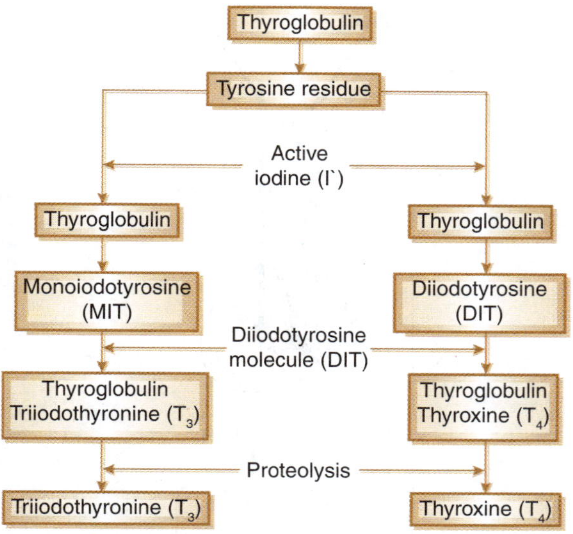

FIGURE 8.3-4 Coupling reaction to form T_3 and T_4.

the TG receptor *megalin* located on the apical membrane. By this process, the colloid enters the cytoplasm in the form of *colloid droplets*, which move through the cytoplasm towards the basal membrane probably as a result of microtubule and microfilament functions (Fig. 8.3-2).

Proteolysis. The colloid droplets fuse with the lysosome vesicles containing proteolytic enzymes. The proteases digest the thyroglobulin molecule releasing T_4, T_3, DIT, MIT and other amino acid constituents into the cytoplasm of the epithelial cells.

- T_4 and T_3 diffuse through the basal border of epithelial cells into the bloodstream via adjacent rich capillary plexus.
- MIT and DIT are rapidly deiodinated within the follicular cells by the enzyme iodotyrosine *deiodinase*. In this way, iodide is retrieved for recycling along with the tyrosine into T_4 and T_3 synthesis (Fig. 8.3-2):

Important Note

In patients with congenital absence of iodotyrosine deiodinase, MIT and DIT get excreted into the urine and symptoms of iodine deficiency appear.

Transport of T_4 and T_3 Secreted T_4 and T_3 circulate in the bloodstream in two forms: bound and free.

1. Bound Form. Most of the circulating T_4 (99.95%) and T_3 (99.5%) is bound to specific binding proteins.

- *Thyroxine-binding globulin (TBG)* is the major binding protein which binds about 70% of T_4 and T_3.
- *Thyroxine-binding prealbumin* (TBPA) or transthyretin (TTR) binds about 15–20% of T_4.
- Thyroxine-binding albumin (TBA) binds about 10% of the T_4.

Binding of the hormone with plasma protein serves following functions:

- It constitutes a reservoir for the supply of free hormones which buffers any acute changes in thyroid gland function.
- It prevents renal loss of hormone in urine, and thereby helps conserve iodide.

T_4 is more tightly bound to plasma protein than T_3. The tight binding of T_4 with plasma proteins shown by its prolonged half-life (approximately seven days).The half-life of T_3 is approximately one day only, due to its lesser affinity for the plasma proteins.

2. Free Form. Only about 0.05% of T_4 and 0.5% T_3 circulate unbound (free form) in the plasma. These free, unbound hormones represent the biologically active hormone. The lower affinity of T_3 for the plasma binding proteins (and thus the higher concentration of unbound T_3) contributes to the greater biologic activity of T_3.

Note. It is important to note that most of the circulating T_3 is not of thyroid origin but diffuses from the tissues, which convert T_4 into T_3 as described below.

Metabolism and Excretion of Thyroid Hormones The major pathways of peripheral metabolism of the circulating thyroid hormone include deiodination, deamination (decarboxylation) and conjugation with glucuronic acid.

1. Deiodination. In the peripheral tissues, T_4 is deiodinated as:

- About one-third of T_4 is deiodinated into T_3 (3,5,3´-tri-iodothyronine) by the enzyme 5´-deiodinase. T_3 so formed remains within the cells to produce metabolic effects but some of it diffuses into circulation to act in other tissues. In this way, 80% of the T_3 present in plasma is formed in the liver, kidney and pituitary.
- Remaining 45% of T_4 is deiodinated to reverse T_3, i.e. RT_3 (3,3´,5´-tri-iodothyronine) by 5-deiodinase. RT_3 is physiologically inert. During fetal life, prolonged fasting and prolonged illness or even after administration of glucocorticoids, a still greater percentage of T_4 is converted into RT_3. On the other hand in obesity, T_3 production is more than the RT_3.

  Note. Since T_4 is deiodinated to T_3, which produces physiological effects, so T_4 itself may be metabiologically inert and hence called a *prohormone*. Therefore, only 13% of circulating T_3 is secreted by thyroid, whereas 87% is formed by deiodination of T_4. Similarly, only 5% of circulating RT_3 is secreted by the thyroid and 95% is formed by deiodination of T_4.
- *T_3 and RT_3* are deiodinated to DIT (T_2) and MIT (T_1). DIT (T_2) is further deiodinated to MIT (T_1) (Fig. 8.3-5).

  Note. Deiodinases that act on thyroid hormones are mainly of three types: D_1, D_2 and D_3.

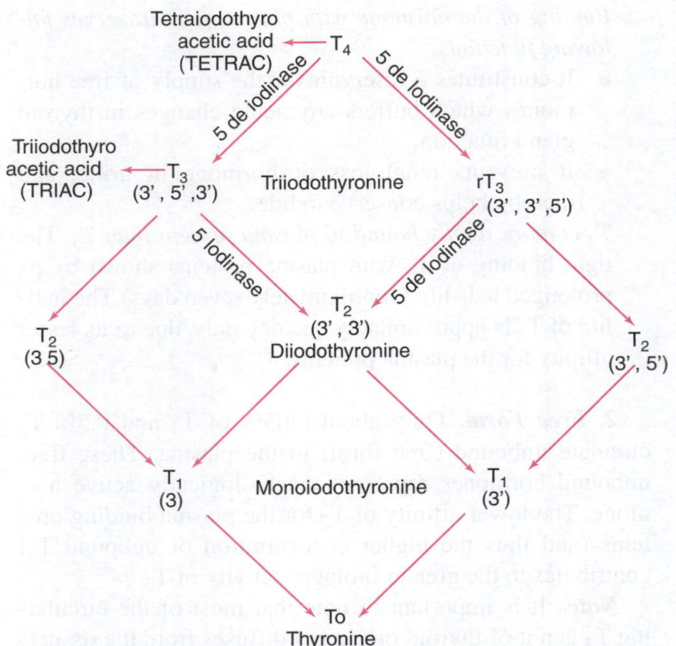

FIGURE 8.3-5 Deiodination of T_4 and T_3 in peripheral tissues.

- D_1, primarily responsible for conversion of T_4 into T_3, is present in high concentration in the liver, kidney, thyroid, pituitary and brown fat, whereas
- D_2 is present in brain (astroglia) and responsible for supply of T_3 to neurons and
- D_3 is present in reproductive tissues and also in brain.

2. Decarboxylation. Very small amounts of T_4 and T_3 are metabolized by decarboxylation to form tetraiodothyroacetic acid (TETRAC) and tri-iodothyroacetic acid (TRIAC).

3. Conjugation. Approximately 15% of thyroid hormones (T_4 and T_3) are conjugated in the liver to form glucuronides and sulphates. The conjugate then is secreted via the bile duct into the intestine. In normal individuals, metabolites of T_4 and T_3 are excreted mainly in the faeces with a small amount appearing in the urine.

Regulation of Thyroid Hormone Secretion

The secretion of thyroid hormones is regulated by:

- Negative feedback mechanism through hypothalamus–anterior pituitary–thyroid gland axis and
- Autoregulation of thyroid gland.

A. Regulation through Negative Feedback Mechanism Operating Through Hypothalamus–Anterior Pituitary–Thyroid Gland Axis The negative feedback mechanism operating through hypothalamus–anterior pituitary–thyroid gland axis (Fig. 8.3-6) play the essential role in controlling secretion of thyroid hormones.

- T_3 appears to be more actively involved than T_4 in the regulation process.

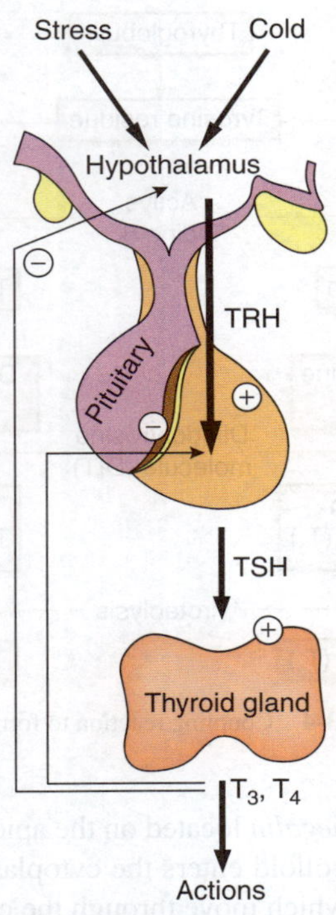

FIGURE 8.3-6 Regulation of thyroid hormone secretion by negative feedback control mechanism through hypothalamo–anterior pituitary–thyroid gland axis.

- The production of thyroid-stimulating hormone (TSH) by pituitary and thyrotropin-releasing hormone (TRH) by hypothalamus is inhibited by T_3 and to a lesser degree by T_4.
- The increased synthesis of TSH and TRH occurs in response to decreased circulatory levels of T_3 and T_4.

Thyroid-Stimulating Hormone. Thyroid-stimulating hormone (TSH) is a dimer (αβ) glycoprotein The α subunit is identical to the α subunit of FSH, LH and hCG, whereas functional specificity of TSH is conferred by β subunit and its:

- Molecular weight: 30,000,
- Biological half-life: 60 min,
- Normal secretion rate: 110 μg/day and
- Average plasma level: 2.3 μIU/ml (range 0.2–0.5 μIU/ml).

TSH secretion is pulsatile; its output starts rising at about 9 p.m., peak reaches at midnight, and then starts declining during the day.

Mechanism of action. TSH binds with plasma membrane receptors of thyroid cells and stimulates adenylyl cyclase with a consequent increase in intracellular cAMP (second messenger), which initiates cascade of reactions to produce biochemical effects (also see page 672).

Action of TSH. TSH, through the mediation of cAMP exerts the following effects on thyroid gland:

1. *Increases the secretion of thyroid hormones* by accelerating all the steps in biosynthesis, which include:
   - Iodide trapping,
   - Conversion of iodide to active iodine,

- Synthesis of thyroglobulin,
- Iodination of thyroglobulin,
- Coupling reaction and
- Proteolysis of thyroglobulin leading to increased secretion of T_3 and T_4.

2. *Increases the number* (hyperplasia) and size (hypertrophy) *of the follicular epithelial cells.*
3. *Increases the vascularity of thyroid gland.*

Important Note

- Removal of pituitary gland is associated with depressed thyroid functions and ultimately results in atrophy.
- Administration of TSH, the effect of which starts within few minutes after the injection, with chronic TSH treatment. The thyroid gland increases in weight and size due to hypertrophy of the cells (goitre).

Regulation of TSH Production

1. *Feedback control by plasma T_4 and T_3.* Day-to-day secretion of TSH depends upon the negative feedback control exerted by plasma levels of free T_4 and T_3 (Fig. 8.3-6):
   - A fall in T_4 and T_3 levels stimulates TSH secretion from anterior pituitary while
   - A rise in T_4 and T_3 levels inhibit TSH secretion.

   Since there exists an established inverse relationship between the plasma levels of thyroid hormones and TSH, therefore, measurement of the plasma TSH levels is a reliable test for assessing the status of thyroid hormones.
2. *Hypothalamic control of TSH.* Hypothalamus adjusts TSH secretion under certain special circumstances, such as exposure to cold, warmth, stress, anxiety, excitement, etc. Hypothalamus exerts its effect by secreting thyrotropin-releasing hormone (TRH).

Thyrotropin-Releasing Hormone. Thyrotropin-releasing hormone (TRH) is a tripeptide secreted by arcuate nucleus of hypothalamus and stored in median eminence from where it is released into the hypothalamo–hypophyseal portal vessels to reach the anterior pituitary.

Mechanism of action. TRH acts on the basophils (thyrotrophs) in the anterior pituitary via the adenylyl cyclase AMP system, and controls the release of TSH.

It is important to note that TRH, and T_3 and T_4 act competitively on pituitary thyrotrophs to control TSH secretion.

Control of TRH. Secretion of TRH by hypothalamus is controlled by:

- *Nervous stimuli* like emotion, stress and exposure to cold, etc. and also by
- *Negative feedback control* exerted by plasma T_3 and T_4 levels on the hypothalamus (Fig. 8.3-6).

B. Autoregulation of Thyroid Gland The secretions of thyroid gland are regulated by food iodine contents. It has been observed that if there is deficiency of iodine content in the diet then the *iodine trapping* mechanism of the follicular cells becomes superefficient and vice versa is also true, i.e. when there is an excess of iodine content in the food then iodine trapping becomes less efficient and organification of the excess amount of iodine does not occur. In this way, iodine availability for thyroxine synthesis remains constant and this phenomenon is called autoregulation of thyroid gland.

Mechanism of Action of Thyroid Hormone

The thyroid hormones do not have any discrete target organs. They affect cellular activity of almost all the tissues of the body. The multitude of thyroid hormone action cannot be explained by a single common mechanism. Basically, they act through genes (transcription and translation effect). Overall scheme of thyroid hormone effects is described (Fig. 8.3-7):

Entry of Thyroid Hormone in the Tissue Cells. Free T_4 and T_3, both enter the cells by a carrier-mediated energy-dependent process. The transport of T_4 is the rate limiting for intracellular production of T_3.

Intracellular production of T_3. Within the cell, most, if not all, of the T_4 is converted into T_3 or RT_3 (Fig. 8.3-7).

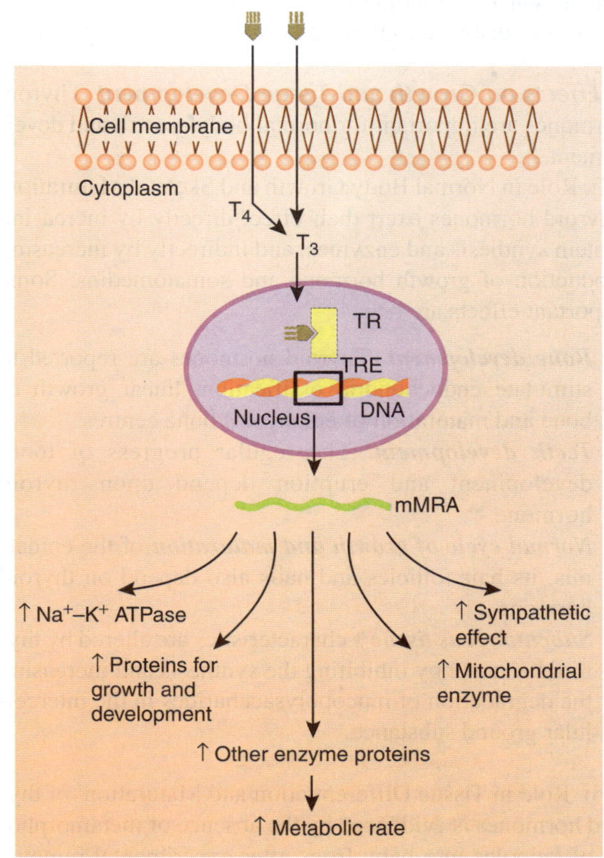

FIGURE 8.3-7 Mechanism of intracellular actions of thyroid hormone.

Effects of T_3 on gene expression. T_3 (and to a much lesser extent T_4), diffuses into the nucleus and binds to three thyroid receptor (TR) subtypes that exist linked to thyroid regulatory elements (TREs) in target DNA molecules, particularly the retinoid X receptor (RXR). This causes activation and inhibition of transcription process resulting in increased synthesis of mRNA. This ultimately results in (Fig. 8.3-7):

- *Increased synthesis of enzymes and specific structural or functional proteins.* This mechanism can explain the anabolic action and other metabolic actions of thyroxine.
- *Increased synthesis of Na^+–K^+–ATPase.* It explains the calorigenic action of thyroxine. Increased metabolic rate has been attributed to increased energy consumption associated with increased Na^+ transport.
- *Increase in the number and activity of mitochondria* in the cells of the body. These increase the rate of ATP synthesis. Extremely high concentrations of thyroid hormones cause uncoupling of oxidative phosphorylation process. As a result, a large amount of heat is produced, but little ATP.

Actions of Thyroid Hormones

As explained above, thyroid hormones bind to the specific thyroid receptors (TRs) on the target cell nuclei and bring about the biochemical action. T_3 is nearly 10 times more potent than T_4 in binding to the receptors. The biochemical functions attributed to thyroid hormones are summarized:

1. Effects on Growth and Tissue Development Thyroid hormones are important for normal body growth and development.

i. Role in Normal Body Growth and Skeletal Maturation. Thyroid hormones exert their effect directly by increasing protein synthesis and enzymes; and indirectly by increasing production of growth hormone and somatomedins. Some important effects are on:

- ***Bone development.*** Thyroid hormones are reported to stimulate endochondral ossification, linear growth of bone and maturation of epiphyseal bone centres.
- ***Teeth development.*** The regular progress of tooth development and eruption depend upon thyroid hormone.
- ***Normal cycle of growth and maturation*** of the epidermis, its hair follicles and nails also depend on thyroid hormone.
- ***Subcutaneous tissue's*** characteristics are altered by thyroid hormone by inhibiting the synthesis and increasing the degradation of mucopolysaccharides in the intercellular ground substance.

ii. Role in Tissue Differentiation and Maturation of thyroid hormones is evidenced by the absence of metamorphosis of tadpoles into baby frogs after experimental removal of thyroid gland in the former. Conversely, administration of T_4 in tadpoles causes early metamorphosis of tadpole into adult dwarf frog, which is not more than the size of the housefly, confirming thereby the role of T_4 in tissue differentiation.

iii. Role in Development of Nervous Tissue. T_3 seems to be necessary for proper axonal and dendritic development as well as normal myelination in the nervous system. The parts of the central nervous system affected are: cerebral cortex, basal ganglia and internal ear (cochlea).This is the reason for mental retardation being a striking feature in a child with congenital hypothyroidism. In such children, the disorder must be detected at the earliest and replacement hormonal therapy should be started, otherwise the mental retardation becomes irreversible.

2. Effect on the Metabolic Rate in General As described in the mechanism of action, the thyroid hormone in general stimulates the metabolic activities and increases the basal rate of oxygen consumption and heat production in most tissues of the body except the brain, retina, gonads, lungs and spleen.

Resting oxygen use in humans ranges from about 150 ml/min in hypothyroid state to about 400 ml/min in the hyperthyroid state (normal 225–250 ml/min).

The magnitude of calorigenic action of thyroxine partly depends on the level of circulating catecholamines.

Increased metabolic rate is associated with increased utilization of many hormones, vitamins and certain drugs. Therefore, patients with hyperthyroidism require a larger vitamin intake. On the other hand, patients with hypothyroidism may show toxic effects at usual doses of certain drugs.

3. Effects on Metabolism The increased O_2 consumption and metabolic rate ultimately depends on an increased supply of necessary substrate for oxidation. Thyroid hormones stimulate the provision of these substrates by their effect on carbohydrate, fat and protein metabolism.

i. Effect on Carbohydrate Metabolism. T_4 and T_3 lead on to overall increase in enzymes, causing:

- Increased glucose absorption from gastrointestinal tract and
- Acceleration in almost all aspects of glucose metabolism, i.e. rapid uptake of glucose by the cells, enhanced glycolysis, enhanced gluconeogenesis and increased insulin secretion and its effects on carbohydrate metabolism.

ii. Effect on Fat Metabolism. Thyroid hormones cause:

- Mobilization of fat from adipose tissue,
- Increase in the levels of fatty acids and enhanced oxidation of free fatty acids by cells and
- Decrease in the quantity of cholesterol, phospholipids and triglycerides in plasma and plasma cholesterol level is lowered due to increased excretion in bile.

Hypothyroidism is associated with elevated plasma cholesterol levels, which can be reversed by thyroid hormone administration.

iii. Effect on Protein Metabolism. *In physiological amounts, the thyroid hormones* function as anabolic hormones. That is, they cause an increase in RNA and protein synthesis leading to positive nitrogen balance.

In high concentrations, thyroid hormones have a catabolic effect leading to negative nitrogen balance. Therefore, muscle weakness and creatininuria are characteristic features of a hyperthyroid patient.

iv. Metabolic Effects Through Other Hormones. T_4 and T_3 potentiate the respective stimulatory effects of epinephrine, norepinephrine, glucagon, cortisol and growth hormone on gluconeogenesis, lipolysis, ketogenesis and proteolysis of the labile protein pool.

v. Effect on Vitamin Metabolism. Thyroid hormones increase the quantity of enzymes. Vitamins are the essential parts of some of the enzymes and coenzymes. Therefore, thyroid hormones cause increased need for vitamins leading to relative vitamin deficiency in hyperthyroidism.

T_4 is essential for conversion of carotene to vitamin A. In hypothyroidism, this reaction is very slow and carotene accumulation in the blood and tissues (carotenaemia) gives a yellow colour to the skin. Carotenaemia can be clinically differentiated from jaundice by the fact that sclera of the eyeballs are not affected in the former condition.

vi. Effect on Water and Electrolyte Balance. Thyroid hormones play a role in regulation of water and electrolyte balance. This fact is clear from the observation that impairment of the thyroid function is associated with retention of water and electrolytes, which can be reversed by hormonal administration.

Note. The overall metabolic effect of thyroid has been aptly described as accelerating the response to starvation.

4. Respiratory Effects Thyroid hormones cannot stimulate O_2 utilization for long without also enhancing oxygen supply, which is accomplished by the following effects of T_4 and T_3.

i. ***Increase in the resting respiratory rate, minute ventilation and ventilatory responses*** to hypercapnia and hypoxia. These actions maintain a normal pO_2 when O_2 utilization is increased and a normal pCO_2 when CO_2 production is increased.
ii. ***Increase in oxygen-carrying capacity of blood*** by slightly increasing the red blood cell mass. This increase in red blood cell mass results from stimulation of erythropoietin production, which arises directly by alteration of its gene expression and indirectly by way of the renal tissue hypoxia that results from increased O_2 use.

5. Cardiovascular Effects Thyroid hormone increases cardiac output, ensuring sufficient oxygen delivery in the tissues. This is accomplished by direct and indirect mechanisms, the latter being probably quantitatively more important (Fig. 8.3-8). In general, the thyroid hormones have the following effects on cardiovascular system:

i. ***Vasodilatation and increased blood flow to tissues*** occurs by two mechanisms:
   - *Indirect mechanism.* Thyroid hormones cause rapid utilization of O_2 and increased production of heat and CO_2. These effects cause vasodilatation and increase in blood flow in most of the tissues especially skin, muscle and heart. Cutaneous vasodilatation is particularly a prominent feature, which helps in dissipation of excessive heat produced.
   - *Direct mechanism.* Thyroid hormones directly decrease systemic vascular resistance by dilating arterioles in the peripheral circulation.
ii. ***Blood volume*** in circulation is increased because of:
   - The effect of vasodilatation produced, as described above and also
   - By activating the renin–angiotensin–aldosterone axis and thereby increasing renal tubular sodium reabsorption.
iii. ***Tachycardia,*** i.e. increased heart rate (at rest, even during sleep) is an important physical sign which is used by clinicians in assessing the function of the thyroid gland. Thyroid hormone produces tachycardia by directly

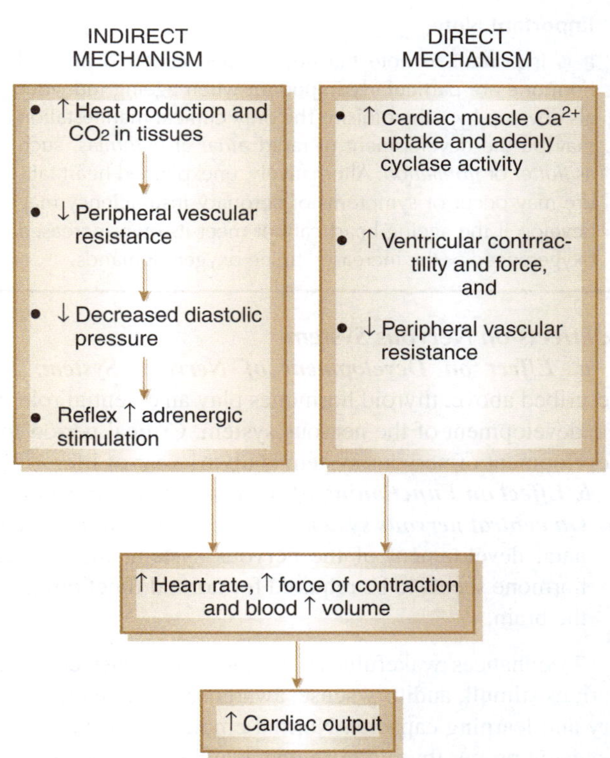

FIGURE 8.3-8 Direct and indirect mechanisms by which thyroid hormones increase cardiac output. The indirect mechanisms are probably quantitatively more important.

increasing the excitability of the heart and indirectly via adrenergic stimulation.

iv. ***Force of cardiac contraction*** is increased by moderate increase in thyroid hormone. The cardiac inotropic effects are partly indirect, via adrenergic stimulation and partly by direct effect of hormones on cardiac muscle. Myocardial calcium uptake and adenylyl cyclase activity are increased and enhance contractile force.
Mechanism: In the cardiac myocytes T_3 is not formed from T_4. When circulatory T_4 enters into the cardiac myocytes, it enhances genes for α myosin heavy chain (αMHC), sarcoplasmic reticulum Ca^{2+}, ATPase and certain K^+ channels. At the same time, thyroid hormone depresses the gene expression for β myosin heavy chain (βMHC). The myosin containing (βMHC) has less ATPase activity as compared to (αMHC). Therefore, αMHC is predominant in hyperthyroidism and there is an increase in speed of contraction.

v. ***Cardiac output*** is increased as a result of increased blood volume, increased heart rate and increased force of contraction which occurs due to both direct and indirect effects of the hormone, as described above.

vi. ***Effect on blood pressure***. *Systolic blood pressure* is increased due to increased strength and rate of heart beat; whereas, *diastolic blood pressure* is decreased due to peripheral vasodilatation. This results into *increased pulse pressure*, but the mean arterial pressure is usually unchanged.

Important Note

It is important to note that the cardiac effects of thyroid hormone are particularly important when ageing individuals develop hypothyroidism. The only clinical manifestation may be the development of rapid *atrial arrhythmias*, such as *flutter* or *fibrillation*. Alternatively, unexplained heart failure may occur or symptoms of coronary insufficiency may develop if the ageing heart cannot meet its own increased oxygen need or the increased tissue oxygen demands.

---

6. Effects on Nervous System

a. Effect on Development of Nervous System. As described above, thyroid hormones play an essential role in the development of the nervous system. Critical period for development of nervous system is up to1 year of life.

b. Effect on Functioning of Nervous Tissue in Adults

i. ***On central nervous system.*** Besides its role during neonatal development of the nervous system, the thyroid hormone seems to be required for normal functioning of the brain.

T_4 enhances wakefulness, alertness, responsiveness to various stimuli, auditory sense, awareness of hunger, memory and learning capacity. Normal emotional tone also depends on proper thyroid hormone availability. *Hypothyroid adults*, therefore, develop:

- Loss of intellectual functions,
- Impairment of memory,
- Somnolence,
- Slowness of sleep,
- Mental and physical lethargy and
- Eventually psychosis (myxoedema madness).

Hyperthyroid adults. Excess of T_4 in adults increases the number of beta-adrenergic receptors and hence potentiates the biological activity of circulating catecholamines. Catecholamines stimulate the reticular activating system (RAS) producing:

- Emotional instability, anxiety, nervousness,
- Overexcitability and nervousness,
- Irritability,
- Insomnia and
- Fatigue with fine rhythmic tremors in hands, tongue and eyeballs.

ii. ***Effects of thyroid hormones on peripheral nervous system.*** Thyroid hormone increases the speed and amplitude of peripheral nerve reflexes.
In hypothyroid adults, therefore, knee-jerk reaction time increases (normal 20 ms) and in thyrotoxicosis decreases.

7. Thyroid Hormone versus Sympathetic Nervous System or Catecholamines

- Certain effects of thyroid hormone, such as the increase in metabolic rate, heat production, heart rate, motor activity and central nervous system excitation are also produced by the adrenergic catecholamines, epinephrine and norepinephrine.
- The exact relationship between thyroid hormone and catecholamines is not known. Most studies show that the thyroid hormone does not increase the level of catecholamines or their metabolites in blood, urine or tissues. In fact, norepinephrine levels—a marker of sympathetic activity are reduced by thyroid hormone.
- Probably, the thyroid hormones produce catecholamine-like effects by increasing levels of cAMP (a beta-adrenergic second messenger), as increased levels of cAMP are found in plasma, urine and muscle after T_4 administration. At least one mechanism for this important effect is that T_3 increases the number of beta-adrenergic receptors in the heart muscle.
- The catecholamines and T_4 potentiate the actions of each other. Further synergism between catecholamines and thyroid hormones is also required for maximal thermogenesis, lipolysis, glycogenolysis and gluconeogenesis to occur.
- Therefore, a useful *adjunct therapy* for hyperthyroidism is treatment with a beta-adrenergic blocking agent, such as propranolol, which is extensively used in severe exacerbation of hyperthyroidism called thyroid storms.

8. Effects on Gastrointestinal Tract Effects of thyroid hormones on gastrointestinal tract (GIT) include:

- Increase in appetite and therefore increase in food intake,
- Increase in rate of secretion of digestive juices and

- Increase in motility of gastrointestinal tract. Excess of thyroid hormone often causes diarrhoea.

9. Effects on Skeletal Muscles

- *Slight increase* in thyroid hormones makes the muscle react with vigour.
- *Excessive quantities* of thyroid hormones weaken the muscles because of increased protein catabolism (Thyrotoxic myopathy). Muscle tremors occurring very rapidly at the rate of 10–15 times per second in hyperthyroidism are due to increased reactivity of neuronal synapses in the areas of the spinal cord that control muscle tone.
- *Lack of thyroid hormones* causes weakness, cramps, stiffness and sluggishness in muscles.

10. Effects on Reproductive System In both women and men, the thyroid hormone plays an important permissive role in the regulation of reproductive functions. The normal ovarian cycle of follicular development, maturation and ovulation; the homologous testicular process of spermatogenesis; and the maintenance of the healthy pregnant state are all disrupted by significant deviations of thyroid hormone levels from the normal range:

- ***In males,*** lack of thyroid hormones causes complete loss of libido and excess of hormones causes impotence.
- ***In females, lack of thyroid*** has varying effects:
  - Menorrhagia and polymenorrhagia and
  - Irregular periods or even amenorrhoea occurs in some women.
- ***In hyperthyroid women,*** there is oligomenorrhoea (reduced bleeding). The effects of thyroid hormones on gonads are due to direct metabolic effects on the gonads as well as indirectly through alterations in the anterior pituitary hormones.

11. Effects on other Endocrine Glands Thyroid hormones also have significant effects on other parts of the endocrine system.

- *Pituitary* production of growth hormone is increased, whereas that of prolactin is decreased.
- *Adrenocortical* secretion of cortisol, as well as metabolic clearance of this hormone, is stimulated, but plasma-free cortisol levels remain normal.
- *Oestrogens and androgens* ratio, in males, is increased. It accounts for occurrence of breast engorgement in males in hyperthyroidism.
- *Parathyroid hormone and 1,25-(OH)$_2$ vitamin D* are decreased as a compensatory consequence of the effects of thyroid hormone on bone resorption. Bone resorption is possibly stimulated by the T_3-induced release of interleukin-6 and -8 from osteoblasts.

12. Effects on Kidney Kidney size, renal tubular epithelium, renal plasma flow, glomerular filtration rate and tubular transport maximum for a number of substances are also increased by thyroid hormone.

APPLIED ASPECTS OF THYROID HORMONES

Abnormalities of Thyroid Gland

- Hyperthyroidism
- Hypothyroidism

Hyperthyroidism

Hyperthyroidism refers to increased secretion of thyroid hormones. Its common causes are:

- *Graves' disease* (described below) and
- *Toxic nodular goitre* (multinodular or solitary nodule). Nodule of thyroid tissue causes large amounts of thyroid hormone secretion. There is no evidence of autoimmune disease.
- *Other causes of hyperthyroidism* are:
  - Thyroiditis (inflammation of thyroid gland),
  - Excessive pituitary secretion of TSH,
  - Ingestion of exogenous T_4 and T_3 and
  - Activating mutations of TRs.

Graves' Disease

Graves' disease or toxic goitre or thyrotoxicosis is the most common cause of hyperthyroidism (Fig. 8.3-9).

Aetiology. It is an autoimmune disease characterized by development of thyroid stimulating antibodies (TSAb) against the TSH receptors, also called long-acting-thyroid-stimulator (LATS). These antibodies bind to TSH receptors and mimic TSH action on thyroid growth and hormone synthesis. The entire thyroid gland undergoes hyperplasia as a result of autoimmune stimulation.

Symptoms and Signs

1. ***General features*** include:
   - Marked increase in basal metabolic rate (BMR),
   - Weight loss, despite an increased intake of food and
   - Increased heat production causes discomfort in warm environments, excessive sweating and a greater intake of water.

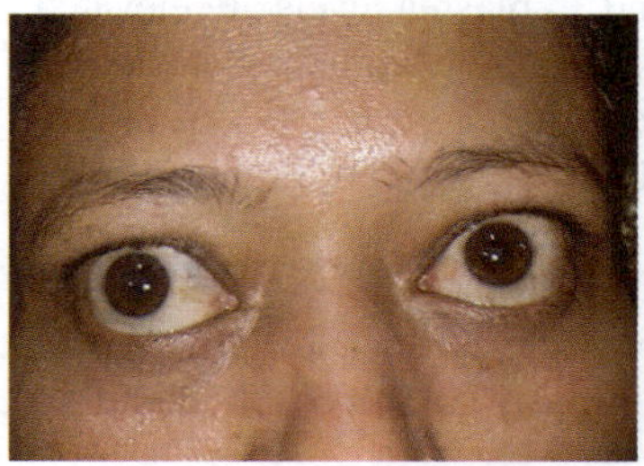

FIGURE 8.3-9 Patient with Graves' disease having exophthalmos.

2. ***Goitre***. Goitre refers to swelling of thyroid gland. Graves' disease is characterized by diffuse goitre, while a single or more nodules indicate toxic nodular goitre.
3. ***Cardiovascular features*** are:
   - Increased pulse rate or sinus tachycardia,
   - Wide pulse pressure (difference between systolic and diastolic pressure) is more than 60 mmHg,
   - Exertional dyspnoea,
   - Arrhythmias (atrial fibrillation is commonest) and
   - Precipitation of angina in patients with ischaemic heart disease.
4. ***Neuromuscular features*** include:
   - Nervousness, irritability,
   - Restlessness, psychosis,
   - Tremors of hand,
   - Muscular weakness and
   - Exaggerated tendon reflexes.
5. ***Gastrointestinal features*** are:
   - Diarrhoea or steatorrhoea and
   - Vomiting.
6. ***Dermatological features:***
   - Perspiration (increased sweating or hyperhidrosis),
   - Loss of hair,
   - Redness of palm and
   - Pretibial myxoedema.
7. ***Reproductive features:***
   - Impotence in males and
   - Oligomenorrhoea or amenorrhoea, abortions and infertility in females.
8. ***Ophthalmological signs:***
   - Lid retraction producing staring look (*Dalrymple's sign*),
   - Lid lag (von Graefe's sign),
   - Wide palpebral fissure,
   - Exophthalmos, i.e. bulging out of eyeballs. Exophthalmos occurs due to cytokine-mediated proliferation of fibroblasts which secrete hydrophilic glycosaminoglycans, leading to increase in interstitial fluid contents combined with chronic inflammatory cells, resulting in marked swelling and ultimately fibrosis of extraocular muscles and rise in retrobulbar pressure. The eyes displace forward (proptosis and exophthalmos) and
   - Diplopia with ocular motility defect because of extraocular muscle involvement.

Investigations

- Both T_3 and T_4 plasma levels are elevated,
- TSH is low or may become undetectable,
- ^{131}I uptake is increased, i.e. >35% at 5 h,
- TRs antibodies may be increased >7 U/L, (N = <7 U/L)
- Serum cholesterol is less,
- ECG shows tachycardia and arrhythmia and
- Ultrasonography of thyroid gland shows diffuse goitre.

Treatment

1. ***Drug therapy*** consists of antithyroid drugs and beta blockers.
   - *Antithyroid drugs*. These drugs block the iodination of tyrosine and hence reduce the synthesis of thyroid hormones. Common antithyroid drugs include carbimazole and propylthiouracil. Carbimazole also has an immunosuppressive action, leading to reduction of serum TR_{Ab} concentration.
   - *Beta blockers*. A nonselective beta-blocker is useful for symptomatic relief but it does not abolish thyrotoxicosis. Propranolol and metoprolol are preferred drugs.
2. ***Surgical subtotal thyroidectomy*** is indicated in large goitre with frequent relapses on drug treatment.
3. ***Radioactive ablation of thyroid*** by ^{131}I is indicated in cases with recurrence following surgery. ^{131}I has long-lasting inhibitory effect on survival and replication of follicular cells.

Hypothyroidism

Hypothyroidism is a clinical syndrome caused by low levels of circulating thyroid hormones.

Aetiology. Depending upon the aetiology, hypothyroidism can be primary or secondary.

Primary hypothyroidism is caused by the disorder of thyroid gland. Causes include:

1. Idiopathic or spontaneous or atrophic hypothyroidism.
2. Goitrous hypothyroidism occurs in:
   - Hashimoto's thyroiditis,
   - Deficiency of iodine,
   - Drug-induced (e.g. para-aminosalicylic acid) and
   - Dyshormonogenesis.
3. Postablative hypothyroidism, i.e.
   - Following surgery or
   - Following ^{131}I administration.
4. Transient due to thyroiditis (self-limiting).
5. Maternally transmitted (iodide, antithyroid drugs).

Secondary hypothyroidism is caused by diseases of anterior pituitary and hypothalamus.

Thyroid hormone resistance: Mutations in the gene that codes TSH receptor β (TRβ) are associated with resistance to the effects of T_3 and T_4. Attention-deficit hyperactivity disorder is a condition associated with thyroid hormone resistance, usually common in hyperactive and impulsive children.

Clinical Features. Clinical features depend upon the age at which deficiency manifests, duration and severity of the disease. Three different clinical entities are:

- Infantile hypothyroidism (cretinism),
- Juvenile hypothyroidism and
- Adult hypothyroidism (myxoedema).

1. ***Infantile hypothyroidism (cretinism)***. It occurs when thyroid deficiency occurs during the first year of life and is characterized by (Fig. 8.3-10) mental retardation, marked retardation of growth, delayed milestones of development, potbelly, protruding tongue, flat nose, dry skin and sparse hair.
   Radiograph of bone shows delayed bone age.
   Treatment should be prompt otherwise mental deficiency will persist.
2. ***Juvenile hypothyroidism*** manifests at adolescence and is characterized by short stature, poor performance at school, delayed puberty and sexual maturation. Other features of adult hypothyroidism are present in variable degrees.
3. ***Adult hypothyroidism*** is also called myxoedema because of the characteristic infiltration of skin by myxoedematous tissue (Fig. 8.3-11). Paradoxically, iodide itself inhibits thyroid functions. In normal individuals, a high dose of iodide acts directly on the thyroid gland and inhibits organification and decreases hormone synthesis. The effect is known as *Wolff–Chaikoff effect*. In hypothyroidism, there is infilteration of body tissues by polymucopolysaccharides, hyaluronic acid and chondroitin sulphate. Infilteration of the dermis causes nonpitting oedema (myxoedema) which is most marked on the skin of the hands, feet and eyelids (periorbital puffiness).Symptoms and signs include:
   - *General features*: Tiredness and weight gain without an appreciable increase in caloric intake (due to lower than normal metabolic rate). Decreased heat production, lower body temperature, intolerance to cold and decreased sweating.
   - *Cardiovascular features*. Adrenergic activity is decreased causing bradycardia. Other features include hypertension, pericardial effusion and precipitation of angina.
   - *Neuromuscular features*. Movement, speech and thought are all slowed, and lethargy, sleepiness, delayed relaxation of ankle jerks, aches and pain are common and pressure palsy of peripheral nerves (e.g. carpal tunnel syndrome) due to entrapment in excess ground substance.
   - *Dermatological features*. Dry thick skin (toad skin), sparse hair, nonpitting oedema due to infiltration by myxoedematous tissue (myxoedema). Lemon yellow tint of the skin occurs due to carotenaemia.
   - *Reproductive features*. Menorrhagia and infertility (common) galactorrhoea and impotence (less common).
   - *Gastrointestinal features*. Constipation (common) and adynamic ileus (less common).
   - *Haematological feature* includes anaemia.

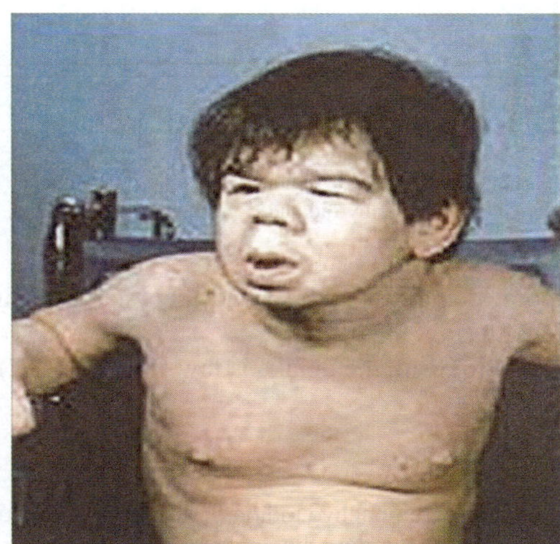

FIGURE 8.3-10 Clinical features of cretinism. Note short stature, pot belly and idiotic look.

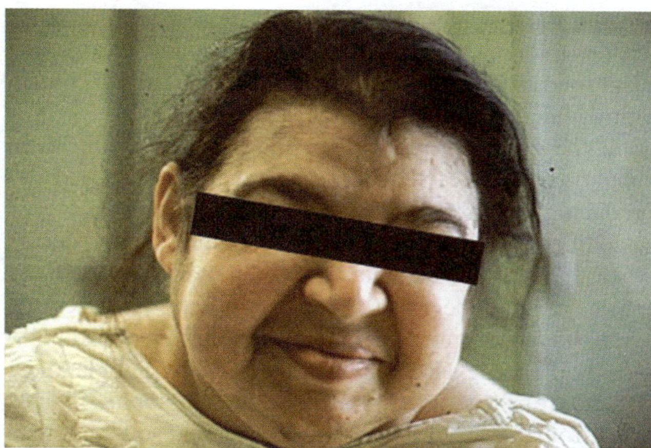

FIGURE 8.3-11 Photograph of a patient with myxoedema showing puffy face, thick lips and periorbital oedema.

Investigations

- Serum T_3 and T_4 levels low,
- Serum TSH levels high in primary, low in secondary hypothyroidism,
- Serum cholesterol high,
- Peripheral blood film shows macrocytic anaemia,
- ECG classically demonstrates sinus bradycardia, low voltage complexes, and ST segment and T wave abnormalities and
- Photomotogram—delayed ankle jerk.

Treatment. Treatment of hypothyroidism is lifelong replacement of thyroid hormones by L-thyroxine.

Goitre

Goitre refers to any abnormal increase in the size of the thyroid gland. The term goitre does not denote the functional status of thyroid gland, because it may be associated with:

- *Euthyroid,* i.e. normal thyroid hormone level,
- *Hypothyroidism,* i.e. low thyroid hormone level and
- *Hyperthyroidism,* i.e. high thyroid hormone levels, as seen in Graves' disease and toxic nodular goitre.

Goitrogenic Substances (Goitrogens). These are the substances that interfere with the production of thyroid hormone and cause thyroid enlargement, i.e. goitre. These include thiocyanates, nitrates and perchlorates and drugs such as thiourea, thiouracil and thiocarbamide, etc. Certain plant foods such as cabbage, cauliflower and turnip contain goitrogenic factors mostly thiocyanates.

If the goitrogen reduces thyroid hormone synthesis to subnormal levels, TSH secretion is increased, chronically producing hypertrophy of thyroid gland (goitre).

Iodine Deficiency Goitre or Endemic Goitre occurs when the daily dietary intake of iodine falls below 10 μg (normal requirement 100–200 μg/day). It decreases the synthesis and secretion of the thyroid hormone leading to increased TSH levels and proliferation of thyroid gland tissue (goitre). It is mostly found in the geographic regions away from the seacoast where the water and soil are low in iodine content. Consumption of iodized salt is advocated to overcome the problem of endemic goitre. In certain cases, administration of thyroid hormone is also indicated.

Thyroid Function Tests

1. Measurement of Basal Metabolic Rate (BMR). Theoretically, it is the physiological test of thyroid functions, since it measures the tissue response (O_2 consumption). However, because of poor sensitivity and specificity, BMR is now seldom used as a thyroid function test.

- Normal values of BMR: ± 20%,
- In hyperthyroidism, BMR may increase to 100% and
- In hypothyroidism, it may decrease to −30 to −40%.

2. Estimation of Protein-bound Iodine (PBI). It reflects the level of circulating T_3 and T_4 bound to plasma protein. However, because of poor sensitivity and specificity, estimation of PBI is no longer considered as a thyroid function test.

- Normal values—6 g/100 ml,
- Decreased levels of PBI are seen in hypothyroidism, pregnancy and acute thyroiditis and
- Increased levels of PBI occur in hyperthyroidism and patients on oral contraceptives.

3. Radioactive Iodine Uptake (RAIU). This test, being a cumbersome and time-consuming procedure, is no longer used nowadays as a routine thyroid function test. To perform this test, 25 curies of radioactive iodine (^{131}I) is given orally in 100 ml water and thyroid uptake is determined by placing an X-ray counter over the neck. An area over the thigh is also counted and count in this region is subtracted from the neck count to correct for nonthyroidal radioactivity in the neck.

- Normal value of RAIU by thyroid (at 24 h) is 20–40%,
- In hyperthyroidism this value may be 60% and
- In hypothyroidism this value may be <20%.

The analysis of radioactive iodine uptake is helpful in understanding the physiology of the thyroid gland. The radioactive iodine uptake in a normal person is plotted in Fig. 8.3-12A.

- In hyperthyroidism, the amount of radioactivity in the thyroid gland rises sharply because iodide is rapidly incorporated into T4 and T3 and then starts declining within 24 h (Fig. 8.3-12B).
- In hypothyroidism, the uptake is low (Fig. 8.3-12C).

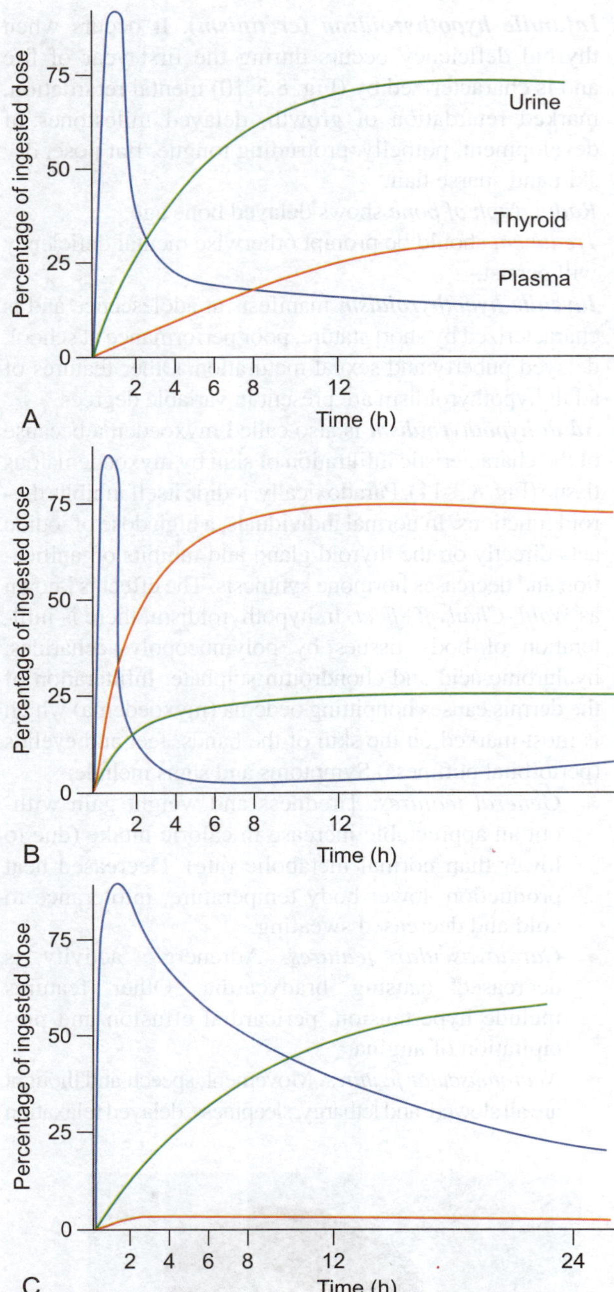

FIGURE 8.3-12 Distribution of radioactive iodine (^{123}I) uptake: **A,** in normal (euthyroid) ; **B,** hyperthyroid and **C,** hypothyroid individual.

Applied Aspects

A large amount of radioactive iodine destroys thyroid tissue; therefore, radioactive iodine therapy is useful in some cases of Graves' disease and thyroid carcinomas.

4. Measurement of Total and Free T_3 and T_4 and TSH Levels in Blood. These tests are considered best and are widely used for the diagnosis of various thyroid disorders. An accurate estimation of thyroid hormones can be done by radioimmunoassay (RIA) or by the ELISA method. Their normal values and changes in hyperthyroidism and hypothyroidism are shown in Table 8.3-1.

Note.

- *Total T_3 and T_4* estimation has the following drawbacks:
- It measures the total amount of the hormone, the major portion of which is bound and does not take part in metabolism.
- The values are liable to be altered with the fluctuations in the levels of thyroid-binding proteins (TBG), such as during pregnancy and other related conditions.
- *Free T_3 and T_4 estimation* truly represents thyroid activity, hence are preferred over total T_3 and T_4.
- *TSH levels* are an important parameter of thyroid disorder which tests the integrity of hypothalamic–pituitary–thyroid axis.

TABLE 8.3-1 Normal Values of T_3, T_4, TSH and Changes in Hyperthyroidism and Hypothyroidism

	Normal values	Hyperthyroidism	Hypothyroidism
• Total serum T_3	0.12 μg/dL	↑	↓
• Total serum T_4	8 μg/dL	↑	↓
• Free serum T_3	0.28 ng/dL	↑	↓
• Free serum T_4	2 ng/dL	↑	↓
• Serum TSH	0.2–5 μIU/ml	↓	↑

5. Ultrasonography of Thyroid Gland. Ultrasonography (B-scan) allows evaluation of an enlarged thyroid gland. It elucidates shape and dimension of nodules in the thyroid gland.

6. Thyroid Scan. A radionucleotide scan of thyroid either by ^{131}I/or ^{99m}Tc is useful in demonstrating functioning thyroid tissue. It detects hot (functioning) and cold (non-functioning) nodule/nodules in the thyroid, in cases with single or multinodular goitre.

7. Antithyroid Antibodies. Detection of antithyroid antibodies is useful in diagnosing autoimmune thyroid disorder, such as Hashimoto's thyroiditis.

8. Fine-needle Aspiration Biopsy (FNAB) is carried out in patients with nodular goitre to detect any malignant process.

Chapter 8.4

Endocrinal Control of Calcium Metabolism and Bone Physiology

INTRODUCTION

Calcium, phosphorus and magnesium belong to a group of seven principal elements which constitute 60–80% of the body's inorganic material. Calcium and phosphorus form important structural components of bones and teeth, while calcium and magnesium are important determinants of neuromuscular excitability. Various hormones involved in the regulation of metabolism of these minerals include:

Calcitropic hormones refer to three hormones, namely, parathyroid hormone (PTH), calcitonin and cholecalciferol (vitamin D_3), which are primarily concerned with the regulation of calcium, phosphate and magnesium metabolism in the body. These hormones act on three organ systems, bones, kidneys, and intestinal tract to maintain calcium and phosphate levels in the face of environmental changes.

Parathyroid hormone-related protein (PTHrP) is the fourth local hormone that acts on the PTH receptor and is important for skeletal development in utero.

Other hormones which also have some effect on calcium metabolism include glucocorticoids, growth hormone, oestrogens and various growth factors.

Discussion in this chapter is limited to regulatory role of PTH, calcitonin and cholecalciferol (vitamin D_3) only. An overview is presented of calcium and phosphate metabolism, as well as of the related structural and functional aspects of bone physiology.

CALCIUM, PHOSPHORUS AND MAGNESIUM METABOLISM

Calcium Metabolism

Physiological and Biochemical Functions

Calcium ions regulate a number of important physiologic and biochemical processes. To ensure that these processes operate normally, the plasma concentration is maintained within a very narrow limit (9–11 mg%). Free, ionized calcium is the biologically active form of calcium. Important physiologic and biochemical functions subserved by calcium are:

1. *Development of bone and teeth.* Calcium along with phosphorus is essential for the formation (of hydroxyapatite) and physical strength of skeletal tissue. Bones which are in dynamic state serve as reservoir of calcium.
2. *Neuromuscular excitation.* Calcium is essential for the transmission of nerve impulse. It interacts with troponin C to trigger muscle contraction. Calcium also activates ATPases and increases the interaction between actin and myosin.
3. *Blood coagulation.* Calcium (factor IV) is involved in several reactions in the cascade of blood clotting mechanism.
4. *Membrane integrity and plasma membrane transport.* Permeability and transport of water and several ions across the cell membrane are influenced by calcium.
5. *Mediation of intracellular action of hormones.* Calcium mediates the intracellular actions of certain hormones by acting as a second messenger (e.g. epinephrine in liver glycogenolysis) and third messenger (e.g. antidiuretic hormone acts through cAMP, and then Ca^{2+}).
6. *Activation of enzymes.* Calcium is needed for direct activation of enzymes, such as lipase (pancreatic), ATPase and succinate dehydrogenase.
7. *Release of hormones and neurotransmitters.* Calcium facilitates the release of certain hormones and neurotransmitters, e.g. insulin, PTH and calcitonin.
8. *Calmodulin-mediated action of calcium.* Calmodulin is a calcium-binding protein. Calcium–calmodulin complex activates certain enzymes, e.g. adenylyl cyclase and calcium-dependent protein kinases.
9. *Regulation of secretory processes.* The microfilament- and microtubule-mediated processes such as endocytosis, exocytosis and cell motility are regulated by calcium.
10. *Contact inhibition.* Calcium is believed to be involved in cell to cell contact and adhesion of cells in tissues. It may also be required for cell-to-cell communication.
11. *Action on heart.* By acting on myocardium, calcium prolongs the systole.

Calcium Distribution in the Body

Calcium is the most abundant mineral in the body. The total content of calcium in an adult man is about 1100 g (27.5 mol). As much as 99% of it is present in the bones and teeth as hydroxyapatite. A small fraction (1%) of the calcium found outside the skeletal tissues performs a wide variety of functions.

Calcium in Bones Calcium in bones is present in two pools:

1. ***Pool of stable calcium*** is much larger (99% of total bone calcium) and is formed by the calcium present in stable mature bones. It represents the calcium pool that is not readily exchangeable, but can be mobilized only through the action of PTH.
2. ***Pool (reservoir) of readily exchangeable calcium*** is much smaller (only 1% of the total bony content) and consists of labile (young) newly formed bone.

Calcium in Plasma Most of the blood calcium is present in the plasma, since blood cells contain very little of it. In the plasma, calcium is present in nondiffusible (40% of total plasma calcium) and diffusible forms. The diffusible form includes further two forms: the ionized calcium (50% of total plasma calcium) and that complexed to HCO_3^-, citrate, etc. (10% of total plasma calcium). The diffusible form of calcium, as the name indicates, is diffusible from blood to the tissues, while the nondiffusible form is not. The nondiffusible form refers to the calcium which is bound to plasma proteins, mostly albumin and to a lesser extent globulin.

Normal values of different forms of plasma calcium are:

Total plasma calcium	: 10 mg% (2.5 mmol/L) (range 9–11 mg%)
• Diffusible calcium	: 6 mg% (1.5 mmol/L)
• Ionized calcium	: 5 mg% (1.25 mmol/L) (50% of total plasma calcium)
• Complexed to HCO_3^-, citrate, etc.	: 1 mg% (0.25 mmol/L) (10% of total plasma calcium)
• Nondiffusible calcium	: 4 mg% (1 mmol/L)
• Bound to albumin	: (i.e. 40% of total plasma calcium)

Dietary Requirement and Sources of Calcium

Dietary requirements of calcium per day are as follows:

• Adult man and woman	: 800 mg/day
• Women during pregnancy, lactation, and postmenopause	: 1500 mg/day
• Children (1–18 years)	: 800–1200 mg/day
• Infants (<1year)	: 300–500 mg/day

Dietary sources of calcium

- *Best sources* are milk and milk products.
- *Good sources* include beans, leafy vegetables, fish, cabbage and egg yolk.

Calcium Balance

The calcium ion is fundamentally important to all biological systems. Therefore, the concentration of calcium must be maintained within specific limits of physiological tolerance in several compartments. The overall calcium homeostasis (calcium balance) or the normal daily calcium turnover is maintained by an interplay of following processes (Fig. 8.4-1):

- Absorption of ingested calcium,
- Exchange of calcium between bone and ECF,
- Secretion of calcium from extracellular fluid (ECF) and
- Excretion of calcium in the faecal matter and urine.

Absorption of Calcium The daily dietary intake of calcium, depending upon the amount of milk and milk products consumed, may vary from 200 to 2000 mg. Unfortunately, in many adults, the daily intake of calcium is below the recommended minimum of 800 mg.

Process of Absorption. The absorption of calcium mainly occurs in the duodenum by an energy-dependent active process. This process involves the activity of calcium-dependent ATPase at brush border of epithelial cells and is regulated by 1,25-dihydroxycholecalciferol.

- Across the brush border, Ca^{2+} is transported via channels known as transient receptor potential vanilloid type-6 (TRPV-6) and binds to an intracellular protein (Calbindin-D_{qK}).
- From the basolateral border of intestinal epithelial cells, absorbed Ca^{2+} is transported into the blood either by Na^+/Ca^{2+} exchanger (NCX_1) or Ca^{2+}-dependent ATPase.

Factors promoting absorption include:

- *1,25-Dihydroxycholecalciferol* directly affects the absorption by its regulatory role.
- *PTH* indirectly promotes the intestinal absorption of calcium by increasing the renal synthesis of 1,25-dihydroxycholecalciferol.
- *Dietary lactose* promotes calcium intake by intestinal cells by some unknown mechanism.
- *Amino acids* lysine and arginine facilitate calcium absorption.
- *Low pH* is more favourable for calcium absorption.

Factors inhibiting calcium absorption are:

- *Phytates and oxalates* present in the diet form insoluble salts with calcium and thereby decrease its absorption.
- *Phosphates* present in high amount in diet result in the formation of insoluble calcium phosphate and prevent calcium uptake. The dietary ratio of calcium:phosphate between 1:2 and 2:1 is ideal for optimum calcium absorption.
- *Free fatty acids* react with calcium to form insoluble calcium soaps. This is particularly observed when fat absorption is impaired.

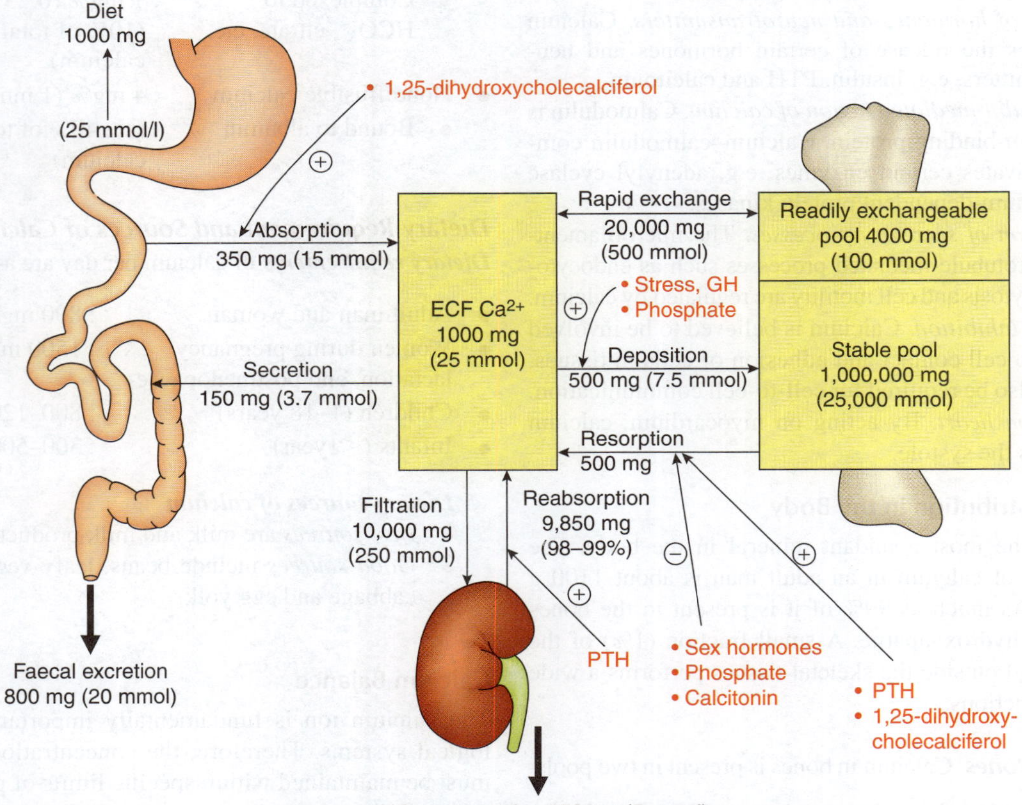

FIGURE 8.4-1 Hormonal maintenance of calcium balance in an adult human ingesting 1000 mg (25 mmol) of calcium per day.

- *High pH* is unfavourable for calcium absorption.
- *Dietary fibre* in high content interferes with calcium absorption.

Adaptative Mechanism for Absorption. The percentage of dietary calcium absorbed from the intestine is inversely related to intake.

- ***Adaptive increase*** in fractional absorption is one mechanism for maintaining normal body calcium start when the dietary intake of calcium is chronically low. The adaptation seems to be produced through greater synthesis of 1,25-dihydroxycholecalciferol.
- ***Adaptive decrease*** in calcium absorption occurs when the diet supplies too much calcium. This adaptation prevents overload and seems to be produced through lesser synthesis of 1,25-dihydroxycholecalciferol.
- ***Normal absorption.*** Normally, at a daily intake of 1000 mg of calcium, about 35% (i.e. 350 mg) is absorbed (Fig. 8.4-1), approximately half passively and half stimulated by vitamin D.

Note. In elderly individuals, both the dietary calcium intake and the absorption of calcium from the intestine are diminished. This decreased calcium input contributes to a declining bone mass and the increased risk of fracture in the aged due to osteoporosis.

Exchange of Calcium between Bone and Extracellular Fluid The extracellular fluid (ECF) contains about 1000 mg of calcium, which is in dynamic equilibrium with the calcium present in the bones.

Two types of exchange occur between the bone and ECF: rapid exchange and slow exchange.

- ***Rapid exchange*** occurs between the ECF and the smaller (1% of the total bony content) readily exchangeable pool of bone calcium. A large amount of calcium (about 20,000 mg per day) moves into and out of the readily exchangeable pool in the bone. The exact significance of this exchange in calcium homeostasis is not properly understood.
- ***Slow exchange*** occurs between the ECF and larger (99% of total bone content) pool of stable calcium. This exchange is the one concerned with bone remodelling by the constant interplay of bone resorption and deposition. This process of bone remodelling results in calcium turnover of about 500 mg/day only. In this remodelling process, a number of factors determine deposition and resorption of bone minerals.

Bone resorption in the remodelling process is stimulated by PTH and inhibited by sex hormones, calcitonin and phosphate (Fig. 8.4-1).

Bone deposition in the remodelling process is promoted by physical stress to the bone provided by walking, sex hormones and growth hormone. Thus, a person suffers from osteoporosis (reduced bone density) if he happens to be immobilized in the bed for long time. In old age, when sex hormones are reduced, there occurs an increased tendency to bone resorption (postmenopausal osteoporosis). Osteoporosis also occurs in Cushing's syndrome and growth hormone deficiency.

Excretion of Calcium The same amount of calcium as absorbed from the gut, i.e. about 350 mg, must ultimately be excreted to maintain balance. Excretion of calcium occurs in the faecal matter as well as urine.

Faecal Excretion of Calcium. About 150 mg calcium is secreted into the intestine through bile, pancreatic juice and intestinal secretions, and excreted in the stools along with the unabsorbed fraction (650 mg) from the diet. In this way, about 800 mg of calcium is excreted in the faecal matter (Fig. 8.4-1).

Urinary Excretion of Calcium. A large amount (about 10,000 mg) of calcium is filtered in the kidneys per day, but 98–99% of the filtered calcium is reabsorbed. About 60% of the reabsorption occurs in the proximal tubules and the remainder in the ascending limb of the loop of Henle and the distal tubule. Distal tubular reabsorption of Ca^{2+} occurs via $TRPV_5$ channels and is regulated by parathyroid hormone. Thus, in a normal healthy adult with calcium intake of 1000 mg, about 150 mg is excreted in the urine (Fig. 8.4-1). Adjustment of this small fraction of filtered calcium that is finally excreted provides a sensitive means of maintaining calcium balance.

Types of Calcium Balance Three types of calcium balance exist:

1. Neutral Calcium Balance. It is seen in normal healthy individuals in which excretion of calcium in the urine and faeces exactly matches (equals) the daily intake of calcium (Fig. 8.4-1). There also exists an internal balance between the entry into and exit from the bone.

2. Positive Calcium Balance. It is seen in growing children, where the intestinal calcium absorption exceeds total excretion of calcium. The excess calcium is deposited in the growing bones, i.e. entry of calcium into bone is more than the exit.

3. Negative Calcium Balance. It is seen in women during pregnancy and lactation. Intestinal calcium absorption is less than the calcium excretion. The deficit comes from the maternal bones, i.e. exit of calcium out of the bone is more than the entry into the bone.

Hormonal Regulation of Plasma Calcium Level

As mentioned earlier, maintenance of plasma calcium level within narrow range (9–11 mg/dL) is essential as it is involved in a number of important physiologic and biochemical processes. Deviations of the ionized calcium from the normal range cause many disorders and can be life-threatening. The hormones regulating plasma calcium levels include:

A. Calcitropic Hormones. The three primarily involved in the calcium homeostasis are:

- Parathyroid hormone (PTH),
- Active form of vitamin D (1,25-dihydroxycholecalciferol) and
- Calcitonin.

Main role of these hormones in calcium metabolism is summarized in Table 8.4-1 and Fig. 8.4-1.

B. Parathyroid Hormone-related Protein (PTHrP). It is a local hormone that acts on the PTH receptors and is important for skeletal development in utero (for details see page 731).

C. Other Hormones. which have some effect on calcium metabolism include:

- *Growth hormone* has stimulatory effect on bone deposition.
- *Sex hormones* have inhibitory effect on bone resorption.
- *Glucocorticoids* have stimulatory effect on bone resorption.
- *Growth factors* have stimulatory effect on bone deposition.

Hypocalcaemia is compensated by (Fig. 8.4-2*):*

- Release of calcium from the bones,
- Increased fractional reabsorption in the kidney and
- Increased absorption from the intestine.

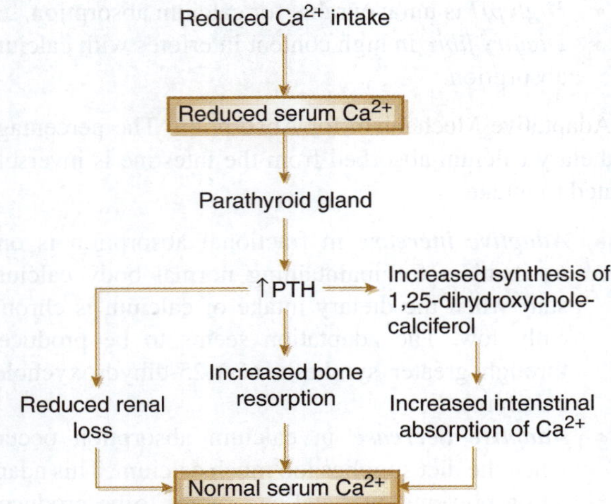

FIGURE 8.4-2 Mechanism of regulation of serum calcium levels in hypocalcaemia.

Phosphorus Metabolism

Physiological and Biochemical Functions

The phosphate ion is also critically important to all biological systems. Important functions subserved by phosphate are:

1. *Development of bone and teeth*
2. *Structural part of:*
   - *High-energy* transfer and storage compounds such as ATP, GTP, creatine phosphate,
   - *Cofactors* such as NAD, NADP and thiamine pyrophosphate.
   - *Second messengers,* e.g. cAMP, inositol triphosphate and
   - *Nucleic acids* (DNA, RNA), phospholipids and phosphoproteins.
3. *Activation of enzymes* by phosphorylation.
4. *Role in carbohydrate* metabolism.
5. *Phosphate buffer system* is important for the maintenance of pH in the blood as well as in the cells.
6. *Important intracellular anion* that balances the certain cations (K^+ and Mg^{2+}) inside the cells.

TABLE 8.4-1 Summary of Calcitropic Hormones That Regulate Calcium Balance

	PTH	1,25-Dihydroxycholecalciferol	Calcitonin
Stimulus for secretion	↓ Serum Ca^{2+}	↓ Serum Ca^{2+} ↑ PTH Serum phosphate	↑ Serum Ca^{2+}
Actions on:			
• Bone	↑ Resorption	↑ Resorption	↓ Resorption
• Kidney	↓ P Reabsorption ↑ Ca^{2+}Reabsorption	↑ P Reabsorption ↑ Ca^{2+}Reabsorption	– –
• Intestine	↑ Ca^{2+}Absorption	↑ Ca^{2+} Absorption	–
Overall effect on:			
• Serum Ca^{2+}	↑	↑	↓
• Serum phosphate	↓	↑	–

Distribution of Phosphate in the Body

An adult body contains about 1 kg phosphate (P) which is distributed as:

- Bones and teeth : 80% (in combination with Ca^{2+})
- Muscles and blood : 10% (in association with proteins, carbohydrates and lipids)
- Chemical compounds : 10% widely distributed in body

Blood Phosphate.

- Plasma levels of (P_1) : 3–5 mg%
- Whole blood : 40 mg% (because RBCs and WBCs have very high content of phosphate)
- Plasma phosphate exists in three forms:
  - Protein bound : 10%
  - Free ions : 40%
  - Complexed with cations (Ca^{2+}, Mg^{2+}, Na^+, K^+) : 50%

Fasting plasma phosphate levels are higher than the postprandial levels. It is because of the reason that after ingestion of carbohydrates, the phosphate from the plasma is drawn by the cells for metabolism (phosphorylation reaction).

Phosphorus Balance (FIG. 8.4-3)

1. Intake and Absorption. Recommended intake is about 800 mg per day. The recommended ratio of Ca^{2+}:P in adults is 1:1 and in infants 2:1. Sources of P are milk, cereals, leafy vegetables, meat and eggs. Ca^{2+} and P are distributed in the majority of natural foods in a 1:1 ratio. Therefore, it is generally held that one should take care of one's protein intake and calcium intake, and this will automatically take care of requirement of phosphorus.

On an average, dietary intake of P in adults is about 1000 mg per day. P is absorbed actively and maximally in duodenum. About 70–80% of P, compared with 30–40% of Ca^{2+}, is absorbed from the gut.

The total plasma phosphorus is about 12 mg/dL, about two third (2/3) in inorganic compound form and remaining one third is present as inorganic phosphorus (P_i). The uptake of P_i occurs by two related sodium-dependent P_i cotransporters (i.e NaP_i-IIa and NaP_i-IIc).

- The low concentration of Na^+ in the enterocyte is established by Na^+–K^+–ATPase on the basolateral membrane. *Factors affecting phosphorus absorption are:*
  - Vitamin D, PTH and GH promote absorption.1,25-cholecalciferol increases P_i absorption via increasing expression of NaP_i-IIa transporter and their insertion onto apical membrane of the enterocytes.
  - Cortisol and heavy metal ions inhibit absorption.

Note. The fraction of dietary phosphate (unlike calcium) absorbed does not change with the change in amount of dietary intake. Therefore, urinary excretion provides the major mechanism for maintaining phosphorus balance.

2. Exchange of Phosphate between Extracellular Fluid and Soft Tissues. The soft tissue stores of phosphate, such as those in the muscle mass, undergo rapid exchange with the ECF pool of phosphate (Fig. 8.4-3). This process plays an important role in the minute-to-minute regulation of plasma phosphate concentration.

3. Exchange of Phosphate between Extracellular Fluid and Bone. About 250 mg of phosphate enters and leaves the bone from 500 mg of ECF pool in the process of bone remodelling.

4. Excretion of Phosphate occurs in faecal matter and urine.

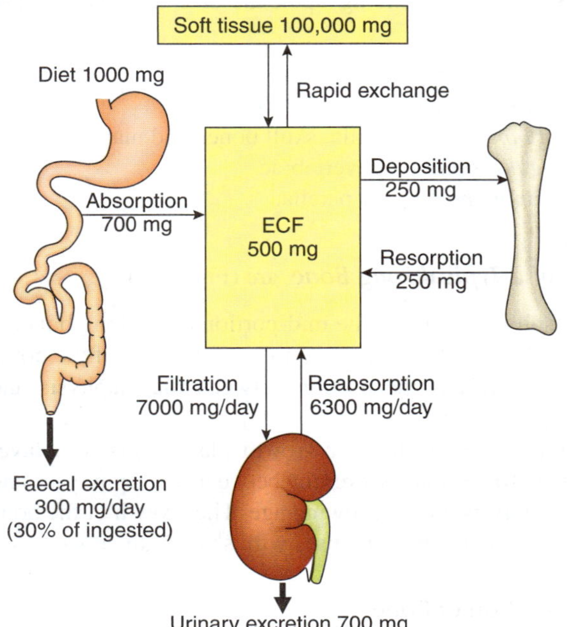

FIGURE 8.4-3 Maintenance of phosphorus balance in an adult human ingesting 1000 mg of phosphorus.

i. ***Faecal excretion*** includes 300 mg (30% of ingested) of phosphate which is not absorbed (Fig. 8.4-3).
ii. ***Urinary excretion.*** About 7000 mg of phosphate is filtered by kidney per day. A larger fraction (90%) of the filtered phosphate is reabsorbed. Like the reabsorption of Ca^{2+}, phosphate reabsorption also takes place in the proximal tubule, the thick ascending limb of the loop and the distal tubule. The proximal tubular reabsorption of phosphate is coupled to Na^+ reabsorption. It increases or decreases with the increase or decrease of Na^+ reabsorption. The sodium-dependent P_i cotransporter involved are NaP_i-IIa and NaP_i-IIc. Thus, in volume expansion, both Na^+ and phosphate

reabsorption decrease. PTH inhibits proximal tubular reabsorption of P_i by inhibiting NaP_i-IIc. The distal tubular reabsorption of phosphate is facilitated by vitamin D.

Thus, in a healthy adult, about 700 mg (10% of total filtered load) is excreted in urine (Fig. 8.4-3).

Regulation of Serum Phosphate Levels

Hypophosphataemia and hypocalcaemia due to dietary or other causes bring about different adaptative changes to normalize the plasma levels. Responses to hypocalcaemia are more immediate than to hypophosphataemia.

As mentioned earlier, hypophosphataemia is mainly compensated by reduced urinary loss and there occurs no change in dietary absorption.

Magnesium Metabolism

The divalent cation, magnesium (Mg^{2+}), is related in some respects to calcium and phosphates.

Functions subserved by magnesium are:

- *Role in formation of bone and teeth.*
- *Serves as a cofactor for several enzymes* requiring ATP, e.g. hexokinase, glucokinase, phosphofructokinase, adenylyl cyclase.
- *Required for proper neuromuscular function.* Low levels of Mg^{2+} lead to neuromuscular irritability.
- *Required for release of PTH* in response to hypocalcaemia and also for the actions of the hormone on its various target tissues.

Distribution of Mg^{2+} in the Body. The body contains a total of 25 g of Mg^{2+}, which is distributed as:

- 10% in bones, in combination with calcium and phosphate and
- 50% in soft tissues and body fluids.

Plasma levels range from 1.8 to 2.4 mg%. About 60% is present in ionized form, 10% in combination with other ions and 30% bound to proteins.

Magnesium Balance. Daily requirement of magnesium is 300–500 mg. Leafy vegetables, nuts and soya bean are rich sources of magnesium. Magnesium is mainly absorbed in the distal part of small intestine (while more Ca^{2+} absorption occurs in proximal parts). No active transport has been demonstrated; only passive and facilitated transport occurs. Consumption of large amounts of calcium, phosphate and alcohol diminish Mg^{2+} absorption. PTH increases Mg^{2+} absorption. On an average, 40% (i.e. 120–200 mg) of intake is absorbed daily. In a steady state, the same amount is excreted in the urine. Magnesium deficiency is compensated by decreased urinary excretion. Adaptative responses to reduced dietary intake of Mg^{2+} are poorly developed as compared to similar responses for hypocalcaemia.

Applied Aspects

Magnesium deficiency causes muscular irritation, weakness and convulsions. These symptoms are similar to that observed in tetany (Ca^{2+} deficiency), which are relieved only by magnesium.

Causes of magnesium deficiency are malnutrition, alcoholism and liver cirrhosis. The low level or Mg deficiency may be observed in uraemia and rickets.

BONE PHYSIOLOGY

Functions and Composition of Bone

Functions of Bone

Bone is a specialized tough connective tissue that forms the skeleton of the body. It subserves the following functions:

1. *Protective function.* The framework formed by the bones protects the vital organs and soft tissues of the body, e.g. thoracic cage protects lungs and heart, and skull protects brain.
2. *Mechanical functions* served by the bones include:
   - *Support* to body.
   - *Attachment* to muscles and tendons.
   - *Movements* are performed at the joints by leverage effects of bones.
3. *Metabolic functions* of bone include their important role in homeostasis of calcium and phosphate metabolism.
4. *Haemopoietic function* includes the formation of blood cells in the red bone marrow.

Types and Parts of a Bone

Types. Bones, depending upon the size and shape, have been classified as:

- *Long bones,* e.g. limb bones
- *Short bones,* e.g. wrist and ankle bones.
- *Flat bones,* e.g. scapula, skull bones and mandible.
- *Irregular bones,* e.g. vertebrae.
- *Sesamoid bones,* e.g. patella.

Parts of a Typical Long Bone are (Fig. 8.4-4.)

- Diaphysis (shaft) is the mid-portion of the long bone.
- Epiphysis is the widened part on either end of the bone.
- Metaphysis is the portion between the diaphysis and epiphysis.
- Epiphyseal cartilage or growth plate refers to a layer of cartilage that is present between the epiphysis and metaphysis during growing age. The growth of the bone stops when epiphysis fuses with shaft of the bone.

Composition of Bone

Bone, a special form of connective tissue, is composed of a collagenous framework (matrix) impregnated with bone

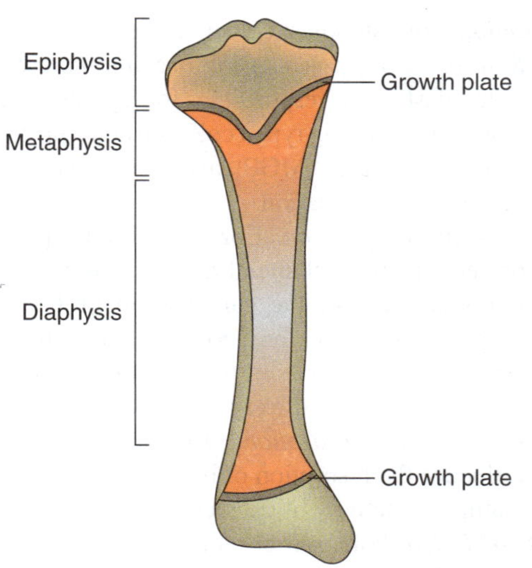

FIGURE 8.4-4 Parts and gross structure of long bones as seen in longitudinal cut section.

salts. The dry, fat free bone consists of one third organic bone matrix, and two thirds minerals (inorganic).

Bone Matrix Bone matrix, also called osteoid, consists of collagen fibres embedded in the gelatinous ground substance.

Collagen fibres are arranged in lamellae. The fibres of one lamellus run parallel to each other, but those of adjoining lamellae run at varying angles to each other. Over 90% of the organic matrix is type I collagen.

Ground substance of a lamellus is continuous with that of adjoining lamellae. It is formed by the extracellular fluid and proteoglycans (which include chondroitin sulphate and hyaluronic acid). These substances are concerned with the regulation and deposition of bone salts.

Bone Salts The bone salts constitute the inorganic component of bone which primarily comprises calcium and phosphate in the form of hydroxyapatite crystals [$Ca_{10}(PO_4)_6(OH)_2$]. Each crystal measures about 400 Å units in length, 100 Å units in breadth and 10–30 Å units in thickness. Adsorbed on the surface of hydroxyapatite crystals are present small amounts of other salts such as sodium, potassium, magnesium and carbonate. The bone salts strengthen the bone matrix.

Structural Considerations

Structure of Bone

Structurally, two types of bones are known: compact or cortical bone, and trabecular or spongy or cancellous bone. In most of the bones, both compact and cancellous forms are present, but thickness of each type varies in different regions of the bone. For example, in long bones, the *epiphyseal region* contains large amount of cancellous bone and outer thin compact bone. While in *diaphyseal regions,* the amount of compact bone is more and cancellous (spongy) bone is very thin (Fig. 8.4-4).

Structure of Compact Bone The compact bone makes the outer layer of most bones and accounts for the 80% of the bone in the body. Histologically, the compact bony tissue is made up of several minute cylindrical structures called *osteons* or *Haversian system* (Fig. 8.4-5). Each osteon is formed by several layers of collagen lamellae (Haversian lamellae) arranged concentrically around a centrally placed canal called the *Haversian canal* which contains the blood vessels, lymph vessels and nerve fibres. In between the concentric layers of collagen tissue are present many *lacunae* (small cavities) which contain *osteocytes.* The osteocytes send long process called canaliculi all around. The canaliculi from neighbouring osteocytes unite to form tight junctions.

The Haversian canals (and therefore the osteons) run along the longitudinal axis of long bones and branch and anastomose with each other. They also communicate with the external surface of the bone through channels that are called *canals of Volkmann*. Blood vessels and nerves pass through all these channels, so that compact bone permeated by a network of blood vessels that provide nutrition to it. The compact bone is lined externally by periosteum and internally by endosteum. Both periosteum and endosteum of the long bones contain osteoprogenitor cells which can differentiate into osteoblasts or osteoclasts.

Structure of Trabecular or Spongy Bone The trabecular or spongy or cancellous bone is present inside the compact bone and makes up 20% of bone in the body. It is made up of spicules or plates or trabeculae which are separated by wide spaces that are filled in by bone marrow. Nutrients diffuse from the bone ECF to trabeculae. The surface to volume ratio is much higher in trabecular bone than the compact bone.

The trabeculae are thin and consist of irregular lamellae of bone with lacunae containing osteocytes. The trabeculae

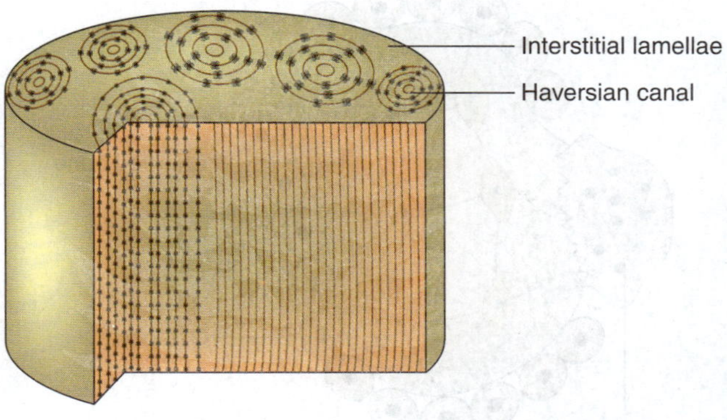

FIGURE 8.4-5 Structure of compact bone.

are covered by a thin layer of connective tissue called *endosteum,* which contains osteoblasts, osteoclasts and osteoprogenitor (stem) cells (Fig. 8.4-6).

Cells of Bone

Osteoprogenitor Cells These are stem cells of mesenchymal origin that can proliferate and convert themselves into osteoblasts whenever there is need for bone formation. They resemble fibroblasts in appearance.

- *In the fetus,* osteoprogenitor cells are numerous at sites where bone formation is to take place.
- *In the adults,* these cells are present over the periosteum as well as endosteum.

Osteoblasts

Bone-forming Cells are called osteoblasts. These are derived from the osteoprogenitor cells. Being concerned with bone formation, they are situated in the outer surface of bone (Fig. 8.4-7), the marrow cavity and epiphyseal plate cells. The differentiation of osteoproginitor cells into osteoblast is by a specific ossification transcription factor, such as Cbfa/RunX2.

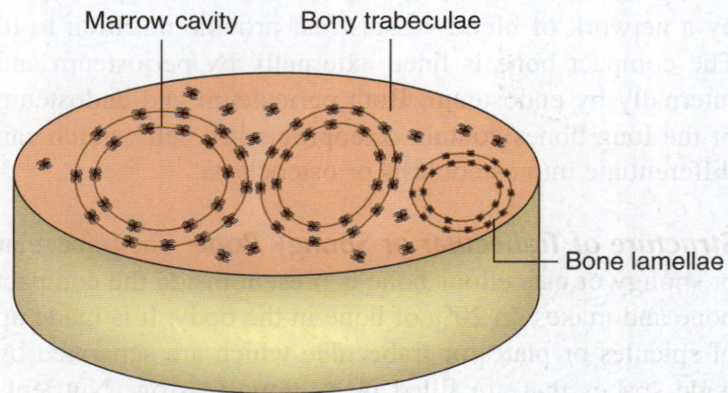

FIGURE 8.4-6 Structure of trabecular bone.

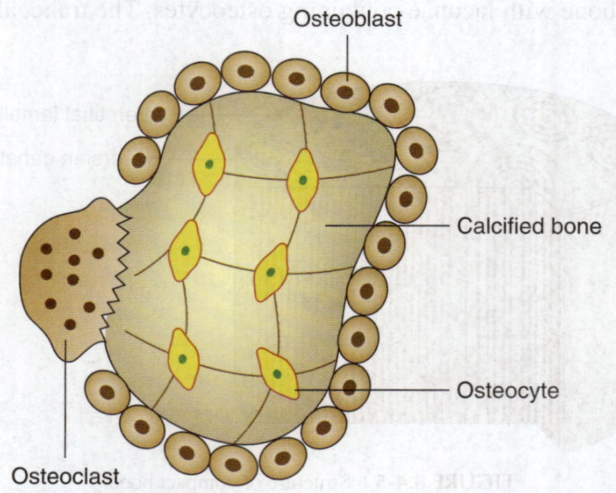

FIGURE 8.4-7 Location of various bone cells.

Functions of osteoblast cells include:

1. *Role in laying down of the organic matrix of bone.* Osteoblasts are responsible for synthesis of bone matrix by secreting type I collagen and a protein called matrix gla protein (MGP), and other proteins involved in the matrix formation.
2. *Role in calcification.* Enzyme alkaline phosphatase present in the cell membranes of osteoblasts plays important role in the calcification of bone matrix. Osteoblasts are believed to shed off matrix vesicles which possibly serve as points around which formation of hydroxyapatite crystals takes place.
3. *Role in bone resorption.* Osteoblasts may indirectly influence the resorption of bone by inhibiting or stimulating the activity of osteoclasts.

Fate of Osteoblasts. After taking part into bone formation, the osteoblasts are converted into osteocytes which are trapped inside the lacunae of calcified bone.

Osteocytes

Cells of mature (or developed) bone are called osteocytes. As mentioned above, they represent osteoblasts, which during bone formation are 'imprisoned' in the lacunae between the bone lamellae (Fig. 8.4-7). The cytoplasmic processes from the osteocytes run into canaliculi and ramify throughout the bone matrix. The processes from neighbouring cells have contact with each other forming tight junction.

Functions of osteocytes are:

- Metabolic activity of osteocytes helps to maintain the bone as living tissue.
- Maintain the integrity of lacunae and canaliculi, and thus keep open the channels for diffusion of nutrients through bone.
- Play an important role in maintaining the exchange of calcium between the bone and extracellular fluid.

Osteoclasts

Bone-removing cells are called osteoclasts. These are giant multinucleated cells found in relation to surfaces where bone removal is taking place. At such locations, these cells occupy pits called *resorption bays* or *lacunae of flowship*. At sites of bone resorption, the surface of an osteoclast shows many folds which are described as a *ruffled membrane* (Fig. 8.4-7).

Osteoclasts are derived from haemopoietic stem cells via monocytes. Probably they are formed by fusion of many monocytes. The bone marrow stromal cells express receptor activator for nuclear factor kappa beta ligand (RANKL) on their surface. When these cells come in contact with monocytes expressing RANK (i.e., RANKL receptor), then two signalling pathways get initiated (Fig. 8.4-8).

Function. Osteoclasts are responsible for bone resorption during bone remodelling. The lysosomal enzymes required for bone resorption are synthesized and released into the bone-resorbing compartment of osteoclasts.

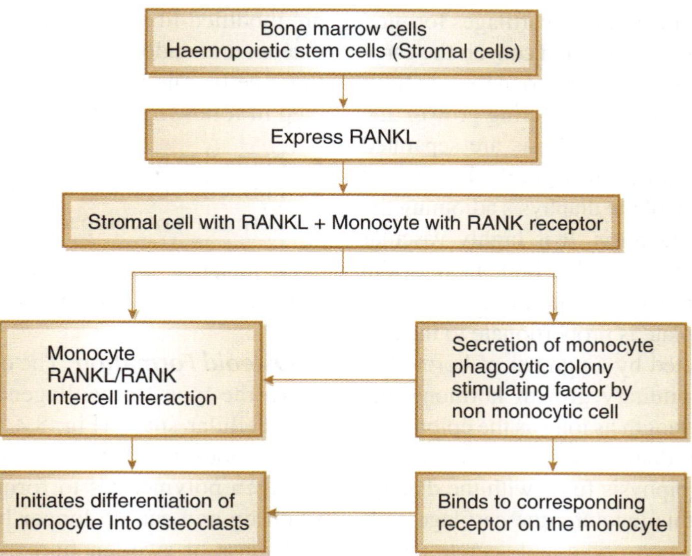

FIGURE 8.4-8 Differentiation of monocytes into osteoclasts. *Note:* Osteoprotegerin (OPG) secreted by the precursor cells controls differentiation of monocytes into osteoclasts by competitively with RANK for binding of RANKL.

Bone Lining Cells Bone lining cells are flattened cells which form a continuous epithelium-like layer on bony surfaces where active bone deposition or removal is not taking place. They are present on the periosteal surface as well as endosteal surface.

Physiological Considerations

The main physiological considerations which need emphasis are:

- Bone growth and
- Bone remodelling.

Bone Growth

All bone is of mesenchymal origin. The process of bone formation is called ossification. There are two mechanisms of bone formation: endochondral bone formation and intramembranous bone formation.

Endochondral Bone Formation. During fetal development, formation of most of the bones is preceded by the formation of a cartilaginous model which is subsequently replaced by bone. This kind of ossification is called endochondral bone formation.

Intramembranous Bone Formation. Formation of some bones, e.g. clavicle, vault of skull and mandibles, is not preceded by formation of a cartilage model, but they are formed directly in a fibrous membrane. This kind of ossification is called intramembranous bone formation.

Steps of Growth of a Long Bone

1. Formation of a Cartilage Model. In the region, where a long bone is to be formed, the mesenchyme first lays down a cartilaginous model of bone.

2. Ossification and Calcification. The ossification is carried out by osteoblasts which enter the central part of the cartilaginous model. This area is called *primary centre of ossification* (Fig. 8.4-9A). Gradually, bone formation extends from the primary centre towards the ends of shaft (Fig. 8.4-9B). Process of formation of bony lamellae from osteoblasts is described separately.

3. Growth in Length and Girth. At about the time of birth, developing bone consists of the bony diaphysis formed by extension of primary centre for ossification and cartilaginous ends. At varying times after birth, *secondary centres*

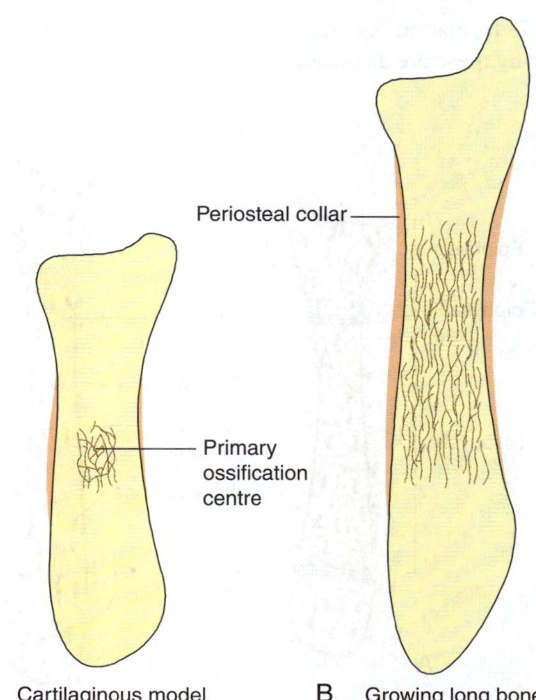

FIGURE 8.4-9 Formation of a long bone: **A,** cartilage model with primary centre for ossification; and **B,** bone growth by extension of primary centre for ossification.

of endochondral ossification appear in the cartilages forming the ends of bones. These centres enlarge and convert the cartilaginous ends into bone. The portion of the bone formed from one secondary centre is called *epiphysis*. During growth, the bone of diaphysis and the bone of epiphysis are separated by a plate of actively proliferating cartilage, the *epiphyseal plate* (Fig. 8.4-10). The portion of the diaphysis adjoining the epiphyseal plate is called metaphysis. It is highly vascular and a region of active bone formation. The bone increases in length as this plate lays down new bone on the end of shaft. The width of the epiphyseal plate is proportionate to the rate of growth. The width is affected by a number of hormones, but most markedly by the pituitary growth hormone and IGF-1. The bone increases in length as long as the epiphyseal plates remain separated from diaphysis (shaft). The growth of the bone stops when the epiphysis fuses with the diaphysis *(epiphyseal closure)*. At this juncture, the cartilage cells stop proliferating, become hypertrophic and secrete vascular endothelial growth factor (VEGF), leading to vascularization and ossification. The epiphyseal closure occurs in an orderly temporal sequence, the last epiphysis closing after the puberty. The normal age at which the epiphysis closes in different bones of the body is well known, and the age of a young individual can be determined by looking at the open and closed epiphysis in radiograph of the skeleton.

Even after bone growth has ceased, the calcium turnover function of bone is most active in the metaphysis which acts as a storehouse of calcium. The metaphysis does not have a bone marrow cavity and is frequently the site of infection.

Bone Formation

Bone formation is carried out by active osteoblasts, which is why these are also called bone-forming cells. Osteoblasts are modified fibroblasts. These cells are found in the periosteum and endosteum. Bone is continuously deposited by these cells. The process of bone formation can be considered in following steps:

- Formation of bone lamellae,
- Formation of trabecular bone and
- Formation of compact bone.

It includes two main processes: osteoid formation and mineralization of bone matrix.

1. Osteoid Formation The osteoblasts synthesize and lay down the type I procollagen molecules into the adjacent extracellular space (Fig. 8.4-11). These cells also secrete a gelatinous matrix in which the fibres get embedded. The collagen polymerizes to form collagen fibres which then swell up and can no longer be seen distinctly. The resultant mass of swollen fibres and matrix is called osteoid (Fig. 8.4-11).

Factors affecting process of osteoid formation include protein intake and a number of growth factors such as TGF-β, IGF-I, IGF-II, PDGF, acidic and basic fibroblast growth factors, etc. Besides these growth factors, insulin, GH, sex hormones (oestrogens, androgen), thyroid hormones, calcitriol and calcitonin also affect the process of osteoid formation.

2. Bone Matrix Mineralization Soon after formation of osteoid, the process of bone matrix mineralization starts.

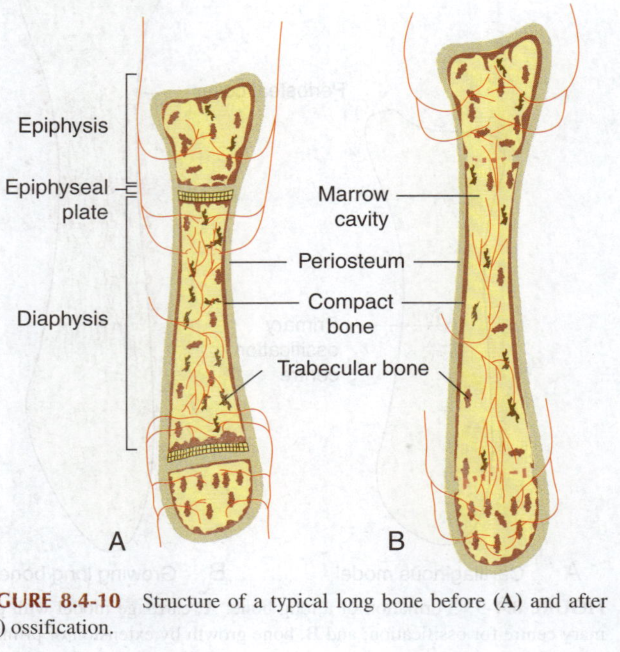

FIGURE 8.4-10 Structure of a typical long bone before (**A**) and after (**B**) ossification.

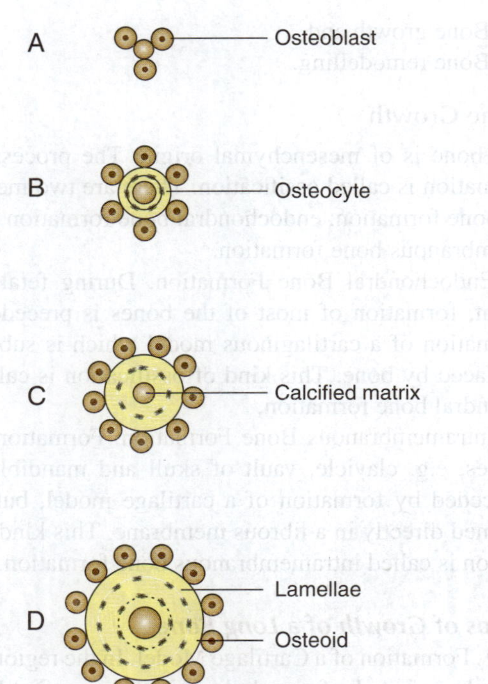

FIGURE 8.4-11 Schematic depiction of process of formation of bony lamellae. For explanation, see text.

It occurs in two phases: an initial slow process of initiation of mineralization followed by rapid mineralization process.

Initiation of Mineralization or Nucleation. The bone matrix is surrounded by a metastatic solution of calcium and phosphate ions (solution in which concentration of Ca^{2+} and Po_4^{3-} exceeds the solubility product of the salt but precipitation is inhibited by certain inhibitors like pyrophosphate). For enucleation to take place, pyrophosphate has to be cleaved into inorganic phosphate by alkaline phosphatase which also has activity of pyrophosphatase. The process of mineralization greatly depends upon the *calcium × phosphate* ion product in extracellular fluid. This product must be above 30/dL for this process to occur.

Rapid Calcification after Enucleation. About 10 days elapse between osteoid formation and initiation of mineralization. However, once mineralization is initiated, i.e. after nucleation, most of the calcium phosphate is deposited within 6–12 h. Thereafter, hydroxide and bicarbonate ions are gradually added to the mineral mixture, and mature hydroxyapatite crystals are slowly formed. After the process of mineralization of bone matrix is completed, the osteoid is converted into a bone lamella (Fig. 8.4-11C).

Formation of a Trabecular Bone After the formation of one bone lamella (as described above; Fig. 8.4-11A–C), another layer of osteoid is laid down by osteoblast. The osteoblasts move away from the bone lamella to line the new layer of osteoid. However, some osteoblasts are caught between the lamella and the osteoid (Fig. 8.4-11D). The osteoid is now ossified to form another lamella. The cells trapped between the two lamellae become osteocytes. In this way, a number of lamellae are laid down one over another and these lamellae together form a trabecula of bone, but many such trabeculae constitute the trabecular or cancellous bone. Within each lamella, mineral fluid containing channels, called *canaliculi,* traverse the mineralized bone. Through these channels, the interior osteocytes remain connected with surface lining cells and with other osteocytes via syncytial cell processes. This system of interconnected cells formed by osteocytes and osteoblasts spreads over all the bone surfaces except small surface area adjacent to osteoclasts. This extensive system of osteocytes and osteoblasts constitutes an osteocystic membrane system which separates bone from ECF. A small amount of fluid called the bone fluid is present between the bone and osteocytic membrane. This arrangement permits transfer of calcium from the enormous surface area of the interior to the exterior of the bone units, and then into the extracellular fluid. This transfer process, which is carried out by the osteocytes, is known as *osteocytic osteolysis.* It probably does not actually decrease bone mass, but it simply removes calcium from the most recently formed crystals.

Conversion of Trabecular Bone to Compact Bone All newly formed bone is cancellous. It is converted into compact bone (Fig. 8.4-12):

- Each space between the trabeculae of cancellous bone comes to be lined by osteoblasts (Fig. 8.4-12A and B).
- The osteoblasts lay down lamellae of bone as already described. The first lamella is formed over the inner wall of the original space and is therefore shaped like a ring (Fig. 8.4-12C).
- Subsequently, concentric lamellae are laid down inside this ring thus forming an *osteon.* The original space becomes smaller and smaller and persists as a *Haversian canal* (Fig. 8.4-12D).

Bone Resorption

Bone resorption, like bone formation, is a continuous process. In bone resorption, destruction of entire matrix of bone occurs resulting in diminished bone mass.

Osteoclasts are the cells responsible for bone resorption. As mentioned earlier, these are giant multinucleated cells formed probably by fusion of circulating monocytes (or bone marrow monocyte precursor cells). These cells contain large number of mitochondria and lysosomes.

Process of bone resorption involves the following steps:

1. Removal of Unmineralized Osteoid Layers. Before osteoclastic resorption can begin, a thin 1–2 µm outer layer of unmineralized osteoid must be removed. This is achieved by collagenase released from lining cells. The lining cells also secrete a molecule that attracts osteoclasts to the site of new denuded bone.

2. Attachment of Osteoclast on denuded bone surface (periosteum or endosteum) is the second step of bone

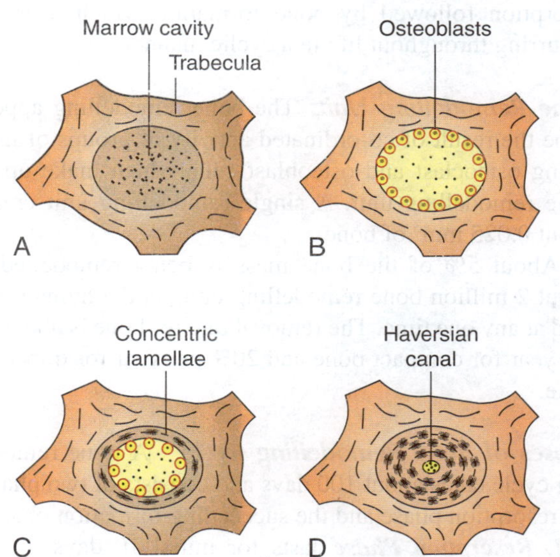

FIGURE 8.4-12 Steps in the conversion of trabecular bone into compact bone.

resorption. This is mediated by the surface receptors called *inteqrins*. At the point of attachment, a ruffled border is created by infolding of the osteoclast's plasma membrane (villi formation). The part of the bone to be resorbed is called bone resorption compartment.

3. Release of Proteolytic Enzymes and Acids. At the site of attachment, the osteoclasts release proteolytic enzymes and lysosomal enzyme and acid from the villi-like projections. Proton pump (i.e. H^+-dependent ATPase) moves from endosomes into the resorption compartment through the cell membrane and acidifies the area (~pH 4.0)

4. Digestion and Dissolution of Bone. The enzymes digest and dissolve organic matrix of the bone, and acids cause dissolution of the bone salts. All the dissolved materials are now released into extracellular fluid, some elements enter the blood. The remaining elements are cleaned up by the macrophages and a shallow cavity is formed in the bone-resorbing compartment. Urinary excretion of organic products released during resorption provides quantitative indices of bone resorption.

Regulation of Bone Resorption. Bone resorption is stimulated by PTH, calcitriol, EGF, PDGF and some other growth factors. The response is mediated through release of prostaglandins, TGFb and IL-I which stimulate osteoclastic activity. Thyroxine and vitamin A also increase bone resorption. Calcitonin acts on osteoclasts through its receptors to *inhibit* their activity.

Note. It is an observation that there is neuroendocrinal regulation of bone mass via leptin. Intracerebroventricular leptin decreases bone formation. This is a consistent observation that obesity protects against bone loss because obese persons are resistant to the effect of leptin.

Bone Remodelling

Definition. Bone remodelling refers to a process of bone resorption followed by bone formation which keeps on occurring throughout life in a cyclic manner.

Bone Remodelling Unit. The bone remodelling appears to be the result of co-ordinated activity of groups of interacting osteoclast and osteoblast cells which make up the bone remodelling unit. A single remodelling unit creates about 0.025 mm^3 of bone.

About 5% of the bone mass is being remodelled by about 2 million bone remodelling units in the human skeleton at any one time. The removal rate for bone is about 4% per year for compact bone and 20% per year for trabecular bone.

Phases of Bone Remodelling Cycle. A bone remodelling cycle takes about 100 days and consists of two phases: the resorption phase and the succeeding formation phase.

1. Resorption Phase lasts for initial 10 days. In this phase, mineralized bone is reabsorbed by osteoclasts releasing calcium and phosphate.

2. Formation Phase lasts for next 90 days and is characterized by reformation of bone by osteoblasts (assimilating calcium and phosphate).

Initiation of Bone Remodelling Cycle. Remodelling occurs in areas of bone that have been structurally weakened by fatigue, by having unusual mechanical stress placed on them or by disease. The osteocytes embedded deep within mineralized bone act as mechanoreceptors that pick up mechanical signals transmitted via interstitial fluid and respond by increasing phospholipase-C, Ca^{2+} and protein kinase C activity. These lead to a stimulation of phospholipase A_2 and production of prostaglandins (PGE_2). PGE_2 in turn reaches the lining cells via the syncytial processes or the canaliculi. The lining cells then initiate recruitment differentiation of osteoclast cells via communication with stromal precursors in the bone marrow. Thus, resorption is the initial process carried out by osteoclast cells, but it is triggered by signals from the osteoblast cells.

Regulation of Bone Remodelling. The paired activity of osteoclast and osteoblast cells in bone remodelling is well regulated. All aspects of the remodelling cycle are influenced by a large number of hormones and growth factors, as well as cytokines from immune cells (Table 8.4-2).

TABLE 8.4-2 Factors Regulating Bone Remodelling

Event	Stimulatory factor	Inhibiting factor
Bone resorption	Parathyroid hormone (constant)	Oestrogen Androgen Calcitonin Transforming growth factor β Interferon Nitric oxide
	Vitamin D, cortisol	
	Thyroxine	
	Prostaglandins	
	Interleukin-1	
	Interleukin-6	
Bone formation	Growth hormone (constant)	
	Insulin-like growth factor	Cortisol
	Testosterone	
	Oestrogen	
	Transforming growth factor β	
	Skeletal growth factor	
	Bone-derived growth factor	
	Calcitonin	
	Parathyroid hormone (intermittent)	

The process of bone remodelling is one example of co-ordinated function of the endocrine and immune systems.

Physiological significance of continuous bone remodelling includes:

- *Bone adjusts its strength* in proportion to the degree of bone stress. For example, in athletes, soldiers and others in whom the bone stress is more, the bones become heavy and strong.
- *Shape of bone can be rearranged* for proper support of mechanical force in accordance with the stress.
- *Old bone becomes relatively weak and brittle.* The development of new bone matrix maintains the toughness of bone.

CALCITROPIC HORMONES

Parathyroid Hormone (PTH)

Functional Anatomy of Parathyroid Glands

Gross Anatomy The parathyroid glands are two pairs of small endocrine glands closely applied to the back of the thyroid gland embedded within its fibrous capsule at the superior and inferior poles. Each gland is slightly oval in shape and is about the size of a split pea, measuring 6 × 4 × 2 mm. The total weight of four normal glands is about 140 mg. Normally, there are four parathyroid glands, but rarely they may be more (6 or even 8).

Histological Structure The parenchyma of the parathyroid gland is made up of cells that are arranged in cords. Numerous sinusoids lie in close relationship to the cells. The cells of the parathyroid glands are of two main types: chief cells and oxyphil cells.

Chief cells, also called as principal cells, are much more numerous than the oxyphil cells. These are small round cells having clear (agranular) cytoplasm and vesicular nuclei. Chief cells secrete the parathyroid hormone (PTH) or parathormone.

Oxyphil cells, in contrast to chief cells, are much larger and contain granules that stain strongly with acidic dyes. These cells first appear at puberty and their function is still not clear.

Structure, Synthesis and Secretion of PTH

Structure. Parathyroid hormone (PTH) is a single-chain polypeptide, containing 84 amino acids and having molecular weight 9500.

Synthesis. PTH is synthesized from a precursor molecule called prepro-PTH, which contains 115 amino acids. The prepro-PTH is degraded to pro-PTH, and finally to active PTH.

Secretion. PTH is released from chief cells by exocytosis in response to decrease in plasma ionized calcium concentration that is sensed by the calcium receptors in the parathyroid cells.

Regulation of PTH Secretion

1. Role of Plasma Ionized Calcium. The secretion of PTH is mainly regulated by circulating levels of ionized calcium which act directly on the parathyroid glands in a feedback fashion. The secretion of PTH is inversely related to the plasma calcium concentration in a sigmoidal fashion (Fig. 8.4-13) indicating that:

- Maximum secretion occurs when plasma ionized calcium levels fall below 3.5 mg%.
- As the plasma ionized calcium concentration rises, PTH secretion progressively diminishes and reaches to a persistent low basal rate when ionized calcium reaches up to 5.5 mg%. Further, rise in plasma ionized calcium levels do not further decrease PTH secretion.

It is important to note that PTH secretion responds to a small alteration in the concentration of ionized plasma calcium within seconds, even if total calcium concentration is kept constant.

2. Role of Serum Magnesium Concentration.

- *Mild decrease* in serum Mg^{2+} concentration stimulates PTH secretion, while
- *Severe decrease* in serum Mg^{2+} concentration inhibits PTH secretion and produces symptoms of hypoparathyroidism (e.g. hypocalcaemia).

3. Role of Plasma Phosphate Concentration. A rise in plasma concentration of phosphate causes an immediate fall in ionized calcium concentration, which in turn stimulates PTH secretion. In addition, high phosphate levels directly increase PTH secretion when ionized calcium concentration is kept constant.

4. Role of Vitamin 1,25-$(OH)_2D_3$. It inhibits transcription of the PTH gene and decreases PTH secretion. It also inhibits proliferation of parathyroid cells and upregulates the Ca^{2+} receptors in parathyroid cells.

Plasma Levels, Half-Life, and Degradation of PTH

Plasma Level of PTH is about 130 pg/ml (approximately 3×10^{-12} M).

Half-life of PTH in plasma is 5–8 min.

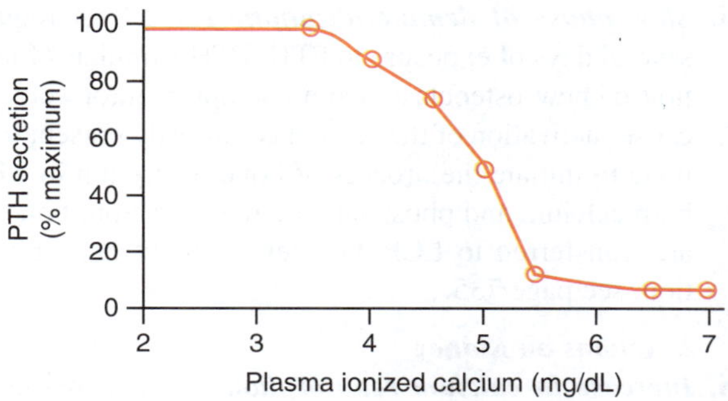

FIGURE 8.4-13 The inverse relationship between parathormone (PTH) and plasma ionized calcium.

Degradation of PTH occurs rapidly in the peripheral tissues. PTH is predominantly split in the liver. The major product is the circulating (6000 molecular weight) carboxy-terminal fragment that is further acted upon in the kidney.

Mechanism of Action and Actions of PTH

Mechanism of Action of PTH PTH acts through its receptors.

PTH Receptors. There are three different types of PTH receptors:

- Parathyroid hormone-related proteins (hPTH/PTHrP) receptors.
- PTH_2 (hPTH-R) are second type of receptors found in brain, placenta and pancreas which do not bind to PHTrP.
- CPTH, a third type of receptor, which reacts with carboxyl terminal of PTH rather than amino terminal.

First two types of receptors (PTHrP and PTH_2) are coupled to Gs proteins.

PTH binds to a membrane receptor protein on the target cells (in bones, kidney and intestine) and activates adenylyl cyclase to liberate cAMP. The cAMP in turn increases intracellular calcium that promotes the phosphorylation of proteins (by kinases).

Actions of PTH The prime function of PTH is to elevate plasma calcium concentration and to decrease the plasma phosphate concentration by acting on three major target organs: directly on bone and kidney, and indirectly on the gastrointestinal tract (Fig. 8.4-14).

1. Actions on the Bone PTH stimulates calcium and phosphate resorption from bones, i.e. causes decalcification or demineralization of bone by two processes which constitute the rapid and slow phases of demineralization.

i. ***Rapid phase of demineralization.*** This phase is also called *osteocyticosteolysis*. In this process, the calcium is transferred from the bone canalicular fluid into osteocytes and then into the extracellular fluid. In this process, phosphate is not mobilized along with calcium.
ii. ***Slow phase of demineralization.*** This effect requires several days of exposure to PTH. PTH stimulates formation of new osteoclasts from osteoprogenitor cells and causes activation of the osteoclasts already present in the bone to initiate the process of bone resorption in which both calcium and phosphate are released from bone and are transferred to ECF. For details about bone resorption, see page 735.

2. Actions on Kidney

i. ***Increase in calcium reabsorption.*** PTH increases the reabsorption of calcium from the ascending limb of loop of Henle and the distal tubules of kidney and helps to prevent hypocalcaemia. However, hyperparathyroidism is characterized by hypercalciuria. This paradoxical effect can be explained by the fact that in hyperparathyroidism, hypercalcaemia produces such a large load of filtered calcium in glomerular filtrate that in spite of increased distal tubular calcium reabsorption, the net excretion of urinary calcium is increased.
ii. ***Inhibition of phosphate reabsorption in the proximal tubule*** is the most dramatic effect of PTH on the kidney. This effect produces phosphaturia and hypophosphataemia. This effect of PTH allows disposition of the extra phosphate released by PTH-stimulated bone resorption.
iii. ***Inhibition of reabsorption of Na^+ and HCO_3^- in the proximal tubule and stimulation of Na^+–H^+ exchanger*** by PTH cause acidification which may prevent the occurrence of metabolic alkalosis, which could result from the release of HCO_3^- during the dissolution of hydroxyapatite crystals in bone.
iv. ***Stimulation of reabsorption of Mg^{2+} by the renal tubules*** caused by PTH helps to conserve this important cation.
v. ***Stimulation of synthesis of 1,25-dihydroxycholecalciferol*** is a very important action of PTH in the kidney.

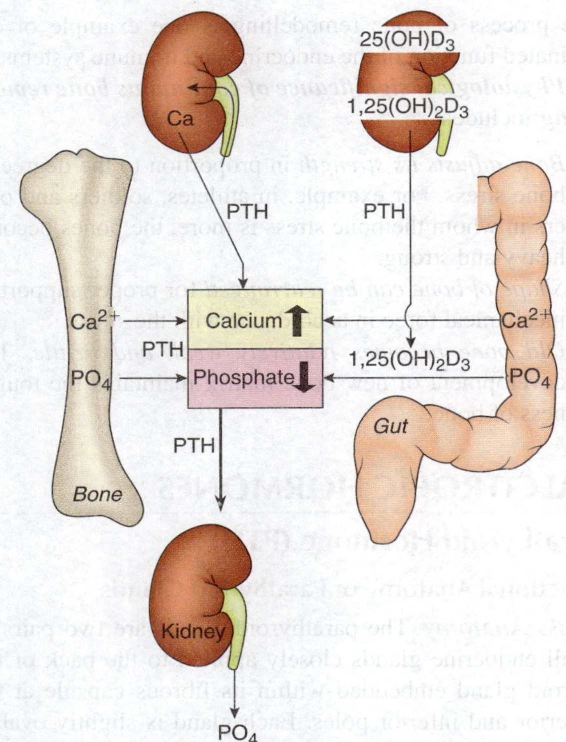

FIGURE 8.4-14 Actions of PTH on bones (stimulation of calcium and phosphate resorption), kidneys (stimulation of calcium reabsorption but inhibition of phosphate reabsorption) and intestine (increase in absorption of calcium and phosphate both). PTH action leads to direct increase in calcium and decrease in serum phosphate level.

3. Actions on Intestines Parathormone greatly enhances both calcium and phosphate absorption from intestine indirectly by increasing synthesis of 1,25-dihydroxycholecalciferol in the kidney.

Vitamin D

The term vitamin D refers to group of closely related steroids produced by the action of ultraviolet light on certain provitamins. There are various forms of vitamin D, such as D_2 and D_3 (most important). The active form of vitamin D, i.e. 1,25-dihydroxycholecalciferol also called as calcitriol, is now considered a hormone because of its following characteristics:

- Site of action is away from site of production. It is produced in the kidney and acts on intestine and bone.
- Acts through receptors present in the specific target organs which include intestine, bone and kidney.
- Feedback control mechanism is used for self-regulation of its synthesis.
- Acts like steroid hormones and increases synthesis of mRNA to increase the concentration of calcium-binding protein in many tissues, especially in intestinal mucosa.
- Acts in association with other hormones such as parathyroid hormone and calcitonin to regulate calcium and phosphate levels in plasma.
- Actinomycin D inhibits its action. This also supports the view that the active form of vitamin D exerts its effect on DNA leading to synthesis of RNA (transcription).
- Its half-life is short, i.e. around 10 h.

Formation of Calcitriol

Calcitriol $1,25(OH)_2D_3$ is the active form of vitamin D_3. Steps involved in its formation are summarized:

Source and Synthesis of Vitamin D_3 Vitamin D_3, the precursor (prohormone) of the hormone 1,25-dihydroxycholecalciferol reaches the blood from two sources (Fig. 8.4-15):

1. Dietary Source. Good dietary sources of vitamin D include fish, fish liver oils and egg yolk. Milk is not a good source of vitamin D. The daily requirement of vitamin D is 400 IU or 10 μg of cholecalciferol. In countries with good sunlight (like India), the recommended dietary allowance for vitamin D is 200 IU (or 5 μg cholecalciferol). Because of its fat solubility, vitamin D absorption from the intestine is mediated by the bile salts.

2. Cutaneous Synthesis. Besides dietary intake, cutaneous synthesis is the other more important source of vitamin D_3 (cholecalciferol) in the body. Vitamin D_3 is synthesized primarily in the specialized skin cells, called *keratinocytes,* which are located in the inner layers of epidermis. The synthesis occurs by the action of ultraviolet (UV) rays on 7-dehydroxycholesterol (an intermediate in the synthesis of cholesterol). First previtamin D_3 is formed

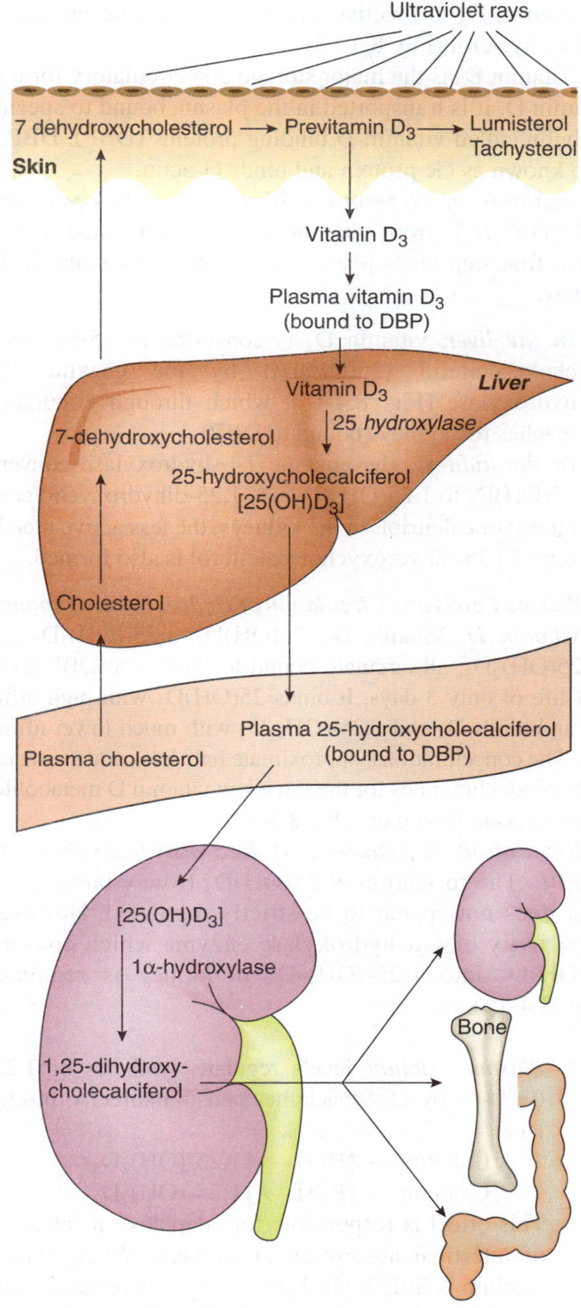

FIGURE 8.4-15 Synthesis and sources of vitamin D_3 and its hydroxylation to form the hormone 1,25-dihydroxycholecalciferol. Main sites of actions of 1,25-dihydroxycholecalciferol are also shown.

which is then converted spontaneously over 3 days to vitamin D_3, in a reaction that is driven by thermal energy from sunshine (Fig. 8.4-15). Although cutaneous synthesis of vitamin D_3 is related in exponential fashion to exposure to UV rays, excessive exposure to the sun, e.g. in fishermen, does not produce vitamin D toxicity, because continuous exposure to sunlight also causes photodegradation of previtamin D_3 to inactive (inert) products like lumisterol and tachysterol (Fig. 8.4-15).

Vitamin D_3 is the major storage and circulatory form of vitamin D. It is transported in the plasma bound to specific globulin called vitamin-D binding proteins (DBP). DBP is also known as Gc protein and binds G-actin.

Synthesis of Hormone 1,25-dihydroxycholecalciferol (1,25(OH)$_2$D$_3$). from vitamin D_3 is accomplished by two steps: first step takes place in the liver and second in the kidney.

- ***In the liver,*** vitamin D_3 is converted to 25-hydroxy-cholecalciferol (25(OH)D_3) by the enzyme 25-hydroxylase (Fig. 8.4-15), which through circulation reaches the kidney (bound to DBP).
- ***In the kidneys,*** the enzyme 1-α-hydroxylase converts 25(OH)D_3 to 1,25(OH)$_2$D$_3$, i.e. 1,25-dihydroxycholecalciferol or calcitriol. In the kidneys, the less active metabolite 24,25-dihydroxycholecalciferol is also formed.

Plasma Levels and Circulation of Hydroxylation Products of Vitamin D. Vitamin D_3, 25(OH)D_3, 1,25-(OH)$_2$D$_3$ and 24,25(OH)$_2$D$_3$, all circulate bound to DBP. The DBP has a half-life of only 3 days. It binds 25(OH)D_3 with high affinity, and binds D_3 and 1,25-(OH)$_2$D$_3$ with much lower affinities. The concentrations, approximate half-lives and estimated daily production rates for the three key vitamin D metabolites in humans are shown in Table 8.4-3.

TABLE 8.4-3 Status of Vitamin D Metabolites in Human

Metabolite of vitamin D	Plasma concentration (ng/ml)	Plasma half-life (days)	Estimated production rate (μg/day)
1,25(OH)$_2$D$_3$	0.03	0.25	1
24,25(OH)$_2$D$_3$	2.00	15–40	1
25(OH)D$_3$	30.00	15	10

Regulation of Synthesis of 1,25-dihydroxycholecalciferol. The formation of 25(OH)D_3 from vitamin D_3 in liver does not appear to be strictly regulated. However, the activity of 1-α-hydroxylase enzyme which converts 25(OH)D_3 into 1,25-(OH)$_2$D$_3$ in kidney is regulated (Fig. 8.4-16) as:

1. ***Plasma calcium*** levels regulate synthesis of 1,25-(OH)$_2$D$_3$ by a feedback mechanism indirectly through PTH.
   - ↓Calcium → ↑PTH → ↑1,25-(OH)$_2$D$_3$
   - ↑Calcium → ↓PTH → ↓1,25-(OH)$_2$D$_3$

   This effect is responsible for adaptative mechanism of intestinal absorption of calcium. When plasma calcium is little high, 1,25-(OH)$_2$D$_3$ is produced and the kidneys mainly convert 25(OH)$_2$D$_3$ into the inactive metabolite 24,25(OH)$_2$D$_3$.
2. ***Plasma phosphate*** level regulates synthesis of 1,25-(OH)$_2$D$_3$ by a feedback mechanism by its direct effect on the enzyme 1-α-hydroxylase.
   - ↓ Phosphate → 1-α-hydroxylase → ↑ 1,25-(OH)$_2$D$_3$ activity
   - ↑ Phosphate → ↓1-α-hydroxylase → ↓1,25-(OH)$_2$D$_3$ activity
3. ***1,25(OH)$_2$D$_3$*** level itself has a:
   - A direct negative feedback effect on its formation,
   - A positive feedback effect on the formation of 24,25(OH)$_2$D$_3$ and
   - A direct action on the parathyroid gland to inhibit the production of mRNA for PTH.
4. ***Other factors*** regarding 1,25(OH)$_2$D$_3$ synthesis are:
   - *Prolactin* increases 1,25(OH)$_2$D$_3$ synthesis.
   - *Oestrogen* increases total circulatory 1,25(OH)$_2$D$_3$, but this effect is probably due to an increase in the secretion of binding protein (DBP).
   - *Hyperthyroidism* is associated with decreased circulating 1,25(OH)$_2$D$_3$ and an increased incidence of osteoporosis.
   - *Metabolic acidosis* depresses the synthesis,
   - *Growth hormone,* HCS and calcitonin stimulate the formation of 1,25(OH)$_2$D$_3$.

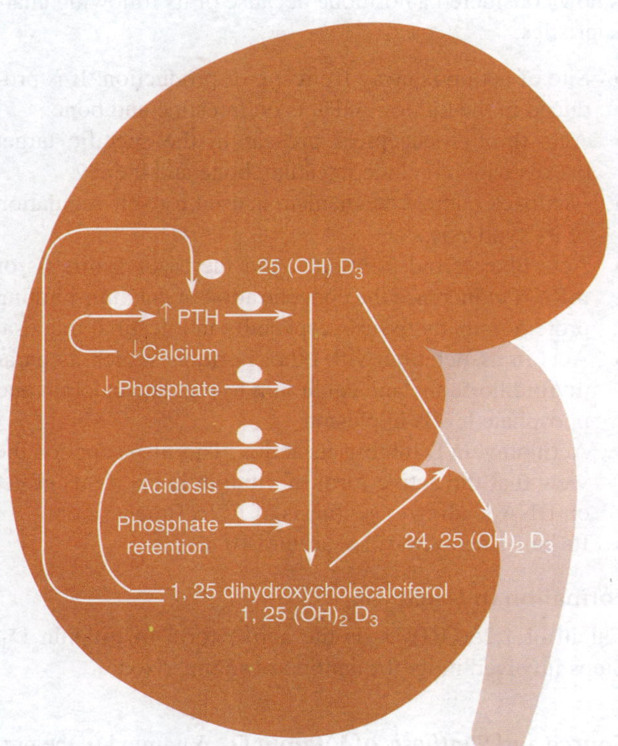

FIGURE 8.4-16 Regulation of synthesis of calcitriol [1,25(OH$_2$)D$_3$] from 25(OH)D$_3$ in the kidney.

Important Note

An 'antiaging protein' also called *α klotho* (named after Klotho—daughter of Zeus in Greek mythology), also has an important role in Ca^{2+} and PO_4^{3-} homeostasis by its effect on 1,25-hydroxycholecalciferol.

Recently, it has been seen that a mice deficient in α klotho protein shows accelerated aging, decreased bone density, mineral density and calcification, hypocalcemia and hyperphosphotaemia. Normally, this protein plays an important role in stabilizing the localization of membrane proteins involved in Ca^{2+} and PO_4^{3-} reabsorption such as $TRPV_5$ and Na^+–K^+ ATPase. It also enhances the activity of fibroblast growth factor-23 (FGF-23) at the receptor. The FGF-23 inhibits the production of 1-α–hydroxylase, resulting in 1,25-dihydroxycholecalciferol reduction.

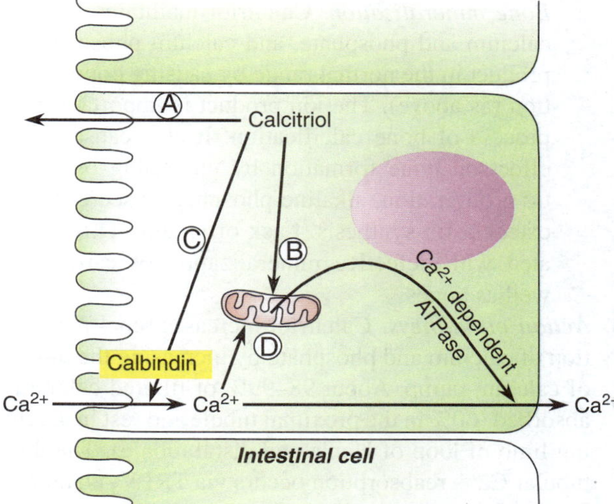

FIGURE 8.4-17 Modes of action of calcitriol in increasing intestinal absorption of calcium: **A,** action at brush borders; **B,** induction of calcium-dependent ATPase; **C,** increased synthesis of calcium-binding proteins, calbindins; and **D,** promotion of entry of calcium into subcellular organelles.

Mechanism of Action and Actions of Calcitriol

Mechanism of Action of Calcitriol Calcitriol (1,25$(OH)_2D_3$) acts by exerting its effect on gene expression in the target cells by binding with the intracellular receptors. The vitamin D receptor is found both in the cytoplasm and nucleus. This mechanism has been described in detail on page 670 (see Fig. 8.1-8).

Actions of Calcitriol

I. Regulation of Plasma Levels of Calcium and Phosphate Calcitriol [1,25$(OH)_2D_3$] is the biologically active form of vitamin D. It regulates the plasma levels of calcium and phosphate by acting at three different sites: intestine, bone and kidney. 1,25-Dihydroxycholecalciferol stimulates gene expression for proteins involved in Ca^{2+} transport (e.g. calbindin-D proteins), mostly found in intestine, kidney and brain.

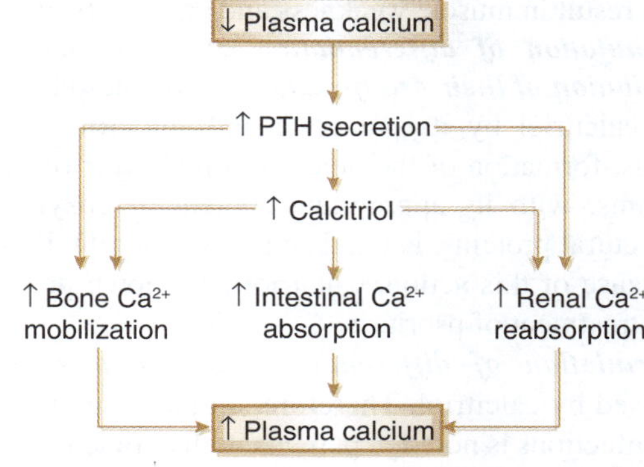

FIGURE 8.4-18 Summary of actions of calcitriol in elevating plasma calcium.

1. ***Action on intestine.*** The major action of calcitriol is to help calcium absorption from the intestine. It appears to perform this function by acting on three levels (Figs. 8.4-17, 8.4-18):
   - Increases calcium permeability at the brush border by causing some changes in the membrane phospholipids,
   - Induces synthesis of calcium-dependent ATPase (which helps to pump calcium out of cell), $TRPV_6$ (transient receptor potential vanilloid type-6) that binds to intracellular protein calbindin-Dk and
   - Induces synthesis of calcium-binding proteins (calbindin). In human intestinal epithelium, two types of calbindins are induced (calbindin-D_qk and calbindin 28k). These molecules may carry calcium across the intestinal cell or they may be important for keeping concentration of free intracellular calcium low (when calcium is being absorbed from the food). The rate of calcium absorption across the duodenum is proportional to the cell content of calbindin.
   - Calcitriol also promotes entry of calcium from cell cytoplasm into subcellular organelles (mitochondrium).
2. ***Actions on bone.*** Calcitriol increases bone resorption as well as bone mineralization.
   - *Bone resorption.* Calcitriol helps bone resorption by PTH. Calcitriol receptors are present in osteoblasts and not on osteoclasts. The formation of receptor–calcitriol complex on osteoblasts originates cytokine signal that stimulates recruitment, differentiation and fusion of precursors into osteoclasts. The osteoclasts cause bone resorption for which PTH is also required.
   - *Osteocyticosteolysis* is also increased by calcitriol.

- *Bone mineralization.* Calcitriol maintains levels of calcium and phosphate, and calcium phosphate ion product in the normal range by causing bone resorption (as above). The ion product is important in the process of bone calcification. It also causes direct effect on bone formation by increasing osteoblastic proliferation, alkaline phosphatase secretion and osteoclastin synthesis. Lack of vitamin D is associated with defective mineralization of cartilage as well as bones.

3. ***Action on kidneys.*** Calcitriol increases renal reabsorption of calcium and phosphate by increasing the number of calcium pump. About 98–99% of filtered calcium is absorbed (60% in the proximal tubule and rest in ascending limb of loop of Henle and distal tubule). The distal tubular Ca^{2+} reabsorption occurs via $TRPV_5$ channels.

II. Other Actions of Calcitriol Besides the above well-known sites of action (intestine, bone and kidney) of vitamin D, the calcitriol receptors have also been found on the cells in a number of tissues. The possible actions of calcitriol in such tissues are summarized:

1. ***Calcium transport into skeletal and cardiac muscles*** is stimulated by calcitriol. Therefore, vitamin D deficiency can result in muscle weakness and cardiac dysfunction.
2. ***Stimulation of differentiation of keratinocytes and inhibition of their proliferation*** is thought to be caused by calcitriol by its paracrine and autocrine function. Thus, formation of the outer cornified layer of the epidermis, with its appropriate content of enzymes and structural proteins, is regulated by vitamin D. Probably, because of this action, calcitriol has shown promise in the treatment of psoriasis.
3. ***Stimulation of differentiation of immune cells*** is caused by calcitriol. Therefore, an increased incidence of infections is noted in patients with deficiency of vitamin D. The role of vitamin D in immunoregulation is evidenced by the fact that macrophages, monocytes and transformed lymphocytes can synthesize $1,25(OH)_2D_3$ from $25(OH)D_3$, and that calcitriol receptors are expressed by promyelocytes, monocytes and activated T-lymphocytes. The possible roles of vitamin D in immune modulation are:
   - Calcitriol stimulates T-helper-2 cells to secrete interleukin-4 (1L-4), and TGF-β and T-helper-1 cells to decrease their production of interleukin-2, γ-interferon and tumour necrosis factor-α TNF-α).
   - Calcitriol decreases the proliferation of T and B lymphocytes as well as immunoglobulin synthesis by B lymphocytes.
4. ***Calcitriol appears to be involved in regulation of growth and production of growth factors*** as the vitamin D receptors are found also in pancreatic islets, anterior pituitary, hypothalamus, placenta, ovary, aortic endothelium and skin fibroblasts.

Calcitonin

Synthesis and Structure

Synthesis. Calcitonin is synthesized in the C-cells or parafollicular cells of the thyroid gland. These cells are of neural crest origin, which during development migrate to the last ectodermal cleft and from these enter the developing thyroid gland. These cells constitute 0.1% of the epithelial cells of the thyroid gland and can be distinguished from ordinary thyroid hormone-producing cells by their large size, pale cytoplasm and small secretory granules.

Calcitonin synthesis proceeds from a large molecule, the preprocalcitonin. In some cells, the primary RNA transcripts encodes preprocalcitonin and directs synthesis of calcitonin.

Structure. Calcitonin is a straight-chain polypeptide with 32 amino acids. Its molecular weight is 3500.

Secretion. Calcitonin is secreted in response to rise in plasma calcium level. The cAMP prompts exocytosis of calcitonin-containing granules.

Regulation of Secretion

1. ***Increase in plasma calcium concentration*** is the major regulator of calcitonin secretion. It is important to note that calcitonin is not secreted until the plasma Ca^{2+} concentration reaches to 9.5 mg% and that above this calcium level, plasma calcitonin is directly proportional to plasma calcium. This provides a feedback mechanism for regulating serum calcium concentration which works exactly opposite to that of PTH (Fig. 8.4-19).
2. ***Gastrointestinal hormones*** such as gastrin, CCK, glucagon and secretin have all been reported to stimulate calcitonin secretion, with gastrin being the most potent stimulus. The elevated gastrin levels in patients with Zollinger–Ellison syndrome and in pernicious anaemia may account for raised plasma calcium levels by secreting calcitonin. However, it is important to note that the dose of gastrin required to secrete calcitonin is much more than the amount of gastrin secreted by food intake. Therefore, it is premature to conclude that calcium in the intestine initiates secretion of a calcium-lowering hormone before calcium is absorbed.

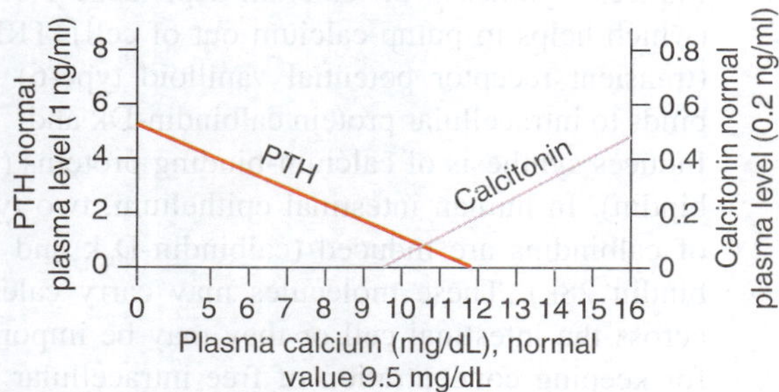

FIGURE 8.4-19 Relationship of plasma calcium concentration with release of calcitonin and parathyroid hormone.

3. ***Other factors*** like β-adrenergic agonist, dopamine and oestrogen also stimulate calcitonin secretion.

Plasma Levels, Half-Life and Degradation

Plasma levels of circulating calcitonin range from 10 to 20 pg/ml, which increase two- to tenfold after an acute increase in the plasma concentration of as little as 1 mg/dL.

Half-life of calcitonin is very short, i.e. less than 10 min.

Degradation. Circulating calcitonin is heterogeneous, and it is largely degraded and cleared by the kidney.

Actions and Physiological Role of Calcitonin

Actions The major effect of calcitonin is to rapidly lower the plasma calcium level. This effect of calcitonin is clearly a physiological antagonist to PTH. However, this effect is transient. Further, with respect to phosphate, it has the same net effect as PTH, it decreases the plasma phosphate. These effects of calcitonin are due to its following actions:

1. ***Action on the bone.*** The main action of calcitonin on the bone is to oppose the bone resorptive action of PTH. Calcitonin inhibits osteoclastic activity due to its direct action on the bone which can occur in the absence of parathyroid gland, GIT and kidneys. Its antiosteoclastic activity is due to the following effects:
   - Calcitonin binds to the plasma membrane receptor on the osteoclast and decreases its activity. The affected osteoclasts rapidly lose their ruffled borders, undergo cytoskeletal rearrangement, exhibit reduced motility, detach from bone surface and are deactivated. Bone resorption is thus decreased.
   - Number of osteoclasts is also reduced.
   - It inhibits the Ca^{2+} permeability of osteoclasts and osteoblast cells and thereby inhibits the active transport of Ca^{2+} from bone cells into the ECF.
2. ***Action on kidney.*** Calcitonin increases loss of calcium and phosphate in the urine. This effect also contributes in producing hypocalcaemia and hypophosphataemia.

Physiological Significance of Calcitonin In adults, the exact physiological significance of calcitonin is uncertain. Since the osteoclast resorption of bone leads to secondary osteoblastic activity, so by reducing resorptive activity, calcitonin also reduces osteoblastic activity. This means that over a long period, calcitonin decreases both osteoclastic and osteoblastic activities. Therefore, effect on blood calcium concentration is transient. Calcitonin thus has a very weak effect on plasma concentration of calcium in human adults. *This fact is confirmed by the following observations*:

- The calcitonin content of human thyroid is low, and after thyroidectomy, bone density and plasma calcium levels are normal as long as the parathyroid glands are intact.
- When a calcium load is injected after thyroidectomy, there occurs only transient abnormalities in calcium metabolism.
- Patients with medullary carcinoma of the thyroid have a very high circulatory calcitonin level but no symptoms directly attributable to the hormone are present. Further, their bones are also normal.
- No syndrome due to calcitonin deficiency has been described.
- From the above observations, it can be concluded that any effect of calcitonin deficiency or excess is easily offset by appropriate adjustments of PTH and vitamin D concentrations.

The Possible Physiological Roles of Calcitonin are:

- ***In children,*** where bone turnover is high, calcitonin may play a role in skeletal development by promoting calcium storage in bones.
- ***Postprandial hypercalcaemia*** may be prevented by calcitonin.
- ***Protects the bones of mother from excess calcium loss during pregnancy*** and lactation when demand for calcium to be used elsewhere dramatically increases.
- ***Calcitonin could participate*** in fetal skeletal development.
- ***Calcitonin may have a functional role in*** the development of accelerated bone loss after menopause. This appears possible because of the fact that plasma calcitonin is lower in women than men and that it declines with aging.
- ***Calcitonin is useful in the acute treatment of hypercalcaemia and in certain bone diseases*** in which a sustained reduction in osteoclastic resorption is therapeutically beneficial.
- ***Calcitonin and CGRP (calcitonin gene-related peptide) may also have paracrine and neurotransmitter function.*** This function seems to be possible because of the discovery of calcitonin and CGRP in a number of locations throughout the body such as pituitary gland, hypothalamus and within cells of neural crest origin. In this regard, calcitonin does exhibit analgesic properties independent of the opioid system.

PTH-related Protein and other Hormones Affecting Calcium Metabolism

PTH-related Protein

Origin and Structure

Sites of Origin. The PTH-related protein (PTHrP) is produced by many different tissues in the body such as skin keratinocytes, lactating mammary epithelium, placenta and fetal parathyroid glands.

Structure. PTHrP has 140 amino acid residues compared with 84 in PTH. The genes for PTHrP and PTH are on paired chromosomes 12 and 11, respectively. However, PTHrP and

PTH have marked homology at their amino terminal ends, with 8 of the first 13 amino acid residues being in the same positions. Because of striking homology between PTHrP and PTH, the PTHrP binds to PTH receptors.

Physiological Roles of PTHrP PTHrP is found in many tissues and may play a physiological role during intrauterine life and early infancy and later during development of different tissues.

1. Regulation of Endochondral Bone Formation. PTHrP is important for endochondral skeletal development. Without PTHrP or functional PTHrP/PTH receptors, the process of orderly progression of the growth plates at either end of the bone is severely disorganized, and the resulting bone becomes very abnormal. At puberty, the sex steroids stop the operation of PTHrP system and the epiphyseal growth plate permanently closes.

2. Role in the Breast Development. PTHrP is produced in large amounts in breast and is involved in breast development and lactation. It is also secreted in large amounts in the milk. The PTHrP swallowed by the infant may thus react with its receptor present in the intestine or it may be absorbed in the infant's bloodstream to fulfil a systemic role.

3. Role in Tooth Development. PTHrP allows normal tooth development and eruption by resorbing alveolar bone.

4. Role in skin development. PTHrP acts as a growth factor for the development of skin and hair follicle.

5. Protective Role in Central Nervous System. The PTHrP is found in the brain (cerebral cortex, hippocampus and granular layer of the cerebellar cortex) where it protects the neurons from toxic overstimulation by glutamate receptors that activate voltage-dependent calcium channels.

Other Hormones and Humoral Factors Affecting Calcium and Bone Metabolism

Certain hormones, other than the calcitropic hormones described above, that also have some effect on calcium metabolism are:

1. Growth Hormone. This increases calcium excretion in urine, but it also increases intestinal absorption of calcium, and this effect seems to be greater than the effect on excretion, with a resultant positive calcium balance. Growth hormone also generates IGF-1 which stimulates protein synthesis in bone.

2. Glucocorticoids. These inhibit bone formation and increase bone resorption by several actions, resulting in osteoporosis.

Glucocorticoids inhibit bone formation by the following effects:

- Decrease collagen synthesis and formation of mature osteoblasts from their undifferentiated precursors.
- Increase apoptosis of osteoblasts and osteocytes which are the functional cells in bone formation.
- Decrease the systemic and local generation of IGF-1 molecules.

Glucocorticoids increase bone resorption by their following effects:

- Increase the levels of immune and inflammatory cytokines that stimulate osteoclast formation and bone resorption by osteoclasts.
- Increase mRNA of collagenase, the enzyme essential for destroying the organic matrix of bone.
- Decrease the absorption of calcium and phosphate from the intestine and also increase the renal excretion of these ions. The resulting hypocalcaemia increases the secretion of PTH, which adds to the bone-resorbing effect of glucocorticoids.

3. Thyroid Hormones. Normal plasma levels of thyroxine is essential for proper skeletal development.

- Congenital hypothyroidism is associated with depressed skeletal development (see page 709).
- Hyperthyroidism may be associated with hypercalcaemia, hypercalciuria and in some instances osteoporosis.

4. Insulin. This is required for bone formation and there is significant bone loss in untreated diabetics.

5. Oestrogens. These prevent osteoporosis, probably by direct effects on osteoblasts. Therefore, incidence of osteoporosis in females increases after menopause.

APPLIED ASPECTS

Some of the important applied aspects with respect to endocrinal control of calcium metabolism and bone physiology are:

- Hyperparathyroidism and hypercalcaemia,
- Hypoparathyroidism and hypocalcaemia and
- Metabolic bone diseases.

Hyperparathyroidism and Hypercalcaemia

Hyperparathyroidism

Hyperparathyroidism is a clinical condition characterized by excessive secretion of parathyroid hormone (PTH). It is of three types: primary, secondary and tertiary.

Primary Hyperparathyroidism

Aetiology. Primary hyperparathyroidism occurs due to excessive secretion of PTH by:

- Single autonomous parathyroid adenoma (most common) and
- Parathyroid carcinoma (rare).

Clinicobiochemical Features

- *Typical manifestations* are hypercalcaemia, hypophosphataemia, hypercalciuria and renal calculi (kidney stones).

- *Features of bone disease* are rarely seen in primary hyperparathyroidism. However, radiographic evidence of subperiosteal bone resorption may be seen in 20% cases.
- *Hypercalcaemia* may produce muscle weakness, lethargy and constipation. Since calcium can stimulate release of gastrin, there may occur hyperchlorhydria and peptic ulceration. Hypercalcaemia may also cause hypertension, cardiac arrhythmias and ECG changes.

Secondary Hyperparathyroidism In this condition, excessive PTH secretion occurs secondary to persistent hypocalcaemia which causes continued stimulation of parathyroid gland. It is actually a compensatory mechanism to restore calcium levels at the expense of bones. Due to continuous stimulation, there occurs hyperplasia of all the parathyroid glands.

Aetiology. Secondary hyperparathyroidism is typically seen in slowly developing renal failure. The plasma calcium level is low in chronic renal failure primarily because the diseased kidneys lose the ability to form 1,25-dihydroxycholecalciferol (calcitriol). However, phosphate retention with resulting hyperphosphataemia also contributes to the decreased plasma calcium in chronic renal failure.

Clinicobiochemical Features. Increased PTH secretion may not always normalize serum calcium level (not to speak of hypercalcaemia). The main characteristic feature of secondary hyperparathyroidism is involvement of bones. Areas of osteoclastic hyperactivity and rampant bone resorption are present next to areas of excessive and disorganized trabecular bone formation. Bone pains, fractures and deformity may result. Alkaline phosphatase and osteocalcin levels are elevated.

Hypercalcaemia

Causes Causes of hypercalcaemia depending on the levels of PTH can be divided into two groups:

1. ***Conditions associated with hypercalcaemia and raised PTH levels***
   - Primary hyperparathyroidism and
   - Chronic renal failure (tertiary hyperparathyroidism).
2. ***Conditions associated with hypercalcaemia and low or undetectable PTH levels***
   - Hypercalcaemia of malignancy,
   - Multiple myeloma,
   - Familial hypercalcaemia,
   - Sarcoidosis,
   - Hyperthyroidism,
   - Thiazide diuretics and
   - Milk alkali syndrome.

Hypercalcaemia of Malignancy Hypercalcaemia is not uncommon in malignancy. Tumours produce hypercalcaemia by two mechanisms:

- ***Local osteolytic hypercalcaemia*** is seen in 20% of the patients which have bone metastasis. The osteolytic factors act locally by eroding the bone. These factors include prostaglandins, IL-I, TNF, TGF-β and vitamin D-like sterols.
- ***Humoral hypercalcaemia of malignancy*** is seen in 91% of the patients who do not have bone metastasis. Hypercalcaemia in these patients with cancers of the breast, kidney, ovary, skin, etc. is caused by raised levels of PTH-related protein (PTHrP). The gene encoding for PTHrP is different from the one coding for PTH. There is, however, marked homology at N-terminal and between PTHrP and PTH.

Familial Hypercalcemia Familial hypercalcaemia occurs due to mutations in the gene for Ca^{2+} receptor (CaR). It occurs in two forms:

- Familial benign hypocalciuric hypercalcaemia is seen in individuals heterozygous for inactivating mutations. It is characterized by a chronic moderate elevation in plasma Ca^{2+} and normal or even raised plasma PTH levels.
- Neonatal severe primary hyperparathyroidism is seen in individuals who are homozygous for inactivating mutations.

Management *Surgery:* Subtotal parathyroidectomy becomes necessary in patients experiencing life-threatening complication of hypercalcemia, who develop parathyroid adenoma/hyperplasia.

Hypoparathyroidism and Hypocalcaemia

Hypoparathyroidism

Hypoparathyroidism refers to a clinical condition characterized by low level of plasma calcium either due to deficient production of PTH or its unresponsiveness. Hypoparathyroidism can be classified into two main groups:

- True hypoparathyroidism and
- Pseudohypoparathyroidism.

A. True Hypoparathyroidism In true hypoparathyroidism, there is deficient production of PTH due to heritable or acquired causes. Depending upon the cause, true hypoparathyrodism may be:

1. ***Postablative or postoperative hypoparathyroidism.*** The most common cause of hypoparathyroidism is either damage to glands or their blood supply or their inadvertent removal during thyroidectomy operation. The incidence is 1% of all the thyroidectomies.
2. ***Infantile hypoparathyroidism.*** It is of two types: transient and persistent.
   - *Transient infantile hypoparathyroidism* occurs in infants born to mothers who were suffering from hyperparathyroidism or hypocalcaemia during pregnancy.

- *Persistent infantile hypoparathyroidism* is seen in Di George syndrome, a congenital immune deficiency disorder associated with parathyroid hypoplasia.

3. ***Idiopathic hypoparathyroidism.*** The exact cause is not known. But, it is being considered as an acquired autoimmune disorder of parathyroid gland. It may occur at any age, but is more common in young individuals.

B. Pseudohypoparathyroidism This is a congenital condition in which PTH production is normal but the target tissues are resistant to its effects. The defect may lie in parathyroid receptors or there may be postreceptor defect. The clinical and biochemical features are similar to hypoparathyroidism, but PTH levels are elevated (since hypocalcaemia produces more production of PTH). Pseudohypoparathyroidism occurs in two forms:

1. The common form in which PTH fails to produce normal increase in cAMP concentration due to congenital reduction of Gs protein and
2. Other less common form in which cAMP production is normal, but phosphaturic action of PTH is defective.

Characteristic Features of Hypoparathyroidism Characteristic features of hypoparathyroidism are:

- ***Hypocalcaemia.*** Total serum calcium may be decreased to 4–8 mg% and the ionized calcium to 3 mg%. A 50% fall in the levels of ionized calcium leads to a clinical condition called *tetany* (described below).
- ***Hyperphosphataemia,*** i.e. an increase in serum inorganic phosphate levels to 6–16 mg%.

Tetany

Tetany refers to a clinical condition resulting from increased neuromuscular excitability.

Causes Causes of tetany include:

1. ***Hypocalcaemia.*** Extracellular calcium plays an important role in membrane integrity and excitability. Thus, when concentration of ionic calcium is reduced to <50% of normal in ECF, cell membrane of neurons becomes more permeable resulting in series of action potentials. Thus, hypocalcaemia is the most common cause of increased neuromuscular irritability leading to tetany.
2. ***Hypomagnesaemia*** also causes tetany, because magnesium ions are also associated with neuromuscular irritability.
3. ***Alkalosis*** which reduces ionic calcium can also produce tetany.

Clinical Features Tetany may be latent or manifest. In manifest tetany, symptoms and signs depend upon the age of the patient.

In children, a characteristic triad of following symptoms may be seen:

- *Carpopedal spasm.* The hands in carpopedal spasm adapt a peculiar posture in which there occurs flexion at metacarpophalangeal joints, extension at interphalangeal and there is apposition of thumb (Fig. 8.4-20). This peculiar posture of hand is called *obstetric hand* or *main d'acconcheur hand.* Pedal spasm is less frequent. In it, the toes are plantar flexed and feet are drawn up.
- *Laryngeal stridor* (loud sound) results from spasm of laryngeal muscles. It may produce asphyxia.
- *Convulsions* and even death may result from the associated asphyxia.
- *Visceral features* of tetany include intestinal cramps, biliary spasm, bronchospasm, profuse sweating, etc. These features are due to increased excitability of autonomic ganglia.

Adult patients have the following features:

- *Paraesthesias*, i.e. tingling sensations in the peripheral parts of limbs or around the mouth is a common feature.
- *Carpopedal spasms* are less common.
- *Laryngeal stridor and convulsions* are very rare.

Latent Tetany. In latent or subclinical tetany, the above-described typical symptoms and signs of tetany are absent, but can be unmasked by following provocative tests:

- ***Trousseau's sign*** (pronounced as 'Troosoz's sign'). Occluding the blood supply to a limb for about 3 min by inflation of a sphygmomanometer cuff (above the systolic blood pressure level) produces characteristic carpal spasm (Fig. 8.4-21) or pedal spasm depending upon the limb tested.
- ***Chvostek's sign*** refers to the twitching of facial muscles produced by tapping the facial nerve at the angle of jaw. This occurs due to increased excitability of nerves to mechanical stimulation.
- Hypocalcemia can cause prolongation of QT interval, which may predispose to ventricular arrhythmias.
- Prolonged hypocalcaemia and hyperphosphataemia may cause calcification of basal ganglia, epilepsy, psychosis and cataract.

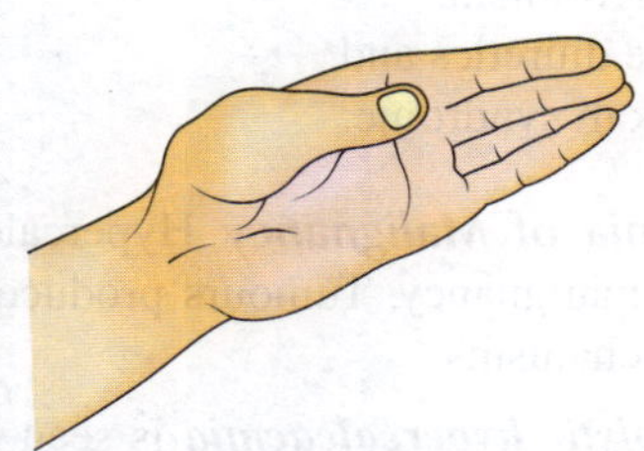

FIGURE 8.4-20 Carpal spasm in a patient with tetany.

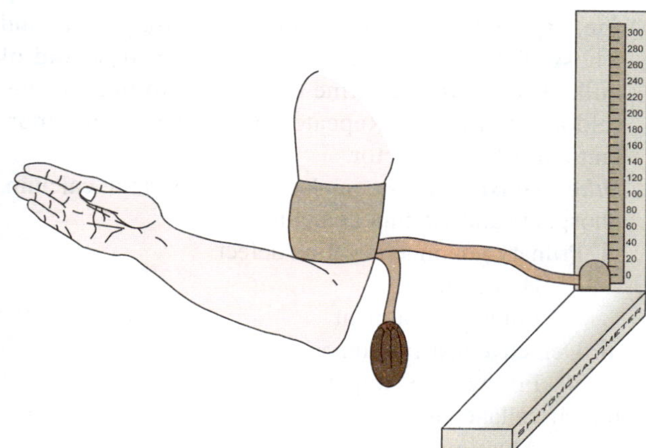

FIGURE 8.4-21 Trousseau's sign to unmask tetany.

Management of Tetany Includes

- *Treatment of hypocalcaemia.* An intravenous injection of 20 ml of 10% calcium gluconate is given to correct hypocalcaemia and relieve tetany.
- For persistent hypoparathyroidism, patients are treated with oral calcium salt and vitamin D analogues (1-α-cholecalciferol or 1,25-cholecalciferol)
- Recombinant PTH is given subcutaneously to treat osteoporosis.
- *Treatment of alkalosis* when present is must.
- *Treatment of the underlying cause* of hypocalcaemia if found will cure the condition.

Metabolic Bone Diseases

The term metabolic bone disease is used for the bone diseases such as rickets, osteomalacia and osteoporosis.

Rickets and Osteomalacia

Rickets (occurring in children) and osteomalacia (occurring in adults) are metabolic bone diseases produced due to deficiency of vitamin D in which there is defective calcification of bone matrix.

Rickets

As mentioned above, in rickets, mineralization of organic bone matrix in growing children is defective. It may also involve cartilaginous matrix of growing end plates of bones.

Causes and Types of Rickets Depending upon the cause, rickets is of following types:

A. Vitamin D Deficiency Rickets is the most common variety. It may occur:

1. ***Nutritional rickets*** is caused by dietary deficiency of vitamin D, either due to poor intake or poor absorption due to high phytate in diet. Vegetarian diet is a poor source of vitamin D.
2. ***Deficient synthesis through skin*** due to inadequate exposure to the sunlight in smoggy cities is particularly known to cause rickets. This disorder usually manifests between the age of 6 months to 2 years, when the growth of bones is very rapid and the baby is fed only on milk and is kept mostly indoor.

B. Vitamin D-resistant Rickets is of rare occurrence. In it, rickets occurs without deficiency of vitamin D. It can be of two types:

1. ***Type I vitamin D-resistant rickets*** is caused by inactivating mutations of the gene for renal hydroxylase resulting in nonformation of 1,25-dihydroxycholecalciferol from vitamin D_3. In such cases, there occurs no response to vitamin D, but a normal response to 1,25-dihydroxycholecalciferol is seen.
2. ***Type II vitamin D-resistant rickets*** occurs due to inactivating mutations of the gene for the 1,25-dihydroxycholecalciferol receptor. In such cases, there is deficient response to both vitamin D and 1,25-dihydroxycholecalciferol.

Pathogenesis of Defective Bone Mineralization in Rickets Vitamin D deficiency leads to poor intestinal absorption of calcium and decreased reabsorption of calcium and phosphates from renal tubules. As a consequence, there is failure of mineralization of organic bone matrix. It is important to note that organic component of bone is normal or somewhat excessive (Fig. 8.4-22). Due to involvement of epiphyseal growth plate in growing bones, the process of ossification at the epiphyseal line is abnormal. Normally, the epiphyseal line is a well-defined narrow strip of 2 mm deep, behind which regular ossification is proceeding. Further, under normal circumstances, the older cartilage cells degenerate and disappear leaving many spaces into which the blood vessels and osteoblasts of the shaft can penetrate. In rickets, this apparently essential preliminary

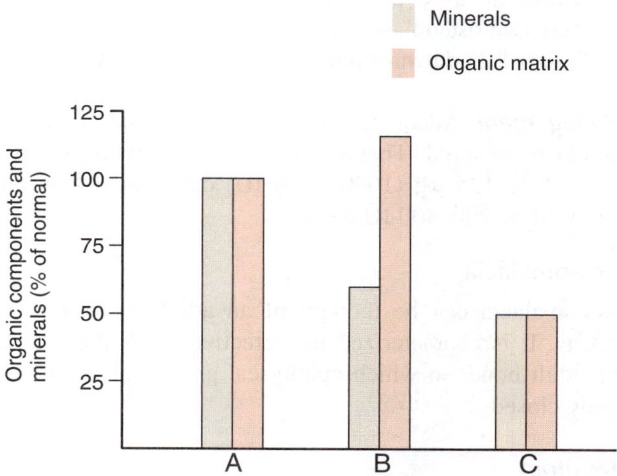

FIGURE 8.4-22 Organic components and mineral contents of bone in: **A**, normal; **B**, osteomalacia; and **C**, osteoporosis.

degeneration does not occur and so ossification is retarded. The cartilage cells persist and go on multiplying and give rise to broad irregular cartilaginous zone which can be felt as a marked project on the surface. The matrix between the cartilage cells and that of new bone itself does not become adequately mineralized resulting in softness of bones.

Clinical Features of Rickets

1. Bony Defects seen in children with rickets are:

- *Craniotabes* is the earliest lesion seen in an infant with rickets. It refers to small rounded areas in the membranous bones of skull which yield under pressure of finger.
- *Widening of wrist* occurs due to epiphyseal widening of lower end of radius bone.
- *Collapse of chest wall* occurs due to flattening of sides of thorax with prominent sternum.
- *Rickety rosary* refers to beading of costochondral junction of ribs.
- *Frontal bossing* and posterior flattening of skull.
- *Harrison's sulcus* refers to indentation of lower ribs at the site of attachment of diaphragm.
- *Bowing of legs* or knock-knee occurs when child starts walking.
- *Kyphosis and pelvic deformities* are also known.

2. General Features

- Infants with rickets are more prone to respiratory and gastrointestinal infections.
- Developmental milestones are delayed.

3. Tetany and Convulsions may occur in cases with marked hypocalcaemia.

4. Biochemical Changes in rickets due to vitamin D deficiency are:

- Low levels of plasma calcium and phosphate.
- Product of plasma Ca^{2+} and PO_4^{3-} is decreased to 30 (normal is 60).
- Serum alkaline phosphatase levels are high due to increased osteoblastic activity.
- Plasma 1,25-dihydroxycholecalciferol is also low or absent.

Management Adequate supply of calcium and vitamin D should be ensured. Therapeutic dose of vitamin D varies from 25 to 125 μg (1000–5000 IU) daily for 6–8 weeks followed by 200–400 IU daily.

Osteomalacia

Osteomalacia can be thought of an adult counterpart of rickets. It is characterized by defective mineralization of the adult bones in which epiphyseal growth plates are already closed.

Aetiology

1. ***Vitamin D deficiency*** is the main cause. The condition is more common in women in child-bearing age, especially in Muslim ladies who use *purdah* and whose diet mainly consists of cereals and devoid of milk. These ladies confine themselves to indoors and seldom see the sun. Repeated pregnancy is an important contributory factor.
2. ***Other causes*** of osteomalacia with normal calcium, phosphate and vitamin D include:
   - i. Primary nonmineralization defect
     - Hereditary
     - Fluoride treatment
   - ii. Defective matrix synthesis
     - Fibrogenesis imperfecta
   - iii. Miscellaneous
     - Aluminium bone disease.

Pathogenesis of Osteomalacia is similar to rickets.

Clinical Features. Clinical features of osteomalacia are almost similar to rickets.

1. Skeletal Abnormalities are dominant features and include:

- Diffuse skeletal pain and bony tenderness are common complaints. Pain may vary from mild backache to severe pain around hip.
- Muscle weakness is also common. A waddling gait may be present due to proximal muscle weakness.
- Bone becomes soft; especially involved are pelvic girdle, ribs and femurs.
- Pseudofractures are seen in flat bones (ribs, scapulae and pelvic rami) or in ends of long bones (e.g. femur).

2. Tetany may occur in few cases with carpopedal spasm.

3. Biochemical features are similar to rickets.

Treatment Treatment is similar to rickets.

Osteoporosis

Osteoporosis is characterized by a reduction of bone mass per unit volume with normal ratio of bone matrix and minerals, i.e. there occurs loss of both bone matrix and mineral component (Fig. 8.4-22).

Pathogenesis Osteoporosis develops due to a mismatch between bone resorption and bone remodelling process; the bone resorption being in excess.

Aetiology Senile osteoporosis is common disease and has become a major public health problem of elderly. All normal humans gain bone mass during adolescence. After a plateau between 20 and 45 year of age, all begin to lose bone mass progressively as they grew older (Fig. 8.4-23). In males, bone loss is usually less significant than females. Further, after menopause, women initially have more rapid bone loss because of additional factor of oestrogen deficiency.

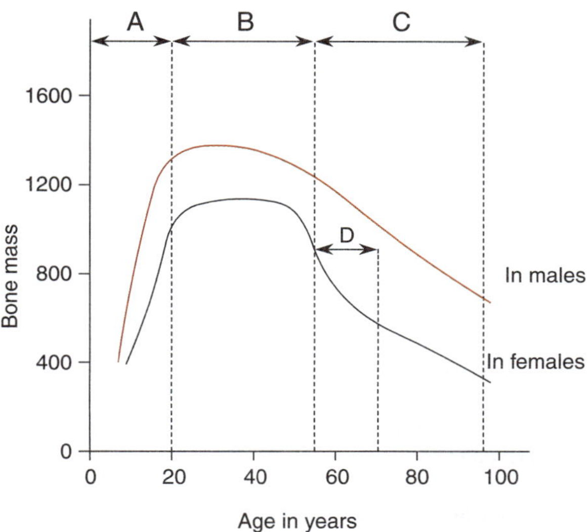

FIGURE 8.4-23 Variation in bone mass (expressed as total body calcium) with age in males and females: **A,** phase of rapid increase in bone mass; **B,** plateau phase; **C,** phase of steady bone loss with advancing age; and **D,** phase of rapid bone loss in women after menopause.

Factors Contributing to Development of Osteoporosis Include:

- ***Immobilization.*** Osteoporosis of immobilization occurs if bones are not subjected to the stress of walking.
- ***Weightlessness.*** Weight bearing is essential for maintenance of bone mass. Weightlessness in space travel produces significant osteoporosis within few months.
- ***Hyperthyroidism*** is associated with more increased osteoclastic activity vis-à-vis bone formation activity, resulting in bone loss.
- ***Cushing's syndrome*** are also associated with increased osteoclastic activity and secondary osteoporosis.
- ***Bone secondaries*** are associated with local release of certain osteoclastic factors which cause osteoporosis.
- ***Chronic renal failure*** is associated with osteomalacia, but in severe cases, osteoporotic bone lesions due to tertiary hyperparathyroidism may also be present.

Characteristic Features of Osteoporosis

1. Bone Density is reduced. In radiographs, the affected bones show clear glass appearance (e.g. ground glass appearance seen in osteomalacia). In severe cases, excessive bone resorption may lead to cyst formation (osteitis fibrosa cystica).

2. Incidence of Fractures is increased; particularly, fractures of the distal forearm (Colles' fracture), vertebral bodies and hips are more common in osteoporosis. All these bones have a high content of trabecular bone, and since trabecular bone is more active metabolically, it is lost more rapidly. Fractures of vertebrae with compression cause kyphosis, producing a typical 'widow's hump' that is common in elderly women with osteoporosis.

3. Biochemical Changes. Serum calcium and phosphate levels are usually normal. There may be increased urine excretion of calcium and hydroxyproline in rapidly developing disease.

Treatment Treatment of osteoporosis should include:

1. ***Calcium intake,*** particularly from natural sources such as milk should be increased.
2. ***Moderate exercise*** may be useful in preventing or slowing the progress of osteoporosis.
3. ***Oestrogen treatment*** is effective in arresting the rapidly developing osteoporosis in women after menopause. Mechanisms by which oestrogen arrest the progress of menopausal osteoporosis are:
   - Oestrogens inhibit secretion of cytokines such as1L-1, 1L-6 and TNFα, and these cytokines foster the development of osteoclasts.
   - Oestrogens also stimulate production of TGFβ, and this cytokine increases apoptosis of osteoclasts.
   - There are oestrogen receptors on osteoblasts, and a direct stimulatory effect on them is also a possibility. However, due to increased incidence of uterine and breast cancer, and cardiovascular diseases oestrogen replacement therapy in postmenopausal women is no longer used.
   - Raloxifene is a selective oestrogen receptor modulator and it has some beneficial effects on bone density. However, the two have some side effects like blood clots.
   - Teriparatide is an analogue of calcitonin and parathyroid hormone can also be used.
4. ***Bisphosphonates,*** such as etidronate, are also useful in osteoporosis. These inhibit osteoclastic activity, increase the mineral content of bone when administered in a cyclic fashion and decrease the rate of new vertebral fractures.
5. ***Fluoride which stimulates osteoblasts,*** making bone more dense, has proved to be of little value in the treatment of osteoporosis.

Osteopetrosis

Osteopetrosis is a rare but severe bone disease, occurs due to defective osteoclast activity. In this disease, osteoclasts are unable to resorb bone; therefore, osteoblastic activity unopposedly increases leading to steady increase in bone density resulting in narrowing and distortion of bony foramina.

Characteristic Features Include

- *Neurological defects* due to compression of nerves when passing through narrowed foramina.
- *Haematological abnormalities* due to crowding of bone marrow cavities.

Cause Osteopetrosis occurs due to lack of a protein encoded by gene early gene c fos and PO-1 transcription factor.

Chapter 8.5

Adrenal Glands

FUNCTIONAL ANATOMY
- General considerations
- Development
- Histological structure
- Blood supply

HORMONES OF ADRENAL CORTEX
- Glucocorticoids
  - Synthesis
  - Plasma levels, transport, metabolism and excretion
  - Mechanism of action
  - Actions of glucocorticoids
  - Regulation of glucocorticoid secretion
- Mineralocorticoids
  - Synthesis
  - Plasma levels, transport, metabolism and excretion
  - Mechanism of action
  - Actions of aldosterone
  - Regulation of aldosterone secretion
- Adrenal sex steroids
  - Synthesis
  - Plasma levels, contribution, metabolism and excretion

APPLIED ASPECTS
- Hyperactivity of adrenal cortex
- Hypoactivity of adrenal cortex

HORMONES OF ADRENAL MEDULLA
- Synthesis and storage
- Secretion of catecholamine hormones
- Circulation, metabolism and excretion
- Mechanism of action
- Actions of catecholamines
- Dopamine
- An integrated response to stress
- Diseases of adrenal medulla

FUNCTIONAL ANATOMY

General Considerations

- There are two adrenal glands, one on either side, situated extraperitoneally at the upper pole of the kidney, hence also called 'suprarenal gland' (Fig. 8.5-1).
- These are also known as 'glands of emergency', as they secrete most vital hormones needed during an emergency.
- Normally, each gland weighs about 5 g and consists of two parts, the adrenal cortex and the medulla, which are absolutely distinct from each other structurally, functionally and developmentally (Fig. 8.5-1).
- The cortex (outer zone), makes up to 80–90% of the gland and is a source of the cortisol hormone.
- The medulla (inner zone), makes up 10–20% of the adrenal gland and is a source of the catecholamine hormones.
- Morphologically and physiologically, the fetal adrenal gland differs strikingly from that of the adult. The adrenal gland is larger at birth than it is during adulthood.

Development

Adrenal Cortex Adrenal cortex is a mesodermal derivative. During fetal life and in a newborn, the adrenal cortex comprises of the outer *neocortex* (15% in volume), which is the progenitor of the adult cortex and the inner *fetal cortex* (85% in volume). The fetal cortex or fetal zone undergoes rapid involution during the first few months of extrauterine life and completely disappears by 3–12 months postpartum. At the same time, the thin outer zone of the neocortex enlarges and differentiates permanently into the three-layered adrenal cortex of the mature human. It is a nuclear receptor with a currently uncertain ligand steroidogenic factor-1 (SF-1), which is essential for the development of the adrenal cortex and expression of the enzymes and steroid hormone biosynthesis. It is axiomatic that all endocrine glands derived from the mesoderm synthesize and secrete steroid hormones.

Adrenal Medulla The adrenal medulla essentially represents an enlarged and specialized sympathetic ganglion derived from the neuroectodermal cells giving rise to sympathetic ganglia. The neural crest gives rise to neuroblasts, which eventually give rise to the autonomic postganglionic neurons, the adrenal medulla and the spinal ganglia. In early fetal life, the adrenal medulla contains only norepinephrine.

Histological Structure

Adrenal Cortex The adrenal gland is covered by a connective tissue capsule from which septa extend into the gland

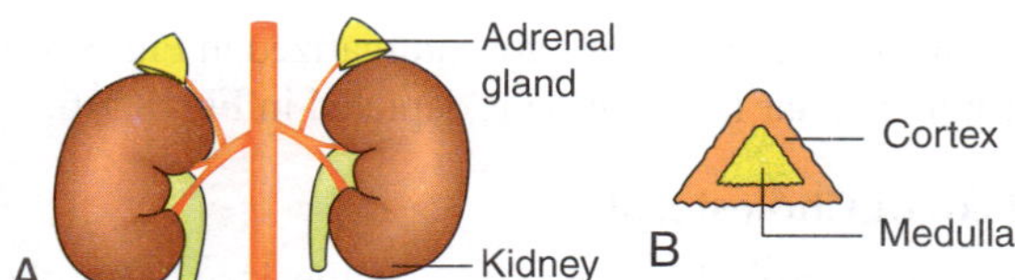

FIGURE 8.5-1 Location (A) and divisions (B) of adrenal glands.

substance. The mature human adrenal cortex consists of three distinct layers or zones of cells (Fig. 8.5-2).

1. ***Zona glomerulosa,*** constituting outer one-fifth of the cortex, is a small zone present under the capsule. It consists of cells that are arranged as inverted U-shaped formations, or acinus-like groups. It is the site of *aldosterone* and *corticosterone* synthesis. Aldosterone is the principal mineral corticoid of the human adrenal cortex.
2. ***Zona fasciculata*** is the widest zone forming middle three-fifths of the cortex. It is made up of cells that are arranged in two cells thick straight columns. Sinusoids intervene between the columns and cells appear clear or vacuolated in stained sections because of high lipid (cholesterol) content.
3. ***Zona reticularis*** forms the inner one-fifth of the cortex. It is made up of a network of compactly arranged cords of cells that branch and anastomose with each other to form a kind of network (hence the name zona reticularis). These cells contain fewer lipids.

Zona fasciculata and zona reticularis constitute a single functional unit where mainly cortisol (and some corticosterone) and androgen (dehydroepiandrosterone, i.e. DHEA) are synthesized.

Adrenal Medulla The adrenal medulla essentially represents an enlarged and specialized sympathetic ganglion. Histologically, it is made up of chromaffin cells, innervated by preganglionic sympathetic neurons.

Chromaffin Cells. The cells forming adrenal medulla show yellow granules in their cytoplasm (i.e. *chromaffin reaction*) and hence called chromaffin cells.

- These cells are columnar or polyhedral and are arranged in all groups or columns that are separated by wide *sinusoids*.
- Functionally, these cells are considered to be modified postganglionic neurons, which do not have axons.
- There are two types of adrenomedullary chromaffin cells, one type of cells constitute 80% of the total cells and synthesize epinephrine (adrenaline), and the second type (remaining 20%) cells synthesize norepinephrine (noradrenaline).
- The epinephrine and norepinephrine is largely stored in the subcellular particles called *chromaffin granules*. These granules are osmophilic, electron dense, membrane-bound vesicles. In addition to the catecholamines, the chromaffin granules also contain proteins, lipids and adenine nucleotides (mainly ATP). One of the proteins localized in the particulate fraction is the enzyme, *dopamine* β-hydroxylase. Soluble acidic proteins found in the granules are called chromogranins.
- The adrenal medulla is now included in the APUD (amine precursor uptake and decarboxylation) cell system or the so-called *diffuse neuroendocrine system*.

Nerve Endings, present in the adrenal medulla, are the *cholinergic preganglionic* sympathetic fibres that synapse directly on chromaffin cells. These fibres traverse the splanchnic nerve and are myelinated (type B) secretomotor fibres emanating mainly from the lower thoracic segments (T_5 and T_9) of the ipsilateral intermediolateral grey column of the spinal cord (Fig. 8.5-3).

Blood Supply (Fig. 8.5-4)

Arterial Blood Supply. The adrenal glands have one of the body's highest rates of blood flow per gram of tissue. The arterial blood to the gland reaches the outer capsule from the superior suprarenal artery (a branch of the inferior phrenic artery), middle suprarenal artery (a branch of the abdominal aorta) and the inferior suprarenal artery (a branch of the renal artery). The arterial blood enters sinusoidal capillaries in the cortex and then drains into medullary veins, which supply blood to the medulla and thus form a *portal system*. This arrangement of portal circulation exposes the medulla to relatively high concentrations of corticosteroids from

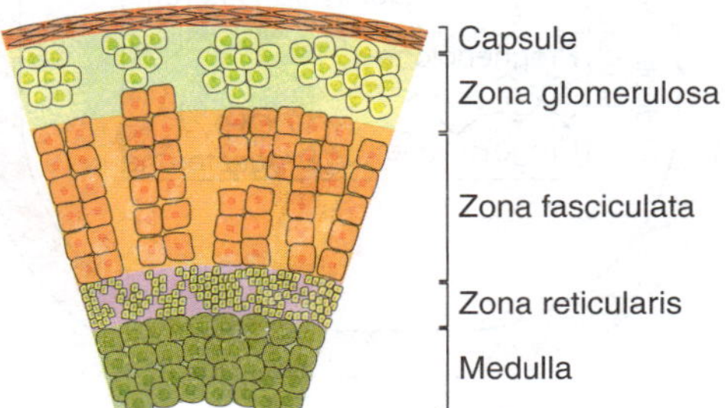

FIGURE 8.5-2 Histological structure of adrenal gland.

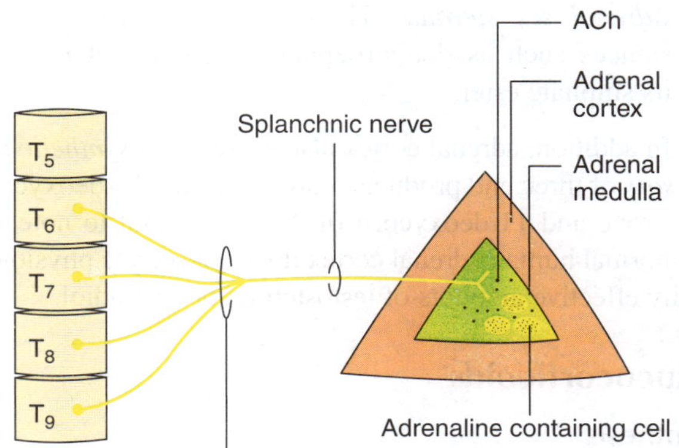

FIGURE 8.5-3 Preganglionic sympathetic fibres synapsing directly on chromaffin cells in the adrenal medulla.

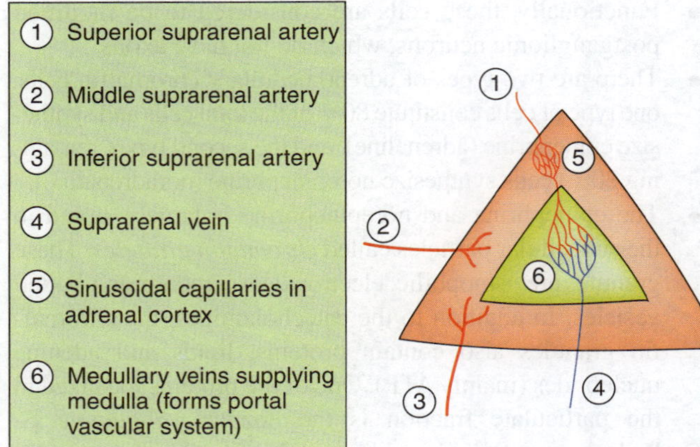

FIGURE 8.5-4 Schematic diagram showing arterial blood supply and venous drainage of adrenal gland. The portal vascular system which exposes the medulla to high concentration constitutes a functional connection between the cortex and medulla.

the cortex. As most of the blood perfusing the medulla is derived from the portal system it is, therefore, partly deoxygenated. There also exists a direct arterial blood supply to the medulla via the *medullary arteries,* which traverse the cortex.

Venous Drainage. The venous blood drains via single central vein, which passes along the longitudinal axis of the gland. The right suprarenal vein drains into the inferior vena cava and left suprarenal vein into the left renal vein.

HORMONES OF ADRENAL CORTEX

Hormones secreted by adrenal cortex, called *corticosteroids*, can be grouped as:

- *Glucocorticoids*, which include *cortisol* and *corticosterone,* which have a widespread effect on glucose and protein metabolism.
- *Mineral corticoids*. Aldosterone is the chief mineralocorticoid. It regulates the sodium balance and ECF volume in the body.
- *Adrenal sex steroids*. These include androgenic substances such as dehydroepiandrosterone (DHEA) and its sulphate ester.

In addition, adrenal cortex also secretes *biosynthetic precursors* of three end products—progesterone, 11-deoxycorticosterone and 11-deoxycortisol. It is important to note that the normal human adrenal cortex does not secrete physiologically effective amounts of testosterone or oestradiol.

Glucocorticoids

Synthesis

The glucocorticoids are synthesized largely by the cells forming zona fasciculata with a small contribution by the cells of zona reticularis of adrenal cortex. The steps involved in the synthesis of glucocorticoids are summarized in Fig. 8.5-5 and their intracellular localization is depicted in Fig. 8.5-6.

Uptake of Cholesterol

The corticosteroid hormones are synthesized from cholesterol, which is actively taken up by the adrenal cells from

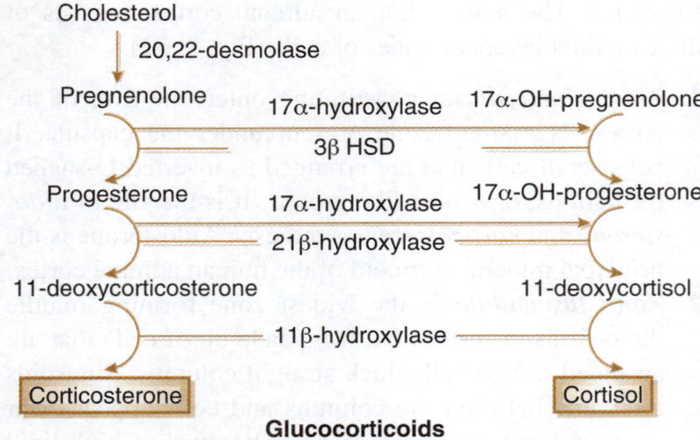

FIGURE 8.5-5 Steps involved in the synthesis of glucocorticoids in the zona fasciculata and zona reticularis.

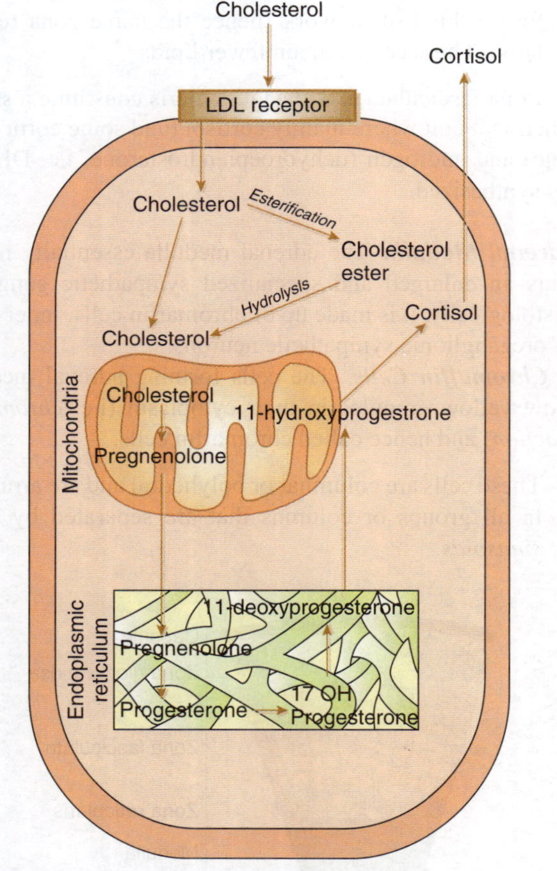

FIGURE 8.5-6 Intracellular localization of steps involved in the synthesis of cortisol.

low-density lipoprotein (LDL) of the blood. Cells of the adrenal cortex are rich in LDL receptors. After entry into the cell by endocytosis, microtubules move the cholesterol to cytoplasmic vacuoles, within which most of the cholesterol is stored as cholesterol ester. A small amount of cholesterol is also synthesized in the adrenal cells from acetyl-coenzyme A (acetyl-CoA). Under basal conditions, corticosteroids are synthesized from free plasma cholesterol but when the production is stimulated by ACTH, the stored esterified cholesterol becomes the most important precursor which is hydrolysed by cholesterol esterase. The free cholesterol enters the mitochondria.

Five oxidative CYP (formerly P450) enzymes (Table 8.5-1) act on various ring carbons of cholesterol to form corticosteroid hormones. As shown in Fig. 8.5-7, the basic steroid structure ring consists of four rings designated as A, B, C and D. The individual carbon atoms comprising the steroid ring are numbered 1–21 (Fig. 8.5-7). Substituent groups in derivative steroid molecules are designated by the number of carbon ring atoms to which they are attached.

Side-chain Cleavage of Cholesterol. This is caused by the mitochondrial enzyme 20,22-desmolase (also known as side-chain cleavage enzyme P450scc). As a result, the cholesterol is converted to pregnenolone, which is a common precursor of all steroid hormones. This is the *rate-limiting step* in the synthesis of corticosteroids.

Conversion of Pregnenolone to 11-deoxycortisol and 11-deoxycorticosterone. This occurs by hydroxylation reactions. These reactions subsequently follow after the formation of pregnenolone and progesterone and occur within the *endoplasmic reticulum* (Fig. 8.5-6). These reactions are catalysed by 17α-hydroxylase, 3 β-01-dehydrogenase and 21-hydroxylase, and convert pregnenolone into 11-deoxycortisol and 11-deoxycorticosterone (Fig. 8.5-5).

Conversion of 11-deoxycortisol to Cortisol. The 11-deoxycortisol is transferred back into the mitochondria (Fig. 8.5-5). This step is very efficient in humans, 95% of the11-deoxycortisol formed is converted into cortisol. The cortisol so-formed rapidly diffuses out of the cell and is not

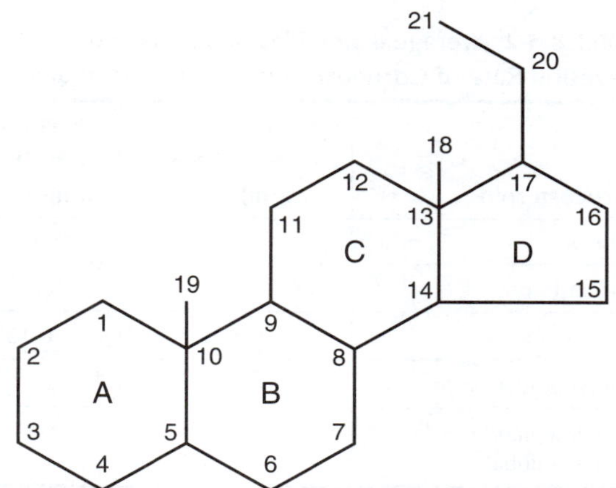

FIGURE 8.5-7 Basic structure of steroid ring. Note, the four rings are designated **A, B, C** and **D**.

stored appreciably in the adrenocortical cell. Hence, during acute need for increased amounts of circulating cortisol, the rapid activation of the entire synthetic sequence from cholesterol is activated by ACTH.

Conversion of 11-deoxycorticosterone to Corticosterone. Under normal circumstances, little corticosterone is formed and cortisol is the dominant glucocorticoid in humans. However, when cortisol synthesis is blocked, the pathway to corticosterone is opened and increased synthesis of corticosterone can provide the glucocorticoid activity necessary for maintaining health. The 11-deoxycorticosterone is converted to corticosterone by the enzyme 11β-hydroxylase.

Plasma Levels, Transport, Metabolism and Excretion of Glucocorticoids

Plasma Levels Plasma levels of glucocorticoids and other corticosteroids are shown in Table 8.5-2. The plasma levels of total cortisol show diurnal fluctuation and range from 10 to 25 μg% with an average of 14 μg%. The rate of secretion of cortisol, which is about 15 mg/day under normal conditions, may increase to 300–400 mg/day under conditions of severe stress.

TABLE 8.5-1 Nomenclature and Location of Enzymes Involved in Synthesis of Glucocorticoids

Trivial name	Code		Location	Action
	Past	*Current*		
20,22-Desmolase	$P450_{SCC}$	CYP-11-A1	Mitochondria	Cleaves the side chain between carbons 20 and 22 of cholesterol
3β-OH-Dehydrogenase	3β-HSD	3β HSD	Endoplasmic reticulum microsome	Catalyses conversion of pregnenolone to progesterone
17α-Hydroxylase	$P450_{C17}$	CYP-17	"	Catalyses the hydroxylation of C-17
21-Hydroxylase	$P450_{C21}$	CYP-21-A2	"	Catalyses the hydroxylation of C-21
11β-Hydroxylase	$P450_{C11}$	CYP-11-B1	Mitochondria	Catalyses the hydroxylation at C-11

TABLE 8.5-2 Average 8 a.m. Plasma Levels and Secretion Rate of Corticosteroids in Adult Humans

Corticosteroid	Plasma concentration (μg/dl)	Secretion rate ↑ (mg/day)
Cortisol	14.0	15
Corticosterone	1.0	03
Aldosterone	0.0006	0.15
Deoxycorticosterone	0.0006	0.20
Dehydroepiandrosterone (DHEA) sulphate	175	20

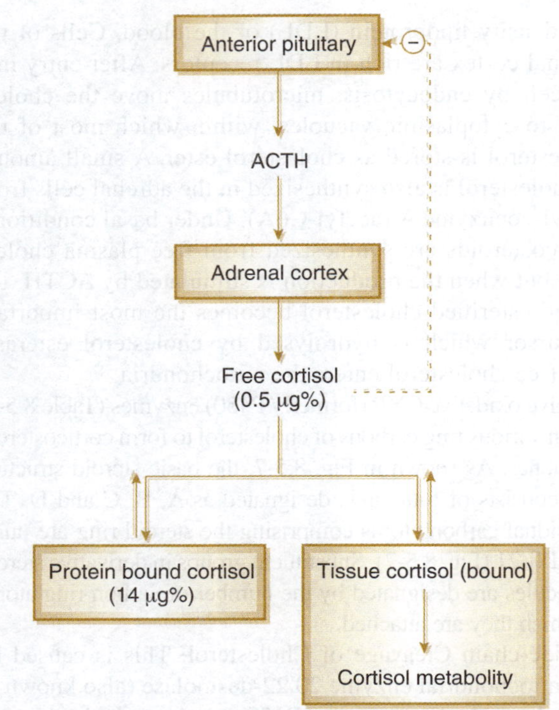

FIGURE 8.5-8 Maintenance of interrelationship between free and bound plasma cortisol.

Transport

Cortisol. In the plasma, cortisol circulates in two forms: bound (90%) and free (10%).

Bound form. Most of the plasma cortisol is bound to specific corticosteroid-binding α_2-globulin (CBG), which is a glycoprotein and is also called transcortin. A small amount (15%) is bound to albumin. The protein binding of the cortisol not only protects it from urinary excretion and degradation, but also serves as a circulatory reserve of the hormone.

Free form of cortisol constitutes only 5–10% of the total plasma cortisol. However, it is the free form which is responsible for the physiological actions of the hormone including the feedback regulation of ACTH.

Interrelationship of Free and Bound Form (Fig. 8.5-8). At the normal levels (average 14 μg/dL), the free form is less than 10% of total plasma cortisol. When the total plasma cortisol increases beyond 20 μg%, the binding sites on transcortin are saturated and there occurs some increase in albumin binding, but the main increase is in the free form.

Transcortin. The normal plasma concentration of transcortin is 3 mg%, and its binding capacity is 20 μg cortisol/dL. It is synthesized in the liver, where its rate of production is increased by the oestrogen. The concentration of transcortin, and therefore of total cortisol, is increased during pregnancy and by oestrogen administration. In the third trimester of pregnancy, transcortin levels are twice that in nonpregnant state. The increased total cortisol is, however, not associated with symptoms of excess cortisol as the levels of (physiologically active) free form of cortisol are normal.

Transcortin levels in plasma are decreased in cirrhosis liver (decreased synthesis), nephrosis (more loss in urine) and in multiple myeloma. Decreased levels of plasma transcortin are associated with decreased total plasma cortisol levels but with no symptoms of cortisol insufficiency, as the levels of free form are normal.

Corticosterone. Like cortisol, it also exists mainly in bound form, but to a lesser degree. That is why its half-life is slightly shorter than cortisol.

Interrelationship between Cortisol and Cortisone. The cortisol is in equilibrium with cortisone via the enzyme 11 β-hydroxysteroid dehydrogenase (HSD). Cortisol is converted to cortisone in the kidney by type 2,11-hydroxysteroid dehydrogenase (type 2,11-HSD) and the cortisone is returned to the plasma, from which it enters cortisol target cells. There cortisone is reconverted to cortisol by type 1,11-HSD (Fig. 8.5-9). The plasma ratio of total cortisone to total cortisol is 0.1:0.2, but because cortisone binds only weakly to transcortin, the plasma ratio of free cortisone to free cortisol is close to 1.0. Further, there is little diurnal variation in plasma cortisone levels. Therefore, in effect, circulating cortisone is something of a prohormone for cortisol, and exogenous cortisone is an effective, though not ideal, replacement in cortisol-deficient individuals.

Metabolism and Excretion Corticosteroids are degraded in the liver and conjugated with glucuronic acid.

Major pathway of cortisol and cortisone metabolism is shown in Fig. 8.5-9. The reduced metabolites of cortisol and cortisone (the cortol and cortolone) are conjugated and excreted in the urine as cortol glucuronide and cortolone glucuronide, respectively.

Minor pathway of cortisol metabolism includes its conversion to 17-ketosteroid derivatives, which are conjugated to sulphates and are rapidly excreted in urine. Approximately 10% of the secreted cortisol is metabolized by this pathway (Fig. 8.5-9).

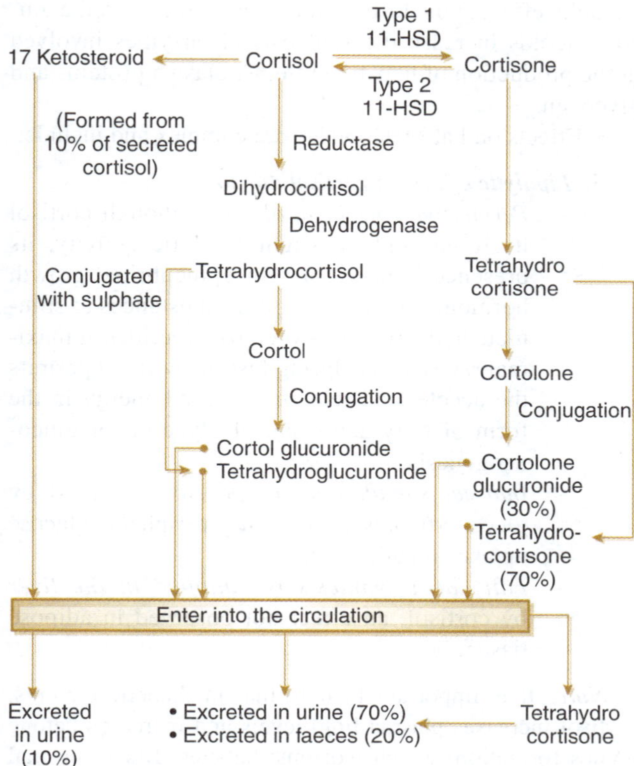

FIGURE 8.5-9 Pathways of metabolism and excretion of glucocorticoids.

***Excretion*.** There is enterohepatic circulation of glucocorticoids. About 70% of the conjugated steroids are excreted in the urine and about 20% in the faeces.

A total of about 22 mg of glucocorticoid derivatives are excreted in urine per day. The average amount of different derivatives excreted in the urine in 24 h is:

- 0.03 mg only as free cortisol (because of protein binding),
- 5 mg as tetrahydrocortisol glucuronide and cortol glucuronide,
- 3 mg as tetrahydrocortisone glucuronide and cortolone glucuronide,
- 6.0 mg as 17-ketosteroids derived from cortisol and cortisone (mostly sulphate conjugate) and
- 7.0 mg as unidentified metabolites.

Important Note

The rate of inactivation and conjugation of glucocorticoids is decreased in liver diseases and during surgery or other stresses. Therefore, in such conditions, the plasma free cortisol level rises higher than it does with maximum ACTH stimulation in the absence of stress.

Mechanism of Action of Glucocorticoids

Like other steroid hormones, the glucocorticoids act through effect on gene expression by binding with specific intracellular receptors called glucocorticoid receptors (GR). For details of mechanism of action see page 684 and Fig. 8.1.8. Glucocorticoid receptors (GR) are of two types: GR-1 and GR-II and are found in many tissues. Most cortisol effects in peripheral tissues are exerted through type II GR, while in the brain the effects are exerted mainly through type I GR. Glucocorticoids, after combining with the GR, alter the protein-synthesizing machinery of the target cells through transcription and translation effect. Altered synthesis of different enzymes in different tissues produces the multiple effects. In addition, glucocorticoids also have nongenomic actions.

Actions of Glucocorticoids

Glucocorticoids are essential for survival.

I. Metabolic Effects of Glucocorticoids Cortisol has major effects on protein, glucose and fat metabolism. By their metabolic effects, the glucocorticoids help to provide fuel molecules in circulation (Fig. 8.5-10). This effect is particularly useful during fasting, exercise and many other stresses. The nocturnal increase in plasma cortisol levels supports the enhancement of gluconeogenesis, lipolysis and ketogenesis, which are necessary for overnight metabolic stability. The different metabolic effects of glucocorticoids are:

1. Effects on Carbohydrate Metabolism. Glucocorticoids exert an anti-insulin effect, which leads to hyperglycaemia by the following actions (Fig. 8.5-10):

i. *Increased gluconeogenesis*. Glucocorticoids increase the rate of glucose production from noncarbohydrate sources by as much as six- to tenfolds by following mechanisms:
- Accelerating the synthesis of hepatic enzymes (e.g. glucose-6-phosphatase) involved in gluconeogenesis.
- Providing more amino acids to the liver for gluconeogenesis by their catabolic effect on muscle protein and inhibitory effect on protein synthesis.
- Providing more glycerol to the liver for gluconeogenesis by increasing lipolysis.

***Note*.** It is important to note that normally increased glucose synthesis is associated with glycogen breakdown. But glucocorticoids promote gluconeogenesis, as well as the storage of carbohydrates as hepatic glycogens. Glycogen synthesis is increased by increasing glycogen synthetase.

ii. *Decreased utilization of glucose in peripheral tissues*. Glucocorticoids inhibit glucose uptake by peripheral tissues like the muscle, skin and connective tissue, lymphoid tissue, bone and adipose tissue. The heart, brain, liver and erythrocytes are spared from this action. In fact, glucose spared by the former group of tissues may be used by the latter group of tissues. This can be valuable in states of stress.

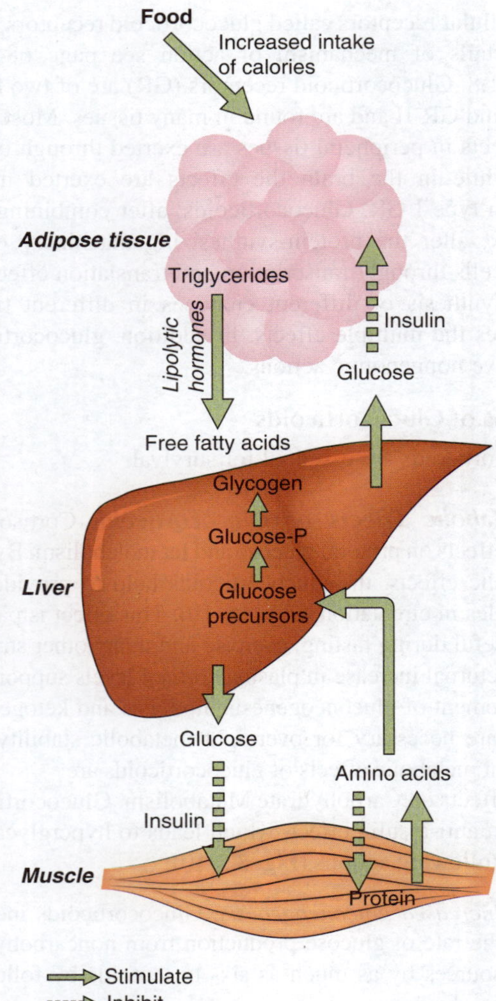

FIGURE 8.5-10 Metabolic effects of cortisol. Note: Cortisol increases intake of calories by increasing appetite; facilitates release of amino acids from the muscle and their use for gluconeogenesis in liver and storage as glycogen; inhibits peripheral utilization of glucose and synthesis of proteins from amino acids and facilitates release of free fatty acids from the adipose tissues.

2. **Effects on Protein Metabolism,** exerted by glucocorticoids are (Fig. 8.5-10):

- ***Catabolic effect.*** Cortisol enhances the release of amino acids by proteolysis in skeletal muscle and other extrahepatic tissues, including the protein matrix of bone. Amino acids so released, especially alanine, form the most important gluconeogenic substrate. The proteolysis in skeletal muscle brings about a negative nitrogen balance.
- ***Antianabolic effect.*** It is the ability of the glucocorticoids to inhibit the de novo synthesis of protein, probably at the translational level.

Note. The only exception to protein catabolic and antianabolic effects of glucocorticoids is the protein anabolic effect at the level of the liver. In the liver, the glucocorticoids increase the synthesis of enzymes involved in the production of hepatic proteins, plasma proteins and glycogen.

3. **Effects on Fat Metabolism** are complex and include:

i. ***Lipolytic effects of cortisol due to:***

- *Permissive role in lipolysis.* Although cortisol itself has only a slight lipolytic activity, its presence is necessary for epinephrine, growth hormone and other lipolytic substances to stimulate hydrolysis of stored triglycerides at maximal rates. Thus, during fasting, cortisol permits the accelerated release of stored energy in the form of fatty acids and of glycerol for gluconeogenesis.
- *Indirect stimulation of lipolysis* is caused by glucocorticoids by blocking peripheral glucose uptake and utilization.
- *Fatty acid synthesis is inhibited in the liver* by cortisol, an effect not observed in adipose tissue.

Note. It is important to note that in diabetic patients, cortisol increases plasma lipid levels and increases ketone bodies formation, which worsens diabetes. But in normal subjects, insulin secretion is increased by raised blood glucose levels and the insulin decreases lipase activity and counterbalances hyperglycaemia.

ii. ***Lipogenic role.*** Glucocorticoids increase differentiation of adipose tissue cells from preadipocytes to adipocytes and stimulate lipogenesis by increasing adipocyte lipoprotein lipase and glucose-6-phosphate dehydrogenase activity. The lipogenic effect varies in different regions of the body. Therefore, in cortisol excess there occurs a selective accumulation of fat in the abdomen, trunk and above (trunked obesity), sparing the extremities which become thin due to loss of muscle mass. The deposition of fat in the face is called 'moonface' and in the suprascapular region it is referred to as *'buffalo hump'* or 'dowager's hump' (features Cushing's syndrome).

Important Note

It is important to note that the fat deposition observed in hypercortisolism reflects increased food intake rather than a change in the rate of lipid metabolism.

- Glucocorticoids increase appetite and food intake by inducing neuropeptide Y (NPY) synthesis and NPY receptors in the hypothalamus and by
- Suppressing CRH release.
- Since cortisol also induces leptin synthesis in adipocytes, the gain in fat mass is eventually limited by the negative feedback of action of leptin on the appetite centre in the hypothalamus.

4. Effects on Electrolyte and Water Metabolism. Glucocorticoids control distribution of body water and electrolytes by their opposing actions:

i. ***Retention of sodium and water*** by following actions:
- *Mineralocorticoid activity* of glucocorticoids is mild but becomes of physiological importance because of the large quantity of cortisol secreted every day. By aldosterone-like activity, the glucocorticoids increase sodium and chloride retention and potassium excretion by the kidney.
- *Aldosterone secretion* is increased by glucocorticoids by increasing the synthesis of angiotensinogens from the liver. The increased aldosterone secretion, in turn, causes excessive retention of sodium and water.

ii. ***Promotion of diuresis***. Glucocorticoids promote diuresis by increasing the inactivation of ADH by liver and by antagonizing the action of ADH at the level of distal convoluted tubules of the kidney.

II. Physiological Actions on Various Organs and Systems

In addition to the metabolic effects noted above, the glucocorticoids affect various organs and systems throughout the body (Fig. 8.5-11):

1. Effects on Muscle

i. ***Contractility and work performance*** of skeletal and cardiac muscle is maintained by the cortisol. The effect on skeletal muscle is exerted at the myoneural junction, by an increase in acetylcholine synthesis. In cardiac muscle, cortisol increases Na^+–K^+–ATPase and β-adrenergic receptors.

ii. ***Decrease in muscle mass and strength*** is caused by an excess of cortisol. This occurs due to decrease in muscle protein synthesis and increase in muscle catabolism.

2. Effects on Bone

i. ***Increased bone resorption.*** Glucocorticoids increase bone resorption transiently by increasing:
- Osteoclastic activity and
- Activity of enzyme collagenase, which is essential for destroying the organic matrix of bone.

ii. ***Inhibition of bone formation*** is the most profound effect of glucocorticoids caused by:
- Decreasing collagen synthesis,
- Inhibiting formation of mature osteoblasts from the undifferentiated cells,
- Increasing rate of apoptosis of osteoblasts and osteocytes,
- Impeding calcium absorption from the intestinal tract by antagonizing the action of 1,25-$(OH)_2$-vitamin D and inhibiting its synthesis and
- Increasing calcium excretion in urine, as GFR increases.

Note. Because of the above effects on bone, *osteoporosis* (which results in skeletal deformity) is a feared and sometimes devastating complication of glucocorticoid therapy that lasts more than a few weeks.

3. Effects on Connective Tissue. Cortisol decreases collagen synthesis, producing thereby:

- Thinning of the skin and
- Thinning of walls of capillaries, which leads to their easy rupture and to intracutaneous haemorrhage.

4. Effects on Vascular System. Cortisol is essential for maintaining normal blood pressure by:

- Sustaining myocardial performance,
- Enhancing the vasopressure effect (responsiveness of arterioles to constrictive effect) of catecholamines (especially norepinephrine) and angiotensin II,
- Decreasing production of vasodilator prostaglandins and
- Maintaining normal blood volume by decreasing the permeability of the vascular endothelium.

Therefore, in the absence of cortisol, the vasopressor action of catecholamines is diminished and hypotension ensues.

5. Effects on Kidney are:
- Increase in glomerular filtration rate (GFR) by increasing glomerular plasma flow,
- Rapid excretion of water load and
- Increase in calcium and phosphate excretion by decreasing their reabsorption in the proximal tubules.

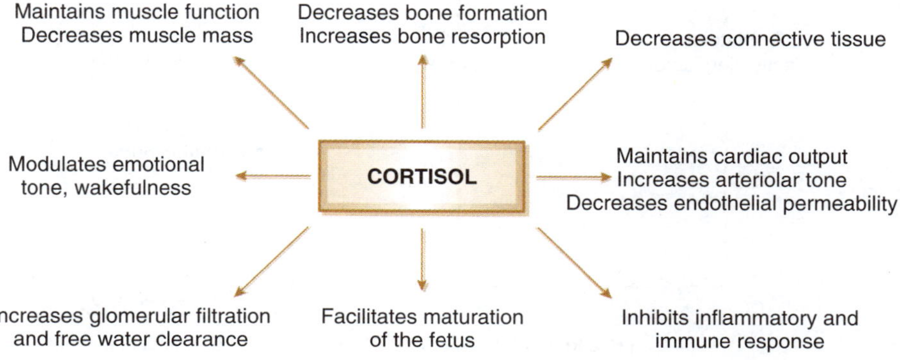

FIGURE 8.5-11 Effects of glucocorticoids on various tissues and organs and systems of the body.

In the absence of cortisol, free water clearance is diminished, because the activity of ADH is not antagonized (also see effect on water and electrolyte metabolism).

6. Effects on Central Nervous System. Glucocorticoid receptors (GR) are present in various parts of the brain, especially in the limbic system. Through these receptors, the glucocorticoids modulate excitability behaviour and mood. Therefore, in the *absence of cortisol (Addison's disease),* there occurs:

- Mood changes in the form of irritability, apprehension and inability to concentrate,
- Increased sensitivity to olfactory and gustatory stimuli (especially salty taste) and
- EEG waves slower than normal rhythm.

Excess of cortisol is associated with:

- Increased brain excitability and insomnia,
- Decreased memory function and
- Decreased threshold for convulsive activity. Because of this reason, glucocorticoids are contraindicated in epilepsy.

7. Effects on Gastrointestinal Tract. The glucocorticoids increase gastric acid secretion and decrease proliferation of gastric mucosal cells. These effects can lead to peptic ulceration following long-term use of cortisol.

8. Effects on Blood Cells and Lymphatic Organs. The excess of glucocorticoids leads to:

- ***Eosinopenia and basopenia,*** due to their increased destruction and increased sequestration in lungs and spleen. The changes in eosinophilic count have been used as an index of change in ACTH secretion.
- ***Lymphopenia,*** i.e. decrease in the number of lymphocytes is caused by inhibiting their proliferation and increasing their destruction in the circulation. This leads to decreased size of lymph nodes, thymus, spleen and other lymphoid tissues.
- ***Neutrophilia,*** i.e. increase in neutrophil count occurs due to their increased release from bone marrow and decreased migration into tissues from the vascular spaces.
- ***Polycythaemia,*** i.e. increased red blood cell (RBC) count occurs due to stimulation of erythropoiesis.
- ***Thrombocytosis,*** i.e. increased platelet count.

III. Anti-Inflammatory and Antiallergic Effects These effects are not produced by the glucocorticoids, which are normally secreted physiologically, but are produced in large doses when administered therapeutically and are thus called the pharmacological actions of glucocorticoids.

1. Anti-inflammatory Effects of glucocorticoids are produced by the following actions (Fig. 8.5-12).

i. ***Glucocorticoids inhibit activation of nuclear factor-kB (a transcription factor)*** by increasing production of IkBa. NF-kB normally exists in the cytosol in bound form with IkBa, which makes it inactive. Inflammation stimuli such as virus, bacteria, cytokines and oxidants-induced signals dissociate NF-kB from IkBa. NF-kB then moves into the nucleus and binds to DNA of the genes to transcript numerous inflammatory mediators resulting in their increased production.

ii. ***Cortisol inhibits the activity of phospholipase A_2,*** which is responsible for arachidonic acid products (such as prostacyclins, prostaglandins and thromboxanes) that may be involved in mediating vascular components of the inflammation, and thus reduce the severity of inflammation by decreasing hyperaemia and capillary

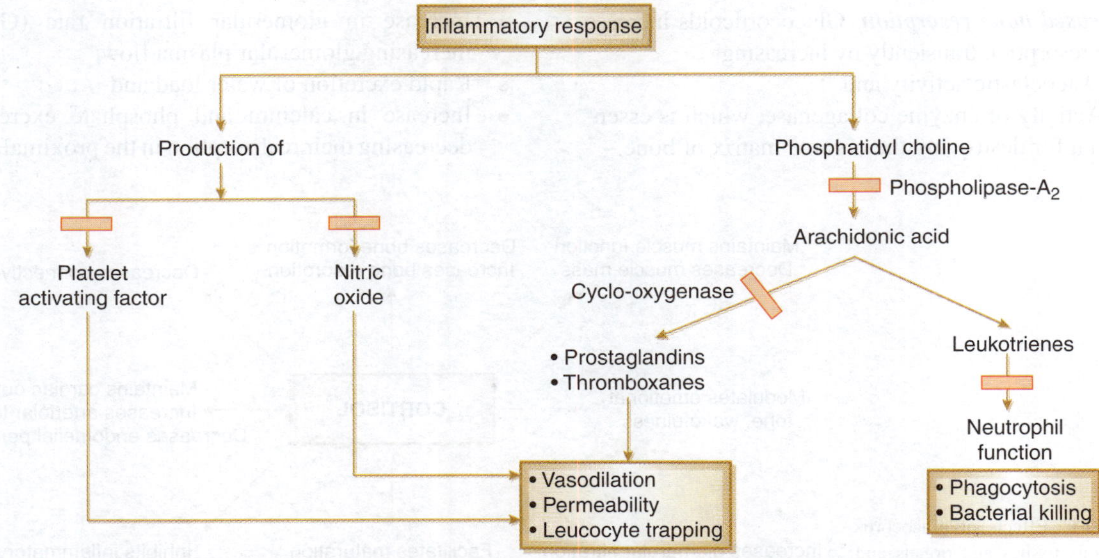

FIGURE 8.5-12 Sites ( ) of action of cortisol in inhibiting inflammatory response.

permeability and thereby preventing exudation, migration and infiltration of leucocytes at the site of injury.

iii. ***Cortisol stabilizes the lysosomal membrane,*** probably by inhibiting the phospholipase A_2, thereby preventing the release of proteolytic enzymes and hyaluronidase, which contribute to tissue damage and swelling.

iv. ***Cortisol inhibits migration of circulating*** leucocytes to the site of inflammation by blocking the leucocyte receptors for chemotactic agents.

v. ***Cortisol inhibits leukotriene*** and thus impairs neutrophil phagocytosis and bactericidal abilities.

vi. ***Cortisol decreases collagen formation*** and the proliferation of fibroblasts and thus impedes the chronic inflammatory responses.

2. Anti-immunity Effect. Cortisol inhibits both cellular and humoral immunity by decreasing the proliferation of T cells (involved in cellular immunity) and B cells (involved in humoral immunity) by producing antibodies. The sites of actions of cortisol in inhibiting immune response are shown in Fig. 8.5-13.

3. Antiallergic Effect. Cortisol reduces the number of circulating basophils and protects against the release of secretory products of granulocytes, mast cells and macrophages, which have vesicles containing serotonin, histamine and hydrolases. This accounts for the fall in blood levels of histamine and histamine-like substances and thereby reducing the histamine-induced features of allergy or hypersensitivity in response to antigen-antibody reaction. It is important to note that cortisol does not affect the combination of antigen with antibodies and has no influence on the effect of histamine once it is released, though it inhibits the intracellular synthesis of histamine.

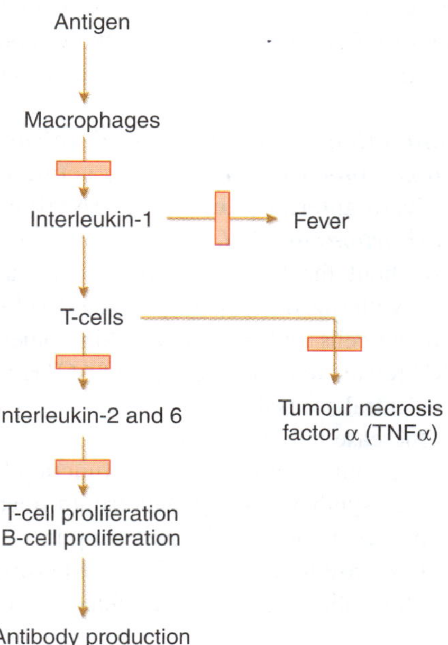

FIGURE 8.5-13 Sites ( ) of action of cortisol inhibiting immune response.

IV. Role of Glucocorticoids in Fetal Life

- ***Maturation of CNS, retina and skin*** is facilitated by the cortisol in utero.
- ***Maturation of lungs.*** During fetal life, oxygen is transferred from the maternal blood through the placenta. In the last weeks of gestation, preparation of the fetal lungs to permit satisfactory breathing immediately after birth is facilitated by cortisol by increasing the activity of key enzymes, such as phosphatidyl acid phosphatase and choline phosphotransferase, which are involved in the biosynthesis of pulmonary surfactants. The pulmonary surfactant lowers the surface tension in pulmonary alveoli and thus permits proper inflation of lungs immediately after birth.
- ***Maturation of gastrointestinal tract.*** In fetal life, maternal glucose is transferred to the fetus through the placenta. The digestive enzyme capacity of the intestinal mucosa changes from a fetal pattern to a mature adult pattern under the influence of cortisol. This maturation process allows the newborn to digest disaccharides present in the milk.

V. Role of Glucocorticoids in Stress Various stresses, e.g. trauma, cold, illness and starvation, are associated with activation of the hypothalamic–hypophyseal–adrenal axis. Increased secretion of glucocorticoids is one of the various mechanisms involved in adaptation to various stresses (see page 766). A variety of stimuli, during stress, act on the hypothalamus and cause release of ACTH from the anterior pituitary via release of CRH, which in turn increases glucocorticoid secretion to as much as 20-fold depending upon the type of stress.

It is important to note that resistance to stress is not increased by the administration of glucocorticoids. How cortisol helps against the stressful conditions is not exactly clear.

Regulation of Glucocorticoid Secretion

The glucocorticoid secretion is regulated by hypothalamic–anterior pituitary–adrenal cortex axis, which exerts its effect through (Fig. 8.5-14):

- Corticotropin-releasing hormone (CRH),
- Adrenocorticotropic hormone (ACTH) and
- Glucocorticoids negative feedback effect.

Note. Since CRH and ACTH are related to regulation of glucocorticoid release, they are described in detail here, rather than along with other hormones of the hypothalamus and anterior pituitary, respectively.

1. Role of Corticotropin-releasing Hormone Corticotropin-releasing hormone (CRH) is secreted by the small cells of the paraventricular nucleus of hypothalamus (the cells which also secrete ADH). It is the important and final mediator of the regulatory inputs of glucocorticoids. CRH is a polypeptide with 41 amino acids.

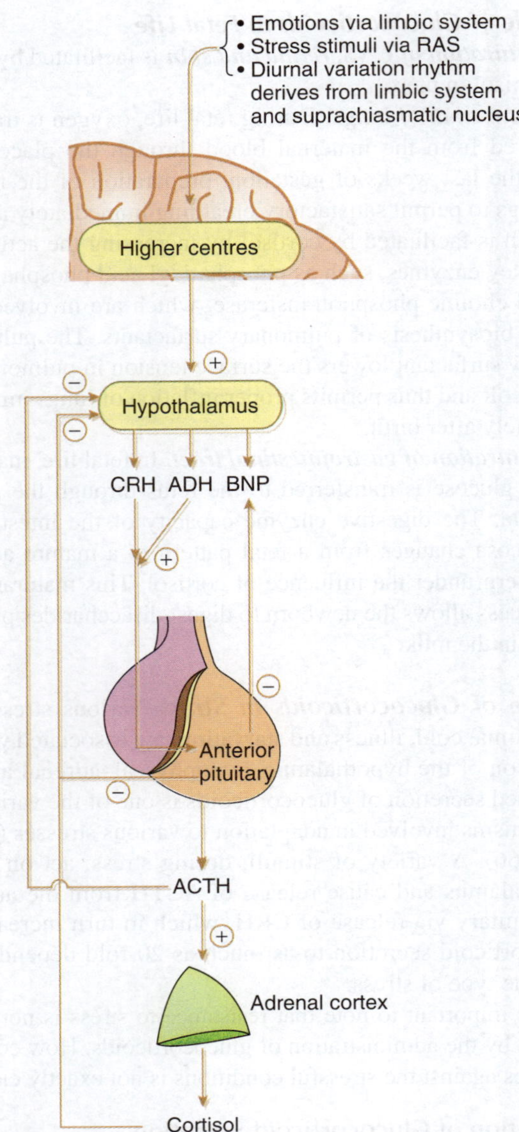

FIGURE 8.5-14 Hypothalamic–anterior pituitary–adrenal cortex axis and negative feedback mechanism controlling glucocorticoid secretion.

Control of CRH Secretion

i. ***Stressful stimuli*** (e.g. pain, anaesthesia, surgery and haemorrhage, etc.), which ultimately increase cortisol secretion within minutes to as much as 20-fold, primarily act on the hypothalamus to increase the secretion of CRH via the reticular activating system (RAS). The tracts from RAS are *cholinergic* and those from the raphe nuclei and the locus coeruleus are catecholaminergic and serotonergic.

ii. ***Circadian rhythm.*** The CRH secretion and thus, ACTH and cortisol secretions, show circadian rhythm (Fig. 8.5-15). If the serotonergic and cholinergic connections between the limbic system and hypothalamus are cut, the circadian rhythm is abolished but the responses to stress are still retained.

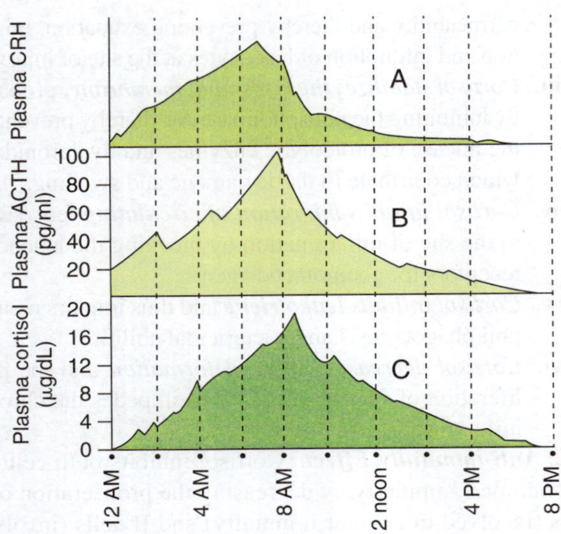

FIGURE 8.5-15 Diurnal variations and pulsatility in secretion of CRH (A), ACTH (B), and cortisol (C). Note, the ACTH peak follows CRH peak and cortisol peak follows ACTH peak by 10 min.

iii. ***ACTH*** acts on the hypothalamus to reduce the secretion of ACTH by short-loop negative feedback mechanism.

iv. ***Glucocorticoids*** exert a long-loop negative feedback effect on CRH secretion (Fig. 8.5-14).

Mechanism of Action of CRH. The CRH reaches the anterior pituitary through the hypothalamic–hypophyseal portal system and acts by cAMP mechanism through the CRH receptors.

Actions of CRH include:

i. ***Stimulation of synthesis and release of ACTH,*** by acting on the *corticotrophs* is the *main function*. A lack of CRH (as in a CRH knockout model) greatly impairs the ACTH diurnal rhythm and its response to stress.

ii. ***Stimulation of synthesis and release of pro-opiomelanocortin products*** by acting on corticotrophs of anterior pituitary via cAMP mechanism.

iii. ***Other actions of CRH.*** CRH receptors are also found throughout the brain and spinal cord and CRH is also synthesized in many peripheral cells including immune cells and cells in the skin. Other actions of CRH related to or independent of ACTH include:

- Central arousal,
- Increase in blood pressure,
- Diminution of reproductive function by decreasing synthesis of gonadotropin-releasing hormones (GnRH) and gonadotropins.
- Decrease in feeding activity and growth and
- Stimulation of release of cytokines in immune cells.

2. *Role of Adrenocorticotropic Hormone* Adrenocorticotropic hormone (ACTH) is secreted by *corticotrophs* which form 20% of the anterior pituitary cells. In the human fetus, ACTH synthesis and secretion begin at 10–12 weeks of gestation, just before the adrenal cortex develops.

Chemistry. ACTH is a straight chain peptide containing 39 amino acids with a molecular weight of 4500.

The 1–24 amino acids in ACTH constitute the active portion of the hormone, which contain full biological activity and the remaining 15 amino acids constitute the tail, which serves the function of stabilization.

Synthesis. ACTH, along with other peptides co-secreted in plasma, are derived from the single precursor pro-opiomelanocortin (POMC) consisting of 241 amino acids. The hormone of this group thus includes (see Fig. 8.2-6):

- ACTH,
- Melanocyte—stimulating hormone (MSH). The alpha- and beta-MSH are produced in the intermediary lobe (which is rudimentary in humans),
- Beta-lipotropin and
- Beta-endorphin.

Mechanism of Action. ACTH acts by combining with the ACTH receptors present on the surface of adrenal cortical tissue cells. The receptor-hormone complex in the presence of calcium activates the cAMP, which is the principal second messenger. The cAMP leads to phosphorylation of key enzymes and histones which result in its biological action.

Actions of ACTH

i. ***Actions on adrenal cortex.*** ACTH is primarily concerned with the growth and functions of the adrenal cortex:
   - It promotes conversion of cholesterol to pregnenolone, which is the precursor of synthesis of all the hormones of the adrenal cortex.
   - It stimulates the secretion of glucocorticoids and the adrenal androgens. But it does not exert direct control on the secretion of mineralocorticoids (aldosterone) from the adrenal cortex.
   - It enhances RNA and protein synthesis in the adrenal glands and thus promotes adrenal cortex growth. ACTH increases the size rather than the number of adrenal cells and in the absence of ACTH, the relevant adrenal zones atrophy.

ii. ***Extra-adrenal actions*** of ACTH occur only with very high levels, which are seen in abnormal conditions. The extra adrenal actions include:
   - *Lipolysis* in the adipose tissue is promoted by ACTH by activating the enzyme lipase.
   - *Stimulation of beta cells of pancreas* to increase the release of insulin.
   - *Stimulation of growth hormone secreting* cells.
   - *MSH-like effect on the melanocytes* of skin resulting in increased pigmentation.

iii. ***Other actions of ACTH.*** ACTH synthesis and receptors for ACTH are also located in some other structures, where its possible roles are:
   - Neuromodulatory or paracrine functions in brain and gastrointestinal tract and
   - ACTH receptor and ACTH secretion occur in lymphocytes, suggesting an important relationship between ACTH and the immune system.

Regulation of ACTH Secretion

i. ***Hypothalamic control on ACTH secretion*** is mainly exerted through CRH (see above). The hypothalamic control is responsible for the following characteristics of ACTH secretion:
   - *Diurnal variation* in the levels of ACTH (and thus of cortisol) is due to variation in CRH release. As shown in Fig. 8.5-15, a large peak in the levels of ACTH and cortisol occurs in the morning (6–8 a.m.) during awakening (plasma level of ACTH range between 20 and 100 pg/ml with an average of 50 pg/ml). Thereafter, the average level decreases markedly (5 pg/ml), just before or after the subject falls asleep. In night workers the rhythm is reversed. The biological clock responsible for diurnal variation in CRH, ACTH and cortisol levels is located either in the limbic system or suprachiasmatic nucleus of the hypothalamus, destruction of any or both of them abolishes the circadian rhythm. The circadian rhythm is diminished or abolished by loss of consciousness, blindness, or constant exposure to either dark or light.
   - *Pulsatile release of ACTH* is also due to pulsatile release of CRH. Up to three pulses per hour, and each pulse lasts about 20 min. Cortisol pulses follow the ACTH pulses. Both, frequency as well as amplitude of ACTH pulses is greater in men than women. Age has little effect on secretion of ACTH.
   - *Release of ACTH in response to stress* is mediated by CRH release (see above) and ADH release. During stress, ADH significantly augments the effect of CRH. In severe stress, the stress-induced hypersecretion of ACTH completely overrides the negative feedback. This hypersecretion cannot be suppressed even if the adrenal cortex secretes cortisol at its maximum levels. Stress may even abolish the diurnal variation of ACTH levels, but pulsatility always persists.
   - *Brain natriuretic peptide (BNP)*, an analogue of the atrial natriuretic hormone (ANH) also inhibits the ACTH release and the ACTH responses to CRH stimulation in humans. BNP is synthesized in the hypothalamus and thus can be considered a corticotroph release-inhibiting hormone.

ii. ***Negative feedback inhibition of ACTH*** is caused by (Fig. 8.5-14):
   - Plasma cortisol levels (long-loop negative feedback) and
   - Plasma ACTH levels (short-loop negative feedback).

3. Negative Feedback Control of Glucocorticoid Secretion Chronically elevated plasma levels of free cortisol (and not the total cortisol, i.e. free plus bound form) exert a direct negative feedback action on its own secretion. This effect is exerted at two levels (Fig. 8.5-14):

- On hypothalamus to decrease formation of CRH and
- On anterior pituitary to decrease formation of ACTH.

Applied Aspects

Two important clinical applications of the negative feedback control of glucocorticoid secretion, which need to be considered are:

i. ***Therapeutic administration of exogenous glucocorticoids*** for a long period suppress the secretion of CRH and ACTH by negative feedback mechanism. This leads to a marked decrease or near absence of secretion of endogenous glucocorticoids from the adrenal cortex. However, the absence is not noticed because the pharmacologic doses of exogenous glucocorticoids continue to perform the physiological functions of glucocorticoids as well. But, when the exogenous glucocorticoids are stopped suddenly, the hypothalamus, pituitary and adrenal cortex cannot recover equally suddenly, leading to *acute adrenal deficiency* characterized by a sudden fall in blood pressure. The individual may even die of *adrenal crisis*. Therefore, to avoid this complication, exogenous steroids should never be stopped suddenly but their doses should be tapered off slowly over a long period.
ii. ***Dexamethasone suppression test.*** This test is based on the ability of dexamethasone (a potent synthetic glucocorticoid) to inhibit ACTH secretion. When the hypothalamic–pituitary–adrenocortical axis is normal, the administration of dexamethasone inhibits the secretion of ACTH and cortisol.

Mineralocorticoids

The mineralocorticoids include:

- Aldosterone. It is the chief mineralocorticoid,
- Deoxycorticosterone (DOC) and
- 18-Hydroxy-deoxycorticosterone (18-OH-DOC) is secreted in small amounts and has some mineralocorticoid activity.

Since aldosterone is the major mineralocorticoid, so discussion in this section is limited to it.

Synthesis

Aldosterone, the chief mineralocorticoid, is synthesized exclusively by the *zona glomerulosa cells*. The steps involved in the synthesis summarized in Fig. 8.5-16, include:

Uptake of Cholesterol for Formation of Corticosterone. This involves the same steps as in the synthesis of glucocorticoids in zona fasciculata (for details see page 740 and Fig. 8.5-5).

Formation of Aldosterone. Some of the corticosterone is hydroxylated and converted to an aldehyde by aldosterone synthase, a mitochondrial P_{450} mixed oxygenase to yield aldosterone, which is rapidly released. The 18-hydroxycorticosterone is not a direct intermediate but a by-product of this enzyme reaction (Fig. 8.5-16).

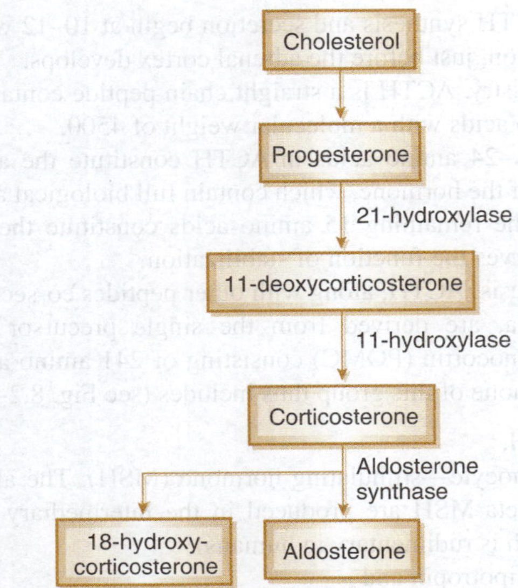

FIGURE 8.5-16 Steps involved in the synthesis of aldosterone.

Plasma Levels, Transport, Metabolism and Excretion

Plasma Levels. Depending upon the dietary intake of sodium, the aldosterone secretion ranges from 50 μg/day (with dietary sodium intake of 150 mEq) to 250 μg/day (with dietary sodium intake of 10 mEq). Plasma levels of aldosterone show diurnal variation with a highest concentration at 8 a.m. (.0006 μg/dL) and lowest at 11 p.m.

The diurnal variation in aldosterone levels is not affected by variation in sodium intake, posture, ACTH suppression by exogenous glucocorticoids, or plasma potassium levels.

Transport. In the plasma, 40% aldosterone circulates in free form and 60% in bound form. Aldosterone is weakly bound to the specific aldosterone-binding globulin, to transcortin and to albumin. Because of the weaker binding of aldosterone as compared to cortisol, its plasma half-life is only 20 min.

Metabolism and Excretion. A total of 90% of aldosterone, like the glucocorticoids, is degraded in the liver and is reduced to *tetrahydroaldosterone*, the major metabolite that is excreted in the urine as aldosterone-3-glucuronide conjugate. A smaller amount of aldosterone is conjugated in the kidney and excreted in urine as 18-glucuronide. 18-glucouronide is converted into free aldosterone by hydrolysis at pH 1.0 and is therefore, usually referred to as *'acid-labile conjugate'*. The aldosterone-18-glucuronide is most commonly measured in the urine for diagnostic purposes. Values of this metabolite in subjects with a normal sodium diet range from 5 to 20 μg/day. Around < 1% of aldosterone is excreted in urine as free form, 5% in the acid-labile conjugate form and 40% in the form of tetrahydro glucuronide.

Mechanism of Action of Aldosterone

The mechanism of action of aldosterone is similar to that of other steroid hormones. It binds to the mineralocorticoid receptor (*type I glucocorticoid receptor*) in target cells (renal tubules, sweat glands, etc.) and the hormone receptor complex migrates to the nucleus, which increases mRNA synthesis and induces or suppresses various proteins described below that mediate the hormone's effects. The aldosterone-stimulated proteins have two types of effects:

- *The rapid effect* is by increasing the activity of epithelial sodium channels (ENaCs). Aldosterone increases the insertion of ENaCs from the cytosolic pool into the cell membrane by activating the SGK gene (serum/glucuronide-regulated kinase).
- *The slower effect* is by increasing the synthesis of ENaCs. The aldosterone does not have an immediate effect. Approximately, 1–2 h is required between exposure to aldosterone and the onset of its action.

Aldosterone also increases the activity of Na^+–K^+ exchanger at cell membrane by rapid nongenomic action.

Actions of Aldosterone

A. Primary Actions of Aldosterone

1. Effects on Renal Tubules. Aldosterone acts on late distal tubules and principal cells of collecting ducts of kidney and causes the following effects (Fig. 8.5-17):

i. *Sodium reabsorption* from the tubular fluid into the renal tubular epithelial cells. The Na^+–K^+ pump operates at the basolateral border and not at the luminal border of tubular epithelial cells and transports Na^+ into blood capillaries. Thus, under the influence of aldosterone, the urinary excretion of Na^+ is decreased and the amount of Na^+ in ECF is increased.

ii. *Potassium excretion*. In the kidney, the active reabsorption of Na^+ occurs in exchange of K^+ and H^+. Thus, aldosterone not only causes reabsorption of Na^+, but excretion of K^+ as well by renal tubular epithelial cells (Fig. 8.5-17). The extent of K^+ excretion is parallel with the rate of delivery of Na^+ to the distal tubule. Thus, a high Na^+ intake will greatly exacerbate urinary K^+ losses caused by aldosterone.

iii. *H^+* excretion. In addition to excretion of K^+, aldosterone also enhances the tubular secretion of H^+ as Na^+ is reabsorbed. Therefore, in aldosterone excess, there occurs mild systemic metabolic alkalosis.

iv. *Ammonium and magnesium* excretion is also increased by aldosterone.

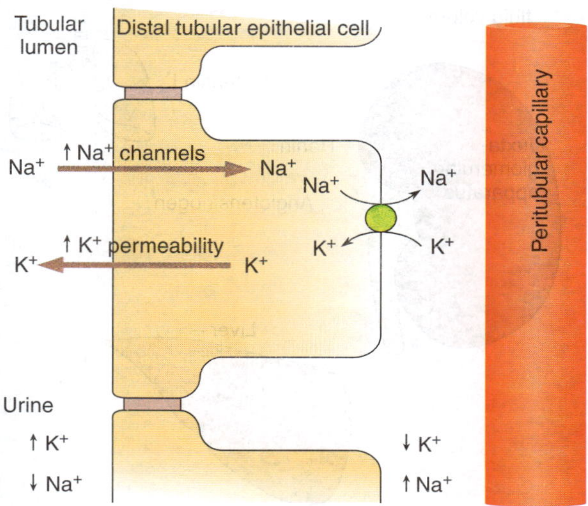

FIGURE 8.5-17 Action of aldosterone on the distal renal tubule.

Mechanism of Action. As mentioned above, aldosterone acts by promoting specific protein synthesis. The *aldosterone-induced protein (AIP) synthesis* increases Na^+ reabsorption by following effects.

- *Membrane permeability* of tubular cells is increased by AIP, increasing passive Na^+ absorption along the electrical and concentration gradients.
- *Increase in number of thiazide-sensitive NaCl cotransporter* is caused by aldosterone in the apical membrane of the distal convoluted tubular (DCT) cells. The NaCl cotransporter increases the inflow of Na^+ from the tubular urine to the renal cells.
- *Increase in the content of Na^+–K^+*–ATPase at the basal (capillary) surface of the renal tubular cells is caused by aldosterone, which pumps the sodium out and then back into the plasma.
- *Increase in the Krebs' cycle enzyme activity* in the mitochondria caused by aldosterone helps to generate energy required for extrusion of Na^+ into the interstitial fluid and capillary blood.
- *Increase in phospholipase activity* caused by aldosterone in the cytosol of cells leads to increased synthesis of fatty acids, which are used in membrane generation.

2. Effects on Sweat Glands, Salivary Glands and Colon

Sweat glands and salivary glands produce primary secretions which contain large amounts of sodium chloride. The sodium chloride is absorbed as the secretion passes through the ducts, and in turn, K^+ and HCO_3^- are excreted. Thus, aldosterone decreases the loss of Na^+ and Cl^- in sweat and salivary secretion.

Colon. The aldosterone stimulates sodium reabsorption from the colon while enhancing potassium excretion in the faeces.

Important Note

Relation of mineralocorticoid to glucocorticoid receptors: It is important to note that mineralocorticoid receptors have higher affinity to glucocorticoids than glucocorticoid receptors to glucocorticoids. Therefore it raises a question: why do glucocorticoids not produce the mineralocorticoid effect in kidney and other target tissue having mineralocorticoid receptors? Because these mineralocorticoid-sensitive tissue contain the enzyme 11β-hydroxysteroid dehydrogenase type 2 (11β-HSD type 2) that converts cortisol to cortisone and corticosterone to its 11 oxyderivatives, and these derivatives do not bind to mineralocorticoid receptors.

- Apparent mineralocorticoid excess (AME) syndrome occurs due to congenital absence or inhibition of enzyme 11b-HSD type 2. In this condition, cortisol has a marked mineralocorticoid effect resulting in a condition like hyperaldosteronism.
- Hyponatraemia, due to salt wasting and hypotension may develop.

B. Secondary Effects of Aldosterone Secondary effects are produced in aldosterone excess or deficiency as a consequence of the described primary action of aldosterone. The secondary effects include:

1. Effects on Plasma Potassium Concentration

i. *Hypokalaemia*, i.e. decrease in plasma K^+ levels may occur in aldosterone excess due to increased urinary excretion of K^+. When plasma K^+ levels fall below 2.5 mEq/L, the hypokalaemia may produce:

- *Muscular weakness* due to decreased excitability of nerves and muscles,
- *Hypokalaemic alkalosis* may occur due to associated increased HCO_3^- reabsorption. Due to metabolic alkalosis, free ionized Ca^{2+} may be decreased leading to tetany and
- *Hypokalaemic nephropathy* may occur in prolonged hyperaldosteronism producing, polyuria, polydipsia and disturbance in concentrating ability of kidney.

ii. *Hyperkalaemia* may occur in aldosterone deficiency, which may lead to:

- *Dehydration* and circulating collapse and
- *Cardiac toxicity,* in the form of weakness of heart contraction and arrhythmia, may even result in death.

2. Effects on Plasma Sodium Levels

i. *Hypernatraemia,* which may occur in aldosterone excess, could lead to:

- *Increase in extracellular fluid (ECF) volume.* Absorption of Na^+ from renal tubules causes simultaneous osmotic absorption of water. This increases the ECF volume.
- *Hypertension* may occur due to Na^+ and water retention.

ii. *Hyponatraemia,* which could occur due to excess Na^+ loss in aldosterone insufficiency, may be associated with:

- *Decrease in ECF* volume due to excessive Na^+ and water loss in urine,
- *Hypotension,* i.e. decreased blood pressure,
- *Hypovolaemic shock* and even
- *Death* may occur.

Therefore, *aldosterone is essential for life*.

Important Note

Aldosterone Escape: As mentioned above, in hyperaldosteronism or when aldosterone is administered for several days to normal individuals, the increased sodium and water absorption by renal tubules leads to an increase in ECF volume and hypertension. However, after 10–15% increase in ECF, *pressure diuresis occurs,* i.e. excretion of sodium and water in urine is increased, in spite of continued action of aldosterone. This phenomenon is called *aldosterone escape* and is probably due to increased secretion of *atrial natriuretic peptide* (ANP).

Regulation of Aldosterone Secretion

Aldosterone secretion is controlled by the following factors (Fig. 8.5-18):

1. Renin–Angiotensin System The principal function of aldosterone is to maintain extracellular fluid (ECF) volume by conserving body sodium. Hence, secretion of aldosterone is influenced by changes in the circulating fluid volume which are sensed in the kidney. The signals arising from the kidney increase aldosterone secretion when ECF volume is decreased and vice versa.

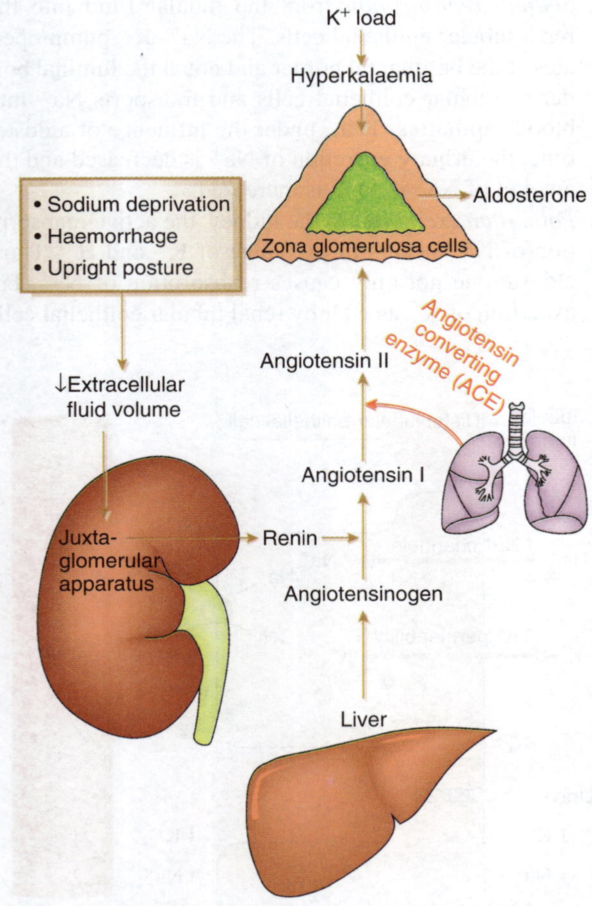

FIGURE 8.5-18 Regulation of aldosterone secretion.

Conditions Associated with Decreased ECF are:

- Sodium deprivation (e.g. dietary restriction),
- Haemorrhage,
- Upright posture for several hours and
- Acute diuresis.

Steps Involved in the Secretion of Aldosterone by Renin–Angiotensin System are:

- *Decrease in ECF volume* leads to decrease in renal arterial blood flow and pressure,
- *Decrease in renal perfusion pressure* causes the juxtaglomerular cells of the afferent arterioles to secrete renin,
- *Renin* catalyses the conversion of angiotensinogen (alpha 2-globulin substrate present in the plasma) to angiotensin I,
- *Angiotensin I* is converted into angiotensin II by the action of angiotensin-converting enzyme (ACE) present in the endothelium of blood vessels, especially in the lungs and
- *Angiotensin II* binds to specific plasma membrane receptors in the adrenal's zona glomerulosa cells and increases the secretion of aldosterone by action on the conversion of cholesterol to pregnenolone and on the conversion of corticoids to aldosterone.

Note. In addition to increasing secretion of aldosterone, angiotensin II also exerts other effects in controlling ECF volume and blood pressure (see page 349).

Aldosterone Secretion may be increased four- to eight-fold by the renin–angiotensin system. The daily aldosterone secretion by this mechanism may vary from 50 mg (with a dietary sodium intake of 150 mEq) to 250 mg (with a dietary sodium intake of 10 mEq).

Factors affecting aldosterone secretion by renin–angiotensin system are:

- *Sympathetic neural activity* enhances renin release in response to hypovolaemia,
- *Local prostaglandins* also stimulate renin release; therefore antiprostaglandin drugs can reduce aldosterone response and
- *Atrial natriuretic peptide* (ANP) reinforces the effects of the renin-angiotensin system on aldosterone secretion.

2. Plasma Potassium Concentration Plasma potassium concentration is a very potent factor in regulating aldosterone secretion. *There exists a vital negative feedback relationship* between plasma potassium concentration and aldosterone secretion, i.e.

- *An increase in plasma concentration* by only 0.5 mEq/L immediately raises plasma aldosterone levels threefold. It is important to note that an increase in dietary potassium from 40 to 200 mEq/day increases plasma aldosterone levels six fold.
- *Decrease in plasma potassium concentration* in potassium depletion lowers aldosterone secretion.

Mechanism of Potassium Effect on Aldosterone Secretion. Potassium is reported to stimulate aldosterone secretion by direct action on the zona glomerulosa cells. It causes depolarization of the cell membrane causing openings of voltage-dependent calcium channels and an increase in intracellular calcium. Hence, calcium channel blockers can inhibit aldosterone secretion.

3. Role of ACTH Unlike secretion of glucocorticoids from zona fasciculata and zona reticularis, the secretion of aldosterone from zona glomerulosa is primarily independent of ACTH control. ACTH plays following roles in mineralocorticoid secretion.

- *Physiologically, ACTH plays an atonic role* in maintaining aldosterone output, i.e. when ACTH is deficient, the zona glomerulosa is less able to respond to its primary stimulus of *angiotensin II* and of potassium.
- The direct stimulating effect of ACTH on aldosterone secretion is mild and transient.
- *Glucocorticoid-remediable aldosteronism (GRA)* is a recently described syndrome which occurs due to autosomal dominant disorder. In this condition there is increased aldosterone secretion and hypertension produced by ACTH. The gene encoding aldosterone synthase and 11β-hydroxylase are 95% identical. In patients with GRA, genes for 11β-hydroxylase and genes for aldosterone synthase get fused. An ACTH-sensitive aldosterone synthase is the product of the hybrid gene. The hyperaldosterone and hypertension in GRA can be remedied by suppressing ACTH secretion with administering glucocorticoids.
- ACTH also stimulates secretion of deoxycortisone (18-OH-DC) from zona fasciculata, which has very mild mineralocorticoid activity.

Adrenal Sex Steroids

Adrenal sex steroids include:

- *Dehydroepiandrosterone* (DHEA), its sulphate ester (DHEA-S) and *androstenedione* are the major androgenic precursor products of the adrenal cortex. They themselves are weak androgens but are converted to the more potent androgen testosterone in peripheral tissues.
- Oestrogen and progesterone are produced in very small amounts. It is important to note that normal human adrenal cortex does not secrete physiologically effective amounts of testosterone and oestrogen.

Synthesis

The adrenal sex steroid precursors are synthesized in the *zona reticularis.*

The steps involved in the synthesis of androgen precursors are summarized in Fig. 8.5-19. The 17-hydroxylated

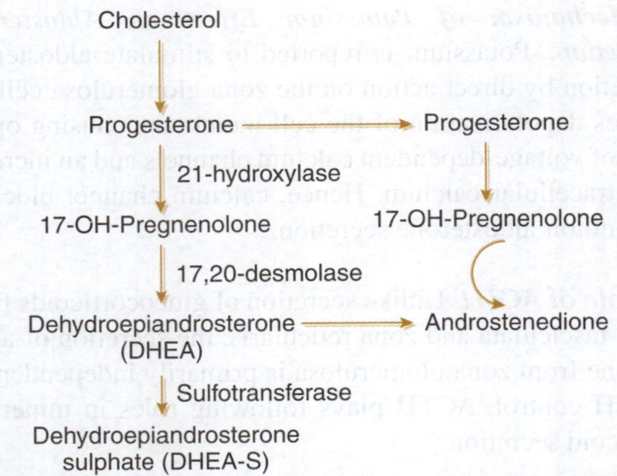

FIGURE 8.5-19 Steps involved in the synthesis of androgen precursors in the zona reticularis.

derivates of pregnenolone and progesterone are the starting points for synthesis of androgen precursors. Fig. 8.5-20, depicting composite synthesis of adrenal cortex hormones, it is 17-hydroxylation is the last reaction common to the synthesis of cortisol and the adrenal androgens. The circumstances that lead to impairment of cortisol synthesis at any point beyond this step, cause accumulation of 17-hydroxypregnenolone and 17-hydroxyprogesterone leading to greatly increased androgen synthesis.

Plasma Levels, Contributiontowards Sex Steroids, Metabolism and Excretion

Plasma Levels. Normal plasma level of DHEA is 150–200 μg% at 25 years of age in both sexes.

Contribution of adrenal glands towards sex steroids and their functions are:

- ***During fetal life,*** the adrenal cortex is hyperplastic and secretes large amounts of DHEA which acts as the main precursor for synthesis of oestrogen by the placenta.
- ***In adult women,*** the adrenal glands supply 50–60% of the androgenic hormone requirement. DHEA-S contributes to increased muscle mass, growth of pubic and axillary hair and libido.
  - The further conversion of androgen precursors to oestrogens in the adrenal cortex is not significant before menopause.
  - After menopause, the oestrogen activity is provided by the oestrogen secreted from adrenal cortex and that arising from conversion of androgen precursors in peripheral tissues.
- ***In adult males,*** since testes produce a large quantity of testosterone, the adrenal androgen precursors are of little biological importance. However, they may be partly responsible for development of male sex organs in childhood.
- ***Tumours of adrenal cortex*** are associated with excessive secretion of adrenal androgens. In prepubertal males, occurrence of such tumours produces precocious pseudopuberty. In prepubertal or in adult females, they cause development of secondary male sexual characteristics (e.g. beard, muscular body and breaking of voice, etc.).

Metabolism and Excretion. The metabolism of androgens, in general, involves reduction of the 3-ketone group and the A-ring in the liver.

- Androsterone and etiocholanolone, the two isomers that are formed as end results of metabolism are excreted in the urine. These metabolites are not specific for the adrenal gland, as they also arise from the gonadal androgens.
- DHEA-S is entirely excreted directly in the urine and is virtually adrenal-specific.

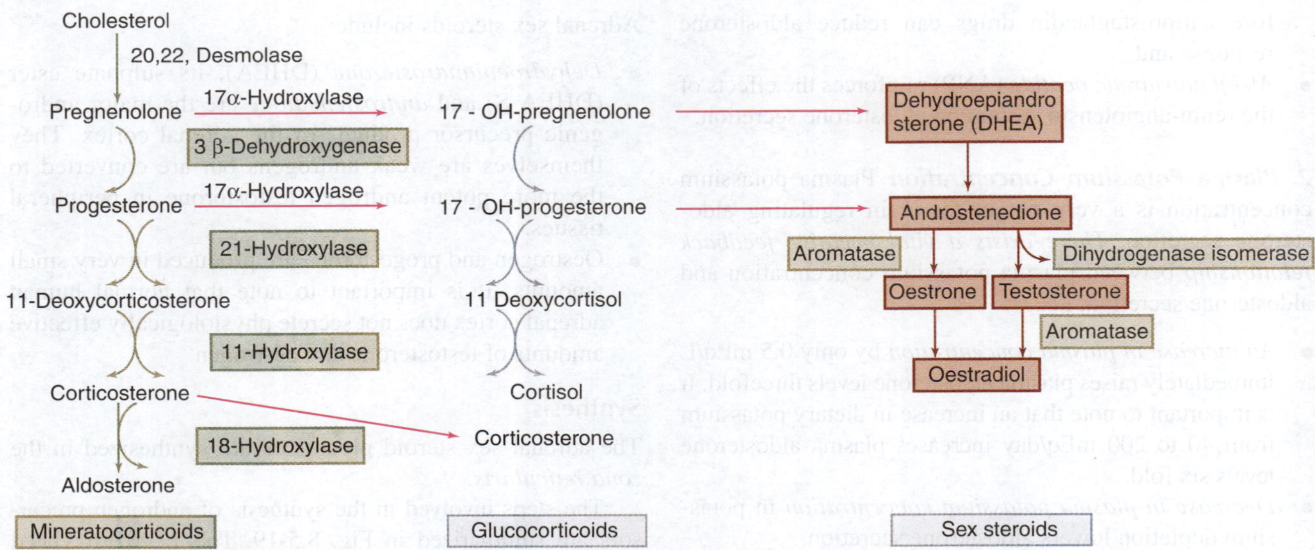

FIGURE 8.5-20 Summary of synthesis of mineralocorticoids, glucocorticoids and sex steroids in adrenal cortex.

- Androsterone, etiocholanolone and DHEA-S are together known as *17-ketosteroids* and constitute the major part of a urinary fraction. Their normal values range from 5 to 14 ng/day in women and 8–20 ng/day in men.
- Normally, two-thirds of the urinary 17-ketosteroids are derived from the adrenal secretions and one-third from gonadal androgen secretions.
- In virilized children or adult women, a large increase in urinary 17-ketosteroid excretion almost always indicates an adrenal abnormality.
- Increased plasma and urinary levels of DHEA-S specifically indicate adrenal abnormality.

APPLIED ASPECTS

The important applied aspects in relation to the adrenal gland, which need mention include:

- Hyperactivity of adrenal cortex and
- Hypoactivity of adrenal cortex.

Hyperactivity of Adrenal Cortex

Disorders of hyperactivity of adrenal cortex include:

- Cushing's syndrome (hypercortisol state),
- Conn's syndrome (hyperaldosteronism) and
- Adrenogenital syndrome (excessive secretion of adrenal androgens).

1. Cushing's Syndrome

Cushing's syndrome refers to the group of clinical conditions occurring due to prolonged excessive levels of glucocorticoids.

Causes Causes of Cushing's syndrome can be divided into two groups:

I. ACTH-dependent Cushing's Syndrome is more common (80% cases and occurs due to hyperplasia of adrenal cortex—secreting excessive glucocorticoids) caused by excess of ACTH in following conditions:

- *Hyperactivity of pituitary* as seen in tumours of pituitary cells, particularly of basophils, which secrete ACTH. The resulting condition of pituitary origin is also called Cushing's disease.
- *Ectopic ACTH production* as seen in benign and malignant nonendocrine tumours, e.g. cancer of lungs or abdominal viscera.
- *Excessive ACTH secretion in hypothalamic disorders* associated with excess of CRH secretion.
- *Excessive ACTH therapy* (iatrogenic).

II. ACTH-independent Cushing's Syndrome is less common (20% cases) and occurs in following conditions:

- *Adrenal origin Cushing's syndrome* is caused by glucocorticoid secreting tumours such as adrenal adenoma and adrenal carcinoma.
- *Excessive glucocorticoid administration* (i.e. iatrogenic) for diseases such as rheumatoid arthritis.
- Abnormal expression of receptors by adrenocortical cells for:
  - Gastric inhibitory peptide (GIP),
  - β adrenergic agonists,
  - Interleukin-I (IL-1) and
  - Gonadotropin-releasing hormone (GnRH).

Characteristic Features Characteristic features of Cushing's syndrome are (Fig. 8.5-21):

1. *Truncal or centripetal obesity.* It occurs due to redistribution of body fat from extremities (which is in the abdominal wall, back and face) producing following characteristic features:
   - *Buffalo hump*, due to collection of fat at upper back,
   - *Moonface*, due to fat collection on the face and
   - *Purple striae or cutaneous abdominal striae or livid stretch marks.* The skin and subcutaneous tissue becomes thin due to protein catabolism. The stretching of abdominal skin due to excessive subcutaneous fat deposition causes rupture of subdermal tissues producing reddish-purple striae.
2. *Muscle weakness* and backache due to protein catabolism.
3. *Sodium and water retention* may cause weight gain, oedema and hypertension.
4. *Hyperglycaemia* occurs due to gluconeogenesis and inhibition of peripheral utilization of glucose. It may lead to glycosuria and adrenal diabetes.

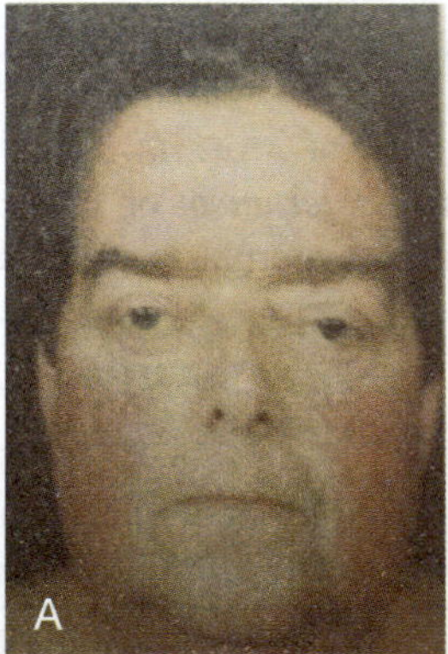

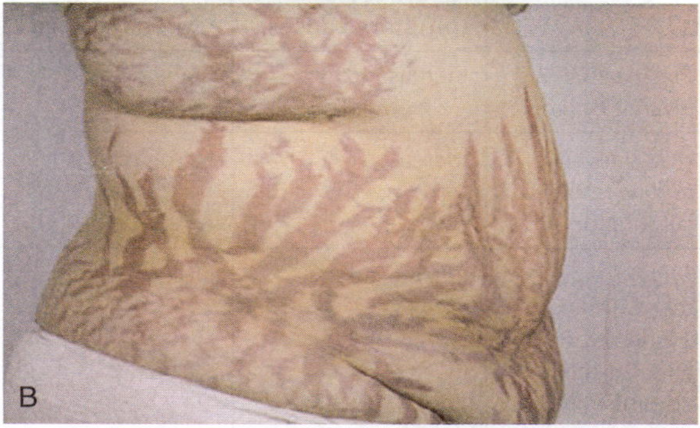

FIGURE 8.5-21 Photograph of a patient with Cushing's syndrome showing moon face (**A**) and truncal obesity and purple striae on the abdomen (**B**).

5. *Hirsutism and menstrual irregularity* may occur due to increased adrenal androgens.
6. *Susceptibility to osteoporosis and bone fracture* is increased due to protein depletion and bone resorption.
7. *Susceptibility to infections* is increased due to immunosuppression.
8. *Psychological, emotional and personality* changes may occur due to CNS effects of glucocorticoids.
9. *Blackening of skin* may occur due to pigmentation caused by MSH-like effects of excessive ACTH.
10. *Susceptibility to peptic ulceration* is increased.

Tests for Cushing's Syndrome

A. Tests to Confirm Diagnosis of Cushing's Syndrome

- *Plasma cortisol level* is raised and there is loss of diurnal pattern, i.e. circadian rhythm is lost.
- *Dexamethasone suppression test* is not able to suppress plasma cortisol level.
- *Insulin-induced hypoglycaemia,* which raises plasma cortisol in normal persons, fails to raise it in Cushing's syndrome.
- The *24-h urinary free cortisol* levels are raised.

B. Tests to Differentiate between ACTH-dependent and ACTH-independent Cushing's syndrome are shown in Table 8.5-3.

Hyperaldosteronism

Hyperaldosteronism refers to overproduction of the hormone aldosterone, a major sodium-retaining hormone.

Causes. Depending upon the cause, hyperaldosteronism may be:

1. *Primary hyperaldosteronism* or *Conn's disease* occurs due to tumour or hyperplasia of zona glomerulosa of adrenal cortex.
2. *Secondary hyperaldosteronism* occurs due to some extra adrenal cause, which stimulates renin–angiotensin–aldosterone system, e.g. nephrotic syndrome, cirrhosis of liver, congestive heart failure and toxaemia of pregnancy.

Characteristic Features of hyperaldosteronism are:

- *Sodium and water retention* leading to hypertension and oedema. It is important to note that marked hypernatraemia and oedema do not occur because Na^+ excretion is soon normalized despite hypersecretion of aldosterone (escape phenomenon, see page 752).
- *Hypokalaemia* may occur due to increased potassium excretion producing muscle weakness and periodic muscle paralysis, whereas prolonged depletion of potassium may cause renal damage producing polyuria.
- *Metabolic alkalosis* may occur due to secretion of more amount of H^+ into renal tubules and metabolic alkalosis may produce hypocalcaemia causing tetany.

Adrenogenital Syndrome

As mentioned earlier, the androgen precursors secreted by the adrenal cortex are of little biological importance under normal circumstances. However, when secreted in large amounts as in *tumour of zona reticularis* of adrenal cortex, the following abnormal features may be produced:

- *In prepubertal males,* the excessive androgens produce precocious pseudopuberty (see page 818).
- *In males,* the oestrogen producing cells may produce female-like secondary sexual characters such as enlargement of breasts (gynaecomastia), atrophy of testes, loss of libido and feminine body.
- *In females,* they cause development of male secondary sexual characteristics, such as beard, muscular body, breaking of voice, male-type hair growth, enlargement of clitoris and amenorrhea.

TABLE 8.5-3 Tests to Differentiate between ACTH-Dependent and ACTH-Independent Cushing's Syndrome

Tests	ACTH dependent (pituitary causes)	ACTH independent (adrenal causes)
• *Plasma ACTH level* at 8 a.m.	Increased	Undetectable
• *ACTH level following* CRH stimulation	Increased	No change
• *Metyrapone test.* Levels of 11-deoxycortisol after 24 h of administration of metyrapone	Decreased	No change

Hypoactivity of Adrenal Cortex

Adrenocortical deficiency (insufficiency), depending upon the site of lesion, can be divided into two types:

i. *Primary adrenocortical deficiency* occurs due to involvement of adrenal cortex and is associated with high ACTH levels due to feedback mechanism. The conditions producing primary adrenocortical deficiency include:
   - Addison's disease and
   - Congenital adrenal hyperplasia.
ii. *Secondary adrenocortical deficiency* occurs due to involvement of pituitary or due to exogenous glucocorticoid administration and is associated with *low ACTH level* due to less production.
iii. Tertiary adrenal deficiency is caused by hypothalamic disorders.

Addison's Disease

Causes. Addison's disease is an important condition of primary adrenocortical deficiency, occurring due to the following causes:

- *Autoimmune disease* causing adrenal cortex atrophy,
- *Tuberculosis, fungal* and *cytomegalovirus* infections producing adrenal cortex destruction, an uncommon but well recognized complication in patients with AIDS,
- *Bilateral adrenalectomy*, but failure to take hormone therapy and
- *Malignant tumours* producing destruction of hormone producing cells in adrenal cortex.

Characteristic Features occur due to chronic deficiency of hormones secreted by all the three zones of the adrenal cortex:

1. *Glucocorticoid insufficiency* produces weight loss, malaise, anorexia, nausea, vomiting, weakness and diarrhoea. Since glucocorticoids are essential for adaptation to stress, therefore in Addison's disease exposure to any type of stress, e.g. even mild infection may be fatal.
2. Mineralocorticoid deficiency produces hyponatraemia, hyperkalaemia, acidosis and decreased ECF volume with hypotension.
3. Loss of androgens causes sparse hair in females.
4. *Increased ACTH secretion* occurs due to feedback mechanism and causes diffused pigmentation of the skin and mucous membranes (because of its MSH-like actions).

   Tests for Addison's disease

   i. Tests to diagnose hypoadrenalism:
      1. Plasma cortisol levels are low.
      2. Plasma aldosterone levels are low or normal.
      3. Serum sodium levels are low.
      4. Serum potassium is high or normal.
      5. Blood glucose is low in severe disease.
      6. Plasma renin activity is high.

   ii. *Tests to differentiate between primary (Addison's disease) and secondary hypoadrenalism:*
      1. *Basal ACTH level.* High in Addison's disease and low in pituitary or hypothalamic disease
      2. *ACTH stimulation test.* 0.25 mg ACTH is given intravenously and blood samples are tested after 30 and 60 min. In Addison's disease, plasma cortisol level does not rise, while in pituitary or hypothalamic disease there occurs a subnormal rise

Treatment of Addison's disease consists of replacement therapy:

- *Glucocorticoid replacement.* Oral prednisolone 20 mg in the morning and 10 mg in the evening is the drug of choice.
- *Mineralocorticoid replacement.* Fludrocortisone 0.05–0.1 mg/day is adequate to maintain blood pressure, electrolytes and renin activity.

Addisonian Crisis or Adrenal Crisis It refers to acute adrenal insufficiency characterized by sudden collapse. The condition becomes fatal if not treated in time.

Causes. Acute adrenal insufficiency may occur in following conditions:

- *Acute precipitation of Addison's disease* under the effect of any stress, e.g. infection, haemorrhage, etc.
- Major surgical operation or trauma.
- Sudden withdrawal of glucocorticoid treatment.

Treatment. It is a medical emergency requiring immediate treatment with:

- Glucocorticoids,
- Mineralocorticoids,
- Fluids, electrolytes and
- Treatment of precipitating factor.

Secondary and Tertiary Adrenal Insufficiency Secondary and tertiary hypoaldosteronism is usually milder than primary adrenal insufficiency. The plasma ACTH level is low, therefore skin pigmentation does not occur.

Hypoaldosteronism. Isolated cases of aldosterone deficiency have also been reported in patients with renal disorders and low circulating renin. This condition is also referred as *hyporeninemic hypoaldosteronism.*

Pseudohypoaldosteronism occurs when aldosterone secretion is normal but there is resistance to its action.

Characteristic Features. The patients of hypoaldosteronism have marked hyperkalaemia.

Congenital Adrenal Hyperplasia

Causes. Congenital adrenal hyperplasia is caused by congenital deficiency of one of the enzymes involved in the biosynthesis of glucocorticoids, particularly *21-hydroxylase deficiency* and deficiency of 11-hydroxylase (Fig. 8.5-20).

Pathophysiological features include:

- *Cortisol and 11-deoxycortisol levels* are decreased due to reduced synthesis.
- *17-Hydroxyprogesterone,* which is substrate for 21-hydroxylase, is raised.
- *ACTH levels are raised* due to feedback mechanism excited by low cortisol levels. ACTH leads to hyperplasia of adrenal cortex.
- *Adrenal androgen (e.g. DHEA) levels* are increased because deficiency of 21-hydroxylase causes excess of 17-hydroxyprogesterone, which serves as a major precursor for adrenal androgens (see Fig. 8.5-19). The increased androgen levels cause sexual abnormalities.

Characteristic features occurring because of above pathophysiological changes are virilism and excessive body growth.

In boys, adrenal hyperplasia leads to a congenital condition known as *macrogenitosomia praecox.* It is characterized by:

- Precocious body growth leading to stocky appearance called *infant Hercules*.

- Precocious sexual development with enlarged penis even at age of 4 years.
- *In female fetus,* high plasma androgen levels cause *masculinized pattern* of development (*virilism*). Sometimes, the female fetus may be born with male-type external genitalia. This condition is called *pseudohermaphroditism*. For details see page 814.

HORMONES OF ADRENAL MEDULLA

The adrenal medulla secretes *catecholamines,* which include epinephrine, norepinephrine and dopamine. About 80% of adrenal medullary catecholamine is epinephrine and the rest is norepinephrine. Apart from catecholamines, the adrenal medulla also contains small amounts of *dynorphins, neurotensin, encephalin, somatostatin* and *substance P*.

Epinephrine circulating in the blood is almost exclusively produced in the medulla, with smaller amounts synthesized in the brain. Humans who have undergone bilateral adrenalectomy excrete practically no epinephrine in the urine, confirming the fact that the medulla is the sole source of circulating epinephrine.

Norepinephrine is secreted by the medulla in small amounts. Norepinephrine is normally a neurotransmitter, but in select circumstances may also function as a hormone. It is widely distributed in neural tissues, which in addition to the medulla include sympathetic postganglionic fibres and central nervous system.

In the brain, the concentration of norepinephrine is the highest in the hypothalamus. The norepinephrine content of tissue reflects the density of its sympathetic innervation. Except for the placenta, which is devoid of nerve fibres, norepinephrine has been demonstrated in almost all tissues. Urinary levels of norepinephrine remain within normal limits even after bilateral adrenalectomy, indicating thereby that the norepinephrine originates from extra-adrenal sources (i.e. the terminals of the postganglionic sympathetic fibres and the brain).

Synthesis and Storage of Catecholamine Hormones

Synthesis of Catecholamines Epinephrine and norepinephrine are synthesized in different cells. The biosynthetic pathway originates with L-tyrosine, which is derived from the diet or from the hepatic hydroxylation of L-phenylalanine by phenylalanine hydroxylase. Conversion of tyrosine to epinephrine occurs in four steps (Fig. 8.5-22):

1. Conversion of Tyrosine to DOPA. The conversion of tyrosine to DOPA (dehydroxyphenylalanine) is catalysed by the enzyme *tyrosine hydroxylase*. This reaction occurs in the chromaffin cell cytoplasm and requires the cofactor tetrahydrobiopterin, molecular oxygen and NADH. This is a rate-*limiting step* in catecholamine synthesis. The subsequent catecholamine products, i.e. DOPA, norepinephrine (NE) and dopamine all inhibit this initial reaction. The enzyme tyrosine hydroxylase is found only in those tissues which

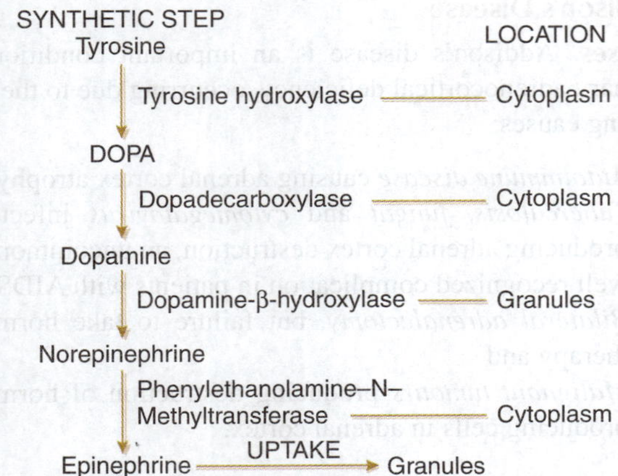

FIGURE 8.5-22 Steps of catecholamine synthesis in the adrenal medulla.

synthesize catecholamines. Nerve impulses increase activity of this enzyme.

2. Conversion of DOPA to Dopamine in the cytosol is catalysed by the enzyme *dopa decarboxylase,* which requires pyridoxal phosphate as a cofactor. This enzyme is not confined only to catecholamine synthesizing tissue.

Dopamine is a naturally occurring precursor of norepinephrine. Dopamine is a weak agonist of α- and β-adrenergic receptors. Dopamine acts through two types of dopaminergic receptors D_1 and D_2.

Effects of Dopamine:

- The main function of dopamine is in the central nervous system. For details, see page 1012.
- The physiologic function of circulating dopamine is unknown, but, injected dopamine produces vasodilation of renal and mesentry by acting on specific dopaminergic receptors.
- On the heart it has a positive ionotropic effect probably by releasing norepinephrine by its action on β adrenergic receptors. Moderate doses of dopamine results in rise in systolic blood pressure but no effect on diastolic pressure.

Important Note

Dopamine is useful in treatment of traumatic and cardiogenic shock, because it causes renal vasoconstriction and relaxes mesangial cells and thus maintains glomerular filtration rate.

3. Conversion of Dopamine to Norepinephrine. Dopamine from the cytosol enters the chromaffin granules by vesicular monoamine transport (VMAT), which can be blocked by the drug reserpine, where it is converted to L-epinephrine by the enzyme *dopamine*-β-hydroxylase (DBH). This reaction requires molecular oxygen and uses ascorbate as hydrogen donor. This enzyme is exclusively present in the granules of these tissues which synthesize catecholamines, e.g. in the granulated vesicles of sympathetic nerve endings and the chromaffin granules of the chromaffin cells of adrenal medulla.

4. Conversion of Norepinephrine to Epinephrine. In about 20% of chromaffin cells, the norepinephrine is the end product and the sequence ends here with its storage. In about 80% of chromaffin cells, norepinephrine diffuses back into the cytoplasm, where it is converted to epinephrine by the enzyme *phenylethanolamine N-methyltransferase (PNMT)* using S-adenosyl methionine as a methyl donor. The enzyme PNMT exists in significant concentration only in the adrenal medulla. Its activity is induced by glucocorticoids (cortisol), which are found in high concentration only in the adrenal portal blood draining the adrenal cortex and supplying the medulla.

Storage of Catecholamines in Storage Granules *(Fig. 8.5-23)*. The epinephrine formed in the cytoplasm is then taken back by the chromaffin granules, in which it is stored as the predominant adrenomedullary hormone. The uptake of dopamine (DA), norepinephrine (NE) and epinephrine (E) by the secretory granules is an active process that requires ATP and magnesium. The catecholamines are stored complexed to calcium, ATP (1 mol of ATP with 4 moles of catecholamine), chromogranins and other factors to prevent excessive increase of intragranular osmotic pressure due to a high concentration of intragranular catecholamines and other molecules. It appears, DA, NE and epinephrine are protected in the granules from the oxidative activity of monoamine oxidase (MAO). Of the three, DA is most vulnerable.

Factors Regulating Catecholamine Synthesis

- *Acute sympathetic stimulation* activates the enzyme tyrosine hydroxylase, possibly by decreasing cytoplasmic catecholamine levels and relieving product inhibition.
- *Chronic stimulation of preganglionic fibres* increases the concentrations of both tyrosine hydroxylase and dopamine-β-hydroxylase, and thus helps to ensure maintenance of the output of both catecholamines when the demand is continuous. The mechanism of induction may involve a cAMP-dependent protein kinase.

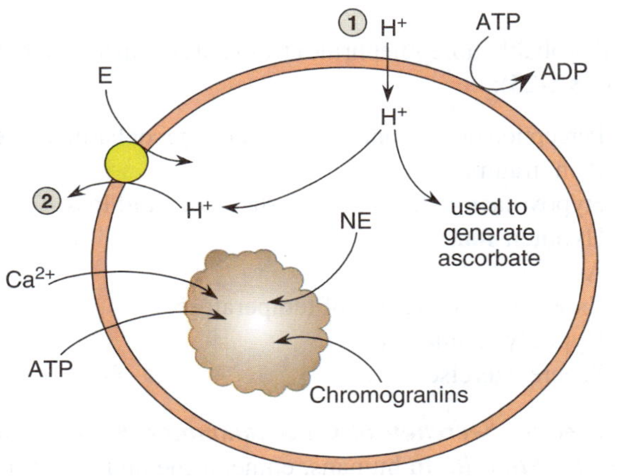

FIGURE 8.5-23 Storage of catecholamines in chromaffin granules.

- *ACTH* acts directly and helps to sustain the levels of the enzymes tyrosine hydroxylase and dopamine-hydroxylase under stressful conditions.
- *Cortisol*, specifically induces the enzyme N-methyl transferase, and therefore, selectively stimulates epinephrine synthesis. The portal circulation system subserves this action, because blood from the cortex has a high concentration of cortisol and it directly perfuses the chromaffin cells.
- *Epinephrine* stimulates its own synthesis. From the medulla, epinephrine diffuses into the cortex, where it stimulates cortisol synthesis by activating the expression of the steroidogenic acute regulatory protein (STAR) gene.

Important Note

- After hypophysectomy, there is decreased synthesis of epinephrine due to decreased plasma levels of glucocorticoids.
- Glucocorticoids are necessary for the development of adrenal medulla. In deficiency of 21 β-hydroxylase enzyme, reduction of glucocorticoids will result in dysplasia of the adrenal medulla. The babies born with 21 β-hydroxylase deficiency have a low circulating level of catecholamines.

Secretion of Catecholamine Hormones

Mechanism of Secretion Secretion from the adrenal medulla is an integral part of the *flight-or-fight reaction* that is evoked by stimulation of the sympathetic nervous system as a response to stress. In other words, adrenal medulla is often activated in association with the rest of the sympathetic nervous system and acts in concert with this system during states of emergency.

Steps involved in the secretion of catecholamines from adrenal medulla are (Fig. 8.5-24):

- Activation of sympathetic nervous system is caused by various stimuli (enumerated above), which are sensed at various higher levels.
- The nerve impulses travelling across the preganglionic sympathetic fibres in greater splanchnic nerve and terminating on the chromaffin cells activate the adrenal medulla by releasing acetylcholine.
- The acetylcholine activates nicotinic receptors on adrenal medullary cells, leading to increase in Na^+ permeability of the cells and their depolarization.
- Depolarization of membrane induces an influx of Ca^{2+} ions, which stimulate exocytosis of the secretory granules.
- Exocytosis of the secretory granules is associated with release of epinephrine, norepinephrine, ATP, the enzyme β-hydroxylase and chromogranin into the circulation. This process involves SNAPs (Synaptosome-associated proteins) and VAMs (Vesicles-associated membrane

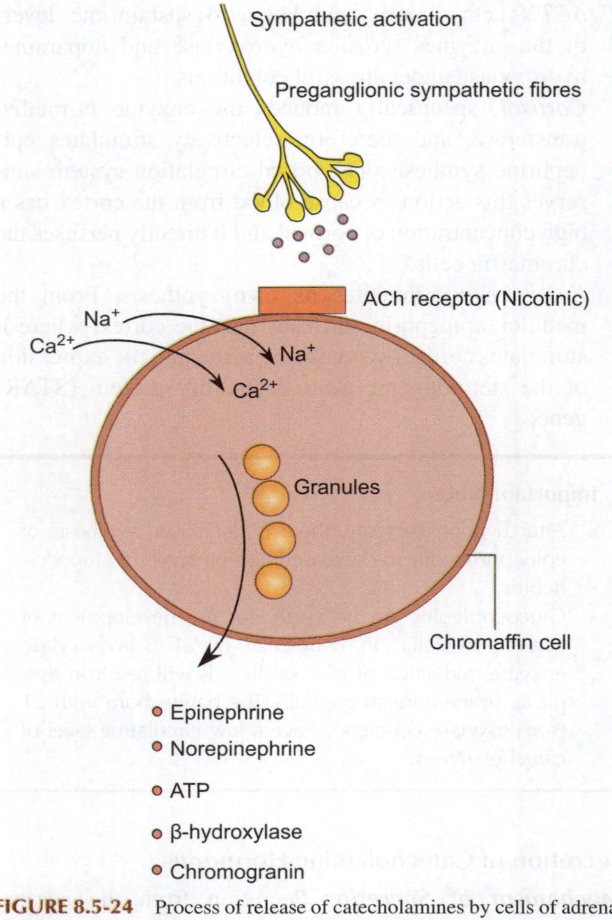

FIGURE 8.5-24 Process of release of catecholamines by cells of adrenal medulla.

proteins). These proteins can be blocked by drugs such as guanethidine and Bretylium. The membranous material of the secretory granules is retained in the chromaffin cells and probably recycled.

Nervous Control of Secretion The catecholamine secretion is entirely controlled by the splanchnic nerves supplying the medulla. These nerves comprise preganglionic sympathetic fibres emerging mainly from lower thoracic segments (T_5–T_9) of ipsilateral intermediolateral grey column of the spinal cord. These fibres, when stimulated, act by releasing acetylcholine close to the adrenal medullary chromaffin cells.

Therefore, the main physiological stimulus for release of catecholamines is acetylcholine. The mechanism of action of acetylcholine is described as above (Fig. 8.5-24).

Physiological and Psychological Stimuli for Release. As mentioned in the beginning, the adrenal medullary activation occurs as a part of a generalized sympathetic response to any emergency situation. Therefore, this has also been called *sympathetic alarm* reaction. The various sensory stimuli associated with rapid release of epinephrine

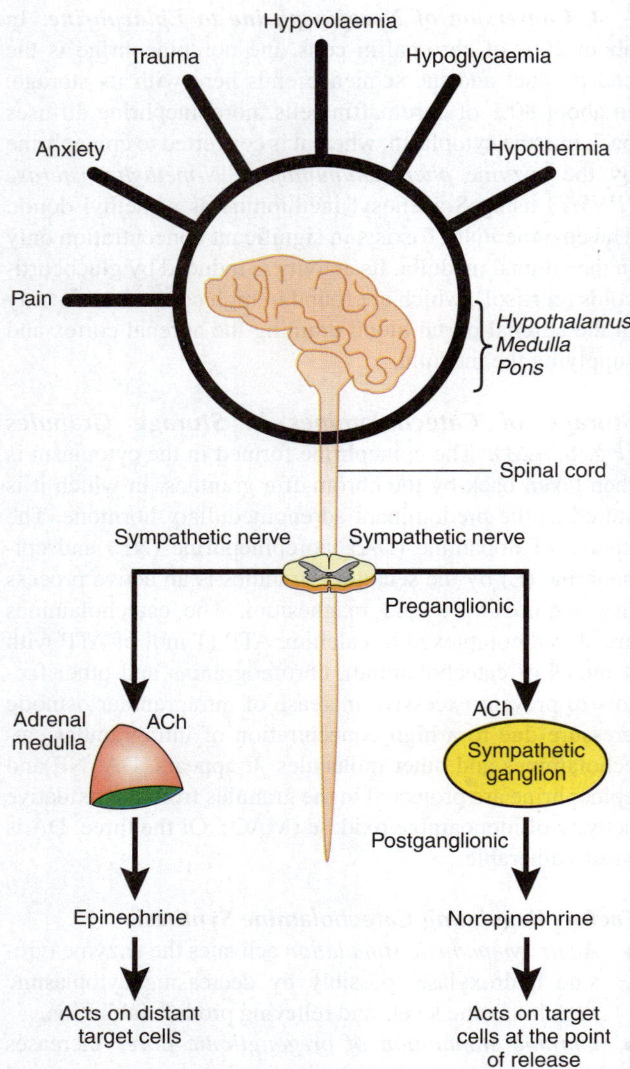

FIGURE 8.5-25 Stimuli associated with secretion of catecholamines from adrenal medulla and sympathetic nervous system. **Note,** adrenal medulla releases primarily epinephrine into the blood stream where it acts on distant targets. The sympathetic ganglia release norepinephrine into the synaptic cleft which acts on the target cell at point of release.

(and probably norepinephrine) from adrenal medulla include (Fig. 8.5-25):

- Perception or even anticipation of danger or harm (anxiety),
- Pain, trauma,
- Hypovolaemia from haemorrhage or fluid loss,
- Hypotension,
- Anoxia,
- Exposure to extremes of temperature,
- Hypoglycaemia and
- Severe exercise.

Selective Secretion of Catecholamines in Response to Specific Stimuli. In humans, epinephrine and norepinephrine appear to be released independently by specific stimuli:

- *Anger and aggressive states,* which are associated with active and appropriate anticipatory behavioural responses to the challenge, i.e. the situations with which the individual is familiar, are associated with increased *norepinephrine secretion.*
- *States of anxiety*, tense but passive emotional displays or threatening situations of unpredictable nature are associated with increased epinephrine secretion.

Stimulation of adrenal medulla also occurs independently of the sympathetic system.

Adrenal medullary stimulation does not always occur as a part of a generalized sympathetic response, e.g. *hypoglycaemia* activates adrenal medulla producing marked increase in catecholamine secretion without any significant increase in sympathetic neural discharge. Conversely, in baroreceptor-mediated cardiovascular reflexes, sympathetic neural system is predominantly involved without activation of the adrenal medulla.

Circulation, Metabolism and Excretion

Circulation

- ***Secreted epinephrine*** and norepinephrine from the adrenal medulla is in the ratio of 4:1. In plasma, about 95% of dopamine and 70% norepinephrine and epinephrine are conjugated to sulphate. Sulphate conjugates are inactive and their function is unsettled.
- ***Basal plasma levels*** (in recumbent humans) of free epinephrine are 30 pg/ml and that of free norepinephrine are 300 pg/ml.
- ***After bilateral adrenalectomy,*** plasma epinephrine levels fall to almost zero but norepinephrine levels remain unchanged.
- ***Variation in plasma levels*** of catecholamines according to physiological or pathological states are quite common. When adrenal medullary secretion increases, the secretion of epinephrine and norepinephrine usually increases in the same proportion. However, the threshold levels at which circulating norepinephrine can produce physiological effects is about 6 times its basal levels, while the threshold level at which epinephrine produces its effects are well achieved during that physiological state (Table 8.5-4, Fig. 8.5-26). Hence, in most of the physiological and pathological conditions increased adrenal medullary secretion results in selective epinephrine mediated effects, in spite of increased secretion of both catecholamines.

Metabolism and Inactivation of Circulating Catecholamines

Plasma Half-life of epinephrine (E) and norepinephrine (NE) is extremely short (1–3 min) and their metabolic clearance rates range from 2 to 6 L/min. The short half-life of catecholamines allows for a rapid turn of their dramatic effects.

Inactivation of Catecholamines released by the sympathetic nerve endings at the synaptic clefts differs from that of the catecholamines released into circulation by the adrenal medulla.

Catecholamines Released at Sympathetic Neuroeffector Junction are inactivated by the following mechanisms:

- *Active neuronal reuptake* into the presynaptic nerve terminals is the most important mechanism of termination of action of NE in the junctional space. This specific reuptake accounts for inactivation of about 85% released NE. Transportation back into the nerve terminal is carried by specific norepinephrine transporter (NET). The NE re-uptaken is either stored in the vesicles (*nonenzymatic inactivation*) or is oxidized by the enzyme monoamine oxidase (MAO) present in the nerve endings (*enzymatic inactivation*).

TABLE 8.5-4 Plasma Concentration of Catecholamines Compared with Their Biological Effective Concentration in Different Physiological and Pathological States

Physiological/ pathological state	Relevant biological action	Plasma epinephrine (pg/ml)		Plasma norepinephrine (pg/ml)	
		Mean value	*Effective range for relevant biological action*	*Mean value*	*Effective range for relevant biological action*
Basal (recumbent) position	–	30	–	300	–
Upright position	↑ heart rate and blood pressure	70	50–125	500	+800
Hypoglycaemia	↑ Plasma glucose	230	150–200	260	+1800
Severe hypoglycaemia	–	1500	–	750	–
Diabetic ketoacidosis	↑ lipolysis and ketosis ↑ Insulin	500	100–400	1200	1800

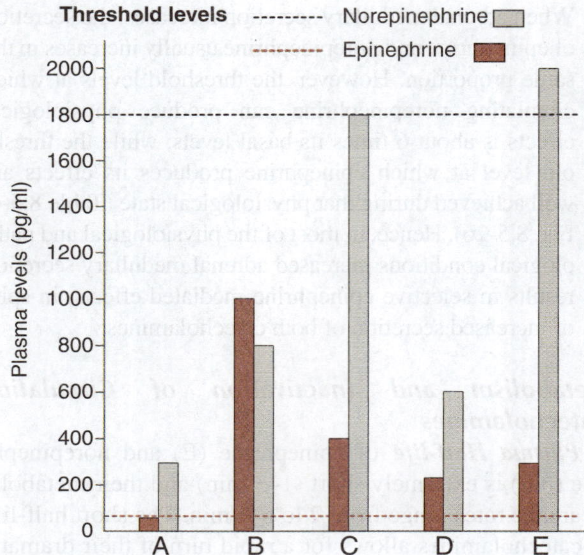

FIGURE 8.5-26 Plasma concentration of epinephrine and norepinephrine in different physiological and pathological states with their threshold levels: **A,** basal levels; **B,** hypoglycaemia; **C,** severe exercise; **D,** surgical stress; and **E,** pheochromocytoma.

- *Dilution by diffusion* out of the junctional cleft.
- *Extraneural uptake.* It accounts for removing the 15% of NE released from adrenergic nerve endings. It is mediated by postsynaptic cells and is followed by intracellular metabolic inactivation by the enzyme monoamine oxidase (MAO) and catechol-O-methyltransferase (COMT).

Circulating Catecholamines (epinephrine and norepinephrine) are metabolized predominantly in the liver and kidney by the enzymes MAO and COMT.

Metabolic Disposition of Catecholamines

Enzymes involved in the metabolic disposition of catecholamines are:

- ***Monoamine oxidase*** (MAO). It is found in very high concentration in the mitochondria of the liver, kidney, stomach and intestine. It catalyses the oxidative deamination of a number of biogenic amines, including the intraneuronal and circulating catecholamines.
- ***Catechol-O-methyltransferase (COMT).*** It is found in the soluble fraction of tissue homogenates with highest levels in liver and kidney. COMT is considered mainly as an extraneuronal enzyme but is also found in the postsynaptic membrane. It metabolizes the circulating catecholamines in the kidney and liver and metabolizes locally released norepinephrine in the effector tissue.

Steps in the Metabolic Disposition of Catecholamines are (Fig. 8.5-27):

- Both norepinephrine and epinephrine are first oxidatively deaminated by the combined action of MAO and AO (aldehyde oxidase to dihydroxymandelic acid (DOMA).
- DOMA is then 0-methylated by the enzyme COMT to vanillyl mandelic acid (VMA).
- Alternatively, the norepinephrine and epinephrine can be first 0-methylated by COMT to produce normetanephrine and metanephrine, respectively.
- The normetanephrine and metanephrine are then oxidatively deaminated by the combined action of MAO and AO to methoxyhydroxyphenylglycol (MHPG) and then to VMA.
- VMA and MHPG are excreted in the urine and bile. These are conjugated to form glucuronides and sulphates.

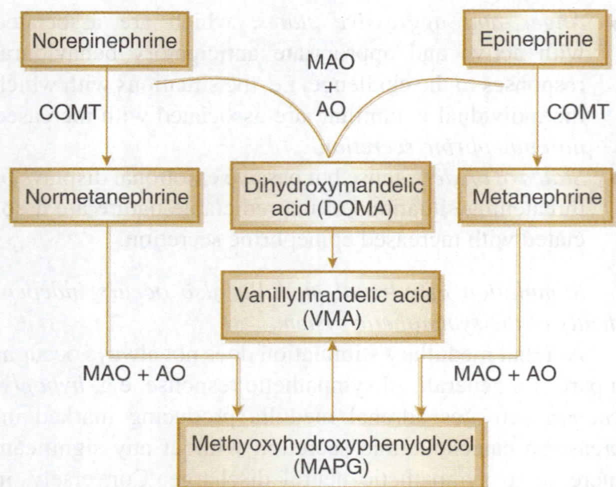

FIGURE 8.5-27 Steps in the metabolic disposition of catecholamines.

Fate of Circulating Catecholamines can be now summarized as:

- Only 2–3% of catecholamines are directly excreted in urine mostly as conjugates.
- About 50% of secreted catecholamines appear in the urine as free conjugated metanephrine and normetanephrine.
- About 35% of secreted catecholamines appear in the urine as VMA and about 12–13% as MHPG.
- In normal humans, about 30 μg of norepinephrine, 6 μg of epinephrine and 700 μg VMA are excreted per day.

Note. It is important to note that:

- Under normal circumstances, epinephrine accounts for a very small fraction of urinary VMA and MOPG; the majority is derived from the norepinephrine and thus reflects the activity of the nerve terminals of sympathetic nervous system rather than that of the medulla.
  - Activity of the medulla can be assessed specifically only by the measurement of plasma epinephrine levels or of urinary free epinephrine excretion.

Adrenergic Receptors and Mechanism of Action of Catecholamines

Adrenergic Receptors Like other amino acids and peptide hormones, catecholamines act through cell membrane and receptors known as adrenergic receptors. Based on their pharmacologic properties, adrenergic receptors are of two types:

Alpha (α) Receptors. These are further of two types (α_1 and α_2). Alpha-adrenergic receptors are sensitive to both epinephrine and norepinephrine. α receptors have multiple subtypes (α_{1A}, α_{1B}, α_{1D}, α_{2A}, α_{2B} and α_{2C}). These receptors are associated with most of the excitatory functions of the body but have one major inhibitory function (i.e. inhibition of intestinal motility).

Beta (β) Receptors. These are further of three types, β_1, β_2 and β_3. Beta-adrenergic receptors respond to epinephrine and in general are relatively insensitive to norepinephrine. These receptors are associated with most of the inhibitory functions of the body but have an important excitatory function (i.e. excitation of myocardium).

Relative potency of two catecholamines varies with each receptor type. In general, epinephrine tends to react more strongly with β receptors and norepinephrine with α receptors but overlap is considerable.

Specific agonists and antagonists have been developed for each receptor type (Table 8.5-5).

Structurally β_1, β_2 and α_2 receptors are similar. All three of these receptors are single unit transmembrane glycoproteins. α_1 receptors differ from these receptors and have a higher molecular weight.

Mechanism of Action and Second Messenger involved are:

- α_1 receptors are coupled to Gq proteins to phospholipase C, leading to the phosphatidylinositol membrane system; and Diacylglycerol (DAG), which mobilize calcium along with protein kinase C, to mediates the hormone effects.
- α_2 receptors are coupled to an inhibitory G-protein; thus hormone binding decreases cAMP levels and protein kinase A activity.
- β_1, β_2 and β_3 receptors are coupled to and stimulate adenylyl cyclase; thus cAMP is the second messenger for their biological effects.

TABLE 8.5-5 Agonists and Antagonists of Adrenergic Receptors

Type of adrenergic receptors	Agonist	Antagonist
α_1	Norepinephrine Phenylephrine Methoxamine	Phenoxybenzamine Phentolamine Prazosin
α_2	Clonidine Apraclonidine Brimonidine	Yohimbine Phentolamine
β_1	Norepinephrine Isoproterenol Dobutamine	Metoprolol Atenolol Betaxolol
β_2	Isoproterenol Albuterol	Propranolol Butaxamine Metaproterenol Salmeterol

Regulation of Adrenergic Receptors. A reciprocal relationship exists between catecholamine concentration and the number and function of adrenergic receptors.

- *Downregulation.* Continuous stimulation of catecholamine release or exposure to catecholamine agonists is associated with a decreased number of adrenergic receptors in target cells and a decreased responsiveness to catecholamines. This phenomenon is called downregulation of receptors.
- *Upregulation.* A sustained decrease in catecholamine secretion (e.g. following sympathectomy) increases the number of receptors and enhances sensitivity to catecholamines. This phenomenon is called upregulation and may account for the *denervation hypersensitivity*, which is observed in sympathetic neuroeffectors following autonomic fibre denervation.
- Rapid desensitization to subsequent doses is produced by acute exposure to catecholamine hormones. This effect is caused by phosphorylation of the various receptors by the hormone-activated protein kinase A or C. Phosphorylation renders the receptors inaccessible to further hormone binding. Receptor desensitization is a form of rapid intracellular negative feedback, which limits hormone actions.

Note. For further details about adrenergic receptors, see page 984.

Actions of Catecholamines

General Considerations

- The catecholamines exert their effects by binding with adrenergic receptors as described above.
- Actions of catecholamines on individual organs and systems are similar to those resulting from stimulation of sympathetic nervous system and are summarized in Table 10.5-2.
- In general, the effects produced by adrenomedullary stimulation last (about 10 times) longer than these produced by sympathetic stimulation, and the effects on metabolism are more pronounced.
- Adrenal medullary stimulation releases predominantly epinephrine (and small amounts of norepinephrine), while sympathetic stimulation mainly releases norepinephrine. So, their effects are different in some tissues owing to the differential existence of two types of adrenergic receptors (alpha and beta).

I. Metabolic Actions of Catecholamines Epinephrine affects metabolic functions more than norepinephrine, via alpha and beta receptors.

1. General Metabolic Effects of Epinephrine. This includes:

- Increased O_2 consumption (by 20–40%) and increased CO_2 output.
- Raised basal metabolic rate (BMR) and respiratory quotient (RQ).
- Increased heat production due to stimulation of cellular oxidative processes.

2. Effect on Carbohydrate Metabolism. Epinephrine produces hyperglycaemia and makes the glucose available for the brain and other tissues to meet the emergency by its following effects:

- *Glycogenolysis* is stimulated in the liver (releasing glucose in circulation) and in the muscle (providing lactate for hepatic gluconeogenesis.
- *Glycogenesis* is reduced in the liver by inhibition of the enzyme glycogen synthase.
- *Gluconeogenesis,* i.e. hepatic production of glucose from lactate, amino acids and glycerol is increased.
- *Insulin secretion* is inhibited. This ensures that glucose will be used mostly by the brain since most of the tissues except brain require insulin for glucose utilization.
- *Glucagon secretion* is stimulated. This amplifies the hyperglycaemic effects of epinephrine.
- *ACTH secretion* is stimulated, which then stimulates cortisol secretion. Cortisol is a potent gluconeogenic hormone, via the hepatic conversion of alanine to glucose.

3. Effects on Fat Metabolism. Norepinephrine has a more potent action on the lipid metabolism than epinephrine, which has a predominant effect on carbohydrate metabolism.

- *Catecholamines* cause increase in lipolysis by stimulating hormone sensitive lipase (via beta receptor, i.e. cAMP) in adipose tissue and muscles. This results in increase in free fatty acids in the circulation which are effectively utilized by the heart and muscle as fuel source.

II. Physiological Actions of Catecholamines

1. Effects on Cardiovascular System

i. *In an isolated heart,* both epinephrine and norepinephrine stimulate β_1 receptors and produce:

- Increase in heart rate by action on SA node,
- Increase in conduction velocity and shortening of functional refractory period by action on AV node,
- Increase in force of contraction by direct effect on ventricular and atrial myocardium.
- In high doses, catecholamines produce multiple pacemaker activity especially in Purkinje fibres and can produce fibrillation, which is why epinephrine and norepinephrine are never administered intravenously.

ii. *In intact heart and blood vessels,* the net effects of epinephrine and norepinephrine are:

Parameter	Epinephrine	Norepinephrine
• Heart rate	↑	↓
• Cardiac output	↑	↓
• Peripheral resistance	↓	↑
• Systolic blood pressure	↑	↑
• Diastolic blood pressure	↓	↑
• Mean arterial pressure	↓ or N	↑

Explanation of the differential effects of epinephrine and norepinephrine

Epinephrine:

- Increases heart rate and force of contraction via β_1 receptors results in increased cardiac output and rise in systolic blood pressure (SBP).
- Causes vasoconstriction in renal, splanchnic and cutaneous vascular bed via β_1 receptors and vasodilation in muscle and liver vessels via $\beta_2$receptors.The net effect is decrease in peripheral resistance and fall in diastolic blood pressure (DBP).
- As a result of rise in SBP and fall in DBP, the pulse pressure (PP) is widened but mean arterial pressure, i.e. MAP (DBP + 1/3 PP) remains unchanged or slightly decreases. Thus reflex effect on baroreceptors is negligible.

Norepinephrine

- Increases heart rate and force of contraction via β_1 receptors results in increased cardiac output and rise in systolic blood pressure (SBP).
- Causes vasoconstriction via α_1 receptors resulting in increased peripheral resistance and increased diastolic blood pressure (DBP).
  - As a result of increased SBP and DBP, mean blood pressure (MBP) is markedly increased, which reflexly by stimulation of baroreceptors (aortic and carotid sinus) decrease heart rate, force of contraction and cardiac output.
  - The net result of norepinephrine effect is decreased heart rate, decreased cardiac output, increased peripheral resistance and increased mean blood pressure. Because of this, norepinephrine and not epinephrine is useful in patients with shock.

2. Effects on Other Systems

On CNS, catecholamines via β receptors activate reticular activating system (RAS) by lowering its threshold and thus lead to arousal and alerting responses producing anxiety, apprehension, and coarse tremors of extremities.

On GIT, epinephrine via β receptors causes relaxation of smooth muscles of wall of the gut decreasing its tone and motility. Via α receptors epinephrine causes contraction of sphincters of gut, the net result is production of constipation.

On Urinary Bladder. Epinephrine produces circumstances conducive for retention of urine by relaxing the detrusor muscles via β receptors and by contracting trigone and sphincters via α receptors.

On Skin. Catecholamines via α receptors act on the pilomotor muscle producing piloerection of hair and by acting on sweat glands of palm and sole, producing localized sweating called adrenergic sweating (e.g. generalized sweating, which is cholinergic).

On Skeletal Muscle. During exercise, epinephrine via β_2 receptors increases blood supply (by causing vasodilation) producing severe contraction and quick fatigue of the skeletal muscles. It also increases glycogenolysis in muscle and releases glucose into circulation.

On Eyes. Epinephrine via α receptors causes dilation of the pupil (mydriasis) by contracting dilator pupillae (radial) muscle; and via β receptors causes relaxation of the ciliary muscle producing flattening of the lens. These effects provide better far vision benefit to the endangered individual.

On Respiration. Epinephrine via β_2 receptors relaxes smooth muscles of bronchioles producing bronchodilation. It also increases rate and force of respiration.

On Blood. Epinephrine produces the following effects:

- *Reduces blood coagulation time* by increasing activity of factor V.
- *Increases RBC count,* haemoglobin content and PCV due to release of RBCs in circulation by causing contraction of spleen.
- *Increases plasma protein concentration* by movement of fluid out of circulation.
- *Neutrophilia* occurs due to release of sequestrated neutrophils into the circulation.

On Secretion of Other Hormones. Catecholamines regulate secretion of a number of hormones:

- *Insulin and somatostatin* secretion is decreased via α_2 receptors (by decreasing cAMP).
- *Glucagon and pancreatic peptide* secretion is increased via β_2 receptors (by increasing cAMP).
- *TRH-induced secretion of TSH* from thyrotrophs is decreased via α_2 receptors (by decreasing cAMP).
- *Thyroid hormone* secretion is enhanced by catecholamines under certain circumstances and peripheral conversion of T_4 to T_3 is stimulated via β_2 receptors.

On Glandular Secretion. Catecholamines cause slight increase in the secretion of *salivary glands* (via α and β_2 receptors), apocrine sweat glands (via β_2 receptors) and lacrimal glands (via α receptors).

On Renin Secretion and Na^+ and K^+ Movement. Catecholamines increase renin secretion by stimulation of β receptors in the kidney. The increase in renin, in turn increases aldosterone secretion, which, in turn enhances sodium retention. This action is augmented by the local catecholamine effects in the kidney on the distribution of blood flow and on renal tubular function.

Influx of potassium into the muscle is stimulated by epinephrine via β_2 receptors. The movement of K^+ into the intracellular space helps to prevent hyperkalaemia.

On nerve fibres. Epinephrine, via α receptors, decreases the latency of action potential in the nerve fibres.

III. Role of Sympathoadrenal System in Various Physiological States

1. Role during Exercise During mild to moderate exercise, mainly the sympathetic nervous system is activated. However, during severe exercise, the adrenal medullary secretion is also increased. Increased sympathoadrenal discharge during exercise plays the following physiological roles:

i. ***Mobilization of stored fuel.*** Catecholamines stimulate:
   - *Glycogenolysis* in muscle for use of glycogen,
   - *Gluconeogenesis* in liver from the lactate that is released by the exercising muscle and
   - *Lipolysis* to provide FFA as alternative fuel which may be required during exercise.

ii. ***Cardiovascular adjustments*** caused by increased sympathoadrenal discharge lead on to massive blood flow to the actively contracting muscles, while maintaining coronary and cerebral blood flow. Increased blood flow is necessary for providing oxygen and fuel (glucose, FFA) for increased muscle metabolism. Adrenergic blockade or autonomic neuropathy impairs cardiovascular responses to exercise and diminishes exercise tolerance.

2. Role during Exposure to Cold Sympathoadrenal system is essential for maintenance of body temperature during exposure to cold. Experimentally, it has been proven that the animals in which both sympathetic nervous system and adrenal glands have been knocked down die because of hypothermia when exposed to cold. However, either the sympathetic nervous system or adrenal medulla is alone incapable of sustaining life. The epinephrine maintains body temperature by conserving body heat, as well as by producing heat:

Heat conservation. During exposure to cold, epinephrine produces constriction of cutaneous vessels and helps to conserve heat. The skin becomes more or less a bloodless sheet of tissue insulating the deeper warmer tissue from the cold environment. Piloerection occurring during exposure to cold in animals with fur or feathers is also mediated through the sympathoadrenal system.

Thermogenesis. The sympathoadrenal system plays an important role in thermogenesis, i.e. heat production by the following mechanisms:

- *Basal metabolic rate (BMR)* is mainly regulated by thyroxine; but epinephrine increases BMR by 7–15%.

- *Nonshivering thermogenesis* is increased by epinephrine. Brown adipose tissue is the site of nonshivering thermogenesis.
- *Chemical thermogenesis* is increased by catecholamines, which in general, stimulates various chemical metabolic processes. For example, catecholamines increase the oxygen consumption beyond that induced by muscular activity. The additional substrate (glucose and FFA) for increased tissue metabolism is provided by catecholamine-induced glycogenolytic and lipolytic actions.

3. Role during Hypoglycaemia Hypoglycaemia is a very potent stimulator of epinephrine secretion from the adrenal medulla, while it does not increase sympathetic neural activity to any significant degree. Plasma epinephrine levels may rise 10- to 50-fold depending upon the severity of hypoglycaemia. By its effects on metabolism described above (page 765), the epinephrine restores plasma glucose levels and glucose delivery to the central nervous system.

An Integrated Response to Stress

Stress, may it be emotional, physical or biological, evokes an integrated response of the sympathoadrenal medullary system and hypothalamic–pituitary–adrenal cortex axis.

Steps involved in stress adaptation by an integrated response of the above system are (Fig. 8.5-28):

Perception of Stress Signals. Stress is perceived by many areas of the brain, from the cortex down to the brainstem including limbic system and reticular-activating system (RAS).

Stimulation of Hypothalamus. Major stresses activate the CRH and ADH neurons in the paraventricular nucleus and adrenergic neurons.

Activation of Hypothalamic–pituitary–adrenal Axis. CRH and ADH release stimulates ACTH release and ultimately elevates plasma cortisol levels.

Activation of Sympathoadrenal Medullary System. Sudden exposure to any type of stress initially produces the sympathetic alarm reaction. Stimulation of adrenergic neurons of hypothalamus ultimately leads to release of epinephrine from adrenal medulla and norepinephrine from the sympathetic ganglia.

Integrated Role of Hormones Released by Hypothalamic–pituitary–adrenal Axis and Sympathoadrenal Medullary System in Stress Adaptation. Together, these hormones help in adaptation to stress by their following actions:

- ***Increase in glucose production.*** Catecholamines rapidly raise plasma glucose by activating glycogenolysis, and cortisol acts more slowly by providing amino acid substrate for gluconeogenesis. Together, they shift glucose utilization towards the central nervous system away from peripheral tissues.
- ***Free fatty acid supply.*** Epinephrine rapidly augments the supply of free fatty acids to the heart and the muscles, and cortisol facilitates the lipolytic role.
- ***Cardiovascular adjustments.*** Catecholamines and cortisol raise blood pressure and cardiac output, and they improve the delivery of substrates to tissues that are critical to the immediate defence of the organism.
- ***Arousal, defensively useful behavioural activation and focussed attention*** result from the adrenergic stimuli to the pertinent brain centres.
- ***Inhibition of activities that are not useful during stress and divert individuals and their resources from defensive responses to danger*** is an important part of adaptation to stress. For example, CRH input to hypothalamic neurons inhibits growth hormone, gonadotropin release and sexual activity. These actions are reinforced by excess of cortisol. In addition, CRH inhibits appetite and feeding behaviour, which are also inappropriate when the individual is facing immediate danger.
- ***Interaction with immune system.*** The hormones produced during stress interact with the immune system to produce a balance between useful local cytokine production at threatened or impenled sites and potentially dangerous systemic effects of these immune system products.

Diseases of Adrenal Medulla

Phaeochromocytoma

Phaeochromocytoma is a rare benign tumour arising from the epinephrine- and norepinephrine-secreting chromaffin cells of adrenal medulla.

Clinical Features are produced by the excess of epinephrine and norepinephrine and include:

- Episodic or nonepisodic hypertension with postural drop.
- Attacks of tachycardia, palpitation, sweating, pallor, headache and chest discomfort.
- Abdominal pain, vomiting, constipation and glucose intolerance.
- Weight loss and weakness.

Tests for Phaeochromocytoma include:

- *24 h urinary excretion* of vanillyl mandelic acid (VMA), metanephrines and catecholamines is increased.
- *Plasma epinephrine* and norepinephrine levels are elevated.
- *Phentolamine suppression test,* i.e. 2.5 mg of phentolamine does not suppress plasma catecholamine at 10 min sample.
- *CT scan and radionuclide studies* to localize any tumour.

Treatment of phaeochromocytoma is surgical excision. However, medical treatment is necessary before and after the surgery, as well as in inoperable cases. Both alpha and beta adrenoreceptor blockers, e.g. labetalol, or combination of phenoxy benzamine and propranolol are used to control hypertension.

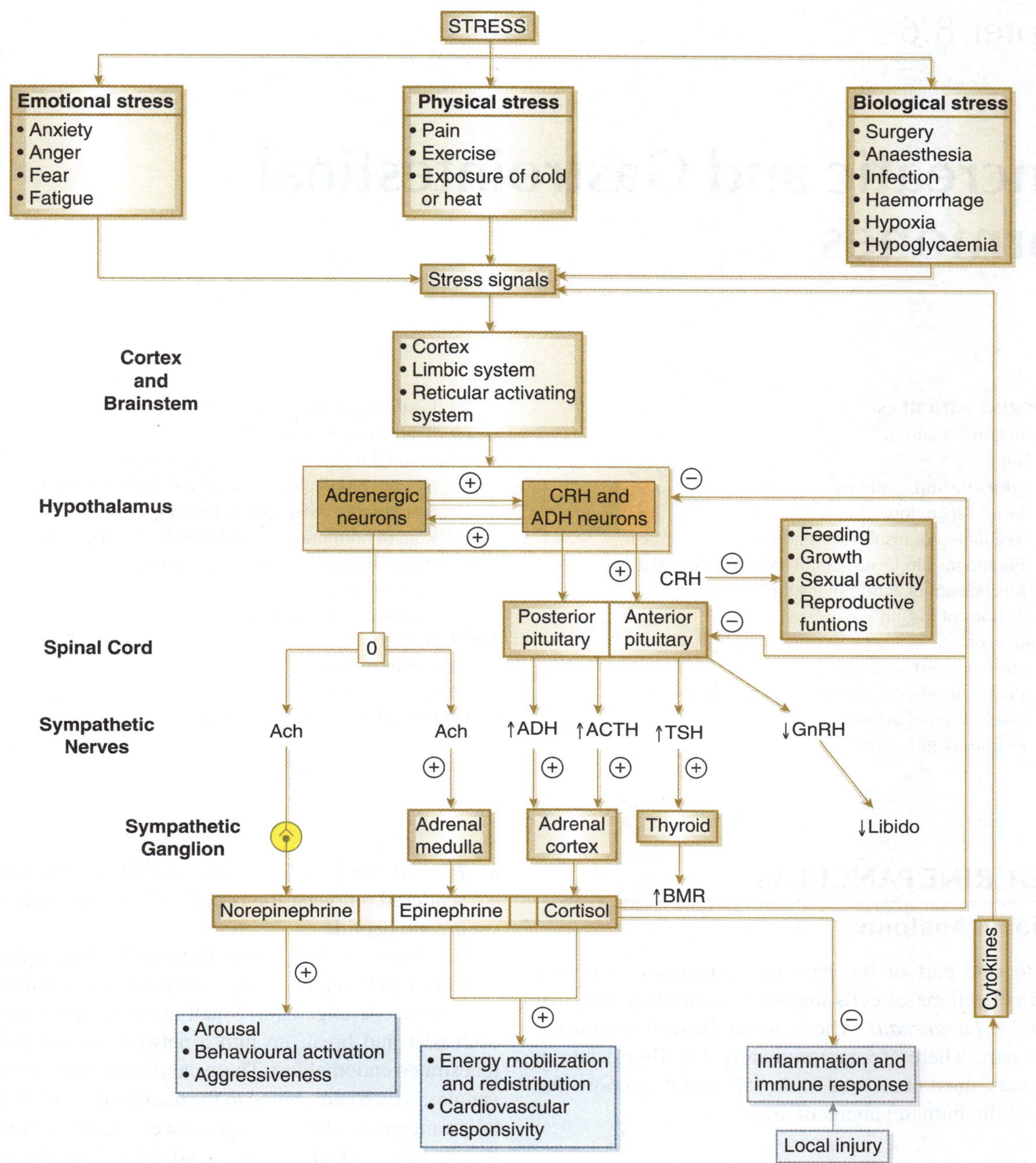

FIGURE 8.5-28 Steps involved in the adaptation to stress by an integrated response of hypothalamic–pituitary–adrenal cortex axis and sympathoadrenal medullary system.

Chapter 8.6

Pancreatic and Gastrointestinal Hormones

ENDOCRINE PANCREAS

Functional Anatomy

The endocrine part of the pancreas comprises numerous rounded collections of cells known as *pancreatic islets* or the *islets of Langerhans*. These are embedded within the exocrine part. There are approximately 1 million islets in the pancreas, most numerous in the tail, and they constitute 1–1.5% of the human pancreatic mass.

Islets of Langerhans The islets are very richly supplied with blood through dense capillary plexus (as in all ductless glands) and innervated by vagal and sympathetic fibres.

Cellular Structure. Each islet contains, an average, 2500 cells which are of four types and arranged as (Fig. 8.6-1):

- *Beta* (β) cells or B cells make up 60–70% of the total cells, and constitute the central core of the islet. These cells secrete insulin.
- *Alpha* (α) cells or A cells form about 20% of the total cells and constitute the outer rim of the islet. These cells secrete glucagon.
- *Delta* (δ) cells or D cells form about 10% of total cells and are intermixed. These are source of somatostatin.
- *PP cells or F cells.* These are also peripherally placed scattered amongst the α cells. These are source of pancreatic peptide.

Gap Junctions link beta cells to each other, alpha cells to each other and beta cells to alpha cells for rapid communication.

Vascular Arrangement. Small arterioles enter the core of each islet and break up into a network of capillaries with fenestrated endothelium. These capillaries then converge into venules, which carry blood to the mantle of the islet. This portal arrangement allows a high concentration of insulin from β cells core, so bathe the α, δ and PP cells of the respective mantles. This type of vascular pattern also suggests the possible paracrine effects of insulin on the other islet cell types.

Pancreatic Islets Have Strategic Location. The proximity of islets to pancreatic acini (of exocrine part) permits them to have local effects on exocrine pancreatic function. Islet hormones are secreted into the pancreatic vein and then into the portal vein, where they join the nutrient stream after meals. This arrangement preferentially exposes the liver, which is the central organ in substrate traffic, to islet hormone concentrations higher than those the peripheral tissues receive. In addition, the liver can extract variable amounts of insulin and glucagon on their first pass through this organ. In this manner, the liver can modulate the hormone's availability to other tissues.

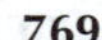

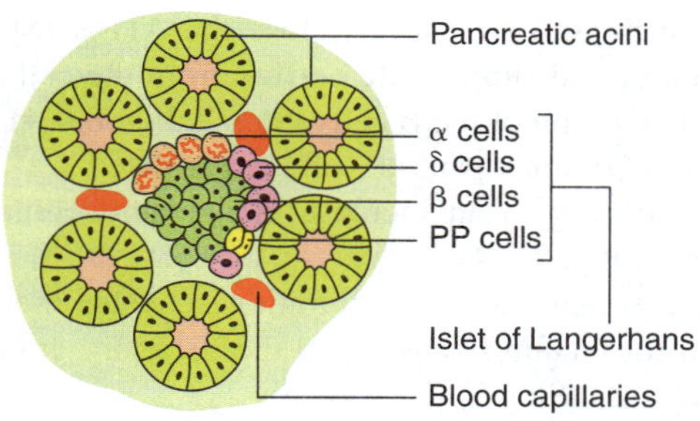

FIGURE 8.6-1 Schematic histological structure of pancreas showing an islet of Langerhans surrounded by exocrine pancreatic acini.

Insulin

Insulin is a polypeptide hormone secreted by the β cells of islets of Langerhans of pancreas. Historically, insulin has several firsts to its credit:

- It was the first hormone to be isolated, purified, crystallized and synthesized.
- The first protein detected to possess hormonal activity.
- The first protein sequences for amino acids to determine the structure.
- The first protein estimated by radioimmunoassay.
- The first protein produced by recombinant DNA technology.

Structure and Biosynthesis

Structure. The human insulin is a protein containing 51 amino acids, arranged in two polypeptide chains: A (having 21 amino acids) and B (having 30 amino acids). These chains are connected to each other by two interchain disulphide linkages, connecting A7 to B7 and A_{20} to B_{19}. In addition, there is an intrachain disulphide link in chain A between amino acids 6 and 11 (Fig. 8.6-2). If the two chains are split apart, functional activity of insulin is lost.

Biosynthesis of Insulin. Beta cells of islets of Langerhans synthesize insulin by the usual protein synthetic machinery. The steps involved are (Fig. 8.6-3):

- The insulin gene (located on chromosome 11) directs the synthesis of *preproinsulin*, an insulin precursor consisting of 108 amino acids with a molecular weight of 11,500.
  - Preproinsulin is cleaved to form *proinsulin* having 86 amino acids and a molecular weight of 9000.
- As the *proinsulin molecule*, containing the A and B chain of insulin and connecting peptide (C-peptide), is guided to Golgi apparatus, disulphide linkages are established to yield the *folded proinsulin* molecule.
- Proinsulin is further cleaved in Golgi apparatus to form the *active hormone insulin* and a connecting peptide (C-peptide).

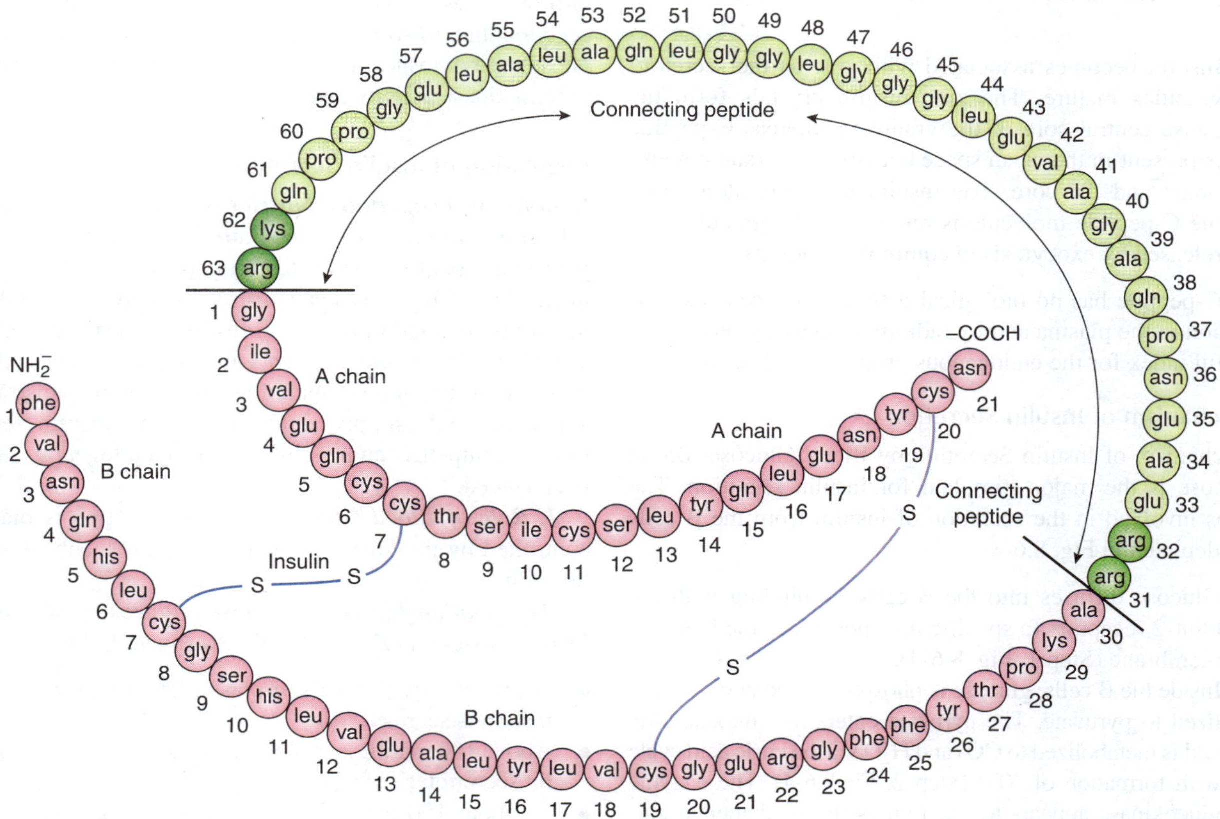

FIGURE 8.6-2 Structure of an insulin molecule.

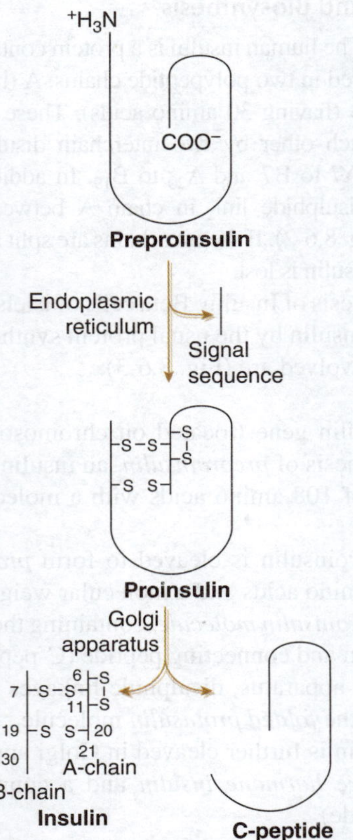

FIGURE 8.6-3 Steps in the synthesis of insulin.

- Insulin becomes associated with zinc as the secretory granules mature. The zinc–insulin crystals form the dense central core of the granules, whereas C-peptide is present in the clean space between the granule membrane and the core. The insulin molecule along with the C-peptide molecule is retained in the granules and released by exocytosis in equimolar amounts.

C-peptide has no biological activity; however, its estimation in the plasma and by radioimmunoassay serves as a useful index for the endogenous production of insulin.

Mechanism of Insulin Secretion

Mechanism of Insulin Secretion by Blood Glucose. Blood glucose is the major stimulant for insulin secretion. The steps involved in the secretion of insulin from the β cells are depicted in Fig. 8.6-4:

- Glucose diffuses into the β cells by binding with the Glut-2 receptors (a specific transporter) on the beta cell membrane (Step 1, Fig. 8.6-4).
- Inside the β cells, glucose is phosphorylated and metabolized to pyruvate. The pyruvate enters the mitochondria and is metabolized to CO_2 and H_2O via the citric acid cycle with formation of ATP (Step 2, Fig.8.6-4). The enzyme glucokinase appears to function as the fundamental glucose sensor that controls the subsequent β cell response.
- The increased ATP levels close the ATP-sensitive K^+ channels and suppress K^+ efflux from the cell causing depolarization of the β cells (Step 3, Fig. 8.6-4).
- Depolarization opens a voltage-regulated Ca^{2+} channels, leading to an increase in the intracellular Ca^{2+} (Step 4, Fig. 8.6-4).
- The elevated Ca^{2+} concentration activates the mechanism for insulin release from the secretory granules by exocytosis (Step 5, Fig. 8.6-4).
- Via the citric acid cycle, pyruvate metabolism also causes an increase in intracellular glutamate. Glutamate also causes release of insulin from secretory granules; this is reason for prolonged second phase of release of insulin in response to glucose.

Mechanism of Insulin Secretion by Fuels Other than Glucose

- A sequence similar to glucose, with specific transporters and enzymatic steps, probably underlies the less prominent stimulation action of other fuels, such as amino acids, ketoacids and fatty acids (Step 6, Fig. 8.6-4).

Mechanism of Insulin Secretion by Glucagon. Glucagon mediates insulin releasing effect by stimulator G (Gs) protein via cyclic AMP. Whereas, inhibitory G proteins mediate the insulin suppressive effects of peptides such as somatostatin (Step 7, Fig. 8.6-4).

Mechanism of Insulin Secretion by Acetylcholine. G-protein linked to phospholipase C mediates the ability of acetylcholine to stimulate insulin release via generation of phosphatidylinositol (IP_3), second messenger and increased protein kinase activity (Step 8, Fig. 8.6-4).

Regulation of Insulin Secretion

I. Role of Exogenous Nutrients Exogenous nutrients (glucose, amino acids, free fatty acids, ketoacids and potassium) control insulin secretion by a feedback mechanism (Fig. 8.6-5). When substrate supply is abundant, insulin is secreted in response. Insulin then stimulates the use of these incoming nutrients and simultaneously inhibits the mobilization of analogous endogenous substrates. When nutrients supply is low or absent, insulin secretion is dampened and mobilization of endogenous fuels is enhanced.

1. Role of Blood Glucose. Insulin secretion is mainly controlled by the level of blood glucose by feedback relationship.

The relationship between plasma glucose and plasma insulin is sigmoidal (Fig. 8.6-6). As shown in Fig. 8.6-6:

- Below 50 mg/dL levels of plasma glucose, virtually no insulin is secreted.
- Above 100 mg/dL levels of plasma glucose, rate of insulin secretion rises rapidly.
- At about 150 mg/dL levels of plasma glucose, a half-maximal insulin secretory response is obtained.

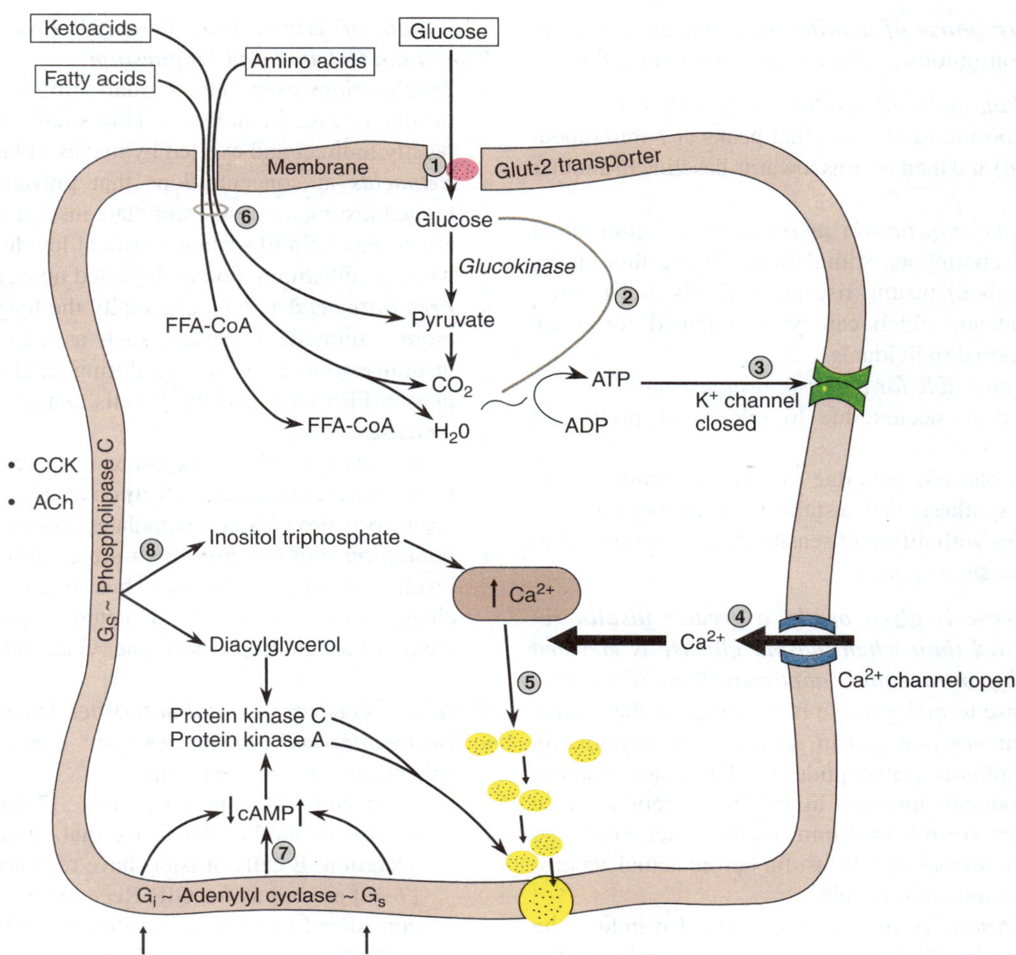

FIGURE 8.6-4 Steps of mechanism of insulin secretion by different stimulants such as glucose (Steps 1 to 5), other fuels (Step 6), peptides such as glucagon (Step 7) and acetylcholine (Step-8).

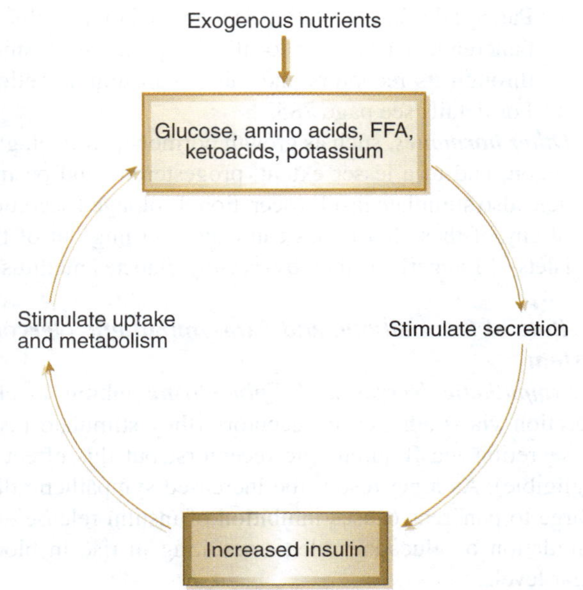

FIGURE 8.6-5 Feedback control of insulin release by exogenous nutrients.

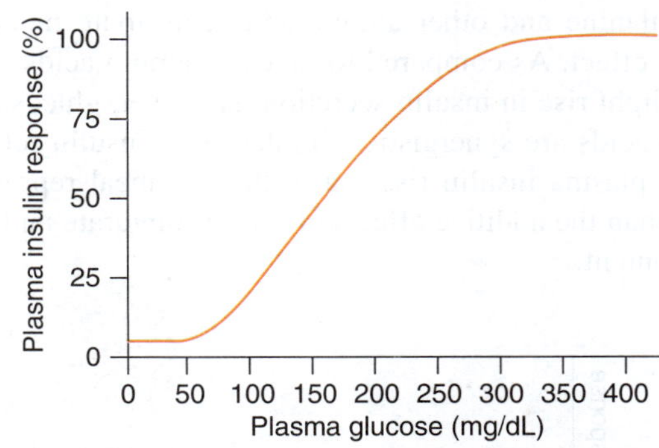

FIGURE 8.6-6 A sigmoidal relationship between levels of plasma glucose and insulin secretion response.

- At a level of about 300 mg/dL, a maximal insulin response occurs.

The rapidly increased insulin secretion above 100 mg/dL levels of plasma glucose in turn reduces blood glucose concentration to fasting level. Reduction of blood glucose causes rapid turning off of insulin secretion (feedback relationship).

Biphasic response of insulin secretion occurs in response to a continuous glucose stimulation (Fig. 8.6-7):

- *An immediate pulse of insulin* is released, within seconds of exposure to glucose, that peaks at 1 min (about 10-fold rise) and then returns towards baseline in another 5–10 min.
- *A second phase of insulin secretion* begins after about 10 min of continuous stimulation. During this phase, plasma levels of insulin rise more slowly and reach a second plateau, which can be maintained for many hours in normal individuals.
  Factors responsible for biphasic response are:
  - Initial peak occurs due to release of preformed insulin.
  - Second phase occurs due to glucose stimulation of insulin synthesis that sustains the secretory phase.
  - Granules with different sensitivity also contribute to the biphasic response.

When glucose is given orally, a greater insulin response is elicited than when plasma glucose is elevated comparably by intravenous administration. This augmented response to oral glucose is attributed to the gastrointestinal hormones like gastrin, secretin, cholecystokinin and gastric inhibitory polypeptide, i.e. GIP (most potent), that cause moderate increase in insulin secretion. Since these hormones are released immediately after meals, so they cause anticipatory rise of insulin before actual absorption of glucose and amino acids.

2. Role of Amino Acids. Amino acids also induce the secretion of insulin. This is particularly observed after the ingestion of protein-rich meal that causes transient rise in plasma amino acid concentration. The basic amino acids, arginine and lysine, are the most potent stimulants; leucine, alanine and other amino acids contribute modestly to this effect. As compared to glucose, amino acids cause only slight rise in insulin secretion. However, glucose and amino acids are synergistic stimulators of insulin release, so the plasma insulin rise that follows a meal represents more than the additive effects of its carbohydrate and protein content.

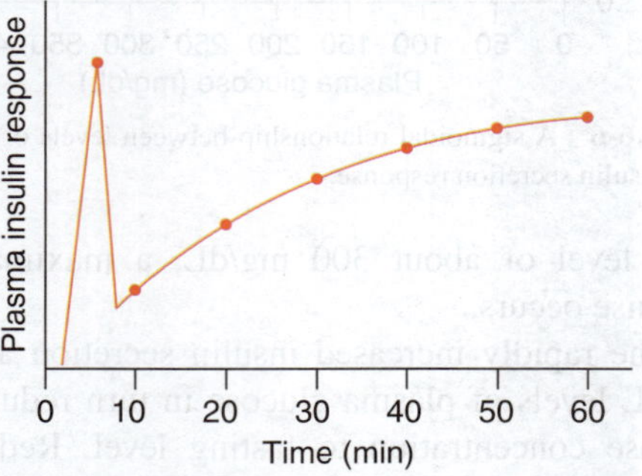

FIGURE 8.6-7 Biphasic insulin response to glucose infusion consists of first phase of rapid release and fall followed by second phase of slow rise.

3. Role of Triglyceride, Ketoacid, Free Fatty Acids, Potassium, Calcium and Magnesium

- ***Tryglycerides*** exert only a small stimulatory effect on insulin release in humans. This small effect may be mostly indirect and exerted by means of GIP.
- ***Ketoacids*** at concentrations that prevail during prolonged fasting modestly stimulate insulin secretion; this effect may help to sustain a critical low level of insulin when β cell stimulation by ingested nutrients is absent.
- ***Free fatty acids*** (FFA), especially the longer chain and more saturated molecules, such as stearate, enhance insulin response to glucose during total fasting when plasma FFA rises and the β cells content of FFA-CoA increases.

  However, long-term exposure of β cells to elevated FFA can have deleterious effects on insulin secretion. This occurs because FFA also stimulates apoptosis of β cells.
- ***Potassium and calcium,*** both are essential for normal insulin response to glucose. Thus, relative insulin deficiency occurs in subjects depleted of potassium, calcium or the calcitropic hormone, vitamin D.

II. Role of Gastrointestinal and other Hormones

- ***Gastrointestinal hormones,*** as mentioned above, enhance the insulin secretion:
  - Glucagon- like polypeptide-1 [7-36] or (GLP-[7-36]) is another gut factor that stimulates insulin secretion. B cells of islets have receptors for GLP-1 [7-36] as well as for GIP. Recently, GLP-1 [7-36] is considered to be more insulinotropic hormone than GIP. They act by increasing Ca^{2+} influx through voltage-gated Ca^{2+} channels.
  - Glucagon also stimulates insulin secretion and pancreatic somatostatin.
  - Pancreatic somatostatin, secreted from D cells of pancreatic islets, acts locally by paracrine fashion through its receptors and inhibits insulin secretion. For details see page 785.
- ***Other hormones,*** such as growth hormone, cortisol, glucagon, and to a lesser extent, progesterone and oestrogen, also stimulate insulin secretion. Prolonged secretion of any of these hormones can cause burning out of the islets of Langerhans thereby causing diabetes mellitus.

III. Role of Sympathetic and Parasympathetic Nervous System

Sympathetic Nerves and Epinephrine inhibit insulin secretion via α-adrenergic receptors (they stimulate insulin secretion via β-adrenergic receptors; but this effect is negligible). As a net result, the increased sympathetic discharge to pancreas causes inhibition of insulin release and stimulation of glucagon release resulting in rise in blood sugar level.

Epinephrine is the most predominant inhibitor of insulin release. In emergency situations like stress, extreme exercise and trauma, the nervous system stimulates the adrenal medulla to release epinephrine. The epinephrine suppresses insulin release and promotes energy-yielding compounds—glucose from liver and fatty acids from adipose tissue.

Parasympathetic Nerves to Pancreas and Acetylcholine (ACh) increase insulin secretion to some extent; ACh stimulates insulin release via generation of phosphatidylinositol second messenger (Step 8 in Fig. 8.6-4). Some of the important factors stimulating and inhibiting insulin secretion are depicted in Table 8.6-1.

Plasma Insulin Levels, Circulation and Degradation

Plasma Levels of Insulin

- Average basal peripheral plasma insulin level is 10 μU/ml.
- After several days of fasting, basal plasma levels of insulin decline over 50%, i.e. become less than 5 μU/ml.
- After prolonged exercise, the plasma insulin levels fall.
- A 3- to 10-fold increase in plasma insulin level is noted after a typical meal. The peak occurs after 30–60 min of initiating the meal.
- Although C-peptide is secreted in amounts that are equimolar to insulin, its basal peripheral plasma levels are approximately fivefold higher, averaging 1 ng/ml. This difference is caused by a lower rate of metabolic clearance for C-peptide.

Rate and Total Amount of Insulin Secretion per Day

- Basal insulin delivery rates to the peripheral circulation in humans are about 0.5–1.25 unit/ h (20–40 μg/h).
- During meals, the delivery rate increases up to 10-fold.
- Total daily peripheral delivery of insulin is about 30 units.

TABLE 8.6-1 Factors Stimulating and Inhibiting Insulin Secretion

Factors stimulating insulin secretion	Factors inhibiting insulin secretion
• ↑ Blood glucose	• ↑ Blood glucose
• ↑ Amino acids (leucine and arginine)	• Somatostatin
• ↑ Fatty acids	• Norepinephrine, epinephrine
• Glucagon	• Galanin
• Intestinal hormones (GIP, GLP-1 [7-36], gastrin, secretin, CCK and others)	• K^+ depletion
• ACh	• Alloxan
• Growth hormones, cortisol	

- If the amount of insulin removed during its first pass through the liver is accounted for (~50% of portal vein insulin), the actual β cell secretory rate becomes approximately 2.5 units/h (60 units/day).

Cycles of Insulin Secretion In addition to the intrinsic low level, 15-min cycles and the brush off insulin secretion stimulated by meals, a higher amplitude insulin cycle exists. This cycle has pulses lasting 2 h that are entrained by glucose and that represent feedback regulation.

The β cell cyclic response (represented by fluctuations in insulin and C-peptide plasma levels) is exaggerated in obesity (Fig. 8.6-8).

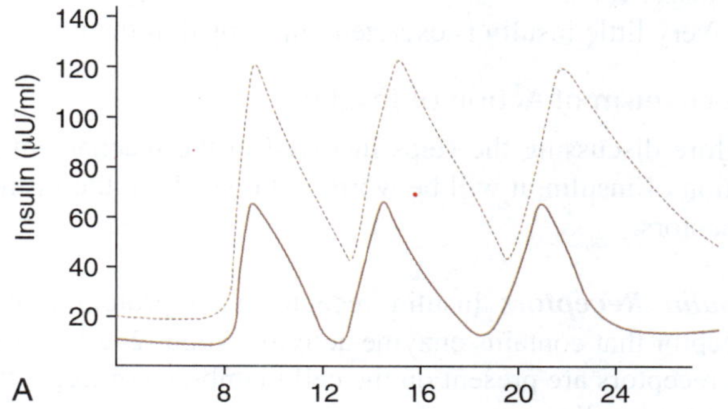

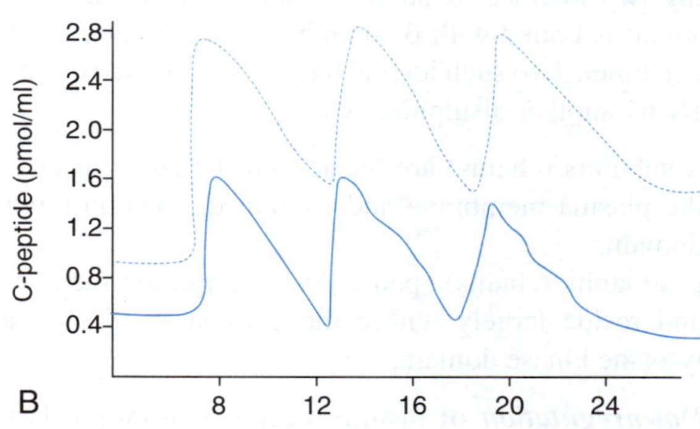

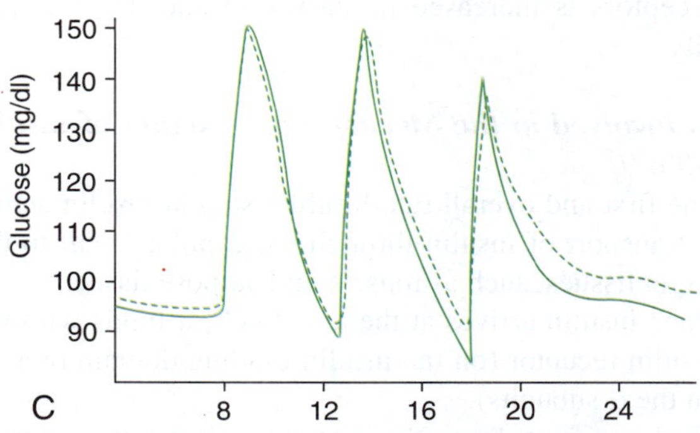

FIGURE 8.6-8 Cyclic response of insulin **(A)**, C-peptide **(B)** and fluctuations of blood glucose level **(C)** observed during 24-h profile in a normal weight (solid lines) and in an obese (dotted line) human.

Circulation and Degradation of Insulin

- *Insulin circulates* unbound to any carrier protein.
- *Half-life of insulin* in plasma is 5–18 min.

Short half-life permits rapid metabolic changes in accordance to the alterations in the circulating level of insulin. This is advantageous for the therapeutic purposes.

- *Metabolic clearance rate* of insulin is about 1000 ml/min.
- A protease enzyme, namely, *insulinase* (mainly found in the kidneys and liver) degrades insulin. It splits the disulphide bonds and separates the A and B chains.
- Degradation of insulin also occurs in association with its plasma membrane receptors after it is internalized by target cells.
- Very little insulin is excreted unchanged in the urine.

Mechanism of Action of Insulin

Before discussing the steps involved in the mechanism of action of insulin, it will be worth to know about the insulin receptors.

Insulin Receptors Insulin receptor is a protein kinase receptor that contains enzyme activity. About 2–3 lac insulin receptors are present on the cell membrane of target tissues for insulin.

Structure (Fig. 8.6-9). The insulin receptor is a tetramer having two identical α subunits and two β subunits. One α subunit is bound with β subunit by a disulphide bond to form a dimer. Two such identical dimers are joined extracellularly by another disulphide bond.

- α subunits (chains) are located on the outer surface of the plasma membrane and contain the insulin-binding domain.
- β subunits (chains) span across the plasma membrane and reside largely within the cytoplasm. These have tyrosine kinase domain.

Downregulation of insulin receptors in target tissues is caused by insulin itself. Therefore, the number of insulin receptors is increased in starvation and decreased in obesity.

Steps Involved in the Mechanism of Action of Insulin (Fig. 8.6-9)

- The first and overall rate-limiting step in insulin action is transport of insulin through the capillary wall to the target tissues, such as muscle and adipose tissue.
- Once insulin arrives at the target cell, it binds with the insulin receptor (on the insulin-binding domain present on the α subunits).
- Binding of insulin to the α-chain activates the tyrosine kinase activity of the β-chains. The activated tyrosine kinase then autophosphorylates the β-chains.

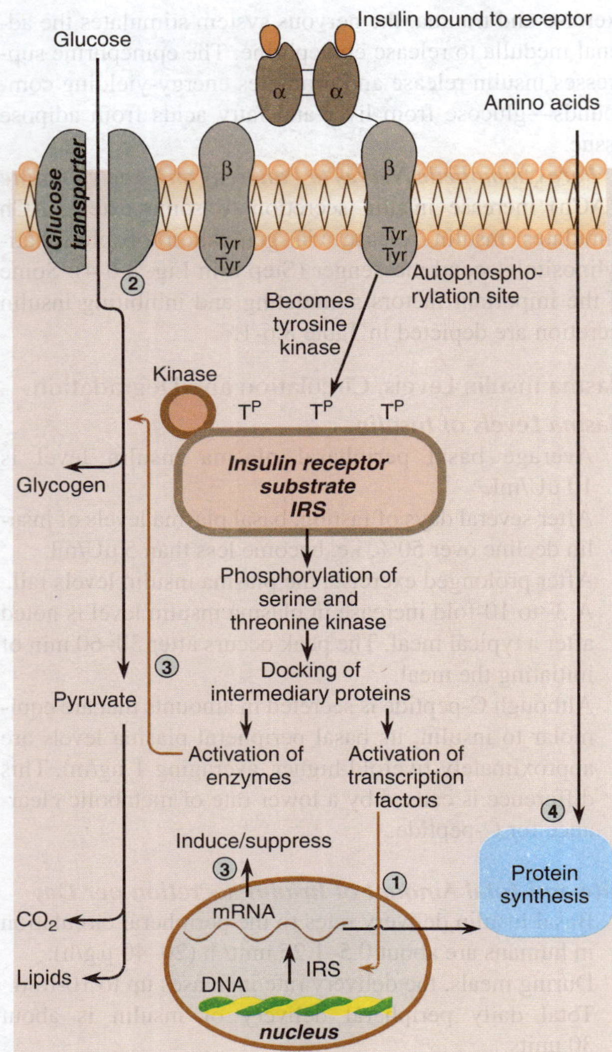

FIGURE 8.6-9 Structure of insulin receptor and mechanism of insulin action on target cell. Note the activity of insulin receptor which ultimately produces following effects of insulin on target cell: (1) Gene expression; (2) translocation of glucose transporters from cytoplasm to plasma membrane; (3) activation or deactivation of various enzymes of glucose and fatty acids metabolism; and (4) protein synthesis through increased mRNAs.

- The phosphorylated receptor then phosphorylates tyrosine residues on intracellular protein substrate or insulin receptor substrates (IRS).
- The IRS tyrosine phosphorylations are followed by various cascades of events that ultimately produce the following effects:

1. Gene Expression in the nucleus of target cell leading to biological action.

2. Translocation of Glucose Transport Proteins to the Plasma Membrane. The glucose transporters are responsible for the insulin-mediated uptake of glucose by the cells. As the insulin levels fall, the glucose transporters move away from the membrane to the intracellular pool for storage and recycle.

3. Activation or Deactivation of Numerous Enzymes in glucose and fatty acid metabolism is brought about by increased mRNAs.

4. Protein Synthesis. Increased mRNA synthesis (transcription) is followed by translation (protein synthesis). In this way, insulin promotes synthesis of enzymes such as glucokinase, phosphofructokinase and pyruvate kinase.

Note. Individuals with 'insulin-resistant' diabetes secrete insulin normally, but their tissues do not respond to their own insulin or the injected insulin. In some of these cases, there is a mutation in the tyrosine kinase domain of the insulin receptor. Insulin binds normally to the mutant receptors, but the tyrosine kinase is inactive, and the downstream consequences of insulin binding do not occur.

Actions of Insulin

The physiologic effects of insulin are divided into rapid, intermediate and delayed actions (Table 8.6-2). The main effects include:

A. Metabolic effects,
B. Effects on ion transport and
C. Role in cell growth and development.

A. Metabolic Effects of Insulin

Insulin plays a key role in the metabolism of carbohydrate, lipids and proteins. The major targets for insulin action are the muscle mass, the liver and adipose tissue.

1. Effects on Carbohydrate Metabolism. In a normal individual, about half (50%) of the ingested glucose is utilized to meet the energy demands of the body (mainly through glycolysis). The other half is either converted to fat (~40%) or glycogen (~10%). This relation is maintained by insulin and is thus severely impaired in insulin deficiency.

TABLE 8.6-2 Principal Effects of Insulin

Rapid (s)
Transportation of glucose, amino acids and fatty acids into the insulin-sensitive cells
Intermediate (min)
(i) Protein synthesis/stimulation
(ii) Inhibition of protein degradation
(iii) Activation of glycolytic enzymes
(iv) Inhibition of phosphorylase and gluconeogenesis
Delayed (h)
Increase mRNA for lipogenic enzyme

As a Net Effect, Insulin Decreases Blood Glucose Concentration by the following mechanisms:

1. ***Insulin increases uptake of glucose in target cells*** by translocating the glucose transporter into the cell membranes.
   - Insulin is required for the uptake of glucose by muscles (skeletal, cardiac and smooth), adipose tissue, leucocytes and mammary glands.
   - Tissues in which glucose transport is not insulin dependent include nervous tissue, kidney, RBC, retina, blood vessels and intestinal mucosa. This property is of critical importance in the nervous system because glucose is the only source of energy and insulin is presented in the blood for about 2 h after each meal. Since transport of glucose into nervous tissue depends on blood glucose level only, therefore, severe hypoglycaemia results in convulsion, coma or even death.
   - Insulin is not required for entry of glucose in hepatocytes (liver); however, insulin-mediated increased utilization indirectly promotes its uptake.
2. ***Insulin promotes glucose utilization***
   - *Glycolysis* (oxidation of glucose) is increased in muscle and liver by insulin.
   - *Glycogen* formation from glucose in muscle and liver is promoted by insulin.
3. ***Insulin decreases glucose production*** by inhibiting:
   - Gluconeogenesis and
   - Glycogenolysis.

Effects of Insulin on Carbohydrate Metabolism in Target Tissues: Liver, Muscle and Adipose Tissue

i. ***Effects on liver*** (Fig. 8.6-10, 8.6-11).
   - ***Increase in glucose uptake.*** Insulin increases the activity of enzyme *glucokinase* which enhances glucose utilization by catalysing its phosphorylation (Fig. 8.6-11). Thus, indirectly, insulin increases glucose uptake by increasing its utilization. In the liver, extracellular glucose levels equilibrate rapidly with intracellular levels by means of Glut-2 transporter (Fig. 8.6-11).
   - ***Promotion of glycogen synthesis.*** Insulin promotes storage of glucose as glycogen by activating the *glycogen synthase enzyme* complex.
   - ***Glycolysis*** is promoted by insulin through activation of enzymes phosphofructokinase and pyruvate kinase.
   - ***Glycogenolysis*** is inhibited by insulin by decreasing glycogen phosphorylase activity and also by decreasing glucose-6-phosphatase levels.
   - ***Gluconeogenesis*** is inhibited by insulin by decreasing the hepatic uptake of precursor amino acids and their availability from muscle (Fig. 8.6-10). Insulin also decreases the levels or activities of the committed gluconeogenetic enzymes, namely, pyruvate

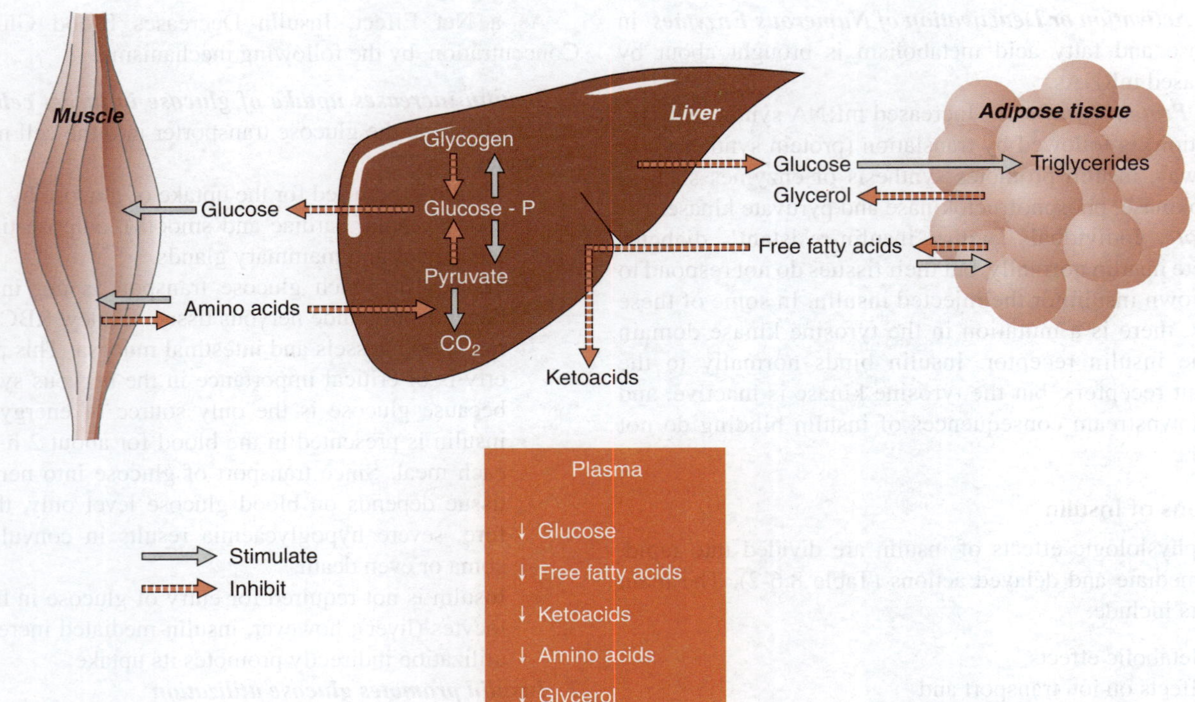

FIGURE 8.6-10 Schematic diagram to illustrate metabolic effects of insulin on carbohydrate (glucose), fats (free fatty acids) and protein (amino acids) resulting in tissue uptake and decrease in plasma levels of substrates.

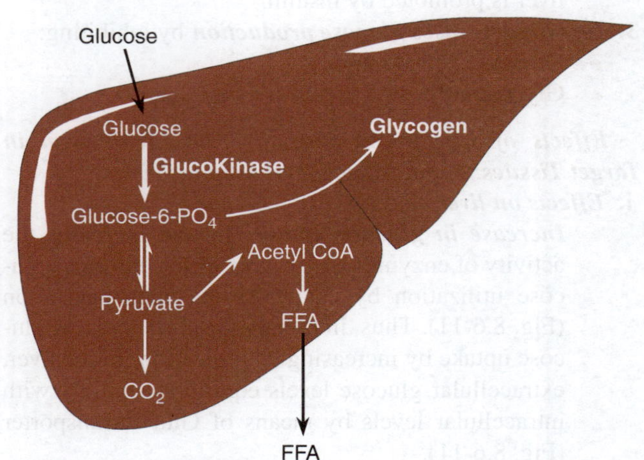

FIGURE 8.6-11 Effects of insulin on carbohydrate metabolism in liver.

carboxylase, phosphoenol pyruvate carboxykinase and fructose-1, 6 biphosphatase. Thus, pyruvate is shunted towards acetyl-CoA which in turn is directed into synthesis of free fatty acids (Fig. 8.6-11).

ii. ***Effects on muscles*** (Fig. 8.6-10, 8.6-12).

- ***Increase in glucose uptake.*** Under resting state, the muscle membrane takes in glucose only during a few hours after meals. This is due to increased amount of insulin secreted after meals. Insulin increases the permeability of muscle membrane for glucose by 10–20-fold by translocating the glucose transporter

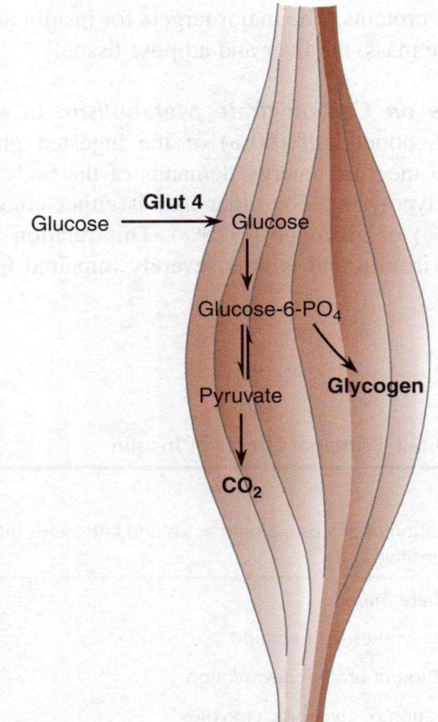

FIGURE 8.6-12 Effects of insulin on carbohydrate metabolism in muscle.

(Glut-4). However, during exercise, permeability of muscle membrane to glucose increases even in the absence of insulin. This is the reason that diabetics are advised regular moderate exercise.

- ***Increase in glycolysis.*** Depending on the insulin concentration, 20–50% of glucose that enters the muscle cell undergoes oxidation, mainly caused by the activation of pyruvate dehydrogenase (Fig. 8.6-12).

Increase in glycogen synthesis. The remainder glucose is deposited as muscle glycogen by insulin activation of glycogen synthase (Fig. 8.6-12).

iii. ***Effects on adipose tissue*** (Fig. 8.6-10, 8.6-13).

- Glucose transport into the adipose tissue cells is stimulated by insulin by translocating the glucose transporter (Glut-4).
- Much of the glucose entering the cells is converted into α-glycerophosphate, which is used in the esterification of fatty acids and permits their storage as triglycerides (Fig. 8.6-13).
- To a minor extent, glucose can also be converted to fatty acids (Fig. 8.6-13).

Glucose transporters. Depending on the transport mechanisms, glucose transporters are of two types:

- ***Sodium-dependent glucose transporters (SGLT1 and SGLT$_2$)*** are responsible for secondary active transport of glucose with sodium ions mainly in the intestine and renal tubules (for details, see page 647 and 510).
- ***Glucose transporters (GLUTs)*** by which glucose enters the cell by facilitated diffusion are further of seven different types named GLUT 1–7 in order of their discovery. Each transporter has been assigned for a special task. Depending on insulin sensitivity of the cells, these GLUTs are:
  - Insulin-sensitive GLUTs: (e.g. GLUT-4) and
  - Noninsulin-sensitive GLUTs: other GLUTs are no insulin sensitive.

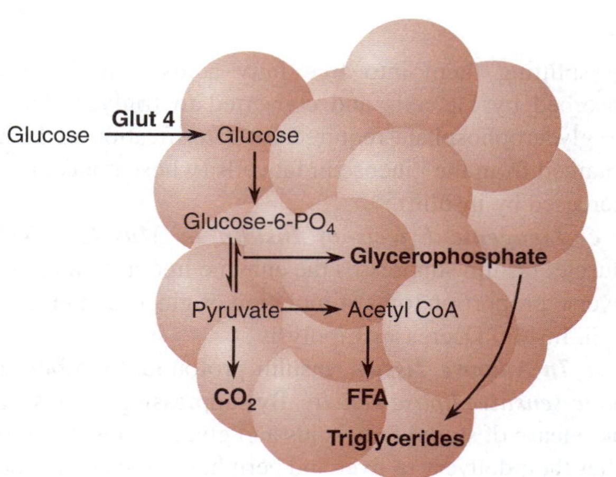

FIGURE 8.6-13 Effects of insulin on carbohydrate metabolism in adipose tissue.

Mechanism of action

- GLUT-4 transporter, present in the muscle and adipose tissue, is stimulated by insulin.
- The molecules of GLUT-4 are present in the cytoplasmic vesicles of insulin-sensitive cells.
  - When insulin receptors of these cells get activated, the vesicles containing GLUT-4 move rapidly towards plasma membrane and fuse with it (insertion of transporter).
  - Activation of insulin receptors causes movement of vesicles to cell membrane by activating phosphatidyl inositol-3 kinase.
  - On cessation of insulin activity, the cell membrane patches containing glucose transporter are endocytosed and ready for next exposure to insulin.
  - Insulin-sensitive tissues also contain GLUT-4 vesicles that move towards cell membrane in response to exercise (insulin-independent GLUT-4). The action of these receptors is triggered by A-5' AMP-activated kinase.
  - The specific functions and major sites of expression of glucose transporter have been summarized in Table 8.6-3.

2. Effects on Lipid Metabolism. The metabolism of both endogenous and exogenous fat is profoundly influenced by insulin.

The net overall effect is to enhance storage and to block mobilization and oxidation of fatty acids by:

- Favouring lipogenesis,
- Decreasing lipolysis and
- Reducing ketogenesis.

Effects of insulin on lipid metabolism in target tissues: liver, adipose tissue and muscle

i. Insulin Increases Lipogenesis

a. Lipogenic Effects on Liver (Fig. 8.6-10, 8.6-14). *Triglycerides synthesis.* When insulin and carbohydrates are available, liver is quantitatively a more important site of fat synthesis than the adipose tissue. As described in effects of insulin on carbohydrate metabolism, insulin promotes storage of glucose as glycogen in the liver cells. However, when glycogen concentration increases to 5–6%, glycogenesis is inhibited and the additional glucose entering is converted to fat in the liver cells.

- First glucose is split to pyruvate (in glycolytic pathway) and pyruvate is converted to acetyl-CoA which is a substrate for fatty acid synthesis.
- Increased citrate and isocitrate formed by citric acid cycle (when excess glucose is being used for energy) activate acetyl-CoA carboxylase to form malonyl-CoA, which is the first stage of fatty acid synthesis.

TABLE 8.6-3 Glucose Transporters, their Functions and Major Sites of Expression

Type of GLUT	Function	Major site of expression
1. Na^+ dependent Secondary active Glucose transporter		
• SGLT-1	Absorption of glucose	Small intestine, renal tubules
• SGLT-2	Absorption of glucose	Renal tubules
2. Facilitated diffusion		
• GLUT-1	Basal glucose uptake	Placenta, brain, RBC, kidney, colon, retina
• GLUT-2	B cell glucose sensor, transport of glucose out of intestinal and renal tubular cells	B cells of islets of pancreas, liver, enterocytes and kidney
• GLUT-3	Basal glucose uptake	Brain, placenta, kidney and many other organ cells
• GLUT-4	Insulin stimulates glucose uptake	Skeletal muscle, cardiac muscle, adipose tissue
• GLUT-5	Exercise-stimulated glucose uptake	Skeletal muscle
• GLUT-6	Fructose transport	Jejunum and sperms
• GLUT-7	Unknown	Brain, leucocytes, spleen
	Glucose-6-phosphate transporter in endoplasmic reticulum	Liver

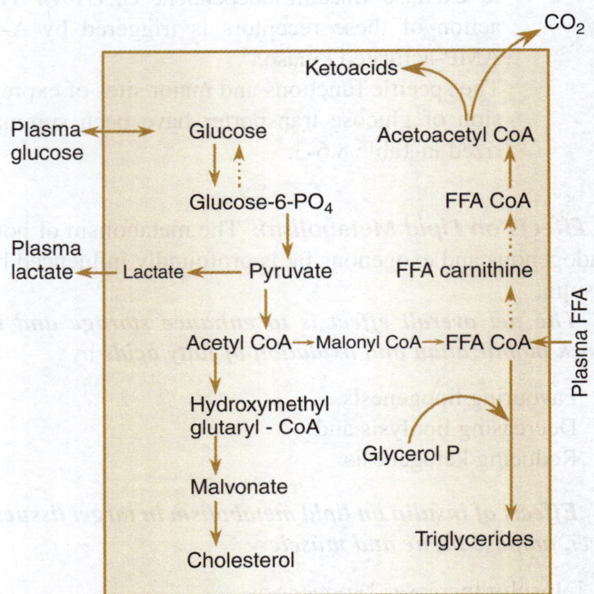

FIGURE 8.6-14 Effect of insulin on lipogenesis in liver.

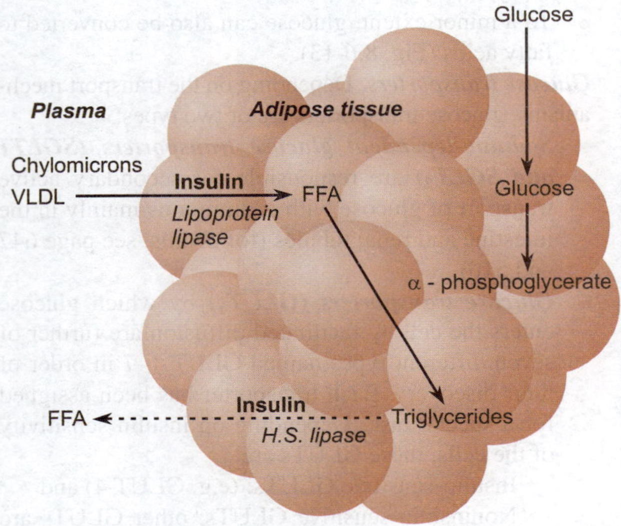

FIGURE 8.6-15 Effects of insulin on fat metabolism in the adipose tissue.

- Insulin favours synthesis of triglycerides from free fatty acids, glycerol-3-phosphate (from glycolysis) and NADPH (from HMP shunt).
- Triglycerides formed in liver cells are released to the blood.

Synthesis of cholesterol. Insulin also favours hepatic synthesis of cholesterol from acetyl-CoA by activating the rate-limiting enzyme hydroxymethylglutaryl-CoA reductase.

b. Lipogenic Effects on Adipose Tissue (Fig. 8.6-15). *Insulin activity promotes deposition of circulating fat into adipose tissue* by activating the key enzyme *lipoprotein lipase* in the capillary wall of adipose tissue. This enzyme favours the uptake of very low-density lipoprotein (VLDL) and chylomicrons into the adipose tissue from circulation by splitting them into free fatty acids. The FFAs are absorbed by fat cells and converted to triglyceride. The α−glycerophosphate required for esterification of FFA is obtained from the glucose in fat cells (whose uptake is also increased by insulin).

c. Lipogenic Effects of Insulin in Muscle. Within muscle, insulin suppresses the enzyme lipoprotein lipase in inverse proportion to its stimulation of glucose uptake.

ii. Insulin Decreases Lipolysis

a. In Adipose Tissue, insulin profoundly inhibits *hormone-sensitive lipase activity*. By suppressing lipolysis and the release of stored fatty acids and glycerol, insulin diminishes their delivery to liver and peripheral tissues. It is noteworthy that abdominal visceral fat is less sensitive to insulin than is subcutaneous fat.

b. In Liver also the mobilization of FFA to peripheral circulation.

c. In Muscle also the insulin inhibits lipolysis of triglyceride stores.

iii. Insulin Reduces Ketogenesis Insulin is the major and perhaps the sole antiketogenic hormone. Its antiketogenic effects are:

- Insulin leads to decreased FFA flow to the liver from adipose tissue. As a consequence, there is marked reduction in the generation of ketoacids.
- Insulin also stimulates the use of ketoacids by the peripheral tissue.
- Under the influence of insulin, FFAs that enter the liver from circulation are shunted away from β oxidation and ketogenesis.
- Antiketogenic action of insulin in the liver may also be mediated by stimulation of malonyl-CoA formation, because malonyl-CoA inhibits the enzyme carnithine acyltransferase. The latter enzyme is responsible for transferring FFAs from cytoplasm into the mitochondria for oxidation and conversion to ketoacids.

iv. Effect of Insulin on Lipoprotein Metabolism. It appears that insulin is required for the utilization of VLDL and LDL. The levels of VLDL and LDL and consequently the concentration of cholesterol are elevated in diabetics, which has been implicated in the pathogenesis of atherosclerosis.

Insulin Regulates Use of Glucose and FFA for Energy Production. From the effects of insulin on carbohydrate and fat metabolism described above, it is obvious that insulin regulates use of glucose and FFA for energy production.

- After a carbohydrate-rich meal, blood insulin level rises and consequently glucose becomes the chief fuel in the muscle. FFA is not used at this time because of low plasma FFA concentration induced by insulin.
- In between the meals, when the blood glucose level tends to fall, insulin secretion also decreases, resulting in greater lipolysis and increased production of FFA. Consequently, FFA becomes the chief fuel.

3. Effects of Insulin on Protein Metabolism.

Insulin is an anabolic hormone; it stimulates protein synthesis and inhibits protein degradation.

Insulin Stimulates Protein Synthesis. Although insulin stimulates the general rate of protein synthesis in vitro, this stimulation is evident in vivo mostly, when amino acids are in abundance after a meal (in the basal state, insulin limits the availability of endogenous amino acids for new protein synthesis). The role of insulin in protein synthesis is:

- It increases the transport of many amino acids (especially valine, leucine, isoleucine, tyrosine and phenylalanine) into the cells by increasing membrane permeability. Thus, plasma amino acids are lowered.
- Insulin increases the translation of messenger RNA on the ribosomes forming new proteins. In the absence of insulin, ribosomes stop working.
- Over a longer period, insulin also increases the rate of transcription of selected DNA genetic sequences in cell nuclei. This results into formation of increased quantities of mRNA causing still more protein synthesis, mainly enzymes for storage of fats, proteins and carbohydrates.
- In the liver, insulin decreases the rate of gluconeogenesis and thus conserves amino acids for protein synthesis.

Insulin Inhibits Protein Metabolism. Insulin inhibits proteolysis. This action is manifested by suppression of the branched chain and aromatic amino acids from muscle and inhibition of their oxidation.

B. Effects of Insulin on Ion Transport

Insulin increases K^+, PO_4^{3-} and Mg^{2+} uptake into the skeletal muscle cell and of K^+ and PO_4^{3-} into hepatic cells from ECF by increasing membrane permeability. Therefore, insulin secreted in response to a carbohydrate load lowers serum K^+, PO_4^{3-} and Mg^{2+} levels, and this hormone is considered to be one of the normal regulators of K^+ balance. This effect of insulin explains the occurrence of hypokalaemia in patients of diabetic acidosis treated with large doses of insulin.

The exact mechanism of hypokalaemia is not yet clear. However, insulin may increase the activity of Na^+/K^+–ATPase so that more K^+ is pumped into the cell. Insulin is very effectively used for temporary relief of hyperkalaemia in patients with renal failure.

Another effect of insulin on electrolytic balance is to increase reabsorption of K^+, PO_4^{3-} and Na^+ by the tubules of the kidney.

C. Role of Insulin in Cell Growth and Development

Insulin is an important factor for growth and development with the following roles:

- ***Anabolic action*** of insulin is as important as growth hormone for promotion of normal growth. Proper growth and development require the presence of both the hormones because anabolic action of one hormone cannot compensate for the other (because of their different modes of action).
- ***Direct stimulatory effect on macromolecules.*** Insulin is not only a general anabolic hormone, but it also stimulates the synthesis of macromolecules in tissues such as cartilage and bone and thereby directly contributes to body growth.
- ***Stimulation of other growth factors.*** The genes for insulin and its receptor are related to genes that encode a variety of tissue growth factors. These growth factors include somatomedins (insulin-like growth factors 1 and 2, i.e. IGF-1 and IGF-2), epidermal growth factor (EGF), nerve growth factor (NGF) and relaxin. Thus,

insulin indirectly contributes to growth by stimulating the transcription of other related gene growth factors, such as IGF-1, and by suppressing the gene for one of the IGF-1-binding proteins.

Note. An insulin-deprived young animal or human has a reduced lean body and bone mass, and it may be profoundly retarded in height and maturation.

The effects of insulin are summarized in Table 8.6-4.

Glucagon

Structure and Synthesis

Structure. Glucagon is secreted by A cells of islets of Langerhans and L cells of lower intestinal tract. Glucagon is a polypeptide composed of 29 amino acids in a single chain and has a molecular weight of 3500. The N-terminal residues 1 to 6 are essential for receptor binding and for biological activity. Unlike insulin, the amino acid sequence of glucagon is the same in all mammalian species.

Synthesis. Glucagon is synthesized from a preproglucagon precursor by islet α cells. It is actually synthesized as proglucagon (molecular weight 9000) which on sequential degradation releases active glucagon. In α cells, human preproglucagon is processed to glucagon and major proglucagon fragment (MPGF). In L cells of lower intestinal tract cells, it is processed primarily to glicentin (a polypeptide consisting of glucagon with additional amino acid residues on either end) and glucagon-like polypeptide-1 and 2 (GLP-1 and GLP-2). Some oxyntomodulin also formed and glicentin-related polypeptide (GRPP) is left (Fig. 8.6-16).

- Glicentin has some glucagon-like activity whereas GLP-1 and GLP-2 have no biological activity, but when GLP-1 is further processed to form GLP-1(7-36), it is a potent stimulator of insulin (see page 772)
- GLP-2 is a mediator in a pathway from NTS to hypothalamus, and an injection of GLP-2 lowers food intake.
- Oxyntomodulin inhibits gastric acid secretion.
- GRPP does not have any established physiological effect.

Secretion. Glucagon is stored in dense granules and is released by exocytosis. This process is inhibited if α cell Ca^{2+} levels are decreased.

Plasma Levels, Circulation and Degradation

- *Circulation of glucagon* in plasma is in unbound form.
- *Basal levels* of glucagon in a normal fasting individual are 100–150 pg/ml.
- *Half-life* of this hormone is 6 min (range 5–9 min).
- *Secretion rate* of glucagon is estimated to be 100–150 μg/day.
- *Ratio of portal vein to peripheral vein* glucagon concentration is about 1.5 in the basal state. This is because glucagon enters the portal vein in relatively high concentration and approximately 50% of which is removed by the liver in a single passage through this organ.
- *Degradation* mainly occurs in the liver. Therefore, in cirrhosis of liver, peripheral blood level of glucagon increases. It is also degraded in tissues and plasma by an aminopeptide. The kidney is the other major site of glucagon degradation. Less than 1% of glucagon filtered by the glomerulus is excreted in the urine.

TABLE 8.6-4 Effects of Insulin on Body Tissues

Liver:
- Increases protein synthesis
- Increases lipid synthesis
- Decreases ketogenesis
- Decreases glucose output due to:
  - Decreased neoglucogenesis
  - Increased glycogenesis
  - Increased glycolysis

Muscle:
- Increases glucose intake
- Increases glycogenesis
- Increases amino acid uptake
- Increases protein synthesis in ribosomes
- Decreases protein catabolism
- Decreases release of gluconeogenic amino acid
- Increases ketone uptake
- Increases K^+ uptake

Adipose tissue:
- Increases glucose entry
- Increases fatty acid synthesis
- Increases glycerol phosphate synthesis
- Increases triglyceride deposition
- Increases activation of lipoprotein lipase
- Inhibition of hormone-sensitive lipase
- Increases K^+ uptake

General: increases growth and development

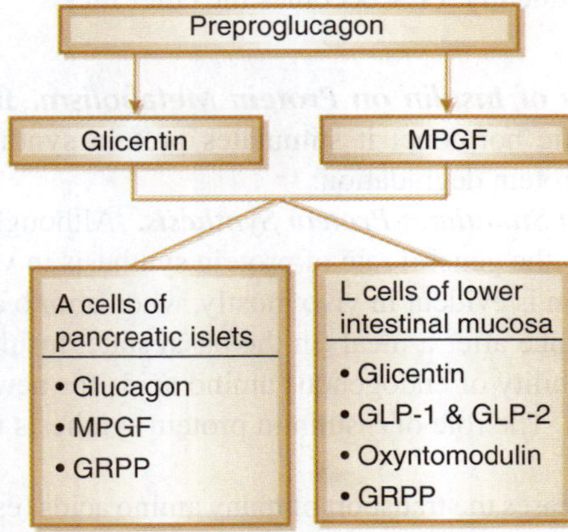

FIGURE 8.6-16 Post-translational processing of preproglucagon in A and L cells.; GRPP, glicentin-related polypeptide; GLP, glucagon-like polypeptide; Oxy, oxyntomodulin; MPGF, major proglucagon fragment.

Mechanism of Action of Glucagon

Glucagon is glycogenolytic, gluconeogenic, lipolytic and ketogenic, and acts on G-protein- coupled receptors. Glucagon binds to the specific receptor on the plasma membrane of target cells and acts through the mediation of cyclic AMP as second messenger. Covalent modification of enzyme activities by phosphorylation is the main mechanism of action (for detail of mechanism see page 671). Glucagon receptors have been identified in variety of tissues. It mostly acts on liver and adipose tissue. It acts competitively at similar points in the liver as insulin. Glucagon may even be viewed as the primary hormone that regulates hepatic glucose production and ketogenesis, and insulin's role may be that of a glucagon antagonist.

Actions of Glucagon

As mentioned above, the actions of glucagon, in almost all respects, are exactly opposite to those of insulin. It promotes mobilization of stored nutrients such as glucose, fatty acids and ketoacids (Fig. 8.6-17) and thus is a hormone of energy release. Its metabolic effects are as follows.

1. Effects on Carbohydrate Metabolism. Glucagon predominately acts on the liver and increases the blood sugar level by following actions:

- ***Increased Glycogenolysis.*** In the liver, glucagon exerts an immediate and profound glycogenolytic effect (breaking down of glycogens through activation of enzyme *glycogen phosphorylase* by cAMP-mediated mechanism). The glucose-1-phosphate released as a result of glycogen phosphorylase activation is prevented from undergoing resynthesis to glycogen by simultaneous inhibition of glycogen synthase. The glucose-1-phosphate is dephosphorylated and glucose is formed.
- ***Increased Gluconeogenesis.*** After the glycogen in liver is exhausted, glucagon increases the rate of gluconeogenesis, i.e. formation of glucose from lactate, pyruvate, glycerol and amino acids. Gluconeogenesis causes a slow but more sustained rise in blood glucose which lasts for hours and days. Glucagon activates multiple enzymes involved in gluconeogenesis, especially the enzyme system converting pyruvate to phosphopyruvate (rate-limiting step in gluconeogenesis). It also increases the entry of amino acids from blood to liver cells and makes them available for gluconeogenesis.

2. Effects on Lipid Metabolism. Glucagon is a powerful *lipolytic agent.* It acts via stimulating cAMP system to activate lipase in adipose tissue which releases FFA and glycerol into the circulation. In the liver, excess of FFAs are oxidized resulting in energy production and ketone body synthesis (ketogenesis). In addition, glucagon also prevents synthesis of triglyceride from FFA by inhibiting the enzyme acetyl-CoA carboxylase. The spared FFAs are directed towards β-oxidation resulting in production of ketoacids. Thus, glucagon is a ketogenic as well as a hyperglycaemic hormone.

3. Effects on Protein Metabolism. Glucagon increases the amino acid uptake of liver, which in turn promotes gluconeogeneis. Thus, glucagon *lowers plasma amino acids.*

4. Calorigenic Effect. Glucagon also has a calorigenic effect. This is not due to hyperglycaemia, but this action requires the presence of glucocorticoids and T_4. It is probably related to increased hepatic deamination of amino acids.

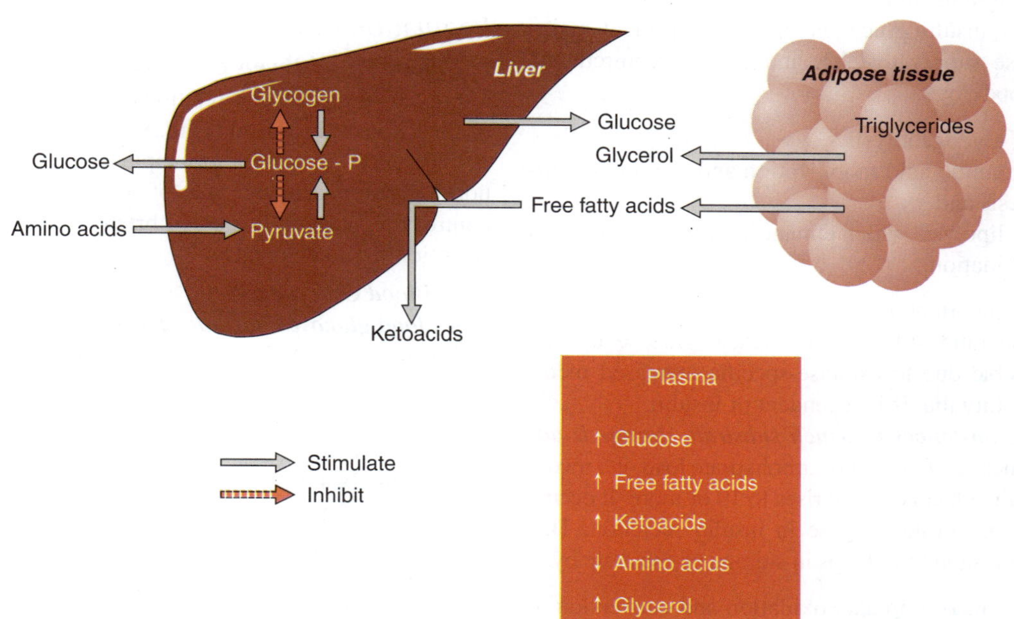

FIGURE 8.6-17 Glucagon causes mobilization of stored energy fuels (glucose, fatty acids and ketoacids) into circulation and hepatic uptake of amino acids for gluconeogenesis; consequently, plasma levels of energy fuels increase and levels of amino acids decrease.

5. *Other Actions of Glucagon.* Other miscellaneous actions of glucagon include:

- Inhibition of renal tubular sodium reabsorption, resulting in natriuresis.
- Modest increase in force of contraction of the heart by activation of myocardial adenylyl cyclase.
- Stimulation of secretion of growth hormone, insulin and pancreatic somatostatin.
- It may also be synthesized in the central nervous system, and it may act locally in the regulation of appetite.
- It is also produced in the gastric and intestinal mucosa by certain cells resembling the α cells of pancreatic islets. The physiological role of the extrapancreatic glucagon secretion is not clear.

Insulin: Glucagon Ratio

Insulin and glucagon are often secreted and act in a reciprocal fashion; when one is needed, the other usually is not. Therefore, the ratio of their concentrations may be more critical than their actual concentration. Together, they co-ordinate the flow and metabolic fate of endogenous glucose, free fatty acids (FFAs), amino acids and other substrates to ensure that energy needs are met in the basal state and during exercise. In addition, they co-ordinate the efficient disposition of the nutrients input from the meals. They accomplish these functions by maintaining a critical ratio.

Under basal conditions, the usual molar ratio of insulin to glucagon in plasma is about 2.0.

Under circumstances that require mobilization and increased use of endogenous substrate such as fasting and prolonged exercise, the insulin–glucagon ratio drops to 0.5 or less. This decreased insulin–glucagon ratio results from both the decreased insulin secretion and increased glucagon secretion. Low insulin:glucagon ratio is helpful in maintaining glucose supply to CNS and energy requirements needs of the body by:

- Increasing glycogenolysis,
- Increasing amino acid mobilization and promoting gluconeogenesis and
- Increasing lipolysis which enhances FFA to muscle and liver for oxidation.

Note. It is important to note that during exercise, low insulin–glucagon ratio still permits muscle glucose uptake, which is possible due to exercise-specific increased membrane permeability that is independent of insulin.

Under circumstances in which substrate storage is advantageous, such as after a pure carbohydrate load or a mixed meal, the insulin–glucagon ratio rises to 10 or more. It occurs mainly due to manifold increase in insulin secretion. This high insulin:glucagon ratio helps in storage of substrate by:

- Increasing glucose uptake, oxidation and conversion to liver and muscle glycogen.
- Suppressing unneeded proteolysis and lipolysis and
- Facilitating clearance of chylomicrons by activation of adipose tissue lipoprotein lipase.

After a pure protein meal, interestingly, only a small change in insulin–glucagon ratio occurs; however, secretion of insulin as well as that of glucagon is increased.

- *Increased insulin secretion* prevents unneeded proteolysis and facilitates muscle uptake of some amino acids and their incorporation into proteins.
- *Increased glucagon secretion* is useful in preventing the decrease in hepatic glucose output and hypoglycaemia that would occur if the extra insulin action were completely unopposed.

Applied Aspects

Macrosomia and GLUT-1 deficiency

Macrosomia refers to a condition of an infant born with light birth weight and large organ size, born to diabetic mother. The condition is caused by:

- Excess circulating antibodies against insulin in the fetus, resulting in pancreatic islet stimulation by raised blood glucose level and raised amino acids in the diabetic mother.
- Fetal macrosomia also occurs when in a pregnant woman antibodies develop against insulin or she is on bovine insulin therapy during pregnancy. Normally, free insulin in the maternal blood is destroyed by protease in the placenta, but antibody-bound insulin is protected and reaches the fetal blood.

The infant with GLUT-1 deficiency has defective glucose transportation across the blood–brain barrier, therefore, there is low CSF glucose, even in the presence of high blood glucose. These individuals develop seizure or severe development growth retardation.

Regulation of Glucagon Secretion

I. Role of Blood Levels of Nutrients

There exists a feedback relationship between blood levels of glucagon and nutrients (Fig. 8.6-18).

The most important principle is the maintenance of normoglycaemia in the face of increased nutrients in the control of glucagon discussed briefly, governing glucagon secretion tissue demands.

1. Blood Glucose Level

Low blood glucose concentration is the most potent stimulus for secretion of glucagon. Hypoglycaemia causes a two- to fourfold increase in plasma levels of glucagon which acts to increase circulating glucose levels (Fig. 8.6-18). Glucagon secretion by α cells increases even when blood sugar falls to just below 70 mg% (normal range 70–110 mg%). Glucagon secretion is stimulated much more by low glucose levels if insulin is absent.

High blood glucose concentration inhibits glucagon secretion (Fig. 8.6-18). Hyperglycaemia lowers glucagon secretion by 50%. The presence of insulin greatly potentiates the suppressive effect of high glucose levels on α cells.

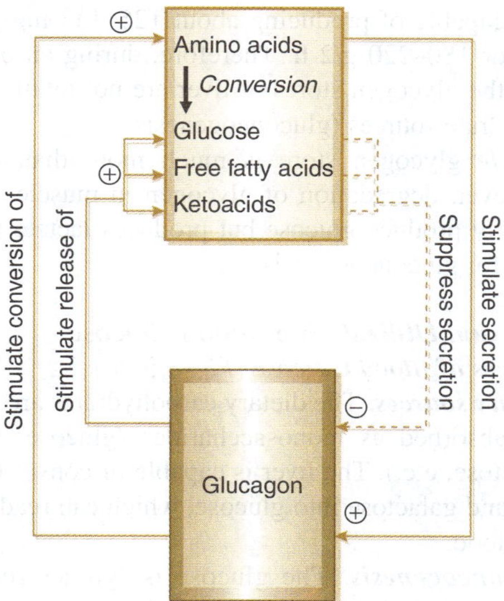

FIGURE 8.6-18 Feedback relationship between glucagon and nutrients. Glucagon stimulates production and release of glucose, free fatty acids and ketoacids, which in turn suppress glucagon secretion, and glucagon in turn stimulates the conversion of amino acids to glucose.

Important Note

The pancreatic B cells also contain GABA; it is suggested that hyperglycaemia induces insulin secretion as well as releases GABA, GABA in turn acts paracrinally on A cells by activating $GABA_A$ receptors and inhibits glucagon secretion. The $GABA_A$ receptors are Cl^- channels, their activation causes Cl^- influx leading to hyperpolarization of A cells.

Secretory pattern of glucagon in response to blood glucose levels is just opposite to insulin. Therefore, during starvation, glucagon secretion increases while that of insulin decreases, and conversely, after a carbohydrate-rich meal, glucagon secretion decreases while that of insulin increases.

2. Plasma Amino Acids. Secretion of glucagon is increased by a protein-rich meal and, most effectively, by amino acids such as arginine and alanine. Since the amino acids increase insulin secretion also, the simultaneous release of glucagon along with insulin prevents the risk of hypoglycaemia, which otherwise would occur after a high protein meal.

There exists a feedback relationship, i.e. amino acids stimulate glucagon secretion, and glucagon in turn stimulates the conversion of amino acids to glucose (Fig. 8.6-18).

3. Free Fatty Acids and Ketoacids. Glucagon stimulates production and release of free fatty acids (FFA) and ketoacids, which in turn suppress glucagon secretion, i.e. there is a feedback relationship (Fig. 8.6-18).

II. Role of Gastrointestinal Hormones Gastrointestinal (GT) hormones such as CCK, gastrin and GIP increase glucagon secretion. This accounts for the enhanced glucagon response to orally ingested nutrients as opposed to the responses to intravenously delivered nutrients.

III. Role of Nervous System *Sympathetic nerve stimulation* to pancreas increases glucagon secretion. The effect is mediated via β-adrenergic receptors and cAMP. Various stresses, fasting, exercise and infection increase the glucagon secretion in part by their stimulatory effect on sympathetic nervous system and partly by release of glucocorticoids.

- Vagal stimulation and acetylcholine also acutely increase glucagon secretion.
- Neurohormone somatostatin inhibits the secretion of glucagon, probably by paracrine or neurocrine effects made possible by the islet microarchitecture.

The principle factors affecting glucagon secretion are summarized in Table 8.6-5.

Hormonal Regulation of Blood Glucose Level

Normal Blood Glucose Levels and Body Glucose Reserves

Normal Blood Glucose Levels. A healthy individual is capable of maintaining the blood glucose level within a narrow range.

- Fasting blood glucose level in a postabsorptive state varies between 70 and 110 mg%.
- Postprandial blood glucose level, i.e. after a large carbohydrate meal or following oral administration of glucose in the dose of 1 g/kg body weight, the blood glucose level increases to about 140 mg% (<150 mg%) in a period of less than 1 h. However, a prompt increase in insulin secretion brings it back to baseline value within 2 h. This response to oral administration of carbohydrate, when plotted on a time scale, is called glucose tolerance curve (Fig. 8.6-19) and is used clinically as a test to study the maintenance of blood glucose levels.

TABLE 8.6-5 Factors Affecting Glucagon Secretion

Stimulators	Inhibitors
• Hypoglycaemia	• Hyperglycaemia
• Amino acids (particularly glucogenic)	• Neurohormones (somatostatins)
• GIT hormones (CCK, gastrin, GIP)	• Secretin
• Stresses: infection, exercise, cortisol, β-adrenergic stimulator, acetylcholine	• FFA, ketoacids
	• GABA, α-adrenergics, phenytoin

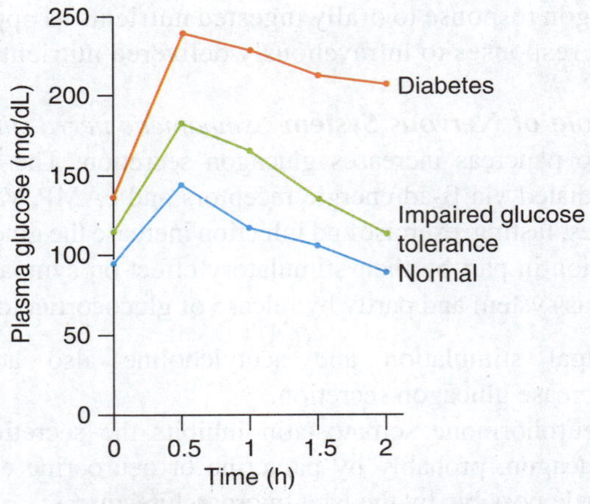

FIGURE 8.6-19 Glucose tolerance curve.

Normal Body Reserves of Glucose

Free Glucose is carbohydrate currency of the body. About 18 g of free glucose is present in an adult human body. This amount is just sufficient to meet the basal energy requirements of the body for 1 h.

Stored Glucose is present in the form of glycogen in liver and muscles.

- *Liver* has about 100 g stored glycogen. An adult liver (weighing about 1.5 kg) can provide only 40–50 g of blood glucose from glycogen that can last only for a few hours to meet the body requirement. However, liver is also capable of producing about 125–150 mg glucose/min or 180–220 g/2 h. Therefore, during an overnight fast, the glycogen stores of liver are not totally noncarbohydrate sources (gluconeogenesis).
- *Muscle* glycogen store is much more than of liver. However, degradation of glycogen in muscle does not directly produce glucose but produces lactate which is used for gluconeogenesis.

Sources and Utilization of Blood Glucose

Sources of Blood Glucose (Fig. 8.6-20)

1. ***Dietary sources.*** The dietary carbohydrates are digested and absorbed as monosaccharides (glucose, fructose, galactose, etc.). The liver is capable of converting fructose and galactose into glucose, which can readily enter the blood.
2. ***Gluconeogenesis.*** The glucose is synthesized in the liver and kidney. Precursors for gluconeogenesis include lactate, glycerol, propionate and some amino acids.
   - Lactate is formed by degradation of glycogen stored in the muscle.
   - Free glycerol and propionate are formed by breakdown of fat in adipose tissue.
   - Amino acids may be derived from dietary sources or from protein breakdown.
3. ***Glycogenolysis.*** Stored glycogen in liver is degraded to glucose, while muscle glycogen after degradation produces lactate which is used for gluconeogenesis as described above.

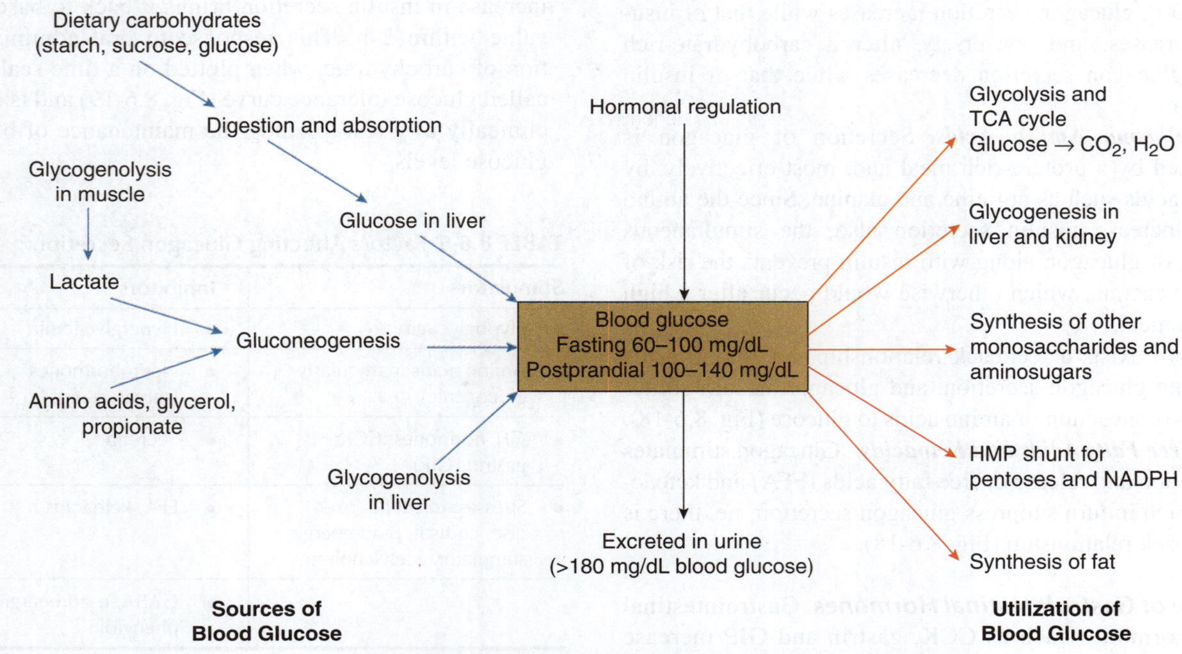

FIGURE 8.6-20 Sources and utilization of glucose.

Utilization of Blood Glucose. The glucose present in the blood is utilized for:

1. ***Provision of energy needs to body tissues.*** The oxidative pathways in which glucose is used include:
   - Glycolysis and tricarboxylic acid (TCA) cycle,
   - Hexose monophosphate (HMP) shunt for pentoses and NADPH and
   - Uronic acid pathway.
2. ***Glycogenesis,*** i.e. synthesis of glycogen in liver and kidney,
3. ***Synthesis of other monosaccharides and amino sugar*** and
4. ***Synthesis of fat.***

Role of Hormones in Regulation of Blood Glucose

Under normal circumstances, various hormones play a significant role in maintaining the blood glucose levels within normal physiological range. This is accomplished by preventing the occurrence of hyperglycaemia and hypoglycaemia.

Prevention of Occurrence of Hyperglycaemia. The occurrence of hyperglycaemia after a pure carbohydrate load or a mixed meal in a healthy individual is prevented by a manifold (4–5 times) increase in insulin secretion. Insulin normalizes the blood glucose levels by:

- Increasing uptake and utilization as chief fuel in the muscles,
- Promoting storage of glucose as glycogen in liver and as triglycerides in the adipose tissue and
- Decreasing glucose production by inhibiting gluconeogenesis and glycogenolysis (for details see actions of insulin on page 775).

Prevention of Occurrence of Hypoglycaemia. Hypoglycaemia, which may occur due to fasting or prolonged exercise, is prevented in a healthy individual by a number of hormones, which include glucagon, epinephrine, growth hormone and glucocorticoids. It is obvious that there is only one hormone, insulin, which prevents hyperglycaemia, whereas at least four hormones are available for prevention of hypoglycaemia. This may be correlated with the fact that moderate and transient hyperglycaemia is harmless and occurs after every meal. However, even moderate hypoglycaemia may lead to serious complications. The brain, retina and germinal epithelium of the gonads are particularly vulnerable to the effects of hypoglycaemia, since they cannot use any fuel other than glucose.

The roles played by different hormones in preventing hypoglycaemia are described:

1. ***Role of glucagon.*** During normal pattern of food intake (consisting of 2–3 meals/day), in between the meals when glucose level tends to decrease, the insulin secretion stops and instead glucagon is poured into the bloodstream under these circumstances.
   - Glucagon promotes hepatic glycogenolysis and gluconeogenesis and thus, glucose is poured into the circulation from the liver (Fig. 8.6-20).
   - At the same time, due to absence of insulin, glucose utilization by muscles is stopped and instead lipolysis in adipose tissue is promoted, and therefore free fatty acids (FFAs) become the chief fuel for muscles.
2. ***Role of epinephrine.*** When starvation period further increases (say many hours), even in the presence of glucagon, blood glucose levels begin to fall. The resulting hypoglycaemia stimulates the sympathetic nervous system through hypothalamus to promote the release of epinephrine from the adrenal medulla. Epinephrine so produced:
   - Increases blood glucose by supplementing the glycogenolytic and gluconeogenic effect of glucagon and
   - Increases FFA production (fuel for muscles) by promoting lipolysis.
3. ***Role of growth hormone and glucocorticoids***. When starvation is more prolonged (say for a few days), along with glucagon and epinephrine, secretion of growth hormone and glucocorticoids is also increased. These hormones, in addition to promoting glycogenolysis, gluconeogenesis and lipolysis, also decrease the peripheral utilization of glucose, thereby sparing glucose for nervous tissue, especially brain.

Somatostatin and Pancreatic Polypeptide

Somatostatin

Structure and Synthesis. Pancreatic somatostatin is a neuropeptide containing 14 amino acids, synthesized by δ cells. It is also synthesized by intestinal cells and was originally discovered as a hypothalamic neuropeptide that inhibits growth hormone secretion.

Regulation of Secretion. Somatostatin secretion is increased after ingestion of food, because increased blood glucose, amino acids, fatty acids and gastrointestinal tract hormones stimulate its secretion. Glucagon, β-adrenergic and cholinergic neurotransmitters also stimulate somatostatin secretion. Insulin and α-adrenergic neurotransmitters inhibit somatostatin secretion.

Mechanism of Action. Somatostatin acts through its receptors; five different types of somatostatin receptors have been identified ($SSTR_1$-$SSTR_5$). Mostly these receptors are GPCR that inhibit adenylyl cyclase activity and exert various effects.

Actions. Somatostatin has the following effects:

- Acts on the islets of Langerhans and inhibits secretion of insulin and glucagon via $SSTR_5$.
- Increases the motility of stomach, duodenum and gall bladder.
- Decreases secretion of hydrochloric acid, pepsin, gastrin, secretin, intestinal juices and pancreatic juice.

- Inhibits the absorption of glucose, xylose and triglycerides across the mucosal membrane.
- *Brain*: Somatostatin is found in various parts of the brain, where it functions as a neurotransmitter with effects on sensory inputs, locomotive activity and cognitive functions (see page 1086). In hypothalamus, it is secreted into portal–hypophyseal vessel and inhibits growth hormone secretion. $SSTR_2$ mediates cognitive and growth hormone inhibition effect.

In a nutshell, actions of somatostatin along with those of insulin and glucagon probably coordinate nutrient input with substrate disposal.

Important Note

Somatostatin analogues are now used therapeutically to alleviate diarrhoea caused by unregulated gastrointestinal hormone secretion. They are also employed to inhibit unregulated release of various peptides and protein hormones by neoplasms.

Pancreatic Polypeptide

Structure and Synthesis. Pancreatic polypeptide has 36 amino acids and belongs to a family of similar molecules including neuropeptide Y in the hypothalamus and gastrointestinal polypeptide Y. It is synthesized by F cells of islets of Langerhans.

Regulation of Secretion. Pancreatic polypeptide is secreted in response to food ingestion via gastrointestinal secretagogues and cholinergic stimulation. Its secretion is also stimulated by hypoglycaemia and inhibited by glucose administration.

Actions and Physiological Importance. Its best known action is to inhibit exocrine pancreatic secretion and slows the absorption of food in humans. Its true physiological importance is not known except that:

- Increased plasma levels of PP serve as markers for the presence of islet cell tumours and their response to treatment.
- A failure of plasma pancreatic polypeptide to increase when plasma glucose is sharply reduced suggests loss of cholinergic pancreatic islet innervation.

APPLIED ASPECTS

Important applied aspects of endocrine pancreas which need mention are:

- Diabetes mellitus and
- Hypoglycaemia

Diabetes Mellitus

Diabetes mellitus, commonly called just diabetes, refers to a clinical syndrome of hyperglycaemia occurring due to deficiency of insulin.

Types and Stages of Diabetes Mellitus

Diabetes mellitus can be classified into following types:

1. *Primary diabetes mellitus* in which the cause is not known. It is of further two types:
   - Insulin-dependent diabetes mellitus (IDDM) or type-I, and
   - Noninsulin-dependent diabetes mellitus (NIDDM) or type-II.
2. *Secondary diabetes mellitus.* It is associated with certain pathological conditions such as pancreatitis, cystic fibrosis, acromegaly and Cushing syndrome.

Stages in the development of diabetes mellitus include:

- *Prediabetics or potential diabetics.* These are the persons with normal blood glucose level but are potential candidates to develop diabetes due to strong genetic predispositions, e.g. first-degree relative of diabetics.
- *Latent diabetics and chemical diabetics.* These persons have normal fasting and postprandial blood glucose levels and normal glucose tolerance test. But their blood glucose becomes abnormally high during stress or after administration of glucocorticoids.
- *Clinical diabetics* have hyperglycaemia, glycosuria and typical symptoms but without complications.
- *Complicated diabetics* are patients with longstanding neglected diabetes with multiple complications.

Insulin-dependent Diabetes Mellitus or Type-I

- Insulin-dependent diabetes mellitus (IDDM), or type-I diabetes, is considered an autoimmune disorder in which antibodies destroy the β cells of islets causing an absolute deficiency of insulin.
- Genetic susceptibility is a major determinant while environmental factors act as a trigger.
- The current view regarding type-1 diabetes is that this is a T cell-mediated disease. The main genetic abnormality is in major histocompatibility complex (MHC) gene located on chromosome 6, though other genes are also involved.

Characteristic features of IDDM are:

- It manifests before 40 years of age (usually between 12 and 15 years) and is also called juvenile onset diabetes. It accounts for 10–20%.
- Patients are usually lean.
- Classical triad of presenting symptoms consisting of polyuria, polydipsia and polyphagia is associated with weight loss.
- Ketosis and acidosis are common complications of this diabetes mellitus.
- Plasma insulin levels are very low or undetectable.

Non-insulin-dependent Diabetes Mellitus or Type-II

Noninsulin-dependent diabetes mellitus (NIDDM) or type-II diabetes is also a genetic disorder. Overeating coupled with underactivity leading to obesity acts as a diabetogenic factor in genetically predisposed individuals. It is supposed to occur due to decrease in insulin receptors on the insulin-responsive (target) cells.

In type-II diabetes, the genetic component is stronger compared to type-I.

In some cases, the defects in individual genes have been identified; these include defect in glucokinase (1%), insulin molecule (0.5%), insulin receptors (1%), GLUT-4 (1%) and insulin receptor-1 (15%) of cases, but the actual genes involved are still not known.

Characteristic features of NIDDM are:

- It manifests after 40 years of age and so is also called as *adult onset diabetes or maturity onset diabetes in young (MODY).*
- It is most common and accounts for 80–90% of diabetic population.
- Most of the patients are obese.
- Symptoms begin gradually and may be ignored and many a times diagnosis is made on urine examination which shows glycosuria.
- Plasma insulin levels are often normal or even elevated.
- Ketoacidosis is not very common.

Obesity (the Metabolic Syndrome) The incidence of obesity is increasing; it relates to the discrepancy between energy consumption and energy expenditure. The risk of type-II diabetes increases 10-fold with body mass index (BMI) >30 kg/m^2 (normal BMI 18.5–24.9 kg/m^2). The susceptibility to obesity and its adverse consequences vary. Metabolic syndrome is mainly a glucose metabolism disorder; therefore, it has special relation with diabetes mellitus. As the body weight increases, there is increase in insulin resistance leading to decreasing ability of insulin to move glucose into muscle and adipose tissues, and glucose release from liver. Hence, obesity is associated with hyperinsulinaemia, dyslipidaemia (increased level of circulating triglycerides and HDL) and development of atherosclerosis. The combination of these findings is commonly referred to as metabolic syndrome or syndrome X. The patients with this syndrome may present as prediabetic or full-fledged type-II diabetes.

IDDM versus NIDDM The comparison between IDDM and NIDDM is given in Table 8.6-6.

TABLE 8.6-6 IDDM versus NIDDM

Feature	IDDM	NIDDM
General features		
Defect	Insulin deficiency due to β cell destruction	Resistance of target tissues to insulin
Prevalence	10–20% of diabetic population	80–90% of diabetic population
Age of onset	<40 years	>40 years
Body weight	Low (thin and lean)	High (obese or normal)
Gene locus	Chromosome 6	Chromosome 1
Family history	Mild or moderate	Very strong
Clinical features		
Duration of symptoms	Weeks (rapid)	Months to year (slow)
Presenting symptoms	Polyuria, polydypsia, polyphagia	Usually patients present with different complications
Complication at the time of diagnosis	Absent	Present (in 10–20% cases)
Acute complication	Ketoacidosis	Hyperosmolar coma
Biochemical features		
Plasma insulin	Decreased or absent	Normal or increased
Autoantibodies	Frequently found	Rare
Ketonuria	Present	Absent
Treatment		
Treatment of choice	Insulin (oral hypoglycaemics not useful)	Oral hypoglycaemics (insulin usually not required)
Mortality if not treated	High	Low

Pathophysiology of Diabetes Mellitus

Pathophysiology of diabetes mellitus revolves around the metabolic alterations associated with insulin deficiency. Most important among them are hyperglycaemia, ketoacidosis, hypertriglyceridaemia and protein catabolism (Fig. 8.6-21):

1. Hyperglycaemia and Its Consequences Hyperglycaemia (elevation of blood glucose concentration) is the characteristic feature of uncontrolled diabetes mellitus. It occurs due to lack of insulin resulting in:

- Decreased peripheral utilization of glucose.
- Increased hepatic output of glucose (owing to glycogenolysis and gluconeogenesis) into the circulation.

Consequences of hyperglycaemia are:

- Glycosuria and its consequences,
- Impaired phagocytic function,
- Hyperosmolar effects and
- Glycosylation of haemoglobin.

i. Glycosuria and Its Consequences

- ***Glycosuria,*** i.e. excretion of glucose into the urine, occurs when the blood glucose level rises above the renal threshold point, i.e. above 180 mg/100 ml.
- ***Polyuria,*** i.e. passage of large amount of urine frequently. It is the result of osmotic diuresis caused by renal excretion of osmotically active glucose molecules.
- ***Loss of electrolytes*** (sodium, potassium and phosphate) in urine also occurs as a side effect of osmotic diuresis.
- ***Cellular dehydration.*** High glucose concentration increases osmotic pressure of extracellular fluid and osmotic transfer of water from cells to extracellular fluid leading to dehydration of cells. In addition to it, osmotic diuresis causes increased loss of water from the body thereby reducing extracellular fluid volume which also causes compensatory dehydration of cells.
- ***Polydipsia,*** i.e. excessive drinking of water, results from activation of thirst mechanism caused by cellular dehydration.
- ***Increased caloric loss*** is the result of loss of glucose in urine.
- ***Polyphagia,*** i.e. excessive eating, occurs due to stimulation of satiety centre caused by deficient utilization of glucose in the hypothalamic ventromedial nuclei. Increased caloric loss also results in compensatory polyphagia.
- ***Loss of body weight*** occurs because of loss of calories in the urine and mobilization of fats and proteins for energy production. Since loss of body weight

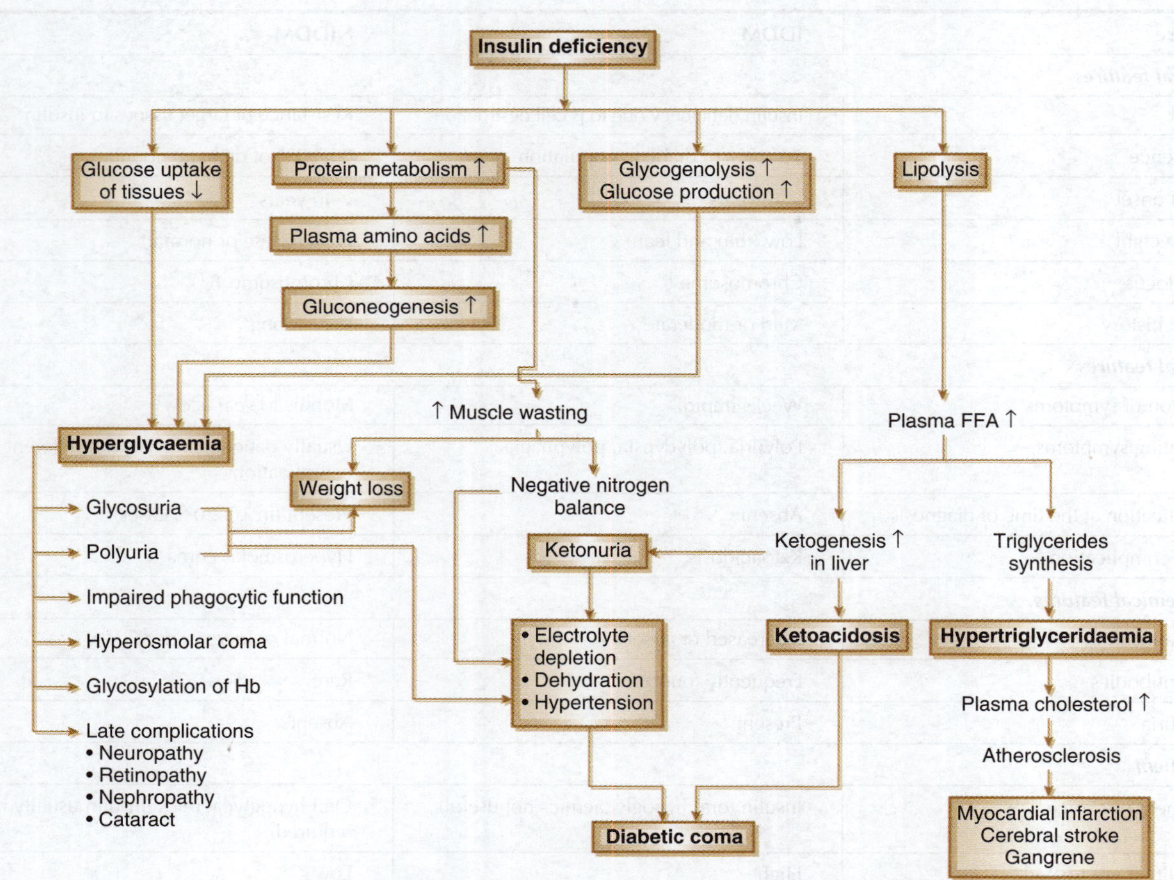

FIGURE 8.6-21 Pathophysiology of diabetes mellitus and its complications.

occurs in spite of excessive food intake, diabetes is called a *condition of starvation in the midst of plenty*.

ii. Impaired Phagocytic Function. Hyperglycaemia impairs all aspects of leucocytic phagocytic function, i.e. adherence, diapedesis, phagocytosis and intracellular killing. Because of impaired phagocytic function, diabetics are more prone to infections compared with the nondiabetics.

iii. Hyperosmolar Effects. Osmolarity of the blood goes on increasing with the increasing blood sugar levels. With the passage of time, a stage may come when glucose production is increased and urinary excretion is decreased, and the plasma glucose level may increase up to 1000 mg%. Under such circumstances the plasma osmolality may be over 375 mOsm/kg. Such a high hyperosmolality may cause dehydration in central nervous system leading to impairment of cerebral functions. Ultimately, a condition called nonketotic hyperosmolar coma may result, which may be even fatal.

iv. Glycosylation of Proteins. Glycosylation of proteins refers to post-translation, nonenzymatic addition of sugar residues to amino acids of proteins.

Glycosylation of haemoglobin. Glycosylated haemoglobin refers to the glucose-derived products of normal haemoglobin (HbA). Among the glycosylated haemoglobins, the most abundant form is HbA_{1C}, which is produced by condensation of glucose with N-terminal valine of each β chain of haemoglobin A (HbA).

- *The rate of production of HbA_{1C}* is directly related to the exposure of RBC to glucose. Thus, the concentration of HbA_{1C} serves as an indicator of the blood glucose concentration over a period approximately to half-life of RBC haemoglobin (i.e. 6–8 weeks).
- *Normally, HbA_{1C}* concentration is about 3–5% of the total haemoglobin.
- *During sustained hyperglycaemia,* as in diabetes mellitus, the concentration of HbA_{1C} may be elevated to 10–20% of the total haemoglobin.
- *Determination of HbA_{1C}* has become an important tool for monitoring of diabetes control and proper regulation of insulin therapy since HbA_{1C} concentration reflects the mean blood glucose level over a 2-month period prior to its measurement.

Note: HbA_{1c} may be erroneously decreased in anaemia and during pregnancy.

Glycosylation of tissue proteins occurs when the blood glucose levels remain elevated for a prolonged duration (years). Glycosylation leads to irreversible changes in the chemical structure of tissue proteins. These chemical changes have been implicated in producing long-term complications of diabetes mellitus, such as:

- Diabetic nephropathy,
- Diabetic retinopathy,
- Diabetic neuropathy and so on.

2. Ketosis, Hypertriglyceridaemia and Their Consequences Since due to insulin deficiency the utilization of glucose is poor, the body turns to fats for obtaining energy by lipolysis. Degree of lipolysis is directly proportional to the deficiency of insulin. As a result of lipolysis, plasma levels of FFAs are increased. FFAs provide energy to the glucose-starved insulin-sensitive tissues like skeletal muscle. Excessive FFAs in plasma leads to:

- Hypertriglyceridaemia and
- Ketosis.

Hypertriglyceridaemia. Conversion of FFAs to triglycerides and secretion of VLDL and chylomicrons is comparatively higher in diabetics. Further, the activity of enzyme lipoprotein lipase is low in diabetic patients. Consequently, the plasma levels of VLDL, and chylomicrons and triglycerides are increased. Hypercholesterolaemia is also frequently seen in diabetics.

Ketosis. Utilization of fats beyond a certain point in the face of impaired carbohydrate utilization leads to formation of ketone bodies in excess. Ketone bodies act as metabolic fuel in the liver. If production of ketone bodies is more than their destruction, there occurs *ketosis* or *ketonaemia*.

Consequences of ketosis include:

- *Cellular dehydration.* Ketone bodies being hyperosmolar remove water from the cells producing cellular dehydration.
- *Ketoacidosis.* Ketone bodies being strong acids dissociate readily and release H^+ ions. In the blood, these H^+ ions are buffered by bicarbonate ions (HCO_3^-) to form carbonic acid. Fall in bicarbonate level in blood leads to acidosis called ketoacidosis. Ketoacidosis develops rapidly in IDDM due to an absolute lack of insulin. This is not commonly seen in NIDDM where there is partial or no loss of insulin (but there is insulin resistance).

Features of ketoacidosis are:

- Rapid, deep respiration (dyspnoea, Kussmaul breathing),
- Acetone smell in patient's breath and
- Urine becomes highly acidic.
- *Electrolyte loss.* When capacity of kidney to replace plasma cations accompanying the organic anions with H^1 and $NH_4{}^1$ is exceeded, Na^1 and K^1 are lost in the urine. The electrolyte and water loss further adds to cellular dehydration.
- *Hypovolaemia and hypotension* may ultimately result from water and electrolytic loss and cellular dehydration.
- *Coma and death.* Depression of consciousness to the level of coma may eventually ensure owing to marked acidosis and dehydration which may finally lead to death.

3. Protein Catabolism Insulin is an anabolic hormone, i.e. it promotes protein synthesis and it also inhibits proteolysis. Therefore, in diabetes, due to insulin deficiency, the protein anabolism is suppressed and catabolism is increased. The amino acids released so are:

- Used in large amounts for energy production and
- Act as substrate for enhanced gluconeogenesis in liver promoted by insulin deficiency.

Consequences of suppression of protein anabolism and increased catabolism include:

- Protein depletion in the body,
- Muscle wasting and
- Negative nitrogen balance.

Clinical Features, Complications and Diagnosis of Diabetes Mellitus

After understanding the pathophysiology of diabetes mellitus, the clinical features, complications and diagnosis of diabetes mellitus can be understood easily.

Clinical Features and Complications of Diabetes Mellitus

Cardinal symptoms include polyuria, polydypsia, polyphagia and weight loss. Occurrence of these symptoms have been explained in pathophysiology.

Biochemical signs include hyperglycaemia, glycosuria, ketosis, ketonuria and ketoacidosis. These have been fully elucidated in pathophysiology.

Complications include:

- *Predisposition to infections* due to impaired phagocytic function and protein depletion.
- *Acute complications* include ketotic coma and nonketotic hyperosmolar coma (for details see pathophysiology).
- *Chronic complications* include:
  - *Atherosclerosis,* i.e. deposition of lipids underneath the tunica intima of blood vessels. The common sites are coronary, cerebral and peripheral arteries. It occurs due to longstanding hyperlipidaemia and hypercholesterolaemia.
- *Microangiopathy,* a vascular lesion in which the capillary basement membrane is thicker, probably due to structural changes caused in tissue proteins by their glycosylation. It is responsible for common complications of longstanding diabetes, which includes:
  - Diabetic retinopathy leading to blindness,
  - Diabetic nephropathy leading to renal failure and
  - Diabetic neuropathy involves autonomic nervous system and peripheral nerves.

Diagnosis of Diabetes Mellitus In clinically suspected cases, diagnosis is confirmed by the following investigations:

1. Urine Examination for Glycosuria. This is a rapid, simple and easy test for diagnosis of diabetes mellitus. Amount of glucose excreted in urine depends upon the severity of disease.

Disadvantage. Glycosuria depends upon the renal threshold level which itself is variable; hence, both overdiagnosis (false positive) and underdiagnosis (false negative) of diabetes are possible. For example, a nondiabetic individual with low renal threshold may pass glucose in the urine (renal glycosuria), while on the other hand, a diabetic with raised renal threshold will have a negative urine test for glucose.

2. Urine Examination for Ketone Bodies. Presence of ketone bodies (acetone) in urine along with glycosuria is almost diagnostic of diabetes mellitus. Other causes of ketonuria are starvation, prolonged fasting, following high fat diet and after repeated vomiting.

3. Fasting and Postprandial Blood Glucose Levels. Samples for estimation of fasting blood glucose is taken after overnight fast and that for postprandial are taken after 2 h of normal diet.

Normal values of plasma glucose are:

- Fasting: 70–110 mg% and
- Postprandial (after 2 h of meals): <140 mg%.

4. Glucose Tolerance Test (GTT). To perform this test, the patient is advised to have normal (unrestricted) carbohydrate diet at least 3 days prior to test. In the early morning, after an overnight fast, the fasting sample of blood and urine are taken. Then 75.0 g of glucose dissolved in 300 ml (a glass) of water is given orally, and blood and urine samples are collected every half an hour for 2½–3 h. Plasma glucose levels are plotted against the time scale and the graph so obtained is known as glucose tolerance curve. The results are interpreted as (Table 8.6-7):

- *In a normal person,* fasting plasma glucose levels range between 70 and 110 mg%, after glucose intake. The peak value of about 140 mg% is reached in an hour or so which returns to fasting level within 2–2½ h (Fig. 8.6-19). Urine does not show the presence of glucose.
- *In diabetes mellitus,* glucose tolerance curve is abnormal. Fasting glucose level is high (≥126 mg%) after

TABLE 8.6-7 Interpretation of Results of Glucose Tolerance Test

	Plasma glucose concentration (mg%)		
	Normal	*Impaired glucose tolerance*	*Diabetes mellitus*
Fasting level	<110	110–126	≥126
Peak postprandial level	<140	>140–<200	≥200

glucose intake peak is also high (≥200 mg%), and does not return to fasting level for a long time (4–6 h) (Fig. 8.6-19). This slow fall of glucose level indicates failure to control due to lack of insulin secretion following sugar ingestion.

- *Impaired glucose tolerance*. The fasting plasma levels between 110 and 126 mg% and peak values (after glucose ingestion) between 140 and 200 mg% are classified as impaired glucose tolerance (Fig. 8.6-19). Such patients are potential candidates to develop diabetes later on. Therefore, they need further supervision and repeated blood sugar estimations at frequent intervals to detect development of diabetes mellitus.

1. ***Glycosylated haemoglobin:*** The rate of formation of HbA_{1C} is directly proportional to ambient blood glucose concentration; a rise of 1% HbA_{1C} fraction indicates an average increase of 2 mmol/L (36 g%) plasma glucose. For details, see page 769.

Management of Diabetes Mellitus

Goals of Therapy. Goals of therapy of diabetes mellitus, irrespective of the type of diabetes are:

- To maintain blood glucose to normal or near normal,
- To maintain ideal body weight as far as possible,
- To keep the patient symptom free and
- To prevent or retard the onset of complications.

Treatment Modalities

1. ***Dietary management*** may be required alone or in association with drug therapy.

   Total energy intake should be specified to keep ideal body weight:
   - *Low energy and weight reducing diet* is recommended for obese patients with NIDDM.
   - *Weight maintenance diet* is prescribed to nonobese patients with NIDDM.

   Dietary constituents recommended for allocation of calories are:

• Carbohydrates	50–60% of calories
• Proteins	10–15% of calories
• Fats	30–35% of calories
• Vitamins and minerals	Adequate

   Frequent small meals should be advised to prevent glycaemic peaks and troughs.

2. ***Oral hypoglycaemic agents (OHA)*** along with dietary management is indicated in patients with NIDDM.
   - *OHA* are divided into two groups: sulphonylurea and *biguanides*. More commonly used drugs belong to second generation of sulphonylurea, e.g. glibenclamide.

3. ***Insulin along with dietary management.*** Insulin is delivered by injections with a very fine and sharp needle. *Indications* of insulin use include:
   - All patients with IDDM (juvenile onset diabetes),
   - Newly detected diabetes with ketoacidosis,
   - Emergencies associated with IDDM and NIDDM and
   - Patients with NIDDM not controlled by oral hypoglycaemic agents.

   Types of insulin: Two types of insulin preparations (short acting and long acting) are commercially available.

   Regimens of insulin therapy include:
   - *Conventional regimen* (single or two injections daily),
   - *Multiple subcutaneous injection regimen* (3–4 injections daily covering the major meals and snacks) and
   - *Continuous subcutaneous insulin* is delivered by insulin pump.

Awareness. It is essential to educate the patients to understand the disorder and learn to handle all aspects of their management comprehensively. Ideally, this can be achieved by multidisciplinary team of doctor, dietician and nurse in the outpatient department.

- Patients requiring insulin need to learn how to measure dose of insulin accurately with insulin syringe or pen, how to inject and how to adjust the dose of blood glucose level.
- Patients on insulin or on oral hypoglycaemic agents should carry a card stating names, address, type of insulin/or antidiabetic drugs and their doses, name, address details of treating physician.
- Self-assessment of glycaemic control particularly in patients with IDDM treated with insulin should be taught to perform capillary blood glucose measurements.
- Lifestyle advice should be recommended to type-II diabetics to reduce the risk of progression.

Gestational Diabetes

During pregnancy, maternal glucose metabolism changes to meet nutritional demand of developing fetus. In second trimester of pregnancy, insulin resistance decreases and at the same time renal threshold for glucose lowers.

- Gestational diabetes develops when pancreas is unable to secrete insulin to compensate insulin resistance.

  The risk factors include: obesity, family history of type-II diabetes.

  Treatment include: strict glycaemic control is required by dietary modification, particularly reducing consumption of refined carbohydrates.

  In patients with established diabetes, during pregnancy:
- Insulin doses must be increased.
- Monitoring is very essential, this includes:
  - Frequent estimation of blood glucose including postprandial measurements,

- HbA_{1C},
- Checks blood glucose periodically during night.

- Regular monitoring of fetus size and screening of fetal abnormalities.

Hypoglycaemia

Hypoglycaemia refers to a clinical condition caused by blood glucose levels below 45 mg% (2.5 mmol/L). The human body has developed a well-regulated system for an efficient maintenance of blood glucose concentration (see regulation of blood glucose page 783). However, still hypoglycaemia (though not common) is observed under some circumstances.

Types and Causes of Hypoglycaemia

Broadly, hypoglycaemia may be divided into two types:

- Hypoglycaemia in nondiabetics and
- Hypoglycaemia in diabetics (more common).

A. Hypoglycaemia in Nondiabetics

1. ***Postprandial hypoglycaemia,*** also known as *reactive hypoglycaemia,* occurs typically after meals within 4 h after ingestion of food. It is caused by transient rise in insulin levels, and symptoms are short lasting. It is more common in patients who have undergone gastric resection. In such patients, rapid movement of swallowed food into the intestine leads to sudden and marked increase in insulin secretion. The patients are advised to eat frequently rather than the three usual meals.
2. ***Postabsorption or fasting hypoglycaemia*** usually does not occur in normal fasting patients. It is seen in patients with:
   - *Insulin-secreting tumours* (adenomas) of pancreatic islets causing *hyperinsulinism, which* is a rare condition. Some adenomas (15%) may be malignant.
   - In some malignant tumours which do not involve pancreatic islets but hypoglycaemia occurs because of increased secretion of IGF-II.
   - *In hepatic failure,* degradation of insulin is less which may result in raised levels of insulin and hypoglycaemia.
   - Hypoglycaemia also occurs in hyperthyroidism and patients who have undergone gastrectomy. Gastrectomy leads to rapid passage of food into the intestine resulting in rapid absorption of glucose, though the plasma glucose level rises rapidly but followed by a rapid fall (hypoglycaemia) due to rise in insulin secretion.
3. ***Hypoglycaemia due to alcohol intake.*** In some individuals who are starved or engaged in prolonged exercise, alcohol consumption may cause hypoglycaemia due to decreased gluconeogenesis.

B. Hypoglycaemia in Diabetics. Hypoglycaemia in diabetics is more common than in nondiabetics. About 4% deaths of IDDM are said to be due to hypoglycaemia.

Causes of hypoglycaemia in diabetics include:

- Overdose of antidiabetic drugs, especially insulin, is comparatively a common cause of hypoglycaemia. This occurs due to difficulty in adjusting the requirement of antidiabetic agents. This is particularly observed in patients who are on an intensive treatment regimen.

Other factors responsible for hypoglycaemia in patients on regular antidiabetic treatment are:

- Intake of too little or no food,
- Heavy exercise,
- Mismatch between insulin administration and food habits,
- Alcohol intake, etc.

Symptoms and Signs of Hypoglycaemia

Symptoms and signs of hypoglycaemia occur due to effects of low levels of glucose per se (mainly on nervous system especially brain) and because of sympathetic stimulation (mainly on CVS, GIT and skin).

1. CNS symptoms are called *neuroglycopenic symptoms*. Since metabolism of brain mainly depends on blood glucose level, it is depressed when glucose level falls below 50–70 mg%. CNS becomes quite excitable (due to facilitation of neuronal activity by hypoglycaemia) which results into hallucinations, extreme nervousness, tremors, confusion, difficulty in concentration, inco-ordination, convulsions, drowsiness and cognitive dysfunctions. When blood glucose levels fall further (<30 mg%), hypoglycaemic coma may develop, which needs to be differentiated from hyperglycaemic coma in diabetics (Table 8.6-8), and needs an emergency treatment by immediate administration of large quantity of glucose intravenously.

Management Treatment of acute hypoglycaemia depends on its severity and whether the patient is conscious and able to swallow. The emergency treatment of hypoglycaemia includes:

- ***In mild cases:*** The subject can be self-treated by fast-acting oral carbohydrate (10–15 g) is taken as glucose drink or tablet followed by snack containing complex carbohydrates.
- ***In severe cases:*** External help is required. If the patient is semiconscious/unconscious, parenteral treatment is required as:
  - Intravenous 75 ml 20% dextrose or intramuscular glucagon (1 mg)
- If patient is conscious and able to swallow, give oral refined glucose as drink or sweets (25 g) or supply glucose gel/jam/honey to buccal mucosa.

Prevention of Hypoglycaemia

- Patient's education regarding potential causes and risk factors inducing hypoglycaemia, and its treatment

TABLE 8.6-8 Hypoglycaemic versus Hyperglycaemic Coma in Diabetics

Sr. No.	Feature	Hypoglycaemic coma	Hyperglycaemic coma
1.	Cause	Regular dose of insulin and no food leading to fall in blood glucose level	Too little or no insulin with regular food intake leading to high blood glucose level
2.	Precipitating factor	Severe unaccustomed exercise	Untreated/hidden infection
3.	Rate of onset	Rapid, develops within minutes	Invariably slow, takes hours or days to develop
4.	Symptoms and signs i) Vomiting ii) Breathing iii) Pulse iv) Skin and tongue v) CNS sign	 • No or occasional vomiting • Laboured breathing • No abnormal smell in breath • Bounding • Moist as no dehydration • Tendon reflexes brisk • Plantar is extensor	 • Frequent vomiting with abdominal pain • Rapid and shallow breathing (Kussmaul) • Air hunger present • Weak/feeble • Dry due to dehydration • Diminished • Plantar is normal (flexor)
5.	Investigations i) Urine ii) Blood	 • No glucose • No ketone bodies • Low blood glucose (usually <30 mg%) • Bicarbonate level normal • pH normal	 • Glycosuria marked • Ketonuria marked • High blood glucose (usually >400 mg%) • Low bicarbonate • Low pH

(accessible supply of glucose), and regular blood glucose monitoring is fundamental to prevent potentially diagnosed side effect of treatment.

- Relatives, friends should also need to be familiar with signs and symptoms of hypoglycaemia and also instructed as to how a situation is to be managed.

2. CVS Symptoms in hypoglycaemia are palpitation, tachycardia and cardiac arrhythmias.
3. GIT Symptoms include nausea and vomiting.
4. Skin Symptoms are sweating and hypothermia.

Compensatory Mechanisms to Fight Hypoglycaemia
See regulation of blood sugar level on Page 785.

GASTROINTESTINAL HORMONES

The glandular cells secreting gastrointestinal hormones are individually scattered in the epithelium of stomach and small intestine and not in the form of clusters of cells as in the endocrine glands. Hence, GIT may be considered as the largest mass of cells that secretes hormones.

The gastrointestinal hormones based on their physio-anatomical similarities can be broadly classified into three groups:

1. Gastrin family of hormones.
2. Secretin family of hormones.
3. Other gastrointestinal hormones.

For details see page 577.

Chapter 8.7

Endocrinal Functions of other Organs and Local Hormones

HORMONES OF THE HEART
- Structure
- Secretion
- Plasma levels, half-life and metabolism
- Natriuretic peptide receptors
- Actions

HORMONES OF THE KIDNEY
- Renin
- 1,25-dihydroxycholecalciferol
- Erythropoietin

PINEAL GLAND
- Functional anatomy
- Melatonin

THYMUS
- Functional anatomy
- Functions

LOCAL HORMONES
- Prostaglandins and related substances
- Acetylcholine
- Serotonin
- Histamine
- Adenosine derivatives
- Plasma polypeptides

In addition to the main endocrinal glands described in previous chapters, the other organs which have endocrinal functions are heart, kidney, pineal gland, thymus and others.

HORMONES OF THE HEART

The heart also acts as an endocrine organ. The muscle cells in the atria, and to a much lesser extent, in the ventricle, contain secretory granules.

The hormones secreted by heart include:

- Atrial natriuretic peptide (ANP),
- Brain natriuretic peptide (BNP) and
- C-type natriuretic peptide (CNP).

Structure

Atrial Natriuretic Peptide (ANP). It was the first natriuretic hormone isolated from the heart. It is a polypeptide and has 28 amino acid residues. It is formed from a large precursor molecule containing 151 amino acid residues.

Brain Natriuretic Peptide (BNP). It was the second natriuretic hormone, first isolated from the porcine brain and hence named as BNP. In humans, it is present in the heart and to a lesser extent in brain also. It is a polypeptide having 32 amino acid residues.

C-type Natriuretic Peptide (CNP). It was the third natriuretic hormone to be isolated in a sequence and so named C-type natriuretic peptide.

In the heart, it is present in a very small amount. It is mainly present in the brain, the pituitary, the kidneys and the vascular endothelial cells. It appears to be primarily a paracrine hormone, as very little amount is present in circulation.

Secretion

Atrial natriuretic peptide secretion is proportionate to the degree to which atria are stretched by increase in central venous pressure. Therefore, ANP secretion is affected by the following conditions:

- *Increase in ECF volume,* following infusion of isotonic saline or ingestion of a high sodium diet increases ANP secretion.
- *Immersion of body in water up to neck* increases central venous pressure by counteracting the effect of gravity on the circulation, and thus increases ANP secretion.
- *Rising from the supine to the standing position* lowers the central venous pressure and thus decreases the ANP secretion.

Plasma Levels, Half-Life and Metabolism

- ***Plasma Levels*** of ANP in normal humans ingesting moderate amounts of sodium are about 5 fmol/ml,

- ***Half-life*** of circulating ANP is very short.
- ***Metabolism.*** ANP is metabolized by the enzyme neural endopeptidase (NEP). Thiorphan inhibits the enzyme neural endopeptidase, and thus when administered, it increases circulating ANP.

Actions

1. Increase in Sodium Excretion by Kidneys. ANP and BNP increase excretion of sodium ion in urine by their following effects:

- Increasing glomerular filtration by dilating afferent arterioles and relaxing mesangial cells and
- Inhibiting Na^+ reabsorption at the level of renal tubules.

2. Role in Escape Phenomenon. See page 752.

3. Lowering of Blood Pressure. ANP lowers the blood pressure by their peripheral and central effects.

i. ***Peripheral blood pressure-lowering effects include:***
- Increase the capillary permeability leading to extravasation of fluid and a decline in blood pressure.
- Relax vascular smooth muscle (VSM) in arterioles and venules. CNP has a greater dilator effect on veins than ANP and BNP.
- Inhibit renin secretion and thus counteract the pressor effects of catecholamines and angiotensin II.

ii. ***Central blood pressure-lowering effect*** is exerted through the ANP-containing neural circuits in the brain which project from the anteromedial part of the hypothalamus to the areas in the lower brainstem that are concerned with neural regulation of cardiovascular system. In general, the effects of ANP in the brain are opposite to those of angiotensin-II. CNP and BNP in the brain probably have functions similar to those of ANP, but have not been elucidated in detail.

Natriuretic Peptide Receptors

Three types of natriuretic peptide receptors (NPR) are known:

1. NPR-A. It has an intracellular guanylyl cyclase domain (Fig. 8.7-1). Atrial natriuretic peptide (ANP) has greatest affinity for this receptor.

2. NPR-B. It also has an intracellular guanylyl cyclase domain (Fig. 8.7-1). CNP has the greatest affinity for this receptor.

3. NPR-C. It has only a small cytoplasmic domain (Fig. 8.7-1). It probably does not trigger any intracellular change. It removes natriuretic peptides from the bloodstream and then releases them later, helping to maintain a steady blood level of the hormones, and is thus also called *clearance receptor*.

HORMONES OF THE KIDNEY

The kidneys secrete three hormones:

- Renin,
- 1,25-Dihydroxycholecalciferol (see page 727) and
- Erythropoietin.

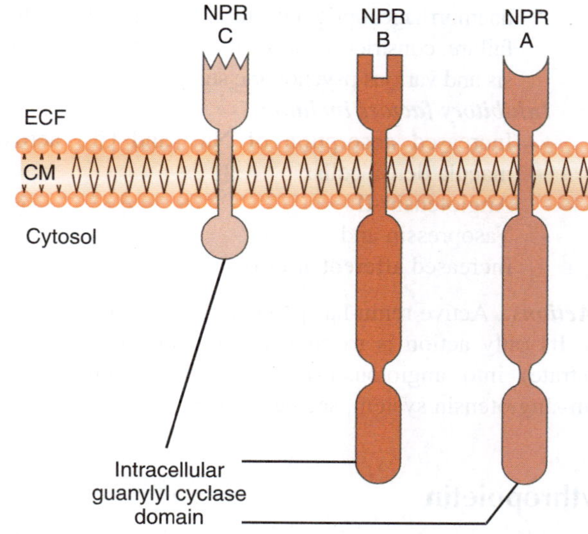

FIGURE 8.7-1 Three types of natriuretic peptide receptors: NPR-A, NPR-B and NPR-C.

Renin

Renin is an aspartyl protease secreted by the granular cells of juxtaglomerular apparatus of the kidneys into the blood stream. It acts in concert with angiotensin-converting enzyme (ACE) to form angiotensin-II from the angiotensinogen, and constitutes the so-called *renin–angiotensin system.*

Structure. Renin is a glycoprotein with a molecular weight of 37,326 in humans. Its molecule consists of two lobes, or domains. The active site of the enzyme is located in a deep cleft between the two lobes.

Synthesis. Renin is synthesized as a large preprohormone. Stages in the synthesis are:

- *Preprorenin.* It contains 406 amino acid residues.
- *Prorenin.* It contains 383 amino acid residues and is formed after the removal of a leader sequence of 23 amino acids from the amino terminal of preprorenin. Some prorenin is converted into renin in the kidneys and some is secreted in the circulation. In addition to the kidney, some other organs such as ovaries also secrete prorenin.
- *Renin.* The active renin contains 340 amino acid residues. It is formed after removal of the prosequence of 43 amino acids from the amino terminal of prorenin. It is important to note that prorenin is secreted by many organs, but the active renin is produced primarily in the kidneys.

Regulation The factors that affect renin secretion are:

- ***Stimulatory factors include:***
  - Increased sympathetic activity via renal nerves,
  - Increased circulating catecholamines,
  - Prostaglandins and
  - Conditions which decrease central venous pressure, such as Na^+ depletion, diuretics, hypotension,

haemorrhage, upright posture, dehydration, cardiac failure, constriction of renal artery or aorta, cirrhosis and various psychologic stimuli.

- ***Inhibitory factors include:***
  - Increased absorption of Na^+ and Cl^- across macula densa cells.
  - Angiotensin-II.
  - Vasopressin and
  - Increased afferent arteriolar pressure.

Actions. Active renin has plasma half-life of 80 min or less. Its only action is to convert angiotensinogen (renin substrate) into angiotensin-I. For further details about renin–angiotensin system, see pages 348, 534.

Erythropoietin

Structure. Erythropoietin (EPO) is glycoprotein with 165 amino acid residues and four oligosaccharide chains that are necessary for its activity in vivo. The gene encoding EPO is located on chromosome 7.

Source. In the fetus and neonate, the major site of production of erythropoietin is liver; but in adults, erythropoietin is mainly (85%) secreted by the juxtaglomerular apparatus of the kidneys with some contribution (15%) from the perivenous hepatocytes in the liver. It is important to note that when renal mass is reduced in adults by renal disease or nephrectomy, the liver cannot compensate and anaemia develops.

Actions. The main role of erythropoietin is to stimulate the bone marrow and cause erythropoiesis (for details see page 141).

Erythropoietin Receptor and Mechanism of Action. The *receptor for erythropoietin* is a linear protein with a single transmembrane domain that is a member of the cytokine receptor superfamily. The gene encoding EPO receptors is located on chromosome 19q. The erythropoietin receptor has three domains (extracellular, transcellular and intracellular).

Mechanism of action. Renal tissue hypoxia leads to increased release of hypoxia-inducible factor-1 (HIF-1), which serves as a transcription factor. HIF-1 binds to hypoxia-response element (HRE) of erythropoietin gene to induce transcription of mRNA for increase synthesis of erythropoietin. Erythropoietin binds to the receptors on the target cells. The receptor has tyrosine kinase activity and it activates a cascade of serine and threonine kinases, resulting in the growth and development of target cells. Thus, erythropoietin increases the number of erythropoietin-sensitive committed stem cells in the bone marrow that are converted to red blood cell precursors and subsequently to mature erythrocytes.

For further details of mechanism of action see page 142

Plasma Levels, half-life and Metabolism. Normal plasma levels of erythropoietin are 50 U/L. Its plasma half-life is about 5 h. It is mainly inactivated in the liver. Loss of even a small portion of the sialic acid residues in the carbohydrate moieties that are part of the erythropoietin molecule shortens its half-life to 5 min, making it biologically ineffective.

Recombinant Erythropoietin. *Epoetin alpha* is a recombinant erythropoietin, which is produced in animal cells. Clinically, it has following uses:

- In treatment of chronic anaemia, which occurs due to erythropoietin deficiency in patients with renal failure and
- To stimulate red cell production in individuals who are banking a supply of their own blood in preparation for autologous transfusions during elective surgery.

Regulation of Secretion of Erythropoietin

1. ***Hypoxia*** is the main factor regulating erythropoietin secretion. For example, occurrence of hypoxia following haemorrhage stimulates erythropoietin secretion which in turn increases erythropoiesis to compensate hypoxia. Conversely, when the RBC volume is increased above normal by blood transfusion, the erythropoietic activity of the bone marrow decreases.
   Mechanism. It has been suggested that the O_2 sensor-regulating erythropoietin secretion in the kidney and liver is a haem protein that in the dioxy form stimulates and in the oxy form inhibits transcription of the erythropoietin gene to form erythropoietin mRNA.
2. ***Other factors*** that affect erythropoietin secretion are:
   - *Cobalt salt and androgens* stimulate erythropoietin secretion.
   - *Alkalosis* that develops at high altitude facilitates erythropoietin secretion.
   - *Catecholamines* via a β-adrenergic mechanism also facilitate erythropoietin secretion.
   - *Adenosine* stimulates and adenosine antagonist (theophylline) inhibits erythropoietin secretion.

PINEAL GLAND

Functional Anatomy

Gross Anatomy and Location. Pineal gland, also known as epiphysis, is a small structure (5 mm × 7 mm) shaped like a pine cone. It is situated in the groove between the two superior colliculi in diencephalic area of brain above the hypothalamus (Fig. 8.7-2). It forms the posterior boundary of the third ventricle and lies under the posterior end of corpus callosum (Fig. 8.7-3). It has a stalk which divides anteriorly into two laminae. The superior lamina contains the habenular commissure while the inferior lamina has the posterior commissure.

Structure. The salient features are:

The pineal stroma has two types of cells: neuroglial and parenchymal.

Parenchymal Cells are large epithelial cells (pinealocytes) with features suggesting that they have a secretory function.

- Like other endocrine glands, the pineal gland has highly permeable fenestrated capillaries.

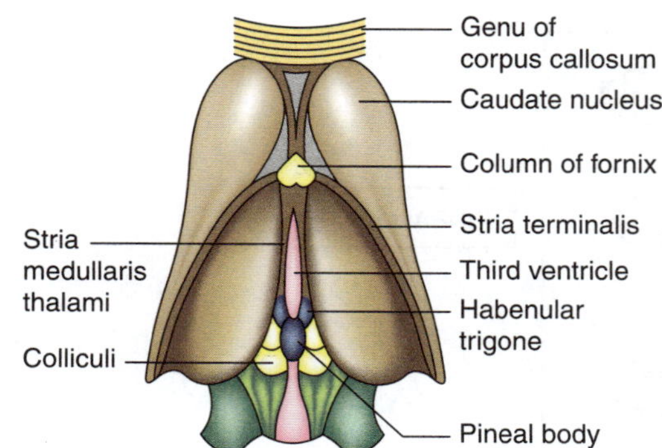

FIGURE 8.7-2 Location of pineal body in the groove between the two superior colliculi.

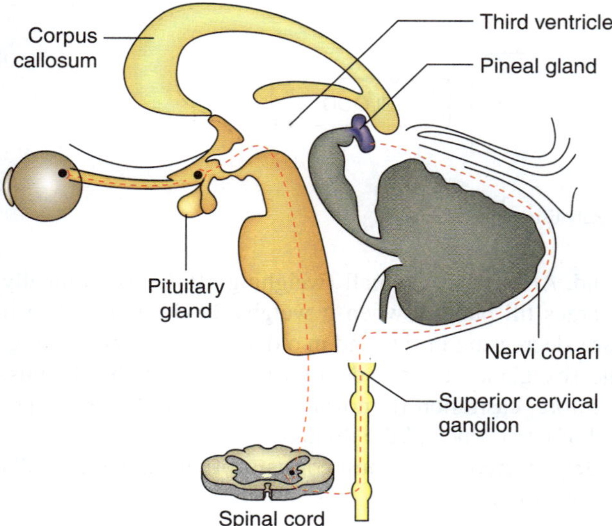

FIGURE 8.7-3 Sagittal section of human brainstem showing pineal gland, its innervation (dotted line). Note, the pineal body forms the posterior boundary of third ventricle and lies under the posterior end of corpus callosum.

- *In infants,* the pineal gland is large, and the cells tend to be arranged in alveoli.
- *In adults,* the pineal gland gets calcified, i.e. small concretions of calcium phosphate and carbonate (*pineal sand*) appear in the tissue. But the epithelial cells exist and secrete some hormonal substance. Because of calcification, the normal pineal gland is often visible on radiographic films of the skull in adults, and a shift of the pineal shadow to one side may indicate a space occupying intracranial lesion on the other side.

Melatonin

Structure, Synthesis, Plasma Levels and Metabolism

Structure and Synthesis. The hormone melatonin is an indole (N-acetyl-5 methoxy-tryptamine). It is synthesized by the parenchymal cells of pineal gland. The enzymes responsible for its synthesis from serotonin are present in pinealocytes. Serotonin—produced from tryptophan—is acted upon by serotonin N-acetylase (the rate-limiting enzyme) to give N-acetylserotonin, S-adenosylmethionine being the methyl group donor to produce melatonin (Fig. 8.7-4).

Plasma Levels of Melatonin show fluctuations with night time rise. The nocturnal plasma levels of melatonin are much higher in children than adults and they decline with age. The average plasma levels of melatonin at various age groups are:

- 1–3 years of age: 250 pg/ml (1080 pmol/L),
- 8–15 years of age: 120 pg/ml,
- 20–27 years of age: 70 pg/ml and
- 67–84 years of age: 30 pg/ml.

Metabolism. In the liver, circulating melatonin is rapidly metabolized by 6-hydroxylation followed by conjugation. More than 90% of melatonin that appears in the urine is in the form of 6-hydroxy conjugates and 6-sulphatoxy melatonin. The exact pathway for melatonin metabolism in brain is not known; perhaps it involves the cleavage of indole nucleus.

Melatonin Receptors and Functions of Melatonin

Melatonin Receptors. Melatonin acts through G-coupled receptors. Two types of melatonin receptors have been identified: MT-1 and MT-2.

- MT-1 receptors possess a high affinity melatonin-binding site compared with MT-2 receptors and are of two subtypes: MT-1a and MT-1b.
- MT-1 receptors inhibit adenylyl cyclase, and MT-2 receptors stimulate phosphoinositol hydrolysis.

Functions of Melatonin

1. ***Role in circadian rhythm of the body.*** The dark–light cycle through suprachiasmatic nuclei (SCN) of hypothalamus initiates neural and humoral signals that entrain a wide variety of well-known circadian rhythms, including diurnal variation in melatonin secretion. The nocturnal peaks in secretion of melatonin in turn appear to be an important hormonal signal entraining other cells in the body for circadian rhythm.
2. ***Effects on the gonads.*** Both inhibitory and facilitatory effects of melatonin on the gonads are described depending upon the species and time of injection of melatonin. This variability in the effect has led to the hypothesis that it is not the melatonin per se but the diurnal change in melatonin secretion that functions as some sort of timing signal which coordinates internal events with the light–dark cycle in the environment.
3. ***Effect on MSH and ACTH secretion.*** An inhibitory effect of melatonin on MSH and ACTH secretion has been reported.

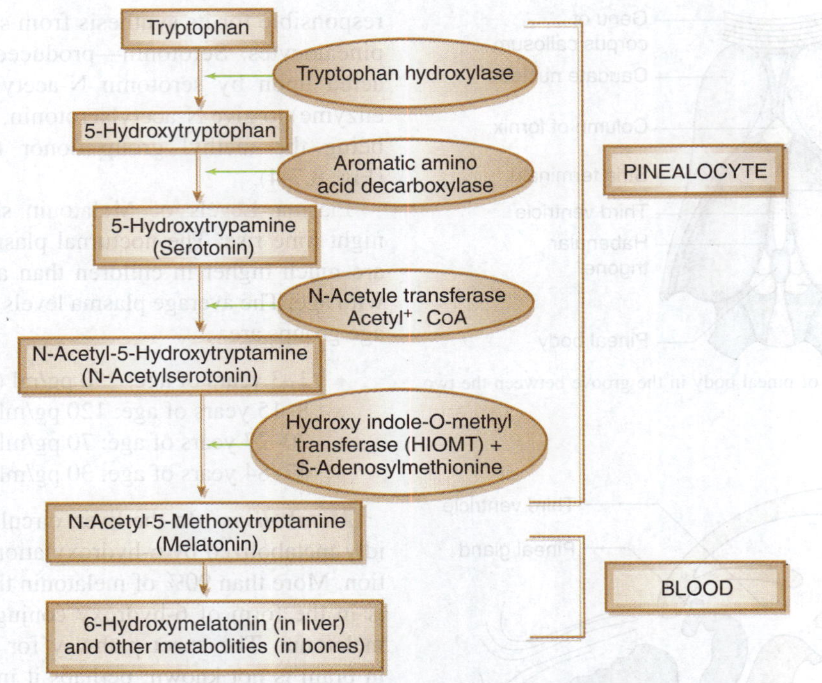

FIGURE 8.7-4 Synthesis and metabolism of melatonin.

4. ***Other actions of melatonin*** include induction of sleep, and inhibition of puberty.

Regulation of Melatonin Secretion

Melatonin Secretion Shows Diurnal Variation in humans and all other species studied to date. It is secreted more during dark period of the day than during the day light hours. This correlates with various internal activities in different periods of the day, i.e. circadian rhythm.

Hypothalamus is Responsible for Circadian Fluctuations of Melatonin Secretion. Hypothalamus exerts its effect through the norepinephrine secreted by postganglionic sympathetic nerves (nerviconari) that innervate the pineal gland. The neural pathway involved is (Fig. 8.7-3):

- ***Retino-hypothalamic fibres*** involved in light–dark cycle synapse in suprachiasmatic nucleus of hypothalamus.
- ***Descending pathways from suprachiasmatic nucleus of hypothalamus*** converge on the intermediolateral grey column of the thoracic spinal cord and end on the preganglionic sympathetic neurons.
- ***Preganglionic fibres*** pass from the spinal cord to superior cervical ganglion.
- ***Postganglionic neurons*** from the superior cervical ganglion project to the pineal in the nerviconari (Fig. 8.7-3).

THYMUS

Functional Anatomy

Thymus is a small lymphoid structure located in the lower part of neck in front of the trachea, below the thyroid gland. At birth, it is small (weighing 10–12 g), gradually enlarges till puberty when it weighs 20–30 g, and then it starts decreasing in size and in old age weighs about 3–6 g. The sex glands exert a depressant effect on the thymus; therefore, castration (removal of gonads) prolongs the period of persistence of the thymus.

Histologically, thymus consists of the inner medulla and outer cortex.

- *Medulla.* It comprises reticular epithelial cells, a few lymphocytes and concentric corpuscles of Hassall.
- *Cortex.* It includes actively multiplying, closely packed lymphocytes and contains no Hassall's corpuscles.

Functions

Thymus has two functions:

- Immunological functions and
- Endocrinal functions.

1. Immunological Functions of Thymus

i. Development of immunologically competent T-lymphocytes is an essential function of the thymus. The lymphocytes produced in bone marrow are processed in the thymus into T-lymphocytes, which pass on to the lymph nodes. The hormone thymosin produced by reticuloepithelial tissue in the thymus stimulates lymphopoiesis. It mainly promotes proliferation of T-lymphocytes. This occurs during the period between 3 months before and 3 months after the birth. Because of this reason, removal of thymus 3 months after birth will not affect the cell-mediated immunity. However, thymectomy in a newborn animal produces:

- Lymphopenia and atrophy of all lymphoid tissue,
- Failure to produce circulating antibodies against the antigens entering the body (e.g. bacteria, viruses, red blood cells, etc.),
- Suppression of delayed hypersensitivity reaction and
- Failure to produce graft rejection.

ii. Maintenance of adequate pool of T-lymphocyte. The hormone thymosin produced by thymus also stimulates lymphopoiesis in the peripheral lymphoid tissue and thus plays a role in maintenance of an adequate pool of T-lymphocytes in adult life. Therefore, removal of thymus in adult animals causes decline of immunological capacity but only after a few months during which the existing pool of competent lymphocytes becomes gradually depleted.

2. Endocrine Function of Thymus. Thymus tissue secretes two hormones, thymosin and thymin.

i. Thymosin. It is a peptide, which, as described above, promotes proliferation of T-lymphocytes in the thymus and peripheral lymphoid tissue.

ii. Thymin, also called thymopoietin, inhibits acetylcholine release at motor nerve endings and thus suppresses neuromuscular activity. Therefore, in hyperactivity of thymus, there occurs myasthenia gravis (see page 83).

LOCAL HORMONES

As described earlier, the endocrine glands secrete hormones into the blood stream which show their actions at some distant places. In contrast, the local hormones are the substances which are produced in many tissues, and when activated in certain circumstances, execute their actions in the same area or in immediate neighbourhood. Commonly produced local hormones are:

- Prostaglandins and related substances, such as thromboxanes, prostacyclin, leukotrienes and lipoxins.
- Other local hormones include acetylcholine; serotonin (5HT); histamine; adenosine derivatives, e.g. AMP, ADP and ATP; and plasma polypeptides, e.g. angiotensin, plasma kinins, etc.
- Local hormones produced in the blood, such as bradykinin, serotonin and angiotensinogen.

Prostaglandins and Related Substances Prostaglandins and related substances include thromboxanes, prostacyclin, leukotriene and lipoxin. These substances are called *eicosanoids*, reflecting their origin from the 20-carbon (eicosa) polyunsaturated fatty acid *arachidonic acid,* linoleic and linolenic acid.

Prostaglandins were so named by Von Euler in 1937, because they were first isolated from prostatic secretion in semen. However, now they are known to be synthesized in almost all tissues of the body.

Structure. Prostaglandins are thus a series of 20-carbon unsaturated fatty acids containing a cyclopentane ring. On the basis of the configuration of this ring, prostaglandins are divided into various groups, e.g. PGA, PGD, PGE and PGF. The number of double bonds in the side chain is indicated by subscript numbers, e.g. PGE_1, PGE_2, etc. Presently, a variety of prostaglandins are identified, but the active forms are PGD_2, PGE_2 and PGF_2.

Synthesis of Prostaglandins and Related Substances

Steps involved in the synthesis of prostaglandins and the related substances are (Fig. 8.7-5):

- *Phospholipids* of the cell membrane are released by the action of phospholipase A_2 and converted into arachidonic acid.
- *Arachidonic acid* is converted into prostaglandin H_2 (PGH_2) by the action of enzymes cyclo-oxygenase 1 and 2 (Cox-1 and 2).
- *PGH_2* is converted into various other prostaglandins, thromboxanes and prostacyclin by various tissue isomerases (Fig. 8.7-5).

Note. In addition to the above-mentioned hormones, arachidonic acid is converted into two more hormones:

- By the action of 5-lipoxygenase into 5-hydroperoxy-eicosatetraenoic acid (5 HPETE), which is converted into *leukotrienes* and
- By the action of 15-lipoxygenase into 15 HPETE, which is then converted into *lipoxins*.

Actions of Prostaglandins and Related Substances

Mechanism of Action. The nonvascular actions of PGs are related to cAMP but vascular actions are independent of cAMP. Thus, the actions of PGs are mediated at least in large part by the serpentine receptors coupled to G proteins (Table 8.7-1). The examples of the tissues in which the effects of the prostaglandins and related substances are predominant are also shown in Table 8.7-1.

Actions of Prostaglandins. PGs have multitudinous and varied actions on almost all tissues of the body. Many of them are discussed in the chapters on the systems in which they play an important role. Some important actions of PGs are:

1. ***Actions on cardiovascular system***
   - Peripheral arteriolar dilatation, especially in splanchnic and muscular bed is caused by PGA_1 and PGA_2.
   - Local vasodilatation, when given into an artery, is caused by PGE_2.
2. ***Actions on kidneys.*** PGA_2 increases renal cortical blood flow and increases urinary excretion of sodium, potassium and water.

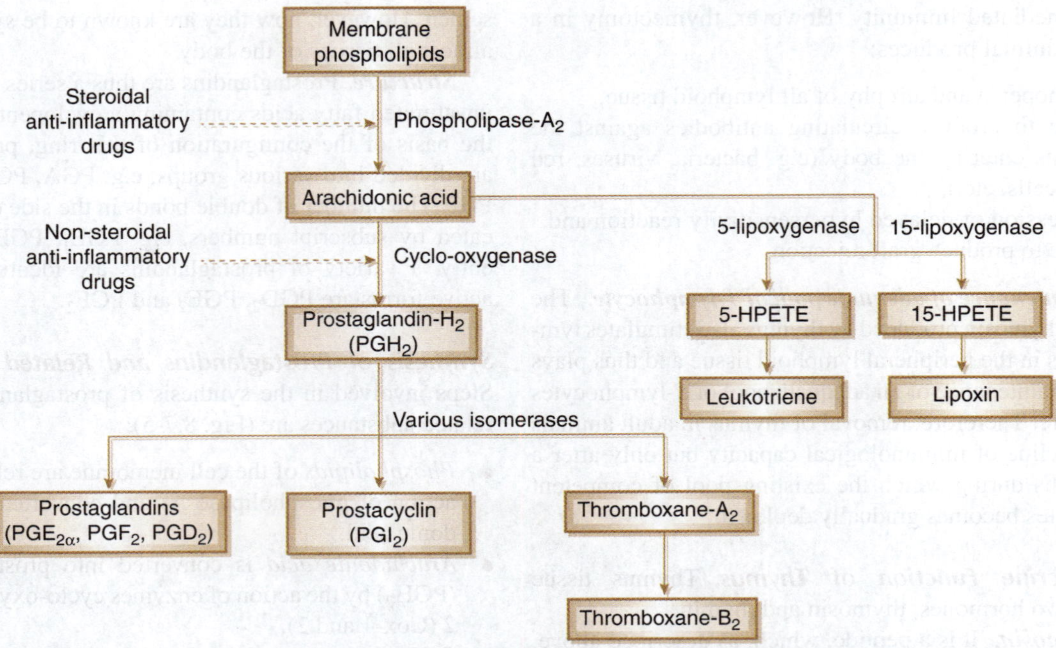

FIGURE 8.7-5 Synthesis of prostaglandins and related substances.

TABLE 8.7-1 Prostaglandins and Related Substances, Their Receptors and Tissues in which Their Effects are Prominent

Substance	Receptors	Tissue
PGD_2	DP_1 and DP_2	Mast cells, airways and brain
PGE_2	EP_1, EP_2, EP_3 and EP_4	Vascular smooth muscle, kidney, platelets and brain
PGF	FP_α and FP_β	Vascular smooth muscle, uterus and airways
Thromboxanes	TP_α and TP_β	Platelets, vascular smooth muscle, macrophages and kidney
Prostacyclin	IP	Endothelium, kidneys, brain and platelets
Leukotriene	Cys LT_1, Cys LT_2 and BLT	Vascular smooth muscle, airways and leucocytes
Lipoxins	LP_α and LP_β	Vascular smooth muscle and lymphocytes

3. *Actions on female reproductive system*

- PGF_{2a} is reported to initiate labour by stimulating contraction of gravid uterus.
- PGF_{2a} is also reported to be responsible for painful uterine contractions during menstruation (dysmenorrhoea).
- PGEs and PGFs promote secretion of hypothalamic gonadotropin-releasing hormone (GnRH).

4. *Role of prostaglandins in inflammation.* Prostaglandins are reported to mediate following effects of inflammation:

- Histamine-induced vascular permeability,
- Pain producing effect of bradykinin by sensitizing cutaneous nerves,
- Can produce pain by their direct action in higher concentration and
- Increase vascular permeability and cellular infiltration.

5. *Actions on blood platelets*

- PGE_1 inhibits platelet aggregation through activation of adenylyl cyclase.
- PGE_2, PGG_2 and PGH_2 promote the aggregation of platelets. Nonsteroidal anti-inflammatory drugs (e.g. aspirin and indomethacin) inhibit this effect by preventing formation of PGG_2 and PGH_2 from arachidonic acid.

6. *Action on bronchial musculature*

- PGE_{2a} causes contraction of bronchial smooth muscles and may precipitate bronchial asthma.
- PGE_3, on the other hand, relaxes bronchial smooth muscles.

7. *Actions on GIT*

- PGE_1, PGEs and PGA_1 inhibit the secretion of gastric HCl.

- PGEs and PGF_{2a} cause inhibition of sodium and water absorption producing profuse watery, cholera-like diarrhoea.
- PGE and PGF increase intestinal motility.

8. ***Metabolic actions of PGs*** in vivo are variable. In vitro, PGE_1 inhibits the ACTH, GH, glucagon and epinephrine-induced lipolysis.
9. ***Actions on nervous system***
   - On CNS, the PGs function as transmitters or modulators of neuron activity.
   - In the ANS, the PGEs stimulate cholinergic neuroeffector junctions and inhibit the release and response to norepinephrine.
10. ***Actions on the eye.*** PGE_2 and PGF_{2a} occur in the iris and produce miosis. Therefore, nonsteroidal anti-inflammatory drugs are used to prevent occurrence of miosis during cataract operation.

Actions of Thromboxane A_2. Thromboxane A_2 is synthesized by platelets. It promotes:

- Vasoconstriction and
- Platelet aggregation

Actions of Prostacyclin. Prostacyclin is produced in vascular endothelium. It produces vasodilatation. The important balance between thromboxane A_2 and prostacyclin in haemostasis is discussed in Chapter 3.5.

Actions of Leukotrienes. Leukotrienes include C_4 (LT C_4), $LTLD_4$, LTE_4 and LTF_4. They are mediators of allergic responses and inflammation. Their release is provoked when specific allergens combine with IgE antibodies on the surfaces of mast cells. They produce:

- Brancho constriction,
- Arteriolar constriction,
- Increased vascular permeability and
- Attract neutrophils and eosinophils.

Receptors for leukotrienes are:

- Cys LT_1. It mediates bronchoconstriction, chemotaxis and increased vascular permeability.
- Cys LT_2. It mediates constriction of pulmonary vascular smooth muscle.
- BLT. It predominantly mediates chemotaxis.

Actions of Lipoxins. Physiological role of lipoxins is uncertain. Their actions include:

- Dilatation of microvasculature (by lipoxin A) and
- Inhibition of cytotoxic effects of natural killer cells (by lipoxin A and lipoxin B).

Other Local Hormones Synthesized in Tissues In addition to prostaglandins and related substances, the other local hormones synthesized in the tissues are:

- Acetylcholine (see page 1008),
- Serotonin (see page 1013),
- Histamine (see pages 179, 1013),
- Substance P (see page 351),
- Heparin (see page 216) and
- Gastrointestinal hormones (see page 587).

Local Hormones Produced in Blood Local hormones produced in blood are:

- Serotonin (see page 206, 350),
- Angiotensinogen (see page 348) and
- Bradykinin (see page 347).

Section 9

Reproductive System

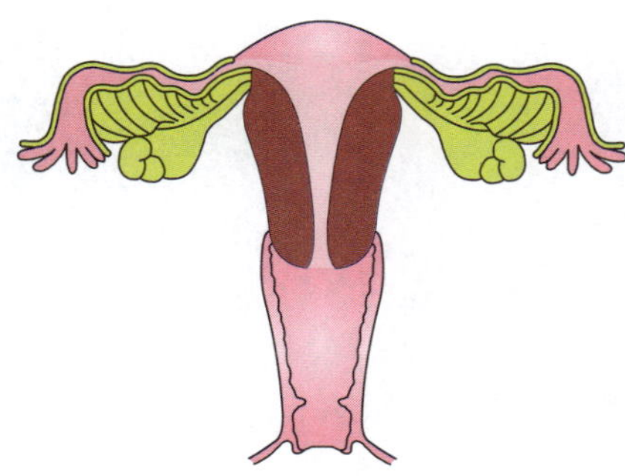

Reproduction is a multidimensional subject with physiological, biochemical, genetic, psychological, emotional, social, economic, moral and many other aspects. The physiology of reproductive system begins with *sex determination,* i.e. genetic differentiation which occurs during fertilization (penetration of the ovum by sperm). An ovum always contains 22+X chromosomes, while a sperm may contain either 22+X or 22+Y chromosomes. Therefore, after fertilization the zygote's chromosomal patterns can be either 44+XX (i.e. female genotype) or 44+XY (i.e. male genotype). The next step in reproductive physiology is *sex differentiation* which begins at about 7 to 8 weeks of intrauterine life when the primitive, bipotential sex gland or gonad (gone=seed) differentiates into either testis or ovary depending upon the genotype (gonadal differentiation). From this point onwards, depending on whether the embryo has a pair of testes or ovaries there will occur development of male or female accessory sex organs (*genital differentiation or phenotype*). After remaining quiescent during childhood, the gonads suddenly awaken into vigorous activity for a period of 3 to 4 years during which gonadal development and maturation reaches to the point where reproduction is possible for the first time. During this phase, there also occurs a sudden spurt of physical growth and the child grows into an adult. This transitional period between the childhood and adulthood is called period of *puberty*, during which the secondary sex characters develop.

The adult *male reproductive physiology* and *female reproductive physiology* involves gametogenic and endocrinal functions of testes and ovaries, respectively. In a sexually active female, the *physiology of pregnancy* involves: fertilization at a proper time and place (fallopian tube), development of the foetus in mother's womb, and finally birth of a new human being, either male or female. After child birth mother continues to provide nourishment by breastfeeding for a further period of 6–9 months (*physiology of lactation*).

The understanding of reproductive physiology is not only important for the promotion of conception and normal foetal growth but also for the prevention of conception (*physiology of contraception*) for population control which is of global concern.

The point when reproductive physiology ends is called *climacteric* (literally meaning, a major turning point). In females it is *menopause*; but in males there is no sharp point.

Chapter 9.1

Sexual Growth and Development

PREPUBERTAL SEXUAL GROWTH AND DEVELOPMENT

In a human embryo, sexual growth involves two processes:

- Sex determination and
- Sex differentiation.

Sex Determination

Sex Determination also known as *genetic differentiation,* refers to the genotype of the foetus, whether male or female. The genotype is determined by the presence of sex chromosomes, hence also known as *chromosomal sex differentiation.*

Human Chromosomes. Each cell (except ovum and sperm) in a normal adult male and female possesses 46 chromosomes (44 autosomes +2 sex chromosomes) usually arranged in an arbitrary pattern (karyotype).

- These chromosomes exist in pairs (22 pairs of autosomes +1 pair of sex chromosomes) and are referred to as diploid (or double number) *chromosomes.*
- *Autosome pairs* are identified by the numbers 1 to 22 on the basis of their morphologic characteristics.
- *Sex chromosomes* are called X and Y chromosomes.
- *The females* possess 44 autosomes plus 2X chromosomes (44+XX).
- The males possess 44 autosomes plus an X chromosome and a Y chromosome (44+XY).

Human Gametes. The mature male gametes are called sperms and mature female gametes are called ova. During gametogenesis, there occurs meiosis (*reduction division*); therefore, the mature sperm and ovum contain half the number of chromosomes, i.e. 23 (22 autosomes + one sex chromosome). This is called *haploid* number.

- Since, the primitive female germ cells (*oogonia*) from which mature ova are formed contain 44+XX chromosomes, so each ovum will contain 22+X chromosomes (Fig. 9.1-1).
- The primitive male germ cells (spermatogonia) from which mature sperms are formed contain 44+XY chromosomes, so half of the normal sperms will contain 22+X and other half will have 22+Y chromosomes (Fig. 9.1-1).

Genetic Sex Determination of the embryo occurs during fertilization, i.e. penetration of the ovum by the sperm as:

- When an ovum (22+X) is fertilized by a sperm containing 22+X chromosomes, the resultant zygote's chromosomal pattern will be 44+XX (*female genotype*).
- When an ovum (22+X) is fertilized by a sperm containing 22+Y chromosomes, the resultant zygote's chromosomal pattern will be 44+XY (male genotype).
- The human Y chromosome is smaller than the X chromosomes. The sperms containing the Y chromosomes are lighter and able to swim faster up in the female

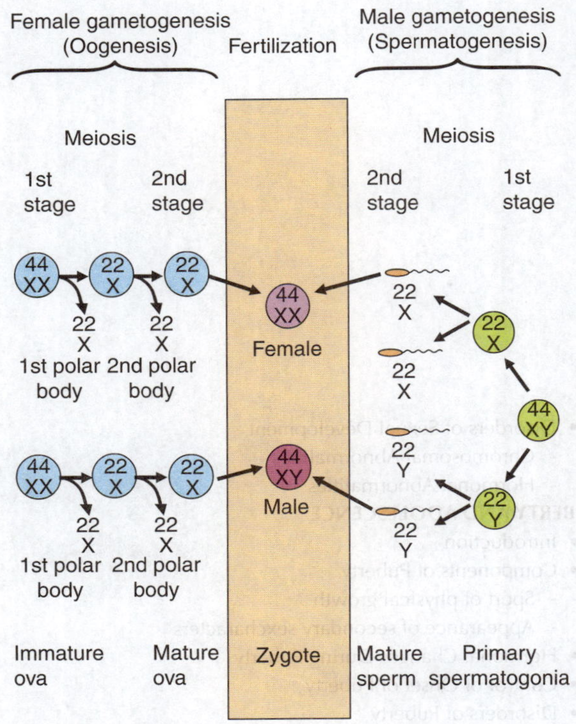

FIGURE 9.1-1 Basis of genetic sex determination.

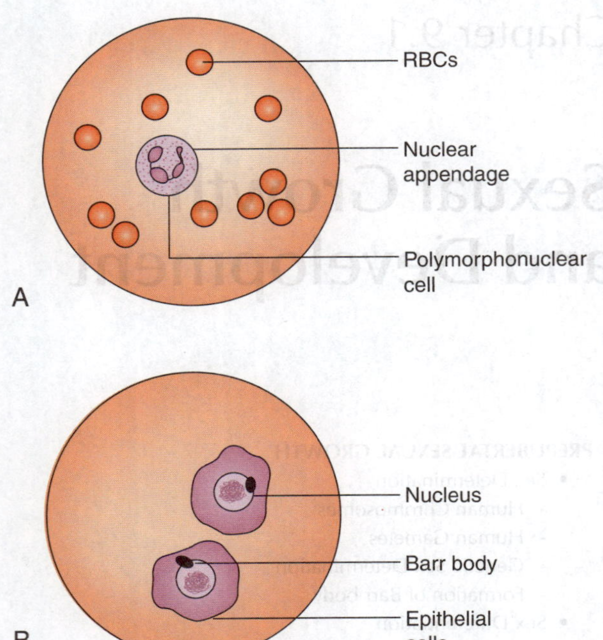

FIGURE 9.1-2 Sex chromatins (Barr body) seen in: **(A)** polymorphonuclear cell and **(B)** epithelial cells of epidermal spinous layer.

genital tract, thus reaching the ovum rapidly. This probably accounts for the fact that the number of males born is slightly greater than the number of females.

Formation of Barr Body During embryonic development, the somatic cells start multiplying immediately after fertilization. It has been seen that one of X chromosomes of somatic cells in the female embryo becomes inactive while the other remains active. The exact details about the inactivation process of X chromosomes are not known, but it may probably be due to the presence of a gene called *Xist* (X-inactivation centre) in the chromosome that produces noncoding mRNA. Formation of *noncoding mRNA* starts inactivation process in the centre of X chromosomes which continues in the subsequent divisions of the cells. The choice to be inactive of one of the X-chromosome is random. Therefore, in an adult female about half of the somatic cells contain an active X chromosome of paternal origin and other half of maternal origin.

The inactive X chromosome of each somatic cell forms a condensed mass called *sex chromatin* or *Barr body*. The Barr body can be seen near the nuclear membrane of the cells (Fig. 9.1-2).

Significance of Barr Body.

1. ***Identification of sex genotype.*** Since Barr bodies are present in the somatic cells of females only, so the sex genotype can be identified by a cytological test. The most suitable cells for this test are:
   - Epithelial cells of epidermal spinous layer,
   - Buccal mucosal cells,
   - Mucosal cells of vagina,- and
   - Polymorphonuclear cells (in about 15% of the polymorphonuclear cells the Barr bodies are seen as drumsticks projecting from the nuclei).
2. ***Identification of abnormal genotypes.*** In the abnormal cells with three or more X chromosomes, there are two or more Barr bodies.

Sex Differentiation

After the sex determination (genotype sex) during fertilization, the normal sex differentiation in the embryo proceeds sequentially. The stages of sex differentiation are:

- Gonadal differentiation,
- Genital differentiation and
- Psychological differentiation.

Gonadal Differentiation

Gonadal differentiation or *gonadogenesis* refers to formation of gonads, i.e. testes in males and ovaries in females. Gonadal sex differentiation is dependent on the genotype of the embryo.

Genital ridge or the urogenital ridge (the condensation of mesenchymal tissue present on each side near the adrenal glands) is the site where gonads develop. The primordial germ cells migrate into the genital ridge, where proliferation of both germinal and nongerminal cells leads to formation of bipotential gonads.

Bipotential gonads. Bipotential gonads are also known as primordial or primitive or indifferent or ambisexual gonads. In a human embryo, these can be identified after 30 days of fertilization. Upto 6 weeks of gestation the bipotential gonads are identical in both sexes and have the rudiments of both male and female gonads.

Structure. The bipotential gonad consists of a medulla, a cortex and primordial germ cells. The germ cells are embedded in the layer of cortical epithelium surrounding a core of medullary mesenchymal tissue (Fig. 9.1-3A, B).

Testicular Differentiation In a genetic male (44+XY) embryo, the bipotential gonads begin to differentiate into testes at approximately sixth week. The Y chromosome plays a key role in the process of testicular differentiation.

Role of Y-chromosome in Testicular Differentiation

- Two transcription genes, one for testicular differentiation and another for formation of Mullerian duct inhibitory substance (MIS) are present on the Y chromosome.
- The gene responsible for testicular differentiation is located near the tip of the short arm of Y chromosome and is called SRY gene (SRY= Sex-determining region of the Y chromosome).
- The SRY gene encodes the *testis determining factor* (TDF) which triggers the testicular differentiation.
- The TDF gene product causes Sertoli cell differentiation. Sertoli cell activity is critically important for all subsequent events in male sexual differentiation.

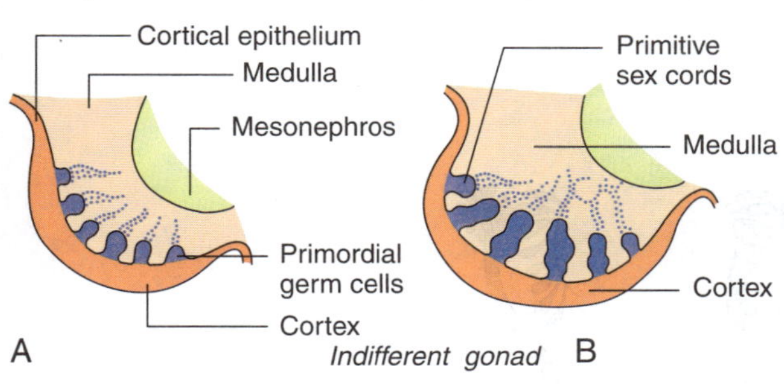

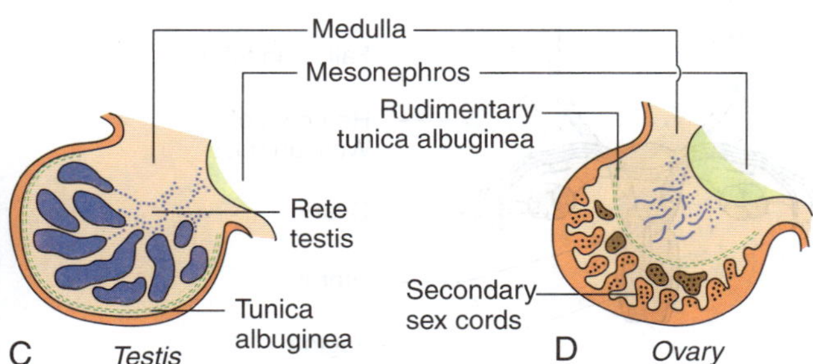

FIGURE 9.1-3 Diagrammatic structure of human bipotential gonad **(A and B)**, and development of testis from the medulla **(C)**, and ovary from the cortex **(D)**.

Process of Testicular Differentiation

- ***At about 6th week*** of gestation, the testicular differentiation begins with the appearance of primitive seminiferous cords (sex cords) from the germinal epithelium covering the medulla of bipotential gonad (Fig. 9.1-3).
- ***At about 7th week of gestation***
  - The solid sex cords are canalized to form seminiferous tubules
  - Meanwhile, a large number of Sertoli cells appear and get organized along the seminiferous tubules.
  - The cortical region (from which female gonad develop) undergoes regression.
- ***At about 8th week*** of gestation, Leydig (interstitial) cells appear in the interstitial spaces of seminiferous tubules and continue to proliferate. The Leydig cells are derived from the sex cords that are not canalized. The membrane of Leydig cells has receptors for human chorionic gonadotropins (HCG) and for luteinizing hormone (LH).
- ***At about 9th week*** of gestation, the Leydig cells synthesize and secrete testosterone in response to HCG secreted by placenta.
- ***At about 14th week*** of gestation, the number of Leydig cells is so much increased that they form more than half of the volume of the testes.
- ***At the end of 16th week*** (4 months), the number of foetal Leydig cells decreases and at term only a few are present.
- ***At about the 35th week*** of gestation, there occurs descent of testes through inguinal canal into scrotum. This marks the final stage of testicular differentiation.

Ovarian Differentiation

- In a genetic female (44+XX) embryo, by about 10th week of gestation, ovarian differentiation can be identified histologically. Since development of ovary requires the presence of XX chromosomes, therefore, with XO chromosomal constitution there may be no ovarian tissue.
- Ovarian differentiation occurs in the absence of TDF.
- The ovaries develop on each side from the cortical region of the bipotential gonad (Fig. 9.1-3C).
- Thecoelomic epithelial cells (cortical cells) proliferate and form granulosa cells which surround the germ cells and commit them to oocyte formation.The Hilar cells form later during the development.
- Meanwhile, the medulla from which testes develop, regresses.
- During 11–12 week of gestation, oogonia undergo meiotic division to form oocyte which is the end point of ovarian differentiation.
- Embryonic ovary, like testis, does not secrete any hormone.
- Hormonal treatment of the mother has no effect on gonadal (as opposed to ductal and genital) differentiation in humans, although it does in some experimental animals.

Genital Differentiation

Genital sex differentiation, also known as *phenotypic sex* differentiation refers to the differentiation of internal genitalia, urethra and external genitalia.

Differentiation of Internal Genitalia

- The internal genitalia differentiate from the *neutral sex anlagen* which develops during the sixth week of gestation along with the development of bipotential gonad.
- The primordia of internal genitalia are a paired set of Wolffian (male) ducts and a paired set of Mullerian (female) ducts. By the seventh week of gestation, the embryo has both male and female primordial ducts (Fig.9.1-4).

Differentiation of Male Internal Genitalia. In the genetic male foetus (44+XY) with functioning testes, testosterone and Mullerian inhibiting substance (MIS) are secreted which result in differentiation of male internal genitalia (Fig. 9.1-4B):

- The testosterone secreted by the Leydig cells stimulate the Wolffian ducts to form the epididymis, vas deferens and seminal vesicles.
- The Mullerian inhibiting substance (MIS) secreted by sertoli cells causes regression of the Mullerian ducts by apoptosis on the side on which it is secreted.

Differentiation of Female Internal Genitalia (Fig. 9.1-4C)

- In the genetic female foetus (44+XX), in the absence of MIS, the female ducts (Mullerian ducts) proliferate and form oviduct (uterine tubes), uterus and upper two-third of vagina. The female internal genitalia are functionally committed to become female as early as 8 weeks.
- In the absence of testosterone, Wolffian ducts degenerate.

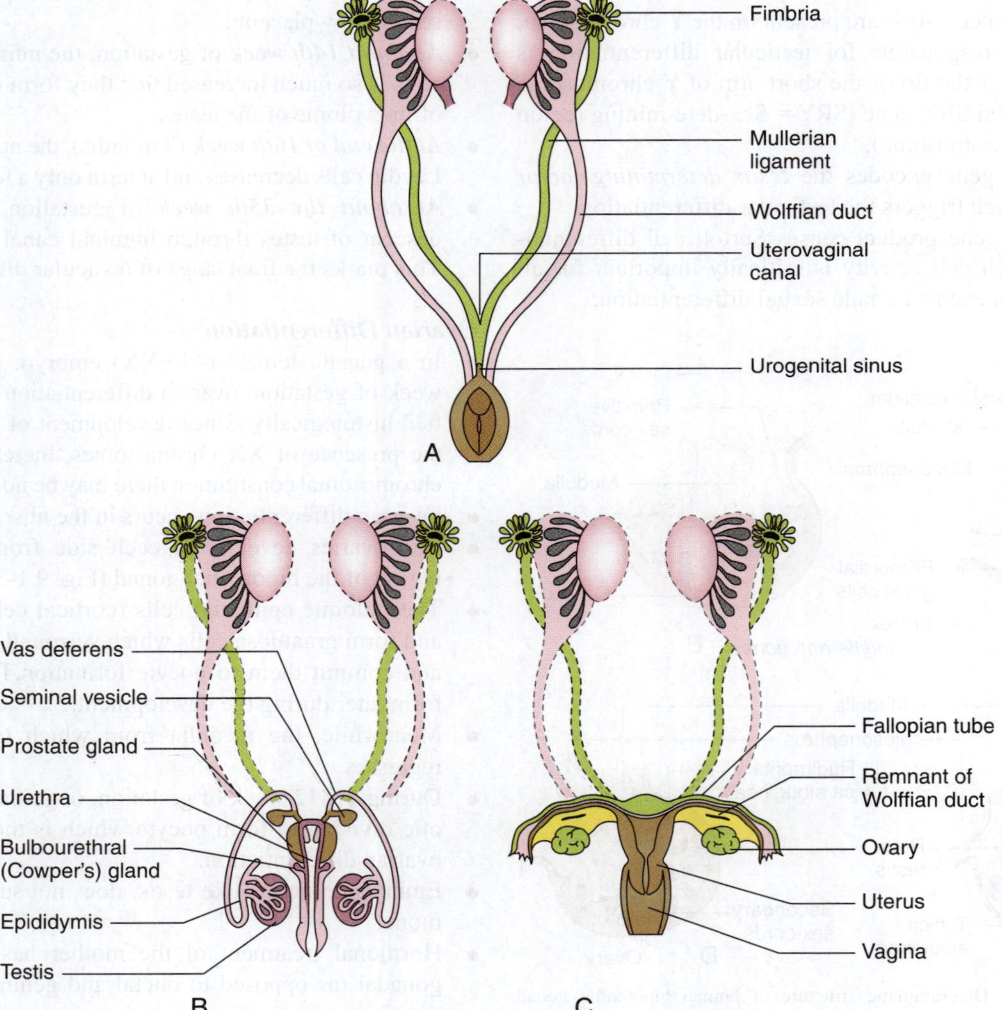

FIGURE 9.1-4 Development of male (B) and female (C) internal genitalia from primordial genital ducts (A).

Note. From the above, it is clear that natural tendency for the foetus is to develop female phenotype. It is the absence of testis and not the presence of ovary which initiates development of female genitalia. Thus, even in a male genotype (XY), if the testis is removed around the seventh week of gestation, the newborn will have female genitalia (according to *Gaudiya Vaishnava doctrine* all persons are fundamentally female, the malehood is merely imposed).

Differentiation of External Genitalia

- In contrast to the internal genitalia, the external genitalia in both sexes develop from *common anlagen*, which are the urogenital sinus, the genital sinus, the genital tubercle, the genital swelling and the genital (urethral) folds (Fig. 9.1-5).
- The external genitalia are bipotential till the eighth week of gestation, i.e. it can develop along either male or female lines.
- *In a male foetus* having functional testis secreting testosterone and dihydrotestosterone (DHT), the external genitalia acquire male characteristics by the 5th month of gestation.
- *In a female foetus*, in the absence of any hormone, external genitalia differentiation occurs along the female line.

The external genitalia derived from the common anlagen in male and female are shown in Table 9.1-1.

TABLE 9.1-1 The Male and Female External Genitalia Derived from the Common Anlagen

Anlagen part	Male derivative	Female derivative
Urogenital sinus	Prostate and prostatic urethra	Urethra
Urethral fold	Penile urethra and shaft of penis	Labia minora
Genital swelling	Scrotum	Labia majora
Genital tubercle	Glans penis	Clitoris

Psychological Differentiation

Psychological sex differentiation refers to normal sexual behaviour in adult male and female. The difference in male and female behaviour is due to some anatomical and functional differences in certain areas of brain of two sexes. It is determined by the effect of androgens on the development of brain in the embryonic stage. It has been studied that:

- A brief exposure of foetal hypothalamus to androgens (from its own testis) during early embryonic period causes male pattern of sexual behaviour during puberty. It occurs due to constant secretion of pituitary gonadotropins.
- Absence of androgenic exposure of foetal hypothalamus in female embryo causes it to stimulate the anterior pituitary in a cyclic way as in adult females.
- Early exposure of female foetus to androgens also produces significant masculinizing effect on sex behaviour in adulthood.

Regulation of Sex Differentiation and Development

From the above discussion it is apparent that the normal sex differentiation and sexual development proceeds sequentially: first chromosomal sex is established at fertilization that determines *gonadal differentiation*. The *genital differentiation* (phenotypic sex) is dependent on *gonadal differentiation*. It is quite obvious that *Y chromosome* plays key role in testicular differentiation or male development. The absence of testicular differentiation results in ovarian differentiation or female like development. The foetal functional testis by secreting Mullerian inhibitory substance (MIS) and testosterone regulates the activity.

Hormonal Regulation of Male Development

The two principal components of male (phenotypic) development *(Wolffian duct differentiation*, and the *virilization of urogenital sinus)* and the development of external genitalia are under control of testosterone and DHT (Fig. 9.1-6).

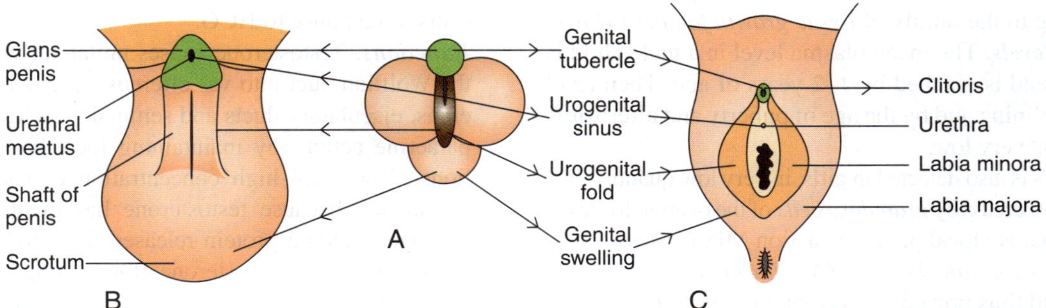

FIGURE 9.1-5 Differentiation of external genitalia in male (**B**) and female (**C**) from common anlagen (**A**).

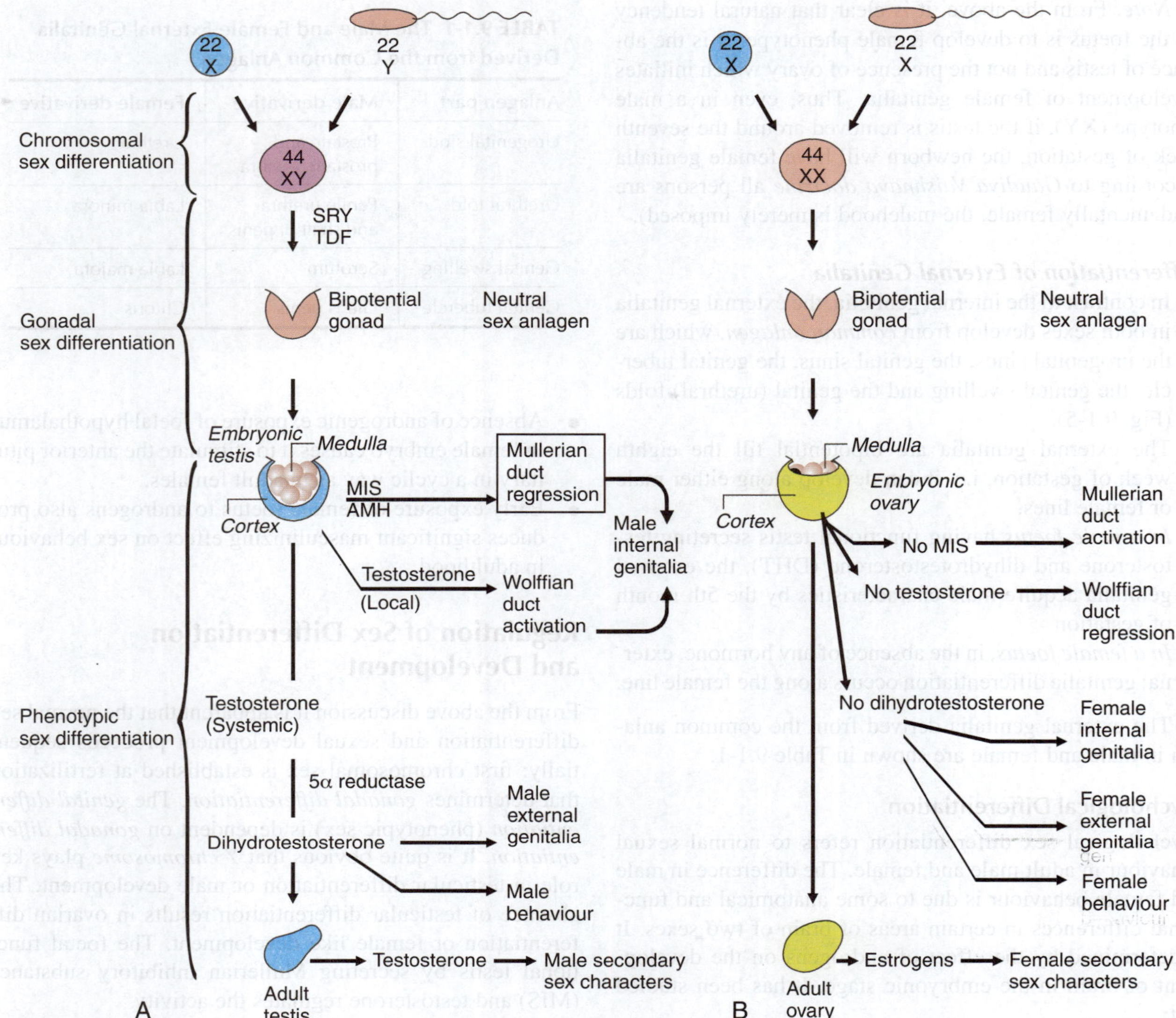

FIGURE 9.1-6 Diagrammatic summary of regulation of normal sex determination, differentiation, and development in male (A) and female (B).

Virilization of male embryo is mediated by three hormones: MIS), testosterone and DHT.

1. ***MIS,*** also called the Mullerian duct regression factor (MRF) or anti-mullerian hormone (AMH), is produced by Sertoli cells of foetal testis. It is polypeptide in nature belonging to the family of *tissue growth factors* (TGF).
   Plasma levels. The mean plasma level in a male child is 4 ng/ml and is reached by 1–2 years of age. Then level starts declining and by the age of puberty and afterwards its level is very low.
   Note. MIS is also detected in girls, in very low quantity. It is probably secreted by *granulosa cells* of the ovarian follicles.
   Functions. By local paracrine action MIS causes:
   - *Regression (involution) of Mullerian duct* by apoptosis and thus prevents development of uterus, oviduct and upper vagina.
   - *Continued growth of Wolffian duct* helps the testosterone in virilization of Wolffian duct and its derivatives.
   - In later embryonic period, it helps in *descent of testis*.
2. ***Testosterone*** is secreted by the Leydig cells of the foetal testis in response to HCG.
   Functions. Testosterone causes unilateral virilization of the Wolffian duct into vas efferens, epididymis, vas deferens, ejaculatory ducts and seminal vesicles by its local paracrine action (by maintaining local high concentrations). The local high concentration of testosterone is maintained because testosterone has great affinity for androgen-binding protein released from Sertoli cells. In the bound form, testosterone flows along the Wolffian duct and released from the binding protein at its site of action.

- In other target organs (prostate and external genitalia), testosterone is first converted into DHT to produce all androgenic effects.

3. ***DHT*** is formed at its site of action from testosterone. The target organs contain an active enzyme 5 α reductase, which converts testosterone into DHT.
   Functions. It causes masculinization of prostate and external genitalia.
   Mechanism of action of androgens. As shown in Figure 9.1-7, testosterone either binds to androgen receptors in the nucleus of target organ directly or following testosterone conversion to DHT. The receptor is common for both (testosterone and DHT), thus resulting in the formation of *hormone receptor complex*, which interact with chromatin.
   Dihydrotestosterone is the most potent natural androgen and is therefore, it is necessary for virilization.
   Note. *Castration* (removal of foetal testis) in an early embryonic stage prevents the formation of male genitalia and thus results in female-like development. However, castration of male foetus at a later stage does not affect male differentiation.

Disorders of Sexual Development

Abnormalities of sexual development occur due to:

- Defect in sex chromosomes leading to genetic abnormalities,
- Hormonal abnormalities leading to defect in gonadal and genital differentiation.

Chromosomal Abnormalities

Chromosomal abnormalities include:

- Trisomy,
- Monosomy,
- Chromosomal abnormality with more than three chromosomes,
- Triploidy,
- Abnormalities in number of chromosome during crossing over process and
- Mosacism.

1. Trisomy Chromosomal abnormalities usually arise during gametogenesis due to *nondisjunction* of sex chromosomes. Nondisjunction is a phenomenon in which a pair of chromosome could not be separated during meiotic division and may go to same pole (Fig. 9.1-8). The resulting gamete then has 24 chromosomes instead of normal 23. At fertilization by this gamete (with 24 chromosomes) the zygote will, therefore, have 47 chromosomes (Fig. 9.1-9); there being three sex chromosomes instead of one of the normal pair (XY or XY). The presence of extra X or Y chromosome gives rise to many syndromes; associated with abnormal development, mental retardation and abnormal growth. Trisomy is presented as:

a. ***Individual with XXX (genotype) pattern of chromosomes*** is referred to as 'superfemale'. However, there is nothing super about them, because there is poor sexual development (infantile), scanty menstruation and mental retardation.
b. ***Individual with XXY pattern of chromosomes*** (Klinefelter syndrome) is an abnormal male due to presence of Y chromosome. It is the most common sex chromosome disorder, has an incidence of 1 in 500 males. It occurs in two forms: the classical form and the mosaic form.
   i. *The classical form* is due to chromosomal nondisjunction phenomenon during gametogenesis (meiotic nondisjunction).
   ii. *The mosaic form* occurs due to chromosomal nondisjunction after fertilization when zygote undergoes mitotic division hence also called *mitotic nondisjunction*.

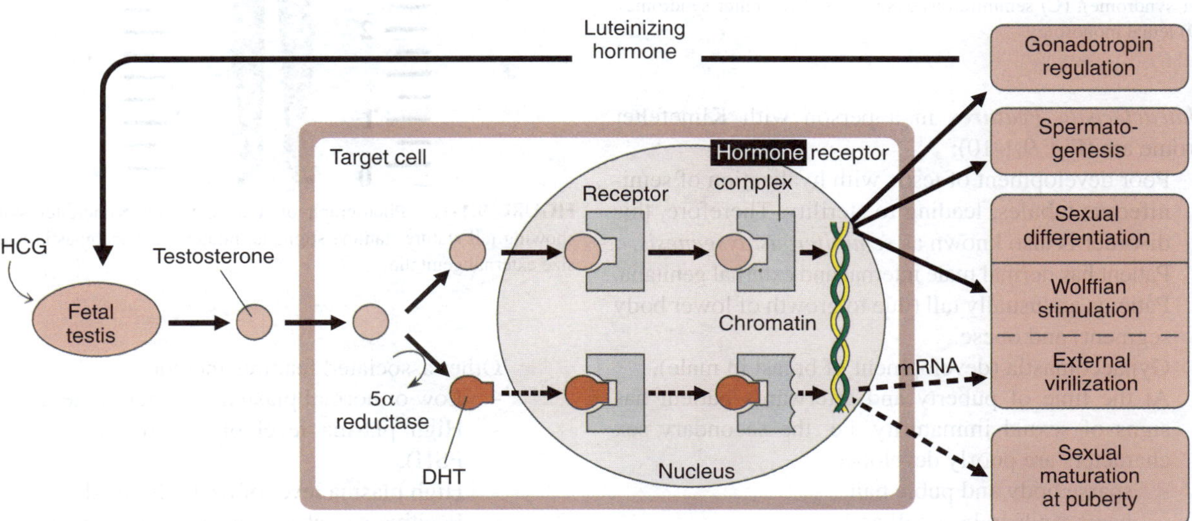

FIGURE 9.1-7 Schematic diagram depicting mechanism of action of androgens secreted by fetal testis.

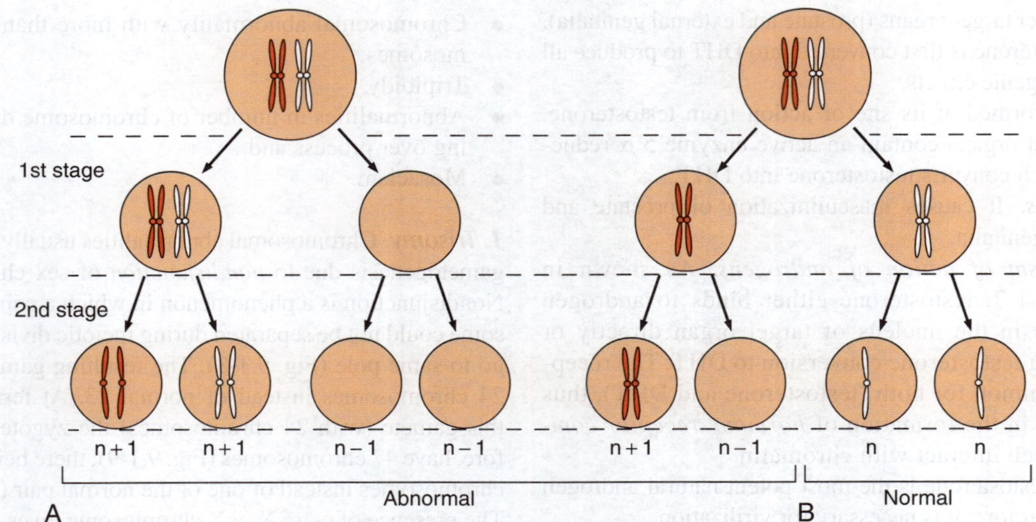

FIGURE 9.1-8 Nondisjunction of sex chromosomes during meiotic division: (A) in 1st stage and (B) in 2nd stage.

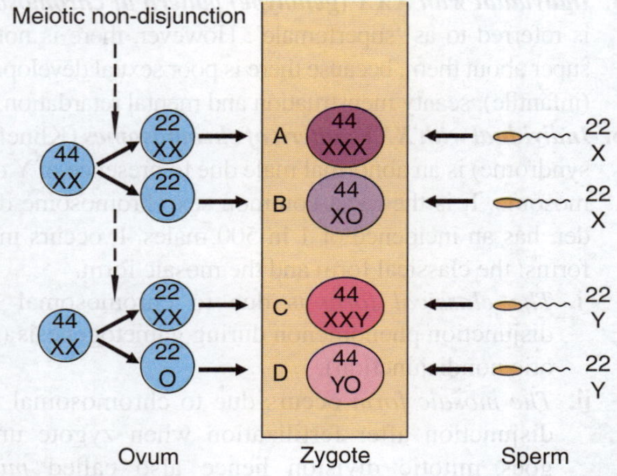

FIGURE 9.1-9 Defects due to maternal nondisjunction of sex chromosomes at the time of meiosis: (A) superfemale; (B) gonadal dysgenesis (Turner syndrome); (C) seminiferous dysgenesis (Klinefelter syndrome); and (D) lethal monosomy.

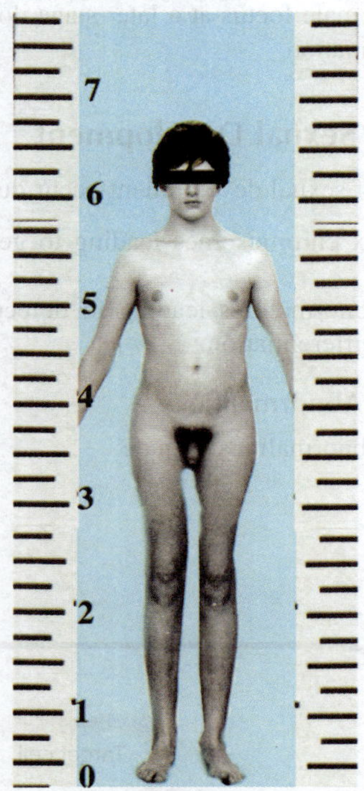

FIGURE 9.1-10 Photograph of a patient with Klinefelter syndrome showing tall stature, famine stigmata, bilateral gynaecomastia and small size external genitalia.

Characteristic Features in a person with Klinefelter syndrome are (Fig. 9.1-10):

- Poor development of testis with hyalization of seminiferous tubules, leading to sterility. Therefore, this disorder is also known as *seminiferous dysgenesis*.
- Patient has normal male internal and external genitalia.
- Patients are usually tall (due to growth of lower body segment) and obese.
- Gynaecomastia (development of breast in male).
- At the time of puberty and afterwards patient has signs of sexual immaturity, i.e. the secondary sex characters are poorly developed:
  - sparse body and pubic hair.
  - penis tends to be small and
  - testes are very small (peanut size).
- Other associated features include:
  - Low or normal plasma testosterone level,
  - High plasma level of gonadotropins (LH and FSH),
  - High plasma level of oestradiol and
  - Positive sex chromatin test (as genetic chromosomal pattern is of female).

Note. *Down syndrome* (also known as mongolism) is an example of autosomal chromosomal trisomy of (21 chromosome).

2. *Monosomy* As shown in Figure 9.1-8, when both chromosomes of a pair go to one gamete, the other gamete resulting from such a division has only 22 chromosomes; and at fertilization the zygote formed will have only 45 chromosomes. Hence, one pair is represented by single chromosome, so, it is called monosomy. Depending upon the presence of X or Y chromosome, there will be either female phenotype (44+XO) or male phenotype (44+YO). The best known example of monosomy disorder is *Turner's syndrome* and other example is individual with 44+YO karyotype.

Turner's Syndrome. Characteristic features of Turner's syndrome are (Fig. 9.1-11):

- Patient's chromosomal pattern (karyotype) is 44+XO; Y chromsome is absent hence patient is phenotypically female.
- Its incidence is 1 in 2500 females.
- There is ovarian dysgenesis because of XO karyotype.
- Normal female internal and external genitalia are present (female phenotype).
- Puberty is delayed. Though there is female type of sexual development but it is characterized by scanty menstruation, amenorrhoea (no menstruation), primary infertility and amastia.
- Other important associated feature is mental retardation.
- Among skeletal abnormalities dwarfism is very common. The characteristic features are webbed neck (folds of skin on the side of the neck present), face is peculiar with low hair line, ptosis (drooping of eyelids), epicanthus (low set ears), micrognathia (small jaw) and co-*arctation* of aorta.

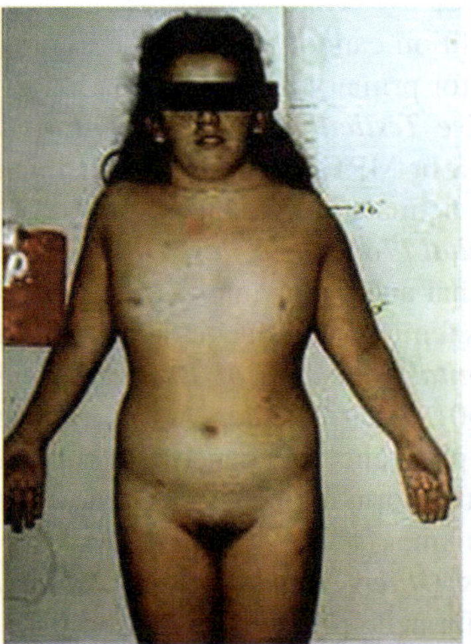

FIGURE 9.1-11 Photograph of a patient with Turner's syndrome (ovarian dysgenesis) showing short stature, webbed neck and underdeveloped secondary sexual characters (sexual infantilism).

Individual with karyotype 44+YO. The condition of monosomy is very lethal and leads to intrauterine death of the foetus.

3. *Chromsomal Abnormalities with More than Three Sex Chromosomes* Such abnormalities are present with either XXXY, or XXXXY, XXYY or XXXX chromosomal patterns. The disorders with these chromosomal patterns are recognized by severe mental retardation.

4. *Triploidy* Sometimes gametes have diploid number of chromosomes, therefore, the zygotes so formed at the time of fertilization will have 46 + 23 = 69 chromosome. This condition is called triploidy. Such foetuses are generally born dead.

5. *Abnormalities in Number of Chromosomes during Crossing-Over Process* These abnormalities are as under:

- Translocation (part of chromosome may get attached to chromosome of different pair).
- Deletion (part of chromosome may be lost).
- Duplication (one chromosome is longer than the normal having duplication of genes and other is shorter than the normal with some missing genes).
- Inversion.

6. *Mosacism* During cell division normally the centromere splits longitudinally so that each chromatid splits longitudinally so that each chromatid becomes separate chromosome, but sometimes centromere splits transversely, thus producing two dissimilar chromosomes (i.e. one chromosome is made up of only short arm of chromatid and other chromosome is only of long arm). Such types of chromosomes are also called isochromosomes (mosacism) and individuals with such chromosomal defects show various types of abnormalities.

Diagnosis of Chromosomal Abnormalities. Early diagnosis (in utero) of these types of disorders is very important. It is made possible by following techniques:

1. Amniocentesis. In this procedure, amniotic fluid is collected by inserting a needle into the amniotic cavity through anterior abdominal wall. The foetal cells present in the amniotic fluid are examined.
2. Chorionic Villus Sampling: In early pregnancy, the foetal cells are obtained by a needle biopsy of chorionic villi.

Hormonal Abnormalities

As discussed in hormonal regulation of sexual development that androgens secreted by foetal testes are essential for male development in genetic male foetus, but, genetic female, when exposed to androgens during 8th–13th week of gestation shows male-like development. The most common developmental disorders due to hormonal abnormalities is pseudohermaphroditism.

Pseudohermaphroditism Pseudohermaphroditism means individual having genotype (gonads) of one sex (either testes or ovaries) and genitalia of other sex. It occurs in two forms:

- Female pseudohermaphroditism and
- Male pseudohermaphroditism.

A. Female Pseudohermaphroditism.

Conditions associated with female pseudohermaphroditism are:

- Congenitalvirilizing adrenal hyperplasia of foetal adrenal glands,
- Excess of maternal androgens and
- Iatrogenic, i.e. following treatment with androgens or with synthetic progestational drugs.

In all the above-mentioned conditions there is exposure to increased levels of androgens to the genetic female foetus.

Characteristic features of female pseudohermaphroditism are (Fig. 9.1-12):

- Genotypically the individual is female (XX).
- Gonads and internal genitalia are feminine like (ovaries, oviduct and uterus are present), but at prepubertal age masculinization occurs in the form of diamond-shaped pubic hair growth and development of penis.
- Increased plasma levels of testosterone and androgens.

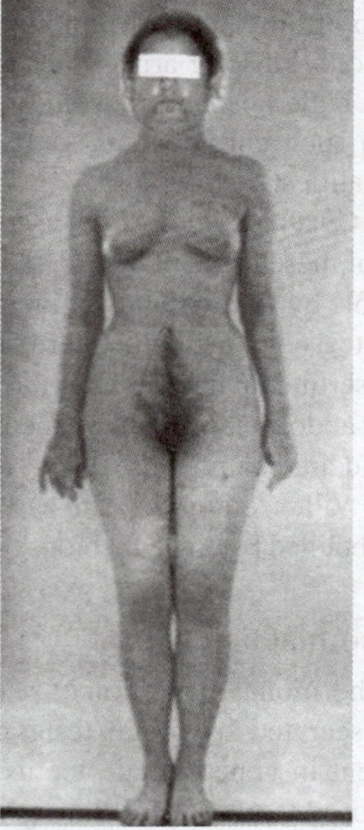

FIGURE 9.1-12 Photograph of a patient of female pseudohermaphroditism (congenital virilizing adrenal hyperplasia showing partial masculinization (diamond shaped pubic hair).

B. Male Pseudohermaphroditism. In this condition, person is genetically male (XY) but have feminisation (female internal and external genitalia). Male pseudohermaphroditism results in following conditions:

- Androgen resistance,
- Defective testicular development,
- Congenital 17 α hydroxylase deficiency,
- Congenital blockade of pregnenolone formation and
- Various other non-hormonal anomalies.

1. Androgen Resistance means androgen levels are normal but cannot exert their full effect on the target tissue. Androgen resistance develops in following circumstances:

When there is deficiency of enzyme α reductase in the target tissue, therefore testosterone cannot be converted into DHT (natural potent androgen), and *when there is mutation of androgenic receptor genes*. The effect varies from mild defect to complete loss of responsiveness of receptors to androgens.

- *In mild defect*, patient is infertile and may or may not be associated with gynaecoamastia.
- *In case of complete loss of responsiveness of androgen receptors* to androgens, patient presents with *testicular feminising syndrome*. In this condition, MIS is present and testosterone is secreted at normal or at high rate. The patient presents with following features:
  - The external genitalia are of female type but vagina ends blindly.
  - There is no female internal genitalia because testicular hormone suppresses Mullerian duct derivatives (no uterus and oviducts), thus at puberty:
    - Nervous system and hypothalamus develop as in normal female (both physically and psychologically), but
    - There occurs primary amenorrhoea due to lack of uterus.

This condition cannot be diagnosed until patient seeks consultation for primary amenorrhoea.

2. Defective Testicular Development. It leads to deficiency of MIS or MRF; which is responsible for feminization in a genetic male individual.

3. Congenital 17α Hydroxylase Deficiency. This enzyme converts adrenal androgens into testosterone. Thus, its deficiency causes feminization due to deficient testosterone.

4. Congenital Blockade of Pregnenolone Formation. (see page 830). The testicular and adrenal androgens are formed from pregnenolone; hence, this congenital blockade of pregnenolone formation is associated with male pseudohermaphroditism.

5. Various Other Non-hormonal Anomalies are also associated with male pseudohermaphroditism.

True Hermaphroditism It is a very rare condition, in which gonads of both sexes are present (an ovary on one side and testis on other side), thus resulting in numerous variations in phenotypic (internal and external genitalia) differentiation (Fig. 9.1-13).

- The external genitalia are variable and predominantly male and female forms are seen.
- The external urethral opening is present on the underside of the penis in predominantly male and in the vagina in predominantly female (hypospadias).
- The gonads may be located at variable sites viz. in the labiosacral fold, in the inguinal canal, or in the abdomen.
- Breast development occurs in 60 to 70% of these patients.
- Chromosomal examination shows mixture of 46 XX and 46 XY constitution.
- Sex chromatin test may or may not be positive.

The true hermaphroditism results due to combined abnormalities.

PUBERTY AND ADOLESCENCE

Introduction

Puberty and adolescence are the phases of growth between childhood and adulthood.

- Puberty refers to the stage of gonadal development and maturation to the point where reproduction is possible for the first time.
- Adolescence refers to the period of sudden spurt of physical growth between childhood and adulthood.

Since these two phases (adolescence and puberty) of growth are overlapping, hence the terms are interchangeable. The total period of growth spurt ranges between 3 and 5 years. It starts from the age of 8 years. The average age of onset of puberty is 12 years in girls and 14 years in boys. The age at which puberty occur varies. In Europe and United states the age of onset of puberty is declining.

Components of Puberty

The two principal components of puberty are: sudden spurt of physical growth and appearance of secondary sex characters.

1. Sudden Spurt of Physical Growth During sudden spurt of physical growth there is increase in height, muscle mass and muscle strength of an individual. The height increases by 7 to 12 centimetres in boys and about 6 to 11 centimetres in girls (Fig. 9.1-14). The increase in height is mainly of the trunk part rather than of limbs.

The muscle mass and muscle stregnth also increases in both the sexes but the increase is far greater in boys as compared to in girls.

2. Appearance of Secondary Sex Characters

Stages of Development of Secondary Sex Characters. The sequence of events of puberty which occurs in 3 to 5 years period have been discussed in 5 stages (Table 9.1-2).

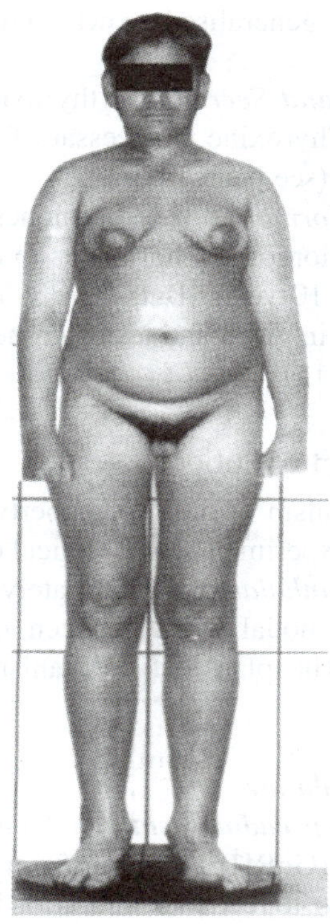

FIGURE 9.1-13 Photograph of a patient with true hermaphroditism showing breast development and underdeveloped male genitalia.

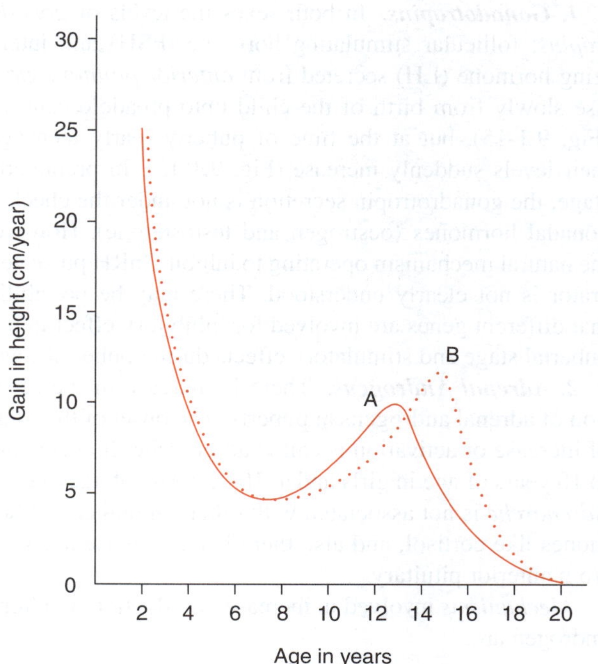

FIGURE 9.1-14 Rate of linear growth from birth onwards.Note, spurt of growth during adolescence in females (**A**) and males (**B**).

TABLE 9.1-2 Sequence of Events During Puberty in Male and Female

Stage of puberty	In females		In males	
	Bone age in years	*Characteristics*	*Bone age in years*	*Characteristics*
Stage 1	Up to 7½	Preadolescent age	7½ years	Preadolescent age
Stage 2	10½	Appearance of breast buds (thelarche)	12	Genital development begins (enlargement of testis)
Stage 3	11½	(i) Axillary and pubic hair appear (pubarche) (ii) Enlargement of breast (elevation) (iii) Sudden increase in height (height spurt)	14	(i) Axillary and pubic hairs start appearing (ii) Enlargement of penis
Stage 4	13	(i) Menstruation starts (menarche) (ii) Breast areola begins to elevate and project	15	(i) Further growth of testis, penis and genitalia (ii) Sudden increase in height (height spurt)
Stage 5	14	(i) Adult genitalia (ii) Secondary sex characters	16½	Adult genitalia and secondary sex characters

Types of Secondary Sex Characters. The secondary sex characters are almost fully developed by the stage 5 of the puberty both in male and females. These can be grouped as (Table 9.1-3):

- Structural,
- Functional and
- Psychological.

Hormonal Changes during Puberty

Besides ovaries and testes, other endocrinal glands (adrenal, thyroid and anterior pituitary), also grow in size and their activity increases at the onset of puberty. The hormonal changes noticed at the time of puberty are:

1. Gonadotropins. In both sexes the levels of *gonadotropins*: follicular stimulating hormone (FSH) and luteinizing hormone (LH) secreted from *anterior pituitary gland* rise slowly from birth of the child upto preadolescent age (Fig. 9.1-15), but at the time of puberty (early teen age) their levels suddenly increase (Fig. 9.1-15). In prepubertal stage, the gonadrotropin secretion is not under the check of gonadal hormones (oestrogen and testosterone). However, the natural mechanism operating to inhibit GnRH pulse generator is not clearly understood. There may be possibility that different genes are involved for inhibitory effect in prepubertal stage and stimulatory effects during pubertal stage.

2. Adrenal Androgens. There is increase in the secretion of adrenal androgens at puberty. The onset of this stage of increase or activation is called adrenarche. It occurs at 8 to 10 years of age in girls and at 10-12 years of age in boys. *Adrenarche* is not associated with other adrenal cortex hormones like cortisol, and also there is no increase in ACTH from anterior pituitary.

Mechanisms involved in increased production of adrenal androgen are:

- Morepregnenolone is diverted to androgen pathway (see page 754) due to changes in enzyme system in the adrenals.
- Release of adrenal androgen stimulating hormone (AASH) from anterior pituitary.

Functions subserved by adrenal androgens at puberty are:

- Growth of pubic and axillary hair in both sexes, and
- Growth of muscle mass and its strength.

3. Growth Hormone. Normally from birth upto prepubertal stage the growth hormone secretion is intermittent (a few peaks every 24 hours) but at the time of puberty, though basal level of growth hormone does not rise but there is increase in the frequency and amplitude of the peaks. It is responsible for generalised growth spurt at adolescence (see page 685).

4. Thyroid Gland Secretions (thyroxine) also increase during puberty. Thyroxine is necessary for normal growth and development (see page 704).

5. Gonadal Hormones (sex hormones). There is slow increase in secretion of sex hormones in children between the age of 7 and 10 years. But, there is rapid rise in oestrogen secretion (in girls) and testosterone in boys in early teenage (Fig. 9.1-15).

Control of Onset of Puberty

The exact mechanism of onset of puberty is still not fully understood, but experimental and clinical observations support that the *hypothalamus* is intimately involved in this process; being a nodal point between nervous and hormonal circuits. The plausible mechanism involved is as (Fig. 9.1-16):

Role of Hypothalamus

- ***From birth to preadolescent age.*** Gonadotropin releasing hormone (GnRH) secretion from hypothalamus is highly sensitive to feedback inhibition by circulating sex hormones (source being adrenal cortex and prepubertal testes). Therefore, from birth to preadolescent age, there

TABLE 9.1-3 Secondary Sex Characters in Female and Male

Group	In female	In male
A. Structural		
i) Body configuration	Narrow shoulders, broad hips (broad pelvis) Thighs converge Arms diverge (wide carrying angle)	Shoulders are broader than pelvis
ii) Skin	Skin is smooth and light	Skin is thick, dark and oily (sebaceous glands secretion thickens and predisposing to acne)
iii) Hair growth on: • Body • Face • Scalp • Pubic region	 Body hair fine and scanty – Thick growth, frontal hairline rounded Concave	 Body hair rough and dark – Moustaches and beard appeared – Frontal hairline indented at the side Convex and extends towards umbilicus (triangle with apex up)
iv) Muscularity	Muscles are soft (+)	Muscle bulk and strength is far greater (+++)
v) Subcutaneous fat	Female distribution of fat due to deposition of fat in breast and hips which gives characteristic curves and contours to the body	
vi) Genitalia and accessory sex organs	Adult type : • Clitoris increases in size, labia majora and minora get enlarged • Breasts are developed • Uterus and vaginal growth increases and their activity starts	Adult type: • Penis and scrotum increase in size and become pigmented, scrotal skin thickens and rugal folds appear • Prostate, seminal vesicles, bulbourethral glands enlarged and their secretion begins
B. Functional		
i) Voice	No change (remains soft and shrill)	Larynx enlarges and vocal cords get thickened, therefore, voice becomes loud, bass (low piched) deep and breaks
ii) Basal metabolic rate (BMR)	Lower	5 to 10% higher than female
iii) RBC count and Hb, concentration	Lower	Higher
iv) Menstrual cycle	Begins	Absent
C. Psychological	Girls are more emotional, shy, introvert and sexually attracted towards males	Behaviour is more aggressive, extrovert, competitive, and interested in opposite sex

is very less or slow release of gonadotropins (FSH and LH) from anterior pituitary.

- ***At the time of puberty*** (12-14 years) hypothalamic cells become more mature and their sensitivity for circulating sex hormones (for negative feedback) decreases much that there is pulsatile release of GnRH from the hypothalamus.

  As a result there occurs an increase in secretion of pituitary gonadotropins (FSH and LH). They act on gonads to release gonadal sex hormones.
- ***Awakening of hypothalamus.*** Hypothalamus at puberty, is also positively stimulated (awakening of hypothalamus) by the critical body mass, visual, external, olfactory and other sensory stimuli.
- ***Role of leptin.*** Leptin (a Greek word meaning thin) is a circulating protein, formed in the fat cells. It is under the influence of Ob gene, hence called product of Ob gene. It acts on the hypothalamus by feedback control mechanism leading to satiety (decreased food intake and increased energy consumption) and thus controls the body weight (see page 958). Therefore, leptin acts as a link between critical body weight and onset of puberty. Certain observations in favour of this fact are:
  - Girls suffering from anorexia nervosa (loss of appetite) stop menstruation, and if they start eating and gain weight, they menstruate again.

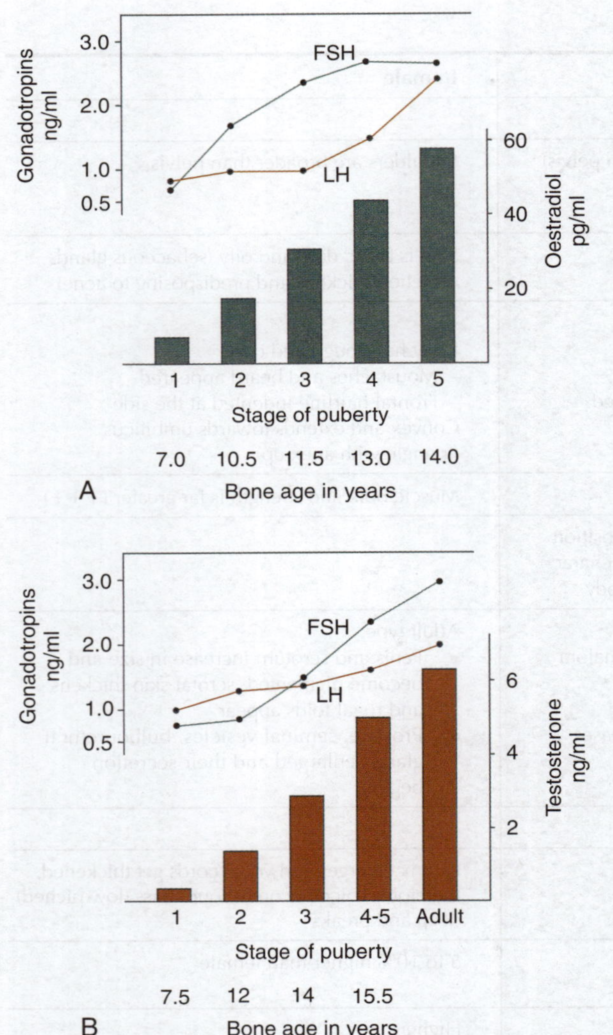

FIGURE 9.1-15 Changes in plasma concentration of gonadotropins and gonadal hormones during different stages of puberty: (A) in girls; and (B) in boys.

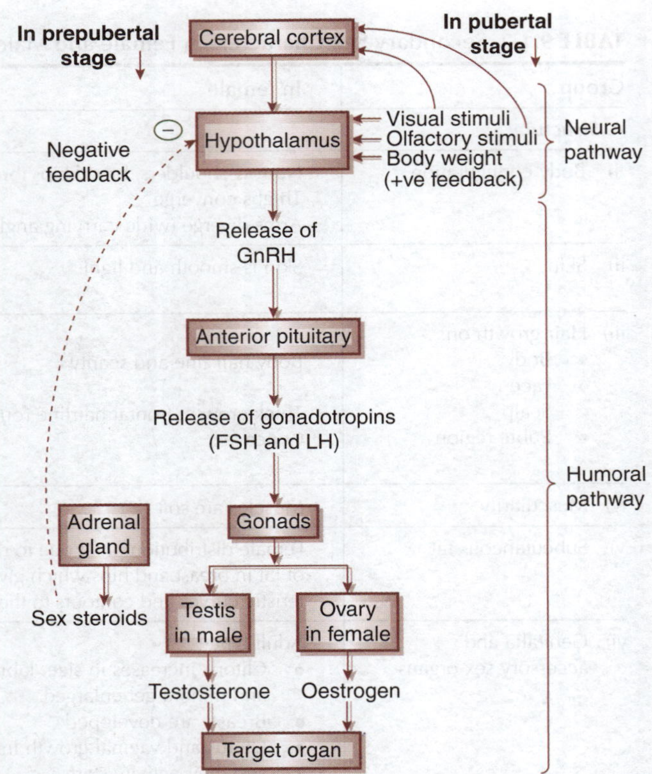

FIGURE 9.1-16 Neurohormonal mechanism of onset of puberty.

- It has been observed in mice that decrease in plasma leptin levels (produced by fasting) is associated with inhibition of onset of puberty, and
- The obese mice (due to defective Ob gene) that cannot produce leptin are infertile.

In both the above cases injection of leptin restores fertility. Also, when leptin treatment is given to immature female mice there is onset of puberty.

Disorders of Puberty

Disorders of puberty are related to the time of its onset, e.g.

- Early onset of puberty (precocious puberty) and
- Late onset of puberty (delayed or absent puberty).

1. Precocious Puberty Precocious puberty refers to onset of puberty in a child before 8 years of age. It is more commonly seen in girls. Precocious puberty is of two types: true precocious puberty and pseudoprecocious puberty.

i. True Precocious Puberty. *In the case of true precocious puberty*, there is early development of secondary sex characters and gametogenesis also starts earlier (Fig. 9.1-17). It operates through normal hypothalamo-pituitary-gonadal axis functioning (early but otherwise normal pubertal secretion of gonadotropins from anterior pitutary) without any other endocrinal disorder. It proceeds isosexually, i.e. there are no disturbing signs of virilization in girls and no feminizing signs in boys.

Causes. Clear cause of precocious puberty may not be found in most of the cases. However, certain conditions related to the disorder are:

- Constitutional or idiopathic, i.e. no cause is known. It is more common in girls.
- Conditions which distrupt the neural pathway for feedback inhibition of GnRH release from hypothalamus. For example:
  - Cerebral disorders involving posterior ventral hypothalamus near the infundibulum which may be tumour, infections, and developmental abnormalities.
  - *Pineal gland tumours* involving hypothalamus.

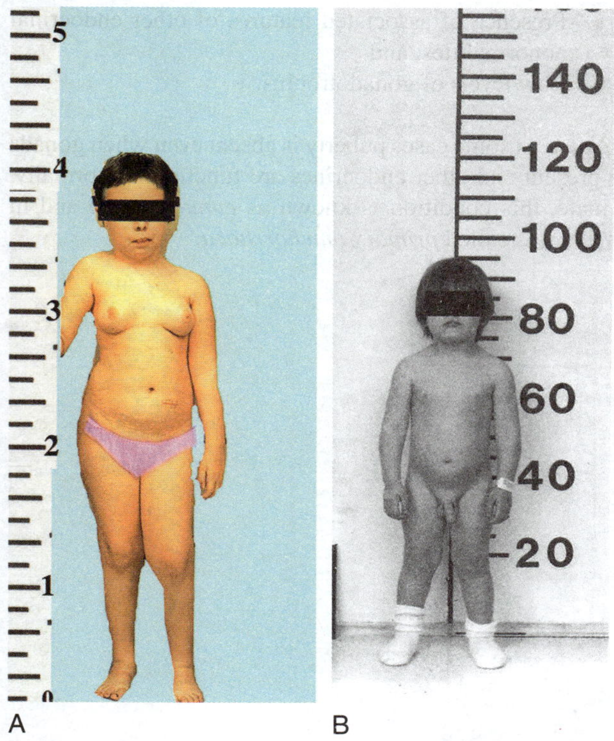

FIGURE 9.1-17 **A,** Photograph of a 7-year-old girl with true precocious puberty (well developed secondary sex characters). **B,** Photograph showing precocious puberty in a male child

In all the above conditions, there is early increased secretion of gonadotropins either due to *decreased inhibition of release of GnRH from the pulse generator* (hypothalamus) or due to chronic stimulation of hypothalamic cells by some irritative focus. Hence the condition is also called *gonadotropin dependent precocious puberty*.

- Precocious puberty also occurs with low or normal gonadotropin levels (hence known as gonadotropin independent precocious puberty). For example, in case when there is increased insensitivity of LH receptors to gonadotropins due to activation/mutations of G proteins which couple receptors to adenylyl cyclase.

ii. Pseudoprecocious Puberty. In pseudoprecocious puberty, there occurs early development of secondary sex characters without gametogenesis. It occurs due to abnormal exposure of sex hormones to immature child. In this type of precocious puberty, child may not remain isosexual and normal sequence of events of puberty are also altered.

Causes. Following conditions involving adrenal or gonads result in pseudoprecocious puberty.

Adrenal conditions are:

- Congenital virilizing hyperplasia (see page 757)
- Androgen secreting tumours in males; and
- Oestrogen secreting tumours in females.

Gonadal conditions are:

- Leydig cell tumour of testis (in males), and
- Granulosa cell tumour of the ovary (in females).

2. Delayed or Absent Puberty

Puberty is considered to be pathologically delayed in case of female, if menarche does not occur by 17 years of age, or in case of male, testicular development and maturation fails to occur by the age of 20 years.

Delayed puberty is more commonly observed in boys than in girls. Usually, it is constitutional or physiological delay and ultimately child catches up. Delayed or absent puberty is a matter of great concern when it occurs in following conditions (Fig. 9.1-18):

- *Failure of hypothalamus/pituitary* to secrete gonadotropins, as in panhypopituitarism or isolated gonadotropin deficiency.
- *Primary gonadal failure*. It refers to developmental failure or gonadal dysgenesis which occurs in Klinefelter

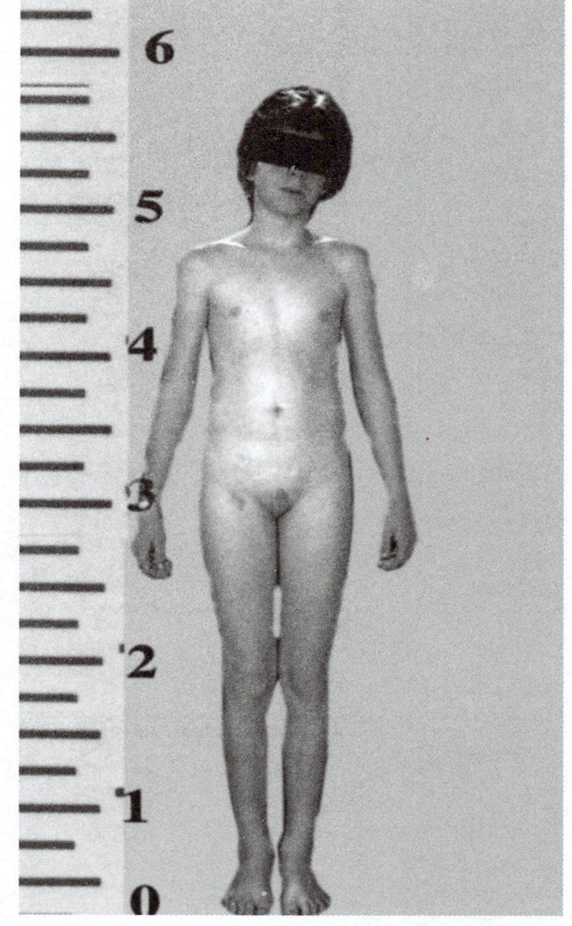

FIGURE 9.1-18 Photograph showing characteristic features of delayed puberty due to gonadotropin failure in a 16-year-old boy.

syndrome in males and Turner syndrome in females (see page 813).

- *Deficiency of enzymes* which are essential for steroid synthesis.
- *Deficiency of specific receptors* in the target tissue.

Features of delayed or absent puberty are:

- Lack of pubertal development,
- Short stature (dwarf),
- Presence of associated features of other endocrinal abnormalities, and
- Low levels of gonadotropins.

Note. In some cases puberty is absent even when gonads are present and other endocrines are functioning normally. In male, this condition is known as *eunuchoidism* and in female, it is called *primary amenorrhoea.*

Chapter 9.2

Male Reproductive Physiology

AN OVERVIEW OF MALE REPRODUCTIVE SYSTEM

The male reproductive system comprises the internal and external genital organs which can be functionally organized as (Fig. 9.2-1):

I. Gonads or Primary Male Sex Glands are a Pair of Testes Gonads or primary male sex glands are a pair of testes which correspond with ovaries in females. The main functions of the testes are to produce sperms and secrete testosterone (male sex hormones).

II. Accessory Sex Glands of Male Reproductive System are

1. ***Seminal vesicles*** are two lobulated glands situated on either side of the prostate between the urinary bladder and rectum.
   - They do not store sperms as their name implies.
   - They secrete a thick alkaline fluid that mixes with the sperms as they pass into the ejaculatory ducts and urethra.
   - The duct of each seminal vesicle joins the ductus deferens to form the ejaculatory duct.
2. ***Bulbourethral (Cowper's) glands*** are two pea-sized glands. Their mucus-like secretion enters the anterior (penile) urethra during sexual arousal.
3. ***Prostate gland*** is the largest accessory gland of the male reproductive system.
   - It lies just below the urinary bladder and the urethra passes through a small hole in the centre of prostate.
   - It secretes a thin milky fluid which forms 30% the volume of semen (a mixture of secretions produced by the testes, seminal vesicles, prostate and bulbourethral glands).
   - Composition and functions of prostatic fluid are described as a component of semen (page 829).

III. Ducts of the Male Reproductive System These include:

1. ***Epididymis***. It is formed by minute convolutions of the duct of the epididymis, so tightly compacted that they appear solid.
   - The efferent ductus transports the sperms from the rete testis to the epididymis where they are stored. The sperms can remain viable for a month in the epididymis.
   - Secretions of epididymis provide nourishment to the spermatozoa and help them to mature.
   - Nonmotile spermatozoa become motile after passing through epididymis.
2. ***Ductus deferens*** or ***vas deferens***. It is the continuation of the tail of epididymis. It ends by joining to the duct of seminal vesicle.
   - It serves as a secondary store house for spermatozoa which will be released at the time of ejaculation.
   - In vasectomy operation for sterilization in males the vas deferens is ligated and sectioned.
3. ***Ejaculatory ducts***. Each ejaculatory duct is a slender tube that arises by the union of the ductus deferens with the duct of seminal vesicle. The ejaculatory ducts open as minute slit-like opening into the prostatic urethra which forms a part of prostatic urethra.
4. ***Urethra***. The male urethra is a muscular tube (18–20 cm long) that conveys urine from the internal urethral orifice of the urinary bladder to the external urethral orifice at the tip of the glans penis. The urethra also provides an exit for semen (sperms and glandular secretions) which is passed by the ejaculatory ducts in its prostatic part.

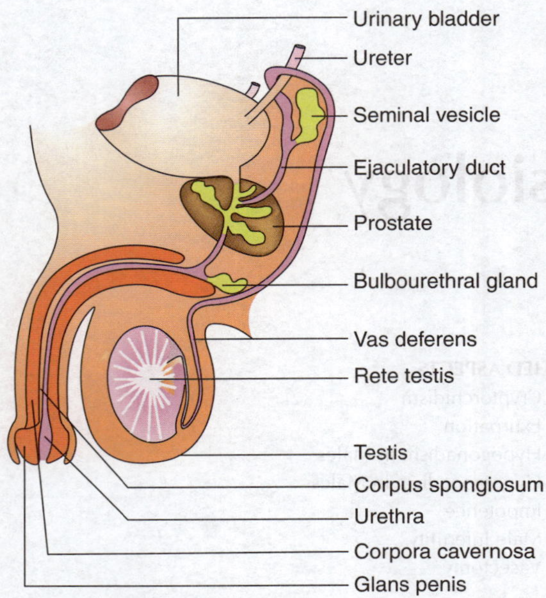

FIGURE 9.2-1 Male reproductive system.

IV. Supporting Structures of the Male Reproductive System

1. ***Spermatic cord***. It suspends the testes in the scrotum and contains structures that pass through the inguinal canal to and from the testis viz. ductus deferens, vessels and nerves of the testis.
   - Its coverings are internal spermatic fascia, cremasteric fascia and external spermatic fascia.
2. ***Scrotum***. It is a cutaneous fibromuscular sac (can be considered an outpouching of the lower part of the anterior abdominal wall) which houses testes, epididymis and the lower ends of the spermatic cords.
   - Internally, scrotum is divided into right and left compartments by the septum of the scrotum.
   - The scrotum maintains the temperature lower than the normal body temperature (about 32°C) which is necessary for normal spermatogenesis.
   - Exposure to cold also inhibits spermatogenesis when exposure to cold occurs, the dartos muscle presents in the scrotum contracts and puts up a thicker investure round the testis and thus keeps them warm.
3. ***Penis***. It is the male copulatory organ and the common outlet for urine and semen. Penis can be divided into three parts: root, body and glans penis. It is composed of three cylindrical bodies of erectile cavernous tissue—the corpora cavernosa and corpus spongiosum.

FUNCTIONAL ANATOMY OF TESTES

Gross Anatomy

Location. The testes are ovoid bodies suspended by spermatic cords into the scrotum, where they are maintained at a temperature lower than the normal body temperature (32°C) necessary for normal spermatogenesis.

Weight. In an adult male, the average weight of each testis is 25 gm (range 10–40 gm). The 90% of the volume of testis is due to the presence of seminiferous tubules. Weight of testis decreases in old age.

Coverings. Each testis from interior to exterior is covered by following three layers (Fig.9.2-2).

i. ***Tunica vasculosa.*** It is the innermost covering made up of loose connective tissue rich in blood vessels.

ii. ***Tunica albuginea.*** It is also called capsule of the testis and consists of closely packed collagen fibres intermingling with many elastic fibres.

   The tunica albuginea, on the posterior part of the testis, expands into a thick mass called *mediastinal testis*. Numerous septa from mediastinal testis project into the tunica albuginea and thus divide the substance of the testis into large number of lobules.

iii. ***Tunica vaginalis*** is the outermost covering composed of mesothelial cells. The tunica vaginalis is a closed sac, partially surrounding the testis. It consists of two layers: the inner visceral layer of tunica vaginalis adheres to the tunica albuginea and the outer parietal layer of tunica vaginalis which lies in close contact with inner surface of scrotum. A small space between these two layers (cavity of tunica vaginalis) is occupied by small amount of fluid.

Coverings of the testis provide protection from trauma and allow free movement of the testis in the scrotum.

Blood Supply *The arterial blood* supply to the testes is by testicular arteries (arise from abdominal aorta). The testicular artery or one of its branches anastomose with artery of ductus deferens. The venous blood is drained by testicular veins emerging from testes and epididymis and join to form a venous network (pampiniform plexus) consisting of 8–12 veins lying anterior to ductus deferens and surrounding the testicular artery in a spermatic cord. The blood in spermatic arteries runs parallel, but in opposite direction to the blood in pampiniform plexus. This anatomic arrangement permits counter current exchange of heat. The pampiniform plexus is a part of thermoregulatory mechanism which maintains constant temperature (lower than normal body temperature).

Lymphatic drainage of the testes to lumbar (lateral aortic) and preaortic lymph nodes.

Nerves (Innervation) of the Testes The autonomic nerves of the testes arise as testicular plexus of nerves on the testicular artery, which contain vagal *parasympathetic fibres* and *sympathetic fibres* from T_7 segment of the spinal cord.

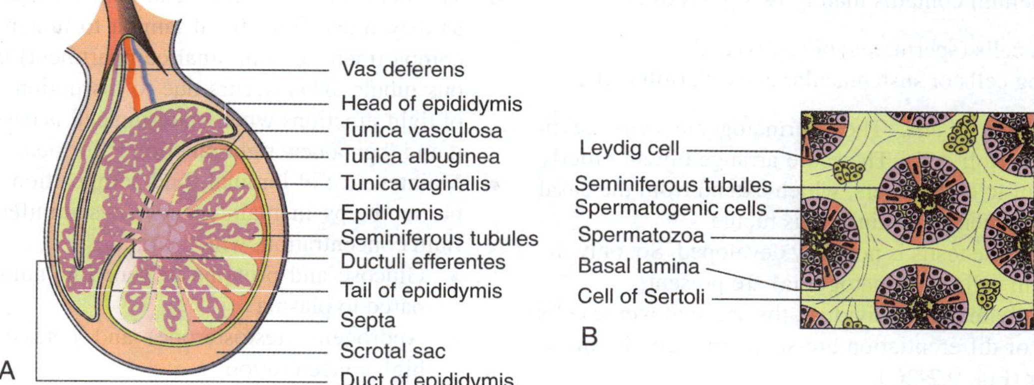

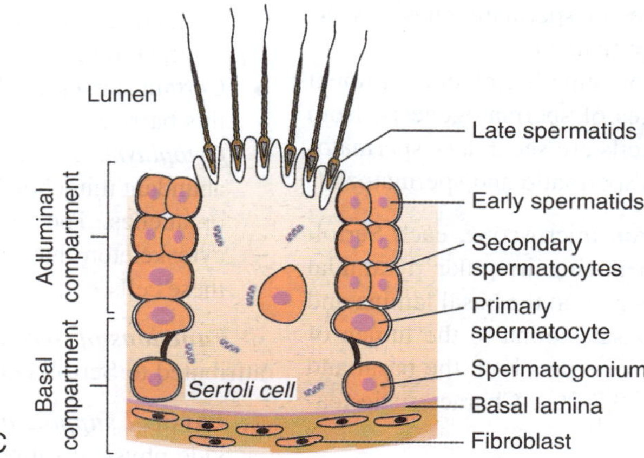

FIGURE 9.2-2 Structure of testis: (**A**) lateral view showing the cut section of testis, epididymis and distal part of spermatic cord; (**B**) histology of testis and (**C**) electron microscopic structure of seminiferous epithelium.

Structure of Testes

Each testis is divided into many lobules by the fibrous septa which project from the mediastinal testis into the tunica albuginea. Each lobule is roughly conical in shape, with its base directed towards the tunica albuginea and apex on mediastinal testis (Fig. 9.2-2A). Each lobule of the testes consists of:

- Seminiferous tubular compartment and
- Interstitial compartment.

Seminiferous Tubular Compartment

The seminiferous tubular compartment of each lobule of the testis contains about two to three seminiferous tubules. The seminiferous tubules constitute about 80 to 90 per cent of the testicular volume.

Gross Description of Seminiferous Tubule Each seminiferous tubule is about 80 centimetre long and 150 μm in diameter. It consists of two parts: the convoluted part and the straight part. The convoluted part forms the loops and continues as two straight ends. Near the apex of the lobules the straight ends join one another to form 20–30 larger straight tubules (tubule recti). The straight tubules pass through the fibrous tissue of mediastinal testis and unite to form a network called rete testis. At the upper end of each testis the rete testis gives of 10–20 efferent ductules which continue into the head of epididymis (Fig. 9.2-2A).

Histological Structure of Seminiferous Tubule Histologically, the wall of seminiferous tubules is comprised of three layers (Fig. 9.2-2B):

1. Outer Capsule or Tunica Propria. It consists of fibroelastic connective tissue containing few muscle like cells (myoid cell). The contraction of myoid cells help in movement of spermatozoa along the wall of the seminiferous tubules.

2. Basment Membrane (Basal Lamina). It is a thin homogeneous lamina lying next to the tunica propria.

3. Epithelial Layer of the seminiferous tubules. This is complex stratified epithelium. Under electron microscope it appears to be arranged in two compartments:

- Basal compartment and
- Adluminal compartment.

The epithelium contains mainly two types of cells:

- The germ cells (spermatogenic cells) and
- Supporting cells or sustentacular cells (Sertoli cells).

Spermatogenic Cells. The spermatogenic cells lie in between the Sertoli cells. These are arranged in an orderly manner in four to eight layers, which extend from the basal lamina to the lumen of seminiferous tubule.

In children, the testis is not fully developed. So, only the primitive germ cells (spermatogonia) are present.

In a sexually mature individual, the spermatogenic cells of all stages of differentiation are seen, arranged in an orderly manner (Fig. 9.2-2C).

- Basal compartment or deep part of epithelium is occupied by cells of early stages of spermatogenesis (spermatogonia and primary spermatocytes).
- Adluminal compartment or superificial compartment contains cells of later stages of spermatogenesis, from periphery to lumen these cells are secondary spermatocytes, early spermatid, late spermatid and spermatozoa.

Sertoli Cells. Under electron microscope, each Sertoli cell appears as a slender cell having irregular pyramidal shape. The base of Sertoli cells rest on the basal lamina and each cell stretches from the basal lamina to the lumen of tubule. Thus, each Sertoli cell occupies both the basal and adluminal compartments (Fig. 9.2-2C). Characteristic features of Sertoli cells are:

- ***Nucleus*** lies near the base and has prominent nucleolus.
- ***Recesses.*** The sides and the apices of the cells are marked by recesses, which are occupied by developing cells of different stages of spermatogenesis (spermatogonia, spermatocytes, spermatids and spermatozoa) from basal to luminal region.
- ***Tight junctions.*** There is no cytoplasmic continuity between the two adjacent Sertoli cells, but plasma membranes of two adjoining cells are connected by tight junctions in the basal region. Hence, the wall of seminiferous tubule is divided into two compartments:

The tight junction forms effective permeability barrier within the seminiferous epithelium, which is defined in man as *blood-testis barrier*.

Significance of blood-testis barrier. It limits the transport of many substances from blood to seminiferous lumen:

- This barrier maintains germ cells in a privileged location, because mature sperm cells are very immunogenic when introduced into the systemic circulation. Thus, blood-testis barrier protects the cells of different stages of spermatogenesis from blood-borne toxic substances and from circulating antibodies.
- It prevents the entry of byproducts of gametogenesis into the blood (that is why autoimmune reactions do not occur). Sometimes breakdown of this barrier leads to autoimmune response against germ cells.
- The maturing germ cells can pass through this barrier as they move from basal lamina to lumen (from basal compartment to adluminal compartment) of seminiferous tubule. This occurs due to disruption (breakdown) of tight junctions when maturing cell is passing through it and then a new tight junction is formed.
- Maintenance of luminal fluid composition. Blood-testis barrier helps in maintenance of seminiferous luminal fluid concentration, which contains:
  - Glucose and proteins in very low amount as compared to plasma
  - Androgens (testosterone) and potassium (K^+) in high concentration
  - It also contains oestrogen, glutamic acid and inositol.
  - It helps in establishing an osmotic gradient that facilitate the movement of fluid and testosterone into the tubular lumen.
- Certain substances like steroids can easily cross through this barrier.

Cytoplasm. The cytoplasm of the Sertoli cells contains abundant mitochondria, endoplasmic reticulum and other organelles. The microfilaments and microtubules form cytoskeleton that is important for cohesive functions of these cells.

Functions of Sertoli Cells Several functions have been attributed to Sertoli cells. These are:

1. ***Physical support and nutrition.*** The Sertoli cells provide physical support to maturing germ cells (the germ cells are present in the recesses on the side walls of the cells), nourish them (being rich in glycogen contents) and also remove waste products from the germ cells.
2. ***Phagocytic function.*** The residual cytoplasmic organelles are cast off from the spermatozoa during conversion of spermatids into sperms. These cytoplasmic byproducts or residues are phagocytized by the Sertoli cells.
3. ***Maintenance of blood-testis barrier*** (see page 824), as described earlier.
4. ***Secretory functions.*** Sertoli cells secrete following hormones and substances:
   - *Mullerian duct inhibitory substance (MIS)* or Mullerian duct inhibition factor (MIF) is secreted by Sertoli cells which help in regression of Mullerian duct in foetus and keep in male sexual development.
   - *Inhibin* is a substance that inhibits spermatogenesis before the onset of puberty by regulating **follicular stimulating hormone** (FSH) secretion by negative feedback at anterior pituitary level.
   - *Androgen binding protein (ABP)* or androgen binding globulin is secreted by Sertoli cells. It has high affinity for testosterone as well as for hydroxytestosterone, thus maintaining high concentration of androgens in the lumen of seminiferous tubules.
   - *Oestrogen.* Small amount of oestrogen is secreted by the testis due to conversion of androgenic precursors to

oestradiol. An enzyme aromatase (CYP-19) involved in this reaction is formed by the Sertoli cells.

- *Transport proteins*, such as transferrins (the iron transporting protein) and ceruloplasmin (copper binding protein) are formed by Sertoli cells which help in transferring iron and copper to tubular cells.
- *Plasminogen activator.* It is required for proteolytic activity for the disruption of tight junctions during migration of maturing germ cells from basal to luminal compartment, and is formed by Sertoli cells.
- *Seminiferous tubular luminar fluid.* Sertoli cells secrete watery, solute rich (K^+ and $HCO^-{}_3$) fluid into the lumen of seminiferous tubules. These cells pump ions into intercellular spaces to create an osmotic gradient that moves water from basal part of Sertoli cells to free luminal surface. This fluid movement provides a driving force for nonmotile spermatozoa.

Interstitial Compartment

The interstitial spaces between the seminiferous tubules constitute about 10 to 20 per cent volume of the testis. The interstitial compartment of each lobule is filled by loose connective tissue containing:

- Blood vessels,
- Lymphatics, and
- *Leydig cells.* The Leydig cells or the so-called interstitial cells are present in groups. They have endocrine function of secretion of male sex hormone (testosterone).

FUNCTIONS OF TESTES

The two principal functions of testes are:

- Gametogenic function (spermatogenesis) and
- Endocrine function.

Spermatogenesis

Spermatogenesis refers to the process of formation of spermatozoa from the primitive germ cells (spermatogonia).

Characteristic Features of Spermatogenesis

- Spermatogenesis begins at puberty and continues throughout adult life to decline in old age.
- The majority of the spermatogonia undergo continuous mitotic division to provide additional stem cells.
- Only a minority of the spermatogonia undergo further differentiation by meiosis, a process unique to germinal epithelium.
- Each differentiating spermatogonium develops into 512 spermatids.
- Spermatogenesis does not occur simultaneously in all the parts of testes. At any one moment, some areas of the seminiferous tubules are active while others are in resting state.
- In humans, it takes an average of 74 days to form a mature sperm from a primitive germ cell.
- The spermatozoa formed in the seminiferous tubules are nonmotile structures.
- The spermatozoa undergo process of maturation while passing through the male genital tract, and acquire the ability of fertilization of an ovum (capacitation) in the female genital tract.

Phases of Spermatogenesis

The phases of spermatogenesis are as follows (Fig. 9.2-3):

1. Phase of Mitotic Division of Spermatogonia. Spermatogonia or the primitive germ cells (44+XY) serve as a pool of undifferentiated stem cells from which develop the spermatozoa. These cells lie near the basal lamina of seminiferous tubules. Three main types of spermatogonia are described:

- *Dark type-A (AD) spermatogonia* (also called type A1) represent a reserve of resting stem cells. They have dark staining oval nuclei. They divide to form more dark type-A cells and also some light type A cells (or A2 cells).
- *Light or pale type-A (AP) spermatogonia* have light staining oval nucleus. They divide to form more light type-A spermatogonia and also some spermatogonia of type-B.
- *Type-B spermatogonia* have spherical nucleus. Each type of spermatogonium divides mitotically 5 times to form 32 type-B spermatogonia. The division occurs in the basal compartment of the seminiferous tubule. Due to incomplete cytokinesis, all cells derived from a single spermatogonium remain connected through cytoplasmic bridges and are synchronized in subsequent cell divisions. The connections remain throughout till the formation of individual spermatozoa.

2. Phase of Formation of Primary Spermatocytes by Mitotic Division. The 32 type-B spermatogonia (44+X+Y) undergo mitosis to form 64 primary spermatocytes (44+X+Y). Primary spermatocytes are large cells with large nucleus having diploid number of chromosomes (2n).

3. Phase of Formation of Secondary Spermatocyte by Meiotic Division. Each primary spermatocyte undergoes meiotic division:

- In the prophase of meiotic division (when chromatids duplicate), each primary spermatocyte is represented as tetraploid number of chromosomes (4n). In this phase they remain for about 22 days.
- After first reduction division (meiosis), the 64 tetraploid primary spermatocytes (4n) are converted into 128 primary spermatocytes with diploid number of chromosomes (2n).
- The 128 primary spermatocytes (meiosis) to form 256 secondary spermatocytes having haploid number of

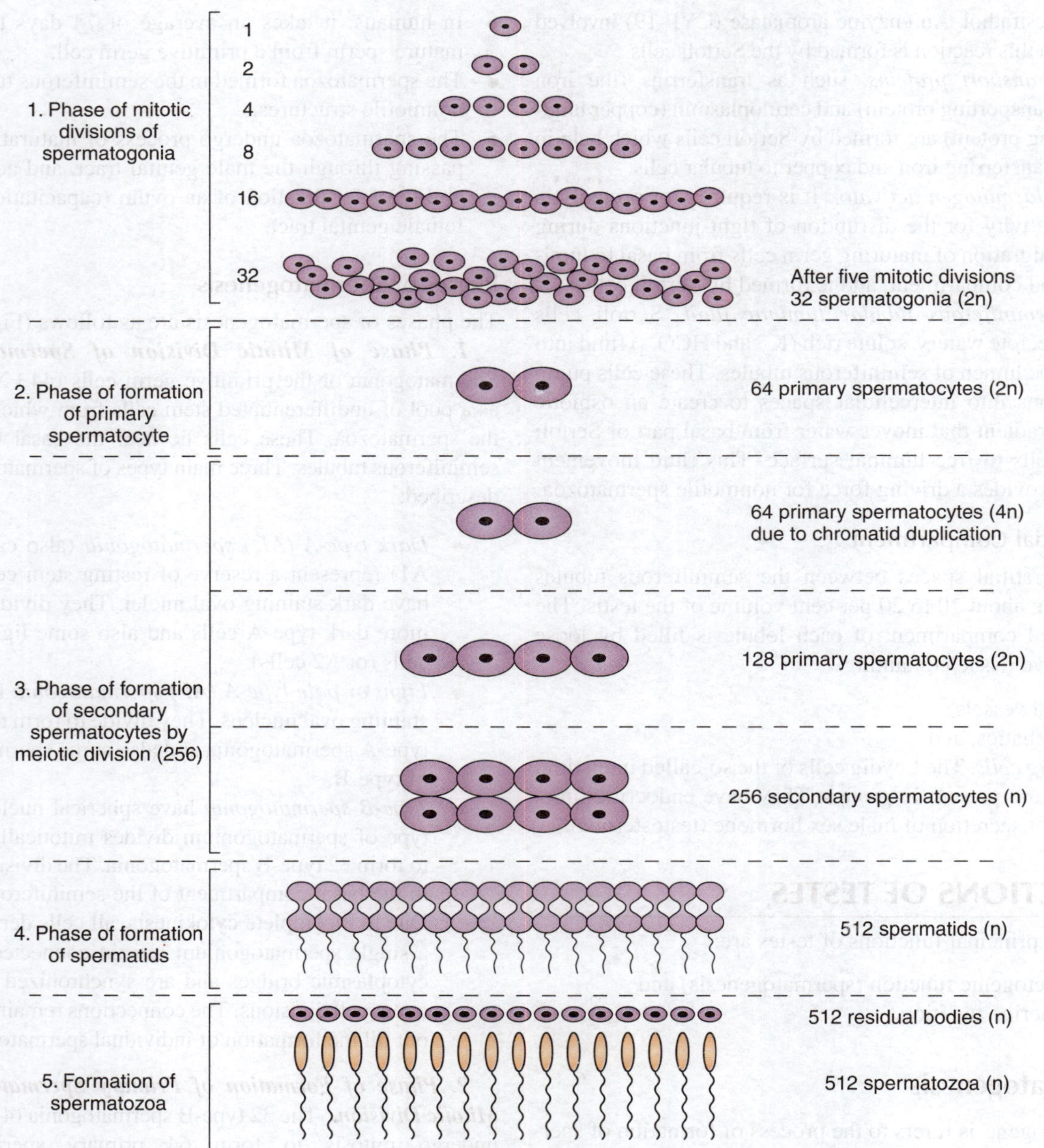

FIGURE 9.2-3 Phases of spermatogenesis.

chromosomes (n), i.e. either 22+X or 22+Y. Therefore, 50% of sperms will have X chromosome and other 50% will have Y chromosome.

- Size of secondary spermatocyte is quite small as compared to primary spermatocyte.

4. Phase of Formation of Spermatid. Each secondary spermatocyte divides mitotically to give rise to two spermatids. Thus, a total of 512 spermatids are formed from a single spermatogonium.

- *Early spermatid* is a small round cell with spherical nucleus containing haploid number of chromosomes.
- *Late spermatids* are formed when the early spermatids undergo changes in the shape and orientation of organelles.

5. Phase of Formation of Spermatozoon (Spermiogenesis)

- The spermatids do not divide further but undergo morphological changes to form sperms or spermatozoa. The spermatid undergoes changes in the shape and orientation of its organelles. The spermatids mature into spermatozoa in the deep folds of the cytoplasm of the Sertoli cells. During this process the components of spermatid which take part in forming spermatozoon are (Fig. 9.2-4):

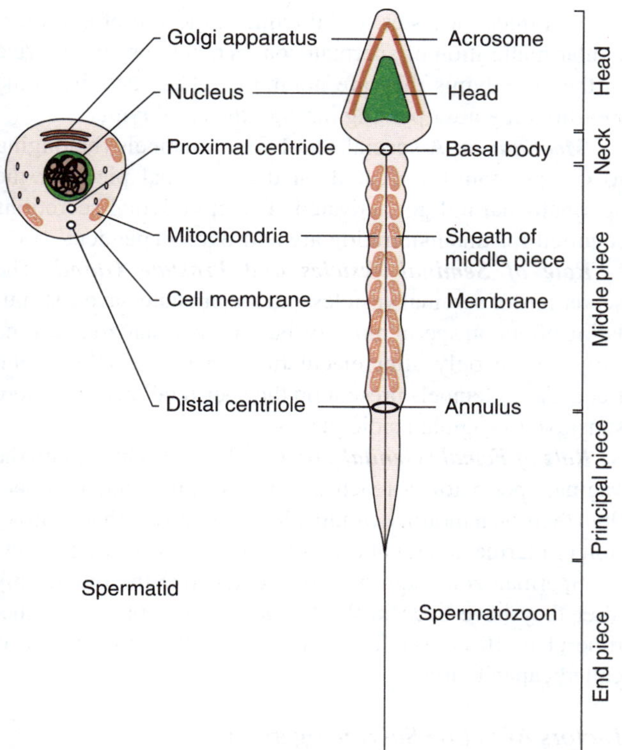

FIGURE 9.2-4 Diagrammatic depiction of derivatives of different parts of spermatozoon from that of spermatid.

- Nucleus undergoes condensation and changes its shape to form head of the spermatozoon.
  - The nuclear proteins are replaced by protamine which surround the chromatins and thus protect them from mutagenic factors.
  - The centriole divides into two parts, the distal part forms the axial filament and the proximal part forms the basal body. In the beginning both the parts lie close to each other but later they migrate away. The region earlier occupied by the centriole later on forms the neck of a spermatozoon.
- *The Golgi apparatus* forms the cap-like structure covering anterior 2/3 of the head (acrosome). It contains proteolytic enzyme (hyaluronidase) and other proteases, which help the sperm in penetration of an ovum during fertilization.
- *Mitochondria* surround the tail part of the sperm lying wrapped in a sheath and provide energy for movements of the spermatozoon.
- *Cell membrane* of the spermatid persists as covering of the spermatozoon. The membranes of late spermatids and of sperms contain germinal angiotensin converting enzyme.(gACE). The specific function of gACE enzyme has yet to be elicited.
- *The cytoplasm and other organelles* (like lipids, ribosomes, etc.) shed off as residual bodies and are phagocytosed by Sertoli cells.
  - The mature spermatozoa are released from the Sertoli cells and become free in the lumen of the seminiferous tubules.

The gametogenic function of testis is maintained by FSH and androgens. The stages from spermatogonium to spermatid are androgen independent. However, the maturation of spermatids to spermatozoa is androgen dependent acting on sertoli cells. FSH acts on sertoli cells and facilitates the last stage of maturation of spermatids and also promotes ABP.

Structure of Spermatozoon A fully formed spermatozoon is an intricate motile cell about 55–65 μm in length. It comprises following parts (Fig. 9.2-5A):

- Head,
- Neck and
- Tail.

1. Head. The head is about 4–5 μm long, flattened from anterior to posterior. It is oval when seen from the front, but appears to be pointed (somewhat like a spear-head) when seen from one side. It is mainly composed of condensed nucleus with a very thin cytoplasmic cell membrane layer around it. It is surrounded by acrosome.

Acrosome is a thick cap-like structure which covers the anterior two-third part of the head. It is formed mainly

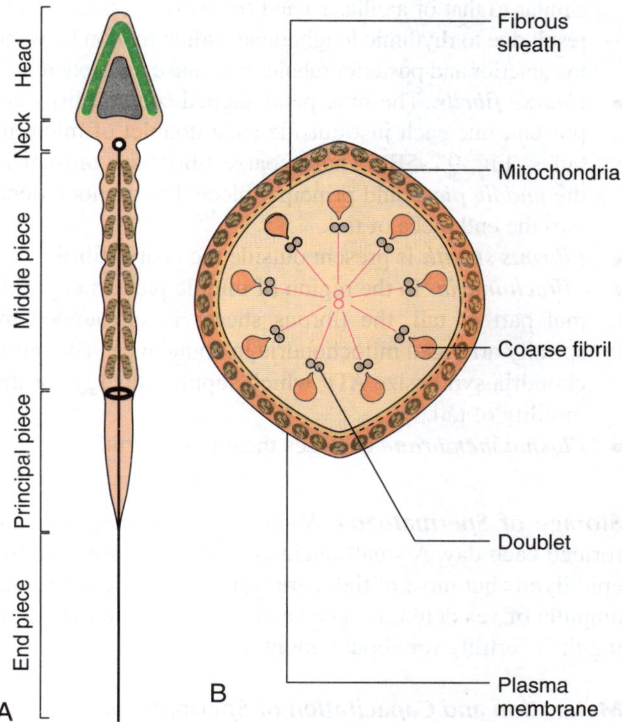

FIGURE 9.2-5 **(A)** Structure of a mature human spermatozoon and **(B)** transverse section of the middle piece of tail part showing its detail structure.

from lysosome-like organelle containing a number of enzymes (hyaluronidase, proteolytic enzymes and acid phosphatase) which help the sperm in penetrating ovum during fertilization.

2. Neck. It is a narrow constricted part. It contains a funnel-shaped basal body and a spherical centriole.

- *Basal body*, it is also called *connecting piece*, because it helps to establish an intimate union between the head and remainder of the spermatozoon through its convex articular surface which fits into a depression called the *implantation* fossa present in the head.

The basal body is made up of nine segmented rod-like structures which become continuous with the axial filaments present in the tail.

3. Tail of the sperm is the motile portion and is also called the flagellum. It can be divided into three parts:

- Middle piece,
- Principal piece and
- End piece.

Structure. The tail of the sperm consists of following components:

- ***Axoneme or axial filament.*** It forms the central skeleton of the tail. The axoneme begins just behind in the neck and extends through the entire length of tail. It is made up of nine pairs (doublets) of microtubules arranged in a circle, surrounding central pair (Fig. 9.2-5B). This structure is similar to that of a cilia. To and fro movements of the tail result due to rhythmic longitudinal sliding motion between the anterior and posterior tubules that make up axoneme.
- ***Coarse fibrils.*** The nine petal-shaped coarse fibrils are present, one each just outside each doublet of microtubules (Fig. 9.2-5B). These coarse fibrils are present in the *middle piece* and principal piece, but do not extend into the end piece of tail.
- ***Fibrous sheath*** is present outside the coarse fibrils.
- ***Mitochondria.*** In the region of middle piece, i.e. proximal part of tail, the fibrous sheath is surrounded by spirally arranged mitochondria in abundance. The mitochondria synthesize ATP which supplies energy for the motility of tail.
- ***Plasma membrane*** encloses the entire sperm.

Storage of Spermatozoa

About 120 million sperms are formed each day. A small quantity of them is stored in the epididymis but most of them are stored in vas deferens and ampulla of vas deferens. They can remain stored maintaining their fertility for about a month.

Maturation and Capacitation of Spermatozoa

Role of Epididymis. The fully formed spermatozoa are released into the lumen of seminiferous tubules, from where they reach the epididymis after traversing the rete testis and efferent ducts of testes. Epididymis is the site of extra testicular maturation of spermatozoa. When the sperms arrive in the epididymis they are nonmotile. They acquire some motility only after passing through the epididymis.

Mechanism. A special set of Ca^{2+} channels (belonging to Catsper family) located on the principal piece of the spermatozoal tail get activated. The epididymal secretions required for this maturation are androgen dependent.

Role of Seminal Vesicles and Prostate Gland. The secretions of seminal vesicles and the prostate have a stimulating effect on sperm motility, but the spermatozoa become fully motile only after ejaculation. In the female genital tract, Ca^{2+} channels present on the sperm tail become more sensitive to vaginal acidic pH (~5)

Role of Female Genital Tract. When introduced into the vagina, spermatozoa reach the uterine tubes much sooner than their own motility would allow, suggesting that contraction of uterine and tubal musculature exert a sucking effect.

Spermatozoa acquire ability to fertilize the ovum only after they have been in the female genital tract for sometime (1 to 10 hours). This final step in their maturation is called capacitation.

Factors Affecting Spermatogenesis

1. Effect of Temperature. The proper spermatogenesis occurs at a temperature lower than the normal body temperature (32°C), which is ensured by following mechanisms:

- Location of testis outside the body cavity in scrotum,
- Evaporative cooling in the scrotum,
- Counter current heat exchanger mechanism operating between the spermatic artery and the vein.

Evidences which highlight the importance of proper temperature during spermatogenesis are:

- *Hot bath* at a temperature of 43 to 45°C for 30 minutes daily result in sterility.
- In atheletes use of insulated atheletic supporters can reduce sperm count due to increased heat around testis.
- *Cryptorchidism* is a condition in which testes are undescended (remain in the abdominal cavity). Such individuals are usually sterile because of thermal damage to spermatogonia.
- *Varicocoele* (dilatation of veins of the pampiniform plexus) occurs due to incompetence of venous valves resulting in retrograde blood flow. In such cases heat exchanger mechanism is disturbed. Such patients are usually sterile.

2. Seasonal Variation in sperm count has been reported. It has been observed that sperm count is greater in the winter season than the summer season, irrespective of the temperature for which scrotum is exposed.

3. Infectious Diseases such as mumps cause degeneration of seminiferous tubules thereby decreasing spermatogenesis.

4. Hormonal Control of Spermatogenesis (see page 833).

Semen

Semen or the seminal fluid refers to the fluid ejaculated during the orgasm at the time of male sexual act.

Characteristic Features

- *Volume*. The average volume of semen per ejaculation is 2.5–3.5 ml after an abstinence of 2 days. Volume of semen decreases with repeated ejaculations.
- *Appearance* of semen is milky due to prostatic secretions.
- *Specific gravity* is about 1.028.
- *Reaction* is alkaline with a pH of 7.5. The alkalinity is due to prostatic secretions. The alkaline semen brings the vaginal pH from 3.5–4 to 6–6.5, the pH at which sperms show optimum motility.
- *Nature* of the semen when ejaculated is liquid but soon it coagulates in vitro or in the vagina, and finally undergoes secondary liquefaction after about 15 to 30 minutes. The clotting of semen soon after ejaculation helps to retain it in the vagina for sometimes. Lysis later on would release the sperms for their free movement into the uterine cavity for fertilization. Mechanism of these changes is:
  - *Mechanism of coagulation of semen*. The fibrinogen present in the semen (contributed by seminal vesicles) is converted into a weak coagulum by the clotting enzyme contributed by the prostatic secretion.
  - *Mechanism of liquefaction*. The coagulum is liquefied after 15–30 minutes by the enzyme fibrinolysin (plasmin). Fibrinolysin is the activated form of profibrinolysin produced in prostate gland (about 2 ml of prostatic fluid at body temperature can liquefy 100–1000 ml of clotted plasma in 18 hours).

Components of Semen and Their Characteristics The semen comprises following components:

1. Spermatozoa

- The normal sperm count varies from 35 million to 200 million per ml of semen with an average of 100 million per ml.
- Fifty per cent or more with counts of 200 million/ml and essentially all of those with counts under 20 million/ml are sterile (although only one sperm is ultimately required for the fertilization of ovum).
- The sperms move at a speed of about 3 mm/min through the female genital tract. They reach the fallopian tubes 30–60 minutes after copulation. The uterine contraction during sexual act facilitates movement of sperms. The sperms remain capable of fertilizing an ovum for 28–48 hours after ejaculation in the female genital tract.

2. Secretions of Seminal Vesicles Secretions of seminal vesicles contribute 60% of the semen volume:

- The secretion from seminal vesicles is mucoid and viscous fluid.
- It is neutral or slightly alkaline in nature.
- It contains fructose, phosphorylcholine, ergothionine, ascorbic acid, flavins and prostaglandins.

  Functions subserved by seminal vesicle secretions are:
  - *Nutrition to sperms* after being ejaculated into female genital tract is provided by the fructose and other nutritive substances from seminal vesicle secretions.
  - *Clotting of semen* soon after ejaculation into the female genital tract occurs due to fibrinogen present in the seminal vesicle secretions.
  - *Fertilization of ovum* may be enhanced by the prostaglandins present in seminal vesicle secretion by the following mechanisms:
    - Increasing the receptive capacity of cervical mucosa for sperms.
    - Increasing the rate of transport of sperms in female genital tract by inducing reverse peristaltic movement of uterus and fallopian tubes.

3. Secretion of Prostate Gland Secretion of prostate gland forms about 10% of the total semen bulk:

- It contributes milky and alkaline fluid part of the semen.
- It contains spermine, citric acid, cholesterol, phospholipids, fibrinolysin, fibrinogenase, zinc, acid phosphatase, phosphate, bicarbonates and hyaluronidase.

  Functions subserved by prostatic fluid component of semen are:
  - *Maintenance of optimum pH for fertilization* (6 to 6.5) is the function of alkaline prostate fluid, which neutralizes the acidity of vaginal secretion. At this pH, the sperms become motile and the chances of fertilization are enhanced.
  - *Clotting of semen* by converting fibrinogen (from seminal vesicles) into a coagulum is caused by the clotting enzymes present in the prostatic fluid.
  - *Lysis of coagulum* is caused by fibrinolysin present in prostatic secretions. The sperms become motile after the lysis of coagulum.

Important Note

Prostate specific antigen (PSA) is a protease secreted by prostate. It hydrolyses the sperm motility inhibitor (semenogelin) in the semen, thus increases sperm motility.

Elevated plasma levels of PSA is an effective screening tool in diagnosis of prostate carcinoma.

4. Secretion of Bulbourethral Gland Secretion of bulbourethral gland and other mucous glands accounts for only a small amount of the semen volume. These secretions provide mucoid consistency to the semen after puberty.

Endocrine Functions of Testes

- The Leydig cells of testes produce male sex hormones known as androgen.
- The Sertoli cells of testes secrete oestrogen, *inhibin* and *activin*.
- The most important testicular hormone is testosterone. Therefore, if not stated otherwise testicular hormone means testosterone.

Secretion and Transport of Androgens

Testes secrete the following androgens (male sex hormones):

1. Testosterone. It is a steroid secreted by the Leydig cells. The Leydig cells are large polyhedral cells lying as cords or groups of cells around large blood capillaries in the interstitial connective tissue between the seminiferous tubules.

- Leydig cells are numerous in newborn male infants and in adult males. So, the androgens are secreted in infancy and after puberty.
- In childhood, Leydig cells are scanty or non-existing. So in childhood, practically no testosterone is secreted approximately until 10–12 years of age.
- The androgen secretion starts decreasing after 40 years and becomes almost zero by the age of 80 years.
- A normal man secretes 300–1000 ng/dL (4–9 mg/day) of testosterone. Plasma testosterone level in adult males is about 0.65 µg%. More than 98% of secreted testosterone is bound to plasma proteins; 65% is bound to albumin, and 33% is bound to testosterone-binding globulin also called sex steroid-binding globulin, i.e. SSBG or gonadal steroid binding globulin, i.e. GBG (because it binds oestradiol as well). A very small percentage of the plasma testosterone is unbound. The free fraction alone is physiologically active in the target tissues, testosterone, acts as a final hormone (for hypothalamus and anterior pituitary) and as prohormone for the skin and male reproductive tract.

2. Androstenedione is an important steroid precursor for blood oestrogens in men.

- It is secreted by the testes at a rate of about 2.5 mg/day.
- It is important to note that the major portions of blood oestradiol and oestrone in normal men are derived from blood testosterone and androstenedione, respectively. Only a small amount of oestradiol is secreted by the Sertoli and Leydig cells of testes.

3. Dihydrotestosterone (DHT) is another important androgen present in the blood.

- Only 20% of the plasma DHT is formed in the testes by the action of 5 α-reductase (from the Sertoli cells) on the testosterone (secreted by Leydig cells).
- About 80% of the plasma DHT is derived from the peripheral conversion of testosterone. In the target tissues such as skin and male reproductive tract (prostate glands, seminal vesicles and epididymis) the testosterone is converted (by 5 α-reductase) into DHT. In these tissues, therefore, DHT is the final hormone and testosterone is the *prohormone*.
- DHT has more than twice the biologic activity of testosterone.

Adrenal cortex also secretes androgens normally testosterone, androstenedione and dehydroepiandrosterone (of these last one is more important). The action of adrenal androgens are unimportant under normal physiological conditions, because their quantity is insignificant. Under abnormal conditions, the excessive secretions of adrenal androgens especially dehydroepiandrosterone (DHEA) may produce musculinizing effects in prepubertal or in adult females and precocious puberty in prepubertal boys (precocious pseudopuberty).

Synthesis of Androgens

Salient points about synthesis of androgens:

- Androgens (C-19 structure) are synthesized in Leydig cells from the cholesterol (C-27 structure).
- The key step in the synthesis of androgens is the conversion of cholesterol to pregnenolone.
- The CYP 11 A 1 enzyme is the rate-limiting enzyme for steroid synthesis in all steroid producing tissues.
- In the developing male foetus, the stimulus for testosterone synthesis is HCG, which is the placental hormone secreted in highest amounts during the first trimester of pregnancy.

Biochemical Pathways of Synthesis of Androgens The enzymatic processes involved in the conversion of cholesterol to androgens are shown in Fig. 9.2-6.

Metabolic Degradation and Excretion of Androgens

Within 25–30 minutes of entry of testosterone into circulation, it is either fixed to the target tissues or degraded in the liver. Testosterone can have one of the following fates:

1. Conversion into DHT occurs in skin and male reproductive tract (prostate gland, seminal vesicles and epididymis) by the enzyme 5 α reductase. DHT crosses the cell membrane of the target cells and produces its effects.

2. Conversion into Oestradiol and Oestrone. Circulating testosterone and androstenedione can be converted to oestradiol and oestrone, respectively, by the action of aromatase (Fig. 9.2-7). Aromatases are membrane bound enzymes found in the brain, skin, liver, mammary tissues, and most significantly in the adipose tissue. Aromatization of circulating androgens is the major pathway for oestrogen formation in the male. Though some oestrogens in males are derived from direct secretion by the testes.

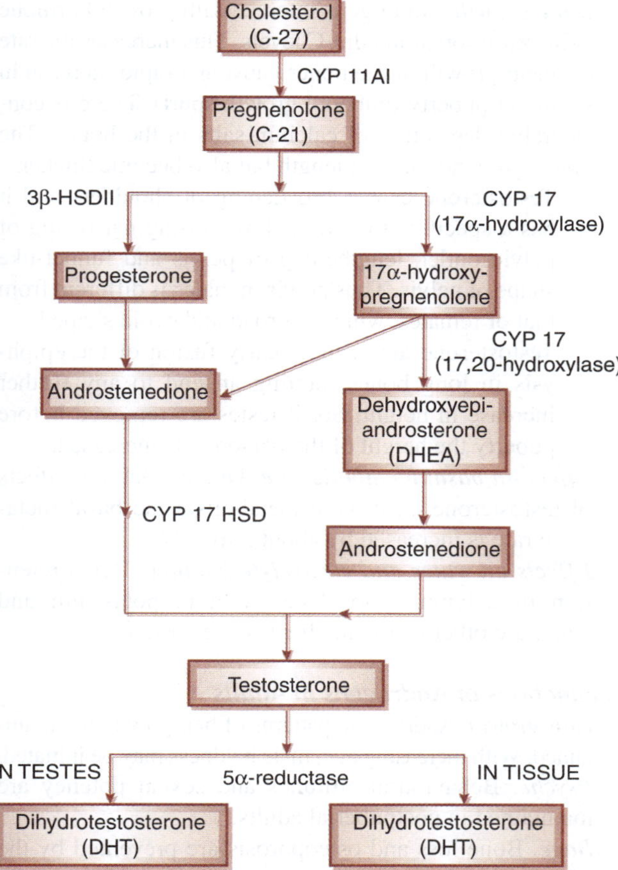

FIGURE 9.2-6 Pathway of formation of androgens from cholesterol.

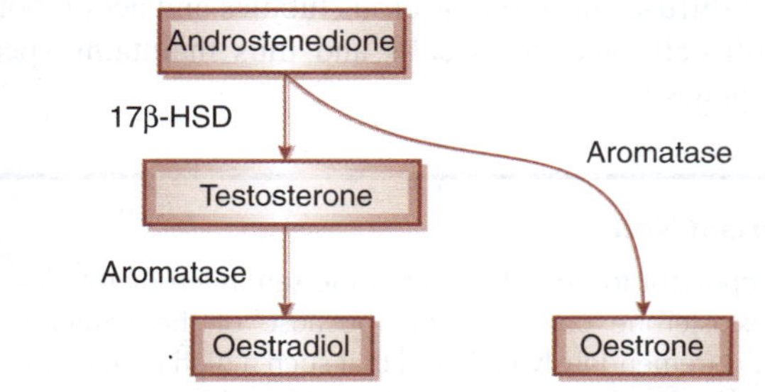

FIGURE 9.2-7 Conversion of androgens to oestradiol and oestrone.

3. Conversion to 17-ketosteroid. The degradation products of testosterone include androsterone, epiandrosterone and etiocholanolone. These three products are grouped together as 17-ketosteroids.

These are conjugated with glucuronic acid or sulphuric acid in the liver and excreted in the bile and urine.

- The excretory rate of urinary 17-ketosteroids in normal men is 15–20 mg/day.
- About two-third of the urinary 17-ketosteroids are of adrenal origin (derived from DHEA) and only one-third are of testicular origin. Excessive secretion of 17-ketosteroids in the urine is an important sign of masculinizing tumours of adrenal cortex.

Note. Because the urinary 17-ketosteroid pool reflects mainly adrenocortical activity, a measurement of the 17-ketosteroid secretion is not a good index of testicular function. The main test for assessing Leydig cell function is measurement of plasma testosterone.

Functions of Androgens

A. Functions of Androgens in Foetal Period (in Utero)

The testosterone is secreted by the foetal testes at about second to fourth month of embryonic life. The functions of androgens in foetal period are:

1. Effect on Sex Differentiation in Foetus

- ***Gonadal sex differentiation*** (as discussed on page 806) is dependent on the genotype of the embryo. In a genetic male embryo (44 + XY), the bipotential gonads begin to differentiate into testes at approximately 6th week of gestation. The Y chromosome plays a key role in the testicular differentiation. In the genetic female (44+XX) embryo, the bipotential gonads differentiate into ovaries by about 10th week of gestation in the absence of testis determining factor (see page 807).
- ***Genital differentiation***

  Differentiation of internal genitalia occurs from the primordia which are a paired set of Wolffian (male) ducts and a paired set of Mullerian (female) ducts. By the 9th week of gestation, the embryo has both male and female primordial ducts (Fig. 9.1-4).

  - The testosterone secreted by the Leydig cells of foetal testes (at about 7th week of intrauterine life) stimulates differentiation of the Wolffian ducts into the epididymis, vas deferens and the seminal vesicles.
  - In the absence of testosterone, Wolffian ducts degenerate and female sex organs develop from the Mullerian ducts in the absence of Mullerian inhibitory substance (MIS).

  Differentiation of external genitalia

  - The external genitalia develop from common anlagen, which are the genital tubercles, genital swelling, genital fold and urogenital sinus (Fig. 9.1-5) (see page 809). The hormone DHT produced by testes in male foetus stimulates the above-listed common anlagen to differentiate into male external genitalia, the penis, scrotum, penile urethra and prostate, respectively (Table 9.1-1) (see page 809) by the 5th month of gestation.
  - In the absence of DHT, the common anlagen differentiate into female external genetalia (Table 9.1-1) (see page 809).

2. Effect on Descent of Testes. The testes developed in the abdominal cavity are pushed into the scrotum through inguinal canal just before birth. Testosterone is necessary for this descent of testes. In a child born with undescended testes (cryptorchidism) administration of testosterone or even gonadotropic hormones (which stimulate the Leydig cells) can cause the testes to descend, if the inguinal canal is large enough to allow the passage of testes.

B. Functions of Androgens at Puberty

1. Effects on External Genitalia

- Testosterone (with or without DHT) causes pubertal enlargement of penis.
- DHT promotes growth. Scrotum increases in size and becomes pigmented. Rugal folds appear in scrotal skin.

2. Effect on Accessory Sex Organs

- Testosterone (with or without DHT) causes enlargement of seminal vesicles.
- DHT promotes growth of prostate and stimulates prostatic secretions.

3. Development of Male Secondary Sexual Characters

- *Body hair*. DHT stimulates the hair follicles and produces the male pattern of hair growth characterized by beard growth, diamond-shaped pubic escutcheon, relatively large amount of body hair and the recession of the temporal hairline (which in some men culminates in baldness).
- *Voice*. The testosterone causes enlargement of larynx and thickening of vocal cords resulting in a deeper low pitched voice (characteristically masculine).
- *Muscle mass and shoulder girdle*. Testosterone causes enlargement of the muscle mass (especially shoulder and pectoral muscles) at puberty.
- *Changes in skin*. The skin becomes thicker all over the body. DHT increases production of sebum by the sebaceous glands with consequent development of acne, especially during puberty.

4. Effects on Psyche

- *Psychological differentiation*. A brief exposure of foetal hypothalamus to androgens (from its own testes) during early embryonic period causes male pattern of sexual behaviour during puberty. It occurs due to constant secretion of pituitary gonadotropins.
- *Libido*. During puberty testosterone initiates sexual drive (libido) and erectile function (potency).
- *Aggresssive behaviour.*Testosterone produces aggressive behaviour and interest in the opposite sex.

5. Anabolic and General Growth Promoting Effects

- ***Testosterone causes nitrogen retention*** in the body (positive nitrogen balance) and causes increased synthesis and decreased breakdown of tissue proteins resulting in accelerated growth of the body and skeletal muscles in particular. Pronounced development of musculature at puberty is one of the most important characteristics of the male. This action of testosterone has led to the misuse of synthetic androgens by athletes and body builders to improve their muscular performance.
- ***Bone growth***. Androgens interact with growth hormone to increase somatomedin-C levels. This increases the rate of linear growth of the bones causing a rapid increase in stature at puberty (pubertal growth spurt). There is considerable deposition of calcium salts in the bones. The bones grow not only in length but also become thicker.
  - Testosterone causes broadening of shoulders and it has a specific effect on pelvis causing narrowing of pelvic outlet, lengthening of pelvis and funnel-like shape of pelvis. Thus pelvis in males is different from that of females, which is broad and ovoid shaped.
  - Testosterone also causes early fusion of the epiphysis in long bones, putting an end to any further increase in height. So, if testes are removed before puberty the height of the person gets increased.
- ***Effect on basal metabolic rate***. Due to anabolic effects of testosterone on protein metabolism the basal metabolic rate is increased by about 5 to 10%.
- ***Effects on water and electrolyte balance***. Renal retention of calcium, phosphate, sodium, potassium and water are other anabolic effects of testosterone.

C. Functions of Androgens in Adults

1. *Hair growth*. Androgenic patterns of hair growth are maintained. With increasing age, male baldness may be initiated.
2. *Psyche*. Behavioural attitudes and sexual potency are maintained in postpubertal adults.
3. *Bone*. Bone loss and osteoporosis are prevented by the androgens in adult males.
4. *Spermatogenesis* is maintained in adulthood by testosterone along with FSH. The testosterone, by paracrine effect diffuses into seminiferous tubules and act on both Sertoli cells and germ cells and thus maintains spermatogenesis.

Important Note

It is important to note that within the seminiferous tubules the testosterone concentration, because of the paracine effect, is tremendously high and that such a high concentration in the local region cannot be achieved by exogenous testosterone therapy by parenteral route. Lack of spermatogenesis due to pituitary failure therefore cannot be corrected by parenteral testosterone therapy.

---

5. *Haematopoiesis*. Testosterone stimulates the production of erythropoietin and also has a direct massive effect on erythropoiesis. These effects account for the greater haemoglobin concentration and RBC count in males.
6. *Effects on circulating and stored body fats*. Testosterone increases circulating levels of low density lipoproteins cholesterol and decreases plasma high density lipoproteins cholesterol.
   - Testosterone favours accumulation of upper body, abdominal, and visceral fat.

7. *Regulation of gonadotropin secretion.* Androgen suppression of LHRH and LH by negative feedback is largely a function of testosterone.

Mode of Action of Androgens

The testosterone may act as the final hormone or prohormone in the target tissues. In skin and male reproductive tract, the testosterone is converted into DHT by 5 α reductase. Humans have two types of 5α reductase encoded by two different genes.

- Type 1-5α reductase; is present in the skin throughout the body, predominantly in the scalp, and
- Type 2-5α reductase; mainly present in the genital skin, prostate and other genital tissues.

The testosterone and DHT, like other steroid hormones, cross the cell membrane of the target tissues and bind with the cytoplasmic androgen receptor (R) to form the androgen-R complex. The androgen-R complex moves to the nucleus to promote greater transcription of mRNA leading to greater synthesis of proteins in the ribosomes. Thus, the testosterone primarily results in increased synthesis of specific proteins required for development of accessory sex organs and muscular growth.

Applied

Congenital 5α reductase deficiency occurs when mutation of gene for 5α reductase, leading to male pseudohermaphroditism. The characterstic features of this condition are:

- Person born with male internal genitlia (with testis) but have external genitalia of female
- These individuals are usually raised as a girl, but at puberty, there is increased secretion of LH and testosterone. Therefore, consequently they develop male body contours and male libido and
- Change the gender identity as boy. Clitoris gets enlarged. The enlargement of penis may occur because of high circulating level of LH and testosterone

Inhibin and Activins

In males inhibin is a testicular factor produced by sertoli cells that inhibits FSH secretion by direct action at the pituitary. Inhibin consists of three polypeptide subunits. One α subunit which is glycosylated and other two nonglycosylated β subunits ($\beta_A$and β_B). The α subunit combines with β_A subunit by disulphide bond to form heterodimer. There are two types of inhibin:

- Inhibin A (ab_A) and inhibin B (ab_B)
- In women inhibins are produced by granulosa cells of ovarian follicles.
- The heterodimers and homodimers of inhibin stimulate FSH secretion rather than inhibiting, therefore these are called as activins.
- Both inhibins and activins belong to TGF β superfamily and act through activin receptors, located at gonads, brain, bone marrow. In embryonic period activins are involved in formation of mesoderm.
- Inhibins and activins bind to α_2 macroglobulin in the plasma and in the tissue bind to glycoprotein known as follistatin. In bound form the physiological activity of both activin and inhibin decreases.

CONTROL OF ANDROGEN SECRETION

See page 834.

Control of Testicular Functions

The two main functions of testes viz. spermatogenesis and secretion of testosterone are controlled by the hypothalamic-hypophyseal-testicular axis.

Control of Spermatogenesis

The hypothalamic-hypophyseal-testicular (seminiferous tubular) axis controlling the spermatogenesis is as follows:

I. Stimulatory Control

1. Role of Hypothalamus. Spermatogenesis begins at puberty and continues throughout adult life to decline in old age. It is believed that at puberty hypothalamic cells become more mature and their sensitivity for circulating sex hormones (negative feedback) decreases so much that there is a pulsatile release (8 to 14 pulses per day) of gonadotropin releasing hormone (GnRH) from the *parvicellular-peptidgeric neurons of hypothalamus.* The GnRH is a decapeptide. It stimulates anterior pituitary to secrete LH and FSH.

2. Role of Anterior Pituitary. The anterior pituitary controls spermatogenesis through the gonadotropic hormones (FSH and LH) and growth hormones. Neither FSH nor LH acts on the spermatogonia. Yet, normal spermatogenesis requires both FSH and LH as described:

3. Role of FSH

- *FSH stimulates cells of Sertoli* which play following roles during spermatogenesis:
  - Sertoli cells help in conversion of spermatids to sperms.
  - They secrete ABP which stabilizes the high supply of testosterone to the developing germ cells in the seminiferous tubular lumen.
  - FSH also promotes the synthesis of inhibin by Sertoli cells.
- FSH indirectly affects testosterone synthesis by increasing the number of LH receptors on the Leydig cells.

4. Role of LH (also Called Interstitial Cell Stimulating Hormone, i.e. ICSH). The LH stimulates Leydig cells to cause testosterone secretion. The testosterone is required for normal spermatogenesis.

5. Role of Growth Hormone. Growth hormone specifically promotes early division of the spermatogonia themselves. In its absence, as in pituitary dwarfs, spermatogenesis is severely deficient or absent.

6. **Role of Testicular Hormones.** Testosterone secreted by Leydig cells by paracrine effect diffuses into seminiferous tubules, where its high local concentration is maintained by ABP. The testosterone acts on both Sertoli cells and germ cells and thus maintains spermatogenesis.

Important Note

- Exogenous testosterone cannot promote spermatogenesis in men lacking Leydig cells, because it is not possible to achieve the required high concentration by parenteral therapy.
- DHT is not required for normal spermatogenesis, therefore, normal sperm development occurs in men with 5 α reductase deficiency.

Oestrogen formed from testosterone by Sertoli cells (when stimulated by FSH) are probably also essential for spermatogenesis.

II. Feedback Inhibitory Control The rapid speed of spermatogenesis is controlled by following negative feedback mechanisms (Fig. 9.2-8):

- Inhibin secreted by Sertoli cells acts directly on the anterior pitutary and inhibits the secretion of FSH.
- Testosterone and oestradiol inhibit LH secretion by negative feedback mechanism:
  - *Oestradiol* exerts the negative feedback effect at both the hypothalamic (GnRH) and pituitary (LH) levels.
  - *Testosterone* has its feedback effect mainly at the hypothalamic (GnRH) level.

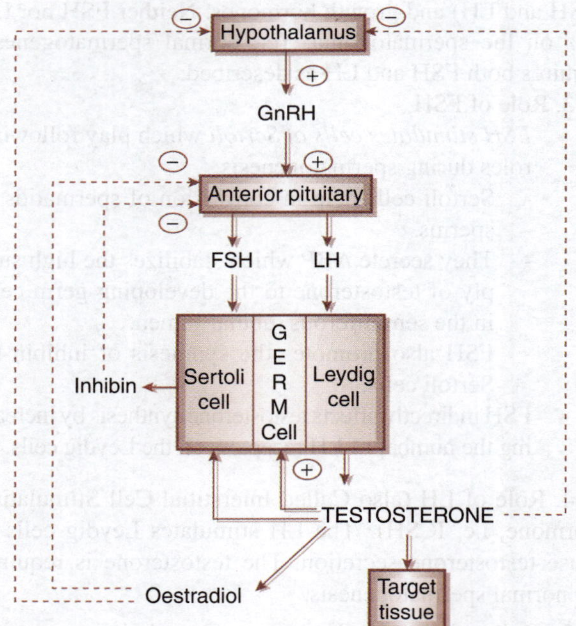

FIGURE 9.2-8 Stimulatory and feedback inhibitory control of spermatogenesis.

Note. Plasma physiologic level of testosterone does not produce significant feedback inhibition of FSH secretion.

Control of Testosterone Secretion

In Foetus During foetal life, human chorionic gonadotropin (HCG) secreted by placenta stimulates the development of Leydig cells in the testes of foetus and causes testosterone secretion.

In Adults

I. Stimulatory Control. The hypothalamic-hypophyseal-testicular (Leydig cell) axis controls the secretion of testosterone in adults as (Fig. 9.2-9).

Hypothalamus produces gonadotropin releasing hormone (GnRH) which stimulates anterior pituitary to secrete FSH and LH.

Anterior pituitary controls secretion of testosterone (steroidogenesis) primarily through LH

- The secretion of LH has been shown to be concordant with the frequency of hypothalamic pulse generator.
- In experimental animals it has been observed that hypophysectomy produces atrophy of Leydig cells which can be restored to normal by administration of LH.

Leydig cells of testes have LH receptors located on their plasma membrane. LH binds to these receptors to activate cyclic AMP synthesis which triggers testosterone synthesis and its secretion.

II. Feedback Inhibitory Control. Plasma testosterone level is maintained at a constant level by a feedback control exerted by testosterone and oestradiol independently to control LH (Fig. 9.2-9):

- Testosterone negative feedback is exerted mainly on the opioidergic neurons that project to GnRH (LHRH) neurons.

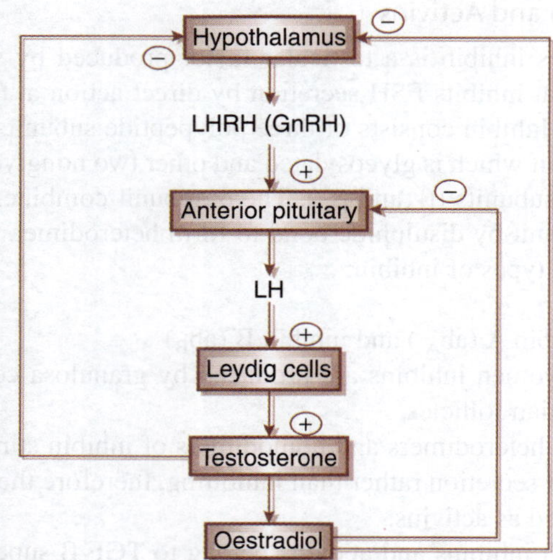

FIGURE 9.2-9 Stimulatory and feedback inhibitory control of secretion of testosterone.

- Testosterone plays a minor role in the inhibition of LH secretion at the level of pituitary.
- Oestradiol exerts negative feedback effects at both hypothalamic and pituitary levels.
- Oestradiol, in contrast to testosterone, exerts a significant direct inhibitory effect on LH secretion at the pituitary level.
- Oestradiol formed by local hypothalamic conversion of testosterone also inhibits LHRH (GnRH).

APPLIED ASPECTS

Some of the important applied aspects, in relation to male reproductive physiology are:

- Cryptorchidism,
- Extirpation,
- Hypogonadism in males,
- Hypergonadism in males,
- Male infertility, and
- Vasectomy.

Cryptorchidism

The testes develop in relation to the lumbar region of the posterior abdominal wall. During foetal life, they gradually descend to the scrotum by the end of the eighth month of gestation.

Cryptorchidism refers to a condition in which the descent of the testes may fail to occur or may be incomplete.

Characteristic features of cryptorchidism are:

- The undescended testes may lie in the lumbar region, in the iliac fossa, in the inguinal canal or in the upper part of scrotum.
- In some cases the testes may complete its descent after birth.
- The incidence of undescended testis, which is 2% at the age of one year and falls to 0.3% after the age of puberty.
- Spermatogenesis often fails to occur in cryptorchidism (due to high temperature of the abdominal cavity) resulting in sterility.
- Androgen secretion from the Leydig cells of testes is unaffected, so male secondary sexual characters develop normally.
- An undescended testis is more likely to develop malignant tumour than a normal testis.

Treatment. Cryptorchidism should be treated as early as possible to prevent male sterility. Surgical correction is advised for correction of undescended testes. However, in some children administration of testosterone or gonadotropic hormone (which stimulates the Leydig cells) can cause the testis to descend provided the inguinal canal is large enough to allow passage of testis.

Extirpation

Extirpation or castration refers to the removal of testes. It will produce following effects:

Effects of Extirpation of Testes before Puberty The removal of testes before puberty results in a clinical condition which is known as *enuchoidism*. It is characterized by:

Permanent sterility as there is no testis so there are no sperms.

Underdevelopment of external genitalia (i.e. penis and scrotum) and accessory sex organs (i.e. seminal vesicles and prostate gland).

Underdevelopment of secondary sexual characters, that is:

- *Hair growth* on face, trunk and in axilla is scanty.
- *Voice is high pitched* like that of child due to underdevelopment of larynx.
- *Muscle mass and shoulder girdle* development is poor.
- *Female like body configuration* occurs due to abnormal deposition of fat on buttocks, hips, pubis and breasts.

Abnormal bone growth due to delay in the union of epiphysis may lead to *increase in height* of the individual, but the bones are weak and thin.

Effects of Extirpation of Testes after Puberty Under such circumstances, some of the male secondary sexual characters and accessory organs (which depend on testosterone) not only for development but also for maintenance are depressed, while some of the masculine features are retained as:

- *Accessory sex organs* are depressed, i.e. seminal vesicles and prostate undergo atrophy.
- *Penis* remains normal in size.
- *Sexual desire* and sexual activity is slightly impaired. Erection occurs but ejaculation is rare because of atrophy of accessory sex organs and lack of sperm.
- *Voice*, usually remains masculine as the growth of larynx is completed during adolescence.
- *Other secondary sexual characters* are not lost.
- *Other body functions* including life span, senility, intelligence, etc. are not affected.

Hypogonadism in Males

Causes. Hypogonadism in males results from absent or deficient testicular functions which may occur in following conditions:

- Congenital nonfunctioning of testes,
- Underdeveloped testes due to absence of HCG in foetal life,
- Cryptorchidism (undescended testes) associated with partial or total degeneration of seminiferous tubules,
- Extirpation of testes and
- Absence of androgen receptors in testes.

Effects of male hypogonadism depend upon whether the testicular deficiency occurs before or after puberty and are similar to those occurring after extirpation before or after puberty, respectively (see page 835).

Frohlich's Syndrome

Frohlich's syndrome also known as adipose genital syndrome or hypothalamiceunuchoidism refers to hypogonadism which occurs due to:

- Hypothalamic disorders,
- Pituitary disorders or
- Genetic inability of hypothalamus to secrete luteinizing hormone releasing hormone (LHRH), i.e. gonadotropin releasing hormone (GnRH).

Features. Under this condition, hypogonadism is often associated with abnormal stimulation of feeding centre. Therefore, the affected person overeats and consequently obesity occurs along with eunuchoidism.

Hypergonadism in Males

Causes. Hypergonadism in males results from excessive secretion of male sex hormones (androgens) as occurs in tumours of Leydig cell.

Features. The occurrence of tumour of Leydig cell is common in prepubertal boys who develop precocious pseudopuberty which is characterized by:

- Rapid growth of musculature and bones,
- But, the height is less due to early closure of epiphysis.
- There is excessive development of sex organs and secondary sexual characters at an early age.
- The tumours can also secrete oestrogenic hormones which can cause overgrowth of breasts (gynaecomastia).

Impotence

Impotence refers to lack of power in male to copulate. It may be:

- *Primary impotence*, which is of rare occurrence.
- *Secondary impotence* may have organic causes or may be followed by drugs or alcohol. Stress and depression are also possible causes.

Male Infertility

Male infertility refers to the inability of sperm to fertilize the ovum.

Causes of male infertility can be grouped as:

1. *Androgen dysfunction with normal sperm count* is seen in:
   - Hypothalamic pituitary defects,
   - Leydig cell defects or
   - Androgen resistance.
2. *Isolated dysfunction of sperm cell production with normal androgen levels* may occur due to:
   - Infection or trauma,
   - Congenital deformation of passages or
   - Formation of nonmotile or otherwise abnormal sperms.
3. *Combined androgen and sperm cell production defects* are:
   - Developmental defects such as Klinefelter's syndrome.
   - Abnormal testicular descent is associated with degeneration of developing sperm cells in the seminiferous tubules due to higher temperature of abdominal cavity or inguinal canal.
   - Acquired testicular defects, such as infections (mumps orchitis) and autoimmune orchitis.
   - Systemic diseases (e.g. chronic liver and kidney diseases).
4. *Failure of deposition of sperms in female genital tract* as occurs in:
   - Obstruction of the vas deferens,
   - Failure of ejaculation during intercourse,
   - Failure of erection during intercourse, and
   - Following vasectomy operation.

Vasectomy

Vasectomy is a surgical procedure for male sterilization (see page 892).

Chapter 9.3

Female Reproductive Physiology

AN OVERVIEW OF FEMALE REPRODUCTIVE SYSTEM

The female reproductive system comprises internal and external genitalia which can be organized as (Fig. 9.3-1):

I. Primary Sex Organs or Ovaries The primary sex organs are a pair of ovaries which correspond with testes in males. The main functions of ovaries are:

- To produce ova and
- To secrete female sex hormones.

II. Accessory Sex Organs The accessory sex organs of females include internal genital organs and external genitalia.

Female Internal Genitalia

The internal genital organs include uterus, fallopian tubes and vagina.

I. Uterus Uterus is a hollow, thick walled muscular organ, situated between the urinary bladder and rectum. It can be divided into two parts (Fig. 9.3-2):

1. Body of the Uterus. It forms upper two-third part of the uterus. Its lower limit is marked by a constriction which corresponds to narrowing of uterine cavity at *internal os*. Body of the uterus can be divided into two parts:

- *Fundus* is the rounded part of the body that lies superior to the opening of the fallopian tubes.
- *Isthmus* is the relatively constricted region of the body (approximately 1 cm long) just above the cervix.

2. Cervix of the Uterus. It is the cylindrical lower part which protrudes into the upper most vagina. It is approximately 2.5 cm long in an adult nonpregnant woman. Its cavity extends from the *internal os* to *external os* which opens into the vagina.

Structure of Uterus

Structure of body of uterus. The wall of body of uterus consists of three layers (Fig. 9.3-3).

1. *Perimetrium* is the external serosal layer.
2. *Myometrium* is the middle muscular layer comprising bundles of smooth muscles amongst which there is a connective tissue.
   - The muscle fibres run in various directions and distinct layers are difficult to define. However, three layers, external, middle and internal are usually described.
   - The muscle cells of the uterus are capable of undergoing great elongation in association with the great enlargement of organ in pregnancy.
   - Contractions of myometrium are responsible for the expulsion of the foetus at the time of child birth.
3. *Endometrium* is the inner layer of uterus which consists of epithelial lining and the stroma (Fig. 9.3-4):
   - *Epithelial lining* is made up of columnar cells. Before menarche (i.e. the age of onset of

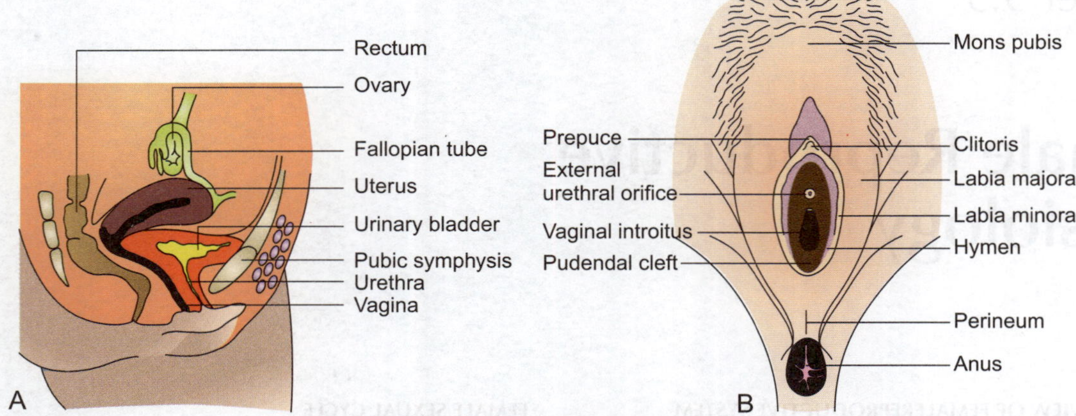

FIGURE 9.3-1 Female reproductive organs: (A) lateral view showing position of internal reproductive organs in relation to pelvic viscera; and (B) female external genitalia.

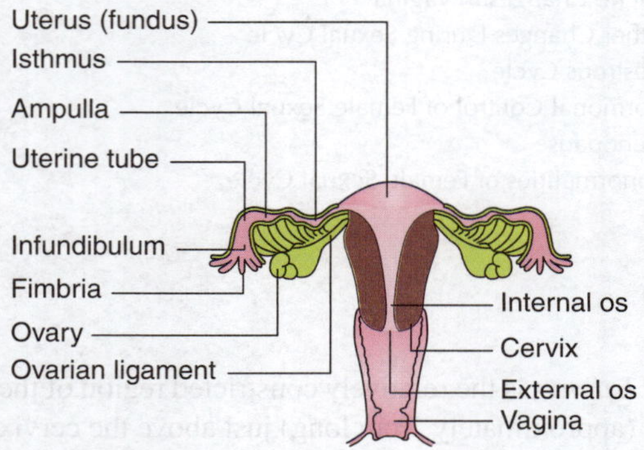

FIGURE 9.3-2 Parts of the uterus and fallopian tube.

menstruation) the cells are ciliated, but thereafter most of the cells may not have cilia.

- *Stroma* of the endometrium, on which the epithelium rests is highly cellular and contains numerous blood vessels and numerous simple tubular uterine glands which are lined by columnar epithelium.

Functional Divisions of Endometrium. Functionally, the endometrium of body of uterus can be divided into two strata:

1. *Stratum functionale* includes superficial two-third thickness of endometrium which undergoes monthly cyclic changes in preparation for the implantation of fertilized ovum and is shed during menstruation. This portion of endometrium is supplied by long and spiral (coiled) arteries.
2. *Stratum basale* is the deeper one-third layer of endometrium. It does not participate in cyclic changes but functions as regenerative layer. This part of endometrium is supplied by short and straight *basal arteries*.

Structure of Cervix of the uterus is somewhat different from that of the body.

1. *Perimetrium* is the outermost serous layer.
2. *Myometrium* layer of the cervix is much less muscular as compared to body of uterus, and contains more connective tissue. During child birth, when the myometrium of body of uterus contracts, the myometrium

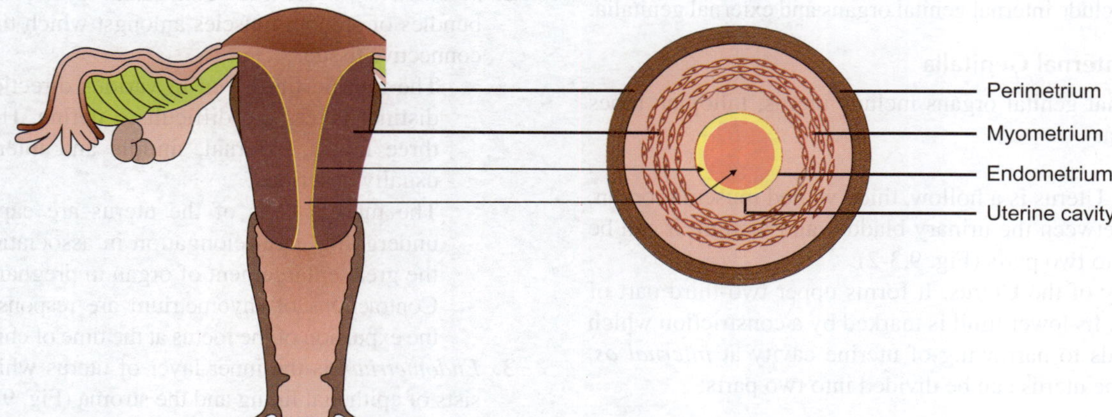

FIGURE 9.3-3 Histological structure of the body of the uterus.

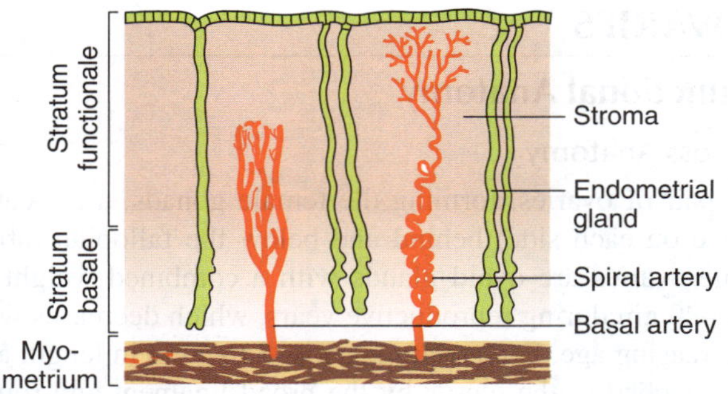

FIGURE 9.3-4 Histological structure of the endometrium.

of cervix dilates, consequently the cervical canal becomes large enough for the foetal head to pass through.

3. *Endocervix* refers to the innermost mucosal layer of cervix in contrast to endometrium of the body of uterus. Endocervix is not shed at the time of menstruation. Endocervix consists of:
   - *Epithelium.* The mucous membrane of the upper two-thirds of cervical canal is lined by *ciliated columnar epithelium*, but its lower one-third epithelium is nonciliated columnar. Near the external os the canal is lined by stratified squamous epithelium which is continuous over the external surface of the part of the cervix projecting into the vagina and with the vaginal epithelium.
   - *Stroma.* The stroma underlying the epithelium of the cervix is less cellular than that of body of uterus.

II. Fallopian Tubes Each fallopian tube (also known as uterine tube) is approximately 10 cm in length and 8 mm in diameter. It has a medial or *uterine end* which is attached to and opens into the uterus and a *lateral end* opens into peritoneal cavity near the ovary.

Parts. Each fallopian tube can be divided into four parts (Fig. 9.3-2):

1. *Uterine or interstitial part* is the most medial part which passes through the thick uterine wall.
2. *Isthmus* is the relatively narrow and thick walled part which is just next to the uterine part. It is about 2.5 cm in length.
3. *Ampulla* is the next thin walled and dilated part of the uterine tube. It is the largest part (7 cm) of the uterine tube.
4. *Infundibulum* refers to the funnel-shaped lateral end of the tube. It is prolonged into a number of finger-like processes known as fimbria. One fimbria is longer than rest of the fimbriae and is attached to the outer pole of ovary.

Structure. Fallopian tubes consist of same three coats as of the uterus viz. endometrium, myometrium and perimetrium.

Functions. The uterine tubes convey ova, shed by the ovaries, to the uterus. Ova enter the tube at its fimbriated end. The sperms enter the uterine tube at its medial end after traversing the vagina and uterine cavity. Secretions present in the tubes provide nutrition, oxygen and other requirements for ova and spermatozoa passing through the tube. Fertilization takes place in the ampulla and the fertilized ovum travels towards the uterus through the tube. The ciliated epithelial cells lining the tube help to move ova towards uterus.

III. Vagina

- The vagina is a musculomembranous tube (about 8 to 10 cm long) located anterior to the rectum and posterior to urethra and urinary bladder.
- Its upper end surrounds the lower part of cervix and its lower end, i.e. vaginal orifice opens into the vestibule of vagina (the cleft between the labia minora).
- No glands open into the vagina. The small amount of secretion present in the vagina is derived partly from the mucous discharge from the cervix and partly from the transudation of fluid from the vaginal epithelium which contains glycogen. Action of bacteria on the glycogen present in the vaginal secretion produces lactic acid which maintains the vaginal pH around 4.5. Acidic environment of vagina prevents the growth of pathogenic organisms.

Structure. The wall of vagina consists of a mucous membrane, a muscle coat and an outer fibrous coat or adventitia.

1. *Mucous membrane* shows numerous longitudinal folds and is firmly fixed to the underlying muscle layer. In an adult female, the vaginal mucosa is lined by stratified squamous epithelium. The epithelial cells are rich in glycogen and this property is oestrogen dependent.
2. *Muscle coat* is made up of an outer layer of longitudinal fibres and a much thinner layer of circular fibres. Many elastic fibres are present among the muscle fibres. The lower end of vagina is surrounded by striated fibres of the bulbospongiosus muscle that form a sphincter for it.
3. *Adventitial coat* surrounds the muscle coat and is made up of fibrous tissue containing many elastic fibres.

Functions. The vagina serves following functions:

- It serves as the excretory duct for menstrual fluid.
- It forms the inferior part of pelvic (birth) canal.
- It receives the penis and ejaculate during sexual intercourse.

Female External Genitalia

The external genital organs include mons pubis, labia majora, labia minora, clitoris, vestibule of vagina, bulbs of vestibule and greater vestibular glands (Fig. 9.3-1B).

The synonymous terms vulva and pudendum include all these parts. The vulva serves:

- As sensory and erectile tissue for sexual arousal and intercourse,
- To direct the flow of urine and
- To prevent entry of foreign material into the urogenital tract.

1. ***Mons pubis*** is the rounded, fatty prominence anterior to the pubic symphysis, pubic tubercle and superior pubic rami.
2. ***Labia majora*** are prominent folds of skin that bound the *pudendal cleft* and thus indirectly provide protection for urethral and vaginal orifices which open into this cleft.
3. ***Labia minora*** are folds of fat free, hairless, pinkish skin. They are enclosed in the pudendal cleft and surround the *vestibule of vagina*. They have a core of spongy connective tissue containing erectile tissue and many small blood vessels.
4. ***Clitoris*** is an erectile organ located where the labia minora meet anteriorly. The clitoris is analogous to male penis, but unlike the penis, the clitoris is not functionally related to the urethra or to urination. It functions solely as an organ of sexual arousal.
5. ***Vestibule*** is the space between the labia minora that contains the opening of urethra, vagina and ducts of greater and lesser vestibular glands. The vaginal orifice is surrounded by a thin fold of mucous membrane called *hymen* which is usually ruptured after first intercourse or otherwise. After child birth, only a few remnants of the *hymen—hymenal* caruncles (tags) are visible.
6. ***Bulbs of the vestibule*** are paired masses of erectile tissue which lie along the sides of vaginal orifice under cover of bulbospongiosus muscles. These are homologous with the bulb of the penis and corpus spongiosum.
7. ***Vestibular glands*** include a pair each of greater vestibular and lesser vestibular glands. These glands secrete mucus into the vestibule during arousal.

OVARIES

Functional Anatomy

Gross Anatomy

A pair of ovaries, forming the female gonads, are located (one on each side) behind and below the fallopian tubes. The ovaries are ovoid glands with a combined weight of 10–20 gm during reproductive years, which decreases with increasing age. Each ovary is about 3 to 5 cm in length and is attached to the uterus by the broad ligament and round ligament of ovary.

Structure Histologically, each ovary consists of following parts (Fig. 9.3-5):

1. Germinal Epithelium. Germinal epithelium refers to the epithelium lining the outer surface of ovary and consists of a single layer of cuboidal cells. This epithelium is continuous with the mesothelium lining the peritoneum, and represents a modification of the latter. The term germinal epithelium is a misnomer, as it does not produce germ cells. The cells of this epithelium bear microvilli and contain numerous mitochondria. They become larger in pregnancy.

2. Cortex. The cortex is the outer thick main part of the substance of the ovary. It consists of following tissues:

- *Tunica albuginea* is the outer condensation of the connective tissue present immediately below the germinal epithelium. The tunica albuginea of the ovary is much thinner and less dense than that of testis.
- *Stroma* of the cortex, present deep to the tunica albuginea, is made up of reticular fibres and numerous fusiform cells that resemble mesenchymal cells.
- *Ovarian follicles* at various stages of development are scattered in the stroma. Each follicle contains a developing ovum. The formation of ova and the development and fate of ovarian follicles are described in oogenesis.

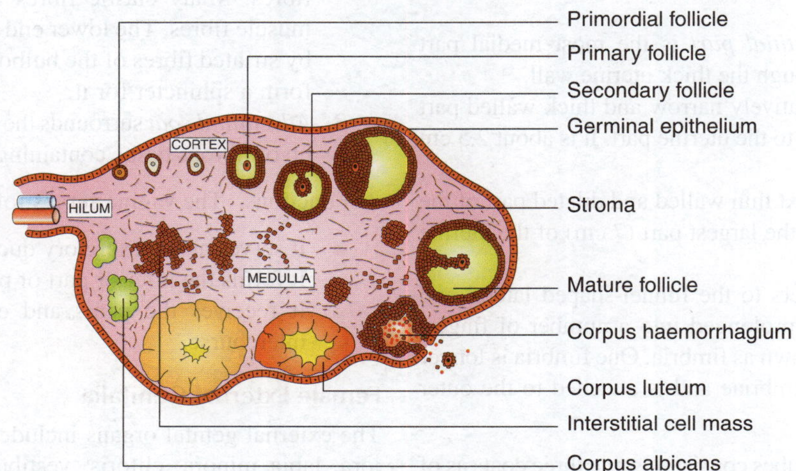

FIGURE 9.3-5 Schematic diagram of the histology of ovary depicting various stages of development of follicles and corpus luteum.

3. Medulla. The medulla is the inner small part of the substance of ovary. It consists of connective tissue in which numerous blood vessels (mostly veins), smooth muscles and elastic fibres are present.

4. Hilum. The hilum refers to the area where ovary attaches to mesentery. It is the site for entry of blood vessels and lymphatic. It also contains some remnants of the mesonephric ducts, and hilus cells that are similar to interstitial cells of the testis. The hilum is continuous with the medulla of the ovary.

Functions of Ovaries

The two principal functions of ovaries are:

- Gametogenic function, i.e. oogenesis,and
- Endocrine function, i.e. secretion of female hormones called ovarian hormones.

Oogenesis

Oogenesis refers to the process of formation of ova from the primitive germ cells.

Phases of oogenesis include:

- Fetal oogenesis,
- Postnatal oogenesis,
- Prepubertal oogenesis and
- Pubertal oogenesis.

1. Foetal Oogenesis

Unlike the foetal testis (in which spermatogenesis begins at puberty), the foetal ovary begins oogenesis by 10 weeks of gestation.

Primitive Germ Cells. When the bipotential gonads differentiate into ovaries in genetic female (44 + XX) embryo (in the absence of testis determining factor, i.e. TDF) by the 10th week of gestation, the primitive germ cells increase in number by mitosis to form oogonia.

Oogonia are the stem cells from which ova are derived. The oogonia proliferate by mitosis to form primary oocytes. The process begins at the 15th week and reaches a peak between 20 and 28 weeks gestation.

- The oogonium is unique in that it is the only female cell in which both X chromosomes are active.

Primary Oocytes formed from the oogonia, enter a prolonged prophase (*diplotene stage)* of the first meiotic division and remain in this state until ovulation occurs after puberty.

Primordial Follicles. The *diploid primary oocytes* become enveloped by a single layer of flat granulosa cells and in this form are called *primordial follicles.* (The granulosa cells are formed by proliferation of coelomic epithelium, i.e. cortical cells). Each primordial follicle is enveloped in a thin membrane called the *basal lamina.* The follicles lack a direct blood supply.

- The primordial follicle is fundamental in reproductive unit of the ovary.
- During peak of development (between 20 and 28. weeks of gestation) the two ovaries contain about 7 million germ cells in the form of oogonia, primary oocytes and primordial follicles.
- Many germ cells undergo atresia (involution) and at term only 2 million germ cells are present, most of which have developed into primordial follicles, some are as oogonia and primary oocytes.

2. Postnatal and Prepubertal Oogenesis

- The number of primordial follicles present in the ovaries at birth rapidly diminishes thereafter.
- By 6 months postpartum all of the oogonia have been converted into primary oocytes and primordial follicles.
- No new ova are formed after birth.
- By the onset of puberty (at about 12–13 years of age) the two ovaries contain about 3,00,000 primordial follicles.

3. Pubertal Oogenesis

- After puberty the oogenesis or formation of ovum occurs in a highly cyclic fashion, once every 28 days till menopause.
- Every month, in each ovary, more than one primordial follicles start undergoing maturation process but only one reaches maturity and the rest undergo atresia at different stages of development. Thus throughout the whole normal reproductive life of about 30 years (from 13 to 42 years) about 450 ova are expelled and the remainder degenerate.
- The different stages of maturation of primordial follicle into graafian follicle (*folliculogenesis)* are described in the ovarian cycle (see page 848).
- The primary oocytes which is in the prophase of first meiotic division since foetal life completes the first meiotic division just before ovulation. As a result *secondary oocyte* containing most of the cytoplasm and *first polar body* are formed. The first polar body soon fragments and disappears.
- The *secondary oocyte* (haploid cell) immediately begins the *second meiotic division* but this division stops at metaphase and is completed only if the mature ovum (ootid) is fertilized by a sperm. In some species, the arrest in metaphase is due to formation of a protein in the ovum known as $PP^{3q\ mos}$ encoded by protooncogene(C-mos). On fertilization $PP^{3q\ mos}$ is destroyed within 30 minutes by Calpain (a Ca^{2+} dependent protease). At that time the *second polar body (polocyte)* is extruded and the fertilized ovum proceeds to form a new individual. Fertilization normally occurs in the ampulla of fallopian tube.

Pubertal Oogenesis versus Spermatogenesis

From the above description of pubertal oogenesis and spermatogenesis (page 825), the following can be concluded:

- In contrast to the male who produces spermatogonia and primary spermatocytes continuously throughout life, the female cannot form oogonia beyond 28 weeks gestation and must function with a declining pool of oocytes.
- Meiosis in the female results in the formation of one viable oocyte. In contrast, each primary spermatogonium in the male ultimately gives rise to 64 spermatozoa.
- Oogenesis in the female begins in *utero* in response to *meiosis-stimulating factor,* whereas in the male, spermatogenesis is arrested at the spermatogonial stage in response to *meiosis-inhibiting factor.*

Endocrine Function of Ovaries

The endocrine function of the ovaries is to produce female sex hormones which include:

- Oestrogens and
- Progesterone.

Oestrogens

Oestrogens are (C-18) steroids. The naturally occurring oestrogens include:

- *Oestradiol.* It is the principal and physiologically most potent oestrogen. Ovarian oestradiol accounts for more than 90% of the circulating oestrogens.
- *Oestrone.* It is a weak ovarian oestrogen.
- *Oestriol.* It is the degradation product of oestradiol and oestrone. It is the weakest of all naturally occurring oestrogens.

Synthesis, Plasma Levels and Transport of Oestrogens

Sites In the normal non-pregnant female, oestrogens are mainly secreted by theca interna and granulosa cells of the ovarian follicles. A small quantity is also produced by adrenal cortex, breast, some areas of brain, placenta (during pregnancy), and by Sertoli cells (in males).

Biosynthesis. The salient points of oestrogen synthesis are:

- Oestrogens are mainly synthesized from cholesterol derived from blood and to a slight extent from acetyl *co-enzyme A.*
- During synthesis progesterone and testosterone are synthesized first and then these are converted into oestrogens.
- The biochemical steps for synthesis of oestrogen are shown in Fig. 9.3-6. There are two pathways (Δ5 pathway and Δ4 pathway) for oestrogen synthesis. The first step, i.e. (the conversion of cholesterol into pregnenolone is common in both the pathways. This reaction is stimulated by gonadotropins (FSH and LH).

Δ5 Pathway. This pathway involves:

- Synthesis of 17 α hydroxypregnenolone and dihydroxyepiandrosterone (DHEA). The reactions are catalyzed by enzymes 17α-hydroxylase and 17, 20-hydroxylase respectively (CYP-17).

Note. CYP-17 is an enzyme which catalyses hydroxylation of C-17 and cleavage of 2 carbon side chain at C-17 of pregnenolone and progesterone.

- Then DHEA (17 ketosteroid) is converted to androstenedione (another androgenic 17 ketosteroid) by an enzyme 3B hydroxysteroid dehydrogenase (3BHSD) and Δ5 reductase.
- Androstenedione is then converted into *testosterone* by17-hydroxysteroid dehydrogenase. This reaction is reversible.
- Testosterone is a precursor for oestradiol formation by aromatase (CYP-19) enzyme.

Δ4 Pathway. In this pathway, progesterone is the initial compound which is formed from pregnenolone by 3 B hydroxysteroid dehydrogenase and Δ5 isomerase.

- Then progesterone is converted to 17α hydroxyprogesterone by 17 α-hydroxylase (CYP-17). 17α-hydroxyprogesterone is another precursor for androstenedione via 17–20 hydroxylase.
- Then both androstenedione and testosterone are converted to oestradiol and oestrone by aromatases (CYP-19).

Mechanism of Biosynthesis of Oestrogen Gonadotropins (FSH and LH) from anterior pituitary stimulate the synthesis of female sex hormones by acting on the receptors.

- Theca interna cells have many Luteinizing hormone (LH) receptors. The LH therefore increases the conversion of cholesterol to androstenedione via cyclic AMP.
- The granulosa cells also possess many FSH receptors. FSH, therefore, facilitates the secretion of oestradiol by acting on these receptors through activation of cyclic AMP, which increases the activity of aromatase enzyme. The mature granulosa cells also acquire LH receptors; therefore, LH stimulates the oestradiol production from granulosa cells also.
- There exists an interaction between theca interna and granulosa cells for oestrogen synthesis (Fig. 9.3-7). The granulosa cells can synthesize oestradiol only when androstenedione is provided to them. The theca interna cells provide supply of androstenedione to granulosa cells.
- In primates, it seems that the oestradiol present in the follicular fluid comes from the granulosa cells.
- The stromal tissue of the ovaries can also synthesize androgens and oestrogens in insignificant amounts.

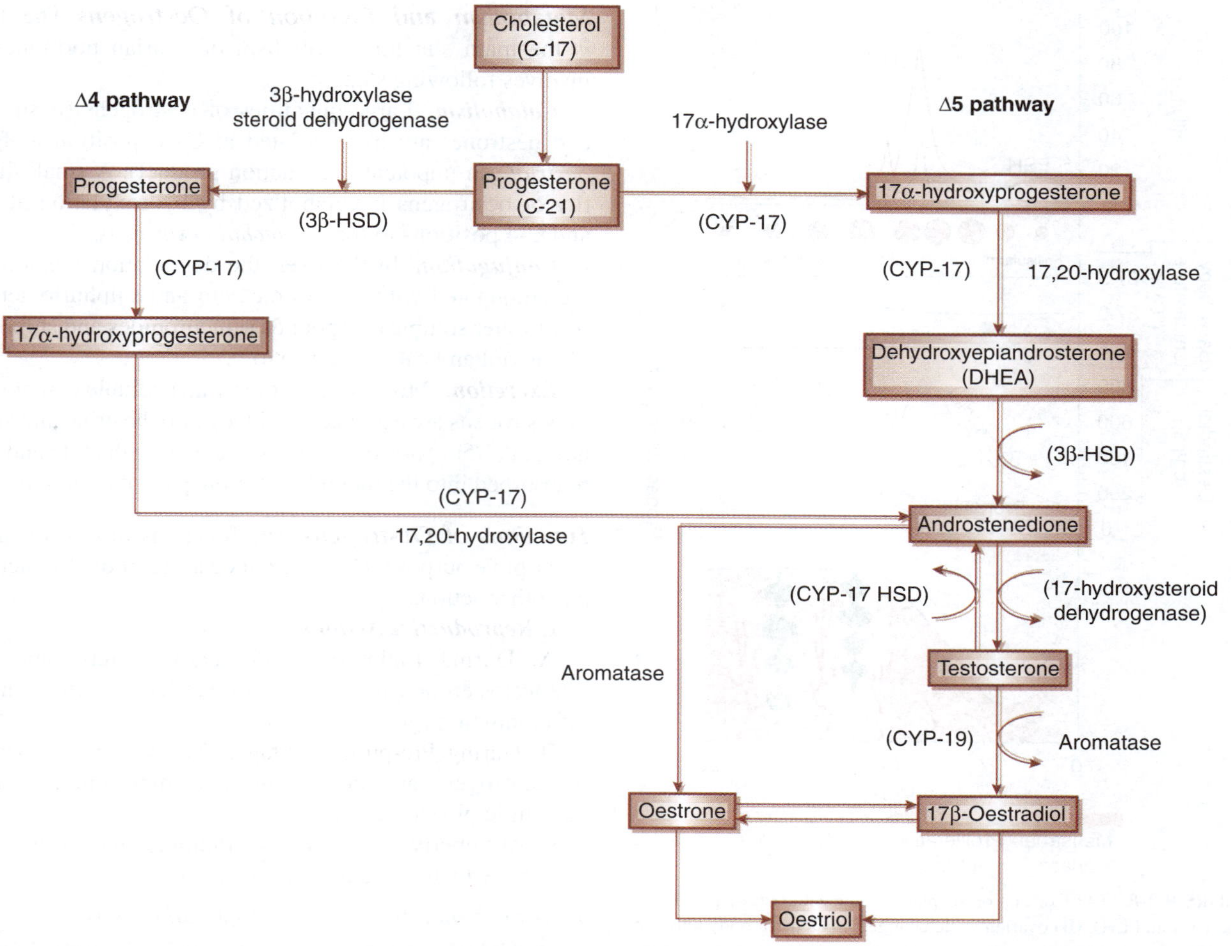

FIGURE 9.3-6 Biosynthesis and metabolism of oestrogen.

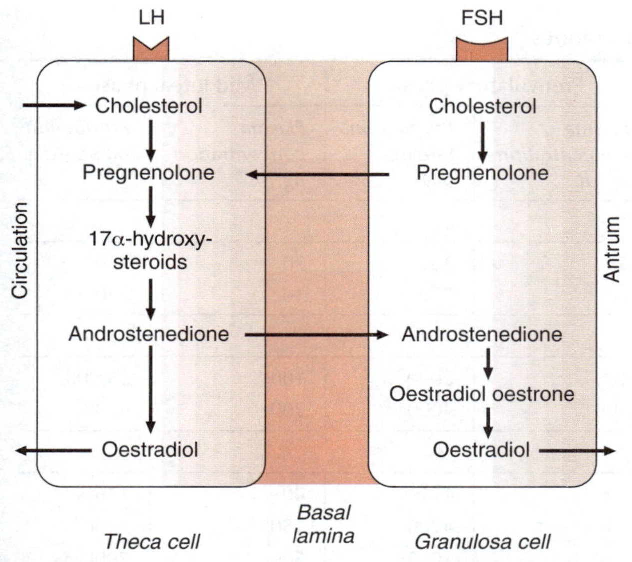

FIGURE 9.3-7 Interaction between theca interna and granulosa cells for synthesis of oestradiol.

Plasma Levels

In a normal adult woman, the plasma levels of oestrogen varies in different phases of the ovarian cycle (Fig. 9.3-8, Table 9.3-1). As shown in Figure 9.3-8D, there are two peaks of oestrogen secretion. The first occurs just before the ovulation (12–13th day of a sexual cycle) and is called *oestrogen surge,* and the second peak occurs in the mid luteal phase. The secretion rate of oestrogen in different phases is:

- In early follicular phase : 36 μg/day,
- Just before ovulation : 380 μg/day and
- Duringmid luteal phase : 250 μg/day.

After menopause the oestrogen level falls to minimum of 50 μg/day.

Transport. In the circulation oestrogens is present in two forms, bound (98%),and free (2%). The oestradiol is mainly bound to plasma proteins: 60% to albumin and 38% to β globulin. The β-globulin is also known as *gonadal steroid binding globulin* (GBG) *protein*. It is the same protein to which testosterone binds.

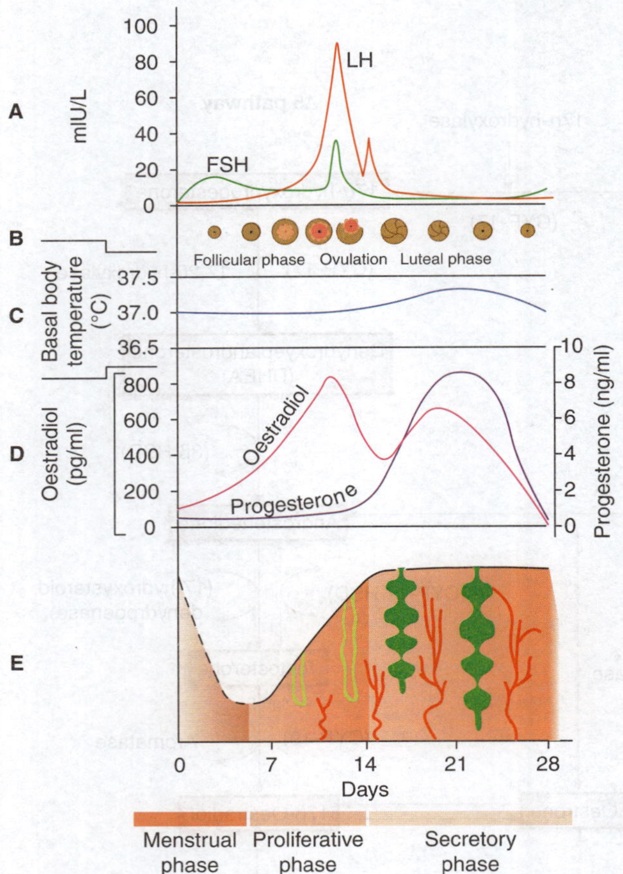

FIGURE 9.3-8 (A) Correlation of plasma concentration of gonadotropins (FSH and LH) ;(B) ovarian cycle changes; ; (C) basal body temperature; (D) ovarian hormones; (E) and endometrial changes during female sexual cycle.

Metabolism and Excretion of Oestrogens The liver is the main site for metabolism of ovarian hormones. It involves following steps:

Catabolism. Large quantities of oestrogens (oestradiol and oestrone) are hydroxylated at C-16 position to form *oestriol* (an unpotent degradation product). A small quantity of oestrogens is catabolized by hydroxylation at C-2 and C-4 positions to form *catechol oestrogens.*

Conjugation. In the liver, the degradation metabolites are conjugated with glucuronic acid and sulphuric acid to form water soluble compounds (glucuronides and sulphates of oestriol and catecholestriole).

Excretion. Most (4/5th) of the water soluble compounds of oestrogens are excreted by kidney into the urine and small amount (1/5th part) of them is secreted into the bile and gets reabsorbed into the blood by enterohepatic circulation.

Functions of Oestrogens The functions of oestrogen for descriptive purposes can be grouped as: reproductive actions and other actions.

I. Reproductive Actions

A. During Embryonic Life. During embryonic life, like testosterone (in males) oestrogen has no effect on sex differentiation (gonadal and genital sex).

B. During Pre-pubertal Stage. During girlhood period, the oestrogens are secreted in very small amount which have little physiological actions.

C. At Puberty. At puberty oestradiol is secreted in larger amounts which cause following changes:

1. *Growth and development of genital organs*

i. ***Ovaries*** increase in size and complete ovarian cycles start which are characterized by folliculosis, ovulation and corpus luteum formation.

TABLE 9.3-1 Plasma Levels and Production Rate of Ovarian Hormones

Hormone	Early follicular phase		Preovulatory phase		Mid luteal phase	
	Plasma concentration ng/dL	*Production rate μg/day*	*Plasma concentration ng/dL*	*Production rate μg/day*	*Plasma concentration ng/dL*	*Production rate μg/day*
Oestrogens (C-18)						
• Oestradiol	6	36	50	380	20	250
• Oestrone	5	50	20	350	10	250
Progesterone						
(C-21)	9	1000	100	2000	1000	25,000
• 17α Hydroxyprogesterone	30	600	200	4000	200	4000
Androgens (C-19)						
• Testosterone	40	144	40	171	40	126
• Androstenedione	150	2600	150	4700	150	3400
• Dehydroepiandrosterone	500	7000	500	7000	500	7000

ii. ***Fallopian tubes*** become functional and show certain changes such as epithelium becomes more cilliated, motility of fallopian tubes also increases at ovulation to transport shedded gametes.

iii. ***Uterus.*** The following changes occur in the uterus:
- *Size.* It enlarges in size, the smooth muscle fibres in myometrial coat increase in number and in size, the contractile protein contents also increase and the muscle fibres become active and excitable.
- *Endometrium* gets thickened due to increase in stroma and blood flow. The rhythmic cyclic changes (proliferative and secretory) occur with the onset of menstrual cycle.

iv. ***Cervix*** also enlarges and with the onset of menstrual cycle, endocervix undergoes cyclic changes (see page 852).

v. ***Vagina*** increases in size. Its epithelial lining increases in height (from 2–3 layer cuboidal epithelium to 10–12 layers cornified squamous epithelium). Vaginal epithelium is quite sensitive to oestrogen and thus show cyclic changes during sexual cycle (see page 853).

vi. ***External genitalia.*** The following changes occur in external genitalia:
- *Increase in size of clitoris,*
- *Labia majora and labia minora* increase in size and get widened.

2. ***Appearance of secondary sex characters.*** Oestrogen is responsible for appearance of secondary sex characters (see page 815):

- In an adult woman, oestrogens along with progesterone regulate the ovarian cycle, menstrual cycle and cyclic changes in cervix, vagina and fallopian tubes (see page 855) in a non-pregnant state.
  - It plays an important role in maintenance of pregnancy and then during parturition (see page 877).
  - It is important for breast development (see page 881).

II. Other Actions. The other functions of oestrogens include the effects on following:

1. ***Effects on bones***

i. Oestradiol accelerates the linear growth of bones at puberty by its osteoblastic activity. The epiphyseal centres are more sensitive to oestrogen than testosterone; for this reason, average height of females is little less than the males.

ii. Oestradiol enlarges the hip and widens the inlet of the pelvic bone to facilitate child birth.

iii. Oestrogens maintain balance between bone formation and bone resorption by following ways:
- It promotes bone formation by deposition of bone matrix by causing Ca^{2+} and HPO_4^{2-} retention and
- Inhibits bone resorption by inhibiting the production of osteoclasts and their activity. These effects are achieved by inhibiting the production of lymphokines such as interleukin-I (IL-1), TNF α, and granulocyte-macrophage colony stimulating factor which promote proliferation of osteoclasts.

Note. Loss of oestrogen actions after menopause shifts the bone balance towards bone resorption, thus causing osteoporosis (see page 735).

2. ***Effects on metabolism***

i. *Protein metabolism*
- Oestrogens cause positive nitrogen balance due to growth promoting effect which causes slight increase in the total body proteins.
- Oestrogens also increase the hepatic synthesis of certain circulating proteins, such as: thyroxine binding globulin, cortisol binding globulins, renin substrate, angiotensinogens, very low density lipoproteins (VLDL),and high density lipoproteins.

ii. *Fat metabolism*
- Oestrogens cause fat deposition in subcutaneous tissues, in the breasts and the thighs.
- Lower the plasma cholesterol level and low density lipids due to increase in number of LDL receptors.

3. ***Water and electrolyte balance.*** Oestrogens like other steroids in general, cause salt and water retention in the body and produce premenstrual tension in some women.

4. ***Effects on vasculature.*** In general oestrogens have vasodilator and anti-vasoconstrictor effects.
   - The vasodilator effect is through local release of vasodilator substances like nitric oxide (NO), prostaglandins E_2 and prostacyclin, and
   - The antivasoconstrictor effect is through inhibition of endothelin-1 release (a vasoconstrictor agent).

Note
- At the end of luteal phase of menstrual cycle there is sudden fall in plasma concentration of oestrogen which results in alterations in the balance of vasodilatation and anti vasconstriction and thus initiates ischaemic necrosis during menstrual phase.
- Loss of vasodilator effect in postmenopausal women leads to increased risk of coronary heart disease.

5. ***Effects on CNS***
   - Oestrogens are responsible for oestrous behaviour in animals and also increase the libido in human females.
   - Oestrogens also act on other areas of the brain and effect the neuronal discharge and thus effect the brain functioning. It has been observed that in mice oestrogen improves the memory and learning. Therefore, deficiency of oestrogen in postmenopausal women is associated with defects in declarative

memory and development of Alzheimer's disease (see page 1127).

6. ***Effects on skin***
   - Oestrogens make the skin soft and more vascular.
   - It makes the sebaceous glands secretions thin and inhibits formation of black heads (comedones) and acne. Therefore, synthetic oestrogens are used as a part of treatment in acne (see page 846).

Mechanism of Action of Oestrogens Oestrogens act by entering into the cell and then bind with cytoplasmic receptors.

Oestrogen Receptors Oestrogen receptors are of two types (ERα and ERβ) and are coded by two different genes located on separate chromosomes.

- *The oestrogen receptor α (ERα)* are mainly present in the endometrium, breasts, pituitary gland and adrenal glands, and in the testes and epididymis in males. Whereas *oestrogen receptors β (ER β)* are located in the ovaries (granulosa cells), bones (osleoclasts), lungs, some areas of brain and in prostate gland and urinary bladder in males.

It has been suggested that the actions of oestrogen which are carried out by circulatory oestrogens and through hypothalamo-pituitary-gonadal axis are mainly mediated through ERα receptors and the actions of oestrogen present in the follicular antrum are mediated through ERβ receptors.

- The receptors contain a heat shock protein (HSP). When oestrogen binds to the receptor the HSP get displaced and *oestrogen receptor complex* so formed is transferred on to the nucleus of the target cell.
- Then the oestrogen receptor get bound to oestrogen response element present on the DNA molecule, and
- Promotes the synthesis of new mRNA and that in turn directs the synthesis of new proteins which modify the target cell activity.

Note. Most of the actions of oestrogens are mediated via genomic receptors (ERα and ERβ). However, some of its effects are so rapid (e.g. effect on brain neuronal discharge and feedback effect on gonadotropins release that they might be mediated through non-genomic receptors present on the plasma membrane.

Synthetic Oestrogens

Types. Various types of synthetic preparations of oestrogen available are:

1. *Ethinyl derivatives* of oestradiol such as *diethylstilbestrol* and *ethinyloestradiol* are the potent oestrogens when given orally (because these are not metabolized in the liver like natural oestrogens).
2. *Plant oestrogens.* Oestrogenic substances also present in plants, these rarely cause adverse effects in human beings but when administered in animal they cause adverse effects.
3. *Nonsteroidal* preparations also have oestrogenic activity.

Therapeutic Uses. The oestrogenic preparations are used under following conditions:

- To reduce menopausal symptoms like hot flushes.
- To prevent postmenopausal osteoporosis.
- To prevent progression to atherosclerosis and incidence of heart attacks and strokes.
- As contraceptive when used along with progesterone.

Side Effects (Adverse Effects). They stimulate growth of endometrium and breast and thus increase the incidence of carcinoma of breast and of uterus. The compounds like *tamoxifen* and *raloxifene* are under trial. It has been suggested that these compounds are effective to check osteoporosis and have cardiovascular effects as that of oestradiol but do not have growth promoting effect on uterus and cervix.

Progesterone

Progesterone is C-21 steroid meant for maintenance of pregnancy and biologically called prostagen or gestagen.

Synthesis, Plasma Levels and Transport of Progesterone

Sites. In a normal adult nonpregnent woman progesterone is mainly secreted by corpus luteum and during pregnancy by the placenta. A small amount is also secreted by adrenal cortex and by testes in case of males.

Biosynthesis. Progesterone is synthesized from cholesterol. Progesterone itself is an important intermediary compound formed during biosynthesis of steroids (oestrogens and androgens). For biosynthesis pathways and steps involved see page 843 and Figure 9.3-6.

Plasma Levels. In a normal adult woman, the plasma levels of progesterone varies with different phases of sexual cycle (Table 9.3-1 and Fig. 9.3-8D).

- ***In early follicular phase,*** plasma concentration of progesterone is very low (about 0.9 ng/ml or 9 ng/dL). About 80–90% of the progesterone is derived from the conversion of adrenal DHEA and androstenedione. But a large amount is also present in the follicular antrum.
- ***In mid-cycle*** (late follicular phase), its level starts rising due to secretion from the granulosa cells and it is mainly 17α- hydroxyprogesterone and
- ***In luteal phase*** it reaches to its peak value, i.e. 18 ng/ml and
- ***At the end of cycle*** its levels fall to its minimum value.
- ***During pregnancy,*** the levels of progesterone further rise (see page 866).
- ***After menopause.*** Progesterone levels fall to its minimum (0.2 ng/ml) or even not detectable.

Transport In the plasma progesterone is present in two forms:

- ***Bound form.*** About 98% of progesterone in the blood is present in bound form with plasma proteins. With albumin (80%) and with corticoid binding protein (CBP) also known as *transcortin* (18%). Hence, progesterone is mostly present in loosely bound form with albumin.
- ***Unbound form*** or free form. Only 2% of circulating progesterone is present in this form.

Metabolism and Excretion of Progesterone

Metabolism. In the liver, progesterone is metabolized to form pregnanediol and 17α-hydroxyprogesterone to pregnanetriol.

- The metabolites then conjugated with glucuronic acid and sulphuric acid to form water soluble substances.

Excretion. The water soluble substance (glucuronides and sulphates) of pregnanediol and pregnanetriol are excreted by the kidney into the urine and small amount is also secreted into the bile.

Functions of Progesterone The physiological actions of progesterone can be grouped as reproductive actions and other actions.

I. Reproductive Actions. Reproductive actions are mainly on the reproductive organs primed by oestrogens and these include:

1. Action on Uterus. Under the influence of progesterone uterus shows following changes:

- *Endometrium*
  - Progesterone slows the proliferation of endometrial cells by decreasing mitotic activity of the cells.
  - The thickness of endometrium also increases.
  - The endometrial glands become tortuous and contain fluid containing glycogen, glycoproteins and glycolipids which provide nutrition to blastula if fertilization occurs.
  - The glandular cells show vacuolation near their bases and the vacuolations move from peripheral part towards the lumen of the gland.
  - The spiral arteries become more coiled.
  - The stroma of endometrium becomes oedematous.

  Thus, progesterone is responsible for secretory phase of the endometrial cycle and prepares the endometrium to receive the zygote.
- *Uterine motility.* Progesterone decreases the uterine motility by following ways:
  - It has antiestrogenic effect on the myometrial cells, decreasing the excitability sensitivity to oxytocin and spontaneous electrical activity and increasing membrane potential.
    - It decreases the synthesis of voltage dependent Ca^{2+} channel proteins, therefore Ca^{2+} uptake decreases.
    - It decreases the number of oestrogen receptors on the myometrium.

2. Endocervix. The cervical secretions become thick and viscid, and ferning pattern disappears.

3. Vagina. Vaginal epithelium becomes thickened, cornified and infiltrated with leucocytes.

4. Fallopian Tubes. Progesterone increases the beating rate of cilia of fallopian tubes towards the uterus. The epithelial cell secretions also increase in amount and are rich in nutritive materials to provide nutrition to a shedded ovum, incoming sperm or to zygote if fertilization occurs.

5. Breast. Progesterone causes lobular and alveolar growth (see page 881) of breast.

6. During Pregnancy. the main function of progesterone is to maintain the pregnancy (see page 866).

II. Other Actions. The other systemic effects of progesterone are:

1. Thermogenic Effect. Progesterone is known as a thermogenic steroid which increases the basal body temperature by 0.5°C in the postovulatory phase.

2. Effect on CNS. Progesterone alters the secretion and release of various neurotransmitters in the hypothalamus and other areas of the brain and thereby decreases the appetite and produces *somnolence*.

3. Effect on respiration. Progesterone increases the sensitivity of the respiratory centre to carbon dioxide stimulation. Due to this fact the $pACO_2$ is slightly less in woman during luteal phase of sexual cycle. Therefore progesterone is used in *Pickwickian syndrome.*

4. Effect on Fat Metabolism.

Progesterone (particularly C-19 progesterone) decreases the serum HDL. Thus, it acts as a proathrogenic agent.

5. Effect on Kidney. Large dose of progesterone produces natriuresis, by blocking action of aldosterone on kidney.

Mechanism of Action

- The effects of the progesterone on its target cell is achieved by acting through its receptors.
- The progesterone receptors are present in the cytoplasm of the target cells and contain a protein called HSP.
- Being lipid progesterone easily enters through bilayer lipid membrane and combines with its receptors.

Then the HSP displaces and thus exposing the DNA binding site.

- Then the receptor progesterone complex get transferred on to the nucleus and binds to a specific site on the DNA molecule, and
- Initiates encoding of gene expression to form new mRNA. The mRNA then directs the apparatus to form new proteins (enzymes and structural proteins) which modify the activities of the target cells.

Note. A synthetic steroid *mifepristone* (RU-486) binds to progesterone receptors and blocks the DNA binding site. Therefore this drug acts as aantiprogesterone drug.

Synthetic Preparations of Progesterone Various synthetic preparations are available under the name *prostagens* and gestagens. Therapeutically these drugs are used in:

- Inevitable abortion and
- As contraceptives when used along with oestrogens.

Other Ovarian Hormones

Besides female sex steroids (oestrogen and progesterone) ovaries also secrete peptide hormones as:

1. Inhibin structurally it is polypeptide, it inhibits the FSH release. For details see page 868.

2. Activin. Structurally, it is also a polypeptide; its action is to activate FSH secretion from anterior pituitary (see page 855).

3. Relaxin is a polypeptide hormone produced by corpus luteum and other sites include: uterus, placenta and mammary glands and in males from the prostate gland.

Its main role is during pregnancy as mentioned:

- It relaxes pubic symphysis and pelvic joints, softens and dilates the uterine cervix and facilitates delivery.

In non-pregnant state it releases from the corpus luteum and endometrium during secretory phase its function is not known.

In males relaxin is present in the semen and helps in sperm motility and penetration of ovum by the sperm.

4. Ovarian Androgens. A small amount of testosterone is also secreted by the ovaries during biosynthesis of oestrogen and progesterone, but the main source of androgens in female is adrenal cortex.

These androgens are responsible for acne vulgaris, libido, and pubic hair.

FEMALE SEXUAL CYCLE

The sexual life span of a female can be divided into three periods:

1. Birth to Puberty. During this period primary and accessory female sex organs remain quiescent. Puberty occurs between 12 and 14 years of age.

2. Puberty to Menopause. With the onset of puberty, the female sexual cycle starts, which repeats every 28 days. The occurrence of first menstrual cycle is called *menarche.* The permanent stoppage of menstrual cycle is called *menopause,* which occurs at the age of about 45 to 50 years. The period between menarche and menopause is called *reproductive period.* During this period females have rhythmical sexual cycles.

3. Postmenopausal Period extends after menopause (45 to 50 years) to rest of the life. During this period the female sexual cycle ceases.

Female sexual cycle refers to monthly rhythmic sexual cycle occurring in females during the normal reproductive period.

Components of human female sexual cycle. During each female sexual cycle, rhythmical changes occur in ovaries and accessory sex organs—uterus, cervix and vagina. The components of female sexual cycle are:

- Ovarian cycle,
- Endometrial cycle,
- Changes in cervix uteri,
- Changes in vagina,
- Other changes during sexual cycle and
- Changes in gonadotropin secretion, i.e. hormonal control of female sexual cycle.

Duration of the female sexual cycle is usually 28 days. But under physiological conditions it may vary between 20 and 40 days. Traditionally first day of the menstrual bleeding is taken as the 1st day to each component of female sexual cycle.

Ovarian Cycle

Ovarian cycle refers to rhythmic changes occurring in ovaries during each female sexual cycle of about 28 days (range 20–40 days). During each cycle, a single mature ovum is released from the ovary. Ovarian changes occurring during the female sexual life completely depend on the gonadotropic hormones (FSH and LH) which are secreted by the anterior pituitary. Both FSH and LH stimulate ovarian target cells by combining with highly specific FSH and LH receptors present on their membranes. FSH and LH activate cyclic adenosine monophosphate (cAMP)—second messenger system in the cell cytoplasm. However, some effects of hormones cannot be attributed entirely to cAMP system. The ovarian cycle can be divided into three phases:

- Preovulatory phase or follicular phase,
- Ovulation and
- Postovulatory phase or luteal phase.

Preovulatory Phase

Preovulatory or follicular phase of the ovarian cycle extends from the fifth day of the cycle till the time of ovulation (which takes place at about 14th day of the cycle). Thus, this phase generally lasts for 8–9 days (but may vary from 10 to 25 days).

- Changes in the ovary during preovulatory phase or follicular phase are mostly under the influence of FSH from the anterior pituitary. LH also helps in maturation of the follicle in the latter part of follicular phase (for details see hormonal control of female sexual cycle; page 854).
- During this phase of each cycle (of about 28 days), some 10–15 primordial follicles start maturing, but only one

follicle matures fully and the rest undergo atresia (atrophy) at different stages of development. The process of maturation of follicle is called folliculogenesis. Phases of folliculogenesis are:

Phases of Folliculogenesis

The follicles at different stages of maturation are (Fig. 9.3-9):

1. Primordial Follicles are the fundamental reproductive units of ovary. At the time of puberty both ovaries contain about 3, 00,000 primordial follicles.

- Primordial follicles are formed in foetal life. Each primordial follicle consists of the primary oocyte in prophase of the first meiotic division surrounded by a single layer of spindle-shaped (flat) cells called the granulosa cells.
- Both the granulosa cells and the primary oocyte are enveloped in a thin membrane called basal lamina (Fig. 9.3-9A).
- The primordial follicles lack a direct blood supply.
- The granulosa cells of the primordial follicle are believed to provide nutrition to the ovum (primary oocyte) throughout the childhood (from birth to puberty). These cells also secrete *oocyte maturation inhibiting factor* (OMIF) which keeps the ovum in immature stage till puberty. At the onset of puberty, under the influence of FSH and LH, the primordial follicles start growing and convert into primary follicles.

2. Primary Follicle. The primary follicle is formed when the primordial follicle undergoes following developmental changes (Fig. 9.3-9B):

- *Granulosa cells*, which are flat (spindle-shaped) in primordial follicle become columnar and undergo mitotic division to form a multilayered stratum granulosum.
- *Oocyte enlarges* and becomes about 20 μ in size.
- *Zona pellucida*, a homogeneous membrane appears consisting of glycoprotein between the granulosa (follicular) cells and the oocyte. With the appearance of zonapellucida, the follicle is now referred to as a multilaminar primary follicle.

3. Secondary Follicle is formed from the primary follicle when following changes occur (Fig. 9.3-9C):

- *Granulosa cells* undergo further proliferation.
- *Oocyte* further increases in size upto 100 μ. Its nucleus becomes larger and vesicular, forming germinal spots.
- *Theca folliculi* or follicular sheath is formed outside the basal lamina from the spindle-shaped cells from the stroma of cortex in ovary. The theca folliculi consist of an inner rim of secretory cells called *theca interna* and an outer rim of thickly packed fibres and spindle-shaped cells called *theca externa* (that merges with the surrounding stroma).

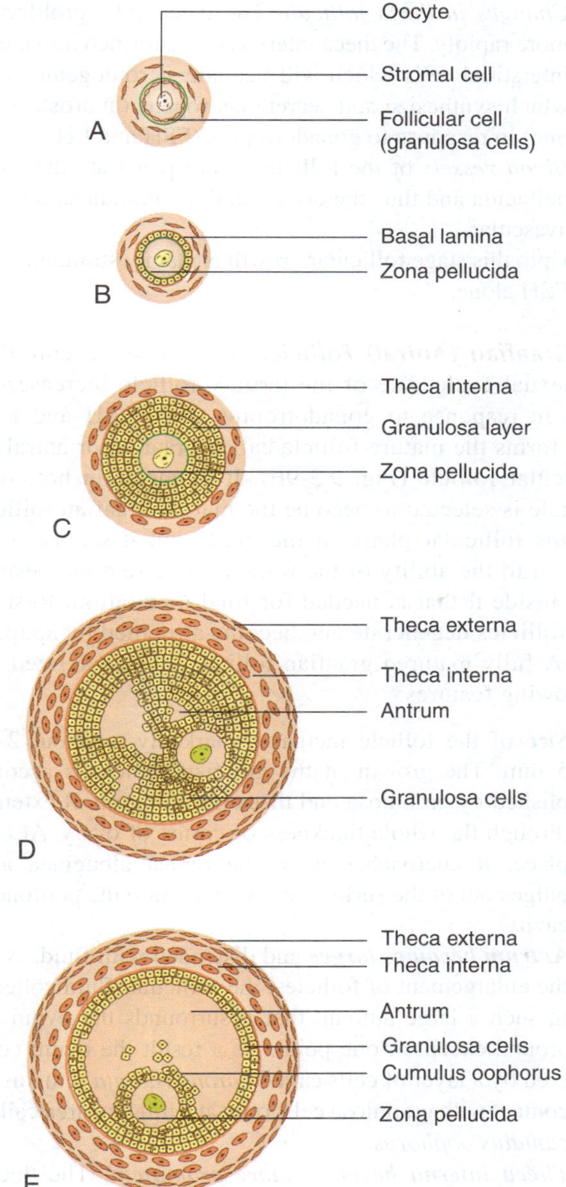

FIGURE 9.3-9 Phases of folliculogenesis.

- *Independent blood supply* consisting of arterioles that do not penetrate the basal lamina is acquired by the secondary follicles.

4. Tertiary Follicle is characterized by following features:

- *Formation of antrum.* After proliferation, the granulosa cells start secreting follicular fluid, this causes cavity to be formed in the stratum granulosum (cavitation), which is called antrum or follicular cavity. The fluid filled in the antrum is called liquor folliculi which also contains oestrogen. The granulosa cells continue to proliferate and the size of follicle is increased (Fig. 9.3-9D).

- *Changes in theca folliculi.* The theca cells proliferate more rapidly. The theca interna is transformed into theca interstitial cells which will become steroidogenic cells which synthesize and secrete androgens (androstenedione) in response to gonadotropins (FSH and LH).
- *Blood vessels* of the follicle do not penetrate the zona pellucida and thus the oocyte and the granulosa remain avascular.
- Upto this stage follicular growth is mainly stimulated by FSH alone.

5. Graafian (Antral) Follicle. After about seventh day of sexual cycle, one of the tertiary follicle increases in size in response to gonadotropins (both FSH and LH) and forms the mature follicle called graafian or antral or vesicular follicle (Fig. 9.3-9E). It is uncertain how one follicle is selected to become the mature graafian follicle in this follicular phase of the cycle, but it seems to be related to the ability of the follicle to secrete the oestrogen inside it that is needed for final maturation. Rest of the follicles degenerate and become atrophied by apoptosis. A fully matured graafian follicle is characterized by following features:

- ***Size*** of the follicle increases markedly to about 2 to 5 mm. The growth of the graafian follicle is accomplished by granulosa and theca proliferation. It extends through the whole thickness of cortex of ovary. At one place, it encroaches upon the tunica albuginea and bulges out of the surface of the ovary into the peritoneal cavity.
- ***Antrum becomes larger*** and distended with fluid. With the enlargement of follicles, the follicular fluid collects in such a large amount that it surrounds the ovum all around except at one point. As a result the ovum covered by a layer of cells called *corona radiata* remains in contact with granulosa cells only at a hill like area called *cumulus oophorus.*
- ***Theca interna becomes more prominent.*** The thickness of theca interna becomes double with rich network of capillaries. The oestrogen secreting cells of theca interna increase and are called the cells of theca glands.
- ***Formation of secondary oocyte.*** Just prior to ovulation, the primary oocyte of the fully matured graafian follicle completes the first meiotic division (which began in foetal life at about 20th, 28th week of gestation, i.e. before birth), and forms the secondary oocyte with a haploid nucleus and the first polar body.

Ovulation

Ovulation refers to release of secondary oocyte from the ovary (following rupture of graafian follicle) into the peritoneal cavity. It usually occurs *14 days after the onset* of menstruation, i.e. *early on day 15* in a normal 28-day cycle (Fig. 9.3-8B).

Process of ovulation involves following sequence of events:

- ***LH surge and ovulatory peak of FSH.*** The ovulation is caused by an LH surge at mid-cycle in response to an elevation in plasma oestradiol concentration (150 picograms per ml).
- ***Onset of LH surge*** (a relatively precise indicator of ovulation) occurs 34 to 36 hours before ovulation.
- ***Peak of the LH surge*** occurs 12 to 24 hours before ovulation (secretion of LH increases 6–10 fold).
- ***Immediately before the LH peak,*** oestradiol levels in the plasma fall.
- ***Ovulatory peak of FSH*** (2–3 fold increase in secretion) occurring 2 days prior to ovulation is thought to be stimulated by progesterone. FSH increases the granulosa cell LH receptors.

Changes in graafian follicle. The LH and FSH produce following changes in graafian follicle before ovulation:

- ***Rapid swelling of the follicle*** is caused by FSH and LH a few days before ovulation. There occurs a rapid growth of new blood vessels into the follicle wall and prostaglandins are secreted into the follicular tissue. Both these cause diffusion of plasma into the follicular fluid and further swelling of the follicle.
- ***Formation of stigma.*** Due to rapid swelling of the follicle, its outer wall is stretched forming a very thin avascular area (stigma) over the most convex point of the follicle which protrudes like a nipple in the peritoneal cavity.
- ***Release of proteolytic*** enzymes from the lysosomes in the theca externa cells is activated by the progesterone.
- ***Dissolution of capsular*** wall and its further weakening is caused by the proteolytic enzymes.
- ***Rupture of graafian follicle.*** The simultaneous stretching and enzymatic dissolution of the follicular wall leads to degeneration of *the stigma.* Within 30 minutes of protrusion, fluid begins to ooze from the stigma followed soon by rupture of follicle with release of ovum (secondary oocyte) surrounded by corona radiata into the peritoneal cavity near the fimbriated end of fallopian tube. Thus, usually only one ovum is released from any one of two ovaries during each sexual cycle. The released ovum enters the fallopian tube through its fimbriated end.

Determination of Ovulation Time Ovulation usually occurs 14 days after the onset of menstruation, i.e. early on day 15 in a normal 28-day cycle. The ovulation time can be determined by following indirect methods:

1. From Basal Body Temperature. The basal body temperature falls slightly (0.3 to 0.5°C) just prior to ovulation and increases slightly after ovulation. Therefore, the time of ovulation can be determined by measuring the morning temperature from rectum or vagina for few days during mid-period of menstrual cycle (Fig. 9.3-8C).

2. From Hormonal Excretion in Urine. The urinary excretion of end products of oestrogen like oestrone, oestradiol and 17 β-oestradiol increases to the peak at the time of ovulation and that of end products of progesterone-like pregnanediol increases after ovulation. Therefore, time of ovulation can be determined by estimating their urinary levels for few days during mid period of menstrual cycle.

3. From Hormonal Levels in Plasma. The plasma content of FSH, LH, oestrogen and progesterone is measured during mid period of menstrual cycle and time of ovulation is determined from following observations:

- LH and oestrogen levels are increased and FSH level is decreased at the time of ovulation.
- Progesterone level is increased after ovulation.

4. By Ultrasound Scanning. the process of ovulation can be recorded.

Anovulatory Cycles

The ovarian cycles during which ovulation does not occur are called unovulatory cycles. If LH surge occurring prior to ovulation is not of sufficient magnitude, ovulation does not occur. First few cycles after puberty may be unovulatory.

Postovulatory Phase

The postovulatory phase also called luteal phase of ovarian cycle is of remarkably constant period of about 14 days. Therefore, retrospectively the time of ovulation can be estimated by subtracting 14 days from the total duration of the menstrual cycle. This phase is characterized by following events (Fig. 9.3-5):

Formation of Corpus Haemorrhagicum. Following ovulation, the outer wall of the graafian follicle collapses and promptly fills with blood forming the so-called corpus haemorrhagicum. Minor bleeding from the follicle into the abdominal cavity may cause peritoneal irritation and fleeting lower abdominal pain (mittelschmerz).

Formation of Corpus Luteum. Soon, the granulosa cells and theca cells of the follicle lining begin to proliferate, and the clotted blood is rapidly replaced with yellowish lipid-rich *luteal cells*. This process is called *luteinization* and the total mass of the cells is now called *corpus luteum*. LH is responsible for luteinization. The lutein cells secrete large amount of progesterone and also oestrogen to a lesser extent. Seven days after ovulation, i.e. by the 22nd day of menstrual cycle the corpus luteum attains adiameter of about 1.5 cm. Growth of corpus luteum depends on its developing blood supply and vascular endothelial growth factor (VEGF) the key component responsible for vasculogenesis. The progesterone secreted by these have a strong negative feedback effect on the anterior pituitary gland to decrease secretion of both LH and FSH. The fate of corpus luteum depends on whether or not pregnancy occurs.

Formation of Corpus Albicans. If there is no fertilization and pregnancy does not occur, the corpus luteum begins to involute (regress) after the 24th day of the sexual cycle and is eventually replaced by a whitish scar tissue, called the corpus albicans. This involution occurs due to falling levels of FSH and LH and also the hormone *inhibin* secreted by the lutein cells. With the involution of corpus luteum, on the 26th day of the normal female sexual cycle, levels of oestrogen, progesterone and inhibin fall. This removes the feedback inhibition of the anterior pituitary consequently the FSH and within a few days LH secretion begins and the next ovarian cycle is initiated.

Corpus Luteum of Pregnancy. However, if the ovum released is fertilized and pregnancy occurs, then the corpus luteum formed during postovulatory phase persists and serves as the major source of oestrogen and progesterone till the 3rd month of pregnancy when the placenta takes over its endocrine function.

Endometrial Cycle (Uterine Cycle)

The endometrial cycle refers to the cyclic changes occurring in the endometrium during active reproductive period (menarche to menopause) in females leading to recurrent monthly bleeding per vaginum (menstruation). These cyclic changes in the endometrium are brought about by the cyclic production of oestrogens and progesterone by the ovaries. Strictly speaking the menstrual cycle is synonymous with the female sexual cycle and includes cyclic changes in all the female reproductive organs. However, in day-to-day practice, the term menstrual cycle is used for cyclic changes in the endometrium. Menstrual is a Latin word meaning mensis, i.e. lunar month of 28 days. Though the menstrual cycle for description purposes is considered to be of 28 days, but the cycle is by no means as regular as the name suggests. The menstrual cycles of 25 to 35 days are also regarded as normal cycles.

Phases of Endometrial Cycle

Conventionally, first day of the bleeding is considered to be the first day of the endometrial cycle. The endometrial cycle of 28 days can be divided into three phases (Fig. 9.3-8E):

- Menstrual phase (1st to 5th day),
- Proliferative phase (6th to 14th day) and
- Secretory phase (15th to 28th day)

For the purpose of better understanding the menstrual phase is described last of all.

Proliferative Phase Extent of proliferative phase, also known as preovulatory phase of endometrial cycle is from day 6th to

14th day. It follows the phase of menstruation, after which only a thin basal layer of original endometrium is left.

Hormone responsible for changes in the endometrium during this phase is oestrogen secreted by the developing graafian follicle in the ovary. Thus, proliferative phase of endometrial cycle coincides with the follicular phase of ovarian cycle.

Changes in endometrium, which occur under the influence of oestrogens during proliferative phase are:

1. Epithelial cells are stimulated to grow and reepithelialise the endometrial surface.
2. Thickness of endometrium, which is less than 1 mm at the end of menstrual phase increases to 3–4 mm at the end of the proliferative phase.
3. Mitosis of the stratum basale regenerates the stroma of stratum functionale.
4. Angiogenesis in the stratum functionale leads to proliferation of blood vessels which become the spiral arterioles that profuse the stratum functionale.
5. Endometrial glands are stimulated to grow. The glands contain glycogen but they are nonsecretory.
6. Ovulation occurs at the end of this phase.

Secretory Phase

Extent of secretory phase (also known as postovulatory phase of endometrial cycle) is from day 15th to 28th day.

Hormones Responsible for changes in the endometrium during this phase are both oestrogens and progesterone secreted by the *corpus luteum* formed after ovulation. Thus, the secretory phase of endometrial cycle coincides with the luteal phase of ovarian cycle.

Changes in the Endometrium, which occur under the influence of oestrogen and progesterone during this phase, are:

- *Additional proliferation of cellular stroma* is caused by oestrogens.
- *Differentiation of the endometrium* is promoted by progesterone causing elongation and coiling of endometrial mucous glands. These glands become secretory and secrete thick viscous fluid containing glycogen.
- *Blood supply* of endometrium further increases as progesterone promotes spiralling of blood vessels.
- *Two characteristic features of endometrium* in secretory phase thus are prominent corkscrew-shaped glands and increased vascularity.
- *Thickness* of endometrium increases to 5–6 mm at the end of secretory phase. Thus, the thickened endometrium with large amounts of nutrients is ready to provide appropriate conditions for implantation of ovum during this phase.
- *If fertilization does not occur* and there is no pregnancy, the corpus luteum in the ovary involutes to form corpus albicans and on day 26th of the menstrual cycle the levels of oestrogen and progesterone fall suddenly and mark the end of secretory phase of endometrial cycle.

Menstrual Phase The menstrual phase of the endometrial cycle is also called the bleeding phase. The average duration of this phase is 3–5 days, but it may be as short as 1 day and as long as 8 days in a normal woman.

Cause of Bleeding and Sequence of Events. About 24 hours before the end of the menstrual cycle, there is a sharp decline in the plasma levels of oestrogen and progesterone, which is responsible for menstrual bleeding. The sequence of events is:

- *Intense spasm of spiral arteries* occurs leading to hypoxia and ischaemia. This effect is mediated via local production of *leukotrienes* and *prostaglandins*.
- *Necrosis of stratum functionale of the endometrium* and of the walls of the sprial arteries occurs as a result of ischaemia.
- *Blood vessels get open up* due to necrosis of their wall resulting in seepage of blood into the surrounding endometrial necrotic tissue.
- *Separation of necrotic tissue* starts gradually from the underlying basal viable tissue and ultimately it is sloughed off. The necrosis and sloughing does not occur simultaneously in whole of the uterus rather it occurs in patches and is completed in 3–5 days.
- *Endometrial debris* contains necrosed sloughed off tissue, blood, serous fluid and large amount of prostaglandins and fibrolysins.
- *Average amount of bloodloss during each* menstrual cycle is 30 ml. Normally, it may vary from slight spotting to about 80 ml and is affected by factors like endometrial thickness and the conditions which affect clotting mechanism. The menstrual blood is predominantly arterial, with only 25% being venous origin.
- *Menstrual blood immediately gets clotted inside the uterine cavity but soon gets liquefied* by fibrolysins present in endometrial debris. This is the reason that menstrual blood does not normally contain blood clots unless the flow is excessive.
- *The prostaglandins* of the endometrial debris cause further spasm of spiral arteries and also produces contractions of myometrium.
- During the menstrual phase about two-third of the superficial endometrium is sloughed off and only a thin basal layer (2mm thick) is left behind.

Cyclic Changes in Cervix

Uterine cervix (cervix uteri) is continuous with the body of the uterus. The mucosal lining of cervix (endocervix) also shows certain cyclic changes during the sexual cycle. These are:

During Menstruation Phase, the mucosa of cervix does not undergo desquamation (shedding off) like that of endometrium.

During Proliferative Phase (oestrogen phase) the secretions of the mucosal cells of endocervix become thin watery and alkaline. At the time of ovulation (14th day of sexual cycle) the cervical mucus is thinnest and its elasticity is maximum. It can be stretched like a long, thin elastic thread upto 8–12 cm (spinnbarkeit effect). The mucus also produces a characteristic fern-like pattern when a drop of mucus is spread on the glass slide and allowed to dry (*Fern test)* (Fig. 9.3-10B).

This characteristic nature of cervical mucus favours the transport of sperms in the female genital tract and makes the conditions favourable for fertilization.

During Secretory Phase under the influence of progesterone, cervical secretions decrease in quantity and become thick, tenacious and cellular, and fern pattern is not seen (Fig. 9.3-10C). These changes make a plug and prevent the entry of sperm through cervical canal.

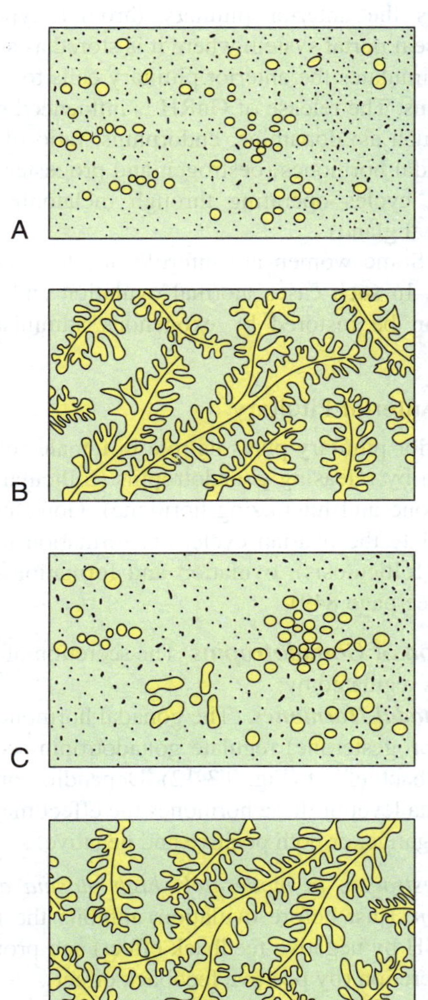

FIGURE 9.3-10 Characteristics of cervical mucus as seen on smear examination during various phases of normal menstrual cycle : **(A)** on 7th day (no fern pattern); **(B)** on 14th day (typical fern pattern); **(C)** on 21st day (fern pattern disappear); and **(D)** 21st day of an unovulatory cycle (fern pattern persists).

Note. *Fern test.* The fern pattern of cervical mucus in proliferative phase and its disappearance in secretory phase is indicative of ovulatory cycle, whereas persistence of fern pattern (Fig. 9.3-10D) throughout the cycle indicates unovulatory cycle.

Cyclic Changes in Vagina

Vaginal canal is lined by stratified squamous epithelium which is highly sensitive to oestrogens (oestradiol). Vaginal epithelium undergoes following cyclic changes in endometrial cycle:

In the Proliferative Phase, vaginal epithelium becomes thickened (by adding up more and more layers of epithelium) and cornified. The cornified cells and maturing cells accumulate glycogen. Vaginal smear at this time shows many large eosinophilic cornified cells having small pyknotic nucleus or it may be absent (Fig. 9.3-11A).

In the Secretory Phase under the influence of progesterone, vaginal epithelium proliferates and gets infiltrated with leucocytes (Fig. 9.3-11B) and the vaginal secretions become thick and viscid.

Other Changes during Sexual Cycle

Hormonal oscillations during sexual cycle though mainly effect ovaries, uterus, cervix and vagina but some changes have also been observed in the fallopian tubes, breast and in the body weight.

1. Changes in Fallopian Tubes are as follows:

i. *During follicular phase,* under the influence of oestrogen there occurs:
- Increase in the number of cilia of epithelial cells and their rate of beating,
- Increase in the number of secretory epithelial cells and
- An increase in the vascularization of fimbria.

ii. *At the time of ovulation,* the motility of fallopian tubes increases.

iii. *During the luteal phase,* under the influence of progesterone, there occurs an increase in the secretion of epithelial cells. This provides nutrition to the ovum, incoming sperm and the zygote if fertilization occurs.

2. Changes in Breast. Some women complain of feeling of fullness and tenderness in the breasts. These symptoms have been related to the proliferation of lobules and duct system under the influence of oestrogen and progesterone. All these symptoms regress during the menstrual phase.

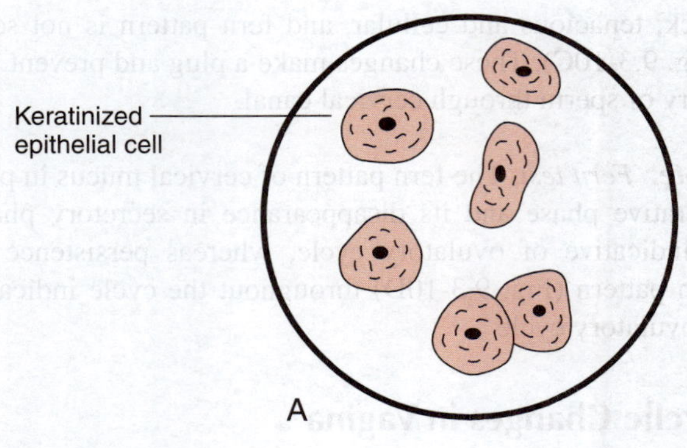

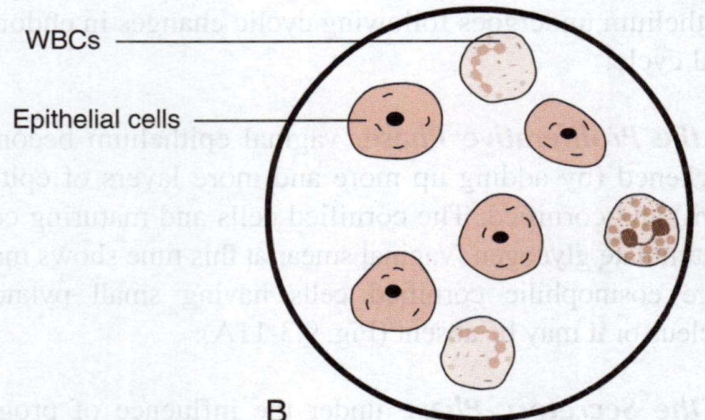

FIGURE 9.3-11 Characteristic features of vaginal epithelium seen on vaginal smear examination during : **(A)** proliferative phase and **(B)** secretory phase of menstrual cycle.

3. Premenstrual Weight Gain. Many women experience feeling of heaviness (premenstrual tension) near the end of cycle. This effect is due to salt and water retention caused by the oestrogen. The feeling of heaviness disappears during the menstruation phase.

Oestrous Cycle

Except primates in all other mammals the sexual cycle is called *oestrous cycle.* It has derived its name from the word oestrous meaning 'heat'. This is the only period when sexual interest is aroused in the female animals. It happens at the time of ovulation and coincides with the male's sexual desire. In oestrous cycle, the underlying endocrinal changes are similar to that of menstrual cycle in primates but bleeding per vaginum does not occur and the duration of cycle also varies from species to species. For example:

- In rat and mouse : 4–6 days,
- In sheep and guinea pig : 14 days,
- In cow : 20 days, and
- In bitches : twice in a year

Two different patterns of oestrous cycles are known in different species:

- *Spontaneous ovulation* occurs in some species such as the dog, rat, guinea pig, cow etc. and
- *Reflex ovulation* is known to occur in some species such as rabbit, ferret and cats in these species ovulation is brought about by *neuroendocrinal reflex* which is aroused by copulation.

Hormonal Control of Female Sexual Cycle

The hypothalamo-hypophyseal-gonadal axis regulates the cyclic changes occurring during female sexual cycle. The role of each component of the axis is (Fig. 9.3-12):

Role of Hypothalamus

Hypothalamus regulates the secretions of gonadotropins (both FSH and LH) through the gonadotropin releasing hormone (GnRH). The GnRH also known as luteinizing hormone releasing hormone (LHRH), is predominantly secreted from the cells of arcuate nucleus and preoptic area. It reaches the anterior pituitary through hypothalamo-hypophyseal portal system where it is stored as small granules. It stimulates the anterior pituitary cells to release gonadotropins. The release of GnRH is influenced by various factors, such as: dopamine, endorphins, ratio of FSH and LH, gonadal hormones (oestrogen and progesterone), dark and light cycles operating through melatonin (released from pineal gland).

Note. Some women are infertile due to hypothalamic disorders. In such cases, normal ovulation and menstrual cycles can be restored by exogenous administration of GnRH.

Role of Anterior Pituitary

The anterior pituitary plays its role in female sexual cycle regulation by releasing gonadotropins (follicular stimulating hormone and luteinizing hormone). Gonadotropins in turn regulate the ovarian cycle, i.e. formation of graafian follicles (folliculosis), ovulation and formation of corpus luteum (see page 849).

Regulation of Gonadotropins The secretion of both FSH and LH is regulated by:

1. Gonadal Hormones. The gonadal hormones (oestrogen and progesterone) regulate gonadotropin secretion by their feedback effect (Fig. 9.3-12). Depending on the relative plasma level of these hormones the effect may be positive or negative, or both positive and negative.

- *Oestrogen, in moderately high plasma concentration,* (just before ovulation) inhibits the release of FSH by negative feedback effect) and promotes LH secretion (by positive feedback effect).
- *High levels of oestrogen and progesterone* in the mid-luteal phase inhibit the secretion of FSH and LH (by negative feedback effect).
- *Low levels of gonadal hormones* (during menstruation phase) increase the secretion of both FSH and LH (by positive feedback effect).

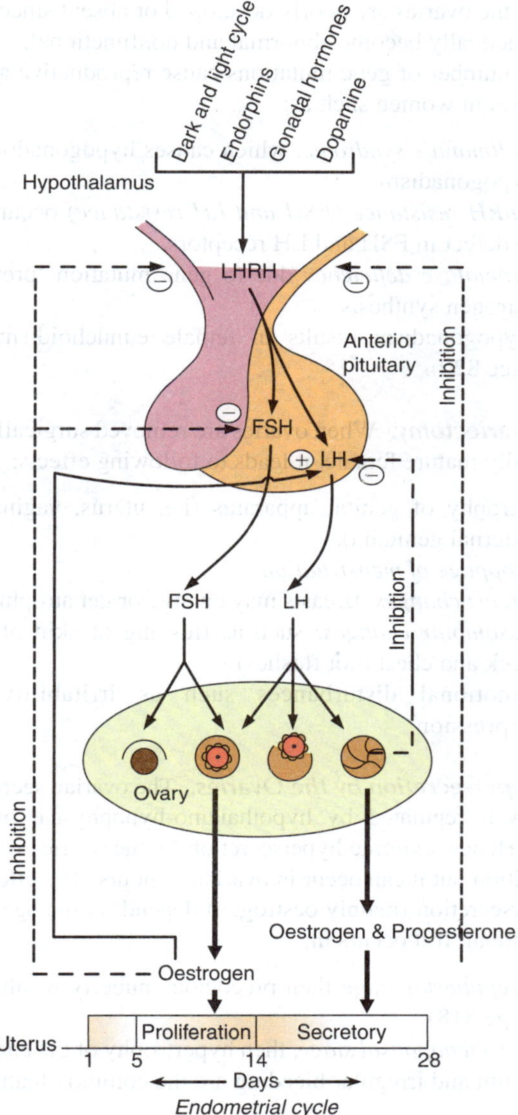

FIGURE 9.3-12 Hypothalamo-hypophysial ovarian axis regulating the female sexual cycle through positive and negative feed-back mechanisms.

The feedback effect (positive or negative) of ovarian hormones is brought about by its action either directly on anterior pituitary or through the hypothalamus (Fig. 9.3-12).

Oral contraceptives are the preparations containing high concentration of oestrogen and progesterone. These drugs inhibit gonadotropin release by negative feedback effect and prevent ovulation.

2. Human Chorionic Gonadotropin (HCG) is a glycoprotein secreted by syncytiotrophoblasts during early pregnancy (12–16 weeks of gestation). Like luteinizing hormone, HCG also maintains the functional state of corpus luteum and thus elevates gonadal hormones resulting in inhibition of gonadotropin release.

3. Prolactin. It is a mammotropic hormone secreted from anterior pituitary during lactation. It inhibits GnRh release and thus lowers the basal secretion of FSH and LH (cause for lactation amenorrhoea).

4. Activin. It is structurally quite similar to inhibin (secreted from ovary). It is synthesized in the cells of anterior pituitary. It stimulates the synthesis and release of FSH by autocrine and paracrine actions.

Role of Ovaries Ovaries play an important role in the regulation of ovarian cycle and endometrial cycle by secreting gonadal hormones (oestrogen and progesterone) (Fig. 9.3-8).

Oestrogen In each sexual cycle, the plasma concentration of oestrogen starts rising from the first day of the cycle and reaches to its peak just before ovulation (at 12th–13th day), called *oestrogen surge.*

- Then within 24 hours burst of LH secretion (LH surge) takes place at mid-cycle and leading to sudden rise in plasma concentration of LH (Fig. 9.3-8A). Thus, oestrogen surge has a positive feedback effect.
- Oestrogen increases the sensitivity and responsiveness of gonadotrophs to GnRH.
- The LH surge is followed (after about 9 hours) by ovulation. Therefore, oestrogen through its positive feedback effect is responsible for *ovulation* due to LH surge.
- Oestrogen is responsible for the proliferative phase of endometrial cycle.

Progesterone

- After ovulation there occurs formation of corpus luteum and the progesterone concentration starts rising. Therefore, in the luteal phase of the ovarian cycle, level of both oestrogen and progesterone are high, but progesterone rises markedly.
- The high levels of gonadal hormones inhibit gonadotropin release by negative feedback effect. Therefore, the levels of FSH and LH are low.
- Progesterone prepares the oestrogen primed endrometrium for implantation. Thus, it is responsible for the secretory phase of endometrial cycle.
- *If fertilization does not occur,* the corpus luteum involutes and levels of oestrogen and progesterone decline.
- Withdrawal of hormones support results in menstruation and at the same time negative feedback effect on anterior pituitary and hypothalamus is also abolished leading to further
- Increase in gonadotropin and next ovarian and endometrial cycle start.

If Fertilization Occurs, then the HCG level rises, which maintain corpus luteum. Therefore, the levels of oestrogen, progesterone remain high and by negative feedback effect gonadotropin levels (FSH and LH) remain low.

Menopause

With advancing age, the human ovaries become unresponsive to gonadotropins and secretion of ovarian hormone declines; resulting in permanent stoppage of menstrual cycle is called menopause. The usual age of menopause is 45–55 years (average 50 years).

- The unresponsiveness of ovary to gonadotropin occurs due to decrease in the number of primordial follicles. Therefore, the ovaries no longer secrete progesterone, and the estrogen level also declines.
- Due to the gonadal hormones negative feedback mechanism, there is a high plasma level of FSH & LH.
- During premenopausal period FSH level increases before a rise in LH, therefore irregular menstrual cycle occurs due to decrease in estrogen, progesterone and inhibin.
- The loss of ovarian functions lead to following symptoms:
  - Hot flushes : The sensation of warmth spreading from trunk region to the face and night sweats. Hot flushes occur in 75% menopausal women. The exact cause of hot flushes is not known, but associated with surge of LH secretion. In menopausal women due to absence of gonadal hormone the peaks of episodic burst of LH secretion increase.
  - It is observed that removal of anterior pituitary, the hot flushes continue that indicated that LH itself is not responsible for hot flushes instead it appears that some estrogen sensitive event in the hypothalamus may initiate both release of LH and episode of flushing.
  - With onset of menopause, risk of disease such as; osteoporosis, Ishemic heart disease and renal disease also increases.

Treatment *Hormonal replacement therapy (HRT)* In postmenopausal women HRT is given to relieve the symptom and to prevent osteoporosis, but is associated with side effects. The typical regimen of HRT is estrogen 1–21 days and progesterone is added from day 14–21 as oral contraceptives. The side effects of HRT include:

- Fluid retention, weight gain, hypertension and thrombosis are matter of concern.
- Transdermal HRT may be more appropriate alternative.
- The time of discontinuation of HRT & duration of therapy is still a matter of debate.

Abnormalities of Female Sexual Cycle

The abnormalities of female sexual cycle are grouped as:

- Abnormalities of ovarian functions, and
- Abnormalities of menstruation.

A. Abnormalities of Ovarian Functions

1. Hypogonadism (hyposecretion of ovarian hormones) means less than normal secretions by the ovaries. It occurs when the ovaries are poorly developed or absent since birth or genetically become abnormal and nonfunctional.

A number of gene mutations cause reproductive abnormalities in women such as:

- *Kallmann's syndrome*. which causes hypogonadotropic hypogonadism.
- *GnRH resistance (FSH and LH resistance)* occurs due to defect in FSH and LH receptors.
- *Aromatase deficiency* due to gene mutation 'prevents' estrogen synthesis
  Hypogonadism results in female eunuchoidism (see page 820).

2. Ovariectomy. When ovaries are removed surgically in a sexually mature female, it leads to following effects:

- Atrophy of genital apparatus (i.e. uterus, vagina and external genitalia),
- *Stoppage of menstruation.*
- *Breast changes.* Breasts may enlarge or get atrophied.
- *Vasomotor changes;* such as flushing of skin of face, neck and chest (hot flushes)
- Emotional disturbances such as irritability and depression.

3. Hypersecretion by the Ovaries. The ovarian secretions are well regulated by hypothalamo-hypophyseal ovarian axis. Hence, extreme hypersecretion by the ovaries is a rare condition but it can occur in ovarian tumours. The effects of hypersecretion (mainly oestrogen) depend on the age of an individual. If it occurs in:

- *Prepubertal stage* then precocious puberty results (see page 818).
- *Postmenopausal stage,* then hypertrophy of the endometrium and irregular bleeding are the common features.

4. McCune – Albert syndrome is a genetic defect in which somatic mutation occurs after initial cell division in the embryo that leads to activation of certain cells, but not others. This condition is associated with multiple endocrinal abnormalities including precocious puberty, amenorrhea and galactorrhea.

B. Abnormalities of Menstruation

1. Anovulatory Cycle' means menstrual cycles occur at normal intervals, but ovulation does not occur. Anovulatory cycles are the normal entity upto 1–2 years after the menarche and few years before menopause. An anovulatory cycle in the fertile period of womanhood is the main cause of female infertility.

2. Amenorrhoea. The term amenorrhoea refers to absence of menstrual bleeding or periods. It is of two types:

- *Primary amenorrhoea* means menstrual bleeding has never occurred and this condition is because of failure of sexual maturation.

- *Secondary amenorrhoea* means cessation of menstrual cycles in a woman who previously has normal and regular cycles. Pregnancy is the most common cause of secondary amenorrhoea. Other conditions which result in secondary amenorrhoea are: emotional disturbances, environmental changes, hypothalamic and pituitary disorders and certain systemic diseases.

3. Hypomenorrhoea. The term refers to scanty menstruation.

4. Menorrhoea. It refers to abnormally profuse bleeding during normal regular cycles.

5. Metrorrhagia. This condition refers to occurrence of uterine bleeding in between the periods.

6. Oligomenorrhoea means infrequent and reduced frequency of menstruation.

7. Dysmenorrhoea is the term related to discomfort menstruation (or painful menstruation). Dysmenorrhoea is very common in young women and it disappears after first pregnancy.

8. Premenstrual Syndrome (PMS). About 7–10 days before the end of cycle some women experience symptoms like irritability, lack of concentration, feeling of depression, heaviness, headache and constipation which is called PMS (see page 845)

Chapter 9.4

Physiology of Coitus, Pregnancy and Parturition

PHYSIOLOGY OF COITUS
- Male Sexual Act
  - Erection of Penis
  - Emission of Seminal Fluid
  - Ejaculation
- Female Sexual Act

PHYSIOLOGY OF PREGNANCY
- Fertilization and Implantation
  - Fertilization
  - Transportation of Ovum
  - Transportation of Sperm in Female Genital Tract
  - Sperm Capacitation
  - Fusion of Gametes
  - Activation of Ovum
  - Implantation
- Placenta and Pregnancy Tests
  - Placenta
  - Formation
  - Placental Membrane
  - Functions
  - Pregnancy Tests
  - Biological Tests
  - Immunological Test
- Physiological Changes in Mother During Pregnancy
  - Genital Organ Changes
  - Breast Changes
  - Weight Gain
  - Haematological Changes
  - Cardiovascular System Changes
  - Respiratory System Changes
  - Urinary System Changes
  - Gastrointestinal System Changes
  - Metabolic Changes
  - Endocrine System Changes
  - Skin Changes
  - Psychological Changes

PHYSIOLOGY OF PARTURITION
- Functional Anatomy
  - Uterus
  - Cervix
- Mechanics of Parturition
  - Uterine Contractility
  - Dilatation of Cervix
- Phases of Parturition
  - Phase 1
  - Phase 2
  - Phase 3
- Control of Parturition
  - Hormonal Factors
  - Mechanical Factors
- Applied Aspects
  - Miscarriage
  - Pre Term Labour
  - Preeclampsia

PHYSIOLOGY OF COITUS

Coitus refers to the process of sexual intercourse by which sperms are deposited into the vagina. Physiologically, coitus involves both male and female sexual act or sexual arousal.

Male Sexual Act or Male Sexual Arousal

The male sexual act is reflexogenic in nature and involves both psychological and physiological components. The male sexual act consists of following three sequence of events:

- Erection of penis,
- Emission of seminal fluid and
- Ejaculation.

I. Erection of Penis or Stage of Excitement In this stage, penis becomes hard, stiff and an elongated structure. Erection of penis is brought about by integrity of the reflex arc, which comprises:

- Sexual stimulation,
- Afferents to the integrating centres,
- Integrating centres,
- Efferents and
- Response.

1. Sexual Stimulation. Sexual stimulation has two components:

- ***Psychological component.*** It is in the form of thought, feeling, watching movie or book picture, etc. The psychological component arises in the cerebral cortex or from limbic system. The impulses from psychic stimulations are carried or descend to the integrating centres located in the spinal cord. The psychic component can *reinforce* or inhibit the integrating centres.

- ***Physical components*** of sexual sensations involve:
  - i. *Sensations from genitalia* (mainly from glans penis). Glans penis contains highly sensitive sensory end organs, which are activated by massaging action of the intercourse.
  - ii. *Sensations from adjacent* areas like scrotum, epithelium of anus and perineal structures.
  - iii. *Sensations from internal structures* like urethra, bladder, prostate, seminal vesicles, testes, vas deferens particularly when these structures are filled with the secretions.

2. Afferents to Integrating Centres. From genitalia and other structures, the afferent impulses are carried by *pudendal nerve* and *sacral plexus* to the sacral part of the spinal cord.

3. Integrating Centres. Integrating centres for reflexogenic erection are located in lumbar segments (L_2 to L_3) and sacral segments (S_2–S_4) of the spinal cord. The lumbar centres are in turn connected to sacral centres.

4. Efferent Pathway for erection is carried through sacral parasympathetic fibres via nervi erigentes to the:

- Smooth muscle fibres of the penile arterioles.
- Erectile tissue (corpora cavernosa and corpora spongiosum of the penis).
- The bulbourethral glands.
- The efferent parasympathetic fibres in pelvic splanchinc nerves (nervi ergentis) release acetylcholine and vasoactive intestinal peptide (VIP) as cotransmitter.
- Nervi erigentes also carry noncholinergic and nonadrenergic fibres, which contain large amount of enzyme *NO synthase* which causes formation of nitric oxide (NO). NO is another potent vasodilator. It activates soluble guanylyl cyclase resulting in increased production of cyclic GMP (cGMP), which is a potent vasodilator.
- Therefore, the substances (neurotransmitters) released are ACh, VIP and nitric oxide.

5. Response. By acting on the effector structures, there occurs:

- Vasodilation of the penile arterioles leading to increased blood flow under pressure resulting in filling of the erectile tissue with blood.
- The blood-filled erectile tissue compresses the central vein of the penis (blocking the venous flow from penis), which further increases the pressure within the sinusoids of erectile tissue, and thus the penis becomes hard rigid structure.
- *Lubrication*: Parasympathetic activity during sexual stimulation causes secretion of mucus from the urethral and bulbourethral glands.

Note. Drugs like sildenafil, tadafil and vardenafil all inhibit breakdown of cGMP, thus used as treatment for erectile dysfunction.

II. Emission of Seminal Fluid In this stage, semen moves into the urethra. Emission is a sympathetic response integrated at upper lumbar spinal segment centres (L_1 and L_2).

- When sexual stimulus becomes very strong then reflexly emission and ejaculation occur. The afferent fibres are mostly from touch receptors present on glans penis (which are stimulated by friction of glans penis and vaginal wall) are carried by internal pudendal nerve to the spinal cord (lumbar segment L_1 - L_2). Efferents are then carried along sympathetic fibres through hypogastric and pelvic sympathetic plexus to initiate emission.
- Emission is carried out by contraction of vas deferens.

III. Ejaculation Ejaculation means deposition of seminal fluid into the vagina of female.

Applied Aspects

Erectile dysfunction (impotance) is the inability of men to get and maintain the erection sufficient for intercourse. It occurs because of vasculogenic, neurogenic, hormonal or psychogenic factors.

Premature ejaculation is a disorder characterized by ejaculation that occurs with minimal sexual stimulation after penetration.

Retrograde ejaculation. In this disorder, semen travels backwards into the urinary bladder rather than out of penile shaft during ejaculation. For neurological dysfunction, the most common cause is damage to penile innervations during prostate surgery.

Female Sexual Act

Female sexual act, similar to male sexual act is reflexogenic and involves psychological and physical components. The three phases of female sexual act are:

- Sexual excitement,
- Orgasm and
- Resolution.

I. Phase of Sexual Excitement The phase of sexual excitement is also called phase of female erection and lubrication. It corresponds to erection of penis in males. This phase is brought about by integrity of the reflex arc which comprises following components:

1. Sexual Stimulation. Sexual stimulation in females like that of males has two components, psychological and physical.

- ***Psychological stimulation.*** The sexual desire in females is aroused by erotic thoughts which originate from the cerebral cortex or limbic system (amygdala). The sexual desire is believed to be increased at the time of ovulation (may be because of high levels of oestrogen). It is also believed that sexual desire in female is produced partly by oestrogen.

- ***Physical component*** of the sexual stimulation consists of sexual sensations aroused from massaging/irritation of external genitalia (vulva, clitoris, labia minora and labia majora) and perineal region. Clitoris is highly sensitive and is responsible for initiation of sexual sensations. Massaging of the breasts and even kissing enforce the sexual sensations.

2. Afferents to the Integrating Centres. The sensory signals are transmitted via pudendal nerve to spinal cord. The impulses are then transmitted to the cerebral cortex and also to the integrating centres for local reflex responses.

3. Integrating Centres. The local reflexes are integrated in sacral segments (S_2, S_3 and S_4) and lumbar segments (L_1 and L_2) of the spinal cord. These integrating centres are also influenced by psychological components.

4. Efferent Pathway. The parasympathetic signals for female erection and lubrication travel by nervi erigentes from sacral plexus to the arteries of external genitalia and Bartholin glands and mucosal epithelial cells of vagina.

5. Response. During sexual intercourse, the erectile tissue (located around introitus and clitoris) is activated by parasympathetic impulses producing:

- Increase in blood flow and accumulation of blood in erectile tissue resulting in increase in the size of external genitalia and vaginal congestion. Congestion of vagina occurs due to transudation of fluid from the vaginal epithelium,
- Vaginal lubrication facilitates the penile insertion. Further vaginal congestion leads to tightening of the vaginal opening around the penis.
- Stimulation also results in copious secretion from Bartholin glands (situated beneath labia minora) and mucous cells in vagina. These secretions further lubricate vagina and help in producing massaging effect on penis.
- With increasing excitement blood flow further increases resulting in deepening of colour of labia majora. Along with local response, systemic effects (as increase in heart rate, respiratory rate and blood pressure) and in general increase in the muscle tone also occur.

II. Orgasm The orgasm results when intensity of sexual stimulation reaches its peak. It is analogous to emmision and ejaculation in males.

During orgasm there occurs rhythmic contractions of peroneal muscles, uterus and vagina, and dilatation of the cervical canal. The intense sexual sensation perceived during orgasm is called climax. This stage lasts for about 15–30 seconds.

It has been observed that in lower animals, oxytocin released from posterior pituitary via amygdala (limbic system-hypothalamus-posterior pituitary stimulation) is responsible for uterine contractions.

III. Resolution Phase Orgasm is immediately followed by resolution phase. This phase is characterized by a sense of satisfaction followed by the relaxed state of mental peacefulness called resolution. The heart rate, blood pressure, respiration and all other parameters come to their normal level and there occurs relaxation of the muscles.

Applied Aspects

Dyspareunia refers to recurrent / presistant genital pain before, during (most common) or after sexual intercourse. This problem is more common in females than males, the more of physical or psychogenic problem.

PHYSIOLOGY OF PREGNANCY

Physiology of pregnancy is mainly concerned with maternal adaptations to provide ideal atmosphere for fertilization, nutrition to the growing foetus, safe child birth and thereafter to fulfil nutritional needs of the newborn. Though mainly reproductive system is involved in pregnancy, but other body systems also undergo adjustments. The physiology of pregnancy, for convenience of description, can be discussed under following headings:

- Fertilization and implantation,
- Formation of placenta and its functions,
- Physiological changes during pregnancy and
- Applied aspects.

Fertilization and Implantation

Fertilization

Fertilization refers to fusion of male and female gametes (i.e. spermatozoon and ovum). It takes place in the middle segment (ampulla) of the fallopian tube. It involves following events:

1. Transport of Gametes Before fertilization, the ovum and sperms reach the ampulla for fertilization.

Transport of Ovum. At the time of ovulation, the ovum is directly expelled into the peritoneal cavity and then enters into the fallopian tube.

Mechanism. The fimbriae of the fallopian tube are internally lined by ciliated epithelium. When ovulation occurs, the fimbriae of infundibulum encircle the surface of ovary, rub it, and pick up the ovum and then direct it towards the ostium by continuous beating of cilia. The

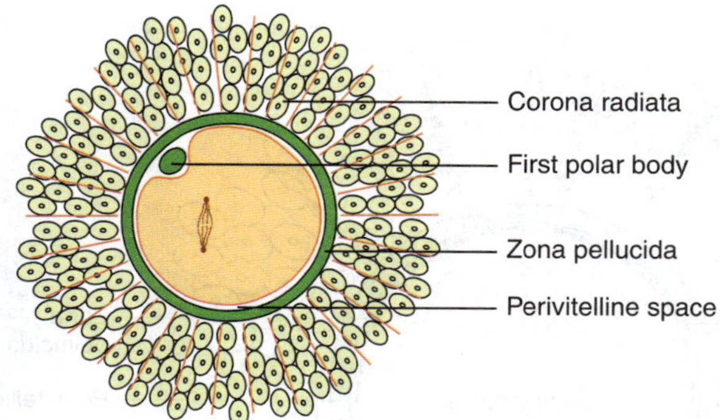

FIGURE 9.4-1 Structure of a mature ovum at the time of ovulation.

contractions of smooth muscle fibres present in the wall of the fallopian tube also help in transport of the ovum. These contractions are increased at the time of ovulation under the influence of oestrogen.

Structure of ovum. The released mature ovum (Fig. 9.4-1) consists of oocyte (containing 23 unpaired chromosomes) surrounded by the inner membranous layer called zona pellucida consisting of glycoproteins and on its outer side surrounded by corona radiata consisting of granulosa cells arranged in multilayers. These cells are held together by matrix composed of hyaluronic acid.

Fate of ovum. The ovum is held up at ampulla isthmic junction for 2–3 days. It remains viable for 6–24 hours after ovulation. During this period, if viable sperm penetrates it, then fertilization takes place and leading on to pregnancy. On the other hand, if fertilization does not occur, the ovum dies out and degenerates.

Transport of Sperms in the Female Genital Tract. After ejaculation, several million sperms (average—200 million sperms per ejaculation) get deposited in the vagina. Out of these about 50-100 sperms manage to reach on to ovum and only one is able to penetrate it. This is because of several factors that affect the transportation and accessibility of the sperm to ovum.

Motility of Sperms. After ejaculation normal sperm shows flagellar movements in the fluid medium at a rate of 1-4 mm/min. Therefore, in 30-60 minutes, they are able to reach the fallopian tube. The motility of sperms in turn depends on:

- pH of the fluid medium,
- Cervical mucus secretions,
- Fluid currents,
- Temperature, and
- Hormones.

i. ***pH of medium.*** Neutral and alkaline pH enhances the activity of sperms, but it is greatly depressed in even mild acidic medium. The vaginal fluid is acidic, hence immediately sperm activity is inhibited and sperms become non-motile. The alkaline semen (pH 7.5) neutralizes the vaginal acidic fluid. Therefore, in less than 60 min after ejaculation sperms again become active and their activity increases in cervix and in the body of uterus for next 25-40 hours.

   Mechanism The principal piece of sperm tail possees special set of proteins (CatSper family) which are alkaline sensitive Ca^{2+} channels, Therefore, the sperms become most active as they pass from vaginal acidic pH (~5) to cervical mucus pH(~8)

ii. ***Cervical secretion.*** The cervical secretion acts as a mechanical barrier for sperms. The nature of cervical secretion depends upon the hormonal concentrations in the plasma. During proliferative phase of menstrual cycle and at the time of ovulation (under the influence of high level of oestrogen) cervical secretion becomes thin and watery, which favours the passage of the sperms. The morphologically abnormal sperms cannot pass through cervical mucus barrier and get entrapped within the fluid.

iii. ***Fluid currents.*** The vaginal and uterine cavity represent a vast sea in which currents are set up by ciliary movements towards exterior (antagonistic direction), which further resists sperm motility.

iv. ***Temperature.*** With rising temperature the activity of sperms increases but their life span is shortened. In ejaculated semen the maximum life span of sperm is 24–48 hours at body temperature. At lower temperature, however, semen can be stored for several weeks and at –100°C sperms can be preserved for many years.

v. ***Hormones.*** Local release of hormones as well as high concentration of certain hormones in the blood affect sperm transport. These include:
   - *Oxytocin.* During coitus, stimulation of female genitalia leads to reflex release of oxytocin from the neuro-hypophysis; oxytocin causes propulsive movements of uterus, which help to aspirate seminal fluid from vagina into the fallopian tube.
   - *Oestrogen.* It makes the cervical secretion thin and watery thus favours transport of sperms.
   - *Prostaglandins.* Prostaglandins present in the semen (contributed by seminal vesicle fluid) also increase female genital tract movements.
   - *Progesterone.* After ovulation, progesterone present in the follicular fluid is released which further stimulates sperm motility.

2. Sperm Capacitation Sperm capacitation refers to the process that makes a sperm to fertilize an ovum. Immediately after ejaculation in female genital tract the sperm undergoes certain changes, which enable it to fertilize an ovum. It takes about 1–10 hours (capacitation period). Sperm capacitation occurs due to removal of certain factors, which normally remain quiescent in male genital tract. These are:

- ***Cholesterol contents of acrosomal membrane.*** In the male genital tract, the acrosomal membrane remains very tough because of high cholesterol contents. Whereas in the female genital tract, the cholesterol contents of acrosomal membrane decreases and it becomes weak leading to easy release of enzymes from the head.

- ***Calcium ions:*** The membrane of sperm becomes permeable to calcium ions. The influx of Ca^{2+} acts by two ways: it makes the flagellar movements of the sperms more strong and whipish (hyperactivation of sperms) and secondly it triggers the release of enzymes from the acrosome.

3. Fusion of Gametes The fusion of ovum and sperm involves the following steps:

i. Chemoattraction. Chemoattraction of the sperms to ovum occurs by substances produced by the ovum. Certain olfactory receptors are expressed by the spermatozoa. A recent view is that ovaries produce certain odorant molecules that interact with these olfactory receptors present on the sperm and is the cause of motility (chemotaxis).

ii. Penetration of Sperm through Ovum Coverings. The sperm passes through two layers (corona radiata and zona pellucida) before it reaches the oocyte.

Penetration of corona radiata (Fig. 9.4-2A). It is made possible by release of enzyme hyaluronidase and other proteolytic enzymes present on the acrosome of the sperm and hyperactivation of the sperm.

- The hyaluronidase polymerizes the hyaluronic acid present in the intercellular matrix holding granulosa cells and
- The proteolytic enzymes digest away the proteins of the structural tissues.

Hyperactivation of sperms (increased flagellar movements) produces penetrating thrust on the ovum due to vigorous lashing of sperm's tail.

Binding of sperm to zona pellucida. After passing through multilayered granulosa cells (corona radiata) many sperms make contact with zona pellucida by binding to receptor protein called *zona pellucida glycoprotein* (ZP_3) (Fig. 9.4-2B). The binding of sperm to ZP_3 triggers acrosomal reaction.

Acrosomal reaction (Fig. 9.4-2C). It involves release of acrosin (protease enzyme) from anterior membrane of acrosome of the sperm. Acrosin opens the penetrating pathway for passage of sperm head into the perivitelline space (space between zona pellucida and oocyte membrane). For effective penetration by the sperm the acrosomal reaction should take place at the zona pellucida because the life span of acrosomal reacted sperm is very short. If it takes place outside zona pellucida, the sperm cannot pass through this membrane.

The acrosomal reaction is also important for actual fusion of sperm cell with oocyte membrane.

iii. Fusion of Sperm with Oocyte (Fig. 9.4-2D). The equatorial region of acrosome is considered to be the site of initial contact between sperm and oocyte membrane (vitelline

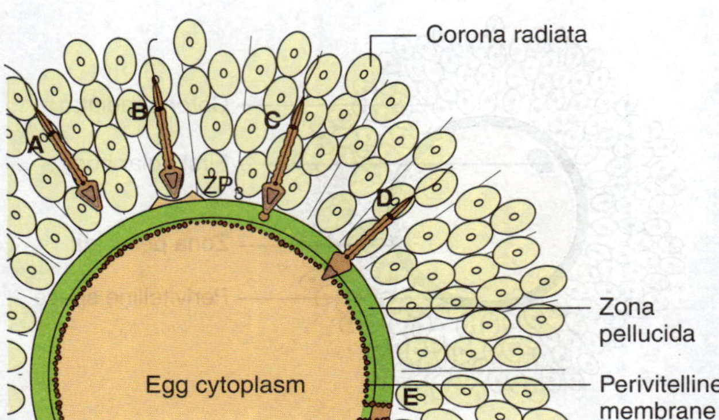

FIGURE 9.4-2 Sequential events of fertilization of an ovum by the sperm: **(A)** penetration of corona radiata; **(B)** binding of sperm to zona pellucida; **(C)** acrosomal reaction; **(D)** fusion of sperm with oocyte; and **(E)** discharge of cortical granules into the perivitelline space producing vitelline block to polyspermy.

membrane). *Fertilin* is a protein present on acrosomal-reacted sperm which interacts with the protein present on vitelline membrane and within 30 minutes the membranes of sperm and oocyte fuse, and genetic material of sperm enters into the oocyte and cause fertilization and embryo begins to develop.

Only one sperm can enter into the oocyte, and further entry of sperms is prevented by the activation of ovum.

iv. Ovum Activation. Fusion of membranes of the gametes leads to ovum activation, which involves following events:

- ***The membrane potential of the ovum decreases*** (depolarization), which is followed by some structural changes in the zona pellucida.
- ***Release of calcium*** from intracellular egg reserve leads to exocytosis of the cortical granules (situated near the oocyte membrane) into the perivitelline space (Fig. 9.4-2E).
- ***Vitelline block to polyspermy.*** The spread of cortical granules along the perivitelline membrane prevents further entry of sperm into the ovum. This is called vitelline block to polyspermy.
- ***Zona blockade to polyspermy.*** The cortical granules contain certain substances like glycosidases and proteases. Glycosidases cause alterations in the ZP_3 receptor protein of the zona pellucida and proteases degrade the ZP_3. Both of these mechanisms cause loss of affinity of sperm for zona pellucida and thus prevent polyspermy. This is called zona block to polyspermy.

Implantation

Implantation of a fertilized ovum involves following steps:

1. Formation of Blastocyst. The fertilized ovum starts dividing immediately and is called morula (16-cell stage) and blastocyst (100-cell stage). On cut section, it shows inner cell mass surrounded by a layer of cells called trophoblast which is covered by zona pellucida (Fig. 9.4-3).

Trophoblast cells layer has great sticking property to the epithelial cells of fallopian tube. As the blastocyst is covered by zona pellucida, the trophoblasts are not exposed and hence the blastocyst is usually not implanted in the fallopian tube. Thus the presence of zona pellucida layer prevents its implantation in the fallopian tube.

2. Transportation of Blastocyst in Uterine Cavity. In next 3-4 days, blastocyst is transported into the cavity of the uterus. The transportation is assisted by fluid currents and ciliary movements of the epithelial cells of the fallopian tube and uterus.

In the cavity of the uterus, blastocyst floats for some time and by this time the zona pellucida layer disappears and trophoblast cell layer is exposed.

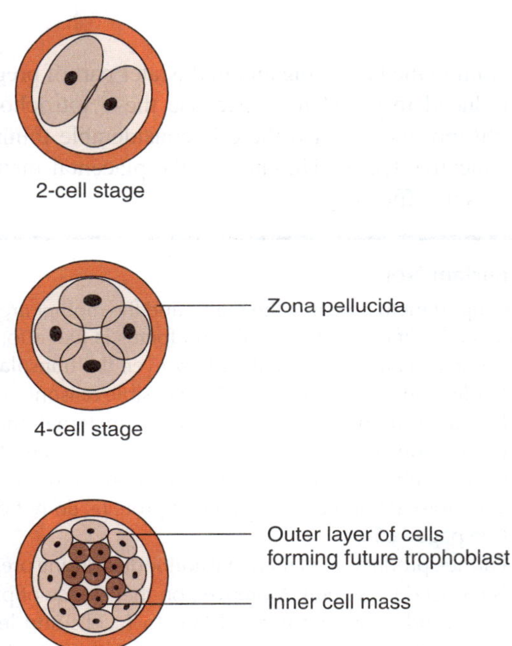

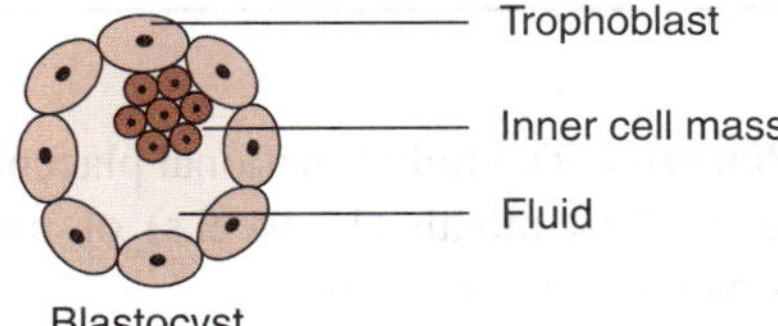

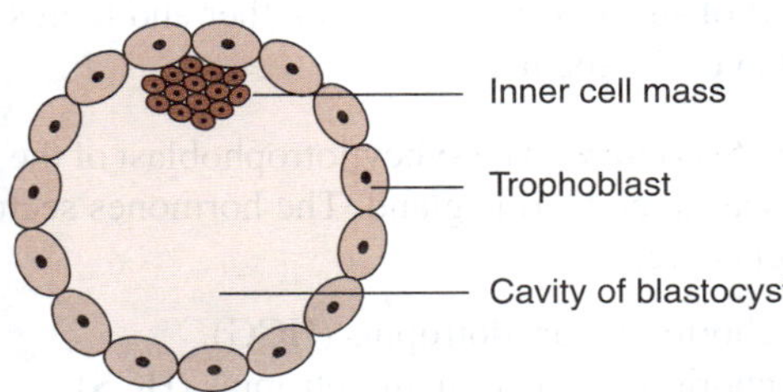

FIGURE 9.4-3 Stages of formation of blastocyst.

Note. Ectopic pregnancy. When the cilia of uterine tube are injured or incapable of movement, then embryo may implants within the fallopian tube itself called ectopic pregnancy. The risk factors for ectopic pregnancy are:

- Chromosomal abnormalities of the conceptus is the most frequent cause of overt miscarriage. Increasing maternal age is associated with an increase frequency of chromosomal abnormalities.
- Congenital or acquired anatomical defects in uterus.
- Endocrine abnormalities leading to alteration of maturation of ova before ovulation, during development and maturation of embryo.

3. Implantation of Blastocyst in the Endometrium. The trophoblasts, due to high sticking property, come in contact with hormonally prepared endometrium of the uterus. The trophoblast layer consists of an inner layer (cytotrophoblast) made of individual cells and an outer layer (syncytiotrophoblast) made up of multinucleated cell mass without distinct boundaries.

The syncytiotrophoblasts secrete proteolytic enzymes that digest and liquefy the endometrium cells. The blastocyst then erodes and burrows into the endometrium—implantation (Fig. 9.4-4).

The blastocyst goes deeper and deeper into the uterus mucosa till whole of it lies within the endometrium. This type of implantation is called endometrial implantation. The normal site of implantation is dorsal wall of uterus.

4. Decidual Reaction. After implantation the endometrium is called decidua. The stroma cells of endometrium get enlarged, become vacuolated and filled with glycogen and lipids. These cells are called decidual cells. Therefore this change in stroma cell is called decidual reaction. The stored glycogen and lipids are the source of nutrition for the embryo till placenta takes up this function.

Placenta and Pregnancy Tests

Placenta

Placenta is a temporary organ formed during pregnancy. It is an important link between the mother and the foetus.

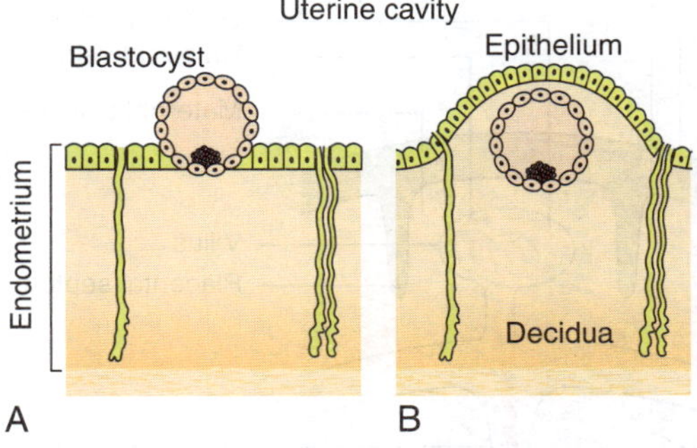

FIGURE 9.4-4 Implantation of blastocyst in the **(A)** endometrium and **(B)** decidual reaction.

Formation of Placenta The decidual part where placenta is to develop is called as *decidua basalis* or *decidual plate*. The part of the decidua that separates the embryo from the uterine cavity is called the *decidua capsularis*, while the part lining the rest of the uterine cavity is called *decidua parietalis*. In region of decidua basalis, the maternal blood vessels proliferate and grow. The syncytiotrophoblast sends cords into the decidua basalis. These cords further grow and send more projections to form *palcental villi*. In the placental villi, the blood capillaries grow from the vascular system of the embryo. The capillaries are covered by thin endothelial cells which are surrounded by mesenchymal tissue (Fig. 9.4-5).

The placental villi are surrounded by blood-filled maternal sinuses (intervillus spaces). The maternal blood flows through uterine arteries into the maternal sinuses and back through the uterine veins of the mother. The foetal blood flows through umbilical arteries into the capillaries of placental villi and back through an umbilical vein into the foetus.

- When fully formed, the placenta is a disc-shaped structure, has a diameter of 15–20 cm and weighs about 500 gm.
- After birth of the baby, the placenta is shed off along with the decidua.

The Placental Membrane The maternal and foetal blood do not mix with each other. They are separated by a placental membrane, made up of the layers of the wall of the villus. From the foetal side these are (Fig. 9.4-6):

- *Endothelium* of foetal blood vessels and its basement membrane;
- Surrounding mesenchymal tissue (connective tissue);
- Cytotrophoblast and its basement membrane and
- *Syncytiotrophoblast*.

All interchanges of oxygen, nutrition and waste products between the maternal blood and foetal blood take place through the placental membrane barrier. The total area of the membrane varies from 4 m^2 to 14 m^2. Its thickness is 0.025 mm in the beginning and in the later part of pregnancy it is reduced to 0.002 mm, because the cytotrophoblastic layer disappears and also there is considerable thinning of the connective tissue. Thinning of the placental membrane increases its efficiency.

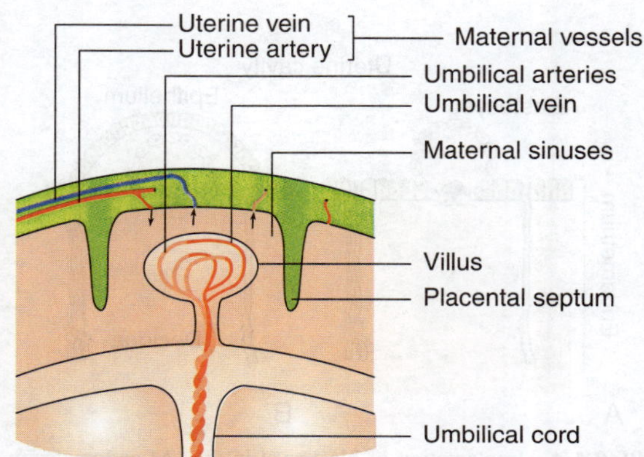

FIGURE 9.4-5 Schematic diagram showing structure of placenta.

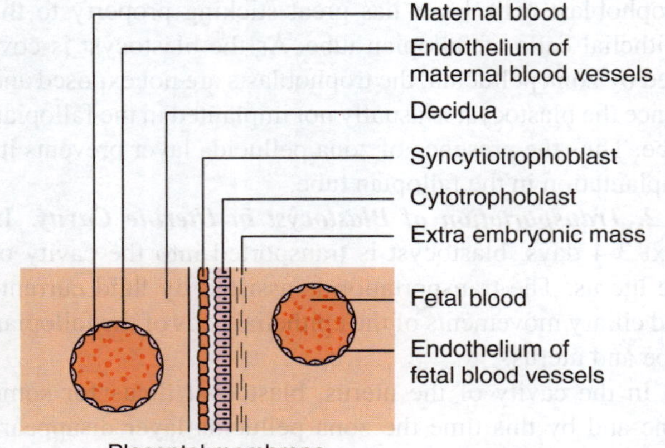

FIGURE 9.4-6 Structure of the placental membrane.

Important Note

It is important to note that the foetus and the mother are two genetically different individuals and foetus is like a foreign tissue (transplant) in the mother. However, the transplant is well tolerated and not rejected. The possible reasons are:

i. Placental trophoblast which separates maternal and foetal tissues does not express polymorphic MHC class I and II genes, rather it expresses HLA-G (monomorphic) genes. Therefore antibodies against foetal proteins do not develop (see page 185).
ii. Further, production of maternal antibodies during pregnancy is reduced in general. Moreover, on the surface of placenta Fos ligand is present which binds to T cells and leads on their apoptosis. For example, a woman with Graves' disease usually becomes euthyroid during pregnancy and shows a decreased level of antithyroid antibodies.

Functions of Placenta The fully functional placenta develops by the end of third month (12 weeks) of pregnancy. Placenta serves mainly three functions:

- Hormone secretion (endocrinal functions of placenta).
- Transport of substances between mother and foetus.
- Protection of the foetus.

A. Hormone Secretion. The syncytiotrophoblast of the placenta serves as an endocrine gland. The hormones secreted by the placenta are:

- Human chorionic gonadotropins (HCG),
- Human chorionic somatomammotropins (HCS),
- Human chorionic thyrotropin (HCT),

- Placental progesterone,
- Placental oestrogens and
- Relaxin.

1. Human Chorionic Gonadotropins. HCG is a polypeptide hormone containing 236 amino acid residues (largest active peptide). It is secreted by syncytiotrophoblast soon after fertilization. It is made up of two subunits—HCG-α (molecular weight—18,000) and HCG-β (molecular weight—28,000). HCG-α is quite similar to α-subunit of LH, FSH and thyroid stimulating hormones (TSH).

Plasma concentration. HCG is produced soon after fertilization and is detected in the maternal blood as early as 6–8 days after conception, and reaches its peak between 60–90 days of gestation. After this the concentration falls to a very low level and just before labour, its level falls to zero (Fig. 9.4-7A). Its approximate peak value in human maternal blood during normal pregnancy is 5 mg/ml. It can be measured by using radioimmunoassay technique.

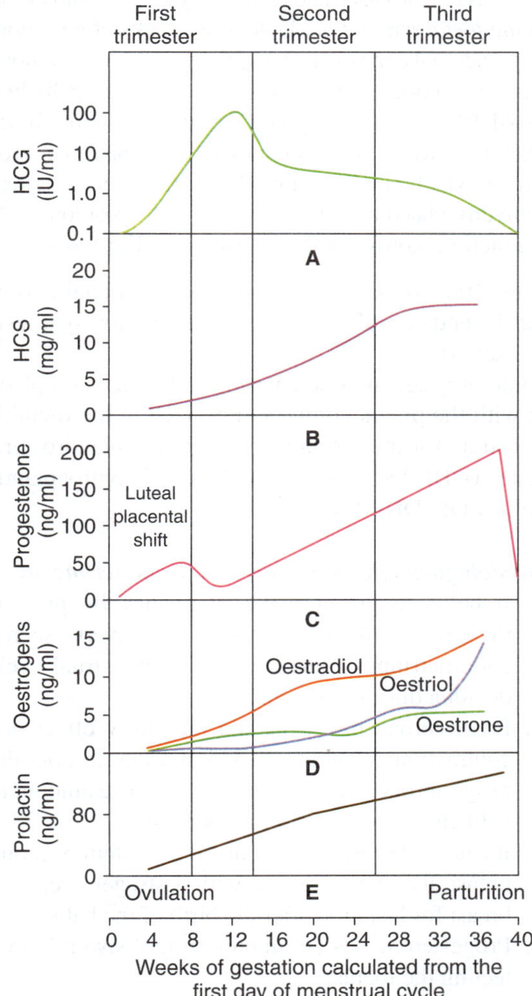

FIGURE 9.4-7 Profile of plasma concentration of hormones during normal pregnancy: **(A)** human chorionic gonadotropin (HCG); **(B)** human chorionic somatomammotropin (HCS); **(C)** progesterone; **(D)** oestrogen; and **(E)** prolactin.

Physiological effects of HCG are:

- HCG is a luteotropic hormone. Its actions are similar to LH of anterior pituitary hence also called second *luteotropic hormone*. It maintains the functions of the corpus luteum up to 7 weeks after conception until foetoplacental unit is able to synthesize its own oestrogen and progesterone.
- HCG converts corpus luteum of menstruation into corpus luteum of pregnancy and stimulates it to secrete 17α-hydroxyprogesterone and lesser amount of progesterone. Blood 17α-hydroxyprogesterone level is an excellent indicator of the activity of corpus luteum of pregnancy. Its peak level is reached 3-4 weeks after conception.
- HCG stimulates foetal testes in male foetus to secrete testosterone prior to foetal pituitary LH secretion. This testosterone and MRF secreted by foetal testes is responsible for development of male genital organs and descent of testes during intrauterine life.
- HCG may also serve as a tropic agent for the adrenal cortex foetal zone to secrete DHEA.

Clinical importance (application) of HCG are:

The presence of HCG in the urine forms the basis of all the pregnancy tests (see page 869). HCG appears in the urine as early as 10 days after gestation with 99% accuracy. Even though it is not absolutely specific for pregnancy because small amounts are also secreted by various gastrointestinal and other tumours in both sexes. Therefore, HCG has been measured as tumor marker in an individual with suspected tumour.

If foetus dies early then HCG disappears from the blood as well as from the urine.

2. Human Chorionic Somatomammotropin. The syncytiotrophoblast cells of placenta also secrete large amount of HCS. HCS is protein in nature and structurally resembles to growth hormone. Its molecular weight is 38,000.

Plasma concentration. The secretion of HCS begins at 5th week of pregnancy. It increases gradually throughout pregnancy and its plasma concentration is directly proportional to the weight of placenta. Its peak reaches at term and peak value is 15 μg/ml (Fig. 9.4-7B). Though large quantities of HCS is present in maternal blood but very little reaches the foetus.

Note. Low maternal HCS levels are indication of placental insufficiency.

Physiological effects of HCS are:

i. *Lactogenic activity.* HCSs have lactogenic activity in lower animals. When administered it causes partial development of breast and also causes lactation. Hence, this hormone was first named as human placental lactogen and was believed to have functions like prolactin. However, in humans its lactogenic action is very weak.

ii. *Growth stimulating activity.* The HCS, being similar to human growth hormone, also shows weak growth stimulating activity. Hence this hormone is also named as human chorionic growth hormone prolactin. It functions as maternal growth hormone of pregnancy and causes deposition of protein in the tissues, and bring about nitrogen, calcium and potassium retention. The growth hormone secretion from anterior pituitary is, however, decreased during pregnancy.

iii. *Insulin sensitivity.* The HCS decreases the insulin sensitivity thus leading to decreased utilization of glucose by the mother. Therefore, larger quantity of glucose is made available to the growing foetus. Glucose is the main substrate used by the foetus.

iv. *Lipolysis.* The HCS promotes release of fatty acids from fat stores of the mother and thus provides an alternate source of energy for metabolism in the mother. Human chorionic somatomammotropic hormone is now considered to be general metabolic hormone that has specific nutritional implications for both the mother as well as the foetus.

3. Human Chorionic Thyrotropin. HCT secreted by the placenta has properties quite similar to that of TSH. The physiological role of this substance is not very clear but its plasma concentration curve is like that of HCG.

4. Placental Progesterone. Progesterone is C-21 steroid hormone.

Synthesis. During early pregnancy it is synthesized by corpus luteum of pregnancy and then by syncytio-trophoblasts of placenta (85% of total contribution). The various facts regarding synthesis of progesterone in placenta are:

- Placental syncytiotrophoblasts do not synthesize cholesterol from acetate which is the main substrate for progesterone synthesis. Therefore, cholesterol is mainly derived from maternal circulation and very little is contributed by the foetus.
- The foetus, placenta and mother, though they are independent, but constitute a functional unit called *fetoplacental maternal unit*.
- The pathways of progesterone synthesis in the feto-placental maternal unit are shown in Fig. 9.4-8.
- In the syncytiotrophoblasts of placenta, pregnenolone is formed from maternal cholesterol.

Pregnenolone is then oxidized by 3β hydroxysteroid dehydrogenase (3β-HSD) to progesterone.

Plasma concentration. During pregnancy plasma concentration of progesterone rises steadily throughout gestation (Fig. 9.4-7C) reaching a maximum plateau at 30–40 weeks of gestation and its level does not fall to zero like other placental hormones. Just before the onset of labour its level decreases.

The initial rise in concentration of progesterone is mainly due to *hydroxyprogesterone* secreted by the corpus luteum and its peak reaches at 3–4 weeks of gestation in response to HCG secretion. Then the level of hydroxyprogesterone starts declining, but plasma concentration as such starts rising. Therefore, the significance of 17α-hydroxyprogesterone level in plasma as well as in urine reflects corpus luteum activity and second steady rise in plasma concentration of progesterone reflects placental trophoblast secretion and is referred as *luteal placental shift*. It occurs at 7th week of gestation. The peak plasma concentration value of progesterone is 190 ng/ml at term.

Fate and metabolism of progesterone. Progesterone synthesized by placenta diffuses back into the maternal circulation and also in the foetal circulation.

- *In the maternal circulation.* The progesterone exerts its physiological effects and is then metabolized in the liver. The principal metabolites of progesterone is *pregnanediol* which is glucuronised and secreted by kidneys into the urine.
- *In the foetal circulation.* Upto 10th weeks of gestation the foetal adrenal cortex (inner zone or foetal zone) cannot synthesize its corticosteroids (cortisol) because 3β hydroxysteroid dehydrogenase (3β HSD) enzyme system is blocked. Therefore, foetal adrenal cortex requires placental progesterone, which circulates into the foetal adrenal cortex and gethydroxylated at C-17, C-21 and C-11 positions to form aldosterone, cortisol and corticosterone (Fig. 9.4-8).

After 10th weeks of gestation, foetal adrenal cortex no longer depends on placental progesterone for synthesis of corticosteroids.

Some of pregnenolone entering in foetus from placenta along with the pregnenolone synthesized in the foetal liver is a substrate for the formation of dehydroepiandrosterone-sulphate (DHEAS) and 16-hydroxy dehydroepiandrosterone (16-OH DHEAS).

Physiological effects of placental progesterone are:

i. It helps to preserve the pregnancy by promoting the growth of endometrium. It converts secretory endometrium of luteal phase of menstrual cycle to decidua during pregnancy.

ii. Progesterone has a marked inhibitory effect on the contractions of uterus. It is important to note that if progesterone is not secreted in adequate amount there is likelihood of threatened abortion.

iii. It causes development of alveolar system of mother's breast. Its synergic action with oestrogen prepares the breast for lactation after the birth of the baby.

iv. Progesterone has an immunosuppressive role in protecting the foetus.

v. By acting as a precursor for corticosteroid synthesis by the foetal adrenal cortex it helps in growth and development of the foetus.

vi. Progesterone antagonizes the effect of aldosterone and thus promotes renal excretion of Na^+ during pregnancy.

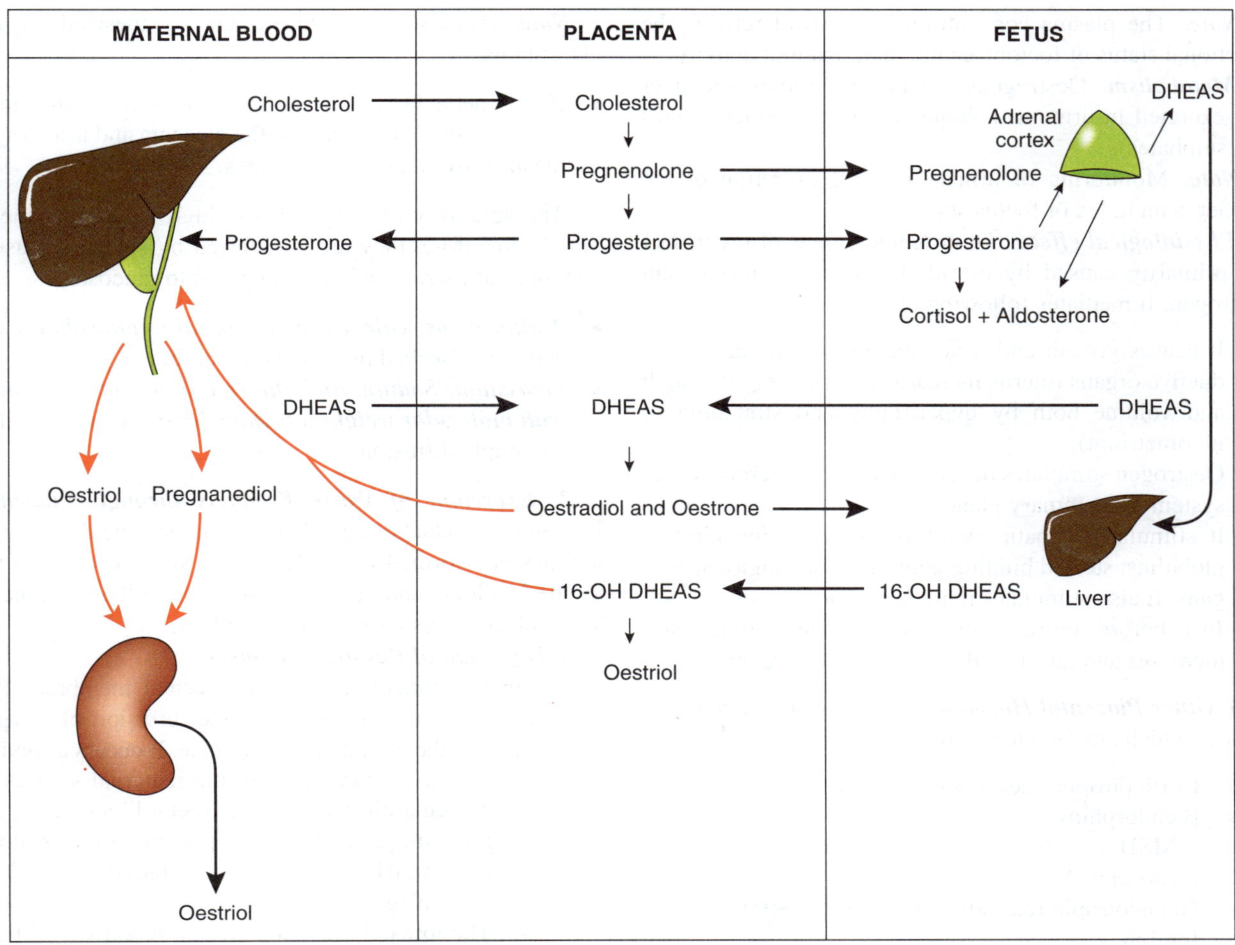

FIGURE 9.4-8 Fetoplacental maternal unit for steroid hormone synthesis.

5. Placental Oestrogens. Placental oestrogens are C-21 steroid hormones quantitatively estriol is the major oestrogen of pregnancy with smaller amount of estradiol and estrone.

Synthesis. During early pregnancy, like progesterone, it is synthesized by corpus luteum and then by the placental syncytiotrophoblasts (90%). However, oestrogen production is different in placenta than that of ovary because; the enzymes 17-hydroxylase and 17, 20-desmolase (CYP 17,20) which are essential for formation of androgen, i.e. dehydroepiandrosterone (DHEA) from cholesterol, are not present in the placenta. Therefore, basic substrate for synthesis of oestrogen is not cholesterol rather it is dehydroepiandrosterone. The steps involved in biosynthesis are shown in Figure 9.4-8.

i. DHEA the principal adrenal steroid is sulphconjugated (sulphated) by sulph kinase in the adrenal cortex of the foetus and of mother to DHEAS.
ii. *In the foetal liver.* The DHEAS is converted to 16-hydroxy dehydroepiandrosterone (16-OH DHEAS) by an enzyme 16-hydroxylase present in foetal liver. This enzyme is also not present in placenta.
iii. *In the placenta.* Placenta obtains DHEAS from the maternal as well as from the foetal circulation. In the placenta DHEAS is deconjugated to DHEA before it is converted into estriol. For the conversion of DHEA to oestriol two types of enzymes are required; 16-*hydroxylase* (which is present in the foetal and maternal liver), and *aromatase* (which is present in the maternal ovary and the placenta).

The enzyme 16-hydroxylase is lacking in placenta. Therefore, estriol is mainly formed by aromatase pathway (Fig. 9.4-8).

Since 16-OH DHEAS is the main substrate for oestrogen, hence estriol is the major placental oestrogen during pregnancy.

The oestrone and oestradiol present in maternal circulation are converted into oestriol in the maternal liver by 16-hydroxylase pathway but amount secreted is very less.

Plasma concentration. Like progesterone, plasma oestrogen (estriol) concentration, rises throughout the gestation. Its peak value (14 ng/ml) and secretory curve parallels as that of progesterone and maximum *plateau* is reached at 30-40 weeks of gestation (Figure 9.4-7D).

Note. The plasma concentration of estriol reflects the functional status of foetoplacental maternal unit activity.

Metabolism. Oestrogens are metabolised in the liver and excreted in urine as soluble conjugates (glucuronides and sulphates).

Note. Monitoring of urinary oestriol excretion of the mother is an index of foetus status.

Physiological effects. Oestrogenic effects of pregnancy are primarily caused by estradiol, which is most potent oestrogen. It mediates following effects:

i. It causes growth and development of maternal reproductive organs (uterus increases in size, weight, length and volume both by hypertrophy and stretching of myometrium).

ii. Oestrogen stimulates development of lactiferous ductal system in mammary glands.

iii. It stimulates hepatic synthesis of thyroxine binding globulins, steroid binding globulins, and angiotensinogens. It also stimulates renin secretion.

iv. Just before term, oestrogen to progesterone ratio increases and uterus is dominated by oestrogen.

6. Other Placental Hormones. A number of other substances which are secreted from placenta are:

- Corticotropin releasing hormone (CRH),
- β endorphins,
- α MSH,
- Dynorphin A,
- Gonadotropin releasing hormones (GnRH),
- Inhibin,
- Leptin,
- Prolactin and
- Prorenin.

Exact role of the above substances during pregnancy is not yet clear. However, substances like GnRH and inhibin act in paracrine fashion to regulate HCG.

B. Transport of Substances between the Mother and the Foetus

1. Transport of Nutrients. The major function of placenta is to provide foodstuffs from mother's blood into the foetus.

During first few weeks after implantation the nutrients are derived from the plasma into the oedematous decidua and from endometrial glandular secretions containing glycogen.

By the 4th week of pregnancy the placenta takes up the nutritive functions. The nutritive materials which are transported from mother's blood into the foetus are:

- *Glucose.* Glucose passes by facilitated diffusion through a carrier molecule present on the trophoblast cells. Glucose level in foetal blood is 20–30% lower than that of maternal blood.

Note. Fructose and sucrose are synthesized in the placenta itself.

- *Fats.* Foetal fat is derived from transfer of free fatty acids and cholesterol across the placenta and is also synthesized from the carbohydrates.

The solubility of fatty acids is high in the cell membranes, therefore, they are transferred by simple diffusion method, but more slowly as compared to glucose.

- ***Amino acids, calcium and inorganic phosphates*** are actively absorbed by placental membrane.
- ***Potassium, Sodium and chloride ions and substances with molecular weight less than 1000*** can cross readily by simple diffusion.

2. Excretion of Waste Products through Placenta. Excretory products, especially urea, uric acid and creatinines etc. formed in the foetus are transported into the mother's blood and then excreted by mother's kidneys. Thus, placenta also acts as foetal kidney.

3. Diffusion of Respiratory Gases

i. ***Oxygen transport*** through placental membrane follows the same principle as the diffusion of oxygen through the pulmonary membrane. It occurs as under:

- Dissolved oxygen from the maternal sinuses of placenta diffuses into the foetal blood along the pressure gradient, (mean pO_2 in mother's blood is 50 mmHg whereas in foetal blood mean pO_2 is 30 mmHg).
- The low pO_2 of foetal arterial blood would have been a serious problem but presence of foetal haemoglobin in the RBCs which has higher affinity for oxygen than adult haemoglobin, and higher haemoglobin concentration of foetal blood (50% greater than mother), shifts the oxygen-haemoglobin dissociation curve to left.
- The foetal blood coming to placenta carries more of CO_2 which is released into maternal blood. Therefore, the pH of maternal blood is slightly acidic as compared to foetal blood. The haemoglobin–oxygen dissociation curve of foetal blood shifts to left and of maternal blood to the right (double Bohr's effect). All the above factors help the foetus to receive sufficient oxygen (Fig. 9.4-9).

ii. ***Transport of CO_2.*** Transport of CO_2 from foetus occurs by diffusion along the pressure gradient. The pCO_2 of foetal blood is 2–3 mmHg higher than that of maternal blood (as CO_2 is continuously being formed in the foetus and eliminated only through placenta). Thus placenta acts as foetal lungs.

4. Transport of Antibodies. Maternal immunoglobulins are transferred by receptor mediated endocytosis into the foetus and are responsible for innate immunity.

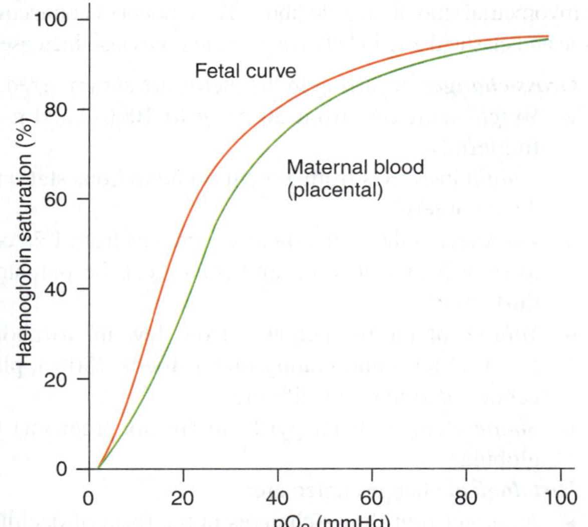

FIGURE 9.4-9 Oxygen–haemoglobin dissociation curve for maternal and fetal blood.

Rh agglutinins are easily transported as compared to ABO agglutinins, that is why the effects of Rh incompatibility are more severe.

5. Transport of Harmful Substances. Certain viruses and many drugs (like nicotine and barbiturates) can easily cross the placental barrier and may produce harmful effect on the foetus. Therefore, as far as possible one should avoid these drugs and smoking during pregnancy. One should also try to remain away from viral infections. HIV virus is also transmitted from mother to foetus.

C. Protection of the Foetus. Placenta protects the foetus in many ways:

- It acts as a barrier for certain harmful substances.
- It provides nutrition to the foetus.
- Its hormonal secretion is responsible for proper growth of the foetus.
- Placental progesterone decreases uterine contractions and thus protects the foetus from being expelled.

Pregnancy Tests

In an adult healthy woman amenorrhoea is the first sign of pregnancy, but it occurs in many other conditions as well. Therefore, detection of early pregnancy is made possible by certain pregnancy tests. The pregnancy detection tests are based on presence of HCG in the urine of pregnant lady. The sensitivity of these tests varies, but usually concentration required to obtain a positive test is about 2500 IU/L and this occurs at about 10–12 days after a missed period. There are two types of pregnancy detection test.

A. Biological Tests

The biological pregnancy tests are based upon the luteinizing activity of HCG. The urine of the pregnant woman is injected either by intraperitoneal or subcutaneous route into the female virigin animal, there occurs ovulation which is detected as haemorrhagic spots on the corpora lutea. Various biological pregnancy tests are summarized in Table 9.4-1.

Note. Although biological tests are very sensitive but nowadays, they are replaced by immunological tests of pregnancy because of convenience and immediate results.

B. Immunological Tests

Immunological pregnancy tests are based on antigenic properties of HCG.

Gravindex Test The kit for this test consists of:

- Gravindex antigen (latex particles coated with HCG), Gravindex antibodies (serum containing antibodies against HCG) and a dark coloured slide.
- The antibodies are prepared by injecting urine of pregnant woman containing HCG into the rabbits. Then after few weeks blood from rabbit is withdrawn and serum is separated (containing anti-HCG antibodies).

TABLE 9.4-1 Biological Tests of Pregnancy

Test	Criteria for positive test
1. Ascheim-Zondek test	
Urine (2-5ml) from pregnant woman is injected (intra-peritoneal/subcutaneous) into an immature mice 2-3 times in a day for 2-3 days.	On third day abdomen is opened and ovaries are examined. Haemorrhagic spots on corpora lutea indicate that ovulation has occurred.
2. Friedman's test	
In an immature female rabbit or in mature adult female rabbit (isolated from male rabbits for a week) urine of pregnant woman is injected.	Abdomen is opened after 24 hours. Detection of haemorrhagic spots on corpora lutea indicate positive test.
3. Hogben's test	
5 ml urine from pregnant woman is injected into the large dorsal lymph sac of the female toad.	After 2–3 hours shedding of ova is observed which indicates positive pregnancy test.
4. Kupperman's test	
3 to 5 ml of urine of a pregnant lady is injected subcutaneously into an immature rat.	After 6 hours ovaries show hyperaemia.
5. Galli-Mainini test	
3 to 5 ml urine is injected into lymph sac of male frog (xenopus).	After 2 hours urine is withdrawn from cloaca of male frog and presence of sperms in the urine indicates +ve pregnancy test.

Procedure. This test is performed on the control and test samples of urine.

Control sample. A drop of urine sample from non-pregnant subject (containing no HCG) is mixed with a drop of antiserum containing HCG antibodies. Then it is mixed with HCG coated latex particles. There will be agglutination, because urine of non-pregnant subject does not contain antigen therefore, antibodies are not neutralized. Thus occurrence of agglutination indicates no pregnancy or pregnancy test is negative.

Test sample. A drop of urine of suspected pregnant lady (containing HCG) is mixed with a drop of antiserum (containing HCG antibodies). Then it is mixed with HCG-coated latex particles. There will be no agglutination, because antibodies have been neutralized by the HCG present in the urine. Therefore, occurrence of no agglutination means positive pregnancy test. The procedure can be summarized as:

Control	Test
A drop of urine of nonpregnant woman (No HCG)	A drop of urine of pregnant woman (HCG)
+	+
A drop of HCG antiserum	A drop of HCG antiserum
+	+
HCG coated latex particles	HCG coated latex particles
↓	↓
Agglutination (–ve pregnancy test)	No agglutination (+ve pregnancy test)

Note. It is important to note that:

- This test is not absolutely specific for pregnancy. It is positive in the presence of certain tumours which secrete HCG.
- Proteinuria may give false-positive results.
- The test becomes negative in later months pregnancy when HCG level falls.

Physiological Changes in Mother during Pregnancy

The normal average duration of pregnancy in human beings is 280 days (40 weeks) and is calculated from the first day of the last menstrual period (LMP), or 256–270 days from the time of ovulation. As pregnancy progresses, growing foetus imposes various types of extra demands on mother's body, which are met with by certain adaptations in almost all the organ systems of the body. These physiological changes include.

I. Changes in Genital Organs

1. Uterus. To accommodate the growing foetus marked increase in the size of uterus takes place. The enlargement is mainly due to hypertrophy and to some extent hyperplasia of the myometrial smooth muscle fibres. The amount of connective tissue and elastic tissue in between muscle fibres also increases.

Gross changes occurring in the uterus are summarized:

- *Weight* increases from 30–50 g to 1000–1200 g at full term.
- *Length* increases from 7.5 cm (in nonparous state) to 35 cm at term.
- *Thickness* of the wall of uterus decreases from 1.25 cm to only 5 mm at term, and foetus can be palpated through it.
- *Volume* of uterus increases from few ml to about 5–7 L at term and mainly due to foetus (50%), placenta and amniotic fluids etc.
- *Shape* changes from pyriform (in nonpregnant) to globular.

Histological changes noted are:

- *Endometrium* shows changes in the form of decidua during initial stages of pregnancy.
- *Myometrium*. The muscle fibres increase in diameter (2 to 7 times) and length (2 to 11 times), and form interlacing network around blood vessels. The contraction of these fibres prevent blood loss from raw surface of placenta after delivery of placenta. Sometimes, if contraction of uterus is not proper then excessive postpartum haemorrhage occurs.

Note. The changes in the uterus occur in first and second months of pregnancy under the influence of oestrogen and subsequent enlargement is due to growing foetus.

2. Ovaries. The corpus luteum enlarges during first 12–16 weeks of pregnancy and then degenerates due to the decreased level of HCG. By this time placenta takes over the functions of secretion of oestrogens and progesterone.

The follicular changes and ovulation do not occur because FSH and LH of anterior pituitary are inhibited.

3. Cervix. The changes in the cervix include:

- Endocervix gets hypertrophied,
- The cervical glands increase in number and their secretions form a plug, that closes the cervical canal and
- The tough cervix becomes soft.

4. Fallopian Tubes. The fallopian tubes are pushed upwards due to increase in the size of uterus. There occurs hyperplasia of the epithelial cells and blood supply also increases.

5. Mammary Glands. Under the influence of various hormones breast enlarges in early pregnancy. Hyperplasia of ductal and alveolar tissue occurs, the areola becomes pigmented and many sebaceous glands become prominent in the areola. Nipples also become larger and pigmented.

II. Weight Gain

A woman may gain total of 10-12 kg of weight during normal pregnancy, which is contributed by (Fig. 9.4-10):

- Foetus: 3 kg
- Placenta and amniotic fluid: 1.5 kg

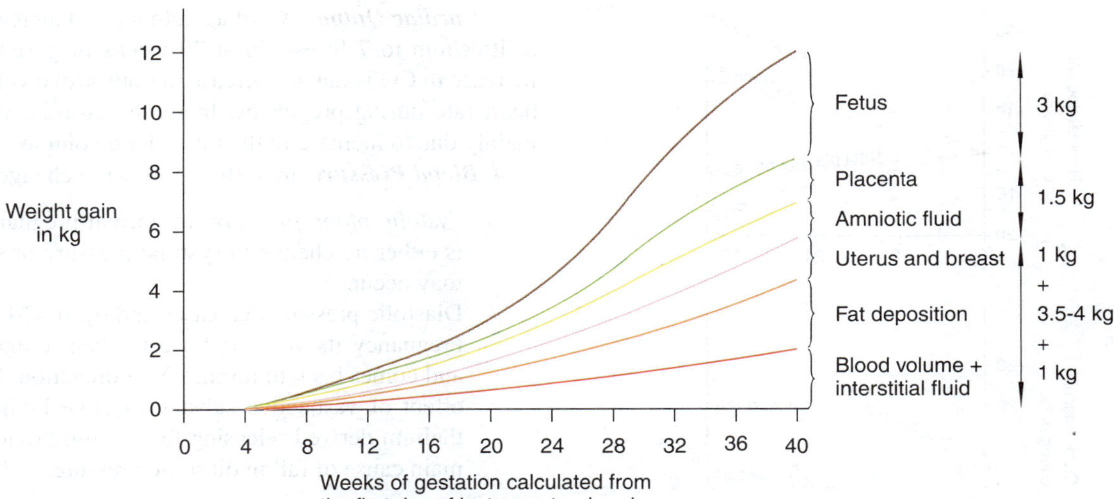

FIGURE 9.4-10 Pattern and components of weight gain during normal pregnancy.

- Uterus and breast enlargement: 1.0 kg
- Increase in blood volume and interstitial fluid: 1.5 kg
- Fat deposition: 3.5 to 4 kg.

Important points about the weight gain are:

- During antenatal examination regular monitoring of body weight is very important. Absence of weight gain in the second or third trimester is a sign of foetal growth retardation and foetal death.
- During early pregnancy weight loss may be observed because of excessive vomiting.
- Due to increased secretion of oestrogen, progesterone, aldosterone and antidiuretic hormone (ADH) during pregnancy Na^+ and H_2O retention occurs.
- Oedema is common, particularly in the lower limbs which is because of pressure of gravid uterus on the femoral vein and also because of Na^+ and water retention.
- Rapid and excessive weight gain raises the suspicion of toxaemia of pregnancy due to excessive fluid retention.

III. Haematological Changes (Fig. 9.4-11A)

1. Blood Volume. The blood volume increases during pregnancy to increase the blood supply to: (i) uterus (to meet its demands), (ii) to skin to dissipate heat generated in the body, and (iii) to the kidney for excretion of extra waste products.

The total blood volume increases by 30%. It begins to increase by 12th week of pregnancy and continues till delivery.

- The plasma volume increases relatively more than that of red cell volume which causes haemodilution thus there is physiological anaemia of pregnancy.

2. The Haemataological Indices show following changes:

- RBC count decreases,
- Hb concentration decreases,
- PCV decreases,
- ESR increases, and
- Reticulocyte count increases.

3. Plasma Proteins show following changes:

The total concentration of plasma proteins decreases from 7.5 to 6 g% due to haemodilution.

- The fibrinogen level increases to 300–400 mg/dL from 200–300 mg/dL
- Serum albumin is markedly decreased,
- Globulins (α and β) are increased.

4. Leucocytes

- Total leucocyte count (TLC) increases and may reach up to 20,000/mm^3.
- DLC. Polymorphonuclear cells are predominantly increased with little change in monocytes, eosinophils and basophils and no change in number of lymphocytes.

5. Platelets

- There occurs slight decrease in platelet count.

6. Coagulation Factors. Pregnancy seems to be a hypercoagulable state due to increase in following coagulation factors:

- Fibrinogen, and
- Factors VII, VIII, IX and X.

The hypercoagulability of the blood plays significant role of haemostasis at the time of separation of placenta during delivery.

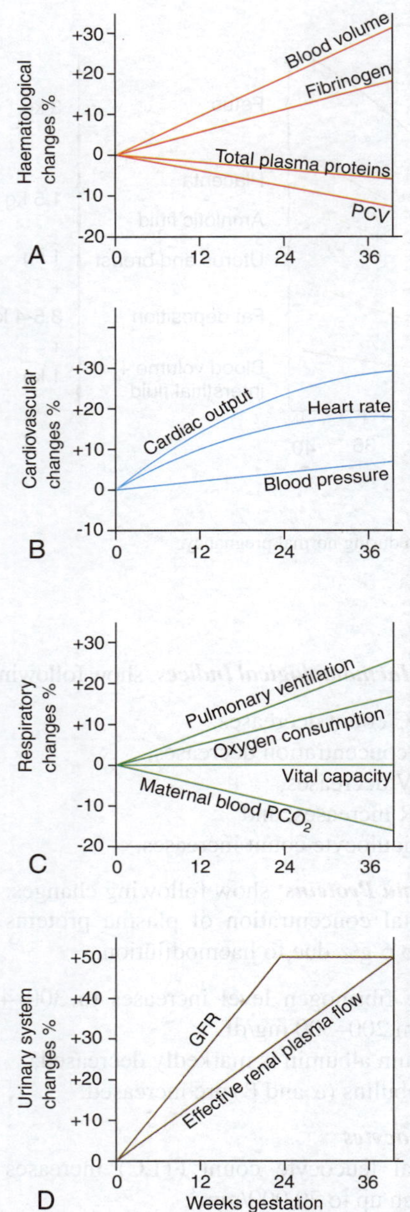

FIGURE 9.4-11 Some physiological changes in the mother during pregnancy: **(A)** haematological changes; **(B)** cardiovascular changes; **(C)** respiratory changes; and **(D)** urinary system changes.

IV. Cardiovascular System Changes (Fig. 9.4-11B)

1. Position of Heart. The gravid uterus pushes the diaphragm upwards resulting change in the position of heart as:

- Heart is displaced laterally, upwards and slightly rotated to its long axis.
- Apex beat of the heart shifts laterally because of the above change in heart's position.
- ECG changes show left axis deviation.

2. Heart Rate. Heart rate also increases by 10–12 beats/min.

3. Cardiac Output. Cardiac output (CO) increases from 5 litres/min to 7 litres/min at 20 weeks of gestation. The increase in CO is due to increase in both stroke volume and heart rate during pregnancy. Increase in stroke volume is mainly due to increase in the total blood volume.

4. Blood Pressure may show following changes:

- *Systolic blood pressure.* In normal pregnancy there is either no change in systolic pressure or some fall may occur.
- Diastolic pressure decreases and by 16–20 weeks of pregnancy its value is lowest. Then it starts rising and comes back to normal. Vasodilatation due to the effect of vasoactive substances (like kinins, endothelium derived releasing factor, nitric oxide) is the main cause of fall in diastolic pressure.

5. Blood Flow. Blood flow to skin, uterus and kidneys increases to meet the demands.

6. Venous Pressure. The gravid uterus exerts pressure on the pelvic veins, abdominal veins and femoral veins, thus increasing the venous pressure. The rise in femoral venous pressure results in oedema in feet (common occurrence), and the increased abdominal venous pressure predisposes to varicose veins, piles and peripheral venous thrombosis.

V. Respiratory System Changes (Fig. 9.4-11C)

1. Anatomical Changes in respiratory system occur due to elevation of diaphragm by the enlarged uterus. It causes increase in transverse diameter of thoracic cage and subcostal angle. These two changes in turn increase the air flow across the bronchial tree.

2. Hyperventilation. High levels of plasma progesterone during pregnancy increase the senstivity of respiratory neurons to CO_2 resulting in hyperventilation. As a result of the maternal blood pCO_2 decrease by 10–15%, pCO_2 becomes about 30 mmHg (normal, 40 mmHg).

3. Ventilatory Functions. The anatomical changes and hyperventilation during pregnancy result in some changes in the parameters of ventilatory functions:

- *Tidal volume* increases,
- *Vital capacity* shows no changes,
- *Inspiratory capacity* increases,
- *Residual volume* decreases,
- *Functional residual capacity* decreases, and
- *Forced expiratory volume* (FEV_1) and peak flow rate do not change.

4. Gas Exchange. Gas exchange across the alveoli is greatly enhanced due to marked increase in the pulmonary blood flow.

5. Oxygen Consumption. Oxygen consumption of body increases by 15% to meet the demands of growing foetus and for the extra work of heart, uterus and other tissue.

VI. Urinary System Changes (Fig. 9.4-11D)

Kidney functions show following changes:

1. Renal Blood Flow. There is marked increase in renal blood flow due to increase in cardiac output and vasodilatation.

2. Effective Renal Plasma Flow (ERPF) increases by 60% during pregnancy.

3. Glomerular Filtration Rate (GFR) increases by 50% due to increase in renal blood flow and solute load.

4. Renal Tubular Absorptive Capacity for sodium and chloride ions also increases by 50% due to high level of steroid hormones secreted by the placenta and the adrenal cortex.

5. Clearance Rate of substances like creatinine, urea etc. increases; therefore the plasma creatinine and plasma urea values decrease during pregnancy.

6. Glycosuria, is a common physiological phenomenon during pregnancy.

7. Proteinuria occurs due to increase in excretion of proteins.

8. Water Balance. During later months of pregnancy excess of water is retained due to:

- *Decreased protein concentration*, specially albumin (proteinuria) leading to decreased colloidal osmotic pressure, and
- Retention of sodium.

9. Acid-base Balance. Hyperventilation during pregnancy results in respiratory alkalosis. Kidneys, therefore, compensate for it by excreting more HCO_3^- ions in the urine.

- Respiratory alkalosis (slight rise in pH) shifts the haemoglobin-oxygen dissociation curve of maternal blood to left.
- Slight rise in pH of blood stimulates the formation of 2,3-DPG, which shifts the Hb-oxygen dissociation curve to the right and facilitates oxygen transfer to the foetus.
- Decreased pCO_2 of maternal blood facilitates transfer of CO_2 from foetus to the mother.

VII. Gastrointestinal System Changes

1. GIT Secretions. Hypochlorhydria is very common due to decreased gastric secretion.

2. GIT Motility decreases under the influence of hormones resulting in delayed gastric emptying

3. Gallbladder Functions. Gall bladder increases in size and empties its contents at a very slow rate.

4. Liver Functions are also altered during pregnancy. The fibrinogen synthesis increases and albumin decreases thus plasma A:G ratio is also altered.

5. Morning Sickness. Anorexia, nausea and vomiting are very common in early pregnancy (first trimester) especially in the morning hours hence known as morning sickness. The cause for the morning sickness is not known.

6. Glucose Tolerance Curve also shows disturbances. It becomes diabetic type due to glucose being rapidly absorbed from the intestine.

VIII. Metabolic Changes

1. The Basal Metabolic Rate (BMR) of the pregnant woman increases by about 15% during later half of the pregnancy.

2. Protein Metabolism. When the diet is balanced and adequate then there is nitrogen retention and positive nitrogen balance. The proteins are deposited in the uterus, breast, in the foetus and in the placenta.

3. Carbohydrate Metabolism shows following changes:

- Blood glucose level increases due to rapid absorption from the gut.
- *Glycosuria* is of common occurrence due to increase in GFR and decrease in renal threshold for glucose.
- *Hepatic glycogen* level decreases.
- Ketosis may occur due to anorexia and excessive vomiting.
- Hyperplasia of β cells of islets of Langerhans of the pancreas occurs leading to increased level of insulin.

4. Fat Metabolism. About 3–4 kg of fat is deposited in the body during pregnancy. There occurs an increase in plasma concentration of cholesterol, phospholipids and triglycerides.

5. Mineral Metabolism depicts following changes:

- ***Calcium and phosphorus.*** In normal pregnancy mother retains about 50 g of extra calcium and 30–40 g of phosphorus. These are deposited in the foetus and also retained in the mother stores (skeleton). These stores act as reservoir for extra demand of Ca^{2+} during lactation. During pregnancy deficiency of calcium occurs, because normally its absorption is poor. Therefore, dietary supplimentation of calcium is very important along with vitamin D.
- ***Iron metabolism.*** Iron requirement tremendously increases during pregnancy and lactation as:
  - About 375 mg of iron is needed for foetal blood formation, and 600 mg (extra) is needed to form mother's own blood and cell mass.
  - During pregnancy non-haemoglobin store of iron varies from 100 to 700 mg.
  - Vitamin K should be supplimented to mother's diet to prevent excessive haemorrhage at the time of delivery.

IX. Endocrine System Changes

Almost all the endocrine glands of the mother react substantially during pregnancy. Firstly due to increased metabolic load on the mother and secondly in response to the hormones produced by the placenta and foetus.

1. Anterior Pituitary. The anterior pituitary gland increases in size by 50% and shows hyperplasia of lactotropes. The anterior pituitary hormones show following changes:

- ***Prolactin.*** Maternal prolactin level increases progressively throughout the pregnancy under the influence of high level of oestrogen (Fig 9.4-7E).

- ***ACTH.*** The plasma concentration of ACTH increases.
- ***Human growth hormone*** by maternal anterior pituitary decreases. This is due to suppression by the chorionic isoform (HCS) of growth hormone.
- ***Gonadotropins and sex hormones.*** Under the influence of high concentration of oestrogen and progesterone during pregnancy the secretion of follicular stimulating hormone (FSH) and luteinizing hormone (LH) from maternal anterior pituitary is suppressed. Therefore, low concentration of FSH and LH inhibits the maturation of graafian follicles in the ovaries.
- ***TSH*** concentration also rises.

2. Posterior Pituitary

- ***Oxytocin*** secretion is inhibited during pregnancy due to high levels of oestrogen and progesterone, but its levels increase during labour.
- ***ADH*** level also increases during pregnancy.

3. Thyroid. The size and secretory activity of thyroid gland increases during pregnancy.

- ***Thyroid binding globulin*** increases which in turn increases the bound fraction of T_3 and T_4. Plasma level of free T_4 remains unchanged. Increased iodide uptake, BMR, and resting pulse during pregnancy are indicators of increased thyroid activity.

4. Parathyroid Functions

- Parathyroid glands show an increase in its size and parathyroid hormone (PTH) secretion.
- Raised level of PTH increases the active form of Vitamin D_3 (1,25 $(OH)_2$ cholecalciferol) and vitamin D_3 binding protein.
- Increased PTH helps in absorption of calcium from the gut and decreases excretion through kidneys; and thereby fullfils the increased requirement of calcium during pregnancy.
- The foetal calcium concentration is more than the maternal levels.

5. Adrenal Cortex. The maternal adrenal glands get enlarged during pregnancy and also there is increase in the width of zona fasciculata. It serves following functions:

- Increased concentration of glucocorticoids is responsible for fat deposition in the adipose tissue and appearance of stria.
- Aldosterone secretion increases progressively and reaches upto 6–8 folds at term. This occurs due to natriuretic effect of progesterone and atrial natriuretic peptide (ANP).
- Normal pregnancy is also associated with increased levels of angiotensinogen, renin and several angiotensins including angiotensin II.
- Other mineral corticoids and deoxycorticosteroid are increased several thousand folds to maintain Na^+ balance and plasma volume.

6. Pancreas. As already mentioned in carbohydrate metabolism, there is β cell hyperplasia leading to increased level of insulin. However, maternal tissue sensitivity to insulin is variable during pregnancy. It increases in first half and decreases in the second half of pregnancy (insulin resistance).

X. Changes in the Skin

1. Hyperpigmentation occurs on the face (butterfly pattern known as chloasma), areola, nipple and midline of abdomen (lineaalba) extending from pubic symphysis to xiphisternum. The hyperpigmentation is related to increased secretion of ACTH and MSH during pregnancy.

2. Stria Gravidarum. These are linear scars present on the lower abdomen due to stretching of skin.

XI. Psychological Changes

The nervous system shows mild changes in the form of: craving for particular types of food item, alterations in the behaviour, emotions and mood. In few cases true psychosis may also develop but cause is not known.

PHYSIOLOGY OF PARTURITION

Parturition is the process by which baby is born. It involves preparation for child birth, act of child birth and recovery from child birth. The uterine myometrium and cervix play an important role for this process. Therefore, a knowledge about the functional anatomy of these structures is mandatory to understand the physiology of parturition.

Functional Anatomy

Uterine Myometrium

The characteristic feature of myometrium is that it consists of two layers of smooth muscle fibres, which are arranged in closely interwoven bundles embedded in the matrix surrounding the blood vessels. The smooth muscle cells are linked with adjacent muscle cells through gap junctions. The number of gap junctions determine the excitability state of the myometrium. The matrix mainly consists of collagen fibres.

The Cervix

It predominantly consists of collagen fibres and ground substance. The ground substance is composed of glucosans such as hyaluronic acid, dermatan sulphate and chondroitin sulphate.

Mechanics of Parturition

From the functional point of view mechanics of parturition mainly involves:

- uterine contractions and
- cervical dilatation.

Uterine Contractions

The uterus, which remains quiescent during period of pregnancy becomes progressively more and more excitable towards the end of pregnancy, until finally it begins strong rhythmical contractions with such a force that expel the foetus.

The uterine activity in a pregnant woman can be studied by recording amniotic fluid pressure changes and intrauterine pressure changes during pregnancy and labour. The characterstic features of uterine activity are:

- ***Upto 30th week (7 months)*** of pregnancy there is very little uterine activity. The uterus undergoes periodic episodes of weak and slow rhythmic contractions called *Braxton-Hicks contractions.*
- ***After 30th week***, the activity gradually increases. The characteristics of these contractions are:
  - *Start of contraction.* The uterine contractions during labour start at the top of the fundus of the uterus and spread on to the body part.
  - *Force of contractions* is high in the fundus and body part of the uterus and comparatively weak in the lower segment near the cervix.
  - *Frequency of contractions* in early labour only once in 30 mintues (1/30 min) and as labour progresses it increases to one in 3 min (1/3 min).
  - *Pressure during contractions* may rise upto 30–35 mmHg and
  - *Period of relaxation* follows each contraction.
  - *Type of contraction.* Uterine contractions are intermittent and are beneficial for the foetus otherwise strong and continuous contractions sometimes impedes blood supply through placenta and would cause foetal death.

Control or Regulation of Uterine Contractility The exact cause of increased uterine activity is not known, but few factors which lead towards parturition are: progressive hormonal changes that cause increased excitability of uterine musculature and progressive mechanical changes. (For details see page 877).

Cervical Dilatation

Throughout pregnancy cervix remains as a rigid structure, but at the time of parturition certain structural and biochemical changes occur and the cervix becomes soft. This is known as cervical ripening. It allows the cervix to stretch when uterine contractions start.

The changes in the cervix which are responsible for its dilatation are:

- Breakdown of collagen fibres,
- Increase in amount of hyaluronic acid, having high water retaining capacity, and
- Decrease in amount of dermatan sulphate.

These changes are mainly under the influence of prostaglandins.

Phases of Parturition

The period of parturition extends from conception to restoration of fertility for the next conception.

For successful child birth, the myometrium and cervix show ordered sequence of events, as discussed in mechanics of parturition. These changes have been divided into four phases: phase 0, 1, 2 and 3 (Fig. 9.4-12).

Phase 0 of Parturition

- This phase corresponds to period of pregnancy, i.e. it extends from conception to initiation of the process of child birth. The average duration of human pregnancy is 270 days from the day of fertilization of the ovum. Since this day cannot be accurately determined, the first day (date) of the LMP is the day from which the duration of pregnancy and expected date of delivery is conventionally calculated and when counted in this way the average period of gestation is 284 days.
- Throughout this phase uterus is quiescent and cervix remains rigid.
- This phase in under the control of progesterone.
- Myometrial tranquility during this phase is attributed to:
  - Depressed uterine smooth muscle contractile response due to decreased intracellular calcium in myometrial smooth muscle cells.
  - Increased degradation of endogenously produced uterotonins by enzymes; e.g. prostaglandins by prostaglandin dehydrogenase, oxytocin by oxytocinase and histamine by diamine oxidase.
  - Inhibition of myometrial cell contractile signal propagation due to sparse oxytocin receptors and paucity of gap junctions between the myometrial cells.

Phase I of Parturition

This phase is the period of preparation for the labour. It commences in the final days of gestation and extends up to the onset of labour. It is difficult to predict the exact date of onset of labour. It may occur any time between 37th and 40th weeks of gestation. During this phase myometrium becomes responsive to oxytocin and cervix undergoes a biochemical remodelling called cervical ripening. Thus, in this phase uterine quiescence is suspended and contractile competency of the uterus is increased and cervix is made ready for dilatation.

Increased Myometrial Excitability to Oxytocin Near Term is attributed to:

- An increase in number of oxytocin receptors on the cells of the uterine smooth muscle during the final weeks of pregnancy.
- An increase in the number and size of gap junctions between the myometrial cells.
- Increased synthesis of contractile proteins in the myometrial cells.

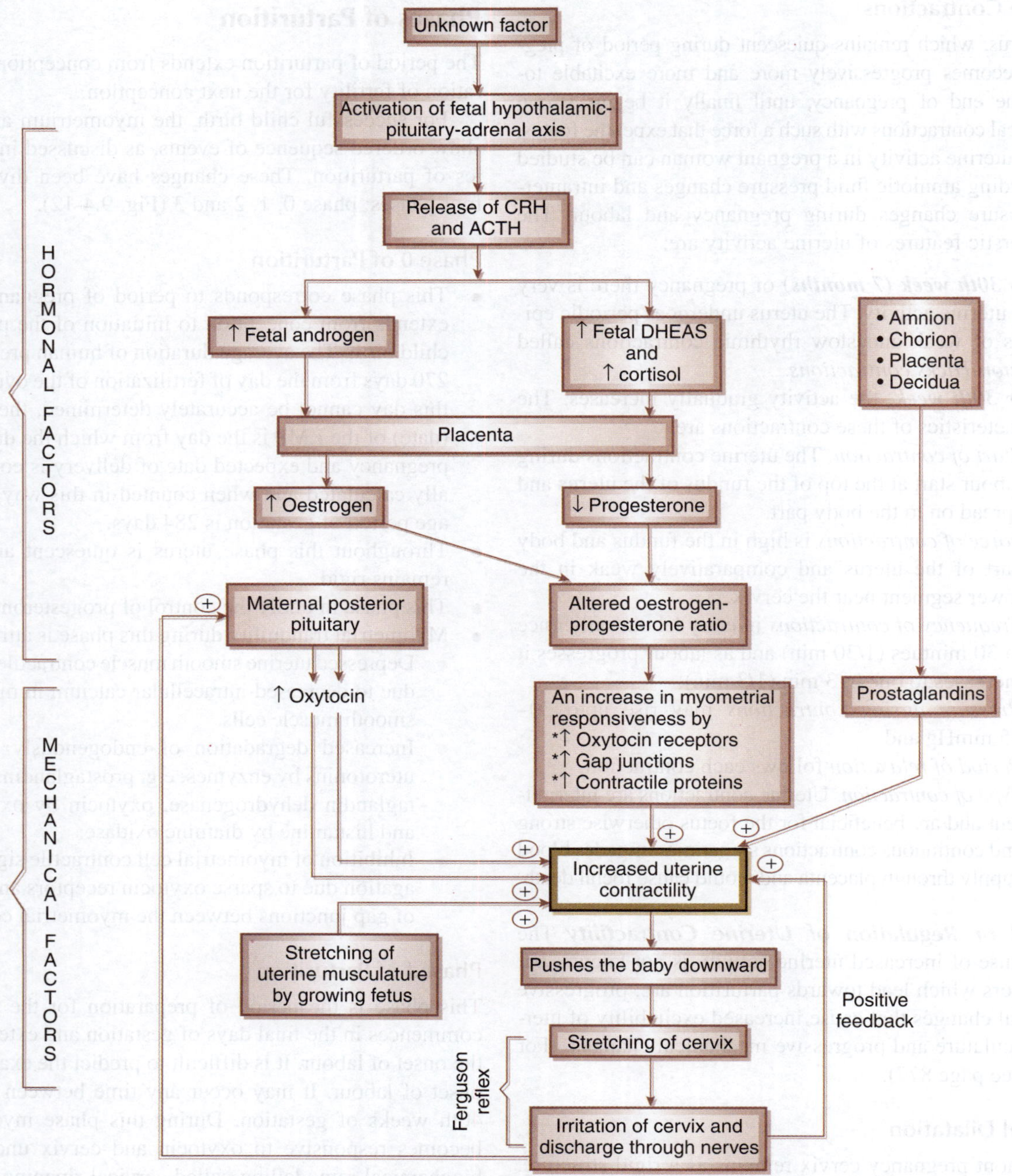

FIGURE 9.4-12 Summary of control of parturition depicting role of hormonal and mechanical factors.

Cervical Ripening, i.e. cervix becomes soft and yielding due to following biochemical changes:

- *Breakdown and rearrangement of collagen fibres*
- Alteration in relative amounts of glycosaminoglycans, i.e. an increase in the content of the hyaluronic acid and decrease in dermatan sulphate content. The above changes in cervix are mediated by the prostaglandins under the influence of oestrogen.

Onset of Labour. The onset of labour marks the end of phase I and beginning of phase II of parturition. The exact cause of onset of labour in human is still not certain. The possible hypothesis is discussed (see page 877).

Phase II of Parturition

This is a phase of active labour. It extends from the onset of labour to delivery of conceptus. It is characterized by powerful uterine contractions which bring about progressive cervical dilatation, foetal descent and finally expulsion of foetus and placenta. This phase is further divided into three stages of labour: stage first, second and third.

Stages of Labour

• ***First Stage*** of labour is characterized by:

- Strong contractions of upper uterine segment which drive the foetus downwards with each contraction.
- Cervical effacement and progressive dilatation, until it is fully dilated to form a birth canal by merging with the lower uterine segment.
- This stage is said to be over when the diameter of external os of cervix is large enough (about 10 cm) to allow the head of foetus to pass into vagina.
- This stage lasts for 8–24 hours in the first pregnancy, but its duration decreases in multipara.

• ***Second Stage of Labour*** is characterized by:

- Fully dilated cervix.
- Rupture of amniotic membranes and loss of amniotic fluid through vagina.
- Strong and more frequent uterine contractions which in association with abdominal muscle contractions (bearing down pains due to neurogenic reflexes from spinal cord to abdominal muscle) lead on to expulsion of foetus through the dilated vagina.
- Duration of this stage varies from one minute (in multipara) to about one hour (in first pregnancy).

• ***Third Stage*** is the stage of separation and expulsion of placenta.

- During the next 10-45 minutes after the birth of baby, the uterus contracts to small size resulting in separation of placenta from its implantation site. Separation of placenta causes bleeding due to opening up of maternal sinuses. The arrangement of smooth muscle fibres in myometrium is such (form figure of 8 around uterine vessels) that their contraction causes constriction of blood vessels and bleeding stops. The prostaglandins released also have some vasoconstrictor effect.
- On an average about 350 ml of blood is lost in normal pregnancy. In some women, uterus fails to contract strongly causing risk of severe bleeding. In such cases, the uterus can be induced to contract by injection of synthetic oxytocin and ergometrine.

Phase III of Parturition

This is the phase of parturient recovery. It begins after the delivery of conceptus and extends till fertility is restored. Oxytocin and endothelin are important hormones regulating the processes which occur during this phase. This phase is characterized by:

- Uterine contraction and retraction to prevent puerperal haemorrhage
- Initiation of lactation and milk ejection to facilitate breastfeeding
- Involution of uterus (i.e. decrease in size and weight) takes place during first 4 to 5 weeks after parturition. Lactation hastens this process.
- The raw surface of endothelium is re-epithelialized and fertility is restored to normal

Control of Parturition

The mechanisms responsible for onset of labour in human are still not understood exactly. However, it has been postulated that parturition in human being closely mimic bovine parturition which has seen reasonably clear in the form of sheep model of parturition. Though the fundamental biomolecular processes of parturition are expected to be similar in all mammalian species, a few important endocrinal differences exist between human and sheep pregnancy before the initiation of parturition. The control of parturition includes the role of (Fig. 9.4-12):

- Hormonal factors and
- Mechanical factors.

A. Hormonal Factors

The hormonal changes that initiate the parturition and that cause increased excitability of uterine musculature are:

1. Activation of Foetal Hypothalamic-pituitary-adrenal Axis. Recently it has been hypothesized that the initial signals for the onset of labour comes from the foetus only. Experimental destruction of foetal pituitary in sheep has been shown to delay the onset of labour.

From sheep model of parturition, it has been postulated that in human some unknown factors are involved in CRH secretion in the foetus resulting in an increase in ACTH secretion few days before parturition. ACTH causes foetal adrenal cortex to secrete large amount of androgens which are converted to oestrogen in the placenta; and DHEAS and cortisol, which may inhibit the conversion of foetal pregnenolone to progesterone.

The above changes lead to an altered oestrogen-progesterone ratio.

2. Role of Altered Oestrogen–progesterone Ratio. The oestrogen and progesterone are secreted progressively in increasing amounts by the placenta during pregnancy. Beginning in the seventh month of pregnancy, the rate of progesterone secretion remains constant whereas the rate of oestrogen secretion continues to rise as described in step I. The progesterone reduces while the oestrogen increases the contractility of the uterine smooth muscle. Therefore, it has been suggested that as the ratio of oestrogen to progesterone is increased during the final week of pregnancy, the uterus begins to contract. The altered oestroen-progesterone ratio also causes:

- An increase in release of oxytocin from maternal posterior pituitary,
- An increase in number of oxytocin receptors in myometrium,
- An increase in prostagladin synthesis and

- An increase in synthesis of myometrial contractile proteins.

3. Role of Oxytocin and Prostaglandins. The altered ratio of oestrogen–progesterone in late gestation seems to be responsible for increase in the number of oxytocin receptors and also for more release of oxytocin from the posterior pituitary of mother. As discussed above the uterine excitability to oxytocin is increased in late gestation due to increase in oxytocin receptors, increase in gap junctions and increase in synthesis of contractile proteins in the myometrial cells.

It has been suggested that the altered oestrogen–progesterone ratio leads to prostaglandin synthesis in human pregnancy from the placenta, amnion, chorion and decidua. The prostagladins enhance the force of oxytocin induced uterine contractions. Administration of drugs like aspirin or indomethacin, which inhibit prostaglandin synthesis, may interfere with the process of labour.

B. Mechanical Factors

Mechanical factors that increase the contractility of uterus include:

1. Stretch of Urterine Musculature usually increases their own contractility (myogenic theory). During pregnancy movements of the foetus cause stretching. As the pregnancy advances with growing foetus stretch further increases leading on to uterine contractility.

2. Positive Feedback Effect. Stretching and irritation of cervix is particularly important in eliciting uterine contractions. The exact mechanism is not known but possibly may be because of positive feedback effect through initiation of the reflex increase in uterine contractility as depicted in Fig. 9.4-12:

The positive feedback mechanism continues until the baby is expelled.

3. Role of Ferguson Reflex. Once labour is started, the uterine contractions dilate the ripened cervix. The cervical dilatation in turn sets of signals in afferent nerves that increase oxytocin secretion from the posterior pituitary. This is called Ferguson reflex.

Clinical application. The obstetricians frequently induce labour by rupturing the membrane so that the head of the baby stretches the cervix more forcefully than usual and thus initiates it, leading to initiation of positive feedback effect and Ferguson reflex.

Summary

The control of parturition is summarized in Fig. 9.4-12.

APPLIED ASPECTS

Miscarriage is defined as pregnancy loss before 20 weeks of gestation, and the medical term is spontaneous abortion. The cause of pregnancy loss may occur in conceptus or in the micro environment of maternal reproductive tract at the time of conception. The causes of recurrent pregnancy loss include:

- Parental chromosome transclocations
- Structural uterine abnormalities such as longitudinal septa and uterine adhesions
- Endocrinal disorders
- Polycystic ovary syndrome
- Thyroid dysfunctions, poorly controlled diabetes
- Autoimmune conditions

Preterm Labour is onset of labour before 37 weeks of gestation. The risk factors and potential mechanism of preterm labour include:

- Multiple gestations and excessive amniotic fluid volume excessively stretches the myometrium may stimulate muscle activity
- Intrauterine infection is associated with high level of cytokine, interleukin-1β, interleukin-6, TNF α and prostaglandins. All these substances stimulate myometrium
- Thrombin recently considered to be an extremely potent uterotonic agent responsible for preterm labour. The increased production of thrombin accompanies bleeding in pregnancy is associated with preterm labour.

Preecclampsia has been defined as triad of hypertension, proteinuria and edema in pregnant women. Preecclampsia typically occurs in third trimester of pregnancy. The presentation of this disorder occurs as:

- *Central nervous system* involvement can manifest as severe headache, visual changes, seizers, stroke and blindness
- *Renal involvement* almost occurs in all cases and can manifest as proteinuria, oligouria or renal failure.
- *Oedema fluid* can accumulate in many sites including hands and feet, face, lungs
- *Hepatic dysfunction* results in hemolysis, deranged liver function tests and low platelet count.

Mechanism of Pathogenesis of Preecclampsia. It was observed that the cytotrophoblast fails to properly invade the maternal blood vessels in preecclampsia. No single mechanism has proven to be wholly responsible for this condition, there are several initiating factors for endothelial dysfunction

Recently it is found that soluble vascular endothelial growth factor (sVEGF) and placental growth factor are markedly elevated in the serum a few weeks before the symptoms. The explanation is that placenta in preecclamptic pregnancies secrete increased amount of δFLt-1 (the soluble antagonist to VEGF) which inhibit the development of small blood vessels.

Treatment. The ultimate treatment of this condition is delivery of pregnancy. If mother is medically supported through timely delivery and postpartum recovery, all deranged physiology will revert back to the normal provided no permanent tissue damage has occurred.

Chapter 9.5

Physiology of Lactation

DEVELOPMENT AND FUNCTIONAL ANATOMY OF BREAST

Breastfeeding is the characteristic feature of all the mammals, including human beings. It has evolved as the best method of nourishing the newborn. The mammary glands (the secondary sex organs) play an important role in lactation process.

Development of Breast

Mammary glands are present in both the sexes; in males they remain rudimentary but in females they are well developed after puberty. The different phases of its development are described:

Breasts in Intrauterine Life (Embryogenesis). At 18–19 weeks of gestation mammary glands develop from a thickened mass of epithelium of the epidermis known as mammary bud (Fig. 9.5-1A).

- From this thickened mass about 16–20 solid outgrowths arise and project into the dermis (Fig. 9.5-1B).
- Then the thickened mass as well as these outgrowths are canalized (Fig. 9.5-1C) to form the rudimentary duct system.
- The secretory element of the gland is formed by proliferation of the terminal part of the outgrowths. It occurs at puberty only.
  - The proximal end of each duct opens into a common pit formed by cavitation of the thickened mass (Fig. 9.5-1D); later on growth of underlying mesodermal tissue pushes the wall of the pit outwards as nipple (Fig. 9.5-1E).

Breasts at Birth. At birth the mammary glands are rudimentary consisting of tiny nipple and few ducts radiating from it.

Breasts at Puberty. From birth to puberty the mammary glands remain quiescent. During puberty following changes occur:

- ***At Thelarche,*** i.e. at the time of puberty (9–11 years of age), before the start of menses. The breast starts developing and get enlarged. During this stage, only duct system proliferates and shows branching.
- ***At Menarche,*** i.e. after the onset of menses, cyclic growth of mammary glands (period of growth followed by quiescence) occurs in each menstrual cycle. The growth period further corresponds to phases of menstrual cycle.

- ***In proliferative phase*** (or oestrogen phase), the duct cells proliferate and continue throughout rest of the cycle.
- ***In luteal phase*** (progestational phase) progesterone stimulates the proliferation of terminal ductules, so there is formation of glandular tissue.
- ***At menstruation*** (bleeding phase) there occurs no proliferation of duct cells as well as of glandular tissue, because levels of both oestrogen and progesterone

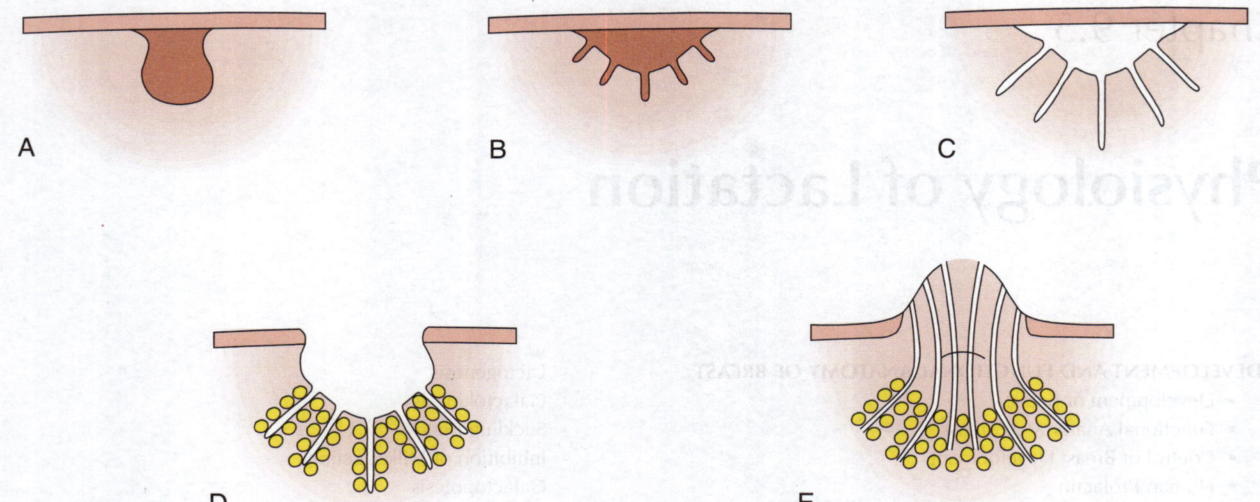

FIGURE 9.5-1 Stages of development of breast in intrauterine life: (**A**) formation of mammary bud; (**B**) outgrowths of mammary bud; (**C**) canalization of outgrowths; (**D**) formation of secretory element and formation of common pit; and (**E**) formation of nipple.

are lowered. Hence, this period is called quiescence period.

With the onset of next menstrual cycle further growth occurs. Thus, there is a progressive growth of breast in successive cycles, along with modelling of the breast by fat deposition in the adipose tissue.

Breasts in Pregnancy During pregnancy remarkable growth of both ductal and glandular systems occurs. It is only during first pregnancy that glandular tissue develops fully.

- ***In first half of pregnancy,*** the duct system proliferates and shows extensive sprouting and branching along with the growth of stroma and deposition of fat.
- ***In second half of pregnancy*** there is enormous growth of glandular tissue.

The extensive growth of mammary glands during pregnancy is known as *mammogenesis* or preparation of breast for lactation.

Breasts during Lactation. After child birth the alveolar cells get enlarged and distended and start forming milk (lactogenesis).

Involution of Breast. After a normal period of lactation (7 to 9 months), the alveolar epithelium undergoes apoptosis and glands revert back to prepregnant stage.

Functional Anatomy of Breast

Gross Anatomy. The fully developed breast is a soft, rounded, elevated structure present over the pectoral region, having central dark pigmented area (areola). The central part of areola, projected above the surface, is called nipple.

Histological Structure. Each mammary gland is covered by overlying skin and underlying it discrete masses of

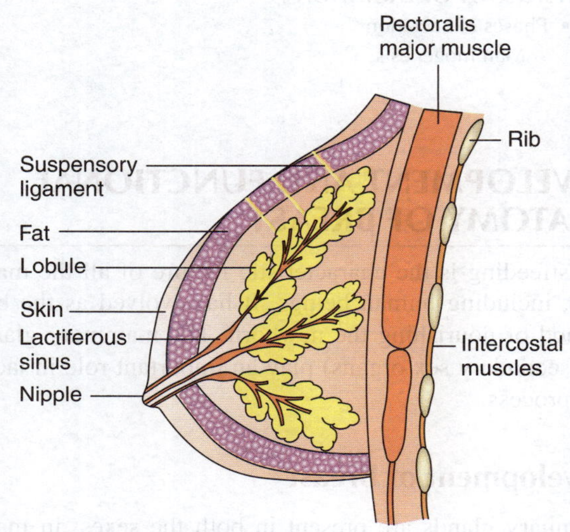

FIGURE 9.5-2 Structure of mammary gland.

glandular tissue is present in the connective tissue consisting of stroma and adipose tissue (Fig. 9.5-2).

- ***The fascia*** covering the mammary gland is connected by suspensory ligaments to overlying skin and underlying muscle.
- ***The mammary glands*** consist of 15–20 lobes and each lobe has a number of lobules.
- ***The glandular tissue*** mainly consists of alveoli having secretory cells.
- ***The secretions*** from these cells are poured by apocrine manner and by exocytosis into the ducts (lactiferous ducts). About 15–20 ducts open at the summit of nipple, and just before opening lactiferous ducts show a dilatation called lactiferous sinus.
- ***The smaller ductules*** are lined by single layer of columnar epithelial cells whereas large ducts are

lined by one or two layers of cells and near the opening at the nipple these are lined by squamous cells.

- ***Around the alveoli,*** ductules and lobules are present in myoepithelial cells (Fig. 9.5-2). They squeeze the contents and pour their secretions into the ductules.
- ***Electron microscopically,*** the secretory cells contain both rough and smooth surface endoplasmic reticulum, numerous mitochondria, prominent golgi apparatus and lysosomes. The proteins are present in the cytoplasm as membrane bound vesicles and fat is stored as large globules.

Control of Breast Development and Growth

Various hormones necessary for full growth and development of mammary glands at various stages are (Fig. 9.5-3):

1. Oestrogen. It is primarily responsible for ductal growth and fat deposition. It also causes thickening of nipples.

2. Progesterone. The development of glandular tissue mainly depends on progesterone. Both oestrogen and progesterone work best with co-operation of hypothalamopituitary-adrenal cortex axis.

3. Other Hormones including growth hormone, thyroxine, cortisol and insulin enhance overall growth and development of mammary glands at all stages.

4. Corpus Luteal and Placental Hormones, particularly oestrogen, progesterone, human chorionic somatomammotropic hormone (HCS, or HPL) are essential for further growth of breast during pregnancy.

5. Prolactin. It is another very important hormone for development of breasts during pregnancy and lactation. It acts on mammary gland tissue which has already grown under the influence of oestrogen and progesterone. It needs to be discussed in detail.

Human Prolactin

Structure, Secretion and Plasma Concentration

Structure and Secretion. Human prolactin is a single peptide chain, secreted by acidophilic cells of anterior pituitary gland.

Plasma Concentration. The prolactin secretion is pulsatile, shows diurnal variations (secretion increases about

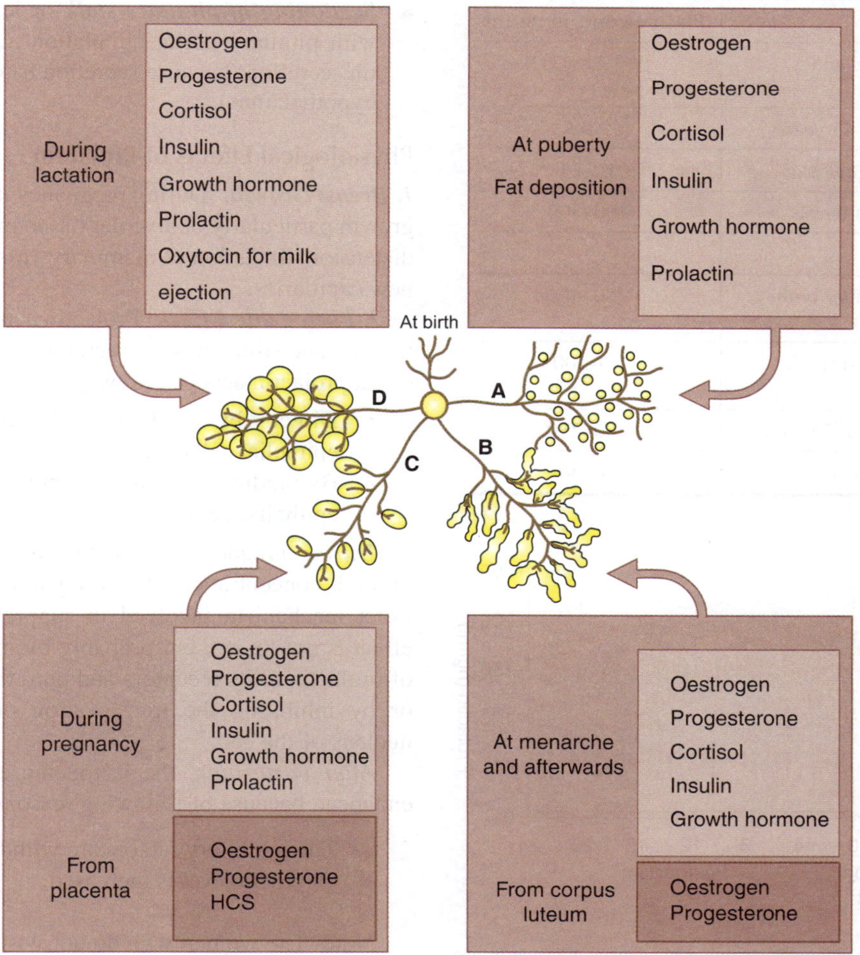

FIGURE 9.5-3 Schematic diagram of hormonal control of breast development during different stages: **(A)** at puberty; **(B)** at menarche and afterwards; **(C)** during pregnancy; and **(D)** during lactation.

one hour after the onset of sleep and continues throughout the sleep period). Its basal average value varies in different conditions (Table 9.5-1).

During pregnancy prolactin secretion starts rising from 8th weeks onwards and peak value (200–400 ng/ml) is reached at term. The sources of prolactin during pregnancy are placenta, amniotic fluid and maternal anterior pituitary gland. The prolactin secretion during pregnancy and during lactation is affected by *oestrogen*. Prolactin secretion parallels with secretion of oestrogen, i.e. 7–8th weeks gestation onwards oestrogen secretion rises along with prolactin (Fig. 9.4-7). This is due to oestrogen inhibition of hypothalamic prolactin inhibitory factor (PIF) (Fig. 9.5-4).

Control of Prolactin Secretion

Hypothalamic Control. Secretion of prolactin from anterior pituitary is controlled by hypothalamus. A PIF formed in the arcuate nucleus of hypothalamus is transported through hypothalamohypophyseal portal system to anterior pituitary where it checks the synthesis and release of prolactin.

PIF has been identified as dopamine. Therefore, the substances like dopamine agonists (bromocriptine) and serotonin antagonists block the secretion of prolactin. Therapeutically bromocriptine is used during postpartum period for reducing prolactin level to inhibit lactation.

TABLE 9.5.1 Showing Range of Plasma Concentration of Prolactin

Condition	Plasma conc. in ng/ml
• Prepubertal period and after menopause	2–8
• Fertile period (16–45 years)	9–14
• Early pregnancy (8 weeks)	10–25
• Late pregnancy (at term)	200–500
• Lactation period	
• Immediately after birth to 10 days	200–400
• 10–90 days (1st week-3 months)	70–200
• 90–180 days (3–6 months)	100–250
• 6 month - 1 year	30–40

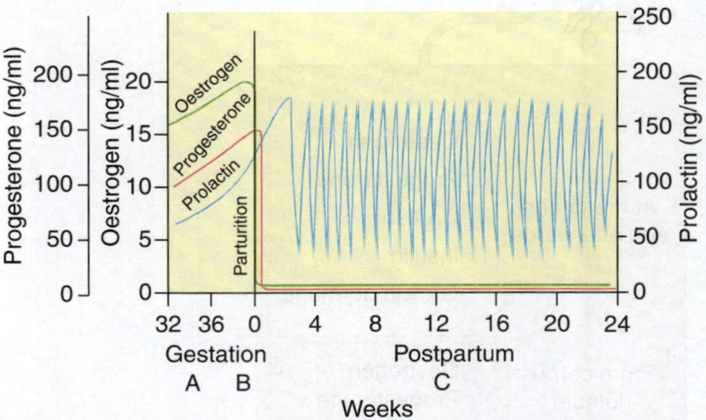

FIGURE 9.5-4 Changes in rate of secretion of oestrogen, progesterone and prolactin: (**A**) in late pregnancy; (**B**) before parturition, and (**C**) during postpartum period.

Factors Enhancing the Release of Prolactin are:

- ***TRH.*** There is prolactin releasing factor for prolactin, but thyrotropin releasing hormone (TRH) also causes release of prolactin from anterior pituitary.
- ***Stress.*** Psychological stress, physiological stress (exercise, pregnancy and lactation) and pathological stress increase prolactin secretion.
- ***Substances*** like; dopamine antagonists (phenothiazine and tranquilizers), adrenergic blockers, serotonin agonists stimulate prolactin release.
- ***Role of oxytocin.*** Oxytocin acts directly on the acidophilic cells of anterior pituitary to stimulate prolactin release.
- ***Sectioning of pituitary stalk*** or lesion which interfere with pituitary portal circulation also increases prolactin secretion (because secretion is tonically inhibited by hypothalamus).

Physiological Effects of Prolactin

1. Breast Growth. During pregnancy it increases the breast growth particularly of alveolar tissue in the form of alveolar distension, dilatation of mammary vessels and formation of new capillaries.

2. Lactogenic Effect. Prolactin acts on the alveolar epithelium and stimulates the secretory activity. For lactogenic effect prolactin acts by two ways:

- Directly by attaching on the surface of the alveolar epithelial cells and
- By binding on to the receptors on the membrane of epithelial cells.

During pregnancy the lactogenic effect is suppressed by high concentration of oestrogen and progesterone. The exact mechanism involved in suppressing the lactogenic effect is not known but probably by inhibiting the binding of prolactin to its receptors and onto the surface of the cell or by inhibiting the translocation of prolactin into the nucleus of the cell.

After parturition, the lactogenic effect of prolactin is enhanced because of following reasons:

- The inhibitory factors are withdrawn,
- Oxytocin level is increased.

Note- The women who do not wish to feed their babies or when baby dies immediately after birth, in these situations, oestrogen is administered to stop lactation.

3. Suppression of Ovarian Cycle in Nursing Mothers. Prolactin inhibits the secretion of gonadotropin releasing hormone from hypothalamus. Therefore, gonadotropin (FSH and LH) secretion from anterior pituitary also decreases. Thus in nursing mothers due to low levels of gonadotropins the ovarian cyclic changes do not occur.

Applied Aspects

Chiari-Frommel syndrome. Though this is a rare condition; it is associated with: (i) persistence of lactation (galactorrhoea), and (ii) amenorrhoea in women, who do not nurse their babies after delivery. Sometimes it is also associated with genital atrophy. The reason is persistent release of prolactin causing suppression of FSH and LH.

Galactorrhoea refers to secretion of breast milk in states not associated with nursing. It occurs due to hyperprolactenemia or hypersensitivity of the breast to normal circulating levels of prolactin. The common causes of hyperprolactinaemia are:

- Medication interfering with dopamine action
- Hyperthyroidism

Treatment: Galactorrhoea can be suppressed by use of dopamine agonist

Chromophobe cell tumour of pitutary gland is characterized by galactorrhoea and high level of prolactin in nonpregnant women.

PHYSIOLOGY OF LACTATION

Phases of Lactation

The physiology of lactation can be divided into four phases:

- Preparation of breast for milk secretion (mammogenesis),
- Synthesis and secretion of milk (lactogenesis),
- Expulsion of milk (galactokinesis) and
- Maintenance of lactation (galactopoiesis).

Mammogenesis

During pregnancy. The breast develops fully and is prepared for milk secretion after delivery (see page 866).

Lactogenesis

Stages of Lactogenesis The process of milk secretion occurs in two stages:

Stage I. In later few weeks of pregnancy, small amount of fluid is secreted in the alveolar cells. It is called colostrum. Its rate of secretion is only 1/100th as that of milk secretion in the postpartum period. Its composition is same as that of human milk except that fats are absent. The stage I secretion occurs due to high plasma levels of prolactin and placental HCS. But due to suppressive lactogenic action of oestrogen and progesterone, free flow of milk never occurs during pregnancy (Fig. 9.5-4).

Stage II. It is the initiation of lactation after child birth. Immediately after the baby is born, sudden loss of oestrogen and progesterone secretion by the placenta allows the lactogenic effect of prolactin. In this stage:

- The secretion rate increases to 500–750 ml/day and
- In next 1–7 days, the breasts begin to secrete milk instead of colostrum.

Human Milk

Types of Human Milk. It is the secretion of mammary glands. Its nature and composition varies with postpartum period. Therefore, the human milk is of three types: colostrum, transition milk and mature milk.

1. ***Colostrum*** is deep yellow coloured fluid secreted by the mammary glands during first few days of postpartum period, it contains:
   - High protein contents (8.5 gm%), rich in immunoglobulins and lactoferrin and
   - Granular bodies (colostrum corpuscles)—consisting of alveolar cells and leucocytes loaded with fats.

   The colostrum is easily coagulated into solid masses.
2. ***Transition milk or intermediate milk.*** It is secreted from 6th day to 15th day of postpartum period. The nature and composition of the secretion changes from colostrum to mature milk. Hence it is called transition milk.
3. ***Mature milk*** is formed from 15th day of postpartum onwards and continues during the whole lactation period (7–9 months).

Composition of Human Milk. Human milk contains 88.5% water and about 11.5% solids. The solids include both organic and inorganic constituents. The composition of mature human milk, colostrum and cow's milk is shown in Table 9.5-2.

Note. Human milk is balanced diet as it contains first class proteins (caseinogen and lactalbumin), carbohydrates fat, mineral salts and vitamins. Therefore, it is an ideal food for the baby.

Formation of Milk. During lactation, the mammary glands are metabolically very active. The milk specific substances amino acids, fatty acids, glucose and Ca^{2+} etc. are derived from plasma into the alveolar cells. The various secretory processes involved in milk synthesis include: (i) fat synthesis and its secretion, (ii) ions and water secretion, (iii) transcytosis of immunoglobulins and other substances from interstitial spaces, and (iv) exocytosis. The hormones like growth hormone, thyroid hormone, parathyroid hormone, insulin and cortisol, of mother increase the capacity of the breast to secrete milk by providing necessary raw materials.

Expulsion of Milk or Galactokinesis. Though milk is secreted continuously into the alveoli of the breast, but it does not flow continuously from alveoli into the duct

TABLE 9.5-2 Composition of Colostrums, Mature Milk and Cow's Milk

Content	*Human Colostrum*	*Human milk*	*Cow's milk*
Water (g)	...	88	88
Lactose (g)	5.3	6.8	5.0
Proteins (g)	2.7	1.2	3.3
Fat (g)	2.9	3.8	3.1
Linoleic acid	...	8.3% of fat	1.65 of fat
Sodium (mg)	92	15	58
Potassium (mg)	55	55	138
Chloride (mg)	117	43	103
Calcium (mg)	31	33	125
Magnesium (mg)	4	4	12
Phosphorus (mg)	14	15	100
Vitamin A (μg)	89	53	34
Thiamine (μg)	15	16	42
Riboflavin (μg)	30	43	157
Nicotinic acid (μg)	75	172	85
Ascorbic acid (mg)	4.4	4.3	1.6

system. It depends upon the suckling reflex and some local mechanisms acting within the breast.

Suckling Reflex It is a neuroendocrinal reflex. The characteristic features and mechanism of suckling reflex (Fig. 9.5-5) are:

- When baby suckles, the sensory nerve endings or receptors located in skin of areola and nipple get stimulated.
- The sensory impulses are transmitted to the hypothalamus through, somatic nerves (from nipple and areola to spinal cord and then to hypothalamus). The activation of hypothalamus causes release of oxytocin and prolactin from pituitary gland.
- The oxytocin is carried to the breasts through blood, where it causes contraction of myoepithelial cells that surround the outer wall of the alveoli, thereby the milk is expressed from alveoli into the ducts at a pressure 10 to 20 mmHg. It is also aided by positive pressure applied by the baby by making an airtight connection around the nipple and then blowing its cheeks.

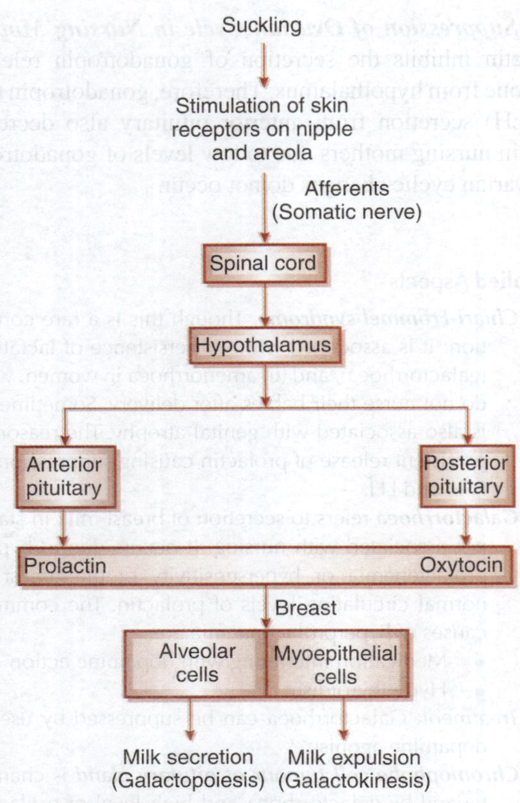

FIGURE 9.5-5 Mechanism of suckling reflex.

Therefore, when baby suckles first, it virtually receives no milk, then within 30 seconds to 1 minute suckling becomes effective and milk begins to flow. This process is called *milk ejection* or *milk expulsion* or *milk let down*.

Note. In case of engorgement of breasts after delivery (which is a very painful condition, suckling becomes difficult). Oxytocin administration leads to free flow of the milk.

- Another important observation is that suckling of one breast causes milk flow in the other breast also.
- Even stimuli such as sight, sound or crying of infant and thought of their infants also cause milk ejection, indicating the psychological component in the neuroendocrine reflex.

Inhibition of Milk Ejection

- Many psychogenic factors in the form of psychological stress, pain etc. inhibit milk ejection by inhibiting oxytocin release.
- Alcohol is also a potent inhibitor of oxytocin.

Maintenance of Milk Secretion or Galactopoiesis

Maintenance of milk secretion or galactopoiesis depends upon the surge in prolactin secretion. After few weeks of child birth, prolactin level falls to its basal value; however, in nursing mothers neuroendocrine reflex causes 10–20 fold surge in prolactin secretion that lasts for one hour (Fig. 9.5-4). Each time when baby suckles, the impulses from nipple and areolar receptors are transmitted by somatic nerves upto the hypothalamus, which cause 1–20 fold surge in prolactin secretion.

The amount of milk production is related to infant's demand.

Importance of Lactation

Breastfeeding is being advocated all over the world because of its advantages both for the baby as well as for the mother.

Advantages of Breastfeeding to the Baby

1. Balanced Diet. Human milk contains proteins, carbohydrates, fat, mineral salts (calcium and phosphorus) and vitamins. So, it is a natural balanced food for the newborn.

2. Protection against Infections. Human milk has high count of lymphocytes, neutrophils and macrophages and high content of lysozymes and immunoglobulins. All these substances due to antiinfection property confer nonspecific as well as specific immunity.

3. Easily Digestible. Human milk because of its following digestive properties can be easily digested by the newborn babies:

- Casein is easily digestible,
- Lactoferrin prevents iron overloading,
- Folate and cobalamin binding proteins assist in absorption of corresponding vitamins,
- Higher concentration of lactose promotes calcium absorption,
- Lipases assist in lipid digestion, because lipid digestion is poor in newborn babies.

4. Growth Factors. Growth promoting factors, like epidermal growth factor, insulin and somatomedin-C are present in the human milk.

5. Other Advantages of Breastfeeding to baby are:

- It is sterile,
- It is convenient to give at right temperature,
- It is inexpensive and
- Chances of allergy to breast milk are rare.

Advantages of Breastfeeding to the Mother

1. Lactational Amenorrhoea. Due to high plasma level of prolactin during lactation, there occurs suppression of FSH and LH. Therefore, after birth of the baby menstruation and ovulation do not start. The period of lactationalamenorrhoea is variable (3 months to 3 years). This is the natural way of contraception and birth spacing.

2. Involution of Uterus. The oxytocin released during each session of breastfeeding also acts on the uterine myometrium, and helps it to involute during postpartum period. The proper involution of uterus protects it against infections.

3. Protection against Breast Engorgement. Breastfeeding does not allow the milk to stagnate, thus preventing the breast engorgement, which is highly painful condition. The stagnant milk acts as a favourable medium for bacterial growth. Therefore breastfeeding protects against infection.

4. Protection against Obesity. Body fat is used for milk synthesis; therefore, there are less chances of becoming obese after pregnancy.

5. Emotional Bonding and psychological satisfaction is enhanced by breastfeeding.

6. Protection against Cancer. The chances of breast cancer are more in those women who have never borne children. This is related to the hormone oestrogen which is responsible for aetiology of breast cancer. Therefore, prolonged lactation provides protection against breast cancer.

Applied Aspects

Hormones and Carcinoma Breast

Breast Cancer is most common malignancy in women. About 35% of carcinoma of breast are estrogen-dependent. The risk of breast cancer is higher in prolonged ovarian hormonal exposure in the form of postmenopausal hormonal replacement therapy.

- About 10% breast cancer is familial, occurs due to mutation involving BRCA 1 and BRCA 2 tumour suppressing genes.
- In non familial breast cancers, molecular studies have identified abnormalities that involve oncogenes, ERBBZ & c-myc, the tumour suppressor gene TP53 and telemerase.
- Environmental factors include: delayed child bearing among better educated women, alcohol intake and smoking.

Treatment. Treatment of breast cancer depends on the stage of the disease at the time of diagnosis.

- Surgical options include, modified radical mastectomy or lumpectomy with local irradiation and chemotherapy (If lymph nodes are also involved)
- The symptoms of estrogen dependent breast carcinoma are relieved by decreasing estrogen secretion. Ovariactomy or tamoxifen (drug inhibiting action of estrogen-most widely used drug) produces remissions
  - Drugs that inhibit aromatase, act by inhibition of estrogen formation are more effective.

Gynecomastia. Breast development in male is called gynecomastia. It occurs due to increased circulating levels of estrogens.

- In newborns gynecomastia is most common, occurs due to transplacental passage of maternal estrogens
- At the time of puberty in normal boys and in men over the age of 50 years it occurs in mild form and is transient.
- In patients with estrogen secreting tumors, androgen resistance, as complication of estrogen therapy and many other conditions such as; eunuchoidism, hyperthyroidism, liver cirrhosis, digitalis therapy and in malnourished prisoners.

Chapter 9.6

Physiology of Contraception

INTRODUCTION
CONTRACEPTIVE METHODS IN FEMALES
- Spacing Methods
  - Rhythm Method
  - Barrier Methods
  - Chemical Methods
  - Intrauterine Contraceptive Devices
  - Lippes Loop
  - Copper T
- Terminal Methods
  - Surgical Methods
  - Tubectomy
  - Laparoscopic Occlusion
  - Medical Termination of Pregnancy
  - Dilatation and Curettage
  - Vacuum Aspiration
  - Prostaglandins
- Pregnancy Vaccines

CONTRACEPTIVE METHODS IN MALES
- Spacing Methods
  - Natural
  - Mechanical Barriers
  - Chemical Methods (drugs)
  - Malepill
  - Testosterone
  - Calcium Channel Blockers
- Terminal Methods
  - Vesectomy
  - No scalpel vas occlusion
- Miscellaneous Methods
  - Hot Baths
  - Suspensories
  - Scrotal Sacks

INTRODUCTION

Aims of Contraception. Contraception refers to prevention of pregnancy. The aims of contraception are:

- The main aim of contraception is family planning to check the enormous increase in population growth, which is the root cause of socioeconomic problems of poor and developing countries, like India.
- Certain contraceptive measures are important to prevent the sexually transmitted diseases like AIDS.
- Contraceptives are also recommended on medical grounds to control the stress of pregnancy, labour and lactation in women suffering from heart diseases, etc.

Methods of Contraceptions can be broadly grouped as:

- Spacing methods and
- Terminal methods.

Both types of contraceptive measures are available for use by females as well as males; therefore, these can be described as:

- Contraceptive methods in females and
- Contraceptive methods in males.

CONTRACEPTIVE METHODS IN FEMALES

Spacing Methods

The spacing methods increase the gap between two pregnancies. These include:

- Rhythm method,
- Barrier methods,
- Chemical methods and
- Intrauterine contraceptive devices.

Rhythm Method

Rhythm method is also known as *calender method* or *safe period method* or natural method. This method of contraception depends on the time of ovulation. In a woman having a regular menstrual cycle, ovulation occurs on 14th day of the cycle. After ovulation, ovum remains viable for 48–72 hours. Similarly, after ejaculation sperms remain alive for 24–48 hours. Thus pregnancy occurs only if coitus is performed during this period. This is the period of high fertility and is called as *dangerous period.*

Therefore, to avoid pregnancy intercourse should be avoided in the dangerous period. Rest of the cycle, i.e. 5-6 days after bleeding phase of menstrual cycle and 5-6 days before the next cycle is the *safe period* (period of least fertility). This method of contraception is successful only if menstrual cycles are regular and woman knows the exact time of ovulation by keeping a record of basal body temperature.

Disadvantage of this method is that it is the most unreliable method when the menstrual cycles are irregular and time of ovulation is variable.

Barrier Methods

Barrier methods of contraception prevent the meeting of ovum and sperms after coitus. These include:

- Mechanical barriers,
- Chemical barriers and
- Combined (mechanical and chemical barriers).

1. Mechanical Barriers The mechanical barriers used as contraceptive are: diaphargm and cervical caps.

Diaphragm. It consists of a flexible rim, made up of a spring to which is attached a cup-shaped synthetic rubber or plastic (Fig.9.6-1A). The diaphragm is available in different sizes. It is inserted into the vagina over the cervix.

Cervical cap. It is smaller as compared to diaphragm (Fig.9.6-1B) and is applied on to the cervix itself.

Note. For proper use of mechanical barriers some spermicidal cream or jelly should be applied in the centre of the device.

Advantages. These devices are inexpensive and usually do not require any medical consultation.

Disadvantages of mechanical barriers include:

- Demonstration by a trained person is needed for the proper use.
- Failures are quite common because chances of displacement of the device are very high.

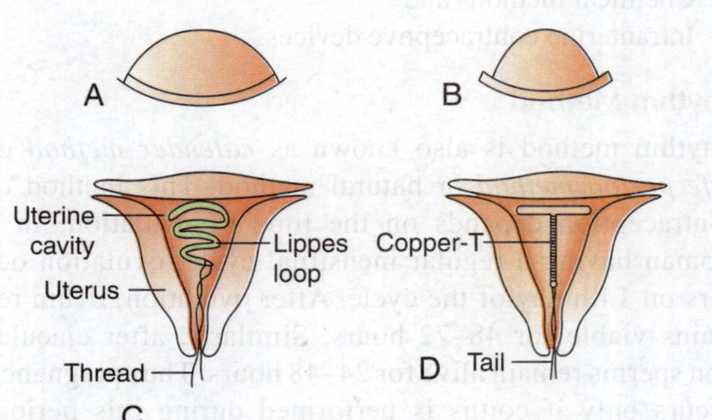

FIGURE 9.6-1 Female contraceptive devices: **(A)** vaginal diaphargm; **(B)** cervical cap; **(C)** Lippe's loop and **(D)** Copper T.

- Some women get cervicitis (inflammation of cervix) and local irritation.

2. Chemical Barriers Chemical barriers refer to spermicidal agents which can destroy the sperms when applied in the female genital tract before coitus. The common sperimicidal agents used are:

- Ricinoleic acid (oldest),
- Nanoxynol - 9 and
- Octoxynol - 3.

These spermicidal agents are available in various forms such as: foam tablets, pastes, creams, jellies, and vaginal sponges. Vaginal sponge is a polyurethane sponge impregnated with nanoxynol-9. It is available by the tradename 'TODAY'.

Advantages. Chemical barriers are inexpensive, well tolerated, and provide good protection.

Disadvantages are that the chemical barriers cause *messiness* and also sometimes may lead to *local irritation* and burning sensation.

3. Combined Methods As mentioned above, mechanical barriers (diaphragm and cervical caps) along with spermicidal agents give good protection.

Chemical Methods

Chemical methods for contraceptions are used in various forms like: locally applied chemicals (in the form of cream, jellies etc.) and taken as drugs (either orally or in injectable form or as implants). The drugs are further of two types, steroidal drugs (oestrogen and progesterone) and nonsteroidal drugs.

Steroidal Drugs

a. Oral Contraceptives. Oral contraceptives are most widely used contraceptive measure by the women all over the globe. These are recommended in women of younger age group (upto 35 years).

Mechanism of action. In general oral contraceptives contain synthetic preparation of oestrogen and progesterone and when taken orally, the plasma concentration of these hormones rises. The raised levels of these hormones by their negative feedback effect act on anterior pituitary to inhibit the release of gonadotropins (FSH and LH) and thus inhibit ovulation.

Types of pills. The oral contraceptives are available in different types of pills:

- Combined pill (classical pill),
- Sequential pill,
- Minipill and
- Postcoital (morning after) pill.

1. Combined Pill or Classical Pill. Composition. It contains both oestrogen and progesterone. Oestrogen (20–50 µg) in combined pills is usually *ethyl estradiol*or mestranol (methoxy derivative of ethyl estradiol) and progesterone (0.5–2 mg) like norethisterone, norgestrel or levonorgestrel.

Availability. The combined pills are available under two brand names; **MALA-N** (packet of 21 tablets) and **MALA-D** (packet of 28 pills, out of which 21 are white coloured of hormones and 7 are brown coloured containing *ferrous fumarate).*

Dosage. The combined pills are taken orally every day at fixed time (preferably at night before going to bed) for 21 days, starting from the 5th day of menstrual cycle to 25th day followed by a gap of 7 days in case of MALA-N. During this gap period bleeding occurs. This bleeding is not a menstrual bleeding as it occurs due to withdrawal of the hormones; therefore, it is called *withdrawal bleeding.*

Mechanism of action. Combined pill acts by three ways:

i. It prevents ovulation,
ii. It prevents implantation, if ovulation occurs and ovum is fertilized by a sperm and
iii. It makes the cervical secretion thick and viscid and thus prevent entry of sperms in the female genital tract.

Note. In combined pills, these days *phase regimens* (biphasic or triphasic) are preferred, because they are more physiological than fixed dose preparations.

2. Sequential Pill. ***Composition.*** These pills contain high dose of oestrogen along with moderate dose of progesterone.

Dosage. Only oestrogen is given starting from the 5th day of menstrual cycle to the 15th day and then followed by both (oestrogen + progesterone) for next 5 days.

Note. Nowadays the sequential pill is not used because of high incidence of *endometrial carcinoma.*

3. Minipill. Minipill (progesterone only) or *micropill.*

Composition. These preparations contain low doses of progesterone (norethisterone—0.35 mg or norgestrel—0.075 mg).

Dosage. The regimen of these pills is that the pill should be taken daily through whole of menstrual cycle.

Mechanism of action. Minipill prevents fertility without inhibiting ovulation. It acts on cervical mucosa (makes it thick), and also decreases motility of fallopian tubes.

4. Postcoital Pill (Morning after Pill). As the name indicates, it is recommended within 72 hours of the unprotected intercourse.

Dosage. Double dose of combined pill (2 pills) should be taken immediately followed by another double dose (two pills) after 12 hours.

Indications. This method of contraception should be used only in emergancy cases like, rape, contraceptive failure and unprotected sex.

Mechanism of action. Possible mechanisms involved are:

- It causes hypermotility of the fallopian tubes and of uterus and thus prevents fertilization and implantation.
- If ovulation and fertilization have occurred, then it prevents implantation of the blastocyst.

Disadvantages. Routinely this method of contraception is not practised because of various side effects like nausea and vomiting.

Advantages and Disadvantages of Oral Contraceptives

Advantages. Oral contraceptives have 100% effectivity.

Disadvantages. Although oral contraceptives are extensively used, but its prolong use leads to certain adverse effects as:

- Hypertension,
- Risk of thromboembolism,
- Metabolic effects like diabetes and obesity and
- Carcinogenic effects (carcinoma breast and carcinoma cervix).

Contraindications

Absolute contraindications for the use of oral contraceptives are:

- Woman having carcinoma of breast or of uterus,
- Liver diseases and
- Hyperlipidaemia.

Relative contraindications. Oral contraceptive should not be given to woman of age group above 35 years.

b. Depot Preparations. Depot preparations are long acting drugs and are highly effective. These are available in three forms :

- Injectable preparations,
- Subdermal implants and
- Vaginal rings.

1. Injectable Preparations. Injectable preparations are oily solutions injected intramuscularly. They are of following types:

i. ***Oily progestrin preparations***. These are available as:
   - *Medroxyprogesterone acetate (DMPA)* is injected intramuscularly every 3 to 6 months. Its dose is 150–400 mg.
   - *Norethindrone enanthate (NET-EN)* is injected intramuscularly every 3 months. Its dose is 200 mg.

Note. These preparations should be injected in first 5 days of menstrual cycle (bleeding phase) to rule out pregnancy.

ii. ***Combined injectable preparations.*** These preparations contain both oestrogen and progesterone. These are given intramuscularly at monthly interval.
   Mechanism of action. These preparations prevent ovulation and alter cervical mucosal secretions.

2. Subdermal Implants. Population council of New York has developed subdermal implants. These are of two types:

i. ***Norplant.*** It consists of six flexible silastic (made of silicon) tubes. Each containing 35 mg progesterone (levonorgestrel).
ii. ***Norplant (R)2.*** It consists of two rods of levonorgestrel.

The subdermal implants are implanted beneath the skin of arm or forearm. Effective contraception is achieved within 24 hours and lasts for 5–6 years.

3. Vaginal Rings. Vaginal rings containing norgestrel are implanted intravaginally. The progesterone is absorbed slowly through vaginal mucosa.

Advantages and Disadvantages of Depot Preparations.

Advantages. As depot preparations are long acting drugs, therefore to avoid daily intake of oral pill, these preparations are preferred, and also

- The contraceptive effectivity lasts for longer period.

Disadvantages of depot preparation are that sometimes they lead to sterility and alterations in menstrual bleeding pattern.

Nonsteroidal Contraceptive Drugs

Centchroman. It is nonsteroidal oral contraceptive drug developed by Central Drug Research Institute (CDRI), Lucknow. It is marketed under the trade name ***Saheli.***

Dose is 30 mg twice in a week for 12 weeks followed by once in a week.

Mechanism of action. It causes:

- Suppression of corpus luteum functions and
- Interferes with motility of fallopian tubes.

Both these effects interfere with implantation.

Advantages of the use of centchroman are:

- Menstrual cycle remains normal and
- There is complete reversibility on its withdrawal.

Intrauterine Contraceptive Devices

Intrauterine contraceptive devices (IUCDs) are inserted into the uterine cavity for long-term contraception. The devices are usually made up of inert materials like plastic, polythene and metal.

Types of IUCDs Basically two types of intrauterine devices are available: nonmedicated and medicated.

a. Nonmedicated IUCDs. These are also known as *first generation IUCDs.* Lippes loop is included in this category.

- ***Lippes loop*** (Fig. 9.6-1C). It is a serpentine or **S**-shaped device made up of plastic to which is attached a fine nylon tail. The plastic used is non-toxic and non-tissue reactive. A small amount of *barium sulphate* is also present in the plastic material to allow its radiographic observation. Lippes loop is available in different sizes.

b. Medicated IUCDs. These are of two types:

- ***Second generation IUCDs.*** These are made up of metal (copper). The copper ions are released slowly and have a strong antifertility effect. This group includes:
  - Copper T-200,
  - Copper T,
  - Some variants of copper T and
  - Newer devices like, NOVA -7, NOVA-T and multi-loaded devices.
- ***Third generation IUCDs.*** These are hormone releasing intrauterine devices. These are filled with progesterone (progesterone reservoir) which is released continuously for one year.
- ***Copper-T.*** Copper-T is the most commonly used IUCD in India. As the name indicates it is made up of copper and its shape resembles the letter T. Like Lippes loop it is also attached with a nylon thread (tail) (Fig 9.6-1D).

Insertion. Copper-T can be inserted into the uterus with the help of plunger (inserter) any time during woman's reproductive period except during pregnancy. Most ideal time for its insertion is during menstruation or within 10 days of the beginning of menstruation, because the diameter of cervical cavity at this time is greater. It can also be inserted during first week after the delivery.

Ideal candidate for IUCDs is the one who:

- Has born one child,
- Has normal menstrual cycle,
- Has no pelvic inflammation and
- Is ready to check the tail of the device.

Mechanism of action. Copper-T acts by following ways:

- *Prevents implantation* and growth of fertilized ovum by evoking aseptic inflammation and thus making endometrium unsuitable for implantation.
- *Sperm phagocytization.* During aseptic inflammatory reaction, large number of neutrophils, macrophages andleucocytes migrate. The sperms get phagocytosed by these cells.
  - Copper ions also affect the enzymes of the endometrium, sperm motility and its capacitation.
  - IUCDs filled with progesterone alter the mucous composition of cervix and make it thick and viscid and thus prevent the entry of sperm through cervical canal.

Advantages, Disadvantages and Contraindications of IUCDs

Advantages of IUCDs are:

- This method of contraception is quite safe, effective and reversible. IUCDs can be easily pulled out or removed when contraception is not required.
- Provides long-term contraception without adverse effects.

Disadvantages of IUCDs are:

- In some cases may cause heavy bleeding.
- The IUCD may come out accidently, when not inserted properly and
- Risks of ectopic pregnancy are there.

Contraindications. Use of IUCD is contraindicated in following conditions:

- In case of suspected pregnancy,
- In women having pelvic inflammation,

- In case of heavy bleeding during menstruation and
- In case of women suffering from carcinoma cervix.

Terminal Methods

Terminal method of contraception means permanent sterilization, which can be achieved either surgically or laparoscopically. Following methods have been employed:

Surgical Methods

1. Tubectomy. Tubectomy is the permanent method of sterilization in female and is recommended only when the family is completed.

Procedure. In tubectomy operation, fallopian tubes are cut and then cut ends are ligated and buried as shown in Fig. 9.6-2.

2. Laparoscopic Occlusion. In this procedure the fallopian tubes are occluded using silicon rubber bands, Fallope rings or Hulka-Clemens clips. This method is much quicker and simple and hospitalization is not required.

Note. Though tubectomy is a permanent method of sterilization, but if necessary then recanalization can be done using plastic tubes. The chances of successful canalization are only 55%.

Medical Termination of Pregnancy

Medical termination of pregnancy (MTP or abortion) is allowed under MTP Act 1971. Medical pregnancy act has laid down following criteria:

- Conditions in which pregnancy can be terminated,
- The person who can do termination and
- Place, where it should be performed.

Indications *Conditions in which pregnancy* can be terminated are:

- *Medical.* When continuation of pregnancy is hazardous to the mother.
- *Eugenic.* When there is substantial risk to the child if born from that pregnancy.
- *Humanitarian grounds.* When pregnancy is the result of rape.
- *Failure of contraceptive measure.*

Methods Medical termination of pregnancy is possible only in first few months of pregnancy (from 7th week to beginning of second trimester). Following procedures have been employed depending upon the duration of pregnancy:

*1. **Dilatation and Curettage (D and C).*** In this procedure, cervix is dilated with dilators and implanted ovum is removed by doing curettage of the endometrium.

*2. **Vacuum Aspiration.*** Like D and C, in this procedure cervix is dilated and then implanted ovum is removed (aspirated) by applying suction. This method is employed only upto 12 weeks of gestation.

*3. **Administration of Prostaglandins.*** In this method prostaglandins are administered into the vagina (intravaginally) which causes uterine contractions resulting in expulsion of the products of conception.

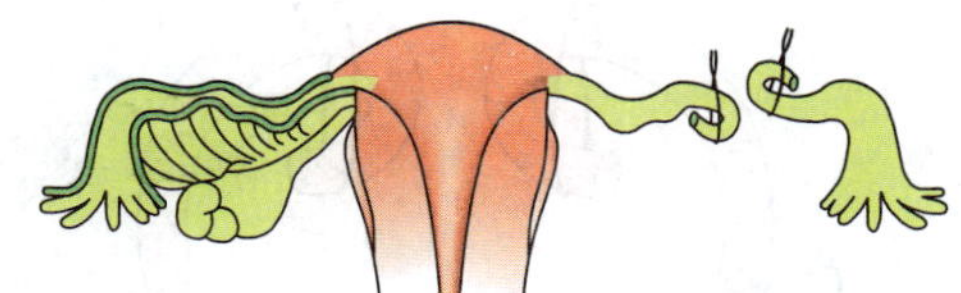

FIGURE 9.6-2 Procedure of tubectomy (female sterilization).

Pregnancy Vaccines

Pregnancy vaccines are under experimental trial. These have not yet been tried in women. Two types of vaccines under considerations are:

- ***Active immunization*** by injecting β *subunit of HCG and tetanus toxoid.* Tetanus toxoid increases the antigenicity capacity. The antibodies produced against β HCG destroy HCG produced by syncytiotrophoblast cells of the foetus.
- ***Vaccine against zona pellucida protein*** is also under trial.

CONTRACEPTIVE METHODS IN MALES

Spacing Methods

The spacing methods of contraception used in males are:

- Natural method,
- Barrier method and
- Chemical methods.

Natural Method or Coitus Interruptus

It is the oldest method of voluntary fertility control. In this method, male withdraws the penis before ejaculation into the vagina and tries to prevent deposition of semen into the vagina. This method needs practice and discipline. The failure rate is high because of following reasons:

- Precoital secretions of the male may contain sperms and even a drop of semen is sufficient to cause pregnancy.
- Slightest mistake in timings of withdrawal may lead to deposition of certain amount of semen.

Barrier Methods

Condom. Condom is the most widely used barrier by the males all around the world. In India it is known by its trade name *Nirodh* (Fig. 9.6-3). It consists of a fine latex sheath and is electronically tested. Various types of condoms available in the market are: dry type, lubricated, and deluxe.

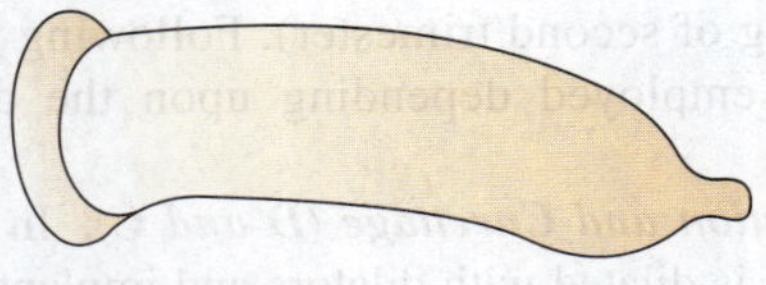

FIGURE 9.6-3 Condom.

Instructions. Instructions to be followed while using a condom are:

- Condom should be worn on erect penis before intercourse,
- Air must be expelled from the teat of the condom,
- It should be held carefully when withdrawing from vagina to avoid spilling of semen in the vagina and
- A new condom should be used for each sexual act.

Mechanism of Action. Condom prevents deposition of semen into the vagina thus does not allow the sperms and the ovum to meet.

Advantages

- They are easily available, safe and inexpensive.
- Their use does not require any medical supervision.
- They also provide protection against sexually transmitted diseases.

Disadvantages

- It may slip off or tear off during coitus due to its incorrect use.
- It interferes with sexual sensations.

Chemical Methods

Antispermatogenic Drugs Few drugs which inhibit spermatogenesis have been available. These include:

1. Male Pill (Gossypol)

- ***Composition.*** Male pill contains Gossypol, a phenolic derivative of cottonseed oil.
- ***Dose.*** The recommended dose is 200 mg/day for two months and followed by 60 mg/week. The drug is taken by oral route.
- ***Mechanism of action.*** Gossypol acts as an effective azoospermic agent. Its exact mechanism of action is not yet known. In 99.9% of cases sperm count decreases to 4 million/ml.
- ***Advantages.*** Male pill contains neither any hormone nor has antihormonal activity, therefore, there is no change in libido and potency of the male.
- ***Disadvantages*** are:
  - Men may become permanently azoospermic after constant use for six months.
  - It also has toxic effects.

2. Hormonal Preparations. Various hormonal preparations which can be used as contraceptive measures in males are:

- ***Testosterone.*** Testosterone (400 mg) when given orally produces azoospermia.
- ***Testosterone with danazol*** (17 α-ethyl testosterone). This preparation is better tolerated and is more effective.
- ***Cyproterone acetate.*** Chemically this drug is related to progesterone. It acts as potent antiandrogenic agent. It produces oligospermia but also causes loss of libido.

3. Tripterygium Wilfordii. This is a special type of wine (prepared from a plant) used in Chinese medicine. The plant contains many active compounds (triptolide, triptiolide, 16-hydroxytriplide and T7/19) which reduce the sperm count, but mechanism of action is not yet known.

4. Calcium Channel Blockers. Calcium channel blockers (e.g. nifedipine) block the Ca^{2+} channels on the cell membrane of the sperms (see page 862) thus prevent the influx of Ca^{2+}. As a result the sperm membrane becomes rigid and loaded with cholesterol. The rigid membrane of sperm prevents its binding to the zona pellucida of the ovum. Because of this effect the patients who are suffering from hypertension and are on nifedipine treatment become sterile.

Terminal Methods

The permanent methods employed for sterilization in males are:

- Vasectomy and
- Vas occlusion using no scalpel technique.

1. Vasectomy Vasectomy is a simple operation in which about 1 cm piece of vas deferens is removed after clamping. Then both the ends are ligated and sutured so that they face away from each other (Fig. 9.6-4). This procedure reduces the risk of recanalization later on.

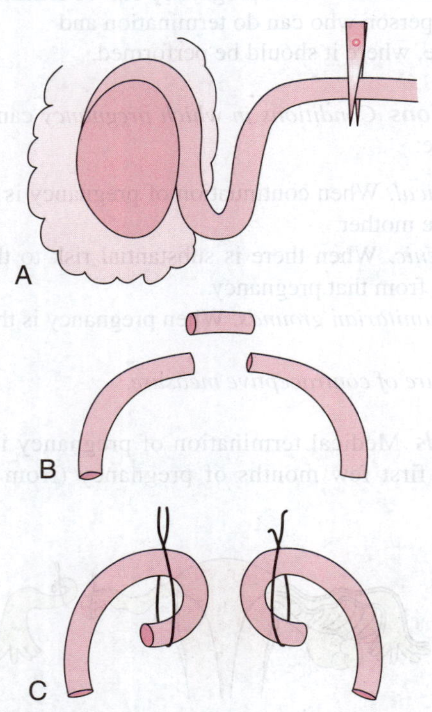

FIGURE 9.6-4 Procedure of vasectomy (male sterilization).

Mechanism of action. After vasectomy sperm production and hormones are not affected but entry of the sperms into the semen is prevented.

Postoperative instructions. Subjects should be advised to follow certain instructions postoperatively. Immediately after vasectomy he is not sterile because the sperms already formed are stored. After about 30 ejaculations semen becomes free from sperms. Therefore, he must use contraceptive measure (condom) postoperatively before he becomes azoospermic.

Advantages of vasectomy are that it is simpler faster less expensive procedure and no hospitalization is required. It is 100% effective.

Disadvantages are:

- *Failure rate* of vasectomy is only 0.15% and that too because of wrong identification of vas.
- *Complications.* Few complications may occur following vasectomy are as under:
  - *Spontaneous* recanalization,
  - Autoimmune response and
  - Psychological effects like
    - diminution of sexual vigour,
    - impotence and
    - headache.

2. No Scalpel Vas Occlusion No scalpel vas occlusion is a newer technique, which is quite safe, convenient and is acceptable to males.

Principle of Occlusion. An elastomer is injected into the vas deferens, it get hardened in situ within 20 mintues and plug the vas (occlude it).

Methods of Vas Occlusion. Vas is occluded by using various types of materials:

- Elastomer plugs,
- SHUG and
- RISUG.

i. ***Elastomer plugs*** are of two types:
- Medical grade polyurethane (MPU) and
- Medical grade silicon rubber (MSR).

MPU and MSR are injected into the vas, which get hardened within 25 mintues forming a plug which acts as barrier for sperms.

Advantages. It is an easy procedure and reversal is possible with 100% efficacy.

ii. ***SHUG.*** It is a preformed, flexible silicon rubber plug which can be inserted into the vas deferens using no scalpel technique.

Advantages. It is preformed plug, therefore, the effect is immediate as the time required for hardening of the material (as in MPU and MSR) is not wasted.

iii. ***Reversible inhibition of sperm under guidance*** (RISUG) is the latest technology. As the name indicates, it is noninvasive and reversible technique. In this method *styrene maleic anhydride* (SMA) is used. SMA is a co-polymer when injected along with dimethyl sulphoxide into the vas deferens; it forms a coating along the inner wall of vas deferens.

Mechanism of action. SMA acts by three ways:
- It blocks the lumen of the vas deferens,
- Its pH is alkaline, therefore, it interferes with acidic pH of the sperms and
- It ruptures the membrane of sperms and destroys them.

Advantages. It can be easily removed by flushing the vas deferens with a *solvent* or by manually squeezing the vas deferens. RISUG has completed phase I and phase II trial stage. Therefore, it seems to be a method of male contraception with 100% efficacy, reversibility and safety.

Miscellaneous Methods

Miscellaneous methods of contraception which can be used in males are:

Thermal Method It is based on the fact that sperms are destroyed by heat (above body temperature). Therefore, following methods are employed:

i. ***Hot baths.*** Daily immersion of testes in hot water (46°C) for few weeks is the effective method of contraception for several months. The effect can be maintained by periodically following hot bath regimen.

Advantages of this method is that it is very cheap and gives pleasant feeling.

Disadvantage is that its reliability is not fully known.

ii. ***Suspensories.*** Men are advised to wear specifically fitted set of briefs, (which hold the testes close to the body) during day time.

iii. ***Insulated scrotal sack.*** It consists of a heating element, thermometer and a control unit (comprising power source and timer). The sack is worn on the waist. In this method external heat is used for short period. Reliability of this method has not yet proved.

Section 10

Nervous System

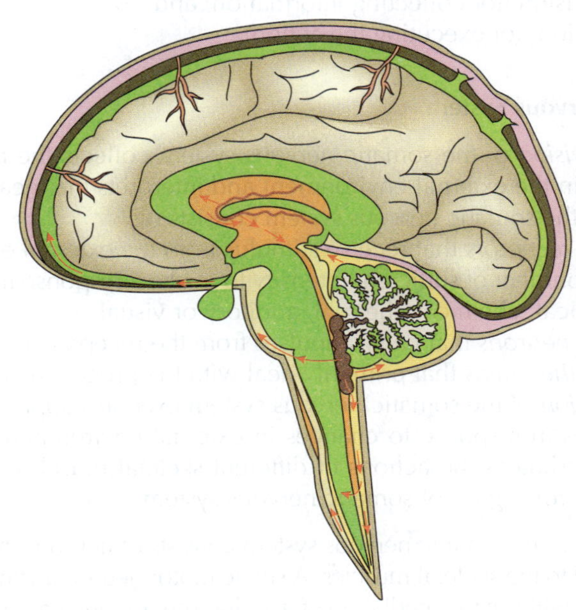

Organization of Nervous System

Nervous system, through sophisticated signalling, acts as a control network within the body. The specialized cells that constitute the functional units of the nervous system are called *neurons*. The neurons are responsible for the reception and response to changes in the internal and external environment. It is estimated that the human nervous system is composed of more than 100 billion neurons which are linked together in a highly intricate manner. Thus, the various parts of the nervous system are interconnected, but for convenience of description, the nervous system can be divided anatomically and functionally into different divisions.

Anatomical Divisions of the Nervous System

The nervous system is broadly classified into two anatomical divisions: the central nervous system and the peripheral nervous system.

1. **Central nervous system (CNS),** which occupies the central axis of the body, includes brain and spinal cord. Brain has three parts:
   - *Forebrain* comprises telencephalon, i.e. central hemispheres (cerebrum) or anterior part of the forebrain, and diencephalon or posterior part of the forebrain. The upper two-third of diencephalon is called thalamus and lower one-third is called hypothalamus.
   - *Midbrain* or mesencephalon and
   - *Hindbrain* or rhombencephalon comprises pons, medulla oblongata and cerebellum.
2. **Peripheral nervous system (PNS)** is the part of nervous system which lies outside the central nervous system. The PNS consists of peripheral nerves and the ganglia associated with them. Peripheral nerves attached to the brain are called *cranial nerves* (12 pairs), and those attached with spinal cord are called *spinal nerves* (31 pairs).

Functional Divisions of the Nervous System

Functionally, the nervous system can be divided into two parts:

- Somatic nervous system and
- Autonomic nervous system.

Both somatic and autonomic nervous systems have two divisions:

- Sensory division (for collecting information) and
- Motor division (for executing the action).

1. Somatic Nervous System

- *Sensory division* of the somatic nervous system collects the information about the changes that take place in the external environment and interprets the meaning of these changes. The sensory division of the somatic nervous system consists of:
  - *Sensory receptors* that receive stimulus from the external environment. A stimulus is a change of environment of sufficient intensity to evoke a response in an organism. The stimulus may be mechanical, chemical, thermal, auditory or visual.
  - *Afferent neurons* that carry impulses from the receptors to the brain and spinal cord.
  - *Parts of the brains* that primarily deal with the processing of information.
- *Motor division* of the somatic nervous system executes appropriate actions with the help of skeletal muscles in response to changes in external environment detected by *the sensory* division. It also co-ordinates the actions of different skeletal muscles of the body. Thus, skeletal muscles are the *effector organs* of somatic nervous system.

Motor division of the somatic nervous system consists of neurons that carry signals away from the brain and spinal cord to the skeletal muscles. A single motor neuron arising in the CNS traverses directly to the skeletal muscle without the mediation of ganglia. The somatic nervous system is under voluntary control.

2. Autonomic Nervous System

The autonomic nervous system (ANS) collects the information about the changes that take place in the internal environment (i.e. internal viscera), interprets these changes, and guides the action and gets the plan executed with the help of smooth muscles of viscera, *cardiac muscles* and *secretory epithelium* of glandular *tissues* (which are effector organs of ANS). In other words, the ANS is responsible for *activities* of the organs of digestion, circulation, excretion, respiration and *reproduction*, as well as of *adrenal medulla, sweat, salivary* and *lacrimal glands*. It also controls the activities of smooth muscles of *iris, ciliary body* and *arrectore spilorum*.

The word autonomous is taken from the Greek words, *'autos'* meaning self and *'nomos'* meaning control. Thus, ANS is an involuntary system.

- *Divisions of ANS*. The ANS has two main divisions: sympathetic and parasympathetic, each having a central and a peripheral component.
  - *Sympathetic division,* also called *thoracolumbar division*, consists of thoracic and lumbar chains of sympathetic ganglia.
  - *Parasympathetic division,* also called *craniosacral division*, consists of the ganglia associated with 3rd, 7th, 9th and 10th cranial nerves.

Understanding the Nervous System

For the purpose of understanding, this section on nervous system has been divided into two subsections:

- **Subsection 10 A: Physiological anatomy and functions of nervous system.** This subsection deals with the anatomy and functions of various parts of nervous system.
- **Subsection 10 B: Neurophysiology.** Neurophysiology or neurophysiological processes include the study of sensory, motor, autonomic and higher functions of the nervous system. Neurophysiology, though a very complex subject, primarily involves following processes:
  - *Reception of changes in internal and external environment.* It is a function of receptors which are of various types.
  - *Transmission of impulses from the receptors to the brain* is the function of afferent neurons. Specialized junctions called synapses are there to transmit impulses from one nerve cell to another. This process is known as *synaptic transmission*. The sensations ascend along the *sensory tracts*.
  - *Relay of sensory impulses* occurs in the thalamus, which is large cluster of nuclei that serves as a relay station.
  - *Processing of the sensation* occurs in the cerebral cortex. The part of the brain that deals primarily with processing of *somatic* sensations is called the *somatosensory cortex*. Similarly, the part of the brain which is involved in processing visual sensation is called *visual cortex*.
  - *Initiation of the response* to a sensation occurs from the concerned area of cerebral cortex, For example, the somatic motor commands are initiated from the motor cortex.
  - *Modulation and coordination of the response* occurs in subcortical centres. For example, the commands from motor cortex are co-ordinated and refined by the *basal ganglia loop system* as well as by the cerebellum.
  - *Execution of response*. The response to a sensation is ultimately conveyed to the effector organs by the efferent nerves. The *efferent nerves* to the skeletal muscles are called *somatic motor nerves*. The response invoked may be involuntary, i.e. in the form of reflexes or voluntary movements.
  - *Storage of information* occurs in the nervous system in the form of memory for future plans.
  - *Emotional and instinctual behaviour* is controlled by hypothalamus and limbic system.
  - *Consciousness and sleep* are special functions of brain. These include activity of reticular-activating system and other systems.
  - *Higher functions of the nervous system* include learning, memory, judgement, language and other functions of the mind.

Chapter 10.1

Physiological Anatomy, Functions and Lesions of Spinal Cord and Brainstem

PHYSIOLOGICAL ANATOMY AND FUNCTIONS OF SPINAL CORD

Gross Anatomy

- The spinal cord (Fig. 10.1-1) extends from the upper border of the first cervical vertebra to the lower border of the first lumbar vertebra.
- Its upper end becomes continuous with medulla oblongata and its lower end called *conus medullaris* becomes continuous with a fibrous cord called *filum terminale*.
- The spinal cord is cylindrical in shape and presents two fusiform-shaped enlargements: the *cervical enlargement* for innervation of upper limbs and *lumbar enlargement* for innervation of lower limbs.
- The cord possesses in the midline anteriorly a deep longitudinal fissure, the *anterior median fissure*, and on the posterior surface a shallow furrow, the *posterior median sulcus*.
- The spinal cord, like the brain, is surrounded by three meninges: the dura mater, the arachnoid mater and the pia mater.

Internal Structure

As seen on cross-section (Fig. 10.1-2), the neural tissue of spinal cord presents inner grey matter and outer white matter. Grey matter is constituted by the nerve cell bodies, dendrites and parts of axons, while white matter is formed by the myelinated and unmyelinated nerve fibres.

[A] Spinal Grey Matter

In transverse section, the grey matter of spinal cord forms an H-shaped mass in the centre of which is present a canal

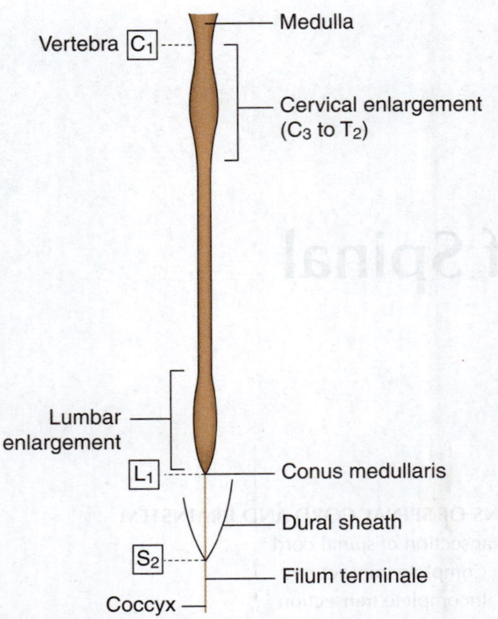

FIGURE 10.1-1 Gross appearance of the spinal cord and its relation with vertebrae.

called the spinal canal. The *spinal grey* matter exhibits following parts:

- ***Dorsal horn*** or posterior grey column refers to the posterior horn-like projection of the H-shaped grey matter in each lateral half of the cord. The dorsal grey column has been subdivided (from anterior to posterior side) into a base, a neck and a head.
- ***Ventral horn*** or anterior grey column refers to the anterior projection of the grey matter in each lateral half of the cord. The ventral grey column has been subdivided into an anterior part the head and a posterior part the base.
- ***Lateral horn*** or intermediate horn or lateral column refers to small lateral projection between the ventral and dorsal grey columns, present in the thoracic segments and first two lumbar segments only.
- ***Grey commissure*** is the part of the grey matter which connects the two (right and left) symmetrical halves of spinal grey matter across the midline. It is traversed by the central canal.

Neurons in Spinal Grey Matter

Neurons in Ventral Horn. The ventral horn neurons of spinal grey matter are involved in motor functions and send motor nerve fibres to the muscles and other effector organs. Functionally, the motor neurons are of four types:

Groups of ventral horn neurons (nuclei in ventral horn grey matter). The above-described neurons of ventral horn are arranged in three mediolateral columns:

1. Medial group,
2. Lateral group and
3. Central group (for details see Chapter 10.9, page 1047).

Neurons in Dorsal Horn The dorsal horn neurons of spinal grey matter are involved in sensory functions. The dorsal horn neurons are of two types:

1. Internuncial Neurons. These are located between the sensory fibres terminating in the dorsal horn and the motor neurons originating in the ventral horn.

2. The Tract Cells. These cells receive impulses from the various receptors of the body through dorsal nerve root fibres. Axons of these cells enter the white matter of the spinal cord on the same or opposite side and constitute either intersegmental tracts or ascending tracts which terminate in various masses of grey matter in the brain. These tracts form a considerable part of white matter of spinal cord.

Groups of Dorsal Horn Neurons (nuclei in dorsal horn grey matter). The above-described neurons of dorsal horn are arranged in four sets of longitudinal neuronal columns. From apex to base of dorsal horn these groups are (Fig. 10.1-3):

1. Substantia Gelatinosa of Rolando. It is a column of small cells which caps the apex of dorsal horn as gelatinous

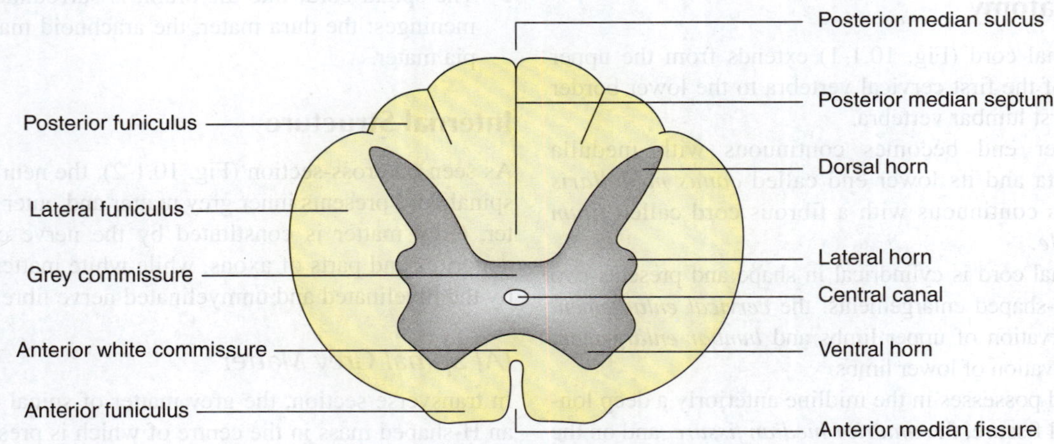

FIGURE 10.1-2 Cross-section of thoracic segment of the spinal cord.

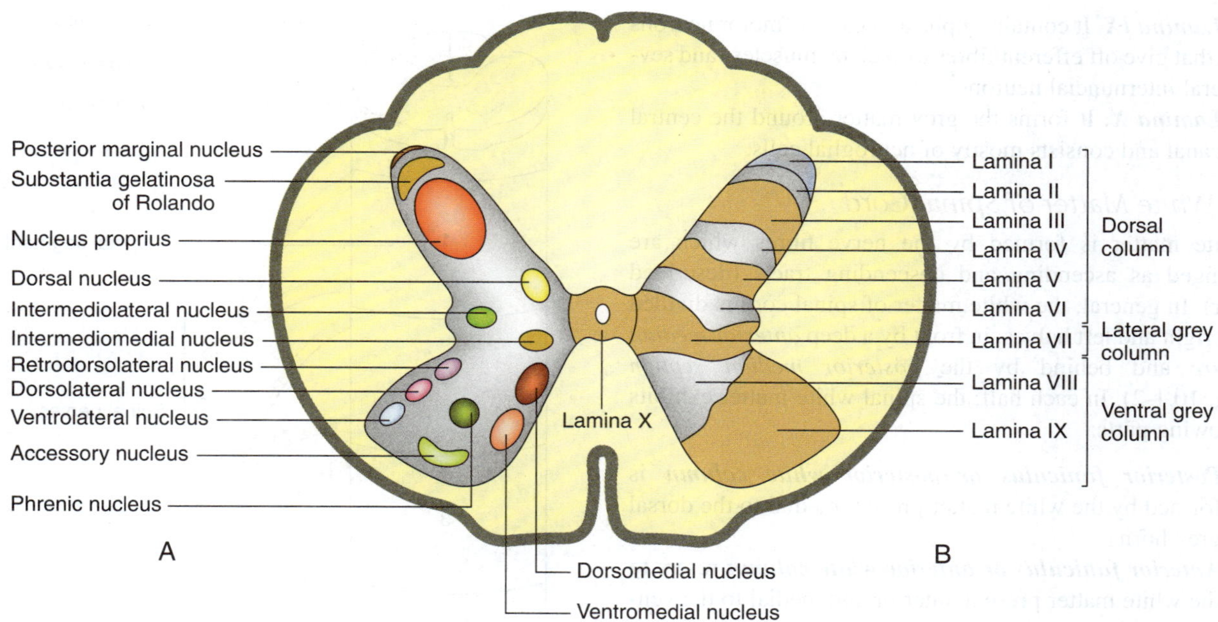

FIGURE 10.1-3 Subdivisions of the grey matter of the spinal cord: **A,** into nuclei; and **B,** into laminae.

material along the entire length of spinal cord. It is continuous above with the nucleus of spinal tract of the trigeminal nerve. The substantia gelatinosa (SG) is traversed by the fibres of the lateral division of the dorsal nerve roots which convey primarily pain and thermal sensations. The SG cell has a role in the 'gate control' of pain.

2. Nucleusproprius. It extends along the entire length of the spinal cord and is composed of internuncial cells and tract cells whose axons form the ascending tracts which occupy the anterolateral white funiculi of white matter of spinal cord.

3. Dorsal Nucleus. Dorsal nucleus also called the thoracic nucleus or Clarke's column extends from C_8 to L_2 segments of spinal cord. It is composed of tract cells which receive proprioceptive, touch and pressure sensations from the trunk and lower limbs. Axons of these cells form the ipsilateral posterior spinocerebellar tract.

4. Posteromarginal Nucleus. It is formed by the marginal cells which cover the substantia gelatinosa at the very tip of the dorsal horn.

Neurons in the Lateral Horn. The lateral horn cells of spinal grey matter also called neurons of the intermediolateral group of visceral efferent neurons which extends from T_1 to L_2 segments and from S_2 to S_4 segments of the spinal cord.

Neurons present in T_1 to L_2 lateral horn. These are preganglionic neurons of sympathetic nervous system. Their axons terminate in relation to postganglionic neurons in sympathetic ganglia.

Neurons present in S_2 to S_4 lateral horn. These are preganglionic neurons of the sacral component of parasympathetic nervous system. Their axons leave the spinal cord through the ventral nerve roots to reach the spinal nerves. They leave the spinal nerves as the pelvic splanchnic nerves which are distributed to some viscera in the pelvis and abdomen.

Divisions of Spinal Grey Matter into Laminae From the point of view of neuronal connections, the spinal grey matter (which has been divided into ventral, lateral and dorsal columns and grey commissure as described above) can be divided into 10 laminae (I to X) called Rexed laminae (Fig. 10.1-3).

- ***Laminae I to VI are confined to dorsal grey column.***
  - *Lamina I* corresponds to posteromarginal nucleus,
  - *Lamina II* corresponds to the substantia gelatinosa,
  - *Laminae III and IV* correspond to nucleusproprius,
  - *Lamina V* corresponds to neck of dorsal grey column and
  - *Lamina VI* corresponds to dorsal nucleus in base of the dorsal grey columns.

Note. Afferent fibres carrying cutaneous sensations end predominantly in laminae I to VI. Proprioceptive impulses reach laminae V and VI. These also receive numerous fibres from the cerebral cortex.

- ***Lamina VII*** is confined to lateral grey column (lateral or intermediate horns). It is composed of autonomic preganglionic neurons.
- ***Laminae VIII and IX*** are confined to ventral grey horn.
- ***Lamina VIII*** occupies most of the ventral horn in thoracic region. It is made of interneurons that receive terminals of vestibulospinal and reticulospinal tracts. Its efferent fibres are projected to lamina IX.

- ***Lamina IX***. It contains alpha and gamma motor neurons (that give off efferent fibres to skeletal muscles) and several internuncial neurons.
- ***Lamina X***. It forms the grey matter around the central canal and consists mostly of neuroglial cells.

[B] White Matter of Spinal Cord

White matter is formed by the nerve fibres which are arranged as ascending and descending tracts (described later). In general, the white matter of spinal cord is divided into right and left halves, in front by a deep *anterior median fissure* and behind by the *posterior median septum* (Fig. 10.1-2). In each half, the spinal white matter exhibits following parts:

- ***Posterior funiculus or posterior white column*** is formed by the white matter present medial to the dorsal grey horn.
- ***Anterior funiculus or anterior white column*** refers to the white matter present anterior and medial to the ventral grey horn.
- ***Lateral funiculus*** is formed by the white matter present lateral to the ventral and dorsal grey columns.
- ***Anterolateral funiculus*** refers to the anterior and lateral funiculi collectively.
- ***Ventral (anterior) white commissure refers*** to the white matter which is present anterior to anterior grey commissure and joins the right and left halves of white matter.
- ***Dorsal (posterior) white commissure*** refers to some myelinated fibres running transversely in the grey commissure, posterior to the central canal.

Note. Tracts of spinal cord are described along with the tracts of the brainstem (see page 908).

Spinal Segments and Spinal Nerves

Spinal Segments

Spinal cord, though a continuous structure, can be considered to consist of 31 spinal segments, each giving attachment to rootlets of the ventral and dorsal root, of each spinal nerve (Fig. 10.1-4). The 31 segments of spinal cord correspond symmetrically to 31 spinal nerves and are named as:

- *8 cervical segments* give attachment to 8 cervical nerves,
- *12 thoracic segments* give attachment to 12 thoracic nerves,
- *5 lumbar segments* give attachment to 5 lumbar nerves,
- *5 sacral segments* give attachment to 5 sacral nerves, and
- *1 coccygeal segment* gives attachment to 1 coccygeal nerve.

Spinal Nerves

Each spinal nerve is a mixed nerve formed by union of two roots: a dorsal (sensory) root and a ventral (motor) root (Fig. 10.1-5).

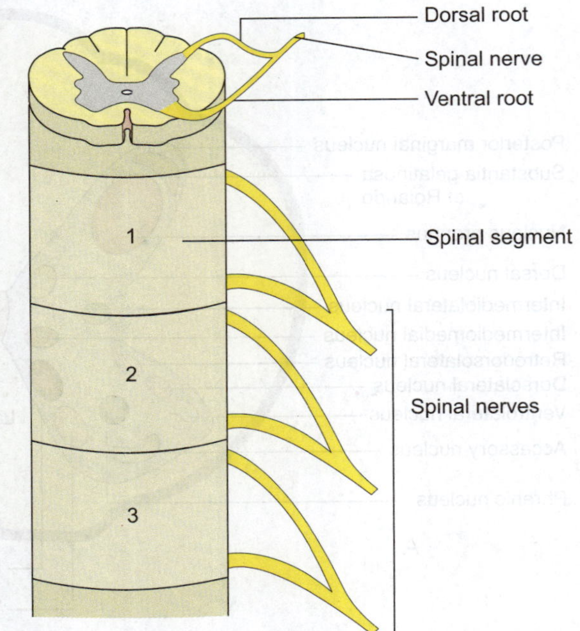

FIGURE 10.1-4 Scheme to illustrate the concept of spinal segments and roots of spinal nerve.

1. Dorsal Nerve Root. The dorsal nerve root is formed by several rootlets which are attached to the surface of the spinal cord along a vertical groove called the posterolateral sulcus. All sensory fibres reach the spinal cord through dorsal nerve roots. Each dorsal nerve root is marked by a swelling called dorsal nerve root ganglion or spinal ganglion. Dorsal root ganglion is composed of T-shaped unipolar neurons with peripheral and central processes.

- ***Peripheral processes*** of dorsal root ganglion cells extend up to sensory receptors in the skin. The area of the skin supplied by a spinal nerve is called dermatome.
- ***Central processes*** of dorsal root ganglion cells constitute the dorsal nerve root which is attached to spinal cord through various rootlets. Each rootlet just before entering the spinal cord divides into medial and lateral divisions.

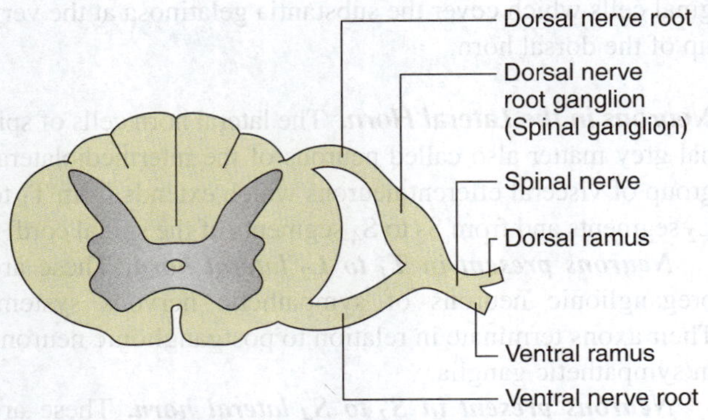

FIGURE 10.1-5 Beginning of spinal nerve and its roots.

Medial division of each rootlet consists of myelinated group I and II fibres which include:

- Proprioceptive fibres from muscles and
- Sensory fibres conveying touch, pressure and vibratory sensations.

Lateral division of each rootlet is composed of thinly myelinated group III fibres and unmyelinated group IV fibres:

- Fast and discriminative pain and temperature sensations are conveyed by group III fibres.
- Slow pain and visceral sensations are conveyed by group IV fibres.

2. Ventral Nerve Root. Ventral nerve root is formed by various rootlets which are attached to the anterolateral aspect of spinal cord opposite the ventral grey column. The ventral nerve root is composed of axons of motor neurons present in the ventral grey horn. The ventral root also contains the autonomic fibres originating from the lateral (intermediate) horn of the spinal grey matter (lamina VII).

Functions of Spinal Cord

Spinal cord serves three groups of functions:

- Sensory functions,
- Motor functions and
- Autonomic functions.

1. Sensory Functions

Entry of Somatic Sensations in Spinal Cord. All the somatic afferent impulses enter the spinal cord through the dorsal nerve root as:

- The fibres mediating *thermal and pain sensations* enter the spinal cord through the lateral division of dorsal nerve root, and
- The fibres conveying all *other sensory impulses* and proprioceptive impulses (touch, deep pressure, joint sense, vibration sense) from muscles, tendons and joints enter the spinal cord through the medial division of the dorsal nerve root.

Onward Transmission of Somatic Sensations. After entering the spinal cord, all the somatic sensations are conveyed to the brain (postcentral gyrus) by following ascending tracts:

Spinothalamic tracts convey sensations from the opposite side as:

- *Ventral spinothalamic tract* conveys gross (crude) touch and tactile sensations and
- *Lateral spinothalamic tract* conveys pain and temperature.

Dorsal column tract sensations. These occupy the dorsal column of the white matter of cord. These are upward continuation of the fibres of the medial division of the dorsal nerve roots of the same side. These tracts mediate sensations of fine touch, tactile localization and discrimination, pressure, vibration sense, sense of position and sense of movement.

2. Motor Functions

Spinal cord performs motor functions through the:

- ***Pyramidal tracts*** which include corticospinal (ventral and lateral) tracts, and
- ***Extrapyramidal tracts*** which include vestibulospinal tract, tectospinal tract, rubrospinal tract, olivospinal tract and reticulospinal tract.
- ***Motor functions*** served by spinal cord are:
  - Control of tone and power of muscles,
  - Control of movement of muscles and joints,
  - Control of deep (tendon) reflexes and
  - Control of superficial reflexes.

3. Autonomic Functions

Visceral afferent impulses in spinal cord travel through dorsal nerve roots to lateral horns of T_1 to L_2 and S_2 to S_4 spinal segments.

Autonomic efferents travelling through spinal cord supply the visceral organs and control the activity of smooth muscles, heart, glands of GIT, sweat glands and adrenals. The spinal cord also regulates the body temperature. In other words, spinal cord helps in maintaining the optimal internal environment of the body through its autonomic function.

PHYSIOLOGICAL ANATOMY AND FUNCTIONS OF BRAINSTEM

The brainstem consists (from below upwards) of the medulla oblongata, pons and midbrain (Fig. 10.1-6).

Medulla Oblongata

Gross Anatomy

The medulla oblongata is conical in shape and connects the pons above to the spinal cord below.

Surface of Medulla (Fig. 10.1-6) Exhibits:

- ***Median fissure,*** present in the centre of anterior surface of medulla, is continuous below with the anterior median fissure of spinal cord.
- ***Pyramids*** are two swellings, one each present on either side of median fissure. These are composed of bundles of nerve fibres that originate in large nerve cells in the precentral gyrus of the cerebral cortex. The pyramids taper below, and have most of the descending fibres which cross over to the opposite side, forming the *decussation of pyramids*.
- ***Olives*** are oval-shaped elevations, present one on each side just posterior to the pyramids. These are produced by the underlying olivary nuclei.

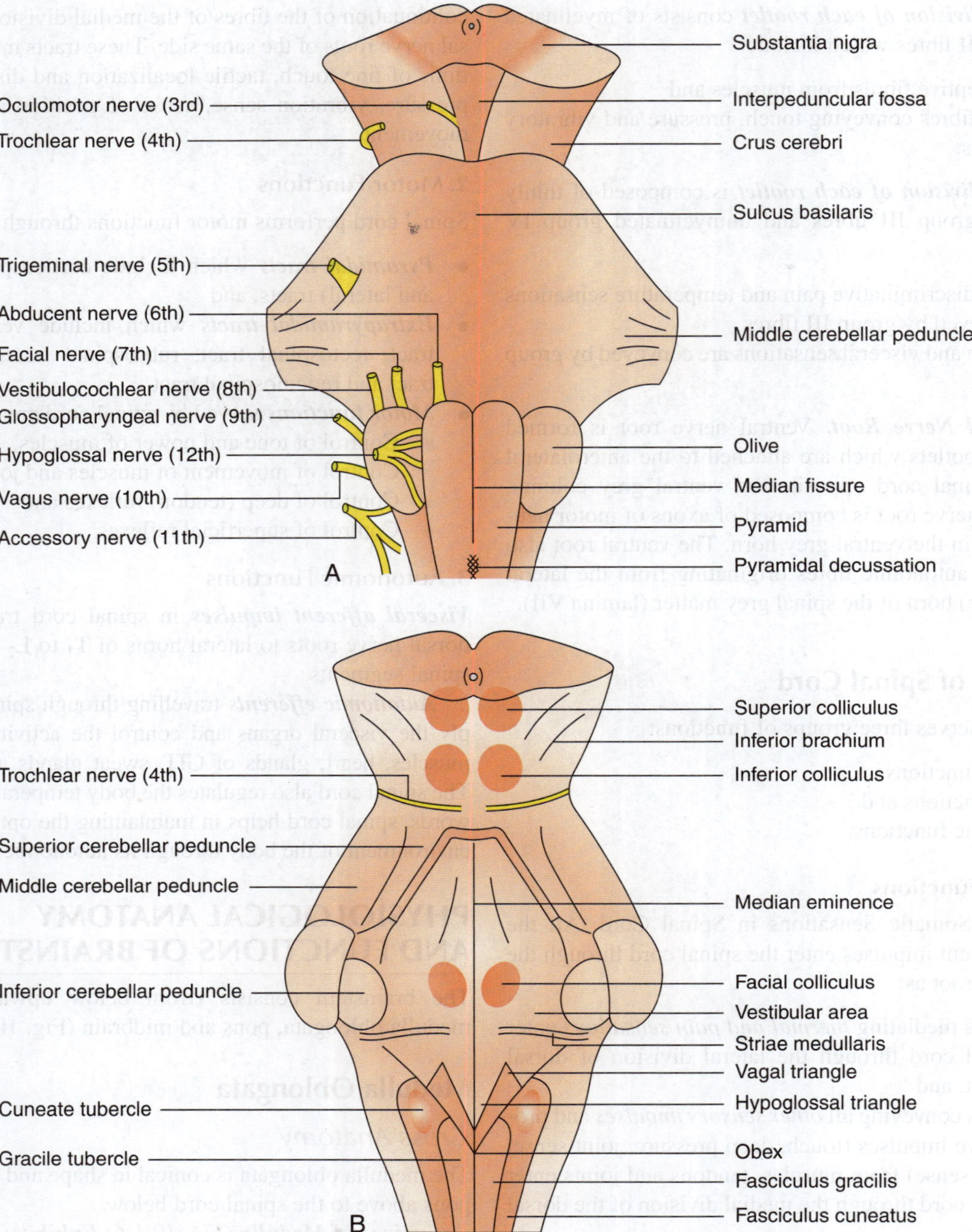

FIGURE 10.1-6 Gross anatomy of brainstem: **A,** ventral aspect; and **B,** dorsal aspect.

- ***Inferior cerebellar peduncles,*** which connect the medulla to cerebellum, are present behind the olives.
- ***Gracilis and cuneatus tubercles*** (produced by the medially placed underlying nucleus gracilis and the laterally placed underlying nucleus cuneatus, respectively) are present on the posterior surface of the inferior part of the medulla oblongata.
- ***Cranial nerves,*** 9th, 10th, 11th and 12th, emerge from the surface of medulla.

Internal Structure

The main features of the internal structure of the medulla oblongata are most easily reviewed by examining cross-sections at following levels:

- Transverse section at the level of pyramidal decussation (Fig. 10.1-7A).
- Transverse section at the level of sensory decussation (Fig. 10.1-7B) and
- Transverse section at the level of olive (Fig. 10.1-7C).

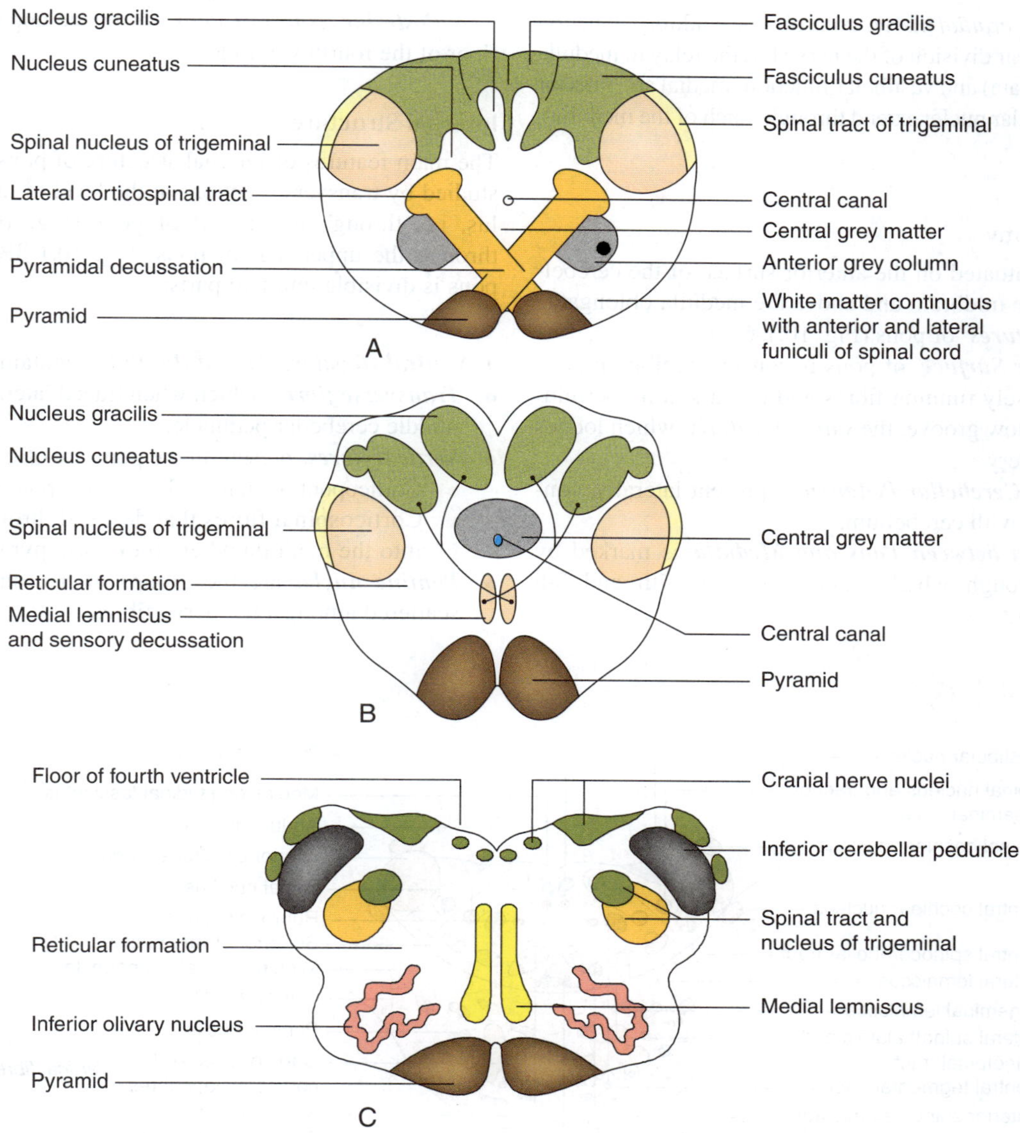

FIGURE 10.1-7 Main features of internal structure of medulla oblongata exhibited by transverse sections at the level of: **A,** pyramidal decussation; **B,** sensory decussation; and **C,** olive.

Note. For detailed description refer to any standard textbook of neuroanatomy.

Functions

1. ***Pathway for ascending and descending tract.*** The medulla oblongata forms the main pathway for the ascending and descending tracts of spinal cord.
2. ***House of vital centres.*** The medulla oblongata houses many important centres which control the vital functions of the body:
   - *Respiratory centres* (inspiratory and expiratory) control the normal rhythmic respiration (page 441).
   - *Vasomotor and cardiac centres* control the blood pressure and functions of heart and vascular system (page 335).
   - *Deglutition centre* controls the pharyngeal and oesophageal phase of deglutition (page 584).
   - *Vomiting centre* is responsible for inducing vomiting in disorders of gastrointestinal tract.
   - *Superior and inferior salivary nuclei,* located in the medulla, control the salivary secretion (page 583).
3. ***Cranial nerve nuclei*** located in the medulla control following functions:
   - *Twelfth cranial (hypoglossal) nerve* controls the movements of tongue.
   - *Eleventh cranial (accessory) nerve* controls the movements of shoulder.
   - *Tenth cranial (vagus) nerve* controls the functions of important viscera viz. heart, lungs and GIT.

- *Eighth cranial nerve* controls the auditory function (cochlear division of the nerve has the relay in medulla oblongata) and vestibular function (medial and inferior vestibular nuclei extend through much of the medulla).

Pons

Gross Anatomy

The pons is situated on the anterior surface of the cerebellum below the midbrain and above the medulla oblongata.

Gross Features of pons (Fig. 10.1-6) are:

- ***Anterior Surface*** of pons is convex, exhibits prominent transversely running fibres and is marked in the midline by a shallow groove, the *sulcus basilaris,* which lodges the basilar artery.
- ***Middle Cerebellar Peduncles,*** present laterally, connect the pons with cerebellum.
- ***Junction between Pons and Medulla*** is marked by a groove through which emerge the 6th, 7th and 8th cranial nerves.
- ***Posterior Aspect of Pons*** forms the upper part of the floor of the fourth ventricle.

Internal Structure

The main features of internal structure of pons can be best studied by transverse sections at the level of facial colliculus, i.e. through lower part of pons (Fig. 10.1-8A) and through the upper part of pons (Fig. 10.1-8B). Internally pons is divisible into two parts:

1. Ventral (Basilar) Part of the Pons contains:

- ***Transverse fibres,*** which when traced laterally form the middle cerebellar peduncle.
- ***Vertical fibres,*** present in the pons are of two types:
  - Corticopontine fibres, which end in pontine nuclei and
  - Corticospinal fibres that descend through the pons into the medulla where they form pyramids.
- ***Pontine nuclei*** are the groups of neurons which are scattered amongst the nerve fibres.

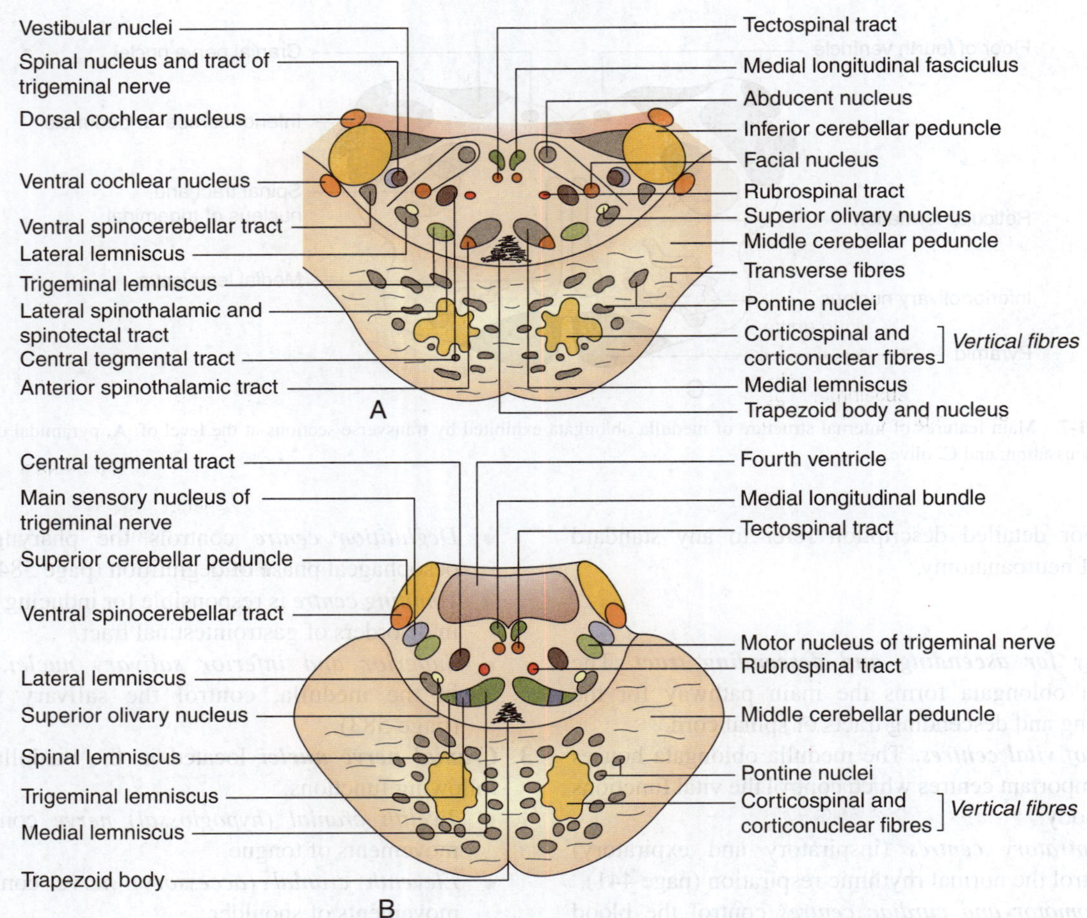

FIGURE 10.1-8 Main features of internal structure of pons exhibited by transverse sections at the level of : **A,** lower part of pons; and **B,** upper part of pons.

2. Dorsal (Tegmental) Part of Pons contains:

- Decussations of trepezoid body,
- Nuclei of 5th, 6th, 7th and 8th cranial nerves,
- Pontine reticular formation and
- A number of descending and ascending tracts.

The most prominent ascending tracts are the four lemnisci: medial, trigeminal, spinal and lateral.

Functions

Pons subserves following functions:

1. ***Connecting pathway between cerebral cortex and cerebellum***. The pontine nuclei receive corticopontine fibres and their axons from the middle cerebellar peduncles which serve as a connecting pathway between cerebral cortex and cerebellum.
2. ***Pathway for ascending and descending tracts*** of spinal cord and medulla oblongata.
3. ***Houses the nuclei*** of 5th, 6th, 7th and 8th cranial nerves.
4. ***Joining station*** for medial lemniscus with fibres of 5th, 7th, 9th and 10th cranial nerves.
5. ***Contains pneumotaxic and apneustic centres*** for regulation of respiration (page 443).

Midbrain

Gross Anatomy

The midbrain is a narrow part of the brain that connects forebrain to hindbrain. Gross anatomical features of midbrain are (Fig. 10.1-6):

Anterior Surface of Midbrain exhibits (Fig. 10.1-6A):

- *Crura cerebri*. These are two large bundles of fibres, one on each side of the middle line.
- *Interpeduncular fossa* in the triangular space between the two crura.
- *Oculomotor nerve* emerges from the medial aspect of crus of the same side.

Posterior Surface of Midbrain exhibits (Fig. 10.1-6B):

- ***Superior colliculi*** are two rounded swellings, one on each side of midline. Each superior colliculus acts as subcort ical centre for visual reflexes and is connected to the lateral geniculate body by a raised band known as superior brachium.
- ***Inferior colliculi*** are two rounded swellings one on each side of the midline located below the superior colliculi. Each inferior colliculus acts as subcortical centre for auditory reflexes and is connected to medial geniculate body by an elevated band known as the *inferior brachium*.

Internal Structure

The main features of internal structure of midbrain can be studied by making two transverse sections—one at the rostral level through the superior colliculi, and the other at the caudal level through the inferior colliculi.

Internally, for convenience of description, the midbrain can be divided into two parts (Fig. 10.1-9):

i. Tectum. Tectum refers to the part of midbrain lying behind a transverse line drawn through the cerebral aqueduct. It consists of superior and inferior colliculi of two sides.

ii. Cerebral Peduncles. Cerebral peduncles (right and left) constitute the part of midbrain lying in front of the line passing through the cerebral aqueduct. Each cerebral peduncle in turn consists of three parts, which from anterior to posterior side are:

- ***Crus cerebri*** (or basis pedunculi). It consists of large mass of vertically running descending fibres from cerebral cortex which include frontopontine fibres (occupying medial one-sixth of crus), corticospinal and corticonuclear fibres (occupying intermediate two-third of crus) and temporopontine, parietopontine and occipitopontine fibres (occupying the lateral one-sixth of crus).

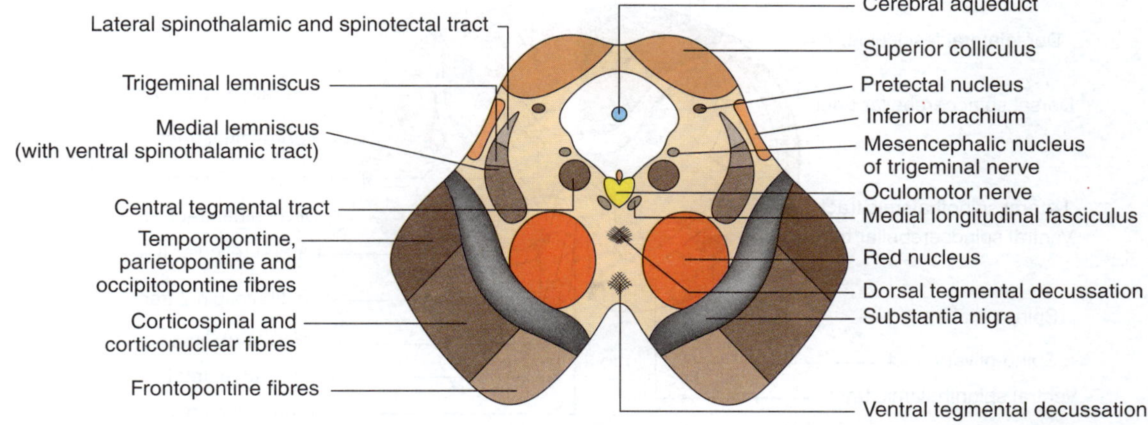

FIGURE 10.1-9 Main features of internal structure of midbrain exhibited by transverse section at the level of superior colliculi.

- ***Substantia nigra*** is a mass of pigmented grey matter (therefore appears dark in colour). Physically, it is considered part of basal ganglia. The connection and functions of substantia nigra are discussed on page 941.
- ***Tegmentum*** of the two sides is continuous across the midline. It contains following important masses of grey matter and nerve fibres:
  - *Red nucleus* is the biggest nucleus present in the upper part of midbrain. Physiologically, the red nucleus is a part of basal ganglia and is involved in regulation of posture (see page 1062).
  - *Nuclei* of 3rd, 4th and 5th cranial nerves.
  - *Reticular formation* of midbrain is continuous below with the reticular formation of pons and medulla.
  - *Fibre bundles* of the tegmentum include medial lemniscus, trigeminal lemniscus, lateral lemniscus, tectospinal and rubrospinal tracts.
  - *Three decussations* take place in the tegmentum due to: crossing of fibres of superior cerebellar peduncle, rubrospinal tracts (Forel's decussation) and fibres of medial longitudinal bundle (Meynert's decussation).

TRACTS OF SPINAL CORD AND BRAINSTEM

The tracts that transmit sensory impulses to the brain are termed *ascending tracts,* and the tracts which are responsible for transmission of motor impulses from the brain to motor neurons reaching muscles and glands are termed *descending tracts*. There are numerous ascending and descending tracts in the spinal cord and brainstem.

Ascending Tracts

Ascending tracts convey impulses arising in various parts of body to different parts of the brain. The ascending tracts present in the spinal cord (Figs 10.1-10 and 10.1-11) can be grouped as:

- Ascending tracts connecting spinal cord with cerebral cortex,
- Ascending tracts ending in the brainstem and
- Spinocerebellar pathways.

I. Ascending Tracts Connecting Spinal Cord with Cerebral Cortex

1. Posterior Column–Medial Lemniscus Pathway

Fasciculus Gracilis and Fasciculus Cuneatus

Location. Fasciculus gracilis and fasciculus cuneatus occupy the posterior white funiculus of the spinal cord, and are, therefore, often referred to as the *posterior column tracts.* Fasciculus gracilis is situated medial to fasciculus cuneatus. The posterior intermediate septum separates the two in the cervical and upper thoracic segments (Fig. 10.1-10).

Origin. These tracts are unique in that they are formed predominantly by the axons of the first-order sensory neurons located in dorsal root ganglia (Fig. 10.1-12).

- Recently, it has been shown that these tracts also contain some fibres that originate in the dorsal grey column (laminae III and IV), i.e. sensory neurons of second order.

Arrangement of Fibres. The fibres derived from the lowest ganglia are situated most medially, while those from the highest ganglia are most lateral. Therefore:

- ***Fasciculus gracilis,*** which lies medially, is composed of fibres from the coccygeal, sacral, lumbar and lower thoracic ganglia; and

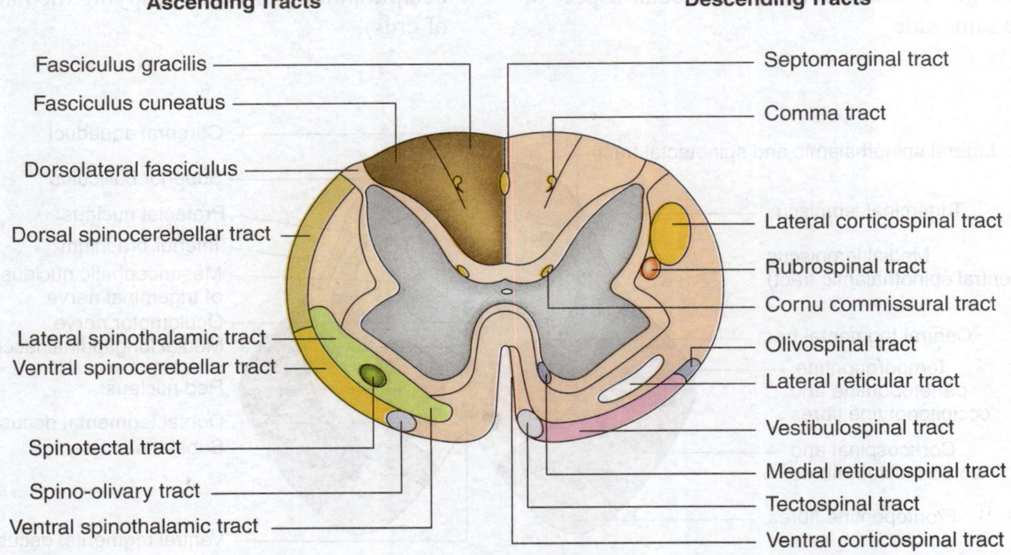

FIGURE 10.1-10 Schematic diagram to show the position of the main ascending and descending tracts of the spinal cord and brain stem.

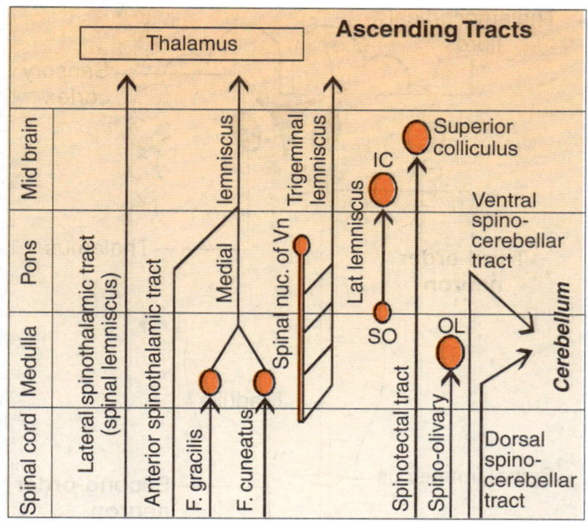

FIGURE 10.1-11 Schematic diagram to show the various ascending tracts of spinal cord and brainstem. SC = superior colliculus; SO = superior olivary nucleus; Vn = vestibular nucleus; OL= olivary nucleus; IC = inferior colliculus.

- ***Fasciculus cuneatus,*** which lies laterally, consists of fibres from upper thoracic and cervical ganglia.

Course. After entering the spinal cord, the fibres ascend through the posterior white funiculus and reach the medulla (Fig. 10.1-12). These fibres do not synapse in the spinal cord. Some fibres of the medial division of the posterior nerve root descend through the posterior white funiculus in the form of fasciculus interfasciculi or comma tract of Schultze.

- Some afferents from spinal ganglia pass through the posterior funiculus to reach the dorsal nucleus and other area of spinal grey matter.

Termination. After reaching the medulla, the fibres of gracilis and cuneatus fasciculi terminate by synapsing with neurons in the nucleus gracilis and nucleus cuneatus, respectively (Fig. 10.1-12).

Medial Lemniscus. The neurons of nucleus gracilis and nucleus cuneatus form the *second-order sensory neurons*. Their axons form the *internal arcuate fibres* which run forwards and medially to cross the midline. The crossing fibres of the two sides constitute the *sensory decussation* or *lemniscus* decussation and then ascend through the medulla, pons and midbrain as *medial lemniscus* (Fig. 10.1-12). The fibres of medial leminiscus terminate in ventral posterolateral nucleus of thalamus.

Third-Order Sensory Neurons. The fibres of medial lemniscus synapse with the third-order sensory neurons located in the thalamus. Axons of the third-order neurons pass through the internal capsule and corona radiata to reach the somatosensory areas of cerebral cortex.

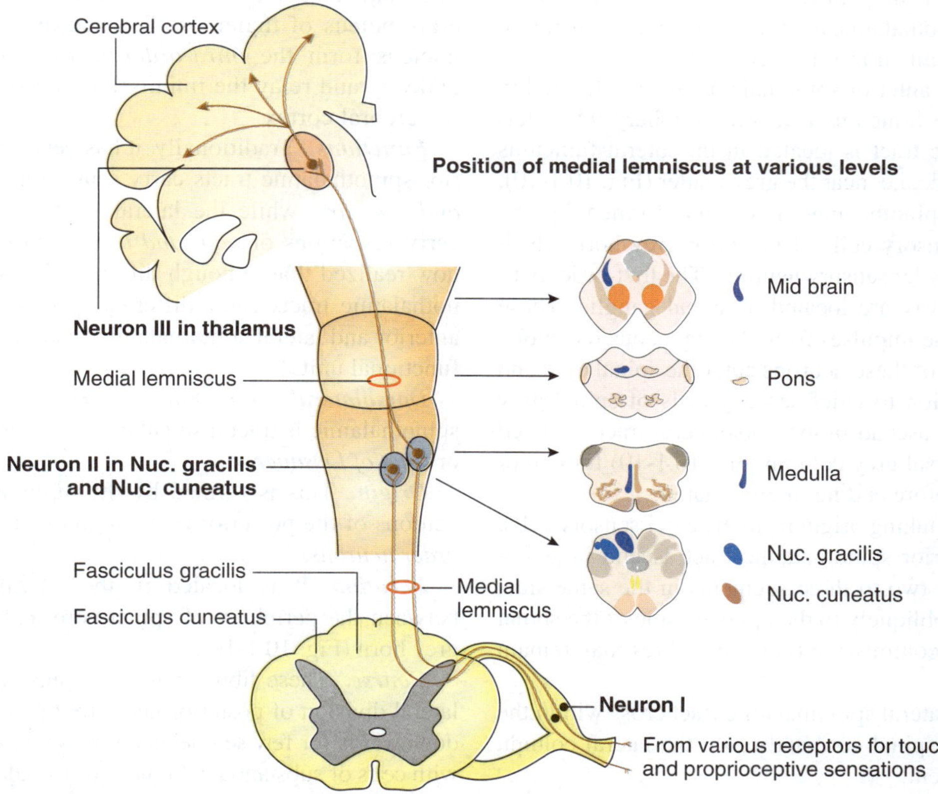

FIGURE 10.1-12 Course of posterior column–medial lemniscus pathway. Note, sensory decussation and position of medial lemniscus at various levels of brainstem.

Functions of Posterior Column–medial Lemniscus Pathway. These fibres carry sensations of some components of touch, vibration and proprioception to the cortex and thus help in following functions:

1. ***Components of sense of touch*** include:
   - Deep touch and pressure,
   - Fine touch, i.e. epicretic tactile sensations,
   - Tactile localization, i.e. ability to localize exactly the part of skin touched,
   - Tactile discrimination, i.e. the ability to recognize as separate two points on the skin that are touched simultaneously.
   - Stereognosis, i.e. the ability to recognize the shape of known objects by touch with closed eyes.
2. ***Proprioceptive impulses*** help in conscious kinaesthetic sensations, i.e. the sense of position of different parts of the body under static conditions as well as rate of change of movement of different parts during body movements.
3. ***Sense of vibrations,*** i.e. ability to detect rapidly changing peripheral conditions. This is the ability to perceive the vibrations conducted to deep tissues through the skin.

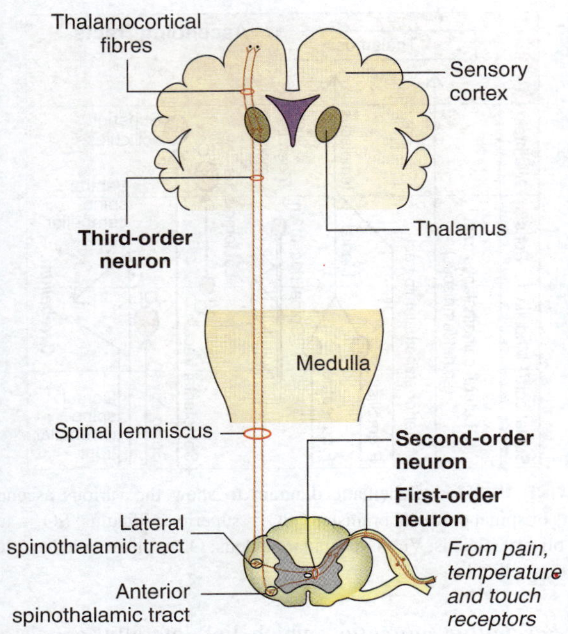

FIGURE 10.1-13 Course of anterior and lateral spinothalamic tracts.

2. Spinothalamic Pathways

Anterior and Lateral Spinothalamic Tracts. The spinothalamic tracts are formed by the axons of the second-order sensory neurons of the pathway of crude touch, and pressure (anterior spinothalamic tract) and pain and temperature (lateral spinothalamic tract) (Fig. 10.1-13).

Location. The anterior spinothalamic tract is located in the anterior white funiculus near the periphery while lateral spinothalamic tract is located in the lateral funiculus towards medial side, i.e. near the grey matter (Fig. 10.1-10).

Origin. The spinothalamic tracts are formed by the axons of chief sensory cells of posterior grey horn which form the second-order sensory neurons. The first-order neurons of this pathway are located in spinal ganglia. These neurons receive the impulses from the cutaneous receptors. Central processes of these neurons enter the spinal cord and terminate in relation to chief sensory cells of spinal grey matter. They may ascend in the dorsolateral tract (situated near the tip of dorsal grey column, Fig. 10.1-10) for one or more segments before ending in grey matter.

Course. After taking origin from the chief sensory cells, the fibres of anterior spinothalamic tract ascend in posterior grey horn for two to three segments in the same side. Then, they cross obliquely to the opposite side of the spinal cord in the white commissure (but some fibres may remain uncrossed).

The fibres of lateral spinothalamic tract cross within the same segment of spinal cord and reach the lateral column of the same segment.

The two tracts also carry about 10% uncrossed fibres and run up in the spinal cord, medulla, pons and midbrain and reach the thalamus. In the brainstem, they form the so-called spinal lemniscus.

Termination. All the spinothalamic fibres running in spinal lemniscus terminate in the ventral posterolateral nucleus of thalamus. The neurons of this thalamic nucleus form the *third-order neurons* of this sensory pathway and relay the impulses to the somaesthetic area of cerebral cortex.

Functions. Traditionally, it has been said that the anterior spinothalamic tracts carry sensations for *crude touch and pressure,* while the lateral tracts have been said to carry sensations of *pain and temperature*. However, it is now realized that although different fibres within the spinothalamic tracts carry different types of sensations, the anterior and lateral spinothalamic tracts constitute a single functional unit.

Dorsolateral Spinothalamic Tract. The dorsolateral spinothalamic is tract also called *fasciculus dorso lateralis* or *tract of Lissauer*.

Origin. This is formed by the fibres arising from the neurons of the posterior root ganglia which form the *first-order neurons*.

Location. It is located in the lateral white column between the periphery of spinal cord and tip of posterior grey horn (Fig. 10.1-10).

Course. These fibres enter the spinal cord through the lateral division of posterior nerve root and pass upwards or downwards for few segments on the same side and synapse with cells of substantia gelatinosa of Ronaldo situated in the posterior grey column. The processes of these cells (*second-order neurons*) cross to the opposite side and ascend in the dorsolateral fasciculus to reach the ventral posterolateral nucleus of thalamus where they synapse.

Functions. This tract carries impulses arising in skin (mainly pain and temperature). Relief of pain after dorsolateral cordotomy may be a result of the cutting of these fibres.

Spino-Cervico-Thalamic Pathway

Functions. It is another pathway through which cutaneous sensations (touch, pressure, pain and temperature) reach the thalamus.

Origin. This tract is formed by the axons arising from neurons located in laminae III to V of spinal grey matter.

Course and Termination. After origin, the fibres ascend through the dorsolateral fasciculus and end in the *lateral cervical nucleus* (which is a small collection of neurons lying among the fibres of the lateral funiculus in spinal segments C_1 and C_2. New fibres arising here project to the ventral posterolateral nucleus of the thalamus.

II. Ascending Tracts Ending in Brainstem

The ascending tracts arising in spinal grey matter and ending in masses of grey matter in different parts of the brainstem are (Fig. 10.1-11) as follows:

1. Spinoreticular Tract

Location. This tract is located in anterolateral white funiculus (Fig. 10.1-10).

Origin. The spinoreticular fibres begin from spinal neurons mainly in lamina VII (also V and VIII).

Course. The fibres are partly crossed and partly uncrossed, and ascend in the ventrolateral part of the spinal cord, intermingling with the spinothalamic tracts.

Termination. These fibres end in reticular formation of medulla and pons:

- In the medulla, the fibres end in nucleus reticularis-giganto-cellularis and lateral reticular nucleus of same side; some fibres terminate in the opposite side.
- In the pons, these fibres terminate in the nucleus reticularis-pontis-caudalis of the same side or opposite side.
- Very few fibres terminate in midbrain.

Functions. The fibres of the spinoreticular tract are the components of ascending reticular-activating system (RAS) and are concerned with arousing consciousness or alertness.

2. Spinotectal Tract

Location. This tract is located in the lateral side of lateral white funiculus anterior to the lateral spinothalamic tract. It is bounded anteriorly by the anterior nerve root (Fig. 10.1-10).

Origin. Fibres of this tract arise from the chief sensory cells of posterior grey column. First appearance of the fibres is in upper lumbar segments. This tract is very prominent.

Course and Termination. After origin from the spinal grey matter, the fibres cross to the opposite side through anterior white commissure to the lateral funiculus. Then the fibres ascend up to the midbrain along with anterior spinothalamic tract and end in the superior colliculus and midbrain reticular nuclei.

Functions. These fibres form alternate route for conduction of *slow pain* and are also concerned with *spinovisual reflexes*.

3. Spino-Olivary Tract

Location. This tract is located in anterolateral part of white funiculus and occupies mostly the anterior white funiculus (Fig. 10.1-10).

Origin, Course and Termination. The origin of the fibres of this tract is not specific. It is also a crossed tract. Its fibres terminate into olivary nucleus of medulla oblongata, from where the neurons project into cerebellum.

Function. This tract is concerned with proprioception.

III. Spinocerebellar Tracts

The spinocerebellar tracts carry proprioceptive impulses arising in the lower part of the body to the cerebellum. Recent investigations have shown that some exteroceptive sensations (e.g. touch) may reach the cerebellum through these pathways. Thus, the spinocerebellar tracts are constituted by the fibres of second-order neurons of the pathway for subconscious kinaesthetic sensation (Fig. 10.1-14). The spinocerebellar pathway is organized into the ventral and dorsal tracts.

1. Ventral Spinocerebellar Tract

Location. It is located in lateral white funiculus of the spinal cord along the lateral periphery (Fig. 10.1-10).

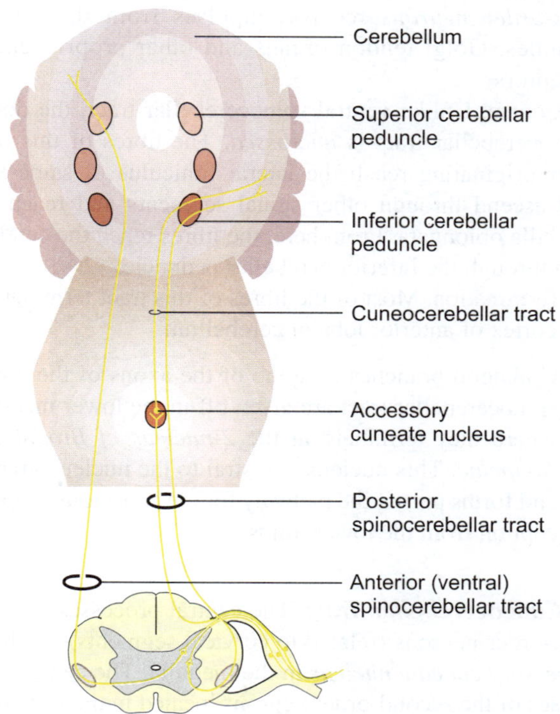

FIGURE 10.1-14 Spinocerebellar tracts.

Origin. The ventral (anterior) spinocerebellar tract, also known as Gower's tract, is constituted by the second-order neurons (of proprioceptive pathway) located in the junctional area between the ventral and dorsal grey column (laminae V, VI, VII) in the lumbar and sacral segments of the cord. These neurons receive impulses from the first-order neurons located in the posterior root ganglia. The peripheral processes of first-order neurons receive impulses from muscle spindles, Golgi tendon organs and other proprioceptive receptors. Some fibres are related to end organs concerned with exteroceptive sensations (touch, pressure).

Course. After origin from the junctional (marginal) cells, the majority of fibres of ventral spinocerebellar tract cross to the opposite side and ascend in the lateral funiculus, anterior to the fibres of dorsal spinocerebellar tract (Fig. 10.1-10) (some fibres ascend in lateral funiculus of the same side also). Then these fibres ascend through spinal cord, medulla, pons and midbrain. Finally, these fibres reach the cerebellum through the superior cerebellar peduncle (Fig. 10.1-14).

Termination. These fibres terminate in the lower limb area of the cerebellar cortex.

2. Dorsal (Posterior) Spinocerebellar Tract

Location. This tract is located in the lateral funiculus along the posterolateral periphery of spinal cord. It is situated posterior to ventral spinocerebellar tract and anterior to entry of posterior nerve root (Fig. 10.1-10).

Origin. The first-order neurons are located in the posterior nerve root ganglia. The peripheral processes of *first-order neurons* receive impulses from the muscle spindles, Golgi tendon organs and other proprioceptive receptors.

Course. Unlike ventral spinocerebellar tract, the dorsal spinocerebellar tract is *uncrossed*. The fibres of this tract after originating reach the lateral funiculus of same side and ascend through other spinal segments and reach the medulla oblongata. From here, the fibres reach the cerebellum through the inferior cerebellar peduncle.

Termination. Most of the fibres of this tract terminate in the cortex of anterior lobe of cerebellum.

- Collateral branches of some of the axons of the dorsal spinocerebellar tract are given off in the lower medulla, where they terminate in the *2-nucleus of Brodal and Aonpeine*. This nucleus is rostral to the nucleus gracilis and forms part of the pathway for the conscious proprioception from the lower limbs.

3. Cuneocerebellar Tract The central processes of some first-order neurons (related to cervical segments) reach the *accessory cuneate nucleus* in the medulla. The central processes of the second-order neurons located in the accessory cuneate nucleus form the cuneocerebellar tract (posterior external arcuate fibres), which enter the inferior cerebellar peduncle of same side to reach the cerebellum.

Functions. This tract brings the *conscious proprioception* impulses from the upper limb. Thus, it may be regarded as the forelimb equivalent of the dorsal spinocerebellar tract.

4. Rostral Spinocerebellar Tract

Origin, Course and Termination. This tract is believed to arise from spinal grey matter in lower four cervical segments (lamina VII) from the neurons which constitute the *nucleus centrobasalis*.

Most of the fibres of this tract are uncrossed. They reach the cerebellum through the inferior and superior cerebellar peduncles.

Functions. This pathway is regarded, functionally, as the forelimb equivalent of the ventral spinocerebellar tract.

The major ascending tracts of spinal cord are summarized in Table 10.1-1.

Descending Tracts

The descending tracts, concerned with the various motor activities of the body, are formed by the motor nerve fibres arising from the brain and descending into the spinal cord and brainstem (Fig. 10.1-15).

Descending Tracts Ending in Spinal Cord

Traditionally, the descending tracts ending in the spinal cord have been divided into two groups:

- Pyramidal tracts and
- Extrapyramidal tracts.

I. Pyramidal Tracts The pyramidal tracts refer to the corticospinal tracts which are constituted by the axons that transmit motor signals directly from the cortex to spinal cord (Fig. 10.1-16).

Origin. Corticospinal tract fibres originate from the following nerve cells in the cerebral cortex:

- Primary motor cortex (area 4)—31%,
- Premotor area (area 8) and supplementary motor area—29% and
- Somatic sensory areas (areas 3, 1, 2)—40%.

All the above fibres form the fibres of upper motor neurons of the motor pathway.

Course and Termination. After originating from the cerebral cortex, the corticospinal tract fibres descend as part of corona radiata and then pass through posterior limb of the internal capsule and then downwards through the brainstem, forming pyramids in the medulla (hence the name pyramidal tracts).

In the lower part of medulla, about 90% fibres of each pyramid decussate in the mid line to reach opposite side.

TABLE 10.1-1 Major Ascending Tracts in the Spinal Cord

Tract	Location	Origin*	Termination	Functions
Fasciculus gracilis and fasciculus cuneatus (tracts of Goll and Burdach)	Posterior white column of spinal cord	Dorsal root ganglia of spinal nerves of the same side	Nucleus gracilis and nucleus cuneatus in medulla of the same side	Joint sense, vibration sense, two point discrimination, stereognosis, conscious kinaesthesia
Spinothalamic tracts • Lateral spinothalamic tract • Anterior spinothalamic tract	Lateral white column Anterior white column	Posterior horn cells of spinal cord of opposite side Posterior horn cells of spinal cord of opposite side	Ventral posterolateral (VPL) nucleus of thalamus Ventral posterolateral (VPL) nucleus of thalamus	Carry pain and temperature from opposite side of the body Carry light touch, pressure, tickle and itch sensation from opposite side of the body
Spinotectal tract	Lateral white column.	Posterior horn cells of spinal cord of opposite side	Superior colliculus of tectum of midbrain	Visuomotor reflexes viz. head and eye movements towards the source of stimulation
Spinocerebellar (anterior and posterior) tracts	Lateral white column (superficially)	Posterior horn cells of spinal cord of same side	Cerebellum	Unconscious kinaesthesia (proprioception)

*Location of cell bodies of neurons from which the axons of tract arise.

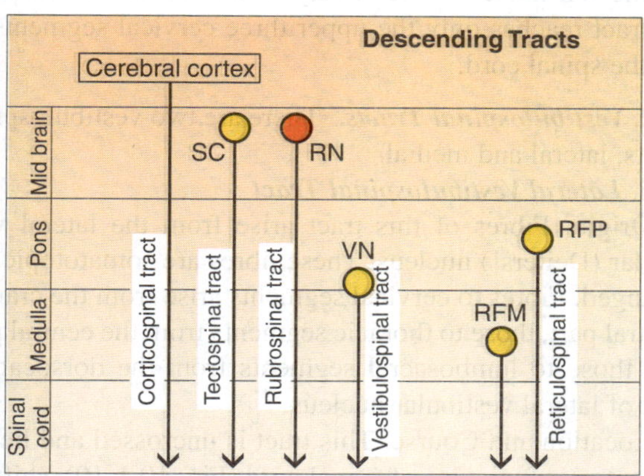

FIGURE 10.1-15 Schematic drawing to show the various descending tracts ending in spinal cord and brainstem. SC = superior colliculus; RN = red nucleus; VN = vestibular nucleus, RFP = reticular formation of pons; RFM = reticular formation of medulla.

From here downwards, the fibres of corticospinal tracts are divided into two separate tracts:

1. *Lateral corticospinal tract* is constituted by 80% of fibres which have crossed to opposite side. The lateral corticospinal tract fibres descend the full length of spinal cord through the posterior part of lateral white funiculus (Figs 10.1-10 and 10.1-16). Most of these fibres terminate in the internuncial neurons of the spinal grey matter. The internuncial neurons carry the impulses to motor neurons situated in the ventral grey horn. Some fibres of the tract terminate directly on ventral horn cells. The axons of the ventral motor neurons supply the skeletal muscles directly by passing through the ventral nerve root. The neurons giving origin to the fibres of pyramidal tract along with their axons constitute the *upper motor neurons*. The ventral motor neurons in the spinal cord along with their axons constitute the *lower motor* neurons.

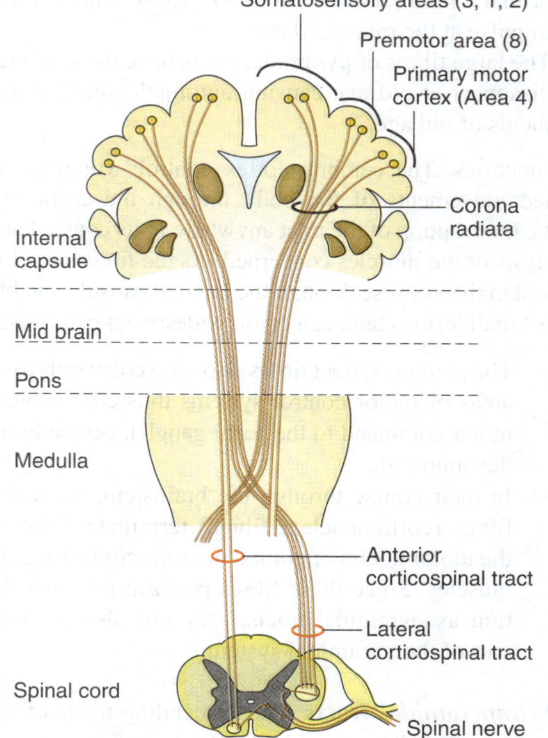

FIGURE 10.1-16 Pathway of corticospinal tracts.

2. *Anterior corticospinal tract* is formed by 20% uncrossed pyramidal fibres. These fibres descend down through the anterior white funiculus of the same side. The anterior corticospinal tract fibres do not reach further than the mid-thoracic region. On reaching the appropriate level of the spinal cord, the fibres of this tract cross the midline (through the anterior white commissure) to reach grey matter on the opposite side of the cord and terminate in a manner similar to that of the fibres of lateral corticospinal tract. Thus, the corticospinal fibres of both the lateral as well as anterior tracts ultimately connect the cerebral cortex of one side with ventral horn cells in opposite half of spinal cord.

Salient Features of Nerve Fibres of Corticospinal Tracts

- Fibres of the corticospinal tract are unmyelinated at birth. Myelination begins in the second postnatal week and is completed by 2 years.
- Most (80%) of the fibres of corticospinal tracts are of small diameter (1–4 μm), while about 20% of fibres are of large diameter (11–22 μm).
- The large-diameter fibres originate from the giant pyramidal neurons (cells of Betz) present in the primary motor cortex (area 4). These fibres transmit impulse at the rate of 70 m/s.
- The large fibres of pyramidal tracts have the tendency to disappear at old age causing automatic shaking movements of old age.

Functions. The cerebral cortex controls voluntary fine-skilled movements of the body through the corticospinal tracts. Interruption of the tract anywhere in its course leads to paralysis of the muscles concerned. As the fibres are closely packed in their course through the internal capsule and brainstem, small lesions here can cause widespread paralysis.

- The pyramidal tract fibres also send collaterals to other areas of motor control systems thus communicating motor command to the basal ganglia, cerebellum and the brainstem.
- In their course through the brainstem, some of the fibres (corticonuclear fibres) terminate directly on the motor nuclei of cranial neurons controlling facial muscles. Since these fibres perform the same function as pyramidal tracts, they are also considered part of the pyramidal system.

II. Extrapyramidal Tracts The descending tracts of spinal cord other than the pyramidal tracts are collectively called extrapyramidal tracts. These include:

- Rubrospinal tract,
- Vestibulospinal tract,
- Reticulospinal tract,
- Tectospinal tract,
- Olivospinal tract and
- Medial longitudinal fasciculus.

1. Rubrospinal Tract

Origin. This tract arises from the large cells (nucleus magnocellularis) or red nucleus in midbrain.

Course. After arising from the red nucleus, the fibres of this tract cross to opposite side in the lower part of segmental of midbrain (ventral segmental decussation). Then, the tract descends through the pons and medulla and follows a course similar to that of lateral corticospinal tract in the lateral funiculus of the spinal cord (Figs 10.1-10 and 10.9-3).

Termination. The fibres terminate mainly on interneurons along with corticospinal fibres.

Functions. This tract exhibits facilitatory influence on the flexor muscles and inhibitory influence on the extensor muscles of the body.

- The red nucleus also receives the corticorubral fibres from the ipsilateral motor cortex. The corticorubrospinal tract thus formed may act as an alternate route of pyramidal system to exert influence on lower motor neurons.
- The rubrospinal tract is most important and much better developed in some animals than in humans. In humans, the red nucleus is relatively small and the rubrospinal tract reaches only the upper three cervical segments of the spinal cord.

2. Vestibulospinal Tracts. There are two vestibulospinal tracts, lateral and medial.

i. ***Lateral Vestibulospinal Tract***

Origin. Fibres of this tract arise from the lateral vestibular (Deiters') nucleus. These fibres are somatotopically arranged. Fibres to cervical segments arise from the cranio-ventral part, those to thoracic segments from the central part and those to lumbosacral segments from the dorsocaudal part of lateral vestibular nucleus.

Location and Course. This tract is uncrossed and lies in the anterior funiculus of spinal cord (Fig. 10.1-10), shifting medially as it descends.

Termination. The fibres extend up to caudal segments of the cord and terminate into neurons of ventral grey column (laminae VII and VIII). Through the interneurons, these are projected to the alpha and gamma neurons of lamina IX; some fibres directly reach the alpha neurons.

Functions. Vestibular nucleus receives afferents from vestibular apparatus mainly from utricles. This pathway is principally concerned with adjustment of postural muscles to linear acceleratory displacements of the body. Lateral vestibulospinal tract mainly facilitates activity of extensor muscles and inhibits the activity of flexor muscles in association with the maintenance of balance.

ii. Medial Vestibulospinal Tract

Origin. The fibres of this tract arise from the medial vestibular nucleus.

Location and Course. This tract descends through the anterior funiculus (within the sulcomarginal fasciculus). The fibres are mostly uncrossed but some fibres are crossed.

Termination. The fibres end in the anterior motor neurons directly or through internuncial neurons (laminae VII and VIII) of the cervical segments of spinal cord.

Functions. This part of the vestibular nucleus receives signals from the vestibular apparatus mainly from the semicircular canals. Functionally, medial vestibulospinal tract is the donor connection of medial longitudinal fasciculus. This tract provides a reflex pathway for movements of head, neck and eyes in response to visual and auditory stimuli.

3. Reticulospinal Tracts

There are two reticulospinal tracts: the medial (pontine) reticulospinal tract and lateral (medullary) reticulospinal tract.

i. Medial (Pontine) Reticulospinal Tract

Origin. It arises in the medial pontine reticular formation.

Course. The tract descends, mostly uncrossed, in the anterior funiculus of spinal cord.

Termination. The fibres terminate in the laminae VII and VIII of spinal grey matter and through internuncial neurons influence alpha and gamma neurons of lamina IX.

ii. Lateral (Medullary) Reticulospinal Tract

Origin. The fibres of this tract originate from the gigantocellular component of medullary reticular formation.

Course. These fibres are mostly uncrossed and a few crossed. This tract descends in the lateral funiculus medial to the lateral corticospinal and rubrospinal tracts (Fig. 10.1-10).

Termination. The fibres terminate in the internuncial neurons of laminae VII, VIII and IX of the spinal cord.

Functions of Reticulospinal Tracts. The reticular formation of the brainstem receives input mostly from the motor cortex through the corticoreticular fibres which accompany the corticospinal tracts. Thus, the cortico-reticulospinal tracts form additional polysynaptic pathways from motor cortex to spinal cord. These tracts are concerned with control of movements and maintenance of muscle tone. The reticulospinal tracts, probably, also convey autonomic information from higher centres to the intermediate region of spinal grey matter and regulate respiration, circulation and sweating.

The pontine and medullary reticular nuclei mostly function antagonistic to each other as:

- Pontine nuclei are excitatory to antigravity muscles and medullary nuclei are inhibitory.
- Pontine nuclei facilitate while medullary nuclei inhibit the control of voluntary and reflex movements and control of muscle tone through gamma neurons.
- Pontine reticular formation favours expiration, while medullary reticular formation favours inspiration.
- Pontine nuclei cause vasoconstriction and medullary nuclei cause vasodilatation.

4. Tectospinal Tract

Origin. Fibres of this tract arise from superior colliculi.

Course. In contrast to other tracts of extrapyramidal system, the fibres cross the midline in the lower part of segmental of the midbrain forming dorsal segmental decussation. Then the tract descends through the pons and medulla into the anterior white funiculus of the spinal cord (Fig. 10.1-10).

Termination. The fibres terminate in upper cervical levels by synapsing on the anterior horn cells through internuncial neurons located in laminae V and VII of the spinal grey matter.

Function. This tract forms the motor limb of the reflex pathway for turning the head and moving the arms in response to visual, hearing or other exteroceptive stimuli.

5. Olivospinal Tract

Origin. This tract of doubtful existence originates from the inferior olivary nucleus.

Course and Termination. The tract fibres descend and terminate ipsilaterally in the anterior horn cells of the spinal cord.

Functions. Exact connections are unknown. Inferior olivary nucleus receives afferent fibres from cerebral cortex, corpus striatum, red nucleus and spinal cord. It influences muscle activity. Probably, it is involved in reflex movements arising from the proprioceptors.

6. Medial Longitudinal Fasciculus

Origin. The medial longitudinal fasciculus (MLF) extends from the midbrain downwards. The fibres of this tract take origin from different area of the brainstem, namely:

- Vestibular nuclei,
- Reticular formation,
- Superior colliculus,
- Interstitial nucleus of Cajal,
- Nucleus of posterior commissure and
- Nucleus of Darkschewitsch.

Course. The MLF (Fig. 10.1-17) in the brainstem is closely related to the nuclei of 3rd, 4th, 6th and 12th cranial nerves. It is also related to the fibres of 7th nerve (as they wind round the abducent nucleus), and to some fibres arising from the cochlear nuclei. Below, the MLF becomes continuous with the anterior intersegmental tract of spinal cord (Fig. 10.1-10) which descends through the posterior part of anterior white funiculus. This tract is well defined only in the upper cervical segments. Below this level, the fibres run along with the fibres of medial vestibulospinal tract.

Termination. Along with the fibres of the medial vestibulospinal tract, the fibres of this tract make connections with ventral horn cells that innervate the muscles of neck.

Functions. MLF plays an important role in the pathway of ocular movements. Its function can be summarized as:

- It ensures harmonious movements of the eyes and neck (head) in response to vestibular stimulation and auditory stimuli.
- It facilitates simultaneous movements of the lips and tongue as in speech.

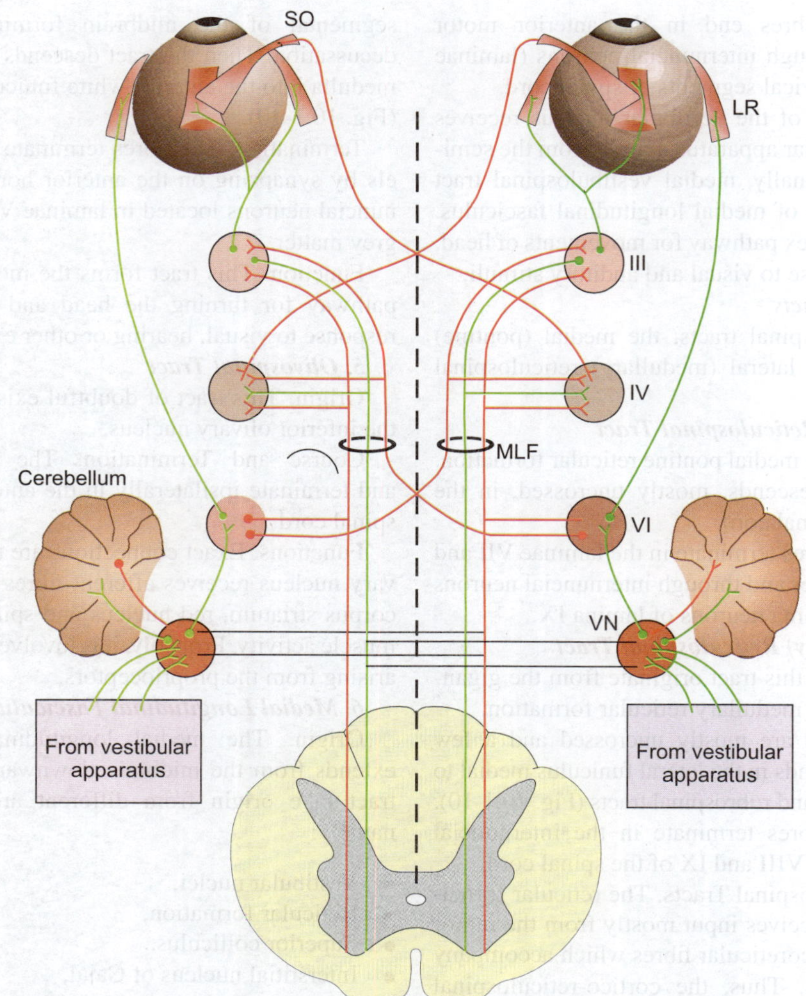

FIGURE 10.1-17 Connections of medial longitudinal fasciculus. SO = superior oblique, LR = lateral rectus, III, IV and VI (nuclei of 3rd, 4th and 6th cranial nuclei), and VN = vestibular nuclei.

Descending Tracts Ending in the Brainstem

Corticonuclear Tracts

Origin. These arise from the cerebral cortex along with the corticospinal tracts (see page 913).

Course and Termination. These fibres descend along with corticospinal tract fibres as part of corona radiata and then pass through posterior limb of the internal capsule. In the brainstem, they cross to the opposite side at various levels and end by synapsing with cells of the cranial nerve nuclei, either direct or through interneurons.

Functions. The nuclei of cranial nerves that supply skeletal muscles are functionally equivalent to ventral horn cells of the spinal cord. These are controlled by corticonuclear fibres.

Cortico-Ponto-Cerebellar Pathway

Origin. This pathway consists of the fibres arising in the cerebral cortex of the frontal, temporal, parietal and occipital lobes.

Course. After originating from the cerebral cortex, the fibres descend through the corona radiata and internal capsule to reach the crus cerebri (Fig. 10.1-10). These fibres synapse with the pontine nuclei of the same side. Axons of the neurons in the pontine nuclei form the transverse fibres of the pons. These fibres cross the midline and pass into the middle cerebellar peduncle of the opposite side and reach the cerebellar cortex.

Functions. This pathway forms the anatomical basis for control of cerebellar activity of cerebral cortex.

Other Fibres Ending in the Brainstem Other fibres arising from the cerebral cortex end in the following masses of grey matter of brainstem:

- Red nucleus (corticorubral fibres),
- Tectum (corticotectal fibres),
- Substantia nigra,

TABLE 10.1-2 Major Descending Tracts of the Spinal Cord

Tract	Location	Origin*	Termination	Functions
Pyramidal tracts				
• Lateral corticospinal (crossed pyramidal) tract	Lateral white column of spinal cord	Primary motor cortex (area 4), pre-motor cortex (area 6) of the opposite cerebral hemisphere *(upper motor neurons)*	Anterior horn cells of the spinal cord *(lower motor neurons)*	Controls conscious skilled movements especially of hands (contraction of individual or small group of muscles particularly those which move hands, fingers, feet and toes)
• Anterior corticospinal (uncrossed pyramidal) tract	Anterior white column	Primary motor cortex (area 4), pre-motor cortex (area 6) of the opposite cerebral hemisphere *(upper motor neurons)*	Anterior horn cells of the spinal cord *(lower motor neurons)*	Same as that of lateral corticospinal tracts
Extrapyramidal Tracts				
• Rubrospinal tract	Lateral white column	Red nucleus of the opposite side located in midbrain	Anterior horn cells of the spinal cord	Unconscious co-ordination of movements (controls muscle tone and synergy)
• Vestibulospinal tract	Anterior white column	Vestibular nucleus	Anterior horn cells of the spinal cord	Unconscious maintenance of posture and balance
Reticulospinal Tracts				
• Medial reticulospinal tract	Anterior white column	Reticular formation in medulla.	Anterior horn cells of the spinal cord	Mainly responsible for inhibitory influence on the motor neurons to the skeletal muscles
• Lateral reticulospinal tract	Lateral white column	Reticular formation in midbrain, pons and medulla.	Anterior horn cells of the spinal cord	Mainly responsible for facilitatory influence on the motor neurons to the skeletal muscles
Tectospinal tract	Anterior white column	Superior colliculus of the opposite side	Cranial nerve nuclei in medulla and anterior horn cells of the upper spinal segments	Controls movements of head, neck and arms in response to the visual stimuli

*Location of cell bodies of neurons from which the axons of tract arise.

- Inferior olivary nucleus (cortico-olivary fibres) and
- Reticular formation (corticoreticular fibres).

The above fibres ultimately form part of extrapyramidal system.

The major descending tracts in spinal cord are summarized in Table 10.1-2.

LESIONS OF SPINAL CORD AND BRAINSTEM

Transection of the Spinal Cord

Transection of the spinal cord can be divided into three types:

- Complete transection,
- Incomplete transection and
- Hemisection.

Complete Transection of Spinal Cord

Common Causes of complete transection are:

- Gunshot injuries,
- Dislocation of spine and
- Occlusion of the blood vessels.

Common Site of involvement is at the mid-thoracic level.

Clinical Stages The effects (symptoms and signs) produced by complete transection of the spinal cord occur in following three stages:

- Stage of spinal shock,
- Stage of reflex activity and
- Stage of reflex failure.

A. Stage of Spinal Shock. Spinal shock refers to cessation of all the functions and activity below the level of the section immediately after injury.

Effects depend on the site of injury; complete transection in cervical region (above C_5) is usually fatal, because of cutting of connections between respiratory centre and respiratory muscles leading to paralysis of respiratory muscles.

In quick transection of spinal cord, the patient feels as it has been cut into two portions, the upper portion (higher centres and mind) is unaffected, but the whole body below the level of injury is deprived of all the sensations and motor activity.

Cause of stage of spinal shock (also called stage of flaccidity) is not known, but it is related to cessation of tonic neuronal discharge from upper brainstem or supraspinal pathway.

Duration and severity of spinal shock depends upon the evolution of animal. Higher the animal, more profound and longer lasting is the spinal shock. This is probably due to encephalization, i.e. greater dependence of spinal cord on higher centres. Therefore, spinal shock lasts for few minutes in frogs, for few hours in cats and dogs, for days in monkey's and in humans it lasts for about 3 weeks.

In higher animals, the entire nervous system is integrated as a functional unit; therefore, damage to any part of the nervous system disturbs its smoothness of working and the functional failure is more severe. This is called *diaschisis*.

Characteristic effects during spinal shock can be summarized:

1. ***Motor effects*** include:
   - *Paralysis of the muscles* occurs below the level of section. Depending upon the site of lesion, when both lower limbs are paralyzed (transection between cervical and lumbosacral enlargements), it is called paraplegia and when all the four limbs are affected (transection below C_5), it is called quadriplegia.
   - *Loss of tone* occurs in the paralyzed muscles. So the muscles become atonic or flaccid. This is called the state of flaccid paralysis.
   - *Areflexia,* i.e. all the superficial and deep reflexes are markedly decreased or lost.
2. ***Sensory effects.*** All the sensations are lost below the level of transections.
3. ***Vasomotor effects.*** The sympathetic vasoconstrictor fibres leave the spinal cord between T_1 and L_2. Therefore, depending upon the site of lesion, the vasomotor effects produced are:
   - Transection of cord below L_2 segment will produce no effect or very little fall in blood pressure.
   - Transection at the level of T_1 segment cuts off all the thoracolumbar sympathetic neurons from the medullary cardiovascular centre. As a result there occurs loss of sympathetic tonic discharge causing arteriolar dilatation leading to a sharp fall in blood pressure (MBP may fall from a normal resting value of 100 to about 40 mmHg). Fall in blood pressure is less marked as the section shifts more distally towards L_2 segment.

   Absence of movements due to paralysis of muscles further retards the circulation and also the venous return producing cold and blue (cyanotic) extremities. Skin becomes dry and scaly and bed sores may develop.

   Note. It is important to note that after paralysis of the muscles, the body temperature becomes subnormal (as muscular contraction is a major source of heat production). When hot bottles are given to raise the body temperature, under such circumstances bed sores develop.

4. ***Visceral effects*** produced are:
   - *Urinary bladder* is paralyzed; however, the sphincter vesicae regain tone early leading to retention of urine.
   - *Rectum* is also paralyzed. Since the bowels become hypotonic, there occurs constipation.
   - *Penis* becomes flaccid and erection becomes impossible.
   - When lesion is at T_6 level, all impulses coming in from the abdominal viscera are cut off from the brain; therefore, gripping sensations or distension of viscera are not appreciated.

B. Stage of Reflex Activity. If the patient survives the stage of spinal shock, gradually he/she gains few functions. That is why this is also called the stage of recovery. After about 3 weeks period, depending largely upon the general health of the patient, the reflex activity begins to return to the isolated segments of spinal cord below the level of lesion. Various developments which take place, in a chronological order, in this stage are:

1. ***Smooth muscles regain functional activity first of all,*** and urinary bladder becomes automatic, i.e. reflex evacuation is gradually established in a perfectly normal manner. Similarly, reflex defaecation is also established.
2. ***Sympathetic tone of the blood vessels is regained,*** next to smooth muscles, when connector cells in spinal cord begin to act independently of the VMC. As a result:
   - *Blood pressure* is restored to normal.
   - *Skin,* which has become dry and scaly, now shows sweating again and becomes more healthy. Bed sores, if any, heal up rapidly.
3. ***Skeletal muscle tone then recovers slowly after 3–4 weeks.*** Recovery of muscle tone is reflex in character and is produced by impulses entering the spinal cord from the muscles.
   - Tone of flexor muscles returns first; therefore, flexors become less hypotonic than extensors leading to '*paraplegia in flexion*' (both lower limbs are in state of flexion).

- In 'spinal man', the limbs cannot support the weight of the body.

  Note. No wasting of muscles is seen, because though the muscles are paralyzed for voluntary movements, they are in constant reflex activity.

4. ***Reflex activity begins to return after few weeks of recovery of muscle tone.*** Recovery of reflex excitability is due to the development of *denervation hypersensitivity* to the mediators released by the remaining spinal excitatory endings and the growing of collaterals from existing neurons with the formation of additional excitatory ending on interneurons and motor neurons.
   - *Flexor reflexes* return first, and to elicit flexor reflex, a painful stimuli is required. The first reflex which usually appears is Babinski's reflex (i.e. *Babinski's* sign is positive).
   - *Extensor reflexes* return after a variable period of 1–5 weeks of appearance of flexor reflexes. Initially, the *knee jerk* appears, and then the *ankle jerk* may return still later. Generally, about 6 months after the occurrence of transection, marked activity appears in the extensor arcs. This results in exaggerated extensor reflexes with the appearance of extensor spasms.
   - Mass reflex can be elicited in some cases by scratching the skin over the lower limbs or the anterior abdominal wall, depending upon the level of lesion. It is characterized by spasm of flexor muscles of both the limbs, evacuation of bladder and profuse sweating below the level of the lesion.

Note. The mass reflex can be utilized to provide paraplegic patients a degree of bladder and bowel control. Patients can be trained to initiate urination and defaecation by intentionally producing mass reflex with the help of a stroke or a pinch on their thighs.

C. Stage of Reflex Failure. The failure of reflex activity may occur when general condition of the patient starts deteriorating due to malnutrition, infections or toxaemia, under such circumstances:

- Reflexes become more difficult to elicit,
- The threshold for stimulus increases,
- Mass reflex is abolished and
- The muscles become extremely flaccid and undergo wasting.

Incomplete Transection of Spinal Cord

In incomplete transection, the spinal cord is gravely injured but does not suffer from complete transection (i.e. a few tracts are intact).

Effects Effects of incomplete transection can be divided into three clinical stages:

- Stage of spinal shock,
- Stage of reflex activity and
- Stage of reflex failure.

A. Stage of Spinal Shock. Features of this stage are similar to those described in stage of spinal shock of complete transection of spinal cord (see page 917).

B. Stage of Reflex Activity. Features of this stage differ remarkably from that of stage of reflex activity of complete transection of spinal cord:

1. **Tone appears in extensor muscles first** (c.f. complete transection in which tone appears in flexor muscles first). This is because of the fact that in incomplete transection, some of the descending fibres in the lateral column of the cord, especially the vestibulospinal and reticulospinal tracts, may escape injury, and both these tracts mainly reinforce activity of extensor motor neurons. Because of comparatively higher tone in extensor muscles, a condition called 'paraplegia in extension' results (c.f. complete transection in which paraplegia in flexion is seen).
2. **Extensor reflexes (stretch reflexes) return first** and flexor reflexes reappear later (c.f. complete transection in which flexor reflexes return first). Extensor reflexes which can be elicited in this stage in incomplete transection and not in complete transection are:
   - ***Phillipson reflex.*** It refers to extension of the opposite limb produced by gentle flexion of one limb. The flexed limb then becomes extended and the opposite one flexed, i.e. the response alternates in each limb producing a steppage movement.
   - ***Extensor thrust reflex.*** It refers to physiological extensor response (i.e. active contraction of quadriceps, and posterior calf muscles with straightening of limb) obtained by pressing the foot upward with the palm of the hand in a patient in whom the lower limb has been passively flexed and allowed to rest on the bed.
   - ***Crossed extensor reflex.*** It refers to occurrence of forcible extension of the opposite limb associated with withdrawal (flexor) reflex produced by noxious stimulus to the sole of foot of one limb.
3. **Mass reflex is not elicited** in incomplete transection (c.f. complete transection in which mass reflex is elicited). This is because the controlling effect of brainstem persists through motor fibres (vestibulospinal and reticulospinal) which have escaped injury.

C. Stage of Reflex Failure. Features of this stage are similar to that of stage of reflex failure with complete transection of spinal cord (see page 919).

Hemisection of the Spinal Cord (Brown-Sequard Syndrome)

Hemisection of the spinal cord refers to a lesion involving one lateral half of the spinal cord (Fig. 10.1-18). It can occur in following accidental injuries. It can also be produced for experimental studies in the animals.

The effects of hemisection of the spinal cord can be described in two stages:

- Immediate effects and
- Late effects.

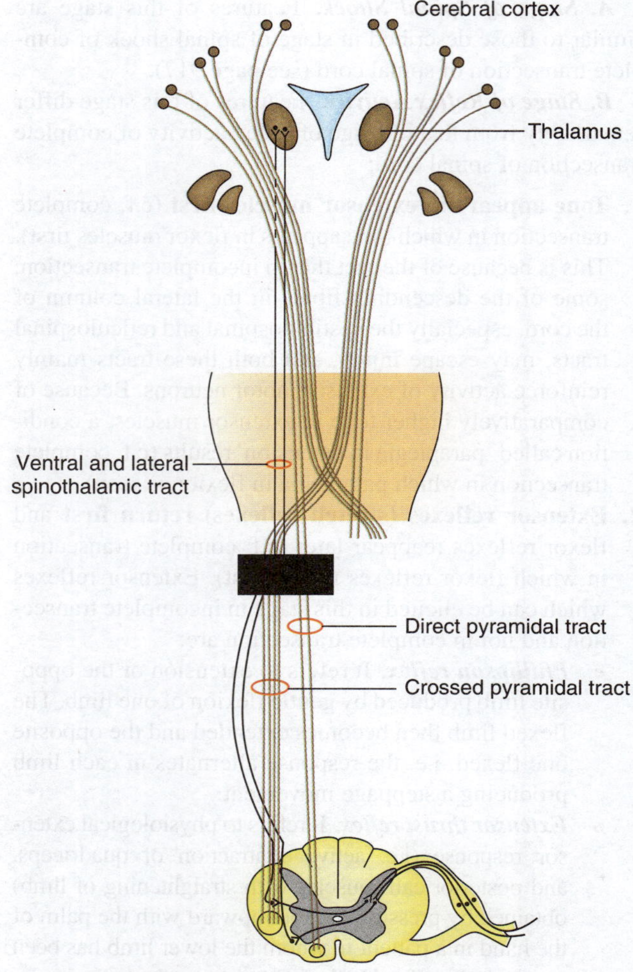

FIGURE 10.1-18 Hemisection of the spinal cord.

Immediate Effects Immediate effects following hemisection of the spinal cord are those of 'spinal shock' (see page 917).

Late Effects If the patient survives, typical motor and sensory changes develop after recovery from the spinal shock. These changes constitute the *Brown-Sequard syndrome* and can be described as:

- Changes at the level of section,
- Changes below the level of section and
- Changes above the level of section.

A. Changes at the Level of Hemisection

I. Changes on the Same Side

1. Sensory Changes. All the sensations are lost (complete anaesthesia) at the level of hemisection on the same side. This occurs because of complete damage to posterior nerve root, posterior horn cells and spinothalamic fibres (which cross to the opposite side).

2. Motor Changes. at the level of hemisection on the same side include:

i. *Complete lower motor neuron* (LMN) type paralysis is seen due to damage to the anterior horn cells. That is:
- Flaccid paralysis of muscles (paralysis with loss of muscle tone),
- All the reflexes are lost,
- Muscle power is lost and ultimately
- Muscles degenerate and undergo wasting due to loss of tone. For detailed features of LMN paralysis, see page 923.

ii. *Complete and permanent vasomotor paralysis* occurs due to damage of the lateral horn cells.

II. Changes on the Opposite Side

1. Sensory Changes. There occurs some loss of pain, temperature and crude touch sensations due to injury to the fibres of spinothalamic tract which cross horizontally in the same segment and may be caught up in the lesion. But tracts of *Gall and Burdach* are not affected, so the sensations carried by these two tracts are not affected.

2. Motor Changes. Usually no motor change occurs. If it occurs, it is very mild and is similar to the effects of lower motor neuron lesion.

B. Changes below the Level of Section

I. Changes on the Same Side

1. Sensory Changes. There is dissociated sensory loss:

- *Injury to uncrossed fibres of tracts of Gall and Burdach* causes loss of fine touch, tactile localization, tactile discrimination, sensation of vibration, conscious kinaesthetic sensation and stereognosis.
- *No injury to spinothalamic tracts* which cross to the opposite side, so crude touch, pain and temperature sensations are not lost.

2. Motor Changes. There occurs upper motor neuron (UMN) type of paralysis due to injury to the pyramidal tracts. Features of UMN paralysis include:

- Increased muscle tone, leading to spastic paralysis,
- Loss of superficial reflexes,
- Exaggeration of deep reflexes,
- Positive Babinski's sign,
- Rigidity of limbs and
- No degeneration and wasting of muscles.

3. Vasomotor Changes. There occurs temporary loss of vasomotor tone due to damage to the descending fibres from the VMC in the medulla to the lateral horn cells. This leads to:

- Dilatation of blood vessels and
- Fall in blood pressure.

However, soon the intact lateral horn cells start acting as supplementary VMC and vasomotor tone returns leading to normalization of blood pressure.

II. **Changes on the Opposite Side**

1. Sensory Changes. Dissociated sensory loss occurs as:

- *Injury to crossed spinothalamic tracts* causes loss of following sensations on the opposite side below the level of lesion: crude touch, pain and temperature.
- *No injury to uncrossed tracts of Gall and Burdach,* so following sensations on the opposite side below the level of lesion are not lost: fine touch, tactile localization, tactile discrimination, vibratory sense, conscious kinaesthetic sensation and stereognosis.

2. Motor Changes. Usually, no motor change on the opposite side below the level of lesion occurs. UMN lesion type paralysis of a few muscles, however, may occur sometimes due to possible damage to some fibres of direct pyramidal tracts of the same side when these fibres cross.

In a nutshell, below the level of lesion there occurs:

- Extensive motor loss but little sensory loss on the same side and
- Extensive sensory loss but little motor loss on the opposite side.

C. Changes above the Level of Lesion

I. **Changes on the Same Side**

1. Sensory Changes. A band of hyperaesthesia, i.e. increased cutaneous sensations are present in one or two segments above the level of section on the same side. This occurs due to irritation of the neighbouring posterior nerve roots above the level of section.

2. Motor Changes. Twitching of muscle in upper one or two segments on the same side may occur due to irritation of the neighbouring anterior nerve roots above the level of section.

II. **Changes on the Opposite Side**

1. Sensory Changes. Either no sensory change or referred hyperaesthesia may be seen one or two segments above the lesion on the opposite side.

2. Motor Changes. No motor change occurs on the opposite side above the level of section.

Regional Peculiarities in Hemisection of Spinal Cord

1. Hemisection in the Cervical Region shows following peculiar changes:

- *Constriction of pupil on the same side,* due to damage to dilator fibres passing via T_1, T_2 and T_3 anterior nerve roots.
- *Loss of following jerks* occur if the lesion involves C_4, C_5 and C_6 segments: biceps, triceps, supinator and pronator jerks.
- *Paralysis of diaphragm* on the same side occurs due to involvement of phrenic nerve (C_3, C_4 and C_5).

2. Hemisection in Lumbar Region may show the following peculiarities:

- Loss of knee jerk and
- Disturbances in the micturition due to involvement of L3 and 4.

3. Hemisection in Lumbosacral Region is associated with loss of control over the sphincters of:

- Urinary bladder and
- Anus.

Complications in Patients with Spinal Cord Transection

Patients with spinal cord transection get immobilized due to paraplegia or quadriplegia and thus may develop following complications:

1. ***Decubitus (postural) ulcers*** occur due to compression of circulation to the skin over bony prominences in bedridden patients by the body weight. These ulcers heal very poorly and are prone to secondary infections.
2. ***Hypercalcaemia, hypercalciuria and calcium stone formation in urinary tract*** may occur due to breakdown of proteins from the bone matrix.
3. ***Urinary tract infections*** are very common owing to urinary stasis associated with paralysis of urinary bladder.
4. ***Septicaemia, uraemia, coma and even death*** may occur as a complication of severe urinary tract infection.

Treatment. High dose of corticosteroid if administered immediately after spinal cord injury has some values, because steroids decrease the inflammatory reaction by suppressing neutrophils activity, and improving capillary permeability.

Lesions of Sensory System in Spinal Cord

Deafferentation (Dorsal Nerve Root Lesion)

Injury to the dorsal nerve root (afferent nerve) produces the following effects:

1. Loss of All Sensations, i.e.

- Loss of exteroceptive senses with anaesthesia and analgesia,
- Loss of conscious muscle sense, producing ataxia,
- Loss of unconscious muscle sense from stretch receptors of muscle spindle, with hypotonia or atonia and
- Loss of visceral senses.

2. Loss of All Reflexes. All the reflexes, superficial as well as deep, are lost.

3. Muscle Tone is lost.

4. Marked Weakness in the Movements of Parts occurs because the higher centres concerned with reflex control of posture are deprived of afferent impulses from joints and muscles.

Syringomyelia

Syringomyelia is a rare disease in which there occurs excessive overgrowth of neuroglial tissue accompanied by cavitation in the grey matter around the central canal of spinal cord. This disease involves the cervical enlargement of the cord more frequently.

Characteristic Features

I. Sensory Features are predominant and occur in the form of dissociated anaesthesia, i.e. loss of pain and temperature with retention of touch sensation as:

1. ***Loss of pain, temperature and crude touch*** sensation occurs due to destruction of the fibres which carry these sensations and are decussating in the grey commissure.
2. ***Fine touch sensation*** is not lost because the fibres carrying this sensation ascend in the dorsal column and escape damage.

Note. The symptoms are bilateral and usually occur in the hands and arms due to the *predilection* of syringomyelin for the cervical enlargement of the cord.

II. Motor Features may also occur due to further spread of gliosis and cavitations:

1. ***Flaccid paralysis of the upper limb muscle*** (LMN type paralysis) may occur initially due to involvement of anterior horn cells.
2. ***Progressive spastic paralysis of the legs*** (UMN type paralysis) may occur later on due to involvement of pyramidal and extra pyramidal tracts.

Tabes Dorsalis

Tabes dorsalis is a disease, usually caused by syphilis, in which there occurs bilateral degeneration of posterior nerve roots and posterior funiculi, especially fasciculus gracilis. It is characterized by the following features:

1. ***Lightening pains*** occur in intermittent attacks due to stimulation of pain fibres in dorsal nerve roots in the initial stages.
2. ***Loss or decrease*** of pain sensibility occurs after sometime producing the following features:
   - *Trophic disturbances* in the form of perforating ulcers of the skin at pressure points. *Charcot joint refers* to deformed joints produced by repeated trauma due to loss of pain sensations. There is no proper support and movements of the joints of the body become uncontrolled.
   - Anaesthesia of central part of face occurs due to involvement of 5th cranial nerve.
   - Anaesthesia at the upper chest, inner border of hands, around the anus and over the legs occurs due to involvement of dorsal nerve roots in cervicothoracic and lumbosacral regions.
3. ***Loss of deep sensations.*** Following sensations are lost on the same side at and below the level of lesion: position sense, vibratory sense, sense of stereognosis and discriminative touch.
4. ***Loss of reflexes.*** Both superficial and deep reflexes are lost in tabes dorsalis mostly because of loss of sensations.
5. ***Sensory ataxia*** occurs due to lack of co-ordination of voluntary involvement. In it the patient walks on a broad base with the legs apart and eyes fixed to the ground for correcting the steps. Typically, the patient raises the legs excessively high and slopes the feet on the ground. *Romberg's sign* is positive.

Multiple Sclerosis

Multiple sclerosis (MS) is a demyelinating disorder having widespread disseminated involvement of white matter of the central nervous system. Because of this, it was also called disseminated sclerosis. It is currently considered to be an autoimmune disease, pathologically characterized by focal inflammation, demyelination and gliosis or scarring. A remitting and relapsing course is the most common, with either complete recovery or residual damage with each attack.

Manifestations of MS depend upon the area of CNS involved. Commonest symptoms reported are:

- Limb weakness (75%),
- Sensory loss (37%),
- Paraesthesia (24%) and
- Optic neuritis (37%).
- Diplopia, vertigo and ataxia are comparatively less common.

Subacute Combined Degeneration of the Spinal Cord

Subacute combined degeneration of the spinal cord is usually associated with pernicious anaemia, due to lack of intrinsic factor which is essential for the absorption of vitamin B_{12}.

In this condition, bilateral degeneration of white fibres of the dorsal column and lateral column of the spinal cord occurs, especially involving the lumbosacral segments. Its manifestations include:

- Loss of position and vibrating senses of the lower extremities and
- Signs of upper motor neuron lesions such as bilateral spasticity, exaggerated tendon reflexes and positive Babinski's sign.

Lesions of Motor System

Lower versus Upper Motor Neuron Lesion Difference between lower motor neuron lesions and upper motor neuron lesions are shown in Table 10.1-3.

Brainstem Lesions

Lesions of Medulla

1. Medial Medullary Syndrome Medial medullary syndrome results from occlusion of the blood supply (anterior spinal artery and its paramedian branches) to medial zone of the medulla. It is characterized by:

- Lower motor neuron paralysis of ipsilateral tongue muscles due to involvement of hypoglossal nerve.

TABLE 10.1-3 Lower versus Upper Motor Neuron Lesions

Lower motor neuron lesion (LMNL)	Upper motor neuron lesion (UMNL)
1. LMNL refers to involvement of neurons (α and γ) of anterior horn of spinal cord and neurons of cranial nerve nuclei	1. UMNL refers to involvement of motor neurons that influence the activity of LMN of spinal cord or cranial nerve nuclei located in brainstem. Thus, in UMNL, the pyramidal and extrapyramidal descending tracts are involved
2. LMN paralysis is typically observed in poliomyelitis, when the polio virus selectively affects the lower motor neurons of spinal cord and brainstem	2. UMN paralysis occurs commonly in vascular accidents or space-occupying lesions.
3. Usually a single or individual muscle is affected	3. Usually a group of muscles are affected
4. Flaccid paralysis of the involved muscle as muscle tone is lost due to involvement of stretch reflex arc	4. Spastic paralysis of the involved muscles as the inhibitory higher control is lost and stretch reflex arc is intact
5. Muscle power is lost and ultimately muscles degenerate and undergo wasting due to disuse (disuse atrophy)	5. No degeneration and wasting of muscles as they are constantly involved in reflex activity (though the voluntary movements are lost).
6. Areflexia, i.e. all the superficial as well as deep reflexes are lost	6. Superficial reflexes {abdominal, cremasteric, anal are lost but deep reflexes are exaggerated (because of increased gamma-motor discharge)}.
7. Babinski's sign is negative, i.e. on stroking the outer edge of sole of the foot with firm tactile stimulus, there occurs plantar flexion (downward movement). It is called floor response (withdrawal reflex) and is considered a normal response	7. Babinski's sign is positive, i.e. on stroking the outer edge of the sole of the foot with firm stimulus, there occurs dorsiflexion of the great toe and fanning out (abduction) of small toes. It is also called extensor response. Positive Babinski's sign indicates involvement of corticospinal tract. In normal infants, this sign is positive prior to myelination of the corticospinal tract (i.e. below 1 year of age)
8. Clonus is absent	8. Clonus is present. It refers to a sustained series of rhythmic muscle jerks when a quick stretch is applied to a tendon. Ankle clonus is usually observed in UMNL by sudden dorsiflexion of the foot.
9. Clasp knife reflex is absent	9. Clasp knife reflex is present, i.e. muscular resistance to passive movement is exaggerated, this resistance is strong at the beginning of movement, but yields suddenly in a clasp knife fashion as more force against resistance is applied. The initial resistance is offered because of the stretch reflex developed in extensor muscles, e.g. triceps of the elbow. The sudden relax of resistance is due to the activation of inverse stretch reflex

- Upper motor neuron paralysis on the contralateral side due to involvement of corticospinal tract.
- Contralateral loss of discriminative senses of the body due to interruption of the medial lemniscus rostral to the decussation.

2. Lateral Medullary Syndrome Lateral medullary syndrome results from the occlusion of posterior inferior cerebellar artery supplying the posterolateral part of the medulla.

Characteristic Features of this syndrome are:

- *Ipsilateral loss of pain and temperature* sensations in the face and forehead area due to interruption of the spinal tract of the trigeminal nerve.
- Contralateral loss of pain and temperature in the rest of the body due to involvement of spinal lemniscus.
- Paralysis of the muscles of the soft palate, pharynx and larynx on the side of lesion due to destruction of the nucleus ambiguus.
- Cerebellar asynergia and hypotonia occur when the inferior cerebellar peduncle is also affected.
- Nystagmus when vestibular nucleus is also affected.

3. Cerebellopontine Syndrome Cerebellopontine syndrome refers to the lesions produced by a tumour in the cerebellopontine angle compressing on the neighbouring structures.

Characteristic Features of this syndrome are:

- ***Involvement of the 7th cranial nerve*** produces:
  - Ipsilateral LMN paralysis of facial muscles of expression,
  - Hyperacusis due to paralysis of stapedius muscle and

- Loss of taste sensation from the anterior two-third of the tongue.
- ***Involvement of 8th cranial nerve*** causes:
  - Persistent tinnitus,
  - Progressive deafness on the affected side and
  - Vertigo.
- ***Cerebellar dysfunctions*** may occur in the forms of:
  - Intention tremors,
  - Dysmetria,
  - Adiadochokinesis and
  - Ataxia on the affected side.
- ***Involvement of the spinal tract of trigeminal*** causes:
  - Ipsilateral loss of pain and temperature of the face and forehead.
- ***Involvement of the spinal lemniscus*** produces:
  - Contralateral loss of pain and temperature of the body.

Pontine Lesions

1. Alternative Trigeminal Hemiplegia Alternating trigeminal hemiplegia is seen in lesions involving the lateral part of mid-pons.

Characteristic Features include:

1. ***Damage to trigeminal nerve*** results in:
   - Ipsilateral absence of all general senses of the face and the forehead and
   - Ipsilateral lower motor neuron (LMN) paralysis of the muscles of mastication.
2. ***Damage to pyramidal tracts*** causes:
   - Contralateral hemiplegia.

2. Raymond's Syndrome Raymond's syndrome, also known as alternating abducent, hemiplegia is characterized by:

1. ***Damage to 6th nerve*** causing:
   - Paralytic convergent squint (esotropia) due to paralysis of lateral rectus muscles and
2. ***Damage to pyramidal tracts*** causing:
   - Contralateral hemiplegia.

3. Millard–Gubler Syndrome Millard–Gubler syndrome results due to lesions of the ventral pons involving 6th nerve fasciculus as it passes through pyramidal tracts and is characterized by:

- Ipsilateral 6th nerve palsy,
- Contralateral hemiplegia and
- Ipsilateral facial nerve palsy.

4. Foville Syndrome Foville syndrome results due to lesions of the lower part of pons and is characterized by same features as Millard–Gubler syndrome except that 6th nerve palsy is replaced by loss of conjugate movement to the same side.

Midbrain Lesions

1. Weber's Syndrome Weber's syndrome occurs in lesions of the midbrain involving fascicular part of the 3rd nerve while passing through cerebral peduncle. It is characterized by:

- Ipsilateral 3rd nerve palsy,
- Contralateral hemiplegia due to damage to corticospinal tracts and
- Facial palsy of upper motor neuron type.

Features of 3rd Nerve Palsy are:

- *Ptosis* due to paralysis of LPS muscle,
- *Deviation*. Eyeball is turned down and out due to unopposed action of superior oblique and lateral rectus muscles.
- Ocular movements are restricted due to paralysis of the muscles supplied by 3rd nerve as:
  - Adduction—due to paralysis of medial rectus,
  - Elevation—due to paralysis of superior rectus and inferior oblique,
  - Depression—due to paralysis of inferior rectus and
  - Extension—due to paralysis of inferior rectus and inferior oblique.
- *Pupil* is fixed and dilated due to paralysis of the sphincter pupillae muscle.
- *Accommodation* is completely lost due to paralysis of ciliary muscles.
- *Crossed diplopia,* elicited on manually raising the eyelid, occurs due to paralytic divergent squint.
- *Head posture*. If the pupillary area is uncovered, head takes a position consistent with the directions of actions of the paralyzed muscles, i.e. head is turned on the opposite side and is tilted towards the same side and chin is slightly raised.

2. Benedikt's Syndrome Benedikt's syndrome results when the lesion involves the intermediate part of midbrain. It is characterized by:

- Ipsilateral third cranial nerve palsy,
- Contralateral loss of pain, touch, temperature, vibratory and proprioceptive senses due to involvement of medial lemniscus and
- Contralateral jerky movements and tremors due to involvement of red nucleus and superior cerebellar peduncle.

Chapter 10.2

Physiological Anatomy, Functions and Lesions of Cerebellum and Basal Ganglia

CEREBELLUM
- Physiological anatomy
  - External features
  - Anatomical parts
  - Anatomical divisions
  - Phylogenetical divisions
  - Functional divisions
  - Histological structure
- Neural circuits and neuronal activity
  - Afferents of cerebellar cortex
  - Neuronal activity of intrinsic cerebellar circuitry
  - Neuronal activity of deep cerebellar nuclei
- Connections of the cerebellum
  - Cerebellar peduncles
  - Afferent connections
  - Efferent connections
- Functions of cerebellum
  - Control of body posture and equilibrium
  - Control of muscle tone and stretch reflexes
  - Control of voluntary movements
  - Other functions
- Cerebellar lesions
  - Common causes
  - Signs of cerebellar dysfunctions
  - Clinical tests

BASAL GANGLIA
- Physiological anatomy
  - Components
  - Corpus striatum
  - Connections
  - Functional neuronal circuits
- Functions of basal ganglia
- Disorders of basal ganglia
  - Parkinson's disease
  - Chorea and athetosis
  - Huntington's disease
  - Hemiballism
  - Wilson's disease
  - Kernicterus
  - Taradive dyskinesia

CEREBELLUM

Physiological Anatomy

Cerebellum, the largest part of hind brain, consists of two lateral parts called the *cerebellar hemispheres* connected in the midline by a narrow central region called the *vermis*.

External Features (Fig. 10.2-1)

Surfaces. The cerebellum has two surfaces:

- *Superior surface* is related to the tentorium cerebelli and
- *Inferior surface* is related to the *hollow* of occipital bone.

Folia. The surfaces of the cerebellum are thrown into numerous transverse folds called folia.

Fissures. The surface of the cerebellum presents three main fissures (Fig. 10.2-1):

1. ***Primary fissure*** lies on the anterosuperior aspect of the cerebellum. It is V shaped, with open being forwards. It forms the posterior limit of the anterior lobe.
2. ***Horizontal fissure*** separates the superior surface of the cerebellum from its inferior surface and thus follows the convex posterior and anterolateral border of the cerebellar hemisphere. It is of no functional significance.
3. ***Posterolateral fissure*** is situated anteriorly on the inferior surface of the cerebellar hemisphere and separates the posterior lobe from the flocculonodular lobe.

Anatomical Parts of Cerebellum

The cerebellum consists of two cerebellar hemispheres, and a median vermis has been divided into many parts which have functional and morphological significance. To show the various parts of cerebellum in a single illustration, it is usual to represent the organ as if it has been opened out (flattened) so that the superior and inferior aspects both can be seen (Fig. 10.2-1).

Parts of Vermis Vermis is so named because it resembles a worm, which is bent on itself to form a complete circle. Superior and inferior surfaces of the vermis are termed as superior vermis and inferior vermis. Proceeding from above downwards the opened up vermis (as seen in Fig. 10.2-1) consists of following parts: lingula, central lobule, culmen, declive, folium, tuber, pyramis, uvula and nodule.

Parts of Hemisphere With the exception of the lingula, each part of the vermis is related laterally to a part of hemisphere as shown in Figs 10.2-1 and 10.2-2.

Anatomical Divisions

Anatomically the cerebellum has been divided into three lobes:

1. ***Anterior lobe*** is that part of cerebellum which lies in front of the primary fissure on the superior surface (Fig. 10.2-1). The parts of vermis and hemisphere forming the anterior lobe are shown in Fig. 10.2-1 and Table 10.2-1.
2. ***Posterior lobe*** is that part of cerebellum which lies between the primary fissure and posterolateral fissure. Thus, it includes both surfaces of the cerebellum (the superior surface rostral to the horizontal fissure and the inferior surface caudal to the horizontal fissure); parts of the vermis and hemisphere forming the posterior lobe are shown in Fig. 10.2-1 and Table 10.2-1.
3. ***Flocculonodular lobe*** is that part of the cerebellum which lies anterior to the posterolateral fissure on the inferior surface. It consists of (Fig. 10.2-1 and Table 10.2-1):
   - *Nodule,* which is rostral part of the vermis and
   - *Floculli,* which are irregular shaped masses attached to nodule on each side. They are almost completely separated from the rest of cerebellum.

Phylogenetical Divisions

Phylogenetically, i.e. according to evolutionary stages, the cerebellum consists of three subdivisions:

1. Archicerebellum. It is the oldest part to develop. It consists of (Fig. 10.2-1):

- Flocculonodular lobe and
- Lingula.

2. Paleocerebellum. Phylogenetically, it is the next part to appear. It consists of (Fig. 10.2-1):

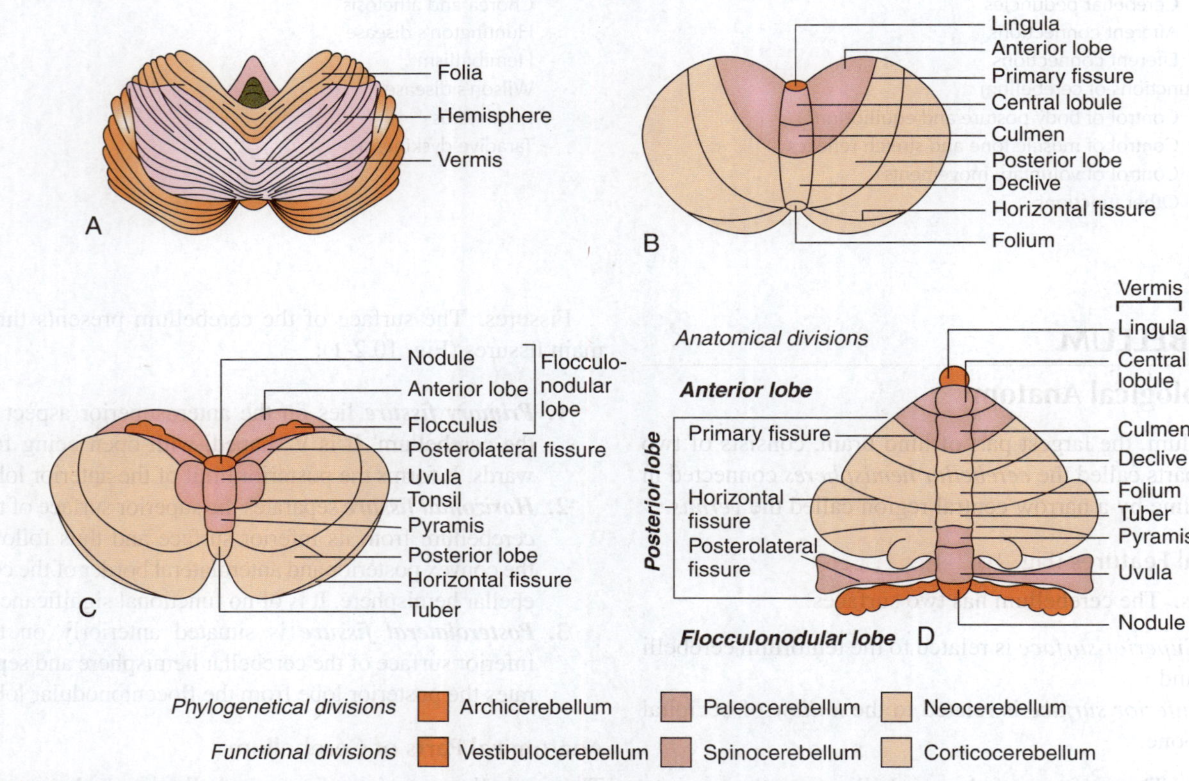

FIGURE 10.2-1 Gross anatomy of cerebellum: **A,** superior surface showing folia; **B** and **C,** superior and inferior surface showing fissures, lobes and parts of vermis; and **D,** schematic diagram to show the parts of vermis and hemisphere in a opened up (unrolled cerebellum).

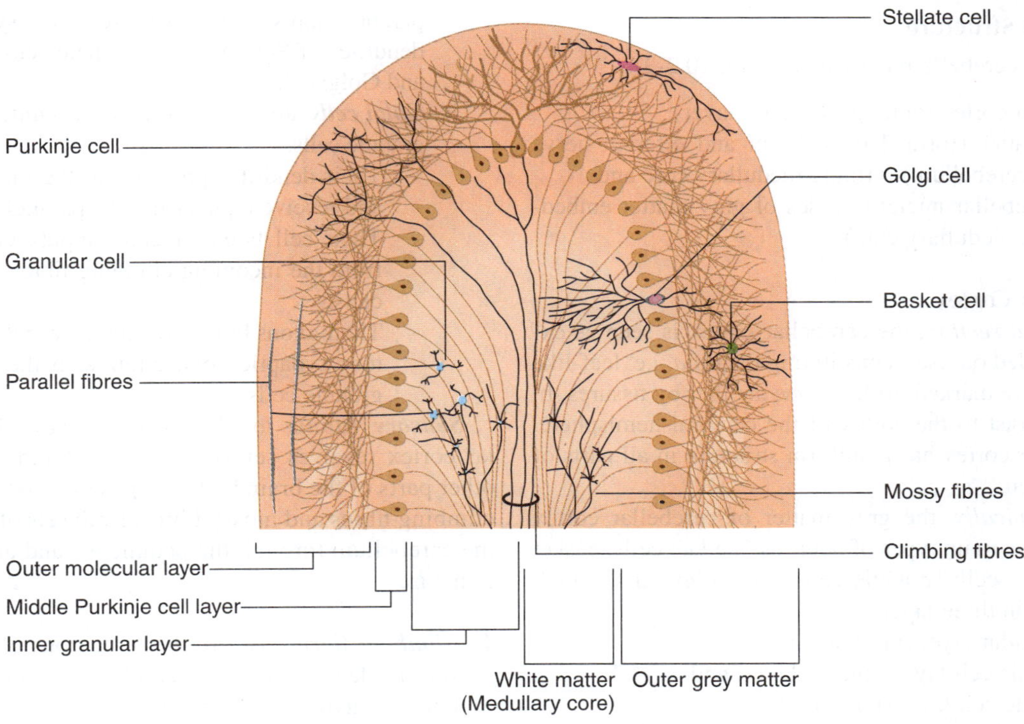

FIGURE 10.2-2 Histology of cerebellar cortex.

TABLE 10.2-1 Lobes of Cerebellum and Parts of Vermis and Hemisphere Forming Them

Lobes of cerebellum	Part of vermis	Part of hemisphere
Anterior lobe	Lingula Central lobule Culmen	No lateral projection Alae Anterior quadrangular lobule
Primary fissure Posterior lobe	Declive Folium	Posterior quadrangular lobule Superior semilunar lobule
Horizontal fissure	Tuber Pyramis Uvula	Inferior semilunar lobule Biventral lobule Tonsil
Posterolateral fissure Flocculonodular lobe	Nodule	Flocculus

- Entire anterior lobe except lingula, and following parts of posterior lobe—pyramis, uvula and paraflocculus

3. Neocerebellum. It is the latest part to develop. It consists of whole of the posterior lobe except pyramis and uvula (Fig. 10.2-1).

Functional Divisions

Functionally, cerebellum is divided into three divisions:

1. Vestibulocerebellum. It includes the flocculonodular lobe, which is its principal component and has vestibular connections only.

- Nucleus fastigial is its effector nucleus.
- It is concerned with control of body posture and equilibrium.

2. Spinocerebellum. It includes the parts forming paleocerebellum, i.e. entire anterior lobe except lingula, and some parts of posterior lobe (pyramis, uvula and paraflocculus).

- *Nucleus interpositus,* i.e. (nucleus globossus and nucleus emboliformis) are its effector nuclei
- It receives proprioceptive inputs from the spinal cord and is concerned with control of axial (trunk) and limb muscles postural reflexes.

3. Corticocerebellum. Corticocerebellum also called as central cerebellum includes whole of the posterior lobe except pyramis and uvula.

- Nucleus dentatus is its effector nucleus.
- It occupies the more lateral regions of the cerebellar cortex and receives information from the cerebral cortex and pons.
- It is concerned with smooth performance of highly skilled voluntary movements.

Histological Structure

Histological, cerebellum consists of (Fig. 10.2-2):

- Cerebellar cortex (outer grey matter layer),
- White matter (formed by afferent and efferent nerve fibres of cerebellum) forming medullary core and
- Deep cerebellar nuclei (masses of grey matter embedded in the medullary core).

I. Cerebellar Cortex

Grossly in cut section, the cerebellar cortex is seen as extensively folded on itself constituting the *folia,* i.e. leaf-like parts which are marked off from one another by fissures. In striking contrast to the cortex of the cerebral hemisphere, the cerebellar cortex has a uniform structure in all parts of the cerebellum.

Microscopically, the grey matter of cerebellar cortex consists of five main types of neurons (stellate cells, basket cells, Purkinje cells, granule cells and Golgi cells) which are arranged in three layers:

- Molecular layer (most superficial),
- Purkinje cell layer (middle layer) and
- Granule cell layer (inner layer).

1. **Molecular layer** is composed of two types of neurons (stellate and basket cells) and unmyelinated nerve fibres
   - **i.** ***Stellate cells*** are star shaped and more superficially located. Their *dendrites* synapse with parallel fibres of granule cells, and their *axons* synapse with dendrites of Purkinje cells.
   - **ii.** ***Basket cells*** are located deep in the molecular layer.
     - They receive inputs from the parallel fibres.
     - Their axons branch and form basket around the cell bodies of Purkinje cells (hence the name).
     - Each basket cell may synapse with about 70 Purkinje cells.

   Nerve fibres present in the molecular layer are parallel fibres (axon of granule cells), dendrites of Purkinje cells, and climbing fibres from inferior olivary nucleus.
2. **Purkinje cell layer.** It is composed of a single layer of large flask-shaped Purkinje cells (biggest neurons in the body).
   - Dendrites of Purkinje cells extend into the molecular layer and provide a huge surface area for axodendritic synapses.
   - Axons of these cells make synaptic connection with the deep cerebellar nuclei in the medullary core. They act as the sole output neurons from the cerebellar cortex, and exert an inhibitory influence to the deep cerebellar and lateral vestibular nuclei.
3. **Granule cell layer** consists of granule and Golgi cells, with their processes, and sensory mossy fibres with their synaptic glomeruli.
   - **i.** ***Granule cells*** are very small, numerous (about 10 billion) spherical neurons. Axons of the granule cells ascend into the molecular layer, and form the parallel fibres that make excitatory synapses with dendrites of Purkinje cells, stellate cells, basket cells and Golgi cells.
   - **ii.** ***Golgi cells*** are large cells and less numerous than the granule cells.
     - Their dendrites project into the molecular layer and receive inputs from the parallel fibres.
     - Their cell bodies receive inputs via collaterals from the incoming climbing fibres and Purkinje cells.
     - Their axons branch extensively and make inhibitory synaptic connection with the dendrites of granule cells.

Sensory Inputs to Cerebellar Cortex. The cerebellar cortex receives sensory inputs (afferent fibres) from other parts of the brain by two types of sensory fibres: the climbing fibres and mossy fibres. Both sets of fibres reach the cerebellum through the peduncles, and are excitatory in nature.

1. ***Climbing fibres*** arise from the neurons of inferior olivary nucleus situated in medulla and reach the cerebellum via olivocerebellar tract.
   - Climbing fibres establish 'one to one' connection with the Purkinje cell dendrites and excite them to discharge.
   - Collaterals of climbing fibres synapse with all other types of neurons in the cerebellar cortex and also the deep cerebellar nuclei.
2. ***Mossy fibres.*** Unlike climbing fibres, the mossy fibres have many sources of origin. These are axons of spinocerebellar, vestibulocerebellar, reticulocerebellar, cuneocerebellar and cortico-ponto-cerebellar tracts.
   - Mossy fibres are named so because they resemble moss plant.
   - Each mossy fibre makes synaptic connections with the dendrites of many granule cells forming synaptic glomeruli. The glomeruli also contain the inhibitory ending of Golgi cells.
   - Each mossy fibre activates about 450 Purkinje cells through, the granule cells and their parallel fibres. Thus, a climbing fibre excites a single Purkinje cell, whereas a mossy fibre through granule cells and parallel fibres fires several thousand Purkinje cells.

     Note. Both the climbing and mossy fibres of sensory inputs exert excitatory influence.
   - Out of five types of neurons in the cerebellar cortex, only the granule cell is excitatory; it releases the excitatory neurotransmitter *glutamate*. The other four types of neurons are inhibitory and release the inhibitory neurotransmitter *gamma aminobutyric acid (GABA)*.

II. White Matter of Cerebellum The cerebellar cortex, i.e. outer grey matter surrounds inner medullary core of white matter (an arrangement opposite to what is seen in spinal cord). White matter is formed by both afferent and efferent fibres. These fibres can be classified in three groups:

1. Projection Fibres of the cerebellum leave or enter the cerebellum and connect it with other parts of central nervous system. These are arranged in three bundles:

- *Inferior cerebellar peduncle* consists of fibres connecting cerebellum with medulla.
- *Middle cerebellar peduncle* contains the fibres which connect cerebellum with pons and
- *Superior cerebellar peduncle* that connects the cerebellum with midbrain.

2. Association Fibres connect different regions of the same cerebellar hemisphere.

3. Commissural Fibres connect the areas of two halves of cerebellar cortex with each other.

III. Deep Cerebellar Nuclei Within the white matter of medullary core of cerebellum are embedded four pairs of masses of grey matter called deep cerebellar nuclei. They lie in close relationship with the roof of the fourth ventricle, and therefore are known as roof nuclei (Fig. 10.2-3).

1. Dentate Nucleus or nucleus dentatus is the largest cerebellar nucleus. Shaped like a purse and made up of a crenated lamina of grey matter, it has an open anterio-median hilum to receive the fibres of superior cerebellar peduncle.

2. Emboliform Nucleus or nucleus emboliformis is an oval mass of grey matter, located just anteromedian to the hilum of dentate nucleus.

3. Globossus Nucleus lies medial to the nucleus emboliformis, and therefore together they are referred to as nucleus interpositus.

4. Fastigial Nucleus or nucleus fastigii is nearly spherical and lies close to the midline just over the roof of fourth ventricle.

Neural Circuits and Neuronal Activity in Cerebellum

Cerebellum executes its functions through excitatory output of the deep cerebellar nuclei to the brainstem and thalamus. Neural connections within the cerebellar cortex, i.e. intrinsic cerebellar circuit (Fig. 10.2-4) is basically concerned with modulating or timing the excitatory output of deep cerebellar nuclei via the fibres of Purkinje cells. This is done in accordance with the signals received by the cerebellar cortex from different parts of the brain and body. The entire process can be discussed, for the purpose of understanding only, under following headings:

- Afferents to cerebellar cortex,
- Neuronal activity of intrinsic cerebellar circuitry and
- Neuronal activity of deep cerebellar nuclei.

Afferents to Cerebellar Cortex

Afferents to cerebellar cortex reach via two types of fibres:

1. Climbing Fibres. These fibres represent terminations of axons reaching the cerebellum from the inferior olivary nucleus. They pass through the granule cell layer, and the Purkinje cell layer to reach the molecular layer. In the molecular layer, each climbing fibre ends on dendrites of single Purkinje cell (Fig. 10.2-4). Because of this, the excitatory effect of climbing fibres on Purkinje cell is very strong. The climbing fibres thus excite the Purkinje cells directly and the deep cerebellar nuclei via the collaterals by releasing the excitatory neurotransmitter aspartate.

2. Mossy Fibres. All the afferent fibres entering the cerebellum, other than the olivocerebellar, are called mossy fibres. These fibres after reaching the granular layer of cerebellar cortex branch profusely and then each branch terminate within a glomerulus (Fig. 10.2-4). The core of each glomerulus is formed by the expanded termination of a mossy fibre called the rosette. About 20 dendrites of

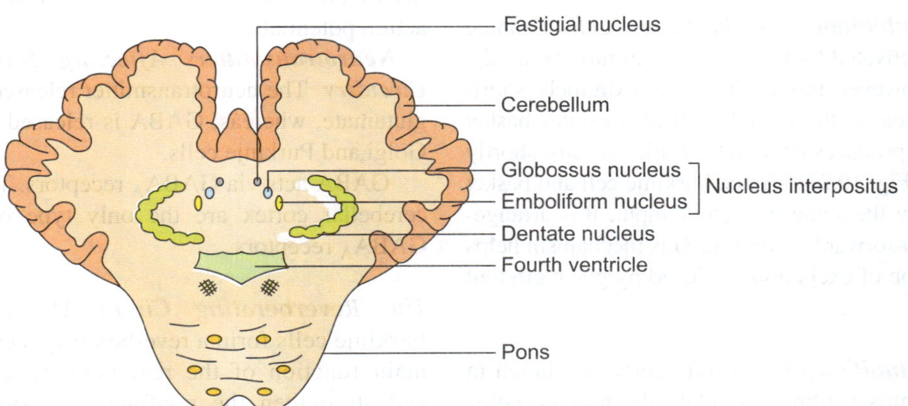

FIGURE 10.2-3 Diagrammatic view of nuclei of cerebellum in relation to roof of fourth ventricle.

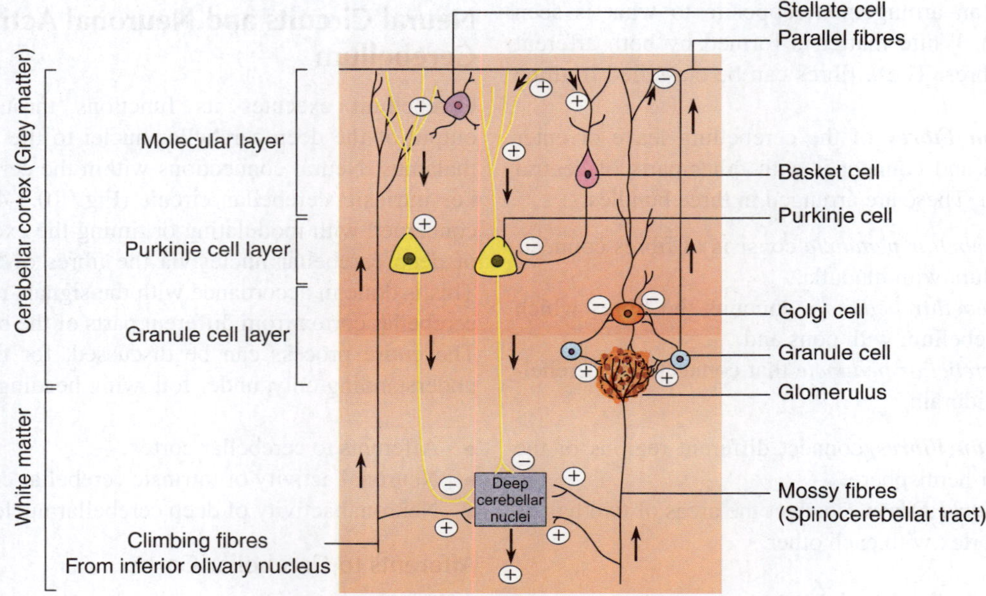

FIGURE 10.2-4 Intrinsic cerebellar circuitry.

granule cells synapse with a rosette in a glomerulus. These synapses are axodendritic. The glomerulus also receives axon terminals of Golgi cells (Fig. 10.2-4).

- In the glomeruli, the mossy fibres release excitatory neurotransmitter glutamate and excite the granule cells and Golgi cells.
- The mossy fibres excite the Purkinje cells indirectly through the granule cells.
- The collaterals of mossy fibres excite the deep cerebellar nuclei directly.

Neuronal Activity of Intrinsic Cerebellar Circuitry

As a result of excitatory input from the climbing fibres or mossy fibres, following activity is set up in the intrinsic cerebellar circuitry.

Feed-forward Inhibition of Purkinje Cells Granule cells, which are activated by mossy fibres, in turn excite the Purkinje cells. However, this excitation is extremely short-lasting. This is because the granule cell also excites basket cell, which in turn produces IPSP in the Purkinje cells, shortly after stimulation (Fig. 10.2-4). Since Purkinje cell and basket cell are excited by the same excitatory input, this arrangement is called feed-forward inhibition. This mechanism helps to limit the duration of excitation produced by given afferent impulses.

Feed-forward Inhibition of Granule Cells As shown in Fig. 10.2-4, the mossy fibres stimulate the granule cells. However, this excitation is short lasting. This is because, the mossy fibre also excites Golgi cell, which in turn inhibits the granule cell. Since the granule cell and Golgi cells are excited by the same excitatory input (from mossy fibres), this arrangement is said to produce feed-forward inhibition of the granule cells.

Feedback Inhibition of Granule Cells As shown in Fig. 10.2-4, the granule cell is excited by the mossy fibres. The axon of granule cell excites the Golgi cell dendrites, whose axon inhibits the granule cell. Thus, excitation of the granule cell is rapidly extinguished by a negative feedback loop. This arrangement is called feedback inhibition of granule cells.

Note. From the above description it is clear that at least three of the identifiable neural circuits inside the cerebellum are meant for ensuring that discharge of the granule cells and Purkinje cells are extremely precise and short lasting (neural sharpening). This helps in accurate timing of action potentials.

Neurotransmitters Affecting Intrinsic Cerebellar Circuitry The neurotransmitter released by granule cell is glutamate, whereas, GABA is released by stellate, basket, Golgi and Purkinje cells.

GABA acts via $GABA_A$ receptors. The granule cells of cerebellar cortex are the only type of neuron that has $GABA_A$ receptors.

The Reverberating Circuit The granule cells and Purkinje cells form a reverberating (echoing) circuit. The main function of the reverberating circuit is to revive and strengthen the nonfunctional synapses, when two neurons discharge by repeatedly and synchronously.

Hebb enunciated this principle, which can be understood by the following example.

Suppose a person is making alternate supinations and pronations of his hand rhythmically. This is made possible by the reverberating circuit of cerebellum. Therefore, this capability is impaired in cerebellar disorders and is called adiadochokinesis. This can be explained as:

As shown in the Fig. 10.2-5, when the person makes supination movement, the signal of descending command from the motor cortex is relayed through the inferior olive to Purkinje cell (PC-1), through the climbing fibres (CF-1). The stimulated Purkinje cell (PC-1) sends a signal to the muscles of supination

When the muscles of supination contract, a set of proprioceptive receptors are stimulated, from where the sensory information is conveyed through the mossy fibre to the granule cell (GrC-1) of the cerebellum. The stimulation of granule cell (GrC-1) sets up excitation in the parallel fibres. Although parallel fibres make synaptic connection with Purkinje cells, but most of these are not functional. Therefore, excitation of parallel fibres initially does not cause excitation of Purkinje cells. It is important to note that excitation of parallel fibres occurs a little while after the excitation of Purkinje cell (PC-1), which has already been explained above, is extremely short lived. Excitation of parallel fibres, a little while after the excitation of

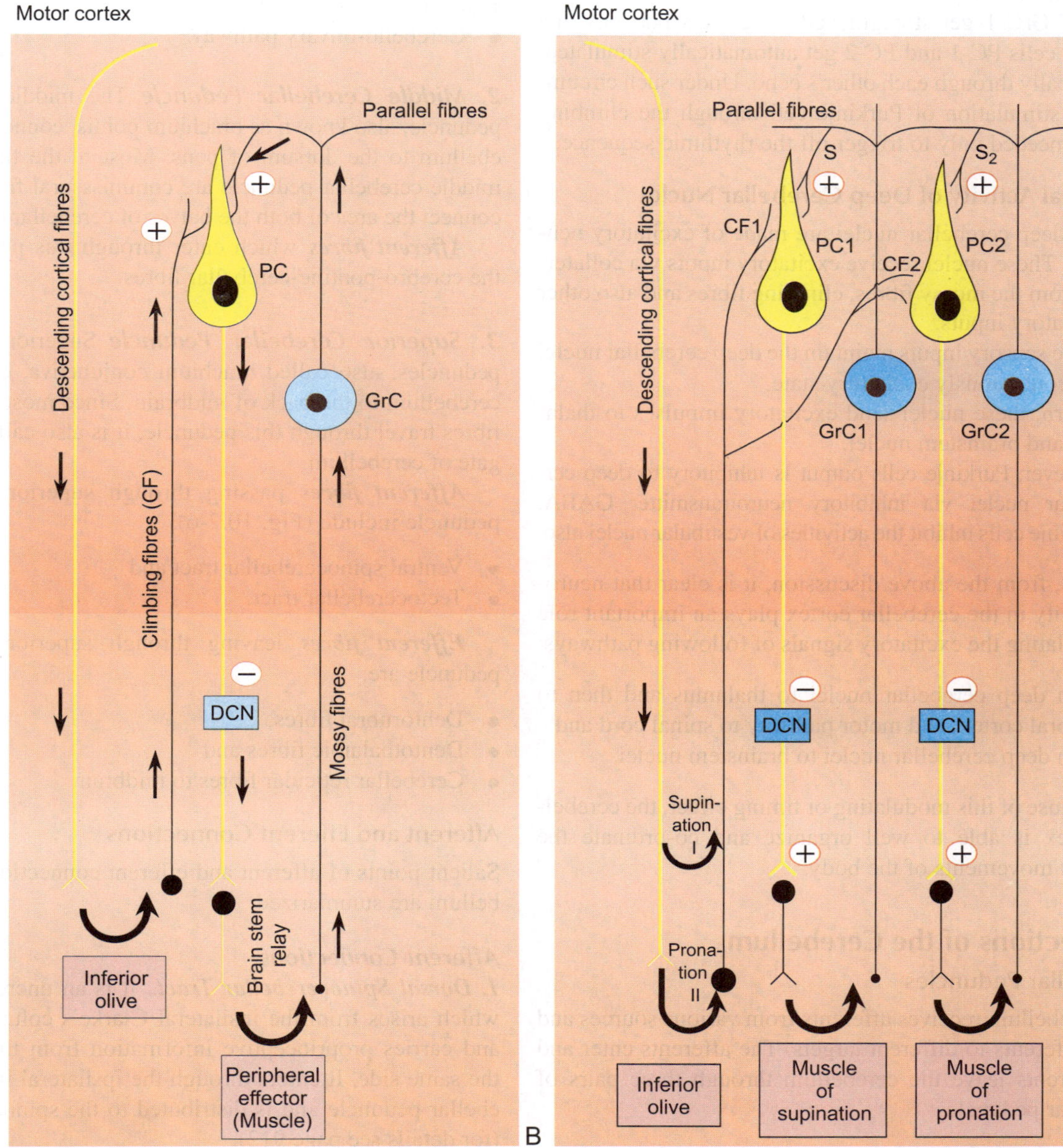

FIGURE 10.2-5 Reverberating circuit: **A,** basic elements; **B,** two sets of reverberating circuits are shown to illustrate their functioning in supination and pronation movements. PC = Purkinje cell; CF = climbing fibre; GrC = granule cell; and DCN = deep cerebellar nuclei.

Purkinje cell can be compared to an echo, which is heard moments after the original sound stops. Because of this similarity, this circuit is called reverberating (echoing) circuit.

Pronation movement (which follows supination) will lead to stimulation of another Purkinje cell (PC-2) through another climbing fibre (CF-2). If the pronation is appropriately timed, the stimulation of PC-2 coincides with the echo of PC-1, i.e. stimulation of parallel fibres of GrC-1.

When supination occurs again, the stimulation of PC-1 coincides with the echo of PC-2, i.e. stimulation of parallel fibres of GrC-2.

When the rhythmic supination and pronation are practised repeatedly, the synaptic connections between PC-1 and parallel fibres of GrC-2; and between PC-2 and parallel fibres of GrC-1 get strengthened. Once this happens, the Purkinje cells PC-1 and PC-2 get automatically stimulated, rhythmically through each other's echo. Under such circumstances, stimulation of Purkinje cell through the climbing fibres is needed only to trigger off the rhythmic sequence.

Neuronal Activity of Deep Cerebellar Nuclei

- The deep cerebellar nuclei are made of excitatory neurons. These nuclei receive excitatory inputs via collaterals from the mossy fibres, climbing fibres and also other excitatory inputs.
- These sensory inputs maintain the deep cerebellar nuclei in a continuously excitatory state.
- In turn, these nuclei send excitatory impulses to thalamus and brainstem nuclei.
- However, Purkinje cells output is inhibitory to deep cerebellar nuclei via inhibitory neurotransmitter GABA. Purkinje cells inhibit the activities of vestibular nuclei also.

Thus, from the above discussion, it is clear that neuronal activity in the cerebellar cortex plays an important role in modulating the excitatory signals of following pathways:

- From deep cerebellar nuclei to thalamus and then to cerebral cortex, and motor pathway to spinal cord and
- From deep cerebellar nuclei to brainstem nuclei.

Because of this modulating or timing effect, the cerebellar cortex is able to well organize and co-ordinate the different movements of the body.

Connections of the Cerebellum

Cerebellar Peduncles

The cerebellum receives afferents from various sources and sends efferents to different targets. The afferents enter and the efferents leave the cerebellum through three pairs of cerebellar peduncles:

1. Inferior Cerebellar Peduncle Inferior cerebellar peduncles, also called as restiform bodies, connect the cerebellum to the dorsolateral aspect of medulla. These constitute the main entrance gates of cerebellum as they contain predominantly afferent fibres.

Afferent fibres passing through inferior cerebellar peduncle are:

- Dorsospinocerebellar tract,
- External arcuate fibres,
- Reticulocerebellar tract,
- Olivocerebellar tract and
- Vestibulocerebellar tract.

Efferent fibres leaving through inferior cerebellar peduncle are:

- Cerebellovestibular pathway,
- Cerebelloreticular pathway and
- Cerebello-olivary pathway.

2. Middle Cerebellar Peduncle The middle cerebellar peduncle, also known as brachium pontis, connects the cerebellum to the dorsum of pons. Most of the fibres of the middle cerebellar peduncle are commisssural fibres, which connect the area of both the halves of cerebellar cortex.

Afferent fibres which enter through this peduncle are the cerebro-pontine-cerebellar fibres.

3. Superior Cerebellar Peduncle Superior cerebellar peduncles, also called brachium conjunctiva, connect the cerebellum to the back of midbrain. Since most of efferent fibres travel through this peduncle, it is also called the exit gate of cerebellum.

Afferent fibres passing through superior cerebellar peduncle include (Fig. 10.2-6):

- Ventral spinocerebellar tract and
- Tectocerebellar tract.

Efferent fibres leaving through superior cerebellar peduncle are:

- Dentorubral fibres,
- Dentothalamic fibres and
- Cerebellar reticular fibres to midbrain.

Afferent and Efferent Connections

Salient points of afferent and efferent connections of cerebellum are summarized.

Afferent Connections

1. Dorsal Spinocerebellar Tract. It is an uncrossed tract, which arises from the ipsilateral Clarke's column of cells and carries proprioceptive information from the limbs of the same side. It enters through the ipsilateral inferior cerebellar peduncle and is distributed to the spinocerebellum (for details see page 912).

2. Ventral Spinocerebellar Tract. The fibres of this tract arise from the marginal cells in the dorsal grey horn of

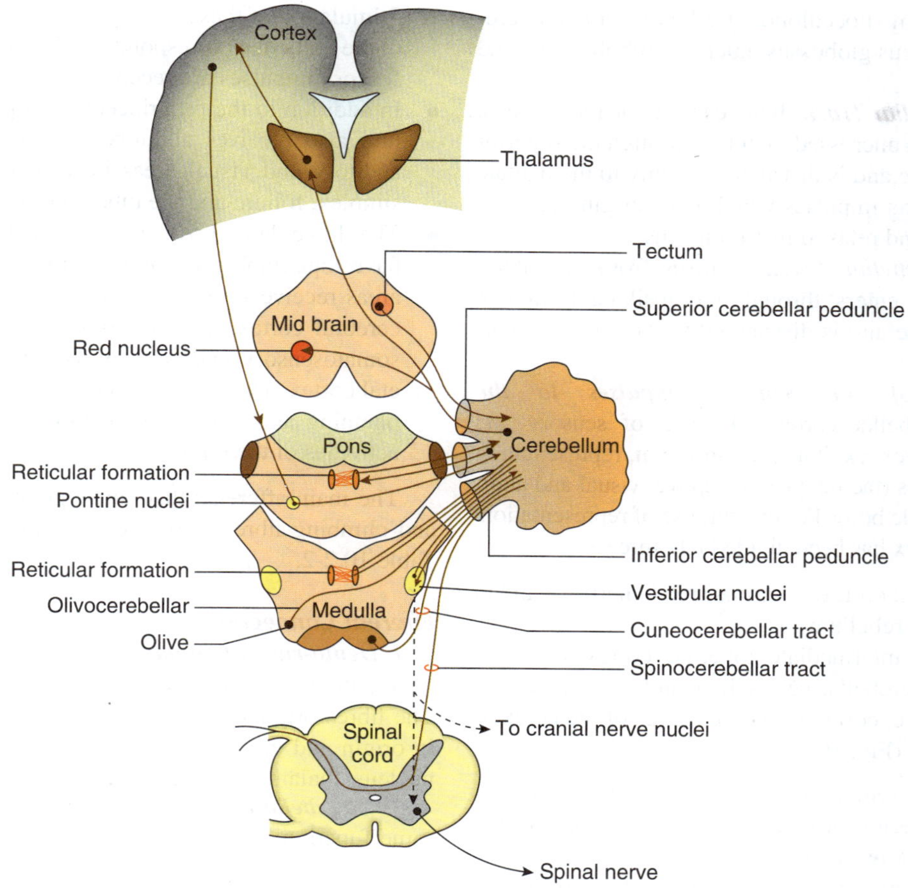

FIGURE 10.2-6 Diagrammatic depiction of main connections of cerebellum.

spinal cord. After taking origin, the fibres cross the midline and ascend in the opposite side. It carries the proprioceptive information from the limbs of the opposite side. It enters the cerebellum through superior cerebellar peduncle, and is distributed to the lower limb area of the cortex of spinocerebellum (details on page 934).

3. Cuneocerebellar Tract. It arises from the accessory cuneate nucleus and carries proprioceptive impulses from the upper limb, upper trunk and neck. It enters through ipsilateral inferior cerebellar peduncle and is distributed to the spinocerebellum.

4. Olivocerebellar Tract. This tract arises from the olivary nucleus and crosses to the opposite side. The olivary nucleus receives afferents from three sources:

- Brainstem nuclei of the same side,
- Spinal cord through spino-olivary tract of same side and
- Cerebral cortex of opposite side

It carries proprioceptive impulses from the whole body and output signals from the cerebral cortex. It enters the cerebellum through the inferior cerebellar peduncle of opposite side and is distributed to all parts of the cerebellar cortex and the deep cerebellar nuclei (for details see page 911).

5. Cortico-ponto-cerebellar Tract. The cortico-pontine fibres arise from the cerebral cortex and end in pontine nuclei from where the pontocerebellar fibres cross to enter the opposite side through the middle cerebellar peduncle. The cortex of each cerebral hemisphere is connected with the opposite half of the cerebellum through this tract. This tract conveys the information to spinocerebellum, about the major signals discharged from the cerebral cortex. Cerebral cortex and the cerebellum work in close co-operation in order to affect the proper coordination of muscular action in voluntary movements (see page 937).

6. Tectocerebellar Tract. It arises from the superior and inferior colliculi of tectum of midbrain, and enters the cerebellum via superior cerebellar peduncle. It carries visual impulses from the superior colliculi and auditory impulses from inferior colliculi (see page 935).

7. Vestibulocerebellar Tract. It arises from the ipsilateral vestibular nuclei and carries information concerning the position and the movements of head. It enters through the inferior cerebellar peduncle and conveys impulses to vestibulocerebellum (flocculonodular lobe) via deep cerebellar nuclei (nucleus globossus, nucleus emboliformis and nucleus fastigii).

8. Rubrocerebellar Tract. It arises from the red nucleus, is both crossed and uncrossed. It enters through the superior cerebellar peduncle and is distributed mainly to the dentate nucleus. It transmits impulses which have originated from the motor cortex and relayed in red nucleus.

9. Reticulocerebellar Tract. It arises from the lateral reticular nucleus, enters through the ipsilateral inferior cerebellar peduncle and is distributed to the whole of cerebellar cortex.

Localization of the Sensory Impulses to the Cerebellum. Cerebellar cortex, like that of sensory and motor cerebral cortex, exhibits point-to-point, representation of sensory impulses (tactile, proprioceptive, visual and auditory) from the whole body. For the purpose of representation, the cerebellar cortex has been divided into three zones:

- *Vermal zone,* i.e. cortex of vermis area (a narrow band in the centre of cerebellum),
- *Paravermal* or intermediate zone, i.e. cortex of medial halves of the cerebellar hemisphere and
- *Lateral zone,* i.e. cortex of lateral halves of the cerebellar hemisphere (Fig. 10.2-7).

Areas of Representation. There is a double representation on the superior surface (anterior area) and on the inferior surface (posterior area).

Anterior area encloses entire anterior lobe and lobulus simplex. In anterior area, the body representation is an inverted ipsilateral projection. Axial parts of the body lie in the vermis, whereas limbs and facial region lie in the intermediate zone of cerebellar cortex.

Posterior area is located primarily in the paramedian lobule. In this area, the body representation is a bilateral projection, less defined and is erect.

- There is same topographical representation of motor areas in the cerebellum as is for the sensory areas.

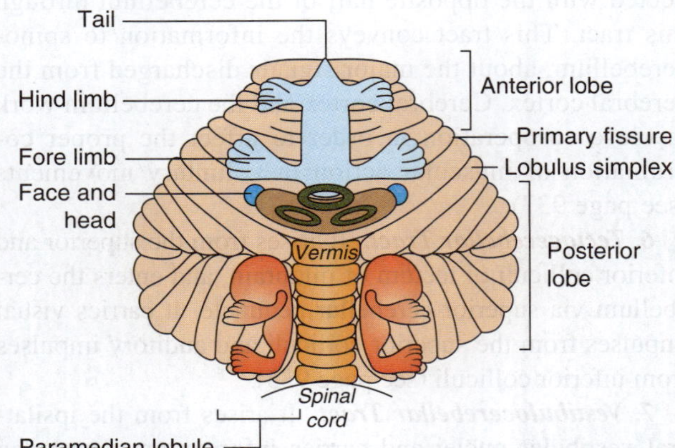

FIGURE 10.2-7 Localization of sensory projection areas on the cerebellar cortex.

Stimulation of these areas produces movements in parts of the body that correspond roughly to those from which sensory impulses are received.

- In addition to the proprioceptive impulses, the cerebellum also receives auditory and visual impulses. The auditory and visual areas lie primarily in the lobulus simplex, folium and the tuber vermis (Fig. 10.2-7).
- The large lateral zones of cerebellar cortex do not have topographical representations of the body. These areas receive signals entirely and exclusively from the cerebral cortex, and premotor areas of frontal cortex, somatosensory and sensory association areas of parietal cortex. These connections play an important role in planning and co-ordinating rapid sequential muscular activities of the body.

The main afferents that converge to form mossy fibres and climbing fibres to the cerebellum are summarized in Table 10.2-2.

Efferent Connections *(Fig. 10.2-6)*

1. Dento-rubro-thalamo-cortical Path. It is a multisynaptic path, synapsing at least in red nucleus and thalamus. The fibres originate from dentate nucleus, which is recent in origin and most well developed in man and so the red nucleus, thalamus and cerebral cortex of opposite side.

2. Cerebello-thalamic-cortical Path. It has also the same function, i.e. controlling or influence over the opposite motor cortex.

3. Cerebelloreticular Path. Anterior horn cells of spinal cord are controlled by the cerebellum through reticulospinal tracts (direct fibres from cerebellum to anterior horn cells do not exist).

4. Cerebellovestibular Fibres pass through the inferior cerebellar peduncle to vestibular nuclei. These efferents control anterior horn cells of the spinal cord through vestibulospinal tract.

5. Cerebello-olivary Fibres reach the inferior olivary nucleus.

6. Some Fibres from the Cerebellum also reach the nucleus of oculomotor nerve and the tectum.

Functions of Cerebellum

Functionally, cerebellum has been divided into three divisions:

- Vestibulocerebellum,
- Spinocerebellum and
- Corticocerebellum.

These three functional divisions play important role in following different functions:

A. Control of Body Posture and Equilibrium

Vestibulocerebellum, which includes flocculonodular lobe as its principal component and nucleus fastigii (as its

TABLE 10.2-2 Principal Afferent System to the Cerebellum

Afferent tracts	Impulses transmitted	Via	Distributed to
1. Dorsospinocerebellar tract	Properioceptive information from limbs of same side	Inferior cerebellar peduncle	Spinocerebellum
2. Ventrospinocerebellar tract	Properioceptive information from limbs of opposite side	Superior cerebellar peduncle	Spinocerebellum
3. Cuneocerebellar tract	Proprioceptive information from upper limb, trunk and neck	Ipsilateral inferior cerebellar peduncle	Spinocerebellum
4. Olivocerebellar tract	Proprioceptive information from whole body and signals from cerebral cortex	Contralateral inferior cerebellar peduncle	Whole cerebellar cortex and deep cerebellar nuclei
5. Tectocerebellar tract	Auditory and visual impulses through superior and inferior colliculi of midbrain	Superior cerebellar peduncle	Spinocerebellar
6. Vestibulocerebellar tract	Vestibular(position and movement of head) information	Inferior cerebellar peduncle	Vestibulo cerebellum (Floculonodular lobe)
7. Pontocerebellar tract	Signals from contralateral cerebral cortex	Middle cerebellar peduncle	Spinocerebellum
8. Rubrocerebellar tract	Signals originated from motor cortex	Middle cerebellar peduncle	Dentate nuclei
9. Reticulocerebellar tract	lateral reticular nuclei	Ipsilateral cerebellar peduncle	Whole of cerebellar cortex

effector nucleus) and vermal region of the cerebellum, are concerned with control of body posture and equilibrium.

Afferents to Cerebellum concerned with the control of body posture and equilibrium include:

- ***Vestibulocerebellar tracts*** which carry input from vestibular nuclei, which convey afferents from the macula of saccule and utricle for static equilibrium and from the ampullary crests of semicircular ducts for kinetic equilibrium.
- ***Spinocerebellar and cuneocerebellar tracts*** carry feedback about tone of muscles or position of the limbs in space.
- ***Reticulocerebellar tracts*** bring feedback about activities of extrapyramidal tracts.

Efferents. The flocculonodular lobe and fastigial nuclei project output fibres through inferior peduncle to vestibular and reticular nuclei of brainstem. The vermal cerebellum sends back the information to spinal cord indirectly through fastigial nuclei.

Mechanism of Action. The efferents from the cerebellum influence the spinal motor neurons to keep the body posture upright through the vestibulospinal and reticulospinal tracts, and regulate the position of eyes in relation to movements of the head by connecting motor nuclei of extraocular muscles (3rd, 4th and 6th cranial nerves) via medial longitudinal fasciculus.

It is important to note that the cerebellum does necessary corrections for maintaining posture and equilibrium, without participation of conscious will and that the corrections made are highly smooth and precise.

B. Control of Muscle Tone and Stretch Reflexes

Spinocerebellum, which includes entire anterior lobe except lingula and some parts of posterior lobe (pyramis, uvula and paraflocculus) as its principal components and nucleus globossus and nucleus emboliformis as its effector nuclei, is mainly concerned with control of muscle tone and anticipatory adjustment of muscle contraction during movement.

Afferents *spinocerebellar, cuneocerebellar* and *olivocerebellar* tracts carry proprioceptive and tactile inputs from the limbs, trunk, neck and other parts of the body. These give feedback about tone of muscles or position of limbs and body. Spinocerebellum also receives auditory and visual impulses through tectocerebellar tract. It also receives the cortical impulses via pontine nuclei.

Efferents. The spinocerebellum is projected into the cerebellar nuclei—fastigii, emboliformis and globossus, Fibres from these nuclei pass through fastigiobulbar, cerebelloreticular and cerebello-olivary tracts and ultimately, to relay to the α and γ motor neurons through the reticulospinal and olivospinal tracts.

Mechanism of Action. Spinocerebellum regulates the postural reflexes by modifying muscle tone. It facilitates the gamma motor neurons in the spinal cord via cerebello-vestibulo-spinal and cerebello-reticulo-spinal tracts. The γ motor neurons reflexly modify the activity of α motor neurons and thus regulate the muscle tone. Thus, cerebellum forms an important site of linkage of α–γ systems responsible for muscle tone.

Proofs. Temporary suppression of anterior lobe activity by surface cooling abolishes discharge from the γ motor neurons, resulting in hypotonia and disturbance in posture. This discharge reappears by warming.

C. Control of Voluntary Movements

Cerebellum is not able to initiate any motor activity, but co-ordinates movements initiated by the motor cortex. Therefore, lesions of cerebellum are associated not with paralysis but with disturbances in the smoothness of movements.

Control of movements by cerebellum includes regulation of time, rate, range (extent), force and direction of muscular activity.

Control of voluntary movements involves co-ordination of activity of the muscles concerned in voluntary movements which can be classified as:

- *Agonists* or prime movers, whose contraction is essentially responsible for the movement of the part,
- *Antagonists* are those which oppose the prime movers,
- *Synergists* are those which assist the prime movers and reduce unnecessary involvements to a minimum and
- *Fixation muscles,* whose contraction causes the fixation of neighbouring joints and maintain the limbs or body in a position appropriate for carrying out the particular movement.

Pathway of Control of Voluntary Movements

Corticocerebellum also called cerebrocerebellum is mainly concerned with integration and regulation of well-co-ordinated muscular activity (though other parts of cerebellum also work in close co-operation in this task). The corticocerebellum includes whole of the posterior lobe, except pyramis and uvula, with dentate nucleus its effector nucleus. Corticocerebellum takes part in smooth performance of highly skilled voluntary movements because of its afferent and efferent connections which form two feedback loops open and close.

1. Open Feedback Loop also known as cerebro-cerebello-cerebral connection or *afferent–efferent circuit* consists of following fibres (Fig. 10.2-8):

1. *Cerebro-ponto-cerebellar tract* which is formed by:

Cortiopontine fibres. These arise from the association areas of the cerebral cortex and project to ipsilateral pontine nuclei. Pontocerebellar fibres from the pontine nuclei pass through middle cerebellar peduncle of the opposite side and terminate in the cerebellar cortex of hemisphere zone (lateral). Thus, whole pathway is called cerebro-ponto-cerebellar tract. This part of the cerebellum does not receive significant proprioceptive input from the spinal cord. Cerebellar cortex in turn connected to the effector nucleus the dentate nucleus.

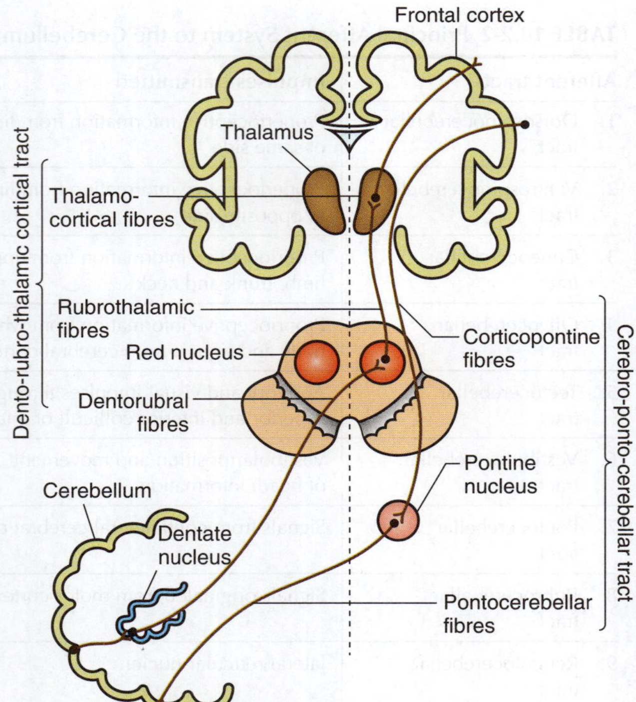

FIGURE 10.2-8 Cerebro-cerebello-cerebral circuit (open-feedback loop).

2. *Dento-rubro-thalamic cortical tract* which includes following fibres:

- *Dentorubral fibres* start from the dentate nucleus and pass via superior cerebellar peduncle to end in red nucleus of opposite side.
- *Rubrothalamic fibres* start from the red nucleus and go to thalamus.
- *Thalamocortical fibres* connect the thalamus to areas 4 and 6 of motor cortex of cerebrum.

Functions. The cerebro-cerebello-cerebral circuit modulates the motor command of pyramidal tract with a programming of movement.

2. Closed Feedback Loop. It is formed by the fibres from the cerebral motor cortex to the paravermal cerebellum to the cerebral motor cortex as (Fig. 10.2-9):

- ***Afferent limb*** is formed by collaterals of corticospinal tracts (which influence the contralateral lower motor neuron of the spinal cord), while descending through the brainstem synapse with the ipsilateral pontine nuclei, inferior olivary nucleus and contralateral reticular nucleus of the medulla.

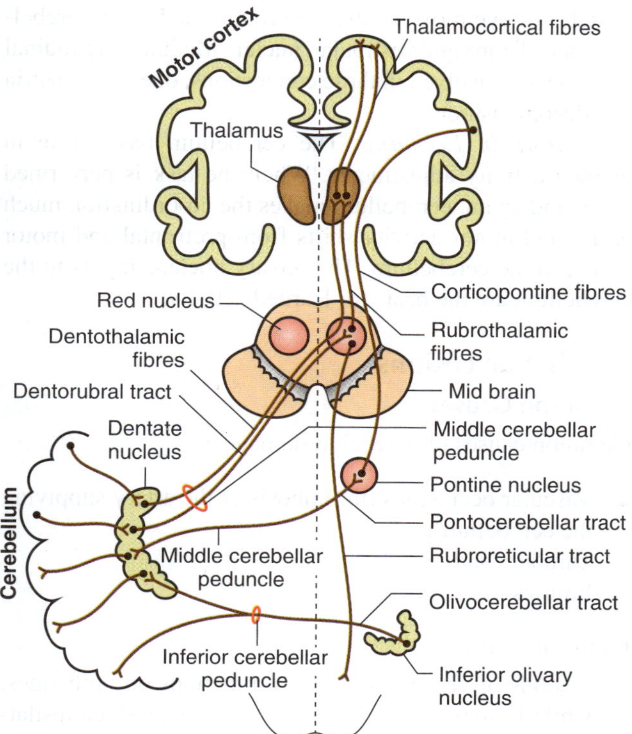

FIGURE 10.2-9 Connections of corticocerebellum (closed circuit).

i. *Pontocerebellar fibres* from the pontine nucleus and *olivocerebellar* fibres from the inferior olivary nucleus reach the contralateral cerebellar cortex; *reticulocerebellar fibres* from the lateral reticular nucleus are projected to the ipsilateral cortex. All the aforesaid fibres are connected to the paravermal (intermediate) region of cerebellum and provide on their way collaterals to the deep cerebellar nuclei.

ii. *Paravermal cerebellar cortex* is in turn connected to the nucleus interpositus and partly to the dentate nucleus.

- ***Efferents from dentate*** nucleus pass through superior cerebellar peduncle, cross the midline and form decussation with the fibres of opposite side. After forming the decussation, these fibres divide into two groups:
  i. *Dentothalamic fibres.* Some fibres arising from dentate nucleus pass through the red nucleus, without having any synapse and terminate in the thalamus. Thalamus in turn projects into the motor cortex via thalamocortical fibres.
  ii. *Dentorubral fibres.* The remaining fibres terminate in the red nucleus of opposite side. From red nucleus, the following tracts arise:
    - *Rubrothalamic tract* terminates in thalamus, from where thalamocortical fibres arise and reach the cerebral cortex.
    - *Rubroreticular tract* terminates into reticular formation which projects into spinal cord via reticulospinal tract.
    - *Rubrospinal tract.* Red nucleus also projects directly into spinal cord through rubrospinal tract.

Mechanism of Action The cerebellum controls the voluntary movements by following actions:

i. Comparator Function. The cerebellum integrates and co-ordinates the patterns of movement involving mostly the distal parts of limbs, especially the hands, fingers and feet by its comparator function.

- When the motor cortex sends impulses through the corticospinal tracts to the lower motor neurons for commanding movements of exploratory nature, it sends messages on way to the paravermal cerebellum about the sequential intended plan of movements for the next fraction of second.
- The cerebellum also gets feedback from the proprioceptive endings of muscles, tendons and joints about what actual movements result.

The paravermal cerebellum (intermediate zone of cerebellar cortex) then compares the intended movement with the actual movement, and through nucleus interpositus sends corrective signals to motor cortex through thalamus and red nucleus. This system of cerebellar *comment* on every command of motor cortex is completed within 10–20 ms.

Thus, the exploratory movement initiated in the motor cortex is corrected by the paracerebellum via the closed-loop circuit (Fig. 10.2-9)

ii. Damping Action. By its comparator action, the cerebellum provides smooth co-ordinate movements of agonist and antagonist muscles of the limbs for the performance of acute purposeful patterned movements. However, all the movements are pendular and have a tendency to overshoot. The corticocerebellum sends impulses to the cerebral cortex to discharge appropriate signals to the muscles so that any extra or exaggeration of muscular activity does not occur and thus prevents the overshooting. In this way, the movements become smooth and accurate. This action of corticocerebellum is called damping action.

iii. Timing and Programming the Movements. When the perfection of movements is fully assured, the planning of sequence of movements and the timing of the learned movements is then maintained from the association cortex to the motor cortex, through lateral zone of cerebellar cortex along with the associated dentate nucleus forming open-loop circuit (Fig. 10.2-8).

- *Planning of sequence of movements.* Lateral parts of cerebellar hemisphere, communicate with the premotor and sensory portion of the cerebral cortex and there is two-way communication between these areas. Plan is transmitted from cerebral cortex to cerebellum and two-way traffic between two areas provides appropriate transition from one movement to the next. This plan is stored in the cerebral cortex in the form of memory. So, after the learning process is over these activities are executed easily and smoothly in sequence.

- *Timing function.* Lateral cerebellar hemisphere also provides appropriate timing for each movement, without which succeeding movements may begin far early or too late.
- *Predicting events.* Cerebellum also plays a role in predicting events, e.g. rate of progression of auditory and visual phenomena. From the changing visual scene, person can predict how rapidly he can approach an object.

It is important to note that all fast skilled movements such as typing, writing, playing of music instruments, etc. is possible because of timing and programming of movements by the cerebellum.

iv. Control of Ballistic Movements. The rapid alternate movements, which take place in different parts of the body, while doing any skilled work like dancing are called ballistic movements. The cerebellum co-ordinates the action of agonist and antagonist muscles, especially when they occur rhythmically. This is explained under 'reverberating circuit' (see page 930).

v. Servomechanism. From the above discussion, it is clear that cerebellum plays an important role in learning of motor skills. Once the skilled works are learnt, the sequential movements could be executed without any interruption. Cerebellum lets the cerebral cortex to discharge the signals, which are already programmed and stored at sensory motor cortex, and does not interfere much. However, if there is any disturbance or interference, the corticocerebellum immediately influences the cerebral cortex and corrects the movements. This action of corticocerebellum is known as servomechanism.

D. Other Functions of Cerebellum

Recent studies have shown that the importance of the cerebellum may extend beyond control of motor activity as:

i. Influence on Autonomic System. It has been postulated that the cerebellum may influence autonomic functions. Electrical stimulation of paleocerebellar cortex produces respiratory, cardiovascular, pupillary and urinary bladder responses. When the anterior lobe is stimulated, the response is sympathetic in nature. On stimulation of tonsils, the response becomes predominantly parasympathetic. Cerebellar influence on autonomic system is probably mediated through the hypothalamus and reticular formation.

ii. Influence on Conduction in Ascending Sensory Pathway may be exerted by the cerebellum through the reticular formation and thalamus.

iii. Control of Eyeball Movements. The oculomotor, trochlear and abducent nuclei, which supply extraocular muscles of eye movements, are brought under the cerebellar control through vestibular nuclei. Medial longitudinal fasciculus is involved in these connections, due to dysmetria and decomposition.

iv. Role in Learning. The cerebellum has a role in learned activity adjustments. When the task is performed again and again, cerebellum makes the co-ordination much easier and motor activity shifts from prefrontal and motor cortex to the cerebellum. The olivary nucleus inputs to the cerebellum are the basis for learned activity.

Cerebellar Lesions

Common Causes

Common causes of cerebellar damage are:

- Vascular occlusions (thrombosis of the artery supplying the cerebellum),
- Tumours and
- Injuries.

General Features

- Lesions of vermis produce dysfunctions on both sides, while lesions of cerebellar hemisphere produce ipsilateral dysfunctions.
- Cerebellar cortex lesions produce abnormalities of movement, which gradually disappear or compensation occurs.
- Lesions of deep cerebellar nuclei produce generalized defects and abnormalities which persist.

Signs of Cerebellar Dysfunctions

Common signs observed in patients with cerebellar dysfunction due to lesions of cerebellum are:

Disturbances in Tone and Posture

1. ***Atonia or hypotonia.*** Hypotonia refers to reduction and atonia to loss of tone in muscles. It occurs due to reduction of the facilitatory neocerebellar output to the descending inhibitory reticular formation.
2. ***Attitude changes*** in unilateral lesions of the cerebellum are:
   - *Rotation of the face towards opposite side* (pulled by the healthy muscles).
   - Lowering of the shoulder on the affected side.
   - Outward rotation and abduction of the leg on involved side.
   - Trunk is bent with concavity towards the affected side; this is because the weight of the body is thrown on the unaffected leg.
3. ***Deviation movement***. The arm held straight out in front of the body, deviates laterally when the eyes are closed. In bilateral lesions, both arms deviate.
4. ***Effect on deep reflexes***. The deep or tendon reflexes become weak and pendular. For example, *pendular knee*

jerk in which after the initial reflex response the leg shakes several to and fro movements before it comes to rest. It occurs due to hypotonia of the quadriceps muscle.

Disturbances in Equilibrium It appears when the flocculonodular lobe is affected, e.g. by the tumour medulloblastoma in children. The patient suffering from disturbance of equilibrium, walks on a wide base, sways from side to side (drunken like gait), and is unable to maintain the upright posture due to involvement of vestibular system.

Disturbances in Movements

*1. **Ataxia,*** i.e. lack of co-ordination of movements, is the hallmark of cerebellar disorder. It is characterized by:

- ***Decomposition of movements,*** i.e. the movements seem to occur in stages at different joints.
- ***Asynergia,*** i.e. lack of co-ordination between the protagonist, synergist and antagonist muscles.
- ***Dysmetria,*** i.e. movements are incorrect in range, direction and force. The movements may overshoot their intended mark (hypermetria) or fall short of it (hypometria). ***Note.*** Ataxia also occurs in certain hereditary conditions, examples are: Friedrich's ataxia (is an autosomal recessive condition occurs below the age of 25 years) and Machado–Joseph disease.

*2. **Intention Tremors*** become evident during purposeful movements, and diminish or disappear with rest. These tremors become more marked as the hand approaches the object, i.e. are observed at the end of movement and are coarse, oscillating, to and fro and rhythmic. These are significantly observed when the efferent pathways of superior cerebellar peduncles are involved.

*3. **Nystagmus*** refers to regular and rhythmic, to and fro involuntary oscillatory movements of the eyes, occurring due to inco-ordination of extraocular muscles. Cerebellar nystagmus occurs during damage to flocculonodular lobes and occurs at rest (when neither the person nor the visual scene is moving).

*4. **Dysarthria*** or scanning speech occurs due to inco-ordination of various muscles and structures involved in speech. The speech is slurred, prolonged and explosive, with pauses at wrong places.

*5. **Astasia*** refers to unsteady voluntary movements.

Clinical Tests for Cerebellar Dysfunctions

Clinically cerebellar dysfunctions can be demonstrated by following tests:

*1. **Finger–nose Test.*** The patient has great difficulty in promptly bringing the finger of outstretched arm to touch the tip of his nose. This is because the intention tremors become more severe as the hand approaches the face.

*2. **Adiadochokinesia,*** i.e. the patient is unable to rapidly perform alternating movements, e.g. supination and pronation of the forearm.

*3. **Rebound Phenomenon.*** When the patient attempts to do a movement against a resistance, and if the resistance is suddenly removed, the limb moves forcibly in the direction towards which the effect was made. This is called rebound phenomenon. It is due to the absence of breaking action of antagonistic muscles.

*4. **Gait Test.*** When the patient is asked to walk on a straight line, he is unable to do so (even with eyes open); he follows a zigzag path due to disturbance of equilibrium.

*5. **Past Pointing,*** i.e. the movement goes beyond the intended point. This is called overshooting and is a manifestation of dysmetria.

*6. **Heel to Shin Test.*** Lying in a supine position, the patient is asked to place his heel on opposite knee, and then slide his heel up and down the shin between knee and ankle. The test is abnormal if heel waves away from the line of shin.

Treatment Ataxia in cerebellar dysfunction can be managed by;

- Supportive therapy which includes physical, occupational and speech therapy.
- Deep brain stimulation of ventral intermediate nucleus of thalamus may be effective in ataxia
- In familial ataxia (due to low level of CoQ-10), coenzyme Q-10 replacement is beneficial to some extent.

BASAL GANGLIA

Physiological Anatomy

Components of Basal Ganglia

According to anatomic definition, basal ganglia are subcortical nuclear masses which include corpus striatum (amygdaloid body and claustrum). They are so named, as they develop in the basal part of cerebral hemisphere. However, from the physiological viewpoint, the term basal ganglia include:

- Corpus striatum,
- Subthalamic nucleus (body of Luys) and
- Substantia nigra.

Corpus Striatum Corpus striatum (Fig. 10.2-10) comprises subcortical masses of grey matter, which are situated in the white core of each cerebral hemisphere. It is divided almost completely by the fibres of internal capsule into two parts:

i. Caudate nucleus (medial part) and
ii. Lenticular nucleus (lateral part), which is further subdivided into two parts:
   - Putamen (outer part) and
   - Globus pallidus (inner part).

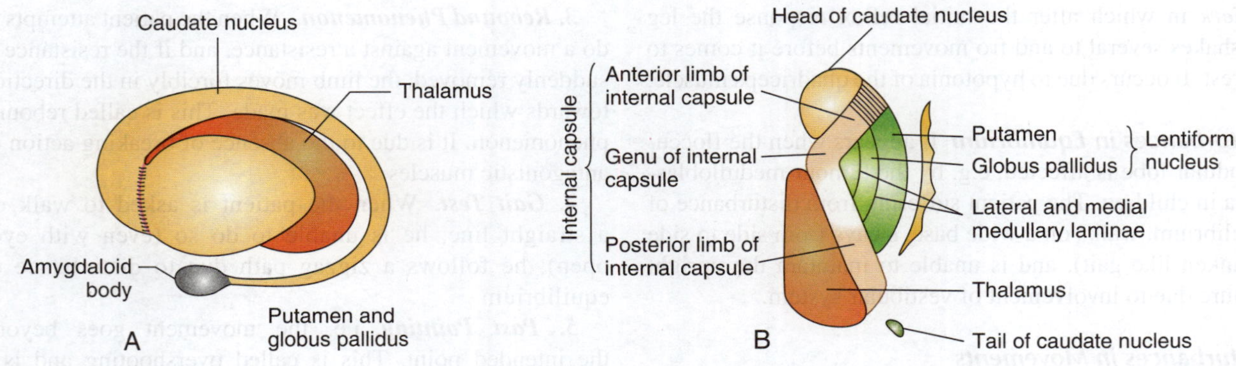

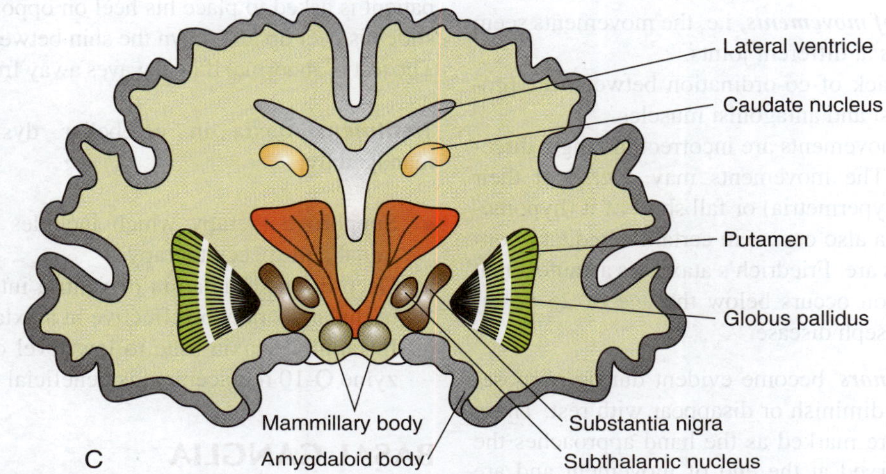

FIGURE 10.2-10 Anatomy of basal ganglia: **A,** lateral view; **B,** horizontal section and **C,** frontal section.

Phylogenetically and Functionally, the corpus striatum can be divided into two parts:

- Neostriatum or striatum and
- Paleostriatum or pallidum.

1. ***Neostriatum or striatum.*** Phylogenetically, the caudate nucleus and putamen are of more recent origin and hence called neostriatum or striatum in short. Functionally and structurally also, the caudate nucleus and putamen are similar. The striatum is divided into:
   - Dorsal striatum and
   - Ventral striatum.
2. ***Paleostriatum*** refers to globus pallidus, which is an older and primitive part. It is also called pallidum, as it is pale (pallid). Pallidum is subdivided into:
   - Dorsal pallidum and
   - Ventral pallidum.

Salient Features of Nuclei of Corpus Striatum *(Fig. 10.2-10)*

Caudate Nucleus. It is a highly curved, comma-shaped band of grey matter. It consists of head, body and a tail. Caudate nucleus is separated from the lentiform nucleus almost completely by the fibres of internal capsule, except lower part of its head where it is continuous with putamen nucleus (part of lentiform nucleus). This area of continuity is known as *fundus striati*. The tail of caudate nucleus ends by becoming continuous with putamen and lies in close relation to the amygdaloid body.

Lenticular Nucleus. It is shaped like a biconvex lens and is triangular in both coronal and horizontal sections. It is divided into two parts by an external lamina of white matter:

- ***Putamen*** is the outer part of lentiform nucleus. It is dark in colour and is roughly quadrilateral.
- ***Globus pallidus*** is the inner small part which is paler in appearance. It is further divided by an internal lamina of white matter into:
  - External segment (GPe) and
  - Internal segment (GPi).

The striatum has four types of neurons; 95% are Gabanergic medium spiny neurons, and remaining 5% striatal neurons are nonspiny, which include: large (cholinergic), medium (somatostatinergic) and small (Gabanergic)

Subthalamic Nucleus Subthalamic nucleus (body of Luys) is a biconvex mass of grey matter, which is situated lateral to red nucleus and dorsal to substantia nigra in the mesencephalon.

Subthalamic nucleus is separated from the ventral nuclei of thalamus by a thin sheet of grey matter known as *zona inserta*.

Substantia Nigra Substantia nigra is a sheet made up of small unpigmented and large pigmented nerve cells. It appears dark in unstained sections as neurons within it contain the pigment neuromelanin. It extends along the entire length of midbrain. Its cranial end reaches close to the subthalamic nucleus. Substantia nigra is divisible into two parts:

1. ***Pars compacta*** is the dorsal part of substantia nigra. Pars compacta of the two sides are continuous with each other across the ventral tegmentum. It contains two types of neurons:
   - Dopaminergic neurons constitute about 75% and
   - Cholinergic neurons are about 25%.
2. ***Pars reticularis*** is the ventral part of substantia nigra. Superiorly, it becomes continuous with the globus pallidus. Most of the neurons in the pars reticularis are GABA-ergic.

Connections of Basal Ganglia

- Striatum (caudate nucleus and putamen) forms the main input side of the basal ganglia.
- Striatum in turn projects mainly to globus pallidus and substantia nigra.
- Pallidum (globus pallidus) is the main output side of the basal ganglia.

Therefore, connections of the basal ganglia (Fig. 10.2-11) can be considered under following three headings:

i. Afferents or input to striatum,
ii. Projections from striatum and
iii. Efferents or output from globus pallidus.

Afferents or Input to Striatum The striatum (caudate nucleus and putamen) is regarded as the input side of the basal ganglia receiving following afferents.

1. ***Corticostriate projections***. These originate from all parts of the cerebral cortex (premotor, supplementary motor cortex and primary somatosensory) and terminate in striatum. These fibres are glutamatergic.
2. ***Thalamostriate fibres***. These originate from centromedian nucleus of thalamus and terminate in striatum.
3. ***Nigrostriate fibres***. These originate from the pars compacta, part of substantia nigra and terminate in the striatum. These are dopaminergic fibres. They are distributed in a typically ordered manner.
4. ***Raphe striate fibres*** are serotoninergic fibres received by the striatum from raphe nuclei in the reticular formation of brainstem.

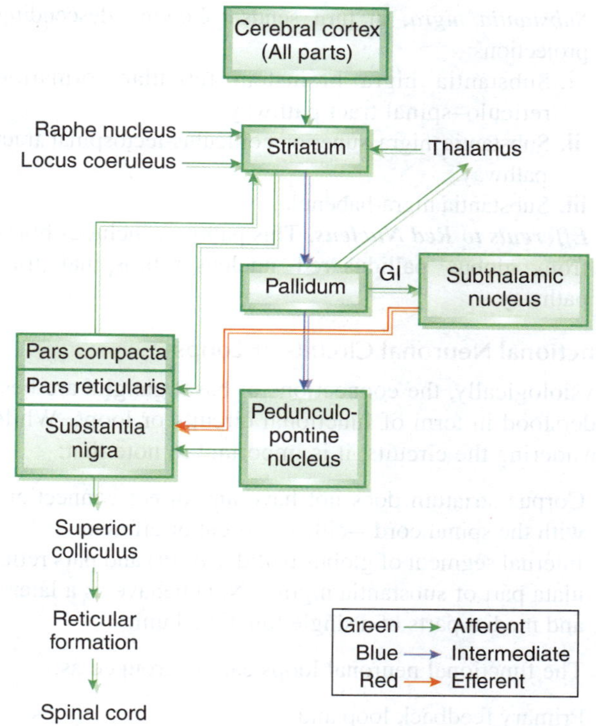

FIGURE 10.2-11 Connections of basal ganglia.

5. ***Locus coeruleus striate fibres*** are noradrenergic fibres received by the striatum from the locus coeruleus.

Projections from Striatum

1. ***Striatum to globus pallidus***. Striatum (caudate nucleus and putamen) which receive most of the afferents gives robust projection to both segments of globus pallidus. These are GABA-ergic inhibitory projections.
2. ***Striatum to substantia nigra***. Striatum also gives GABA-ergic inhibitory impulses to pars reticulata of the substantia nigra.

Efferents or Output from Globus Pallidus The pallidum (globus pallidus) is the output side of basal ganglia. The efferents of pallidum are as follows:

1. ***Efferents to thalamus***. These fibres are called thalamic fasciculus or ansafascicularis. They arise from the internal segment of globus pallidus (GP_1) and go to ventroanterior, ventrolateral and centromedian nuclei of thalamus. From thalamus, fibres project on to prefrontal and premotor cortex.
2. ***Efferents to subthalamic nucleus***, which in turn project to substantia nigra.
3. ***Efferents to substantia nigra***. The pallidum projects to the substantia nigra. These fibres take three routes:
   - Some reach the substantia nigra directly,
   - Others go via subthalamic nucleus and
   - Still others via pedunculopontine nucleus.

Substantia nigra, in turn sends following descending projections:

i. Substantia nigra brainstem reticular formation reticulo–spinal tract pathway.

ii. Substantia nigra superior colliculus-tectospinal tract pathway.

iii. Substantia nigra-habenula.

4. ***Efferents to Red Nucleus.*** This pathway includes fibres from globus pallidus–red nucleus–rubrospinal tract pathway.

Functional Neuronal Circuits or Loops

Physiologically, the connections of basal ganglia are best understood in term of functional circuits or loops. While considering the circuits, it is important to note that:

- Corpus striatum does not have any direct connections with the spinal cord—either afferent or efferent.
- Internal segment of globus pallidus (GPi) and pars reticulata part of substantia nigra (SNpr) behave as a lateral and medial parts of a single functional unit.

The functional neuronal loops can be grouped as:

1. Primary feedback loop and
2. Additional feedback loop.

1. Primary Feedback Loop or Cortex-Basal Ganglia-Motor Cortex Circuit The primary functional neuronal circuit or loop is formed by (Fig. 10.2-12):

- Afferents from all parts of cerebral cortex to striatum (excitatory glutamatergic)
- Projection of striatum to globus pallidus and substantia nigra (GPi and SNpr). (GABA-ergic inhibitory)
- Efferents from GPi and SNpr to thalamus (GABA-ergic inhibitory).
- Projections from thalamus to motor cortex and striatum.

Functions. Cortex-basal ganglia-cortex neuronal circuit, provides a negative feedback loop to control the activity of motor cortex

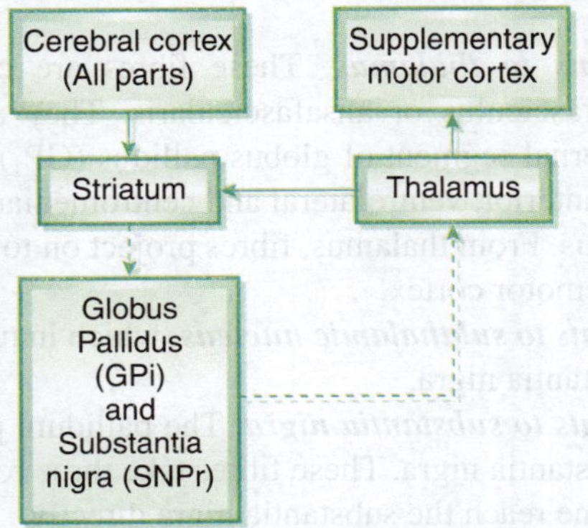

FIGURE 10.2-12 Pathway of primary feedback loop (cortex–basal ganglia–cortex neuronal circuit)

Parts. The primary feedback loop (cortex-basal ganglia-cortex neuronal circuit) consists of two parts, i.e. two distinct loops built into it:

- Caudate loop and
- Putamen loop.

i. *Caudate loop* or circuit is shown in Fig. 10.2-13A. This loop passes through caudate part of pallidum (GPi) and caudal part of substantia nigra (SNpr) and ventrolateral parts of thalamus.

Functions. Caudate loop plays a role in cognitive control of motor activity (thinking process of brain). It also plays a role in the control of eye movements.

ii. *Putamen loop or circuit*. As shown in Fig. 10.2-13B, the putamen loop passes through rostral part of GPi and SNpr, and ventroanterior part of thalamus.

Function. Putamen loop is mainly responsible for motor control of body movements.

2. Additional Feedback Loop In the primary feedback loop, the connections between the striatum and globus pallidus are direct. However, there are two additional indirect feedback loops:

I. *Indirect pathway via subthalamic nucleus*

As shown in Fig. 10.2-14, this pathway contains three inhibitory neurons:

- One from striatum to the external segment of globus pallidus (GPe),
- Another from GPe to subthalamic nucleus and
- The third from internal segment of globus pallidus (GPi) to thalamus.

As shown in Fig. 10.2-14, the striatum disinhibits the subthalamic nucleus (STN). The STN in turn stimulates GPi, which then releases its inhibitory output to thalamus. The overall effect of this circuit is therefore inhibitory.

II. *Indirect pathway involving pars compacta,* part of substantia nigra. As shown in Fig. 10.2-15, in this pathway, pars compacta part of substantia nigra (SNpc), projects to striatum (nigrostriatal pathway). The nigrostriatal pathway utilizes dopamine as a neurotransmitter. The SNpc is inhibited by the striatum through the striatonigral pathway. The SNpc in turn exerts both, facilitatory as well as inhibitory, effects on the striatum through the dopamine as:

- *Dopamine exerts an excitatory effect* which it acts through D_1 dopamine receptors, present as the excitatory cholinergic interneuron of striatum.
- *Dopamine exerts inhibitory effect* when it acts through D_2 receptors present on the excitatory cholinergic interneuron.

Functions of Basal Ganglia

Control of Voluntary Motor Activity

Basal ganglia control the voluntary movements, which are initiated by the motor cortex. During lesions of basal

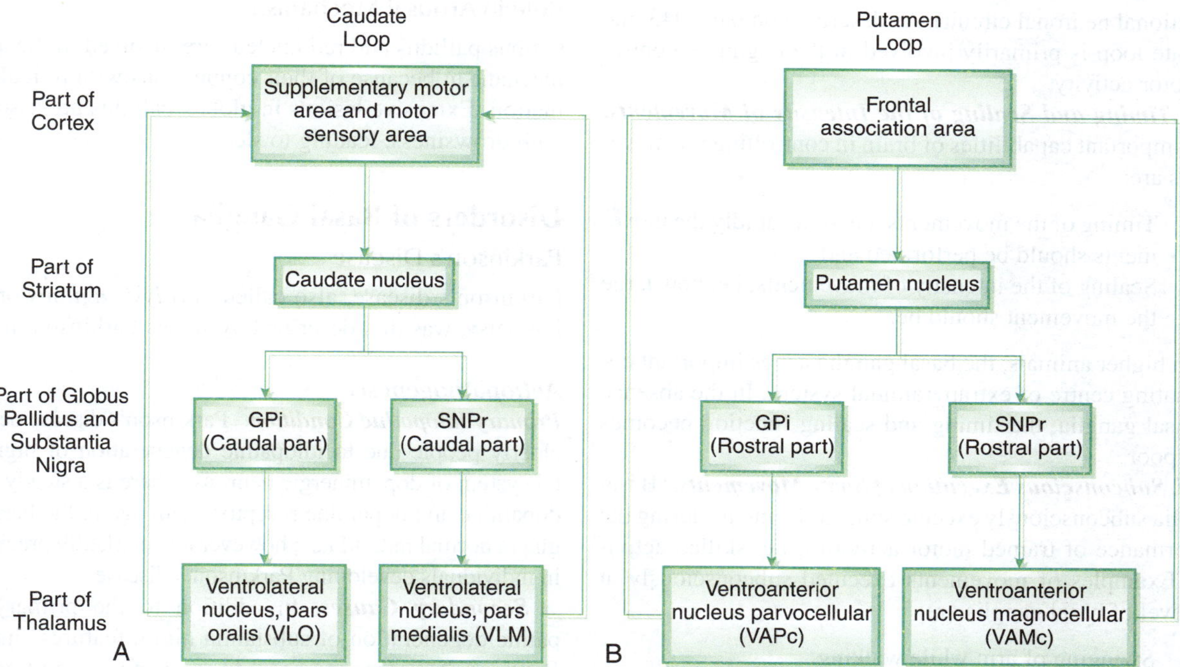

FIGURE 10.2-13 **A:** Pathway of caudate loop; and **B:** pathway of putamen loop.

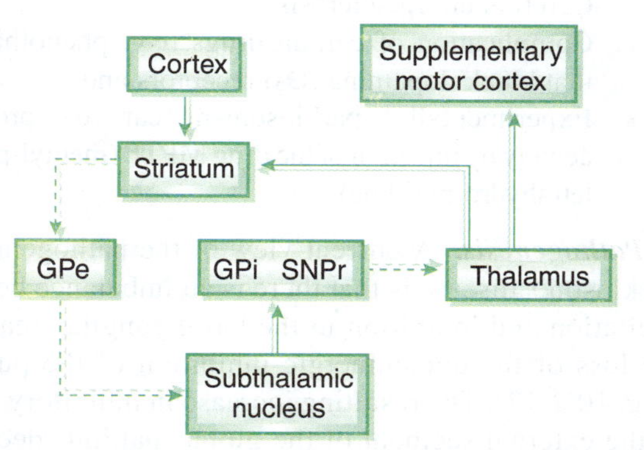

FIGURE 10.2-14 Indirect pathway of feedback loop involving subthalamic nucleus.

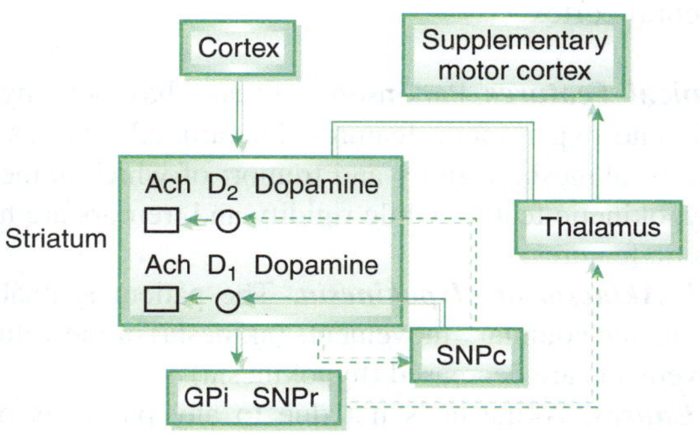

FIGURE 10.2-15 Indirect pathway of feedback loop involving substantia nigra pars compacta (SNpc).

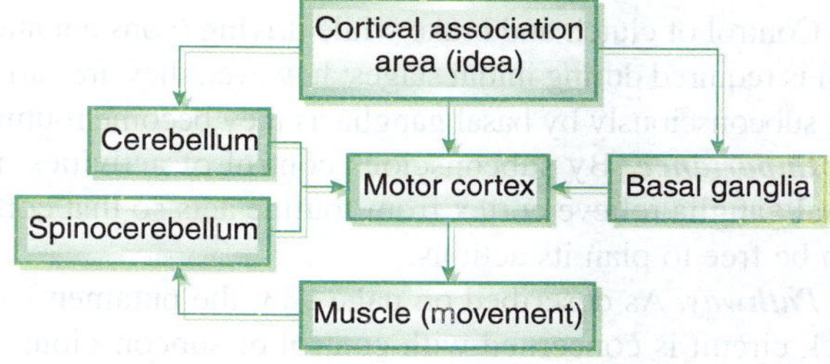

FIGURE 10.2-16 Planning and programming of movement.

ganglia, the controlling mechanism is lost and so movements become inaccurate and awkward.

Role of basal ganglia in control of voluntary motor activity includes:

- Cognitive control of motor activity,
- Timing and scaling of intensity of movements and
- Subconscious execution of some movements.

i. Cognitive Control of Motor Activity. Physiological studies have shown that neural discharge in basal ganglia, like cerebellum, begins well before the movements begin. Therefore, it is believed that basal ganglia, like the cerebellum, are involved in the planning and programming of the movement (Fig. 10.2-16).

Most of the motor actions occur as a consequence of thoughts generated in mind. This process is known as cognitive control of motor activity.

Pathway. The cognitive control of motor activity is executed by the basal ganglia through the feedback loops (functional neuronal circuit). As described on page 943, the caudate loop is primarily involved in the cognitive control of motor activity.

ii. Timing and Scaling of the Intensity of Movements. Two important capabilities of brain in controlling the movements are:

- Timing of the movements, i.e. how rapidly the movements should be performed and
- Scaling of the intensity of movements, i.e. how large the movement should be.

In higher animals, the basal ganglia act as important co-ordinating centre of extrapyramidal system. In the absence of basal ganglia, the timing and scaling function becomes very poor.

iii. Subconscious Execution of Some Movements. Basal ganglia subconsciously execute some movements during the performance of trained motor activities, i.e. skilled activities. Examples of movements executed subconsciously at the level of basal ganglia are:

- Swinging of arm while walking,
- Crude movement of facial expression that accompany emotions and
- Movements of limbs while swimming.

Control of clutch and brake while driving (constant attention is required during initial stages; however, they are carried out subconsciously by basal ganglia as they become routine).

Importance. By subconscious control of activities, the basal ganglia relieve cortex from routine acts so that cortex can be free to plan its actions.

Pathway. As described on page 943, the putamen feedback circuit is concerned with control of subconscious execution of some movements, during the performance of trained motor activities as listed above.

Control of Reflex Muscular Activity

The basal ganglia exert inhibitory effect on spinal reflexes and regulate activity of muscles, which maintain posture. Visual and labyrinthine reflexes are important in the maintenance of posture. The co-ordination and integration of impulses for these activities depend upon basal ganglia.

Control of Muscle Tone

Muscle spindles and the gamma motor neurons of spinal cord (which are responsible for maintaining the tone of the muscles) are controlled by basal ganglia, especially substantia nigra.

Pathway includes projection from cortical inhibitory area-striatum-pallidum-substantia nigra-reticular formation-spinal cord.

Proof. In lesion of basal ganglia, muscle tone increases. Rigidity (lead-pipe type) is a characteristic feature of Parkinson's disease.

Role in Arousal Mechanism

Globus pallidus and red nucleus are involved in the arousal mechanism because of their connections with reticular formation. Extensive lesions in globus pallidus are associated with drowsiness, leading to sleep.

Disorders of Basal Ganglia

Parkinson's Disease

Parkinson's disease, also called *paralysis agitans* or shaking palsy, was first described by James Parkinson in 1817.

Aetiopathogenesis

Primary Idiopathic Condition. Parkinson's disease occurs in elderly people due to idiopathic degeneration of nigrostriatal system of dopaminergic neurons. There is a steady loss of dopamine and dopamine receptors with age in the basal ganglia in normal individuals; however it is markedly precipitated in individuals developing Parkinson's disease.

Secondary Causes. In addition to the primary idiopathic degeneration of substantia nigra, features similar to Parkinson's disease can occur in some other conditions. The term *Parkinsonism nigra* is used to denote such a condition, which may occur due to following causes:

- Viral encephalitis,
- Cerebral arteriosclerosis,
- Complication of certain drugs (e.g. phenothiazine) that block dopamine (D_2) receptors and
- Experimentally, parkinsonism can be produced acutely by injection of the drug MPTP (methyl-phenyl-tetrahydro-pyridine).

Pathogenesis. A current view of the pathogenesis of Parkinson's disease is that there is an imbalance between excitation and inhibition in the basal ganglia created by the loss of the dopaminergic inhibition of the putamen (Fig. 10.2-17). The resulting increase in inhibitory output to the external segment of the globus pallidus decreases inhibitory output from the subthalamic nucleus, and this increases the excitatory output from this nucleus to the internal segment of globus pallidus. This in turn increases the inhibitory output from this segment to the thalamus, causing a reduction in excitatory drive to the cerebral cortex.

Clinical Features Parkinson's disease has both hypokinetic and hyperkinetic features. Its cardinal features are a triad of akinesia, rigidity and tremor; of which akinesia is a hypokinetic feature while rigidity and tremors are hyperkinetic features.

1. Akinesia or Hypokinesia. The patient is unable to initiate the voluntary movements (akinesia) or the voluntary movements are decreased (hypokinesia).

Causes. Akinesia is not due to any paralysis or decrease in muscle power; the sensory system is also normal.

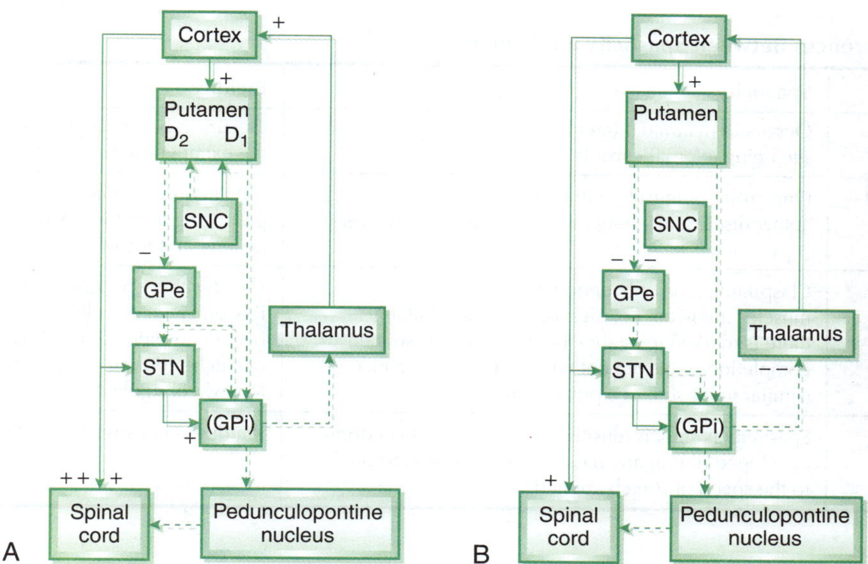

FIGURE 10.2-17 Basal ganglia-thalamo-cortical circuitry: **A,** in normal; and **B,** in Parkinson's disease. Solid arrows indicate excitatory output and dashed arrows inhibitory output. Number of plus (+) and minus (−) signs indicate relative increase and decrease in excitation and inhibition of outputs. GPe (external segment of globus pallidus), GP (internal segment), SNC (substantia nigra compacta), SIN (subthalamic nucleus).

Difficulty in initiating voluntary movements is because of hypertonictiy of the muscles.

Manifestations of akinesia or hypokinesia include:

- Delayed motor initiative, as evidenced by prolonged reaction time.
- Slow performance of voluntary movements (bradykinesia).
- Mask-like facial expression due to decrease in movements of facial muscles.
- Absence of normal associated movements, e.g. swinging of arms during walking.
- Shuffling or festinant type gait, in which patient is bent forward and walks quickly with short steps as if trying to catch up centre of gravity or preventing himself from falling.
- Retropulsion, i.e. when a walking patient is suddenly pulled backwards, he begins to walk backwards and is unable to stop.

2. Rigidity refers to increase in tone of the muscles.

Characteristic features of rigidity occurring in Parkinson's disease are:

- It occurs due to increased tone in both the protagonists and antagonist muscles.
- Mainly large proximal group of muscles of limbs, e.g. biceps and knee flexors are affected.
- Usually, there occurs uniform resistance to flexion giving a feeling as if lead pipe is being bent (lead-pipe rigidity).
- Sometimes, there is a series of catches during passive motion of the limbs (cogwheel rigidity).
- Due to rigidity, posture becomes that of flexion attitude in which: back is flexed, arms are abducted and flexed and the knees are bent.
- In advanced cases, the rigidity may increase to such an extent that a statue-like appearance is produced with complete absence of movements.
- Rigidity differs from spasticity seen in lesions of pyramidal tracts (see Table 10.2-3).

Cause of rigidity. An increased discharge of γ-efferents supplying the muscle spindle causes rigidity. This fact is confirmed by the observation that local injection of 1% procaine solution into the affected muscles decreases rigidity by abolishing the γ-discharge.

Neural mechanism. As described on page 942, the striatum (caudate nucleus and putamen) is under the influence of both excitatory (cholinergic) fibres and inhibitory (dopaminergic) fibres. Under normal circumstances, there exists a balance between the excitatory and inhibitory influences. In patients with Parkinson's disease, lack of dopaminergic activity due to degeneration of neurons in the substantia nigra shifts the balance towards excitatory cholinergic fibres. As a result, hyperkinetic features of Parkinson's disease appear.

Proof. The above facts can be confirmed by the following observations:

- Administration of physostigmine (which increases the action of acetylcholine) leads to increase in rigidity and tremors.
- Administration of reserpine (which depletes dopamine stores in dopaminergic nerve endings) increases rigidity and tremors.

TABLE 10.2-3 Differences Between Spasticity and Rigidity

Feature	Spasticity	Rigidity
1. Lesion	Occurs in pyramidal tract lesions, commonest site being internal capsule	Occurs in basal ganglia lesion, therefore, called the extrapyramidal rigidity
2. Muscles involved	One group of muscles either agonist or antagonist (usually antigravity muscles) are involved	Both agonist and antagonist muscles are involved producing a uniform hypertonia often resulting in general attitude of flexion of the limbs and trunk
3. Characteristics of hypertonia	Clasp-knife type of hypertonia is seen in muscles involved, i.e. on passive flexion initially there is marked resistance but then there is sudden completion of movement without much resistance (similar to closure of a pocket knife).	Usually, there occurs a uniform resistance to flexion giving a feeling as if lead pipe is being bent (lead-pipe rigidity) Sometime there is a series of catches during passive motion of the limb (cogwheel rigidity)
4. Relation of hypertonia to stretch	Spasticity is stretch sensitive, i.e. degree of hypertonia developed during any passive stretch is proportional to the speed of stretch applied.	Rigidity is not stretch sensitive

- Administration of phenothiazines (which block D_2 dopamine receptors) leads to increase in rigidity and tremors.

*3. **Tremors.*** Tremors (i.e. involuntary, rhythmic and oscillatory movements of the distal parts of limbs and head) seen in Parkinson's disease have following characteristics:

- The tremors are present at rest, but disappear during activity. It is hallmark of Parkinson's disease and so popularly known as resting (static) tremors.
- Frequency of tremors ranges from 4 to 6 times/s.

It is frequently seen as frill-rolling movements of the hand, i.e. rhythmic contraction of thumb over first two fingers.

- Tremors are suppressed during sleep and exaggerated by stress anxiety and excitement.

The tremors are observed as rhythmic movements of pronation and supination in fingers, hands, lips or tongue.

Neural mechanism. The tremors seem to occur due to pacemaker activity in the nucleus ventralis intermedius of the thalamus. Thalamic neurons exhibit an intrinsic autorhythmicity, and probably it gets unmasked due to increase in the inhibitory input from the pallidum. The thalamic pacemaker activity induces oscillation in the long-loop reflex pathways, which originate from muscle spindle. The reflex path runs through the thalamus up to the cortex and then loops back to extrafusal muscle fibres along the corticospinal tract.

Treatment

Drug Treatment

1. ***L-dopa*** is used in the treatment of Parkinson's disease. It can cross the blood–brain barrier and reaches the brain tissue, where it is concentrated into dopamine and thus compensates its deficiency.
   - Drug dopamine is not used as it cannot cross the blood–brain barrier.
   - Along with L-dopa, carbidopa (sinemet) is also used. Carbidopa prevents the conversion of L-dopa into dopamine in the liver and thus prevents side effects, which can occur due to excessive dopamine content in liver.
   - Carbidopa cannot cross blood–brain barrier and thus in the brain L-dopa is converted into dopamine.
   - L-dopa in low doses diminishes rigidity and in high doses reduces tremors.
2. ***Dopamine agonists,*** such as apomorphine, bromocriptine, pramiprexole and ropinirole also have effective role in some patients with Parkinson's disease.
3. ***Catechol-O-methyltransferase (COMT) inhibitors*** such as entacapone, when given along with L-DOPA, act by blocking the breakdown of L-DOPA and increases its concentration in the brain.
4. ***Monoamine oxidase-B (MAO-B) inhibitors*** (e.g. selegiline) also prevents breakdown of dopamine

Surgical Treatment

- Palliditomy-Surgical destruction of globus pallidusinterna (GP_i) or of subthalamic nucleus (thalamomotomy)
- Ventrolateral nucleus of thalamus can also ameliorate the symptoms of Parkinson's disease by restoring the output balance towards normal.
- Implantation of dopamine-secreting tissue in or near to basal ganglia,
- Transplant of adrenomedullary tissue of the patient's own, also works effectively for some time and
- Fetal striatal tissue transplantation are better taken up and make connections with hosts basal ganglia

Chorea and Athetosis

Chorea is characterized by rapid, jerky and involuntary movements (dancing movements). It occurs due to damage to caudate nucleus. Chorea is seen frequently in children as a complication of rheumatic fever.

Athetosis is characterized by slow, rhythmic, twisting, worm like and confluent writhing movements of the extremities, affecting chiefly the fingers and the wrists. It occurs due to damage to putamen. Athetosis may occur in children following birth injuries.

Huntington's Disease

Cause. It is a genetic disease of nervous system, characterized by trinucleotide repeat expansion. It is inherited as an autosomal dominant disorder, usually occurring between 30 and 50 years of age. The abnormal gene responsible for the disease is located near the end of short arm of chromosome. The abnormal gene codes for a protein called huntingtin, which is comparatively less soluble and form toxic aggregates in the nuclei of the cell Huntington disease is also related with increased activity of tissue caspase-1 in the brain, due to mutation or knocked out gene for apoptosis-regulating enzyme.

Site of Lesion. There occurs damage to GABA-ergic and cholinergic neurons of striatum (caudate and putamen) that project to pallidum. The loss of GABA-ergic pathway to the external pallidum releases inhibition, permitting the hyperkinetic features of the disease to develop.

Characteristic Features of Huntington's disease are:

- An early sign is jerky trajectory of the hand when reaching to touch a spot.
- Later, hyperkinetic choreiform movements appear, and gradually increase until they incapacitate the patient.
- Speech becomes slurred and then incomprehensible.
- There occurs progressive loss of memory (dementia).

It is a gradually progressive disease, with no effective treatment, which ultimately leads to death.

Treatment

1. *Tetrabenazine*. Administration of tetrabenazin is efficiently used to reduce chorioform movements (the characteristics of Huntington's disease). This drug binds with vesicular monoamine transporters (VMAT), and thus inhibits uptake of monoamines into the synaptic vesicles and also acts as dopamine receptor antagonist.

Hemiballism

Cause. It is a rare disease caused by damage of subthalamic nucleus. Common cause of damage is haemorrhage in the nucleus. Damage to the subthalamic nucleus reduces inhibitory output from GPi SNpc to thalamus (Fig. 10.2-14). This leads to disinhibition of thalamic output, resulting in hyperkinetic movements, mediated by corticospinal tracts.

Characteristic Features. The most important feature of hemiballism is: spontaneous attacks of flail-like, intense and violent movements affecting whole of the opposite half of body.

Wilson's Disease

Wilson's disease, also known as hepatolenticular degeneration, is caused by copper toxicity, resulting from impaired biliary excretion of dietary copper. It is genetic autosomal recessive disorder occurring due to mutation of copper-transporting ATPase gene (ATP7β) located on the long arm of chromosome 13q.

- *Liver* involvement is in the form of cirrhosis.
- In affected individual, copper accumulates in the periphery of the cornea and causes characteristic yellow rings (Kayser–Flescher's rings). Toxic effects are most pronounced in the liver and brain.
- *In brain,* the lesions are widespread. However, the changes are more marked in lenticular nucleus, particularly putamen resulting in symptoms of Parkinsonism, i.e. muscular rigidity, tremors and akinesia.

In this condition, the copper content of substantia nigra is high and plasma level of ceruloplasmin (copper-binding protein) is low.

Treatment *Chelating agents* such as penicillamine and trienthine are used to decrease copper in the body in Wilson's disease.

Kernicterus

Kernicterus refers to damage of globus pallidus caused by indirect bilirubin, which crosses the blood–brain barrier. It occurs in haemolytic disease of newborn, which results due to Rh antibodies. In this condition, death is very common. However, if the child survives, it may show rigidity, chorea, athetosis and mental deficiency (also see page 156).

Taradive Dyskinesia

Taradive dyskinesia is another basal ganglia disease, caused by neuroleptic drugs such as phenothiazide or haloperidol, used as medical treatment for psychiatric disorders. Prolonged use of these drugs produces biochemical abnormalities in the striatum by blocking dopaminergic transmission

Characteristic Features are

- Involuntary movements of face and tongue and
- Cog wheel rigidity

Treatment *Clozapine* is an atypical effective neuroleptic drug used as substitute for traditional neuroleptic drugs to avoid risk of development of taradive dyskinesia.

Chapter 10.3

Physiological Anatomy, Functions and Lesions of Thalamus and Hypothalamus

THALAMUS

Physiological Anatomy

The thalamus proper (i.e. dorsal thalamus) along with ventral thalamus (old name subthalamus), epithalamus and hypothalamus constitutes the diencephalon. The diencephalon along with the cerebral hemispheres forms the so-called forebrain. It is important to note that:

- The thalamus proper is now called *dorsal thalamus*.
- The *ventral thalamus* is the new name for the subthalamus.
- The *reticular nucleus,* earlier included in the dorsal thalamus, is now considered a part of ventral thalamus (on functional grounds).
- The *subthalamic nucleus* is now included among the basal ganglia (page 941) to which it is closely related functionally. It is not included in the ventral thalamus (old name subthalamus).
- The *medial and lateral geniculate bodies* are now considered as an integral part of dorsal thalamus.

Earlier, they have been considered distinct from the other regions of the thalamus and have been grouped together as metathalamus.

External Features

The dorsal thalamus is a large ovoid structure placed immediately lateral to the third ventricle. It has an anterior and a posterior end and four surfaces viz. dorsal, ventral, medial and lateral.

- *Anterior end* (or pole) lies just behind the interventricular foramen.
- *Posterior end* (or pole) is expanded and is called pulvinar. It lies just above and lateral to the superior colliculus.
- *Dorsal or superior surface* of the thalamus is convex and triangular in outline. It forms the part of floor of the central part of lateral ventricle (Figs 10.3-1, 10.3-2).
- *Ventral or inferior surface* of the thalamus is related to the hypothalamus anteriorly (Fig. 10.3-1) and to the ventral thalamus posteriorly (Fig. 10.3-2).
- *Medial surface* forms the greater part of the lateral wall of third ventricle and is lined by ependyma. The medial surfaces of the two thalami are connected by a short bar of grey matter called the *interthalamic adhesion*. Inferiorly, the medial surface is separated from the hypothalamus by *hypothalamic sulcus* (Fig. 10.3-1).
- *Lateral surface* of thalamus is related to the posterior limbs of internal capsule.

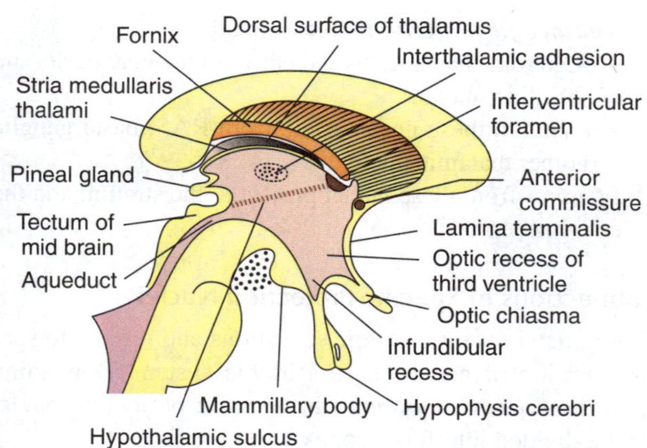

FIGURE 10.3-1 Median section through the brain showing medial surface of thalamus and hypothalamus.

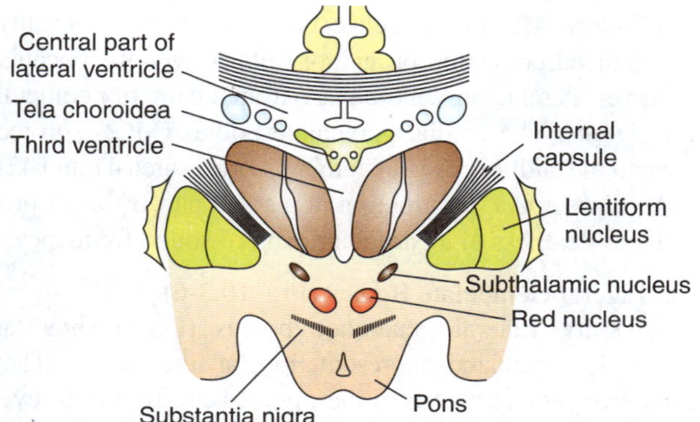

FIGURE 10.3-2 Coronal section through the brain passing through the basilar part of pons showing the relations of ventral surface of thalamus and subthalamic structures.

Internal Structure

Like other parts of brain, the thalamus consists of grey matter (mainly) and white matter (Fig. 10.3-3).

White Matter White matter is scanty in thalamus and includes:

- *Stratum zonale,* a thin layer of white matter covering the superior surface of thalamus.
- *External medullary lamina* is a thin layer of white matter covering the lateral surface of thalamus. It consists of thalamocortical and corticothalamic fibres.
- *Internal medullary lamina* is a Y-shaped sheet of white matter placed vertically in the grey matter of thalamus. It consists mainly of internuclear thalamic connections.

Grey Matter Grey matter of thalamus in divided into three masses of nuclei by the Y-shaped internal medullary lamina (Fig. 10.3-3):

- Anterior part,
- Lateral part and
- Medial part.

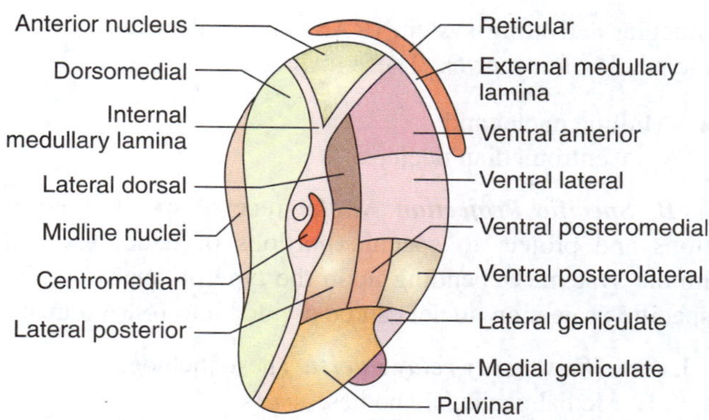

FIGURE 10.3-3 Horizontal section of right thalamus (superior aspect) showing nuclear subdivisions.

Classification of Thalamic Nuclei

Anatomical Classification of Thalamic Nuclei Anatomically, thalamic nuclei can be classified as (Fig. 10.3-3):

1. Anterior Group of Nuclei. The mass of grey matter enclosed within the bifurcation of the internal medullary lamina is called *anterior nucleus*.

2. Lateral Group of Nuclei. The mass of grey matter present in the lateral part of thalamus is subdivided into ventral and dorsal group of nuclei, each containing three nuclei:

(i) *Ventral group of nuclei* includes:
- Ventral anterior nucleus,
- Ventral lateral (lateroventral) nucleus and
- Ventral posterior (posteroventral) nucleus which is further divided into two parts:
- Ventral posterolateral nucleus and
- Ventral posteromedial nucleus
- Medial and lateral geniculate bodies are present in the posterior zone of ventral groups of nuclei.

(ii) *Dorsal group of nuclei* are:
- Lateral dorsal nucleus,
- Lateral posterior nucleus and
- Pulvinar.

3. Medial Group of Nuclei

- Dorsomedial nuclei, present in the medial part of thalamus,
- Centromedian nucleus and other interlaminar nuclei present within the internal medullary lamina and
- Midline nuclei that lie between the medial part of thalamus and the ependyma of the third ventricle.

Functional Classification of Thalamic Nuclei Functionally, the thalamic nuclei can be grouped under two divisions:

- Nonspecific projection nuclei and
- Specific projection nuclei.

A. ***Nonspecific Projection Nuclei*** are those which receive impulses for diffuse secondary responses from the reticular-activating system (RAS) and project diffusely to the whole of neocortex. These include:

- Midline nuclei and
  - Centromedian nucleus.

B. Specific Projection Nuclei receive specific sensations and project to specific portions of neocortex and limbic system. Depending upon the type of sensation, the specific projection nuclei can be divided into four groups:

I. ***Specific sensory relay nuclei.*** These include:
1. Medial geniculate bodies,
2. Lateral geniculate bodies and
3. Posteroventral group of nuclei.

II. ***Motor control nuclei.*** These include:
1. Ventrolateral group of nuclei and
2. Ventral anterior nucleus.

III. ***Visceral efferent control nuclei.*** These include:
1. Anterior group of nuclei and
2. Dorsomedial nucleus.

IV. ***Integrative and perceptual function control nuclei:***
1. Pulvinar nucleus,
2. Lateral posterior nucleus and
3. Dorsal lateral nucleus.

Connections of Thalamus

Afferent and efferent connections of the various thalamic nuclei based on their functional classification are as (Fig. 10.3-4):

Connections of Nonspecific Projection Nuclei

These are functionally associated with *diffuse thalamic projection* which produces marked changes in the electrical activity of the cerebral cortex when they are stimulated.

Nonspecific projection nuclei include:
- Centromedian nucleus and other intralaminar nuclei and
- Midline nuclei.

Afferents to these nuclei come from RAS, basal ganglia and other thalamic nuclei.

Efferents from these nuclei project to the stratum and the entire neocortex.

Connections of Specific Projection Nuclei

These nuclei receive specific sensations and project to specific portion of neocortex and limbic system. Depending upon the type of sensation, the specific projection nuclei can be divided into four groups:

I. Specific Sensory Relay Nuclei

1. Medial Geniculate Bodies (Fig. 10.3-5)

Afferents. Medial geniculate bodies receive a 'topically' organized projection of auditory fibres from the cochlear nerve, lateral lemniscus and also from the inferior colliculi.

Efferents. The medial geniculate bodies (MGB) project on to the auditory area of cerebral cortex (area 41 and 42).

Applied aspect. Destruction of a small part of MGB produces deafness of a particular band of sound frequency.

2. Lateral Geniculate Bodies (Fig. 10.3-6)

Afferents. Lateral geniculate bodies (LGB) show an orderly organized representation of the retina. They receive projections from the optic tracts from both eyes (temporal fibres of the same side and nasal fibres of the opposite side). They also receive projections from the superior colliculi. In the LGB, the macula is represented in the caudal two-thirds, whereas the remaining retina is represented in the rostral one-third (see page 1151).

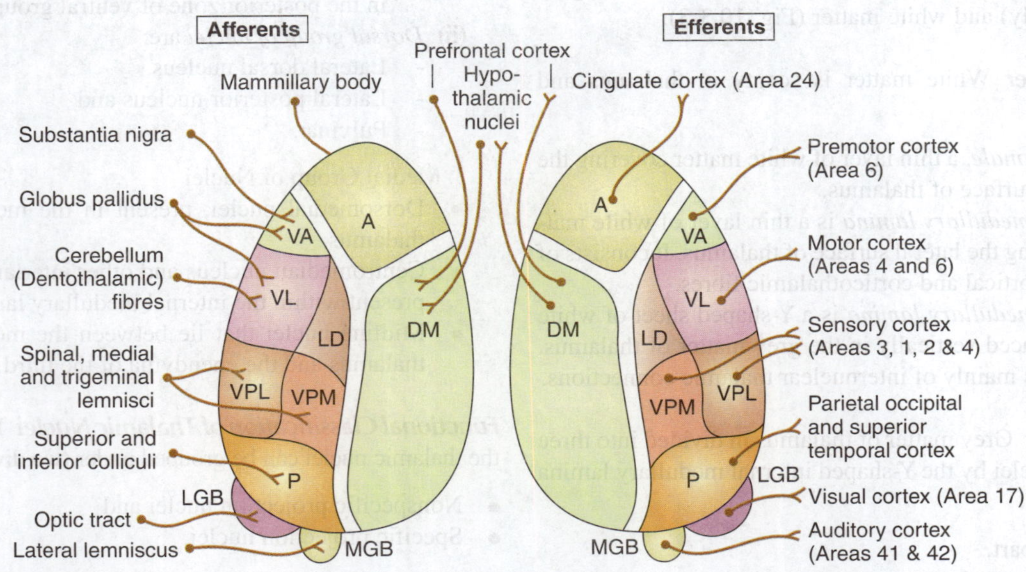

FIGURE 10.3-4 Afferent and efferent connections of some of thalamic nuclei. A: anterior nucleus; VA: ventral anterior nucleus; VL: ventral lateral nucleus; VP: ventral posterior nucleus; P: pulvinar; LGB: lateral geniculate body; and MGB: medial geniculate body.

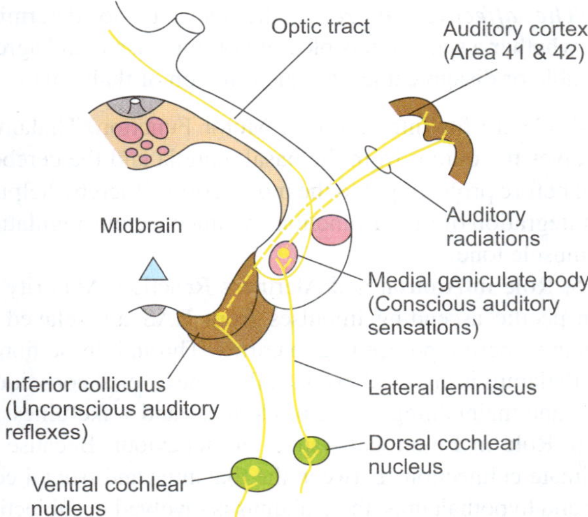

FIGURE 10.3-5 Connections of medial geniculate body.

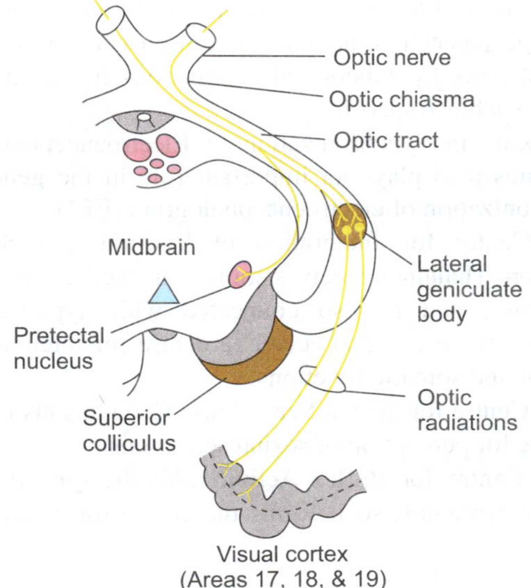

FIGURE 10.3-6 Connections of lateral geniculate body.

Efferents from LGB (optic radiations) project topographically on the visual cortex of occipital lobe (areas 17, 18 and 19).

3. Ventral Posterior Nucleus (Fig. 10.3-4)

Afferents. The ventral posterior nucleus has two divisions: ventral posterior lateral (VPL) and ventral posterior medial (VPM). VPL and VPM are the sites of termination of ascending somatic afferent tracts.

- *The medial lemniscus* carrying afferent fibres from the gracile nucleus, cuneate nucleus and spinothalamic afferents terminate in the VPL. Thus, VPL receives somatosensory impulses (touch, pressure, pain, proprioceptive, temperature and kinaesthetic) from the trunk and limbs, i.e. the whole body except face.
- *The trigeminal lemniscus* carrying afferents from face and taste fibres terminate in the VPM. Thus, VPM receives somatosensory impulses from the face along with sensations of taste.
- *In the ventral posterior nucleus,* a topographic representation of the body can be demonstrated.

Efferents. Ventral posterior nucleus is the main sensory nucleus and its efferents go to the sensory cortex, areas 3, 1, 2 (postcentralgyrus) via posterior limb of internal capsule.

II. Motor Control Nuclei

1. Ventral Lateral Nucleus (Fig. 10.3-4)

Afferents. Ventrolateral (VL) nucleus is the chief motor nucleus of the thalamus. It acts as a relay station for cerebellar impulses. It receives the dentothalamic fibres from the dentate nucleus of the opposite cerebellar hemisphere. It also receives fibres from the globuspallidus via thalamic fasciculus.

Efferents from VL nucleus project on the primary motor cortex and premotor cortex (area 4 and 6), via posterior limb of internal capsule.

These relay proprioceptive information and voluntary motor functions.

2. Ventral Anterior Nucleus (Fig. 10.3-4)

Afferents. The ventral anterior (VA) nucleus is involved in the programming of movements controlled by the basal ganglia. Its afferents come from the globuspallidus, cerebellum and substantianigra.

Efferents from VA go to the premotor cortex (area 6).

III. Visceral Efferent Control Nuclei. The nuclei concerned with visceral efferent control mechanism are:

1. Anterior Nucleus (Fig. 10.3-4)

Afferents. Anterior (A) nucleus belongs to the Papez circuit of limbic system (see page 1082). It is concerned with recent memory and emotions. It receives afferents from the hippocampus directly via fornix and relayed through mammillary body (mammillothalamic tract).

Efferents from anterior nucleus go to the cingulate gyrus (area 24) of the cerebral cortex.

2. Dorsal Medial Nucleus The dorsal medial nucleus has reciprocal connections with the prefrontal cortex and hypothalamus. Its point to point interconnections with the prefrontal cortex imply important functions in thinking, memory, judgement and in emotional behaviour.

IV. Integrative and Perceptual Function Control Nuclei

***1. Pulvinar Nucleus** (Fig. 10.3-7)*

- ***Afferents.*** Pulvinar nucleus is concerned with integration of visual, auditory and other sensations. It receives afferents from the superior and inferior colliculi.
- ***Efferents*** go to the parietal, occipital and superior temporal cortex (auditory and visual association areas).

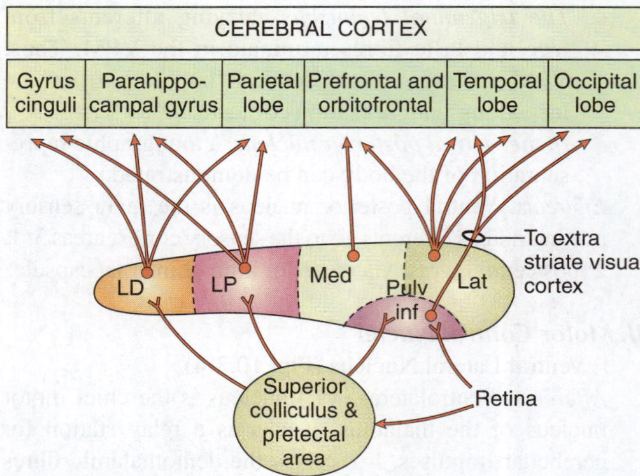

FIGURE 10.3-7 Scheme to show the connections of lateral group of thalamic nuclei. LD: Lateral dorsal; LP: lateral posterior; Med: medial; Pulv: pulvinar; and Lat: lateral.

2. Lateral Posterior Nucleus (Fig. 10.3-7)

- ***Afferents***. It receives fibres from the superior colliculus.
- ***Efferents*** from the lateral posterior nucleus reach the cerebral cortex of the superior parietal lobule. They also reach the cingulate and parahippocampal area.

3. Dorsal Lateral Nucleus (Fig. 10.3-7)

- ***Afferents.*** It receives afferents from the superior colliculus.
- ***Efferents.*** Projections reach the cingulate gyrus, the parahippocampal gyrus and parts of the hippocampal formation. Some fibres reach the cortex of parietal lobe.

Functions of Thalamus

1. Sensory Relay Centre. Almost all the sensory impulses (except olfactory) reach the thalamic nuclei, which relay them to the cerebral cortex by a series of projection fibres collectively termed the thalamic radiations (ascending thalamocortical system). Because of this, the thalamus is usually considered the head ganglion of all the sensory system.

2. Centre for Integration of Sensory Impulses. The thalamus is not only a great relay station for all sensations, but also forms a major centre for integration and modification of peripheral sensory impulses before the impulses are projected to specific areas of cerebral cortex. This function of thalamus is called processing of sensory information. Because of this, the thalamus is usually considered as a functional gateway of cerebral cortex.

3. Crude Centre for Perception of Sensations. In addition to processing and relaying of sensations, the thalamus also acts as a crude centre for sense perception. Pain sensation is perceived in the thalamus itself. Usually, the sensations have two qualities: the discriminative nature and the affective nature.

- ***The discriminative nature*** is the ability to recognize type, location and other details of the sensation. It is the function of the cerebral cortex.
- ***The affective nature*** is the capacity to determine whether a sensation is pleasant or unpleasant and agreeable or disagreeable. It is the function of thalamus.

4. Centre for Integration of Motor Function. Thalamus receives the output from the basal ganglia and the cerebellum before projecting it to the motor cortex, thereby helping in integration of motor functions by unconscious regulation of muscle tone.

5. Role in Arousal and Alertness Reaction. Majority of nonspecific ascending impulses from RAS are relayed to thalamus before proceeding to cortex. Through these fibres, the thalamus is involved in controlling the level of consciousness and maintaining a state of alertness and wakefulness.

6. Role in Emotional Aspect of Behaviour. Because of intimate connections between the thalamus and frontal cortex and hypothalamus, the thalamus is involved in subjective feeling of various emotions. Thus, it acts as a part of limbic system. It also forms a part of the Papez circuit and is concerned with recent memory and emotions.

7. Role in Language. Thalamus is also concerned with language (speech) function. Integration between different cortical parts by subcortical connections in the thalamus helps to achieve speech.

8. Role in Synchronization of Electroencephalogram. Thalamus also plays an important role in the genesis of synchronization of electroencephalogram (EEG).

9. Centre for Integration of Visceral and Somatic Function. Thalamus receives somatic as well as autonomic sensations, and is also connected with hypothalamus. Because of this, it also acts as a centre for integration of visceral and somatic functions.

10. Centre for Sexual Sensations. Thalamus also acts as a centre for perception of sexual sensations.

11. Centre for Reflex Activity. All the sensory fibres relay in thalamus, so it forms the centre for many reflex activities.

Applied Aspects

Thalamic Syndrome

The thalamic syndrome is a disturbance of emotional responses to sensory experience.

Cause. Thalamic syndrome is produced by damage to posteroventral and posterolateral nuclei as a result of thrombotic blockage of thalamogeniculate branch of posterior cerebral artery.

Symptoms and Signs in thalamic syndrome occur on the opposite side of the body. These include:

I. Sensory Symptoms due to involvement of posteroventral nucleus are:

1. ***Astereognosis*** occurs due to loss of tactile localization, tactile discrimination and stereognosis.

2. ***Thalamic phantom limb,*** i.e. patient is unable to locate the position of limbs with closed eyes and searches for the limb in air. This occurs due to loss of kinaesthetic sensations.
3. ***Thalamic overreaction,*** i.e. the threshold for pain, touch and temperature is decreased and the sensations become exaggerated and disagreeable.
4. ***Amelognosis***. It is illusion felt by the patient that his/her limb is absent.

II. Motor symptoms due to involvement of posterolateral nucleus are:

1. ***Ataxia, decreased muscle*** tone and profound muscular weakness occur due to damage to cerebellar afferents.
2. ***Involuntary movements,*** any of the following may be associated:
   - Involvement of fibres coming from globuspallidus leads to chorea (quick jerky movements) or athetosis (slow writhing and twisting movements).
   - Intention tremors are usually associated with thalamic syndrome.
3. ***Thalamic hand or athetoid hand*** refers to the abnormal posture of hand occurring in patients with thalamic syndrome. It is characterized by moderate flexion of the wrist with hyperextended fingers.

Korsakoff's Syndrome

Korsakoff's syndrome refers to lesions of mediodorsal nucleus of thalamus characterized by difficulty in remembering new information.

Frontal Lobotomy

For relief of intractable pain, connections of the dorsal nuclei of thalamus with the frontal lobe are divided surgically especially by an operation called *frontal lobotomy,* after which the patient feels the pain, but does not show a disagreeable response.

HYPOTHALAMUS

Physiological Anatomy

External Features

The hypothalamus, though a very small part of brain (a few cubic cm in size and weighing about 10 g), plays a very important role of regulating all vegetative and most endocrine processes in the body. It is the most important organ of integration in the homeostatic control of internal environment. It is a bilateral diencephalic structure, diffuse nuclear mass situated below the thalamus.

Boundaries of hypothalamus are (Fig. 10.3-1):

- ***Superiorly,*** hypothalamic sulcus separates it from the thalamus.
- ***Inferiorly,*** it is related to the structures in the floor of third ventricle viz. tuber cinereum, infundibulum and the mammillary bodies, which are considered its parts.
- ***Medially,*** it forms part of the wall of third ventricle.
- ***Laterally,*** it is in contact with the internal capsule.
- ***Anteriorly,*** it extends up to anterior commissure and lamina terminalis.
- ***Posteriorly,*** the hypothalamus merges with the ventral thalamus at a vertical plane just caudal to the mammillary bodies.

Subdivisions and Nuclei of Hypothalamus

For convenience of description, the hypothalamus can be divided (Fig. 10.3-2) as:

- ***From medial to lateral*** into two zones:
  - Medial zone and
  - Lateral zone.
- ***From anterior to posterior,*** the hypothalamic nuclear mass is arranged in four regions:
  - Preoptic region,
  - Supraoptic region,
  - Tuberal region and
  - Mammillary region.

Hypothalamic Nuclei Nuclear masses of hypothalamus present in different regions of the hypothalamus are (Fig. 10.3-8):

1. ***Preoptic region.*** It is located behind the lamina terminalis. It contains preoptic nucleus.
2. ***Supraoptic region.*** It lies above the optic chiasma and rostrally continuous with preoptic area. It forms the anterior nucleus group which includes:
   - Suprachiasmatic,
   - Supraoptic anterior and
   - Paraventricular nucleus.
3. ***Tuberal region.*** It is the widest region of the hypothalamus and forms the middle nuclear group which includes dorsomedial, lateral, tuberal, ventromedial and arcuate (infundibular or tuberal) nucleus.

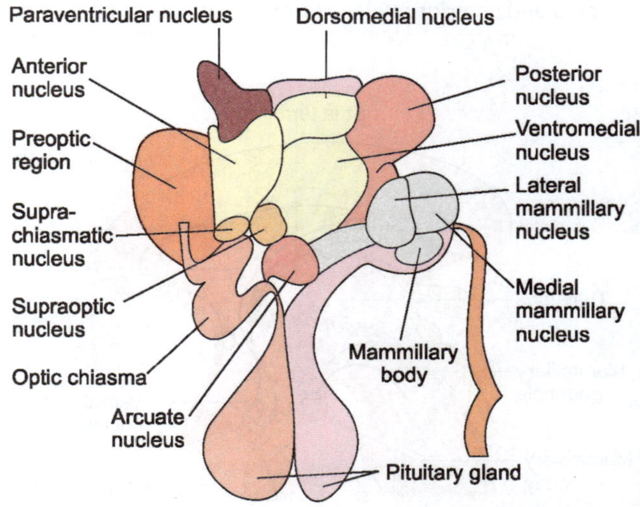

FIGURE 10.3-8 Nuclei of hypothalamus.

4. ***Mammillary region.*** It forms the *posterior nuclear* group, which includes the posterior and mammillary nucleus.

Connections of Hypothalamus

The hypothalamus serves as the main integrator of the autonomic nervous system and is concerned with visceral functions, and is, therefore, connected to other areas having a similar function. These include the various parts of the limbic system, the reticular formation and autonomic centres in the brainstem and spinal cord.

Apart from its neural connections, the hypothalamus also acts by releasing secretions into the bloodstream and into the CSF.

Afferent Connections

1. From Other Parts of Limbic System. Hypothalamus receives afferents from other parts of limbic system in the form of following nerve fibre bundles (Figs 10.3-9 and 10.3-10):

- ***Medial forebrain bundle*** forms the major pathway of the hypothalamus. It consists of both ascending and descending fibres. The descending fibres begin in the anterior olfactory areas (anterior perforated substance, olfactory tubercle and pyriform cortex) and run through the lateral zone of hypothalamus, to reach the tegmentum of midbrain. These fibres end in hypothalamic nuclei and raphe nuclei of the reticular formation of the midbrain. These fibres are related to basic emotional drives and to the sense of smell.
- ***Fornix*** is the main projection for the hippocampal formation and ends in the mammillary body, and on the arcuate nucleus some hippocampal fibres are carried to medial forebrain bundle which relays them in septal nuclei.
- ***Stria terminalis*** arises from the amygdaloid body, reaches over the thalamus and terminates in the preoptic area and anterior nucleus of hypothalamus. Some fibres from the amygdaloid body also pass the hypothalamus through the ventral amygdalofugal tract.
- ***Medial hypothalamic tract*** runs from restricted region of hippocampus to the arcuate nucleus. This pathway and stria terminalis are the only two major afferent pathways running directly to medial hypothalamus. Other afferent fibres take indirect route in medial forebrain bundle and lateral hypothalamus to reach the medial hypothalamus.
- ***Cingulate gyrus*** establishes connections with the hypothalamus through its projections to the hippocampus.

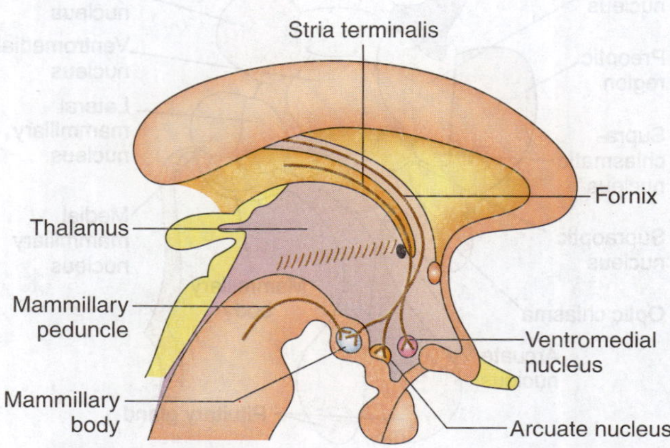

FIGURE 10.3-9 Some afferent connections of hypothalamus.

2. From Brainstem, the afferents reach to hypothalamus via the following nerve bundles:

- ***Mammillary peduncle.*** It is a bundle of fibres that connects the tegmentum of the midbrain to the mammillary body. The fibres in it carry gustatory and general visceral impulses from the spinal cord and brainstem centres (nucleus of tractus solitarius and dorsal nucelus of vagus) to the hypothalamus.
- ***Dorsal longitudinal fasciculus of Schutz*** arises from the periaqueductal grey matter and spreads over dorsal and caudal region of hypothalamus. These fibres also carry visceral impulses to hypothalamus.
- ***Medial forebrain bundle.*** As mentioned above, the medial forebrain bundle consists of both descending and ascending fibres. The ascending fibres arise from the midbrain and project to the lateral hypothalamic and preoptic nuclei. These fibres also carry visceral impulses to the hypothalamus.
- ***Catecholaminergic pathways from the locus coeruleus*** ascend monosynaptically to cerebrum and cerebellum. On way to cerebellum, they project fibres to thalamic nuclei, hypothalamus, septal area, amygdaloid body and hippocampus. These projections modify the degree of alertness. Ascending catecholaminergic fibres are distributed to supraoptic and paraventricular nuclei, and possibly regulate the output of the releasing hormones of the hypothalamus.
- ***Serotoninergic pathways*** ascending from the raphe nuclei of the pons and lower midbrain terminate in the hypothalamus, septal nuclei, amygdaloid body and neocortex. Presumably, they regulate the sleep–wake cycle, because total insomnia develops when the serotonin stores are depleted by the use of the drug reserpine.

3. From Neocortex. Corticohypothalamic fibres have been described to exist in humans that interconnect the prefrontal and posterior orbitofrontal regions with preoptic, paraventricular and ventromedial nuclei of hypothalamus. Some authors, however, deny such neocortical projections to the hypothalamus.

4. From Globus Pallidus. The pallidohypothalamic fibres from globuspallidus go to diffused area of hypothalamus.

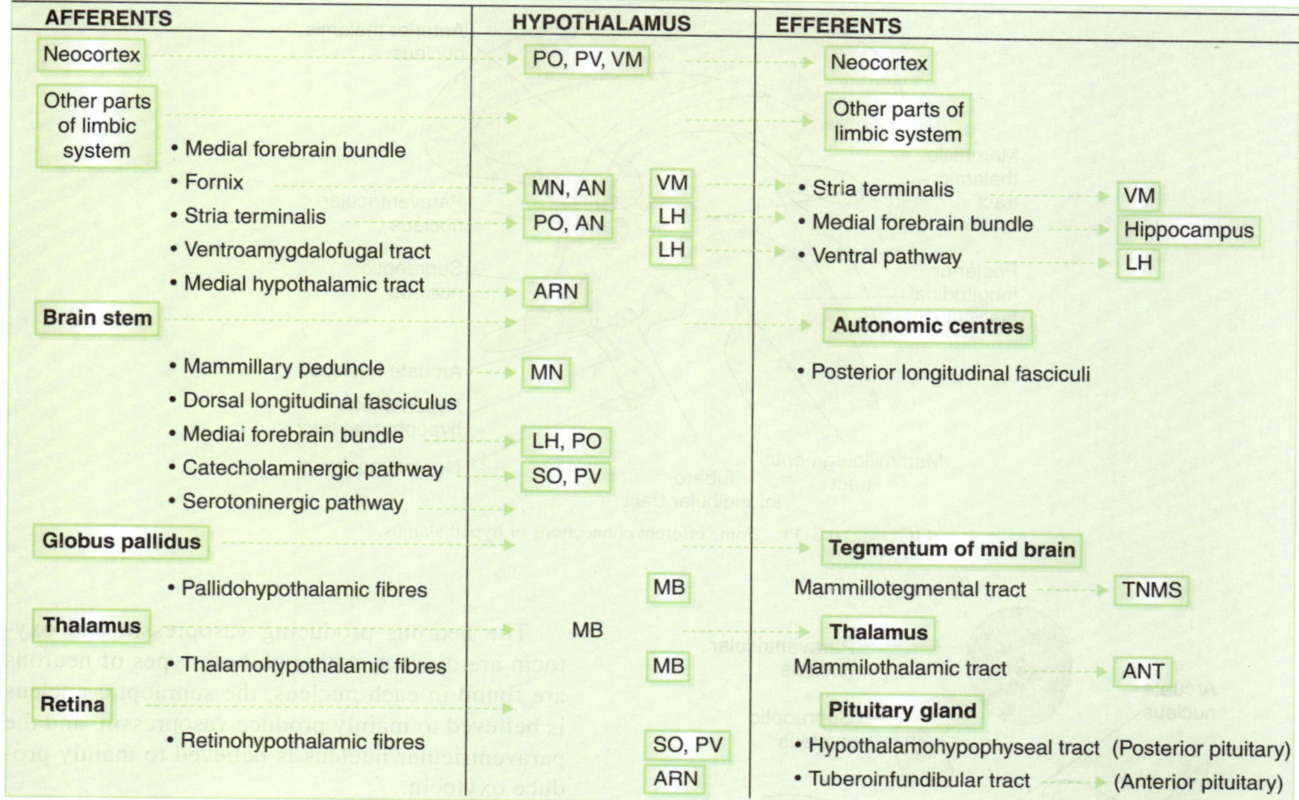

FIGURE 10.3-10 Simplified scheme of main afferent and efferent connections of hypothalamus. PO = preoptic; PV = paraventricular; VM = ventromedial; MN = medial nucleus; AN = anterior nucleus; LH = lateral hypothalamus; SO = supraoptic; ARN = arcuate nucleus; MB = mammillary body.

5. From Thalamus. The thalamohypothalamic fibres from the dorsomedial and midline nuclei of thalamus go to diffused area of hypothalamus.

6. From Retina. The retinohypothalamic fibres are projected from the ganglionic cells of the retina to suprachiasmatic nucleus of hypothalamus through the optic nerve and optic chiasma. This pathway possibly explains the influence of light on the hormonal regulation of reproductive cycle by the hypothalamus.

Efferent Connections. Efferents from the hypothalamus go to (Figs 10.3-10 and 10.3-11):

1. Autonomic Centres. *Posterior longitudinal fasciculus* runs from the autonomic nuclei in hypothalamus and goes to the autonomic nuclei in the brainstem and spinal cord. Centres in the brainstem receiving such fibres include the nucleus of *solitary tract,* the dorsal nucleus of the vagus, the nucleus ambiguus and the parabrachial nucleus. Fibres descending to spinal cord end in neurons in the intermediolateral grey column.

2. Other Parts of Limbic System. The hypothalamic nuclei provide reciprocal connections to other parts of limbic system mainly through:

- ***Stria terminalis,*** which connects ventromedial nucleus with amygdaloid nucleus.
- ***Medial forebrain bundle,*** which connects lateral hypothalamus with septal nuclei where they relay and then project to hippocampus.
- ***Ventral pathway,*** which connects lateral hypothalamus with amygdaloid nucleus.

3. Thalamus. The *mammillothalamic tract* (bundle of Vicqd'Azyr) connects the mammillary body to the anterior nucleus of thalamus which in turn is connected with gyrus linguli thus forming a component of Papez circuit of the limbic system. These fibres are responsible for those emotions and aspects of behaviour that are related to preservation of the individual and species.

4. Tegmentum of Midbrain. The mammillotegmental tract arises from the mammillary body and terminates in the ventral and dorsal tegmental nuclei of midbrain.

5. Neocortex. Fibres from hypothalamus project widely to the neocortex. They play a role in maintaining the cortical arousal.

6. Pituitary Gland. Influences from the hypothalamus are conveyed to pituitary gland (hypophysis cerebri) in two different forms:

i. *Hypothalamo–hypophyseal tract* (Fig. 10.3-12). It is composed of axons of the large neurosecretory cells of

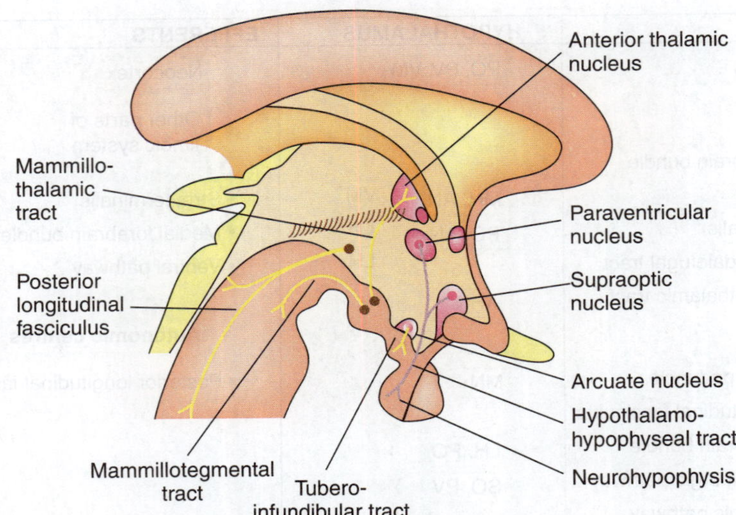

FIGURE 10.3-11 Some efferent connections of hypothalamus.

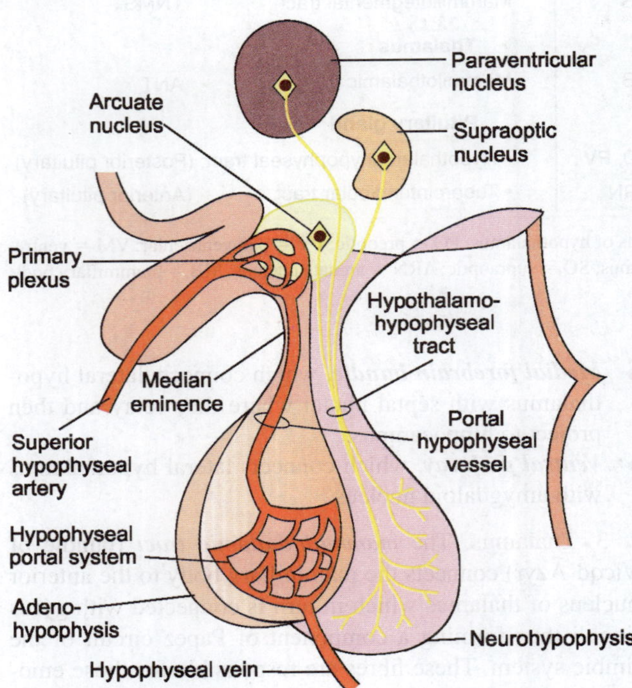

FIGURE 10.3-12 Neural and vascular connections of hypothalamus with posterior (neurohypophysis) and anterior (adenohypophysis) lobes of pituitary gland (hypophysis cerebri).

the supraoptic and paraventricular nuclei of hypothalamus. The fibres of this tract are unmyelinated and pass to posterior lobe of pituitary (neurohypophysis) through the infundibular stem of hypothalamus and form a series of dilated terminals known as *Herring bodies* which come in contact with the capillary bed of the neurohypophysis. The neurosecretory cells of supraoptic and paraventricular nuclei secrete *vasopressin* (ADH) and *oxytocin*.

The neurons producing vasopressin and oxytocin are distinct. Although both types of neurons are found in each nucleus, the supraoptic nucleus is believed to mainly produce vasopressin, and the paraventricular nucleus is believed to mainly produce oxytocin.

- Afferents from the nipple of the breast, stimulated by suckling by the baby, increase the discharge rate of neurons in the paraventricular nuclei leading to release of oxytocin from the posterior pituitary.

ii. ***Tuberoinfundibular tract*** (tubero-hypophyseal tract). It consists of fibres arising from the arcuate nuclei of the tuberal region of the hypothalamus, and extend to the median eminence and infundibular stem where the fibres come in close contact with the capillary plexus of the *hypophyseal portal system* (Fig. 10.3-12). The neurons of hypothalamic nuclei synthesize certain *releasing* or *inhibiting factors* (or hormones) which are conveyed as membrane-bound vesicles by the tuberoinfundibular tract to the hypophyseal portal vessels. These hormones are carried by the portal vessels to the anterior pituitary (adenohypophysis) where they regulate the secretion of anterior pituitary hormones.

Functions of Hypothalamus

Autonomic Functions Sherrington described the hypothalamus as the *head ganglion* of the autonomic nervous system.

- ***Anterior hypothalamus*** is the parasympathetic area. It has an excitatory effect on this system.
- ***Posterior hypothalamus*** is the sympathetic area and has an excitatory effect on it.

Autonomic functions subserved by the hypothalamus are:

i. Cardiovascular Regulation. Hypothalamus regulates the cardiovascular system through cardiovascular control centres in the reticular regions of medulla and pons.

- Stimulation of posterior and lateral nuclei of hypothalamus increases the heart rate and arterial blood pressure and produces cutaneous vasoconstriction.
- Stimulation of preoptic area decreases the heart rate and arterial blood pressure and produces cutaneous vasodilatation.

ii. Regulation of Pupil Size

- Stimulation of posterior and lateral hypothalamus causes dilatation of pupil, while
- Stimulation of anterior and medial parts of preoptic and supraoptic areas produce constriction of pupil.

iii. Regulation of Peristaltic and Secretomotor Functions of Alimentary Tract

- *Stimulation of posterior and lateral hypothalamus* diminishes the secretion and motility of gastrointestinal tract (ergotropic function).
- *Stimulation of anterior and medial hypothalamus* increases peristalsis and secretomotor functions of alimentary tract (trophotropic function).

Endocrinal Functions

i. Control of Anterior Pituitary. The hypothalamus controls the functions of anterior pituitary by secreting certain 'releasing' and 'inhibiting' hormones which reach the anterior pituitary by a neurovascular link through the tuberoinfundibular tract and hypophyseal portal vessels as described on page 680.

Hypothalamus does the following functions through the releasing hormones:

- Controls the metabolism by controlling thyroid gland (see page 703).
- Through its influence over the adrenal cortex, controls the metabolism of different foodstuffs and maintains electrolyte balance (see page 747).
- Keeps the gonads inhibited till the physical growth is complete. After physical growth is complete, this inhibition is removed so that gonads start functioning and gametes are produced (propagation of species). Gonadal hormones acting on the brain bring about physiological changes for mating of male and female.
- Controls the formation of milk by the breasts by controlling prolactin secretion (see page 882).

ii. Regulation of Posterior Pituitary Functions. The hypothalamus regulates the posterior pituitary functions through the hypothalamic–hypophyseal tract (for details see page 691).

Neural control of posterior pituitary with the secretion of antidiuretic hormone (ADH) by the supraoptic and paraventricular nuclei helps in regulation of water balance by controlling water excretion by kidneys (see page 692).

iii. Regulation of Uterine Contractility and Regulation of Milk Ejection from the Breast. Stimulation of paraventricular nucleus of hypothalamus causes its cells to secrete the hormone oxytocin. Oxytocin increases the contractility of uterus. It also contracts the myoepithelial cells that surround the alveoli of breast and cause milk ejection. At the end of pregnancy, especially large quantities of oxytocin are secreted. Oxytocin helps to promote labour contractions.

When the baby suckles the breast, signals from nipple to hypothalamus cause reflex oxytocin release which causes expulsion of milk through nipples. For details see page 884.

Regulation of Sleep–Wake Cycle The hypothalamus plays an important role in sleep–wake cycle:

- *Anterior hypothalamus* is considered a *sleep facilitatory centre,* as its stimulation leads to sleep.
- *Posterior hypothalamus* acts as *waking centre,* as its stimulation causes wakefulness.
- *Sleep is also considered to occur as a negative phenomenon,* i.e. inhibition of wakefulness centre in the posterior hypothalamus by the anterior hypothalamus also contributes to occurrence of sleep. Lesions in the posterior hypothalamus produce severe coma (for details see page 1105).

Control of Circadian Rhythm Circadian rhythm refers to rhythmic fluctuations in certain physiological parameters of the body. These are called circadian rhythms because they often show 24-h cycles (circadian around a day). Many of the rhythms are co-ordinated with each other.

Common rhythmic variations in homeostatic regulatory mechanism are:

- Rhythmic secretion of ACTH (see page 749),
- Rhythmic secretion of growth hormone (see page 683),
- Rhythmic secretion of melatonin (see page 798),
- Sleep–wake cycles (as described above),
- Body temperature rhythm (see page 1240) and
- Rhythmic gonadotropin secretion (see page 816, 854).

Basis of circadian rhythm. The circadian rhythms are *internally driven*. The *suprachiasmatic nuclei* of hypothalamus is the main site of most circadian rhythms in the body. These are believed to contain the 'biological clock', which regulates the circadian rhythm according to the 24-h light–dark cycles. The suprachiasmatic nuclei receive important inputs from:

- The eyes via retinohypothalamic fibres (page 797) and
- The lateral geniculate nuclei.

Effect of environmental factors on circadian rhythm. Environmental factors such as light–dark cycles, temperature, meal timing, etc. only provide *hints* and are required only to set a circadian rhythm cycle of 24 h. Otherwise, the circadian rhythms are internally driven and can occur in the absence of environmental factors as evidenced below:

- Normally, rats show locomotor activity in the dark (at night) and inactivity in the day time. These cycles of activity and inactivity continue even when the rats are put permanently in darkened laboratory for a few days with no exposure to light.
- The cycles of activity and inactivity can be disrupted by bilateral lesions of suprachiasmatic nuclei.

Physiological significance of circadian rhythm

- The circadian rhythm enables *homeostatic mechanism* to be utilized immediately and automatically. For example, there is a rhythm in the urinary excretion of ACTH.
- The circadian rhythms have effects on the body's resistance to various drugs. For example, difference in the sensitivity of dose of a potentially lethal drug depends markedly on the time the drug is given.

Disturbances of circadian rhythm can occur during high speed jet travel. One may travel several thousand kilometres within a few hours. As a result, the traveller's external clock (day or night) does not coincide with the internal biological clock. That is, the body may be in rest (night) phase while it is day time in the country of destination. It results in irritability, mental depression or even physical illness. The symptoms subside in a few days. The condition is called jet lag.

Regulation of Food Intake The regulation of food intake is an essential vegetative function of the hypothalamus which maintains the body weight of an individual relatively constant over a long period. To regulate the food intake, hypothalamus has two centres, namely, the *feeding centre* and *satiety centre* located in the tuberal region.

Feeding Centre. The lateral hypothalamic nucleus subserves as the feeding centre or hunger centre. When this is stimulated, in animals it creates a sensation of hunger and leads to increased food intake (hyperphagic). This causes obesity. The destruction of feeding centre leads to loss of appetite (anorexia).

Normally, the feeding centre is always active and its activity is inhibited by satiety centre after food intake.

Satiety Centre. Satiety is opposite to hunger, i.e. it is a feeling of fulfilment after food intake. The *ventromedial nucleus* of hypothalamus acts as satiety centre. Stimulation of this in animals causes sensation of food intake (fulfilment). Destruction of satiety centre leads to hyperphagia.

There are the following hypothesis regarding regulation of food intake:

- Glucostatic theory,
- Lipostatic theory,
- Gut peptide theory and
- Thermostatic theory.
- ***Glucostatic theory.*** The cells of satiety centre act as glucoreceptors (also called glucostats); therefore, the activity of satiety centre is governed by glucose utilization of these cells. The satiety centre activity decreases when the glucose supply is inadequate leading to less or no inhibition of feeding centre, resulting in its inactivation and the individual feels hungry. On the other hand, when there is adequate supply of glucose, the satiety centre cells' activity increase leading to inhibition of feeding centre and there is feeling of fulfilment.

Important Note

Polyphagia in diabetes mellitus is explained by the glucostatic theory. There is inadequate glucose utilization by glucoreceptors of satiety centre (due to deficiency of insulin).

- ***Lipostatic theory.*** The neurons of feeding centre respond to levels of fatty acids and amino acids. The body fat depots initiate either neural or hormonal signals that are related to the hypothalamus and control the food intake:
    - Leptin (Greek word, means thin) is a circulating protein hormone produced by the adipose cells. By its action on hypothalamus, it decreases release of Neuropeptide y resulting in a decrease in food intake.

Important Note

Leptin acts through leptin receptors, mainly present in brown adipose tissue and brain microvasculature. Leptin controls the size of body fat; therefore, obesity occurs due to defective leptin receptor gene (Ob gene).

- ***Gut peptide theory.*** According to the gut peptide hypothesis, presence of food in gastrointestinal tract (GIT) releases certain polypeptides and GIT hormones (like CCK,/glucagon, GRP, peptide YY and somatostatin) that act on the hypothalamus to inhibit food intake. Circulating CCK plays a major role through its receptors (CCK_A and CCK_B) present in the hypothalamus.
- ***Thermostatic theory.*** Body temperature (core) regulates food intake. Fall in body temperature increases, and rise decreases the food intake.

The balanced activity of satiety and feeding centres is responsible for the normal food intake.

Role of Neurotransmitters in Food Intake. *Food intake is increased* by the stimulation of α_2-adrenergic receptors in medial hypothalamus and centrally acting opioids.

Food intake is decreased by the stimulation of β-adrenergic and dopaminergic in lateral hypothalamus and by stimulation of serotonergic pathways.

Role of Hypothalamic Peptides. Principal hypothalamic polypeptides (neuropeptide Y, orexin-A and orexin-B, melanin-concentrating hormone (MCH) and ghrelin) increase the food intake, whereas α MSH, CART (cocaine- and amphetamine-regulated transcript) and CRH decrease food intake.

Regulation of Sexual Behaviour and Reproduction In animals, the hypothalamus plays an important role in maintaining the sexual function, especially in females. A decorticate female animal will have regular oestrous cycle provided the hypothalamus is intact.

A pathway of sex regulation has been identified as amygdala—stria terminalis–preoptic area–tuberal region of hypothalamus. The tuberal region of hypothalamus maintains the basal secretion of gonadotropin-releasing hormone (GnRH), and its connection with the preoptic area is essential for the cyclical surge of gonadotropin before ovulation.

Proof. Electrical stimulation of preoptic area produces ovulation in experimental animals and destruction of neural links between the preoptic and tuberal region prevents ovulation. For details see page 850.

Role in Emotional and Instinctual Behaviour The emotional and instinctual behaviour is mainly regulated by limbic cortex (for details see page 1083). The hypothalamus along with the limbic structures is concerned with affective nature of sensory impulses, i.e. whether the sensations are pleasant or unpleasant. These affective qualities are also called a reward and punishment. The two centres in hypothalamus involved in such a behaviour and emotional changes are called reward centre and punishment centre.

Reward and Punishment Centres

- ***Reward centre*** is located along the course of medial forebrain bundle, especially in lateral and ventromedial nucleus of hypothalamus. Electrical stimulation of this area encourages the animal to seek more of such stimulation.
- ***Punishment centre*** is located in medial hypothalamus (periventricular zone). The electrical stimulation of this area leads to pain, fear, defence, escape reactions and the other elements of punishment. The experimental animal avoids further stimulation of this area.
- ***Role of reward and punishment centres.*** Almost anything that we do is related in some way to reward and punishment. If we do something that is rewarding, we continue to do it. If we do something that is punishing, we cease to do it.

Therefore, *reward and punishment centres constitute one of the most important of all the controllers of our bodily activities, our drives, our aversions and our motivation.*

Sensory experience that is causing neither reward nor punishment is remembered hardly at all; the animal becomes habituated to such sensory experience and then ignores it. But when the sensory experience causes either reward or punishment, the cortical response becomes progressively more and more intense. Thus, *reward and punishment centres help in selecting the information that we learn.*

Rage. Strong stimulation of punishment centres produces a violent and aggressive emotional state called rage. Normally, it is kept in check by counterbalancing activity of ventromedial nuclei of hypothalamus, hippocampus, amygdala and anterior portion of limbic cortex.

Rage reaction is characterized by:

- Development of a defence posture,
- Extension of limbs,
- Lifting of tail,
- Hissing and splitting,
- Piloerection,
- Wide opening of eyes,
- Dilation of pupil and
- Severe savage attack, even on mild provocation.

Sham rage. Normally, animals and humans maintain a balance between the rage and the opposite state, i.e. calm emotion. This occurs due to reciprocal connections between hypothalamus and cerebral cortex. When the connection between cerebral cortex and hypothalamus is severed by decortication, the experimental animal exhibits an outburst of rage on mild peripheral stimulation. This is known as *sham rage,* since the emotions associated with are absent. Thus, sham rage is due to release of hypothalamus from the cortical control, and it can be abolished by lessening the caudal hypothalamus.

Role in Regulation of Body Temperature The hypothalamus acts as a principal integrating centre for heat regulation. By adjusting a balance between heat production and heat loss, it helps to maintain body temperature at 37°C. Hypothalamus accomplishes this function by two centres:

i. Heat Loss Centre. Anterior hypothalamus, especially preoptic area, acts as heat loss centre.

- Increase in the temperature of blood flowing through this area increases the activity of temperature-sensitive neurons which results in cutaneous vasodilatation and increased sweating causing more heat loss.
- Lesions of anterior hypothalamus abolish the physiological response to heat exposure.

ii. Heat Gain centre. The posterior hypothalamus acts as a heat gain centre. Electrical stimulation of posterior hypothalamus results in cutaneous vasoconstriction and shivering.

A lesion of the posterior hypothalamus abolishes not only body response to cold but to heat as well, because this area is the final integration centre for all thermoregulatory signals. Final efferent signals for heat production or heat loss emerge from the posterior hypothalamus.

Regulation of body temperature is discussed in detail in Chapter 12.4 (see page 1240).

Role in Regulation of Water Balance Hypothalamus regulates the water balance of the body by two mechanisms (Fig. 10.3-13):

- *Through thirst centre* by controlling water intake and
- *Through osmoreceptors* in supraoptic nucleus by controlling water loss.

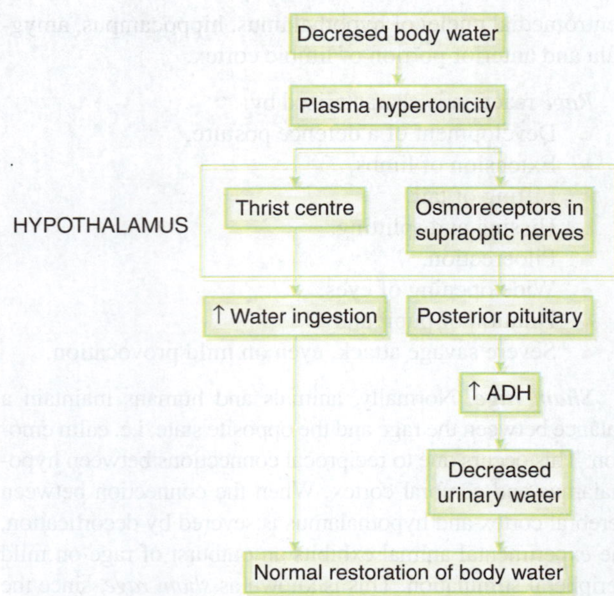

FIGURE 10.3-13 Mechanism of regulation of water balance by hypothalamus.

i. Through Thirst Centre. Thirst centre located in the lateral nucleus of hypothalamus is stimulated by plasma hypertonicity (which occurs when the water content of the body is reduced). This causes intense desire for water and the animal drinks large quantities of water. It has been observed that:

- Discrete lesions of thirst centre abolishes fluid intake and the animal dies of dehydration.
- Electrical stimulation of this area in conscious animals (through chronically implanted electrodes) causes the animal to drink water as long as the stimulation continues.
- Injection of hypertonic saline in this area induces the animal to drink large amount of water. However, injection of isotonic saline, distilled water and even hypertonic urea do not induce drinking. These experiments suggest that the thirst centre monitors plasma osmolality and is separate from the osmoreceptors involved in ADH release.

Further, it has been observed that the sensation of thirst is satisfied simply by the act of drinking, even before sufficient water is absorbed from the gastrointestinal tract to correct the plasma osmolality. Oropharyngeal and upper gastrointestinal receptors appear to be involved in this response. However, relief of the thirst sensation via these receptors is short lived. Thirst is completely satisfied only when the plasma osmolality, blood volume and arterial pressure are corrected.

- Decrease in ECF volume also stimulates thirst by an independent pathway. Haemorrhage leads to increased drinking even when there is no increase in osmolality of plasma. The effect of decreased ECF volume on thirst is mediated via the renin–angiotensin system (see page 534). Renin secreted in response to hypovolaemia results in an increase in circulating angiotensin II that acts on subfornical organ (a specialized receptor area in diencephalon) and organum vasculosum of lamina terminalis (OVLT). Both the areas are highly permeable and are part of circumventricular organs and located outside the blood–brain barrier.
- Baroreceptors located in heart and blood vessels also play role in thirst mechanism.

ii. Through Osmoreceptors in Supraoptic Nucleus. The increased plasma osmolality also stimulates osmoreceptors in supraoptic nucleus. The stimulated neurons of supraoptic nucleus in turn send impulses to posterior pituitary gland to secrete hormone ADH. This hormone reaches the kidney tubules through blood and causes increased absorption of water from the collecting ducts of the kidneys. Thus, water loss is decreased. When body has excess water, exactly opposite events occur.

iii. Other Factors Regulating Water Intake Include:

- ***Parandial drinking:*** Increased intake of liquids during eating is considered to be learned or a habit, but it may be associated with:
  - Increased plasma osmolality occurring due to absorption of food and
  - Action of certain GIT hormone

If protein intake is high, the metabolic products of protein cause osmotic diuresis; therefore, to maintain water balance, intake of water increases.

- ***Psychological factors*** also play an important role in water intake. It has been observed that in patients of psychosis or some hypothalamic disease, dehydration causes hypernatremia, but they cannot increase their water intake on stimulation of thirst centre.
- ***Local factors.*** Dryness of the pharyngeal mucus membrane causes sensation of thirst.

Dehydrated animals, such as dogs and cats, can drink lots of water to make up the water deficit but stop drinking even before the water is absorbed and plasma osmolality is still higher. This observation suggests that some gastrointestinal metering mechanism is also involved.

For further details of water balance control of body fluid osmolality, see page 543.

Applied Aspects

Lesions of Hypothalamus Lesions of hypothalamus include:

- Tumour,
- Inflammation (or encephalitis),
- Ischaemia due to vascular disorder and
- Damage due to surgical operations in this area.

Disturbances in Hypothalamic Lesions Lesions of hypothalamus may result in a variety of disturbances:

- Autonomic disturbances,
- Disturbances of body temperature regulation,
- Sleep disturbances due to lesions in mammillary body and anterior hypothalamus,
- Endocrine abnormalities, e.g. hypogonadism and hypothyroidism,
- Disturbance in sexual functions due to involvement of mid–hypothalamus,
- Disturbance of body water balance due to damage to supraoptic nuclei or infundibular stalk, characterized by excessive thirst and polyuria and
- Emotional disturbances leading to sham rage due to lesions in ventromedial and posterolateral parts.

Clinical Conditions in Hypothalamic Lesions Lesions of hypothalamus may produce any of the following specific clinical conditions:

*1. **Diabetes Insipidus*** occurs due to deficiency of ADH occurring in tumour or sham lesions of anterior hypothalamus in which supraoptic nuclei are damaged. It is characterized by excessive thirst and polydipsia.

*2. **Narcolepsy.*** It is a hypothalamic disorder with abnormal sleep pattern. Patient gets sudden attacks of unresistable desire of sleep during day time. The duration of sleep is usually short—from few seconds to about 20 min.

*3. **Cataplexy.*** Cataplexy refers to sudden emotional outburst of anger, fear or excitement associated with narcolepsy. The attack lasts for few minutes. In this, consciousness is not lost.

Chapter 10.4

Physiological Anatomy and Functions of Cerebral Cortex and White Matter of Cerebrum

CEREBRAL CORTEX

External Features

Poles, Surfaces and Borders of Cerebral Hemisphere

Cerebrum consists of two cerebral hemispheres which are separated from each other in the upper part by a median longitudinal fissure in which the *falx* cerebri (a fold of dura mater) invaginates. In the lower part, the two cerebral hemispheres are connected by the largest white commissure called *corpus callosum*.

Each cerebral hemisphere has three poles, three surfaces and three borders:

Poles. Three poles of each hemisphere are:

- Frontal pole anteriorly,
- Occipital pole posteriorly and
- Temporal pole that lies between the frontal and occipital poles, and points forwards and somewhat downwards.

Surfaces. Three surfaces of each hemisphere are:

- *Superolateral surface*,
- *Medial surface* and
- *Inferior surface* which is further subdivided into an anterior orbital part and a posterior tentorial part.

Borders. Three borders of each hemisphere are:

- *Superomedial border* which separates the superolateral surface from the medial surface.
- *Inferolateral border* intervenes between the superolateral surface and inferior surface.
- *Medial border* separates the medial surface from the inferior surface. From front to backwards, it is divided into three parts: medial orbital border, hippocampal border and medial occipital border.

Sulci and Gyri

The surface of cerebral hemisphere is covered by a thin layer (2–4 mm thick) of grey matter called the cerebral cortex. The entire surface of cerebral hemisphere is folded with intervening grooves of fissures. The folds or convolutions are called gyri, and the intervening fissures are called sulci. The cerebral cortex follows the irregular contour of the sulci and gyri of the hemisphere and extends into depth of the sulci. As a result of the folding of the cerebral surface, the cerebral cortex acquires a much larger surface area (about 2200 cm^2) than the size of the hemisphere would otherwise alone.

Lobes of Cerebral Hemisphere

Each cerebral hemisphere is divided into four lobes. The boundaries separating one lobe from the other on the

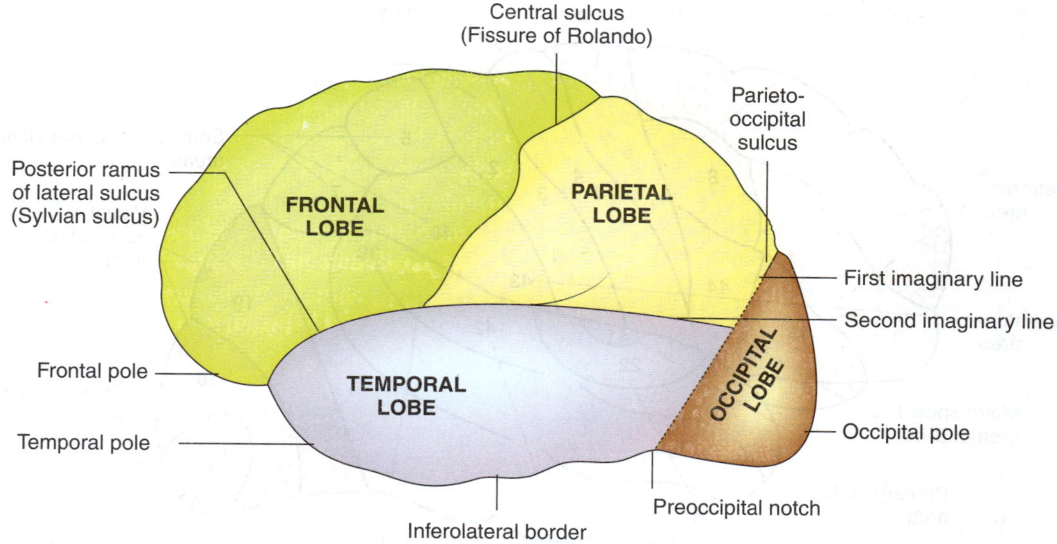

FIGURE 10.4-1 Superolateral surface of cerebral hemisphere to show different lobes, poles and borders.

superolateral surface of cerebral hemisphere are formed by three prominent sulci and two imaginary lines (Fig. 10.4-1).

Sulci, which separate the lobes, are:

- Central sulcus or fissure of Rolando,
- Posterior ramus of lateral or sylvian sulcus and
- Parieto-occipital sulcus.

Imaginary lines which complete the subdivisions of the hemisphere into lobes are:

- *First imaginary line* connects the upper end of parieto-occipital sulcus to the parieto-occipital notch, and
- *Second imaginary line* is a backward continuation of the posterior ramus of lateral sulcus to meet the first imaginary line.

The Four Lobes of each cerebral hemisphere as seen on superolateral surface (Fig. 10.4-1) are:

- ***Frontal lobe.*** It lies in front of the central sulcus and above the posterior ramus of lateral sulcus. It is concerned with motor functions.
- ***Parietal lobe.*** It lies between the central sulcus and parieto-occipital sulcus and upper part of first imaginary line. Below, it is separated from the temporal lobe by the posterior ramus of lateral sulcus and its continuation (the second imaginary line). It is concerned with sensory functions.
- ***Temporal lobe.*** It lies below the posterior ramus of lateral sulcus and its continuation the second imaginary line. Behind, it is separated from the occipital lobe by the lower part of the first imaginary line. It is concerned with hearing.
- ***Occipital lobe.*** It lies behind the parieto-occipital sulcus and its continuation the first imaginary line. It is concerned with vision.

Cortical Functional Areas

On the basis of number and thickness of cortical laminae and cell type (cytoarchitecture), Brodmann divided the cortex into 47 areas.

The concepts regarding the different functional areas of cerebral cortex have undergone considerable modifications in recent years. It has been seen that motor and sensory functions are strictly not separated. Many motor fibres arise outside the motor cortex from areas which are regarded as partly sensory. However, in clinical work, reference continues to be made to classical subdivisions.

Classically, cortical functional areas are subdivided into (Fig. 10.4-2):

- ***Motor areas*** include:
  - Primary motor area (Brodmann's area 4),
  - Premotor area (area 6),
  - Frontal eye field (area 8) and
  - Supplementary motor area.
- ***Sensory areas*** include:
  - Primary somaesthetic areas (areas 3, 1 and 2),
  - Secondary (supplementary) somaesthetic area and
  - Somaesthetic association areas (areas 5, 7 and higher association area 40).
- ***Auditory areas*** include:
  - Primary auditory area (area 41) or auditory area I,
  - Auditory association area (area 42) or auditory area II and
  - Higher auditory association area (area 22).
- ***Visual areas*** include:
  - Primary visual area (area 17) or visuostriate area of visual area I,
  - Visual association area 18 (peristriate area) and
  - Visual association area 19 (parastriate area).

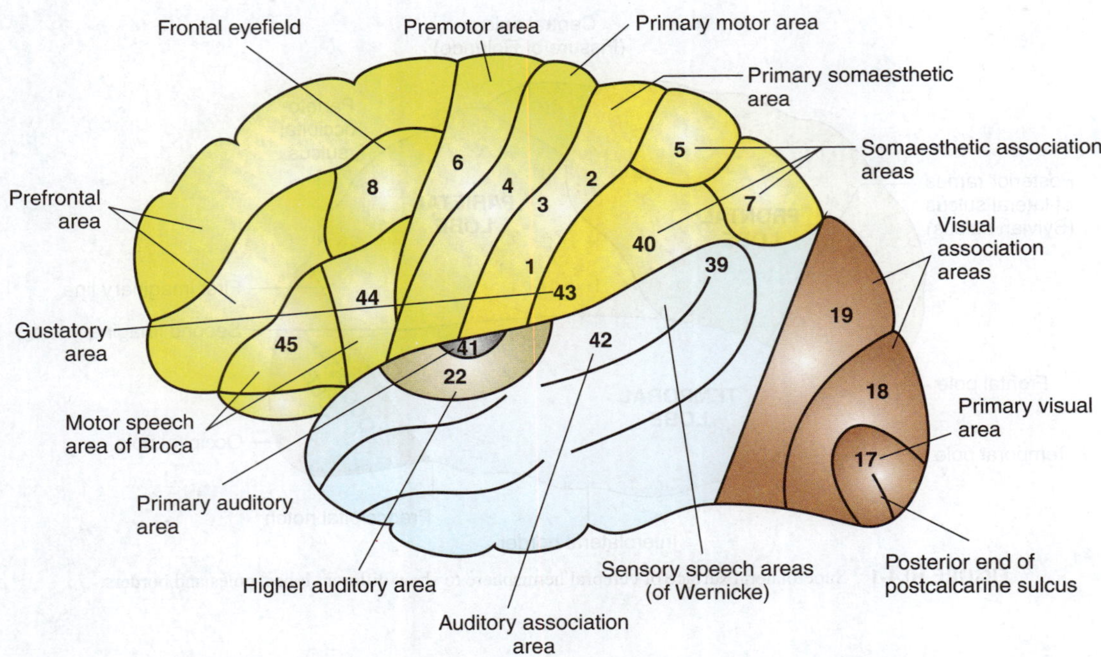

FIGURE 10.4-2 Different areas on the lateral surface of the human cerebral cortex.

- ***Speech areas*** include:
  - *Motor speech* area comprises:
    - Anterior area (Broca's area) or areas 44, 45 and
    - Superior area.
  - *Sensory speech areas* comprise:
    - Area 39 (or reading centre),
    - Area 40 and
    - Area 22 (Wernicke's area).
- ***Smell area*** is:
  - Area 28.
- ***Gustatory area*** is:
  - Area 43.

Note. The different cortical functional areas are described along with the description of various lobes of cerebral cortex.

Phylogenetical Divisions of Cerebral Cortex

The cerebral cortex, also known as pallium, is divided phylogenetically into three parts: allocortex, mesocortex and neocortex.

1. Allocortex or old cortex forms about 10% of the entire cortex and can be further subdivided into:

- ***Archipallium*** (ancient cortex), which includes hippocampus and dentate gyrus.
- ***Paleopallium*** (old cortex) comprises uncus and part of parahippocampal gyrus, which belong to the piriform area of olfactory cortex.

Since most of the allocortex is located around the peripheral margin of the diencephalon in the form of a ring, it is also called *limbic cortex*. This ring of limbic cortex functions as a two-way communication linkage between neocortex and lower limbic structures. Along with the thalamus and hypothalamus, the limbic cortex is concerned with emotional and instinctive behaviour.

2. Mesocortex, which is the transitional zone between allocortex and neocortex, comprises the cingulate gyrus, part of parahippocampal gyrus and *subiculum*.

3. Neocortex, also called an isocortex, comprises rest of 90% of the cerebral cortex in human brain. The actual extent of neocortex has increased with the evolution of mammals. The comparative ratio of allocortex and neocortex in rat, cat, monkey and humans is shown in Fig. 10.4-3.

Histological Structure of Cerebral Cortex

Histologically, the allocortex is composed of three distinctive layers, while the neocortex is composed of six layers named I to VI from outside to inside (Fig. 10.4-4).

Histologically, the cerebral cortex is composed of nerve cells and fibres. Three types of cells may be identified in the cerebral cortex:

1. Pyramidal Cells. About two-third of all cortical neurons are pyramidal cells. These cells have triangular cell bodies, with the apex generally directed towards the surface of cortex. Axon arises from the base of the cell and a large dendrite arises from the apex, and other dendrites arise from the basal angles. The processes of pyramidal cells extend vertically through the entire thickness of cortex. These cells are present in layer II, III and V of the neocortex.

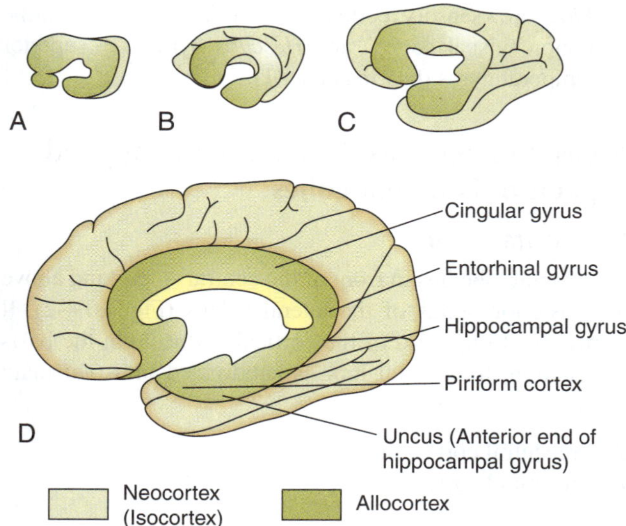

FIGURE 10.4-3 Relative extent of allocortex and neocortex in different mammals: **A,** rat; **B,** cat; **C,** monkey; and **D** human.

2. Stellate or Granule Cells. These cells form about one-third of the total neurons. These cells have small cell bodies from where the dendrites arise in all directions. Layer IV is packed with such cells and is best developed in primary sensory cortex.

3. Fusiform Cells. These are comparatively few in number. Such cells have spindle-shaped cell bodies, and are present in layer VI.

Laminae of Neocortex The six laminae of neocortex numbered I to VI are (Fig. 10.4-4):

I. Molecular or Plexiform Layer. It mainly consists of transverse nerve fibres dispersed with occasional horizontal cells.

- The transverse fibres are derived from the apical dendrites of pyramidal cells, axons of stellate and *Martinotti* cells (pyramidal cells with short axon) of deeper layer which ascend and ramify horizontally in this layer.
- The horizontal cells of Cajal are small pear-shaped or fusiform.

II. External Granular Layer. It contains numerous stellate or granule cells, and a lesser number of small pyramidal cells. It is traversed by afferent and efferent projection fibres. Dendrites of cells of this layer pass into the molecular layer. The axons end in the deeper layer. Some axons enter the white substance of the hemisphere.

III. Outer Pyramidal Layer. It consists mainly of pyramidal neurons and some stellate and basket cells. The pyramidal cells are of two types: the *small cells* lie in the superficial zone and *medium-sized* cells occupy the deeper zone.

IV. Internal Granular Layer. This layer consists of densely packed stellate cells. The inner zone of this layer is traversed by a prominent aggregation of transversely running fibres called external band of Baillarger.

V. Inner Pyramidal (Ganglionic) Layer. This layer consists of large pyramidal cells. It is specially developed in

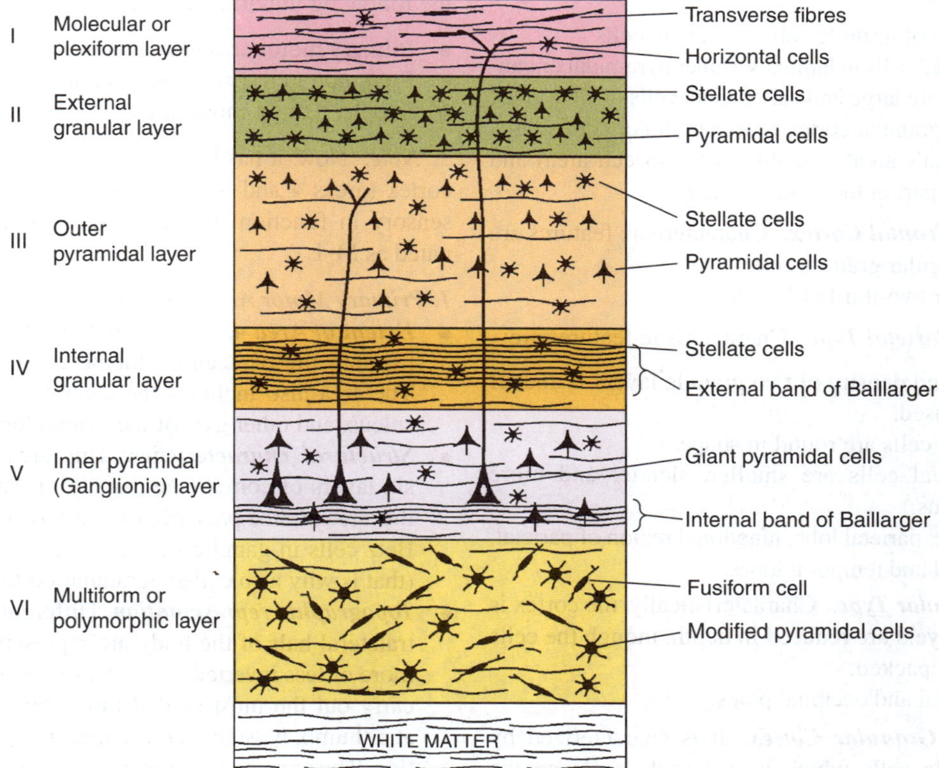

FIGURE 10.4-4 Histological structure of neocortex.

the motor cortex, where these cells are called giant cells or Betz cells. This layer is traversed by a prominent aggregation of transversely running fibres called *internal band of Baillarger.*

VI. Polymorphous or Multiform Layer. This layer contains neurons of various sizes and shapes, many of which are probably modified pyramidal cells. Many spindle-shaped cells called fusiform cells are present in this layer. This layer also contains cells of Martinotti, whose axons project vertically towards the outer surface of the cortex to ramify in the molecular layer. This layer merges with the white matter of the cerebral cortex.

Important Notes

- Most of afferent fibres from the specific nuclei of thalamus make synapses in laminae I to IV.
- Afferent projections from the nonspecific thalamic nuclei and from ascending reticular system terminate in all laminae of cortex.
- Laminae II and IV are concerned with sensorial modalities.
- Laminae III to V are meant for somatomotor or visceromotor activities.
- Laminae I and VI are engaged for integration of association of sensorimotor behaviour.

Types of Neocortex Depending upon the local variations in the histological layers, the neocortex can be divided into five types:

- ***Type 1 or Agranular Cortex.*** It is characterized by:
  - Absence of granule cells or stellate cells.
  - Pyramidal cells in lamina V (inner pyramidal or ganglionic) are large and called giant cells or Betz cells.

    Sites. Agranular cortex is seen in motor cortex (area 4), Broca's area (area 44, motor speech area) and anterior part of the island of Reil.
- ***Type 2 or Frontal Cortex.*** Characteristic features are presence of triangular granule cells.

  Sites. Anterior two-third of frontal lobe.
- ***Type 3 or Parietal Type.*** Characteristic features are:
  - Depth and density of two granule layers II and III is increased.
  - Granule cells are round in shape.
  - Pyramidal cells are smaller, slender and more numerous.

    Sites are: parietal lobe, junctional region of parietal, occipital and temporal lobes.
- ***Type 4 or Polar Type.*** Characteristically, the cortex is narrow and all layers are reduced in depth, though the cells are more densely packed.

  Sites are frontal and occipital poles.
- ***Type 5 or Granular Cortex.*** It is characterized by excess of granule cells which have largely replaced the pyramidal cells in layers III and V.

  Sites are: sensory cortex (postcentral gyrus), calcarine region (visual cortex) and *Heschl's* gyrus, i.e. superior temporal gyrus (hearing area 41).

Areas, Connections, Functions and Applied Aspects of Different Lobes

[A] Frontal Lobe

The frontal lobe lies in front of the central sulcus and above the posterior ramus of the lateral sulcus (Fig. 10.4-2). It forms about one-third of the cortical surface. On the basis of function, the frontal lobe is subdivided into two main areas:

- Precentral cortex and
- Prefrontal cortex.

I. Precentral Cortex

Precentral cortex refers to posterior part of the frontal lobe that includes lip of central sulcus, precentral gyrus and posterior part of superior, middle and inferior frontal gyri. Stimulation of different points in this area causes activity of discrete skeletal muscles. Therefore, precentral cortex is also called excitomotor area of cortex. Stimulation of motor area also causes some sensory perception.

Therefore, nowadays the motor cortex and sensory cortex are together known as *sensorimotor cortex.*

Areas in Precentral Cortex The precentral cortex includes the following important areas:

- Primary motor area (Brodmann's area 4),
- Premotor area (Brodmann's areas 6, 8, 44 and 45) and
- Supplementary motor area.

Note. Now, it has been suggested that the sensorimotor cortex (areas 4 and 6) is primarily motor and secondarily sensory in function; hence, these areas have been designated as M-1.

1. Primary Motor Area (area 4)

- ***Extent of Area 4.*** It lies in the precentral gyrus extending into the paracentral lobule on the medial surface. The area also includes the anterior wall of the central sulcus, and other gyri of the frontal lobe (Fig. 10.4-5).
- ***Structural characteristics.*** This area contains all the six layers of cortex (see page 964). Special features of this area are the presence of giant pyramidal cells called Betz cells in ganglionic layer and a thin granular layer (that is why also called agranular cortex).
- ***Topographic representation.*** Different parts of the contralateral half of the body are represented separately in more or less inverted order. Those parts of the body that carry out the most skilled movements, e.g. the fingers and thumb, have the largest areas of cortical representation. The areas for tongue, jaw and facial movements lie in the inferior part of the motor cortex; those for the arm,

trunk and leg are arranged in sequence in the motor area, which extends to the vertex, and on to the medial surface of the cerebral hemisphere. The parts in the paracentral lobule are for the foot and perineum. Thus, the body is represented upside down (however, the face is not represented in inverted manner) (Fig. 10.4-6A).

- ***Electrical stimulation of this area reveals***:
  - Above-described motor homunculus (topographical representation).
  - Motor cortex is organized in terms of movements rather than individual muscles (i.e. stimulation reveals discrete isolated movements on the opposite side of the body).
  - Stimulation of the points representing upper parts of the face, pharynx and the vocal cords produces bilateral responses.
- ***Functions.*** From the above, it is clear that this area is centre for volition, i.e. it is concerned with initiation of voluntary movements of the contralateral half of the body and initiation of speech.
- ***Area 45,*** also called as suppressor area, forms a narrow strip anterior to area 4. It inhibits movements initiated by area 4.

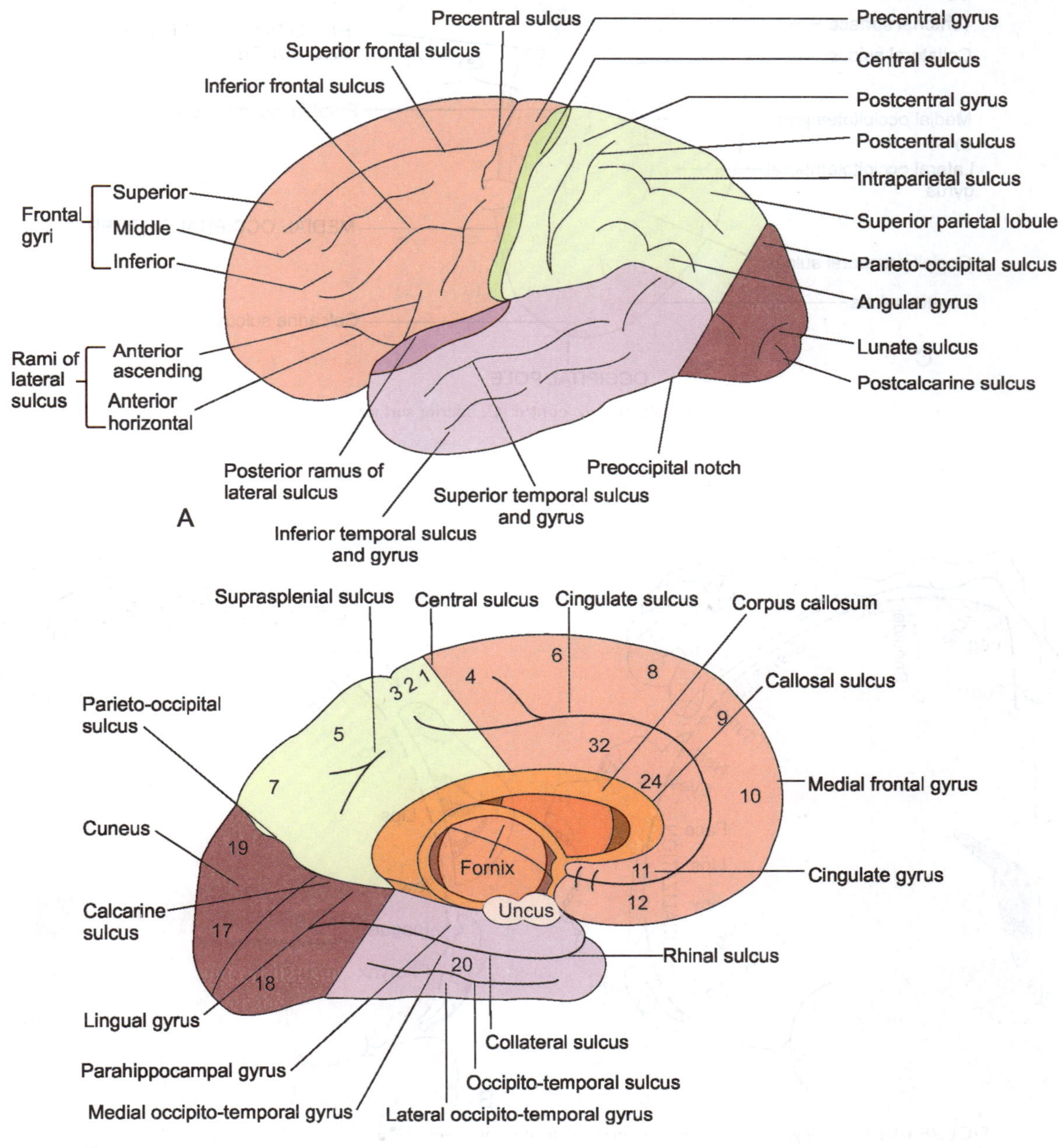

FIGURE 10.4-5 Left cerebral hemisphere showing lobes, sulci and gyri: **A,** superolateral surface; **B,** medial surface; and

Continued

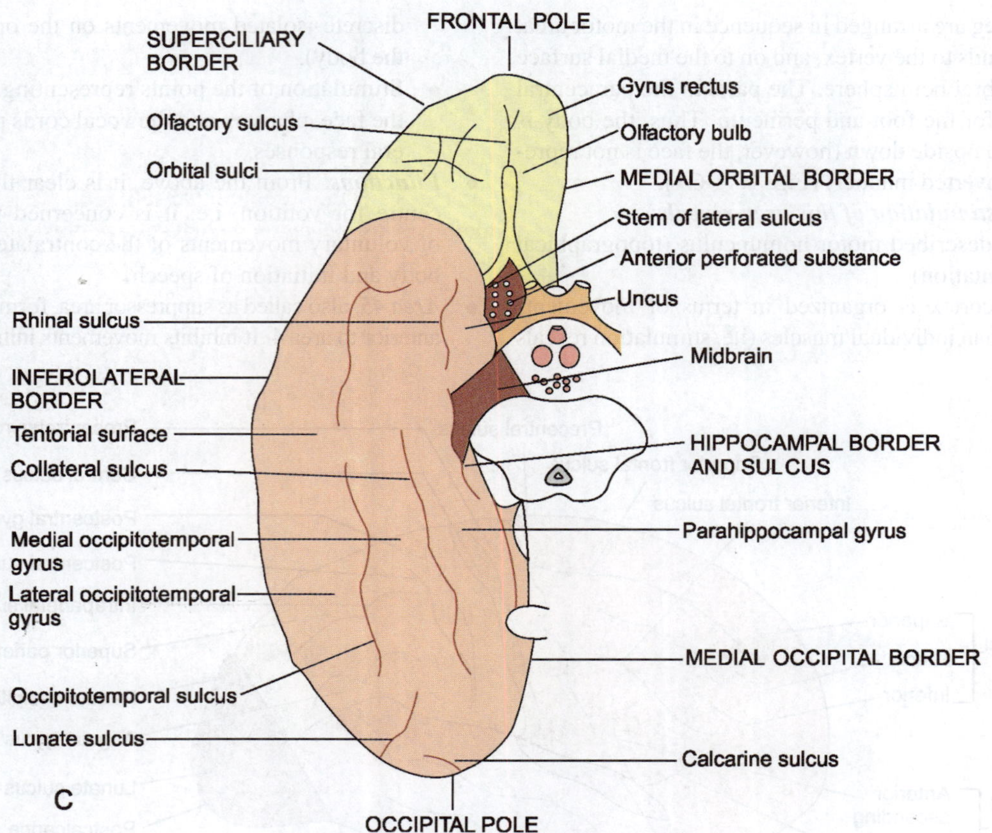

FIGURE 10.4-5, cont'd C, inferior surface.

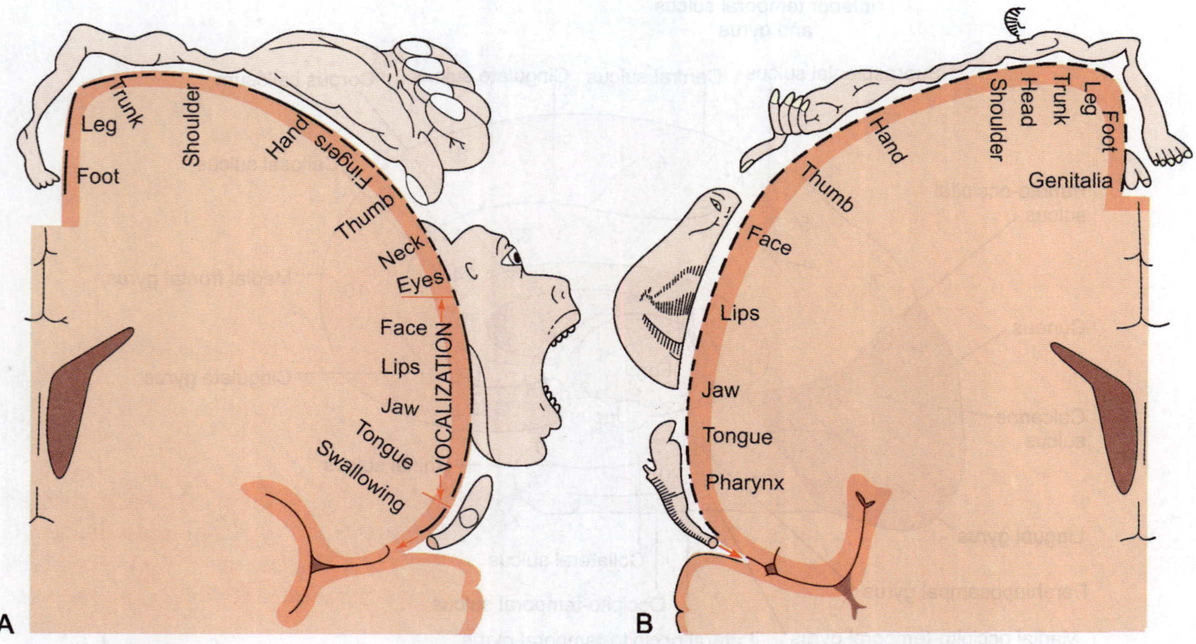

FIGURE 10.4-6 Topographical representation (homunculus) of motor (A) and sensory (B) areas in cerebral cortex.

2. Premotor Area. Premotor area lies anterior to the primary motor area and includes Brodmann's areas 6, 8, 44 and 45.

Structurally, it is similar to primary motor cortex except for the absence of giant pyramidal cells in ganglionic layer.

Area 6. ***Location.*** It abuts on the primary motor cortex area both above and behind, and thereby includes the posterior parts of the superior, middle and inferior frontal gyri. This area is divided into two parts, upper 6a and lower 6b. Cells from this area contribute fibres to pyramidal tracts.

- ***Topographical organization*** of this area is roughly the same as that of primary motor cortex.
- *Functions.* Area 6 co-ordinates the voluntary action of area 4 and extrapyramidal system and is, therefore, involved in the integration of voluntary movements. Thus, the skilled movements are accurate and smooth.
- ***Electrical stimulation*** of area 6a in humans causes same effects as that of stimulation of area 4. However, the strength of stimulus must be stronger while stimulating area 6.
  - Stimulation of area 6a causes generalized pattern of movements like rotation of head, eyes and trunk towards the opposite side.
  - Stimulation of area 6b produces rhythmic, complex co-ordinated movements involving the muscles of face, buccal cavity, larynx and pharynx.
- ***Lesions of area 6*** in monkeys lead to loss of skilled movements. Recovery may occur, but the movements become awkward. This also produces a grasping reflex. Lesions involving area 6 along with area 4 produce severe symptoms of hemiplegia with spastic paralysis.

Area 8. It is also called frontal eye field.

- ***Location.*** It lies anterior to area 6.
- ***Afferents*** to this area come from the occipital lobe and dorsomedial nucleus of thalamus.
- ***Efferents*** from area 8 go to nuclei of third, fourth and sixth cranial nerves.
- ***Function.*** It is concerned with control of eye movements.
- ***Electrical stimulation*** of area 8 causes conjugate movements of eyeballs to the opposite side, opening and closure of eyelids, pupillary dilation and lacrimation.
- ***Lesions*** of this area turn the eyes towards the affected side. Conjugate movements of the eyes are absent. Pupil and eyelids are not affected.

Areas 44 and 45 or Broca's motor speech area.

- ***Location.*** It is special region of premotor cortex situated in inferior frontal gyrus. Area 44 is situated in pars triangularis and 45 in pars opercularis of the gyrus.
- ***Functions.*** This area, especially in dominated hemisphere (left hemisphere in right handed person), is concerned with movements of those structures which are responsible for the production of voice and articulation of speech, that is, it causes activation of vocal cords, simultaneously with movements of mouth and tongue during speech.
- ***Lesions of this area*** cause motor aphasia, i.e. inability to speak the word, though vocalization is possible.

3. Supplementary Motor Area ***Location.*** Supplementary motor area is located in medial surface of frontal lobe rostral to primary motor area (Fig. 10.4-5).

Topographical organization. In this area, components of the upper body are located dorsal to those of the lower body.

Functions. This area in association with premotor area provides attitudinal movements, fixation movement of different segments of the body and positional movements of head and eyes.

Connections of Precentral Cortex

Afferents to Precentral Cortex come from following sources:

1. ***Fibres from adjacent regions*** include those from:
   - Somatic sensory area of parietal cortex,
   - Adjacent areas of frontal cortex anterior to motor cortex and
   - Subcortical fibres from auditory and visual cortices.
2. ***From opposite hemisphere.*** Subcortical fibres passing through corpus callosum connect corresponding areas of cortices in the two sides of brain.
3. ***Fibres from thalamus*** include:
   - Tracts from ventrolateral and ventroanterior nuclei of thalamus which in turn receive from cerebellum and basal ganglia. They cause co-ordination between functions of motor cortex, basal ganglia and cerebellum.
   - Fibres from intralaminar nuclei of thalamus to cause general level of excitability of motor cortex.

Efferents from Precentral Cortex include:

1. ***Corticospinal tract*** (pyramidal tract) is the most important tract through which the motor cortex controls the activity of the anterior horn cells in the spinal cord. About 30% of fibres arise from primary motor area, 30% from premotor and supplementary motor areas and 40% from the somatic sensory area of parietal lobe.
2. ***Collaterals from pyramidal tracts*** and large number of fibres from motor cortex go to deeper regions of cerebrum and brain stem as follows:
   - ***Adjacent areas of cortex.*** Axons of Betz cells send collaterals to adjacent areas of cortex. These collaterals inhibit adjacent areas (lateral inhibition) and sharpen the boundaries of excitatory signals.
   - ***Basal ganglia.*** Large number of fibres go to caudate nucleus and putamen from where additional pathway goes to brainstem.

- ***Red nucelus.*** Some fibres go to red nuclei and then to spinal cord through rubrospinal tracts.
- ***Reticular substance.*** Some fibres go to reticular substance of brainstem, from where fibres pass to spinal cord through reticulospinal tract.
- ***Vestibular nuclei.*** Some fibres go to vestibular nuclei, from where through the vestibulospinal tract they reach the spinal cord.
- ***Pontine nuclei.*** Large number of fibres synapse in pontine nuclei and pass to the cerebellum (pontocerebellar fibres).
- ***Inferior olivary nuclei.*** Collaterals also go to inferior olivary nuclei and then to cerebellum through olivocerebellar tract.

II. Prefrontal Cortex

Location. Prefrontal cortex, also called prefrontal lobe or orbitofrontal cortex, is the anterior part of frontal lobe lying anterior to areas 8 and 44 (Fig. 10.4-5).

Major areas. Prefrontal cortex has different Brodmann's areas such as 9–14, 23, 24, 29, 32 and 44–47 located as:

- ***Areas 9–12*** lie in superior frontal gyrus and also extend on to the adjacent medial surface of the hemisphere.
- ***Area 13*** is located in the orbital part of the inferior surface of the frontal lobe.
- ***Area 24*** is situated in the precallosal part of the cingulate gyrus on medial surface.
- ***Area 32*** lies in the cingulate gyrus.
- ***Areas 44–47*** lie in the inferior frontal gyrus.

Connections of prefrontal cortex shown in Fig. 10.4-7 are:

Afferents to prefrontal cortex come from:

i. *Dorsomedial nucleus of thalamus* project on to areas 9–12 on the lateral and adjacent medial surface and areas 44–47 in the inferior frontal gyrus. Since the dorsomedial nucleus of thalamus in turn receives afferents from the posterior hypothalamus, therefore, the impulses which reach the prefrontal lobe via the medial nucleus represent a resultant of hypothalamic and thalamic activity.

ii. *Anterior nuclei of thalamus* project on to cingulate gyrus (areas 23, 24, 29 and 32). Since the anterior nucleus of thalamus receives afferents from the mammillary bodies of the hypothalamus, they in turn receive the afferents from the hippocampus via the fornix. The hippocampus is thus ultimately projected to inhibitory area 24.

The prefrontal lobe thus forms a closed circuit connection with the thalamus called *Papez circuit* (Fig. 10.10-4). This circuit is responsible for resting EEG and plays an important role in the genesis of emotions.

Efferents from prefrontal cortex go to:

i. *Thalamus.* Fibres from areas 9 and 10 go to ventral and medial thalamic nuclei.

ii. *Tegmental reticular formation.* Fibres from areas 9 and 10 also go to reticular formation in the tegmentum.

iii. *Pontine nuclei.* Fibres from area 10 pass to the pontine nuclei as frontopontine tract and thence to the cerebellum.

iv. *Caudate nucleus.* The inhibitory areas 8 and 2, 4, 5 discharge to the caudate nucleus.

v. *Mammillary bodies.* Fibres from area 13, the hippocampus, uncus and amygdala project via the fornix to the mammillary bodies of the hypothalamus.

Functions of Prefrontal Cortex

1. Centre for Planned Actions. Prefrontal association areas in close association with motor cortex plan complex patterns and sequence of motor movements.

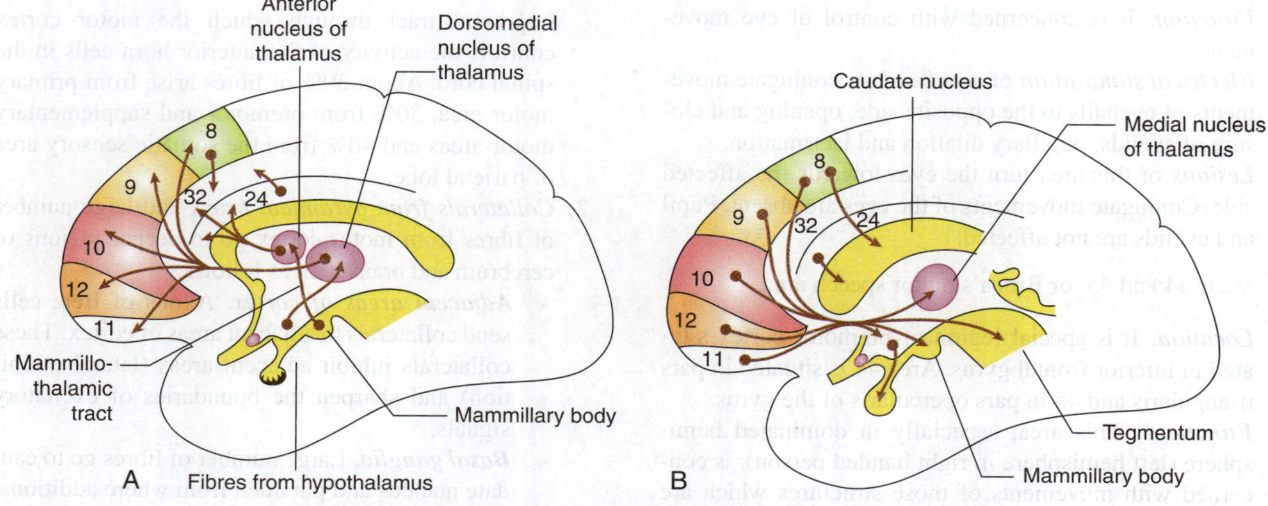

FIGURE 10.4-7 Connections of prefrontal lobe: **A**, afferents; and **B**, efferents.

2. Centre for Higher Functions. This forms the centre for higher functions like emotions, learning, memory and social behaviour. It is responsible for various autonomic changes during emotional conditions because of its connections to hypothalamus and brainstem.

3. Seat of Intelligence. Short-term memories are registered in prefrontal cortex. It can keep track of many bits of information and also has ability to recall this information bit by bit for subsequent thoughts. It is therefore called seat of intelligence or an organ of mind.

4. Control of Intellectual Activities. The prefrontal cortex has the following intellectual abilities:

- To prognosticate.
- To plan the future.
- It allows the person to concentrate on central theme of thought. It helps in depth and abstractness of thought and thereby in elaboration of thought.
- It allows to delay action in response to incoming sensory signals so that sensory information can be weighed until the best response is obtained.
- It allows to consider the consequence of motor actions before their performance.
- It plays role in solution of complicated mathematical, legal and philosophical problems.
- It allows to correct avenues of information in diagnosis of rare diseases.
- It allows to control one's activity according to the moral laws.

Frontal Lobe: Applied Aspects

Frontal Lobe Syndrome Frontal lobe syndrome refers to symptom complex occurring due to injury or ablation of prefrontal cortex.

Prefrontal leucotomy, i.e. cutting the connection between the thalamus and prefrontal lobe, also results in frontal lobe syndrome. Bilateral prefrontal lobectomy (extirpation) also results in similar condition. In the past, these operations were performed in patients with severe mental illness. However, nowadays, due to availability of tranquilizers and other drugs (which can control mental illness), these operations are not conducted because of the associated complications.

Characteristic features of frontal lobe syndrome are:

- *Flight of ideas,* which results in difficulty in planning.
- *Emotional instability,* there occurs lack of restraint leading to hostility, aggressiveness and restlessness.
- *Euphoria,* i.e. a false sense of wellbeing and failure to realize or indifference to seriousness of other's feelings or emotions.
- *Impairment of memory* occurs for recent memory only. The memory of remote events is not lost.
- *Loss of moral and social sense* is common and there is loss of love for family.
- *Lack of attention and power of concentration* associated with restlessness is a common feature.
- *Lack of initiative following marked depression* of intellectual activity leads to reduced mental drive.
- *Functional abnormalities* may occur in the form of:
  - Hyperphagia, i.e. increased appetite,
  - Loss of control over urinary or rectal sphincters,
  - Disturbances in orientation and
  - Slight tremor.

[B] Parietal Lobe

Parietal lobe (Fig. 10.4-1) lies between the central sulcus and parieto-occipital sulcus, and upper part of first imaginary line. Below, it is separated from the temporal lobe by the posterior ramus of lateral sulcus and in continuation of it the second imaginary line.

Areas of Parietal Lobe

Functionally, parietal lobe can be divided into three parts:

- Primary sensory area (which corresponds to Brodmann's areas 3, 1 and 2),
- Secondary sensory area and
- Sensory association areas (Brodmann's areas 5 and 7).

Note. Since stimulation of sensory area also produces some motor response and stimulation of motor area also causes some sensory perception, therefore, nowadays the sensory and motor cortex is combinedly called somatosensory cortex, and:

- Primary sensory area (areas 3, 1 and 2) is called primary somatosensory (sensorimotor) area or first somatosensory area (SI) and
- Secondary sensory is called second somatic sensory area (SII).

Primary Sensory Area (First Somatic Sensory Area)

Location. The first somatic sensory area (SI) occupies the posterior wall of the central sulcus, the postcentral gyrus and the postcentral part of the paracentral lobule (Fig. 10.4-5).

Major areas. It includes Brodmann's areas 3, 1 and 2.

Structurally, the primary sensory cortex is granular cortex which is densely packed with stellate cells, with a few small and medium-sized pyramidal cells.

Topographical organization. The primary sensory cortex receives sensory inputs from the opposite half of the body. The representation of the body within this area is similar to that already noted in primary motor cortex (page 968, Fig. 10.4-6B).

The sensations derived from the skin are appreciated in the anterior part of the area and proprioceptive sensations in the posterior part of the area.

Electrical stimulation of primary sensory area (SI) produces vague sensations like numbness and tingling.

Lesions. If lesions occur only in the sensory cortex without involvement of thalamus, the sensations are perceived but the discriminative functions are lost. If thalamus is also affected by lesion, there occurs loss of sensations in the opposite side of the body.

Secondary Sensory Area

Location. Secondary sensory area, also called second somatic sensory area (SII), is situated in postcentral gyrus below the area of face of first somatic sensory area. Most of it is buried in the superior wall of the sylvian fissure (lateral cerebral sulcus).

- *Topographical representation*. The secondary sensory (SII) area receives sensory impulses from primary sensory area (SI) as well as from thalamus directly. Like SI, the SII area also manifests a dermatomal (point-to-point) sequence of representation (although there is more overlap). Thus, the body is represented twice in the somatic sensory cortex, i.e. in area SI as well as in area SII.
- Neurons in the anterior part of area SII respond to touch whereas neurons in the posterior part can be excited by touch, auditory, visual and nociceptive stimuli.

Lesions of SII produce deficits in discrimination power, whereas sensory processing in SI is not affected.

Sensory Association Areas The sensory association areas include areas 5 and 7. Area 40 is a higher association area.

Area 5. It lies posterior to area SI in the parietal lobe and contains neurons which react to passive or active rotation of a joint or joints. Few neurons respond to tactile stimuli like the other areas in SI and SII; area 5 also displays a columnar organization (point-to-point representation).

Area 7. It is located in superior parietal lobule deep into the intraparietal sulcus extending close up to the occipital lobe. This area is concerned with more elaborate process of discrimination between the stimuli.

Area 40. This is higher association area, located in supramarginal gyrus, and is concerned with stereognosis, i.e. recognition of common objects placed in the hand without looking at them. A lesion affecting area 40 produces tactile agnosia (astereognosis and tactile aphasia).

Connections of Parietal Lobe

Afferent Connections of Somatosensory Area

First somatic sensory area (SI) receives afferent projections from posteromedial (VPM) and posterolateral (VPL) parts of the ventral posterior nucleus of thalamus, which convey exteroceptive and proprioceptive impulses from the contralateral side but from both sides of face.

- *Area 3* neurons respond to light touch and receive a dense input from the thalamus.
- *Areas 1 and 2* neurons respond to deep stimuli such as pressure and joint movements and receive few thalamic fibres.
- None of the neurons of primary sensory cortex are influenced by nociceptive (painful) stimuli.
- Sensory area in the paracentral lobule receives the sense of distension from the bladder and rectum.
- The lower part of postcentral gyrus acts as a taste receptive centre.

Second somatic sensory area (SII) receives afferent projection from area SI as well as directly from the thalamus.

Sensory association area receives impulses from area SI and SII.

Efferents from Somatosensory Area

- Pyramidal cells of the sensory area contribute fibres to corticospinal, corticobulbar and corticonuclear tracts. These fibres, presumably modulate the sensory input at the root entry zone of posterior grey column of the spinal cord, and nuclei gracilis and cuneatus of the lower medulla.
- All somatosensory areas (particularly SI) send fibres to the caudate nucleus and putamen.
- Area SI also sends efferent fibres:
  - Back to its own thalamic projection nuclei and
  - To the tectum, pons and cerebellum.

Association Fibres from the Sensory Cortex

- Through association fibres the sensory cortex is connected with other cortical areas.
- Association fibres interlinking the areas SI, SII, area 5 and area 4 are involved in somatic sensations (Fig. 10.4-8).

Commissural Fibres from the Sensory Cortex

- Commissural fibres are mostly axons of pyramidal cells of layer III and connect the corresponding somatosensory areas with those of the opposite hemisphere.
- Area SI projects to the contralateral areas SI and SII.
- Area SII projects only to area SII of the opposite hemisphere.

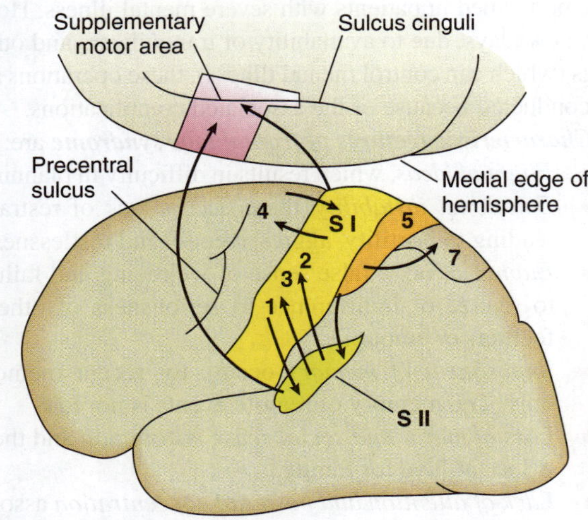

FIGURE 10.4-8 Connections of parietal lobe areas involved in somatic sensations.

Functions of Parietal Lobe

First somatic sensory area (SI) (areas 3, 1 and 2) localizes, analyses and discriminates different cutaneous and proprioceptive senses:

- *Area 3* receives cutaneous sensations of touch, pressure, position and vibratory senses (pain and temperature have slight representation in the primary sensory area).
- *Area 1* receives projections from cutaneous and joint senses.
- *Area 2* is primarily concerned with deep senses from muscles and joints.

Second somatic sensory area (SII) receives sensory impulses from SI and from thalamus directly. Though the exact role of this area is not clear, it is concerned with perception of sensation. Thus, the sensory parts of the body have two representations in area SI and area SII.

Sensory association areas (areas 5 and 7) are associated with more elaborate process of discrimination between the stimuli, thus helping in differentiating the relative intensity of different stimuli. Therefore, warm objects are distinguished from warmer, cold from colder, rough from rougher, etc.

Higher association area (area 40) helps in recognition of common familiar objects placed in the hand without looking at them (stereognosis).

Inferior part of postcentral gyrus contains centre for taste and general sensations from tongue. Lesion of this part causes loss of taste and general sensations of opposite half of the tongue.

Angular gyrus helps in recognition of spatial relationship by:

- Tactile localization, i.e. the precise point stimulated is accurately localized.
- Tactile (two-point) discrimination, i.e. two points of a compass placed close together are recognized as two and not as one.
- Accurate estimation of the extent and direction of small joint displacements.

[C] Temporal Lobe

Temporal lobe (Fig. 10.4-1) lies below the posterior ramus of lateral sulcus and its continuation the second imaginary line. Behind, it is separated from the occipital lobe by the lower part of first imaginary line which connects the upper end of parieto-occipital sulcus to the parieto-occipital notch.

Areas of Temporal Lobe

The major areas in the temporal lobe are (Fig. 10.4-5):

- Primary auditory area (areas 41 and 42) and
- Auditory association area (areas 22, 21 and 20).

Primary Auditory Area Primary auditory area, also called audiosensory area, includes Brodmann's areas 41 and 42 and forms the centre for hearing.

Location. It is situated in the middle of the superior temporal gyrus on the upper margin and on its deep or insular aspect (Heschl's or transverse temporal gyrus). Heschl's gyrus can be seen only when the lips of the lateral sulcus are widely separated (Fig. 10.4-2).

Connections *of this area* are:

- *Afferents* are received from:
  - Medial geniculate body via auditory radiations and
  - Pulvinar of thalamus.
- *Efferents* are sent to:
  - Medial geniculate body,
  - Superior colliculus and
  - Pulvinar.

Functions. This area perceives the nerve impulses as sound, i.e. auditory information such as loudness, pitch, source and direction of sound.

Auditory Association Area Auditory association area corresponds to Brodmann's areas 22, 21 and 20.

Area 22

- ***Location.*** Area 22 also called Wernicke's area is a sensory speech centre situated in the posterior part of superior temporal gyrus behind the areas 41 and 42 (Fig. 10.4-2), in the categorical hemisphere, i.e. dominant hemisphere.
- ***Functions.*** It is concerned with:
  - Interpretation of the meaning of what is heard and
  - Comprehension of spoken language and the formation of ideas that are to be articulated in speech.

Areas 21 and 20

- ***Location.*** Areas 21 and 20 are located in the middle and inferior temporal gyrus, respectively.
- ***Functions.*** These areas receive impulses from primary area and are concerned with interpretation and integration of auditory impulses.
- ***Lesions*** of these areas impair auditory, short-term memory without impairing visual memory.

Applied Aspects

Unilateral Removal of Temporal Lobe Unilateral removal of temporal lobe causes no deafness. This is because each ear is bilaterally represented in the auditory pathway from the medulla upwards and projects about equally to the two cerebral hemispheres. Thus, the removal of one auditory cortex has only a slight effect on auditory acuity (sharpness of hearing).

Temporal Lobe Syndrome Temporal lobe syndrome, also known as *Kluver-Bucy syndrome,* is produced in animals particularly monkeys after removal of bilateral temporal lobe along with amygdala and uncus.

Characteristic Features of this syndrome are:

- ***Aphasia,*** i.e. disturbances in speech.
- ***Visual agnosia,*** i.e. inability to recognize the objects in spite of good vision.
- ***Auditory disturbances*** in the form of frequent attacks of tinnitus, auditory hallucinations with sounds like buzzing, ringing or humming.

- ***Hyperphagia and omniphagia,*** i.e. animal starts eating more and eating that diet which it was not eating previously.
- ***Hypersexuality*** is noted in male animals due to damage to amygdaloid nuclei and piriform cortex.
- ***Increased oral activity,*** i.e. animal starts repeatedly putting up in their mouth to all the moveable objects present in the surrounding.
- ***Hypermetamorphosis,*** i.e. animal starts responding to every stimulus, whether it is experienced before or not.
- ***Dreaming states,*** i.e. the animals are not aware of their own activities and have the feeling of unreality.

Clinical significance. In humans with bilateral temporal lobe diseases or lesions, various above-mentioned symptoms are seen.

[D] Occipital Lobe

Occipital lobe lies behind the parieto-occipital sulcus and its continuation down an imaginary line (Fig. 10.4-1). It is concerned with vision.

Areas of Occipital Lobe

Occipital lobe is mostly formed of sensory and association areas and has only slight motor function. It contains visual cortex having three areas (Figs 10.4-2, 10.4-5):

- Primary visual cortex (area 17),
- Visual association area (area 18) and
- Visual association area or occipital eye field (area 19).

Primary Visual Cortex is also called striate area (area 17). It lies on the medial surface of the occipital lobe in and near the calcarine sulcus occupying parts of lingual gyrus and cuneus. It also extends to the superolateral surface of the occipital lobe limited in front by the lunate sulcus.

It receives the fibres of the optic radiations which bring impulses from parts of both retinae, and these parts are represented within the area in a specific orderly manner. It constitutes the centre of vision.

Peristriate Area, also called visual association area (area 18), lies in the walls of lunate sulcus.

Parastriate Area (area 19) is also a visual association area. It lies in the cortex in front of the lunate sulcus.

Modified Nomenclature of Visual Areas Recently, a modified nomenclature recognizing five visual areas has been described:

V1 : First visual area in area 17,
V2 : Second visual area occupying the greater part of area 18, but not the whole of it,
V3 : Third visual area occupying a narrow strip over the anterior part of area 18,
V4 : Fourth visual area within area 19 and
V5 : Fifth visual area at the posterior end of superior temporal gyrus.

Connections

Afferents to visual cortex come from the lateral geniculate body in the form of optic radiations. The right visual cortex receives impulses arising from the temporal half of right retina and nasal half of the left retina; and the left visual cortex receives those arising from the temporal half of the left retina and nasal half of the right retina.

Thus, there is a point-to-point projection of the retina in the visual cortex in such a way that the right visual cortex is concerned with perception of objects situated to the left of the vertical median line in the visual fields and left visual cortex with the objects situated to the right half.

Efferents from visual cortex go to:

- ***Various parts of the cerebral cortex*** in both hemispheres, in particular they reach the frontal eye field which is concerned with eye movements.
- ***Superior colliculus,*** the pretectal region and the nuclei of cranial nerves supplying muscles that move the eyeballs also receive efferents from the visual cortex.
- ***Corticogeniculate*** projection has also been evidenced physiologically.
- ***Thalamus*** (pulvinar) also receives efferents from the visual cortex.

Functions

- ***Primary visual area (area 17)*** is concerned with perception of visual impulses.
- ***Visual association areas (area 18 and area 19)*** are concerned with interpretation of visual impulses. These are involved in the recognition and identification of objects in the light of past experience.
- ***Occipital eye field area (area 19)*** is concerned with the movements of eyeball. Therefore, like other sensory areas, the visual area is also to be regarded as partly motor in function.

WHITE MATTER OF CEREBRUM

Passing through, between and around the subcortical masses of grey matter of cerebrum are tracts of white fibres. The white fibres of cerebrum are of three types (Fig. 10.4-9):

- Association fibres,
- Commissural fibres and
- Projection fibres.

I. Association Fibres

Association fibres connect the different gyri of the same hemisphere. These are of two types (Fig. 10.4-10):

1. ***Short association fibres,*** which connect the adjacent gyri are innumerable.
2. ***Long association fibres,*** which connect the widely separated gyri are arranged in five groups:
   - ***Superior longitudinal fasciculus.*** It connects the frontal region to the temporal and occipital region.

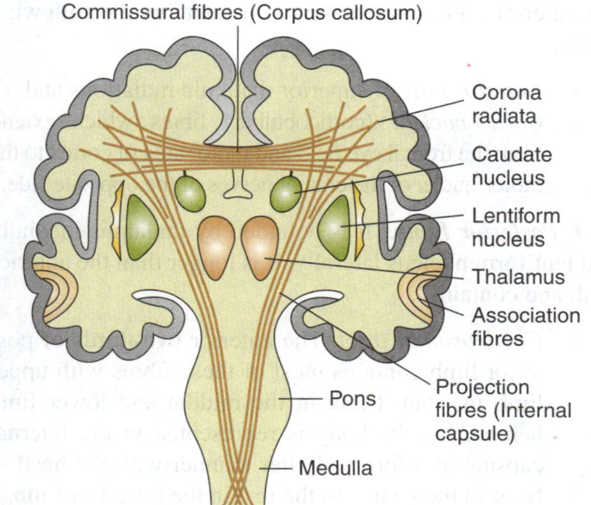

FIGURE 10.4-9 Frontal view of coronal section of brain showing the position of the association, commissural and projection fibres.

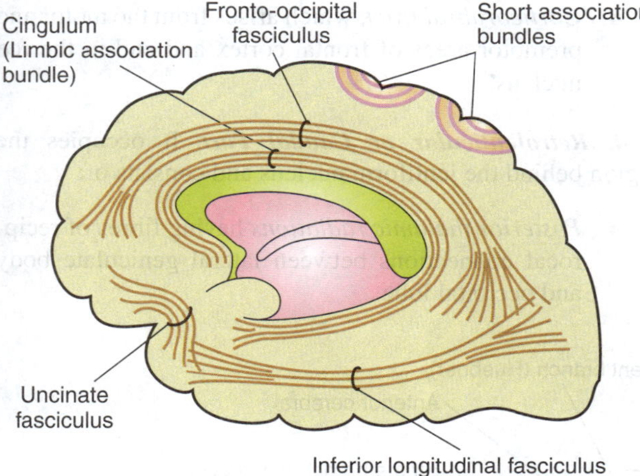

FIGURE 10.4-10 Short and long association fibres.

- *Inferior longitudinal fasciculus.* It runs from the occipital pole to the temporal lobe.
- *Cingulum.* It runs from below the rostrum of the corpus callosum to the temporal lobe.
- *Fronto-occipital fasciculus.* It also runs from the frontal pole to the temporal and occipital regions. It lies in a deeper plane than the superior longitudinal fasciculus.
- *Uncinate fasciculus.* It connects the anterior speech area (Broca's area) and orbital surface of the frontal lobe with the cortex over the temporal pole.

II. Commissural Fibres

Commissural fibres connect the corresponding parts of two cerebral hemispheres with each other. There are five bundles of commissural fibres (Fig. 10.4-11):

- Corpus callosum,
- Anterior commissure,
- Posterior commissure,
- Habenular commissure and
- Hippocampal commissure.

III. Projection Fibres

Projection fibres connect the cerebral hemispheres with other parts of CNS, e.g. thalamus, brainstem and spinal cord.

Projection fibres include the afferent and efferent tracts contained in corona radiata and internal capsule.

- ***Afferent projection fibres*** include thalamic radiations, which according to their disposition have been named as:
  - Anterior thalamic radiations,
  - Superior thalamic radiations,
  - Posterior thalamic radiation (including optic radiations) and
  - Inferior thalamic radiation (including auditory radiations).
- ***Efferent or motor*** projection fibres include:
  - Corticobulbar and corticospinal tracts (pyramidal system),
  - Corticopontine fibres,
  - Corticorubral fibres and
  - Corticothalamic fibres.

Corona Radiata Corona radiata (fountain of fibres) refers to that part of projection fibres that radiates from the upper end of internal capsule to cerebral cortex (Fig. 10.4-9). It contains both the ascending and descending fibres.

Internal Capsule Internal capsule is a thick curved band of projection fibres (ascending and descending) that occupy the space between the thalamus and caudate nucleus medially, and the lentiform nucleus laterally. Superiorly, it fans out as corona radiata and inferiorly, the fibres descend into the crus cerebri.

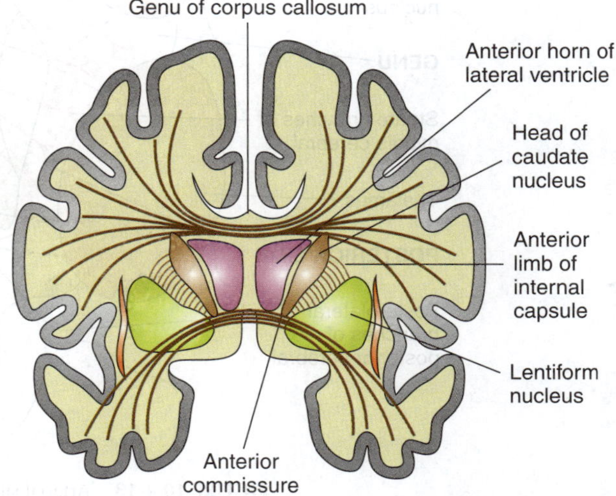

FIGURE 10.4-11 Genu of corpus callosum and anterior commissure.

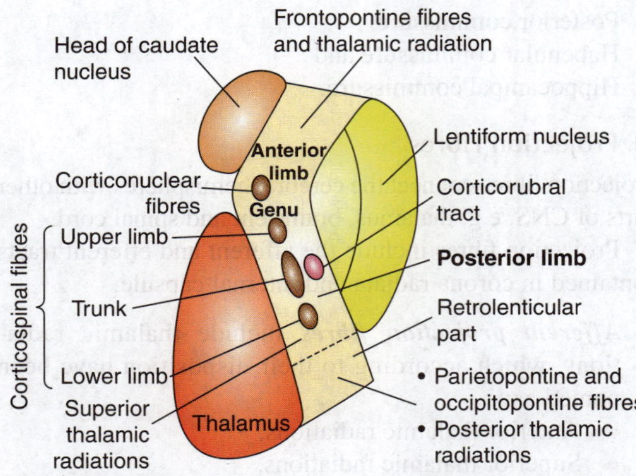

FIGURE 10.4-12 Parts of internal capsule; disposition of motor fibres and thalamic radiations passing through it.

Subdivisions of Internal Capsule are (Fig. 10.4-12):

1. Anterior Limb. It is short and lies between the head of caudate nucleus and lentiform nucleus.

It consists of:

- Anterior thalamic radiations, containing reciprocal connections between the dorsomedial and anterior nuclei of thalamus and prefrontal cortex and gyrus cinguli.
- Corticopontine (frontopontine) fibres from the frontal cortex to nuclei pontis.

2. Genu. It is the region of the band in the capsule situated medial to the apex of the lentiform nucleus. It connects the anterior and posterior limbs. It contains the following fibres:

- *Anterior part* of superior thalamic radiations and
- *Corticonuclear* (corticobulbar) fibres which extend from the frontal eye field and motor area of cortex to the motor nuclei of the cranial nerves of the opposite side.

3. Posterior Limb. It is bounded by thalamus medially and lentiform nucleus laterally. It is longer than the anterior limb and contains:

- *Corticospinal tract.* The anterior two-thirds of posterior limb contains most of these fibres with upper limb in front, trunk in the middle and lower limb behind, i.e. the body is represented in the internal capsule in a fore and after manner with the head in front in the genu and the rest in the posterior limb.
- *Corticopontine* (parietopontine) fibres.
- *Superior thalamic radiations* which comprise the fibres having reciprocal connections between the ventral nuclei of thalamus and the parietal lobe.
- *Corticorubral tract,* which arises from the motor and premotor areas of frontal cortex and end in the red nucleus.

4. Retrolenticular or Caudal Part. It occupies the region behind the lentiform nucleus and consists of:

- *Posterior thalamic radiations* having fibres of reciprocal connections between lateral geniculate body and occipital lobe.

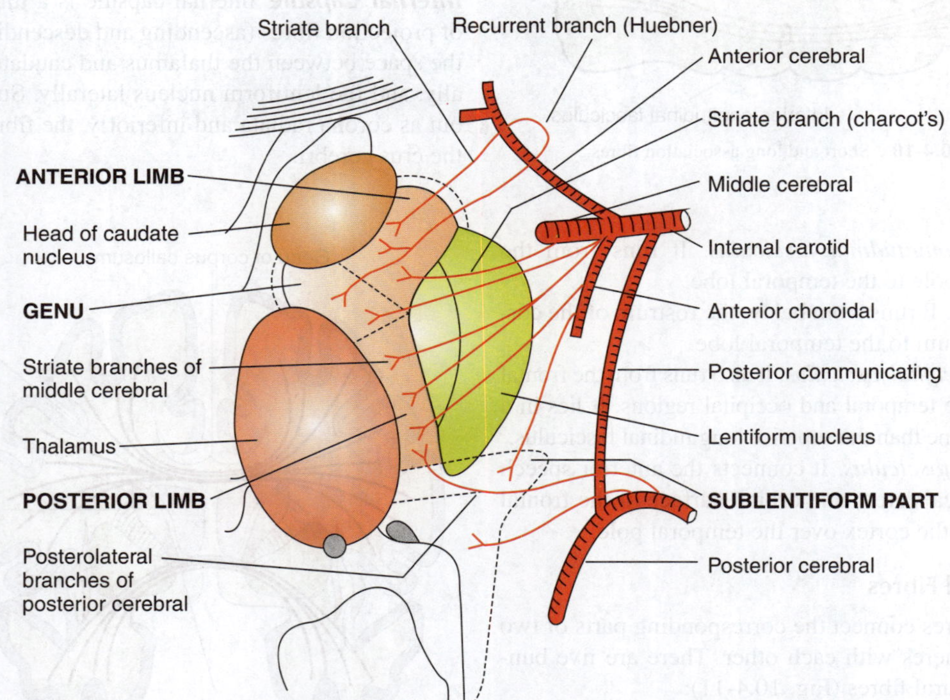

FIGURE 10.4-13 Arterial supply of internal capsule (schematic).

- *Optic radiations* (geniculocalcarine tract) extending from the lateral geniculae body to visual cortex.
- Corticopontine (parietopontine, occipitopontine and temporopontine) fibres.

5. Sublentiform Part. It occupies the region beneath the posterior part of the lentiform nucleus and consists of:

- *Auditory radiations* which originate in the medial geniculate body and terminate in the Heschl's convolutions on the superior surface of the superior temporal gyrus (auditory area).
- *Inferior thalamic radiations* having fibres of reciprocal connections between the medial geniculate body and the temporal lobe.
- *Corticopontine* (parietotemporopontine) fibres.

Blood Supply of Internal Capsule The internal capsule is supplied by the branches of middle cerebral, anterior cerebral and posterior cerebral arteries (Fig. 10.4-13).

Applied Aspects

Internal capsule fibres are densely crowded in a narrow area. Pyramidal fibres being compressed in this little space are particularly vulnerable to effects of even a pinpoint vascular lesion.

- Damage to internal capsule from infarction and haemorrhage is a common form or stroke, resulting in loss or decrease in sensations and movements of the opposite half of the body (hemianaesthesia and hemiplegia).
- Most common cause of hemiplegia is the thrombosis or rupture of one of the striate branches of middle cerebral artery which passes through the anterior perforated substance to supply the internal capsule. One of the lateral striate arteries, which is the largest of the perforating branches, is said to be particularly prone to such pathological conditions and is commonly called the artery of the cerebral haemorrhage (Charcot's artery) (Fig. 10.4-12). Usually all tracts are involved causing complete contralateral hemiplegia with associated sensory loss.
- Thrombosis of the anterior choroidal artery (Fig. 10.4-13) involves the optic radiations producing contralateral hemianopia and hyperacusia.
- Thrombosis of the recurrent branch of anterior cerebral artery (Huebner artery) (Fig. 10.4-13) results in contralateral paralysis of the face and upper limbs on account of the involvement of corticonuclear fibres and adjacent pyramidal fibres for the superior extremity.

Chapter 10.5

Autonomic Nervous System

ANATOMICAL CONSIDERATIONS

Autonomic Nervous System: Divisions

The autonomic nervous system (ANS) collects the information about the changes that take place in the internal environment (i.e. internal viscera), interprets these changes and guides the actions and gets the plan executed with the help of smooth muscles of viscera, cardiac muscles and secretory epithelium of the glandular tissues (which are the effector organs of ANS). In other words, ANS is responsible for activities of the organs of digestion, circulation, excretion, respiration and reproduction, as well as of adrenal medulla, sweat, lacrimal and salivary glands. It also controls the activity of smooth muscles of iris, ciliary body and arrectores pilorum.

The word autonomous is taken from Greek words the *autos* meaning 'self' and the *nomos* meaning 'control'. Thus, ANS is an involuntary system. Since it controls the vegetative functions, it is also called vegetative system.

Divisions of ANS

Autonomic nervous system has two main physiological as well as anatomical divisions, sympathetic and parasympathetic, each having a central and a peripheral component.

- ***Sympathetic division,*** also called thoracolumbar division, consists of thoracic and lumbar chains of sympathetic ganglia.
- ***Parasympathetic division,*** also called craniosacral division, consists of the ganglia associated with 3rd, 7th, 9th and 10th cranial nerves.

Somatic versus Autonomic Nervous System Sensory division of somatic nervous system collects information about the changes that take place in the external environment, while that of autonomic nervous system collects the information about the changes that take place in the internal environment (viscera).

- ***Effector organs*** of somatic nervous system are skeletal muscles, while that of ANS are smooth muscles, cardiac muscles and secretory glandular epithelium.
- ***General arrangement of somatic and autonomic nervous system*** (Fig. 10.5-1) shows that:
  - *Afferent (sensory) neuron* of somatic system having cell body in the dorsal root ganglion terminates in dorsal horn while that of ANS terminates in intermediolateral horns.
  - *The interneuron* (connector neuron) of somatic system has cell body in the dorsal horn and terminates in the ventral horn, while that of ANS has cell body in intermediolateral horn and terminates in the autonomic ganglia.
  - *Efferent (motor) neuron* has cell body in the ventral horn and its axon carries impulses of skeletal muscles (effector organ). The postganglionic neuron in ANS has cell body outside the CNS in the autonomic ganglion and its axon terminates in visceral effector.
  - There is a single efferent neuron in somatic system, which extends from CNS to effector organ. While in ANS there are two efferent neuron chains between CNS and the effector organ: first efferent neuron (preganglionic neuron) has its cell body in CNS, while the second efferent neuron (postganglionic neuron) has its cell body outside CNS in the ganglion (Fig. 10.5-1).

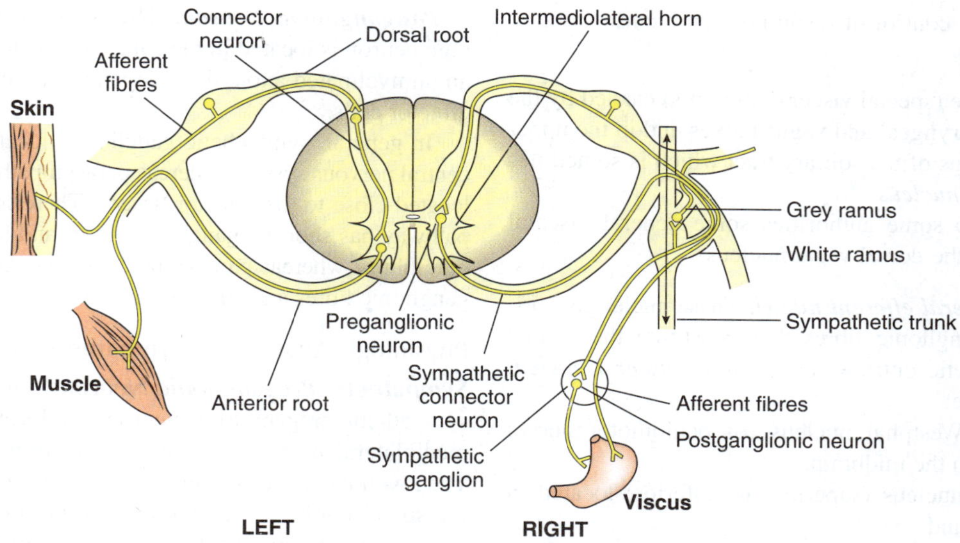

FIGURE 10.5-1 General arrangement of somatic parts of nervous system (on the left) compared with autonomic parts of nervous system (on the right).

- Somatic motor system innervates the skeletal muscles, while the ANS innervates the smooth muscles, cardiac muscles and secretory glandular epithelium.
- *Neurotransmitter* released at efferent (motor) neuron ending in somatic system is acetylcholine, while in ANS the neurotransmitter released between pre and postganglionic neuron is also acetylcholine, but that between postganglionic and effector organ depends on the component of ANS (see page 983).
- Somatic system activity always causes muscle excitation, while ANS can cause both excitation and inhibition.
- Somatic motor activity is always voluntary, while ANS motor activity is usually involuntary.

General Organization of the Autonomic Nervous System

The autonomic nervous system (ANS) is organized as:

I. Autonomic Areas in the Cerebral Hemispheres The autonomic areas controlling visceral functions located in the cerebral hemisphere are:

- Structures included in limbic system (see page 1082),
- Prefrontal cortex,
- Hypothalamus and
- Part of thalamus.

Higher brain centres, such as the limbic cortex, parts of the cerebral cortex, can influence the activity of autonomic nervous system by sending signals to the hypothalamus and lower brain area.

Hypothalamus is the site of integration of somatic, autonomic and endocrine functions. Such an integration is essential for the maintenance of homeostasis during exposure to stresses like extreme hot, extreme cold, stress of surgical operation, stress of injuries, haemorrhage and so on.

Since hypothalamus plays an important role in the regulation of autonomic activity, it has been called the main ganglion of the ANS. However, it is now known that the limbic cortex is equally important in the regulation of the ANS.

II. Autonomic Centres in the Brainstem These are located in the reticular formation and in the general visceral nuclei of cranial nerves.

Autonomic Centres in Reticular Formation

- *Gigantocellular* nucleus and
- *Parvocellular nuclei.*

Stimulation of gigantocellular nucleus and the upper part of the ventral reticular nucleus causes depression of vasomotor activity, while stimulation of other areas has a pressure effect,

These effects are mediated through connections between the reticular formation and autonomic centres in the brainstem and spinal cord, but the pathways concerned are not well defined.

General Visceral Nuclei of Cranial Nerves. These include both general visceral afferent and efferent nuclei.

- ***General visceral afferent nucleus*** is represented by the *nucleus of solitary tract* present in the medulla. It receives fibres carrying general visceral sensations through the vagus and glossopharyngeal nerves. Through these afferents and through connections with the reticular formation, nucleus plays an important role in reflex control of respiratory and cardiovascular functions.

Fibres of taste (special visceral afferents) carried by the facial, glossopharyngeal and vagus nerves end in the upper part of the nucleus of the solitary tract which is sometimes called *gustatory nucleus*.

According to some authorities some general visceral afferents end in the dorsal vagal nucleus.

- ***General visceral efferent nuclei.*** These nuclei give origin to preganglionic fibres that constitute the cranial parasympathetic outflow. *The general visceral efferent nuclei* include:
  - Edinger–Westphal nucleus (of oculomotor nerve) situated in the midbrain,
  - Salivary nucleus (superior and inferior) located in the pons and
  - Dorsal nucleus of vagus, present in the medulla.

III. Autonomic Centres in the Spinal Cord These are located in the intermediolateral grey column of spinal cord at two levels:

1. Neurons present in the thoracic and upper two or three lumbar segments of spinal cord (T_1 to L_3) constitute the preganglionic neurons of sympathetic nervous system (thoracolumbar outflow).
2. Neurons present in the second, third and fourth sacral segments of spinal cord (S_2 to S_4) are the preganglionic neurons of the sacral part of parasympathetic system, which along with the cranial part constitute the craniosacral outflow.

IV. Peripheral Part of ANS This is made up of all autonomic nerves and ganglia throughout the body. It is important to stress here that there is no nerve in the body which is totally made of autonomic fibres. Hence, it is not possible to speak of autonomic nerves. In fact, autonomic fibres are intimately related to different cranial and spinal nerves.

Neurons of ANS

It is believed that ANS has both afferent and efferent components. The visceral afferents are sometimes called *autonomic afferents*; however, many disagree and consider the autonomic nervous system essentially an efferent (motor) system for the visceral organs, blood vessels and secretory glands. Unlike in motor nerves, where a single motor neuron travels all the way from spinal cord or cranial nuclei to the muscle, the autonomic efferent pathway from the spinal cord or cranial nuclei is made of two neurons: the preganglionic and postganglionic.

Preganglionic Neurons. The cell body of the preganglionic neuron is located in either the brainstem or spinal cord. The axon of this visceral motor neuron projects as a thinly myelinated preganglionic fibre to an autonomic ganglion.

Postganglionic Neuron. The body of the postganglionic neuron is located in the autonomic ganglion and sends an unmyelinated axon, the postganglionic fibre, to visceral effector cells.

In general, sympathetic ganglia are located close to the central nervous system, whereas parasympathetic ganglia are located close to the effector tissues. Therefore, sympathetic pathway has short preganglionic fibres and long postganglionic fibres, whereas parasympathetic pathway has long preganglionic fibres and short postganglionic fibres.

Physiologic Anatomy of Sympathetic Nervous System

Sympathetic Preganglionic Neurons The cell bodies of sympathetic preganglionic neurons are located in the intermediolateral horn of the spinal cord from level T_1 to L_2. The myelinated axons of these visceral motor neurons leave the spinal cord via the ventral root and then pass via the white rami communicantes to the paravertebral ganglia of the sympathetic trunk (Fig. 10.5-1). After reaching the sympathetic trunk, preganglionic fibres may pass to one of the following three destinations:

- They may terminate in the ganglion at the level of entrance by synapsing with an excitor cell in the ganglion (Fig. 10.5-2).
- They may travel up or down in the sympathetic trunk to terminate in the ganglia located at a higher or lower level (Fig. 10.5-2).
- They may travel through the sympathetic trunk, and exit without synapsing via splanchnic nerve and terminate in a prevertebral ganglion (Fig. 10.5-2).

Preganglionic fibres that innervate the adrenal medulla travel through the sympathetic trunk exit without synapsing via greater splanchnic nerve and end directly on the cells of suprarenal medulla. These medullary cells may be regarded as modified sympathetic excitor cells that secrete epinephrine and norepinephrine into the blood stream. These secretory cells of the adrenal medulla are derived embryologically from nervous tissue and are analogous to postganglionic neurons.

Sympathetic Ganglia Sympathetic ganglia are of three types:

- Paravertebral ganglia,
- Prevertebral or collateral ganglia and
- Peripheral or terminal ganglia.

1. Paravertebral Ganglia. Paravertebral ganglia are arranged as enlargements along the entire length of two sympathetic trunks (right and left placed on either side of vertebral column throughout its length). Paravertebral ganglia of sympathetic trunk are divided into:

- *Cervical ganglia.* These are three in number: superior, middle and inferior.
  - *Thoracic ganglia.* These are 11–12 in number.
  - *Lumbar ganglia* are four in number.

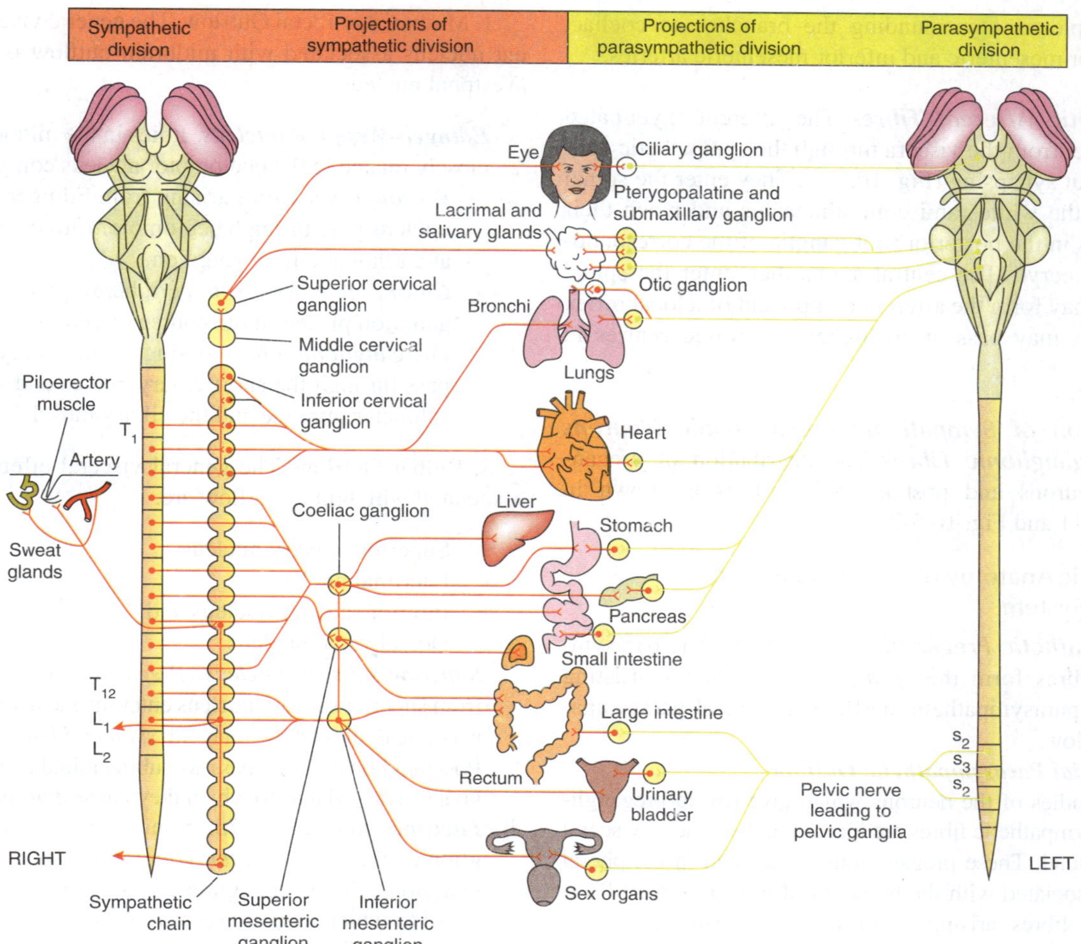

FIGURE 10.5-2 Efferent parts of autonomic nervous system: parasympathetic (on the left) and sympathetic (on the right).

Note. In all, there are 22 or 23 ganglia on each trunk.

The inferior cervical ganglion and the first thoracic ganglion are often fused to form a large stellate ganglion.

The two sympathetic trunks end below by joining together to form a single ganglion, the *ganglion impar*.

2. Prevertebral or Collateral Ganglia are three in number (coeliac ganglion, inferior mesenteric ganglion and superior mesenteric ganglion).

3. Peripheral or Terminal Ganglia are located within or close to structures innervated by them. Heart, bronchi, pancreas and urinary bladder are innervated by the terminal ganglia.

Postganglionic Sympathetic Neurons Sympathetic postganglionic neurons are located primarily in ganglia on the sympathetic trunks. Some are located in the prevertebral ganglia and the peripheral autonomic plexus (Figs 10.5-1 and 10.5-2). Axons arising from these neurons behave in one of the following ways:

- *The axons may pass through a grey ramus communicantes* and re-enter ventral root to reach a spinal nerve (Fig. 10.5-1). The grey rami communicantes are grey in colour because the postganglionic fibres are unmyelinated fibres. In the spinal nerve, the postganglionic fibres travel through its branches to innervate sweat glands and arrectores pilorum muscles of the skin in the region to which spinal nerve is distributed.
- *The axons may reach a cranial nerve* through a communicating branch and may be distributed through it as in the case of spinal nerve.
- The axons may pass into a vascular branch and may be distributed to branches of the vessel.
- Some fibres from these plexuses may pass to other structures in the neighbourhood of the vessel.
- *The axons of postganglionic neurons arising* in sympathetic ganglia may travel through the vascular branches and through autonomic plexus to reach some viscera (e.g. the heart).
- *The axons of postganglionic neurons located in peripheral autonomic plexus innervate neighbouring viscera.* These fibres often travel to the viscera in plexuses along blood vessels. For example, fibres for the gut travel

along plexuses surrounding the branches of coeliac, superior mesenteric and inferior mesenteric arteries.

Sympathetic Afferent Fibres The afferent myelinated fibres travel from the viscera through the sympathetic ganglia without synapsing (Fig. 10.5-1). They enter the spinal nerve via the white rami communicantes and reach their cell bodies in the posterior root ganglia of the corresponding spinal nerve. The central axons then enter the spinal cord and may form the afferent component of a local reflex arc. Others may pass up to higher autonomic centres in the brain.

Distribution of Sympathetic Preganglionic Neurons and Postganglionic Fibres The distribution of preganglionic neurons and postganglionic fibres is shown in Table 10.5-1 and Fig. 10.5-2.

Physiologic Anatomy of Parasympathetic Nervous System

Parasympathetic Preganglionic Neurons The parasympathetic fibres form the *craniosacral outflow,* consisting of cranial parasympathetic outflow and sacral parasympathetic outflow.

I. Cranial Parasympathetic Outflow

The cell bodies of the neurons which give rise to preganglionic parasympathetic fibres are located in the general visceral efferent nuclei. These preganglionic fibres end in peripheral ganglia associated with the branches of cranial nerves. Postganglionic fibres arising in these ganglia supply smooth muscles or glands. Cranial parasympathetic outflow can be further divided into:

- Midbrain or tectal outflow and
- Bulbar outflow.

1. Midbrain or Tectal Outflow. The general visceral efferent nucleus associated with midbrain outflow is Edinger–Westphal nucleus.

Edinger–Westphal nucleus. It lies in the midbrain and is closely related to the oculomotor nucleus complex.

- *Preganglionic fibres* arising from Edinger–Westphal nucleus pass through oculomotor (3rd cranial) nerve and relay in ciliary ganglion.
- *Ciliary ganglion* is a peripheral parasympathetic ganglion placed in the course of oculomotor nerve.
- *Postganglionic fibres* arising in the ciliary ganglion pass through the short ciliary nerves and supply the sphincter pupillae and the ciliary muscle.

2. Bulbar Outflow. The general visceral efferent nuclei associated with bulbar outflow are:

- Superior salivary nucleus,
- Lacrimal nucleus,
- Inferior salivary nucleus and
- Dorsal vagal nucleus.

i. ***Superior salivary nucleus.*** *Preganglionic fibres* arising from superior salivary nucleus enter the facial (7th cranial) nerve and ultimately relay in *submandibular ganglion.* Postganglionic fibres pass to submandibular and sublingual salivary glands to which they are secretomotor.

ii. ***Lacrimal nucleus*** of 7th cranial nerve sends preganglionic fibres to the *pterygopalatine* (sphenopalatine) ganglion. The postganglionic fibres reach the lacrimal gland to which they are secretomotor.

iii. ***Inferior salivary nucleus*** sends preganglionic fibres into the glossopharyngeal (9th cranial) nerve. These fibres relay in the otic ganglion, from where the postganglionic fibres go to parotid gland to which they are secretomotor.

TABLE 10.5-1 Distribution of Preganglionic Neurons and Postganglionic Fibres

Segmental level of preganglionic neurons	Area of distribution	Final distribution of postganglionic fibres
T_1 and T_2	Head and neck	Dilator pupillae muscle, Superior and inferior, Muller's muscles of eyelids, blood vessels and sweat glands.
T_3 and T_4	Thoracic viscera	Heart, oesophagus, trachea, bronchi and lungs
T_5 to T_9	Upper limb	Blood vessels, sweat glands and arrectores pilorum muscles
T_{10} to L_2	Lower limb	Blood vessels, sweat glands and arrectores pilorum muscles.
T_6 to T_{12}	Upper abdominal viscera	GIT, liver, spleen capsule, adrenal medulla and urinary tract
L_1 and L_2	Lower abdominal viscera	Bladder, uterus and fallopian tubes (or testis, vas deferens, seminal vesicles and prostate)
T_1 to T_{12}	Thoracic and abdominal parieties	Blood vessels, sweat glands and arrectores pilorum muscles

iv. *Dorsal (motor) nucleus of the vagus.* About 75% of all parasympathetic fibres arise from dorsal nucleus.

Preganglionic fibres travelling in the vagus nerve end in ganglia (or nerve plexuses) closely related to the visceral organs, such as heart, lungs, bronchi, oesophagus, stomach, small intestine and large intestine up to two-third of transverse colon.

Postganglionic fibres arise in these ganglia, and run a short course to supply smooth muscles and glands in these organs.

II. Sacral Parasympathetic Outflow

1. Preganglionic fibres. Cell bodies of the preganglionic neurons, which constitute the sacral parasympathetic outflow, are located in the intermediolateral grey horn of second, third and fourth sacral segments (S_2, S_3 and S_4) of spinal cord (Fig. 10.5-2). Their axons form the preganglionic fibres, which pass out through the ventral spinal root of corresponding nerves. These axons leave the spinal nerves to form the pelvic splanchnic nerves, which end in the pelvic autonomic plexuses.

2. Postganglionic fibres. The postganglionic neurons are located in the pelvic autonomic plexuses close to or within the viscera. Their axons (postganglionic fibres) run a very short course to supply the concerned pelvic viscera. These fibres also supply the rectum, the sigmoid colon, the descending colon and the left one-third of transverse colon.

Parasympathetic Afferent Fibres

The afferent myelinated fibres travel from viscera to their cell bodies located either in the sensory ganglia of the cranial nerves or in the posterior root ganglia of the sacrospinal nerves. The central axons then enter the central nervous system and take part in the formation of local reflex arc, or pass to higher centres of the ANS.

The afferent component of ANS is identical to the afferent component of somatic nerves and forms part of the general afferent segment of the entire nervous system. The nerve endings in the autonomic afferent component may not be activated by such sensations as heat or touch but instead by stretch or lack of oxygen. Once the afferent fibres gain entrance to the spinal cord or brain, they are thought to travel alongside, or are mixed with the somatic afferent fibres.

PHYSIOLOGICAL CONSIDERATIONS

Autonomic Neurotransmitters and Receptors

Neurotransmitters of ANS *(Fig. 10.5-3)*

Parasympathetic Fibres

1. Preganglionic fibres: acetylcholine
2. Postganglionic fibres: acetylcholine

Sympathetic Fibres

1. Preganglionic fibres: acetylcholine

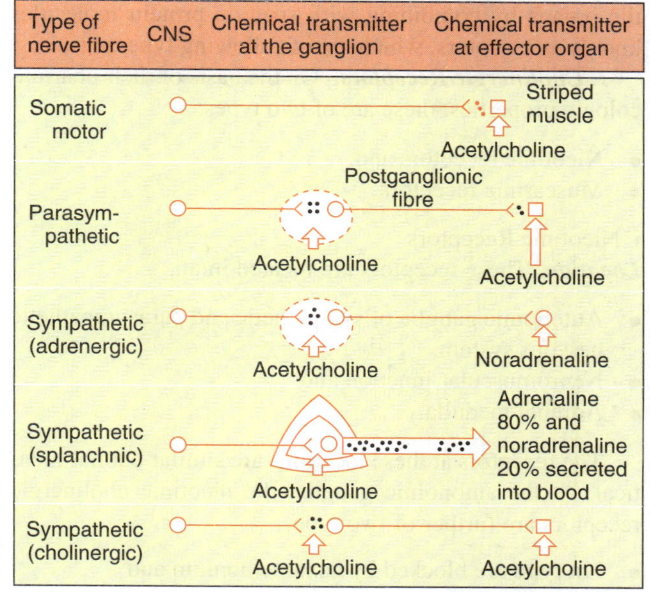

FIGURE 10.5-3 Neurotransmitters of peripheral somatic and autonomic nervous system.

2. Postganglionic fibres:

   Adrenergic fibres: norepinephrine (mainly) or epinephrine. All postganglionic sympathetic fibres other than cholinergic.

Note. The catecholamines present in plasma are Norepinephrine, epinephrine and dopamine and the source of dopamine comes from the adrenal medulla whereas norepinephrine mainly releases from the nerve endings, which diffuses into the bloodstream. Norepinephrine has prolonged effect compared with acetylcholine.

Cholinergic fibres: the postganglionic sympathetic cholinergic nerve fibres supplying sweat glands, blood vessels in heart and skeletal muscles.

Thus:

- All preganglionic fibres (sympathetic as well as parasympathetic) release acetylcholine.
- All postganglionic parasympathetic fibres release acetylcholine.
- Most postganglionic sympathetic (adrenergic) fibres release norepinephrine.
- A few postganglionic sympathetic (cholinergic) fibres release acetylcholine

Note. Acetylcholine released from the nerve endings acts locally, and usually does not circulate in the blood. The effect of acetylcholine is of short duration because of high concentration of acetylcholine esterase at cholinergic nerve endings.

For details about neurotransmitters, see page 1006.

Autonomic Receptors The autonomic neurotransmitters (acetylcholine and norepinephrine) produce their effects on the organs by combining with specific protein molecules known as receptors, which are of following types:

1. Cholinergic Receptors. On the basis of their pharmacologic properties, these are of two types:

- Nicotinic receptors and
- Muscarinic receptors.

i. Nicotinic Receptors

Location. These receptors are located in/at:

- Autonomic ganglia of sympathetic and parasympathetic nervous system,
- Neuromuscular junction and
- Adrenal medulla.

The receptors at these locations are similar but not identical. At the autonomic ganglia, the nicotinic cholinergic receptors are further of two types.

- **Nn type** are blocked by hexamethonium and
- **Nm type** are located at neuromuscular junction and are blocked by D-Tubocurare

Activation. Nicotinic receptors are activated by:

- Acetylcholine (Ach) and
- Nicotine.

Effect. These receptors produce excitation.

Blockage. Ganglion blockers (e.g. hexamethonium and trimethaphan) block the nicotinic receptors for Ach in the autonomic ganglia, but not at the neuromuscular junction.

Mechanism of action. The nicotinic receptors are ion-gated channels for Na^+ and K^+, Ach binds to α subunit of the nicotinic cholinergic receptors.

ii. Muscarinic Receptors

Location. Muscarinic receptors are located in the:

- Heart,
- Smooth muscles (except vascular smooth muscle) and
- Glands.

Types: The muscarinic receptors are divided into subtypes, i.e. M_1–M_5. M_2 and M_3 are main subtypes; M_2 receptors are present mainly in the heart and M_3 are located on smooth muscles and glands.

Activation. These receptors are activated by:

- Acetylcholine (Ach) and
- Muscarine.

Effect produced by their stimulation.

- *Inhibitory in the heart,* e.g. decreased heart rate and decreased conduction velocity in AV node.
- *Excitatory* in smooth muscle and glands (e.g. increased gastrointestinal motility and increased secretion).

Blockage. Muscarinic receptors for acetylcholine are blocked by atropine.

Mechanism of action

- *In heart at SA node,* these receptors cause inhibition of adenylyl cyclase, which leads to opening of K^+ channels, slowing of the rate of spontaneous depolarization and decreased heart rate.
- *In smooth muscle and glands,* these receptors act by formation of IP_3 and increase in intracellular Ca^{2+}.

2. Adrenergic Receptors. On the basis of their pharmacologic properties, adrenergic receptors are of two types:

- *Alpha (α) adrenergic receptors* (which are of further two types: α_1 and α_2) and
- *Beta (β) adrenergic receptors* (which are of further three types: β_1, β_2 and β_3).

i. α_1 Receptors

Location. α_1 receptors are located on:

- Vascular smooth muscles of skin and splanchnic regions.
- Gastrointestinal and bladder sphincters and
- Radial muscles of the iris.

Effect. These receptors produce excitation, e.g. contraction or constriction.

Catecholamine sensitivity. α_1 receptors are equally sensitive to norepinephrine and epinephrine, but only norepinephrine is present in concentrations that are high enough to activate α_1 receptors.

Mechanism of action. These receptors act by the formation of inositol 1,3,5-triphosphate (IP_3) and increase in intracellular Ca^{2+}.

ii. α_2 Receptors

Location. α_2 receptors are located in:

- Presynaptic nerve terminals,
- Platelets,
- Fat cells and
- Walls of the gastrointestinal tract.

Effect. Often produce inhibition (e.g. relaxation or dilatation).

Mechanism of action. α_2 receptor causes inhibition of adenylyl cyclase and decrease in cyclic adenosine monophosphate (cAMP).

iii. β_1 Receptors

Location. β_1 receptors are located in the:

- Sinoatrial (SA) node,
- Atrioventricular (AV) node and
- Ventricular muscles of the heart.

Effect. These receptors produce excitation (e.g. increased heart rate, increased conduction velocity and increased contractility).

Catecholamine sensitivity. β_1 receptors are sensitive to both norepinephrine and epinephrine, and are more sensitive than the α_1 receptors.

iv. β_2 Receptors

Location. β_2 receptors are located on:

- Vascular smooth muscle of skeletal muscle,

- Bronchial smooth muscle,
- Walls of the gastrointestinal tract and
- Bladder.

Effect. These receptors produce relaxation (e.g. dilation of vascular smooth muscle, dilation of bronchioles and relaxation of bladder wall).

Sensitivity to epinephrine is more than to norepinephrine. These are more sensitive to epinephrine than the α_1 receptors, e.g. when small amounts of epinephrine are released from the adrenal medulla, vasodilation (β_2 effect) occurs, when larger amounts of epinephrine are released from the adrenal medulla, vasoconstriction (α_1 effect) occurs.

Mechanism of action. Same as for β_1 receptors.

v. β_3 Receptors.

These receptors are located on the adipose tissue and causes lipolysis. *Mechanism of action: β_3 receptors cause increase in cyclic AMP (cAMP).*

Note. The type of adrenergic receptors present in various organs and the effects produced by their stimulation are depicted in Table 10.5-2.

TABLE 10.5-2 Responses of Effector Organs to Sympathetic and Parasympathetic Stimulation

S. No.	Effector organ	Parasympathetic effect	Sympathetic effect	
			Receptor type	*Response*
1.	***Eyes***			
	• Dilator pupillae muscle	–	α_1	Contraction (mydriasis)
	• Sphincter pupillae muscle	Contraction (meiosis)	–	–
	• Ciliary muscle	Contraction (produces accommodation for near vision)	–	
2.	***Heart***			-
	• SA node	↓ Heart rate and vagal arrest	β_1	↑ Heart rate
	• Atria	↓ Contractility, ↓ Conductivity	β_1 and β_2	↑ Contractility ↑ Conductivity
	• A-V node and conduction system	↓ Conduction velocity	β_1 and β_2	↑ Conduction velocity
	• Ventricles	↓ Contractility	β_1 and β_2	↑ Contractility
3.	***Arterioles***			
	• Coronary		α_1 and α_2 β_2	Constriction Dilatation
	• Cutaneous and mucosal	No supply	α_1 and α_2	Constriction
	• Skeletal muscle	No supply	α_1 β_2	Constriction Dilatation
	• Cerebral	Dilatation	α_1	Constriction
	• Pulmonary	Dilatation	α_1 β_2	Constriction Dilatation
	• Abdominal viscera	No supply	α_1	Constriction
	• Renal	No supply	$\alpha_1$andα_2 $\beta_1$andβ_2	Constriction Dilatation
	• Salivary glands	Dilatation	$\alpha_1$andα_2	Constriction
4.	***Systemic veins***	No supply	α_1 and α_2 β_2	Constriction Dilatation
5.	***Lungs***			
	• Bronchial muscles	Contraction	β_2 α_1	Relaxation Inhibition
	• Bronchial glands	Stimulation	β_2	Stimulation
6.	***Salivary glands***	Stimulation (profuse watery secretion)	α_1	Stimulation (thick viscous secretion)
7.	***Stomach***			
	• Motility and tone	increases	α_1, α_2 and β_2	Decreases
	• Sphincters	Relaxation	α_1	Contraction
	• Secretion	Stimulation	α_2	Inhibition

Continued

TABLE 10.5-2 Responses of Effector Organs to Sympathetic and Parasympathetic Stimulation—cont'd

S. No.	Effector organ	Parasympathetic effect	Sympathetic effect	
			Receptor type	*Response*
8.	***Gall bladder***	Contraction	β_2	Relaxation
9.	***Liver***	–	α_1 and β_2	Glycogenolysis
10.	***Pancreas*** • Exocrine glands • Endocrine glands	 Stimulates secretion –	 α_1 α_2 β_2	 Inhibits secretion Inhibits insulin secretion Stimulates glucagon
11.	***Spleen capsule***	–	α_1 β_2	Contraction Relaxation
12.	***Adrenal medulla***	Secretion of epinephrine and norepinephrine	–	–
13.	***Urinary bladder*** • Detrusor muscle • Sphincter	 Contraction Relaxation	 β_2 α_1	 Relaxation (usually) Contraction
14.	***Uterus***	Variable	α_1 β_2	Contraction (pregnant) Relaxation (nonpregnant)
15.	***Male sex organ***	Erection	α_1	Ejaculation
16.	***Lacrimal glands***	Secretion		
17.	***Skin*** • Pilomotor muscle • Sweat glands	 – Generalized (cholinergic sweating)	 α_1 α_1	 Contraction (erection of hair) Localized (adrenergic) sweating
18.	***Nasopharyngeal glands***	Secretion	–	–
19.	***Adipose tissue***	–	α_1 and $\beta_1\beta_3$	Lipolysis, release of FFA
20.	***Juxtaglomerular cells***	–	β_1	Increased renin secretion
21.	***Pineal gland***	–	β_1	Increased melatonin synthesis
22.	***Skeletal muscles***	–	β_2	Increased glycogenolysis
23.	***Basal metabolic rate***	–	β_2	Increased
24.	***Mental activity***	–		Increased

3. Nonadrenergic and Noncholinergic Transmitters. Some autonomic fibres release neuropeptide besides classical neurotransmitters. These include:

i. ***Adenosine triphosphate (ATP)*** The small vesicles of postganglionic noradrenergic fibres contain ATP. The low-frequency stimulation causes ATP release.

ii. ***Neuropeptide Y*** is another transmitter present in large vesicles of postganglionic sympathetic endings supplying to the vasculature of viscera, skin and skeletal muscles that releases on high-frequency stimulation in addition to norepinephrine.

iii. ***Galanin, vasoactive intestinal peptide (VIP), calcitonin gene-related peptide (CGRP) or substance P*** are released along with acetylcholine on sympathetic stimulation to sweat glands.

Functions of Autonomic Nervous System: Effects of Autonomic Nerve Impulses on Effector Organs

General Principles

- ANS controls the various vegetative functions which are beyond voluntary control and thus plays an important role in maintaining the constant internal environment (homeostasis).

- Most of the visceral organs have dual innervation, i.e. are supplied by both sympathetic and parasympathetic divisions of ANS. The two divisions produce antagonistic effects on each organ and provide a very fine degree of control over the effector organ. When the fibres of one division supplying to an organ are sectioned or affected by lesion, the effects of fibres from other division on the organ become more prominent.
- Some of the visceral organs are innervated by one division of ANS only, e.g.
  - Uterus, adrenal medulla and most of the arterioles are innervated by sympathetic division only.
  - Glands of stomach and pancreas are innervated by parasympathetic division only.
- In the case of sphincter's muscles, both adrenergic and cholinergic innervations are excitatory, but one supplies the constrictor component of the sphincter and other the dilator.
- *Effects of acetylcholine,* i.e. of localized cholinergic discharge, are generally discrete and short lasting, because Ach is rapidly removed from the nerve endings, due to high concentration of acetylcholine esterase at cholinergic nerve endings.
- *Effects of norepinephrine* are more prolonged than Ach, as it spreads further. In the blood, epinephrine and dopamine come from the adrenal medulla, while norepinephrine diffuses from the adrenergic nerve endings.

  Epinephrine versus norepinephrine (also see page 764).
- Epinephrine acts equally on α and β receptors, and has a special property of stimulating β_2 receptors. While norepinephrine acts mainly on α receptors, and also on β_1 receptors but has no action on β_2 receptors.

Effects of Stimulation of Sympathetic and Parasympathetic Division of ANS Responses of effector organs to autonomic nerve impulses are summarized in Table 10.5-2.

Differences between Sympathetic and Parasympathetic Systems

As summarized in Table 10.5-2, sympathetic and parasympathetic systems produce antagonistic effects on each organ of the body. The main differences between sympathetic and parasympathetic systems are depicted in Table 10.5-3.

APPLIED ASPECTS

A few important considerations about applied aspect of autonomic nervous system are:

- Disease/syndrome due to dysfunction of ANS.
- Autonomic drugs,
- Autonomic failure and
- Autonomic function tests.

Diseases/Syndrome of Autonomic Dysfunctions

1. Organophosphate Poisoning Organophosphates are cholinesterase inhibitors present in pesticides. Acute pesticide (organophosphate) poisoning occurs due to rapid absorption of organophosphates from gut, lungs, skin and conjunctiva.

Mechanism: Organophosphate pesticide, e.g. parathion, malathion, nerve gases (like soman serine) when bind to the enzyme, it undergoes hydrolysis and leads to the following signs and symptoms.

Signs and Symptoms of organophosphate poisoning occur due to excessive activation of autonomic/muscarinic activity. These include:

- *GIT:* excessive salivation, vomiting, gastric erosions and hematemesis
- ***Respiration:*** bronchial constriction, pulmonary haemorrhage, pulmonary oedema and ultimately respiratory failure.
- *CNS* signs include cognitive disturbances, convulsions, seizures and even coma.
- *CVS:* tachycardia and arrhythmia leading to cardiac failure.
- ***Renal system:*** acute oliguria leading to renal failure.

Management: As poison is most toxic and lethal, hence early diagnosis and management is mandatory. The treatment is mainly supportive as:

- Maintenance of patent airway by endotracheal intubation with assisted ventilation.
- Oxygen therapy to overcome hypoxia only when there is respiratory failure.
- Fluids: intravenous fluid therapy under CVP monitoring to compensate fluid loss.
- Removal of poison from GIT by gastric lavage.
- Haemodialysis is done for renal failure.
- Specific treatment includes:
  - Atropine (muscarinic cholinergic receptor antagonist) should be given parentally to control the signs.
  - Cholinesterase regenerator (pralidoxime)
  - Benzodiazepine can be used to control the seizures.

2. Mushroom Poisoning There are many poisonous varieties of mushrooms which can be confused with edible fungi and may be eaten by mistake resulting in mushroom poisoning or mycetium. About 95% of mushroom poisoning is caused by the ingestion of *Amanita phalloids*. This variety of mushroom contains toxins (phallatoxin and amatoxins)

Signs and Symptoms occur due to excessive activation of muscarinic cholinergic synapses. The major signs of mushroom poisoning occur within 2–3 h include:

- Nausea, vomiting, vasodilation, sweating, diarrhoea and urinary urgency occur within 2–3 h.
- After about 12 h, the stage is marked by severe hepatocellular and renal damage.
- The final stage (after 72 h) is characterized by acute renal failure, hepatic necrosis, sepsis and coma.

TABLE 10.5-3 Main Differences between Sympathetic and Parasympathetic System

Feature	Sympathetic system	Parasympathetic system
Location	Cell bodies of preganglionic neurons are located in intermediolateral horn of T_1–L_2 or L_3 spinal segments, so also called thoracolumbar outflow	Cell bodies of preganglionic neurons are located in: • *Cranial nuclei* associated with 3rd, 7th, 9th and 10th cranial nerves (cranial outflow) and • Intermediolateral horn of S_2 to S_4 spinal segments (sacral outflow). So, it is also called craniosacral outflow.
Components and ganglia	• Components are consolidated • Ganglia are linked up to form a chain	• Components are isolated. • Ganglia remain isolated.
Preganglionic fibres	Are short, myelinated and end in paravertebral or prevertebral ganglia	Are long, myelinated and end on short postganglionic neurons located on or near the viscera.
Postganglionic fibres	• Long • Nonmyelinated	• Short • Myelinated
Neurotransmitter • Preganglionic fibres • Postganglionic fibres	 • Cholinergic • Mostly adrenergic	 • Cholinergic • Cholinergic
Area of effect	Preganglionic fibres branch, enter several ganglia and transmit nerve impulse to many postganglionic fibres. So, sympathetic activity is spread over many segments	Preganglionic fibres do not branch; each enters a single ganglion and transmits nerve impulses to a single postganglionic fibre. Therefore, parasympathetic activity is localized, i.e. target is usually a single organ or system.
Functions	Mass sympathetic discharge usually occurs in threatening situation, i.e. it prepares the individual to cope with the emergency. It causes flight or fight reactions characterized by: • Dilatation of pupil • Increased heart rate • Increased blood pressure (providing better perfusion of the vital organs and muscles). • Constriction of cutaneous arterioles (which limits blood loss from wounds, if any) • Increased alertness and arousal due to decreased threshold in the reticular formation. • Increased blood glucose and FFA levels (supplying more energy). Because of these actions, sympathetic system is also sometimes called *catabolic nervous system*.	Unlike sympathetic nervous system, the functions of parasympathetic system are discrete and each function is separately regulated. This system is concerned with vegetative aspect of day-to-day living. For example, its action favours: • Digestion and absorption of food, increased activity of intestinal musculature and increased gastric secretion and pyloric relaxation. • Micturition, • Pupillary constriction and • Bradycardia Since parasympathetic system decreases the rate of metabolism, it is also called *anabolic nervous system*.

Antimuscarinic Syndrome occurs due to ingestion of a separate variety of mushroom (*Amantia muscaria*). This variety of mushroom also contains an alkaloid that blocks muscarinic cholinergic receptors.

The Classical Symptoms of Antimuscarinic Syndrome are:

- Red as beet, i.e. flushed skin,
- Hot as hare, i.e. hyperthermia,
- Dry as bone, i.e. no sweating & dry mucous membrane,
- Blind as bat, i.e. blurred vision and cycloplegia and
- Mad as halter, i.e. confusion and delirium.

Diagnosis of Mushroom Poisoning: The diagnosis is made on clinical history of ingestion, identification of mushroom (if possible) and measurement of amatoxin in blood by radioimmunoassay.

Management includes:

- Gastric lavage and activated charcoal may be given to absorb the poison.
- Supportive treatment by I.V. fluids.
- Antidotes of amatoxin such as penicillin G and silibinin inhibit uptake of amatoxin by the liver cells
- Thiocitic acid (a Krebs cycle coenzyme) also has a role.
- Atropine: rapid onset of muscarinic poisoning can be effectively treated with atropine.
- Antimuscarinic syndrome can be treated with physostigmine (a cholinesterase inhibitor), that acts peripherally and centrally.

- If patient is agitated, then sedation with benzodiazepine or an antipsychotic drug treatment.

Autonomic Drugs

Autonomic drugs exert their effects by action on the autonomic receptors directly or indirectly. These include:

- Sympathomimetic drugs,
- Sympatholytic drugs or sympathetic blockers,
- Parasympathomimetic drugs and
- Parasympatholytic drugs or parasympathetic blockers.

Sympathomimetic Drugs Sympathomimetic drugs also called adrenaline-like drugs, when administered in the body produce effects similar to the effects of sympathetic nerve stimulation. These can be divided into two main groups:

Directly acting sympathomimetic drugs. These drugs act directly on the α- and/or β-adrenergic receptors. Examples of these drugs are: adrenaline, noradrenaline, phenylephrine, isoproterenol and albuterol.

Indirectly acting sympathomimetic drugs. These drugs enhance the actions of naturally occurring norepinephrine (NE) in body by any of the following mechanisms:

- By displacing NE from the storage sites in the sympathetic nerve endings, e.g. amphetamine.
- By inhibiting the reuptake of NE by noradrenergic nerve endings and hence increasing the NE concentration in sympathetic sites, e.g. imipramine.
- By acting as monoamine oxidase (MAO) inhibitor agent and hence decreasing the catabolism of NE in sympathetic nerve terminals.

Sympathetic Blockers Sympathetic blockers or sympatholytic drugs block the actions of sympathetic neurotransmitters. Mechanisms by which sympatholytic drugs act are:

- Prevention of synthesis and storage of NE, e.g. reserpine.
- Prevention of release of NE, e.g. guanethidine.
- Blockage of α receptors, e.g. phentolamine
- Blockage of β receptors, e.g. propranolol, metoprolol, timolol, etc.
- Blockage of transmission of nerve impulse through sympathetic ganglion (ganglion blockers), e.g. hexamethonium and pentolinium.

Parasympathomimetic Drugs Parasympathomimetic drugs, also known as acetylcholine like drugs, when administered in the body produce effects similar to the effect of parasympathetic nerve stimulation. Depending upon their mechanism of action, parasympathomimetic drugs are of following types:

- ***Drugs acting on muscarinic receptors,*** e.g. pilocarpine and methacholine.
- ***Drugs prolonging the action of acetylcholine,*** e.g. neostigmine and physostigmine, which inhibit the activity of acetylcholine esterase.

Parasympathetic Blockers Parasympathetic blockers, also called parasympatholytic drugs, block the actions of parasympathetic neurotransmitters by blocking the muscarinic receptors. Examples of parasympathetic blockers are atropine, homatropine, scopolamine, cyclopentolate and tropicamide.

Autonomic Failure

Types. Autonomic failure is of two types:

Primary autonomic failure from the unexplained (primary) autonomic neuronal degeneration. It was previously known as orthostatic hypotension because this is the chief presenting feature of the disorder.

Secondary autonomic failure occurs secondary to some general medical disorders. Diabetes mellitus is the most common cause of secondary autonomic dysfunction.

Features of autonomic failure (primary or secondary) are:

- *Cardiovascular features* include tachycardia and orthostatic hypotension.
- *Sudomotor features* are anhidrosis and heat intolerance.
- *Gastrointestinal features* include constipation, occasional diarrhoea and dysphagia.
- *Urinary features* are nocturia, frequency, urgency, incontinence and retention of urine.
- *Reproductive organ problems* include erectile and ejaculation failure.
- *Ocular features* include miosis and enophthalmos.

Horner's Syndrome Horner's syndrome refers to ipsilateral *oculo-sympathetic paresis* due to any cause. Its common causes are Pancoast's tumour of the lung, malignancy of cervical lymph nodes pressing on the cervical sympathetic chain.

Clinical Features of Horner's syndrome are:

- ***Ptosis*** (drooping down of upper eyelid) due to paralysis of Muller's muscle of upper eyelid.
- ***Miosis*** (small pupil) due to paralysis of dilator pupillae muscle.
- ***Facial anhidrosis,*** i.e. reduced sweating on the ipsilateral face and neck.

Autonomic Function Tests

The tests of autonomic functions are broadly divided into two categories: noninvasive and invasive tests.

The noninvasive tests include:

A. Tests of Cardiovascular Autonomic Function

1. Valsalva's Manoeuvre. After closing both the nostrils patient is made to blow into a tube connected to sphygmomanometer and maintain air pressure at 40 mmHg for

15 s. The ECG recording is done during 15 s following the Valsalva manoeuvre. Normal response consists of tachycardia during strain and bradycardia after release (Fig. 10.5-4) (see page 377).

Valsalva ratio. The ratio between longest R-R interval (after the strain) and shortest R-R interval (during the strain) is known as the Valsalva ratio. Normal Valsalva ratio is >1:20. In autonomic neuropathy, Valsalva ratio is <1:20.

2. Heart Rate Variation during Deep Breathing. While recording ECG, patient is asked to inhale deeply for 5 s followed by exhalation for 5 s alternately for six times. The ratio between longest R-R interval during expiration and the shortest R-R interval during inspiration (E/1 ratio) in each respiratory cycle is calculated, and averaged for the total record. Normal ratio is >1:20 (Fig. 10.5-5). In autonomic dysfunction E/1 ratio is <1:2.

3. Heart Rate Response to Standing. Normally, a change of posture from supine to standing results in mild increase in HR. The ratio between the HR on standing and in supine posture is >1:4. In autonomic neuropathy this ratio is 1:0, i.e. there occurs no change in HR with posture change.

4. Heart Rate Variability (HRV) refers to beat-to-beat variation of heart rate. The sympathetic and vagal discharges directed to sinuatrial node are usually synchronous with each cardiac cycle. These discharges can be modulated by central and peripheral oscillators. These modulating effects of neural mechanism on heart rhythm is inferred with the help of HRV analysis.

5. Cold Pressor Test (CPT) measures the function of sympathetic neural control of cardiovascular system. Blood pressure is recorded while dipping the hand in cold water at temperature 8–10°C. Rise in blood pressure should be more than 15mmHg from basal value is considered to be a normal response.

6. Blood Pressure Response to Standing. Normally, a change of posture from supine to standing leads a slight fall in systolic blood pressure (SBP), which is never more than 10 mmHg. In autonomic dysfunction, this fall in SBP on change of posture is 10 mmHg or even more. This is called *orthostatic hypotension.*

7. Blood Pressure Response to Sustained Hand Grip. Patient is asked to maintain hand grip or a hand grip dynamometer at 30% of the maximum voluntary contraction for 5 min. Blood pressure is recorded just before and at the end of hand grip. Normally, the diastolic blood pressure (DBP) shows an increase by more than 15 mmHg. In autonomic dysfunction, the rise in DBP is always less than 10 mmHg.

B. Test of Sudomotor Function

1. Evaluation of ***sweating response to heat exposure*** tests the sudomotor functions. This test is performed by exposing the patient to electric heater till his body temperature is raised by 1°C; and the sweating response is studied by demarcating the area of sweating with the help of iodine starch or alizarin red, or quinizarin powders which change colour when moist.
2. ***Galvanic skin response (GSR)*** is based on change in skin electrical resistance. It is an electrodermal response that determines change in the electrical conductivity of skin, caused by increased activity of sweat glands. The sympathetic activity increases the conductance that is measured from the finger tips by placing electrodes on middle distal phalanges, index and middle finger. The wave-like increase in skin conductance begins 1–2 s after the onset of stimulus and peak reaches within 5 s.

C. Tests of Pupillary Functions Pupillary function tests are specifically useful in detecting sympathetic denervation of iris (e.g. in Horner's syndrome). Commonly performed tests are:

1. ***Cocaine test.*** Cocaine prevents the reuptake of NE at the adrenergic synapse and thus when 4% cocaine is instilled in both eyes, the normal pupil will dilate but the Horner's pupil will not.
2. ***Adrenaline test.*** When adrenaline 1 in 1000 strength or 1% noradrenaline is instilled in both the eyes, Horner's pupil dilates more than the normal due to denervation hypersensitivity in the involved eye.

D. Tests of Bladder Function In autonomic dysfunction, a cystometrogram reveals:

- Absence of accommodation of urinary bladder in response to bladder filling and
- Absence or poor voluntary bladder contraction when asked to micturate. The bladder capacity may be increased to 1 L in advanced cases of autonomic neuropathy.

Invasive tests include:

- Intravenous recording of postganglionic sympathetic activity.
- Response of autonomic nervous system to infusion of pressor agents.
- Estimation of plasma catecholamine levels.

Noninvasive methods are commonly used due to their ease of performance.

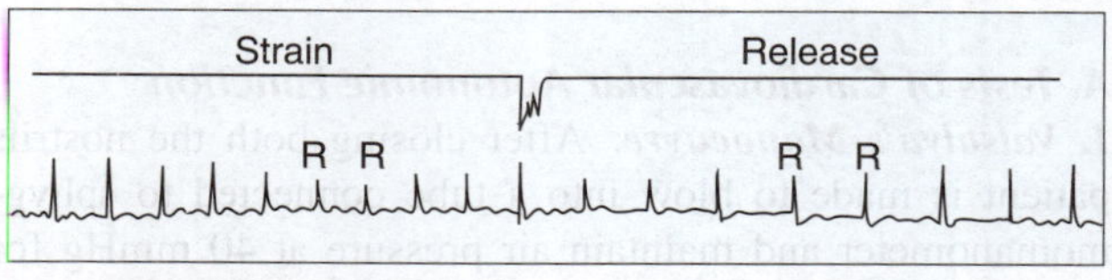

FIGURE 10.5-4 Effect of Valsalva manoeuvre on heart rate.

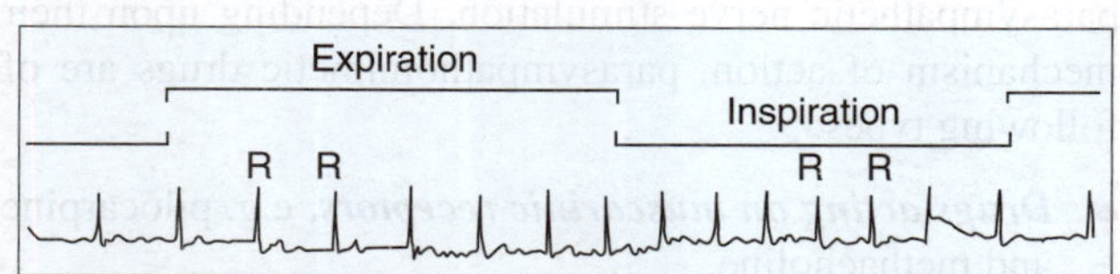

FIGURE 10.5-5 Heart rate variations during deep breathing.

Chapter 10.6

Meninges, Cerebrospinal Fluid, Blood–Brain Barrier and Cerebral Blood Flow

MENINGES OF THE BRAIN

The brain is enclosed within the cranial cavity by three concentric connective tissue layers: pia mater, arachnoid mater and dura mater, which constitute the meninges of the brain (Fig. 10.6-1).

Pia Mater Pia mater, covering closely and continuously the external surface of the brain, is a thin and highly vascular membrane. Folds of pia mater enclose tufts of capillaries called choroid plexuses to form telachoroidea in relation to ventricles of brain.

Arachnoid Mater Arachnoid mater is connected to the pia mater by many filamentous fibres. Subarachnoid space between these two layers is filled with cerebrospinal fluid (CSF).

Dura Mater Dura mater is composed of two layers: outer endosteal and inner meningeal. These are fused except where folds form (e.g. falx cerebri) or venous sinuses (e.g. superior sagittal sinus) are enclosed between them. *Subdural space* separates the dura mater from arachnoid mater. The arachnoid mater has minute protrusions (*arachnoid villi*), which pass through fenestrae in the dura mater and project into the venous sinuses to allow escape of CSF into venous sinuses.

CEREBROSPINAL FLUID

Cerebrospinal fluid (CSF) cushions the brain, and along with blood–brain barrier, the buffering function of neuroglia and the regulation of CNS circulation controls the extracellular environment of neurons. Within the substance of brain in the *ventricular system,* there are series of spaces filled with CSF.

Composition, Volume and Pressure of CSF

Composition of CSF. The extracellular fluid within the CNS communicates directly with the CSF. Thus, the composition of CSF indicates the composition of the extracellular environment of the neurons in the brain and spinal cord. The composition of CSF vis-a-vis blood is depicted in Table 10.6-1. The CSF differs from blood in having a lower concentration of K^+, glucose, and protein and a higher concentration of Na^+ and Cl^-. CSF normally lacks blood cells. The increased concentration of Na^+ and Cl^- enables the CSF to be isotonic to blood, despite the much lower concentration of proteins in the CSF.

CSF Volume and Pressure. The cranial cavity contains about 140 ml CSF, 100 ml blood and 200 ml of extracellular fluid in the brain which weighs about 1350 g. Thus, the extracellular fluid space in the cranial cavity totals approximately 440 ml.

The volume of CSF within the cerebral ventricles is approximately 40 ml, and that in the subarachnoid space is about 100 ml. The pressure in the CSF column is about 120–180 mm H_2O when a person is recumbent. Rate of CSF formation (about 0.35 ml/minute) is independent of CSF pressure as well as systemic blood pressure.

Formation, Circulation and Absorption of CSF

Formation of CSF. The CSF is mainly formed by the choroidal plexuses, which are covered by specialized ependymal cells. The *choroidal plexuses* are located in the cerebral

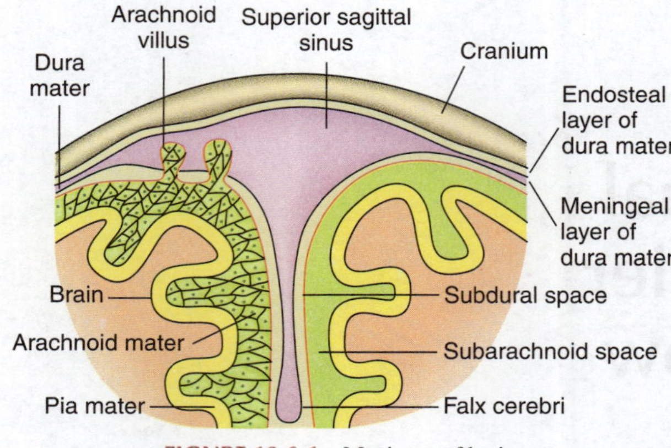

FIGURE 10.6-1 Meninges of brain.

TABLE 10.6-1 Composition of CSF vis-à-vis Blood

Constituent	Lumbar CSF	Blood
Na^+ (mEq/L)	148	136–145
K^+ (mEq/L)	2.9	3.5–5
Mg^{2+}	2.2	1.6
Ca^{2+}	2.3	4.7
$HCO^-{}_3$	25	24.8
PCO_2 (mmHg)	50	40
Osmolality (mosm/kg H_2O)	289	289
Cl^- (mEq/L)	120–130	100–106
Glucose (mg/dL)	50–75	70–100
Protein (mg/dL)	15–45	6.8×10^3
pH	7.3	7.4
Inorganic P (mg/dL)	3.4	4.7
Urea (mg/dL)	120	15.0
Creatinine (mg/dL)	1.5	1.2
Uric acid (mg/dL)	1.5	5.0
Urea (mg/dL)	0.2	175.0

ventricles (lateral, third and fourth). About 500 ml of CSF is secreted per day.

Mechanism of Formation of CSF: Cerebrospinal fluid is formed continuously by choroid plexus in two stages:

- In first stage, plasma is passively filtered across the capillary endothelium of the choroid.
- In the next stage, ions and water are secreted actively across choroid endothelium.
- HCO_3^-, Cl^- and K^+ enter the CSF via channels located on the apical membrane of the epithelial cells.
- Water is secreted through aquaporins to maintain osmotic gradient.

Circulation of CSF (Fig. 10.6-2). CSF formed in the lateral ventricles passes through the interventricular foramina (of Monro) into the third ventricle. Thence, the fluid flows through the cerebral aqueduct (aqueduct of Sylvius) into the fourth ventricle. From fourth ventricle, some CSF passes into the central canal of spinal cord, but most escapes into the subarachnoid space (surrounding the brain and spinal cord) through the median aperture (foramen of Magendie) of fourth ventricle and the two lateral apertures of fourth ventricle (foramina of Luschka).

Subarachnoid cistern refers to the regions where subarachnoid space is distended to form pools of CSF. An example is the *lumbar cistern,* which surrounds the lumbar and sacral spinal roots below the level of termination of spinal cord. The lumbar cistern is the target for lumbar puncture, a procedure used clinically to sample the CSF.

Absorption of CSF. A large part of CSF is removed by bulk flow, through the valvular *arachnoid villi* into the dural venous sinuses in the cranium. Unlike rate of formation, the absorption rate of CSF is a direct function of the CSF pressure.

- At normal average CSF pressure (112 mm H_2O), the filtration and absorption is equal and at pressure 68 mm H_2O CSF absorption is zero (Fig. 10.6-3).

Functions of CSF

i. Protection to CNS by acting as a 'water jacket', as it absorbs shock in the event of blow, due to following effects:

- The duramater is attached to the cranial bone firmly and there is no subdural space.
- The arachnoid mater is being held to duramater by surface tension of the thin layer of fluid present between two layers.
- The brain within the arachnoid is supported by the blood vessels, fibrous arachnoid trabecular and various nerve roots.
- The net weight (Dry weight 1400 g in air) reduces to 50 g in water bath of CSF (i.e. brain is suspended in the CSF due to its buoyancy effect). Therefore, when there is blow on the head, the arachnoid slides over the duramater and brain moves, but its movement is checked by the CSF cushion and arachnoid trabeculae.

ii. Removal of Waste Products of brain metabolism.

iii. Regulates Extracellular Environment for the neurons of central nervous system.

iv. Transports hormones and hormone-releasing factors.

Clinical Applications

Head Injuries

Causes. The brain injury occurs most commonly when skull is fractured and bone is driven into the neural tissue (depressed fracture), or

- Due to blow on the head, brain is accelerated and driven against the skull or tentorium at the point just opposite to the blow is struck (contrecoup injury) or

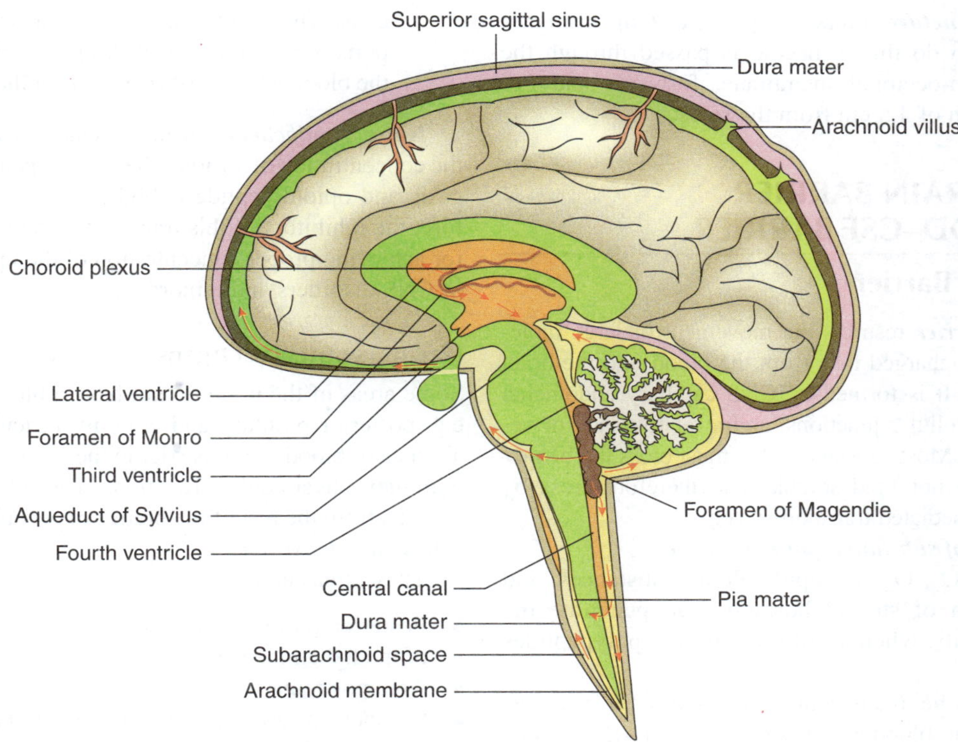

FIGURE 10.6-2 Circulation of cerebrospinal fluid. Arrows indicate the direction of flow.

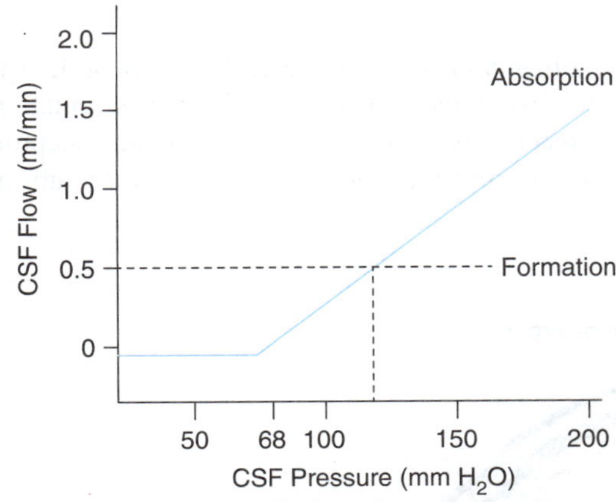

FIGURE 10.6-3 CSF formation and absorption.

- When movement of brain is so strong to tear the delicate bridging veins from the cortex to bone.

Hydrocephalus. Hydrocephalus refers to an abnormal accumulation of CSF in the cranium.

Causes of hydrocephalus include:

- Obstruction to CSF circulation,
- Excessive production of CSF and
- Interference with absorption of CSF.

Types of Hydrocephalus are:

- *Internal or noncommunicating hydrocephalus* occurs when obstruction is within the ventricular system or in the roof of fourth ventricle. It results in the dilatation of the ventricles.
- *External or communicating hydrocephalus* occurs when obstruction is in subarachnoid space or arachnoid villi. In it excess fluid is mainly in the subarachnoid space. The arachnoid granulations often suffer from moderate obstruction in patients suffering from cerebral meningitis or haemorrhage into the subarachnoid space.

Signs and Symptoms

- *Acute hydrocephalus* due to intraventricular bleeding may cause stupor and coma.
- *Subacute hydrocephalus* (develops over few days) produces progressive drowsiness and lethargy and incontinence.
- *Chronic hydrocephalus* (developing over few weeks) causes movement difficulties and incontinence.

Management of Hydrocephalous Include

- Ventriculostomy for ventricular drainage for symptomatic relief.
- Ventricular CSF shunting is the best treatment for chronic hydrocephalus.

Lumbar and Cisternal Puncture

Lumbar puncture refers to tapping of CSF from lumbar cistern. CSF examination is required in many disorders of CNS. It is performed by inserting a needle in between the L_2 and L_3 or L_3 and L_4 vertebrae.

Cisternal puncture refers to tapping of CSF from cisterna magna. To do this, a needle is passed through the posterior atlanto-occipital membrane, forwards and upwards, to a depth of 4.5 cm from the surface.

BLOOD–BRAIN BARRIER AND BLOOD–CSF BARRIER

Blood–Brain Barrier

Blood–brain barrier restricts the movement of large molecules and highly charged ions from the blood into the brain and spinal cord. It is formed by CNS capillary endothelial cells, their intercellular junctions, and a relative lack of vesicular transport. Most substances that must cross the blood–brain barrier are not lipid soluble, and therefore cross by specific carrier-mediated transport system.

Penetration of substances into the brain:

- Water, CO_2, O_2 and lipid-soluble substances, and free form of steroid hormone can penetrate the brain easily, whereas all proteins and polypeptides do not.
- Glucose, the main source of energy for neurons, crosses the blood–brain barrier very slowly but can be transported into CSF rapidly by specific glucose transporters (GLUT-1). In brain two forms of GLUT-1 exist, i.e. GLUT-1 55K and GLUT-1 45K. Both forms are though encoded by same gene, but differ due to the extent they are glycosylated . For details of glucose transporters see page 777.
- P-Glycoprotein is a multidrug nonspecific transporter present in the apical membrane of the endothelial cells. This multidrug nonspecific transporter transports a large number of drugs or peptides back into the blood which cross cerebral capillaries.

Note: *Significance*: In the absence of this transporter, the concentration of various chemotherapeutic agents, analgesic and opioid peptide is higher than in control. Therefore, the inhibitors of this transporter can be of great value for achieving proper concentration of therapeutic treatment of CNS disorders and tumors.

Circumventricular Organs (Fig. 10.6-4)

Some areas of the brain do not have a blood–brain barrier, e.g. posterior pituitary and circumventricular organs. The absence of blood–brain barrier in these regions is consistent with their physiological functions. These leaky regions are isolated from the rest of the brain by specialized ependymal cells called *tanycytes.*

These areas are:

- Posterior pituitary (neurohypophysis) and ventral part of medial eminence,
- Area postrema,
- Organosum vasculosum of lamina terminalis (OVLT) and
- Subfornical organs (SFO).

Functions Being outside the blood–brain barrier, they function as:

- ***Neurohemal organs.*** The secreted polypeptides (neurohormones) by the neurons enter into the circulation.
- ***Chemoreceptor zone.*** They also contain receptors for many different type of peptides and other substances.

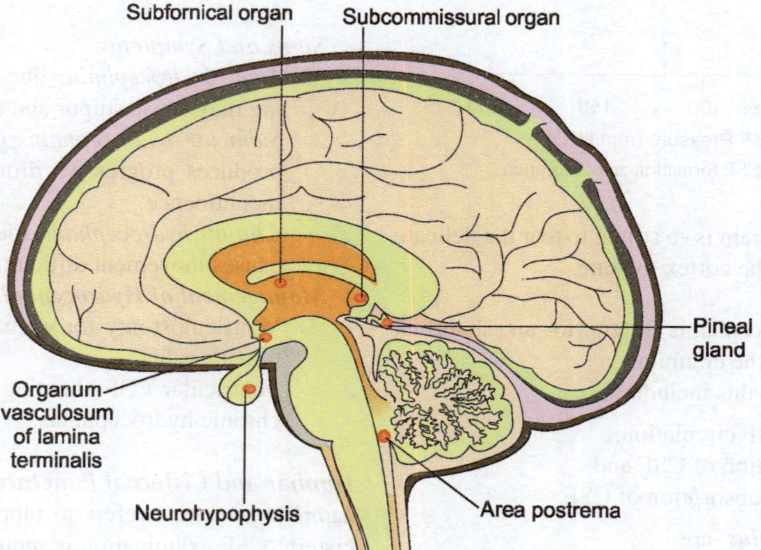

FIGURE 10.6-4 Circumventricular organs.

The circulating substances act on these receptors and thus trigger change in brain activity, e.g.

- Vomiting induced by chemotherapy.
- Angiotensin II act on OVLT (osmoreceptor) to increase water intake.

Disruption of blood–brain barrier occurs in a variety of pathological situations such as brain tumours and bacterial meningitis, etc. This fact can be exploited radiologically by introducing into the circulation a substance that normally cannot penetrate the blood–brain barrier. If the substance can be imaged, its leakage into the region occupied by the brain tumour can be used to demonstrate the distribution of tumour.

- ***Kernicterus.*** The blood–brain barrier is immature at birth; therefore, in severely jaundiced infants with high levels of the bilirubin (due to hepatic-bilirubin-conjugating system immaturity), bilirubin enters the brain and damages the basal ganglia leading to kernicterus.
- ***Crigler–Najjar syndrome.*** Congenital deficiency of glucuronyl transferase leading to high levels of free bilirubin in blood causes encephalopathy but does not cause brain damage.

Blood–CSF Barrier The capillaries that traverse the choroidal plexuses are freely permeable to plasma solutes. However, a barrier (blood–CSF barrier) exists at the level of epithelial cells that make up the choroid plexuses. This barrier is responsible for carrier-mediated active transport.

Relationship between intracranial fluid compartments and the blood–brain barrier and blood–CSF barrier is shown in Fig. 10.6-5.

CEREBRAL BLOOD FLOW

Functioning of the brain is closely related to the level of cerebral blood flow. Total cessation of blood flow to the brain causes unconsciousness within 5–10 s because of the decrease in oxygen delivery and the resultant cessation of metabolic activity.

Normal cerebral blood flow in an adult averages 50–65 ml/100 g or 750–900 ml/min. Thus, the brain receives approximately 15% of the total resting cardiac output.

Details of cerebral blood flow are given at page 371.

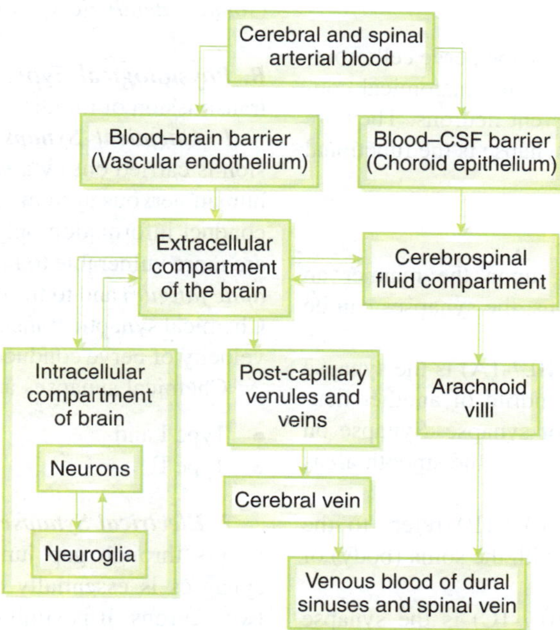

FIGURE 10.6-5 Structural and functional relationship between intracranial fluid compartments and blood–brain and blood–CSF barriers. The tissue elements indicated in parentheses form the barrier. Arrows indicate direction of fluid flow under normal conditions. Substances entering the neurons and glial cells (i.e. intracellular compartments) must pass through the cell membrane.

Chapter 10.7

Synaptic Transmission

SYNAPSE: DEFINITION AND TYPES

Definition

The synapse is the anatomic site where the nerve cells communicate among themselves. There is no anatomical connection or continuity between different neurons. They are connected only functionally. So, a synapse is the functional junction between two neurons.

Types of Synapses

A. Anatomical Types Depending upon the manner an axon terminates on the other neurons, the synapses can be of following types (Fig. 10.7-1):

1. Axo-dendritic Synapse (Fig. 10.7-1A) is the synapse between axon of a neuron with dendrite of another neuron. It is the most common type of synapse. Synapse on dendrites may be located on spines or on the smooth areas between spines (Fig. 10.7-2).

2. Axo-somatic Synapse (Fig. 10.7-1B) refers to the synapse between axon of a neuron with the soma (body) of another neuron.

3. Axo-axonic Synapse (Fig. 10.7-1C) is the synapse between axon of a neuron with axon of another neuron. It is a less common type of synapse. An axo-axonal synapse may be located either on the initial segment (of the receiving axon) or just proximal to an axon terminal.

In some parts of the brain (e.g. thalamus) some synapses are seen in which the presynaptic element is a dendrite instead of an axon. Such synapses may be *dendro-axonic* or *dendro-dendritic*. In yet others, the soma of the neuron may synapse with the soma of a neuron (*somato-somatic synapse*) or with a dendrite (*somato-dendritic synapse*).

B. Physiological Types Depending upon the process of transmission of impulse, the synapses can be classified as:

1. Chemical Synapses are those in which transmission is carried out by a *neurotransmitter*. Most synapses in human nervous system are of this type. Chemical synapses conduct information only in one direction. These synapses are more vulnerable to fatigue on repeated stimulation (*synaptic fatigue*) and to the effects of hypoxia and pH changes. Chemical synaptic transmission is definitely slower than the velocity of nerve conduction resulting in the synaptic delay.

Chemical synapses are of two types:

- Type I and
- Type II.

2. Electrical Synapses are those in which transmission occurs through gap junctions. Transmission at electrical synapses is essentially an electronic conduction between two neurons. It is similar to the process of nerve conduction. The electrical synapses can conduct in both directions. The speed of transmission at electrical synapses is the same as that of nerve conduction.

Electrical transmission is seen in a few locations (e.g. within the retina and olfactory bulb) in human nervous system. It is found mainly in invertebrates and lower vertebrates.

3. Conjoint Synapse refers to a synapse where both the chemical and electrical transmissions coexist.

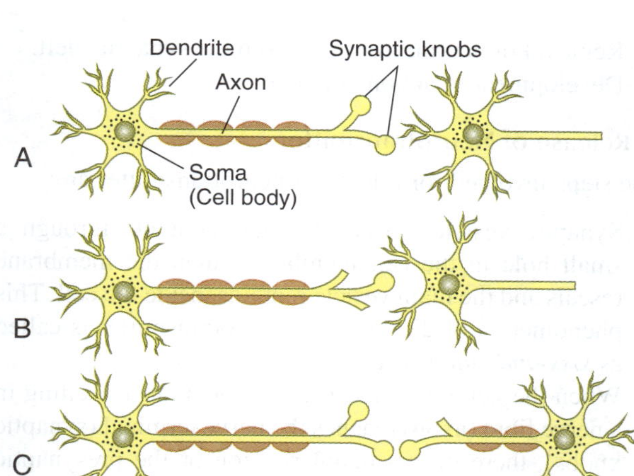

FIGURE 10.7-1 Types of synapses depending on the manner, an axon terminates on the other neuron: **A,** axo-dendritic synapse; **B,** axo-somatic synapse; and **C,** axo-axonic synapse.

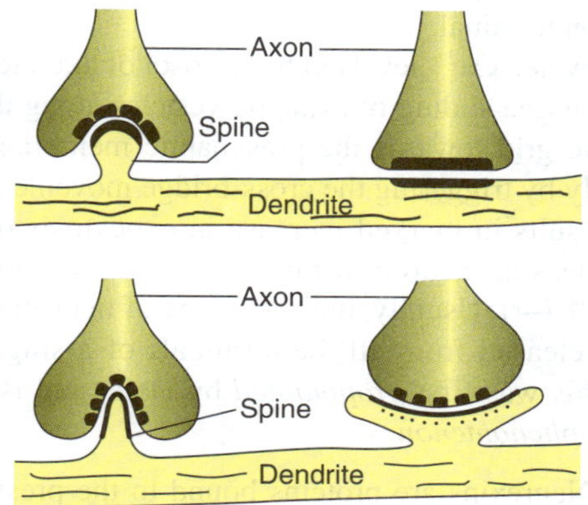

FIGURE 10.7-2 Variations in the orientation of axo-dendritic synapses.

CHEMICAL SYNAPSE

Structure of a Chemical Synapse

As mentioned earlier, the synapse is the functional junction between two neurons. A typical chemical synapse between the axon of one neuron and dendrite of other neuron exhibits the following characteristics (Fig. 10.7-3):

Synaptic knob or button. As the axon of neuron approaches the synapse, it loses the myelin sheath and divides into a number of fine branches which end in small swellings called the *synaptic knobs* or *synaptic buttons,* which make synapse with the soma or dendrite of the postsynaptic neuron. Each synaptic knob contains large number of mitochondria and synaptic vesicles containing neurotransmitter. Mitochondria provide ATP required for synthesis of neurotransmitter.

There are three types of synaptic vesicles:

- *Small clear vesicles* contain acetylcholine, glycine or GABA.
- *Small vesicles with dense core* contain catecholamines.
- *Large vesicles with dense core* contain neuropeptides as transmitters.

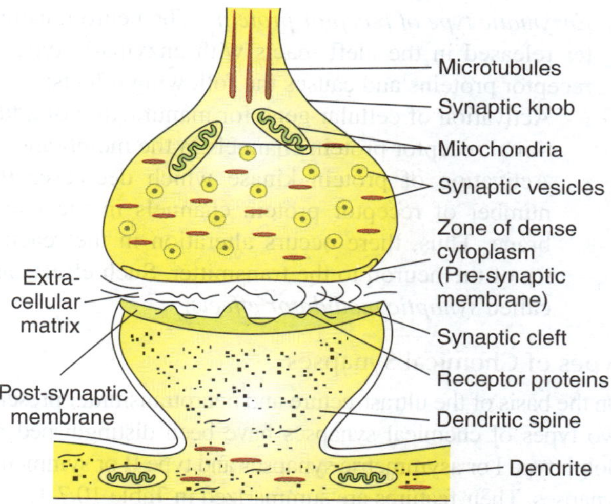

FIGURE 10.7-3 Structure of a chemical synapse.

Besides the neurotransmitter, the vesicles also contain other proteins to bind the neurotransmitter to the vesicle. The microtubules present in the synaptic knob transport the vesicles along the axons up to the presynaptic grid. Cross-bridges have been observed between the vesicles and the microtubules suggesting that the mechanism of transport of the vesicles along the microtubules may be similar to the sliding of actin on myosin filament.

Presynaptic membrane refers to the axonal membrane lining the synaptic knobs. On the inner aspect of presynaptic membrane are present *zones of dense cytoplasm,* which presumably form a *presynaptic vesicular grid* for organized channelling of the vesicles to the presynaptic membrane at a site opposite to the receptors on the postsynaptic membrane.

Synaptic cleft is a small gap (20–40 nm wide) between the pre- and postsynaptic membranes. It is filled by the extracellular fluid containing some glycoproteins. A neurotransmitter is released into this cleft from the presynaptic membranes. Enzymes present in the cleft destroy the neurotransmitter. The extracellular matrix may be acting as an adherent between synaptic neurons. Postsynaptic process is the name given to the region of receiving neuron (e.g. dendritic spine) where the synaptic knob synapses.

Postsynaptic membrane is the membrane lining the postsynaptic process. On the inner aspect of postsynaptic membrane is present a *zone of dense cytoplasm* which constitutes the active zone of a synapse. Postsynaptic membrane contains large number of receptor proteins which protrude outwards in the synaptic cleft. A neurotransmitter released in the synaptic cleft binds with these receptor proteins to cause the effect.

Receptor proteins are of two types:

1. *Ion channel receptor proteins*. These line the ion channels (Na^+, K^+, Cl^-, etc.) and the neurotransmitter released in the cleft causes opening of the channels by reacting with these receptor proteins.

2. *Enzymatic type of receptor proteins*. The neurotransmitter released in the cleft reacts with enzymatic type of receptor proteins and causes the following effects:
   - Activation of cellular gene for manufacture of additional receptor protein channels in the membrane.
   - Activation of protein kinase which decreases the number of receptor protein channels in the membrane. Thus, there occurs alteration in the reactivity of the neuron to the transmitter. Such effects are called *synaptic modulator effects*.

Types of Chemical Synapses

On the basis of the ultrastructure and neurotransmitter present, two types of chemical synapses have been distinguished by Golgi: type I or asymmetric synapses and type II or symmetric synapses. Their features are summarized in Table 10.7-1.

Process of Chemical Synaptic Transmission

Most synapses within the CNS use chemical transmitters. The sequence of events which occurs during chemical synaptic transmission is:

- Release of neurotransmitter.
- Development of the excitatory postsynaptic potential (EPSP) or inhibitory postsynaptic potential (IPSP).
- Removal of neurotransmitter from the synaptic cleft.
- Development of action potential.

TABLE 10.7.1 Features of Two Types of Chemical Synapses

Feature	Type I or asymmetric synapses	Type II or symmetric synapses
• Structure	Asymmetric	Symmetric
• Synaptic cleft	Wider (about 30 nm)	Narrower (about 20 nm)
• Thickening of postsynaptic membrane	Marked	Less marked
• Dense extra-cellular material in the synaptic cleft	Present	Absent
• Shape of vesicles	Small spherical and dense cored	Flat or elongated
• Neurotrans-mitters released	Acetylcholine, glutamate or serotonin is released by spherical vesicles. Dense cored vesicles release noradrenaline, adrenaline or dopamine	GABA, glycine
• Type of effect	Mostly excitatory	Mostly inhibitory
• Type of synapse	Usually axo-dendritic	Usually axo-somatic

A. Release of Neurotransmitter

The steps involved for release of neurotransmitter are:

- Synaptic vesicles discharge their contents through a small hole in the cell membrane, then the membrane reseals and the main vesicle remains inside the cell. This phenomenon of discharge of neurotransmitter is called as *kiss-and-run discharge*.
- When the nerve impulse (action potential) travelling in a nerve fibre (axon) reaches the nerve terminal (synaptic knobs), there occurs depolarization of the presynaptic terminal.
- As a result of depolarization, the voltage-gated Ca^{2+} channels present on the presynaptic membrane open up increasing its permeability to Ca^{2+} ions. Consequently, the Ca^{2+} ions present in the ECF of synaptic cleft enter the axon terminal.
- The elevated Ca^{2+} levels in the cytosol of axon terminal stimulate the sliding of synaptic vesicles along the presynaptic grid towards the presynaptic membrane, presumably by triggering the cross-bridge movements.
- This results in marked increase in exocytosis of vesicles releasing neurotransmitter into the synaptic cleft (Fig. 10.7-4). Usually, only one type of neurotransmitter is released from all the terminals of a single neuron. This was first *propounded* by Dale, and is called *Dale's phenomenon*.

Note: Neurexins are proteins bound to the presynaptic membrane which bind neurexin receptor located on the postsynaptic membrane. There are more than 1000 different types of neurexins that provide synapse specificity. The proteins involved during the process of vesicle docking and fusion with nerve endings are:

- V snare protein (SNAP), responsible for fusion of vesicle to cell membrane.
- Synaptobrevin responsible for docking the vesicle membrane with t-snare protein (syntexin) in the cell membrane.
- Multiprotein complex regulated by small GTPases such as Rab 3 (Fig. 10.7-5)
- After being released from the presynaptic terminal, the transmitter diffuses across the synaptic cleft and binds to the postsynaptic receptors. The time lapse (<1 ms) occurring between arrival of nerve impulse at the presynaptic terminal and the effect of neurotransmitter on postsynaptic membrane is called *synaptic delay*.

B. Development of Excitatory Postsynaptic Potential (EPSP) and Inhibitory Postsynaptic Potential (IPSP)

Binding of the neurotransmitter to the postsynaptic receptors causes the opening of channels through which ions can flow. Both excitatory and inhibitory receptors exist on the postsynaptic membrane.

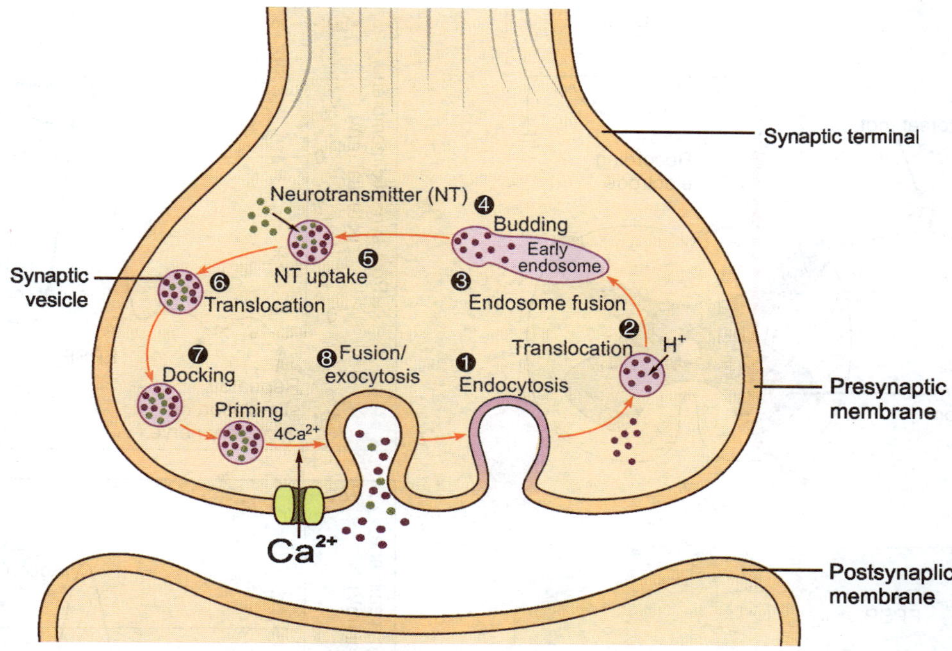

FIGURE 10.7-4 Steps of release of neurotransmitter at synaptic cleft and synaptic vesicle cycle in the pre synaptic terminal: 1, endocytosis; 2, vesicle formation; 3, endosomal fusion; 4, budding; 5, neurotransmitter uptake; 6, translocation; 7, docking; 8, exocytosis.

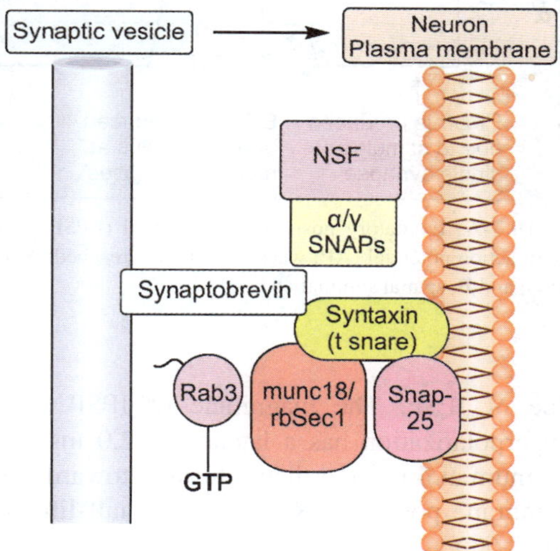

FIGURE 10.7-5 Proteins involved during process of synaptic vesicle docking and fusion in nerve endings.

Excitatory Postsynaptic Potential Excitatory postsynaptic potential (EPSP), i.e. depolarization of the postsynaptic membrane is produced by the excitatory neurotransmitters. The most common excitatory neurotransmitter within the CNS is *glutamate*. The magnitude of the EPSP is 8 mV. The depolarization starts with a latency of 0.5 ms, rises to its peak in 2.0 ms and then declines with a half-life of 4.0 ms (Fig. 10.7-6B).

Recording of EPSP. The EPSP is a local response. It can be studied by inserting a microelectrode into ventral horn cell of the spinal cord and stimulating the sensory nerve fibres in the dorsal root (Fig. 10.7-6A).

Ionic Basis of EPSP. The excitatory neurotransmitter binds with a specific receptor protein and opens the ligand-gated Na^+ channels on the postsynaptic membrane. As a result, the Na^+ ions diffuse inward and depolarize the membrane. However, since a very small area of postsynaptic membrane develops increased Na^+ permeability, the amount of Na^+ influx is able to produce only a brief depolarization followed by a slower decline to resting potential.

Conduction of EPSP. The EPSP does not transmit over the cell. However, it can depolarize the adjacent membrane. This occurs passively due to local currents which are setup.

Summation of EPSP. The EPSP is a graded response. It does not follow all-or-none law like action potential. It shows temporal and spatial summation.

- ***Temporal summation*** occurs when repeated stimuli are applied at very short intervals (i.e. before the EPSP due to previous stimulus has decayed). The next stimulus adds to the previous postsynaptic potential producing a large response (Fig. 10.7-7A).
- ***Spatial summation*** occurs when postsynaptic membrane receives impulses from a large number of presynaptic terminals simultaneously. The effect of all the impulses is added up and enough transmitter substance is released to cause a greater response (Fig. 10.7-7B).

Both types of summations occur simultaneously in the neuronal pool. When the temporal or more commonly spatial summation brings the membrane potential of the cell to the firing level, an action potential is fired and propagated in the postsynaptic neuron.

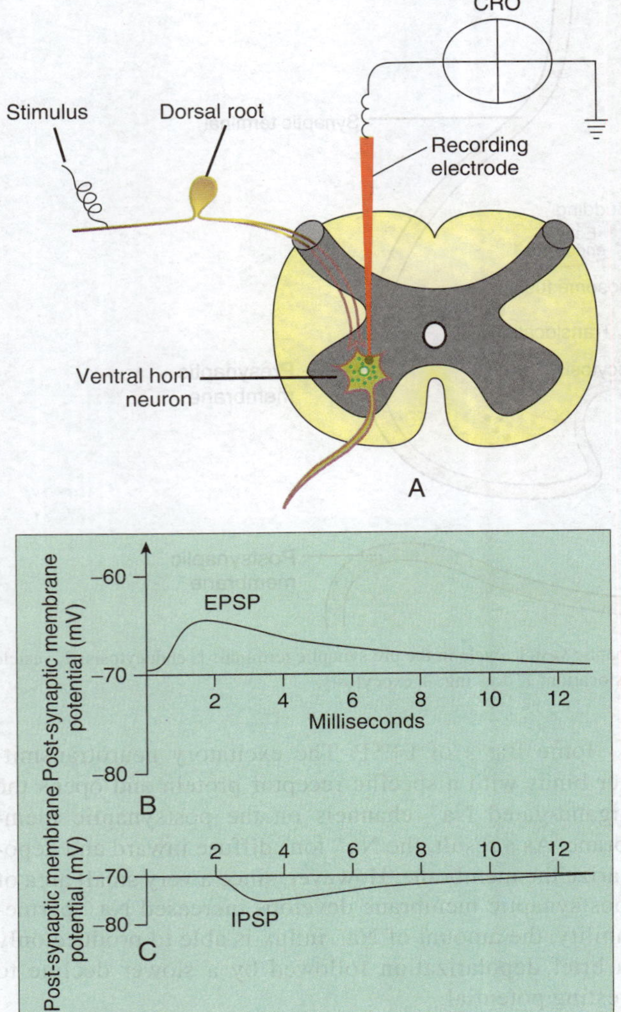

FIGURE 10.7-6 Excitatory postsynaptic potential (EPSP) and inhibitory postsynaptic potential (IPSP): **A,** method of recording of EPSP and IPSP; **B,** the record of EPSP; and **C,** the record of IPSP.

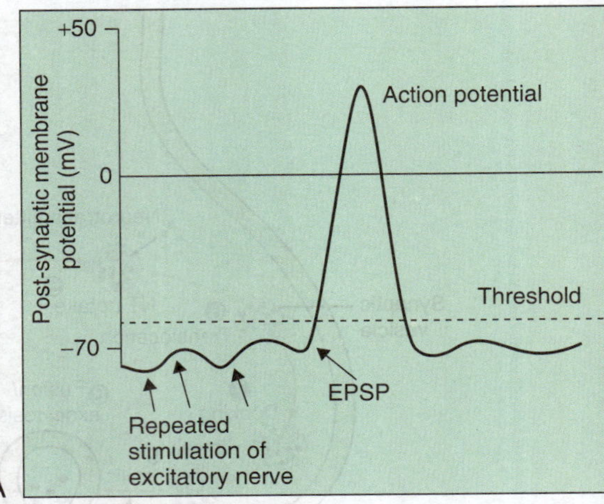

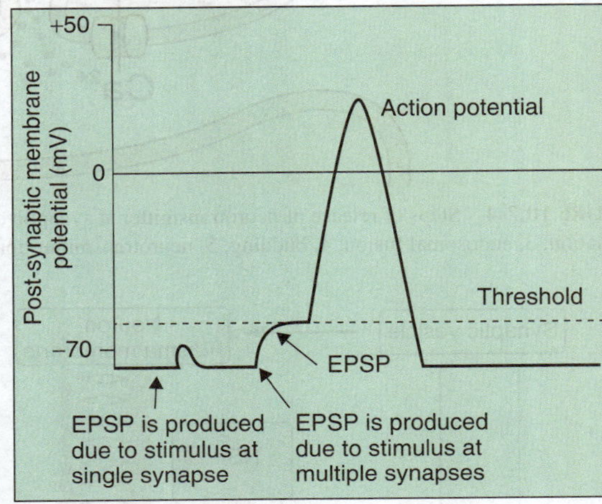

FIGURE 10.7-7 Excitatory postsynaptic potential (EPSP) summation resulting in action potential (AP) when threshold is reached: **A,** temporal summation; and **B,** spatial summation.

Inhibitory Postsynaptic Potential Inhibitory postsynaptic potential (IPSP), i.e. hyperpolarization of the postsynaptic membrane, is produced by the inhibitory neurotransmitters released in the synaptic cleft. The most common inhibitory neurotransmitters within the CNS are *glycine* and γ-aminobutyric acid (GABA). IPSP is produced by stimulation of certain presynaptic fibres which regularly initiate a hyperpolarizing response in spinal motor neurons.

Ionic Basis of IPSP. The inhibitory transmitter released at the synaptic cleft causes opening of either K^+ channels or Cl^- channels in the postsynaptic membrane, leading to diffusion of large number of K^+ ions from the neuron to the extracellular fluid or large number of Cl^- ions to diffuse to the interior of the neuron. This causes postsynaptic membrane potential to become more negative (*hyperpolarization*). This change in potential is called IPSP.

Value of IPSP. The magnitude of IPSP is −2mV. The hyperpolarization has a latency of 2.0 ms, attaining its maximum at 4 ms and then returning towards the resting membrane potential (RMP) with a half-life of 3 ms (Fig. 10.7-6C).

Recording of IPSP can be made by a technique similar to that of recording of EPSP (Fig. 10.7-6A).

Summation of IPSP. Spatial and temporal summation also occurs, as seen with EPSP (Fig. 10.7-7). This type of inhibition is called postsynaptic (or direct) inhibition.

Arrangement of Neurons Involved in Production of EPSP and IPSP Afferent fibres in the dorsal nerve root mostly have EPSP-producing terminals (page 1006 Fig. 10.7-18). Both afferents A and B release EPSP-producing neurotransmitter. Stimulation of afferent B produces IPSP because of the intervention of Golgi bottle neuron that releases an inhibitory chemical transmitter (glycine) near the ventral horn cells. The Golgi bottle neurons are small plump cells present in the grey matter of the spinal cord, inserted in the pathway between the dorsal root afferents and the ventral horn cells (an interneuron).

C. Inactivation of Neurotransmitter from the Synaptic Cleft

The neurotransmitter released in the synaptic cleft from the presynaptic terminal is soon inactivated in one of the three ways:

- Diffusion of the transmitter out of the cleft, or
- Enzymatic degradation of the transmitter, e.g. dissociation of acetylcholine by acetylcholinesterase or
- Active transport back into the presynaptic terminal (transmitter reuptake), e.g. active reuptake of norepinephrine at sympathetic postganglionic nerve endings.

The amount of chemical transmitter present in a synaptic knob is exhausted within a few seconds to a few minutes of maximal neuronal activity. However, synthesis of the chemical transmitter at the nerve terminal goes on continuously and new vesicles are formed as quickly as they are used up.

The inactivation of the neurotransmitter is essential so that in response to a single electrical impulse, there is release of a transient pulse of the neurotransmitter in the synaptic cleft. Persistence of the transmitter in the synaptic cleft would have produced prolonged stimulation of the postsynaptic neuron in response to a single electrical impulse in the presynaptic neuron.

D. Development of Action Potential

The development of action potential (AP) from EPSP can be considered in three steps:

- Synaptic integration,
- Generation of the initial segment spike and
- Generation of propagated signals, i.e. action potential.

Synaptic Integration. Synaptic integration refers to the phenomenon of summation (temporal as well as spatial as described above) of both EPSP and IPSP produced at the postsynaptic membrane. It is the net algebraically summated potential which determines whether synaptic transmission will occur or not. For example, if there are five presynaptic neurons of which three produce EPSP (+ 8 mV each), and the other two produce IPSP (−2 mV each), the summated potential will be $(+8 \times 3) + (-2 \times 2) = +20$ mV and synaptic transmission will occur. On the other hand, if only one produces EPSP (+8 mV) and the other four produce IPSP (−2 mV each), then the summated potential will be equal to zero and no synaptic transmission will occur.

It is important to note that after giving out the summated output (i.e. after synaptic integration), the entire soma-dendritic tree is quickly resorted to its resting potential by the *soma-dendritic (SD) spike,* i.e. the action potential that travels retrogradely over the soma and dendrites (as described below). It allows fresh summation of subsequently generated EPSPs and IPSPs.

Generation of Initial Segment Spike. The summated potential (EPSP and IPSPs) produced by the excitatory and inhibitory neurotransmitters spreads passively to the initial segment which comprises axon hillock and the proximal part of the unmyelinated nerve fibres. If the summated potential is large enough to depolarize the initial segment of neuron to threshold level of about 6–10 mV (the threshold of initial segment is lowest as compared to the other parts of the nerve fibre), a spike potential called the *initial spike* (IS) is generated (Fig. 10.7-8). The magnitude of IS is 30–40 mV from the threshold level.

Generation of Propagated Signals, i.e. Action Potential. The IS spike requires a relatively low degree of depolarization for its own production (due to low threshold value of initial segment), but once initiated, it itself produces a further depolarization of 30–40 mV by opening the voltage-gated channels on the axon hillock (the sodium channels are plenty in axon hillock than in any other part of the soma). Thus, the IS spike in turn triggers the generation of the action potential (AP) spike (Fig. 10.7-8). Once generated, the AP travels in both directions, i.e. peripherally in the axon as a nerve impulse and also retrogradely over the cell membrane of soma and dendrites. This backward conducted AP is called the *soma-dendritic (SD) spike*. The SD spike (as described above) helps to clear the existing EPSP so that the cell is ready to react to another set of stimuli.

Inhibition at Synapses

Four different types of inhibitions known to occur at synapses in the CNS are:

- Postsynaptic inhibition,
- Presynaptic inhibition,

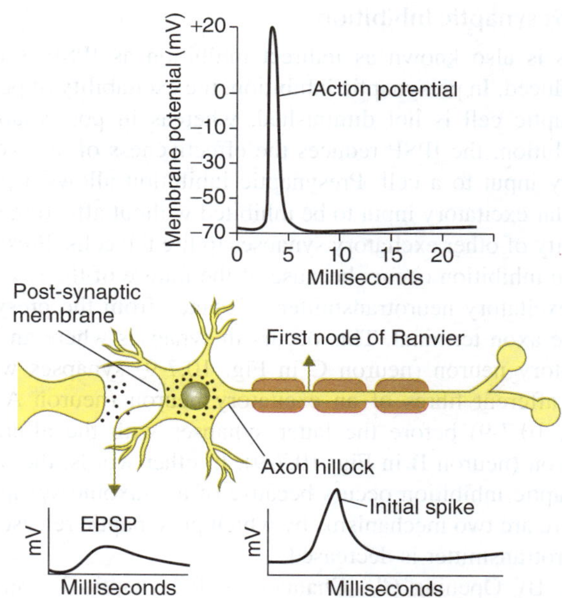

FIGURE 10.7-8 Summated postsynaptic potential producing initial spike (IS) and action potential (AP).

- Feedback inhibition and
- Feed-forward inhibition.

1. Postsynaptic Inhibition

The postsynaptic inhibition, i.e. inhibition of the postsynaptic membrane, can occur by the following mechanisms:

i. Direct Postsynaptic Inhibition by Development of Inhibitory Postsynaptic Potential (IPSP) (as described above, page 1000) occurs due to release of inhibitory neurotransmitters.

ii. Postsynaptic Inhibition without Development of IPSP can occur due to some short-circuiting mechanism as described:

In some neurons, the concentration differences for K^+ and Cl^- ions are such that the Nernst potential of these ions are equal to the resting membrane potential (RMP) of the neuron. Therefore, even if either K^+ or Cl^- channels open, there is no net transfer of ions in either direction and no EPSP can develop. But when the neuron is excited through other synapse causing inflow of Na^+ ions, the rapid flux of K^+ and Cl^- ions (because K^+ and Cl^- channels are open) would nullify EPSP produced. Greater influx of Na^+ is therefore required to overcome K^+ or Cl^- flux and cause excitation (may be 5–20 times the normal). This tendency of K^+ or Cl^- ions to maintain potential to RMP level (when channels are wide open) masks the effect of sodium current flow by excitatory synapse, thus causing inhibition.

iii. Postsynaptic Inhibition due to Refractory Period. Sometimes, the postsynaptic membrane can be refractory to the excitation because it has just fired and is in its refractory period, i.e. existing EPSP has not been still cleared by the soma-dendritic (SD) spike.

2. Presynaptic Inhibition

This is also known as indirect inhibition as IPSP is not produced. In presynaptic inhibition, the excitability of postsynaptic cell is not diminished, whereas in postsynaptic inhibition, the IPSP reduces the effectiveness of all excitatory input to a cell. Presynaptic inhibition allows a particular excitatory input to be inhibited without affecting the ability of other excitatory synapses to fire the cells. Presynaptic inhibition occurs because of the failure of the release of excitatory neurotransmitter substance from the presynaptic axon terminal. This occurs in synapses where an inhibitory neuron (neuron C in Fig. 10.7-9) synapses with the afferent fibres of an excitatory neuron (neuron A in Fig. 10.7-9) before the latter synapses with the afferent neuron (neuron B in Fig. 10.7-9). In other words, the presynaptic inhibition occurs because of axo-axonic synapse. There are two mechanisms by which presynaptic release of neurotransmitter is decreased:

i. By Opening Cl^- Channels of Presynaptic Terminal. The inhibitory neuron (neuron C in Fig. 10.7-9) releases an inhibitory neurotransmitter (i.e. GABA) which binds to

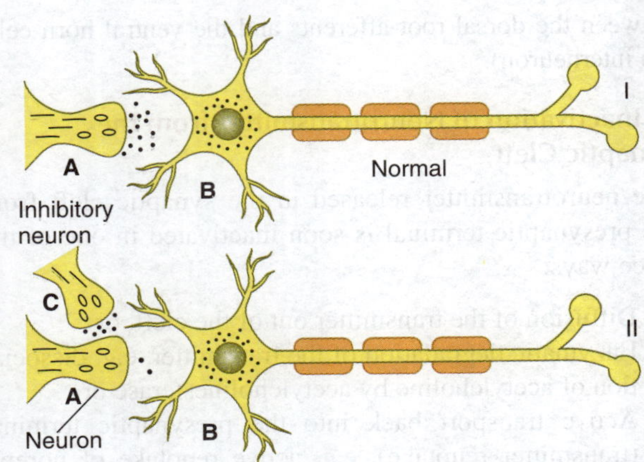

FIGURE 10.7-9 Presynaptic inhibition produced by an inhibitory neuron (C) which synapses with presynaptic axon terminal (A), i.e. by axo-axonic synapse. I: Normal excitatory neurotransmitter released by presynaptic terminal (A); and II: Reduced excitatory neurotransmitter released by presynaptic terminal (A) due to effect of inhibitory neuron (C).

GABA-gated Cl^- channels on the presynaptic neuron terminal (neuron A in Fig. 10.7-9). Increase in Cl^- permeability results in hyperpolarization of the presynaptic axon terminal (neuron A). When an action potential (AP) arrives at the presynaptic terminal, the size of AP is reduced because of the increased Cl^- conductance. Because of smaller size of AP, less Ca^{2+} enters the nerve terminal, and thus the amount of excitatory neurotransmitter released is markedly decreased.

ii. By Activation of G Protein. When the inhibitory transmitter GABA released from the inhibitory neuron (neuron C in Fig. 10.7-9) binds to a receptor called a *GABA receptor,* it activates a *G protein*. The G protein aids in reducing the amount of excitatory neurotransmitter released from the presynaptic terminal (neuron A) by acting in one of two ways:

- ***By opening K^+ channels.*** The G proteins may open K^+ channels that reduce the size of AP reaching the nerve terminal by hyperpolarizing the presynaptic nerve terminal.
- ***By directly blocking the Ca^{2+} channels.*** The G protein may directly block the opening of Ca^{2+} channels that normally occurs when the AP reaches the nerve terminal; consequently, less Ca^{2+} enters the presynaptic terminal and the amount of excitatory neurotransmitter release is diminished.

3. Feedback Inhibition

The feedback inhibition, also known as *Renshaw cell inhibition,* is known to occur in spinal alpha motor neurons through an inhibitory interneuron (the Renshaw cell, Fig. 10.7-10). In feedback (or recurrent) inhibition, a neuron inhibits those very neuron(s) that excite it. In other words, a neuron is inhibited by its own output (that is why it is called negative feedback inhibition). In this way, firing of an action potential by a motor neuron of the spinal cord is followed by a phase of

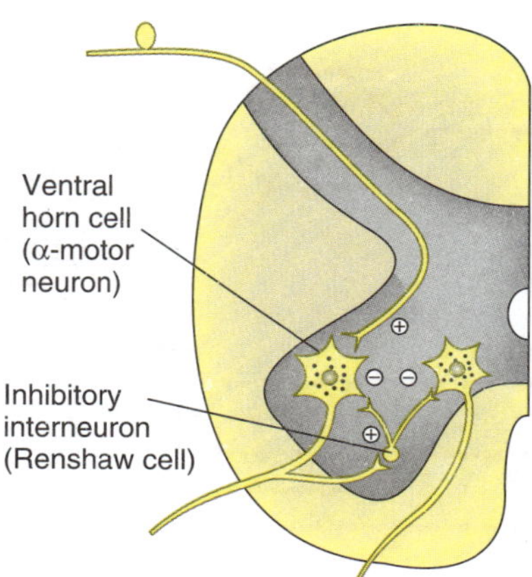

FIGURE 10.7-10 Renshaw cell when excited by a recurrent branch of an alpha motor neuron produces feedback inhibition of the soma of the same and other motor neurons.

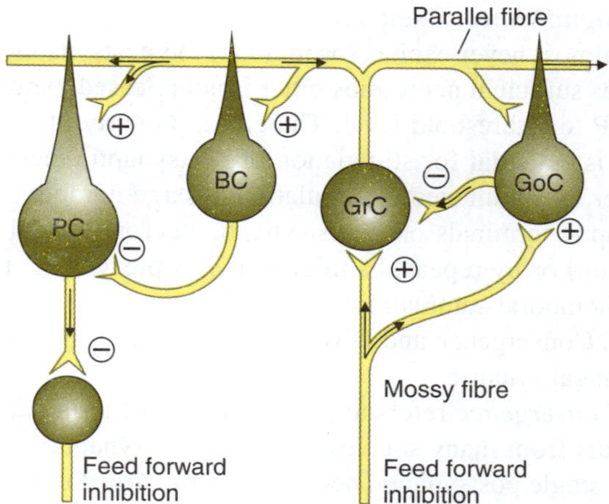

FIGURE 10.7-11 Feed-forward inhibition of Purkinje cell (PC) by basket cell (BC). Note that both Purkinje cell and basket cell are excited by the granule cell (GrC).

hyperpolarization (inhibition) of not only the same motor neuron but also many others in the neighbourhood. The feedback inhibition is thus basically a postsynaptic inhibition but is classified separately because the inhibitor Renshaw cells are activated by a collateral of the ventral horn cell rather than an afferent neuron. This type of feedback inhibition is also seen in other parts of CNS as well. It serves to limit the excitability of the motor neurons.

4. Feed-forward Inhibition

Feed-forward inhibition is seen in cerebellum. In this type of inhibition, a neuron is connected through two pathways: one excitatory and other inhibitory. For example, in cerebellum, the granule cell (Gr C) excites Purkinje cells (PC), which is soon inhibited by the basket cell (BC), which in turn was also excited by the granule cell (Fig. 10.7-11). This type of arrangement in the cerebellum limits the duration of excitation produced by any given afferent volley, i.e. allows a brief and precisely timed excitation.

Significance of Synaptic Inhibition

In central nervous system (CNS), the synaptic inhibition offers a type of restriction over neurons and muscles to react properly and appropriately. Thus, the inhibition helps to select the exact number of impulses and to omit or block the excess ones. When the inhibitory system at synaptic level is destroyed, for example, by a poison like strychnine, there occurs continuous and convulsive activity even with slight stimulation. In the nervous disorders like Parkinsonism, the inhibitory system is impaired resulting in rigidity.

Properties of Synaptic Transmission

Some characteristic features of synaptic transmission are described briefly:

1. One-way Conduction. The chemical synapse allows only one-way conduction of an impulse, i.e. from the presynaptic to the postsynaptic neuron and never in the opposite direction. This is called the law of dynamic polarity or Bell–Magendie law.

Cause. One-way conduction occurs because only the presynaptic nerve terminals contain the chemical neurotransmitter, whereas the postsynaptic membrane contains the specific receptor sites. Therefore, an impulse conducted antidromically in an axon dies out at the soma due to absence of the chemical transmitter in the cell body.

Significance. The axons can conduct impulse in either direction with equal ease. However, the synapses act like a valve and are responsible for the orderly conduction of impulse in one direction only.

2. Synaptic Delay. Synaptic delay refers to a time lapse which occurs between arrival of nerve impulse at the presynaptic terminal and its passage to the postsynaptic membrane. Normally, synaptic delay occurs by approximately 0.5 ms (almost always less than 1 ms).

Causes of synaptic delay include time taken for:

- Release of neurotransmitter,
- Diffusion of transmitter through synaptic cleft to postsynaptic membrane,
- Action of neurotransmitter to bind with receptors on the postsynaptic membrane and to cause the opening of ion channels and
- Diffusion of ions causing changes in resting membrane potential (i.e. development of EPSP or IPSP).

Significance. When an impulse passes through a chain of neurons, it is delayed at every synapse. The synaptic delay is one of the causes for the latent period of the reflex activity. The number of neurons involved in the reflex can be estimated from the duration of reaction time of a reflex action.

3. Summation Property of Synapse. A synapse exhibits property of both temporal and spatial summation of EPSP and IPSP (see page 999).

Significance. Excitation of a single presynaptic terminal almost never excites (or inhibits) the postsynaptic neuron as sufficient neurotransmitter is not released to raise the EPSP to a threshold level. Therefore, property of summation is essential for stimulation of postsynaptic membrane either by simultaneous stimulation of large number of presynaptic terminals on a postsynaptic neuron (spatial summation) or by repeated stimulation of a presynaptic terminal (temporal summation).

4. Convergence and Divergence property is present in a chemical synapse.

Convergence refers to a phenomenon of termination of signals from many sources (i.e. many presynaptic neurons on a single postsynaptic neuron). Information coming from large number of presynaptic neurons is integrated to decide the onward effect. For example, ventral horn cells of the spinal cord receive convergent signals from corticospinal tract, reticulospinal tract, rubrospinal tract and sensory afferent from dorsal root, etc. (Fig. 10.7-12).

Divergence. One presynaptic neuron may terminate on many postsynaptic neurons. Thus, a single impulse is converted to a number of impulses going to a number of postsynaptic neurons which may travel in the same tract or into multiple tracts (Fig. 10.7-13). This causes magnification and therefore helps in amplification of an impulse. This phenomenon is known as divergence.

5. Occlusion Phenomenon. The term occlusion describes the situation in which response to stimulation of two presynaptic neurons is less than the sum total of the response obtained when they are stimulated separately. For example, when two presynaptic neurons (say A and B) are stimulated separately, each stimulates 10 postsynaptic neurons (making a total of 20), but when stimulated simultaneously, they stimulate less than 20 postsynaptic neurons (say 15). This happens because of the fact that some postsynaptic neurons are common to both the presynaptic neurons (Fig. 10.7-14). Thus, occlusion is due to overlapping of afferent fibres in their central distribution.

6. Subliminal Fringe Effect. An afferent nerve fibre divides into many hundred branches. Of these, a large number may terminate on one efferent neuron, while a smaller number terminate on other efferent neuron lying nearby. When an afferent neuron is stimulated, the efferent (postsynaptic) neuron that has many presynaptic terminals is excited to threshold level and action potential (AP) is fired. Others in the peripheral zone (fringe area) are excited to subthreshold level only, i.e. their excitability is increased but an AP is not fired. This is known as *subliminal fringe effect* (subliminal means below threshold and fringe means border). Thus, the postsynaptic neurons

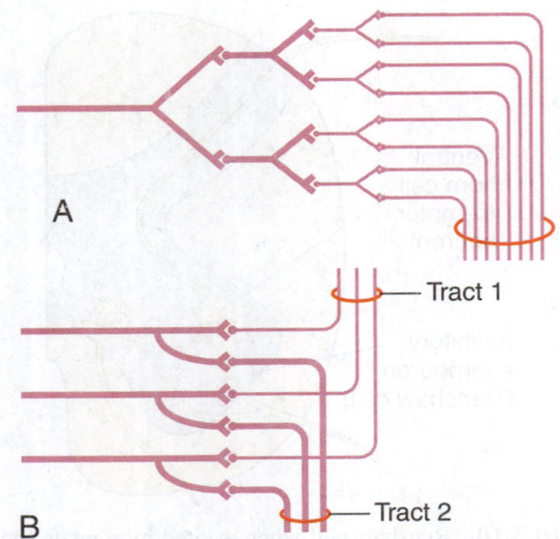

FIGURE 10.7-13 Phenomenon of divergence: **A,** divergence in same tract; and **B,** divergence into multiple tracts.

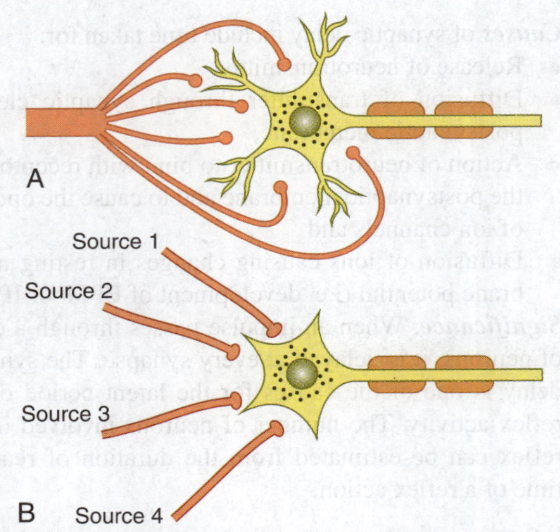

FIGURE 10.7-12 Convergence of signals on a single neuron: **A,** convergence from a single source; and **B,** convergence from multiple sources (e.g. ventral horn cell of spinal cord).

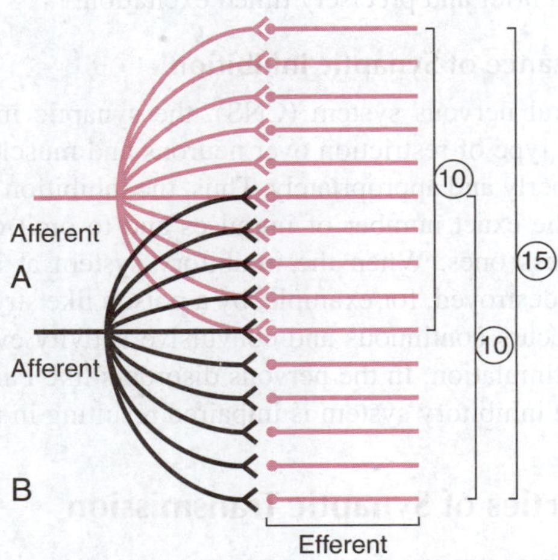

FIGURE 10.7-14 Occlusion phenomenon: stimulation of afferent neuron **A** and **B** each excites 10 efferent neurons. Simultaneous stimulation of neuron **A** and **B** together excites 15 efferent neurons because 5 efferent neurons are common to both.

that are fired are said to be in discharging zone and those which are not fired are said to be in subliminal fringe (i.e. not in the discharging zone).

Because of subliminal fringe effect, the response obtained by the simultaneous stimulation of two presynaptic neurons is greater than the sum total response obtained when they are separately stimulated. This is exactly opposite to occlusion and can be explained as below. Suppose separate stimulation of afferent neurons 'A' and 'B' each causes depolarization of five efferent neurons and subliminal fringe effect in two efferent neurons, then a total of 10 efferent neurons are stimulated. But when neurons A and B are stimulated simultaneously, the number of postsynaptic neurons stimulated is more (say 12) (Fig. 10.7-15). This is because of the fact that two efferent neurons which are excited subliminally both by the neuron A and B summate to produce threshold stimulation. This is another example of spatial summation.

Physiological significance. As a result of summation, occlusion and subliminal fringe effect, the patterns of impulses in peripheral nerves are usually altered as they pass through synapses on the way to brain. One such effect is phenomenon of referred pain (see page 1031).

7. Facilitation. When presynaptic axon is stimulated with several consecutive individual stimuli, each stimulus may evoke a larger postsynaptic potential than that evoked by previous stimulus. This phenomenon is known as facilitation.

Mechanism. Each succeeding stimulus increases the duration of action potential in the presynaptic neuron, so the voltage-gated Ca^{2+} channels can remain open for a prolonged period liberating more neurotransmitter by exocytosis from the presynaptic neuron. In facilitation, therefore, normally a subliminal stimulus from a presynaptic neuron primes the postsynaptic neuron, so that another subliminal

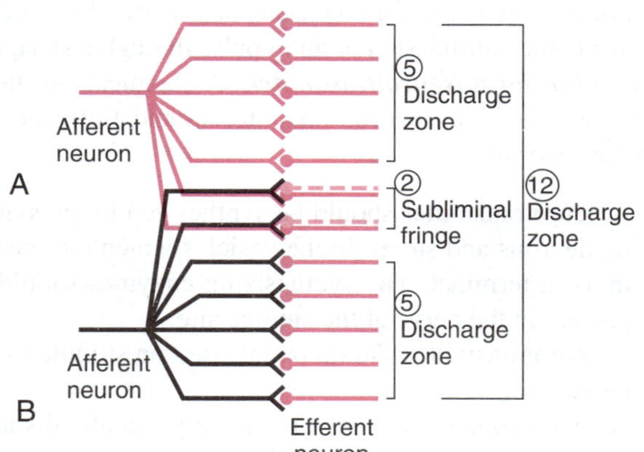

FIGURE 10.7-15 Subliminal fringe effect: stimulation of afferent neuron **A** and **B** each excites five efferent neurons and subliminal fringe effect on two efferent neurons (which are common to both **A** and **B** neurons). Simultaneous stimulation of neuron **A** and **B** together excites 12 efferent neurons because the subliminal fringe effect on 2 neurons gets summated to produce threshold stimulation.

stimulus can evoke a discharge from the postsynaptic neuron. Hence, the first stimulus is supposed to facilitate the effect due to prolonged exposure of postsynaptic neuron to the neurotransmitter.

8. Synaptic Fatigue. When the presynaptic neuron is stimulated separately, the rate of impulse discharge in the postsynaptic neuron is initially high but within a few seconds there occurs a gradual decrease and finally disappearance of the postsynaptic response. This phenomenon is called *synaptic fatigue* or *habituation*. Fatigue is a temporary phenomenon. Therefore, fatigue and recovery from fatigue constitute an important short-term mechanism for modulating sensitivities of different neuronal circuits.

Mechanism. Fatigue mainly occurs due to *exhaustion of chemical neurotransmitter,* as at high rate of impulse transmission, the synthesis of chemical transmitter fails to keep pace with rate of release at presynaptic terminals. Other factors contributing to fatigue are:

- Progressive decreased release of neurotransmitter due to a gradual inactivation of Ca^{2+} channels which decrease the intracellular Ca^{2+},
- Accumulation of waste products and
- Refractiveness of postsynaptic membrane to transmitter substance.

9. Synaptic Plasticity and Learning. Plasticity refers to capability of being easily moulded or changed. Synaptic transmission can be increased or decreased on the basis of past experience. The changes in synaptic transmission can occur due to alterations at pre- or postsynaptic location. Plastic changes in synaptic transmission known are:

- Post-tetanic potentiation,
- Long-term potentiation,
- Synaptic fatigue or habituation (see page1005),
- Sensitization and
- Low-frequency depression.

i. ***Post-tetanic potentiation***. When a presynaptic neuron is stimulated with a single stimulus, followed by stimulation with a volley of stimuli (says 100/s) for 2 s and then again with a single stimulus, the second stimulus evokes a larger postsynaptic response than the first stimulus. The phenomenon is called post-tetanic potentiation. This occurs due to the fact that a brief tetanizing stimulus in the presynaptic neuron results in an increase in intracellular Ca^{2+} due to increased Ca^{2+} influx (Fig. 10.7-16).

ii. ***Long-term potentiation***. When the post-tetanic potentiation gets much more prolonged and lasts for days, it is called long-term potentiation. It occurs due to an increase in the intracellular Ca^{2+} in the postsynaptic neuron rather than the presynaptic neuron. This phenomenon commonly occurs in the hippocampus.

iii. ***Sensitization***. Sensitization refers to prolonged occurrence of increased postsynaptic responses after a stimulus

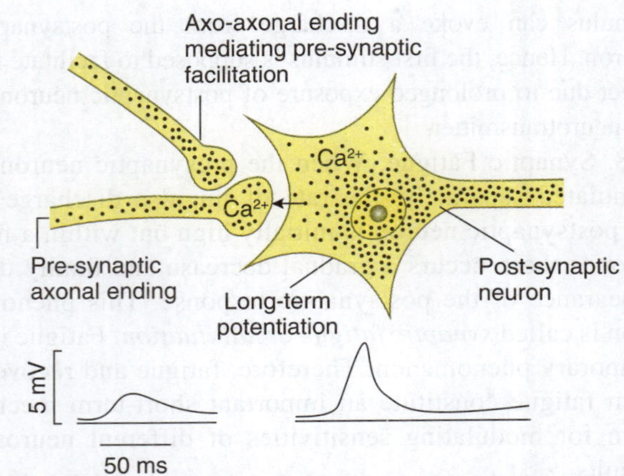

FIGURE 10.7-16 Synaptic plasticity: presynaptic and postsynaptic sites producing changes in the strength of synaptic transmission.

is paired once or several times with a noxious stimulus. It is basically *presynaptic facilitation* of an impulse that occurs due to Ca^{2+}-mediated changes in adenylyl cyclase that results in greater production of cAMP.

10. Reverberation. Reverberation refers to the phenomenon of passage of impulse from presynaptic neuron and again back to presynaptic neuron to cause a continuous stimulation of presynaptic neuron. Nervous system is a network of fibres and in this network it is possible that a branch of axon of a neuron may establish connection with its own dendron. This causes reverberation of impulse through same circuit again and again (Fig. 10.7-17). This is prevented to some extent by phenomenon of fatigue.

11. Reciprocal Inhibition. Reciprocal inhibition refers to a phenomenon in which an afferent signal activates an excitatory neuron to a group of muscles and simultaneously activates inhibitory signals to other, usually antagonistic muscles. For example, during flexion of a joint, the afferent stimulus causes excitation of the neurons supplying the flexor muscles of the joint and at the same time a branch of afferent fibre excites an inhibitory interneuron which synapses with motor neuron supplying the extensor muscles of the joint (Fig. 10.7-18).

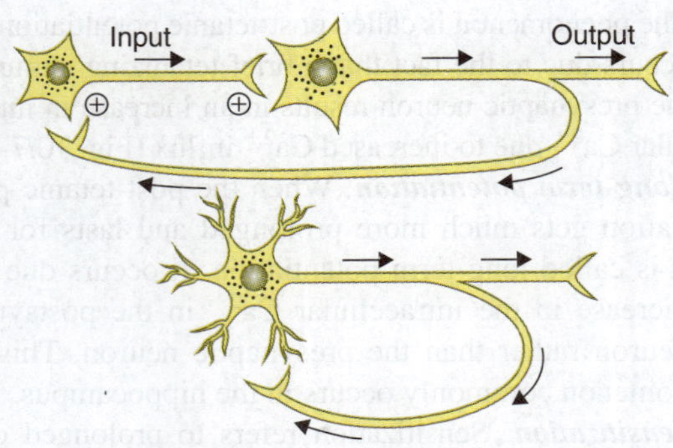

FIGURE 10.7-17 Reverberating circuit.

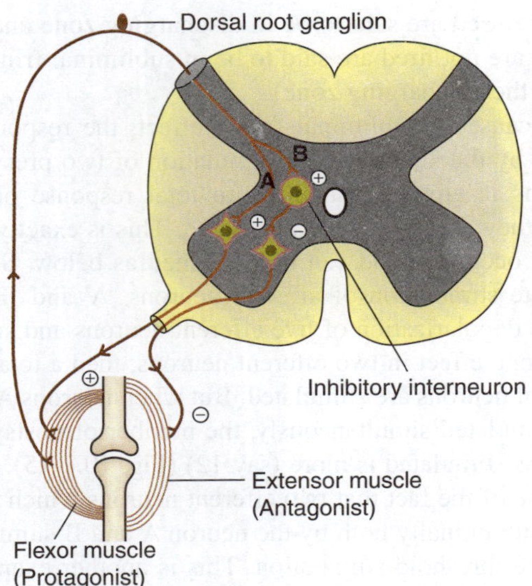

FIGURE 10.7-18 Neuronal arrangement of reciprocal inhibition. An afferent stimulus producing contraction of flexors of a joint (through A) and causes inhibition of extensors (through B) by intervention of an inhibitory neuron.

12. After Discharge. After discharge of a synapse refers to a phenomenon in which a single instantaneous input results into sustained output signals (i.e. a series of repetitive discharges). Input signals only for 1 ms and output signal lasts for many milliseconds.

13. Effect of Acidosis and Hypoxia. The CNS neurons cannot sustain lack of oxygen. Synaptic transmission is particularly vulnerable to the effect of acidosis and hypoxia. This may explain why the first site of fatigue of the synaptic chain is located in the brain.

NEUROTRANSMITTERS

Definition

Neurotransmitters are the chemical substances which are responsible for transmission of an impulse through a synapse.

Criteria for a Neurotransmitter. A chemical substance to be qualified as a neurotransmitter should fulfil the following criteria:

- A neurotransmitter should be synthesized by presynaptic neurons and stored in the vesicles which are present in axon terminal. The synthesizing enzymes should be present in the nerve at the storage site.
- A neurotransmitter should be released on stimulation of nerve.
- A neurotransmitter travels a very small distance between presynaptic membrane and postsynaptic membrane.
- A neurotransmitter is associated with an enzyme or enzyme system for its inactivation.
- A neurotransmitter when applied extrinsically should mimic the effects of the nerve stimulation.

- Drug, which modifies the response to nerve stimulation, should also modify the proposed transmitter action in a similar way.

Extended Definition of Neurotransmitter also includes, in addition to the principal neurotransmitters, the following chemical substances:

- ***Neuromediators*** or ***neurohormones***. These chemical substances are synthesized in neurons and poured into the bloodstream through terminals resembling synapses in structure. Similar chemical substances are also poured into the cerebrospinal fluid or into the intercellular spaces to influence other neurons in a diffuse manner.
- ***Neuromodulators*** are the chemical substances which are associated with synapses but do not influence synaptic transmission directly, but influence the effects of transmitters or of neuromediators. Several peptides found in the nervous system probably act as neuromodulators. These include substance P, vasoactive intestinal polypeptide (VIP), somatostatin, cholecystokinin and many others.

General Characteristics of Action of Neurotransmitters

- The neurotransmitter released from the presynaptic membrane diffuses through the synaptic cleft to postsynaptic membrane. The postsynaptic cell may be a neuron, muscular cell or glandular cell.
- On the postsynaptic membrane, the neurotransmitter combines with a receptor protein. The receptor of the effector cell may be associated with:
  - Ion channels that alter the membrane potential of the cell, or
  - An enzyme that results in the formation of a second messenger in the effector cell.
- Action of neurotransmitter occurs within milliseconds; therefore, changes induced are fast and direct.
- A neurotransmitter can activate both postsynaptic and presynaptic receptors.
- The neurons may release more than one transmitter which interact often both presynptically and postsynaptically with specific receptors and produce effects. The balance between various transmitters released may vary under different conditions so that differential release of one or other mediator may result from varying impulse patterns.

Classification

At present, more than 50 substances have been reported to fulfil the criteria as a neurotransmitter. Generally, these substances can be classified in two ways:

Biochemical Classification Biochemically, neurotransmitters can be divided into two groups:

A. Small Molecule Neurotransmitters. These act rapidly and cause acute response. These are synthesized and packed into synaptic vesicles in the axon terminal. Important small molecule neurotransmitters with their site of release given in *parentheses* are as:

I. *Acetylcholine (Ach):*
- Neuromuscular junction,
- All preganglionic autonomic neurons,
- All postganglionic parasympathetic neurons,
- Postganglionic sympathetic neurons to sweat glands and skeletal muscle blood vessels,
- Some amacrine cells of retina and
- Many parts of CNS.

II. *Biogenic amines*
- Catecholamines: epinephrine (EP), norepinephrine (NE), dopamine.
- Serotonin (5hydroxytryptamine, 5HT) and
- Histamine.

III. *Amino acid neurotransmitters*
- Gamma-aminobutyric acid (GABA),
- Glycine,
- Glutamic acid or glutamate and
- Aspartic acid or aspartate.
- Adenosine triphosphate (ATP)

B. Neuropeptide Transmitters. These are large molecules, slowly acting and have prolonged effect. These neurotransmitters include:

- Neuroactive peptides.
- Pituitary peptides.
- Peptides acting on the gut and brain.
- Neuropeptides from other tissues.

In general, neuropeptides are colocalized with one of the small molecule neurotransmitters (Table 10.7-2).

TABLE 10.7.2 Small Molecule Neurotransmitters and Their Colocalization with Various Neuropeptides

Neurotransmitters	Neuropeptide
1. Acetylcholine	Substance P, vasoactive intestinal peptide (VIP), somatostatin, GnRH, enkaphlin, calcitonin gene-related protein (CGRP) and neurotensin
2. GABA	Substance P, somatostatin, cholecystokinin and TRH
3. Glycine	Neurotensin
4. Glutamate	Substance P
5. Norepinephrine	Enkaphlin, neuropeptide-Y, somatostatin, vasopressin and neurotensin
6. Epinephrine	Enkaphlin, neuropeptide-Y, neurotensin and substance P
7. Dopamine	Enkaphlin, somatostatin and cholecystokinin
8. Serotonin	Cholecystokinin, NPY, substance P and VIP

Physiological Classification Some of the neurotransmitters cause excitation of postsynaptic neurons, while others cause inhibition. Thus, physiologically, neurotransmitters can be divided into two groups:

- Excitatory neurotransmitters and
- Inhibitory neurotransmitters.

1. ***Excitatory neurotransmitters*** can cause an action potential (if the target cell is another neuron), contraction (if the target cell is a muscle) or secretion (if the target cell is a gland).

   In the CNS, the excitatory neurotransmitters produce a depolarization of the postsynaptic membrane called the excitatory postsynaptic potential (EPSP). The most common excitatory neurotransmitter within the CNS is glutamate. Other excitatory neurotransmitters are acetylcholine, aspartic acid, etc.
2. ***Inhibitory neurotransmitters*** reduce or block the activity of the postsynaptic cell. They produce a hyperpolarization of the postsynaptic membrane called the inhibitory postsynaptic potential (IPSP). The most common inhibitory neurotransmitters within the CNS are *glycine* or *gamma-aminobutyric* acid (GABA). Other inhibitory neurotransmitters include dopamine.

Receptors

The action of neurotransmitter on its target depends on the type of receptor on which it acts rather than on the properties of the mediator. The receptors on which these neurotransmitters act are discussed along with individual neurotransmitter. The main general characteristics of the receptors are:

- Each chemical mediator has potential to act on many subtypes of receptors. For example, norepinephrine acts on α_1, α_2, β_1, β_2 and β_3 subtypes of adrenergic receptors. This makes the effect of the ligand on the cell more selective.
- For many secreted neurotransmitters, the receptors are present on presynaptic as well as on the postsynaptic membrane. The presynaptic receptors are of two types: autoreceptors and heteroreceptors
  - *Autoreceptors* inhibit further secretion of the neurotransmitters by feedback control (e.g. norepinephrine acts on α_2 presynaptic receptors and inhibits its further secretion).
  - *Heteroreceptors* are another type of presynaptic receptors which are activated by different ligands rather than secreted by nerve endings on which the receptor is located (e.g. norepinephrine acts on cholinergic nerve endings to inhibit the release of Ach).
- All the receptors and their subtypes are basically divided into two main groups: ionotropic and metabotropic receptors.
  - *Ionotropic receptors* are ligand-gated membrane channels. When the ligand binds to the receptor, the membrane channel opens (activation) and increases the ion conductance. The activation is for a brief period (few milliseconds); therefore, these receptors are meant for fast synaptic transmission.
  - *Metabotropic receptors* are G protein-coupled transmembrane receptors (GPCR). When the neurotransmitter binds to the receptors, the activated receptor initiates production of second messenger that modulates the voltage-gated channels present on the neuronal membrane.
- On the postsynaptic membrane, receptors are concentrated in clusters close to the endings of presynaptic neuron that secrete specific neurotransmitter for them. This is because of presence of specific binding proteins (neurexins).
- ***Desensitization.*** The receptors become unresponsive if they are exposed to the neurotransmitter for prolonged period. Desensitization is further of two types:
  - *Homologous desensitization* refers to unresponsiveness to one particular type of ligand only, but responsive to other types of ligands
  - *Heterologous desensitization* refers to when the cell becomes unresponsive to other types of ligands also.

Principal Neurotransmitters

A. Small Molecule Neurotransmitters

I. Acetylcholine

Acetylcholine (Ach) is a principal neurotransmitter released by many neurons in the nervous system.

Cholinergic Neurons. Cholinergic neurons, i.e. neurons which secrete Ach at their nerve endings include:

- Nerve endings at the neuromuscular junction,
- Preganglionic parasympathetic nerves,
- All preganglionic sympathetic nerves,
- All postganglionic parasympathetic nerves,
- Postganglionic sympathetic cholinergic nerves, those which innervate:
  - Sweat glands and
  - Skeletal muscle blood vessels (sympathetic vasodilator nerves),
- Endings of some amacrine cells of the retina and
- Many parts of the brain (especially cerebral cortex, thalamus and forebrain nuclei). Ach is specifically released by large pyramidal cells and many neurons of basal ganglia.

Cholinergic Receptors. Ach receptors are of two types: nicotinic and muscarinic (see page 984).

i. ***Nicotinic receptors*** (which respond to low doses of nicotine) are present on postsynaptic membrane of:
   - All autonomic (sympathetic as well as parasympathetic) ganglia and
   - Postsynaptic membrane at neuromuscular junctions in skeletal muscle.

ii. ***Muscarinic receptors*** (which respond to mushroom poison muscarine) are present on postsynaptic membranes of:
- Smooth muscles,
- Cardiac muscles and
- Glandular cells.

Ach synthesis, Storage, Release and Removal

- ***Ach synthesis and storage.*** Ach is synthesized within the mitochondria in the presynaptic terminal from acetyl coenzyme A (CoA) and choline by a reaction catalysed by the enzyme choline acetyltransferase. After formation, Ach is stored temporarily in synaptic vesicles with ATP and proteoglycin for later release.
- ***Release of Ach by the nerve terminal*** (see page 80).
- ***Removal of Ach from synaptic cleft*** (see page 82).

The biochemical events at cholinergic synapse are (Fig. 10.7-19):

- Choline is transported into presynaptic terminal by a Na^+-dependent choline transporter (CHT).
- Acetylcholine is synthesized from choline and acetyl coenzyme A (CoA) by enzyme choline acetyltransferase (ChAT) in the cytosol.

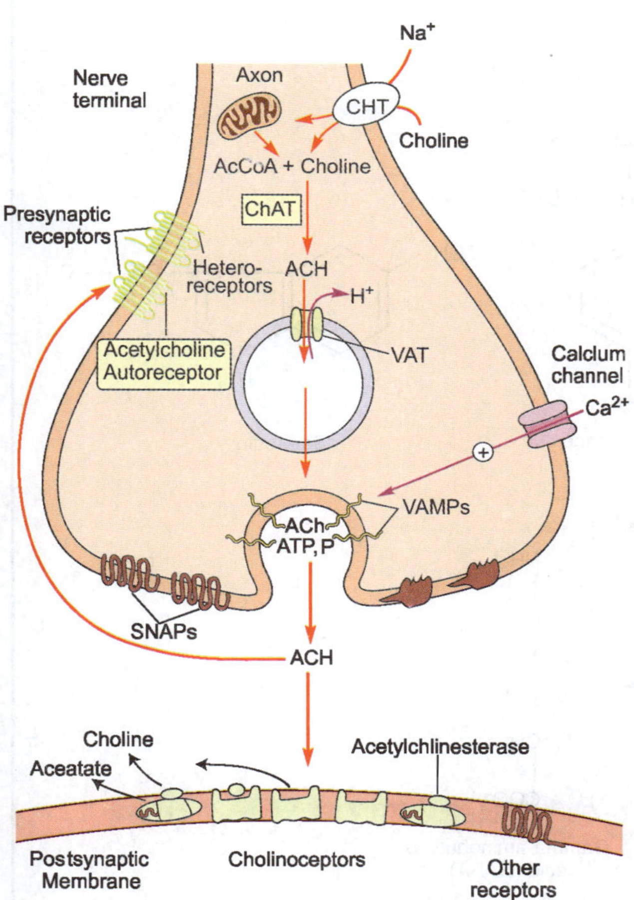

FIGURE 10.7-19 Biochemical events at a cholinergic synapse.

- Ach is then transported from cytosol into the vesicles by vesicle-associated transporter (VAT) along with a peptide (P) and ATP.
- Release of Ach from the nerve terminal occurs on opening of voltage-gated Ca^{2+} channels.
- Influx of Ca^{2+} leads to fusion of vesicles containing Ach to the surface of the membrane (exocytosis).
- Expulsion of Ach and cotransmitter into the synaptic cleft involves synaptosome-associated protein (SNAPs) and vesicle-associated membrane protein (VAMPs).
- Released Ach acts on muscarinic G protein-coupled protein (GPCR) on postsynaptic target (e.g. smooth muscles) and on nicotinic receptors (autonomic ganglia and neuromuscular junction).
- Ach is metabolized rapidly by enzyme acetylcholinesterase in the synaptic cleft.
- Presynaptic autoreceptors and heteroreceptors modulate Ach release.

Actions of Ach. Acetylcholine is very quick in action and in most instances it is excitatory. It produces the excitatory function of synapse by opening the ligand-gated Na^+ channels. At very few places (vagus supplying heart), Ach acts as a inhibitory transmitter.

Muscarinic versus nicotinic actions of Ach on the postsynaptic receptors are summarized in Table 10.7-3.

Role of Ach in function of brain. Both muscarinic and nicotinic receptors are found in the CNS; however, most of these are muscarinic. The cell bodies of cholinergic neurons in the brain are concentrated in relatively few areas, but their axons are widely distributed.

TABLE 10.7.3 Muscarinic versus Nicotonic Actions of Ach

Features	Muscarinic action	Nicotinic action
1. Site of action	• Postsynaptic membranes in cardiac muscles, smooth muscles and glandular cells	• All autonomic ganglia • Neuromuscular junctions in skeletal muscles
2. Characteristics of action	• Actions resemble those of mushroom poison muscarine • Actions are slow in onset • Actions are prolonged	• Action resembles the drug nicotine • Actions are quick in onset • Actions are of brief duration
3. Actions are antagonized by	• Atropine which combines with Ach receptors at the sites of muscarinic action	• Hexamethonium at autonomic ganglia and • Tubocurarine at skeletal muscles

- Cholinergic neurotransmission has been most thoroughly studied in cerebral cortex where it acts as an excitatory neurotransmitter. The release of Ach in the cortex is proportional to the level of cortical excitability, being increased by a variety of convulsants and decreased by anaesthesia.
- Its role in memory and malfunction in Alzheimer's disease has aroused a considerable interest recently in anti-cholinesterase drugs like tacrine and donepezil.
- Cholinergic projections are also involved in motivation, perception and cognition (see page 1089).
- Cholinergic neurons in the pons and lateral tegmental nuclei project through the pons–midbrain reticular formation to the thalamus and are involved in the attention and arousal function of RAS (see page 1105).
- In the basal ganglia, Ach is a principal excitatory neurotransmitter (see page 940).
- The ponto-geniculo-occipital (PGO) spike system responsible for REM sleep is cholinergic (see page 1107).

II. Biogenic Amines

1. Catecholamines

- Catecholamines include epinephrine (adrenaline), norepinephrine (noradrenaline) and dopamine.
- Epinephrine (EP) is not a common neurotransmitter in the brain or peripheral nervous system but is the major hormone secreted by the adrenal medulla.
- The biogenic amines are the basic *by R-NH$_2$* group. Catecholamines contain a catechol ring (a six-sided carbon ring with adjacent hydroxyl group), and an amine ring (Fig. 10.7-20).

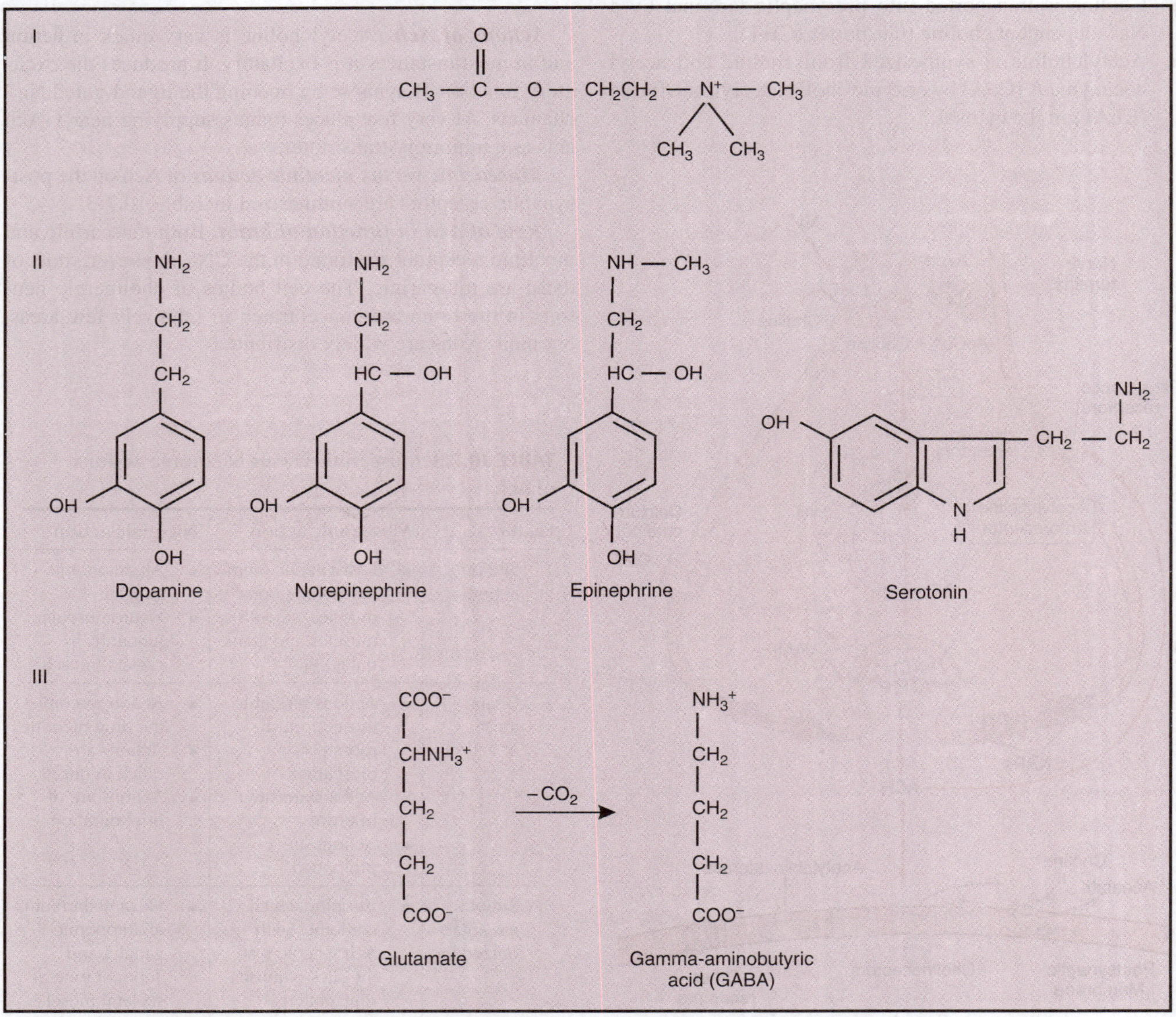

I

$CH_3-C(=O)-O-CH_2CH_2-N^+(CH_3)_3$

II

Dopamine   Norepinephrine   Epinephrine   Serotonin

III

Glutamate $\xrightarrow{-CO_2}$ Gamma-aminobutyric acid (GABA)

FIGURE 10.7-20 Structures of various neurotransmitters: **I**, acetylcholine; **II**, biogenic amines; and **III**, amino acids.

Biosynthesis, Metabolism and Excretion. The three catecholamines, epinephrine (EP), norepinephrine (NE) and dopamine (DA), are synthesized from the amino acid phenylalanine (Fig. 10.7-21). For details, see page 758.

Norepinephrine and Epinephrine

Adrenergic neurons refer to those neurons which either secrete epinephrine (adrenaline) or norepinephrine (noradrenaline) at their nerve endings.

Epinephrine is produced almost exclusively in the adrenal medulla, with small amount being synthesized in the brain.

Norepinephrine is released by adrenal medulla and following noradrenergic nerve endings in peripheral and central nervous system:

- Postganglionic sympathetic neurons. It is the primary neurotransmitter released from postganglionic sympathetic neurons except those supplying the sweat glands and blood vessels of skeletal muscles.
- Neurons of cerebral cortex and hypothalamus.
- Noradrenergic neurons of pons and medulla oblongata constitute two major systems: locus coeruleus system and lateral tegmental system. From these neurons, the axons descend to *spinal cord* and *cerebellum,* and ascend to innervate the nuclei of hypothalamus (supraoptic, paraventricular and periventricular), thalamus and most of the neocortex. Norepinephrine primarily acts as a modulator in these regions.

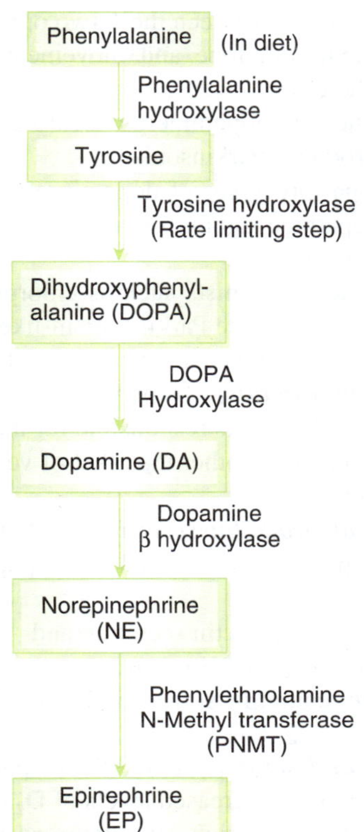

FIGURE 10.7-21 Synthesis of catecholamines from the amino acid phenylalanine.

Regulation of NE release. There is a presynaptic regulation of NE release mediated by presynaptic α-receptors and a positive feedback mechanism mediated by presynaptic ß-receptors. Such combined effects control the need-oriented release of neurotransmitter.

Removal and metabolism of NE. Norepinephrine is removed from the synapse by *re-uptake* or is *metabolized* in the presynaptic terminal by monoamine oxidase (MAO) and catechol-O-methyl transferase (COMT). The metabolites are: dihydroxymandelic acid (DOMA), normetanephrine (NMN) and 3-methoxy-4-hydroxy-phenyl-glycol (MOPG). For details, see page 761 (Fig. 8.5-10).

Distribution of noradrenergic neurons in the CNS is shown in Fig. 10.7-22.

Actions. For detailed action of epinephrine and norepinephrine on different systems of the body, see page 763.

- In general, norepinephrine is mainly an excitatory neurotransmitter; only at a few places, it is inhibitory.

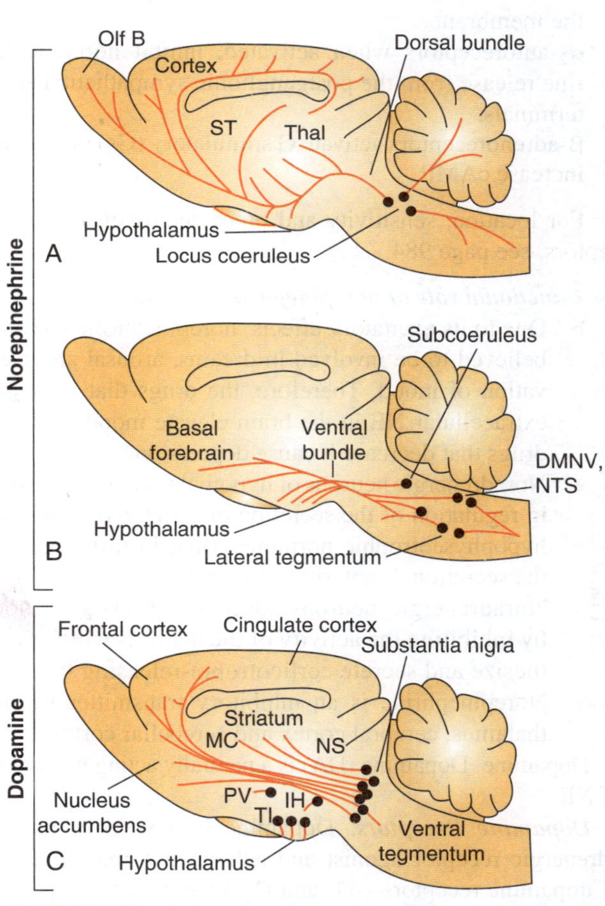

FIGURE 10.7-22 Aminergic pathways in central nervous system. Two principal noradrenergic systems. Locus coeruleus **(A)** and lateral tegmental **(B)**; and dopaminergic pathway **(C)**. Olf B = olfactory bulb, ST= striaterminalis, Thal = thalamus, DMNV = dorsal motor nucleus of vagus, NTS = nucleus tractussolitarius (nucleus of solitary tract), NS = nigrostriatal system, PV = periventricular system and MC = mesocortical system.

- Epinephrine and norepinephrine produce different effects due to the existence of two types of adrenergic receptors: alpha and beta, each further subdivided into alpha-1 and alpha-2, and beta-1, beta-2 and beta-3, respectively.
- Epinephrine acts equally on both alpha and beta receptors, while norepinephrine acts on alpha receptors (see page 984).
- Their receptor action is linked for the second messenger cAMP, cGMP, etc.

Adrenoreceptors Epinephrine and norepinephrine act on both types (α and β) of adrenoreceptors. Both α and β receptors have subtypes: α_{1A}, α_{1B}, α_D, α_{2A}, α_{2B}, α_C, β_1 and β_2.

Adrenoreceptors are metabotropic receptors:

- α_1-adrenoreceptors are coupled to Gq protein and leads to formation of IP_3 and DAG, which mobilize intracellular Ca^{2+} stores and activate protein kinase C.
- α_2-adrenoreceptors activate G inhibitory (Gi) protein to inhibit adenylyl cyclase and decrease cAMP. α_2-adrenoreceptors activate G protein-coupled inward rectifier K^+ channels and cause hyperpolarization of the membrane.
- α_2-autoreceptors when activated, inhibit norepinephrine release from the postganglionic sympathetic nerve terminals.
- β-adrenoreceptors activate G stimulatory (Gs) protein to increase cAMP.

For location, sensitivity and other details of adrenoreceptors, see page 984.

Functional role of norepinephrine in CNS

- Due to its excitatory effects, norepinephrine (NE) is believed to be involved in dreams, arousal and elevation of mood. Therefore, the drugs that increase extracellular NE in the brain elevate mood, and the drugs that decrease it cause depression.
- Noradrenergic neurons of hypothalamus are involved in regulation of the secretion of ADH, oxytocin and hypophyseotrophic hormones (that in turn regulate the secretion of anterior pituitary).
- Noradrenergic neurons suppress ACTH secretion by inhibiting the activity of the neurons which synthesize and secrete corticotropin-releasing factor.
- Norepinephrine is an inhibitory transmitter in the thalamus, cerebral cortex and cerebellar cortex.

Dopamine Dopamine (DA) is a naturally acting precursor of NE.

Dopamine Receptors. Dopamine is a weak α and ß adrenergic receptor agonist and acts on two main classes of dopamine receptors—D_1 and D_2. Five different types of dopamine receptors have been cloned, but these basically fall into two major classes:

- D_1 receptors (D_1 and D_5) and
- D_2 receptors (D_2, D_3 and D_4).

All dopamine receptors are metabotropic:

- *D_1* receptors activate adenylyl cyclase via Gs protein and
- *D_2* receptors inhibit adenylyl cyclase via Gi protein. The brain contains more of D_2 receptors.

Dopaminergic neurons have their cell bodies in the midbrain. They project from the substantia nigra to the (Fig. 10.7-22C):

- Striatum (nigrostriatal tract),
- Olfactory tubercle,
- Nucleus accumbens and
- Limbic system area.

Note. Highest concentration of dopamine is present in the basal ganglia, limbic system and chemoreceptor trigger zone (CTZ) in the medulla. It does not cross the blood–brain barrier.

Metabolism of dopamine. Dopamine is metabolized by MAO and COMT (details see on page 762).

Functional Roles of Dopamine in CNS

1. ***Control of movements.*** Dopamine serves as a central neurotransmitter for control of movement of the corpus striatum, which has been described as the chemical factory of the CNS, modulates muscle tone and voluntary movements by influencing extrapyramidal motor system, which can be inhibited by nigrostriatal neurons releasing dopamine and is stimulated by the intrastriatal release of acetylcholine from excitatory neurons. The functional balance between these two opposing systems maintains optimum tone and movement of voluntary muscles. Therefore:
   - Deficiency of dopaminergic neurons (nigrostriatal tract) produces Parkinsonism.
   - Levodopa (precursor of dopamine) and *bromocriptine* (dopamine agonist) overcome the akinesia of Parkinsonism.
   - Dopamine antagonists such as chlorpromazine and haloperidol produce Parkinsonism-like symptoms in human beings and catalepsy in animals.
2. ***Induction of vomiting.*** Dopamine also mediates the activity of (CTZ) and is responsible for the induction of all types of vomiting other than that of vestibular origin (see page 604).
3. ***Inhibition of prolactin secretion and stimulation of GnRH***. Dopamine is released in hypothalamus and causes:
   - Inhibition of prolactin secretion and
   - Stimulation of GnRH release.
4. ***Retina*** also contains some inhibitory dopaminergic neurons.
5. ***Dopamine and schizophrenia.*** Schizophrenia type of psychosis involves increased levels of D_2 receptors.
   - Amphetamine, which stimulates secretion of NE and dopamine (DA), produces schizophrenia when administered in high doses.

- Several drugs used as tranquilizers reduce the content of dopamine in the brain neurons and are effective in relief of schizophrenia (see page 1091).

Note. It is possible that there exist different cotransmitters for dopamine in different areas which affect its activity differently.

2. Serotonin

Synthesis and Metabolism. Serotonin (5 hydro-oxytryptamine, 5HT) is synthesized from tryptophan (an essential amino acid). It is inactivated by monoamine oxidase (MAO) to form 5-hydroxy indole acetic acid (5-HIAA), which is excreted in urine. In the pineal gland, 5HT is converted into melatonin.

Sites of Secretion. 5HT is present in brain and non-neural cells.

- *In the brain,* serotonergic neurons have their cell bodies in the brainstem and they project to portions of hypothalamus, limbic system, neocortex and spinal cord.
- *Non-neural cells* that contain serotonin are blood platelets (highest concentration, mast cells and GIT enterochromaffin cells and myenteric plexus).

Serotonergic Receptors. Serotonergic receptors have been classified into seven major types ($5HT_1$–$5HT_7$) and they are further of subtypes:

- $5HT_1$: $5HT_{1A}$, $5HT_{1B}$, $5HT_{1C}$, $5HT_{1D}$, $5HT_{1E}$ and $5HT_{1F}$,
- $5HT_2$: $5HT_{2A}$, $5HT_{2B}$ and $5HT_{2C}$ and
- $5HT_5$: $5HT_{5A}$ and $5HT_{5B}$.

Location and main functions:

- 5HT receptors are presynaptic as well as postsynaptic.
- $5HT_{2A}$ cause smooth muscle contraction and platelet aggregation.
- $5HT_{2C}$ regulates food intake in response to leptin.
- $5HT_3$ is present in GIT and area postrema, and is related to vomiting.
- $5HT_4$ receptors are present in GIT (responsible for peristalsis) and also in brain.
- $5HT_6$ and $5HT_7$ are distributed in the limbic system.

Effects of 5HT. General considerations are:

- Some 5HT receptors are excitatory, while others are inhibitory. In general, 5HT has an excitatory effect on motor pathways and an inhibitory effect on the sensory pathways.
- Effects of 5HT generally have as low onset indicating that it works as a neuromodulator (which often modify the postsynaptic cell's response to specific neurotransmitters).
- The activity of serotonergic neurons is lowest or absent in sleep and highest during states of alert and wakefulness. The increased 5HT activity causes increase in motor responsiveness and suppresses sensory systems to screen out distracting stimuli.

Functional Roles of 5HT in CNS

1. ***Regulation of carbohydrate intake and hypothalamic-releasing hormones.*** Serotonergic pathways function in regulation of carbohydrate intake and hypothalamic-releasing hormones, and they have been implicated in alcoholism and other obsessive–compulsive disorders.
   Norepinephrine and 5HT both are involved in food intake and control of body temperature.
2. ***Pain inhibition.*** Serotonin inhibits impulses of pain sensation in posterior grey horn of spinal cord. The presence of descending serotonergic neurons in the brainstem and spinal cord is essential for the analgesic action of morphine.
3. ***Hallucinations and 5HT.*** LSD (lysergic acid diethylamide), the most potent hallucinogenic drug known, activates the serotonergic neurons.
   Several chemical substances related to 5HT, such as *psilocybin*, a hallucinogenic agent found in some mushrooms, have potent psychic effects.
4. ***Depression of mood*** (see page 1090).

3. Histamine

Histamine is formed by decarboxylation of the amino acid histidine.

Sites of Secretion. Histamine is secreted in brain and non-neural cells.

- *In the brain*, histaminergic neurons have their cell bodies mainly in the posterior hypothalamus and their axons project to all parts of the brain, including the cerebral cortex and spinal cord.
- *Non-neural cells* that contain histamine are of gastric mucosa and heparin-containing mast cells.

Histamine Receptors are of four types: H_1 H_2 H_3 and H_4. All the three types of receptors are found in the brain and peripheral tissues:

- H_1 receptors activate phospholipase C,
- H_2 receptors increase intracellular cAMP and
- H_3 receptors are presynaptic, and they mediate inhibition of the release of histamine via a protein.
- H_4 receptors are recently described receptors and they play a role in regulating cells of immune system.

Functional Role of Histamine in CNS. Histamine is an excitatory neurotransmitter. The exact function of diffuse histaminergic system is not known as yet. It is believed that histamine plays an important role in arousal and sexual behaviour, regulation of secretion of some anterior pituitary hormones, drinking and pain threshold.

4. Adenosine Triphosphate (ATP)

ATP has recently been identified as a small molecule neurotransmitter. It is co-localized and is co-released from synaptic vesicles of noradrenergic postganglionic neurons. The ATP receptors are **P** receptors and are further of three subtypes: $\mathbf{P_{2X}}$, $\mathbf{P_{2Y}}$ and $\mathbf{P_{2U}}$.

- $\mathbf{P_{2X}}$ receptors are ligand-gated ion channels involved in rapid synaptic responses in autonomic nervous system. $\mathbf{P_{2X}}$ receptors are widely distributed throughout the body, but mainly in the dorsal horn cells, thus ATP has a role in sensory transmission.
- $\mathbf{P_{2Y}}$ and $\mathbf{P_{2U}}$ receptors are metabotropic, which are GPCR.

III. Amino Acid Neurotransmitters

Excitatory amino acid neurotransmitters that cause neuronal depolarization include glutamic acid (glutamate) and aspartic acid (aspartate).

Inhibitory amino acid neurotransmitters that cause neuronal hyperpolarization include: gamma-aminobutyric acid (GABA) and glycine.

1. Glutamic Acid Glutamic acid (glutamate) is the most prevalent *excitatory neurotransmitter* in the brain and dorsal sensory nerve terminals.

Synthesis, Storage and Release and Removal. In the CNS neurons, glutamate is mainly derived from either glucose, via the Krebs' cycle, or from glutamine which is synthesized by glial cells and taken up by the neurons. *In the first pathway* (Fig. 10.7-23), the α-glutarate produced by Krebs' cycle is converted into glutamate by enzyme GABA transaminase (GABA-T). *In the second pathway,* the glutamate released from nerve terminal by exocytosis is transported into the glial tissue by a transporter (glutamate reuptake transporter), and converted into glutamine by the enzyme glutamine synthase. Glutamine then diffuses back into the nerve terminal and gets hydrolysed by the enzyme glutaminase. The released glutamate is also taken directly from synaptic cleft into the nerve terminal by a membrane transporter.

It is stored in the synaptic vesicles. Vesicular glutamate transporter is responsible for maintaining its high concentration in the vesicles and released by calcium-dependent exocytosis. The action of glutamate is mainly terminated by carrier-mediated *re-uptake* into the nerve terminals and neighbouring glial cells.

Glutamate Receptors present on the postsynaptic neurons are:

- ***Inotropic glutamate receptors*** which when stimulated increase the conductance of Na^+ and Ca^{2+} into the cell leading to depolarization.

  There are three subtypes of ionotropic glutamate receptors, each named after the specific agonists:

  - AMPA (α-amino-3 hydroxy-5 methylisoxazol-4-proprionate),

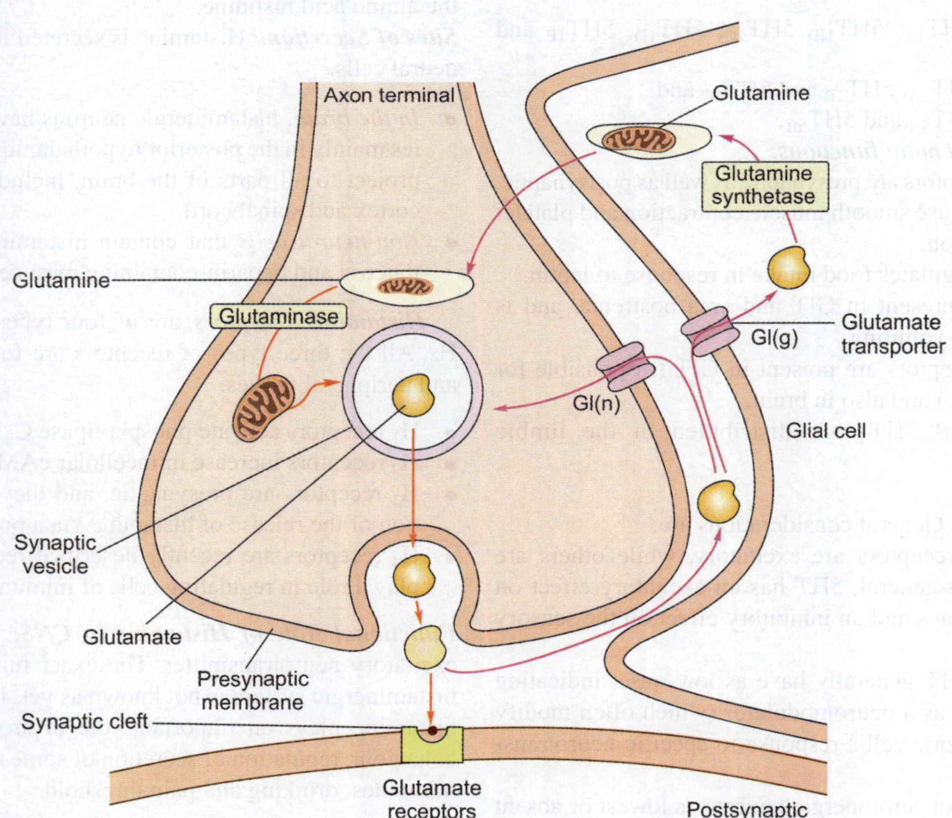

FIGURE 10.7-23 Biochemical events at a glutamatergic synapse. Glutamate released into the synaptic cleft by Ca^{2+}-dependent exocytosis. Released Glu can act Glutamate on ionotropic and G protein-coupled receptors on the postsynaptic neuron.

- Kainate (kainati, a seaweed acid) and
- NMDA (N-methyl-D-aspartate).

Distribution

- Neurons of CNS have both AMPA and NMDA receptors.
- Whereas, kainate receptors are located on:
  - Presynaptic GABA-secreting nerve endings and
  - Postsynaptically in hippocampus, cerebellum and spinal cord.

Action

NMDA receptors are involved in memory and learning (see page 1125).

- ***Metabotropic glutamate receptors*** (mGlUR) stimulate the phosphoinositol turnover and diacylglycerol (DAG) or decrease in intracellular cAMP. Eight different subtypes of mGLuR are known (mGLuR1–8). These receptors are located on both presynaptic and postsynaptic sites and are widely distributed in the brain.

Action: mGLuR are involved in synaptic plasticity.

2. Aspartic Acid Aspartic acid or aspartate seems to be the chief excitatory transmitter of cortical pyramidal cells.

3. Gamma-Aminobutyric Acid Gamma-aminobutyric acid (GABA) is the major inhibitory neurotransmitter in the whole CNS, i.e. spinal cord, brainstem, cerebral cortex and cerebellum.

- ***Synthesis.*** It is formed by decarboxylation of glutamic acid by the enzyme glutamate decarboxylase (GAD) pyridoxalphosphate; a vitamin B complex derivative is cofactor for GAD.
- ***Removal*** of GABA from the synaptic cleft occurs chiefly by its re-uptake via GABA transporter, and transported into the synaptic vesicles by vesicular GABA transporter.
- ***GABA receptors***. There are three subtypes of GABA receptors: $GABA_A$, $GABA_B$ and $GABA_C$.
  - $GABA_A$ receptors are pentameric, made up of combination of α, β, γ, δ and ϵ subunit.
  - $GABA_A$ and $GABA_B$ are ionotropic receptors and allow entry of Cl^- into the neurons.
  - $GABA_C$ receptors are metabotropic GPCR and act by:
    - Increasing conductance in K^+ channel,
    - Inhibiting adenylyl cyclase and
    - Inhibiting Ca^{2+} influx.

GABA produces presynaptic inhibition, i.e. indirect inhibition (see page 1002) by these types of receptors.

Thus, due to effect of GABA on postsynaptic membrane, K^+ comes out of synapse and Cl^- enters in. This leads to hyperpolarization which is known as inhibitory postsynaptic potential (IPSP) (see page 1002).

4. Glycine Glycine has inhibitory as well as excitatory effects:

- Glycine is an inhibitory neurotransmitter found primarily in the grey matter of spinal cord and brainstem.
- It produces direct inhibition (postsynaptic inhibition) in the spinal cord and acts by increasing Cl^- conductance by acting on glycine receptor which functionally resembles GABA receptors.
- Agents, such as strychnine and tetanus toxin, that antagonize the postsynaptic inhibitory action of glycine produce convulsions and muscular hyperactivity.
- Glycine when binds to NMDA receptors it makes them more sensitive to glutamate action. Therefore, it facilitates pain transmission by NMDA receptors.

B. Neuropeptide Transmitters (Large Molecule Neurotrasmitter)

Neuropeptide transmitters are slowly acting and have a prolonged effect in contrast to small molecule transmitters, which act rapidly and cause short-lasting acute response. These cannot be synthesized in the cytosol of the axon terminal but are typically synthesized in the soma as integral components of large proteins. These large molecules are cleaved in the cell body and packaged into vesicles in the Golgi apparatus either as active peptidergic agent or as a precursor of the neuroactive substance. The vesicles are delivered to axon terminals, and the transmitter is released into the synaptic cleft.

Mechanism of Action. The peptides can alter ion channel function and modify cell metabolism or gene expression, and these actions can be sustained for minutes, hours, days or presumably even longer.

Types of Neuropeptides. Many of the peptides function in communication network within the neural, endocrine and immune systems. These are:

1. Neuroactive Peptides. These include releasing hormones from hypothalamus such as TRH, LH-releasing hormone and somatostatin.

2. Pituitary Peptides. These include ACTH, beta-endorphin, vasopressin and oxytocin.

- ***Vasopressin (ADH) and oxytocin.*** Besides acting as hormones (see page 693), they are also present in the neurons that project to the brainstem and spinal cord. They appear to be involved in control of CVS.

3. Peptides Acting on the Gut and Brain. These include leucine, enkephalin, methionine, substance P, cholecystokinin, VIP, neurotensin, insulin, glucose and opioid polypeptides.

- ***Opioid peptides***
  - Enkephalins are peptides that bind to opoid receptors are called opioid peptides.
  - Enkephalins are two closely related pentapeptides: met-enkephalin and leu-enkephalin.
  - Enkephalins are mainly found in nerve endings of GIT, many parts of brain and substantia gelatinosa of spinal cord.

- Endogenous opioid peptides are synthesized as large precursor molecules. For details see page 1036.
- ***Enkephalins*** act on three types of receptors which occur in discrete locations in CNS:
  - In areas that contain the pathway which conveys pain information,
  - In parts of the brain involved in mood and
  - In parts of the brain involved in emotions.
- ***Opioid receptors***
  - Opioid receptors are μ, k and δ. They differ in their physiologic effects and affinity for various opioid peptides. Opioid receptors are GPCR, and act by inhibiting adenylyl cyclase. μ receptors increase K^+ conductance; k and δ receptors close the Ca^{2+} channels. By all, these effects they cause hyperpolarization of central neurons and primary afferents.
- ***Substance P.*** Substance P is a polypeptide containing 11 amino acids, which belongs to tachykinin family of polypeptides. Other members of this family are neurokinin A and neurokinin B. It is the transmitter released by:
  - Primary pain nerve endings in spinal cord,
  - Hypothalamus and
  - Nigrostriatal system of basal ganglia.

Receptors. There are three types of neurokinin receptors, NK_1–NK_3. Substance P binds preferably to NK_1 receptors. Activation of these receptors lead to increased production of IP_3 and DAG.

The actions of substance P are:

- Acts as mediator for transmission of pain in dorsal horn.
- In hypothalamus, it may play a role in neuroendocrine regulation.
- In the skin, it acts as a mediator released by nerve endings and is responsible for axon reflex (see page 338).
- In intestine, it is involved in peristalsis.
- NK_1 receptor antagonists have been used as antidepressants and antiemetics in patients undergoing chemotherapy.
- ***Cholecystokinin (CCK) and vasoactive intestinal polypeptide (VIP).*** These are also found in brain, the former in the hypothalamus and the latter in the cerebral cortex. *Opioid polypeptides* have an important role in the inhibition of pain signals in the brain and spinal cord.

4. Neuropeptides from Other Tissues. These include angiotensin II, bradykinin, bombesin and neuropeptide-α. *Neuropeptide*-Y is closely related to pancreatic polypeptide and is present in many parts of the brain and ANS. It increases the vasoconstrictive effect of norepinephrine. Its level in the circulation from sympathetic nerves increases during severe exercise.

Chapter 10.8

Somatosensory System

GENERAL SENSORY MECHANISM

Introduction

Sensations

Sensory division of the human nervous system is concerned with collection of the information about outside world, and changes occurring within the body itself. Sensation refers to conscious perception of sensory information reaching the brain. Sensations may be broadly classified into two groups:

1. Special Senses. These include visual sensations, auditory sensations, gustatory (taste sensation), and olfactory (smell) sensations. These have been discussed in detail in different chapters of Section 11.

2. Somaesthetic Senses. These, depending upon their point of origin, can be classified into three types:

A. ***Exteroceptive sensations*** also known as cutaneous sensations arise from the surface of the body and can be divided into two groups:

i. *Epicratic sensations* are mild or light sensations, which are perceived more accurately. These include:

- *Fine touch* or tactile sensation is the light touch sensation arising from the surface of the body.
- *Tactile localization* is the ability to locate the area of skin where tactile stimulus is applied.
- *Tactile discrimination* is the ability to locate the two adjacent areas of skin where tactile stimuli are applied.
- *Temperature sensation with fine range*, i.e. between 25°C and 40°C.

ii. *Protopathic sensations* are primitive or crude type of exteroceptive sensations. These include:

- Pressure sensation,
- Pain sensation and
- Temperature sensation with a wider range, i.e. below 25°C and above 40°C.

B. ***Visceral sensations*** arise from the viscera, i.e. internal organs and thus are called visceral sensations.

C. ***Proprioceptive and kinaesthetic sensations*** arise from the muscles, tendons and joints. These include:

i. *Proprioceptive sensations*: These are concerned with the physical state of the body, i.e. the sense of position, tendon and muscle sensations, deep pressure and sense of equilibrium.

ii. *Kinaesthetic sensations* or kinaesthesia: It is the conscious recognition of rate of movement of different parts of the body. Kinaesthetic sensations include both:

- Conscious kinaesthetic sensations, and
- Unconscious kinaesthetic sensations.

Components of Sensory System

The sensory division of the human nervous system includes following components (Fig. 10.8-1):

1. Sensory Receptors. These are specialized cells that transduce stimulus energy into neural signals.

2. Afferent Neurons. These carry sensory impulses to the sensory cortex and constitute the neural pathway. Sensory neural pathway consists of:

- First-order neurons,
- Second-order neurons and
- Third-order neurons.

3. Sensory Cortex. It includes the sensory areas of cerebral cortex. It is formed by fourth-order sensory neurons. The information received in the sensory cortex results in a conscious perception of the stimulus, i.e. a sensation.

Receptors

Sensory receptors are specialized cells that receive stimuli from the external or internal environment, and transduce these signals into neural signals. A *stimulus* is a change of environment of sufficient intensity to evoke a response in an organism. The external stimuli may be mechanical, chemical, thermal, auditory or visual.

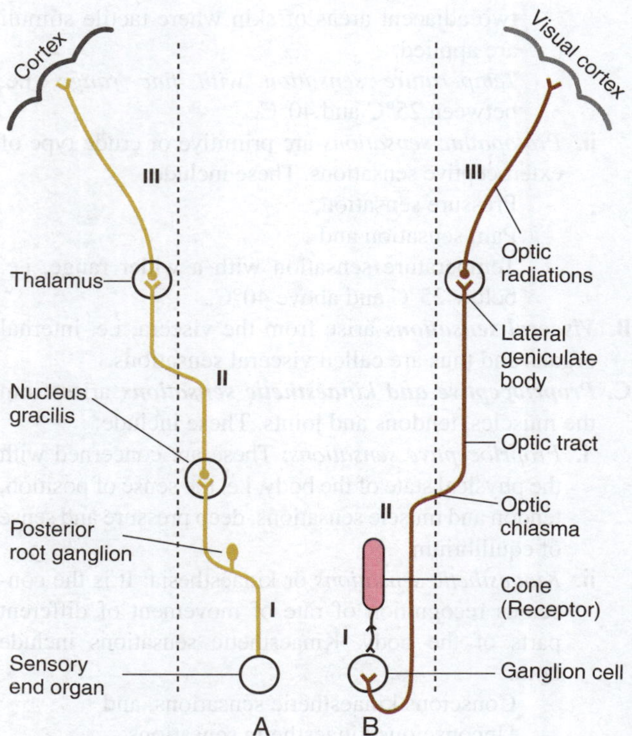

FIGURE 10.8-1 Pathway of somatic (**A**) versus visual sensations (**B**).

Classification of Receptors

Receptors can be variously classified:

A. Depending on the Source of Stimulus (Sherrington's Classification)

1. ***Exteroceptors,*** i.e. the receptors which receive stimuli from immediate surrounding outside the body, e.g.
   - *Cutaneous receptors* for pain, touch and temperature.
2. ***Enteroceptors***, i.e. the receptors which receive stimuli from within the body. These include:
   - *Chemoreceptors* that measure blood gases,
   - *Baroreceptors* that measure blood pressure,
   - *Proprioceptors* that measure the position of the limbs or the force of muscle contraction,
   - *Osmoreceptors* that respond to osmotic pressure of plasma and
   - *Glucoreceptors* that respond to arteriovenous blood glucose difference.
3. ***Telereceptors,*** i.e. the receptors that receive stimuli from the distance, e.g.
   - Visual receptors,
   - Cochlear receptors and
   - Olfactory receptors.

B. Depending on Type of Stimulus Energy

1. ***Mechanoreceptors***, i.e. those receptors which respond to mechanical stimuli. These include:
   - **i.** *Cutaneous receptors (in epidermis and dermis) for cutaneous tactile sensibility, e.g.*
     - Free nerve endings,
     - Merkel's discs (expanded nerve endings),
     - Ruffini's endings (spray endings),
     - Meissner's corpuscles (encapsulated nerve endings),
     - Krause's corpuscles (encapsulated nerve endings) and
     - Hair end organs.
   - **ii.** *Cutaneous receptors for deep tissue sensibility, e.g.*
     - Free nerve endings,
     - Merkel's discs,
     - Ruffini's endings and
     - Pacinian corpuscles (encapsulated nerve endings).
   - **iii.** *Muscle and joint receptors, e.g.*
     - Muscle spindles or stretch receptors,
     - Golgi tendon receptors and
     - Joint receptors.
   - **iv.** *Hair cells, e.g.*
     - Hair cells in organ of Corti (cochlear) or auditory receptors and
     - Hair cells in vestibular apparatus or vestibuloreceptors for equilibrium.
   - **v.** *Baroreceptors* of carotid sinus and aortic arch for detecting level of arterial blood pressure.
2. ***Thermoreceptors,*** which detect environmental temperature, e.g.:
   - Cold receptors and
   - Warm receptors.

3. ***Photoreceptors*** or electromagnetic receptors, i.e. rods and cones of the retina that respond to light stimuli.
4. ***Chemoreceptors*** which detect change in chemical composition of the environment in which they are located, e.g.
   - Taste receptors,
   - Olfactory receptors,
   - Osmoreceptors in supra optic nuclei of hypothalamus,
   - Aortic and carotid body receptors that detect the level of arterial pO_2, pCO_2 and pH,
   - Glucoreceptors,
   - Chemoreceptors on the surface of medulla for detecting the level of blood pCO_2 and
   - Chemoreceptors in hypothalamus detecting the levels of blood glucose, fatty acids and amino acids.
5. ***Nociceptors***, i.e. the receptors which respond to extremes of mechanical, thermal and chemical stimuli producing pain.

C. Depending on the Type of Sensations

- Touch receptors,
- Cold receptors,
- Heat receptors,
- Pain receptors,
- Taste receptors,
- Olfactory receptors,
- Auditory receptors and
- Light receptors.

D. Depending on the Rate of Adaptation

1. ***Slowly adapting receptors***, i.e. tonic or static receptors that fire action potentials continuously during stimulus application, e.g. pain receptors, cold receptors and muscles and joint receptors.
2. ***Rapidly adapting receptors***, i.e. phasic or dynamic receptors, which fire action potentials at a decreasing rate during stimulus application, e.g. Pacinian corpuscles and olfactory receptors.

E. Clinical or Anatomical Classification of Receptors

1. ***Superficial receptors***, i.e. those present in skin and mucous membrane.
2. ***Deep receptors***, i.e. those present in muscles, tendons, joints and subcutaneous tissue.
3. ***Visceral receptors***, which are present in the visceral organs.

Sensory Transduction

Sensory transduction refers to the phenomenon of transduction of environmental signals into neural signals by the receptors. Steps of sensory transduction are:

- Arrival of stimulus to receptor,
- Production of generator or receptor potential and
- Production of action potential in sensory nerve.

Arrival of Stimulus to Receptor The stimulus arriving at the given sensory receptor may be in the form of:

- ***Mechanical force*** causing depression of the skin, which stimulates mechanoreceptors,
- ***Light or electromagnetic wave,*** which stimulates photoreceptors of the retina,
- ***Chemical,*** e.g. a molecule of NaCl on the tongue which stimulates chemoreceptors,
- ***Cold or warm temperature***-stimulating thermoreceptors and
- ***Sound energy***-stimulating auditory receptors, and soon and so forth.

Production of Receptor Potential When a stimulus excites the receptor, it changes the potential across the membrane of the receptors. This change in the potential is called receptor or generator potential.

Mechanism of Development of Receptor Potential *(Fig. 10.8-2)* The change in membrane potential in a receptor is caused by a change in permeability of membrane of the unmyelinated terminals to Na^+. The resultant influx of Na^+ causes development of generator or receptor potential.

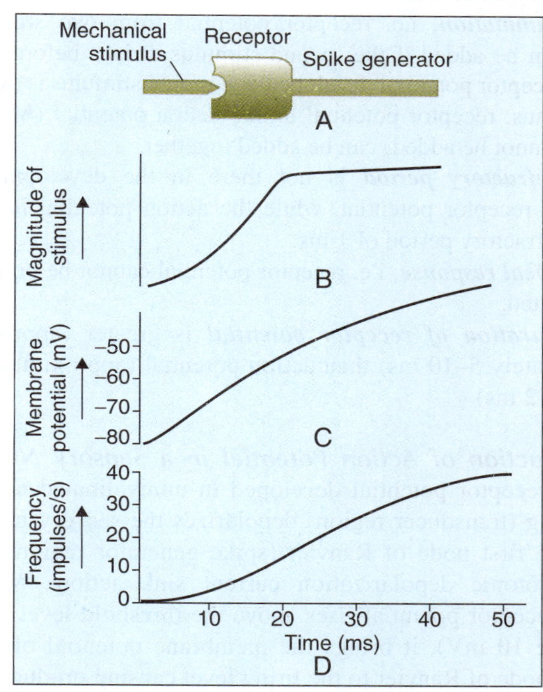

FIGURE 10.8-2 Mechanism of development of generator potential, and its relationship with the intensity of stimulus: **A,** Stimulus to mechanoreceptor causes its deformation which opens up channels which are permeable to Na^+ causing membrane depolarization; **B,** the magnitude of stimulus intensity; **C,** the receptor potential (generator potential) follows the time course; and **D,** the action potential. Note: The magnitude of generator potential and frequency of action potential are proportionate to the magnitude of the stimulus.

The different stimuli initiate change in the membrane permeability by following mechanisms:

- ***Mechanical deformation*** of the receptor causes its stretching and opens the ion channels (Fig. 10.8-2A).
- ***Chemical stimulus*** opens the ion channels by direct effect on the membrane.
- ***Change in temperature*** of the membrane changes the permeability of the membrane.
- ***Effect of light*** on the photoreceptors changes the membrane permeability.

Opening up of ion channels in the sensory receptors allows current to flow. Usually the current is inward, which produces depolarization of the receptor. The exception is in the photoreceptors, where light causes hyperpolarization.

Properties of Receptor Potential The receptor potential is not action potential. It is similar to excitatory postsynaptic potential (EPSP) in synapse, end plate potential (EPP) in a neuromuscular junction and electrotonic potential in a nerve fibre. The important properties of receptor potential are:

1. ***Graded response:*** Receptor potential is a graded response, i.e. its amplitude increases with the increasing velocity of stimulus application, and increasing strength of stimulus. Thus, unlike action potential it does not obey all or none law.
2. ***Summation***, i.e. receptor potential from two stimuli can be added if the second stimulus arrives before the receptor potential developed due to first stimulus is over. Thus, receptor potential unlike action potential (which cannot be added) can be added together.
3. ***Refractory period*** is not there in the development of receptor potential, while the action potential has a refractory period of 1 ms.
4. ***Local response***, i.e. receptor potential cannot be propagated.
5. ***Duration of receptor potential*** is greater (approximately 5–10 ms) than action potential (approximately 1–2 ms).

Production of Action Potential in a Sensory Nerve

The receptor potential developed in unmyelinated nerve ending (transducer region) depolarizes the sensory nerve at the first node of Ranvier (spike generator region) by electrotonic depolarization current sink action. When the receptor potential rises above the threshold level (i.e. above 10 mV), it brings the membrane potential of the first node of Ranvier to the firing level causing production of action potential, which is propagated in the nerve fibre (Fig. 10.8-2D). Thus, the first node of Ranvier (spike generator region) converts the graded response of the receptor into action potential. Greater the magnitude of receptor potential, greater is the rate of discharge of action potentials in the nerve fibre.

Recording of Receptor Potential and Action Potential

For the purpose of demonstration, the receptor potential can be recorded from Pacinian corpuscles, because:

- It is a large-sized receptor,
- It can be easily dissected from the mesentery of experimental animals and
- Its anatomical configuration allows study with the microelectrode.

Structure of Pacinian Corpuscle. A Pacinian corpuscle consists of concentric lamellae of connective tissue, surrounding an unmyelinated terminal portion of a nerve fibre. The myelin sheath of the sensory nerve fibre begins inside the corpuscle. Therefore, the first node of Ranvier is located inside the corpuscle but the second node of Ranvier is mostly outside the corpuscle (usually near the point at which the nerve fibre leaves the corpuscle) (Fig. 10.8-3A).

Technique of Recording. Recording electrodes (connected to a cathode ray oscilloscope CRO) are placed on the nerve fibre, one on the unmyelinated ending, and other on the second node of Ranvier (Fig. 10.8-3A).

- When a mild pressure is applied on the corpuscle, a mild nonpropagated depolarizing potential called the generator or receptor potential can be recorded.
- When the pressure is increased in steps, the magnitude of receptor potential is increased (Fig. 10.8-3B).
- The depolarized segment of the unmyelinated nerve ending produces electrotonic depolarization (current sink action) in the first node of Ranvier.
- When the magnitude of receptor potential is sufficient (above 10 mV), an action potential is generated in first node of Ranvier, which is propagated in the nerve fibre (Fig. 10.8-3B).
- If still greater pressure is applied on the receptor, the frequency of discharge is proportionately increased.

Demonstration of Site of Receptor Potential The receptor potential originates from the unmyelinated nerve ending and not from the corpuscle or from first node of Ranvier can be demonstrated experimentally as:

- When pressure is applied to the naked unmyelinated nerve ending after removal of the connective tissue of the corpuscle, the receptor potential is still produced but it decays more slowly (Fig. 10.8-3C).
- When pressure is applied to the naked unmyelinated nerve ending after blockage of the first node of Ranvier (by pressure or drug, e.g. narcotics), the receptor potential response persists but action potential cannot be recorded (Fig. 10.8-3D).
- When the sensory nerve is cut and allowed to degenerate, neither the receptor potential nor the action potential can be recorded (Fig. 10.8-3E).

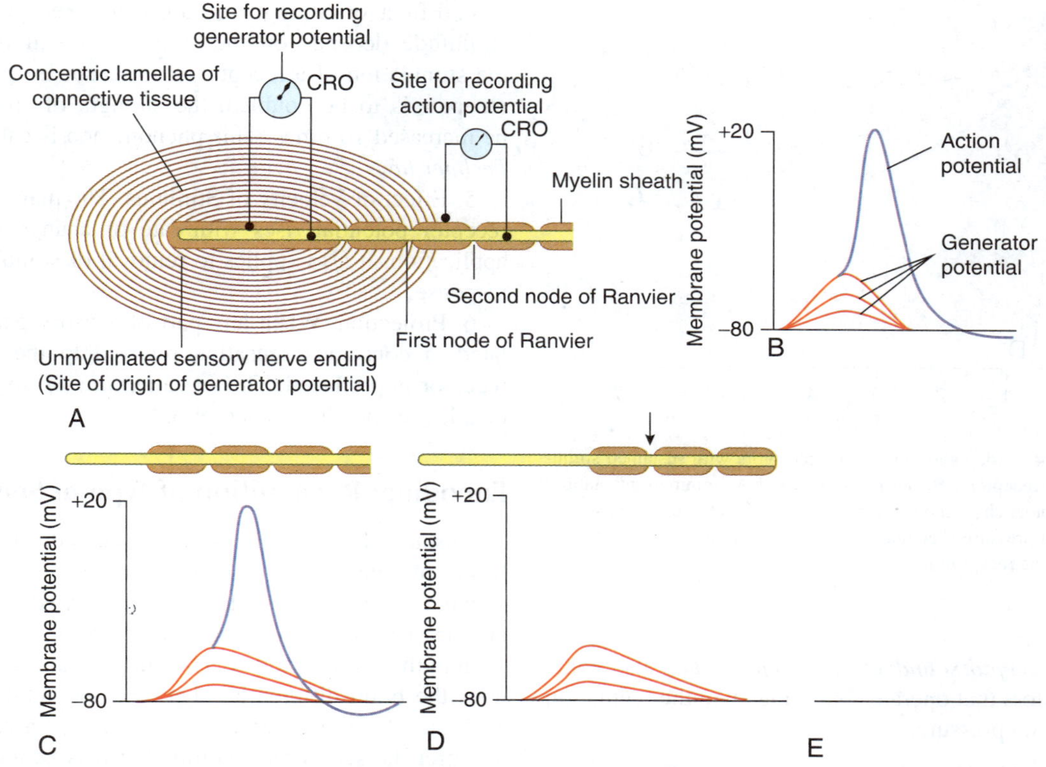

FIGURE 10.8-3 Recording of receptor potential from Pacinian corpuscle: **A,** placement of recording electrodes; **B,** record of receptor potential and action potential produced by graded pressure to the Pacinian corpuscle; **C,** same response as in B after the removal of connective tissue capsule indicates that receptor potential originates from the unmyelinated nerve endings, and not the capsule; **D,** blockage of first node of Ranvier abolishes conduction of receptor potentials produced; and **E,** no response is produced when sensory nerve is cut.

Properties of Receptors

1. Specificity of Response. Each receptor is easily stimulated (has low threshold) by only one type of appropriate (adequate) specific stimulus. This specificity of response by a particular receptor is also called law of adequate stimulus. Although each receptor is exquisitely sensitive to its adequate stimulus, receptors can respond to other forms of energy if the intensity is high enough. For example:

- ***Adequate stimulus*** for rod and cones of retina is light. Therefore, retina can detect the presence of a single photon of light. Pressure on the eyeball can also stimulate retinal receptors, but the threshold of these receptors to pressure is much higher than the threshold of the pressure receptors in skin.
- ***Adequate stimulus for Ruffini's receptors*** is warm water at low intensity of stimulus producing a specific response. The warm water at very high stimulus intensity can also stimulate naked nerve ending of pain, but the response produced is not complete.

2. Production of Receptor Potential on Stimulation. As described in detail above, each receptor produces receptor or generator potential, when stimulated by adequate stimulus. When the receptor potential rises above the threshold, the action potential is produced in the nerve fibre attached to the receptor (for details see page 1023).

3. Adaptation. When a receptor is continuously stimulated with the same strength of stimulus, the receptors respond at a very high impulse rate at first, but the frequency of action potential in its sensory nerve decreases progressively, till finally many of them no longer respond at all in some of the receptors (Fig. 10.8-4). This property is called adaptation. Depending on the rate of adaptation, the receptors are of two types:

Tonic receptors. These are slow and incompletely adapting receptors. These receptors keep on firing action potentials continuously during the stimulus application. Such receptors are important for life as they keep the brain constantly appraised of status of the body and its relation to its surroundings. Examples of such receptors are:

- *Muscle spindles* are tonic receptors which continue to discharge as long as the muscle is stretched and thus are helpful in prolonged postural adjustments.
- *Pain and cold receptors* are tonic receptors which keep on giving warning to brain about the noxious stimuli till they are present.

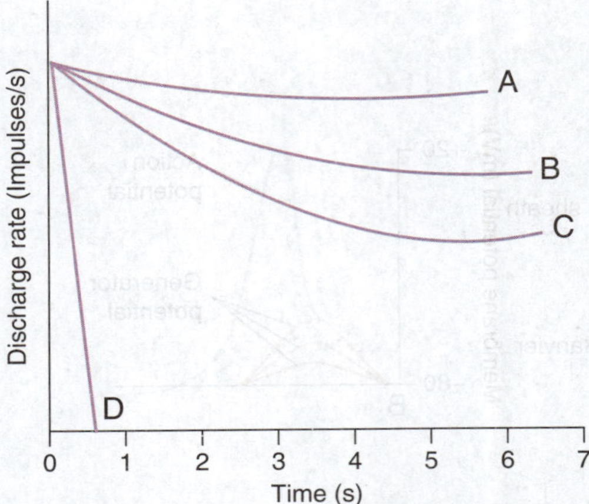

FIGURE 10.8-4 Adaptation in sensory receptors with sustained stimulation: **A,** pain receptors; **B,** muscle spindles show minimal adaptation; **C,** thermoreceptors show moderate adaptation; and **D,** touch (Meissner's corpuscles) and pressure (Pacinian corpuscle) receptors show most rapid adaptation (phasic receptors).

- *Baroreceptors and chemoreceptors* are also tonic receptors that operate continuously in the regulation of blood pressure.

Note. Imagine, if the above receptors would have showed marked adaptation, the life would have not been possible.

Phasic receptors. These are rapidly adapting receptors, which fire action potentials at a progressively decreasing rate, during stimulus application. These transmit signals only when the stimulus strength is changed. Therefore, number of impulses transmitted is directly proportional to the rate at which the changes take place. Thus, the receptor potential in them is short and decays rapidly. Examples of phasic receptors are:

- ***Meissner's corpuscles, Pacinian corpuscle and olfactory receptors.***
  Function of adaptation is to decrease the amount of sensory information reaching the brain.
  Mechanism of adaptation varies in different receptors, for example:
  - *Rods and cones* adapt by changing their chemical composition,
  - *Mechanoreceptors* (Pacinian corpuscles) adapt due to redistribution of fluid.

Basically, sensory adaptation takes place via two major mechanisms:

- *Failure of transducer mechanism to maintain* a receptor potential despite continued stimulus application and
- *Failure of spike generator* to sustain a train of action potentials despite the presence of receptor potential. The decreased excitability of spike generator membrane may be attributed to an increase in the membrane conductance to K^+ or the activity of the electrogenic Na^+–K^+ pump, or the inactivation of Na^+ channels.

4. **Effect of Strength of Stimulus.** Receptor potential amplitude depends on the strength of stimulus. During the stimulation of a receptor, if the response given by the receptor is to be doubled, the strength of stimulus must be increased 10 times. This phenomenon is called *Weber–Fechner law*.

5. **Effect of Velocity of Stimulus.** The magnitude of the receptor potential rises with rate of change of stimulus application. It also applies to removal of stimulus, e.g. off response.

6. **Projection.** When any part of sensory path is stimulated, a conscious sensation referred to the location of receptor is produced. This is called *law of projection* (for details see encoding of sensation).

Encoding: Recognition of Type of Sensation

As discussed above, the sensory receptors transduce all forms of sensory stimuli into a common type of neural signal, i.e. action potentials which are carried by the peripheral nerves and sensory tracts in the spinal cord and brainstem to the sensory cortex. The question that arises is: how does the brain differentiate between the action potentials generated from a touch receptor and a pain receptor and interpret the sensation accordingly? It is believed that the sensory receptors themselves act as peripheral analysers. The intensity, location and quality of a stimulus are encoded as:

1. Encoding of Stimulus Intensity

The brain interprets different intensities of sensation (i.e. whether the touch is light or heavy; pain is mild, moderate or severe) by the following two mechanisms:

- By frequency of action potentials generated in the sensory fibres and
- By the number of recruitment of sensory units.

A. By Frequency of Action Potential Generated in Sensory Nerve Fibres

The encoding of intensity of stimulus is related to the rate of impulse discharge in the sensory nerve fibres as explained:

i. The magnitude of receptor potential is directly proportional to the logarithmic increase in the intensity of stimulus. For example, if the response given by a receptor is to be doubled, the strength of stimulus must be increased 100 times.

ii. The frequency of action potential produced in a sensory nerve is directly proportional to the magnitude of receptor potential (Fig. 10.8-5).

iii. From the above statements (i) and (ii), the frequency of action potential (S) in a sensory nerve is directly proportional to the logarithmic increase in intensity of stimulus (I), i.e.

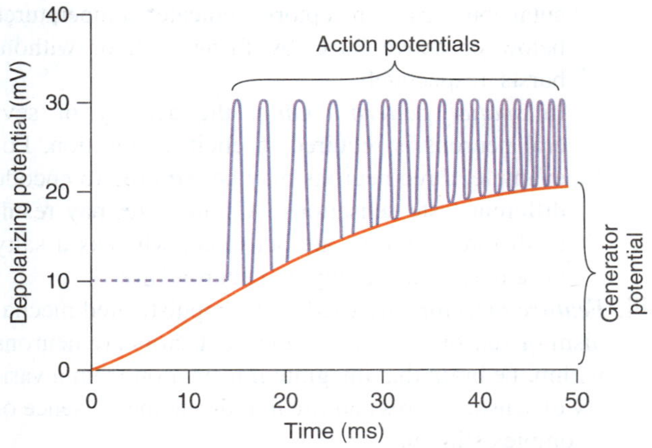

FIGURE 10.8-5 Relationship between intensity of stimulus, magnitude of receptor potential and frequency of action potential.

S = k log I + C, where K and C are constants.

The above equation is called 'Weber–Fechner law', which states that the magnitude of sensation felt is directly proportional to the log of intensity of the stimulus.

B. By Number of Recruitment of Sensory Units. A single afferent neuron with all its receptor endings makes up a *sensory unit* (Fig. 10.8-6). When the strength of stimulus is increased, it spreads over a large area activating more and more receptors in the neighbouring area and thus more and more *sensory units are recruited* to convey the impulse to brain. This increase in the recruitment of sensory units is interpreted as increase in the intensity of the stimulus.

2. Encoding of Stimulus Location

The stimulus location is recognized accurately due to point-to-point representation of the body in the somatosensory cortex. Therefore, when the sensory fibres are experimentally stimulated anywhere in their course to the cortex, the conscious sensation produced is referred to the location of the receptor. This principle is called the *law of projection*. Because of this, after amputation of a limb, sometimes a patient complains of intense pain in the absent limb (*phantom limb*).

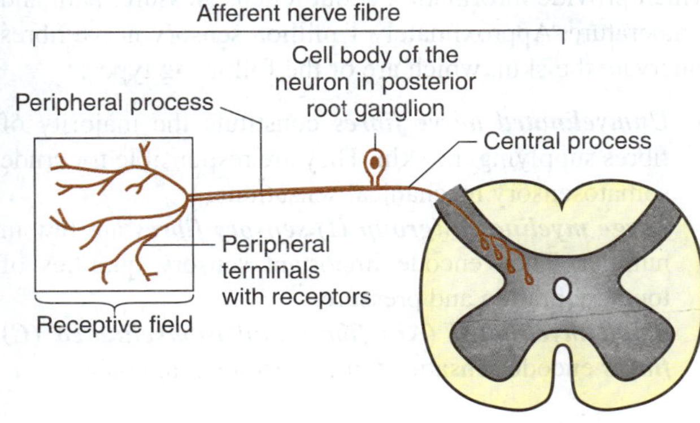

FIGURE 10.8-6 Sensory unit and receptive field.

These sensations are produced due to irritation of the damaged nociceptive and proprioceptive afferents at the stump of the amputated limb. The sensations evoked are projected to the area where receptors used to be located.

This mechanism of encoding, called *topographic representation,* is also used by visual sensation in addition to the somatosensory system to localize the point of stimulus application. This mechanism of encoding by topographic representation is influenced by:

- Receptive field of neurons and
- Phenomenon of lateral inhibition.

Receptive Field of Neuron. Each sensory neuron receives information from a particular sensory area called its receptive field (Fig. 10.8-6). Generally, the receptive fields of neighbouring neurons overlap and interdigitate with the areas supplied by others.

The smaller the receptive field the more precise the encoding of stimulus localization. For example, the ability to distinguish between two adjacent mechanical stimuli to the skin *(two-point discrimination)* is greater on the fingertips and lips where the receptive fields are much smaller and overlap considerably than on the hands and back where the receptive fields are large and widely separated.

Lateral Inhibition. Lateral inhibition is a phenomenon by which stronger inputs are enhanced and the weaker inputs of adjacent sensory units are simultaneously inhibited. Stimulus localization can be made more precise by lateral inhibition as explained: When two stimuli are applied to the skin, in the absence of lateral inhibition they can be recognized as separate only if they are applied in receptive fields that are separated from each other by a nonstimulated receptive field (Fig. 10.8-7A), otherwise the stimuli will produce an equal discharge in all these neurons (Fig. 10.8-7B).

- With lateral inhibition, the neuron with the receptive field in the centre is presynaptically inhibited by collaterals from the neurons with receptive fields located laterally. As a result, the receptive field in the centre does not fire and two stimuli are perceived (Fig. 10.8-7C).

3. Encoding of Stimulus Quality

In general, since action potentials are similar in all nerves, then why does stimulation of a touch receptor cause a sensation of touch and not of warmth? Similarly, stimulation of photoreceptors causes a sensation of light and not of hearing. Stimulus quality is encoded by the following mechanisms:

i. *Labelled line mechanism.* It is the mechanism in which the stimulus quality is encoded by the particular neural pathway that is stimulated. The basic sensory modalities are encoded by this mechanism. Each fibre or collection of neurons linked by related sensory fibres is referred to

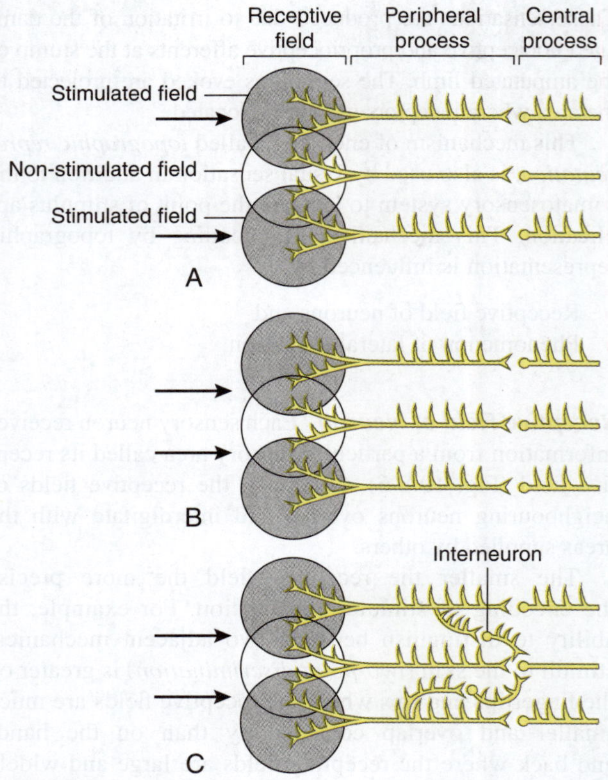

FIGURE 10.8-7 Two stimuli can be perceived distinct in the absence of lateral inhibition if they stimulate receptive fields that are separated from each other by a nonstimulated receptive field (**A**). Otherwise the stimuli produced equal amount of discharge in all the three neurons (**B**). With lateral inhibition, the neurons with receptive field in the centre are presynaptically inhibited by collaterals from the neurons located laterally. As a result, the receptive field in the centre does not fire and two stimuli are perceived (**C**).

as a *labelled line*. For example, action potentials travelling along the fibres and neurons that comprise the anterolateral system (spinothalamic tract) are perceived as pain, whereas action potentials carried over the dorsal column–medial lemniscus system are distinguished as touch or pressure. Further (i) the sensation of touch is elicited whether the receptors on skin are excited by mechanical deformation or by electrical stimulation, and (ii) the same type of sensation results no matter where along the sensory pathway the stimulus is applied.

The specificity of the sensory pathway from the receptors to the sensory cortex has been called *Muller's doctrine of specific nerve energies.*

ii. ***Pattern of activity within the neural pathway*** that carries information to the brain, which is used to encode stimulus quality is a more complex mechanism. The two types of pattern coding are:

- In *temporal pattern coding*, the same neuron can carry two different types of sensory information depending upon its pattern of activity. For example, cutaneous cold receptors indicate temperatures below or above 30°C by firing with or without bursts, respectively.
- In *spatial pattern coding*, the activity of several neurons is required to elicit a sensation. For example, three neurons may be required to encode different taste sensations. A sour taste may result if all three neurons are activated, whereas a salty taste may result if only two neurons fire.

iii. ***Feature detectors*** are used in the sophisticated mechanism of sensory coding. Feature detectors are neurons within the brain that integrate information from a variety of sensory fibres and fire to indicate the presence of a complex stimulus.

- For example, the location of an object in space can be encoded by cortical cells receiving information from a single eye. However, special feature detectors receiving information from both eyes are required to specify the depth of an object in the space.
- Similarly, the location of sound in space requires integration of information from both ears by feature detectors within the brainstem.

SOMATOSENSORY SYSTEM

Somatosensory system can now be discussed in view of the general sensory mechanism under the following headings:

- Somatic sensations,
- Pathways in somatosensory system,
- Role of thalamus in somatosensory system and
- Somatosensory cortex.

Somatic Sensations

Somatic sensations include sensations of:

- Touch, pressure, two-point discrimination, vibration, stereognosis,
- Temperature,
- Pain and
- Proprioception and kinaesthesia.

Cutaneous sensations. The skin contains receptors which provide information about touch, pressure, pain and temperature. Approximately 1 million sensory nerve fibres innervate the skin, which are of the following types:

- ***Unmyelinated nerve fibres*** constitute the majority of fibres supplying the skin. They are responsible for crude somatosensory mechanical sensations.
- ***Large myelinated (group II) sensory fibres*** are few in number. They encode important sensory qualities of touch, vibration and pressure.
- ***Small myelinated (Aδ) fibres and unmyelinated (C) fibres*** encode sensations of temperature and pain.

Cutaneous receptors can be grouped as:

- Mechanoreceptors,
- Thermoreceptors and
- Nociceptors.

Touch, Pressure, and Vibration Sensations

Mechanoreceptors Mechanoreceptors provide information about touch pressure and vibration stimuli to skin. In general, these receptors consist of an unmyelinated axon surrounded by lamellated connective tissue corpuscles. These include (Fig. 10.8-8):

1. Pacinian Corpuscles

Structure. Pacinian corpuscle, about 1 mm in diameter, consists of an onion-like concentric lamellae of connective tissue surrounding an unmyelinated terminal portion of a nerve fibre. The myelin sheath of the sensory nerve fibre begins inside the corpuscle. Therefore, first node of Ranvier is located inside the corpuscle but the second node of Ranvier is mostly outside the corpuscle (Fig. 10.8-3A, 10.8-8A).

Location. Pacinian corpuscles are located in the skin, subcutaneous tissue, mesentery and in the neighbourhood of tendons and joints.

Function. They *detect tissue vibration* or other extremely rapid changes in the mechanical state of the tissue.

Receptive Field, Stimulus and Adaptation. Receptive field of Pacinian corpuscles is large. They respond to deformation caused by mechanical pressure. The Pacinian corpuscle is a very *rapidly adapting* receptor, so only a few action potentials are generated, regardless of stimulus intensity. The deformation of the nerve terminal is not maintained during continuous stimulus application because the inner lamellae become rearranged. This is called adaptation. That is why we do not feel seat pressure when sitting. A *vibratory stimulus*, however, produces a steady discharge of the Pacinian corpuscle. Each time the stimulus is removed and applied, the Pacinian corpuscle discharges another action potential.

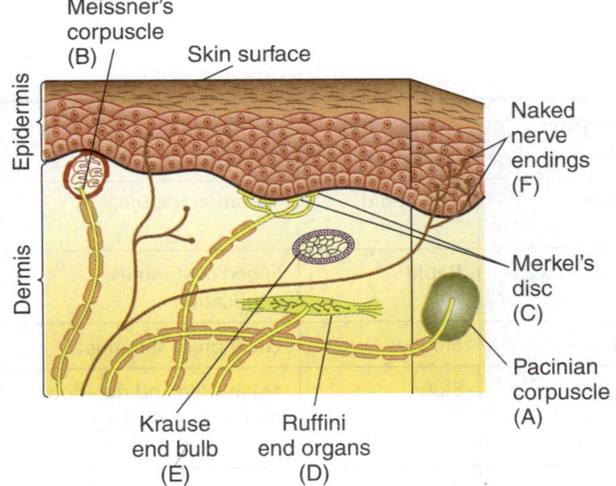

FIGURE 10.8-8 Sensory receptors: **A,** Pacinian corpuscle; **B,** Meissner's corpuscle; **C,** Merkel's disc; **D,** Ruffini end organs; **E,** Krause end bulb; and **F,** free nerve endings.

2. Meissner's Corpuscles

Structure and Location. They are small encapsulated receptors supplied by A-beta type (group II) of myelinated nerve fibres (Fig. 10.8-8B). They are present in nonhairy parts of skin and are abundant at fingertips, lips, nipples and orifices of the body.

Receptive Field, Stimulus, Function and Adaptation. These can be stimulated only by deformation of the small region of the skin lying just above the receptors; therefore, they have a *small receptive field.* They are used to detect rate of stimulus application. They are sensitive to movements of light objects over the surface of the skin. The ability to detect the rate of deformation when the skin is moved over an object is especially important to blind individuals using Braille. Meissner's corpuscles rapidly adapt to a maintained or slowly applied stimulus.

3. Merkel's Discs

Structure and Location. Merkel's discs are unique because the transducer is not on the nerve terminal but on the epithelial cells that make up the disc (Fig. 10.8-8C). The epithelial sensory cells form synaptic connections with branches of a large single group II afferent myelinated fibre. They are present in areas where Meissner's corpuscles are present, i.e. in abundance at fingertips, lips, nipples and orifices of the body.

Receptive Field, Stimulus, Function and Adaptation. Merkel's discs are *slowly adapting* receptors with a *small receptive field* that is used to detect the *location of a stimulus*. They, along with Meissner's corpuscles play an important role in localizing touch sensations and also in determining the texture of what is felt. Therefore, they are also called *tactile receptors*.

4. Ruffini's End Organs

Structure and Location. They are multibranched encapsulated endings (Fig. 10.8-8D). The receptor is located on the terminal of a group II axon that is covered by a liquid-filled collagen capsule. Collagen strands within the capsule make contact with the nerve fibres and overlying skin. They are present in the deeper layers of skin and also in the deeper tissues.

Receptive Field, Stimulus, Function and Adaptation. Ruffini's end organ is a *slowly adapting* receptor with a *large receptive field,* which is used to detect the *magnitude of stimulus*. Since they adapt very little, they continuously signal the state of deformation of the skin and deeper tissues. They are present in joint corpuscles where they detect the degree of joint rotation.

5. Hair End Organs

Structure and Location. Each hair and its basal nerve fibre form the hair end-organ.

Stimulus and Function. Hair end-organ is stimulated by slight movement of hair. These receptors mainly detect the movement of objects on the surface of the body.

6. Krause's End-Bulbs

Structure and Location. They are spherical mechanoreceptors (Fig. 10.8-8E). Their afferent fibres belong to the Aδ group. They are present in conjunctiva, in the papillae of lips and tongue, in the skin of genitalia and in the sheath of nerves.

Stimulus and Function. They detect touch and pressure.

7. Free Nerve Endings

Structure and Location. These are terminal branches of thin myelinated Aδ or unmyelinated C fibres (Fig. 10.8-8F). They are present everywhere in the skin and in many other tissues.

Stimulus and Function. As mechanoreceptors, they detect touch and pressure.

Salient Features of Mechanoreceptors. Salient features of main mechanoreceptors are summarized in Table 10.8-1.

Functions of Touch and Pressure Mechanoreceptors

1. Detection of Touch, Pressure, and Vibration Sensations by Mechanoreceptors. Touch, pressure and vibration are considered to be different forms of the same sensation.

- ***Pressure*** is felt when the force applied on the skin is sufficient to reach the receptors located in the deeper layers of skin.
- ***Touch*** is felt when the force is insufficient to reach the deeper layers.
- ***Vibrations*** are felt when there are rhythmic vibrations in the force.
- ***Detection of touch, pressure or vibration sensation by a mechanoreceptor*** depends, among other factors, on whether they are rapidly adapting or slowly adapting receptors.
- ***Slow-adapting mechanoreceptors,*** in general, are meant for sensing sustained pressure. They are of no use in detecting vibrations. These include Merkel's discs and Ruffini's end organs.
- ***Rapid-adapting mechanoreceptors,*** in general, are meant for detecting rapid fluctuation in pressure (vibration). They are of not much use in signalling sustained pressure. These include Pacinian corpuscles, Meissner's corpuscles, Krause's end-bulbs and hair end organs.

2. Two-point Discrimination. It is the ability to distinguish two touch stimuli separately. It depends upon the interaction of touch sensibility and parietal lobe. The minimum distance by which two touch stimuli can be perceived as separate stimuli varies from 2–3 mm on the lips and fingertips to over 60 mm on the back of the trunk. The difference in the distance between the two points seems to be related to the density of touch receptors in different parts of the body.

3. Stereognosis. Stereognosis refers to the ability to recognize familiar objects such as a key, coins, pen, pencil, spoons, etc. by merely handling them without looking at them. Touch and pressure receptors are involved in this sensation, but the cerebral cortex (somatic sensory association area) plays a major role.

Astereognosis, i.e. loss of stereognosis is an early sign of damage to the parietal lobe when the touch–pressure sensation is normal.

Neural Transmission

Type of Nerve Fibres. The touch-pressure sensation from the mechanoreceptors is carried to CNS by:

- A(β and δ) sensory fibres and

TABLE 10.8-1 Salient Features of Cutaneous Mechanoreceptors

Receptors	Main descriptive feature	Receptive field size	Adaptation sensation	Encoded
Pacinian corpuscles	Onion-like capsule surrounding unmyelinated nerve ending	Large	Very rapid	Vibration, tapping
Meissner's corpuscles	Small encapsulated, present in nonhairy skin	Small	Rapid	Speed of stimulus application
Merkel's disc	Transducer is on epithelial cells	Small	Slow	Location of stimulus
Ruffini's end organs	Multibranched Encapsulated Liquid-filled collagen corpuscle	Large	Slow	Magnitude and duration of stimulus (pressure)
Hair end organs	Hair and its basal nerve	Small	Rapid	Movement of object on the surface of body
Krause's end bulbs		Small	Rapid	Touch and pressure

- Unmyelinated C fibres also conduct some touch impulses.

Spinal cord tracts which carry touch-pressure sensations are two lemniscus systems (dorsal column and ventral spinothalamic tract).

Dorsal column carries sensations of:

- Fine touch (touch with low threshold excitation),
- Detailed tactile localization,
- Two-point discrimination and
- Stereognosis.

Lesions of dorsal column are therefore associated with elevation of touch threshold and loss of above sensations.

Ventral spinothalamic tracts carry sensations concerned with gross tactile sensations of crude touch.

Lesions of ventral spinothalamic tract are therefore associated with slight touch deficit. The touch localization remains normal.

Proprioceptive and Kinaesthetic Sensations

Proprioceptive and kinaesthetic sensations arise from the muscles, tendons and joints. These include:

1. Proprioceptive Sensations. These are concerned with the physical state of the body, i.e. sense of position, tendon and muscle sensations, deep pressure and sense of equilibrium.

2. Kinaesthetic Sensations. Kinaesthesia is the conscious recognition of rate of movement of different parts of the body. Kinaesthetic sensations include:

- Conscious kinaesthetic sensations and
- Unconscious kinaesthetic sensations.

Receptors Concerned The receptors concerned are called *proprioceptors* and include:

- Muscle spindle or stretch receptors (see page1048),
- Joint receptors located in the joint capsules and ligaments around the joints. Ruffini's end organs are the most important receptors for this function. A few Pacinian corpuscles are also involved.
- Golgi tendon organ(see page1057), and
- Vestibular receptors (see page 1074).

Neural Transmission

Type of Nerve Fibres. Sensations from the above-mentioned receptors are carried by the myelinated nerve fibres (group I and II) in the peripheral nerves.

Neural pathway involved is:

- *Conscious sense of position, vibration and deep pressure* is carried by axons from joint receptors and Pacinian corpuscles. These enter via posterior root, branch and enter the *dorsal column* on the same side. From the spinal cord, ultimately these sensations reach the somatosensory cortex.
- *Unconscious proprioceptive information* arising from the muscle spindles, Golgi tendon organs and joint receptors travel through group Ia and Ib fibres in peripheral nerves and through spinocerebellar tracts and dorsal column in the spinal cord. From the nuclei gracilis and cuneatus, fibres concerned with unconscious proprioception reach the cerebellum as external arcuate fibres. Spinocerebellar tracts enter the cerebellum through the inferior peduncle.

Temperature Sensation

Thermoreceptors

Structure. Thermoreceptors refer to a special type of free nerve endings, which are responsible for detecting temperature sensation. Separate receptors with discrete receptive fields exist for encoding warm and cold sensations and are called warm receptors and cold receptors, respectively. Free nerve endings of unmyelinated C fibres form the *warm receptors* and those of *small myelinated* Aδ fibres form the *cold receptors.*

Location. Thermoreceptors are located in the skin of all parts of the body. However, density of thermoreceptors is greatest in the lips, moderate in the fingertips, and least in the skin of trunk.

Receptive Fields. The receptor fields of thermoreceptors (unlike those of mechanoreceptors) do not show any overlap, probably because precise localization of thermal stimulus is rarely important to the body. Because of the lack of overlap, it is possible to delineate distinct *hot spots* (areas having warm receptors) and *cold spots* (areas having cold receptors) on the skin that respond to warmth and cold, respectively. In any area of the body, number of cold spots is about 4–10 times the number of hot spots.

Stimulus. Thermoreceptors respond to the temperature of subcutaneous tissue surrounding them and not to the environmental temperature as such. Because of this reason cold metal objects feel colder than wooden objects of the same temperature. The metal being a good conductor conducts heat away from the skin more rapidly and cools the subcutaneous tissue to a greater degree than the wood. Similarly, the alcohol-induced cutaneous vasodilatation gives a feeling of warmth, even when the person is exposed to extreme cold.

The Salient Features of Response Exhibited by Warm and Cold Receptors Are:

Warm Receptors They are activated when skin temperature is between 30 and 43°C (Fig. 10.8-9A).

- The steady state firing rate of warm receptors reaches a peak at temperatures of approximately 42°C (Fig. 10.8-9A).
- Warm receptors transiently increase their firing rate when skin temperature increases, and decrease their firing rate when skin temperature decreases (Fig. 10.8-9B). This is because the sensation produced by a small change in temperature depends on the current skin temperature. For example, a stimulus of 35°C feels warm if the skin is at 30°C, and cool if the skin is at 40°C.

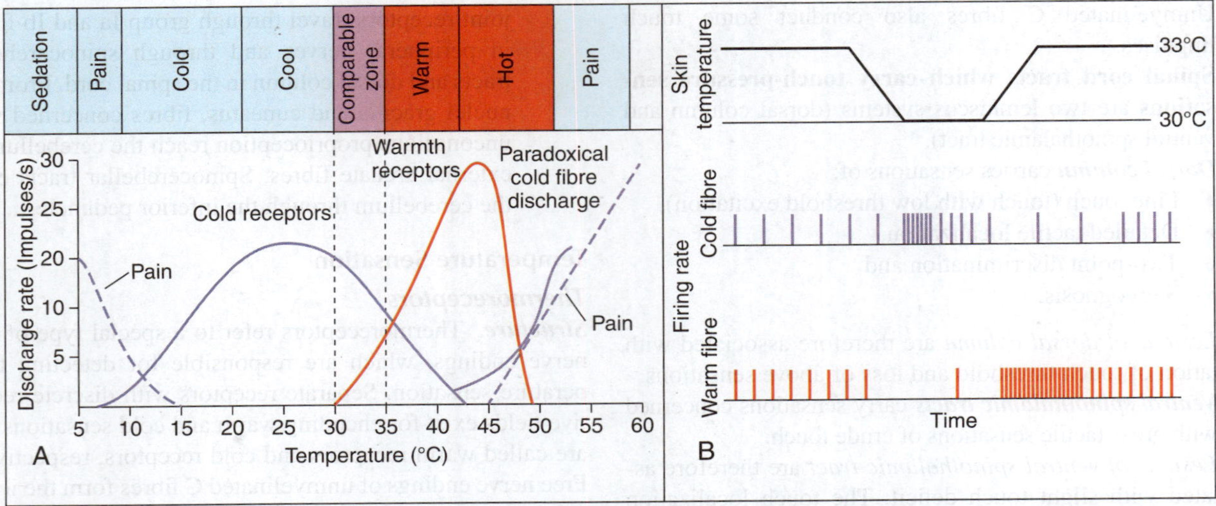

FIGURE 10.8-9 **A,** Impulse discharge rate of cold and warm receptors as a function of temperature; and **B,** spikes train illustrating the dynamic response of warm and cold receptors to a change in temperature. When the temperature decreases, cold fibres increase their firing rate transiently and then adapt to firing rate. Similarly, when temperature increases warm fibres transiently increase their firing rate before adapting to rate indicated by the graph.

Cold Receptors

- They are activated when the skin temperature is between 10 and 40°C (Fig. 10.8-9A).
- The steady state firing rate of cold receptors reaches a peak at temperatures between 25°C and 30°C (Fig. 10.8-9A).
- Cold fibres transiently increase their firing rate when temperature decreases, and transiently decrease their firing rate when skin temperature increases (Fig. 10.8-9B).
- Paradoxically, temperatures between 45°C and 50°C stimulate cold fibres as well as pain fibres producing mixed sensations of cold and pain (Fig. 10.8-9A).
- Cold temperature below 10°C stimulates only pain receptors (Fig. 10.8-9A).
- Thus, between 30°C and 40°C both cold and warm receptors are stimulated, which help the person in fine gradation of temperature. Therefore, between 30°C and 40°C (neutral or comfort zone), complete perceptual adaptation occurs (i.e. awareness of temperature disappears).
- At moderate cold, the receptor activated is TRAM 8 (Transient potential channel and M signifies menthol ingredient present in mint that gives a cool taste)
- At temperature 34°C TRPV4 (Transient potential channel and V refers to vanilloids) receptors activate a group of chemical complexes by heat, acid and chemicals capsaicin (ingredient of hot pepper).
- At temperatures between 35°C and 39°C, TRPV3 (Transient potential channel vanniloid) are activated.

Adaptation Thermoreceptors show moderate degrees of adaptation (Fig. 10.8-4C). Therefore:

- On exposure to cold, when skin temperature begins to fall, initially the person feels much colder than at a later stage, even when exposed to the same cold environments. This is because when the temperature decreases, cold fibres increase their rate of firing and then adapt to the firing rate (Fig. 10.8-9B).
- Similarly, on sudden exposure to hot environment, the feeling of warmth is more intense in the beginning. This is because, when the temperature increases, warm receptors increase their firing rate before adapting to the rate indicated in the graph (Fig. 10.8-9B).

Neural Pathway The impulses from cold receptors are carried by Aδ myelinated fibres, and those from the warm receptors are carried by unmyelinated fibres in the lateral spinothalamic tract. In the CNS, the lateral spinothalamic tract and the medial lemniscus carry impulses to the thalamus. Ultimately, impulses reach the somatosensory cortex.

Pain Sensation

Definition and Purpose

Definition. Pain refers to an unpleasant sensory and emotional experience associated with actual or potential tissue damage. The word pain has been derived from a Greek word *Poena* meaning 'penalty or punishment'.

Purpose. Pain sensation is different from other sensations because its purpose is not to inform the brain about the quality of a stimulus, but rather to indicate that the stimulus is physically damaging. Therefore, though the pain sensation is unpleasant, it is useful in the following ways:

- It makes one aware of a harmful agent in close contact with the body, and the body gives preferential treatment to this information.
- It causes the individual to react to remove the pain stimulus to prevent further damage to the tissues.

- Pain receptors are nonadaptable receptors; therefore, they keep the person apprised of the damaging stimulus as long as it persists. Thus, the pain sensation has a protective function.

Pain Receptors, Stimuli and Chemical Mediators of Pain

Nociceptors. Nociceptor is the name given to receptors of pain to indicate that they respond to noxious stimuli. The noxious stimuli can be damaging or potentially damaging mechanical, chemical and thermal stimuli.

Structure. Nociceptors refer to special types of free nerve endings of two types of nerve fibres:

- Aδ myelinated nerve fibres and
- C unmyelinated nerve fibres.

The differences between the two types of nociceptors are given in Table 10.8-2.

Location. High density of pain receptors is present in the superficial layers of skin and in many deeper tissues, like the periosteum, joints, arterial wall and falx and tentorium in the cranium. Parenchyma of liver and alveoli of lungs are insensitive to pain, but the liver capsule, bronchi, and parietal pleura are very sensitive to pain. Most other deeper tissues have relatively sparse pain nerve endings, but widespread tissue damage always results in pain, even in these areas.

Types. Nociceptors can be broadly grouped as somatic nociceptors and visceral nociceptors.

1. ***Somatic nociceptors*** are free nerve endings of Aδ and C fibres as mentioned above. Depending upon the response to different noxious stimuli, the types of nociceptors are:
   - *Unimodal nociceptors,* which respond exclusively to one modality, such as noxious chemical or heat stimulation.
   - *Polymodal nociceptors* are sensitive to several varieties of noxious stimuli.
   - *Silent nociceptors* are activated only in inflammation or tissue damage. Up to 40% of C fibres and 30% Aδ fibres are silent nociceptors.

Different variety of receptors are located on the nociceptive nerve endings, activated by noxious, thermal, mechanical or chemical stimuli. These receptors mainly belong to nonselective cation channels called transient potential channels (TRP channels) and include (Fig. 10.8-10):

- $TRPV_1$ receptors: (Transient potential channel and V refers to chemical vanilloids) activated by intense heat, acid and capsaicin (an active ingredient of hot pepper)
- $TRPV_3$: Transient potential channel present in keratinocytes of skin
- $TRPA_1$: Transient potential channel and A represents ankyrin (activated by noxious mechanical, and cold thermal stimuli)
- ASIC: Acid-sensing ion channels that are activated by pH changes.
- Some nociceptive endings release intermediate molecules, which activate receptors on nerve endings;
  - Purinergic receptor (P_{2X} and P_{2Y})—ATP releases on mechanical stimuli, that acts on these receptors.
  - Tyrosine receptor kinase A (TrkA)—activated by nerve growth factors, which are released as a result of tissue damage.
  - B_1 and B_2 receptors—activated by bradykinin.
  - Prostanoid receptors—activated by prostaglandins.
  - Cytokine receptors

TABLE 10.8-2 Characteristic Features of Aδ Fibres and C-Fibre Nociceptors

S No. Feature	Aδ fibre nociceptors	C-fibre nociceptors
1. Number	Less	More
2. Myelination	Myelinated	Unmyelinated
3. Diameter	2–5 m	0.4–1.2 μm
4. Conduction velocity	12–30 m/s	0.5–2 m/s
5. Specific stimulus	Most sensitive to pressure (mechanoreceptor)	Most sensitive to chemical agents like: • Local anaesthetics, • Histamine, • Kinins and • Prostaglandins
6. Impulse conduction	Conduct impulses only in response to noxious stimuli (fast component of pain)	Conduct impulses in response to thermal and mechanical stimuli and slow component of pain
7. Sensitivity to electrical stimulus	More	Less

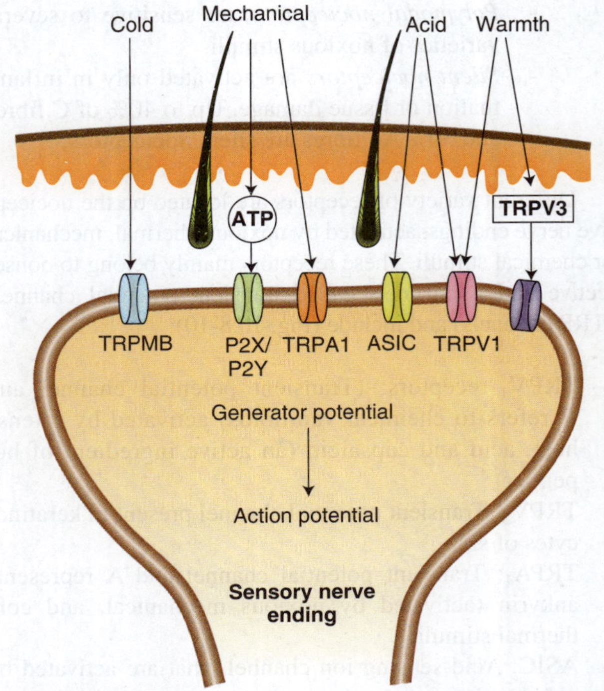

FIGURE 10.8-10 Receptors on receptive unmyelinated nerve terminals in the skin.

All these receptors mediate inflammatory pain.

2. ***Visceral nociceptors:*** Visceral pain is not produced by many tissue-damaging stimuli such as localized cutting, clamping or burning. However, widespread inflammation, ischaemia, mesenteric stretching, or spasm or dilatation of hollow viscera produce pain. There is little evidence for specialized pain receptors in viscera. Visceral pain is often due to excessive tension on nerve endings in the smooth muscles, i.e. probably stretch receptors produce pain when stimulated to high firing rates by intense stimuli. For example, pain due to uterine contractions during childbirth, or pain due to colic of alimentary, biliary or urinary tracts.

Pain Stimuli. Pain receptors are activated by three types of noxious stimuli: mechanical, thermal and chemical.

- ***Mechanical and thermal stimuli*** tend to elicit fast pain. *Fast pain* is felt when a needle is stuck into the skin, when the skin is cut with a knife or when the skin is acutely burned. It is also felt when the skin is subjected to electric shock. Fast, sharp pain is not felt in most of the deeper tissues. Mechanical and thermal stimuli, however, can also elicit slow pain.
- ***Chemical stimuli*** usually tend to elicit slow suffering type of pain that occurs after tissue injury, although this is not always the cause.

As mentioned earlier, pain sensation is associated with actual or potential tissue damage caused by noxious stimuli. Damaged tissue releases certain chemicals which act on nociceptors and cause pain sensations. Chemical mediators of pain include:

- *K^+, ATP and ADP* are released following cell death.
- *Bradykinin* is formed by the reaction of certain circulating globulins with proteolytic enzymes released by dying cells. It is most powerful in causing tissue damage pain.
- *Leukotrienes* are released from mast cells.
- *Serotonin* is released from platelets.
- *Histamine* is released from mast cells.
- Accumulation of *lactic acid* in tissues due to anaerobic mechanism during ischaemia also stimulates nociceptors and causes pain.
- *Prostaglandins* are mediators of pain, fever and inflammation. These are synthesized by enzyme cyclo-oxygenase, which is induced in peripheral tissues by cytokines, growth factors and other inflammatory stimuli.
- Activation of a nociceptive nerve terminal stimulates the axon reflex and releases *substance P* and *calcitonin gene-related peptide* (CGRP) from other terminals of the same nociceptive nerve fibre.
- Prostaglandins and substance P enhance the sensitivity of pain endings but do not directly excite them.
- Nociceptin.

Classification of Pain Basically pain is classified as; physiological pain (acute pain) and pathological pain (chronic pain).

- ***Physiological or acute pain*** has a sudden onset, recedes with healing process and is also termed as *'good pain'* as it is an important protective mechanism. Withdrawal reflex is an example of protective role.
- ***Pathological pain or chronic pain*** is also considered as *'bad pain'* because it persists for long period. Chronic pain occurs due to injury (neuropathic pain), inflammation, and ischemia and persists for a long time even after recovery and is usually unresponsive to analgesic agents.

Qualitative Types of Pain Sensations Qualitatively pain sensations are of two types: fast pain and slow pain.

1. Fast Pain. Fast pain is a sharp, well-localized, pricking sensation that results from activation of the nociceptors on the Aδ fibres. The fast pain sensations travel faster and thus appear within 0.1 ms after the application of the stimulus. It is carried by Aδ fibres, which have a small receptive field and a topographic representation in the cortex.

***Accompaniments of fast pain** are:*

- *Withdrawal reflex,* which causes the individual to move the involved body part away from the source of painful stimulus.
- *Sympathetic response,* i.e. increased blood pressure, tachycardia and mobilization of body energy supply.

2. Slow Pain. Slow pain is a poorly localized, dull, throbbing, burning sensation that results from activation of nociceptors on the C fibres. It appears after one second or more following the application of stimulus. It is carried by C type of nerve fibres, which are unmyelinated fibres.

Accompaniments of slow pain are:

- *Emotional perception* in the form of unpleasantness, and in long-standing cases irritation, frustration and depression.
- *Autonomic symptoms* in the form of nausea, profuse sweating, vomiting, and lowering of blood pressure.
- *Generalized reduction in skeletal muscle tone.*

Clinical Types of Pain In clinical practice, pain sensations can be classified as:

- Somatic pain,
- Visceral pain,
- Referred pain,
- Radiating pain and
- Projected pain.

1. Somatic Pain. Somatic pain, as the name indicates, arises from the tissues of the body other than viscera. It is of two types:

- ***Superficial somatic pain*** arises from the skin and superficial tissues. Its features are usually similar to the *fast pain*.
- ***Deep somatic pain*** arises from the muscles, joints, bones and fascia. Usually, its features are similar to that of *slow pain*.

Clinical conditions associated with somatic pain. Common conditions that are associated with pain stimuli in day-to-day clinical practice are:

- *Injuries*, which can be in the form of mechanical trauma, chemical injuries (e.g. those caused by acid burns) and thermal injuries.
- *Tissue ischaemia:* Blockage of the blood flow to the tissues causes severe pain. Pain is caused due to accumulation of lactic acid in the tissues due to anaerobic mechanisms during tissue ischaemia. Other agents such as bradykinin and proteolytic enzymes released due to tissue damage caused by ischaemia may be more important cause of pain.
- *Inflammation* of the tissues caused by infecting agents (bacteria, virus and other organisms) is very important cause of pain in clinical practice. Chemical mediators released due to tissue damage are responsible for eliciting pain.
- *Muscle spasm:* It causes pain due to direct stimulation of mechanosensitive pain receptors as well as indirectly by producing tissue ischaemia due to spasm of blood vessels.

2. Visceral Pain.

Visceral nociceptors see page 1030.

Features of visceral pain are:

- *Poorly localized,* because pain receptors in viscera are comparatively few.
- *Unpleasant* because of emotional perception.
- *Autonomic symptoms* in the form of nausea, vomiting, profuse sweating and lowering of blood pressure.
- *Reflex contraction of skeletal muscle* of abdominal wall, clinically known as guarding, is a common association, especially when inflammation of viscera involves peritoneum. It is a protective reflex which helps to protect the underlying inflamed structures from unintentional injury.
- *Radiates* or is referred to other site(see referred pain).

Common causes of visceral pain are:

1. *Inflammation* of the viscera, e.g. appendicitis, cholecystitis, pancreatitis, etc.
2. *Overdistension of hollow viscera*, e.g. intestinal distension in intestinal obstruction, urinary bladder distension in urinary obstruction, etc.
3. *Spasm of hollow viscus:* Pain is caused due to mechanical stimulation of pain endings and ischaemia. For example, pain due to uterine contraction during child birth, pain due to colics of alimentary, biliary or urinary tracts.
4. *Chemical stimuli:* Damaging substances may leak from gastrointestinal tract into the peritoneal cavity, e.g. gastric acid leaking through perforated gastric or duodenal ulcer.
5. *Ischaemia,* as occurring in tractions on mesentery. Pain is due to acidic metabolic end products or tissue degenerative products such as bradykinin and proteolytic enzymes.

Neural Pathway. Visceral pain sensation is carried by unmyelinated type C afferent fibres in the sympathetics (from most of the viscera) and in the parasympathetic (from many pelvic viscera) nerves. Their cell bodies are located in the dorsal roots and the homologous cranial nerve ganglion.

In the central nervous system, visceral pain fibres travel along with somatic pain fibres in the spinothalamic tract and medial lemniscus.

3. Referred Pain. Referred pain as the name indicates is that pain which originates due to irritation of a visceral organ and is felt not in the organ but in some other somatic structure (usually skin) supplied by the same neural segment.

Characteristic features of referred pain are:

1. Such a pain is said to be referred to the second structure. For example:
   - In *myocardial ischaemia,* pain is referred to the left shoulder and arm.
   - Pain due to *stone in lower part of ureter* is usually referred to the corresponding testis and inner thigh.
   - *Inflammation of diaphragm* secondary to pleurisy or severe cholecystitis produces pain at the tip of shoulder.

2. Because the *skin is topographically mapped* and the viscera are not, the pain is identified as originating on the skin and not within the viscera.
3. Pain is usually referred to a structure with *common embryonic origin* and hence is innervated by a common neural segment. This principle is called the *dermatomal rule*. For example, embryologically, the heart and the left arm have the same segmental origin. Similarly, the testes and kidney develop from the same primitive urogenital ridge.

Theories of referred pain are:

1. *Convergence theory:* According to this theory, when the first-order neurons carrying pain sensation from a somatic area and a visceral organ converge on a common second-order neuron (Fig. 10.8-11A), the brain is unable to identify the source of pain. Since somatic pain is far more common, the brain interprets all pain as somatic pain even when the source is actually visceral.
2. *Facilitation theory:* According to this theory, the visceral irritation is inadequate for producing pain by itself. However, it facilitates pain fibres from somatic structures (Fig. 10.8-11B), so that even minor somatic irritation produces perceptible pain.

4. Radiating Pain. Sometimes, visceral pain is experienced both locally and also at a distant point (referred pain). In fact, pain seems to spread from the local area to the distant site. This is called radiating pain. Examples of radiating pain are:

- In appendicitis, pain starts in the right iliac fossa and radiates towards centre of abdomen.

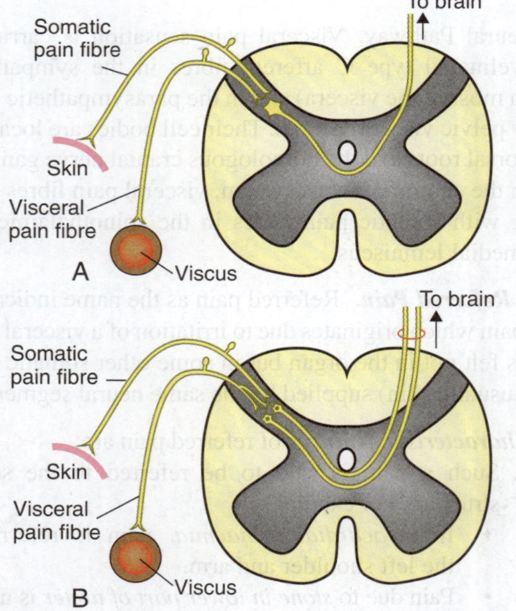

FIGURE 10.8-11 Theories of referred pain: **A**, convergence theory; **B**, facilitation theory.

5. Projected Pain. When the sensory fibres carrying pain sensations are stimulated anywhere in their course to the sensory cortex, the pain sensations evoked are projected to the area where receptors are located. This is called *projected pain*. It should not be confused with referred pain in which pain originating in visceral organs is referred to sites on the skin. Projected pain follows the *law of projection* (see page 1022). Examples of projected pain are:

- After amputation of a limb, sometime the patient complains of intense pain in the absent limb (phantom limb). The pain sensations are produced due to irritation of nociceptive fibres at the stump but are projected to the area where receptors used to be located.
- Striking the elbow causes pain to be projected to the hand.

6. Hyperalgesia. Hyperalgesia refers to enhanced painful response to a stimulus. It is of two types:

i. ***Primary hyperalgesia.*** In it, the noxious stimuli produce more severe pain than expected. It occurs over an area of tissue damage. The pain threshold is lowered, so that even non-noxious stimuli (e.g. touch) produce pain (*allodynia*). The movement-related symptoms of osteoarthritis and touch-evoked pain of herpetic neuralgia are both examples of mechanical allodynia. Primary hyperalgesia is due to release of alogenic pain-producing substances like histamine, 5HT, plasma kinin and prostaglandins from the damaged tissues.

Several other changes occurring that lead to chronic pain are:

- NGF released by damaged tissue reterogradely transported to cell bodies of dorsal root ganglia and increases production of substance P, and also affects expression of tetadoxin-resistant Na^+ channels (NaV;18) on dorsal root ganglia and increases their activity.

ii. ***Secondary hyperalgesia*** refers to occurrence of far more severe pain than expected in response to noxious stimulus applied to normal healthy skin. In this condition, there is no lowering of pain threshold. Secondary hyperalgesia has been explained to result due to phenomenon of subliminal fringe. Primary pain afferents from an area of tissue damage not only stimulate the appropriate second-order neurons to threshold level producing pain and primary hyperalgesia, but also excite the second-order neurons belonging to nearby area to subthreshold level. Hence, application of noxious stimulus produces more intense pain in this area.

Note. Nociceptin is an opioid-like polypeptide, and has no binding affinity for opioid receptors. It causes hyperalgesia when injected intracranially in experimental animals. It probably has a role in pain transmission.

Causalgia. Causalgia is a condition in which spontaneous burning pain sensation occurs after a long time in the area of even trivial injuries. It is also accompanied by *hyperalgesia* and reflex sympathetic dystrophy.

Reflex sympathetic dystrophy means sympathetic discharge reflexly causes pain in the injured skin area. The exact cause is not known, but research in the animals reveals that:

- In the affected area, the skin becomes thin, hair growth increases and nerve injuries lead to sprouting of the sympathetic nerve fibres. The overgrowth of sympathetic (noradrenergic) endings enters into the dorsal root ganglia of the spinal nerves. Therefore, discharge of these noradrenergic endings stimulates the altered circuitry of nerve fibres in the skin.
- Use of α-adrenergic blocker helps in relief of causalgia type pain.
- Excessive activation of NMDA receptors on spinal motor neurons leads to increased activity in pain pathways.
- Increased activation of neuroglia (microglia) near afferent nerve terminals by release of neurotransmitters from sensory afferents, which in turn leads to release of proinflammatory substances (cytokines) that act presynaptically on pain processing by PK_{2X} receptors and increase the excitability of postsynaptic neurons. Therefore, antagonists of PK_{2K} receptors may be used therapeutically to alleviate chronic pain.

Properties of Pain Sensations In general, properties of pain sensation are:

1. ***Threshold and intensity.*** Pain is not felt when the intensity of stimulation is low (i.e. subthreshold stimulus). However, when intensity increases, more and more pain is felt according to Weber–Fechner law (page 1023). When intensity of stimulus is very high, pain even spreads to neighbouring areas.
2. ***Adaptation.*** Since pain receptors do not show any adaptation, so pain continues as long as receptors are stimulated. In some instances, the activation of pain receptors becomes progressively greater as the pain stimulus continues, this is called *hyperalgesia*.
3. ***Localization of pain.*** In general, pain sensations are poorly localized. Superficial pain is comparatively better localized than deep pain. Visceral pain is most of the time referred to the area other than the area overlying the viscus.
4. ***Emotional accompaniment.*** Pain sensation is usually associated with unpleasantness. Long-standing pain causes irritation, frustration and even depression.
5. ***Influence of rate of damage on intensity.*** If rate of damage (extent of damage in time) is high, intensity of pain is high and vice versa. Therefore, slowly growing tissue-damaging agents, e.g. cancer, at early stage may not produce pain at all.
6. ***Qualitative types.*** Qualitatively pain sensation is of two types, fast and slow. Each type having its typical features as described above (page 1030).
7. ***Muscular response.*** Acute pain may be associated with skeletal muscle spasm in the affected area, e.g. spasm of the muscles around fractured area. This has a beneficial effect as it causes immobilization of the part and the part gets rested automatically.
8. ***Reflex response.*** Fast pain evokes a *withdrawal reflex* and a sympathetic response (see page 1030). Slow pain is associated with autonomic symptoms (see page 1031).

Neural Pathway and Perception of Pain Sensations

Two separate pathways exist for transmission of fast and slow pain to the brain.

Pathway for the Fast Pain

- ***In peripheral nerves.*** Fast pain signals are transmitted from Aδ fibres at velocities between 6 and 30 m/s to dorsal root ganglion and then enter the spinal cord at dorsal root of spinal nerve (formed by axons of cells of dorsal root ganglion) (Fig. 10.8-12).
- ***In the spinal cord***, Aδ fibres ascend or descend for one or two segments in the tract of Lissauer lying immediately posterior to the dorsal horn and then terminate into neurons of lamina I. These neurons give rise to fibres that immediately cross to the opposite side of the cord through anterior commissure (Fig. 10.8-12) and then

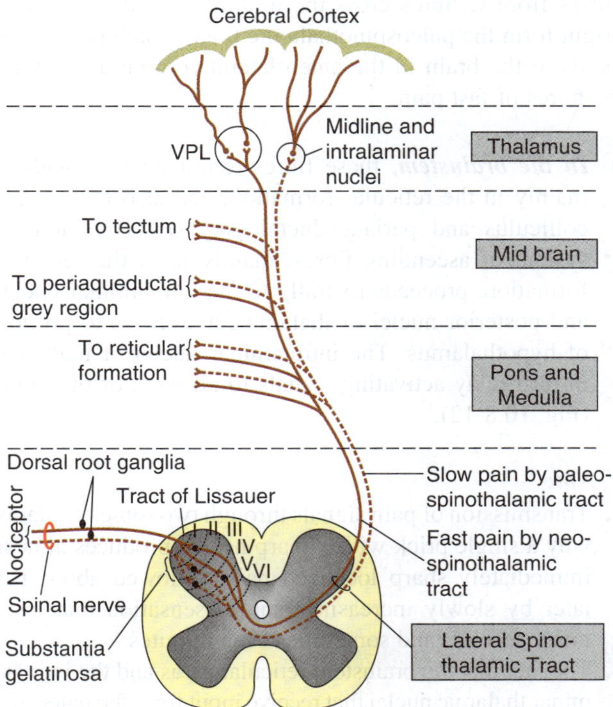

FIGURE 10.8-12 Neural pathway of fast and slow pain.

pass upwards to the brain in the anterolateral columns as *neospinothalamic tract.*

In the brainstem, a few fibres from the neospinothalamic tract terminate in the reticular formation, but most of them pass upwards to the thalamus (Fig. 10.8-12).

- ***In the thalamus,*** most of the fibres project to the ventral posterolateral (VPL) nucleus. From here, thalamic neurons project to the primary sensory cortex (Fig. 10.8-12).

Importanat Note

This system is primarily used in the localization of pain stimuli. When tactile receptors are also stimulated along with fast pain fibres, localization of fast pain is exact. If only pain receptors are stimulated, localization is poor.

Pathway for Slow Pain

- ***In peripheral nerves,*** slow pain impulses are carried by slow-conducting unmyelinated fibres at velocities ranging from 0.5 to 2 m/s to the dorsal root ganglion and then enter the spinal cord at dorsal root of spinal nerve (formed by axons of cells of dorsal root ganglion) (Fig. 10.8-12).
- ***In the spinal cord,*** the C fibres terminate in the laminae II and III of the dorsal horn. Laminae II and III are together known as substantia gelatinosa.

From here, fibres go to lamina V of dorsal horn. Axons of neurons of lamina I of dorsal horn which receive impulses from C fibres cross the midline near their level of origin form the paleospinothalamic tract, which passes upwards to the brain in the anterolateral column along with the fibres of fast pain.

- ***In the brainstem,*** these fibres terminate very widely, mainly in the reticular formation, and also in superior colliculus and periaqueductal grey (PAG) region. A system of ascending fibres, mainly from the reticular formation, proceeds rostrally to the intralaminar nuclei and posterior nuclei of thalamus, as well as to portion of hypothalamus. The intralaminar nuclei of thalamus in turn relay activating signals to all parts of the brain (Fig. 10.8-12).

Note

1. Transmission of pain signals through two routes explains why a single prick with a sharp needle produces almost immediately sharp localized pain, followed about 1 s later by slowly increasing painful sensation that lasts many seconds and sometimes even minutes.
2. The fact that the brainstem reticular areas and the intralaminar thalamic nuclei that receive input from the paleospinothalamic pathway are part of the brainstem-activating or alerting systems may explain why individuals with chronic pain syndromes have difficulty in sleeping.

Perception of Pain Sensations. Perception of pain is the phenomenon by which noxious stimuli reach consciousness. It involves two components:

- Nociceptive component and
- Affective (cognition and attention) component.

1. Nociceptive Component of Pain Perception involves the neural pathway of pain as described above.

The role of somatic sensory cortex (SI) in pain perception is not entirely clear. Complete removal of SI cortex does not eliminate the perception of pain. Such lesions do, however, interfere with ability to interpret the quality of pain and to determine its precise localization. Therefore, it is believed that pain perception occurs at subcortical levels, i.e. in the thalamus and in the reticular formation of the brainstem. However, somatosensory cortex helps in exact and meaningful interpretation of quality and localization of pain.

2. Affective (Cognitive and Attention) Component of Pain Perception is the psychological component. It involves the activity of spinothalamic tracts–limbic system pathway. *Cognitive perceptions* are those abilities that recognize, discriminate, memorize or judge afferent information. It involves patient's ability to relate a painful experience to another event, e.g. pain experienced in a pleasant environment elicits a less intense response than experienced in a setting of depression.

Attention plays role in the perception of pain on the basis that only a fixed number of afferent stimuli can reach cortical centres. Therefore, if a patient in pain concentrates on a separate and unrelated image, e.g. getting deeply involved in a music or an interesting movie on television, it is possible that he will perceive lesser intensity of pain than otherwise. The biofeedback and hypnosis, for their positive impact on pain, operate on this principle.

Pain Suppression Systems in CNS The degree of reaction to painful stimuli varies from individual to individual, mainly because of existence of pain suppression systems in the central nervous system. The pain suppression consists of two major components:

- Spinal pain suppression system and
- Supraspinal pain suppression system.

A. Spinal Pain Suppression System. There exists a pain inhibitory complex in dorsal horn of spinal cord which blocks the pain signals at the initial entry point to the spinal cord.

Gate Control Hypothesis has been put forward by Metzak and Wall in 1965 to explain the working of spinal pain suppression system. According to this hypothesis, the dorsal grey horn acts as a gate for transmission of pain sensation and this gate can be partly or completely closed by:

- Segmental suppression and
- Supraspinal suppression.

1. ***Segmental suppression:*** It has been observed that activation of large myelinated touch fibres (Aβ) reduces pain. It is called the gating of pain and occurs because after

entering the spinal cord, the Aβ fibres give collaterals that cause *presynaptic inhibition* (primary afferent depolarization) of pain carrying both type C and Aδ fibres, where they synapse in the dorsal horn (Fig. 10.8-13). This is done by blocking calcium channels in the membranes of nerve terminals. Although poorly understood, such circuitry probably explains the relief of pain achieved by following manoeuvres:

- Rubbing or massage or pressure in the vicinity of painful area.
- Local application of warmth or cold.
- Local application of counterirritants, i.e. stimulation of skin.
- Acupuncture and
- Transcutaneous electric nerve stimulation (TENS) in which pain site or the nerves leading from it are stimulated by electrodes placed on the surface of skin.

2. ***Supraspinal suppression*** is caused by the supraspinal suppression system described below.

B. Supraspinal Pain Suppression System. There exist three different supraspinal descending pain modulation pathways:

- Descending serotonergic and opioid inhibitory system,
- Descending purinergic inhibitory system and
- Descending adrenergic inhibitory system.

1. Descending Serotonergic and Opioid Inhibitory System: It is the most important supraspinal pain inhibitory system. Components of this system (Fig. 10.8-14) are:

i. ***Raphe magnus nucleus (RMN).*** It is a thin midline nucleus located in the lower pons and upper medulla. Its neurons receive innervation from the periaqueductal grey (PAG) reticular formation, hypothalamus and frontal cortex. Neurons of RMN contain both serotonin (5HT) and substance P. The *serotonergic neurons* of the RMN project down the dorsolateral column to influence the neurons in dorsal horn of spinal cord, which are excited by primary nociceptive afferents. The serotonergic fibres are believed to exert their effect by *postsynaptic inhibition*. The drug amitriptyline alleviates pain by increasing the levels of serotonin. The function of substance P in these neurons and their relationship with serotonin is uncertain. Inhibition of pain fibres in the spinal cord inhibits withdrawal reflex evoked by application of noxious stimuli. Other sensory modalities like touch and temperature are not affected.

ii. ***Periaqueductal grey (PAG) area in the midbrain.*** It inhibits pain by stimulating the raphe magnus nucleus (RMN) (Fig. 10.8-15). Neurons of PAG have opioid receptors on their surface membranes. In general, four types of opioid receptors have been described **n**, **K**, **5** and **o**. When *opioid receptors* are stimulated by exogenously administered opioid compounds (analgesics) or by endogenous opioid neurotransmitters (endorphins and enkephalins) found in the brain, the pain suppression circuitry is activated and this leads to reduced pain perception.

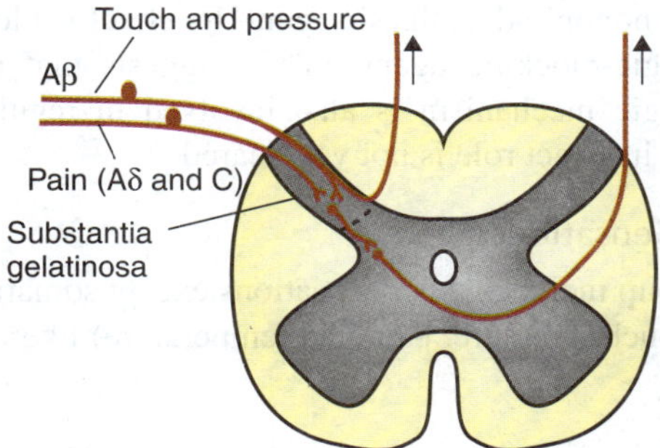

FIGURE 10.8-13 Spinal pain suppression system. **Note:** The collateral from Aβ fibres from touch receptors cause presynaptic inhibition of pain afferent Aδ and C fibres.

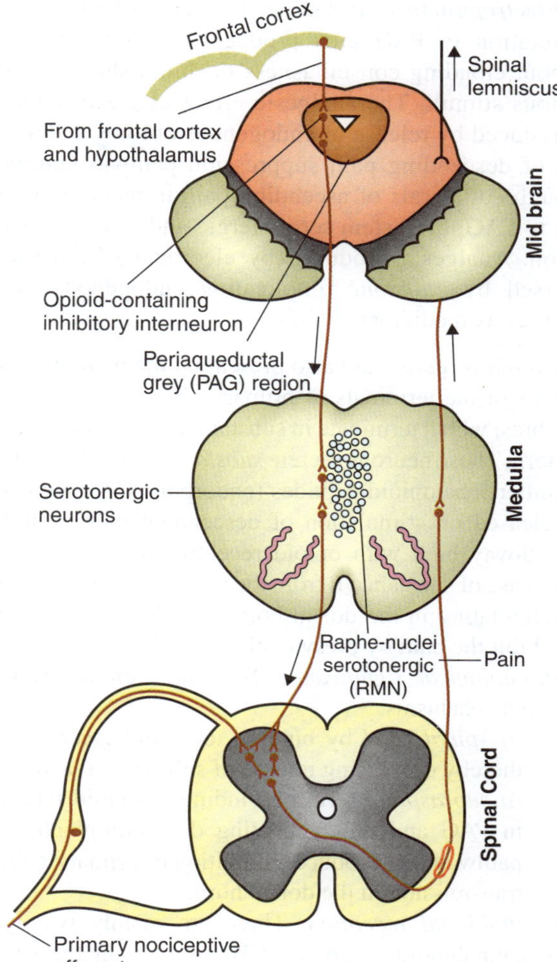

FIGURE 10.8-14 Supraspinal serotonergic and opioid pain inhibitory system.

Electropuncture. It has been observed that electrical stimulation in PAG area produces profound analgesia without clouding consciousness or diminishing the non-noxious stimuli. The analgesic effect of electropuncture is produced by release of endogenous opioids and activation of descending pain suppression pathway indirectly through collaterals of ascending pain transmission pathway to PAG, brainstem serotonergic and catecholanergic region. Analgesia produced by electrical stimulation is reversed by *naloxone,* implicating endogenous opioid peptides as mediators.

- *Opioid receptors* are also present on the membrane surface of the terminals of primary afferent pain-carrying fibres, which terminate in substantia gelatinosa of dorsal horn. These neurons secrete *substance* P as a neurotransmitter. The opioid peptides (endorphin and enkephalin) released on stimulation of descending pain inhibitory pathway bind with opioid receptors and decrease the release of substance P from the primary afferent neurons terminating in the dorsal horn (Fig. 10.8-15), and thus inhibit the pain by presynaptic inhibition.
  Physiological significance. Morphine relieves pain by two mechanisms:
  - *At spinal level* by binding to opioid receptors and thereby decreasing release of substance P and
  - *At supraspinal level* by binding to opioid receptors in PAG and thus activating descending inhibitory pathway that produces inhibition of primary afferent transmission in the dorsal horn.
- *Cannabinoid receptors.* There are mainly two types of cannabinoid receptors: CB_1 present on the central neurons and CB_2 on the peripheral neurons. Some non-neural cells also possess these receptors. An endogenous ligand analogous to these receptors (anandamide) exerts its analgesic effect by binding to these receptors.

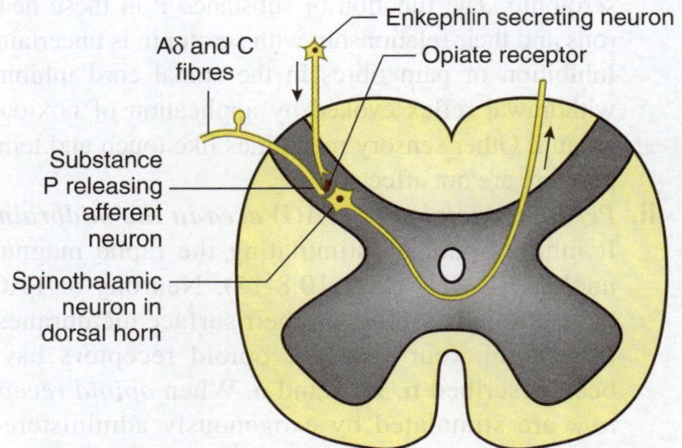

FIGURE 10.8-15 Location of opioid receptors on terminals of primary pain afferent neurons, and their relationship with enkephalin secreting neuron in dorsal horn (mechanism of presynaptic inhibition of pain fibres by opioid peptides).

iii. *Hypothalamus and frontal cortex* also play role in pain suppression. Neurons descending from hypothalamus and frontal cortex stimulate both the above-described brainstem centres of pain inhibition, i.e. PAG as well as RMN (Fig. 10.8-14).

The descending serotonergic and opioid pain inhibitory system is stimulated in following situations:

Stress induced analgesia occurs:

i. *When limbic system is stimulated.* Limbic system is the seat of emotions. Fibres from limbic system supply the PAG. This explains why a soldier wounded in the battlefield may feel no pain during the heat of battle, also called stress induced analgesia. In this condition;
- Release of norepinephrine from brainstem catacholminergic neurons and amygdala (the part of limbic system) is involved in motivational-affective response to pain.
- Release of cannabinoids, such as 2-archidonoyl glycerol (2AG) and anadomide may have a role in stress-induced analgesia.

ii. *Autofeedback.* When the spinothalamic tract (STT) is stimulated, the collaterals from STT stimulate the descending inhibitory pathway (Fig. 10.8-15).

2. Descending Purinergic Inhibitory System, comprising specifically of adenosine, has been recognized. Adenosine exhibits both pre- and postsynaptic actions and produces antinociception by indirect interaction with excitatory amino acid release. Role of adenosine on pain suppression system is corroborated by the following two observations:

- Significant decrease in circulating blood and CSF adenosine levels in patients with neuropathic pain and
- Effective attenuation of neuropathic pain following low-dose infusion of adenosine.

3. Descending Noradrenergic Inhibitory System. Fibres of this system originate from the *locus coeruleus* and medullary reticular formation and descend in dorsolateral fasciculus. Environmental factors, such as stress, may activate this descending inhibitory mechanism. Norepinephrine-depleting agents, including reserpine and α_2-antagonists, and lesions within the noradrenergic system, all interfere with morphine analgesia.

4. Acetylcholine. Epibatidine, a cholinergic agonist, is a strong nonopioid analgesic agent. Its effect is blocked by cholinergic-blocking agents. This suggests that nicotinic cholinergic mechanism is also involved in regulation of pain but its exact role is not yet cleared.

Other Sensations

This group includes other sensations except somatic sensations (touch, pressure, pain and temperature) like:

- Itch,
- Tickle and
- Synthetic senses.

Itch (Pruritue). It is an irritative skin condition which occurs due to mild stimulation (especially when something moves across the skin).

Characteristic Features are:

1. It occurs only in the skin, eyes and certain mucous membranes but not in the deep tissue and viscera.
2. It originates due to stimulation of *itch receptors* which are naked nerve endings of unmyelinated C fibres. The receptors are stimulated by two ways:
   - By repeated local mechanical stimulation of skin and
   - By certain chemical agents, e.g.
   - Bile salts (raised plasma concentration of bile salts during pregnancy),
   - Histamine (in urticaria, severe itching results due to release of large quantity of histamine from antigen–antibody complex) and
   - Kinins.

   Kinins produce their effect by activation of GPCRs (B_1 and B_2). B_2 receptors are protease-activated receptor-2 (PAR-2) that produce both nociceptive and pruitogenic response.
3. The pathway for itch sensation like pain is carried by fibres into the spinal cord and then conducted by lateral spinothalamic tract.
4. Scratching relieves the itching. The mechanism is same as gate control hypothesis in pain sensation, i.e. scratching stimulates large, fast-conducting afferents which cause presynaptic inhibition of fibres in the dorsal horn cells.
   - Antihistaminics and
   - B_2 antagonists are effective in reducing pruritis and reduce scratching behaviour (occurs in response to activation of PAR-2 receptors).

Tickle. Tickle is another variable of touch sensation. It is regarded as a pleasurable feeling compared with itching (which gives annoying feeling) and pain (is an unpleasant feeling).

Synthetic Sense. The combinations of various cutaneous sensations produce different experiences that are entirely different from primary sensation. Therefore, the new experience is regarded as synthetic sense.

Pathways in Somatosensory System (Transmission of Sensations)

Neurons of Sensory Pathway

Pathways in somatosensory system are formed by a chain of three neurons, which ultimately reach the sensory cortex:

First-order Neurons These are the primary afferent neurons that receive the transduced signals from the sensory receptors and carry them to the spinal cord or brainstem. The cell bodies of the primary afferent neurons are located in *dorsal root ganglia.* These are T-shaped unipolar neurons with peripheral and central processes. The peripheral processes reach the sensory receptors and form the sensory part of *spinal nerves* (which are mixed nerves). Central processes constitute the *dorsal nerve root* of the spinal nerve (and also see page 902).

Type of Sensory Fibres. The fibres of first-order neurons in the spinal nerves and dorsal nerve root comprise Aα, Aβ, Aδ and C type fibres, and are often referred to group I, II, III and IV, respectively, by the sensory physiologists (Table 10.8-3). Aα and β fibres are not present in sensory pathways. For further details about types of fibres, see page 74.

Second-order Neurons The second-order neurons are located in the spinal cord or brainstem. They receive information from one or more primary afferent neurons and transmit it to the thalamus. *In spinal cord,* the neurons involved in sensory functions are present in dorsal horn of spinal grey matter. The grey matter of *dorsal horn* is divided into laminae. For details, see page 901, before proceeding further. Axons of the second-order neurons form the *ascending sensory tracts* described below.

Third-order Neurons Third-order neurons of the sensory pathway are located in specific nuclei of thalamus. From here, the encoded sensory information ascends to sensory cortex through the thalamic radiations.

Sensory Nerves and Dermatomes

Sensory Nerves All sensory fibres reach the CNS through their cranial equivalents.

Dorsal Nerve Roots in Spinal Cord (Fig. 10.1-5): Different types of sensory fibres forming sensory part of spinal nerve carry different type of sensations (Table 10.8-3). Each dorsal nerve root is attached to the spinal cord through

TABLE 10.8-3 Type of Sensory Fibres

Sensory group	Fibre type	Origin
Ia	Aα	Annulospinal endings on intrafusal muscle fibres
Ib	Aα	Golgi tendon organs
II	Aβ	Flower-spray endings on intrafusal muscle fibres. Touch and pressure receptors
III	Aδ	Receptors for pain (fast), cold and crude touch receptors
IV	C	Pain (slow) and temperature receptors

various rootlets. Each rootlet just before entering the spinal cord divides into medial and lateral divisions.

- ***Medial divisions*** of each rootlet consists of myelinated group I and II fibres which include:
  - Proprioceptive fibres from muscles and
  - Sensory fibres conveying touch, pressure and vibratory sensations.
- ***Lateral division*** of each rootlet comprises:
  - Thinly myelinated group III (Aδ) fibres that carry fast and discriminative pain and temperature sensations and
  - Unmyelinated group IV (type C) fibres which carry slow pain and visceral sensations.

Dermatomes Dermatome refers to the area of skin supplied by one dorsal root (spinal cord segment). It is important to note that dermatomes are quite different from the peripheral nerve fields, because fibres from one dermatome may be present in different peripheral nerves.

During the embryo stage, the body is divided into orderly metameres. In the postnatal life, owing to excessive growth of limbs, the metamere arrangement, except in the trunk, is no longer present. Therefore, dermatomes are remnants of orderly metameric arrangement, which has survived only in the trunk, where the dermatomes consist of a series of 12 narrow overlapping bands running from the vertebral column to the midventral line (Fig. 10.8-16). The bands slope down as they pass around the body. Apparently, the dermatomes are not arranged in an orderly way, as the L_5 dermatome in the leg is at a more distal site than the S_4 dermatome, which is near the anus (Fig. 10.8-17). However, this apparent complexity of the dermatomes in man is simplified if the man is visualized as a quadruped animal (like monkey, the ancestor of man) (Fig. 10.8-17). The knowledge of dermatomes is utilized to know the level of spinal cord injury or the level of spinal tumour or other lesions by mapping the area of altered sensation produced.

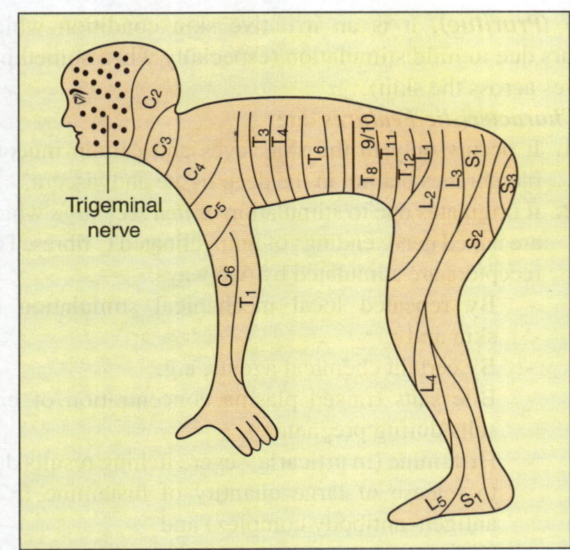

FIGURE 10.8-17 Dermatomes in man visualised as quadruped animal (like ancestors), to clarify the apparent complexity and to memorize the various dermatomes.

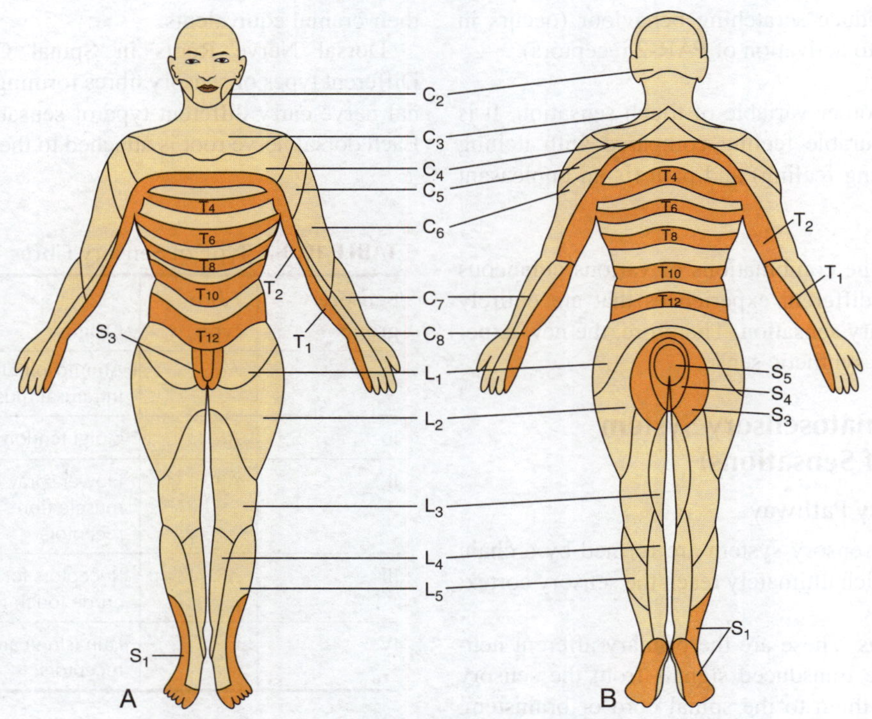

FIGURE 10.8-16 Dermatomes as seen from front (**A**) and back (**B**).

Plasticity of Dermatomes. The dermatomes were originally marked by Sherrington in the later years of 19th century. This is a landmark discovery for which Sherrington may be considered the father of neurology. Much later, Kirk and Denny Brown reported that under some conditions, dermatomes may alter their area of supply to a slight extent. This phenomenon is called plasticity of dermatomes.

Ascending Sensory Tracts

The major ascending sensory tracts in the spinal cord have been grouped as:

- Dorsal column sensory pathway,
- Anterolateral sensory pathway and
- Dorsolateral column sensory pathway.

The ascending sensory tracts are summarized below (for details see page 908):

Dorsal Column Sensory Pathway Dorsal column sensory pathway (Fig. 10.1-12) in man is well developed and wholly myelinated.

First-order neurons are formed by Aα(Ia) and Aβ(II) fibres that enter the spinal cord at medial division of dorsal nerve roots. These carry sensations of fine touch, tactile localization, two-point discrimination, vibration, pressure with intensity discrimination and sense of position and proprioception. These fibres run in the spinal cord through *dorsal column* as fasciculus gracilis and fasciculus cuneatus (Fig. 10.8-18) to end in the *nucleus gracilis* and *nucleus cuneatus*, respectively. Many fibres of the dorsal columns, on their way up, terminate or relay in the dorsal grey horn.

Second-order neurons arise from the nucleus gracilis and nucleus cuneatus located in medulla oblongata. These decussate in the medulla as *internal arcuate fibres* and ascend up in the brainstem as medial lemniscus. The fibres of *medial lemnisci terminate* in the *ventroposterior lateral* (VPL) nucleus of thalamus.

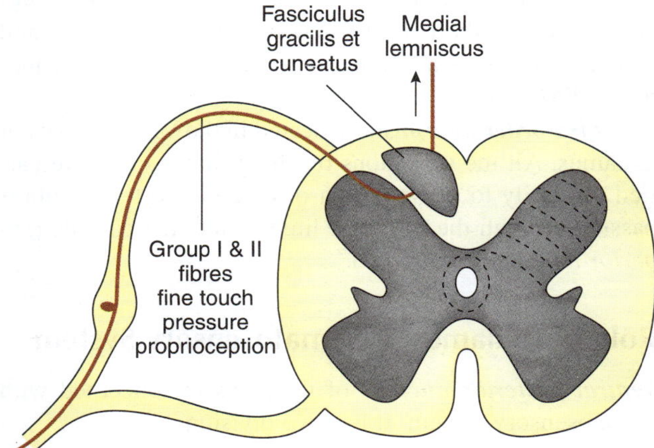

FIGURE 10.8-18 Dorsal column sensory pathways. Fibres carrying touch, pressure and proprioceptive sensations are arranged as fasciculus gracilis and fasciculus cuneatus in dorsal column of spinal cord.

Third-order neurons are from the *ventroposterior lateral nucleus* of thalamus. These ascend to the sensory cortex through the thalamic radiations.

Spatial Orientation of Nerve Fibres in Dorsal Column. In the dorsal column, fibres coming from lower parts of the body are in the centre, while those coming from progressively higher segmental level form successive layers laterally.

Functions of Dorsal Column Pathway. See page 910.

Effects of Damage to Dorsal Column Pathway. Sensations of fine touch, tactile discrimination, vibration sense, joint and position sense are carried by dorsal column pathway. Therefore, damage to this pathway will produce the following effects:

- ***Sensory ataxia,*** i.e. imbalance due to damage to the sensory pathway. In it, it is difficult for the person to detect the position without the help of visual apparatus in an erect position. If this person is asked to stand and close his/her eyes, the body cannot maintain balance properly and tends to fall in one direction (Romberg's sign).
- ***Loss of sensations*** of fine touch, tactile discrimination and vibration sense on the affected side.

Anterolateral Pathway.

First-order neurons of anterolateral pathway are formed by Aδ(III) and (IV) fibres which enter the spinal cord as lateral division of the dorsal nerve root. These carry sensations of pain, temperature and crude touch. After entering the spinal cord, these fibres separate into short ascending and descending branches, which constitute the *dorsolateral tract of Lissauer*. They finally terminate on the *nucleus proprius* of the spinal cord, one or two segments rostral and caudal to the point of entry of the dorsal root. Some sensory afferents end on the short interneurons in the *substantia gelatinosa,* which connects them to nucleus proprius (Fig. 10.8-12).

Second-order neurons arise from the nucleus proprius and cross in the anterior commissure of the spinal cord to the opposite side in anterior and lateral white column in which they run upward to the brain as anterior and lateral spinothalamic tracts, respectively.

Anterior spinothalamic tract mainly carries sensation of crude touch, tickle, itch, etc. Higher up in the brainstem, the anterior spinothalamic tract joins the medial lemniscus of thalamus.

Lateral spinothalamic tract consists of the fibres carrying pain and temperature sensation, and higher up in the brainstem is called the spinal lemniscus (Fig. 10.8-12).

Note. In addition, there are spinoreticular (to the reticular system of the brainstem) and spinotectal (to the tectum) pathways.

Anterolateral pathways terminate in two areas:

- Throughout *reticular nuclei* of brainstem.
- Spinal and medial lemnisci terminate in the *ventrobasal complex* and *intralaminar* nuclei of thalamus. Generally, tactile signals and temperature signals

terminate in ventrobasal complex. Pain signals only partly project to ventrobasal complex of thalamus. Instead, most of them enter the reticular nuclei of brainstem and then to intralaminar nuclei of thalamus.

Third-order neurons arise from the ventrobasal complex of thalamus and carry tactile signals to the somatic sensory area of the cortex along with the fibres of dorsal column.

Characteristics of Transmission in Anterolateral Pathway. In general, anterolateral system is a crude type of transmission than the dorsal column system, as depicted by the following characteristics:

- ***Velocity of transmission*** is about one-third compared with that of dorsal column system (8–40 m/s).
- ***Spatial organization*** in the pathway is poor, causing poor degree of localization of sensation.
- ***Gradation of intensities*** judged is far less accurate compared with those of dorsal column system.
- ***Ability to transmit repetitive signals*** is also poor.

Dorsolateral Column Pathway Dorsolateral column pathways carry proprioceptive impulses arising from the muscles and joint receptors of the lower part of the body to the cerebellum. Recent investigations have shown that some exteroceptive sensations, e.g. touch, may also reach the cerebellum through these pathways.

First-order neurons are located in the posterior root ganglia. Their peripheral processes receive impulses from muscle spindles, Golgi tendon organs and other proprioceptive receptors. Some fibres are related to end organs concerned with exteroceptive sensations (touch and pressure).

Second-order neurons are located in the junctional area between the ventral and dorsal grey column (laminae V, VI and VII) in the lumbar and sacral segments of spinal cord. Their axons form the:

- Ventral spinocerebellar tract and
- Dorsal spinocerebellar tract.
- ***Note.*** For details, see page 911.

Pathway of Sensations from Face and Oral Cavity The sensations of touch, pain and temperature from the face and oral cavity, including teeth, and proprioceptive information from the jaw muscles are carried by trigeminal nerve.

First-order neurons are located in the *trigeminal ganglion*, which is equivalent to dorsal nerve root ganglia in the spinal cord. The peripheral processes of these neurons form three divisions of the trigeminal nerve: ophthalmic, maxillary and mandibular, which innervate different areas of the facial skin (Fig. 10.8-19). The central processes of these neurons of trigeminal ganglia terminate in different components of trigeminal sensory nucleus as (Fig. 10.8-20):

- ***Principal sensory trigeminal nucleus,*** located in the pons, receives fibres carrying *tactile* sensations.

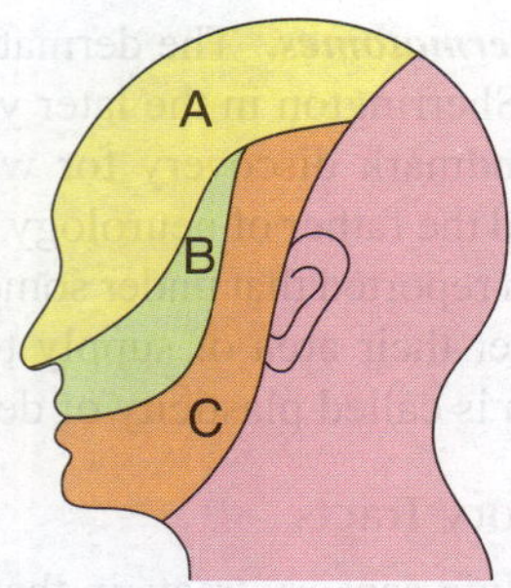

FIGURE 10.8-19 The areas of face innervated by three divisions of trigeminal nerve: **A,** ophthalmic; **B,** maxillary; and **C,** mandibular.

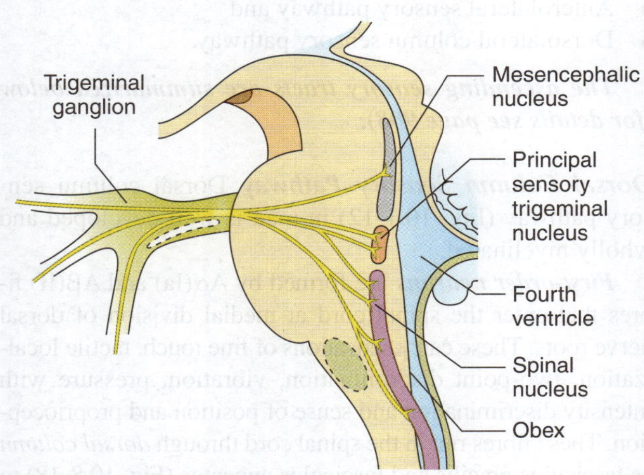

FIGURE 10.8-20 Termination of central processes of trigeminal ganglion in three components of sensory nucleus of trigeminal nerve.

- ***Spinal nucleus*** is elongated and extends down to the upper spinal cord. It receives fibres carrying *pain* and *temperature* sensations.
- ***Mesencephalic nucleus,*** which extends from the pons into midbrain, receives fibres carrying *proprioceptive* information.

Second-order neurons are located in the above-described three components of the sensory trigeminal nucleus. Axons of these neurons cross to the opposite side and ascend as *trigeminal lemniscus* to the ventroposterior medial (VPM) nucleus of thalamus.

Third-order neurons are located in the VPM nucleus of thalamus. All the sensations reaching this nucleus are carried primarily to sensory area of cerebral cortex by fibres passing through the posterior limb of internal capsule *(superior thalamic radiations)*.

Role of Thalamus in Somatosensory System

Ventral posterior nucleus of thalamus is concerned with somatosensory system. It has two divisions:

- Ventral posterior lateral (VPL) nucleus and
- Ventral posterior medial (VPM) nucleus.

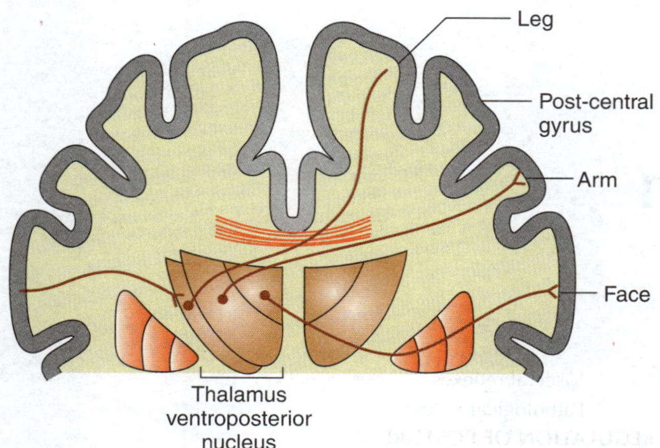

FIGURE 10.8-21 Topographic representation of the body in ventral posterior nucleus of thalamus and thalamic projections to sensory cortex.

For details, see page 948.

Topographic representation of the body can be demonstrated in ventral posterior thalamic nucleus as (Fig. 10.8-21):

- *Face region:* Fibres carrying sensations from the face terminate in the most medial part of the nucleus,
- *Arm region* is represented in the middle part of nucleus and
- *Leg region* in the lateral most part of the nucleus.

Somatosensory functions of thalamus. Thalamus acts as a:

- Sensory relay centre,
- Centre for integration of sensory impulses and
- Crude centre for perception of sensations.

In short, pain sensations are perceived in the thalamus itself. All other sensations are transmitted to the cerebral cortex by third-order neurons arising from the thalamus (for details, see page 952).

Somatic Sensory Cortex

Somatic sensory cortex is described under the following headings:

- Areas,
- Topographical organization of the body in somatic sensory cortex,
- Connections and
- Functions.

For details, see page 971.

Chapter 10.9

Somatic Motor System

INTRODUCTION
COMPONENTS OF SOMATIC MOTOR CONTROL SYSTEM
- Highest level of motor control
- Middle level of motor control
- Lowest level of motor control

SKELETAL MUSCLES: THE EFFECTOR ORGAN OF SOMATIC MOTOR SYSTEM
- Motor unit
- Muscle sensors
- Muscle tone

REFLEX ACTIVITY
- General consideration
  - Anatomical aspects
  - Classification of reflexes
  - Animal preparations for study of reflexes
  - Properties of reflexes
- Spinal cord reflexes
  - Stretch reflex
  - Golgi tendon reflex
  - Withdrawal reflex
- Clinical reflexes at a glance
  - Superficial reflexes
  - Deep reflexes
  - Visceral reflexes
  - Pathological reflexes

REGULATION OF POSTURE
- Mechanisms involved in regulation of posture
  - Postural reflexes
  - Static reflexes
  - Statokinetic reflexes
- Role of different regions of nervous system in maintenance of posture
  - Role of spinal cord
  - Role of brainstem
  - Role of cerebellum
  - Role of basal ganglia
- Mechanism of standing in man

VESTIBULAR APPARATUS AND EQUILIBRIUM
- Functional anatomy
- Vestibular receptors
- Vestibular pathways
- Mechanism of functioning of vestibular apparatus
- Functions of vestibular apparatus
- Maintenance of equilibrium
- Applied aspects

INTRODUCTION

Effector Organ. The motor activity, be it in the form of walking, physical labour, skilled work like typing or even expression of thoughts and feelings through gesture of speech, is a result of highly coordinated movements produced by the skeletal muscles. The skeletal muscles thus form the *effector organ* of the somatic motor system.

Motor Unit and Motor Neuronal Pool. The skeletal muscle activity basically depends upon the pattern and rate of discharge of motor neurons supplying the muscles. A *motor unit* consists of single motor neuron and the muscle fibres that it innervates. For fine control (e.g. muscles of the eye), a single motor neuron innervates only a few muscle fibres. For larger movements (e.g. postural muscles), a single motor neuron may innervate thousands of muscle fibres. All the motor neurons for a given muscle make up the *motor neuron pool* for the muscle. The force of muscle contraction is graded by recruitment of additional motor units (size principle). The *size principle* states that as additional motor units are recruited, more motor neurons are involved and more tension is generated.

Lower Motor Neurons and Final Common Pathway. Thus, the somatic motor activity depends ultimately upon the pattern and rate of discharge from the alpha motor neurons situated in the ventral (grey) horn of spinal cord and its homologous neurons in the motor nuclei of the cranial nerves present in the brainstem. The *alpha motor neurons* are also known as lower motor neurons. The lower motor neurons form the only pathway through which the signals from other parts of the nervous system reach the muscles. Therefore, the *lower motor neurons* constitute the so-called *final common pathway* of motor system.

Somatic Motor Activity, in General, Comprises voluntary movements, reflex responses, rhythmic motor activities and control of posture and equilibrium.

1. ***Voluntary movements,*** like typing, playing musical instruments, writing, drawing, painting etc., represent the most complex motor activity. Such movements are

characterized by being purposeful and initiated at will. These movements can improve with training and once learned they can be executed with minimal voluntary attention. In other words, the motor system 'learns by doing', and performance improves with repetition. This involves the *synaptic plasticity.*

2. ***Reflex responses*** are rapid, stereotyped and involuntary activities. They are purposeful but not under voluntary control. They are produced in response to specific stimuli, e.g. withdrawal reflex in response to a nociceptive stimulus.
3. ***Rhythmic motor activities*** like walking, running, and chewing combine features of the voluntary as well as reflex responses. These movements are initiated and terminated voluntarily. However, once initiated, these relatively stereotyped repetitive movements may continue in almost reflex response-like pattern.
4. ***Control of posture and equilibrium.*** The maintenance of upright posture is a prerequisite for any goal and direction-oriented phasic movement. It is impossible to separate postural adjustments from voluntary movement in any rigid way, but it is possible to differentiate a series of postural reflexes that not only maintain the body in an upright, balanced position but also provide the constant adjustments necessary to maintain a stable postural background for voluntary activity.

Medial versus Lateral Motor System. The skeletal muscles, which are the effector organs for motor activity, have been organized into two groups: medial proximal and lateral distal. The *medial proximal group* comprises the axial and girdle muscles, whose actions involve the axis and proximal limbs. Their activity determines posture, progression and equilibrium. The *lateral distal group* of muscles are the muscles of digits and distal segments of limbs. They are responsible for skilled voluntary movements. There exists a topographical organization of these groups in the central nervous system as medial and lateral motor nervous systems.

Medial motor system. Phylogenetically, medial motor system is old. It includes following tracts:

- Anterior corticospinal tract,
- Fibres of corticobulbar tract other than those belonging to lateral system,
- Lateral and medial vestibulospinal tracts,
- Reticulospinal tract and
- Tectospinal tract.

The fibres of medial motor system terminate on the motor neurons situated in the medial part of ventral grey horn of spinal cord (via interneuron). Axons of medial group of motor neurons of spinal cord supply the axial and proximal limb muscles (medial proximal group of muscles), which are concerned with posture of the body. The corticobulbar fibres of the medial system innervate the axial muscles of upper part of trunk and are involved in the maintenance of posture and equilibrium. These fibres are also involved in the movements of chewing and movements of eyebrows.

Lateral motor system. Phylogenetically, the lateral motor system is new. It includes the following tracts:

- Lateral corticospinal tract,
- Rubrospinal tract and
- A part of corticobulbar tract.

The fibres of the lateral motor system terminate in the motor neurons situated in the lateral part of ventral grey horn in spinal cord (directly or via interneurons) and on the equivalent motor neurons of cranial nerve nuclei in brainstem. Axons of these motor neurons supply the muscles of digits and distal segments of the limbs and regulate the skilled voluntary movements.

The corticobulbar fibres of the lateral system are concerned with movements of expression in lower part of face and movements of tongue.

Control of Somatic Motor Activity. The voluntary actions and postural movements are carried out not only by the simple contraction and relaxation of skeletal muscles but also the adjustment of tone in these muscles. The execution, planning, coordination and adjustments of the movements of the body are under the influence of different parts of the nervous system which together constitute the somatic motor system, which is organized as three-tier system consisting of highest level of motor control, middle level of motor control and lowest level of motor control.

1. *Highest level of motor control* involves activities of various areas of cerebral cortex. It is mainly concerned with generation of the idea of voluntary movements (motor plan) and issuing the motor commands for their execution.
2. *Middle level of motor control* involves activities of various subcortical centres such as basal ganglia, some brainstem nuclei and cerebellum. The middle level of motor control is concerned with developing and perfecting each motor programme and subprogramme for bringing out a motor act. It also supervises the implementation of a motor programme.
3. *Lowest level of motor control* is exerted by cranial nerve nuclei in brainstem and spinal cord. The spinal cord contains the final common pathway through which a movement is executed.

Role of Sensory Receptors in Motor Control Activity. Feedback signals to CNS from the proprioceptors in muscles, joints, skin and other sensory receptors are used to adjust the motor commands during somatic motor activity.

Plan of Study of Somatic Motor Control System. In view of the above background, the somatic motor control system is discussed in detail under the following headings:

- Components of somatic motor control system,
- Skeletal muscles: The effect or organ of somatic motor system,
- Reflexes and
- Regulation of posture and equilibrium.

COMPONENTS OF SOMATIC MOTOR CONTROL SYSTEM

The somatic motor control system is organized as a three-tier system consisting of (Fig. 10.9-1):

- Highest level of motor control,
- Middle level of motor control and
- Lowest level of motor control.

These components of the somatic motor control system work in concert to exert their control over skeletal muscles and their coordinated activity.

I. Highest Level of Motor Control

Cerebral Cortex

The highest level of motor control is exerted through motor cortex and two major descending pathways emerging from the motor areas.

Motor Cortex

Areas of motor cortex include (Fig. 10.9-2):

- *Primary motor cortex* (Brodmann's area 4). It is located in the frontal lobe within the precentral gyrus. It is somatotopically organized. It is organized in terms of movements rather than individual muscles, e.g. stimulation reveals discrete isolated movements on opposite half of the body.
- *Premotor cortex.* It is located immediately anterior to the lateral portion of the primary cortex. It includes Brodmann's areas 6, 8, 44 and 45.
- *Supplementary motor cortex* is located in medial surface of frontal lobe rostral to the primary motor area (Figs 10.4-5 and 10.9-2)

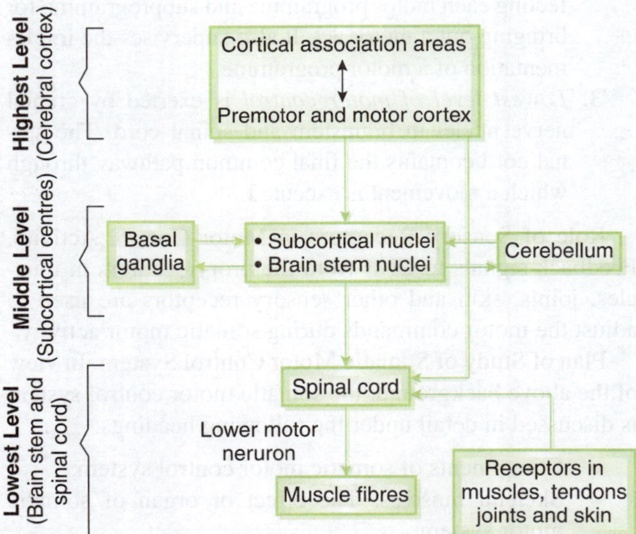

FIGURE 10.9-1 Integration of highest, middle and lowest level of somatic motor control system.

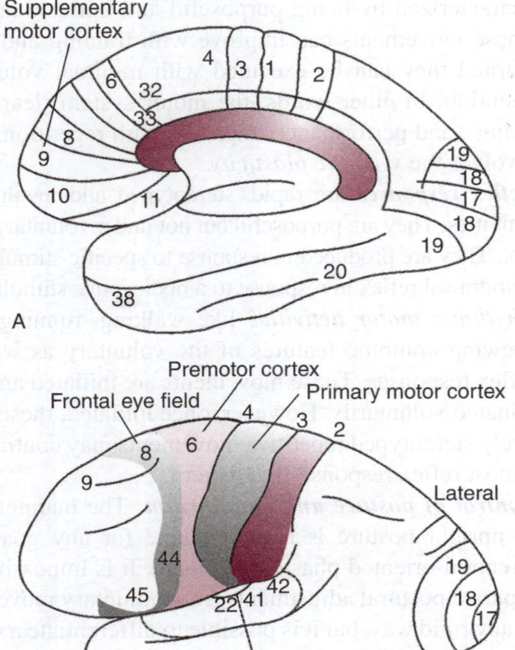

FIGURE 10.9-2 Medial (above) and lateral (below) view of human cerebral cortex to show the motor cortex.

Note: For details of motor cortex, see page 966.

Functional role of motor cortex in control of voluntary movements is summarized:

Supplementary motor cortex is responsible for generating the idea for a movement. There it plans the movements. Lateral cerebellum and basal ganglia are also involved in the planning and programming of movements. This is evidenced from the fact that all these areas involved in planning show electrical activity before the primary motor cortex. Basal ganglia play their cognitive role through the *caudate loop* (motor association → cortex → caudate nucleus → thalamus → cortex) (see page 943 and Fig. 10.2-13A).

Primary motor cortex is responsible for execution of movement. Programmed patterns of motor neurons are activated in the motor cortex. Excitation of upper motor neurons in the motor cortex is transferred in large part via the corticospinal tracts to spinal cord and the corresponding corticobulbar tracts to motor neurons in the brainstem, where the lower motor neurons are activated and cause voluntary movement.

Premotor cortex coordinates the voluntary activity:

- *Area 6* coordinates the proximal and axial muscles during a motor task. Therefore, it is involved in the integration of voluntary movements. It ensures that the skilled movements are accurate and smooth.
- *Area 8,* also called frontal eye field, is involved in coordination of eye movements.

- *Areas 44 and 45*, also called Broca's motor speech areas (especially in dominant hemisphere, e.g. left hemisphere in right-handed person), are engaged in coordination of the activity of musculature involved in speech, e.g. activation of vocal cords simultaneously with movements of mouth and tongue during speech.
- *A head rotation area* associated with frontal eye field is functionally linked to area 8 and serves to enable movements of the head correlated with eye movements.
- *An area related to the control of fine movements of the hand* is located within the premotor cortex, just anterior to the hand region of area 4. When this area is damaged, the muscles of the hand are not paralyzed, but certain hand movements are lost; this is called *motor apraxia*.

Plasticity property of motor cortex. The motor system 'learns by doing', and performance improves with repetition. This involves synaptic plasticity. The motor cortex shows plasticity. This has been confirmed by positron emission tomography (PET) and functional MRI (fMRI) in intact experimental animals and humans. For example, the finger areas of the contralateral motor cortex show enlargement as a pattern of rapid finger movement is learned with the fingers of one hand; this change is detectable at 1 week and maximal at 4 weeks.

Descending Motor Pathways from Motor Cortex

A. ***Pyramidal tracts*** include the tracts which are constituted by the axons that transmit motor signals directly from the cortex to spinal cord (*corticospinal tracts*) and cranial nerve nucleus (*corticobulbar tracts*). *Corticospinal tracts* include 31% fibres arising from the primary cortex (area 6), 29% from premotor area (area 4) and supplementary cortex, and 40% arising from the somatic sensory cortex (areas 3, 1 and 2). Corticospinal fibres are divided into two tracts (Fig. 10.1-16 see page 912):

Lateral corticospinal tract is constituted by the 80% of fibres which cross the midline in the medullary pyramids. These fibres end directly in neurons in the ventral horn that innervate the distal limb muscles which are responsible for making skilled precision movements (e.g. the muscles that move the fingers and hands and the muscles that produce speech) (*lateral motor system*).

Anterior corticospinal tract is formed by 20% uncrossed fibres which descend ipsilaterally in the ventral white column of the spinal cord. These fibres ultimately cross the midline but only at the level where they synapse. This pathway phylogenetically is oldest and does not synapse directly with ventral horn cells, but an interneuron is always interposed in between. These interneurons synapse on neurons in the *medial portion of ventral horn* that controls the axial (trunk muscles) and proximal limb muscles that are concerned with posture and equilibrium (*medial motor system*).

B. ***Extrapyramidal tracts.*** These are large number of fibres arising from the motor cortex which do not enter the corticospinal tracts but relay in the various basal ganglia, red nucleus, reticular formation of brainstem and vestibular nuclei. Ultimately, they constitute the reticulospinal (or corticoreticulospinal), vestibulospinal (or corticovestibulospinal), rubrospinal (or corticorubrospinal), tactospinal (or corticotactospinal) and olivospinal tract. All these are combinedly called the extrapyramidal tracts. Thus, in contrast to pyramidal tracts, the extrapyramidal tracts constitute multisynaptic pathway affecting the contralateral side of spinal cord (Fig. 10.9-3).

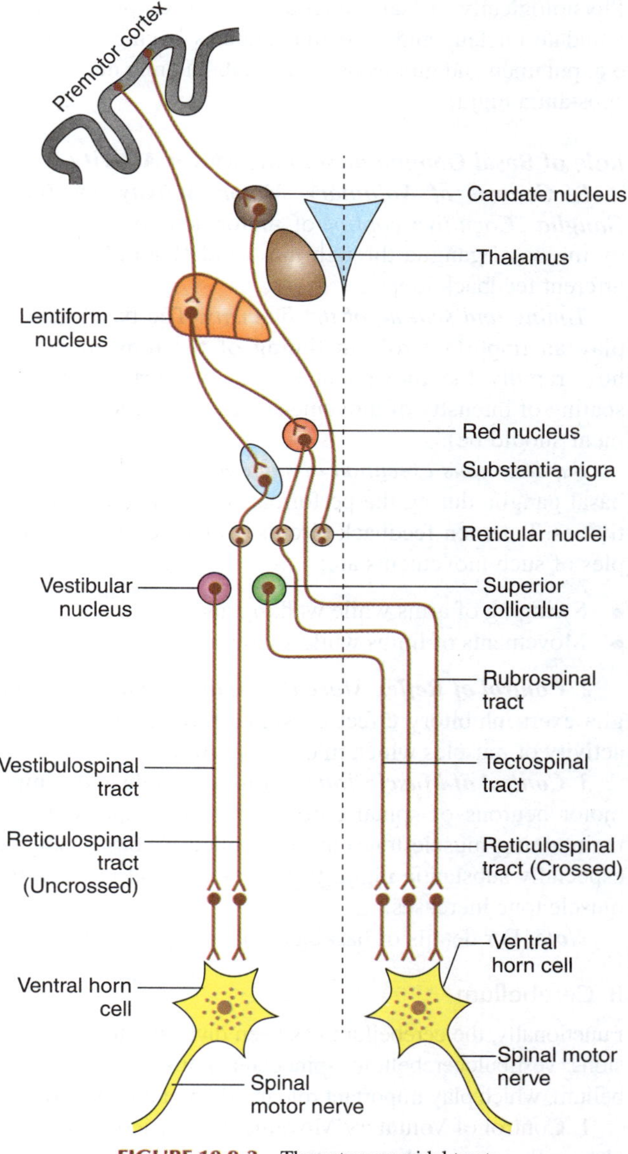

FIGURE 10.9-3 The extrapyramidal tracts.

Functions. Extrapyramidal pathways are chiefly concerned with regulation of muscle tone and posture and equilibrium.

Note. For details of corticospinal tract, see page 912 and for details of extrapyramidal tracts, see page 914.

II. Middle Level of Motor Control

The middle level of motor control specifies the postures and movements necessary to carry out the desired acts. It is concerned with developing and perfecting each motor programme and subprogramme for bringing out a motor act. It also supervises the implementation of motor programmes.

The middle level of motor control involves activities of basal ganglia, cerebellum and brainstem.

A. Basal Ganglia

Physiologically, basal ganglia include corpus striatum (caudate nucleus and lenticular nucleus having two parts, e.g. putamen and globus pallidus), subthalamic nucleus and substantia nigra.

Role of Basal Ganglia in Somatic Motor Activity

1. Control of Voluntary Motor Activity by Basal Ganglia. *Cognitive control* of motor activity is executed by the basal ganglia through the 'caudate loop' (a part of afferent feedback loops).

Timing and scaling of the intensity. The basal ganglia play an important role in timing of the movement (i.e. how rapidly the movement should be performed), and scaling of intensity of movement (i.e. how large the movement should be).

Subconscious execution of some movements is done by basal ganglia during the performance of trained motor activities. Putamen feedback circuit is involved in it. Examples of such movements are:

- Swinging of arms while walking and
- Movements of limbs while swimming.

2. Control of Reflex Muscular Activity. The basal ganglia exert inhibitory effect on spinal reflexes and regulate activity of muscles which maintain posture.

3. Control of Muscle Tone. Muscle spindle and gamma motor neurons of spinal cord (which are responsible for maintaining muscle tone) are controlled by basal ganglia, especially substantia nigra. In lesions of basal ganglia, the muscle tone increases.

Note. For details of basal ganglia, see page 939.

B. Cerebellum

Functionally, the cerebellum has been divided into three divisions: vestibulocerebellum, spinocerebellum and corticocerebellum, which play important role in different motor activities.

1. Control of Voluntary Movements. Corticocerebellum, also called cerebral cerebellum, is intimately associated with control of timing, rate, range (extent), duration, direction and strength of a movement. Corticocerebellum performs this function through the following neuronal circuits:

- *Open feedback loop* or cerebro-cerebello-cerebral circuit (Fig. 10.2-8), and
- *Closed feedback loop* formed by fibres from the cerebral motor cortex to paravermal cerebellum to the cerebral cortex (Fig. 10.2-9).

Mechanism of action. The cerebellum controls the voluntary movements by following actions:

i. ***Comparator function.*** The cerebellum receives inputs from the command neurons about the sequential intended plan of movements for the next fraction of second. It also gets feedback (afferents) from the proprioceptive endings of muscles, tendons and joints about what actual movements result. All these information are integrated and the corrective signals are sent to the motor cortex. This happens through the closed feedback loop.

ii. ***Damping action.*** Corticocerebellum sends impulses to the cerebral cortex to discharge appropriate signals to the muscles so that any extra or exaggeration of muscular activity does not occur and thus overshooting is prevented. This action of corticocerebellum is called damping action.

iii. ***Timing and programming of the skilled movements*** is done by corticocerebellum through open feedback loop (Fig. 10.2-8), which modulates the motor command of pyramidal tracts through two-way communication.

iv. ***Servomechanism.*** Cerebellum lets the cerebral cortex to discharge the signals which are already programmed and stored at sensory motor cortex, and does not influence much. However, if there is any disturbance or interference, the corticocerebellum immediately influences the cerebral cortex and corrects the movements. This action of corticocerebellum is known as servomechanism.

2. Control of Body Posture and Equilibrium is done by vestibulocerebellum (see page 934).

3. Control of Muscle Tone and Stretch Reflex is the function of spinocerebellum (see page 935).

Note. For details about cerebellum, see page 925.

C. Brainstem

Reticular formation and vestibular nuclei are important components of the motor control system present in the brainstem.

Reticular Formation. The *motor control centres* within the reticular formation are a relay station for all descending motor commands, except those requiring the greatest precision, which are transferred directly from the cortex to spinal cord.

- The motor control centres receive and modify the motor commands to the proximal and axial muscles of the body responsible for maintaining normal posture tone.

- These neurons are prevented from firing too rapidly by inhibitory input derived from the cerebral and cerebellar components of motor control system. The amount of inhibition is increased to reduce postural tone and is decreased to enhance postural tone. The withdrawal of inhibition, called release of inhibition, is frequently used to increase neuronal activity within the CNS.

Vestibular Nuclei. Vestibular nuclei, located within the brainstem and cerebellum, receive information from *vestibular receptors* via vestibular nerve fibres (8th cranial nerve). Vestibular system reflexes:

- Maintain tone in antigravity muscles,
- Coordinate the adjustments made by the limbs and trunk to maintain balance and
- Adjust the position of the eyes to maintain visual fixation when the position of head changes.

III. Lowest Level of Motor Control

The lowest level of motor control is exerted by motor nuclei of cranial nerves and spinal cord. The spinal cord contains the *final common pathway* through which a movement is executed. Organized in the spinal cord are patterns of movements that involve nearly all muscles in the body. By selecting the proper motor neurons for a particular task and by reflexly adjusting the amount of motor neuron activity, the spinal cord contributes to the proper performance of a motor task. The spinal cord activity ranges from a simple withdrawal reflex to coordinated movement of all four extremities.

Spinal Cord

Motor Neurons

Motor neurons of spinal cord present in ventral horn are:

1. Alpha Motor Neurons. These are the largest neurons which give rise to myelinated axons that average about 14 μm in diameter and conduct action potentials very rapidly. The axons of alpha motor neurons leave the spinal cord through the ventral nerve roots of spinal nerves and innervate the extrafusal fibres of the skeletal muscles. These are responsible for contraction of muscles in upper limbs, trunk and lower part of the body.

2. Gamma Motor Neurons. These are much smaller and give rise to smaller axons that average about 5 μm in diameter and conduct action potentials at a slower velocity than the alpha motor neurons. These neurons innervate the intrafusal fibres of the muscle spindles and are responsible for maintenance of muscle tone.

3. Interneurons. These are about 30 times more numerous than motor neurons, are highly excitable and may have a spontaneous firing rate as high as 1500 per second. The interneurons actually receive the bulk of synaptic input that reaches the spinal cord, either as incoming sensory information or signals descending from higher centres in the brain.

4. Renshaw Cells are particular variety of interneurons that receive input from collateral branches of the axons of alpha motor neurons. Their axons carry the impulses back to the cell bodies of the same alpha motor neurons. These are inhibitory neurons that play an important role in synaptic inhibition at the spinal cord.

Arrangement of Motor Neurons in Ventral Horn The motor neurons responsible for the contraction of skeletal muscles are arranged topographically in the ventral grey horn of the spinal cord in three mediolateral column groups:

1. Medial Group. It extends along most of the length of spinal cord. The neurons situated in the medial part of ventral grey horn innervate the muscles near the midline of the body called *axial muscles and the muscles in the proximal portions of limbs*. These muscles are involved in the adjustment of posture and gross movements. Medial group of neurons extends along the most of the length of spinal cord.

2. Lateral Group. This group of neurons is confined to the cervical and lumbosacral enlargements and supplies the muscles in distal portions of the limbs called distal muscles. These distal muscles are involved in the well-coordinated skilled voluntary movements.

3. Central Group. This group of neurons is represented by the phrenic and accessory nuclei (in the cervical region) and by the lumbosacral nucleus (in the lumbosacral region).

Motor Functions Motor functions served by spinal cord are:

- Control of movement of muscles and joints,
- Control of tone and power of muscles,
- Control of deep (tendon) reflexes and
- Control of superficial reflexes.

SKELETAL MUSCLES: THE EFFECTOR ORGAN OF SOMATIC MOTOR SYSTEM

Motor activity, be it in the form of walking, physical labour, skilled work like typing, performing surgical operations or even expression of thoughts and feelings through gesture or speech, is a result of highly coordinated movements produced by the skeletal muscles. The skeletal muscles thus form the effector organ of the somatic motor system. The physiology of skeletal muscle has been discussed in Chapter 2.3. However, certain aspects that need elaboration of skeletal muscle as effector organ and are relevant to complete the study of somatic motor system are:

- Motor unit,
- Muscle sensors (proprioceptors) and
- Muscle tone.

Motor Unit

The motor unit is the functional module used by the motor control system to carry out a movement. The movement produced by a skeletal muscle basically depends upon the pattern and ratio of discharge of motor neurons supplying the muscle. A *motor unit consists* of single motor neuron and the muscle fibres that it innervates.

Note. It is suggested that before proceeding further, details about motor unit should be read (see page 93).

Muscle Sensors

Muscle sensors refer to the proprioceptors present in the muscles, tendons of muscles, joints, ligaments and fasciae. Proprioceptors are the receptors which give information about change in position of different parts of the body in space, especially joints or tension of muscles at any given moment. The muscle sensors are:

- Muscle spindle,
- Golgi tendon organ,
- Pacinian corpuscle and
- Free nerve endings.

In addition to the above proprioceptors, the labyrinth also contains proprioceptors (see page 1074).

1. Muscle Spindle Muscle spindles are *stretch receptors* present in the skeletal muscles. These are meant for proprioceptive mechanism and so are a type of proprioceptors. Each skeletal muscle contains muscle spindles of variable number depending upon the task performed. Muscles involved in precision movements contain many more spindles than muscles used to maintain posture. For example, hand muscles have approximately 80 spindles, which is 20% of the number of spindles contained in back muscles weighing 100 times as much.

Structure (Fig. 10.9-4). Each muscle spindle consists of 3–10 small muscle fibres (called intrafusal muscle fibres), encapsulated in a thin connective tissue capsule containing fluid. The muscle spindles are present in between and parallel to the extrafusal fibres (large force-generating muscle fibres). Either end of the muscle spindle is attached to the endomysium of the extrafusal muscle fibres.

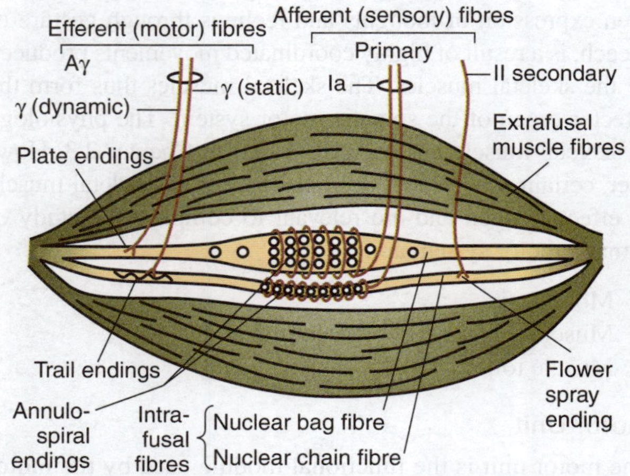

FIGURE 10.9-4 Structure of a muscle spindle.

Intrafusal muscle fibres consist of a central noncontractile portion which does not contain actin and myosin filaments and is thus devoid of striations. Portions on either side of the central part are contractile (as they contain actin and myosin filaments) and are called striated poles. The central part of each intrafusal fibre is the sensory portion. Stretching or contraction of the polar striated regions of the intrafusal fibre causes the stretching of this central noncontractile sensory portion. Intrafusal fibres are of two types:

- ***Nuclear bag fibres:*** Each spindle contains about 2–5 nuclear bag fibres which are about 30 μm in diameter and 7 mm in length. In these fibres, many nuclei are congregated into an expanded bag in the central portion, hence the name.
- ***Nuclear chain fibres*** are 15 μm in diameter and 4 mm in length. In these fibres, nuclei are arranged in a single file in the central part in the form of a chain, hence the name. Approximately, 6–10 nuclear chain fibres exist in each typical spindle.

Nerve Supply of the Muscle Spindle. The muscle spindle is innervated by both sensory and motor nerve fibres. It is the only receptor in the body which has got motor nerve supply also.

i. Sensory Nerve Supply. The central noncontractile portion of each intrafusal fibres is the receptor portion. Sensory fibres supply this area. There are two types of sensory fibres:

- ***Group Ia fibres,*** also known as primary sensory endings, supply central receptor portions of both nuclear bag as well as nuclear chain fibres. Since these fibres spirally wind round the intrafusal fibres, these are also called annulospiral endings. They have diameter of about 17 μm and carry impulses at the rate of 70–120 m/s.

  The primary endings supplying both the nuclear bag as well as nuclear chain intrafusal fibres are stimulated when the muscle spindle is stretched. But the pattern of response is different: a *dynamic response* is shown by nerve endings supplying the nuclear bag fibres and a static response is shown by the nerve endings supplying the nuclear chain fibres (see below).
- ***Type II fibres,*** also known as secondary sensory endings, innervate the receptor portion of mainly nuclear chain fibres on one side of the primary endings. They are also known as flower spray endings. They have a diameter of about 8 μm. These nerve endings respond mainly to sustained stretching, and therefore measure the muscle length.

ii. Motor Supply. The efferent fibres to the muscle spindle are called *gamma fibres* because their axons belong to the Aγ group of fibres. Gamma efferent fibres control the sensitivity of the receptors to stretch. There are two types of gamma fibres:

- ***Dynamic gamma fibres*** primarily innervate the striated poles of nuclear bag fibres where they end as motor end plate, hence also called *plate endings.* These fibres increase the sensitivity of the Ia afferent fibres to stretch. That is, the Ia afferent firing rate for a given *velocity of stretch* is increased by the discharge of the dynamic gamma fibres.
- ***Static gamma fibres*** primarily innervate the striated poles of nuclear chain fibres where they end as a network of branches called *trail endings.* They increase the tonic activity in the Ia afferent fibres at any given muscle length. Sometimes, they also give a branch to some nuclear bag fibres which have characteristics similar to those of nuclear chain fibres (so-called static nuclear bag fibres).

Functions of Muscle Spindle

1. Role in Stretch Reflex. Muscle spindle forms the receptor organ of stretch reflex and thus plays a key role in stretch reflex (for details see page 1053).

2. Role in Maintaining Muscle Tone. Muscle spindle plays an important role in maintaining the muscle tone by controlling the discharge from gamma motor neurons (for details see page 1057).

3. Role in Maintaining Skeletal Muscle at a Certain Physiological Length. Most important function of muscle spindle is to act as a comparator of the extrafusal fibre length. At a normal resting extrafusal fibre length, there is a slight discharge in the type Ia afferents. When the muscle length is passively increased (i.e. when muscle is stretched passively), type Ia discharge is increased. The reflex increase in α-motor neuron discharge causes contraction of the extrafusal fibres and restores their original length. Thus, the muscle spindles, through the stretch reflex, act as a feedback device to maintain the skeletal muscle at a certain physiologically useful length. This action of muscle spindles (particularly in the antigravity muscles) is of fundamental importance in the maintenance of standing posture.

4. Role as Proprioceptor. Muscle spindle plays the role of proprioceptor in following sensations:

- ***Unconscious proprioceptive sensations*** are carried from the muscle spindles to the spinal cord, where the second-order neurons constitute the dorsal and ventral spinocerebellar tracts.
- ***Conscious kinaesthetic sensations*** are carried from the muscle spindles in the dorsal columns to ultimately reach the somatic sensory cortex. This function of muscle spindle is similar to that of joint receptors.

2. Golgi Tendon Organ The Golgi tendon organs are high threshold stretch receptors present in the tendons. They are supplied by group Ib afferent fibres and detect muscle tension (for details see page 1057).

3. Pacinian Corpuscle Pacinian corpuscles are pressure receptors situated in fasciae throughout the muscles, tendons, joints and periosteum. They are supplied by *group II afferent fibres* and detect *vibration.*

4. Free Nerve Endings Free nerve endings are basically pain receptors situated in the muscles, tendons, fasciae and joints. They are supplied by *group III and IV afferent fibres* and detect noxious stimuli.

Muscle Tone

Definition. Muscle tone is defined as resistance offered to active or passive stretch. In other words, muscle tone refers to sustained partial state of contraction of the muscle under resting condition, i.e. a state of partial tetanus. The muscle tone is present in all the muscles, but is well pronounced in the extensor muscles, i.e. antigravity muscles.

Basis of Muscle Tone. The muscle tone is purely a function of myotactic (stretch reflex), occurring due to low frequency and asynchronous discharge of γ-motor neurons. The discharge is out of phase with each other which ultimately merges to produce smooth muscle contraction.

Anomalies of Muscle Tone are hypotonia and hypertonia.

1. ***Hypotonia*** refers to decrease in muscle tone. The hypotonic or also called flaccid muscle offers little or no resistance to stretching. The muscles are generally hypotonic when the rate of γ-efferent discharge is low, i.e. when stretch reflex becomes hypoactive.

   Causes of hypotonia include:

   i. *Destruction of efferent or afferent pathway* of stretch reflex:
      - Destruction of efferent (motor) nerve to a muscle by injury or poliomyelitis.
      - Destruction of afferent pathway may be seen in tabes dorsalis, a syphilitic affection of the dorsal nerve root of spinal cord.

   ii. *Stimulation of inhibitory areas* of brain located in medulla.

   iii. *Inhibition* or destruction of facilitatory areas of brain located in pons.

   iv. *Decreased γ-motor discharge during sleep.*

   v. *Effects of certain drugs* like barbiturates and tranquilizers in high doses.

   vi. *Destruction of cerebellum* also produces hypotonia rather than hypertonia (see page 938).

   vii. Hypothyroidism.

2. ***Hypertonia*** refers to increase in muscle tone. The hypertonic or spastic muscle offers high resistance to stretch. The muscles are generally hypertonic when the rate of γ-efferent discharge is high, i.e. when stretch reflex becomes hyperactive.

Causes of hypertonia *include:*

- Stimulation of facilitatory area of brain.
- Destruction of any of the inhibitory areas of brain.
- Other factors which increase the γ-efferent discharge are anxiety, unexpected movements and stimulation of skin by noxious agents.

Types of hypertonia: Hypertonia is of two types:

- *Spasticity* refers to hypertonia which is confined to only one group of muscles. For example, lesions of internal capsule and upper motor neuron lesions produce spasticity.
- *Rigidity* refers to hypertonia which involves both groups of muscles, i.e. extensor as well as flexors equally. For example, lesions of basal ganglia produce rigidity.

REFLEX ACTIVITY

General Considerations

A reflex is an involuntary response to a peripheral nervous stimulation. In other words, it is a mechanism by which sensory impulse is automatically converted into a motor effect through the involvement of CNS. It is a type of protective mechanism which tries to protect the body from irreparable damage. For example, when the hand is placed inadvertently on a hot object, it is immediately withdrawn reflexly. Thus, the hand is protected from getting burnt.

Anatomical Aspects

Reflex Arc

The pathway for a reflex activity is called reflex arc. It forms the functional unit of nervous system for a reflex and consists of (Fig. 10.9-5):

- Afferent limb,
- Centre and
- Efferent limb.

1. Afferent limb of each reflex arc consists of a receptor and an afferent or sensory nerve.

- ***Receptor*** is a modified nerve ending which receives the stimulus and after getting stimulated (depolarized) sends information to the CNS through the afferent neurons.
- ***Afferent neuron*** carries sensory input from the receptor to the centre. The afferent neurons enter the CNS via the dorsal roots or cranial nerves and have their cell bodies in the dorsal root ganglia or in the homologous ganglia on the cranial nerves.

2. Centre. This is the part of CNS (spinal cord or brain) where afferent limb ends and either synapses directly with efferent motor neuron or establishes a connection with the efferent neuron via interneurons (internuncial or intercalated neurons). Thus, the number of synapses (connection between afferent and efferent neurons) may vary from one (in the simplest form of reflex) to many hundred.

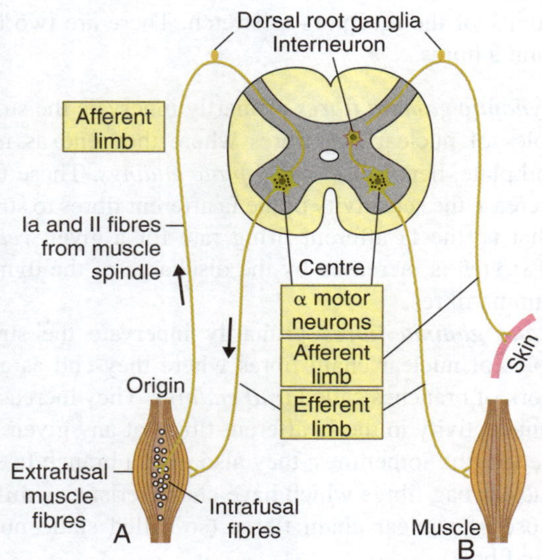

FIGURE 10.9-5 Components of reflex arc in a monosynaptic (**A**) and disynaptic (**B**) reflex.

3. Efferent Limb of a reflex arc consists of an efferent or motor nerve and an effector organ.

- ***Efferent nerve*** transmits motor impulses from the centre to the effector organ. Since the connection between afferent and efferent neurons is usually present in the CNS, therefore, activity in the reflex arc is modified by the multiple inputs converging on the efferent neuron.
- ***Effector organ*** may be in the form of a muscle or a gland which shows the response to the stimulus.

Classification of Reflexes

Reflexes can be classified in different ways:

I. Depending upon the Number of Synapses *(Fig. 10.9-5)*

1. ***Monosynaptic reflexes*** are those which contain only one synapse, e.g. stretch reflexes (biceps, triceps or knee jerk).
2. ***Disynaptic reflexes*** have two synapses, i.e. one interneuron is placed between afferent and efferent neurons of the reflex arc, e.g. inverse stretch reflex.
3. ***Polysynaptic reflexes*** are characterized by more than one interneuron placed between afferent and efferent neurons of the reflex arc, e.g. withdrawal reflex, cross flexor reflex and cross extensor reflex.

II. Anatomical Classification Depending upon the location of reflex arc centre, the reflexes can be classified as:

1. ***Cortical reflexes.*** In these reflexes, the centre is located in cerebral cortex.
2. ***Cerebellar reflexes*** have the centre of reflex arc in cerebellum.
3. ***Midbrain reflexes:*** The centre of reflex arc in such a reflex is located in midbrain.

4. ***Bulbar or medullary reflexes:*** In these reflexes, the centre is located in the medulla oblongata.
5. ***Spinal reflexes*** have the centre of reflex arc in spinal cord. Depending upon the segments involved, the spinal reflexes can be divided into three groups:
   - ***Segmental reflexes.*** In such reflexes, the efferent neuron begins in the same segment of the spinal cord where the afferent neuron ends.
   - ***Intersegmental reflexes.*** In these reflexes, the efferent neuron ends in a segment of spinal cord and the efferent neuron begins in some other segment of spinal cord.
   - ***Suprasegmental reflexes.*** The centre for such reflexes lies above the spinal cord.

III. Physiological Classification

1. ***Flexor reflexes.*** These reflexes occur in response to nociceptive (pain) stimuli and are characterized by flexion of the joints, e.g. thorn prick to the sole is immediately followed by reflex flexion of the knee and hip joints. These reflexes are also called *withdrawal reflexes.*
2. ***Extensor reflexes.*** Stretch reflexes are extensor reflexes. These are the basis of muscle tone and posture of the body. These are also called *antigravity reflexes.*

IV. Inborn Versus Acquired Reflexes

1. ***Inborn or unconditional reflexes*** are present since birth and do not require any previous learning or training, e.g. reflex salivation when any object is kept in mouth.
2. ***Acquired or conditional reflexes*** develop after birth. Such reflexes are acquired after conditioning, i.e. after previous learning or training, e.g. reflex salivation by the sight, smell, thought or hearing of a known edible substance.

V. Clinical Classification Clinically, reflexes are classified into:

- Superficial
- Deep,
- Visceral and
- Pathological reflexes.

Animal Preparations for Study of Reflexes

The reflexes can be studied in:

- Spinal preparation and
- Decerebrate preparation.

1. Spinal Preparation. In it, the spinal cord is transected at cervical region and respiration is maintained by respiratory pump. When spinal cord is transected in the thoracic region, artificial respiration is not required since diaphragmatic breathing continues. Such preparation allows study of properties of spinal reflex.

2. Decerebrate Preparation. In decerebrate preparation, the transection is taken in the brainstem between superior and inferior colliculi.

Properties of Reflexes

1. Adequate Stimulus. Reflex response is obtained only when a precise stimulus for a given reflex activity is applied. The precise stimulus that involves a reflex response is called *adequate stimulus* for that particular reflex. For example, scratch reflex in a dog is initiated only by multiple linear touch stimuli. If multiple stimuli are widely separated, the reflex is not initiated.

2. Delay. All reflex activity is associated with delay. Delay refers to the time interval between application of stimulus and starting of the response. It is attributed to synaptic delay and to time required for passage of impulse along the nerves. Therefore, delay is minimum in a monosynaptic reflex.

3. One-way Conduction. During any reflex activity, the impulses are transmitted in only one direction through the reflex arc as per Bell–Magendie law. The impulses pass from receptors to the centre and then from the centre to effector organ.

4. Summation of stimuli, both temporal and spatial, plays an important role in the facilitation of responses during the reflex activity as explained:

- ***Temporal summation.*** Application of a subminimal (subthreshold) stimulus to a nerve fibre does not elicit reflex response. However, when the nerve fibre is stimulated repeatedly with subthreshold stimuli in quick succession (taking care of refractory period of the nerve), response does occur. This occurs due to summation of EPSPs produced by subthreshold stimuli, a phenomenon called temporal summation.
- ***Spatial summation.*** When an efferent nerve fibre supplying a muscle is stimulated with subthreshold stimulus, a reflex response is not elicited. However, when two or more nerve fibres supplying the same muscle are stimulated simultaneously with subthreshold stimuli, a reflex contraction of the muscle is obtained due to the phenomenon of spatial summation.

5. Occlusion refers to a phenomenon by which stimulation of two neighbouring nerves simultaneously evokes lesser response than sum total of the responses obtained when each nerve is separately stimulated. This can be demonstrated in a flexor reflex involving a muscle which is innervated by two motor nerves, say A and B. For example, electrical stimulation of nerve A causes development of tension of 8 T units (an arbitrary unit). Stimulation of the nerve B with the same electric shock causes development of tension of 8 T units. When both nerves, A and B, are stimulated simultaneously with the same electric shock, the tension developed is about 12 T, i.e. it is less than the sum of tensions produced (8 T + 8 T = 16 T) by the two nerves separately. This phenomenon is called occlusion. This occurs because of the fact that there is overlapping of the nerve fibres during the distribution, i.e. fibres are supplied by both A and B nerves (Fig. 10.9-6).

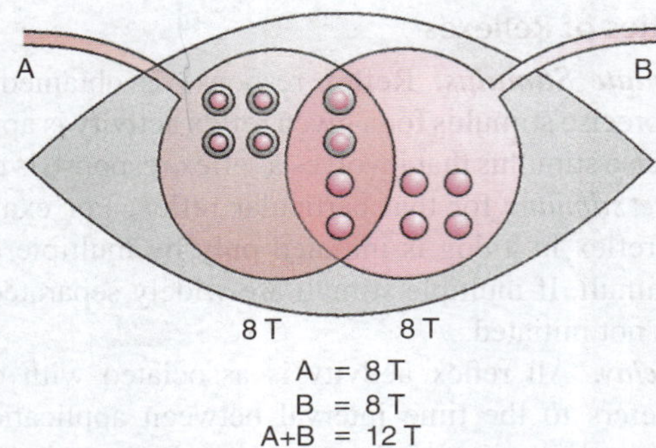

FIGURE 10.9-6 Occlusion occurs due to overlapping in the distribution of nerve fibres.

6. Subliminal Fringe refers to a phenomenon by which simultaneous stimulation of two nerves (say A and B) with weak shock evokes greater response than the sum total of the responses when each nerve is separately stimulated with the weak shocks. Thus, a subliminal fringe phenomenon appears to produce opposite effect to that of occlusion phenomenon. Phenomenon of subliminal fringe can be explained as:

Each afferent nerve on entering the spinal cord stimulates two groups of neurons: one group is stimulated adequately and second group subminimally. Each weak stimulus, therefore, produces action potential in the nerves of group one neurons. The neurons belonging to second group are also excited but only subminimally (so this group is common). When both A and B are simultaneously stimulated, the action potential also develops in the second group of neurons and therefore response obtained is greater (Fig. 10.9-7).

7. Recruitment. When an excitatory nerve is stimulated with a stimulus of constant strength for a long time, there occurs a progressive increase in the response of reflex activity. This is due to the progressive increase in the number of motor neurons activated. This phenomenon is called recruitment. However, there is a limit to the number of motor neurons which can be recruited. So, beyond a certain limit, the prolongation of stimulation does not increase the response and a plateau is reached.

8. Irradiation. When the sensory stimulus is too strong, impulse spreads to many neighbouring neurons in the centre and produces a wider response. It is due to transmission of impulse through large number of collaterals of afferents and their interneurons.

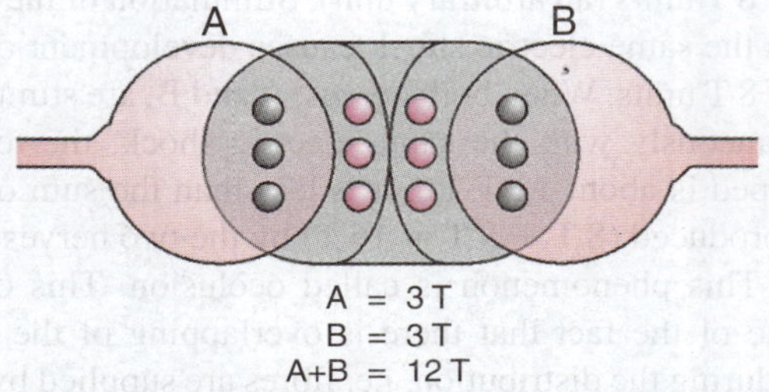

FIGURE 10.9-7 Subliminal fringe.

9. Final Common Pathway. Efferent pathway of the reflex arc is formed by α-motor neurons that supply the extrafusal muscle fibres. All neuronal influences (excitatory and inhibitory) affecting muscular contraction ultimately funnel through the motor neurons; therefore, they are called common final pathway. Numerous inputs converge on them and determine the activity in the final common path (Fig. 10.9-8). If an α-motor neuron is stimulated, skeletal muscle fibres contract, if the α-motor neuron is not stimulated, the skeletal muscle fibres relax. Thus, the α-motor neuron forming the final common pathway serves both as an integrating centre and an efferent pathway.

10. Facilitation. When a reflex is elicited repeatedly at proper intervals, the response becomes progressively higher for first few occasions, i.e. each subsequent stimulus exerts a better effect than the previous one. This is due to facilitation occurring at the synapse.

11. Inhibition. During a reflex activity, impulses through sensory fibres from protagonist muscles inhibit the action of antagonist muscles. For example, when flexor muscles of a joint are stimulated, extensor muscles are inhibited. The inhibitory activity exerted by interneurons is responsible for such a reciprocal inhibitory effect.

12. After Discharge. When a reflex action is elicited continuously for some time, and then the stimulation is stopped, the reflex response (contraction) may continue for some time even after cessation of the stimulus. This is called after discharge. This occurs because of the fact that the centre continues to discharge even after stoppage of stimulus. This is mainly because of the internuncial neurons which continue to transmit impulses to the centre even after cessation of stimulus. This happens because the motor neurons are stimulated through multiple internuncial pathways, and some of them take longer time to reach the motor neurons.

13. Fatigue or Habituation. When a particular reflex is elicited repeatedly at frequent intervals, the response is reduced progressively and then disappears all together. This is called fatigue or habituation. The first site of fatigue is synapse, then the motor endings and lastly the muscle.

14. Rebound Phenomenon. The reflex activity can be inhibited for some time by some method. However, once the inhibitory effect is over, the reflex activity reappears and becomes more powerful. This is called rebound phenomenon. Its cause is still not known.

15. Fractionation. The force of a muscle contraction is much higher when it is stimulated directly through motor nerve compared with when it is stimulated reflexly through a sensory nerve. This is due to phenomenon of occlusion of the motor neurons when a sensory nerve is stimulated. Because of occlusion, number of motor neurons stimulated is lesser.

16. Sensitization. When an injurious stimulus is repeatedly applied, intensification of response occurs. This is

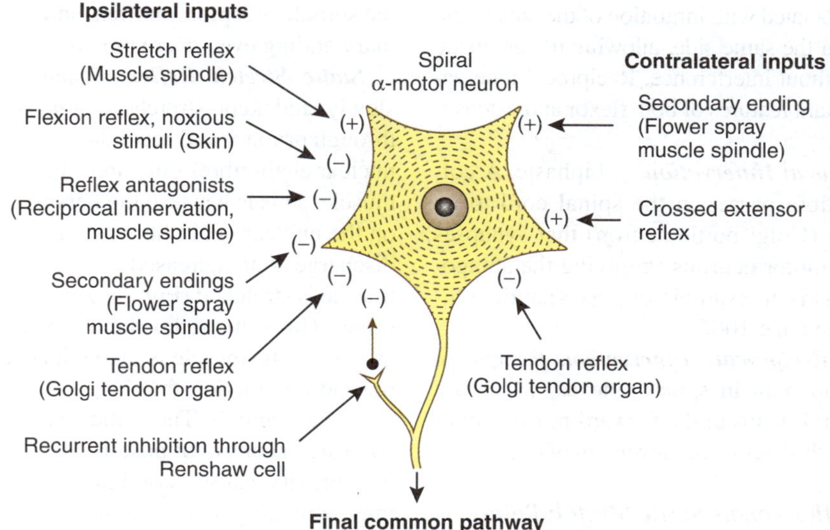

FIGURE 10.9-8 The inputs converging on the body of alpha (α) motor neuron (final common pathway).

known as sensitization. Sensitization, in fact, is the presynaptic facilitation of an impulse.

Spinal Cord Reflexes

Spinal cord reflexes enhance the ability of the motor control system to produce a coordinated movement. According to the receptors from which they originate, the spinal cord reflexes can be categorized into muscle reflexes and cutaneous reflexes.

- ***Muscle reflexes.*** Two important reflexes which originate in muscles are:
  - Stretch reflex and
  - Lengthening reaction or Golgi tendon reflex.
- ***Cutaneous reflexes.*** The most important of the cutaneous reflexes is:
  - Withdrawal (flexor, pain) reflex.

1. Stretch Reflex

Stretch reflex, also known as myotactic, refers to reflex contraction of a muscle that is stretched.

- ***Type.*** It is the best known monosynaptic reflex in the body.
- ***Stimulus*** that evokes the reflex response is 'stretch' to the muscle.
- ***Reaction time,*** i.e. the time between the application of the stimulus and the response for a stretch reflex is 19–24 ms. Stretch reflex is the quickest of all the reflexes.
- ***Central delay,*** i.e. the time taken for the reflex activity to traverse the spinal cord, in a stretch reflex (being monosynaptic) is only 0.6–0.9 ms.
- ***Stretch reflex*** *is well developed* in antigravity muscles such as extensor group of muscles of legs and flexor groups of muscles of arm.
- ***Examples*** of stretch reflexes are knee jerk, ankle jerk, biceps jerk, and triceps jerk (see page 1061).

Reflex Arc of Stretch Reflex *(Fig. 10.9-5)*

1. Afferent limb consists of receptor and afferent nerve.

- ***Receptor*** for stretch reflex is muscle spindle. As a sensory receptor, the muscle spindle detects the degree and rate of muscle stretch. For detailed structure of muscle spindle, see page 1048.
- ***Afferent nerve.*** As described earlier (nerve supply of muscle spindle), two types of nerve fibres, group Ia fibre and group II fibres, supply the muscle spindle (see page 1048). The afferent nerve fibres emerging from the muscle spindle travel along the spinal nerve and enter the spinal cord through the dorsal root and send branches to every α-motor neuron that goes to the muscle from which the Ia originated.

2. Centre. The centre for stretch reflex is the ventral grey horn area where the afferent nerve ends and synapses directly with the α-motor neuron. Thus, an α-motor neuron is the final common pathway, serving as both integrating centre and efferent pathway.

3. Efferent Limb consists of the efferent nerve and an effector organ.

- ***Efferent nerve.*** The axons of α-motor neurons (with which the afferent fibres synapse directly) form the efferent nerve fibres which leave the spinal cord through the ventral root and supply the skeletal muscle fibres.
- ***Effector organs.*** Both extensor and flexor muscles exhibit stretch reflexes, and thus form the effector organs.

Reciprocal Innervation in Stretch Reflex The stretch reflex is characterized by reciprocal innervation, i.e. excitation of one group of muscles is associated with inhibition of the antagonistic group of muscles on the same side, allowing the agonistic muscles to contract without interference. Reciprocal innervation is one of the important features of both flexor and extensor reflexes.

Pathway of Reciprocal Innervation is biphasic. A collateral from each Ia fibre passes in the spinal cord to an inhibitory interneuron (Golgi bottle neuron) that synapses directly on one of the motor neurons supplying the antagonist muscles. Thus, this is an example of postsynaptic inhibition (Fig. 10.7-18 see page 1006).

Significance of Reciprocal Innervation. Reciprocal innervation is very important in spinal reflexes, which are involved in locomotion. It helps in the forward movement of one limb while causing the backward movement of other limb.

Dynamic Stretch Reflex versus Static Stretch Reflex

Dynamic Stretch Reflex. When the muscle is stretched suddenly, the length of spindle receptor also increases suddenly (as the intrafusal fibres forming muscle spindle are attached in parallel with extrafusal fibres of the muscle). Sudden increase in length of spindle receptor stimulates the primary nerve ending powerfully. The primary nerve endings supplying the nuclear bag fibres show a dynamic response, i.e. they discharge most rapidly while the muscle is being stretched (Figs 10.9-9, 10.9-10B) and transmit strong signals to the spinal cord, and it causes instantaneous, very strong reflex contraction of the same muscle from which the signals originated. This is called dynamic stretch reflex, the function of which is to oppose sudden change in length, e.g. knee jerk and ankle jerk. Dynamic stretch reflex is over within fraction of a second, because primary nerve endings supplying nuclear bag fibres are stimulated actively only when there is a rapid change of length, i.e. they are stimulated only when the length is actually increasing. As soon as the length stops increasing, the rate of impulse discharge through those endings returns back to normal. Further, when the muscle contracts reflexly, the spindle receptors shorten, and the discharge through primary ending even decreases momentarily (Fig. 10.9-10C).

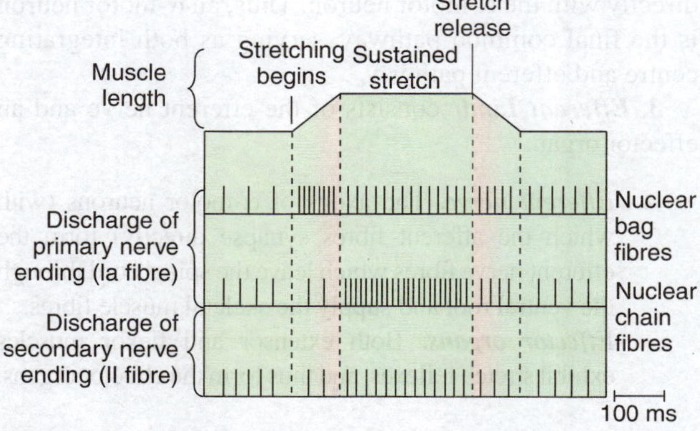

FIGURE 10.9-9 Response of primary (Ia) and secondary (II) nerve endings of muscle spindles to muscle stretch.

Static Stretch Reflex. When the muscle is stretched slowly and kept stretched, signals are continuously sent through primary and secondary nerve endings supplying the nuclear chain fibres only and cause reflex contraction of the muscle. This is because the nerves from the primary ending on the nuclear chain fibres show a static response, i.e. they discharge at an increased rate throughout the period when a muscle is stretched (Fig. 10.9-9). This is called static stretch reflex. This static reflex therefore causes muscle contraction as long as the muscle is maintained at excessive length. The muscle contraction thus opposes the force that is causing the excess length. The static stretch reflex plays an important role in control of posture, e.g. when the person is standing, gravity causes continuous stretch on the antigravity muscle making them to remain in a contracted state as long as gravity is causing the stretch.

Note. From the above, it is clear that a primary nerve ending responds to both changes in length (static stretch reflex) as well as changes in the rate of stretch (dynamic stretch reflex). The response of primary endings to the phasic as well as static events in the muscle is important because the prompt, marked phasic response helps to dampen oscillations caused by conduction delays in the feedback loop regulating the muscle length.

Role of Gamma Motor Neurons

1. Role of γ-efferent Discharge in Adjusting the Spindle Sensitivity by Preventing Unloading. As discussed above, the firing rate of primary nerve endings (Ia fibres) increases when the muscle is stretched (Fig. 10.9-10B), and causes reflex contraction of the muscle by increased α-motor neuron activity. Contraction of the extrafusal muscle fibres makes the muscle spindle slack and decreases the firing rate of Ia fibres (Fig. 10.9-10C). The decreased rate of Ia afferent discharge that occurs during muscle contraction is called *unloading of muscle spindle,* and is functionally disadvantageous because the CNS stops receiving information about the rate and extent of muscle shortening. However, by the activity of γ-motor neurons, this unloading is prevented (Fig. 10.9-10D). The γ-motor neurons cause the striated poles of intrafusal fibres of muscle spindle to shorten along with shortening of extrafusal fibres during muscle contraction. As a result of contraction of the striated polar regions of intrafusal fibres, the central receptor region of the intrafusal fibres remains stretched during muscle contraction, and unloading does not occur. In this way, the γ-motor neuron activity adjusts the sensitivity of the muscle spindle so that it will respond appropriately during muscle contraction as well. Further, the γ-motor neurons control both dynamic as well as static activity of muscle spindle as described.

- ***Dynamic gamma motor neurons*** primarily innervate the striated poles of nuclear bag fibres (Fig. 10.9-4).

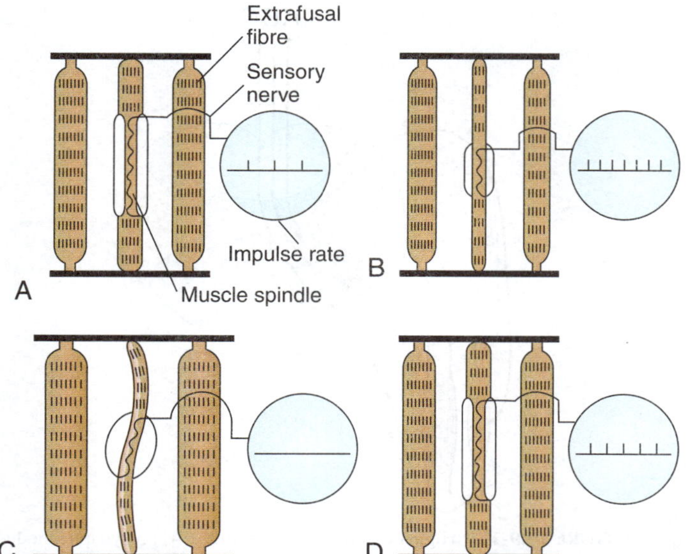

FIGURE 10.9-10 Firing rate of primary nerve endings (Ia) under different conditions: **A,** muscle at rest; **B,** muscle stretched; **C,** muscle contracted; and **D,** muscle contracted with increased gamma (γ) efferent discharge.

Thus, when they are fired, only nuclear bag fibres shorten. Because the nuclear bag fibres are responsible for the phasic (i.e. velocity-sensitive) portion of Ia afferent response to stretch, stimulation of the dynamic γ-fibres increases phasic activity without affecting static activity.

- ***Static γ-fibres*** primarily innervate the striated poles of nuclear chain fibres (Fig. 10.9-4). When they are fired, only the nuclear chain fibres shorten. Because the nuclear chain fibres are responsible for the static (i.e. length-sensitive) component of Ia afferent response to stretch, stimulation of the static γ-fibres increases static activity without affecting phasic activity.

Note. The above-described γ-motor neuron-mediated change in length of intrafusal fibres forms the so-called *length servomechanism,* which is a system of negative feedback device that operates to maintain muscle length during body movements and thus helps in regulation of posture (see page 1062).

2. Role of Coactivation of Alpha and Gamma Motor Neurons. During a normal voluntary movement (e.g. *lifting a weight*), the active shortening of the extrafusal fibres would relieve tension on the muscle spindles (i.e. unload the spindle) and hence tend to decrease Ia discharge. However, during voluntary contraction, the motor control system causes α–γ *coactivation,* preventing the unloading of muscle spindle that would occur during muscle contraction. Thus, increased γ-discharge along with the increased α-discharge during voluntary movement maintains constant Ia discharge. The constant level of Ia input to the CNS during a voluntary movement indicates that motor command is being carried out.

Note. The α–γ coactivation also forms the so-called *follow-up servomechanism* during voluntary movements.

For example, during voluntary movement of weightlifting, if the weight to be lifted is underestimated by the CNS, the motor command system does not activate a sufficient number of α-motor neurons to lift the weight and the extrafusal fibres fail to contract to desired length. However, because of γ-motor neuron activity, the intrafusal fibres contract stretching the central receptor region of the intrafusal fibres, resulting in increased Ia afferent activity. This is called *loading of muscle spindle.* The increased Ia activity indicates that the motor command is not being carried out. The CNS uses this information to readjust its command to the spinal cord. Even before the CNS responds to the information provided by the Ia fibres, the increased Ia activity directly stimulates the α-motor neurons of spinal cord causing forceful muscle contraction sufficient to lift the unexpected weight. This change in α-motor neuron activity at the spinal cord level (without the higher motor command system) forms the 'follow-up servomechanism', which ensures that the extrafusal fibres contract to the desired length in spite of mismatched motor command.

3. Role of Gamma Loop. It is theoretically possible that the CNS is capable of initiating movements directly by stimulating only γ-motor neurons, using a pathway called the gamma loop (Fig. 10.9-11). The loop begins with γ-motor neuron, which discharges to cause intrafusal muscle fibre contraction. This leads to an increase in Ia afferent fibre activity, which in turn causes increased γ-motor neuron discharge via a monosynaptic reflex causing muscle contraction.

Although the gamma loop can elicit movement on its own, it normally does not do so. However, because of coactivation,

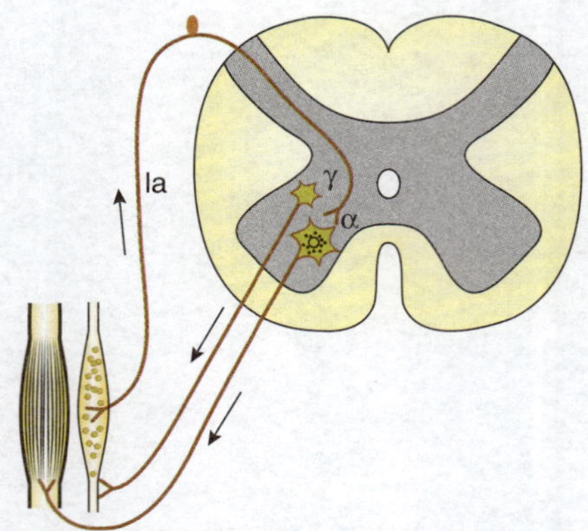

FIGURE 10.9-11 The gamma loop system of initiating muscle contraction directly through stimulation of γ motor neurons.

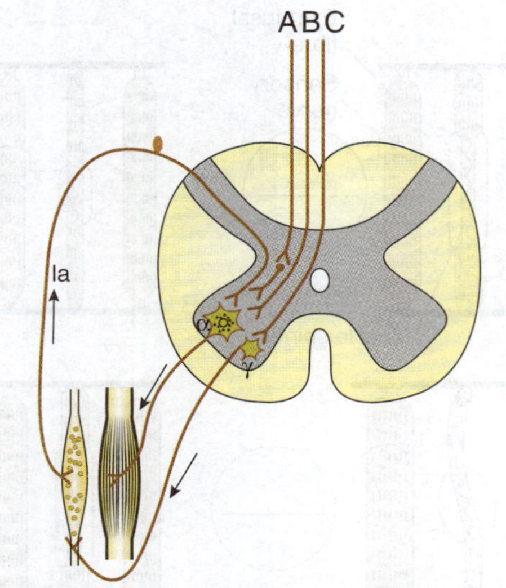

FIGURE 10.9-12 Higher control of stretch reflex: **A,** presynaptic modulation of Ia sensory input; **B,** direct action on alpha motor neurons; and **C,** modulation of gamma motor neuronal activity (centrifugal control).

the gamma loop is activated during all movements and thus contributes to the excitability and firing rate of the α-motor neurons.

Higher Control of Stretch Reflex From the above discussion, it is clear that stretch reflex involves three types of nerve fibres:

- Afferent fibres(Ia type),
- Gamma motor efferents and
- Alpha motor efferents.

Though the stretch reflex is a spinal reflex, the activity in the reflex arc can be modified (inhibited or facilitated) by higher centres through their influence on the above-cited nerve fibres involved in stretch reflex.

1. Control of Afferent (Ia Type) Discharge The afferent fibres carry input arising from the activity of muscle spindle. The higher centres control it by presynaptic modulation of the sensory input (Fig. 10.9-12A).

2. Control of Gamma Efferent Discharge

i. *Direct modulation of gamma neuronal activity (centrifugal control).* The motor neurons of the γ-efferent system are regulated to a large degree by descending tracts from a number of areas in the brain (Fig. 10.9-12C). Via these pathways, the sensitivity of the muscle spindles and hence the threshold of the stretch reflexes in various parts of the body can be adjusted and shifted to meet the needs of postural control. Some of the important brain areas that facilitate or inhibit the stretch reflex are (Fig. 10.9-13):

- ***Facilitatory reticular formation*** is a large area in the brainstem which discharges spontaneously in response to afferent input. This increases discharge of γ-motor neurons and stretch reflex becomes hyperactive.
- ***Inhibitory reticular formation*** is a small area which does not discharge spontaneously. It acts by inhibiting γ-efferent neuron discharge, thereby decreasing the spindle sensitivity.

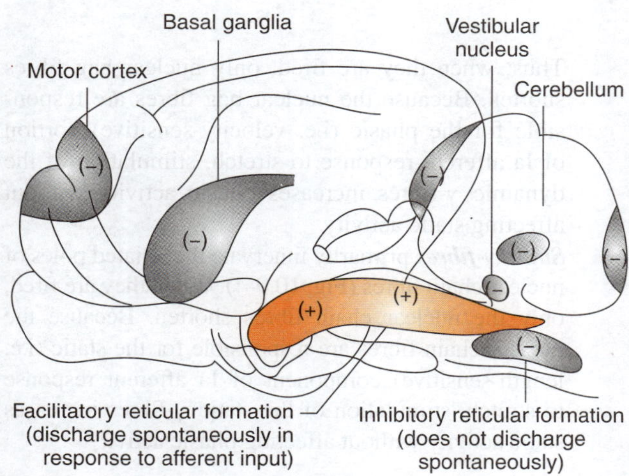

FIGURE 10.9-13 Brain areas that have facilitatory (+) and inhibitory (−) effect on stretch reflex.

- ***Cerebral motor cortex*** and cerebellum reflexly inhibit the stretch reflex by stimulating the inhibitory reticular formation.

ii. *Other factors which influence γ-efferent discharge*

- ***Anxiety*** causes an increased discharge, a fact that probably explains the hyperactive tendon reflexes sometimes seen in anxious patients.
- ***Unexpected movement*** is also associated with a greater γ-efferent discharge.
- ***Stimulation of skin,*** especially by noxious agents, increases γ-efferent discharge to ipsilateral flexor muscle spindles and decreases that to extensors and produces the opposite pattern in opposite limb. This fact is sometimes used as reinforcement to elicit deep tendon reflexes (such as knee jerk), which are not being elicited otherwise. For it, the individual is

asked to pull the hands apart when the flexed fingers are hooked together; this facilitates the knee jerk (*Jendrassik's* manoeuvre). It is contributed to increased γ-efferent discharge initiated by afferent impulses from the hands.

3. Control of Alpha Motor Efferent Discharge Alpha motor neurons form the efferent pathway of stretch reflex. All neural influences (excitatory or inhibitory) affecting muscle contraction ultimately funnel through the α-motor neurons; therefore, they form the so-called *final common pathway.* Numerous inputs converge on them and determine the activity in final common path (Figs 10.9-8, 10.9-12B).

Functions of Stretch Reflex

i. Role in Maintaining Muscle Tone. The muscle tone refers to partial state of contraction of the muscle under resting condition. It is the function of stretch reflex, which is under the influence of discharge from the gamma motor neuron. In the brainstem, there are two areas—facilitatory area is the pons and inhibitory area is the lower part of medulla. These areas send the impulses to gamma motor neurons. Facilitatory area is intrinsically active, so it continues to discharge facilitatory impulses causing constant activation of gamma motor neurons. This causes stretching of the muscle spindle fibres resulting into slight reflex contraction of the extrafusal fibres of muscle under resting state (producing muscle tone). Inhibitory area in the medulla becomes active only if it receives impulses from cerebellum or cerebral cortex.

ii. Role in Maintaining Posture. Static component of stretch reflex, the fundamental posture control mechanism, is especially prominent in medial extensor muscles and antigravity muscles. For example, when a person is standing upright, gravity tends to stretch the quadriceps muscle. This stretching elicits a stretch reflex resulting into sustained contraction of quadriceps as long as the stretch is there. This maintains the extension around the knee joint and upright posture.

iii. Role in Control of Voluntary Movement. A stretch reflex helps the motor command system in performing voluntary movements. During activity generated by the motor command system, the group Ia fibres from the muscle spindle inform the motor control system about the changes in muscle length. The constant level of Ia input to the CNS during a movement indicates that the motor command is being carried out. An increase in activity of Ia indicates that motor command is not being carried out. The CNS uses this information to readjust its command to the spinal cord. In addition, the Ia activity is also used at the spinal cord level to adjust the α-motor neuron activity as per need. Thus, the Ia activity provides the α-motor neuron with a source of excitatory input in addition to that coming from the higher centres.

2. Golgi Tendon Reflex (Disynaptic Reflex)

The Golgi tendon reflex, also called 'inverse stretch reflex', is a disynaptic reflex. The receptors involved are the Golgi tendon organs.

Golgi Tendon Organs Golgi tendon organs (Fig. 10.9-14) are high threshold stretch receptors located in the tendons and musculoaponeurotic junction. They are placed in series between the muscle fibres and the tendon (in contrast to muscle spindles which are located in parallel to muscle fibres) and are thus stretched whenever the muscle contracts. Usually, 10–15 muscle fibres are connected in series with one Golgi tendon organ. Each Golgi tendon organ basically consists of a group of nerve endings covered by a capsule of connective tissue. In a given muscle, the Golgi tendon organs are less numerous than muscle spindles.

- The Golgi tendon organs are supplied by *Ib type sensory nerve fibres.* The nerve fibres supplying the Golgi tendon organ ramify into many branches. Each branch ends in the form of a knob.
- The Golgi tendon organs have neither muscle fibres nor an efferent innervation.

Pathway and Activity of Reflex (Fig. 10.9-15)

- When a muscle contracts, the muscle tension increases. The Golgi tendon organ detects the muscle tension and sends impulses through afferent (group Ib) fibres which enter the spinal cord through dorsal root.
- In the spinal cord, the group Ib afferents stimulate the inhibitory interneurons.
- The inhibitory interneurons in turn release inhibitory mediator glycine which inhibits α-motor neurons and cause relaxation of the muscle that was originally contracted.
- At the same time, due to reciprocal innervation, the antagonistic muscles are excited.
- The Golgi tendon reflex thus displays reciprocal innervation but lacks after discharge and irradiation.

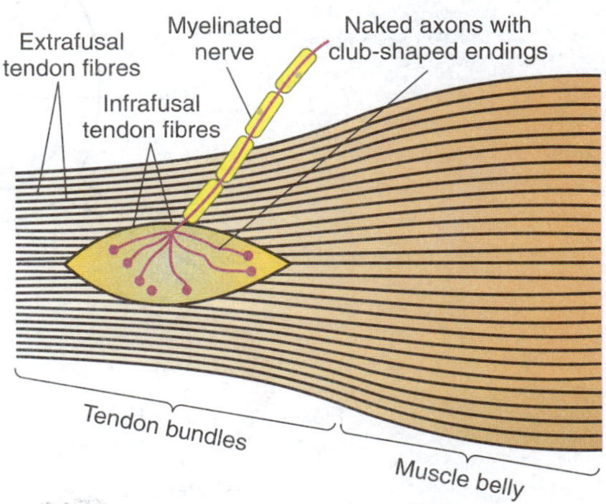

FIGURE 10.9-14 Structure of Golgi tendon organ.

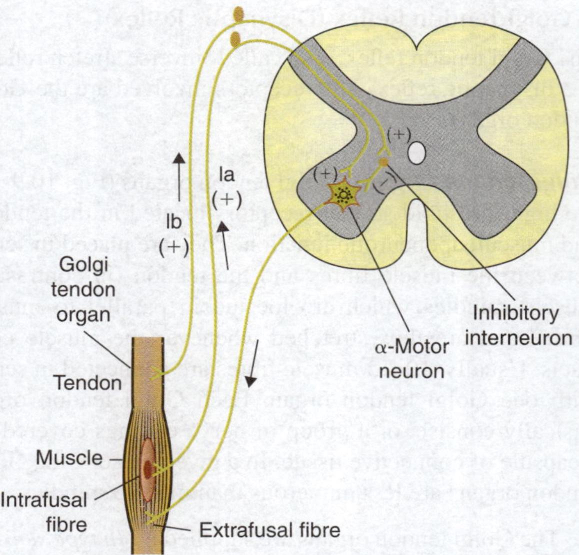

FIGURE 10.9-15 Pathway of stretch and inverse stretch reflex.

Physiological role or the functions of Golgi tendon reflex are:

- ***Protective function.*** Historically, this reflex has been described as a protective reflex in which a strong and potentially damaging muscle force reflexively inhibits the muscle, causing the muscle to lengthen instead of trying to maintain the force and risking damage.
- ***Regulation of tension during normal muscle activity*** is a more important role of this reflex. This reflex has been described as *autogenic inhibition* which indicates that the force generated when the muscle contracts is the stimulus for its own relaxation.

Clasp-knife reflex refers to an exaggerated form of the Golgi tendon reflex, which can occur with disease of the corticospinal tracts (hypertonicity or spasticity). For example, when the arm is hypertonic, the increased sensitivity of the muscle spindles in the extensor muscles (triceps) causes resistance to flexion of the arm. Eventually, tension in the triceps increases to the point at which it activates Golgi tendon reflex, causing triceps to relax and the arm to flex closed like a jack knife, hence the name clasp-knife reflex. The physiological name for it is *lengthening reaction,* because it is the response of a spastic muscle to lengthening.

3. Withdrawal Reflex (Polysynaptic Reflex)

Definition and Receptors

Definition. Withdrawal reflex, also known as flexor reflex, is a cutaneous reflex that occurs in response to nociceptive (pain) stimuli and is characterized by removal of a body part from painful stimulus.

Receptors for withdrawal reflex are *nociceptors* located in free nerve endings of Aδ and C fibres.

Pathway (Reflex Arc) of Withdrawal Reflex. Withdrawal reflex is a polysynaptic reflex consisting of the following pathways (Fig. 10.9-16):

- The pain fibres carrying impulses, upon entering the spinal cord, synapse on many interneurons. Some of these also convey information to CNS. Others form several reflex pathways.
- Polysynaptic reflex paths branch in a complex fashion. The number of synapses in each of their branches is variable (Fig. 10.9-17).
- A branch from some of the axons of interneuron in the reflex pathway feeds back on themselves forming the *reverberating circuits,* which are responsible for after discharge (Fig. 10.9-17).

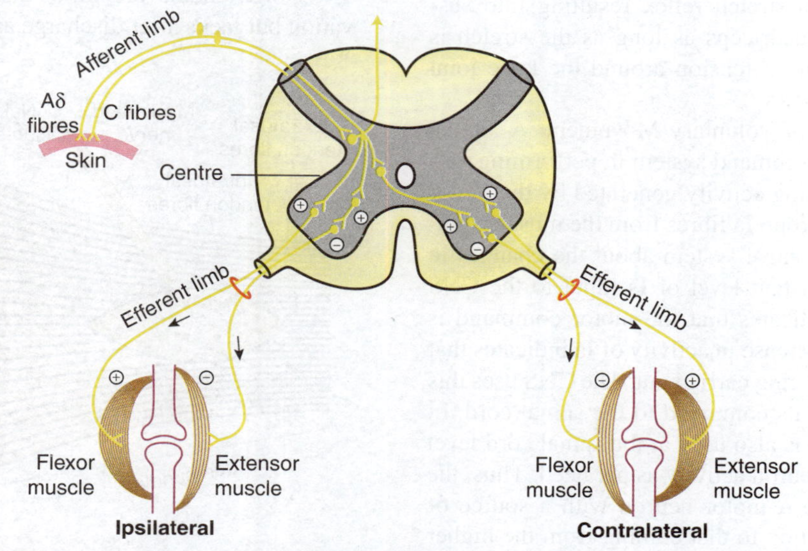

FIGURE 10.9-16 Reflex arc of a polysynaptic reflex (withdrawal reflex or crossed extensor reflex).

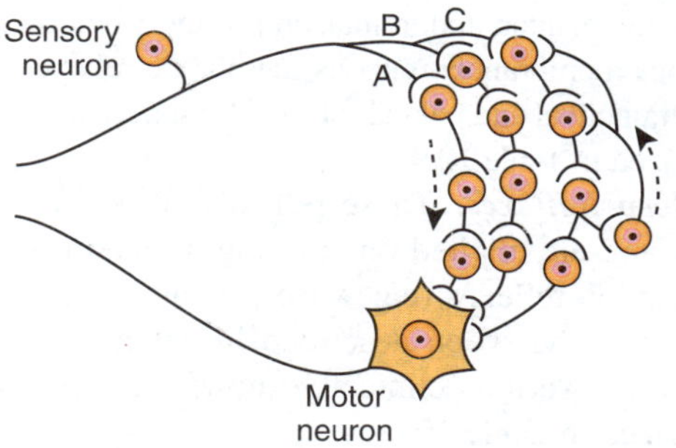

FIGURE 10.9-17 Schematic depiction of connections between afferent and efferent neurons in the spinal cord. The dorsal root fibre has been shown to activate pathway **A** with three interneurons, pathway **B** with four interneurons and **C** with four interneurons. Note that one of the interneurons in the pathway C connects to a neuron that feedbacks on to previously excited neuron forming reverberating circuits.

- The interneurons form several pathways of different lengths to ultimately end on α-motor neurons as follows (Fig. 10.9-17):
  - Some of the interneurons project onto α-motor neurons on the ipsilateral side and stimulate the flexors which withdraw the limbs.
  - Some of the interneurons form inhibitory pathway and terminate on α-motor neurons supplying the extensor muscles on the ipsilateral side producing their relaxation. This is called reciprocal innervation, which ensures that the flexion movement is not impeded by contraction of the extensors.
  - Some of the interneurons cross to the opposite side of spinal cord and end on the α-motor neurons supplying the extensors on contralateral side. In case of need, this pathway produces extension of the opposite limbs (crossed extensor reflex).

Effector Organs The effector organs of the withdrawal reflex are the skeletal muscles that cause withdrawal of the limb. Although they are called flexors, these muscles are flexors in the physiologic, not anatomic, sense. For example, the muscles that cause the fingers to open to drop a hot coal, although anatomically referred to as extensors, are considered flexors, because they are involved in the withdrawal reflex.

Response in Withdrawal Reflex The reflex response to a painful stimulus varies from just withdrawal of the affected part to withdrawal of the whole body depending upon the strength of painful stimulus and location of the stimulus. The different types of responses observed in a withdrawal reflex are as follows:

• ***Local Sign*** refers to the ability of the reflex to confine to the portion of body affected by the noxious stimulus. For example, if the medial surface of a limb is stimulated, the response will include some abduction, whereas stimulation of the lateral surface will produce adduction and flexion. The reflex response in each case generally serves to effectively remove the limb away from the irritating stimulus. Therefore, if an individual accidently touches a hot stove, it is likely that he or she will jerk only the hand away from the stove (one-limb response).

• ***Flexor Response.*** When a noxious stimulus is applied to a limb, the typical response is in the form of contraction of flexors and inhibition of extensors leading to flexion of the stimulated limb and its withdrawal from the irritating stimulus.

• ***Crossed Extensor Reflex Response*** (two-limb response). When a strong stimulus is applied to a limb, the response includes not only flexion and withdrawal of the limb but also extension of the opposite limb. This crossed extensor response is produced by the interneuronal pathway that crosses to the opposite side of spinal cord. In lower limbs, crossed extensor reflex allows one limb to support the body while the other is raised off the ground.

• ***Shifting Reaction (Four-Limb Reflex Response).*** It is difficult to demonstrate this response in normal animals but is easily demonstrated in spinal animals (produced by a transverse section in the lower region of spinal cord) in which the modulating effects of stimulus from the brain have been abolished. Application of electric shock to one hind limb of a spinal animal will produce a response in all the four limbs as:

- Flexion of the hind limb to which stimulus is applied,
- Extension of the contralateral hind limb,
- Extension of the ipsilateral forelimb and
- Flexion of the contralateral forelimb.

• ***Widespread Withdrawal Response*** is obtained when the noxious stimulus is very strong. For example, if an individual picks up a hot coal, not only will the fingers open and drop it, but the entire arm will withdraw and the individual may even leap away from the fire.

Mechanism of Varied Grades of Withdrawal Response Irradiation of the stimulus and recruitment of motor units are the mechanisms involved in the varied grades of response in withdrawal reflex.

Irradiation refers to spread of excitatory impulses up and down the spinal cord to more and more motor units leading to activation of a large number of impulses. This occurs when the noxious stimulus is strong enough that impulses spread to many neighbouring neurons in the centre and produce wider response.

Recruitment of Motor Units refers to progressive increase in number of motor units activated by spreading interneuronal activity. Of course, there is a limit to the number of motor units that can be recruited. So, beyond a certain limit, prolongation of stimulation does not increase the response and a plateau is reached.

Characteristics of Withdrawal Reflex

1. Long Latency. The withdrawal reflex has a relatively long latency, i.e. has a higher reaction time. *Reaction time* is the interval between application of stimulus and onset of response. It is determined in part by the time taken by the impulse transmission in afferent and efferent limbs of the reflex arc (*peripheral delay)* and in part by the time spent by the impulse in traversing the spinal cord (*central delay*). The long latency in withdrawal reflex is because of peripheral delay (as the afferent pathway uses small, slowly conducting fibres) as well as due to central delay (as it involves many synapses).

> It is important to note that in case of stretch reflex, the central delay is less than 1 ms, indicating that it is a monosynaptic reflex (MSR). In case of flexor reflex, the central delay is much longer.
>
> In crossed extensor response, the central delay may be longer than 20 ms, reflecting the huge number of interneurons involved in the reflex.

2. Response Outlasts Stimulus, i.e. withdrawal reflex shows after discharge. *After discharge* refers to the continuation of reflex withdrawal of the limb even after the sensory receptor has stopped firing. It is produced by *reverberating circuits* (i.e. a branch from the axon of one interneuron in the reflex pathway feeds back onto previously excited neurons, re-exciting them and prolonging alpha motor neuron firing).

3. Patterned Response. The crossed extensor reflex produces a patterned response, i.e. the affected limb always flexes while the contralateral limb extends.

4. Summation. See page 1051.

5. Occlusion. See page 1051.

6. Subliminal Firing. See page 1052.

7. Recruitment. See page 1052.

8. Irradiation. See page 1052.

9. Reciprocal Inhibition. See page 1006.

Function of Withdrawal Reflex Withdrawal reflex is a protective reflex initiated by a potentially harmful (nociceptive) stimulus. The flexor response takes the limb away from the source of irritation. A withdrawal reflex is associated with a crossed extensor reflex, which helps to support the body and is of physiological significance in the context of regulation of posture. Withdrawal reflex is prepotent, i.e. it pre-empts all other reflex activities taking place at that time in the involved spinal cord segment.

Clinical Reflexes

Clinically, the reflexes can be grouped as:

I. Physiological Reflexes

1. Superficial Reflexes. These reflexes are initiated in response to stimulation of receptors on skin (cutaneous reflexes, e.g. plantar, abdominal, cremasteric, bulbo-cavernous) or mucous membranes (mucous membrane reflexes), e.g. corneal, conjunctival and palatal reflex. The superficial reflexes are summarized in Table 10.9-1.

2. Deep Reflexes. These reflexes are basically stretch reflexes and are elicited on stroking a tendon, so they are called tendon reflexes (e.g. knee jerk and ankle jerk). The stretch reflex has been described in detail on page 1053; however, the various clinically known stretch reflexes are summarized in Table 10.9-1.

3. Visceral Reflexes are elicited from the visceral organ or at least one part of the reflex arc is formed by autonomic nerve, e.g. carotid sinus reflex (see page 340), micturition reflex (see page 562) and occulocardiac reflex. A few of the clinically known visceral reflexes are summarized in Table 10.9-1.

II. Pathological Reflexes The pathological reflexes are abnormal reflexes, which are not found normally. They are elicited in pathological conditions, e.g.

- Babinski sign,
- Mass reflex,
- Clonus and
- Pendular Movements.

1. Babinski Sign. It is the abnormal plantar reflex, i.e. instead of plantar flexion of great toe there occurs dorsiflexion of great toe and abduction (fanning out) of small toes and also accompanied with flexion of knee and dorsiflexion at the ankle joint. The abnormal plantar response is called *extensor plantar or Babinski sign positive. Significance.* Babinski sign is present in the following conditions:

- Upper motor neuron lesion (UML). It is the most important sign.
- Physiologically, it is present in infants (below age of 1 year) due to nonmyelination of pyramidal tracts and also during deep sleep.

2. Mass Reflex. This reflex can be elicited in patients with spinal cord lesions. When the skin (on any portion in the midline) is stimulated by gentle pinpricks, there occurs evacuation of bowel or bladder, flexion of lower limb and sweating of skin below the level of lesion.

Significance. Patients suffering from spinal cord injuries are particularly trained to elicit mass reflex to evacuate bowel and bladder.

3. Clonus. Clonus means series of rapid and jerky movements which occur due to involuntary contraction of the muscle in response to sudden rapid and constant stretch. Clonus signifies hyperflexia and hypertonia associated with increased gamma efferent activity. Clonus is seen in calf muscles (producing ankle clonus) and quadriceps (patellar clonus).

Ankle clonus. To elicit ankle clonus, support the slightly bent knee on one hand and hold the foot and suddenly dorsiflex

TABLE 10.9-1 Characteristic Features of Clinical Reflexes

Reflex	Method to elicit	Response	Spinal segment/cranial nerve and centre involved
I. Superficial reflexes *(a) Cutaneous reflexes*			
1. *Plantar reflex*	Strike the outer aspect of the sole of the foot with a blunt object (e.g. key) and move towards the ball of small toes	Plantar flexion of the foot and toes	L_5 to S_1
2. *Abdominal reflex*	Lightly stimulate the wall of abdomen by stroking with key or some blunt object from out to inside (parallel to costal margin) in upper quadrants and (parallel to inguinal ligament) in lower quadrants of the abdomen	Contractions of the underlying abdominal muscle *Note.* The reflex is difficult to elicit in elderly individuals, obese persons and in multipara	T_7 to T_{12}
3. *Cremasteric reflex*	Stimulate the skin of upper and inner part of the thigh	Pulling upwards of scrotum and testicles due to contraction of cremasteric muscles. This reflex may not be elicited in elderly individuals	L_1 and L_2
4. *Scapular reflex*	Stroke the skin of interscapular region	Contraction of supra- and infra-spinatus muscles	C_5 to T_1
5. *Anal reflex*	Gently stimulate the skin of perianal region	Contraction of external and internal anal sphincters	S_2 to S_4
6. *Bulbocavernous reflex*	Gently pinch the dorsum of glans penis	Contraction of bulbocavernous muscle	S_3 to S_4
(b) Mucous membrane reflexes			
7. *Corneal reflex*	Touch the cornea with wisp of cotton from lateral aspect	Closure of eye of same and of opposite side	*Afferents*: Via ophthalmic division of Vth (trigeminal) cranial nerve. *Centre*: In the pons. *Efferents*: Via facial nerve to orbicularis oculi muscle
8. Conjunctival reflex	Touch the conjunctiva with wisp of cotton	Closure of the eyes	Pathway is same as for corneal reflex
9. *Palate reflex*	Touch on the either side of posterior pharyngeal wall with a swab stick	The contraction of the palate	*Afferents:* 9th cranial nerve *Centre:* Nucleus ambiguus *Efferents:* 10th cranial (vagus) nerve
II. Deep reflexes (tendon reflexes)			
1. *Knee jerk*	The subject is in lying or in sitting position. Place the left hand under the knee (to be tested). Tap the tendon of the quadriceps midway between its origin and insertion with knee hammer	Observe the extension of knee due to contraction of quadriceps femoris muscle. Sometimes, if unable to elicit, then apply reinforcement (Jendrassik's manoeuvre, page 1056	Femoral nerve (L_2, L_3 and L_4)
2. *Ankle jerk*	With foot slightly everted and dorsiflexed, strike on the tendo-Achilles.	Plantar flexion of the foot occurs due to contraction of calf muscle	S_1 and S_2
3. *Triceps jerk*	Keep the forearm of the subject to rest across his/her chest. Then tap the triceps tendon with broader side of the patellar hammer.	Contraction of triceps with extension of the elbow	C_6 and C_7

Continued

TABLE 10.9-1 Characteristic Features of Clinical Reflexes—cont'd

Reflex	Method to elicit	Response	Spinal segment/cranial nerve and centre involved
4. *Biceps jerk*	Keep the position of elbow at right angle with forearm and the forearm is semi-pronated. The examiner then places his/her thumb or index finger on the tendon of the biceps muscle and then strikes on the finger (kept on biceps tendon) with pateller hammer	Contraction of biceps with flexion of elbow	C_5 and C_6
5. *Supinator*	Tap the lower end of the radius at styloid process, keeping the position of elbow same as for biceps jerk.	Supination of forearm and flexion of elbow	C_5 and C_6
6. *Jaw jerk*	Ask the subject to open the mouth slightly. Then place one finger firmly below the lower lip and tap on the finger in a downward direction	Contraction of masseter muscle causes closure of the jaw	Afferent and efferents are carried by trigeminal nerve. Centre lies in the pons

the ankle and maintain the stretch for some time. This causes series of rhythmic plantar flexion at ankle joint. *Patellar clonus.* The patient's leg is extended, then the patella is suddenly pushed downwards towards the foot. Repeated contraction of quadriceps results in rhythmic movements of leg.

Clonus occurs due to:

- The stretch reflex–inverse stretch reflex sequence. The basis of this sequential event is synchronized discharging of motor neurons without involving Golgi tendon discharges.
- The muscle spindles of tested muscle become hyperactive and their discharges lead to excitation of all the motor neurons supplying at one time and cause contraction of the muscle.
- The muscle contractions (extrafusal fibres) results in stoppage of spindle discharges (relaxation of muscle) but as the stretch on the muscle is maintained causing spindle activation and again muscle contraction.

4. Pendular Movements. In patients of cerebellar dysfunctions, while eliciting tendon jerk, slow oscillatory movements develop instead of brisk movement. Such movements are called pendular movements and are a manifestation of hypotonia and lack of restrictive effect.

REGULATION OF POSTURE

- Physiologically, posture refers to subconscious adjustment of tone in different muscles so as to maintain balance during displacement of the body caused by gravity or acceleration.
- The erect posture is a prerequisite to most of the somatic motor activities of man and other higher animals.
- In humans, maintenance of an erect posture is more difficult than the quadruped animals, because the tall body has to be maintained in erect posture over a small base provided by two feet.
- Largely, the posture is maintained through reflex adjustments of tone in proximal extensor muscles. As gravity is the main force tending to displace the body, the proximal extensor muscles are also called antigravity muscles. Since a standing human being can fall in any direction, the muscles which oppose the fall act as antigravity muscles, depending upon the direction of fall. Therefore, any of the muscles of trunk and limbs can act as antigravity muscles.
- Maintenance of an erect posture during movements of the body and more so while performing physical work (*dynamic posture*) is more complicated than maintenance of posture while standing still (*static posture*). This uphill task is accomplished by a very complex and coordinated reflex activity occurring in response to afferent input from muscle joints, vestibular and visual receptors.
- For the purpose of understanding, the regulation of posture can be discussed under two main headings:
  - Mechanisms involved in maintenance of posture and
  - Role of different regions of nervous system in maintenance of posture.

Mechanisms Involved in Maintenance of Posture

At any given moment, in any position of the body (static or dynamic), the posture is maintained by alteration in the tone of different muscles which is controlled by a stretch reflex. The stretch reflex is a spinal reflex influenced by supraspinal control. The input to higher centres involved in the control of muscle tone through certain reflexes (called postural reflexes) significantly contributes to the maintenance of tone and hence the posture. Thus, the two main mechanisms involved in maintenance of posture are:

- Muscle tone and
- Postural reflexes.

Role of Tone in Antigravity Muscles in Maintenance of Posture

Largely, the posture is maintained through reflex adjustments of tone in the antigravity muscles. The basic postural reflex involved in the control of muscle tone is stretch reflex described in detail on page 1053.

Posture control is required not only for holding the body in an erect position but also for fixation of the body parts over adjoining body segments. The centre of gravity of head passes in front of the centre of gravity of atlanto-occipital joint. Thus, the head has got always a tendency to roll forwards. To hold the head in an erect position, cervico-occipital muscles are to be maintained in a state of constant tension. A similar problem is encountered in maintaining the equilibrium of the body in an erect position.

In the upright position, gravity tends to displace the body downward, stretching quadriceps muscles as the legs flex at the knees. The muscle stretch evokes discharge from the muscle spindles of the quadriceps leading to its reflex contraction. This ensures that the knee joints, i.e. the main weight-bearing joints, do not give way under the effect of gravity. This maintains the leg as a pillar of support and thus counteracts the gravitational displacement of the body.

In general, the antigravity muscles of the body are endowed with a somewhat higher muscle tone than the other muscles of the body.

In humans, flexors of upper extremity and extensors of lower extremity are the main antigravity muscles. Retractors of neck, the elevators of joint, supraspinatus, the extensors of back, rectal muscles of abdominal wall, extensors of knee and ankle are the muscles that exhibit greatest degree of tone. When these muscles completely relax (as in unconscious person), the body collapses.

Various postural reflexes (described below) influence the medial motor system and the motor neurons of antigravity muscles. The inputs to this system through the postural reflexes significantly contribute to the maintenance of tone. Thus, tone is the result of activity of various medial system pathways that descend to excite both alpha and gamma motor neurons, which innervate antigravity muscles and their spindles. Spinal transection interrupts this activity in the descending medial system and hence abolishes tone of the antigravity muscles (proximal extensors) below the level of transection. The two pathways of medial system that are most important in maintenance of tone are the *lateral vestibulospinal tract* and *pontine reticulospinal tract*. Thus, spinal shock can be produced by any transection caudal to the origin of vestibulospinal tract from lateral vestibular nucleus. However, if the transection is just rostral to this nucleus, then in contrast to spinal shock, the tone of antigravity muscles is actually enhanced and an exaggerated antigravity muscle posture is obtained. This phenomenon is called decerebrate rigidity (see page 1070).

Maintenance of Muscle Tone

Stretch Reflex, as mentioned earlier, plays the main role in maintenance of muscle tone (page 1057). Though the stretch reflex is a spinal reflex, supraspinal control modifies the reflex in an intact animal.

Centre for Muscle Tone. The centre for muscle tone lies in anterior motor neurons (α-motor neurons) of spinal cord, which are stimulated through a constant γ-motor neuron discharge. Activity of gamma and alpha motor neurons is modified by both extrapyramidal and pyramidal fibres which terminate on them (directly or through interneurons). Mainly, the extrapyramidal system is responsible for maintaining tone. It consists of basal ganglia, motor nuclei of reticular formation of brainstem, vestibular nuclei and descending fibres conveying impulses to spinal cord. From cerebral cortex (area 6), also some fibres descend and merge with the extrapyramidal nuclei.

Supraspinal control on muscle tone is (Fig. 10.9-18) exerted by facilitatory and inhibitory areas in the brainstem through gamma motor neurons.

Bulboreticular facilitatory area is located in the pons and discharges facilitatory impulses to spinal motor neurons. This area in turn receives facilitatory impulses from vestibular nuclei, facilitatory portion of cerebral cortex,

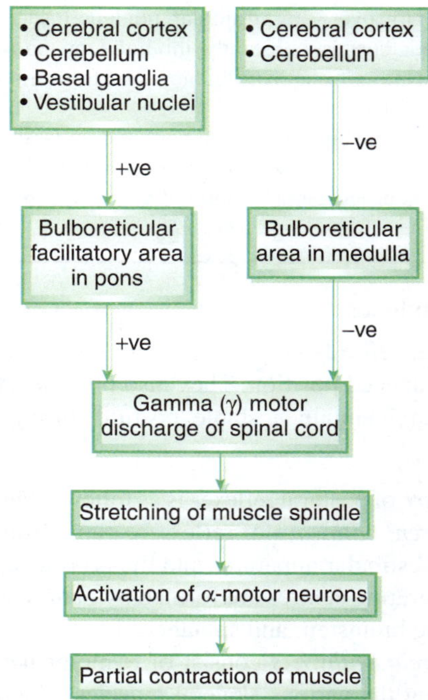

FIGURE 10.9-18 Flowchart depicting control of muscle tone.

cerebellum and basal ganglia. The facilitatory area continues to discharge impulses causing constant activation of gamma motor neurons. This causes stretching of the muscle spindle fibres resulting into reflex partial contraction of the muscle under resting state, thus producing muscle tone.

- ***Bulboreticular inhibitory area*** is located in the lower part of medulla. This area has no intrinsic activity of its own. It becomes active only if it receives impulses from cerebellum or cerebral cortex and in turn inhibits bulboreticular facilitatory area to some extent. But without support from cerebrum or cerebellum, this area cannot inhibit the activity of facilitatory area.
- ***Role of cerebellum.*** Cerebellum is the site of alpha–gamma linkage. Therefore, in the presence of cerebellum, the muscle tone is maintained through both the alpha (nonmyotatic) and gamma (myotatic) activity. However, in the absence of cerebellum, muscle tone is maintained by alpha (nonmyotatic) activity only. This can be demonstrated by classical and ischaemic decerebrate rigidity.

Important Note

Normally, the muscle tone is due to tonic discharge of gamma motor neurons to the muscles due to predominant effect of descending fibres of facilitatory reticular formation. Thus, muscle tone is normally not under the tonic control of alpha motor neurons (tonic control of motor neurons should not be confused with the stimulation of α-motor neurons through corticospinal fibres during voluntary phasic contraction). It is important to note that tonic control of α-motor neurons is exerted almost entirely through vestibulospinal pathway. However, the vestibular nucleus (especially the Deiter's nucleus) is constantly inhibited by corticospinal fibres as well as festigiovestibular fibres from the cerebellum (Fig. 10.9-19).

Under certain abnormal conditions and under experimental situation when the vestibular nucleus gets disinhibited, there occurs exaggeration of muscle tone that is α-led rather than γ-led.

Postural Reflexes

The postural reflexes help to maintain the body in an upright and balanced position. They also provide adjustments necessary to maintain a stable posture during voluntary activity.

Reflex arc of postural reflexes is as follows (Fig. 10.9-20):

- *Afferent pathways* of reflex arc come from the eyes, the vestibular apparatus and the proprioceptors.
- Integrating centres are formed by neuronal networks in the brainstem and spinal cord.
- *Efferent pathways* consist of α-motor neurons supplying the various skeletal muscles which form the effector organs.

Types of postural reflexes. Broadly, postural reflexes are of two types:

- ***Static reflexes:*** These are elicited by gravitational pull and involve sustained contraction of muscles.
- ***Statokinetic reflexes:*** These reflexes, also called phasic reflexes, are elicited by acceleratory displacement of the body. They maintain a stable postural background for voluntary activity.
- Both these types of postural reflexes are integrated at various levels in the CNS from the spinal cord to cerebral cortex and are affected largely by pyramidal pathways.

A. Static Reflexes

Static reflexes are primarily involved in adjustments to displacements produced by gravity. These are of three types:

- Local static reflexes,
- Segmental static reflexes and
- General static reflexes.

I. Local Static Reflexes As the name indicates, the local static reflexes exert their effect on the same limb from which the stimulus was initiated. Some of the important local static reflexes include:

- Reflex control of antigravity muscle tone,
- Positive supporting reaction and
- Negative supporting reaction.

1. Reflex Control of Antigravity Muscle Tone. The most important of the local static reflexes is basic stretch reflexes (which has been described in detail on page 1054) controlling tone in those extensor muscles which keep the body upright (*antigravity muscles*).

Muscle tone in antigravity muscles is best illustrated in decerebrate preparations (see page 1070), where it produces decerebrate rigidity. The hypertonicity in decerebrate preparations has a characteristic extensor distribution, resulting in a caricature (i.e. exaggerated mimicry) of the normal posture.

2. Positive Supporting Reflexes. Positive supporting reflex or reaction is characterized by simultaneous reflex contractions of both extensors and flexors of a limb (i.e. both the protagonists and antagonists) converting it into a solid rigid pillar. The positive supporting reaction plays an important role of *steading the ankle joint in standing position.* At the ankle joint, both dorsiflexion and plantar flexion are possible, but neither of them is desirable during standing position. The dorsiflexion of the foot would tip the body forward, while plantar flexion would throw the body backward (Fig. 10.9-21). The stabilization of ankle joint in intermediate position is possible by simultaneous contraction of extensor and flexors of foot brought about by the positive supporting reaction. Afferent impulses from the stimulated

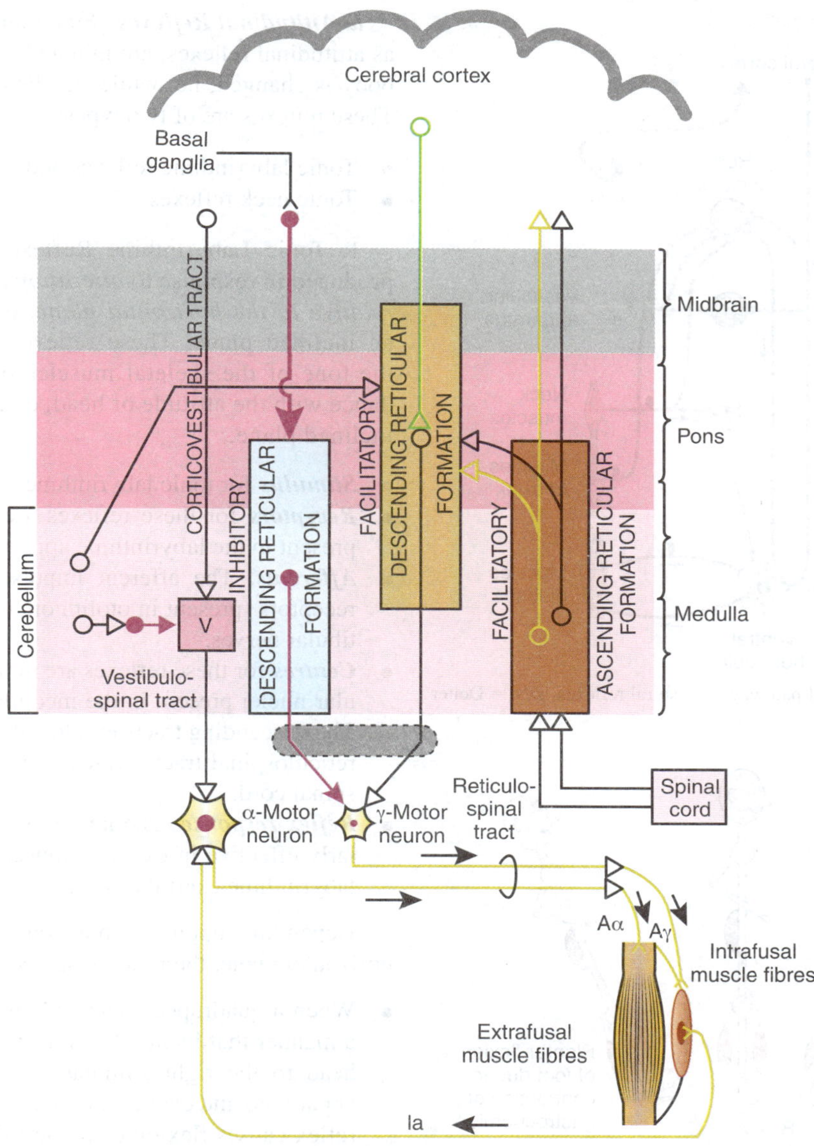

FIGURE 10.9-19 Supraspinal control of muscle tone (solid circles and arrows indicate inhibitory signals and open circles and arrows indicate facilitation). V = vestibular nuclei.

skin of sole (touch–pressure receptors) and the muscles (proprioceptors) cause reflex contraction of both flexor and extensor muscles acting on the ankle joint, converting the leg and ankle joint into one solid pillar.

3. Negative Supporting Reaction. Negative supporting reaction refers to disappearance of positive supporting reaction. It is also an active phenomenon initiated by stretch of the extensor muscles. This helps the limbs to be used for activities other than supporting the body weight.

Demonstration of Local Reflexes. The centres of the local static reflex are located in spinal cord. These can be demonstrated in spinal animal (see page 1070).

II. Segmental Static Reflexes The segmental static reflexes are characterized by a bilateral reflex response when stimulus is applied to one limb. The best example of segmental static reflexes is *crossed extensor reflex response component of withdrawal reflex.* In this reflex, a strong stimulus to one limb produces flexion in the ipsilateral limb and extension in the contralateral limb (see page 1069).

Role of Crossed Extensor Reflex in Control of Posture

- In the lower limb, this reflex allows one limb to support the body while other is raised off the ground. For example, when due to painful stimulus one limb is flexed reflexly, the extensor of the other limb compensates and sees to it that the body is not thrown off balance.
- The crossed extensor reflex also plays an important role during walking. During walking, on one side the flexors are active and the extensors are inhibited, while the reverse is seen on the other side.

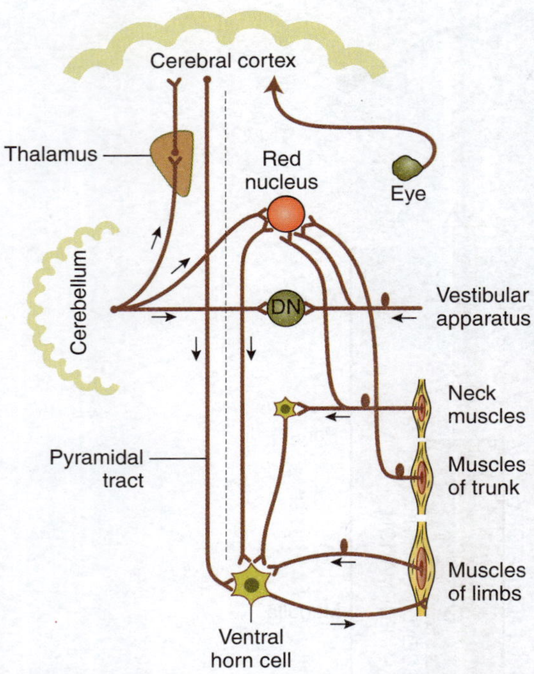

FIGURE 10.9-20 Neuronal pathway of postural reflexes. DN = Deiter nucleus.

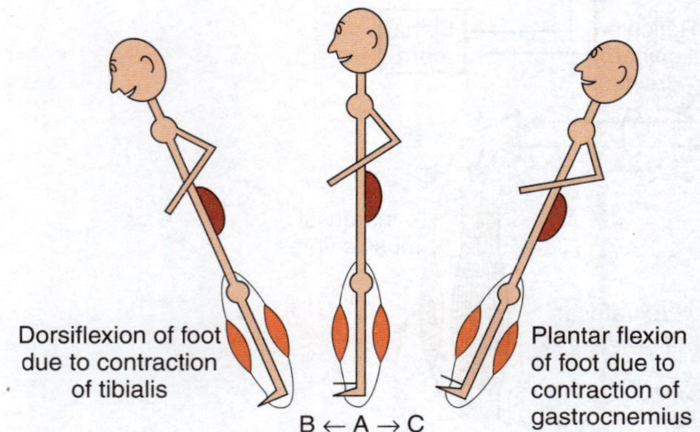

FIGURE 10.9-21 Role of positive supporting reaction in stabilizing the ankle joint: **A,** simultaneous contraction of flexors and extensors of foot to stabilize ankle joint; **B,** dorsiflexion at foot produces forward fall; and **C,** plantar flexion at foot produces backward fall.

Demonstration of Static Segmental Reflex. The centres for these reflexes are situated in the spinal cord. These can be best demonstrated in a *spinal animal* (see page 1070).

III. General Static Reflexes General static reflexes are characterized by a generalized effect from the many muscle groups in the body in response to a stimulus that arises at one side of the body. For example, numerous postural adjustments occur in response to changes in the head position. Broadly, general static reflexes can be divided into three groups:

- Attitudinal or Statotonic Reflexes,
- Long-loop stretch reflexes and
- Righting reflexes.

a. Attitudinal Reflexes. Statotonic reflexes, also known as attitudinal reflexes, are initiated when the attitude of the body is changed, i.e. while standing on an inclined plane. These reflexes are of two types:

- Tonic labyrinthine reflexes and
- Tonic neck reflexes.

1. Tonic Labyrinthine Reflexes. These reflexes are produced in response to *alteration in the position of head relative to the horizontal plane,* e.g. while standing on an inclined plane. These reflexes decrease or increase the tone of the skeletal muscles of the limbs in accordance with the attitude of head, e.g. while standing on an inclined plane.

- ***Stimulus*** for tonic labyrinthine reflex is gravity.
- ***Receptors*** for these reflexes are in the otolith organs, present in the labyrinthine apparatus.
- ***Afferents.*** The afferent impulses generated from the receptors (present in otolith organ) travel along the vestibular nerves.
- ***Centres*** for these reflexes are in the vestibular and reticular nuclei present in the medulla oblongata. *Efferents.* The descending tracts employed are vestibulospinal and reticulospinal tracts which end on α-motor neurons of spinal cord.
- ***Reflex response.*** The labyrinthine reflexes are particularly effective in extensor muscles. The impulses from labyrinthine exert the same effect on all the four limbs.

Depending upon the position of head in relation to horizontal plane, the reflex response produced is:

- When a quadruped stands on an inclined plane in such a manner that its *head sets tilted to right.* Tilting of the head to the right stimulates the labyrinth (vestibular apparatus) and evokes the tonic labyrinthine reflex. The reflex causes flexion of the left limbs and extension of the right limbs, thereby lending some amount of postural stability on the inclined plane (Fig. 10.9-22A).
- When the quadruped stands on the inclined plane in such a manner that the *head is tilted backwards,* the tonic labyrinthine reflexes cause reflex flexion of the forelimbs and reflex extension of the hind limbs (Fig. 10.9-22B).

2. Tonic Neck Reflexes. These reflexes are produced in response to alteration in the position of head relative to the body.

- ***Stimulus*** for tonic neck reflexes is stretch of neck muscles.
- ***Receptors*** of tonic neck reflexes are probably pacinian corpuscles in the ligaments of the cervical joints, particularly atlanto-occipital joint and also *muscle spindles* of neck muscles.
- ***Centre*** for these reflexes lies in the medulla oblongata.

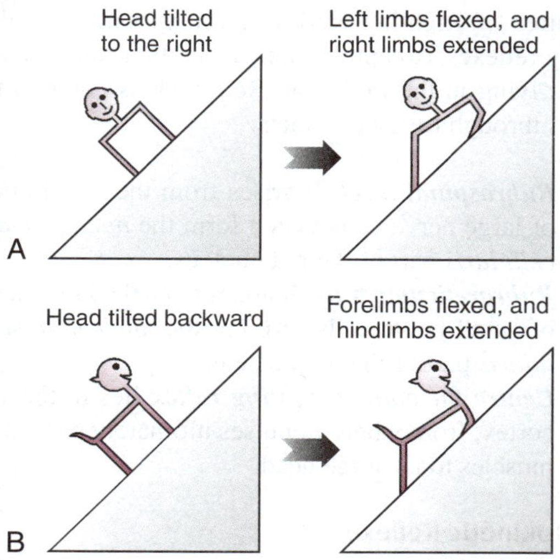

FIGURE 10.9-22 Reflex response of tonic labyrinthine reflexes: **A,** when head is tilted to right; and **B,** when head is tilted backwards.

- ***Efferent*** paths are the long corticospinal tracts. *Reflex response* obtained depending upon the position of the head in relation to the body is:
  - *Ventroflexion (turning down) of head* causes flexion of the forelimbs and extension of the hind limbs (Fig. 10.9-23A).
  - *Dorsiflexion (turning up) of head* causes extension of the forelimbs and flexion of the hind limbs.
  - *Turning of head sideways,* i.e. towards right or left produces flexion of the ipsilateral limbs and extension of contralateral limbs (Fig. 10.9-23B).

Combined Response of Tonic Neck and Labyrinthine Reflexes. Under normal circumstances, when the position of head is changed, the tonic neck and labyrinthine reflexes are simultaneously evoked such that they produce algebraic sum of separate responses:

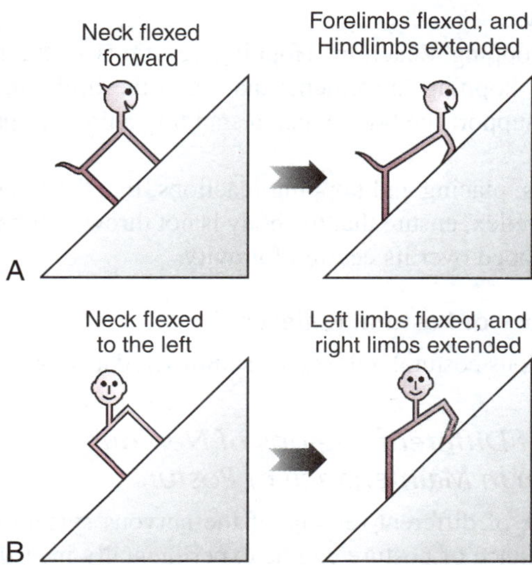

FIGURE 10.9-23 Reflex response of tonic neck reflexes: **A,** when neck is flexed forward; and **B,** when neck is flexed to the left.

- ***On dorsiflexion*** of the head, labyrinthine impulses produce increased tone in extensors of all the four limbs, while impulses from neck extend forelimbs and flex hind limbs. Therefore, the actual result observed is extension of forelimbs (as both reflexes tend to increase extensor tone) and little change in hind limbs (because two reflexes are exerting antagonistic influences).
- ***On ventroflexion*** of the head, labyrinthine impulses produce increased tone in the flexors of all the four limbs, while impulses from neck flex forelimbs and extend hind limbs. Therefore, the actual result observed is flexion of the forelimbs (as both reflexes tend to increase flexor tone) and little change in the hind limbs (because two reflexes are exerting antagonistic influences).

Role of Tonic Neck and Labyrinthine Reflexes. The tonic neck and labyrinthine reflexes bring about a redistribution of muscle tone in all the limbs and ensure that the body is not thrown off balance even when standing on an inclined plane.

- ***In quadruped animals,*** tonic neck and labyrinthine reflexes occur when standing on an inclined plane and not while standing on a level plane.
- ***In man,*** the tonic labyrinthine reflex is active during the erect posture. This is because in an erect posture, the vestibular apparatus is thrown about 30° backwards. This results in slight flexion of the upper limbs and extension of the lower limbs. When the head is tilted 30° forwards, the tonic labyrinthine reflex ceases but the concomitant flexion of the neck triggers the tonic neck reflex which has the same effect on the limbs. As in quadrupeds, in man too, the tonic neck and labyrinthine reflexes are observed when the trunk is not upright.

However, similar to other postural reflexes, these reflexes too can be suppressed voluntarily.

b. Long-loop Stretch Reflexes. The long-loop stretch reflexes, also called *functional stretch reflexes,* are polysynaptic reflexes with their reflex arc centred in the cerebral cortex. These reflexes are continuously active in the erect posture and bring about a continuous correction of the sways that occur from moment to moment during standing. The human body behaves like an inverted pendulum hinged at the ankle joint. For example, when the body sways forwards, there occurs stretching of the gastrocnemius muscle. This initiates monosynaptic stretch reflex as well as long-loop polysynaptic reflex which bring about reflex contraction in the gastrocnemius muscle resulting in correction of forward sway. In addition, the visual inputs which suggest that the body is swaying also initiate long-loop postural reflexes.

The two long-loop reflexes (one proprioceptive, and the other, visual) ensure that the body is not thrown off balance when tipped over its centre of gravity. The importance of these two reflexes can be realized in patients with lesions of dorsal column such as tabes dorsalis. *Sensory ataxia* seen in such patients is accentuated on closing of the eyes (Romberg's sign). The Romberg's sign is pathognomonic of sensory ataxia and helps to differentiate it from cerebellar ataxia, in which this sign is absent.

c. Righting Reflexes. Righting reflexes help to correct the position of the body when it goes off balance and falls down. In other words, righting reflexes help to maintain head and body into an erect position under all circumstances. For example, if an animal is laid on its side or back, the head at once rights itself, body follows and the animal finally resumes the upright posture. Decerebrate animal, though remains in the upright position, it can never actively resume the upright posture as it has no righting reflexes.

The righting reflexes consist of a chain of reactions following one another in an orderly sequence. Each reflex causes the development of the succeeding one as follows:

1. ***Head righting reflex,*** also called labyrinthine righting reflex, is initiated when the animal's head is in lateral position. The impulses arising from the saccules reflexly stimulate the appropriate muscles to bring the head back to the upright position.
2. ***Body righting reflexes or body-on-head righting reflex.*** When an animal lies on the ground, the side in contact with the ground is constantly stimulated while the other side is not. This differential stimulation of the deep structures in the body wall reflexly rights the head. The head can thus be righted even after bilateral labyrinthectomy.
3. ***Neck righting reflex or 'neck-on-body' righting reflex.*** As a result of labyrinthine righting reflex and body-on-head righting reflexes, the head is righted but the body remains in the lateral position. This leads to twisting of neck, which in turn involves a further reaction, the neck righting reflex. This reflex brings thorax and lumbar region successively into the upright position.
4. ***Body-on-body righting reflex.*** When the body is lying on the ground and the righting of the head is prevented, the differential stimulation of the body surfaces provides the necessary cues for righting the body directly. This is called body-on-body righting reflex.
5. ***Limbs righting reflex.*** Impulses arising from the limb muscles are responsible for attainment of appropriate posture of limbs.
6. ***Optical righting reflexes.*** Optical impulses also cause righting of the head. This has been confirmed by the fact that in animals with visual cortex intact, righting of head can take place with eyes open even after denervation of the labyrinths and neck muscles. In humans, optical righting reflexes are far more important than the labyrinthine righting reflex.

Centres of Righting Reflexes. *Chief centre* for all the righting reflexes, except the optical righting reflexes, is *red nucleus* lying in the midbrain. Red nucleus controls these reflexes through following tracts:

- ***Rubrospinal tract.*** It arises from the small number of large nerve cells which form the *nucleus magnocellularis* part of the red nucleus.
- ***Rubroreticular tract.*** It arises from the large number of small nerve cells forming the *nucleus parvocellularis* part of the red nucleus.
- ***Centre for optical righting reflex*** lies in the visual cortex, from where impulses ultimately pass to neck muscles to right the head.

B. Statokinetic Reflexes

Statokinetic reflexes are elicited by angular (rotatory) and linear acceleratory (progressive) stimuli to the labyrinthine receptors of vestibular apparatus.

These are programmed reflexes that depend on the motor cortex. Ultimately, these reflexes are mediated by lateral vestibulospinal tracts. These include:

1. Vestibular Placing Reaction. This reflex is evoked by linear acceleration through stimulation of receptors in the utricle and saccule. This reflex response is an adaptive reaction that prepares the animal for appropriate support by the limbs on surface contact. Thus, as soon as the foot comes in contact with any firm surface, the foot is reflexly placed on the surface and the leg muscles are adjusted so as to support the body.

2. Visual Placing Reaction. The placing response as described above can be initiated by visual cues as well and is then labelled as visual placing reaction. Many postural reflexes mediated by vestibular system can be stimulated by visual stimuli. Thus, the visual system frequently compensates for lesions of the vestibular apparatus or its central pathways.

3. Hopping Reaction. Hopping reactions occur in the form of hopping movements that keep the limbs in position to support the body when a standing animal in pushed laterally.

Thus, placing and hopping reactions, like the long-loop stretch reflex, ensure that the body is not thrown off balance when tipped over its centre of gravity.

Summary of Postural Reflexes

The various postural reflexes are summarized in Table 10.9-2.

Role of Different Regions of Nervous System in Maintenance of Posture

The role of different regions of the nervous system in the maintenance of posture can be experimentally investigated (usually in a cat) by producing transection in the neuraxis at various levels.

TABLE 10.9-2 Various Postural Reflexes

Reflex	Stimulus	Response	Receptors	Integrating centre in CNS
A. Static reflexes				
1. Local static reflexes				
i. Stretch reflex	Stretch	Contraction of antigravity muscles	Muscle spindles	Spinal cord and midbrain
ii. Positive supporting reflex	Contact of skin of the sole of foot with ground	Contraction of flexors and extensors of the limb	Touch and pressure receptors from skin of sole of foot Proprioceptors from distal flexors	Spinal cord
iii. Negative supporting reaction	Stretch of extensor muscles	Disappearance of positive supporting reaction	Proprioceptors in extensors	Spinal cord
II. Segmental static reflexes				
Crossed extensor reflex	Painful stimulus	Contraction of flexors of the ipsilateral limb and extensors of contralateral limb to support the body	Nociceptors	Spinal cord
III. General static reflexes				
1. Attitudinal reflexes				
i) Tonic labyrinthine reflex	Gravity (alteration of position of head relative to horizontal plane)	Extensor rigidity	Otolith organs	Vestibular and reticular nuclei present in the medulla oblongata
ii) Tonic neck reflex	Stretch of neck muscles due to alteration of position of head relative to body	Flexion of forelimbs and extension of hind limbs on ventroflexion of head (turning down). Extension of forelimbs and flexion of hind limbs on upward turning of head. Flexion of ipsilateral limbs and extension of contralateral limbs on turning the head sideways	Pacinian corpuscles in the ligaments of cervical joint (atlanto-occipital joint), and muscle spindles of neck muscles	Medulla
2. Long-loop stretch reflex	Stretch of the muscle due to swaying of body	Continuous moment to moment corrections of sways which occurs during standing	Muscle spindles (monosynaptic reflex) Visual receptor (long-loop reflex)	Spinal cord Cerebral cortex
3. Righting reflexes				
i) Labyrinthine righting reflex	Gravity	Brings the head in upright level	Otolith organs in saccules of labyrinth	Midbrain
ii) Body righting reflex (body on head righting reflex)	Pressure on side of body (differential stimulation of deep structures of the body wall)	Righting of head	Exteroceptors	Midbrain
iii) Neck righting reflex (neck on body righting)	Stretch of neck muscles	Righting of thorax and shoulders and then pelvis	Muscle spindles	Midbrain
iv) Body on body righting reflex	Pressure on side of the body	Righting of body even when righting of head is prevented	Exteroceptors	Midbrain
v) Limbs righting reflex	Stretch of limb muscles	Appropriate posture of limbs	Muscle spindles	Midbrain
vi) Optical righting reflex	Visual cues	Righting of head	Eyes	Cerebral cortex

Continued

TABLE 10.9-2 Various Postural Reflexes—cont'd

Reflex	Stimulus	Response	Receptors	Integrating centre in CNS
B. Statokinetic reflexes				
i) Vestibular placing reaction	Linear acceleration	Foot placed on supporting surface in position to support body	Receptors in utricle and saccule	Cerebral cortex
ii) Visual placing reaction	Visual cues	Foot places on supporting surface	Eyes	Cerebral cortex
iii) Hopping reactions	Lateral displacement while standing	Hops, maintains the limb in position to support the body	Muscle spindle	Cerebral cortex

Role of Spinal Cord: Spinal Animal

Spinal Animal The role of spinal cord in the maintenance of posture can be studied in a spinal animal. The spinal animal can be produced by a transection in the spinal cord at cervical region and respiration is maintained artificially by the respiratory pump. In this way, most of the cord functions can be studied in a spinal animal. If spinal cord is transected below the origin of phrenic nerve in the mid-thoracic region then diaphragmatic respiration continues and so the artificial respiration is not required.

Effects of spinal cord transection. As described earlier, the effects produced by complete spinal cord transection occur in three stages:

- Stage of spinal shock,
- Stage of reflex activity and
- Stage of reflex failure.

Note. For details, see page 917.

Posture in Spinal Animal during Stage of Reflex Activity. Except the basic stretch reflex and supporting reflexes which are integrated in spinal cord (Table 10.9-2), all other postural reflexes are absent, as they require the integrity of upper motor neurons coming from various levels of neuraxis.

Postural characteristics of a spinal animal thus are:

- ***Stretch reflex*** (page 1053) and *supporting reaction* (page 1064) though present but are very weak and cannot support the weight of the animal. Therefore, the animal cannot stand on its legs.
- ***Muscle tone*** returns first in flexor muscles; therefore, flexors become less hypotonic than extensors producing *paraplegia in flexion* (both lower limbs are in state of flexion).

Role of Brainstem: Bulbospinal Animal or Decerebrate Animal

Decerebrate Animal Decerebrate animal is one in whom the brainstem is transected at intercollicular level (between superior and inferior colliculi).

Characteristic Features of a decerebrate animal are:

1. ***Decerebrate rigidity,*** i.e. spasticity in all the antigravity muscles occurs immediately after decerebration. This will be discussed later.
2. ***No spinal shock:*** Spinal shock does not develop with lesion at this level or any other higher level.
3. ***Postural reflexes present in decerebrate animal*** are those which have their integration centre in the spinal cord or medulla or pons. These include:
   - *Stretch reflexes.* These are strongly positive. Decerebrate rigidity is basically due to harmoniously operating group of stretch reflexes.
   - *Positive supporting reaction.* This can be elicited by application of pressure on the pads of fingers or toes. The afferent impulses from the skin and interossei muscles (which are stretched) cause reflex contraction of both extensors and flexors of the limb, converting limb into a rigid pillar. All the joints are locked. Limbs support the weight of the body and the degree of tone is adequate to maintain the upright posture, but is not sufficient to take up upright position.
   - *Negative supporting reaction.* This can be elicited by passive plantar flexion which releases the limbs from positive reaction.
   - *Crossed extensor reflex.* This can also be demonstrated, i.e. when one forelimb is flexed, the other forelimb is adjusted (page 1065).
   - *Tonic neck and tonic labyrinthine* reflexes are also present (for details, see page 1066). Therefore, in decerebrate animals, posture of limbs and trunk can be adjusted accordingly with the help of these reflexes.
4. ***Righting reflexes are absent;*** therefore, decerebrate animal can stand on its four legs but slight displacement causes the decerebrate animal to topple over.

Decerebrate Rigidity Decerebrate rigidity refers to marked increase in the tone (hypertonia) of extensors, i.e. antigravity muscles occurring immediately after decerebration of the animal.

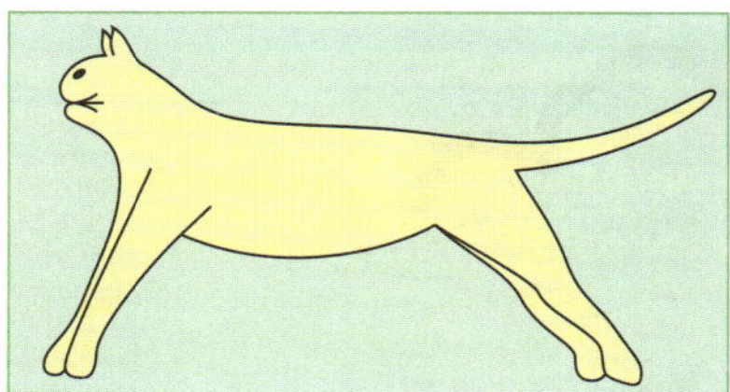

FIGURE 10.9-24 Characteristic features of decerebrate rigidity in cat.

Characteristic Features of Decerebrate Rigidity. Characteristic features of decerebrate rigidity (Fig. 10.9-24) are:

- Hyperextension of all the four limbs,
- Dorsiflexion (hyperextension) of tail and head,
- Extreme hyperextension of the spine (opisthotonus) produces concave configuration of the back,
- The animal can be made to stand on four limbs but easily toppled by a slight push and
- Postural reflexes, which can be elicited in decerebrate rigidity are described above.

Mechanism of Decerebrate Rigidity. Depending upon the mode of production, the decerebrate rigidity is of two types:

- Classical decerebrate rigidity and
- Ischaemic decerebrate rigidity.

Mechanism of Classical Decerebrate Rigidity. Classical decerebrate rigidity refers to the decerebrate rigidity that occurs following transection of brainstem at intercollicular level. It is produced by exaggerated stretch reflex due to increased activity of gamma motor neurons as explained:

- As mentioned earlier (page 1056), the gamma motor drive to muscles is maintained by descending impulses from facilitatory reticular formation (FRF) as well as inhibitory reticular formation (IRF) with the former predominating.
- IRF or bulboreticular inhibitory arc has no intrinsic activity but is kept activated by descending supraspinal fibres mostly from the basal ganglia, cerebral cortex and cerebellum.
- FRF or bulboreticular facilitatory area, in contrast, gets facilitatory inputs mainly from the ascending sensory stimuli which relay through ascending reticular formation. It also receives facilitatory corticobulbar extrapyramidal projections.
- Transection at the mid-collicular level cuts off all facilitatory and inhibitory corticobulbar extrapyramidal pathways. Hence, following decerebration, the IRF, having no intrinsic activity, becomes less active since none of it is driven by cerebellum only. While FRF, which is mainly derived by ascending sensory stimuli, remains strongly active.
- Thus, the resulting release of spinal gamma motor neurons from the descending inhibitory reticular formation and continued effect of facilitatory reticular formation markedly increases muscle spindle sensitivity to stretch resulting in rigidity of muscles (Fig. 10.9-25).
- This rigidity is lost by deafferentiation (cutting of afferents from muscle). This proves that decerebrate rigidity is due to increased activity of gamma motor neurons causing exaggerated stretch reflex.
- The rigidity observed after classical decerebration is actually a form of spasticity. When a spastic muscle is stretched passively, initially great resistance is offered by the muscles. However, if still more force is used, the resistance suddenly disappears. This type of response is called *clasp-knife* effect. The initial intense resistance is due to the exaggerated stretch reflex and the sudden decrease in resistance is due to activation of the Golgi tendon reflex.
- In humans, similar spasticity is observed in the extensors of lower limb and flexors of upper limb in patients with hemiplegia due to vascular lesions in the internal capsule leading to destruction of pyramidal and extrapyramidal tracts.

Mechanism of Ischaemic Decerebrate Rigidity Ischaemic decerebration is obtained by ligating the common carotid artery and basilar arteries in which cerebral cortex is rendered ischaemic and nonfunctional. This safer alternative method of decerebration was attempted as classical decerebration was frequently associated with the death of the experimental animal.

- The rigidity observed after ischaemic decerebration is different from that observed in classical decerebration and occurs due to an entirely different reason. The ischaemic decerebrate rigidity is in fact due to disinhibition of α-motor neurons, i.e. exaggerated α-motor neuron discharge. The increased α-motor neuron drive results in direct stimulation of extrafusal fibres (*α-rigidity*).
- This rigidity is not lost by deafferentiation (cutting off afferents from muscles). This proves that ischaemic decerebrate rigidity is not due to increased γ-motor neuron activity but is due to increased α-motor neuron activity.

Classical versus Ischaemic Decerebrate Rigidity Differences between classical and ischaemic decerebrate rigidity are summarized in Table 10.9-3.

Role of Midbrain: Mesencephalic Animal or High Decerebrate Animal

Mesencephalic or high decerebrate animal is one in whom the brainstem is transected at the rostral border of midbrain.

Characteristic Features of a mesencephalic animal are:

1. ***Decerebrate rigidity,*** similar to that of bulbospinal animal, is present but it disappears when the limb is performing a reflex activity.

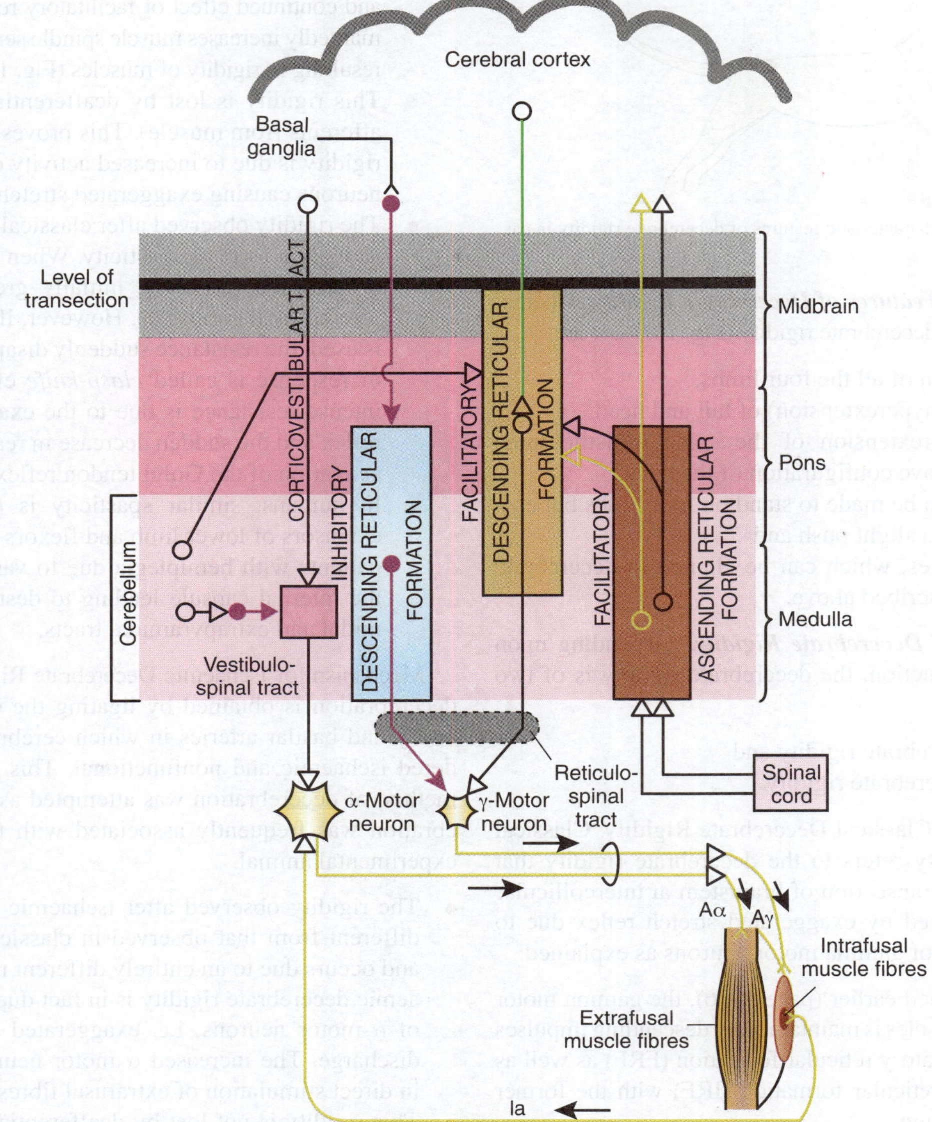

FIGURE 10.9-25 Supraspinal control of stretch reflex. Note the pathway cut in the transaction at mid-collicular level producing decerebrate rigidity.

TABLE 10.9-3 Differences between Classical and Ischaemic Decerebrate Rigidity

Classical decerebrate rigidity	Ischaemic decerebrate rigidity
1. *Produced by* transection of brainstem between superior and inferior colliculi	Ligating both the common carotid arteries and basilar artery at the junction of pons and medulla
2. *Rigidity observed* is type of spasticity which exhibits clasp-knife effect	Rigidity produced is due to marked muscle tone which does not exhibit clasp-knife effect
3. *Rigidity is mainly due to* increased activity of gamma motor neurons, hence also called γ-rigidity	Increased alpha motor neuron activity, hence also called α-rigidity
4. *Deafferentiation, i.e. cutting off posterior nerve root,* abolishes rigidity, proving that it is reflex in origin	Does not abolish rigidity, indicating that hypertonia is induced directly and not reflexly
5. *Local injection of procaine into nerve trunk.* Reduced spasticity	Does not reduce rigidity
6. *Systemic administration of chlorpromazine* reduces spasticity	Has no effect on rigidity
7. Removal of anterior lobe of cerebellum increases rigidity	Has no effect

2. ***No spinal shock,*** similar to bulbospinal animal.
3. ***Animal cannot only stand*** but also typical quadrupedal walking movements can be reflexly performed.
4. ***Righting reflexes*** having integration centre in the midbrain are present. These include:
   - Labyrinthine righting reflex,
   - Neck righting reflex,
   - Body-on-head righting reflex and
   - Body-on-body righting reflex.

   For details of these reflexes, see page 1068. The chief advance in postural regulation in mesencephalic animal over bulbospinal animal lies in the presence of righting reflexes. By means of the righting reflexes, the midbrain animal can bring its head right way up and get the body into the erect position under all circumstances.
5. ***Pupillary light reflexes*** having an integration centre in the midbrain are present (for details, see page 1171).
6. ***Nystagmus,*** the reflex response to rotational acceleration, can be elicited (see page 1078).

Role of Cerebellum

Spinocerebellum regulates the postural reflexes by modifying muscle tone. It facilitates the gamma motor neurons in the spinal cord via cerebello-vestibulo-spinal and cerebello-reticulo-spinal tracts. The gamma motor neurons reflexly modify the activity of alpha motor neurons and thus regulate the muscle tone. Thus, cerebellum forms an important site of linkage of α–γ systems responsible for muscle tone (for details, see page 935).

Unilateral cerebellar disease in humans causes:

1. *Atonia* or hypotonia in the skeletal muscles of the same side.
2. *Attitude changes* include:
   - Rotation of the face towards opposite side,
   - Lowering of shoulder on the affected side,
   - Outward rotation and abduction of the leg on involved side and
   - Trunk is bent with concavity towards the affected side; this is because the weight of the body is thrown on the unaffected leg.
3. *Deviation movement.* Arm held straight out in front of the body deviates laterally when the eyes are closed.
4. *Deep or tendon reflexes* become weak and pendular.

Role of Basal Ganglia: Decorticate Animal

Decorticate animal is one in whom the whole cerebral cortex is removed but the basal ganglia and brainstem are left intact.

Postural Characteristics of a Decorticate Animal. ***Moderate rigidity*** is present due to loss of the cortical area that inhibits spinal γ-motor neurons discharge via reticular formation. It is seen only when the animal is at rest. It commonly occurs on the hemiplegic side after haemorrhage or thrombosis in the internal capsule.

Decorticate animal does not have such intense hypertonia as a decerebrate preparation. This is because the basal ganglia that are intact in decorticate animal activate the descending inhibitory reticular formation and thereby prevent hypertonia.

Typical posture in a decorticate man consists of full extension of legs, arms lying across the chest, with semi-flexion at elbow, slight pronation of forearm and flexion of wrist and fingers (Fig. 10.9-26).

Postural reflexes. In decorticate man or animal, the following reflexes can be elicited:

- Typical neck reflexes (page 1066),
- Righting reflexes (page 1068),
- Postural reflexes which are seriously disrupted by decortication are:
  - Hopping reactions and
  - Placing reactions.

Note. It is easier to maintain a decorticate animal than a midbrain animal because temperature regulation and integration of visceral homeostatic mechanism are present in the hypothalamus.

Mechanism of Standing in Man

As mentioned earlier, a tall human has to stand over a narrow base of feet; therefore, maintenance of an erect posture is more difficult than the quadruped animals. Mechanisms that play important role in erect standing posture are:

Reflex Adjustment in Muscle Tone of Antigravity Muscles undoubtedly plays the most important role in making the man stand erect. From this statement, it may be presumed that a continued contraction of most of the trunk and leg muscles keeps the posture upright. However, electromyographic studies have revealed very little muscle activity in a person standing quietly in upright position.

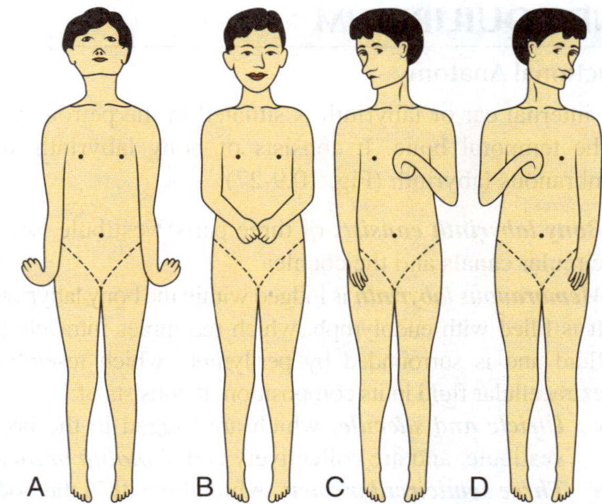

FIGURE 10.9-26 Decerebrate (**A**) and decorticate (**B, C** and **D**) rigidity in humans.

Configuration of Hip and Knee Joints is such that they are kept extended by the gravity itself. However, a little activity of the antigravity muscles is required to maintain the very precarious balance. This explains the little muscle activity revealed by electromyographic studies.

The Effect of Gravity has to be opposed by reflex contraction of some of the antigravity muscles all the time, otherwise a standing man may fall in any direction (forwards, backwards or sideways). The different antigravity muscles which oppose the fall under various circumstances are:

- ***Extensors of the trunk and flexors of the legs*** contract sufficiently to restore the balance when the body sways forward.
- ***Rectiabdominis and leg extensors*** contract to restore the balance when the body sways backward.
- ***Contralateral external oblique abdominal muscles*** maintain the balance when the body leans sideways.
- ***Head has a tendency to sway more than the trunk:*** Since the centre of gravity of head passes in front of the centre of gravity of atlanto-occipital joint, therefore, the head always has got a tendency to roll forwards. To hold the head in an erect position, the cervico-occipital muscles are to be maintained in a state of constant tension.

Reflex changes in antigravity muscles described above are induced by:

- ***Stretch receptors*** in the trunk and leg muscles,
- ***Visual afferents*** also play an important role in reflex maintenance of upright posture in man. This is why, when the eyes are closed, the upright posture is less steady and there occurs more swaying (bending) of the trunk.
- ***Vestibular afferents*** help in maintaining the erect position of head.

VESTIBULAR APPARATUS AND EQUILIBRIUM

Functional Anatomy

The internal ear or labyrinth is situated in the petrous part of the temporal bone. It consists of bony labyrinth and membranous labyrinth (Fig. 10.9-27).

- ***Bony labyrinth consists*** of three parts: vestibule, semicircular canals and the cochlea.
- ***Membranous labyrinth*** is lodged within the bony labyrinth. It is filled with endolymph, which resembles intracellular fluid and is surrounded by perilymph, which resembles extracellular fluid in its composition. It consists of:
  - ***Utricle and saccule,*** which are lodged in the bony vestibule, and are collectively called *otolith organs.*
  - ***Three semicircular ducts,*** which lie within the body of semicircular canals.
  - ***Duct of cochlea,*** which lies within the bony cochlea.

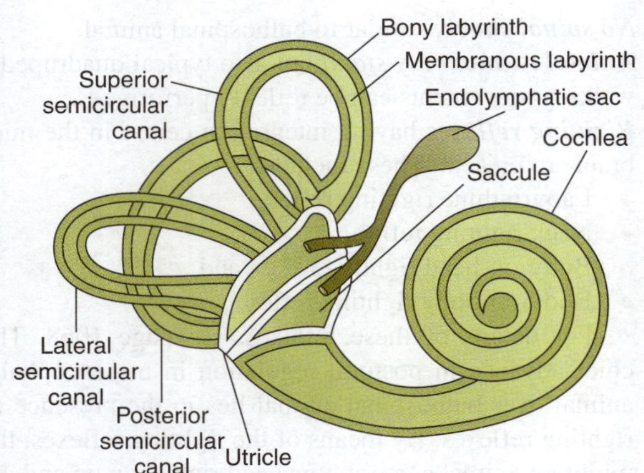

FIGURE 10.9-27 Vestibular apparatus: semicircular canals and otolith organs.

Vestibular Apparatus The semicircular canals, and the utricle and saccule collectively form the vestibular apparatus. The vestibular apparatus plays important role in maintaining posture and equilibrium.

Semicircular Canals. The three semicircular canals are arranged at right angles to each other, so that all the three planes are represented as (Fig. 10.9-28):

- ***Anterior semicircular canal*** is vertical and placed at right angles to the long axis of the petrous bone. Thus, it lies in a plane that points forward and outward at about 45° from the sagittal plane.
- ***Posterior semicircular canal*** is also vertical but is placed parallel to the long axis of the petrous bone. Thus, it lies in a plane that points backward and outward at about 45° from the sagittal plane.
- ***Lateral semicircular canal*** is set in a horizontal position making an angle of about 30° with the horizontal plane.

It is important to note that:

- The right anterior and left posterior canals lie in one plane, while the left anterior and right posterior canals lie in the other plane.
- One end of each semicircular canal is dilated and is called *ampulla*. The ampulla contains the receptor organ known as *crista ampullaris* (Fig. 10.9-29).
- The semicircular canals open into the utricle by means of five orifices. The ampullary end of each canal and narrow end of horizontal canal open independently, while narrow ends of anterior and posterior canals open jointly by a common orifice.

Otolith Organ refers to the combined two vestibular sacs called the utricle and saccule.

- ***Utricle*** is the larger of the two vestibular sacs in which open the three semicircular canals. It is indirectly connected to the saccule and ductus endolymphaticus by the

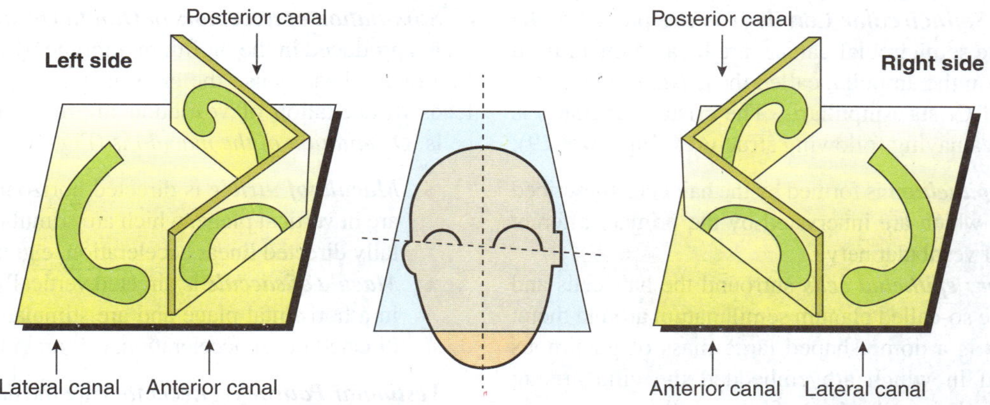

FIGURE 10.9-28 Position of semicircular canals when head is tilted forward at 30°.

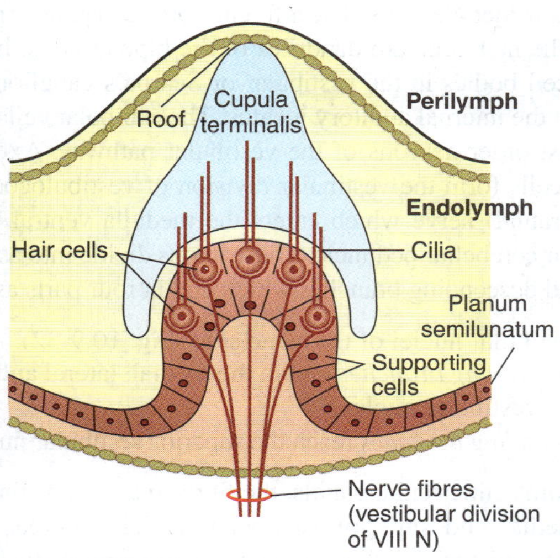

FIGURE 10.9-29 Structure of crista ampullaris.

ductus utriculosaccularis. The *ductus endolymphaticus,* after being joined by the ductus utriculosaccularis, passes on to end in a small bag-like structure called *endolymphatic sac* (Fig. 10.9-27).

- ***Saccule*** is a globular sac that is connected to utricle indirectly through the ductus utriculosaccularis, and cochlea via the *ductus reunion* (Fig. 10.9-27).

Vestibular Receptors

The receptor cells of the vestibular system are called hair cells, which are slowly adapting mechanoreceptors.

- The hair cells of the semicircular canals are located in a mass of tissue within the ampulla called *crista ampullaris.*
- The hair cells of the utricle and saccule are located in a mass of tissue called the *macula*.

Hair Cells *(Fig. 10.9-30)* The vestibular hair cells are of two types:

- ***Type I hair cells*** are flask shaped. These make synaptic contacts with afferent nerve fibres only.
- ***Type II hair cells*** are cylindrical in shape and make synaptic contacts both with afferent and efferent nerve fibres.
- ***Cilia of hair cells*** (Fig. 10.9-30): The apex of each hair cell has a cuticular plate from which arise about 40–60 cilia. These cilia are called *stereocilia,* which are motile.

A large nonmotile cilium located at one end of the cell is called *kinocilium.*

Activity of Hair Cells. Hair cells are polarized cells. The membrane potential of hair cells is about −60 mV. When the stereocilia are bent towards the kinocilium, the cell depolarizes and membrane potential is decreased to about −50 mV. When the stereocilia are bent away from the kinocilium, the cell hyperpolarizes. The changes in the activity of hair cells are conveyed to central nervous system by afferent fibres which form the vestibular part of 8th cranial nerve. The mechanoelectrical transduction in vestibular hair cells is same as that occurring in auditory hair cells (see page 1182).

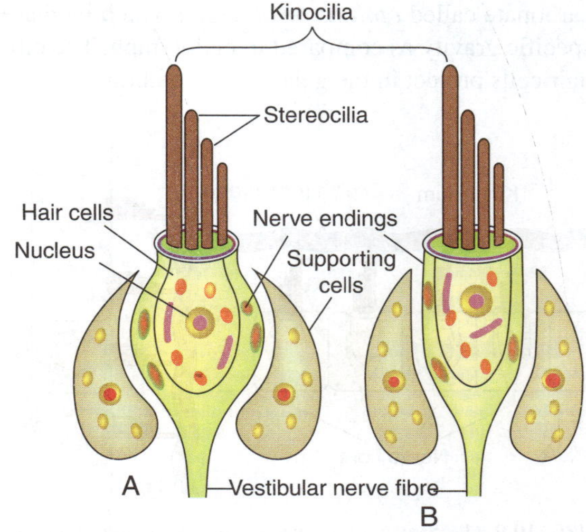

FIGURE 10.9-30 Structure of hair cells: **A,** type I and **B,** type II.

Receptors in Semicircular Canals The receptors, i.e. the hair cells of the semicircular canals, are located on a raised mass of tissue in the ampulla, called the *crista ampullaris*.

Structure of Crista Ampullaris. The crista ampullaris is a ridge-like area having following structures (Fig. 10.9-29):

- ***Neuroepithelium*** is formed by the hair cells (described above), which are innervated by the primary afferent fibres of vestibular nerve.
- ***Secretory epithelial cells*** surround the hair cells and form the so-called planum semilunatum around them.
- ***Cupula*** is a dome-shaped large mass of gelatinous material in which are embedded the cilia arising from the hair cells. At its free end, the cupula is in loose contact with the wall of ampulla. As a result, it forms a compliant seal that closes the lumen of the canal, preventing free circulation of endolymph.

Stimulation of Receptors in Semicircular Canals. The movements produced in the endolymph by the angular movements of head pushes the cupula backwards, causing the cilia of hair cells to bend. Depending upon whether the stereocilia are pushed towards or away from the kinocilium, the hair cell depolarizes or hyperpolarizes.

It is important to note that cupula is unaffected by linear acceleration force, as it has the same specific gravity as the endolymph.

Receptors in Otolith Organs The receptors (hair cells) of the otolith organs (utricle and saccule) are located in a raised mass of tissue called macula.

Structure of Macula. The macula consists of (Fig. 10.9-31):

- ***Neuroepithelium*** of macula like that of crista ampullaris is formed by hair cells (both type I and II).
- ***Supporting cells*** are present around the hair cells.
- ***Otolith membrane.*** It is a flat gelatinous membrane covering the hair cells. This contains crystals of calcium carbonate called *otoliths or otogonia* which increase its specific gravity as compared to endolymph. The cilia of hair cells project in the gelatinous membrane.

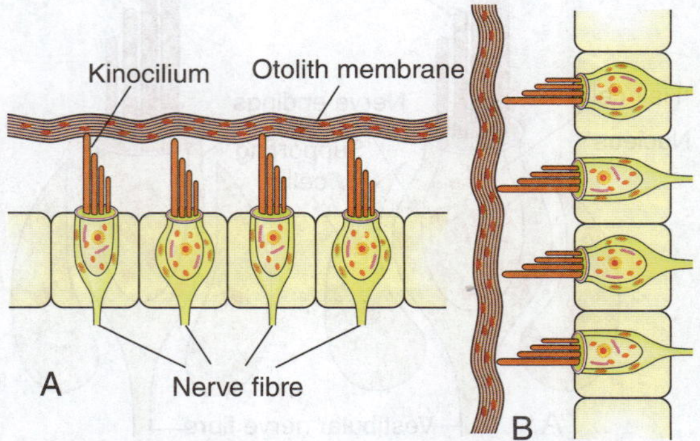

FIGURE 10.9-31 Structure of macula of: **A,** utricle (horizontally placed); and **B,** saccule (vertically placed).

Stimulation of Receptors in Otolith Organs. The movements produced in the otolith membrane by linear acceleration of the head cause the cilia of hair cells to bend. This leads to excitation of vestibular afferents supplying these cells. *Orientation of the macula* is (Fig. 10.9-31):

- ***Macula of utricle*** is directed horizontally so its cilia are in vertical plane, which are stimulated by horizontally directed linear acceleration, e.g. moving in a car.
- ***Macula of saccule*** is directed vertically, so its cilia are in a horizontal plane and are stimulated by vertically directed linear acceleration, e.g. moving in a lift.

Vestibular Pathways *Receptors* are the hair cells located in the crista ampullaris of semicircular canal and maculae of utricle and saccule.

First-order Neurons. The afferent fibres carrying impulses from the hair cells are dendrites of the bipolar cells, having their cell bodies in the vestibular or Scarpa's ganglion situated in the internal auditory meatus. These bipolar cells form the first-order neurons of the vestibular pathway. Axons of these cells form the vestibular division of vestibulocochlear (8th cranial) nerve which enters the medulla ventral to the inferior cerebellar peduncle. These axons divide into ascending and descending branches which end in four parts as:

- Vestibular nuclei of the same side (Fig. 10.9-32).
- *Descending branches* end in the medial, lateral and inferior vestibular nuclei.
- *Ascending branches* reach the superior vestibular nucleus.

From semicircular canals, the fibres mainly terminate in the medial and superior vestibular nuclei, whereas from saccule and utricle, they project predominantly to lateral vestibular nuclei.

Note. For all practical purposes, the four vestibular nuclei are treated as a single functional unit.

Vestibular Nuclei. The vestibular nuclei contain cell bodies of the second-order neurons of the vestibular pathway.

Afferent Connections. In addition to the main afferents from vestibular apparatus, the vestibular nuclei also receive inhibitory fibres from the cerebrum and cerebellum (Fig. 10.9-32).

Efferent Connections. Efferents from vestibular nuclei are:

- ***Vestibulospinal tracts*** (anterior and lateral) end directly and also via short interneurons around the ventral horn cells. The inputs from the vestibular nuclei are *excitatory to antigravity* alpha motor neurons.
- ***Vestibulo-ocular tract.*** These are the fibres which ascend through the *medial longitudinal fasciculus* and terminate in the nuclei of 3rd, 4th and 6th cranial nerves. These fibres are concerned with movements of eyeballs in relation to the position of the head.
- ***Vestibulocerebellar fibres*** pass through the inferior cerebellar peduncle and terminate in flocculonodular lobe and fastigial nuclei in the cerebellum of both sides.

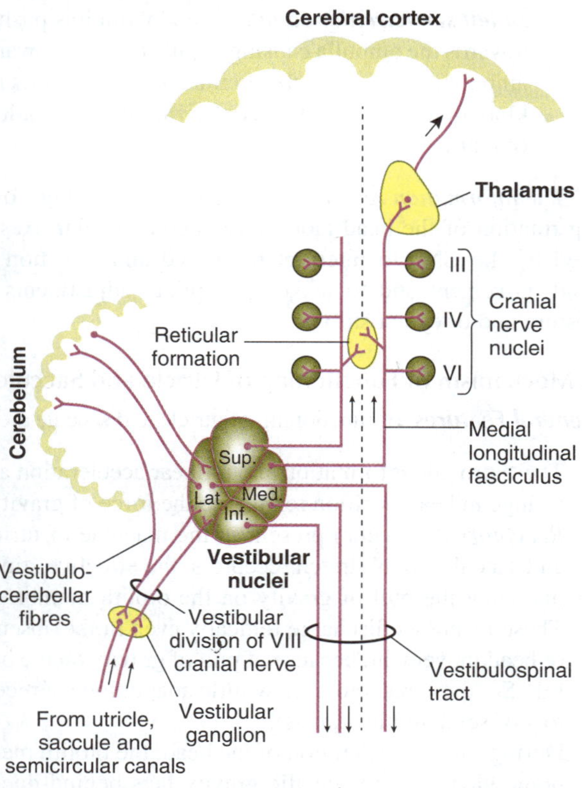

FIGURE 10.9-32 Neural pathway from vestibular apparatus.

- ***Vestibuloreticular spinal tract.*** Some fibres from the vestibular nuclei reach the reticular formation of brainstem, ultimately forming the vestibulo-reticulo-spinal tract.
- ***Vestibulo-rubro-spinal tract.*** Some fibres from the vestibular nuclei reach the red nucleus forming the vestibulo-rubro-spinal tract.
- ***Vestibulo-thalamo-cortical fibres.*** Some fibres from the vestibular nuclei pass via medial lemniscus to the opposite thalamus and thence to the opposite temporal lobe.

Mechanism of Functioning of Vestibular Apparatus

A. Mechanism of Functioning of Semicircular Canals

Salient Features of Functioning of Semicircular Canals

- *Receptors* of semicircular canals are stimulated by rotatory movements or *angular acceleration* of the head.
- *Semicircular canals are oriented* in three different planes, so movement of the head in any direction generates a unique pattern of activity within the semicircular canals. The three axes of the semicircular canals are those activated while:
  - Nodding the head up and down (as in signifying yes). This movement occurs along transverse axis.
  - Shaking the head from side to side (as in signifying no). This movement occurs along the vertical axis.
  - Tilting the head so that ear touches the shoulders. This movement occurs along the anteroposterior axis.
- Receptors of horizontal canals are stimulated during rotation of head in vertical axis, while receptors of vertical canals are stimulated during rotation of head in anteroposterior or transverse axis. However, the mechanism of stimulation of receptors is same in all the canals.
- Receptors of semicircular canals are stimulated only at the beginning and at the stoppage of rotatory movements. During continued rotation at a constant speed, these receptors are not stimulated rather they are adapted as explained.

Mechanism of Stimulation and Adaptation of Receptors of Semicircular Canals. Mechanism of stimulation and adaptation of receptors of semicircular canals is explained below during rotation of head in vertical axis:

1. At the Beginning of Movement

Movements to the right (i.e. clockwise rotation along the vertical axis) stimulates the hair cells in the right horizontal canal and inhibits these in the left horizontal canal. As shown in Fig. 10.9-33, when the head begins to move, the horizontal canals move in clockwise direction but the endolymph within the semicircular canals lags behind because of inertia. This phenomenon causes relative displacement of endolymph in the direction opposite to that of the rotation of the head. That is, the endolymph is pushed in the anticlockwise direction (Fig. 10.9-33B).

- ***In right semicircular canal,*** the endolymph is pushed towards the ampulla causing the cupula to move towards ampulla. As a result, the stereocilia are pushed towards the kinocilium, leading to depolarization (stimulation) of hair cells.
- ***In left semicircular canal,*** the endolymph is pushed away from the ampulla causing the cupula to move away from the ampulla. As a result, the stereocilia are pushed away from the kinocilium, leading to hyperpolarization (inhibition) of hair cells. This combination of excitation of one ampulla and inhibition of ampulla from other canal forms the basis of the direction of movement. At the beginning of movement, frequency of discharge from excited hair cells may increase to a frequency of 100–500 impulses per minute from a resting discharge of 50–100 impulses per minute.
- ***Movements to the left*** (i.e. counterclockwise movements), on the other hand, stimulate the hair cells in the left horizontal semicircular canal and inhibit those in the right horizontal canal by the same mechanism as explained above.

2. After 15–20 s of Continuous Movement at a Constant Velocity, there Occurs Adaptation of Receptors. After 15–20 s of continued movement of head at a constant velocity, the endolymph also takes up the same rate of movement as its canals and

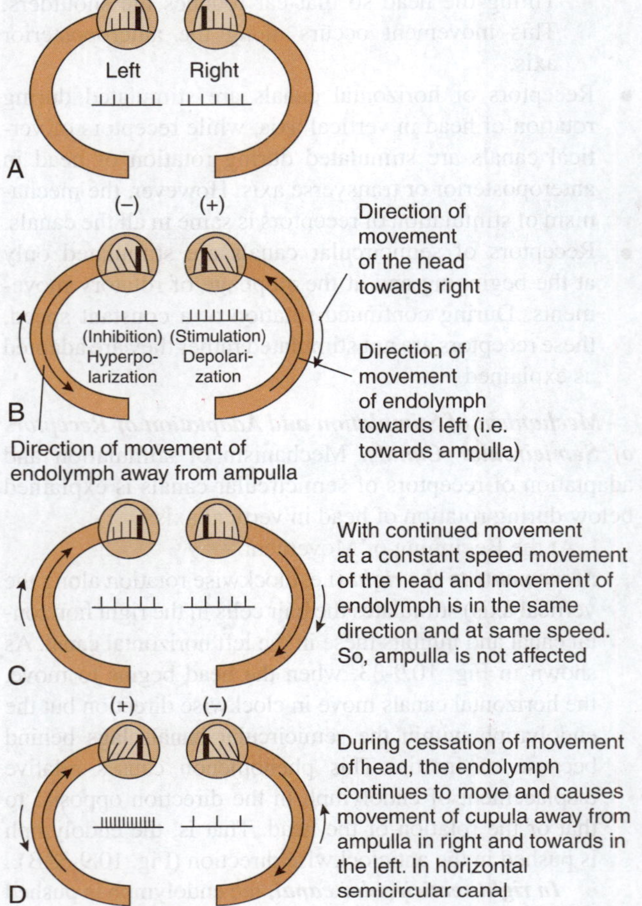

FIGURE 10.9-33 Mechanism of stimulation of receptors in horizontal (lateral) semicircular canal during rotation of head towards right: **A,** resting position; **B,** when head begins to rotate to right; **C,** after 15–20 s of continued movement of head at a constant speed; and **D,** when the head stops moving.

the cupula return to their original resting position. So, hair cells are no more excited or inhibited and return to their resting membrane potential and resting discharge of about 50–100 impulses per minute (Fig. 10.9-33C). Thus, the receptors in semicircular canals show signal changes in motion (acceleration) but are insensitive to movements at a constant angular velocity. This state of insensitiveness of receptors during a constant angular velocity is referred to as *state of adaptation of receptors.*

3. When the Head Stops Moving. When the head stops moving, i.e. during cessation or deceleration of movement, the endolymph within the canals continues to move. That is, the endolymph is now pushed in the opposite direction (Fig. 10.9-33D):

- ***In right semicircular canal,*** the endolymph is pushed away from the ampulla causing the cupula to move away from the ampulla. As a result, the stereocilia are pushed away from the kinocilium, leading to hyperpolarization (inhibition) of hair cells.
- ***In left semicircular canal,*** the endolymph is pushed towards the ampulla causing cupula to move towards ampulla. As a result, stereocilia are bent towards the kinocilium, leading to depolarization (stimulation) of hair cells.

The information received from semicircular canals during rotation of the head along three perpendicular axes is used by the CNS to interpret the speed and direction of head movement and to make appropriate adjustments in posture and of eye positions.

B. Mechanism of Functioning of Utricle and Saccule

General Features of functioning of utricle and saccule are:

- These provide information about linear acceleration and change in head position relative to the force of gravity.
- *Receptors* (hair cells) present in the maculae of utricle and saccule act as stretch receptors, the effective stimulus being the pull of gravity on the otolith membrane. These receptors discharge tonically even in the absence of head movement, because of pull of gravity on the otolith. So, these receptors show little adaptation (of receptors of semicircular canals).
- During linear acceleration of the head, the otolith membrane having more specific gravity lags behind due to inertia. This causes cilia of hair cells embedded in otolith membrane to bend. This leads to excitation of vestibular afferents supplying these cells.

Functioning of Utricle. As mentioned earlier, the macula of utricle is directed horizontally and so its cilia are in vertical plane (Fig. 10.9-31). These vertically oriented cilia are stimulated by horizontally directed linear acceleration, e.g. moving in a car. These hair cells are also stimulated during dorsiflexion or ventroflexion of the head, i.e. by nodding the head up and down (as in signifying yes).

Functioning of Saccule. As mentioned earlier, macula of saccule is directed vertically and so its cilia are in the horizontal plane (Fig. 10.9-31). These horizontally oriented cilia are stimulated by vertically directed linear acceleration, e.g. moving in a lift up or down. These hair cells are also stimulated when the head is tilted sideways, e.g. if the head is tilted laterally to the right, the otolith membrane of macula of right saccule hangs downwards and pulls on its macula which is maximally stimulated, and the otolith membrane of left saccule points upwards and rests on the macula; this being the position of minimal stimulation of the nerve endings.

Vestibular Reflexes

1. Vestibulo-ocular Reflex (VOR) The vestibulo-ocular reflex maintains visual fixation during movements of the head by producing reflex nystagmus and postrotatory nystagmus as described:

Nystagmus. For example, when the head is rotated to the left, the eyes move slowly towards the right in order to keep the image on the fovea. When the eyes have rotated as far as they can, they are rapidly returned to the centre of the socket. These reflex movements of the eyes are called nystagmus. Thus, nystagmus has two components of the movements:

- ***Slow components,*** i.e. slow movement of the eyes to maintain visual fixation is initiated by receptors in the semicircular canals. When the head rotates to the left, receptors in the left horizontal canal are stimulated. Their axons activate reflex movements of the eyes towards the right through the impulses reaching the nuclei of 3rd, 4th and 6th cranial nerves.
- ***Quick component.*** When slow movement of eyeballs is limited, the eyeballs move to a new fixation point in the direction of rotation of head. This movement to a new fixation point occurs with a jerk. So, it is called the quick component. The quick component of nystagmus is due to impulses from the vestibular nuclei to the ocular muscle.

Postrotatory nystagmus occurs after the body has been rotated and the movement ceases. This is due to movement of cupula in the opposite direction caused by the endolymph when rotation is stopped. Thus, the postrotatory nystagmus rotates in a direction opposite to the original nystagmus and continues until the cupula returns to its resting position. It can be demonstrated by Barany chair.

Applied Aspect

Nystagmus present in the resting state is a sign of pathology. There are two types of nystagmus: (i) congenital nystagmus, which is seen at birth and (ii) acquired nystagmus, which occurs in later life. Acquired nystagmus is seen in various clinical conditions like:

- Fracture of temporal bone affecting semicircular canals,
- Damage to flocculonodular lobe of cerebellum or to fastigial nucleus, and also
- Associated with multiple sclerosis, head injury, brain tumours and during stroke.

Treatment: For acquired nystagmus, the best treatment is to treat the underlying cause.

- Surgery: Some cases of acquired nystagmus are successfully treated by rectus muscle surgery.
- Botox: For short term, nystagmus can be corrected by injection of botox (botulinum toxin) to paralyse the ocular muscles.

2. Otolith Reflexes

Otolith organs initiate a reflex that prevents leg injuries when an individual walks downstairs or jumps from a platform. When making such a descent, the muscles of the leg begin to contract before the feet reach the ground to cushion the force of impact.

- The otolith receptors responsible for this reflex are stimulated by the linear acceleration of the head that occurs during descent.
- Individuals lacking otolith reflexes are prone to leg injuries because of the large contact force that occurs during descent (e.g. stepping off a bus).

Functions of Vestibular Apparatus

1. Role in Maintenance of Equilibrium. The otolith organs detect change in position of head and help in maintenance of equilibrium under static condition.

- The otolith organs also detect linear acceleration of the head and help in maintenance of equilibrium during such movements.
- Semicircular canals detect angular acceleration and help in maintaining equilibrium during dynamic phase. They also have a predictive function.
- When the person is in dynamic state, they predict ahead of time that the person is likely to fall off balance and help nervous system to do adjustments to prevent a fall.

2. Role in Maintenance of Posture. The vestibular apparatus plays important role in maintenance of posture through vestibular reflexes, which include:

- Vestibular placing reaction,
- Righting reflexes,
- Vestibulo-ocular reflex and
- Vestibulo-otolith reflex.

Maintenance of Equilibrium

Equilibrium refers to maintenance of line of gravity constant at rest and during movement by adjusting the tone of different muscles, while the term posture signifies an unconscious adjustment of tone of different muscles so as to maintain balance during rest as well as during movements.

Role of Various Parts of Neural System in Maintaining Equilibrium

1. Role of Vestibular Apparatus (as Described Above)

2. Role of Cerebellum

- ***Uvula of cerebellum*** gets impulses from macula of utricle and saccule and helps in maintaining equilibrium under static conditions.
- ***Flocculonodular lobe of cerebellum*** gets impulses from the semicircular canals and helps in maintaining equilibrium during rapid changes in direction of motion.

3. Role of Brainstem. Main role is played by four pairs of vestibular nuclei present in the brainstem:

- ***Superior vestibular*** nuclei receive signals from semicircular canals and send impulses to:
  - *Medial longitudinal fasciculus* to cause corrective movements of eyes and

- *Medial vestibular tract* to cause appropriate movements of the neck and head.
- ***Medial vestibular nuclei*** receive signals from semicircular canals and send signals to:
  - *Medial longitudinal fasciculus* to cause corrective movements of eyes and
  - *Vestibulospinal tract* to cause appropriate movements of head and neck.
- ***Lateral vestibular nuclei*** receive signals from otolith organs and in turn send:
  - Through lateral vestibulospinal tract to spinal cord for controlling body movements.
- ***Inferior vestibular nuclei*** receive signals from semicircular canals and utricle and in turn send signals to:
  - Cerebellum and
  - Reticular formation of brainstem.

4. Role of Other Factors is Maintenance of Equilibrium. ***Neck proprioceptors*** transmit information about orientation of head with respect to the body to vestibular and reticular nuclei of brainstem and cerebellum.

Neck reflexes must function opposite to vestibular reflexes to maintain equilibrium of the entire body. When vestibular apparatus is destroyed, then the bending of head produces muscular reflexes (called neck reflexes) in the forelimbs.

Body exteroceptors and proprioceptors transmit information from other parts of the body besides neck. This also plays an important role in maintenance of equilibrium. For example, pressure from foot pad informing whether weight is more forward or backward on the feet. This information is useful for maintenance of equilibrium.

Visual receptors also play an important role in maintenance of equilibrium. It has been noted that after complete destruction of vestibular apparatus and loss of proprioceptive information, a person can still use visual mechanism effectively to maintain balance. But in such cases, if the eyes are closed or the person is moving rapidly, balance is lost.

Applied Aspects

The important applied aspects in relation to vestibular apparatus which need special emphasis are:

- Vestibular dysfunctions and
- Experimental stimulation of semicircular canal.

A. Vestibular Dysfunctions

1. Motion Sickness

Aetiopathogenesis: Motion sickness is a symptom complex occurring due to excessive and repeated stimulation of vestibular apparatus while travelling in automobile, ship, aircraft or spacecraft. The psychological factors, like anxiety about the unfamiliar mode of travel, may be additional factors in causation of motion sickness.

The disease occurring during travelling by ship is referred to as *sea sickness.*

Characteristic features of motion sickness are:

- Unpleasant sensation of rotation accompanied by nausea, vomiting, sweating, pallor, salivation, headache, disorientation and even diarrhoea. Most of the symptoms and signs are the effects of vestibular stimulation on the medullary autonomic centres.

Prevention. Motion sickness can be prevented by taking antiemetic drugs such as *Avomine* and by avoiding greasy and bulky food before travelling.

- Space motion sickness is usually experienced by the astronauts when they are first exposed to microgravity environment. The symptoms of nausea, vomiting and dizziness experienced usually wear off after a few days, and may occur in reentry into the gravity force. These symptoms occur due to mismatched neural signal inputs by the vestibular apparatus and other gravity sensors.

2. Benign Paraoxysmal Positional Vertigo (BPPV). An important common vestibular disorder that is characterized by episodes of vertigo associated with turning of the head in particular position. This occurs due to separation of otoconia from the otolith membrane, which get lodged into cupula or semicircular canal.

Treatment. Usually symptoms of BPPV disappear after a few weeks. Canalith repositioning a simple slow manoeuvre is advised to maintain position of head so that otoconia move from semicircular canal back into the vestibule (utricle).

3. Meniere's Disease

Aetiopathogenesis. It is caused by overdistension of the membranous labyrinth, probably due to oversecretion *(endolymphatic hydrops).*

Characteristic features. Meniere's disease originates in the labyrinth and typically present as a triad consisting of:

- Fluctuating deafness of sensorial type,
- Tinnitus which may be very troublesome and
- Episodic attacks of rotatory vertigo.

The disease is usually unilateral to start with and the common age of onset is 35–50 years and comes in attacks. Patient usually has nausea, vomiting and fullness of ear in addition to the above-listed triad.

Treatment The symptoms of Meniere's disease can be controlled by reducing fluid retention by dietary changes like low salt/salt-free diet.

- Vestibular suppressants such as melizine (antihistaminic drug) are useful. It acts by decreasing excitability of labyrinth, and also blocks conduction in middle ear–vestibular–cerebellar pathway.
- In patients with frequent attacks, the implantation of a small tube or shunt into the abnormally swollen endolymphatic sac is done.

4. Labyrinthectomy

Bilateral labyrinthectomy, i.e. removal of labyrinthine apparatus on both sides, is characterized by:

- *Equilibrium* is maintained by visual sensation. The individual cannot right himself when blindfolded.
- *Postural reflexes* are severely affected.
- *Muscle tone* is decreased but there is no permanent loss.
- *Hearing* loss is also there.

Unilateral labyrinthectomy, i.e. removal of labyrinthine apparatus on one side, is characterized by following immediate and permanent effects. *Immediate effects* occurring due to unopposed action of intact labyrinth are:

- *Oblique deviation of the eyeballs*, i.e. one eyeball is rolled upwards and outwards and the other downwards and inwards,
- *Nystagmus,*
- *Rotation and lateral flexion of the head*, so that occiput is turned to the side of lesion and
- *Flexion of limbs* on the side of lesion and extension of limbs on the opposite side.

Permanent effects are:

- Nystagmus,
- Reciprocal changes in the tone and head rotation persist and
- Rotation of the trunk decreases.

B. Experimental Stimulation of Semicircular Canals

The semicircular canals can be stimulated by two methods:

- Rotational movement by Barany chair and
- Caloric stimulation.

1. Stimulation by Rotational Movement Using Barany Chair

- ***Method.*** The subject is made to sit in the chair with head tilted forward at 30°. The chair is rotated at 30 rpm for 20 s.
- ***Effects.*** *During rotation* with eyes open, *nystagmus* occurs continuously throughout the period of rotation. *After rotation* in Barany's chair for 20 s at 30 rpm, following effects are noted:
    - *Postrotatory nystagmus* occurs for about 30 s.
    - *Dizziness,* i.e. feeling of unsteadiness occurs immediately after stoppage of rotation. It is associated with feeling of rotation in the opposite direction.
    - *Vertigo,* i.e. feeling of rotation even after stoppage of rotation.
    - *Nausea and vomiting* may occur after rotation for a longer period.

2. Caloric Stimulation. The semicircular canals can be stimulated by introducing hot (40°C) or cold (30°C) water into the external auditory meatus.

- ***Mechanism.*** The transmission of change in temperature into labyrinth alters the specific gravity of the endolymph. As a result, the cupula is set into motion and the hair cells are stimulated.
- ***Effects.*** Caloric stimulation produces the same effects as rotational movement, i.e. there occurs:
    - Vertigo,
    - Dizziness and
    - Nystagmus.

If cold water is poured into the right ear, the patient develops left jerk nystagmus (rapid phase towards left), while the reverse happens with warm water. It can be remembered by the mnemonic 'COWS' (cold-opposite-warm-same).

- ***Clinical aspects***

1. Caloric stimulation is used as a clinical test for diagnostic purpose.
2. While irrigating the ear canal for treatment of ear infections, it must be ensured that fluid used is at the body temperature level, otherwise annoying symptom of caloric stimulation will occur.

Chapter 10.10

Limbic System and Physiology of Emotional, Behavioural and Motivational Mechanisms

LIMBIC SYSTEM

Physiological Anatomy

Components of Limbic System The term limbic has been derived from the word 'limbus' which means a ring. Thus, the term limbic system is applied for those parts of the cortex (limbic cortex or limbic lobe) and subcortical structures that form a ring around the brainstem. Previously, this area was called rhinencephalon because of its relation to olfaction. It is now known to play, apart from olfaction, a role in functions like behavioural activity, emotions, motivational drives, memory and regulation of viscera, and so it is also referred to as 'visceral brain'. Components of limbic system are (Fig. 10.10-1):

- ***Limbic cortex*** or the so-called limbic lobe surrounds the subcortical structures of the limbic system. Phylogenetically, limbic cortex is an older part of the cerebral cortex (allocortex) having primitive histological structures, i.e. only three layers (page 964). Rest of the cerebral cortex is greatly developed (neocortex) and in most areas has six layers (page 965). Limbic cortex is composed of (Figs 10.10-1, 10.10-2):
  - Orbitofrontal cortex,
  - Subcallosal gyrus,
  - Cingulate gyrus,
  - Parahippocampal gyrus and
  - Uncus.
- ***Subcortical structures*** included in the limbic system are:
  - Hypothalamus,
  - Septum,
  - Paraolfactory area,
  - Anterior nuclei of thalamus,
  - Amygdala,
  - Portions of basal ganglia and
  - Hippocampus.

Connections

Bundles of axons connecting the various components of limbic system are (Fig. 10.10-3):

- Fornix (see page 954),
- Mammillothalamic tract (see page 955),
- Stria terminalis (see page 955),
- Stria medullaris thalami and
- Medial forebrain bundle (see page 954).

Papez circuit refers to a closed circuit formed by connections between the cingulate gyrus (located in the prefrontal lobe), hippocampus, mammillary bodies and anterior nucleus of thalamus (Fig. 10.10-4). This circuit is

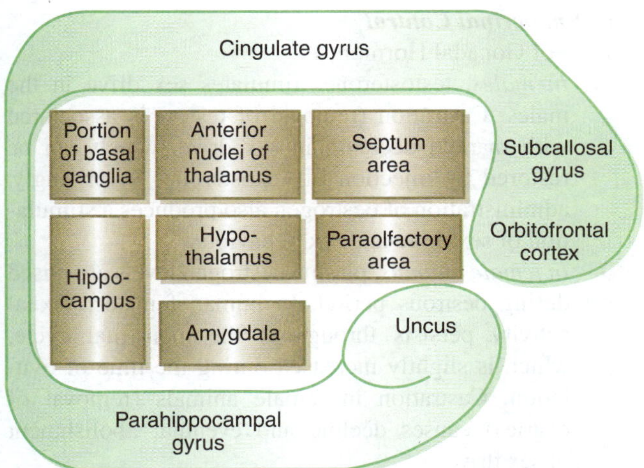

FIGURE 10.10-1 Diagrammatic representation of the structures forming limbic system.

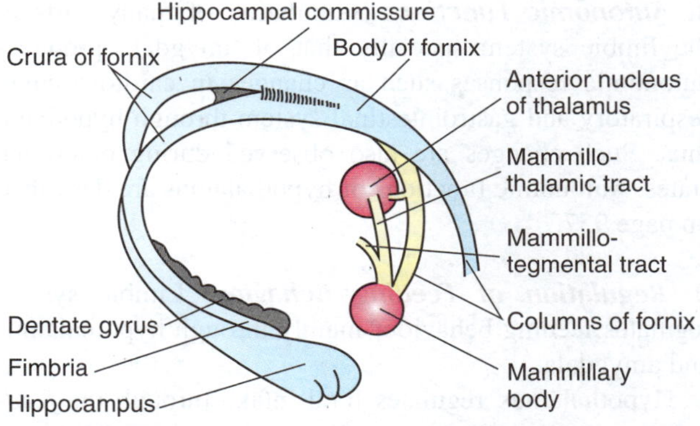

FIGURE 10.10-3 The fornix and related pathways of the limbic system.

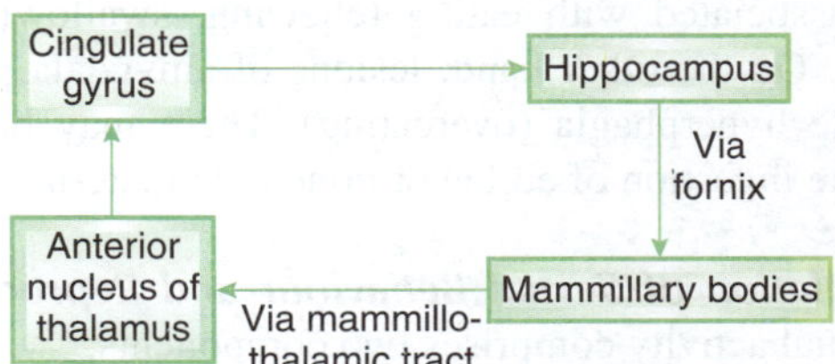

FIGURE 10.10-4 The Papez circuit.

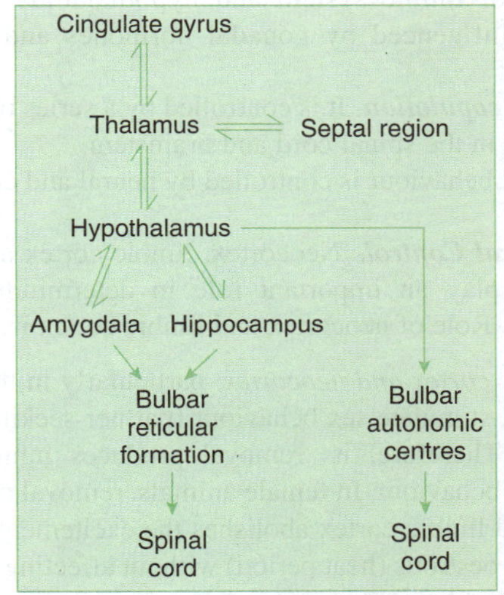

FIGURE 10.10-5 Efferent projection of limbic system.

responsible for resting EEG (page 1098) and for those emotions and aspects of behaviour that are related to preservation of the individual and species.

Efferent projection of limbic system is shown in Fig. 10.10-5.

Characteristic features of limbic system connections are:

- *Limbic system has very little connection with the neocortex.* Because of this, emotional and instinctual behaviour is not under voluntary control, especially in lower animals. Thus, from a functional point of view, neocortical activity does modify emotional behaviour but it cannot be turned on and off at will.
- *Prolonged after discharge* is shown by the anatomic closed circuit of the limbic system following a sensory experience. Therefore, the emotional responses are usually prolonged, i.e. continue long after the end of the stimuli that produce them.

Functions of Limbic System

Most of the functions of limbic system are intimately related to the functions of hypothalamus which have been described in Chapter 10.3, page 956. These include:

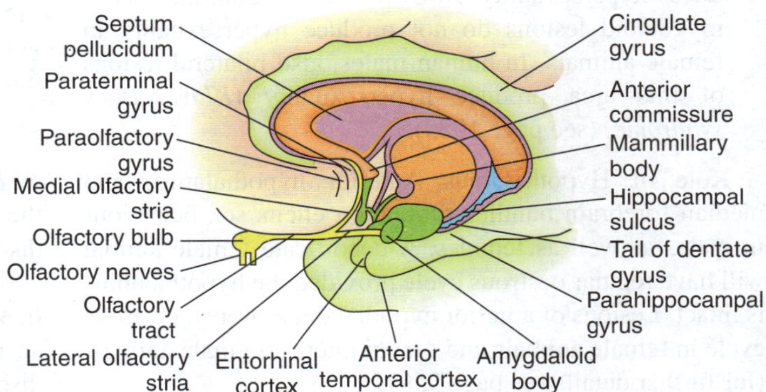

FIGURE 10.10-2 Medial surface of right cerebral hemisphere showing limbic cortex (limbic lobe) and other components of limbic system.

1. Autonomic Functions Stimulation of many parts of the limbic system specially that of amygdala produces autonomic responses such as changes in cardiovascular, respiratory and gastrointestinal system through hypothalamus. Such changes are also observed during emotional states. Autonomic functions of hypothalamus are described on page 957.

2. Regulation of Feeding Behaviour Limbic system regulates feeding behaviour mainly through hypothalamus and amygdala.

Hypothalamus regulates food intake through the *feeding centre* and *satiety centre* (for details see page 958).

Amygdala. Stimulation of amygdala produces movements associated with eating (chewing, swallowing and licking). On the other hand, lesions of amygdala produce moderate hyperphagia (overeating). There may be indiscriminate ingestion of edible or nonedible materials.

3. Regulation of Sexual Behaviour and Reproduction The sexual activity comprises two components:

Sexual Behaviour. The basic sex drive (urge to copulate) is an instinctual behaviour as food intake. It is the function of limbic system and hypothalamus which in turn are influenced by gonadal hormones and cerebral cortex.

Act of copulation. It is controlled by a series of reflexes integrated in the spinal cord and brainstem.

Sexual behaviour is controlled by neural and endocrinal factors.

i. Neural Control. Neocortex, limbic cortex and hypothalamus play an important role in determining sexual behaviour. Role of neocortex and limbic cortex is:

- *Limbic cortex and neocortex,* particularly in the frontal region, stimulate sex behaviour (partner-seeking behaviour). Therefore, its removal produces inhibition of sexual behaviour. In female animals, removal of neocortex and limbic cortex abolishes the excitement reaction during oestrous (heat period) without affecting the other aspects of heat.
- *Piriform cortex overlying amygdala* inhibits sex drive in males. Therefore, its destruction in male animals produces hypersexuality. However, amygdaloid and periamygdaloid lesions do not produce hypersexuality in female animals. In human males, also bilateral lesions of this area produce hypersexuality (*Klüver–Bucy syndrome)* (see page 1085).

Role of Hypothalamus. Anterior hypothalamus and median forebrain bundle stimulation elicits sex behaviour in males as well as females. A decorticate female animal will have regular oestrous cycle provided the hypothalamus is intact. Lesions of anterior hypothalamus abolish oestrous cycle in female animals and sexual interest in male animals (for further details see page 959).

ii. Endocrinal Control

Role of Gonadal Hormones

- *In males,* testosterone stimulates sex drive in the males. Castration (removal of testes) is associated with marked decrease in sex drive, which can be restored by injection of testosterone. Surprisingly, administration of oestrogen also produces a stimulation of sex drive and sex behaviour.
- *In female animals*, plasma oestrogen levels are raised during oestrous period. In human females, sexual activity persists throughout the menstrual cycle, which is slightly increased during the time of ovulation. Castration in female animals (removal of ovaries) causes decline and eventual abolishment of sex drive.

Role of Encephalization. In humans, sex behaviour is largely encephalized, i.e. the perception that sexual act produces pleasure is a big cause of sex behaviour. Therefore, menopausal women (akin to castrated female animals) continue to have sex behaviour. Further, sex behaviour is strongly influenced, in humans, by social customs, rules and social taboos.

Role of Pheromones. Pheromones are chemicals which by their smell act as sex attractants in animals. It has been observed that in monkey, sexual drive is greater in the male when exposed to a female at the time of ovulation than when exposed to a female at other time of ovarian cycle. Certain fatty acids present in the vaginal secretions during ovulation are supposed to attract the male monkey by their smell.

The role of pheromones in human sexuality is, however, uncertain.

4. Maternal Behaviour Maternal behaviour, as demonstrated in rat, is the function of cingulate gyrus and retrosplenial portion of the limbic cortex. In animals, maternal behaviour is primarily neurogenic, i.e. it depends on olfactory, auditory, visual and thermotactile stimuli arising from the young ones. Prolactin and oxytocin, though absolutely not essential, have been reported to facilitate maternal behaviour. Maternal behaviour, in rats, is manifested by nest building, suckling, and licking the pups and retrieving the pups when separated. In general, the maternal behaviour is concerned with the nursing (breastfeeding) and protection of the offspring by the mother.

5. Emotional Behaviour Emotional behaviour is one of the most important functions of limbic system. It has been discussed separately in 'physiology of emotions'.

6. Motivational Behaviour Motivational behaviour is also an important function of the limbic system and has been discussed separately as 'physiology of motivation'.

Summary of Different Components of Limbic System

1. Hypothalamus Hypothalamus and its functions are described on page 956. *Areas of hypothalamus associated with behavioural control* functions are:

- Increased level of general activity, leading to *rage and aggression.* It occurs when lateral hypothalamus is stimulated.
- *Sexual arousal* occurs when most anterior and posterior portion of hypothalamus is stimulated.
- *Feelings of reward, tranquillity and pleasure* are appreciated when reward centre is stimulated.
- *Fearing, feeling of punishment and aversion* are felt when punishment centre is stimulated.

Lesions of hypothalamus are associated with:

- Extreme passivity and loss of drive,
- Excessive eating and drinking and
- Rage and violent behaviour.

2. Amygdala Amygdala is a large aggregate of cells located above the inferior horn of the lateral ventricle and is embedded in the uncus. It consists of two subdivisions: a corticomedial nuclear group and a basolateral group of nuclei. In humans, basolateral nuclei of amygdala are very well developed and they play an important role in behavioural activities not generally associated with olfactory stimuli.

Afferents to amygdala come from all portions of limbic cortex as well as from neocortex and, therefore, it is called the 'window' through which the limbic system sees the place of the person in the world.

Efferents from amygdala are varied and extensive, reaching the cortex, hippocampus, septum, thalamus and hypothalamus.

Stimulation of amygdala produces following effects:

1. *Autonomic effects through hypothalamus.* These include:
   - Changes in heart rate (increase or decrease),
   - Changes in blood pressure (increase or decrease),
   - Changes in gastrointestinal secretion and motility,
   - Defaecation and micturition,
   - Pupillary dilatation,
   - Piloerection and
   - Secretion of anterior pituitary hormones.
2. *Involuntary movements* which can be elicited are:
   - Tonic movements as raising of head or bending of the body,
   - Clonic rhythmic movements,
   - Circling movements
   - Clonus and
   - Movements associated with olfaction and eating (chewing, swallowing, etc.).
3. *Behavioural effects* are:
   - Reaction of reward and punishment (rage and escape),
   - Sexual activities include erection, copulatory movements, ovulation, uterine activity and premature labour.

Bilateral destruction of temporal pole is associated with destruction of amygdala which leads to *Klüver–Bucy syndrome* characterized by:

- Extreme orality, i.e. excessive tendency to examine objects orally,
- Loss of fear,
- Decreased aggressiveness,
- Tameness,
- Changes in eating behaviour,
- Psychic blindness and
- Excessive sexual drive.

3. Hippocampus Hippocampus is formed due to projection of the hippocampal sulcus into the floor of the inferior horn of lateral ventricle.

Connections. Hippocampus has many indirect connections to many portions of cerebral cortex.

Stimulation of hippocampus can evoke rage, passivity and excessive sexual drive. It is also hyperexcitable, and weak stimuli can produce epileptic seizures.

Functions of hippocampus are:

- Like amygdala, it is an additional channel through which incoming signals can lead to appropriate behavioural pattern.
- It is suggested that hippocampus also provides the signal for memory consolidation, e.g. the transformation from short-term to long-term memories of verbal and symbolic type.

Lesions of the hippocampus lead to *anterograde amnesia,* i.e. a profound inability to form new memories based on any type of verbal symbolism (language).

4. Limbic Cortex Limbic cortex acts as an association area for control of behaviour:

- ***Anterior temporal cortex*** has gustatory and olfactory association,
- ***Parahippocampal gyrus*** has complex auditory association, and complex thought association derived from Wernicke's area of the posterior temporal lobe.
- ***Posterior cingulate cortex*** has sensory motor association.

Lesions of different parts of limbic cortex produce certain symptoms that suggest their functions, e.g.

- *Bilateral destruction of anterior temporal cortex* leads to Klüver–Bucy syndrome as described above.
- *Bilateral lesions in the posterior orbitofrontal cortex* lead to insomnia and restlessness.
- *Bilateral destruction of anterior cingulate and subcallosal gyri* evokes an extreme rage reaction.

PHYSIOLOGY OF EMOTIONS

Components of Emotions

Emotions refer to an aroused state involving intense feeling, autonomic activation and related behaviour which accompany many of our conscious experiences. Emotions have two major components: mental and physical. The components of emotions are explained below by considering the example of response of an individual to sudden very loud noise.

I. Mental or Sensory Component Mental or sensory component of emotions comprises cognition, affect and conation.

Cognition. It refers to a phenomenon by which one becomes aware (sees) and recognizes a situation. For example, when an individual hears a sudden very loud noise, and from his/her experience recognizes it to be bomb blast. This is called cognition. Thus, mere seeing but not recognizing is not cognition.

Affect. It is a German word which means development of a feeling. In the above example, the person after cognizing the loud sound as bomb blast is frightened; this feeling of frightening is called affect.

Conation. It is the force that directs or urges to take some action. For example, the desire to run away from the site of loud noise after getting frightened is conation.

II. Physical or Expressive or Peripheral Component

Physical or Expressive or peripheral component of the emotions is the motor side of emotional behaviour. It consists of two subcomponents—somatic and autonomic:

- ***Somatic*** part of the physical component of emotions basically comprises changes in the skeletal muscles. The accomplishment of the act of running away from site of noise in the above example constitutes the somatic part of the physical component.
- ***Autonomic part*** of the physical component of emotions involves the coordinated activity of sympathetic and parasympathetic nervous system. For example, occurrence of tachycardia, raised blood pressure, increased respiration rate, etc. after getting frightened from the sudden loud noise constitute the autonomic part of the physical component.
  - ***Sympathetic expression.*** Fear (as in the above example) is associated with sympathetic expression which is characterized by an increase in heart rate, increase in respiration rate, cutaneous vasoconstriction, sweating (cold sweat), piloerection, pupillary dilatation and dryness of mouth.
  - ***Parasympathetic expression*** is noticed during grief or pleasure.

Note. In many instances, the somatic part of the physical component of emotions may be absent. For example, after getting insulted and provoked, one may beat the insulter (somatic part present). While the other individual may feel enraged, develop high blood pressure plus tachycardia but restrains oneself and does not show any somatic side of expression (indeed, this is common in civilized societies).

Functions Served by Peripheral Component of Emotions

1. ***Preparatory function,*** i.e. the body is prepared for action. It involves:
   - *General arousal,* which prepares the organism as a whole for action and
   - *Specific arousal,* which prepares the organism for a particular behaviour. For example, *sexual arousal* involves:
     - General arousal in the form of tachycardia that prepares for physical exertion and
     - Specific arousal in the form of tumescence.

Theories of Genesis of Emotions

Physical changes are secondary to emotional feelings or vice versa have been the matter of debate. Following theories have been put forward from time to time in this regard; the genesis of emotions as explained by Arnold is as under:

Arnold Theory. According to this theory of genesis emotions (Fig. 10.10-6):

- By *cognition* one becomes aware and recognizes a situation.
- By *unconscious evaluation,* the situation is judged as to be harmful or beneficial.
- *Affect* is conscious reflection of unconscious appraisal. A feeling is thus generated consciously in response to unconscious evaluation of a situation. Such a feeling may be in the form of fear, joy, grief or rage.

Thus, according to Arnold's theory, emotions have their own logic and that the peripheral component of emotions results from unconscious evaluation of situation as potentially harmful or harmless. Therefore, in response to a particular situation, different individuals react differently, e.g. in response to a bomb blast by terrorist attacks:

- Some will be frightened,
- Proterrosist persons will have a feeling of joy,
- Antiterrorists will develop a feeling of rage and so on.
  - Further, Arnold pointed out that autonomic responses are not an essential component of emotions.

Emotional Behaviour

Different emotions produce different sets of behaviour. Physiological basis of most emotional behaviours has been studied extensively in animals and little bit in humans.

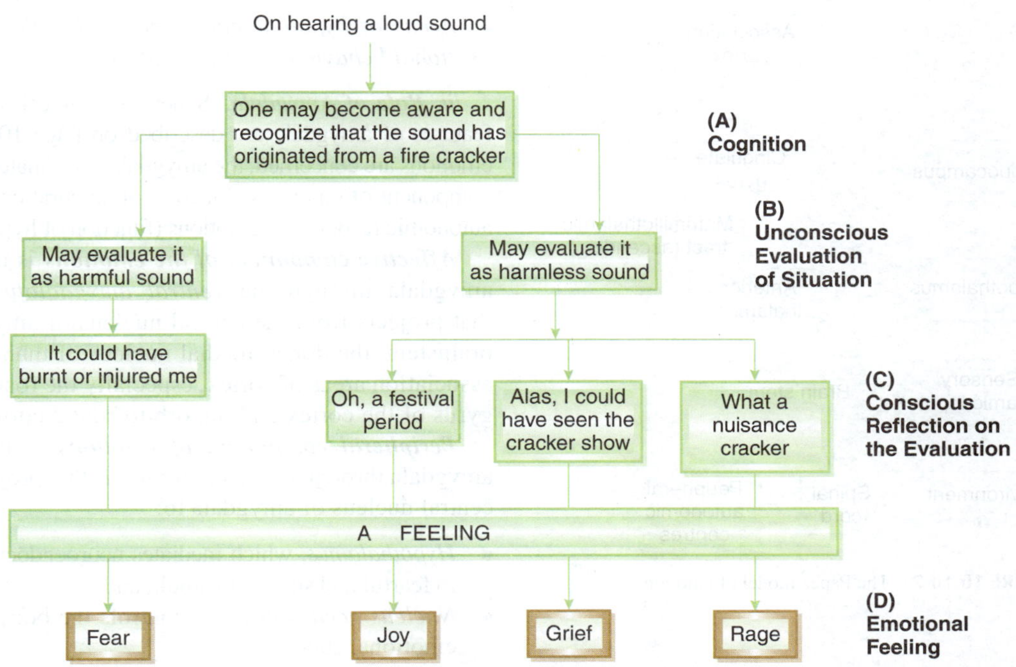

FIGURE 10.10-6 Steps of Arnold's theory of emotions: **A,** cognition; **B,** unconscious evaluation of situation; **C,** conscious reflection on the evaluation; and **D,** emotional feeling.

Behaviour is considered an expression of emotions. Some of the emotional behaviours are:

- Rage, fear and placidity (see page 959),
- Sexual behaviour (see page 1084) and
- Feeling of reward and punishment (see page 1089).

Neural Substrate of Emotions

1. Role of Central Nervous System

i. Role of Cerebral Cortex. Cerebral cortex, especially the frontal, cingulate, and parahippocampal cortices, plays an important role in *affective component* of *emotions*:

- Detailed processing of conscious experience of emotional feeling occurs in cerebral cortex.
- Cortical mechanisms also provide the means by which memory and imagination too can evoke emotional feeling.
- Cortex also provides the mechanisms that direct the motor responses to the external event during emotional behaviour, e.g. to approach or avoid a situation.
- Cortical mechanisms also provide the means which account for the modulation, direction, understanding or even inhibition of emotional behaviour. For example, once we know that an explosive sound came from only a fire cracker, the fear subsides by cortical suppression of reflex emotional responses.

Lesions of cerebral cortex concerned with emotions are associated with emotional disturbances as:

- *Lesions of orbitofrontal cortex* reduce the normal aggressiveness and emotional responsiveness.
- *Lesions of ventromedial frontal cortex* have normal autonomic response mechanism, i.e. show normal galvanic skin responses (sweating measured electrically) to *startle* stimuli, such as unexpected loud noises or bright lights. However, when they are shown emotionally disturbing pictures, they fail to show the expected autonomic response to these emotionally charged stimuli.
- *Lesions of anterior cingulate cortex* reduce the emotional response to chronic intractable pain. Such patients experience pain as a sensation and exhibit appropriate autonomic reactions, but the sensation is not perceived as intensely unpleasant.

ii. Role of Hypothalamus. Hypothalamus and other components of limbic system are intimately concerned with physiology of emotions. Functions of all these components have been described on page 1085. However, their role as neural substrates of emotions is described below even at the cost of repetition.

Hypothalamus has been considered the main seat of emotions. Papez suggested a model of emotional expression and experience on the basis of clinical and to some extent anatomical facts (Fig. 10.10-7).

- *Sensory input* from environment passes through the thalamus to the hypothalamus.
- *Ascending output from hypothalamus* passes on through the mammillothalamic tract to the anterior thalamus and on to the cingulate cortex.
- *Output from cingulate cortex* interacts with the sensory cortical signals in the association cortex.

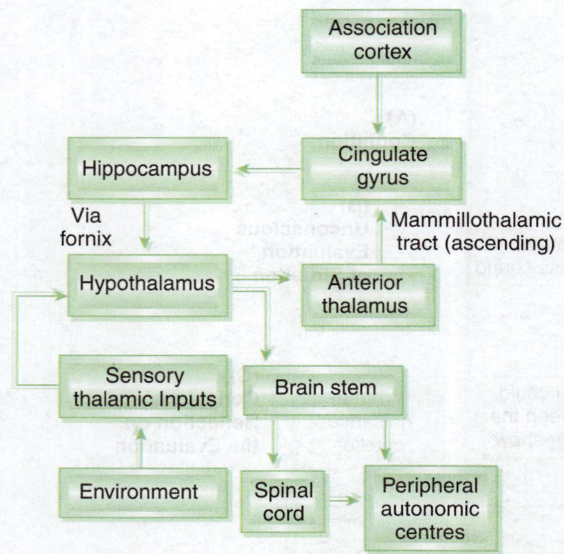

FIGURE 10.10-7 The Papez model of emotions.

- Thus, the sensory information from the cortex, particularly those from the frontal lobe, is lent an emotional flavour and reaches the hippocampus.
- *Hippocampus* projects onto the hypothalamus through the fornix and thus completes the so-called Papez circuit (Fig. 10.10-4).
- *Descending projections from hypothalamus* pass through the brainstem down to the spinal cord and out into peripheral autonomic nervous system. The output of the peripheral autonomic nervous system produces the manifestation of emotional expressions.
- *Areas of hypothalamus concerned with various emotional behaviour* (See page 959).

iii. Role of Amygdala. Salient anatomical and functional features of amygdala are described on page 1085. As far as emotions are concerned, the amygdala coordinates the affective component of emotions (function of cerebral cortex) with the autonomic response to emotions (function of hypothalamus).

Affective component of the emotions is influenced by amygdala through the *ventral amygdalofugal pathway* that projects from the central nucleus of amygdala to the brainstem, the dorsal medial nucleus of thalamus and the association areas of cortex, especially the rostral cingulate gyrus of the cortex and the orbitofrontal cortex.

Peripheral component of emotions is influenced by amygdala through the *stria terminalis* that projects from the central nucleus of amygdala to:

- *Hypothalamus*, which mediates neuroendocrinal response to fearful and stressful stimuli, and
- *Nucleus accumbens* that controls the body language in emotional states.

Summary of role of amygdala in emotions. Various anatomical projections from the central nucleus of amygdala, neuroendocrinal response and the peripheral signs of emotions produced are summarized in Table 10.10-1.

Concepts of extended Papez circuit. Recently, a concept of extended Papez circuit has been described in which the focus has been shifted to the main role of amygdala in emotions (Fig. 10.10-8). The Papez circuit of emotions, described by James Papez in 1937, points out that the circuit is completed by projection of hippocampus to hypothalamus through the fornix (Fig. 10.10-7).

TABLE 10.10-1 Summary of Role of Amygdala in Emotions

Sr.	Anatomical projection from central nucleus of amygdale	Neuroendocrinal response on stimulation	Peripheral signs of emotions
1.	Lateral hypothalamus	Sympathetic stimulation	Increased heart rate, increased blood pressure and pupillary dilatation
2.	Dorsal motor nucleus of vagus, nucleus ambiguus	Parasympathetic stimulation	Bradycardia, urination, defaecation
3.	Parabrachial nucleus	Increased respiration	Panting, respiratory distress
4.	Ventral tegmental area, locus coeruleus and dorsal lateral tegmental nucleus	Activation of catecholamines	Behavioural and electroencephalographic arousal
5.	Nucleus reticularis, pontis caudalis	Increased reflexes	Increased startle
6.	Central grey area	Cessation of behaviour	Social interaction
7.	Trigeminal and facial motor nucleus	Jaw movements and mouth opening	Facial expression of fear
8.	Paraventricular nucleus of hypothalamus	ACTH release	Corticosteroid release (stress response)

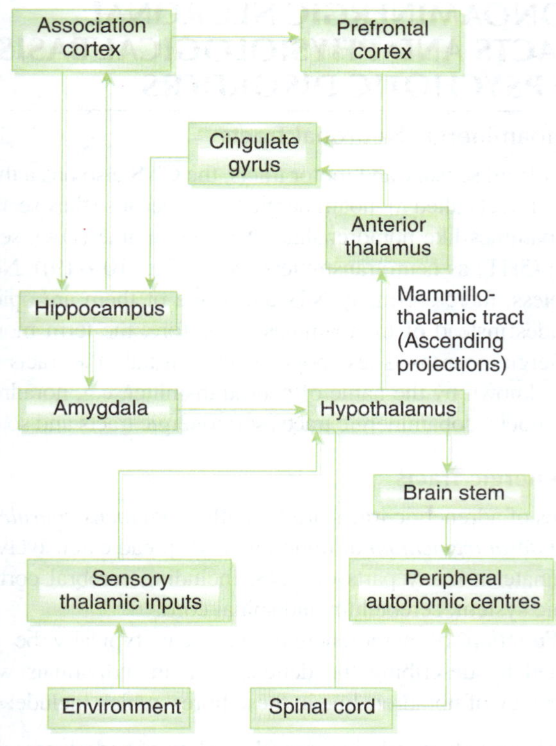

FIGURE 10.10-8 The extended Papez circuit of emotions.

2. Role of Peripheral Nervous System Autonomic as well as somatic motor peripheral nervous system is involved in the peripheral expression of the emotions.

i. ***Autonomic nervous system*** is the chief mediator of the emotional output. There is some degree of specificity in the pattern of autonomic expressions depending upon the type of emotion in question and also whether the autonomic response is primary, i.e. independently determined or secondary to the somatomotor behaviour. Cannon described the emotional response to an emergency or involving diffuse sympathetic activation and outpouring into the blood of excitatory substances, i.e. the catecholamines.

ii. ***Somatic motor nervous system*** is involved in the somatic part of the physical component of emotions, which basically comprises changes in skeletal muscles.

PHYSIOLOGY OF MOTIVATION

Motivation is that component of behaviour which is responsible for accomplishing a particular task.

Neural Mechanism of Motivation

Neural mechanisms involved in motivation are based on the concept of reward and punishment. It has been elucidated by the effects of self-stimulation of brain.

Concept of Reward and Punishment

Almost anything that we do is related in some way to reward and punishment. If we do something that is rewarding, we continue to do it. If we do something that is punishing, we cease to do it.

Reward and Punishment Centre. It appears that conditions which result in stimulation of reward centre produce motive to do a job. For details about *reward and punishment* centres, see page 959.

Experiment to demonstrate activity of reward and punishment centres. This experiment demonstrates that the animal itself regulates the stimulation of reward and punishment centres (self-stimulation). The *Hess technique* of experiment is: a rat is placed in a cage having a bar (lever) that can be pressed by the rat. The electrical connections are made in such a way that on pressing the bar a stimulus may be applied to the brain of rat through an electrode (Fig. 10.10-9). Following observations are made:

- *When no stimulus is applied* to the brain on pressing the bar, the animal presses it occasionally (at random).
- *When stimulation is applied to the reward centre* (located along the course of medial forebrain bundle, especially in lateral and ventromedial nucleus of hypothalamus), on pressing the bar the animal presses the bar repeatedly at a rate much above the rate of random pressing. It has been reported that stimulation of reward centre produces a *pleasure sensation* (feeling of complete relaxation).
- Further, it has been observed that even if a painful barricade is placed between the rat and bar (lever), the rat ignores the pain to cross the barrier to press the bar. This means that the rat must have developed a strong motive to derive pleasure sensation.

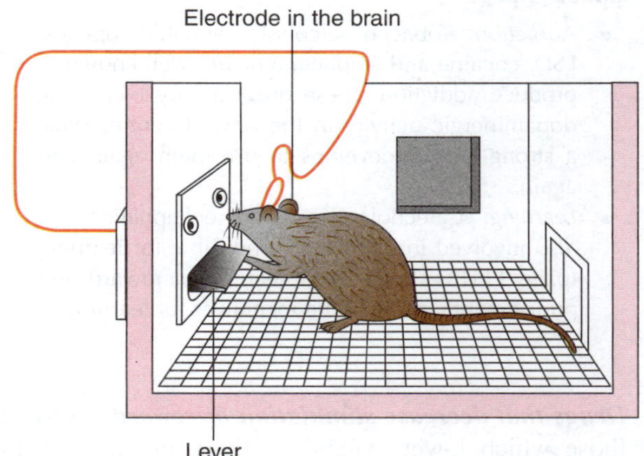

FIGURE 10.10-9 Experimental set-up to demonstrate reward and punishment centres by self-stimulation.

- Instead of painful barrier, if a complicated maze is made between the rat and bar (lever), the rat learns to cross the maze. This means that development of a motive is a strong factor for learning. From this, it can be concluded that if there is no motive to do a job, people will not do the job nor they will learn to do the job.
  - It has been observed that self-stimulation increases when the animal is deprived of food and decreased by castration (restarted by the administration of sex hormones).
  - When stimulation is applied to punishment centre (located in medial hypothalamus, periventricular zone) on pressing the bar, the animal avoids further stimulation of this area. The pressing rate of bar is decreased much below the rate of random pressing. It has been reported that electrical stimulation of punishment centre leads to pain, fear, defence, escape reactions and the other elements of punishment.

Role of Neurotransmitters

Neurotransmitters involved in the pathway that stimulate the *reward centre* are:

- Catecholamines (norepinephrine and dopamine),
- Morphine and
- Enkephalin.

Drugs that increase stimulation of reward centre are those which increase synaptic activity in catecholamine pathway, e.g.

- *Amphetamine,* which causes increased release of dopamine.
- *Nicotine and alcohol* increase the amount of dopamine.
- *Cocaine* inhibits the re-uptake of dopamine and norepinephrine.

Applied Aspects

- *Addiction.* Tobacco, alcohol, cannabis, opiates, LSD, cocaine and amphetamine are well known to produce addiction. These drugs act by increasing dopaminergic activity in the reward centre. Thus, a strong motive develops to use them again and again.
- *Learning.* Catecholamines and enkephalins are also involved in pathways responsible for learning (page 1118). Therefore, it seems that reward and punishment constitute the incentives for learning.

Drugs that decrease stimulation of reward centre are those which lower synaptic activity in the catecholamine pathway, e.g. chlorpromazine hydrochloride (Largactil).

MONOAMINERGIC NEURONAL TRACTS AND PHYSIOLOGICAL BASIS OF PSYCHOTIC DISORDERS

Monoaminergic Neuronal Tracts

Apart from sensory and motor tracts, the CNS also has a third kind of tract called monoaminergic tracts (because they secrete monoamines like noradrenaline (NA), dopamine (DA), serotonin (5HT) as neurotransmitters (NTs) (Fig. 10.7-19)). Nevertheless, there are many NTs and some of them are opioid peptides instead of monoamines. Therefore, the term monoaminergic neurons is less popular now. In fact, the tracts are better known by the name of neurotransmitter, e.g. noradrenergic tracts, dopaminergic tracts, serotonergic tracts and so on.

Adrenergic Tracts

Fibres of adrenergic tracts arise chiefly from *locus coeruleu s* and *lateral tegmentum* of midbrain, and spread extensively to terminate in many parts of CNS, including cerebral cortex, limbic system, cerebellum and spinal cord.

Function of noradrenergic fibres can typically be explained by describing the deficits seen in individuals with deficiency of noradrenaline in these fibres, which include:

- Abnormal mood, i.e. mood is down, and depression develops,
- Increase in hunger and appetite and
- Increased sleep.

Dopaminergic Tracts

Two major dopaminergic pathways arise from the midbrain:

- *Nigrostriatal*, from substantia nigra of midbrain to corpus striatum, and
- *Mesolimbic*, from mesencephalon to nucleus accumbens which is situated little cranial to corpus striatum.

Functions of dopaminergic pathways are understood from the abnormalities of these tracts:

- Damage of nigostriatal pathway or dopaminergic receptor deficiency causes *Parkinsonism* (for details see page 944).
- Excessive dopaminergic activity in mesolimbic fibres leads to schizophrenia.

PHYSIOLOGICAL BASIS OF PSYCHOTIC DISORDERS

1. Depression

In a normal person, the mood usually swings, i.e. with bad news (e.g. failure in examination) the mood is down and with good news (e.g. distinction in examination), the mood is elated. However, when mood chronically remains down without any specific reason, then the condition is called as depression.

Signs and Symptoms are:

- Chronic depression of mood,
- Lack of interest,
- Suicidal tendency,
- Excessive sleep and overeating.

Causes. The physiological basis of this disorder is decreased activity of either noradrenergic or serotoninergic fibres. The defect may be at the receptor level or there is deficiency of neurotransmitters (noradrenaline or serotonin).

Treatment. Drugs that increase the excitatory effects of NA are effective in treating depression; these include monoamine oxidase (MAO) inhibitors, tricyclic antidepressants and drugs that enhance the action of serotonin. Manic-depressive conditions (bipolar disorder) can be effectively treated by lithium compounds that diminish the actions of NA and serotonin.

2. Mania

In this condition, mood remains chronically elated without any specific reason. It is due to overactivity of noradrenergic fibre activity.

3. Schizophrenia

Schizophrenia is another common psychotic disorder in which there is false perception of sensations (hallucinations), though there is no anatomical lesion in the sensory pathway.

Cause. Schizophrenia is thought to be associated with excessive activity of dopaminergic mesolimbic pathway (mainly due to overactivtiy of D_2 receptors). Evidence supporting this theory derives from the fact that schizophrenic symptoms are reduced by drugs such as chlorpromazine and haloperidol that diminish dopamine release at axon terminals (drugs that block D_2 receptors). Recently developed antipsychotic agents are effective, but they bind to D_2 receptors to a limited degree; however, they bind effectively to D_4 receptors. This effect leads to a possibility that schizophrenia is associated with D_4 receptor abnormality.

Characteristic Features of schizophrenia are:

- Hallucinations, auditory as well as visual,
- Delusions of grandeur, intense fear, or paranoia and
- Withdrawal from the society, i.e. patient prefers extreme isolation, avoids company with persons and has no interest in the surroundings.

Treatment. As mentioned above, the drugs which decrease the dopamine concentration in the central nervous system are used. But the main drawback of these drugs is that they cause deficiency of dopamine, which precipitates parkinsonism.

Agranulocytosis is a potential side effect most of the antipsychotic drugs. However, certain drugs that do not cause agranulocytosis, but effectively reduce the symptoms of schizophrenia are risperidone, aripiprazol, olanzapine and palliperidone.

Chapter 10.11

Reticular Formation, Electrical Activity of the Brain, and Alert Behaviour and Sleep

RETICULAR FORMATION AND RETICULAR ACTIVATING SYSTEM
- Neuronal aggregates of RF
  - Reticular nuclei
  - Functional neuronal aggregates
- Reticular pathways
  - Cortico-reticulospinal pathways
  - Cerebello-reticular connections
  - Visceral control pathways
  - Reticular activating system (RAS)
- Neurotransmitters of reticular formation
- Functions of reticular formation

ELECTRICAL ACTIVITY OF THE BRAIN
- Evoked cortical potentials
  - Stimulus-related potentials
  - Event-related potentials
  - Clinical uses of evoked potentials
- Electroencephalogram
  - Technique of EEG recording
  - Normal EEG
  - Neurophysiological basis of EEG.
  - Variations in the EEG waveforms with age
  - Abnormal EEG waveforms

WAKEFULNESS AND SLEEP
- Wakefulness
  - Neural substrate for wakefulness
  - Chemical mediators of wakefulness
- Sleep
  - Sleep-wake cycle and factors affecting sleep
  - Types and stages of sleep
  - Non-REM
  - REM sleep
  - Sleep cycle
  - Genesis of sleep
  - Physiological significance of sleep
  - Sleep disorders

RETICULAR FORMATION AND RETICULAR ACTIVATING SYSTEM

Reticular formation (RF) refers to the complex network of neurons and nerve fibres which occupy the midventral portion of the brainstem around the central cavity and is exclusive of the specific nuclei and tracts. In other words, it is formed by neurons and processes left over after all well-defined named nuclei and pathways have been accounted for. Phylogenetically, it represents the old reticular core of the brain. The brainstem reticular formation (RF) comprises the medullary RF, pontine RF and midbrain RF. Structurally, brainstem reticular formation consists of:

- Neuronal aggregates,
- Afferent connections and] Reticular pathway
- Efferent connections.

Neuronal Aggregates of RF

Reticular Nuclei A number of reticular nuclei have been described. The limits of such nuclei are ill-defined (and often controversial), and their functional significance is often obscure. These can be divided into three longitudinal columns (in each half of the brainstem):

- ***Nuclei of median column*** lie next to the middle line and are called *nuclei of raphe*, e.g. raphe nuclei in the midbrain.
- ***Nuclei of medial column*** lie laterally to the nuclei of median column. These are made of large cells and so also called *magnocellular nuclei*, e.g. nucleus giganto-medullaris in the medulla and pontine tegmental nuclei.
- ***Nuclei of lateral column*** lie laterally to the nuclei of medial column. These are made of small neurons and so also called *parvocellular nuclei*. Examples of such nuclei are central nucleus of medulla and central nucleus of pons.

Functional Neuronal Aggregates Functional neuronal aggregates, though not anatomical entities, have been described to have fairly well-defined physiological functions. These include:

- Cardiac centres
- Respiratory centres,

- Vasomotor centres,
- Salivatory centres and
- Chemoreceptor neurons.

Reticular Pathways

Connections of RF are:

- Afferent connections
- Efferent connections, which include:
  - Descending projections and
  - Ascending projections.

The afferent and efferent connections of the RF form several pathways. Some of the major pathways are:

- Cortico-reticulospinal pathways
- Cerebello-reticular connections,
- Visceral control pathways and
- Reticular activating system (RAS).

Cortico-reticulospinal Pathways

Afferents of this pathway to neurons of RF come from the motor and other areas of cerebral cortex.

Areas of reticular formation which receive impulses from the cerebral cortex are:

- Bulbo-reticular inhibitory area located in the lower part of the medulla (see page 1056) and
- Bulbo-reticular facilitatory area located in the pons (see page 1056).

Cortico-reticulo-cerebellar and Cortico-reticulo-basal Ganglia Connections Some afferents from cerebral cortex, after relaying in reticular formation project to the cerebellum and basal ganglia. The influence of the cerebellum and basal ganglia on the motor function has been described in Chapter 10.9.

Visceral Control Pathways Certain centres in the reticular formation regulate respiration, heart rate and blood pressure. These effects are mediated through connections between the reticular formation and autonomic centres in the brainstem and spinal cord, but the pathways concerned are not well defined.

Reticular Activating System Reticular activating system (RAS) also known as ascending reticular activating system (ARAS) is a complex polysynaptic pathway that projects diffusely from the brainstem reticular formation to the cerebral cortex.

Collaterals to RAS funnel from the following sources (Fig. 10.11-1):

- Long, ascending sensory pathways such as spinothalamic tracts are the important sources of collaterals to RAS. The fibres of the tracts, which convey slow pain, send the richest collateral connections to the RAS.

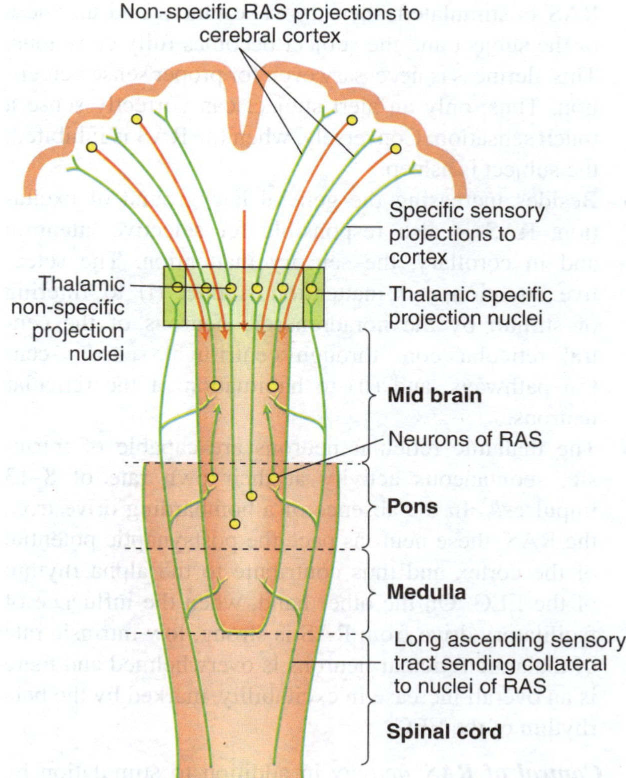

FIGURE 10.11-1 Diagrammatic depiction of reticular activating system (RAS) vis-a-vis specific sensory projections.

- In addition to long ascending sensory tracts, collateral to the RAS also funnel from the trigeminal, auditory, visual and olfactory pathway systems.

Efferent Projections from RAS are:

- Majority of RAS fibres end in nonspecific thalamic nuclei (intralaminar and midline nuclei), and from there are projected diffusely and nonspecifically to the whole neocortex (Fig. 10.11-1).
- Another part of RAS bypasses the thalamus to project diffusely to the cortex.

The RAS fibres occupy the core portion of the brainstem (Fig. 10.11-1). Whereas the specific fibres occupy the lateral parts of the brainstem.

Stimulation of RAS. The reticular activating system (RAS) is stimulated by impulses funnelled into it through the collateral described above. Thus, the RAS is a *non-specific system* which can be excited by any sensation. Whereas, the classic sensory pathways are specific in that the fibres in them are activated by only one type of sensory stimulation.

Functions of RAS are:

- RAS sends a strong facilitatory drive to the central neurons, raising their background excitability and increasing their responsiveness to specific stimuli. Thus, when

RAS is stimulated, there is wakefulness and alertness of the subject and the subject becomes fully conscious. This alertness is necessary even for proper sense perception. Thus, only an alert subject can correctly sense a touch sensation. Conversely, when the RAS is inhibited, the subject is asleep.

- Besides increasing the general background of excitation, RAS is also responsible for selective attention and in corollary, the sensory inattention. The selective attention and inattention is due: (i) to filtering of stimuli by the noradrenergic neurons of the central reticular core through centrifugal sensory central pathways, and (ii) to habituation of the reticular neurons.
- The thalamic reticular neurons are capable of intrinsic, spontaneous activity at their own rate of 8–13 impulses/s. In the absence of a bombarding drive from the RAS, these neurons pace the postsynaptic potential of the cortex and thus contribute to the alpha rhythm of the EEG. On the other hand, when the influence of facilitatory drive from RAS is strong, low intrinsic rate of thalamic reticular neurons is overwhelmed and there is an overall increase in excitability, marked by the beta rhythm of the EEG.

***Control of RAS** activity* in addition to stimulation by sensory collaterals is:

- The neural activity of the central core and consequently of the RAS are under feedback influence of the corticofugal impulses to the reticular formation. *Facilitatory feedback impulses* come from the motor cortex while centrifugal *inhibition* is from the limbic cortex.
- Under the specific *inhibitory influence* of the raphe neurons, the RAS drive and the intrinsic thalamic activity are both considerably reduced and EEG characteristic of sleep sets in.

Applied Aspects of RAS which need mention are:

- ***Lesions of RAS*** in experimental animals produce interminable sleep and coma. In humans also, lesions in the RAS (e.g. tumours) cause prolonged sleep.
- ***Many agents producing sedation,*** hypnosis, and anaesthesia (e.g. benzodiazepine and barbiturates) act by preventing synaptic transmission in RAS and thus inhibiting the RAS.

Neurotransmitters of Reticular Formation

Some of the systems employing different neurotransmitters which have been identified in reticular formation are:

- ***Large cholinergic neurons*** of midbrain and pontine reticular formation project to the cerebral cortex via relays in the thalamus.
- ***Small adrenergic neurons*** spread over the entire length of reticular formation and also project extensively to the cerebral cortex via relays in the intralaminar nuclei of the thalamus.
- ***Noradrenergic neurons*** from several areas of the reticular formation project to cerebellum.
- ***Dopaminergic neurons*** of midbrain reticular formation and substantia nigra project to several basal ganglia.
- ***Serotonergic neurons*** of the raphe nuclei in the lower pontine and medullary reticular formation project to thalamus and cerebral cortex besides projecting to the hypothalamus and limbic structures.

Serotonergic neurons in the raphe nuclei of medullary reticular formation also project to the substantia gelatinosa of the spinal cord where they control transmission of pain impulses.

In the serotonergic system, a neuroactive peptide usually coexists in the same neuron. Serotonergic neurons, having different peptides accompanying them may project to different cells, or different combinations of transmitters may control the activity of the same cell differently. One of the substances may act as a transmitter, and the other as a modulator.

The possibilities for different ways in which combinations of neurotransmitters may exert their effect are virtually endless.

Functions of Reticular Formation

1. Sleep-wakefulness. The RAS of reticular formation is the neural substrate of the consciousness and sleep–waking cycle (for details see page 1112).

2. Selective Attention and Sensory Inattention. The reticular formation is also responsible for selective attention and sensory inattention, through the corticofugal control of sensory input and due to habituation.

3. Conditioning and Learning. Reticular formation is an integral part of the neural substrate for conditioning and learning (for details see page 1118).

4. Control of Muscle Tone and Regulation of Postural Reflex Changes. Reticular formation modulates the tone of extensor (antigravity) muscles. The pontine (medial) reticulospinal tract has an excitatory and the medullary (lateral) reticulospinal tract has an inhibitory influence on extensor muscle tone (for details see page 1063).

5. Autonomic Functions. The visceral regulating centres are an integral part of the reticular formation. The influence of higher neurons over the viscera and autonomic functions are mediated through the visceral centres in reticular formation.

6. Modulation of Pain. Serotonergic neurons of the modulatory raphe nuclei form a part of the endogenous pain relief system. By affecting the transmission of pain impulses through the substantia gelatinosa of the spinal cord, these neurons modulate the perception of pain (for details see page 1035).

7. Control of Neuroendocrine System. The reticular formation projections play a role in the control of neuroendocrine systems in the hypothalamus.

ELECTRICAL ACTIVITY OF THE BRAIN

Evoked Cortical Potentials

Evoked potential refers to surface electrical activity recorded from the surface of the scalp in response to a specific and adequate stimulus—auditory, visual or somatosensory. Stimulation by a specific adequate stimulus produces two types of electrical activity in the cerebral cortex known as primary evoked potential and diffuse secondary response. It is important to note that the evoked potential recorded is barely discernible amidst the backdrop of EEG waves (the noise). In order to identify the evoked potential, the technique of averaging is used in order to enhance the signal-to-noise ratio.

Primary Evoked Potential. This is the initial, brief (lasting for few milliseconds) and localized response over the specific sensory cortex. For example, in the foot area of the postcentral gyrus, if an electrical shock is administered over the foot or over the occipital lobe after photopic stimulation, the primary evoked potential is characterized by (Fig. 10.11-2):

- Latency of about 5–12 ms (average 10 ms).
- First there appears a surface positive wave which is followed by a small negative wave.
- The primary evoked potential is highly specific in its location and can be observed only where the pathway from a particular sensory organ ends, i.e. it is produced by conduction of sensory signals through the specific sensory pathways.

Secondary Diffuse Response is characterized by:

- Latency of about 20–80 ms (average 50 ms), i.e. it appears at about 50 ms of sensory stimulus.
- Positive–negative wave sequence of the secondary diffuse response is frequently larger and more prolonged than the positive–negative wave sequence of primary evoked potential.
- The surface-positive diffuse secondary response, unlike the primary, is not highly localized. It can be recorded at the same time from most of the cerebral cortex. It is due to spread of impulses through the RAS to the cerebral cortex.

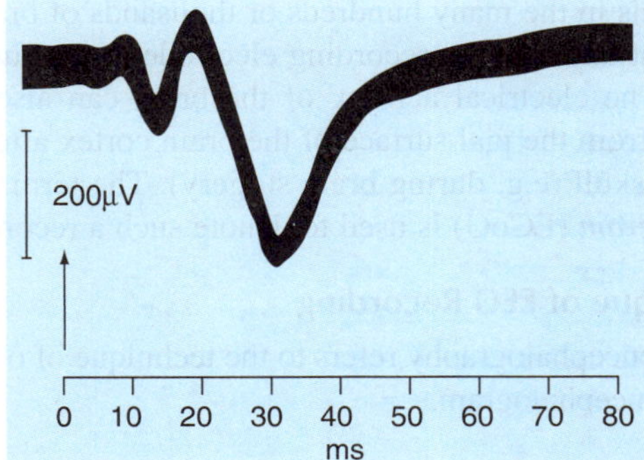

FIGURE 10.11-2 Response evoked in contralateral sensory cortex by stimulation of sciatic nerve in a cat. The upward deflection is surface negative.

Types of Evoked Potentials

Depending on the type of stimulus the evoked potential can be:

- Visual evoked potential (VEP),
- Brainstem auditory evoked potential (BAEP),
- Somatosensory evoked potential (SEP) and so on.

Depending upon the latency of response, evoked potential can be classified into:

- Stimulus-related potentials (short-, mid- and long latency) and
- Event-related or endogenous potentials.

Stimulus-related Potentials Stimulus-related potential refers to a series of waves that relates to the sensory modality. For example, the auditory stimulus-related response has been divided into three sequential time periods:

- Early latency response,
- Mid-latency response and
- Long latency response.

1. Early Latency Response (ELR) to an auditory stimulus is characterized by a latency of < 10 ms and is named as 'brainstem auditory evoked potential' (BAEP)'

Waves of ELR. Early latency response consists of a series of waves named I–VII (Fig. 10.11-3).

- *Wave I* represents the volume conducted electrical activity from the auditory nerve,
- *Wave II* from the pons and
- *Wave III* from the midbrain.

Interpeak latency (IPL) indirectly reflects the neural conduction in the corresponding segment of the central auditory pathway as:

- I–III IPL, i.e. interpeak latency between waves I and III is a measure of conduction in the more caudal segment of the brainstem auditory pathway, i.e. the auditory nerve and pontomedullary portion.
- III–V IPL is a measure of conduction in the more rostral (pontine and midbrain) portions of the pathway.

2. Mid-latency Response (MLR) to an auditory stimulus is characterized by a latency of 10–50 ms. It is considered to represent the electrical activity arising in the thalamocortical radiations, the primary auditory cortex and the early association cortex.

3. Long Latency Response (LLR) to an auditory stimulus is characterized by a latency of more than 50 ms. The neural generators of long latency response are unknown. It is a negative–positive complex comprising (Fig. 10.11-4):

- A large negative wave (N_1) and
- A large positive wave (P_2).

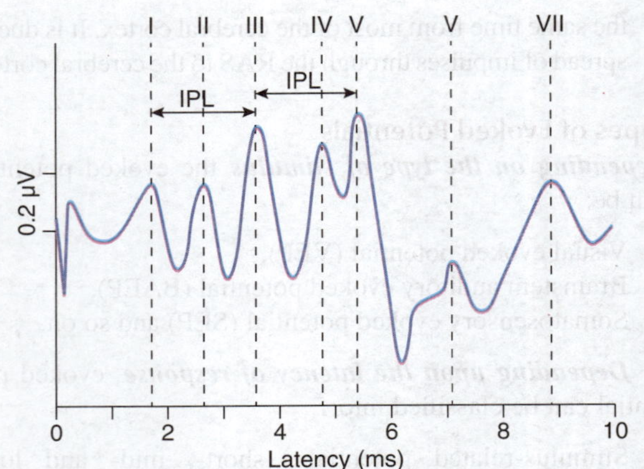

FIGURE 10.11-3 Early latency response to an auditory stimulus of 60 dB at 10/sec (brainstem auditory evoked potential).

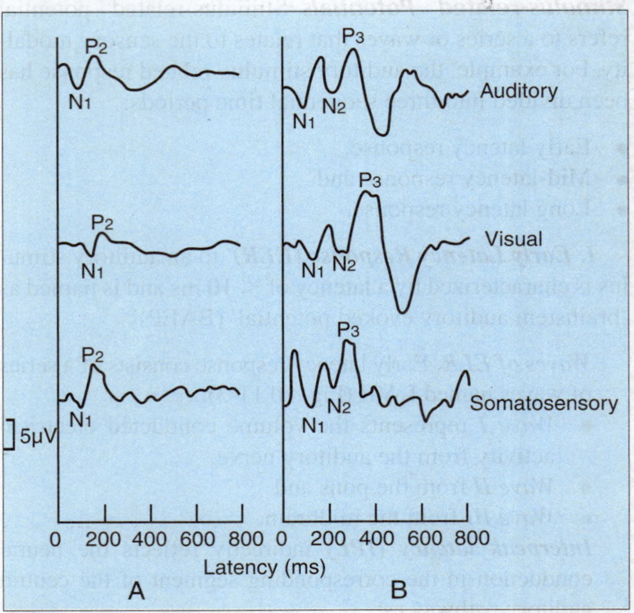

FIGURE 10.11-4 Stimulus-related (**A**) and event-related (**B**) long latency potential evoked by auditory, visual and somatosensory stimuli.

The visual and somatosensory stimuli too elicit a similar response (Fig. 10.11-4). All these responses are stimulus evoked and reflect the functional integrity of the sensory pathways in the CNS. Unlike the event-related potentials (discussed below), they are largely independent of the subject's attention or level of arousal.

Event-related Potentials (ERPS) Event-related potentials (ERPs) are dependent upon the subject's attention or level of arousal (c.f. stimulus-related potential, as described above). The ERPs are elicited only when the subject is required to distinguish one stimulus (the target) from the other (the nontargets). The ERPs primarily depend upon the setting, in which the target stimulus occurs and are relatively independent of the physical characteristics of that stimulus. Thus, ERPs are related to the cognitive events associated with the distinction of target from nontarget stimuli. Long latency response in event-related potentials is also a negative–positive complex comprising (Fig. 10.11-4):

- A negative wave (N_2) and
- A positive wave (P_3).

Clinical Uses of Evoked Potentials

Stimulus-related Evoked Potentials reflect the functional integrity of the sensory pathways from receptor to cortex. Therefore, any delay in conduction as depicted by delayed peak or interpeak latencies would be of diagnostic value. The lesions interrupting the conduction pathways can be inflammations, demyelinating disorders, degenerative lesions and tumours. For example in patients with optic neuritis due to multiple sclerosis (a demyelinating disorder), the abnormal visually evoked potentials (VEP) is diagnostic.

Event-related Evoked Potentials are related to cognitive behaviour. Therefore, considerable interest has developed in the possible clinical use of these potentials in the evaluation of patients who suffer from disorders of cognition. The use of ERPs in the clinical assessment of dementia and delirium is fairly well established by now. *Dementia* refers to an abnormal deterioration of intellect affecting several areas of cognitive functions, such as abstraction, orientation, judgement and memory more than 50%. Cases of dementia are due to age-related, senile dementia of Alzheimer's type. ERPs in patients with dementia are characterized by prolonged latency and reduced amplitude of P_3 component (Fig. 10.11-5).

Electroencephalogram

The term electroencephalogram (EEG) (introduced by the German psychiatrist Hans Berger) refers to record of spontaneous electrical activity of the brain taken from the surface of scalp (c.f. evoked potential which is the surface electrical activity recorded in response to a specific and adequate stimulus). The spontaneous electrical activity of the brain is due largely to graded or summated postsynaptic potentials in the many hundreds or thousands of brain neurons that underlie the recording electrode at the surface of scalp. The electrical activity of the brain can also be recorded from the pial surface of the brain cortex after opening the skull (e.g. during brain surgery). The term *electrocorticogram* (ECoG) is used to denote such a record.

Technique of EEG Recording

Electroencephalography refers to the technique of obtaining electroencephalogram.

Bipolar Versus Unipolar Electroencephalogram

Bipolar electroencephalogram is the record of potential variations between a pair of scalp (cortex) electrodes.

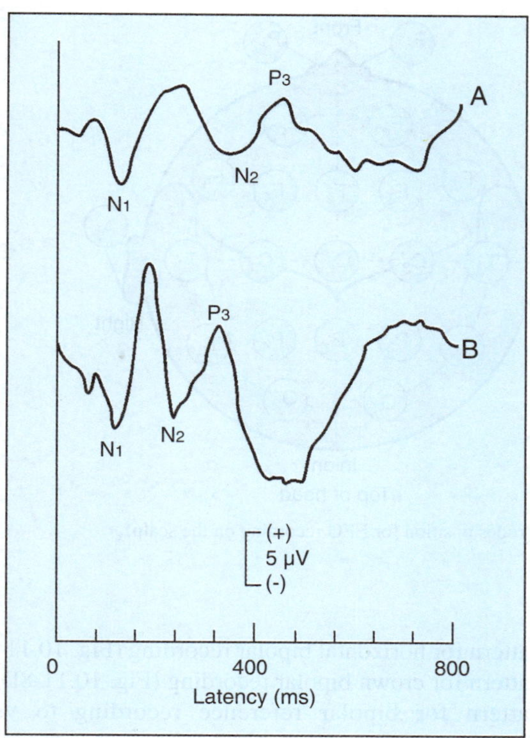

FIGURE 10.11-5 Event-related potential (ERP) in a patient with dementia (**A**) shows prolonged latency and reduced amplitude of P_3 component as compared to a normal subject (**B**).

Unipolar electroencephalogram is the record of potential variation between an active scalp (cortical) electrode and a theoretically indifferent electrode placed on some part of the body (distant from the cortex such as earlobe).

Thus, the electroencephalography basically involves record of potential difference between a pair of scalp electrodes (bipolar electroencephalography) or between an active scalp electrode and an indifferent electrode (unipolar electroencephalography). The electrodes are connected to a cathode ray oscilloscope (CRO) via a suitable amplifier. The modern EEG machine has 8–16 channels, which can simultaneously record electrical activity from areas of many scalp electrodes.

Location of Electrodes Different techniques such as Illinois, Montreal, AIRD or Cahn methods have been described to determine the electrode attaching positions. The most popular method is the *International 10–20 system (Montreal method)* recommended by the International Federation of Societies for Electroencephalography and Clinical Neurophysiology. This system is based upon measurement from four standard points on the head: the nasion, the union and the left and right preauricular points. This system is named '10–20 system', because electrodes are spaced either 10 or 20% of the total distance between a given pair of skull landmarks as (Fig. 10.11-6):

- The longitudinal line of the head is divided into portions of 10, 20, 20, 20, 20 and 10%, respectively, on the basis of nasions and inions (Fig. 10.11-6A).
- The transverse line of the head is divided into portions of 10, 20, 20, 20, 20 and 10% on the basis of left and right preauricular points (Fig. 10.11-6B).
- The whole area of scalp is then divided into various points on the basis of lines passing through the above described points on the longitudinal and transverse lines (Fig. 10.11-6C). These points have been given electrode numbers (Fig. 10.11-7A), international symbols (Fig. 10.11-7B) and names (Table10.11-1).

EEG Recording Modes Before an EEG signal comes to the input of the amplifier through the electrode, the electrode position of the channels are determined by the montage selector. The method of combining the electrode positions is called *montage*. Each montage includes a predetermined connection format. The predetermined combinations of electrode connections are called patterns. EEGs used in

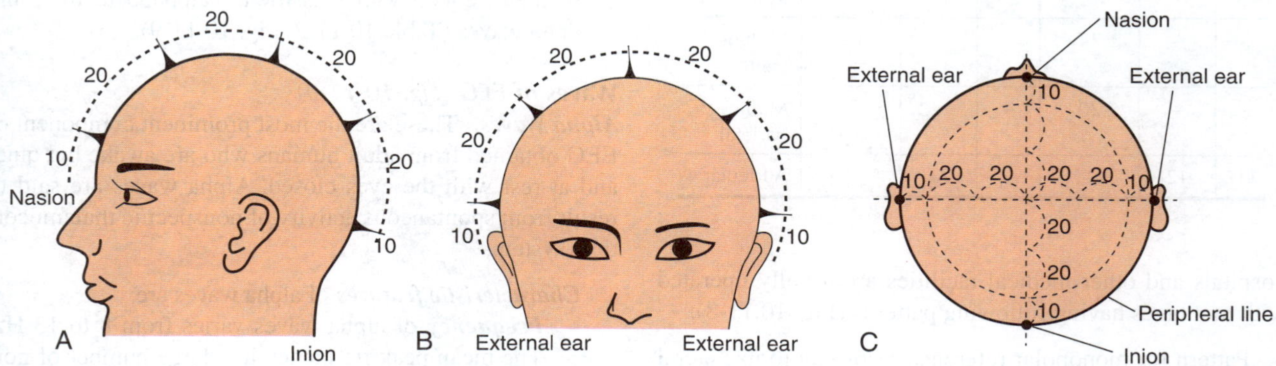

FIGURE 10.11-6 Reference points in International '10–20 System of electrode position for EEG recording: divisions of longitudinal nasion–inion line (**A**); transverse left and right earline (**B**); and various points on the scalp on the basis of lines passing through (**C**).

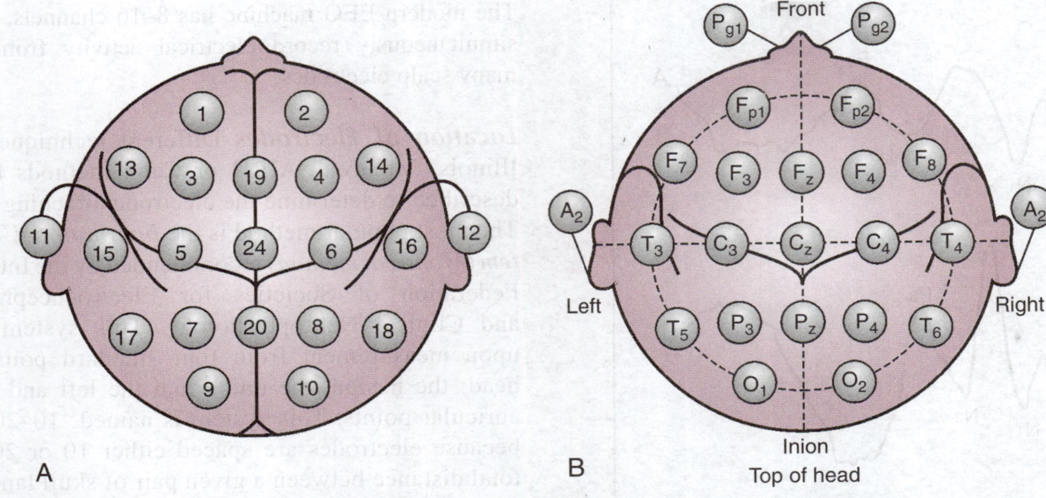

FIGURE 10.11-7 Number **(A)**, symbols **(B)** for different electrodes position for EEG recording on the scalp.

TABLE 10.11-1 Name, Number and Position of Electrodes on the Scalp for Recording Electroencephalogram

Electrode number			International symbol			Name
Left	*Right*	*Midline*	*Left*	*Right*	*Midline*	
1	2	–	FP_1	FP_2	–	Frontal pole
3	4	–	F_3	F_4	–	Frontal
5	6	–	C_3	C_4	–	Centre
7	8	–	P_3	P_4	–	Parietal
9	10	–	O_1	O_2	–	Occipital
13	14	–	F_7	F_8	–	Anterior temporal
15	16	–	T_3	T_4	–	Middle temporal
17	18	–	T_5	T_6	–	Posterior temporal
–	–	19	–	–	F_Z	Midline frontal
–	–	24	–	–	C_Z	Midline central
–	–	20	–	–	P_Z	Midline parietal
11	12	–	A_1	A_2	–	Auricular

hospitals and other medical facilities are usually operated with montages having following patterns (Fig. 10.11-8):

- Pattern for monopolar reference recording to ipsilateral ears (Fig. 10.11-8A),
- Pattern for vertical bipolar recording or parasagittal chains (Fig. 10.11-8B),
- Pattern for horizontal bipolar recording (Fig. 10.11-8C),
- Pattern for crown bipolar recording (Fig. 10.11-8D and
- Pattern for bipolar reference recording to vertex (Fig. 10.11-8E).

Normal Electroencephalogram

The electroencephalogram (EEG) consists of waves which are oscillations in the electrical potential of the brain having the following characteristics:

- The oscillations differ in the frequency and amplitude at different points on the scalp and during different stages of mental alertness.
- *Frequencies* of brain waves range from 1 to over 50 cycles/s.
- *Amplitude* of brain waves may vary from 50 to 200 μV.
- Much of the time, brain waves are *irregular* and no general pattern is obtained. At other times, distinct patterns do appear.
- Different waves recorded in a normal person, depending on their frequency are classified as alpha, beta, theta and delta waves (Table 10.11-2, Fig. 10.11-9).

Waves of EEG *(Fig. 10.11-9)*

Alpha Waves. These are the most prominent component of EEG obtained from adult humans who are awake but quiet and at rest with the eyes closed. Alpha waves are said to result from spontaneous activity of nonspecific thalamocortical system.

Characteristic features of alpha waves are:

- ***Frequency*** of alpha waves varies from 8 to 13 Hz. The mean peak frequency in a large number of normal adults is 4.2 Hz.
- ***Amplitude*** of these waves slowly waxes and wanes, but the average amplitude is about 50 μV.

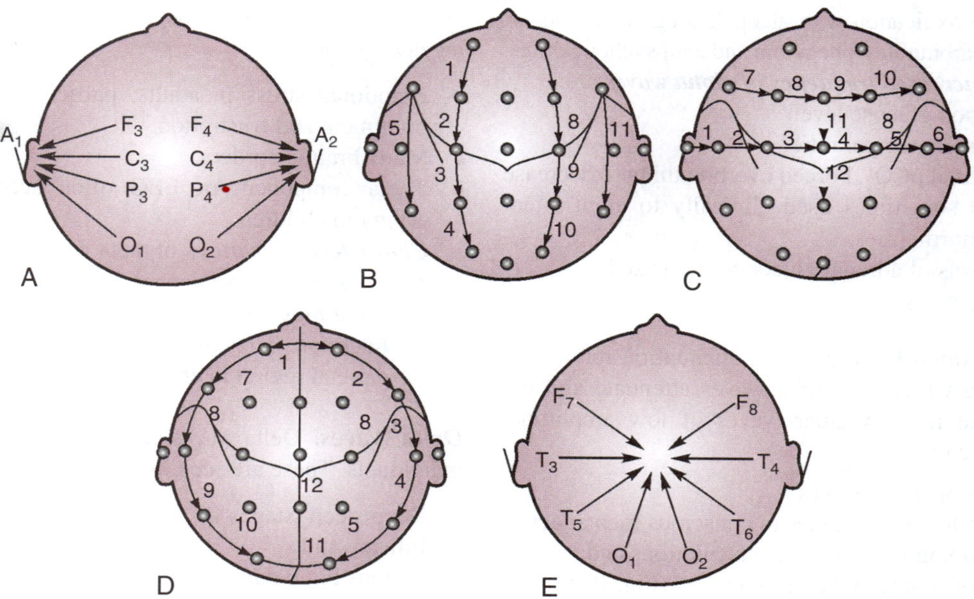

FIGURE 10.11-8 Montages, i.e. patterns of predetermined combination of electrode connections used commonly for EEG recording in hospitals: **A,** for monopolar reference recording to ipsilateral ears; **B,** for bipolar vertical recording; **C,** for horizontal bipolar recording; **D,** for crown bipolar recording; and **E,** for bipolar reference recording to vertex.

TABLE 10.11-2 Classification of Brain Waves Depending on Frequency of Oscillations

Frequency (in Hz)	Type of EEG wave	Amplitude (in μV)
1–4	Delta (δ)	20–200
4–7	Theta (θ)	10
8–13	Alpha (α)	50
14–30	Beta (β)	5–10

- ***Location.*** Alpha waves are most marked in the parieto-occipital area of the scalp, though these are observed sometimes from other locations as well.
- ***Disappear*** during sleep.

Causes of decreased frequency of alpha waves are:

- Old age, due to decreased cerebral perfusion leading to decreased cerebral metabolism,
- Low blood glucose level,
- Low body temperature,
- Low levels of adrenal glucocorticoids,
- High arterial partial pressure of CO_2 and
- Sleep.
- The frequency and magnitude of alpha rhythms is also reduced in encephalopathies (metabolic, toxic or due to hyponatraemia and vitamin B_{12} deficiency)

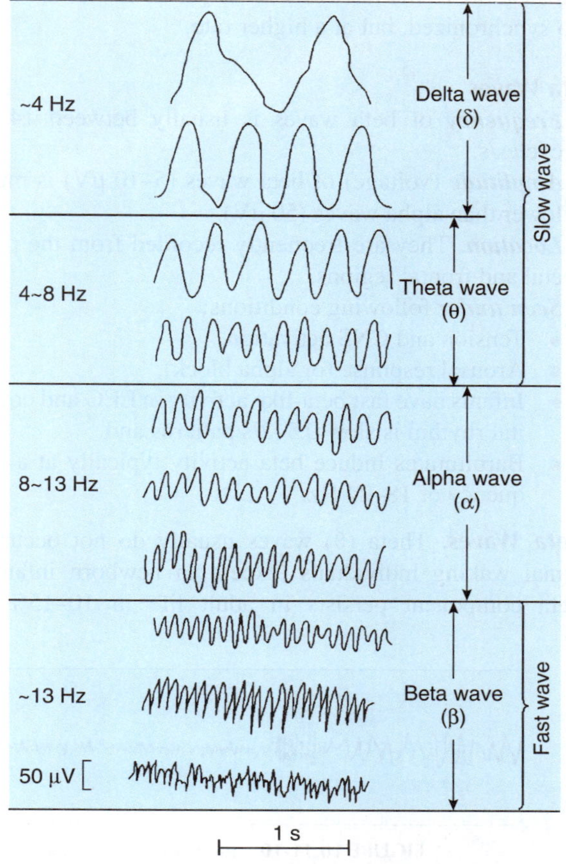

FIGURE 10.11-9 Different types of normal EEG waves.

- Acute intoxification with alcohol, drugs like amphetamine, barbiturates, phenytoin and antipsychotic drugs.

Causes of increased frequency of alpha waves are:

- High blood glucose level,
- Rise in body temperature,
- Low arterial pCO_2. Forced overbreathing to decrease pCO_2 is sometimes used clinically to elicit latent EEG abnormalities.
- High levels of adrenal glucocorticoids and
- Alerting states.

Alpha Block *Alpha block* or alpha attenuation refers to a phenomenon in which the alpha waves attenuate and are replaced by the fast, irregular waves of low amplitude. Alpha block occurs when:

- The persons open their eyes,
- When the individual engages in conscious mental activity such as doing mathematical calculations and
- When any form of stimulation is applied (Fig. 10.11-10).

The term *aroused* or *alerting response* is also used to denote an alpha block, since it is correlated with arousal or alerting response.

The term desynchronization has also been suggested for alpha block, because it represents breaking up of the obviously synchronized neural activity necessary to produce regular alpha waves. However, the term desynchronization is misleading as the fast EEG activity seen in alert states is also synchronized, but at a higher rate.

Beta Waves

- ***Frequency*** of beta waves is usually between 14–30 cycles/s.
- ***Amplitude*** (voltage) of beta waves (5–10 μV) is much lower than alpha waves (50 μV).
- ***Location.*** They are frequently recorded from the parietal and frontal regions.
- ***Seen under*** following conditions:
  - Tension and CNS activation,
  - Arousal response (or alpha block),
  - Infants have fast beta-like activity in EEG and occipital rhythm is slow 0.5–2/s patterns and
  - Barbiturates induce beta activity typically at a frequency of 18–24 Hz.

Theta Waves. Theta (θ) waves usually do not occur in normal waking individuals (except in newborn infants). Theta component persists in adult life in 10–15% of normal subjects. Usually theta waves are seen under following conditions:

- Emotional stress in adults, particularly during disappointment and frustration.
- Many brain disorders.
- Theta component of EEG often accentuates during crying in children.

Characteristic features of theta waves are:

- ***Frequency*** is between 4–7 Hz.
- ***Amplitude*** (10 μV) is slightly larger than alpha waves.
- ***Location.*** They are recorded from the temporal and parietal region in children.

Delta Waves. Delta waves do not occur in normal waking individuals. These are seen in following conditions:

- Deep sleep (stages III and IV of non-REM sleep),
- Infancy and
- Serious brain damage.

Characteristic features (Fig. 10.11-9) are:

- ***Frequency*** is less than 4 Hz,
- ***Amplitude*** is very high (20–200 μV),
- ***Can be produced*** by overbreathing,
- ***Occurs strictly*** in the cortex independent of activities in lower regions of the brain, therefore, they occur in sleep when cortex is released from the activating influence of lower centres.

Neurophysiological Basis of EEG

The neurophysiological basis of EEG has not been fully elucidated. Some of the important points in this regard are:

Cortical Grey Matter Along with its Thalamic Connection plays an important role in the EEG. Largely, the activity recorded in the EEG is that of rhythmically discharging cell bodies in the most superficial layers of cortical grey matter. Thalamus discharge synchronizes this activity.

Current Flow in the Fluctuating Dipoles formed by the cell bodies and dendrites of the cortical cells accounts for the potential changes recorded as EEG. The dendrites are the sites of nonpropagated hypopolarizing and hyperpolarizing local potential changes. The cell dendrites relationship is, therefore, that of a constantly shifting dipole. Hence they become sites of current sink. The dense dendritic tree is present in a particular (vertical) orientation and this results in the brainwave patterns (Fig. 10.11-11).

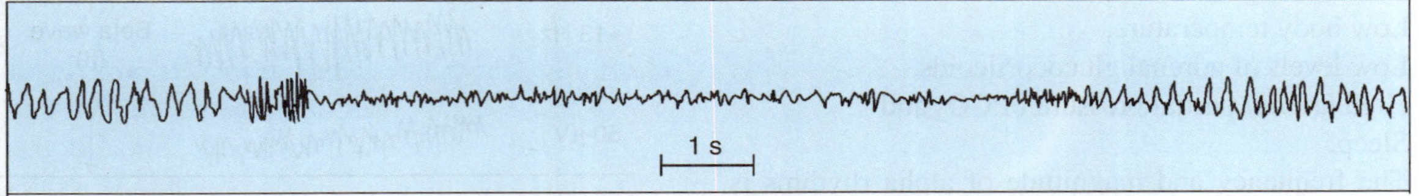

FIGURE 10.11-10 Electroencephalography depicting alpha block produced by olfactory stimulus in a rabbit.

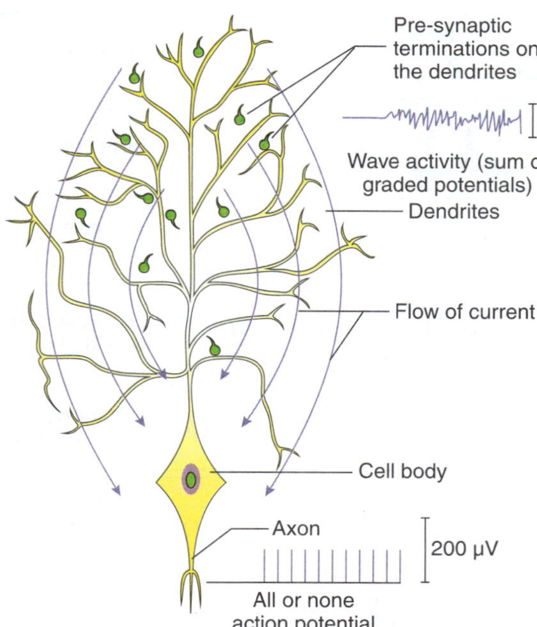

FIGURE 10.11-11 Electrical activity recorded from vertically oriented dendritic tree of pyramidal cells in the cerebral cortex compared to that recorded from an axon.

In general, when the sum of the dendritic activity is positive relative to the cell, the cell is hyperpolarized and less excitable and when it is negative the cell is depolarized and hyperexcitable. Thus, the EEG is due to graded potentials which are summated postsynaptic potentials in the brain neurons (Fig. 10.11-11).

Synchronizing mechanisms. Synchronizing activity of neighbouring cells and rhythmic discharge from thalamus are responsible for the synchronizing mechanism.

1. ***Synchronizing activity of neighbouring cells*** is due to:
   - The effect of parallel neural processes on each other in a volume conductor (Fig. 10.11-12).
   - The interconnection of neurons by inhibitory pathway.
2. ***Rhythmic discharge from thalamus*** also responsible for synchronization of EEG waves is evident from following observations:
   - Stimulation of certain thalamic nuclei of the frequency of about 8 cycles/s produces on EEG record with similar frequency in greater part of the ipsilateral cerebral cortex. The amplitude of the waves also waxes and wanes, i.e. alpha rhythms are produced.
   - Large lesions of the thalamus produce disturbances in the synchronized activity of the EEG on the side of lesion.

Desynchronizing mechanisms. Desynchronization, as mentioned earlier in alpha block, refers to replacement of a rhythmic EEG pattern with irregular low voltage activity (arousal reaction). It occurs due to sensory stimulation of the reticular activating system (RAS) as is evident from the following observations:

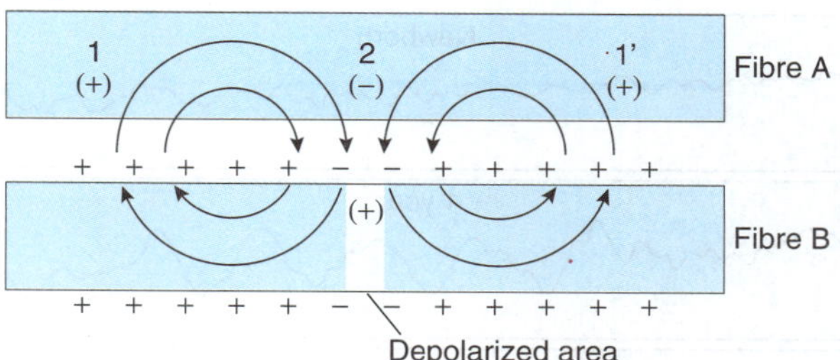

FIGURE 10.11-12 The electrical property of two parallel placed nerve fibres. Note that current flows into the depolarized area of active fibre B from the surrounding membrane as an impulse passes along the nerve. At points 1 and 1' on the membrane of inactive fibre A positive charges build-up. Thus the membrane becomes slightly hypopolarized in these two regions. At point 2 of the fibre A positive charges are removed, so the membrane undergoes a slight depolarization at this point.

- Stimulation of specific sensory system up to midbrain only (up to where reticular formation is present) produces desynchronization; and the stimulation of these systems above the midbrain does not produce desynchronization.
- Large lesions of the midbrain that interrupt the medial lemnisci and other ascending specific sensory systems fail to prevent the desynchronization produced by specific sensory stimulation below the midbrain level.
- High frequency stimulation of reticular formation in the midbrain features like that of nonspecific projection nuclei of the thalamus produces desynchronization and arousal in sleeping animals.
- Lesions in the midbrain tegmentum that disrupt the RAS without damaging the specific systems are associated with a synchronized EEG pattern that is unaffected by sensory stimulation.

Variations in the EEG Wave Formation with Age The EEG, wave forms at rest in humans and varies with age as (Fig. 10.11-13):

- *In infants* (up to 1 year of age) the occipital rhythm is slow (0.5–2 Hz) than those of adults (8–13 Hz).
- *In children*, the occipital rhythm speeds up and, the adult alpha pattern gradually appears during adolescence.
  - In children of 4 years of age, theta and alpha waves of 7–8 Hz appear.
  - In 9-year-old children, an alpha wave of about 10 Hz appears in the occipital region.
  - After 15 years of age, the EEG waveforms become almost the same as those of adults.
- In adults (between 15 and 60 years) the EEG wave forms and the typical adult alpha pattern is seen. However, even during these ages, the slow waves decrease as the age rises and the fast waves increase *over 60 years of age*, the slow waves increase again as the age increases.

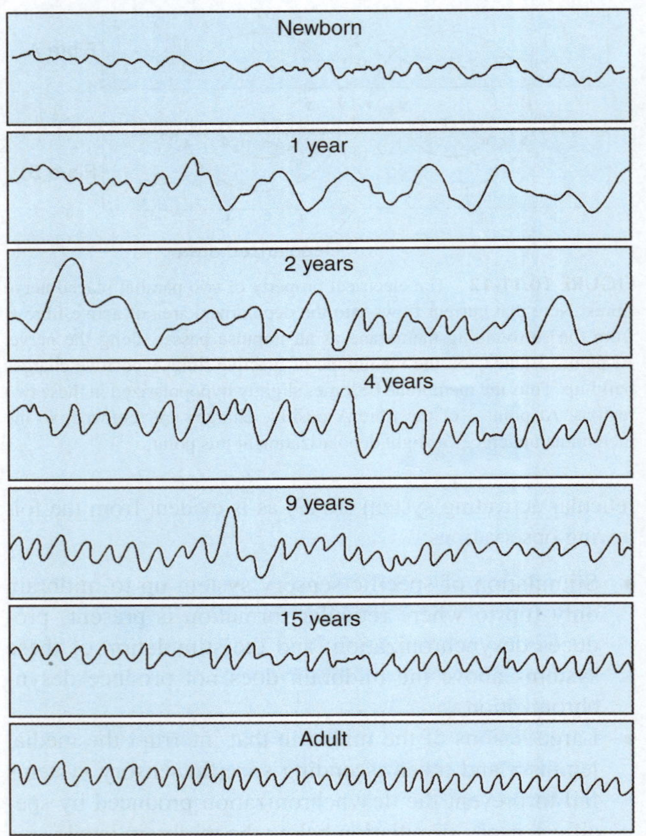

FIGURE 10.11-13 Variations in the EEG wave forms with age.

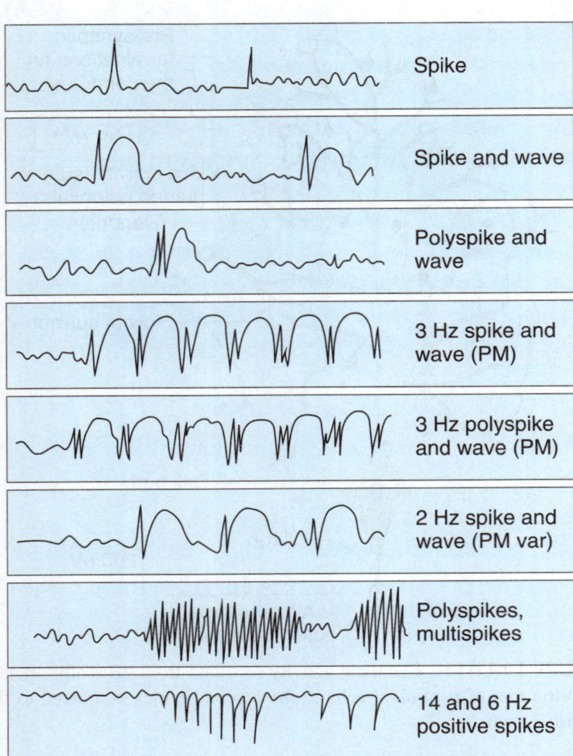

FIGURE 10.11-14 EEG waveform of epilepsy. PM = petit mal.

Applied Aspects

Abnormal EEG Waveforms

1. Epilepsy Epilepsy is a syndrome in which there are recurring seizures due to damage to the brain.

Electroencephalographic inspection is indispensable to the diagnosis of epilepsy. Epileptic seizure represents highly synchronized but abnormal neuronal activity. The waveforms of epilepsy (Fig. 10.11-14) include idiopathic abnormal waves such as a spike, sharp wave and spike and slow wave complexes. Between these abnormal waves, an irregular slow wave appears and the background waveform is disturbed. An abnormal wave sometimes appears isolated in the limited part or continues all over the waveform. The generating condition and form are different case by case. A general spike slow wave complex of 3 Hz appears in the case of absent petit mal. Autonomic nerve fit is characterized by a positive spike of 14 or 6 Hz. Nod spasm is characterized by seriously abnormal rhythm and is called a wasting syndrome and seen in babies. Serious fit is usually accompanied by a spasm and consciousness is lost. The EEG waveform shows continuous spikes or sharp waves.

Epileptic seizures are of two types, partial and generalized.

(i) *Partial seizures* usually occur due to involvement of a small group of neurons due to causes like; head injury, infection, tumour or stroke. The partial seizures are further of two subtypes; simple and complex.

- Simple partial seizure, in which there is no loss of consciousness. The typical seizure is characterized by localized jerky movements in one hand progressing to clonic movements of the entire arm, lasting for about 60–90 s and

The seizure is always preceded by typical aura comprising of abnormal sensations. The time period for normal neurological activity to return back after the seizure is called the postictal period.

- Complex partial seizure is not associated with altered consciousness.

(ii) *Generalized seizures*. In this type, there is simultaneous widespread electrical activity in both the cerebral hemispheres. Generalized seizures are also of further two subtypes; convulsive and nonconvulsive, depending on tonic and clonic movements.

- Tonic–clonic seizure formerly called *grand mal epilepsy* or convulsive generalized seizure is characterized by tonic phase (in which there is sudden onset of contractions of the limb muscles for about 30 s) followed by clonic phase (alternating contraction and relaxation of limb muscles causing jerky movements) lasting for 1–2 min. **EEG** changes during tonic phase show fast activity and slow wave activity (each slow wave preceded by spike) occurs during clonic phase.

- Absence seizure formerly called *petit mal epilepsy* is a nonconvulsive generalized seizure, characterized by momentary loss of consciousness only. There is no typical aura and postictic period. EEG changes show doublets (3/s), each comprised a typical spike and wave pattern lasting for 10 s. This pattern of EEG occurs due to activation of low threshold T-type Ca^{2+} channels of thalamic neurons.

Pathophysiology: Epilepsy occurs due to release of glutamate from astrocytes. The current view suggests that there are structural basis for increase in excitability due to reorganization of astrocytes along with sprouting of dendrites and new synapse formation.

- Genetic mutation-Mutation of certain ion channels have been associated with idiopathic epilepsy which occurs in different forms:
  - *Childhood absence epilepsy (CAE)* is associated with mutation of a subunit gene (responsible for GABA receptors called as GABA B_3).
  - *Inherited form* of generalized epilepsy with fever (febrile seizures) is associated with mutation of sodium channel subunit gene called SCNIA and SCNIB mutations.

Treatment: The basis of therapeutic measures for epilepsy is to reduce excitability, by enhancement of inhibitory neuronal transmission (increase release of GABA).

The anticonvulsant drugs include:

- Gabapentin acts by decreasing Ca^{2+} influx into the cells and reduces glutamate release.
- Topiramate blocks voltage-gated Na^{+} channels associated with glutamate receptors resulting in potentiation of inhibitory effect of GABA.
- Ethosuxamide reduces low threshold T-type Ca^{2+} currents in thalamic neurons, therefore, effectively used for treatment of absence seizures.
- Phenytoin and valproate act on voltage-gated Na^{+} channels to reduce glutamate release, thus block firing of neurons.

Surgery: The seizures associated with temporal lobe are treated by surgical treatment.

Vagal nerve stimulation is effective in partial seizures.

Activation. Activation is made to detect latent epilepsy, which cannot be detected by ordinary EEG recording. A flash stimulus, hyperventilation, sleep or drug administration is used to induce an epileptic attack.

2. Consciousness Dysfunction A slow wave appears in the case of consciousness dysfunction according to the degree of seriousness. In the serious case, a general slow wave or delta-wave prevails in the EEG waveform. In the more serious cases, the waveform becomes flat or sometimes disappears. However, there are many exceptions. Disturbances of consciousness include coma, syncope and stupor.

(i) ***Coma***. Coma refers to a permanent state of sleep which is characterized by a loss of consciousness from which arousal cannot be elicited. It is produced by lesions blocking the connection between the ascending RAS and the thalamus.

O_2 consumption of the brain is reduced in coma. This is in marked contrast to normal sleep, in which there is no change in brain O_2 consumption from the waking state.

During state of coma, stimulation of sensory pathways can cause a momentary desynchronization of the EEG but does not produce any behavioural changes.

(ii) ***Syncope*** (fainting) refers to a transient pathologic loss of consciousness.

(iii) ***Stupor*** is the more persistent loss of consciousness, from which arousal can be obtained.

3. Organic Brain Dysfunction An abnormal wave appears when brain functional trouble occurs due to cerebral tumour, brain–blood vessel trouble (bleeding, clogging, artery/vein leakage, hardened brain artery, etc.) or brain injury caused by an external wound of the head. In the case of brain tumour, e.g. no waveform is generated from the tumour part, but a slow wave is generated from the surrounding organization (Fig. 10.11-15). The EEG waveform shows the slow wave according to the seriousness of the brain functional trouble. When there is a tumour near the brain surface, a slow wave appears in accordance with that part and the waveform is of the irregular multiform. On the contrary, if there is a tumour deep in the brain, a monorhythmic high-amplitude slow wave like that of under the cortex or brainstem is seen. The slow wave increases as the tumour becomes serious.

4. Brain Death Labelling brain death is important to fulfill the desire to obtain organs for transplant operations and to remove the life-support system. *Criteria for labelling brain death* are; when the brain cells stop activity, the patient falls into a comatose state and finally respiration stops, the pupils are dilated, the EEG waveform becomes flat in all channels and finally disappears. Most patients die in this state.

WAKEFULNESS AND SLEEP

Wakefulness

The reticular activating system (RAS) of the reticular formation is the neural substrate of the consciousness and sleep–waking cycle. As described earlier, RAS is a complex polysynaptic pathway that projects diffusely from the brainstem reticular formation to the cerebral cortex, both directly as well as via the thalamus (for details

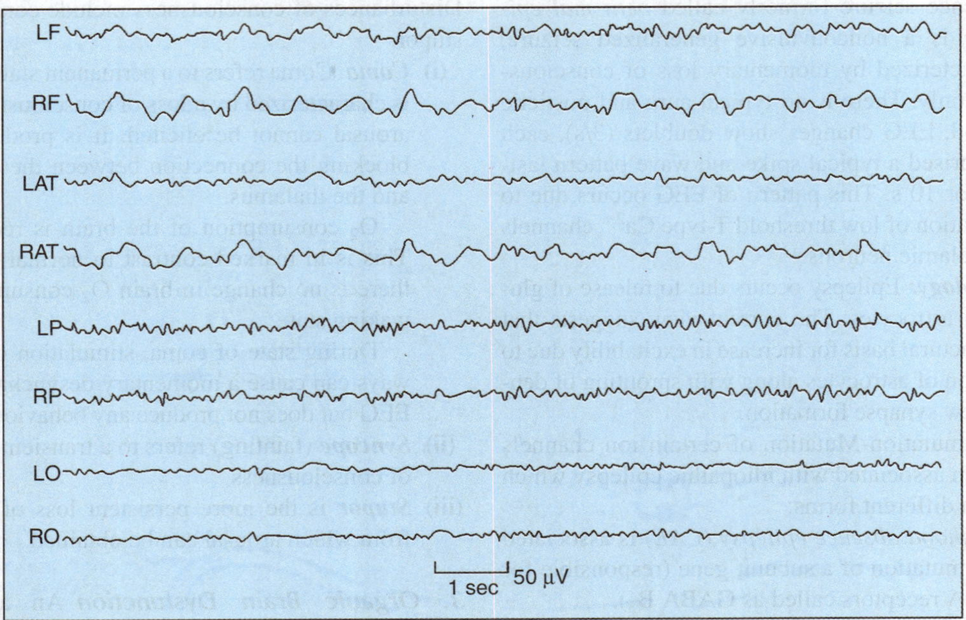

FIGURE 10.11-15 EEG waveform of brain tumour.

see page 950). The RAS is stimulated by impulses funnelling into it through the collaterals from the specific sensory pathways. The RAS, in turn sends a strong facilitatory drive to the cerebral cortex, raising the background excitability and increasing the responsiveness of central neurons to specific stimuli. According to Dr Magoun, an American brain physiologist, projection of nonspecific stimuli by RAS to cortex is responsible for wakefulness and alertness of the subject and the subject becomes fully conscious. When such impulse projection becomes less frequent, it is called sleep. When the pulse activity stops, it is called a dead sleep.

Neural Substrate for Wakefulness

In addition to the projections from the RAS, the wakefulness and consciousness are maintained by a continuous sensory input to the cortex from visceral as well as somatic systems via the nonspecific thalamic system, subthalamus, hypothalamus and basal forebrain. This is proved by *cerveau isolé* (transections separating the cerebrum, from the brainstem and spinal cord) which produces a sleep-like state with cortical slow waves. The neural substrates of wakefulness generating systems are described briefly:

1. Reticular Activating System (RAS), as discussed above, is mainly responsible for the tonic maintenance of the cortical activation and behavioural arousal of the wakefulness. The cortical activation and behavioural arousal are controlled by two different mechanisms:

- Cortical activations without behavioural arousal are produced by the central tegmentum of midbrain.
- Behavioural arousal without cortical activation is produced by the ventral tegmentum of midbrain.

2. Thalamus. The nonspecific thalamic system formed by the ventromedial, intralaminar and midline nuclei are involved in the activation of the entire cerebral cortex. These nuclei get tonic drive from the reticular formation, and in turn, project diffusely to cerebral cortex.

3. Hypothalamus and Subthalamus. The ascending impulses from midbrain reticular formation also relay to cerebral cortex through posterior hypothalamus and subthalamus. In addition, the posterior hypothalamus also acts as the waking centre, as its stimulation causes wakefulness. Conversely, lesions of posterior hypothalamus result in coma.

4. Basal Forebrain. It comprises the nucleus basalis of Meynert (substantia innominata), nuclei of the diagonal band and septum. The basal forebrain receives impulses from the reticular formation, and in turn, project to the cerebral cortex and is responsible for cortical activation of wakefulness.

Chemical Mediators of Wakefulness

Chemical mediators of wakefulness include:

- Neurotransmitters,
- CSF-borne peptides and
- Blood-borne peptides.

Neurotransmitters

1. Catecholamines. Norepinephrine neurons of the locus coeruleus and brainstem, which project diffusely to the forebrain, including the cortex, play an integral role in the

cortical activating system. This fact is corroborated by the following observations:

- ***L-dopa*** (a precursor of catecholamine) has been reported to cause improvement in comatose states due to cerebral lesions.
- ***Reserpine,*** a drug which depletes catecholamines in nerve terminals induces drowsiness.
- ***Amphetamine,*** a sympathomimetic amine, produces intense arousal and cortical activation.
- ***Cocaine*** also produces increased arousal and alertness. It acts by blocking reuptake of norepinephrine at the nerve terminals.

2. Acetylcholine. Cholinergic neurons, which contribute to wakefulness and cortical activation, can be divided into two major groups:

i. ***Neurons located in the caudal mesencephalic oral pontine reticular formation.*** These project forward into the forebrain, particularly into the medial intralaminar thalamic nuclei, and also into the lateral hypothalamus and the frontal cortex.
ii. ***Neurons located within the basal forebrain*** consist of substantia innominata or to nucleus basalis of Meynert, nuclei of diagonal band and septum. These project to the entire cerebral cortex in a widespread manner.

Role of cholinergic neurons in wakefulness is also corroborated by following observations:

- *Cholinergic agonists and anticholinesterases* (e.g. neostigmine) promote cortical activation and wakefulness.
- *Acetylcholine antagonist* like atropine produces a decrease in vigilance due to loss of cortical activation.
- *Alzheimer's disease*, which is associated with loss of cholinergic innervation of cerebral cortex and degeneration of cholinergic neurons of the basal forebrain, in addition to dementia is also characterized by sleep disturbances.

3. Histamine. The histamine-containing neurons are located in posterior hypothalamus. These account for:

- Arousing effect produced by intraventricular administration of histamine and
- Sedative effect produced by antihistaminic drugs.

4. Glutamate. It is an excitatory neurotransmitter released from cerebral cortex in highest quantities during cortical activation of spontaneous waking or that induced by stimulation of the midbrain reticular formation.

CSF-borne Peptides It has been presumed that wakefulness promoting factors (probably peptides) are present in CSF; since CSF taken from a waking donor animal is reported to produce wakefulness and cortical activation in the recipient animal. Some of the CSF-borne peptides, which have been known to produce wakefulness include:

- Substance P,
- Hypothalamic releasing factors and
- Vasoactive intestinal peptide (VIP).

Blood-borne Peptides Blood-borne peptides that act as wakefulness promoting factors are:

- ***Epinephrine and histamine.*** These do not cross the blood–brain barrier but act on the circumventricular organs that lie outside the blood–brain barrier and mediate cortical arousal.
- ***Glucocorticoids.*** These readily cross the blood–brain barrier and act directly on the neurons to enhance arousal in stress.

Sleep

Sleep refers to a state of unconsciousness from which the individual can be aroused by sensory or other stimuli. When asleep, an individual is not aware of the environment and is unable to perform activities that require consciousness. During sleep, the stimulus pulse transfer becomes less frequent between the reticular formation and cerebral cortex.

Factors Affecting Sleep. Sleep time remains fairly stable from day-to-day even under widely varying conditions, and is only modestly affected by variations in activity and sensory stimulation. However, the factors which minimize sensory stimulation and favour the onset of natural sleep are:

- Darkened room,
- Comfortable surrounding temperature,
- Silence,
- Physical and mental relaxation,
- Satiation of a basic urge such as hunger or sex and
- Low-frequency stimulation, such as by patting, rocking in a cradle or sitting in a moving vehicle.

The above described factors have only a modest effect, if any. The only behavioural factor that reliably and substantially increases sleep is prior sleeplessness. On the other hand, anxiety and emotional stimuli by release of epinephrine cause activation of RAS and make sleep more difficult.

Types and Stages of Sleep

Sleep is of two types: non-REM sleep and REM sleep, which alternate in a sleep cycle. The presence of sleep can be assessed by behavioural analysis and more accurately by electrical records of physiological activities during sleep. ***Behaviourally***, sleep is defined by four criteria:

- Reduced motor activity,
- Decreased response to stimulation,

- Stereotypic postures (in humans, e.g. lying down with eyes closed) and
- Relatively easy reversibility (distinguishing it from coma and hibernation).

Polysomnography refers to electrical records of physiological indicators of sleep, which include:

- *Electroencephalography* (EEG) that measures the collective activity of cortical neurons. EEG changes of sleep are described in detail.
- *Electromyography* (EMG), which monitors the muscle activity. The motor unit potential shows a gradual diminution as sleep approaches.
- *Electro-oculography* (EOG) that monitors the eye movements. EOG shows slow eye movements (SEMs) as sleep approaches. These generally disappear within several minutes of the EEG changes. Rapid eye movements are recorded during REM sleep.

Non-REM Sleep Non-REM sleep, i.e. non-rapid eye movement sleep is also known as: *Slow wave sleep* (SWS), because in this type of sleep brain waves are very slow.

In normal adults, sleep mostly begins with non-REM sleep. It is a rest type of sleep which a person experiences during the first hour of sleep after having been awake for many hours. The non-REM sleep alternates with REM sleep during the sleep cycle.

The non-REM sleep is discussed under following headings:

- Stages and EEG patterns of non-REM sleep,
- Physiological changes during non-REM sleep,
- Behavioural changes during non-REM sleep and
- Intellectual changes during non-REM sleep.

Stages and EEG Patterns of Non-REM Sleep

Stage of Wakefulness. As described above, the state of wakefulness and consciousness results due to stimulatory impulses from RAS to cerebral cortex.

EEG pattern during wakefulness is characterized by asynchronous and low amplitude brain waves called beta waves (Fig. 10.11-16A).

State of Quiet, Wakeful rest with Eyes Closed. State of quiet, wakeful rest with eyes closed is the period in between the stage of wakefulness and stage of sleep.

EEG pattern during quiet wakeful resting stage, as described earlier (page 1098), is characterized by alpha waves, which are highly synchronized, large waves having a frequency of 8–13 cycles/s (Fig. 10.11-16B).

State of Non-REM Sleep When an individual from the state of quiet rest with eyes closed enters the state of non-REM sleep, the consciousness is reduced. The non-REM sleep, also known as slow-wave sleep progresses in an orderly way from light to deep sleep in four stages:

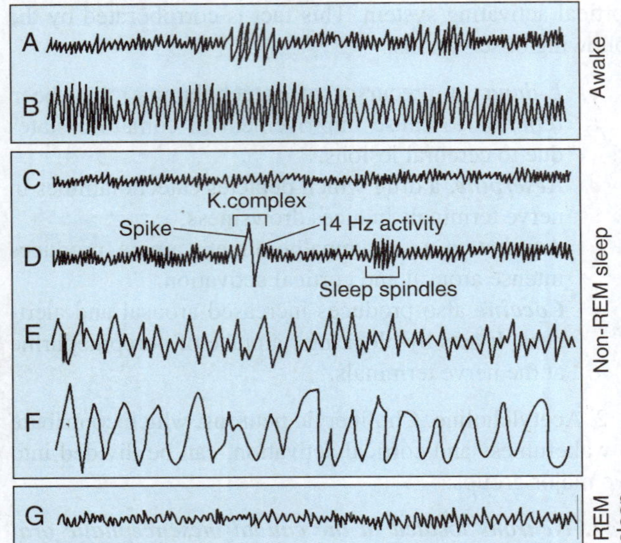

FIGURE 10.11-16 EEG patterns of wakefulness and different stages of sleep: **A,** during wakefulness, **B,** during stage 1 of non-REM sleep; **D,** during stage 2 of non-REM sleep; **E,** during stage 3 of non-REM sleep; **F,** during stage 4 of non-REM sleep; and **G,** during stage of REM sleep.

- ***Stage 1 of non-REM sleep*** (stage of very light sleep). EEG pattern in this stage is characterized by low amplitude mixed frequency activity (Fig. 10.11-16C). There is still considerable sensitivity to sensory stimuli. However, the mild-to-moderate stimuli are often unable to produce a full arousal; instead they produce a sharp electronegative wave at the vertex called *vertex sharp wave* or *V-wave*.
- ***Stage 2 of non-REM sleep*** also called stage of light sleep is characterized by appearance of sleep spindles. These are bursts of alpha-like 10–14 Hz, 50 μV waves which periodically interrupt the alpha rhythm (Fig. 10.11-16D).
  - Auditory stimuli during this phase readily evoke the K-complexes in the EEG. They also occur spontaneously during this stage. The K-complex consists of one or two high-voltage waves followed by a brief 14 Hz activity (Fig. 10.11-16D).
- ***Stage 3 of non-REM sleep*** or stage of moderate deep sleep in characterized by an EEG that display high amplitude slow (0.5–2 Hz) waves called delta waves (Fig. 10.11-16E).
- ***Stage 4 of non-REM sleep*** or stage of deep sleep produces an EEG pattern dome-like very slow, large wave called *delta waves* (Fig. 10.11-16F). Thus, the characteristics of deep sleep are a pattern of rhythmic slow waves, indicating marked *synchronization*.

Physiological Changes during Non-REM Sleep

- Muscle tone decreases progressively.
- Heart rate and blood pressure are decreased.
- Respiration rate is also decreased.

- Eyes begin slow, rolling movement until they finally stop in stage 4 (deep sleep) with eyes turned upwards.
- Body metabolism is lowered.
- Pituitary shows pulsatile release of growth hormones and gonadotropin.

Behavioural Changes during Non-REM Sleep. Behaviourally, the non-REM sleep is characterized by:

- Progressive reduction in consciousness.
- An increasing resistance to being awakened, it is more difficult to wake-up a person from stages 3 and 4 than from stages 1 and 2 of non-REM sleep.
- It is more difficult to wake-up a young person than the elderly from sleep, because the elderly person spends very little time in stages 3 and 4 of non-REM stage.
- When awakened, the person does not report dreaming.
- Response to visual stimuli is present in <15% of the time during stages 1 and stage 2.
- Auditory reaction times become longer as stage 1 sleep approaches. At the sleep onset the auditory response is absent.
- There is some response to meaningful stimuli even in sleep, which indicates that sensory processing continues at some level after the onset of sleep. This is apparent from the *discriminate responses* during sleep to meaningful versus nonmeaningful stimuli. Examples of discriminate responses are:
  - Lower arousal threshold for one's own name versus someone else's name
  - A sleeping mother is more likely to hear her own baby's cry than the cry of an unrelated infant.
  - A captain wakes-up to the cry of 'iceberg' in the midst of the din and bustle of a ship.

Intellectual Functions during Non-REM Sleep

- *Thoughts* become illogical and incoherent towards the onset of sleep.
- *Retrograde amnesia* occurs during transition from wakefulness to sleep. This is because sleep inactivates the consolidation of short-term into long-term memory. Examples of retrograde amnesia include:
  - Inability to grasp the instant of sleep onset in memory,
  - Not remembering the ringing of alarm clock,
  - Morning amnesia for coherent sleep talking and
  - Poor recall of midnight dreams.
- *Memory* for the few minutes before sleep is lost, if sleep persists for approximately 10 min. Patients suffering from syndromes of excessive sleepiness may experience similar memory problems in the daytime if sleep becomes intrusive.

REM Sleep REM sleep, i.e. 'rapid eye movement' sleep is also called 'fast wave (desynchronized) sleep, or 'paradoxical sleep' or 'dream sleep' or 'deepest sleep' (as explained below). In adults, the REM sleep follows non-REM sleep while their entry into sleep occurs via REM sleep.

EEG Pattern of REM Sleep. During REM sleep, EEG is characterized by a high-frequency and low-amplitude pattern (β rhythm), i.e. some desynchronized pattern that is seen in the waking state (Fig. 10.11-16G). Hence, REM sleep is also called 'fast wave sleep' or 'desynchronized sleep'. However, the individual clearly is unresponsive to environment stimuli, and thus is asleep. Further, it is usually more difficult to awaken in REM sleep than in non-REM sleep. Because of the EEG pattern of wakefulness, the REM is also called 'paradoxical sleep'.

In cats, REM sleep is also associated with ponto-geniculo-occipital (PGO) waves. The PGO waves are not detectable in humans by scalp EEG, but are recordable by depth EEG recordings. These waves originate in pons and pass rapidly to lateral geniculate body and then to the cerebral cortex and hence the name PGO. These waves activate the reticular inhibiting area in the medulla producing hypotonia.

Behavioural Changes during REM Sleep

- *Arousal*. As mentioned above, it is difficult to arouse an individual from REM sleep as it is from deep sleep.
- However, when awakened from REM sleep, the individual is immediately alert and aware of the environment. *Dreaming* occurs during REM sleep, so it is also called 'dream sleep'. There is vivid dream recall from approximately 80% of arousals from REM sleep.

Physiological Changes during REM Sleep

- *Rapid eye movements* are the hallmark of this state of sleep and that is why the name REM sleep. Rapid eye movements (saccadic eye movements) are bursts of small jerky movements that bring the eye from one fixation point to another to allow a sweeping of visual images of dreams.
- *Heart rate and respiration rate* become irregular.
- *Muscle tone* is reduced due to inhibition of spinal motor neurons via brainstem mechanisms. Snoring during sleep results from partial obstruction of airways caused by relaxed tongue (due to muscular atonia) in supine position.
- *Twitching of limb* musculature occurs occasionally. Because muscle tone is reduced tremendously during REM sleep, frequency and intensity of muscle twitching does not produce injuries or awaken the individual.
- *Middle ear muscles* are also active during REM sleep.
- *Penile erection* in males and engorgement of clitoris in females may occur during REM sleep.
- *Impaired thermoregulation*. Sweating or shivering during sleep in response to ambient temperature occurs in non-REM sleep and ceases in REM sleep.
- *Teeth grinding* (*bruxism*) may be seen in children.

Sleep Cycle

In a normal adult, the average sleep period of about 7–8 h is divided into approximately 5 cycles during which non-REM sleep and REM sleep alternate with each other. There is an orderly progression of sleep states and stages during a typical sleep cycle as described below (Fig. 10.11-17).

- *Sleep onset* in normal adults usually occurs with non-REM sleep.
- *Stage 1 (very light sleep)* of non-REM sleep is initiated after a state of drowsiness as soon as an individual falls asleep.
- *Stage 2 (light sleep), stage 3 (moderate deep sleep)* and stage 4 (deep sleep) of non-REM sleep are then reached progressively during the next hour or so. After approximately 15 min deep sleep, the depth of sleep starts to decrease progressively from stage 4 to 1.
- *State of REM sleep* is then reached (after about 90 min of non-REM sleep during the first sleep cycle). After the end of REM sleep (5 min), the first cycle is completed and is followed by the next sleep cycles (about 5 cycles during normal sleep of about 7 h).
- Transition from sleep to the awake state occurs either at the end of REM sleep or at the end of the 2nd stage of non-REM sleep of the last sleep cycle.

Duration of Sleep Cycles and Sleep Stages The average duration of each sleep cycle is about 90 min (range 70–120 min). Duration of different sleep stages is different in different cycles as (Fig. 10.11-18):

- Duration of non-REM sleep, which is about 85 min (out of total 90 min) in first cycle decreases progressively in the subsequent sleep cycles.
- About 25% of the entire sleep period is passed in REM sleep
- Duration of REM sleep, which is about 5 min (out of total 90 min) in first cycle increases progressively in the next cycle.
- Duration of deeper stages (3 and 4) of non-REM sleep is maximum during first cycle and then decreases progressively and may even disappear altogether from the later cycles.
- Duration of 2nd stage of non-REM sleep increases progressively from 1st cycle onwards and may even occupy most of the non-REM portion of later cycles. About 50% of the entire sleep period is spent in the 2nd stage of non-REM sleep.
- As morning approaches, the individual may be periodically awakened during later sleep cycles.
- The approximate duration (%) of different stages of sleep during 1st cycle and during the entire sleep is as (Table 10.11-3):

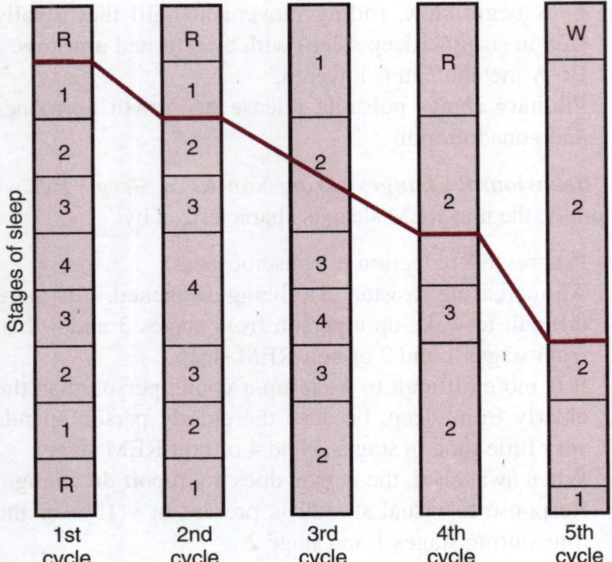

FIGURE 10.11-18 Duration of different stages of non-REM sleep and REM sleep. Note all the five sleep cycles have been shown of equal duration just for comparative depiction of duration in percentage of different stages. However in reality the cycle varies in duration. R = REM sleep, W = wake.

Variations in Sleep Cycles Variations in sleep cycle, from the typical adult pattern depicted in Fig. 10.11-17 and 10.11-18, occur under certain circumstances. In adults,

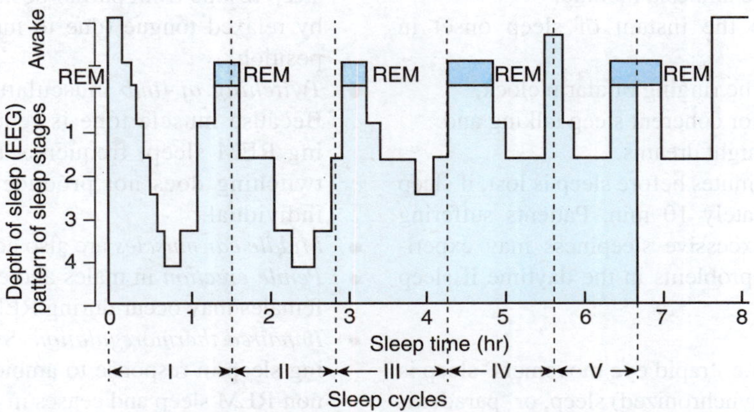

FIGURE 10.11-17 Typical sleep cycles in an adult individual.

TABLE 10.11-3 Approximate Duration of Different Stages of Sleep in First Sleep Cycle and during Entire Sleep

Stage of sleep	1st cycle (%)	Entire sleep (%)
Non-REM sleep		
Stage 1	5	4
Stage 2	20	50
Stage 3	30	6
Stage 4	40	15
REM sleep	5	25

onset of sleep with REM sleep occurs under special circumstances such as in jetlag, chronic sleep deprivation, narcolepsy, acute withdrawal of REM suppressing drugs and endogenous depressions.

Variations in Total Sleep Duration Average sleep time per day differs according to the age:

- During infancy: 16 h,
- During childhood: 10 h,
- During adulthood: 7–8 h and
- During old age: < 8 h.

Variation in Time Period of Different Stages of Sleep: Effect of Age

- Prematurely born infants spend about 80% of their sleep time in REM sleep.
- Full-term infants spend only 50% of their sleep time in REM sleep.
- The total time spent in REM sleep is reduced to about 1.5–2 h by puberty and remains unchanged thereafter.
- From the above, it is clear that the reduction in sleep time from 16 h in infants (8 h REM and 8 h non-REM sleep) to 10 h during childhood (2 h REM and 8 h non-REM sleep) occurs almost entirely by a reduction of the amount of time spent in REM sleep (Fig. 10.11-19).
- In adulthood, reduction in total sleep time to 8 h (2 h REM and 6 h non-REM sleep) from 10 h in childhood is by a reduction in the time spent in deep stages of non-REM sleep (Fig. 10.11-19).
- *In old age*, there is very high variability in the type and duration of sleep. By the age of 60, slow wave sleep (SWS) may no longer be present, particularly in men. Women appear to maintain SWS later in life than men. REM sleep as a percentage of total sleep is maintained well in healthy old age.

Effect of Prior Sleep Deprivation

- *Following differentially deprived of REM or slow wave sleep*, a preferential rebound of that stage of sleep will occur when natural sleep is resumed.

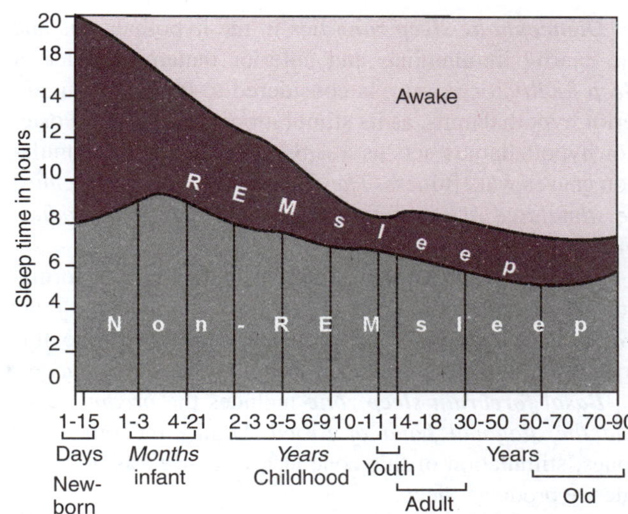

FIGURE 10.11-19 Variation of total period of wakefulness, non-REM sleep and REM sleep with age.

- *Following a total sleep loss of one or more nights*, slow wave sleep tends to be recovered first. REM sleep tends to recover only after the recuperation of slow wave sleep.
- *Recovery sleep*, whether following differential or total sleep loss, is usually deeper than basal sleep, i.e. it has a higher arousal threshold throughout non-REM and REM sleep.

Effect of Temperature. Sleep in general and REM sleep in particular is disrupted by extremes of temperature.

Effect of Circadian Rhythms. The distribution of sleep stages is affected by the time of the day/night at which sleep occurs first. Since REM sleep peaks in the morning hours, therefore, if sleep onset is delayed until morning, REM sleep will tend to predominate and may even occur at the onset of sleep.

Effect of Drugs

- *Benzodiazepines* (such as diazepam) reduce non-REM sleep (SWS).
- *Barbiturates, tricyclic antidepressants and monoamine oxidase* inhibitors (MAOIs) reduce REM sleep.
- *Alcohol* intake immediately before sleep produces REM suppression early in the night.

Genesis of Sleep

The sleep state does not result from the passive withdrawal of arousal due to fatigue of reticular activating system (RAS) as thought earlier. Now, it is established that the sleep is produced by an active process which is different for non-REM sleep and REM sleep.

Genesis of Non-REM Sleep The non-REM sleep is generated by interaction of neurons, which are grouped as:

- Diencephalic sleep zone,
- Medullary synchronizing zone and
- Basal forebrain sleep zone.

Diencephalic sleep zone lies in the hypothalamus and the nearby intralaminar and anterior thalamic nuclei. *A sleep facilitatory centre* is considered to be located in anterior hypothalamus, as its stimulation causes sleep. Posterior hypothalamus acts as a *waking centre*, as its stimulation causes wakefulness. *The diencephalic sleep zone must be stimulated at low frequency (about 8 Hz) to produce sleep.*

Medullary synchronizing zone is in the reticular formation of medulla oblongata at the level of *nucleus of the tractus solitarius* (NTS). Like diencephalic sleep zone, this zone also produces sleep when stimulated at *low frequency*.

Basal forebrain sleep zone includes the *preoptic area and the diagonal band of Broca*. Unlike the other two zones, stimulation of this zone at low, as well as high frequency produces sleep.

Activity of Non-REM on Cells. *The non-REM on cells is due to GABAergic inhibitory neurons that mediate sleep-inducing action of the above-described sleep zones*. These cells are thought to produce sleep by inhibiting the *histaminergic cells in the posterior hypothalamus as well as cells of nucleus reticularis pontis oralis in the midbrain that mediate arousal*. They are maximally active in non-REM sleep and inactive during waking and REM sleep (Fig. 10.11-20). Many non-REM on cells are activated by heat and thus may mediate the *sleep-inducing effects of elevated temperature*.

Mechanism of Production of Sleep Spindles and Slow Waves of Non-REM Sleep. The non-REM sleep is characterized by EEG spindles and slow waves that are produced by synchronized postsynaptic potentials in the cortical neurons. These synchronized synaptic potentials are generated by the rhythmic firing of thalamic relay neurons that project to the cortex (Fig. 10.11-20). The rhythmic firing of relay neurons is a result of action of GABAergic inhibitory neurons in the nucleus reticularis that forms a shell around the thalamus.

Genesis of REM Sleep Rapid eye movement sleep is generated by the interaction of neurons in the caudal midbrain and pons with the neurons in the medulla and forebrain.

REM sleep as described earlier is characterized by:

- Blockage of EEG spindles and slow waves,
- Occurrence of PGO waves,
- Muscle atonia and
- Phasic motor action.

Genesis of the above components of REM sleep is discussed.

Role of Cholinergic Neurons of Midbrain and the Adjacent Dorsal Pons. These cells form an important component of the midbrain arousal system and are maximally active during waking and REM sleep. Their activity contributes to the blocking of the slow waves of EEG acetylcholine (ACh), and other transmitters released by these cells depolarize the GABAergic inhibitory neurons in the reticularis nucleus. This depolarization prevents the hyperpolarization that activates the low-threshold Ca^{2+} channels, which in turn initiate the rhythmic firing of the reticular neurons. In the absence of rhythmic firing of the reticular neurons, the thalamocortical relay cells fire only asynchronously, and this asynchronous activity results in the low-voltage EEG, characteristic of waking and REM sleep.

Role of Nucleus Reticularis Pontis Oralis. The nucleus reticularis pontis oralis (RPO) forms another important neuronal machinery for genesis of REM sleep. Three classes of neurons in the RPO of particular interest are:

1. ***Cholinergic PGO-on Cells.*** The discharge of these neurons produces the so-called ponto-geniculate-occipital

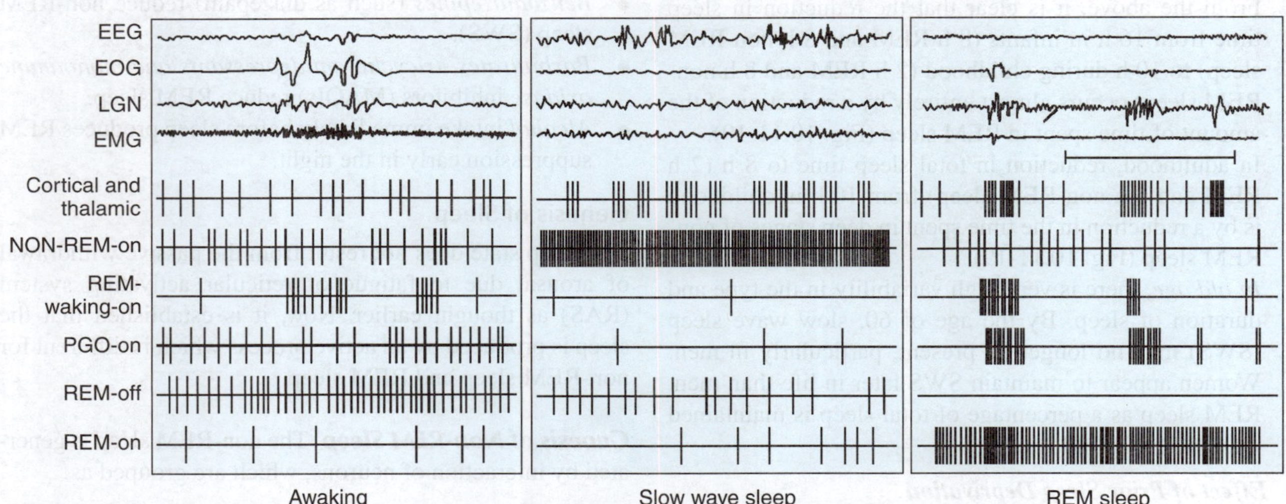

FIGURE 10.11-20 The pattern of activity of key cell groups during waking and slow wave and REM sleep. Each vertical line represent an action potential. EEG: electroencephalogram, EOG: electro-oculogram depicting eye movement, LGN: recording from lateral geniculate nucleus showing ponto-geniculo-occipital (PGO) spikes activity during REM sleep, and EMG: electromyography of dorsal neck cell.

(PGO) spikes that are characteristic of REM sleep (Fig. 10.11-20). The term PGO spikes come from the fact that they originate in the lateral pontine tegmentum and pass rapidly to the lateral geniculate body and thence to the occipital cortex.

Regulation of PGO-on cells. The PGO-on cells are regulated by serotonergic REM-off cells (Fig. 10.11-20) in the raphe nuclei of brainstem, noradrenergic neurons in the locus coeruleus and histaminergic neurons in the posterior hypothalamus. All these neurons contribute to wakefulness and block the activity of PGO-on cells during waking. However, in the transition from non-REM to REM sleep all these neurons remain silent and allow the PGO-on cells to begin discharging in bursts generating PGO spikes. It appears that cessation of activity in these three cell groups may contribute to changes in EEG, autonomic tone and muscle tone during REM sleep.

2. ***REM-waking-on-cells*** of RPO fire at high rate during active waking as well-during REM sleep (Fig. 10.11-20) and at low rate during non-REM sleep. Some of these cells project to the motor neurons in the spinal cord, and others project to the motor neurons that drive the extraocular muscles.
   - *Burst firing of REM-waking-on cells* during waking mediates movements of the head, neck, limbs and eyes.
   - *Burst firing of REM-waking-on cells* during REM sleep produces rapid eye movement and muscle twitches, breaking through the concurrent inhibition of motor neurons.
3. ***REM-on-cells***. REM-on-cells of RPO show high level of activity during REM sleep but have very little or no activity during waking and non-REM sleep (Fig. 10.11-20). Although few in number, these cells play a key role in REM sleep.
   - *One subtype of REM-on-cells* is GABAergic and is responsible for inhibition of activity in serotonergic and noradrenergic cells during REM sleep.
   - *Another subtype of REM-on-cells* is possibly glutamatergic and is responsible for loss of muscle tone in REM sleep.

   Important points to be noted are:
   - *Reserpine*, a drug which depletes serotonin and catecholamines, blocks slow wave sleep and some aspects of REM sleep but increases PGO spike activity.
   - *Barbiturates* decrease the amount of REM sleep.

Chemical Mediators of Sleep

Neurotransmitters employed by neurons forming the neural substrate of sleep as discussed above include:

- Serotonin,
- Acetylcholine and
- Noradrenaline.

Endogenous sleep producing substance. For nearly a century, sleep researchers have searched for substances that might be responsible for induction of sleep. However, no endogenous substance is yet widely accepted as causing sleep. The substances that have been identified by experiments on sleep-deprived animals as sleep-producing substances (S/S) are:

- *Muramyl dipeptide* (MDP), a chemical related to substances found in bacterial cell walls,
- *Interleukin-1* (IL-1), a cytokine that may mediate the effects of muramyl dipeptides as well as immune response,
- *Adenosine,*
- *Delta sleep-inducing peptide* (DSIP), a substance isolated from the blood of sleeping rabbits,
- *Prostaglandin* D_2 and
- Arginine vasotocin (AVT).

Physiological Significance of Sleep

Sleep is an indispensable phenomenon. Its physiological significance is highlighted.

1. ***Sleep may serve as a period of body's rest and metabolic restoration*** as evidenced by the following physiological changes during non-REM sleep.
   - Pulsatile release of growth hormone and gonadotropins from the pituitary and
   - Decrease in blood pressure, heart rate and respiration.
2. ***Sleep is necessary for certain forms of learning***. In experimental animals, learning sessions do not improve performance until a period of slow wave sleep (SWS) or SWS plus REM sleep has occurred. However, it is not known why sleep is necessary, and there is as yet no clinical correlate to this experimental observation.
3. ***REM sleep is necessary for mental well-being***. The correlation between dreaming and REM sleep indicates that the brain is highly active at this time. This may allow for the expression, through dreams, of concern in the subconscious and for long-term chemical and structural changes that the brain must undergo to make learning and memory possible.
4. ***REM sleep plays important role in homeostatic mechanism.*** It is evident from the observation that when the experimental animals are completely deprived of REM sleep for long periods, they lose weight in spite of increased caloric intake and finally die.

Applied Aspects

Sleep–Wake Cycle and Factors Affecting Sleep

Sleep and wakefulness, like many of the body's regulatory mechanisms, have a circadian rhythm of about 24 h. A newborn infant has many cycles of sleep and wakefulness in 24 h, but after the age of 2 years a single sleep–wake cycle is established. In a normal adult, the sleep–wake cycle consists of 7–8 h of sleep and 16–17 h of wakefulness.

Control of Sleep–Wake Cycle Sleep–wake cycle, like other circadian rhythms, is endogenous. The biological clock controlling the circadian rhythms is *suprachiasmatic nucleus* of the anterior hypothalamus. The circadian rhythms are endogenous and can persist without environmental cues; however, under normal circumstances, the rhythms are modulated by external timing cues called *zeitgebers* (time givers) that adapt the rhythm to the environment. Sunlight is a powerful timing cue. Light entrains this rhythm by means of *retinohypothalamic tract*. Although the suprachiasmatic nucleus regulates the timing of sleep, it is not responsible for sleep itself.

Neurochemical Mechanisms Transition between sleep and wakefulness manifests as circadian rhythm. The RAS of the brainstem is composed of a group of neurons (locus coeruleus and raphe nuclei) that releases norepinephrine, serotonin or acetylcholine. When the activity of these neurons increase, there is decreased activity of acetylcholine containing neurons of the pontine reticular formation. This pattern of neuronal activity is responsible for the awake state, whereas reverse of this pattern is responsible for REM sleep.

Non-REM sleep occurs, when there is greater even balance (i.e. increase in GABA and decrease in histamine) that promotes Non-REM sleep via deactivation of the thalamocortical neurons (Fig. 10.11-21). Posterior hypothalamic neurons produce orexin that is considered to be an important factor for switching between sleep and awake state.

Sleep Disorders

1. Insomnia refers to an inability to have sufficient or restful sleep despite an adequate opportunity for sleep. It is a subjective problem that occurs at one time or another in almost all adults. Insomnia can be relieved temporarily by sleeping pills, especially benzodiazepines. Prolonged use of these drugs can be habit-forming and can compromise daytime performance.

2. Fatal Familial Insomnia is a serious disorder characterized by worsening insomnia, impaired autonomic and motor functions, dementia and eventually death. It is a progressive disease that occurs in both an inherited and a sporadic form.

3. Narcolepsy refers to an irresistible urge to sleep. As mentioned in the sleep cycle, in adults the sleep onset occurs with non-REM sleep, which is followed by REM sleep. However, in narcolepsy, REM sleep is entered directly from the waking states. Narcolepsy may manifest as:

- ***Episodes of sudden sleep.*** The individuals go to sleep while performing daytime tasks.
- ***Cataplexy.*** In some narcoleptics, the profound reduction in muscle tone characteristic of REM sleep can occur without loss of consciousness. During such an attack, called cataplexy, the individual suddenly becomes paralyzed, falls to the ground and is unable to move.
- ***Dream-like state during wakefulness*** is another mode of manifestation of narcolepsy. Narcoleptics describe it as a hallucination.

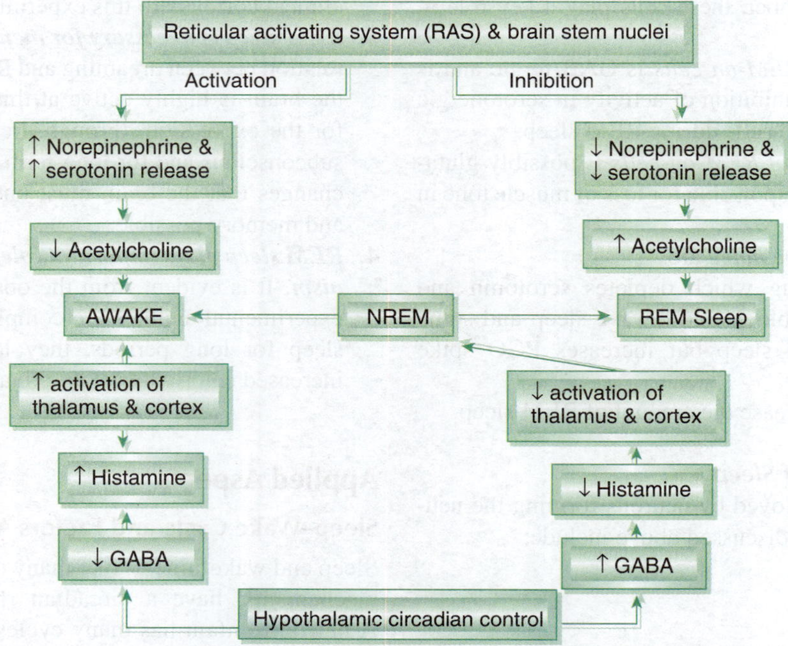

FIGURE 10.11-21 Alternating activity of brainstem and hypothalamic neurons influencing sleep and wake cycle.

4. Some Sleep Disorders Associated with Non-REM Sleep (Slow Wave Sleep), or more specifically, occurring during arousal from slow wave sleep are:

- ***Sleepwalking (somnambulism).*** Episodes of sleepwalking are more common in children than in adults and occur predominantly in males. These episodes may last for several minutes. Such individuals walk with their eyes open and avoid obstacles, but when awakened, they cannot recall the episode.
- ***Bed-wetting*** (nocturnal enuresis), i.e. involuntary voiding of urine, occurs in some children during slow wave sleep.
- ***Nightmares (pavor nocturnus or episodes of night terror).*** During a nightmare that occurs in slow wave sleep, the individual wakes up screaming and appear terrified. However, no reason for acute anxiety is recalled. By contrast, terrifying dreams that occur during REM sleep are graphically remembered.

5. REM Behaviour Disorder. It is a newly recognized condition in which REM sleep is not associated with inhibition of muscle tone. Consequently, such persons act out their dreams, i.e. they thrash about and may even jump out of bed, ready to do battle with imagined aggression. The generalized or localized muscle contraction associated with vivid visual imagery, i.e. the motor response to some of the dream events is referred to a *hypnic myoclonia*.

Chapter 10.12

Some Higher Functions of Nervous System

LANGUAGE AND SPEECH

- Neurophysiology of language and speech
  - Components of sound-based language
  - Wernicke's theory of language
  - Development of speech
  - Mechanism of speech and speech centres
- Speech disorders
  - Dysarthria
  - Aphasia

LEARNING AND MEMORY

- Learning
  - Incidental learning
  - Reflex learning
- Memory
  - Implicit memory
  - Explicit memory
  - Mechanism of memory
- Interhemispheric transfer of learning and memory
  - Applied aspects
  - Drugs facilitating learning and memory
  - Amnesia
  - Alzheimer's disease and senile dementia

HIGHER INTELLECTUAL FUNCTIONS OF THE PREFRONTAL ASSOCIATION CORTEX

- Thought process
- Working memory and intellectual functions
- Episodic memory

LANGUAGE AND SPEECH

Neurophysiology of Language and Speech

Communication through language is a unique faculty, which places the humans much above the animals. Language refers to that faculty of nervous system which enables the humans to understand the spoken and printed words, and to express ideas in the form of speech and writing. There are two aspects of communications: language input (the sensory aspect) and language output (the motor aspect). Sensory aspect of language includes the visual, auditory and proprioceptive impulses, while the motor aspect includes the mechanisms concerned with expression of spoken (sound) language and written language.

Components of Sound-based Language

Before understanding neurophysiology of language, it will be worthwhile to become familiar with the different components of sound-based language which include phonemes, morphemes, syntax, lexicon, semantic, prosody and discourse. These components are applicable not only to sound based but also to sign languages. For example, a morpheme in sign language would be the smallest meaningful movement.

Phonemes refer to the fundamental sounds in a language whose linking together in a particular order forms morphemes.

Morphemes, a combination of phonemes, are the smallest meaningful units of words. Morpheme may be a word itself or some morphemes may combine to form a word.

Words are made of syllables which include consonants and vowels. Use of syllables is a unique characteristic of human language.

Lexicon refers to collection of all words in a given language.

Syntax refers to linking together of different words by the use of verbs and appropriate choice of verb tenses, i.e. making a sentence (called rules of grammar in popular usage)children develop syntax independent of formal training, which suggests that there is an innate basis for the development of human language.

Semantic refers to understanding the meaning of lexiconsand syntaxes.

Discourse refers to linking together of sentences in such a way that they constitute a meaningful narrative.

Prosody refers to rise and fall of the pitch of the voice in speaking that can modify the literal meaning of words and sentences.

Wernicke's Theory of Language

To explain the mechanism of speech, Wernicke put forward a theory of language production in the brain (a neurological model of language, which was later revived by Gestiwind.

This theory was formulated on the basis of defects in language observed in patients with lesions of different parts of the cortex. According to this theory, utterance arises in Wernicke's area and is passed on to Broca's area via the arcuate fasciculus. After the sentence is formulated in Broca's area, it is transferred to the motor cortex where the articulation is programmed by activation of appropriate muscles in mouth and face, etc. The essentials of this theory have survived more than a hundred years. However, modifications have been made in it regarding the areas in which lesions produce the distinct varieties of aphasia.

Development of Speech

Development of speech involves coordinated activity of three important areas of cerebral cortex, namely Wernicke's area, Broca's area and motor areas of the categorical (dominant) hemisphere.

Development of speech in a child occurs in two stages:

First Stage. In this stage, there occurs an association of certain words with visual, tactile, auditory and other sensations, aroused by objects in the external world, which is stored in the memory.

Second Stage. This stage of development of speech involves establishment of new neuronal circuits. When a definite meaning has been attached to certain words, pathway between the auditory area (area 41) and motor area for the muscles of articulation which helps in speech (area 44) is established. And, the child attempts to formulate and pronounce the words, which are learnt.

Mechanism of Speech and Speech Centres

Speech is of two types: spoken and written.

- ***Spoken speech*** involves both understanding of spoken words as well as expressing ideas in the form of spoken words.
- ***Written speech*** also involves both understanding of written words as well as expression of ideas in the form of written words. Mechanism of speech involves coordinated activities of central speech apparatus and peripheral speech apparatus. The central speech apparatus consists of cortical and subcortical centres. The peripheral speech apparatus includes larynx or sound box, pharynx, mouth, nasal cavities, tongue and lips. All the structures of peripheral speech apparatus work in coordination with respiratory system, under the influence of motor impulses from the respective motor areas of the cerebral cortex.

Mechanism of speech and the centres concerned with can be described separately for:

- Understanding of speech and
- Expression of speech.

Understanding of Speech (Sensory Aspects of Communication) Different mechanisms are involved in the understanding of a spoken speech and written speech.

Understanding of Spoken Speech. Understanding of the spoken words is accomplished by the following activities:

1. **Hearing of the spoken words** requires an intact auditory pathway from the ears to primary auditory areas.
   - ***Primary auditory areas*** also called auditory sensory areas include the Brodmannle area 41 and 42 and form the centre for hearing.
     - *Location.* Primary auditory areas are located in the middle of superior temporal gyrus on the upper margin and on its deep or insular aspect (Fig. 10.12-1).
   - ***Connections.*** *Afferents* are received from the medial geniculate body (via auditory radiations), and pulvinar of thalamus.

     Efferents are sent to medial geniculate body, superior colliculus and pulvinar.
   - ***Functions.*** This area perceives the nerve impulses as sound, i.e. auditory information such as loudness, pitch, source and direction of sound.
2. **Recognition and understanding of the spoken words** is carried by *auditory association areas* (21 and 20) located in the middle and inferior temporal gyrus, respectively (Fig. 10.12-1).These areas receive impulses from primary area and are concerned with interpretation and integration of auditory impulses
3. **Interpretation and comprehension of the speech ideas.** This involves the activities of *Wernicke's area.* Wernicke's area (area 22) is a *sensory* speech centre, located in the posterior part of the superior temporal gyrus, behind the areas 41 and 42 (Fig. 10.12-1) in the categorical hemisphere, i.e. dominant hemisphere. ***Functions*** of this area are:
   - Interpretation of the meaning of what is heard and
   - Comprehension of the spoken language and the formation of idea that are to be articulated in speech.

Understanding of Written Speech. Understanding of the written speech is accomplished by following activities (Fig. 10.12-2).

1. **Perception of written words** requires an intact visual pathway from eyes to primary visual cortex.

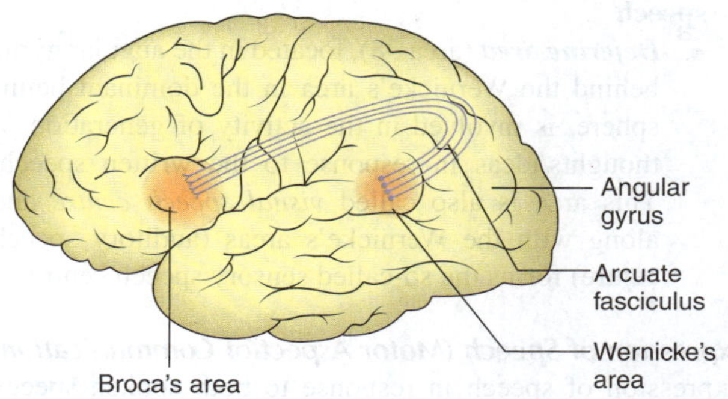

FIGURE 10.12-1 Lateral surface of left (categorical) hemisphere showing location of primary areas of language.

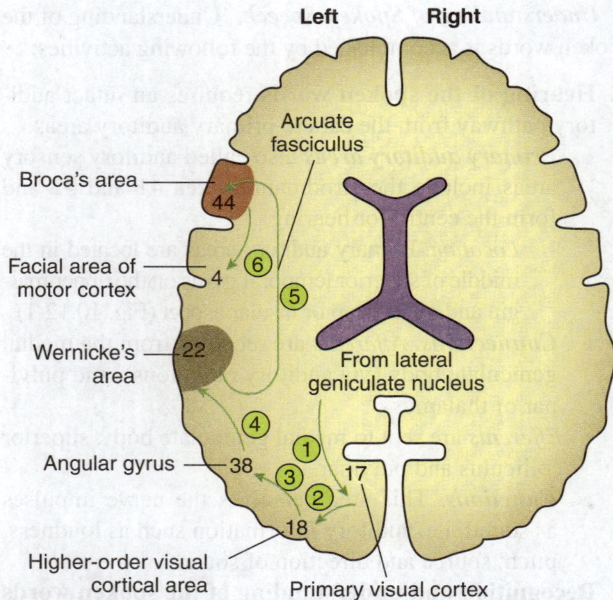

FIGURE 10.12-2. Neural pathway in brain involved in the understanding and expression of written speech.

- ***Primary visual cortex,*** also called as striate area (area 17), or the centre of vision lies on the medial surface of occipital lobe in and near the calcarine sulcus occupying parts of lingual gyrus and cuneus. It also extends to the superolateral surface of the occipital pole limited by the lunate sulcus.
  Afferents to area 17 are fibres of the optic radiations, which bring impulses from parts of both retinae, and these parts are represented within the area in a specific orderly manner.
  Functions. Primary visual cortex is concerned with perception of visual impulses.

2. **Interpretation of written speech**
   - ***Visual association areas*** (area 18 and 19), located in the walls and in front of lunate sulcus, are concerned with the interpretation of written words. These areas are involved in the recognition and identification of the written words in the light of past experience.
3. **Generation of thoughts/ideas in response to written speech**
   - ***Dejerine area*** (area 38), located in the angular gyrus behind the Wernicke's area in the dominant hemisphere, is involved in the activity of generation of thoughts/ideas in response to the written speech. This area is also called *visual speech centre* and along with the Wernicke's areas (auditory speech centre) forms the so-called sensory speech centre.

Expression of Speech (Motor Aspect of Communication)

Expression of speech in response to both spoken speech and written speech can be in the form of spoken speech or written speech or both. It involves the activities of *motor speech centres,* which include Broca's area (area 44) and Exner's area.

1. Expression in the Form of Spoken Speech. Expression in the form of spoken speech involves the activities of motor speech (Broca's area) area.

Broca's area or motor speech area (area 44) is a special area of the premotor cortex situated in inferior frontal gyrus.

Functions. This area, especially in the dominant hemisphere (left hemisphere in right handed person) processes the information received from the sensory speech centres (Wernicke's area and Dejerine's area) into a detailed and coordinated pattern for vocalization, which is then projected to motor cortex for implementation. Thus, Broca's area is concerned with the movements of those structures which are responsible for the production of voice and articulation of speech, i.e. it causes activation of vocal cords simultaneously with movements of mouth and tongue during speech, lesions of this area cause motor aphasia.

Note:

- In adulthood, if person learns a second language, by fMRI it is observed that, a separate area lying adjacent to the Broca's area is involved for this action.
- Another observation revealed that if a person learns a second language in early life, then only single area is involved for both languages.

2. Expression in the Form of Written Speech. Expression in the form of written speech is the function of Exner's area (Fig. 10.12-2).

Exner's area (motor writing centre) is situated in the middle frontal gyrus in the categorical (dominant) hemisphere in the premotor cortex. It processes the information received from Broca's area into detailed and coordinated pattern; and then along with the motor cortex (area 4) initiates the appropriate muscle movements of the hand and fingers to produce written speech.

Concept of Dominant Hemisphere for Language

In human cerebral cortex, the interpretive functions of Wernicke's area, the angular gyrus, and the frontal motor speech areas (i.e. the ability to understand or express oneself by spoken or written speech) are more highly developed in one hemisphere called the *dominant hemisphere*. How one hemisphere comes to be dominant is not yet understood. It is important to note that:

- In approximately 95% of all individuals, the left hemisphere is dominant regardless of handedness.
- Since the motor area concerned with the hand movements is closely associated with the centre for speech, this explains the right handedness in over 90% of the individuals.
- Right hemisphere dominance is seen in only 15% of left handers.

- About 70% of left handers also have left hemisphere dominance.
- The area in the nondominant hemisphere that corresponds to Wernicke's area is also involved in language function. It is responsible for understanding the emotional content or intonation of spoken language. It also serves equally important functions of understanding and interpreting nonverbal, visual or auditory experiences such as recognition of visual patterns or faces and interpretation of music.

Concept of Categorical and Representational Hemisphere

Presently, it is believed that left hemisphere is not really dominant over the right hemisphere. In fact, the two halves of the brain have independent capabilities of consciousness, memory storage and control of motor activities and speech. The corpus callosum and anterior commissure connect the two halves of brain. By these connections, information stored in one hemisphere is made available to the other hemisphere and then the activities of two hemispheres are coordinated.

As summarized below, some specialized higher functions are allowed to each hemisphere. Therefore, the terms 'dominant' and 'nondominant' have been replaced by *categorical* and *representational* hemisphere, respectively.

Functions Allotted to Left Hemisphere in Right-Handed Person

- Right hand control,
- Spoken language,
- Written language,
- Mathematical skills,
- Scientific skills and
- Reasoning.

Functions Allotted to Right Hemisphere in a Right-handed Person

- Left hand control,
- Music awareness,
- Three-dimensional awareness,
- Art awareness,
- Insight and
- Imagination.

Speech Disorders

Dysarthria

Dysarthria is a disorder of speech in which articulation of words is impaired, but the comprehension of spoken and written speech is not affected. It may be due to paresis, or in coordination of the muscles involved in the production of speech as seen in lesions of pyramidal tract, cranial nerves, cerebellum or basal ganglia.

Aphasia

Aphasia refers to, inability to understand spoken or written speech or inability in expressing the spoken or written speech in the absence of mental confusion or motor deficit. Depending upon the site of lesion, the aphasia may be:

- Sensory aphasia,
- Motor aphasia or
- Global aphasia.

Sensory Aphasia

Site of lesion. Sensory or receptive aphasia, also known as Wernicke's aphasia is the result of lesion in the Wernicke's area.

Characteristic features of sensory aphasia are:

1. *Difficulty in understanding the meaning of speech.* In this condition, the affected individuals are capable of hearing or identifying written or spoken words, but they do not comprehend the meaning of the words.
2. *Motor speech* is intact, and the patients talk very fluently (or rather excessively), that is why, it is also called *fluent aphasia*. However, the speech does not make much sense and is often associated with:
   - *Anomia,* i.e. inability to find an appropriate word to express a thought.
   - *Neologism,* i.e. using or creating new words or new meanings for established words.
   - *Paraphasias,* i.e. production of unintended words or phrases during effort to speak.
   - *Conduction aphasia* is another form of fluent aphasia. In this condition patient can speak well, has good auditory comprehension, but cannot put words together. Earlier it was thought that due to lesion of arcuate fasciculus (that connects Wernicke's area to the Broca's area), but the latest view is that lesion occurs near the auditory cortex in the perisylvian fissure.
3. *Impairment in reading and writing.* Since the patient cannot comprehend the written words (*word blindness*) he/she is unable to read aloud or copy print into writing.

Motor Aphasia

Site of lesion. Motor aphasia, also known as Broca's aphasia results from lesions involving the Broca's motor speech area (area 44) in the frontal lobe.

Characteristic features of Broca's aphasia are:

1. *Comprehension of written or spoken* speech is good.
2. *Difficulty in speaking.* The affected individual is able to formulate verbal language in his mind but cannot vocalize the response. The defect is not in the control of musculature needed for speech but rather in the elaboration of the complex patterns of neural and muscle activation, i.e. *effect* which defines the motor aspect of language.
3. *Speech is nonfluent,* i.e. the patient utters only a few words with great difficulty. Because of this, motor aphasia is also known as *nonfluent aphasia* or *expressive aphasia.*
4. *Inability to write* (*agraphia*)

Global Aphasia Global aphasia refers to total inability to use language communication.

Site of lesion. This condition is produced as a result of loss of both Wernicke's and Broca's areas. In this situation, speech becomes scanty and fluent. In case of deaf subjects, if a lesion occurs in the categorical hemisphere, then these individuals are unable to communicate in sign language.

Common Cause of Aphasia Aphasias are mostly produced by thrombosis or embolism of a blood vessel in the dominant hemisphere. Aphasias are commonly associated with right sided motor and sensory deficit but may also occur independently, when the lesion is restricted to cortical association area.

LEARNING AND MEMORY

Learning

Learning and memory are closely related. Learning is impossible without memory and memory has no meaning without learning. In fact, learning and memory are two sides of a coin. Learning refers to a neural mechanism by which the individual changes his or her behaviour on the basis of past experience. Two patterns of learning are:

- ***Reflex learning,*** in which the learning is associated with an immediate behavioural changes and
- ***Incidental learning,*** in which the behavioural changes are not immediately apparent. The individuals acquire information about the world while attending incidentally to sensory inputs, and thereby develop the potential to behave differently. The two broad classes of reflex learning are:
  - Nonassociative learning and
  - Associative learning.

[A] Nonassociative Learning

In nonassociative learning, the subject learns about the properties of a single stimulus. It results when an animal or person is repeatedly exposed to a single type of stimulus. Two forms of nonassociative learning are common in everyday life: habituation and sensitization.

Habituation

Habituation refers to decrease in response to a benign (neutral type) stimulus, when the stimulus is presented repeatedly. When the stimulus is applied for the first time it is novel and evokes reaction. This response is called *orientation reflex* or 'what is it' response. However, due to habituation lesser and lesser response is evoked on repeated stimulation. Eventually, the subject totally ignores the stimulus and thus gets habituated to it. The response presumably diminishes because the individual learns that the stimulus is not important. For example, when a new clock is presented to a subject, at first the ticking noise may be annoying and may cause some difficulty in sleeping. However, after several nights the clock is no longer noticed.

It is important to note that presentation of another, usually noxious stimulus results in recovery of the habituated response, i.e. *dishabituation*. Dishabituation is a major criterion to demonstrate that habituation has indeed occurred.

Cellular basis of habituation has been studied in lower animals like snail (Aplysia). Habituation of the gill withdrawal reflex occurs when the siphon of the snail is touched repeatedly, and the snail does not withdraw its gill anymore. Habituation is associated with a decrease in neurotransmitter released at the synapses, which in turn is due to the inactivation of Ca^{2+} influx at the axon endings (Fig. 10.12-3). However, the mechanism of inactivation of Ca^{2+} channels is not known.

Sensitization

Sensitization is opposite to habituation. In it, repeated application of a distinctly pleasant or unpleasant (strong) stimulus produces greater and greater response. For example, an animal responds more vigorously to a mild tactile stimulus, after it has received a painful pinch. Similarly, a spanking can lead to a greater likelihood that a child will obey a parent's admonition. Thus, in sensitization, learning occurs in a direction opposite to that seen in habituation, presumably so that the behaviour becomes directed toward

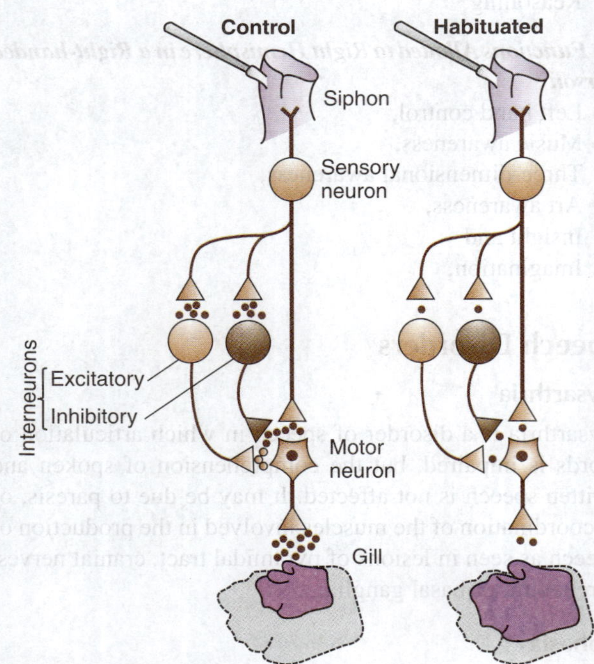

FIGURE 10.12-3 Cellular mechanism of habituation as studied in the gill-withdrawal reflex of marine snail (Aplysia) (presynaptic inhibition).

escape from the stimulus. Moreover, a sensitizing stimulus can override the effects of habituation, i.e. can cause dishabituation (as described above).

Cellular mechanism of sensitization has also been studied in lower animals like Aplysia (snail). After a painful stimulus is applied to the tail repeatedly, the snail subsequently withdraws its gill much more vigorously in response to an innocuous touch on the siphon. The sensitization is associated with increased release of neurotransmitters from the axonal endings of the sensory neuron. This results due to presynaptic facilitation of synaptic transmission brought about by a third neuron called the facilitatory neuron (Fig. 10.12-4). The transmitter released by the presynaptic interneuron, is serotonin (5-HT). Here it binds to two serotonin receptors on the sensory nerve terminals (Fig. 10.12-5) One engages a G protein (G s), which increases the activity of adenylyl cyclase. The adenylyl cyclase converts adenosine triphosphate (ATP) to cyclic adenosine monophosphate (cAMP), thereby increasing the level of cAMP in the terminal of sensory neuron. The cAMP activates the cAMP-dependent protein kinase A (PKA) by attaching to its inhibitory regulatory subunit, thus releasing its active catalytic subunit. The catalytic subunit of PKA acts along three biochemical pathways to cause increased release of neurotransmitter at axonal nerve ending of sensory neurons.

- In *pathway 1,* the catalytic subunit phosphorylates K^+ channels, thereby decreasing the K^+ current. This prolongs the action potential and increases the influx of Ca^{2+}, thus augmenting transmitter release.
- In *pathway 2,* vesicles containing transmitter are mobilized to the releasable transmitter pore at the active zone and the efficiency of exocytotic release machinery is also enhanced.
- In *pathway 3,* L-type Ca^{2+} channels are opened. Serotonin acting through a second receptor, engages the G protein (Go) that activates a phospholipase-C (PLC), which in turn stimulates intramembranous diacylglycerol to activate protein kinase-C (PKC).

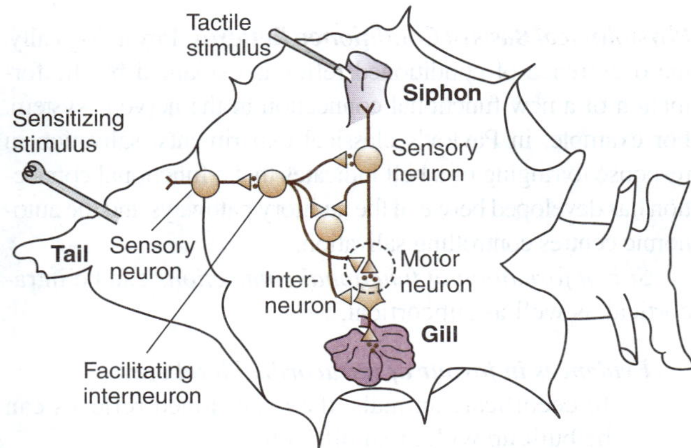

FIGURE 10.12-4 Cellular mechanism of short-term sensitization as studied in the gill-withdrawal reflex (presynaptic facilitation).

As shown in Fig. 10.12-5, the pathways 2-2a and 3-3a involve in the joint action of PKA and PKC.

[B] Associative Learning

In associative learning, the subject learns about the relationship between two stimuli or between a stimulus and behaviour. Two forms of associative learning have been distinguished based on the experimental procedures used to establish the learning:

- Classical conditioning and
- Operant conditioning.

Classical Conditioning

Classical conditioning involves learning a relationship between two stimuli. Classical conditioning is also termed Pavlovian conditioning, conditioned reflex type I, respondent conditioning or type-S conditioning.

Characteristic features of a classical conditioned reflex are:

- A conditioned reflex is reflex response to stimulus that previously elicited little or no response, *acquired by repeatedly pairing the stimulus with another stimulus* that normally does produce the response. Thus, in classical conditioning, a temporal association is made between a neutral conditioned stimulus (CS) and an unconditioned stimulus (US) that elicits an unlearned response. It is *peculiar to the individual* and refers to the fact that certain conditions must be present if this class of response is to develop. It depends for its appearance on the *formation of new functional connections in CNS.*
- *Reinforcement,* i.e. a process of following a conditioned stimulus (CS) with the basic unconditioned stimulus (US) is must for retaining a conditioned reflex, otherwise it will *extinct*.

Pavlov's experiment to demonstrate classical conditioned reflex is:

- When food, i.e. an unconditional stimulus (US) is presented to a hungry dog, it produces salivation (anunconditioned response) or
- If a bell is rung (a conditioned stimulus (CS)), just before the food (US) is presented, the dog learns to associate the bell (CS) with the food (US).
- Eventually, ringing the bell (CS) alone causes salivation.
- Of course, if the food fails to appear consistently when the bell is rung, the conditioned response fades away, a process called *extinction* or *internal inhibition*. Thus, a conditioned reflex needs to be reinforced frequently, otherwise it dies out.

Prerequisites for Development of Conditioned Reflex

- ***Alertness and good health.*** The animal must be alert and in good health.
- ***Timing of conditioned (CS) and unconditioned (US) stimuli*** is critical in classical conditioning. The CS

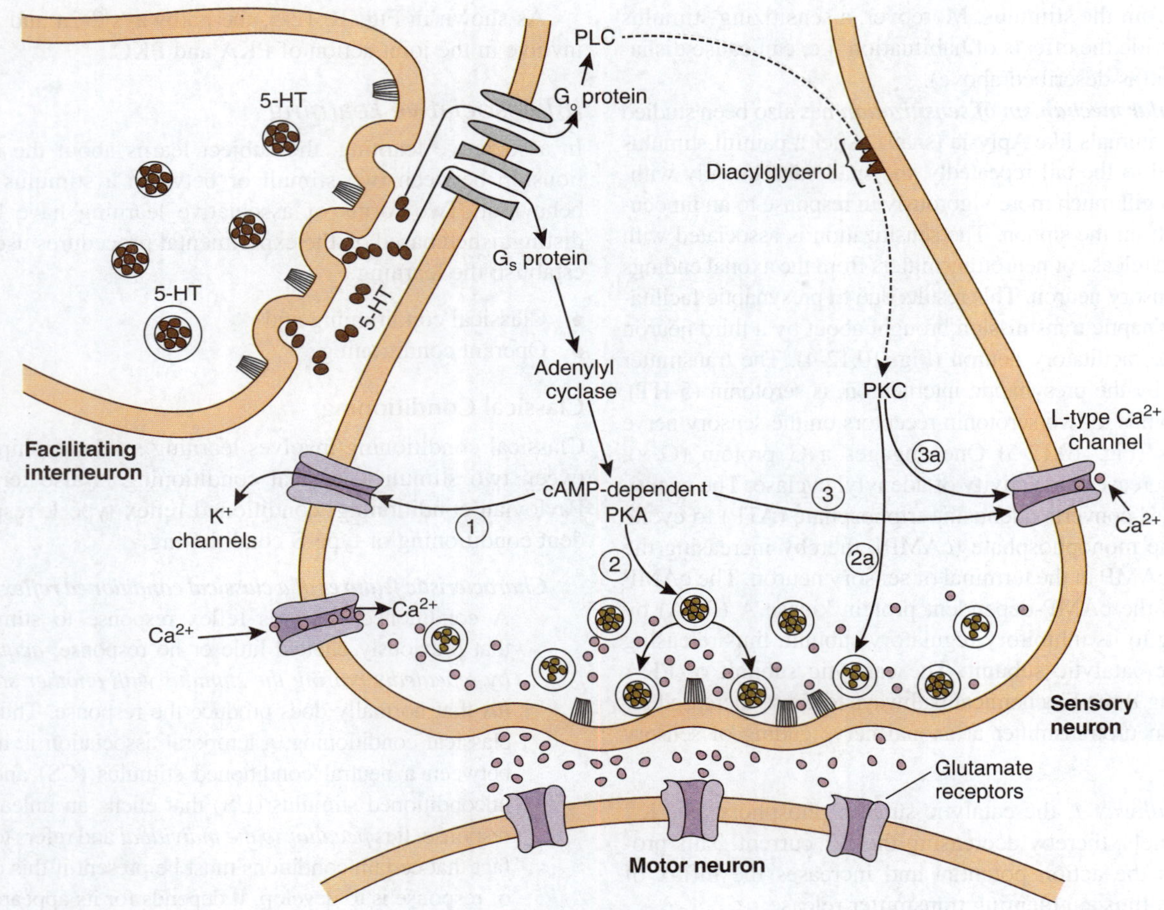

FIGURE 10.12-5 Pathways involved in increased release of neurotransmitter (responsible for sensitization).

must precede the US, often within an interval of about 0.5 s. If the CS follows US, no conditioned response is developed.

- ***Duration of conditioned stimulus (CS).*** The CS must be allowed to continue to act so as to overlap the US. Almost any stimulus, if suitably employed may become the CS.
- ***Reinforcement.*** For a conditioned reflex to continue, it is essential that CS should always be followed by US. As described above, when US fails to follow CS consistently, the conditioned reflex fades away soon. This phenomenon is known as *extinction* or *internal inhibition*.
- ***No external inhibition.*** When the animal is disturbed by an external stimulus immediately after the CS is applied, the conditioned response may not occur. This is called external inhibition.
- ***Type of unconditioned stimulus (US).*** The conditioned reflexes are difficult to form when the US proves a pure motor response; since the motor responses are also under voluntary control.
- ***Pleasant and unpleasant versus neutral unconditioned stimulus (US).*** Conditioned reflexes are relatively easily formed when the US is associated with a pleasant or unpleasant effect than when associated with a neutral effect. For example, stimulation of the brain reward system is a powerful US; this is called pleasant or *positive reinforcement*. Similarly, stimulation of the avoiding system or a painful shock to the skin is also a powerful US; and this is called an unpleasant or *negative reinforcement*.

Physiological Basis of Conditioned Reflexes Physiologically, the occurrence of conditioned reflex is explained by the formation of a new functional connection in the nervous system. For example, in Pavlov's classical experiments, salivation in response to ringing of a bell indicates that a functional connection has developed between the auditory pathways and the autonomic centres controlling salivation.

Site of formation of functional connections can be intracortical as well as subcortical.

Evidences in favour of intracortical level are:

- In decorticate animals, the conditioned reflexes can be built up with great difficulty.
- Presence of sensory cortex is must to understand a complex sensory conditioned stimulus.

Evidence in favour of subcortical level. Nondiscriminative conditioned reflexes to simple sensory stimuli can be formed in the absence of whole neocortex. This indicates that the new functional connections can also be formed at subcortical level.

Cellular Mechanism of Conditioned Reflex Classical conditioning involves presynaptic facilitation of synaptic transmission that is dependent on activity in both the presynaptic and postsynaptic cells. Cellular mechanism of classical conditioning has also been studied in gill withdrawal reflex. As shown in Fig. 10.12-6, when the unconditioned stimulus (to the tail of a snail) and the conditioned stimulus (on mantle shelf) are timed so that the CS just precedes the US, then the modulatory interneurons engaged by the US will activate the sensory neurons immediately after the CS has activated the sensory neurons. This sequential activation of the sensory neurons during a critical interval by the CS and US leads to greater presynaptic facilitation than when the two stimuli are not appropriately paired. This novel feature unique to classical conditioning is called *activity dependence*.

There are presynaptic and postsynaptic components to activity-dependent facilitation that produce the large increase in transmitter release that occurs with classical conditioning. Further, it is important to note that classical conditioning requires the activation of NMDA receptors for glutamate present on the motor cell, as opposed to the non-NMDA receptors that are activated during sensitization.

Presynaptic components include:

- Activation of adenylyl cyclase by Ca^{2+} influx, representing the CS and
- Activation of serotonergic receptors coupled to adenylyl cyclase, representing the US.

Postsynaptic component includes:

- A retrograde signal indicating that the postsynaptic cell has been adequately activated by US.

Operant Conditioning

Operant conditioning is also termed as instrumental conditioning, type II conditioning, type-R conditioning or trial-and-error conditioning. It involves associating a specific behaviour with a reinforcement event. In it, the organism's behaviour is instrumental in conditioning. Therefore, the organism learns which of its actions are responsible for the occurrence of reinforcement event.

Operant conditioning is of two types:

- ***Reward conditioning.*** In it a naturally occurring response is strengthened by positive reinforcement (reward).
- ***Adversive conditioning.*** In it a naturally occurring (innate) response is weakened by a negative reinforcement (punishment).

Experiment to Demonstrate Operant Conditioning. A hungry animal (e.g. rat) is placed in a cage with a lever (bars) protruding in the cage. Because of naturally occurring (innate) response, the rat will randomly press the lever.

- If pressing of lever is not associated with any event the pressing of the lever will be at a random rate.
- If pressing a lever is associated with a positive reinforce, i.e. reward (e.g. food) the rate of pressing the lever will be much more than the random rate (*reward conditioning*).
- If pressing of lever is associated with a negative reinforce, i.e. punishment (e.g. electric shock), the lever-pressing rate will be much less than the random rate (*aversive conditioning*).

Neural Mechanism of Operant Conditioning Because operant and classical conditioning involve different kinds of association–classical conditioning involves learning an association between two stimuli, whereas operant conditioning involves learning the association between a behaviour and a reward–one might suppose the two forms of learning are mediated by different neural mechanisms.

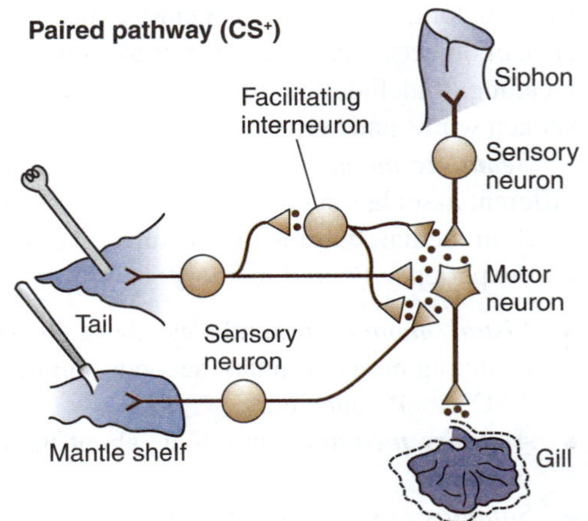

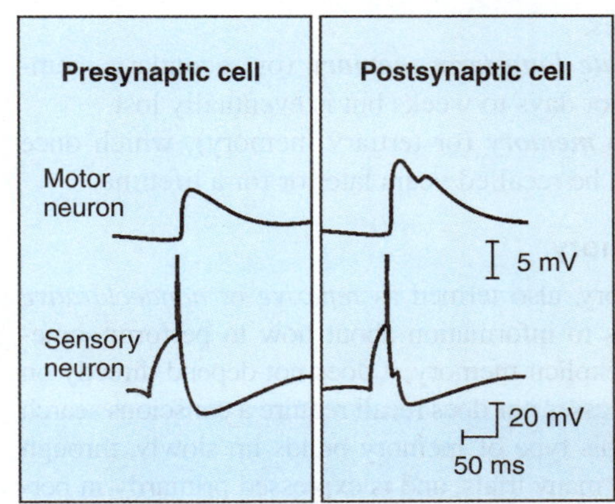

FIGURE 10.12-6 Cellular mechanism of conditioned reflex.

However, the laws of operant and classical conditioning are quite similar, suggesting that the two forms of learning may use the same neural mechanisms.

Memory

As mentioned earlier, memory and learning are closely related to each other. Memory refers to the acquisition, storage and retrieval of sensory information; while learning is the change in behaviour based on the sensory information stored in the brain. Brain has different sites and mechanisms for handling different types of information.

Types of Memory

Memory can be classified in two ways:

I. Physiologically, on the Basis of How Information is Stored and Recalled

The memory can be classified as implicit memory and explicit memory.

Implicit memory, also called nondeclarative or reflexive memory refers to information about how to perform something. It is not associated with awareness and does not involve processing in the hippocampus in most instances.

Explicit memory, also termed as declarative or recognition memory, refers to factual knowledge of people, places and things and what these facts mean. It is associated with consciousness or at least awareness, and is dependent for its retention on the hippocampus and other parts of the medial temporal lobes of brain.

II. Depending upon Permanency of Storage

Depending upon permanency of storage, memory is short-term, intermediate long-term and long-term memory.

1. ***Short-term memory,*** also termed as *primary memory,* lasts for seconds to hours. Example of short-term memory includes memory of a new telephone number after calling the operator or after looking into directory. Most of the times such a telephone number is forgotten after few minutes.
2. ***Intermediate long-term memory*** (or secondary memory) lasts for days to weeks but is eventually lost.
3. ***Long-term memory*** (or tertiary memory), which once stored, can be recalled years later or for a lifetime.

Implicit Memory

Implicit memory, also termed as *reflexive* or *nondeclarative memory,* refers to information about how to perform something. Unlike explicit memory, it does not depend directly on conscious processes nor does recall require a conscious search of memory. This type of memory builds up slowly, through repetition over many trials, and is expressed primarily in performance, not in words. Examples of implicit memory include motor skills, habits, behavioural reflexes and the learning of certain types of procedures and rules, which once acquired, become unconscious and automatic. It also includes priming in which recall of words and objects is improved by prior exposure to them. An example is improved recall of a word by a subject with amnesia when presented with first few letters of it. Most forms of implicit memory are acquired through different forms of reflexive learning which comprise:

1. *Nonassociative learning*, that includes:
   - Habituation and
   - Sensitization.
2. *Associative learning*, that includes:
   - Classical conditioning and
   - Operant conditioning.

Different forms of reflexive learning, which comprise implicit memory, have been described above (page 1129). These involve different brain regions:

- Memory acquired through *fear conditioning,* which has an emotional component is thought to involve *amygdala.*
- Memory acquired through *operant conditioning* requires the *striatum* and *cerebellum.*
- Memory acquired through classical conditioning, sensitization and habituation involves changes in the sensory and motor systems involved in the learning.

Explicit Memory

Explicit memory, also termed as *declarative* or *recognition memory,* refers to factual knowledge of people, places and things, and what these facts mean. This is recalled by a deliberate conscious effort. Explicit memory is highly flexible and involves the association of multiple bits and pieces of information. In contrast, implicit memory is more rigid and tightly connected to the original stimulus conditions under which the learning occurred.

Explicit memory can be further classified as *semantic memory* (a memory of facts) and *episodic memory* (a memory for events and personal experience).

Semantic (Factual) Memory The semantic memory is that form of long-term explicit memory that embraces knowledge of objects, facts and concepts as well as words and their meaning. It includes the naming of objects, the definition of spoken words and verbal fluency.

Semantic memory is stored in a distributed fashion in different association cortices. For example, the word alarm clock immediately brings its features in our mind from our past experience (stored memory) as follows:

- ***Visual memory*** reminds us about its shape, needles depicting hours, minutes, seconds and markings for 1 to 12 O'clock hours, etc.
- ***Auditory memory*** reminds us about its sound (ringing of alarm);
- ***Somatos ensory memory*** reminds us that it is made of a plastic or metallic box, having a smooth, transparent

glass. The visual, auditory and somatosensory memory which reminds us about different attributes is stored in different areas of neocortex. Whenever the information about the features of an alarm clock has to be recalled, the recall is built up from distinct bits of information, each of which is stored in specialized (dedicated) memory stores of neocortex. Thus, there is no general semantic memory store, i.e. semantic knowledge is not stored in a single region.

Damage to a specific cortical area leads to loss of specific information, and therefore a fragmentation of knowledge as exemplified:

- ***Associative visual agnosia*** results from damage to the posterior parietal cortex. In it, patient cannot name objects but can identify them by selecting the correct drawing and can faithfully reproduce detailed drawings of the object.
- ***Appreciative visual agnosia*** occurs in damage to occipital lobes and surrounding region. In it, patients are unable to draw objects but they can name them if appropriate perceptual cues are available.

Episodic (Autobiographical) Memory. Episodic memory refers to memory of events and personal experiences. For example, we use episodic memory when we recall that last Sunday I visited my friend's house in Kailash colony of New Delhi.

Episodic Memory is Stored in Association Areas of Prefrontal Cortex. These prefrontal areas work with other areas of the neocortex to allow recollection of when and where a past event occurred. Therefore, particularly striking symptom in patients with frontal lobe damage is *source amnesia,* i.e. tendency to forget how information was acquired. Since the ability to associate a piece of information with the time and place it was acquired is at the core of how accurately we remember the individual episodes of our lives, a deficit in source information interferes dramatically with the accuracy of recall of episodic knowledge.

Mechanism (Physiological and Cellular or Molecular Basis) of Memory

Studies of memory retention and disruption of memory have revealed that both explicit and implicit memories are stored in stages by different mechanisms. Input to the brain is processed into *short-term memory* before it is transformed through one or more stages (intermediate long-term memory) into more permanent long-term storage.

Mechanism of Implicit Memory

As mentioned earlier, most forms of implicit memory are acquired through different forms of reflexive learning (habituation and sensitization), and associative learning (classical and operant conditioning). Short-term storage of implicit memory for these simple forms of learning result from *changes in the effectiveness of synaptic transmission*:

- ***Habituation*** *involves an activity-dependent presynaptic depression of synaptic transmission*, resulting from the decrease in neurotransmitter released at the synapses.
  - Cellular basis of habituation is described on page 1129.
- ***Sensitization*** *involves presynaptic facilitation of synaptic transmission,* which is associated with increased release of neurotransmitters from the axonal ending of the sensory neuron.
  - Cellular mechanism *of sensitization* is described on page 1130.
- ***Classical conditioning*** *involves presynaptic facilitation of synaptic transmission that is dependent on activity in both the presynaptic and postsynaptic cell.*
  - *Physiological basis and cellular mechanism of classical conditioning* is described on page 1132.

Mechanism of Long-term Storage of Implicit Memory

The process by which transient short-term memory is converted into a stable long-term memory is called consolidation. *Consolidation of long-term implicit memory* for simple forms of learning involves three processes:

- Gene expression,
- New protein synthesis and
- Growth (or prunning) of synaptic connections.

Molecular biological analysis of long-term storage, of implicit memory reveals that it involves the cAMP–PKA–MAPK–CREB pathway.

Mechanism of Explicit Memory Both semantic and episodic types of explicit memory are the result of at least four related but distinct types of processing; encoding, consolidation, storage and retrieval.

Mechanism of Short-term Explicit Memory ***Encoding*** refers to the process by which newly learned information is attended to and processed when first encountered. The extent and nature of this encoding are critically important for determining how well the learned material will be remembered at later times. For a memory to persist and be well remembered, the incoming information must be encoded thoroughly and deeply.

Neural Substrate for Encoding of Explicit Memory As mentioned earlier, the explicit memory is associated with consciousness (or at least awareness) and is dependent for its retention on the *hippocampus* and other parts of *medial temporal lobes* of the brain.

Studies with human patients and with experimental animals suggest that knowledge stored as explicit memory is processed as (Fig. 10.12-7):

- Sensory information is first acquired through processing in one or more of the three polymodal association cortices

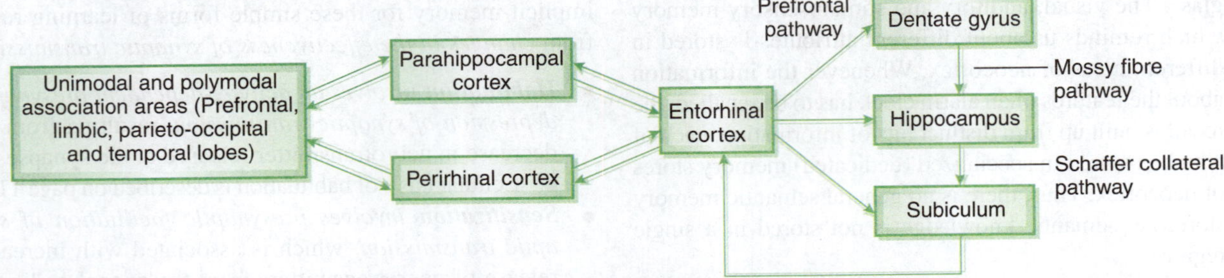

FIGURE 10.12-7 Neural substrate for encoding of explicit memory (the input and output pathways of the hippocampal formation).

(the *prefrontal, limbic* and *parieto-occipital-temporal cortices*) that synthesize visual, auditory and somatic information.

- From polymodal association cortices, the information is conveyed in series to the *parahippocampal* and *perirhinal cortices*, then the *entorhinal cortex,* the dentate gyrus, the hippocampus, the subiculum and finally back to the entorhinal cortex.
- From the entorhinal cortex the information is sent back to parahippocampal and perirhinal cortices and finally back to polymodal association areas of the neocortex.

Physiological processes in the neural substrate associated with storage of short-term explicit memory (*hippocampus*) are:

- Continuous neural activity in reverberating circuits,
- Activation of synapses on presynaptic terminals that typically result in prolonged facilitation, i.e. long-term potentation (LTP) or prolonged inhibition, i.e. long-term depression (LTD) and
- Accumulation of calcium in axon terminals may eventually lead to enhanced synaptic output from the terminal.

Long-term Potentiation (LTP). The long-term potentiation involves protein synthesis and growth of presynaptic and postsynaptic neurons and their connections. LTP is a rapidly developing postsynaptic potential that occurs in response to repeated stimulation of presynaptic neuron. It last for a prolonged period (for days).

- ***Mechanisms***: There are different mechanisms for development of LTP. Though LTP develops in different parts of the nervous system but it has been studied in great detail in the hippocampus, specifically for connections of pyramidal cells of cortical area 3 region (CA_3) and of CA_1 region via collaterals called (Schaffer's collaterals). The underlying mechanisms depend on changes in following types of receptors; N-methyl-D-aspartate receptors (NMDA), which are Na^+- dependent receptors and α-amino-3-hydroxy-5-methylisoxizal-4-propionic acid (AMPA) receptors or Na^+- independent receptors. The sequence of events is (Fig. 10.12-8):
  - At resting membrane potential, glutamate releases from the presynaptic neuron.
  - Glutamate binds on to NMDA receptors as well as to non-NMDA or AMPA receptors.
  - LTP initiated by NMDA receptors increases intracellular Ca^{2+}, either in presynaptic or in postsynaptic neurons, whereas in activation of AMPA receptors there is increased Na^+ and K^+ flow (because of the presence of Mg^{2+} on NMDA receptors that blocks their flow through these receptors).
  - However, depolarization triggered by the activation of AMPA receptors relieves the Mg^{2+} blocked in the NMDA receptors and Ca^{2+} enters into the postsynaptic neurons.
  - The increase in cytoplasmic Ca^{2+}, activates Ca^{2+}/Calmodulin kinase, protein kinase C(PKC) and tyrosine kinase, which together induce LTP.
  - The Ca^{2+}/Calmodulin kinase II phosphorylates the AMPA receptors, increasing their conductance and causing movement of more AMPA receptors to the synaptic membrane from the cytosolic storage site.
  - As there is an initiation of LTP, nitric oxide releases by the postsynaptic neuron; that passes retrogradly to the presynaptic neuron and causes long-term quantitative increase in the release of glutamate.

In hippocampus, LTP occurs in mossy fibres that connect granule cells in the dentate cortex. LTP is induced due to increase in Ca^{2+} in the presynaptic neuron rather than in the postsynaptic neuron in response to tetanic stimulation and is independent of NMDA receptors. The increased influx of Ca^{2+} in presynaptic neuron activates Ca^{2+}/Calmodulin-dependent adenylyl cyclase that increases cAMP.

Long-term Depression (LTD). Long-term depression is just opposite to LTP. It is characterized by a decrease in synaptic strength, due to slower stimulation of presynaptic neurons and is associated with lesser rise in the intracellular Ca^{2+}. LTD was first noticed in hippocampus, but subsequently it was observed in many other regions of CNS also. It is also observed in same fibres in which LTP is present.

Mechanism of Intermediate Long-Term Memory Intermediate long-term memory can result from temporary chemical or physical changes in either the presynaptic or postsynaptic membrane that can persist for a few minutes to

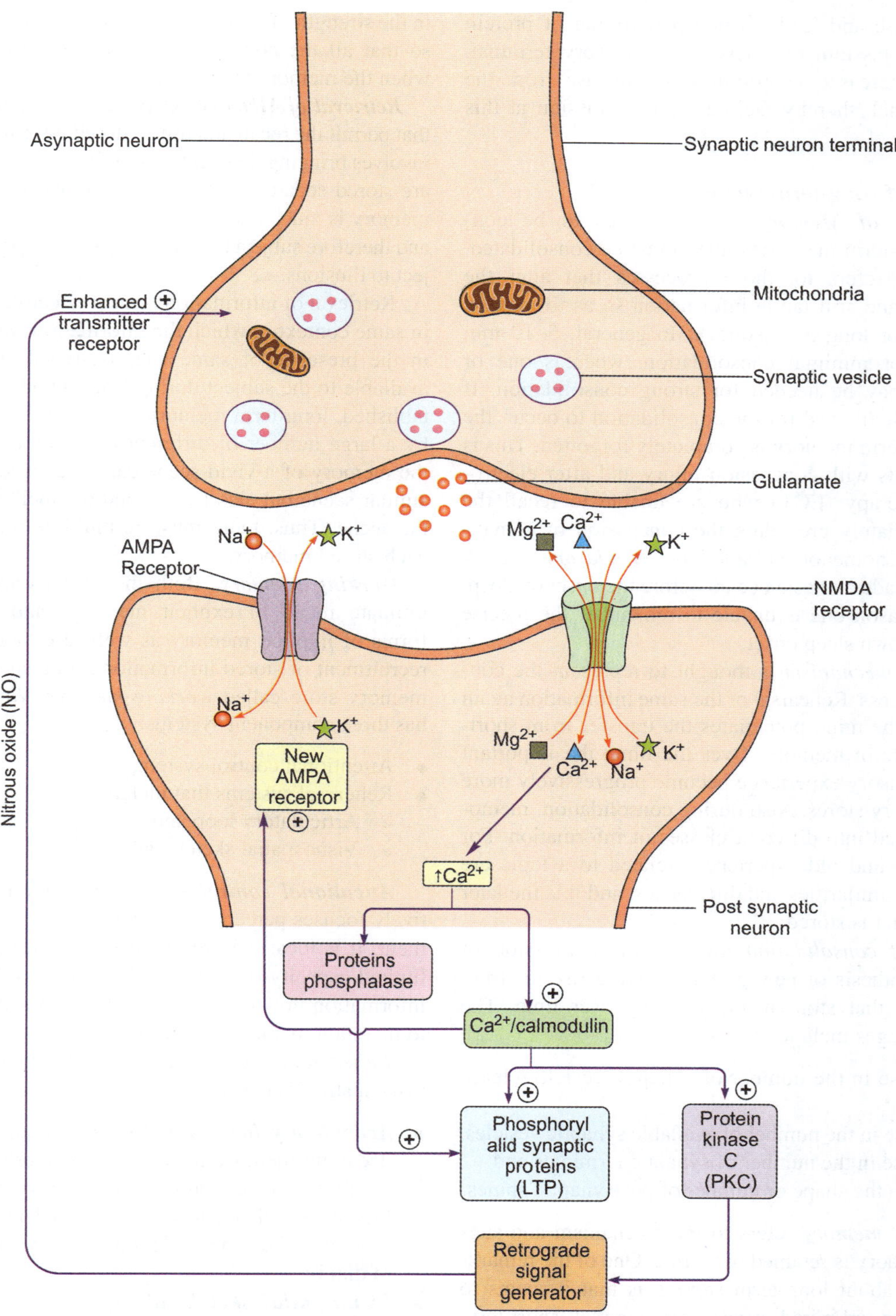

FIGURE 10.12-8 Production of LTP in Schaffer collaterals in the hippocampus.

several weeks. The newly stored sensory information is still labile during this stage, which is converted into long-term memory after the process of consolidation is complete.

Physiological process in the neural substrate associated with intermediate long-term memory is that of synaptic facilitation and has been studied in the snail *Aplysia*. As shown in figs 10.12-4, 10.12-5, stimulation of a facilitator terminal at the same time as activation of another sensory input causes serotonin to be released at synaptic sites on the sensory terminal. Stimulation of serotonin receptors activates adenylyl cyclase in the main sensory terminal, resulting in formation of cyclic-AMP, which causes the release of a protein kinase and leads to phosphorylation of protein that blocks potassium channels in the sensory terminal, resulting in increased neurotransmitter release from the sensory terminal, thereby facilitating transmission at this synapse.

Mechanism of Long-term Memory

Consolidation of Memory. For memories to be converted to long-term memories, they must be consolidated. Consolidation refers to, those processes that alter the newly stored and still labile information so as to make it more stable for long-term storage. In general, 5–10 min is required for minimal consolidation, whereas one or more hours may be needed for strong consolidation. If this time is not allowed for the consolidation to occur, the data in short-term memory is completely forgotten. This is seen in patients with concussion injury and after electroconvulsive therapy (ECT) who are unable to recall the events immediately preceding the concussion or convulsion. This phenomenon is called *retrograde amnesia*. A similar retrograde amnesia occurs before the onset of sleep. This is the reason one is unable to remember the precise time of one's own sleep onset.

Rehearsal mechanism is thought to represent the consolidation process. Rehearsal of the same information again and again in the mind potentiates the transfer from short-term to long-term memory. Over the time, the important features of sensory experience become progressively more fixed in memory stores. Also during consolidation, memories are codified into different classes of information. For example, new and old experiences related to a topic are compared for similarities and differences, and it is the later information that is stored.

Process of consolidation involves the expression of genes and synthesis of new proteins, giving rise to structural changes that store memory stably over time. The structural changes include:

- An increase in the number of synaptic vesicle release sites,
- An increase in the number of available synaptic vesicles,
- An increase in the number of synaptic terminals and
- Changes in the shape or number of postsynaptic spines.

Storage of memory refers to the mechanism and sites by which memory is retained over time. One of the remarkable features about long-term storage is that it seems to have an almost unlimited capacity. In contrast, short-term working memory is very limited.

Neural Substrate for Long-term Storage Memory. While the encoding process for short-term explicit memory involves the hippocampus, long-term memories are stored in the various parts of neocortex. Apparently, the various parts of the memories—visual, olfactory, auditory, etc. are located in the cortical regions concerned with these functions, and the pieces are tied together by long-term changes in the strength of transmission at relevant synaptic junctions so that all the components are brought to consciousness when the memory is recalled.

Retrieval of Memory Retrieval refers to those processes that permit the recall and use of stored information. Retrieval involves bringing different kinds of information together that are stored separately in different storage sites. Retrieval of memory is much like perception; it is a constructive process and therefore subject to distortion, much as perception is subject to illusions.

Retrieval of information is most effective when it occurs in same context in which the information was acquired and in the presence of same cues (retrieval cues) that were available to the subject during learning. However, once established, long-term memories can be recalled or accessed by a large number of different associations. For example, the memory of a vivid scene can be evoked not only by a similar scene but also by a sound or smell associated with the scene. Thus, there must be multiple routes or keys to each stored memory.

Working Memory. Both the initial encoding and the ultimate recall of explicit memory (and perhaps some forms of implicit memory as well) are thought to require recruitment of stored information into a special short-term memory store called *working memory*. Working memory has three component systems:

- Attentional control system,
- Rehearsal systems that include:
  - Articulatory loop and
  - Visuospatial sketch pad.

Attentional control system or (central executive) actively focuses perception on specific events in the environment. It is located in the prefrontal cortex and has a very limited capacity (less than a dozen items). It regulates the information flow to two rehearsal systems that are thought to maintain memory for temporary use.

Rehearsal systems include the articulatory loop and the visuospatial sketch pad.

- ***Articulatory loop*** is a storage system with a rapidly decaying memory trace where memory for words and numbers can be maintained by subvocal speech. It is this system that allows one to hold in mind, through repetition, i.e. a new telephone number as one prepares to dial it.
- ***Visuospatial sketchpad*** represents both the visual properties and the spatial location of object to be remembered. This system, allows one to store the image of the face of a person one meets at a dinner party.

The two rehearsal memory systems are thought to be located in different parts of the posterior association cortices. The information processed in either of these systems has the possibility of entering long-term memory.

Interhemispheric Transfer of Learning and Memory

Much information is transferred between the two hemispheres through the corpus callosum, although some is transmitted through other commissures (e.g. the anterior commissure or hippocampal commissure).

Experiment to demonstrate importance of corpus callosum for interhemispheric transfer of information is (Fig. 10.12-9):

- An experimental animal (cat or monkey), with an intact optic chiasma and corpus callosum, and the left eye closed is conditioned to a visual discrimination task (Fig. 10.12-9 A_1).
- When the animal is asked to perform the same task with left eye open and right eye closed, the task can still be performed (Fig. 10.12-9 A_2) indicating that both hemispheres have learned the task. Conclusion is that either interocular transfer has occurred due to intactoptic chiasma or corpus callosum (Fig. 10.12-9 A_3).
- When the optic chiasma is transected before the animal is trained (Fig. 10.12-9 B_1), the result is the same (Fig. 10.12-9 B_2), concluding that learning is transferred via corpus callosum (Fig. 10.12-9 B_3).
- When both the optic chiasma and corpus callosum are cut before training (Fig. 10.12-9 C_1), then information is not transferred (Fig. 10.12-9 C_2), and each hemisphere must learn the task independently. This confirmed the fact that the learning is transferred via corpus callosum (Fig. 10.12-9 C_3).

Similar results about failure of intercortical transfer of learning and memory is also seen in human patients, who have had a surgical transection of the corpus callosum to prevent interhemispheric spread of epilepsy. Studies in subject indicate that the transfer of visual memory occurs in the posterior part of the corpus callosum while transfer of auditory and somaesthetic memory occurs in the anterior part of the corpus callosum.

Further, functional capabilities of the two hemispheres when compared by exploring the performance of individuals with a transected corpus callosum have yielded following results:

- Right hemisphere specializes in spatial task, facial expression, body language and speech into notion.
- Patients with a transected corpus callosum lack coordination. For example, when they are dressing, one hand may button a shirt while other tries to unbutton it.
- From this experiment, it can be concluded that the two hemispheres can operate quite independently when they are no longer interconnected.

Applied Aspects

- Drug facilitating memory,
- Amnesia,
- Alzheimer's disease and senile dementia,
- Confabulation and
- Stranginess and familiarity

Drugs Facilitating Memory

Learning and memory is reported to improve in animals when a variety of CNS stimulants are administered immediately, before or after the learning sessions.

Common CNS stimulant that facilitates learning and memory are: caffeine, amphetamine, physostigmine, nicotine, pemoline, strychnine and pentylenetetrazol.

Mechanism of action. CNS stimulants act probably by facilitating consolidation of memory. For example, physostigmine acts by inhibiting acetylcholinesterase and hence, preventing breakdown of acetylcholine, while nicotine stimulates cholinergic receptors.

Amnesia

Amnesia refers to loss of memory. It is of two types: antegrade amnesia and retrograde amnesia.

- ***Antegrade amnesia*** refers to inability of an individual to establish new long-term memories of those types of information that form the basis of intelligence. This usually occurs in lesions involving hippocampus.
- ***Retrograde amnesia*** refers to inability of an individual to recall past memories. Amnesia is much greater for events of recent past than those of remote past. Memories of distant past are rehearsed so many times that the memory traces are deeply engrained and elements of these memories are stored in the widespread areas of the brain. Retrograde amnesia occurs in lesions involving the temporal lobe (*temporal lobe syndrome*).

Alzheimer's Disease and Senile Dementia

Senile Dementia Senile dementia refers to a clinical syndrome in elderly people that is characterized by progressive impairment of memory and cognitive capacities. There are a number of diseases that are manifested by dementia in mid and late life.

Common causes of dementia in the elderly are:

- Alzheimer's disease,
- Cerebrovascular disease,
- Lewy body dementia,
- Parkinsonism,
- Prion diseases, etc.

Alzheimer's Disease Alzheimer's disease is the most common cause of dementia in the elderly persons.

Pathophysiology. Both genetic and environmental factors may be responsible to the etiology of disease. Alzheimer's disease is a prototypical neurodegenerative disease. It is characterized by a series of abnormalities in the brain that selectively affect neurons in specific regions, particularly in the neocortex, the entorhinal area, hippocampus, amygdala,

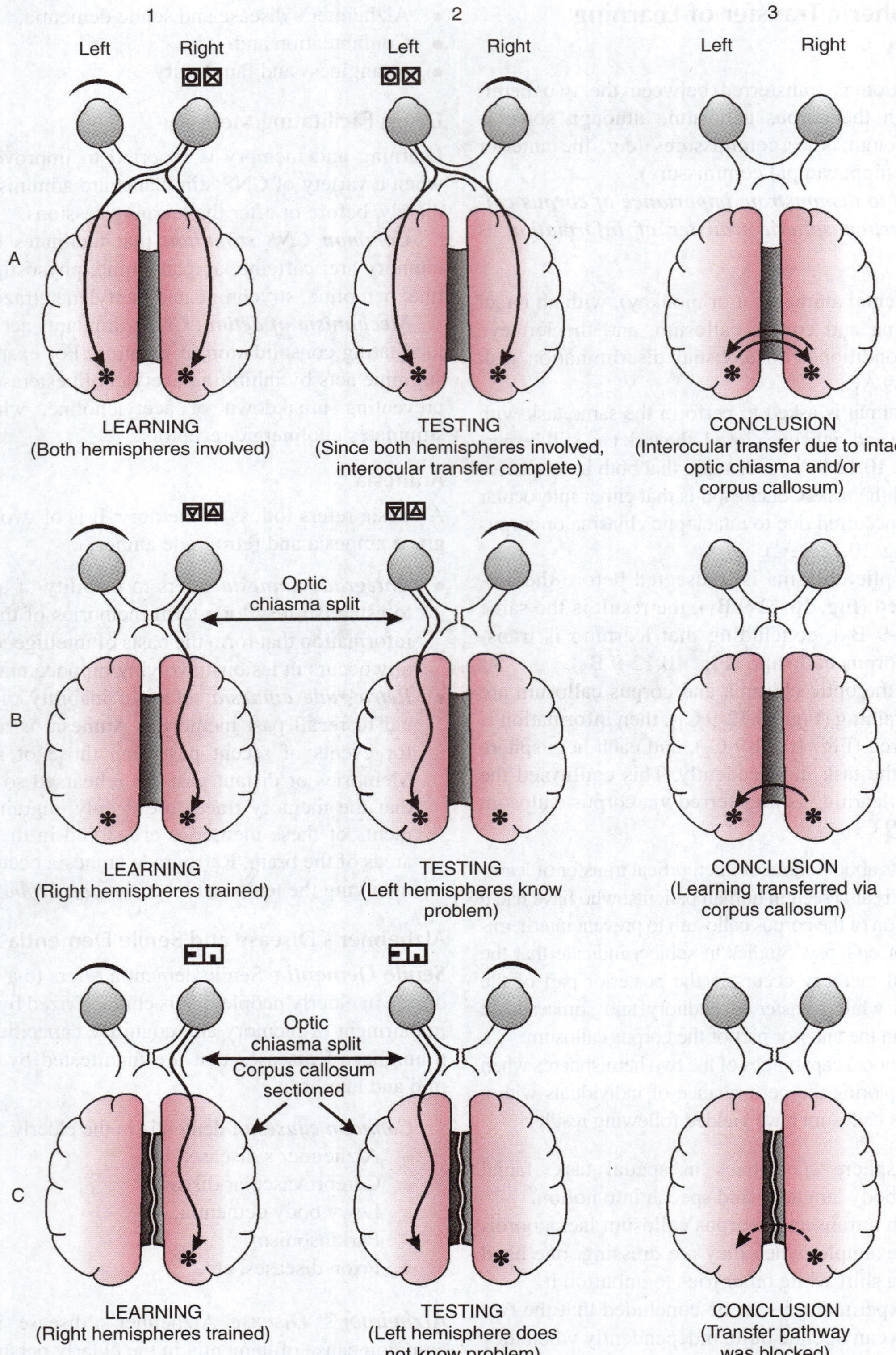

FIGURE 10.12-9 Experiment to demonstrate importance of corpus callosum for interhemispheric transfer of learning and memory (for details see text).

nucleus basalis, anterior thalamus, locus coeruleus and raphe complex. There is a severe loss of cholinergic neurosis in the affected areas. The major cholinergic pathways involved in Alzheimer's disease are shown in Fig. 10.12-10.

Familial form of disease seen in early onset disease, and is caused by mutation in the genes for amyloid precursor protein, presenilin I and II. It is transmitted as an autosomal dominance. Each mutation leads to over production of β–amyloid protein. Recently, it is found that mutation of α–2 macroglobulin gene is associated with late onset disease.

Alzheimer's disease is associated with cytoskeletal abnormalities in the affected nerve cells, most important being accumulation of neurofibrillary tangles in the neuronal cytoplasm made up of hyperphosphorylated *tau* protein that binds to microtubules. Amyloid plaque (fibrillar peptides) deposits surrounded by altered nerve fibres and glial cells are one of the hallmarks of Alzheimer's disease.

Note. The β–amyloid plaques are the products of amyloid precursor protein (APP), a normal transmembrane protein that projects into the extracellular fluid from nerve cells. This protein is hydrolysed at three sites by α, β and γ secretase. The polypeptides formed after hydrolization by γ-secretase are toxic. These polypeptides get aggregated and stick on to AMPA receptors and Ca^{2+} channels and thus prevent Ca^{2+} influx, and also induce inflammatory reaction and formation of intracellular tangles (Fig. 10.12-11).

Characteristic features of Alzheimer's disease are:

- Loss of recent memory in an otherwise alert individual,
- Impairment in other areas of cognition such as language, problem solving, judgement, calculation, attention, perception and so on.

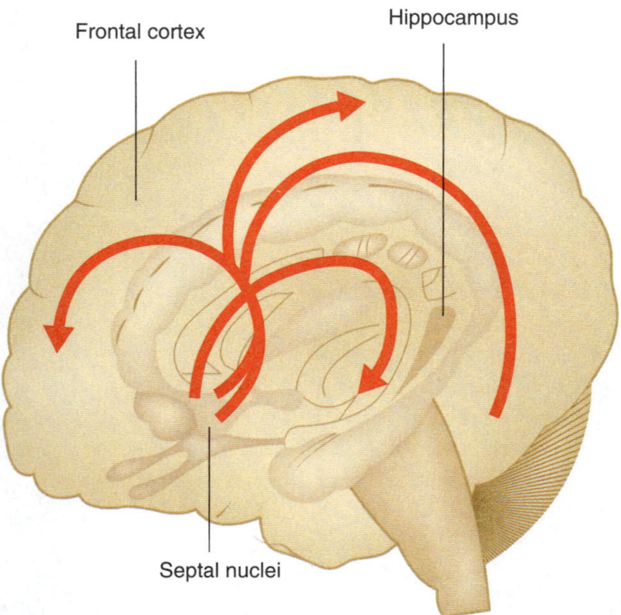

FIGURE 10.12-10 Major cholinergic pathways involved in Alzheimer's disease.

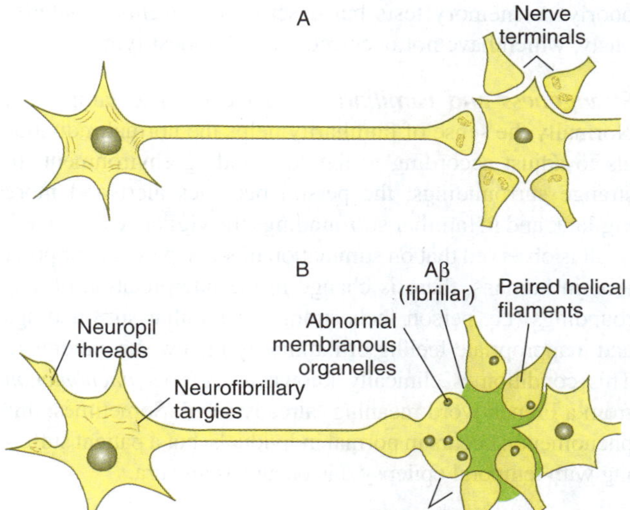

FIGURE 10.12-11 Comparison of neuron: **A,** in normal individual and **B,** with abnormalities associated with Alzheimer disease.

- Psychiatric symptoms begin to appear as the disease progresses.
- Extra pyramidal and akinetic hypertonic symptoms also appear in later stages.
- There may occur loss of spatial orientation.
- Finally, patient has to lead a vegetative life without memory, without thinking power, speechless, inability to understand anything, *apraxia* (inability to perform voluntary movements) and *agnesia* (inability to recognize objects in spite of intact sensory modality).

Treatment. There is no effective treatment for Alzheimer's disease, as yet *physostigmine*, which inhibits cholinesterase causes some improvement. Presently, focus is on treating associated symptoms such as depression, agitation, sleep disorders, hallucinations and delusions.

- Memantine is a NMDA-receptor antagonist that prevents glutamate-induced excitability in brain is useful for treating patients with moderate to severe Alzheimer.
- R-flubiprofen is useful in blocking the production of β–amyloid protein.
- Vaccines that allow the body immune system to produce antibodies against these proteins are under trial.

In prospective study, it is mentioned that if a person is doing frequent effortful mental activities like solving crossword and puzzles, the onset of cognitive dementia slows down. Explanation is based on the fact that hippocampus and its connections have plasticity.

Confabulation

Confabulation occurs in patients with lesion of ventromedial part of frontal lobe. In this condition, individuals perform poorly on memory tests but describe the events spontaneously, which have not occurred (called honest lying).

Strangeness and Familiarity Strangeness and familiarity. Normally the sense of familiarity helps the normal individuals to adjust according to the surrounding environment. In strange surroundings, the person becomes alert and more vigilant, and in familiar surroundings the vigilance is relaxed.

It is observed that on stimulation of some parts of temporal lobe in humans, there is change in the interpretation of surroundings (i.e. person feels strange in familiar surroundings and inappropriate feeling of familiarity in new surroundings). This condition is clinically known as *dejs vu phenomenon* from a French word meaning 'already seen'. Sometimes, this phenomenon occurs in normal individuals, but a patient suffering with temporal epilepsy this occurs as an aura.

HIGHER INTELLECTUAL FUNCTIONS OF THE PREFRONTAL ASSOCIATION CORTEX

Prefrontal cortex refers to the portion of frontal lobes in front of the motor cortex. This area, like other association areas, is better developed in man than in any other species. The function of the prefrontal cortex is complex and multifactorial, and is typically explained by describing the deficits seen in individuals in whom the prefrontal lobotomy has been performed for tumour of this region. The functions thought to be performed by prefrontal cortex are:

1. Role in Thought Process Prefrontal cortex gathers information from widespread area of the brain to develop solutions to problems, whether they require motor or nonmotor responses. Without this function, thoughts lose their logical progression, and the individual loses the ability to focus attention and is easily distracted in the sequence of thoughts. Hence, any activity involving a number of steps in sequence cannot be performed properly. In other words, there occurs *inability to progress towards goals* or *to carry through sequential thoughts*.

2. Site of Working Memory and Intellectual Functions Prefrontal cortex is considered the site of 'working memory'. Working memory refers to the ability to hold and sort bits of information to be used in problem-solving function. By combining these stored bits of information, an individual can prognosticate, plan for the future, delay a response while further information is gathered, consider the consequences of actions before they are performed, correlate information from many different sources and control actions in accordance with societal or moral laws. All of these are considered as *intellectual functions* of the highest order and seem to be definitive for the human experience.

The patients with lesions of prefrontal cortex have great difficulty in abstract thinking, e.g. planning for future or considering the consequences of a particular motor activity beforehand. The patient cannot act within the norm of social or moral behaviour.

3. Role in Episodic Memory Patients with prefrontal lesions show a difficulty in remembering the temporal sequence of events, i.e. he cannot remember how long ago, he saved an event or picture card (episodic memory, i.e. a memory for events and personal experience).

Section 11

Special Senses

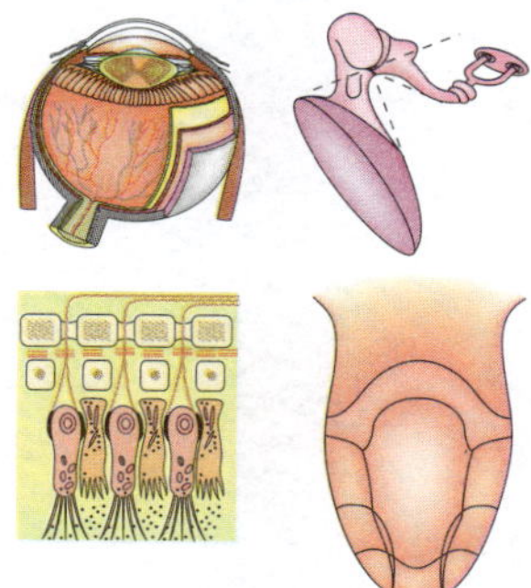

As we have studied, the sensory division of the human nervous system is concerned with collection of the information about the outside world and the changes occurring within the body itself. The term *sensation* refers to the conscious perception of sensory information reaching the brain. The sensations have been broadly divided into general and special sensations.

General sensations. These, depending upon their point of origin can be classified into three main groups:

- *Exteroceptive sensations,* i.e. those arising from the skin, e.g. touch and temperature sensation,
- *Visceral sensations,* i.e. those arising from the viscera and
- *Proprioceptive and kinaesthetic sensations,* i.e. those arising from the muscles, tendons and joints.

Special sensations. There are a few organs in the body which collect information of special significance to us from the external environment and are, therefore, called the organs of special senses. These organs of special senses have developed in the heads of animals, along with corresponding neural systems in the brain during the involutionary process of encephalization. These special sensory systems include:

- *The sense of vision,* which allows the animal to detect and analyse light,
- *The sense of hearing,* that makes possible the detection and analysis of sound and
- *The chemical senses of taste and smell* which are responsible for appreciation of chemical signals in the environment.

General versus Special Sensations

- ***Location of receptors.*** Receptors for general sensations are located throughout the body, e.g. touch, pain, pressure and temperature sensations, while the receptors for special senses are located at one place in the head near the nervous system, e.g. receptors for vision, hearing, taste and smell.

- ***Response of receptors.*** The receptors for general sensations get easily stimulated by different stimuli; however, they respond maximally to an adequate stimulus. Further, the receptors response is nonspecific to different stimuli. While, the receptor for special senses are specialized and respond only to one type of stimulus. Further, the receptor response is more complex and makes co-ordination within the CNS.

This section is devoted to special sensations, while the general sensations have been discussed in Chapter 10.8 on the Somatosensory System.

Chapter 11.1

Sense of vision

INTRODUCTION AND FUNCTIONAL ANATOMY

Introduction

Sense of vision, the choicest gift from the Almighty to the humans and other animals, is a complex function of the two eyes and their central connections. The eyeballs are able to perform their function with the help of following physiological activities:

- Maintenance of clear media of the eye,
- Maintenance of normal intraocular pressure (IOP),
- The image forming mechanism,
- Physiology of vision,
- Physiology of binocular vision,
- Physiology of pupil and
- Physiology of ocular motility.

Before discussing the details of the above physiological considerations, it will be worthwhile to be conversant with the broad outlines of functional anatomy of the eyeball and related structures.

Functional Anatomy

There are two eyeballs, each being suspended by *extraocular muscles* and fascial sheaths in a quadrilateral pyramid-shaped bony cavity called *orbit.* Each eye is protected anteriorly by two shutters called the *eyelids.* The anterior part of the sclera and posterior surface of the eyelids is lined by a thin membrane called *conjunctiva.* For smooth functioning, the cornea and conjunctiva are to be kept moist by tears, which are produced by the lacrimal gland and drained by lacrimal passages, which together form the *lacrimal apparatus.* The eyelids, the eyebrows, the conjunctiva and lacrimal apparatus are collectively known as the *appendages of the eye.* A brief account of anatomy of the eyeball and its related structures is given.

The Eyeball

Each eyeball (Fig. 11.1-1) is a cystic structure kept distended by the pressure inside it. Although generally referred to as a globe, the eyeball is not a sphere but an oblate spheroid.

Dimensions of an Adult Eyeball

Anteroposterior diameter	: 24 mm
Horizontal (transverse) diameter	: 23.5 mm
Vertical diameter	: 23 mm
Circumference	: 75 mm
Volume	: 6.5 ml
Weight	: 7 gm

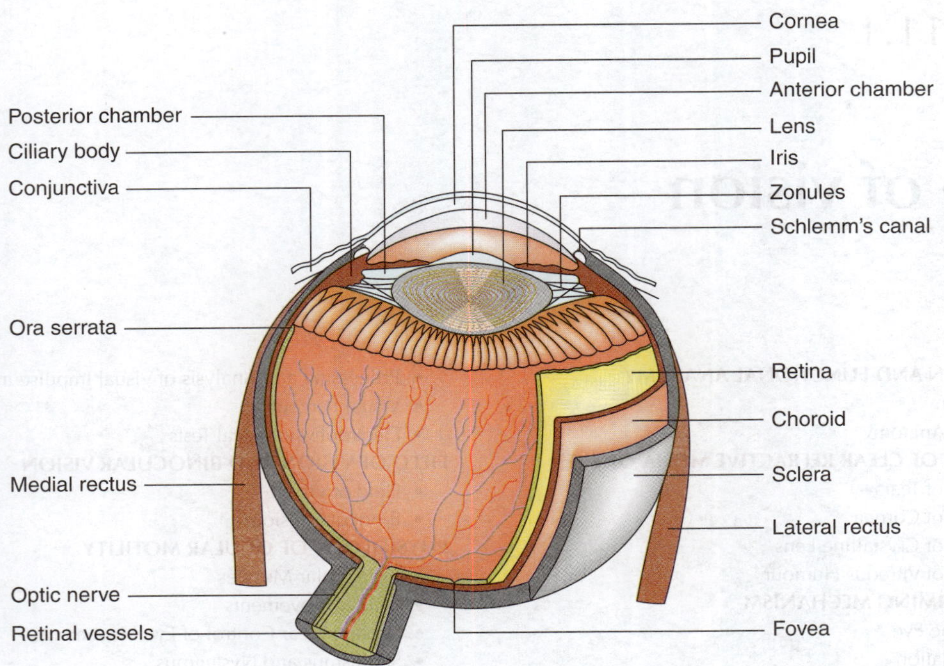

FIGURE 11.1-1 Gross anatomy of eyeball.

Coats of the Eyeball The eyeball comprises three coats: outer (fibrous coat), middle (vascular coat) and inner (nervous coat).

1. The Outer Fibrous Coat. The fibrous coat (Fig. 11.1-1) is a dense strong wall which protects the intraocular contents. Anterior one-sixth of this fibrous coat is transparent and is called cornea. The posterior five-sixth opaque part is called sclera. Junction of the cornea and sclera is called limbus.

Cornea. The cornea is a transparent, avascular, watchglass-like structure with a smooth shining surface. The average diameter of the cornea is 11–12 mm. Its thickness in the central part is 0.52 mm and in the peripheral part 0.67 mm.

Sclera. The sclera is a strong, opaque, white fibrous layer. It is a relatively avascular structure about 1 mm in thickness. It is pierced by nerves and vessels entering in the eyeball. Histologically, sclera consists of three layers: episcleral tissue, sclera proper and lamina fusca.

2. The Middle Vascular Coat. The middle vascular coat (Fig. 11.1-1) also known as uveal tract, from anterior to posterior, can be divided into three parts: iris, ciliary body and choroid. The blood supply of uveal tract is derived from the short posterior ciliary arteries, long posterior ciliary arteries and anterior ciliary arteries.

Iris. Iris is a coloured, circular diaphragm with a central aperture of 3–4 mm size known as pupil. The pupil regulates the light reaching the retina. The pupil constricts and dilates by the contraction of sphincter pupillae and dilator pupillae muscles of the iris, respectively. The sphincter pupillae is supplied by the parasympathetic nerves while the dilator pupillae is supplied by the sympathetic nerves.

Ciliary Body. The ciliary body is the middle part of the uveal tract. In cut section, it is triangular in shape with base forwards. Anteriorly, the iris is attached to about the middle of the base of the ciliary body. Posteriorly, the ciliary body becomes continuous with the choroid. The ciliary body can be divided into two parts: anterior known as pars plicata and posterior known as pars plana.

The ciliary body contains a nonstriated muscle called the ciliary muscle which is supplied by parasympathetic fibres and takes part in the process of accommodation of the eye.

There are about 70–80 finger-like projections from the pars plicata part of the ciliary body. These are called *ciliary processes* and are the site of aqueous humour production—a watery fluid which maintains the IOP of the eyeball.

Choroid. Choroid is a dark brown highly vascular layer situated in between sclera and retina. It supplies nutrition to the outer layers of retina. The inflammations of choroid invariably involve the underlying retina.

3. The Inner Nervous Coat (Retina). Retina, the innermost tunic of the eyeball, is a thin, delicate, transparent membrane. It is the most highly developed tissue of the eye. It is concerned with the visual functions (details on page 1144).

Interior of the Eyeball Interior of the eyeball consists of anterior and posterior chambers containing the aqueous humour, the lens and the vitreous.

Anterior and Posterior Chambers. *Anterior chamber* is the space bounded anteriorly by the back of cornea and posteriorly by the anterior surface of iris. *Posterior chamber* is the space between the front of crystalline lens and back of iris. Through pupil, anterior and posterior chambers communicate with each other. *Aqueous humour* is a watery fluid present in the anterior and posterior chambers of the eyeball.

Crystalline Lens The lens is a transparent, biconvex, crystalline structure placed between the iris and the vitreous. It is suspended from the ciliary body by the suspensory ligaments or zonules of Zinn. Refractive power of the lens is about 15–16D. Lens is elastic in nature and its power changes with accommodation. Elasticity of the lens gradually decreases with the age. It is an avascular structure and derives its nutrition from the aqueous humour.

Vitreous Humour Vitreous humour is an inert, transparent, jelly-like structure that fills the posterior four-fifth of the cavity of eyeball. It serves the optical function. It consists of 90% water, some salts and mucoproteins.

Extraocular Muscles, Appendages of Eye, and Orbit

Extraocular Muscles

A set of six extraocular muscles (4 recti and 2 obliques) control the movements of each eye (see page 1166).

Appendages of the Eye

Eyebrows. The two eyebrows are arched structures placed horizontally over the superciliary ridge of the frontal bone, separated from each other by a smooth hairless prominent area known as glabella. The surface of the eyebrows is covered by hair which project obliquely from the skin and form an important part of the eyebrows. They protect the eyeball from sweat, dust and other foreign bodies.

Eyelids. The eyelids are mobile tissue curtains placed in front of the eyeballs. These act as shutters protecting the eyes from injuries and excessive light. These also perform an important function of spreading the tear film over the cornea and conjunctiva.

Eyelashes are short curved hair present on the lid margins (free edges of the eyelids).

Conjunctiva. The conjunctiva is a translucent mucous membrane which lines the posterior surface of the eyelids and anterior aspect of the eyeball upto limbus.

Parts. Conjunctiva consists of following parts:

1. ***Palpebral conjunctiva*** lines the posterior surface of the eyelids.
2. ***Bulbar conjunctiva*** covers the anterior part of eyeball upto the limbus.
3. ***Fornices.*** Superior and inferior conjunctival fornices are the cul-de-sac formed at the junction of bulbar conjunctiva with the palpebral conjunctiva.
4. ***Plica semilunaris*** is a pinkish crescentic fold of conjunctiva present in the medial canthus.

Orbit. The bony orbits are quadrangular truncated pyramids situated between the anterior cranial fossa above and the maxillary sinuses below. Seven bones take part in its formation. It has four walls (medial, lateral, superior and inferior), a base and an apex.

MAINTENANCE OF CLEAR REFRACTIVE MEDIA OF THE EYE

The main prerequisite for visual function is the maintenance of clear refractive media of the eye. The major factor responsible for transparency of the ocular media is their avascularity. The structures forming refractive media of the eye from anterior to posterior are:

- Tear film,
- Cornea,
- Aqueous humour (see page 1169)
- Crystalline lens and
- Vitreous humour.

Physiology of Tears

Lacrimal Apparatus The lacrimal apparatus (Fig. 11.1-2) comprises the structures concerned with the formation (main lacrimal gland and accessory lacrimal glands) and drainage (lacrimal passages: puncta, canaliculi, lacrimal sac and nasolacrimal duct) of tears.

Tear Film and Its Functions

Tear Film Tear film refers to the fluid covering the cornea and conjunctiva. Tears are composed of 98% water and 1.5% sodium chloride (which gives the tears their salty flavour). It also contains antibacterial substances like

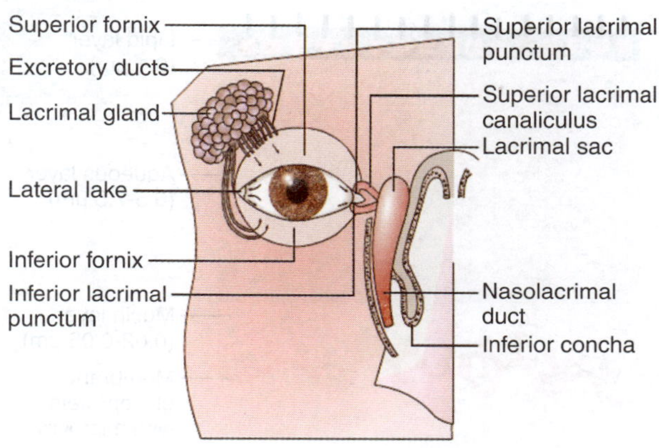

FIGURE 11.1-2 The lacrimal apparatus.

lysozyme, betalysin and lactoferrin. Anatomically, the precorneal tear film has been described to consist of three layers, which from posterior to anterior (Fig. 11.1-3) are:

1. ***Mucous layer.*** It consists of mucus secreted by conjunctival goblet cells.
2. ***Aqueous layer.*** It is formed by tears secreted by the main and accessory lacrimal glands.
3. ***Lipid layer.*** This, outermost layer, is formed by secretions of meibomian, Zeiss and Moll's glands.

Functions of the Tear Film

1. It keeps the cornea and conjunctiva moist.
2. It provides oxygen to the corneal epithelium.
3. It washes away debris and noxious irritants.
4. It prevents infection due to presence of antibacterial substances.
5. It facilitates movements of the lids over the globe.

Physiology of Cornea

Cornea forms the main refracting medium of the eye. It is a transparent watchglass-like structure, the anterior surface of which is bathed with tears, and endothelial surface is bathed in aqueous humour.

Histological Structure Histologically cornea consists of the following five layers (Fig. 11.1-4):

1. ***Epithelium.*** It is of stratified squamous type and consists of 5 to 6 layers of cells.
2. ***Bowman's membrane.*** It is an acellular structure which consists of condensed collagen fibrils. Once damaged, it does not regenerate and leaves behind a faint corneal scar.
3. ***Stroma (substantia propria).*** It forms the 90% of corneal thickness. It mainly consists of collagen fibrils arranged in sets of regular lamellae, lying parallel to the surface. The corneal lamellae are embedded in ground substance. The ground substance consists of acid mucopolysaccharides, chondroitin sulphate (Type A and C) and keratin sulphate. Scattered between the lamellae are the corneal corpuscles (keratocytes) and a few wandering leucocytes and macrophages.
4. ***Descemet's membrane.*** It is a thin but strong homogeneous elastic membrane. It is secreted by endothelial cells and is essentially their basement membrane. It readily regenerates after an injury.
5. ***Endothelium.*** It consists of a single layer of flattened polygonal cells. It does not regenerate in human.

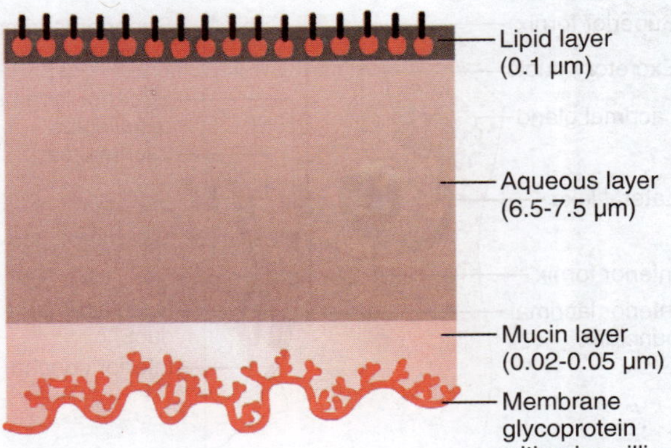

FIGURE 11.1-3 Structure of tear film.

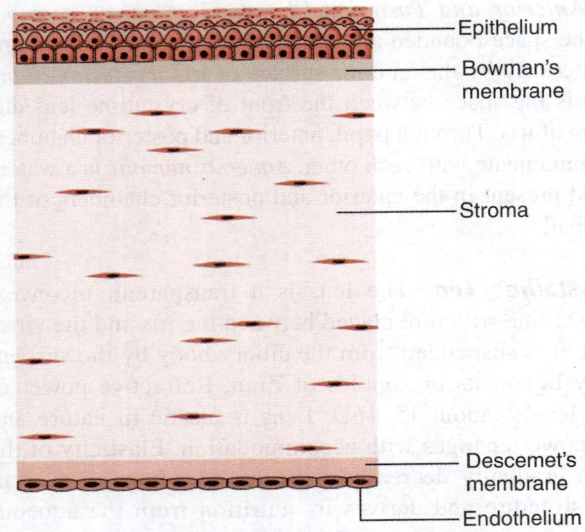

FIGURE 11.1-4 Microscopic structure of cornea.

Corneal Transparency The main physiologic function of the cornea is to act as a major refracting medium, so that a clear retinal image is formed. Maintenance of corneal transparency of high degree is a prerequisite to perform this function.

Factors Responsible for Corneal Transparency

1. ***Anatomical factors*** contributing to corneal transparency are:
   - Avascularity of cornea
   - Absence of pigment in the cornea
   - Demyelinated nerve supply
   - Regular arrangement, nonkeratinization andhomogenicity of refractive index of corneal epithelium.
   - A peculiar regular arrangement of the stromal lamellae (lattice theory)
   - Paucity of cells in the stroma
   - Regular arrangement of endothelial cells.
2. ***Relative dehydration of stroma.*** The normal cornea maintains itself in a state of relative dehydration which is essential for the corneal transparency. The water content of the normal cornea is approximately 80%. It is kept constant by a balance of factors which draw water in the cornea and the factors which prevent the flow of water in the cornea.

Factors maintaining relative corneal dehydration are:

- *Stromal swelling pressure,* it is the pressure (60 mmHg) exerted by the glycosaminoglycans (GAGs).
- Barrier function of epithelium which is largely impermeable to water.
- Endothelial active pump system pumps fluid and electrolytes from the stroma to the aqueous. It includes Na^+-K^+-ATPase pump system.
- Special intercellular junctions in the endothelium also act to some extent as barrier for the fluid.
- IOP should be optimum to control fluid transport in the cornea.

Source of Nutrition

- ***Peripheral cornea*** receives its nutrients via the blood stream of perilimbal plexus.
- ***Central cornea*** is avascular and nutrients enter by either simple diffusion or active transport through aqueous
- humour. Oxygen is derived directly from air through the tear film. It is an active process undertaken by the epithelium.

Metabolism

- ***Cornea requires energy to*** maintain its deturgescence and also for epithelial cell renewal.
- ***Energy in the form of ATP*** is provided by the metabolism of glucose. The most actively metabolizing layers of cornea are epithelium and endothelium, the former being 10 times thicker than the latter requires a proportionately large supply of metabolic substrate. About 65% of corneal metabolism occurs via glycolysis and the remainder by way of Krebs' cycle and HMP shunt.

Physiology of Crystalline Lens

Structure of Lens The lens is a transparent, biconvex, crystalline structure. Its diameter is 9–10 mm and thickness varies with age from 3.5 mm (at birth) to 5 mm (at extreme of age). It consists of following layers (Fig. 11.1-5) :

1. Lens Capsule. It is a thin, transparent, hyaline membrane surrounding the lens.

2. Anterior Epithelium. It is a single layer of cuboidal cells which lies deep to the anterior capsule. In the equatorial region, these cells become columnar, which are actively dividing and elongating to form new lens fibres throughout the life.

3. Lens Fibres. These form the main bulk of the lens and are arranged compactly as nucleus and cortex of the lens.

- ***Nucleus*** is the central part containing the oldest fibres. It consists of different zones: embryonic nucleus, foetal nucleus, infantile nucleus and adult nucleus.
- ***Cortex*** is the peripheral part which comprises the youngest fibres.

4. Suspensory Ligaments of Lens (zonules of Zinn). These consist essentially of a series of fibres by which lens is suspended from the ciliary body.

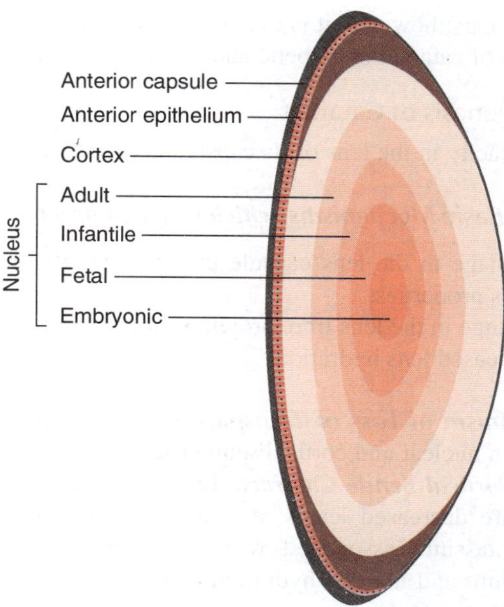

FIGURE 11.1-5 Structure of crystalline lens.

Lens Transparency Factors that play a significant role in maintaining outstanding clarity and transparency of lens are:

- Avascularity,
- Tightly packed nature of lens cells,
- The arrangement of lens protein,
- Semipermeable character of lens capsule,
- Same index of refraction in all parts of the lens,
- Pump mechanism of lens fibre membranes that regulate the electrolyte and water balance in the lens, maintaining relative dehydration and
- Auto-oxidation, high concentration of reduced glutathione in the lens maintains the lens proteins in a reduced state and ensures the integrity of the cell membrane pump.

Metabolism

Lens Requires a Continuous Supply of Energy (ATP) for active transport of ions, amino acids, maintenance of lens dehydration and for a continuous protein and GSH synthesis. Most of the energy produced is utilized in the epithelium which is the major site of all active transport processes. Only about 10–20% of the ATP generated is used for protein synthesis.

Source of Nutrient Supply. The crystalline lens, being an avascular structure is dependent for its metabolism on chemical exchanges with the aqueous humour

Pathways of Glucose Metabolism. Glucose is very essential for the normal working of the lens. Metabolic activity of the lens is largely limited to epithelium and cortex, while the nucleus is relatively inert. In the lens, 80% glucose is metabolized anaerobically by the glycolytic pathway, 15%by pentose hexose monophosphate (HMP) shunt and a small proportion via oxidative Krebs' citric acid cycle. Sorbitol pathway is relatively inconsequential in the normal lens; however, it is extremely important in the production of cataract in diabetic and galactosaemic patients.

Pathogenesis of Cataract

Any opacity in the lens or its capsule is called cataract.

Three Basic Mechanisms which cause cataract are:

- Damage to the lens capsule that changes its membranous properties,
- Change in the lens fibre protein synthesis and
- Increased lens hydration.

Mechanism of Loss of Transparency. It is basically different in nuclear and cortical senile cataracts.

1. Cortical Senile Cataract. Its main biochemical features are decreased levels of total proteins, amino acids and potassium associated with increased concentration of sodium and marked hydration of the lens, followed by coagulation of proteins.

The probable course of events leading to senile opacification of cortex may be as shown in the flowchart:

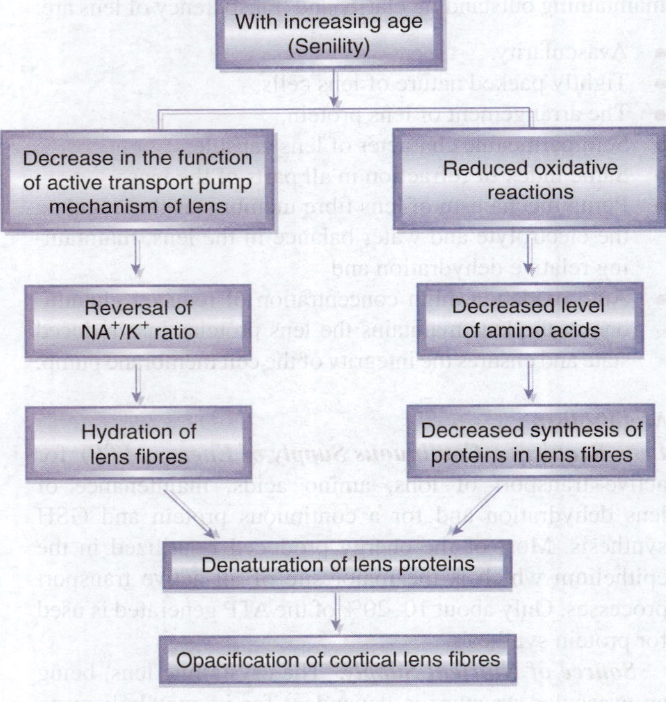

2. Nuclear Senile Cataract. In it the usual degenerative change is intensification of the age-related nuclear sclerosis associated with dehydration and compaction of the nucleus resulting in a hard cataract. It is accompanied by a significant increase in water insoluble proteins. However, the total protein content and distribution of cations remain normal. There may or may not be associated deposition of pigment urochrome and/or melanin derived from the amino acids in the lens.

Physiology of Vitreous Humour

Vitreous humour is an inert, transparent, colourless, jelly-like structure that fills the posterior four-fifth of the cavity of eyeball and is about 4 ml in volume

Structure. The normal youthful vitreous gel is composed of a network randomly oriented collagen fibrils interspersed with numerous spheroidal macromolecules of hyaluronic acid. The collapse of this structure with age or otherwise leads to conversion of gel into solution. The vitreous body can be divided into two parts: *cortex* (peripheral part) and *nucleus* (the main vitreous body)

Biochemical Composition. The vitreous body is composed of three major structural components: water, collagen-like fibres and hyaluronic acid, GAGs and a few other minor components.

Metabolic Activities. Cortical vitreous, though represents only 2% of the total vitreous volume is the metabolic centre of vitreous body. Hyalocytes present mainly in this part of vitreous are involved in the production of hyaluronic acid.

Functions. The vitreous gel mainly serves the *optical function*. In addition, it mechanically stabilizes the shape and volume of globe, and is a pathway for nutrients to reach the lens and retina.

THE IMAGE FORMING MECHANISM

The functioning of the eye as an optical instrument can be compared with a close circuit colour television camera (Fig. 11.1-6), in which:

- ***Eyelids*** act as shutter of the camera.
- ***Cornea and crystalline lens*** act as the focusing system of the camera.
- ***Iris*** acts as a diaphragm which regulates the size of the aperture (pupil) and therefore the amount of light entering the eye.
- ***Choroid and pigment epithelium of retina*** help in forming the darkened interior of the camera.
- ***Neural retina*** acts as a light sensitive plate or film on which images of the objects in the environment are focused. The light rays striking the retina generate potentials in the rods and cones. Thus the eye converts energy in the visible spectrum into action potentials in the optic nerve.
- ***Optic nerve and its connections*** convey the impulses generated in the retina to the occipital region of the cerebral cortex where they produce sensation of vision.

To understand the image forming mechanism of eye (i.e. optics of eye) and its abnormalities, it is imperative to have some knowledge about the light and geometrical optics.

Optics of the Eye

As an optical instrument, eye can be compared to a camera with retina acting as a unique kind of 'film'. The focusing

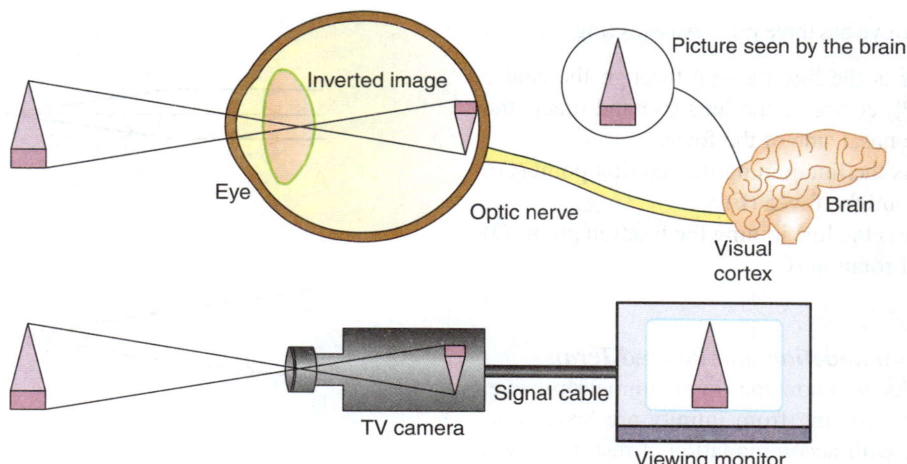

FIGURE 11.1-6 The sense of sight in many ways similar to a close circuit colour TV system. It is superior in all respects except ease of replacement.

system of eye is composed of several refracting structures; these include (the numbers in parentheses are their refractive indices)—(*i*) cornea (1.37), (*ii*) aqueous humour (1.33), (*iii*) crystalline lens (1.42) and (*iv*) vitreous humour (1.33). These constitute a homocentric system of lenses, which when combined in action form a very strong refracting system of a short focal length. The total dioptric power of the eye is about +60 D out of which about +44 D is contributed by cornea and +16 D by the crystalline lens.

Cardinal Points of the Eye

Listing and Gauss, while studying refraction by lens combinations, concluded that for a homocentric lens system, there exist three pairs of cardinal points, which are: two principal foci, two principal points and two nodal points, all situated on the principal axis of the system. Therefore, the eye, forming a homocentric complex lens system, when analyzed optically according to Gauss' concept can be resolved into six cardinal points (schematic eye). The cardinal data of the ***schematic eye*** is as follows (Fig. 11.1-7A):

- Total dioptric power is +58 D, of which cornea contributes +43 D and the lens +15 D.
- The principal foci F1 and F_2 lie 15.7 mm in front of and 24.4 mm behind the cornea, respectively.
- The principal points P1 and P_2 lie in the anterior chamber 1.35 mm and 1.60 mm behind the anterior surface of cornea, respectively.
- The nodal points N1 and N2 lie in the posterior part of lens 7.08 mm and 7.33 mm behind the anterior surface of cornea, respectively.

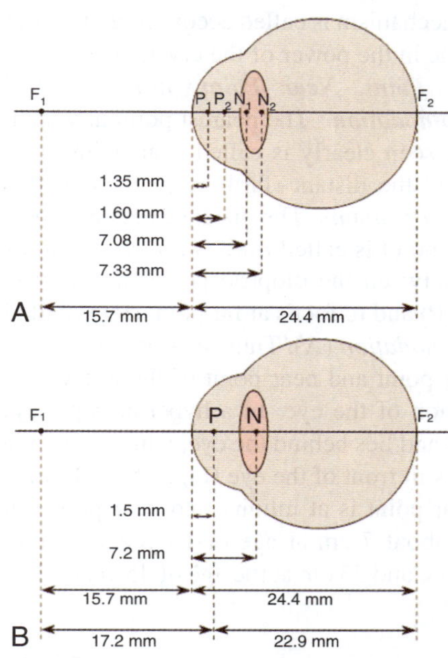

FIGURE 11.1-7 Cardinal points of: **(A)** schematic eye and **(B)** Listing's reduced eye.

The Reduced Eye

Listing's reduced eye. The optics of eye otherwise is very complex. However, for understanding, Listing has simplified the data by choosing single principal point and single nodal point lying midway between two principal points and two nodal points, respectively. This is called Listing's reduced eye. The simplified data of this eye (Fig.11.1-7B) are:

- Total dioptric power +60 D.
- The principal point (P) lies 1.5 mm behind the anterior surface of cornea.
- The nodal point (N) is situated 7.2 mm behind the anterior surface of cornea.
- The anterior focal point is 15.7 mm in front of the anterior surface of cornea.
- The posterior focal point (on the retina) is 24.4 mm behind the anterior surface of cornea.
- The anterior focal length is 17.2 mm (15.7 + 1.5) and the posterior focal length is 22.9 mm (24.4 - 1.5).

Axes of the Eye The eye has three principal axes (Fig. 11.1-8).

1. The *optical axis* is the line passing through the centre of the cornea (P), centre of the lens (N) and meets the retina (R) on the nasal side of the fovea.
2. The *visual axis* is the line joining the fixation point (O), nodal point (N) and the fovea (F).
3. The *fixation axis* is the line joining the fixation point (O) and the centre of rotation (C).

Accommodation

Definition of Accommodation and Related Terms

Accommodation. As we know that in an emmetropic eye, parallel rays of light coming from infinity are brought to focus on the retina, with accommodation at rest. Our eyes have been provided with a unique mechanism by which we can even focus the diverging rays coming from a near object on the retina in a bid to see clearly (Fig. 11.1-9). This mechanism is called accommodation. In it there occurs increase in the power of the crystalline lens.

Far Point, Near Point, Range and Amplitude of Accommodation. The nearest point at which small objects can be seen clearly is called near point or *punctum proximum*and the distant (farthest) point is called far point or *punctum remotum*. The distance between the near point and the far point is called *range of accommodation*. The difference between the dioptric power needed to focus at near point (P) and to focus at far point (R) is called *amplitude of accommodation* (A). Thus, A = P – R.

Far point and near point of the eye vary with the static refraction of the eye. In a hypermetropic eye, far point is virtual and lies behind the eye, while in myopic eye it is real and lies in front of the eye (Fig. 11.1-10). In an emmetropic eye, far point is at infinity and near point varies with age; being about 7 cm at age of 10 years, 25 cm at the age of 40 years, and 33 cm at the age of 45 years. Thus, the amount that the eye can alter its refraction is greatest in childhood and slowly decreases until it is lost in middle age.

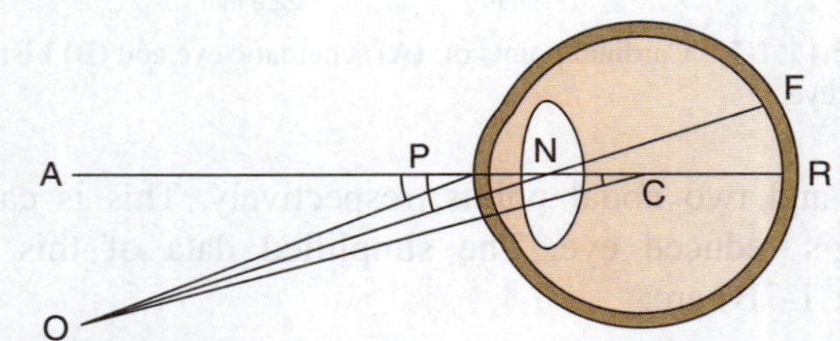

FIGURE 11.1-8 Axes of the eye: AR, optical axis; OF, visual axis; and OC, fixation axis.

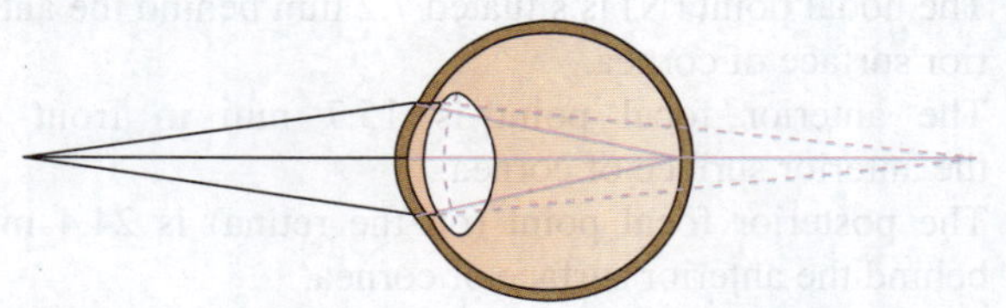

FIGURE 11.1-9 Effect of accommodation on divergent rays entering the eye.

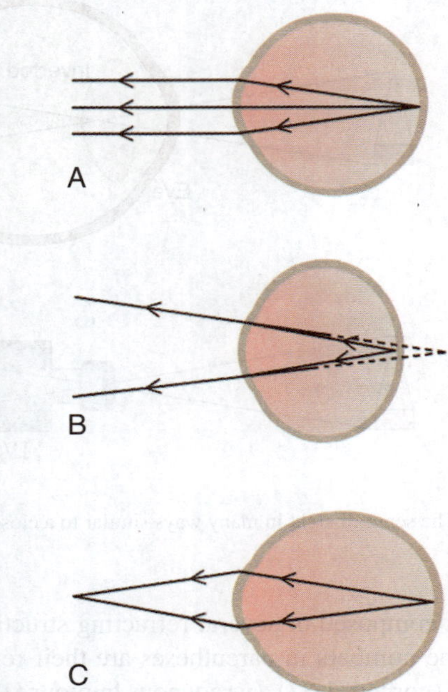

FIGURE 11.1-10 Showing far point in **(A)** emmetropic eye;**(B)** hypermetropic eye and **(C)** myopic eye.

Mechanism of Accommodation As we know, accommodation is a process by which one can focus the objects at different distances in a bid to have a clear vision. Its mechanism varies from species to species. Just for an interest examples of a few species are:

- Some fishes retract their lenses to focus on distant objects.
- Snakes and frogs have a mechanism to move the lens forward for near vision.
- Horses, by moving their heads, tilt the retina so that different regions lie at appropriate distances behind the lens. In man the process of accommodation is achieved by a change in the shape of the lens.

Theories of Mechanism of Accommodation in Human the Relaxation Theory. This theory was first proposed by:

- Thomas Young and elaborated by Helmholtz in 1885, by whose name it is known generally. The importance given to the lens capsule was emphasized by Fincham in 1937. The main points of the relaxation theory are:
    - When the eye is at rest (unaccommodated), the malleable substance of young lens is compressed in its capsule (which is elastic structure) by tension of the zonules. The surfaces of the compressed lens are less curved and these change the dioptric power in lens.
    - Zonules are kept under tension by a pull executed on them by the elastic choroid (Helmholtz original

assumption). However, recently it is being assumed by many workers that the zonules are kept under tension by the relaxation of fibres of the ciliary muscle.

- Contraction of the ciliary muscle causes the ciliary ring to shorten and move forward the equator of the lens. It also pulls the choroid forward. As a result the zonules are relaxed *(basic mechanism of relaxation theory)*, the tension on the capsule is relieved and the lens attains a more spherical shape. As the refractive index of lens (1.39) is more than the refractive index of aqueous and vitreous, increase in convexity of the lens increases its dioptric power and thus allows the near objects to be focused clearly on the retina.

Ocular Changes in Accommodation The changes which take place in the eye during accommodation can be summarized as:

*1. **Slackening of the Zonules.*** Zonules are normally tense and keep the lens flat. They slacken during accommodation due to contraction of ciliary muscle.

*2. **Changes in the Curvature of Lens Surface.*** The principal change in the lens during accommodation is seen in the anterior surface of the lens. At rest the radius of curvature of the anterior surface of the lens is 11 mm and that of posterior surface is 6 mm. In accommodation the curvature of posterior surface remains almost the same, but the anterior surface changes, so that in strong accommodation its radius of curvature becomes about 6 mm in the periphery and 3 mm in the central part which bulges more. The central part of the anterior surface bulges more because the anterior capsule is thinner here (Fig. 11.1-11) as compared to the peripheral part. The posterior capsule is the thinnest region and so the posterior surface has a greater curvature even in the unaccommodated lens.

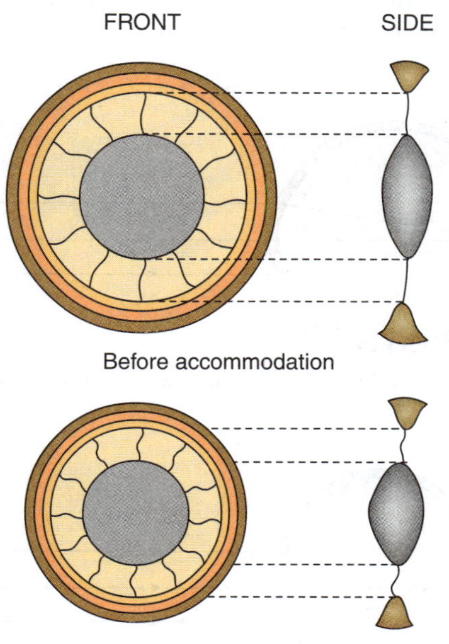

FIGURE 11.1-11 Changes in the ciliary body ring zonules and shape of lens during accommodation.

*3. **Anterior Pole*** of the lens moves forward carrying the iris with it, resulting in shallowing of the anterior chamber in the centre.

*4. **Axial Thickness*** of the lens is increased owing to forward movement of the anterior pole (posterior pole remaining fixed).

*5. **Changes in the Tension of Lens Capsule*** have also been studied. During accommodation the anterior capsule becomes slack.

*6. **Lens Sinks Down*** because the accommodated lens is held less firmly by its zonular attachment, it is influenced by the force of gravity and tends to sink within the globe.

*7. **Changes within the Lens Substance.*** In addition to the changes in curvature of the lens, the changes in the lens substance also create a change in the refractive power of the lens. The internal changes are brought about by changes in curvature of the various portions of lens having different indices of refraction.

*8. **Pupillary Constriction and Convergence of Eyes.*** In addition to the changes in the lens and zonular system, the pupil constricts and the eyes converge, almost simultaneously. These changes occur in a bid to achieve clear vision for near objects. The pupillary constriction is a synkinesis and not a true reflex, for it does not depend on either accommodation or convergence alone for its appearance.

*9. **The Choroid*** is stretched forward by the ciliary muscle contraction.

*10. **The Ora Serrata*** moves forward about 0.05 mm with each dioptre of accommodation.

Optical Aberrations of the Eye

The eye, in common with many optical systems in practical use, is by no means optically perfect; the lapses from perfection are called aberrations. Fortunately, the eyes possess those defects to so small a degree that, for functional purposes, their presence is immaterial. It has been said that despite imperfections the overall performance of the eye is little short of astonishing. Physiological optical defects in a normal eye include the following:

1. Diffraction of Light Diffraction is bending of light caused by the edge of an aperture or the rim of a lens. Even a perfect lens, free from aberrations, will not focus light to a point due to diffraction. The actual pattern of a diffracted image point produced by a lens with a circular aperture or pupil is a series of concentric bright and dark rings (Fig. 11.1-12). At the centre of the pattern is a bright spot known as the Airy disc after Sir George Airy who was the first to report it.

2. Spherical Aberrations Spherical aberrations occur owing to the fact that spherical lens refracts peripheral rays

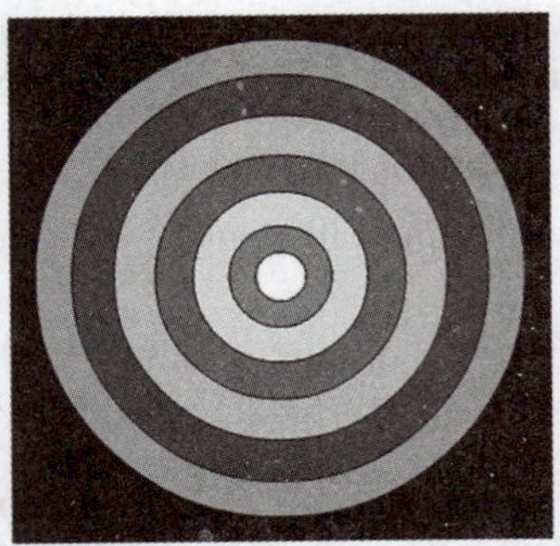

FIGURE 11.1-12 The diffraction of light. Light brought to a focus does not come to a point, but gives rise to blurred disc of light surrounded by several dark and light bands (the Airy disc).

more strongly than paraxial rays which in the case of a convex lens brings the more peripheral rays to focus closer to the lens (Fig. 11.1-13).

The factors which contribute in diminishing the spherical aberrations of human eye are:

- Peculiar curvature of the cornea, i.e. flatter periphery than the centre.
- Peculiar structure of the crystalline lens wherein the central portions have a greater density and are arranged in layers of greater curvature than the peripheral portion.
- Iris blocks the peripheral rays to enter the eye and thus in ordinary circumstances refraction of only paraxial rays of light takes place.

3. Chromatic Aberrations Chromatic aberrations result owing to the fact that the index of refraction of any transparent medium varies with the wavelength of incident light. In human eye, which optically acts as a convex lens, blue light is focused slightly in front of the red (Fig. 11.1-14). In other words, the emmetropic eye is, in fact, slightly hypermetropic for red rays and myopic for blue and green rays. This fact forms the basis of bichrome test used in subjective refraction.

Common Defects of the Image Forming Mechanism

Emmetropia Emmetropia (optically normal eye) can be defined as a state of refraction, when the parallel rays of light coming from infinity are focused at the sensitive layer of retina with the accommodation being at rest (Fig.11.1-15).

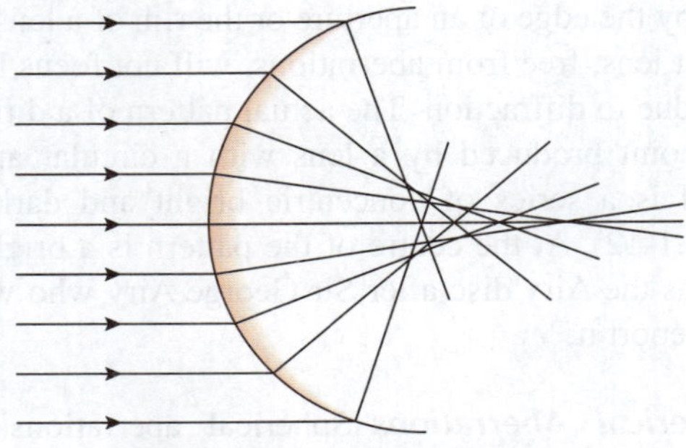

FIGURE 11.1-13 Spherical aberration.

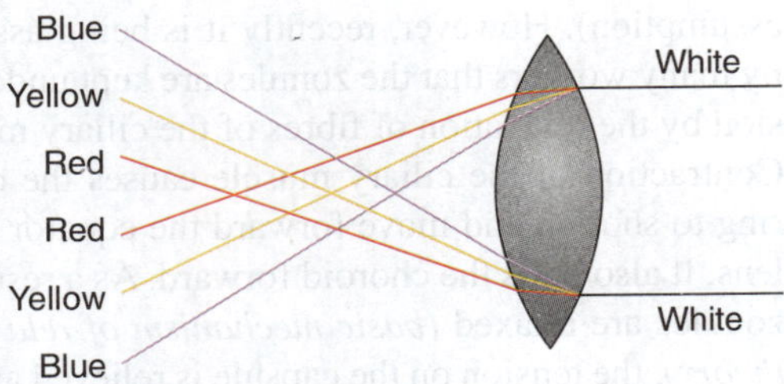

FIGURE 11.1-14 Chromatic aberration.

Ametropia Ametropia (a condition of refractive error), is defined as a state of refraction, when the parallel rays of light coming from infinity (with accommodation at rest), are focused either in front or behind the sensitive layer of retina, in one or both the meridia. The ametropia includes myopia, hypermetropia and astigmatism.

Hypermetropia Hypermetropia (hyperopia) or long sightedness is the refractive state of the eye wherein the parallel rays of light coming from infinity are focused behind the retina with accommodation being at rest (Fig.11.1-16).

Mechanism of Production. Aetiologically, hypermetropia may be axial, curvatural, index, positional and due to absence of lens.

1. ***Axial hypermetropia*** is by far the most common form. In this condition, there is an axial shortening of eyeball. About 1 mm shortening of the anteroposterior diameter of the eye results in 3 dioptres of hyper metropia.

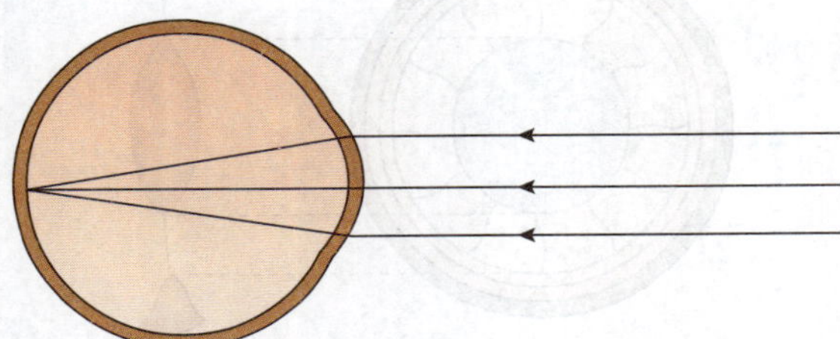

FIGURE 11.1-15 Refraction in an emmetropic eye.

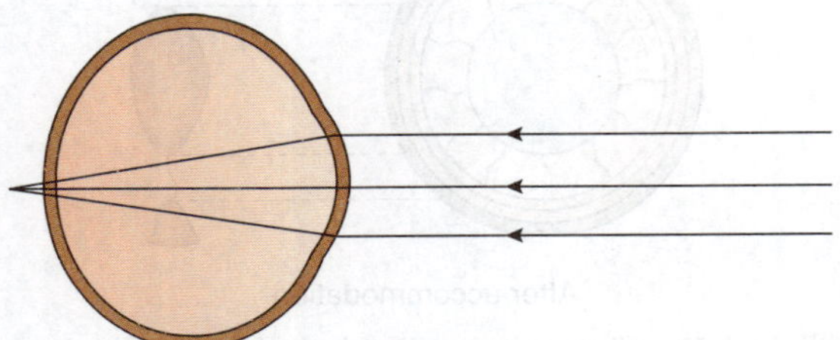

FIGURE 11.1-16 Refraction in hypermetropic eye.

2. *Curvatural hypermetropia* is the condition in which the curvature of cornea, lens or both is flatter than the normal. About 1 mm increase in radius of curvature results in 6 dioptres of hypermetropia.
3. *Index hypermetropia* occurs due to change in refractive index of the lens in old age. It may also occur in diabetics under treatment.
4. *Positional hypermetropia* results from posteriorly placed crystalline lens.
5. *Absence of crystalline lens* either congenitally or acquired (following surgical removal or posterior dislocation) leads to aphakia—a condition of high hypermetropia.

Characteristic Features

- ***Far-sightedness.*** Persons with mild to moderate hypermetropia, in their young age, can see the distant objects clearly using their accommodation. This is why hypermetropia is also called far sightedness or long sightedness.
- ***Near point*** of vision moves further away and the patient may have sometimes problem in near vision, when most of the accommodation is used for correcting for vision. Because of this hypermetropia requires presbyopic correction at younger age.
- ***Asthenopic symptoms.*** Due to sustained accommodation (i.e. prolonged muscular effort), individuals may develop mild headache, eyeache, feeling of tiredness and discomfort in reading. All these symptoms are collectively called asthenopic symptoms.
- ***Accommodative convergent squint*** may develop in children with moderate to high hypermetropia (usually by the age of 2–3 years) due to excessive use of accommodation.

Optical Correction. Basic principle of teartment of hypermetropia is optical correction with convex (plus) lenses, so that the light rays are brought to focus on the retina (Fig. 11.1-17).

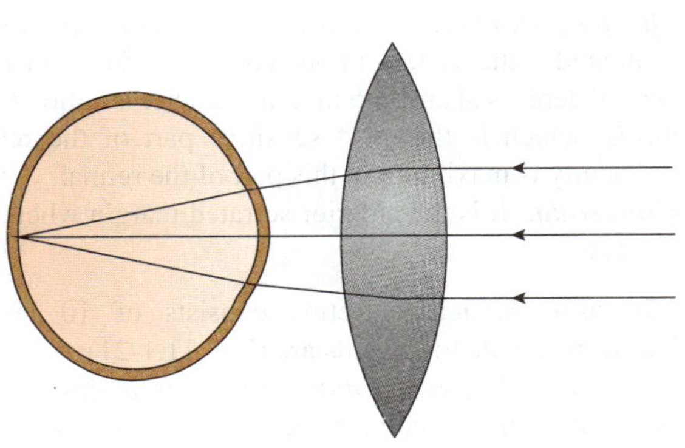

FIGURE 11.1-17 Refraction in hypermetropic eye corrected with convex lens.

Myopia

Myopia or short-sightedness is a type of refractive error in which parallel rays of light coming from infinity are focused in front of the retina when accommodation is at rest (Fig. 11.1-18).

Mechanisms of Production

1. ***Axial myopia*** results from increase in anteroposterior length of the eyeball. It is the most common form.
2. ***Curvatural myopia*** occurs due to increased curvature of the cornea, lens or both.
3. ***Positional myopia*** is produced by anterior placement of crystalline lens in the eye.
4. ***Index myopia*** results from increase in the refractive index of crystalline lens associated with nuclear sclerosis.
5. ***Myopia due to excessive accommodation*** occurs in patients with spasm of accommodation.

Characteristic Features

- ***Short sightedness.*** Far point of vision is a finite point in front of the eye (at infinity in emmetropes). Therefore, the myopic persons cannot see the distant objects. This is why myopia is also called *short sightedness.*
- ***Accommodation*** in uncorrected myopia is not developed normally, since they need not accommodate to see the near objects clearly. For this reason, they may suffer from convergence insufficiency, exophoria and early presbyopia as they grow older.

Optical Correction. Basic principles of treatment of myopia is optical correction with concave (minus) lenses, so that the clear image is formed on the retina (Fig. 11.1-19). A myopic patient may not need glasses for near vision in old age, because his near point may be at a reading distance (which recedes back in emmetropic presbyopes).

Astigmatism

Astigmatism is a type of refractive error wherein the refraction varies in the different meridia. Consequently, the rays of light entering the eye cannot converge to a point focus

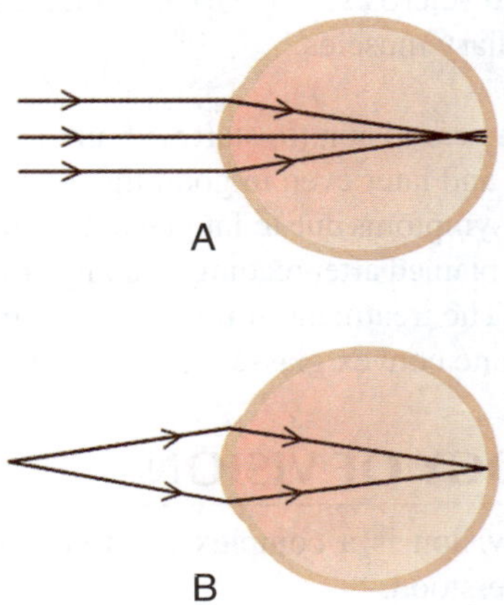

FIGURE 11.1-18 Optics of myopia: (A) parallel rays are focussed in front of retina; and (B) divergent rays from an object situated at a far point of the eye are focused at the retina.

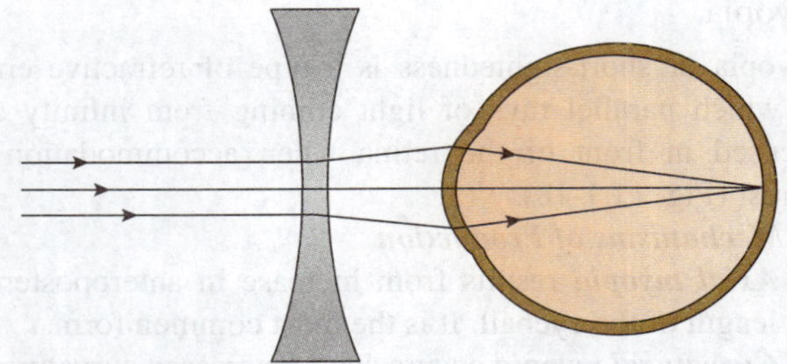

FIGURE 11.1-19 Refraction in a myopic eye corrected by concave lens.

but form focal lines. Broadly, there are two types of astigmatism: regular and irregular.

Regular Astigmatism. he astigmatism is regular when the refractive power changes uniformly from one meridian to another (i.e. there are two principal meridia).

Irregular Astigmatism. It is characterized by an irregular change of refractive power in different meridia. There are multiple meridia which admit no geometrical analysis.

Presbyopia

Presbyopia (eyesight of old age) is not an error of refraction but condition of physiological insufficiency of accommodation, leading to failing vision for near. To understand the condition of presbyopia, a working knowledge about accommodation is mandatory see page 1141.

Since, we usually keep the book at about 25 cm, so we can read comfortably up to the age of 40 years. After the age of 40 years, the near point of accommodation recedes beyond the normal reading or working range. This condition of failing near vision due to age-related decrease in the amplitude of accommodation or increase in punctum proximum is called presbyopia.

Pathophysiology of Presbyopia. Decrease in the accommodative power of crystalline lens with increasing age, leading to presbyopia, occurs due to: (i) decrease in the elasticity and plasticity of the crystalline lens (which results from age-related sclerosis); and (ii) age-related decrease in the power of ciliary muscles.

Symptoms

- Difficulty in near vision (to start with in the evening and in dim light and later even in good light).
- Asthenopic symptoms due to fatigue of the ciliary muscle are also complained after reading or doing any near work.

Treatment. The treatment of presbyopia is the prescription of appropriate convex glasses for near work.

PHYSIOLOGY OF VISION

Physiology of vision is a complex phenomenon which is still poorly understood.

The main mechanisms concerned with vision are:

- ***Initiation of vision*** (phototransduction), a function of photoreceptors (rods and cones),
- ***Processing and transmission of visual sensation,*** a function of the image processing cells of retina and visual pathway.
- ***Visual perceptions,*** a function of visual cortex and related areas of cerebral cortex. It is based on the activities of serial processing stations in the visual pathway and parallel processing pathways. The visual perceptions are the functional elements of the vision, i.e. the sensations which result from stimulation of retina with light. These are of four kinds, namely the light sense, the form sense, the contrast sense and the colour sense. Further, different cortical areas make different contributions to the processing of motion, depth, form and colour.

For the purpose of understanding, the description of physiology of vision can be organized as:

- Retina, photoreceptors and visual pigment,
- Phototransduction,
- Processing and transmission of visual impulse in retina,
- Processing and transmission of visual impulse in visual pathway,
- Processing and analysis of visual impulse in the visualcortex and
- Concept of serial and parallel processing of visual information.

Retina, Photoreceptors and Visual Pigments

Before embarking on the complex physiological processes concerning initiation and transmission of visual sensation, a brief description of the retina, photoreceptors and visual pigments will be useful.

Retina

Gross Anatomy Retina, the innermost tunic of the eyeball is a thin, transparent membrane. It is concerned with the visual functions. Grossly, retina exhibits three distinct areas: optic disc, macula lutea and peripheral retina (Fig.11.1-20):

Optic Disc. It is a well-defined, circular, pink coloured disc of 1.5 mm diameter. It has only nerve fibre layer, so it does not excite any visual response. It produces *blind spot* in the field of vision.

Macula Lutea (Yellow Spot). It is a comparatively dark area situated at the posterior pole temporal to the optic disc. Its central depressed area 1.5 mm in diameter is called *fovea centralis,* which is the most sensitive part of the retina. Visual acuity is maximum in this part of the retina.

Oraserrata. It is the anterior serrated margin where the retina ends.

Microscopic Structure Retina consists of 10 layers, which from outside to inwards are (Fig. 11.1-21):

1. Layer of Pigment Epithelium. It is a single layer of hexagonal cells containing melanin pigments. It serves following *functions:*

- Absorbs stray light, and thereby reduces light scatter.

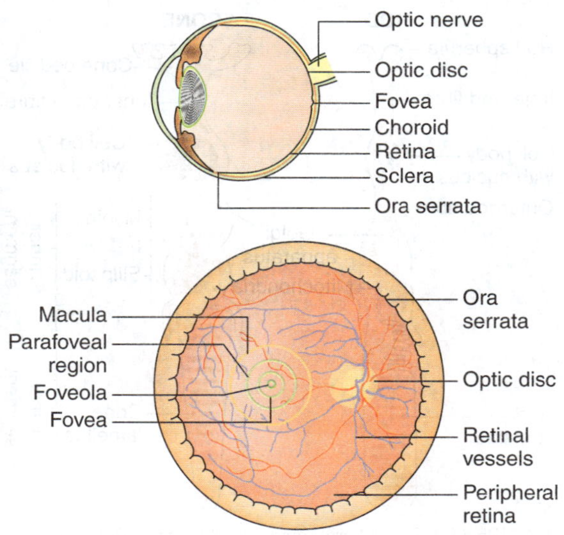

FIGURE 11.1-20 Gross anatomy of retina.

- Phagocytose the ends of the outer segments of rods which are continuously shed.
- Reconvert the metabolized photopigment into a form that can be reused after it is transported back to photoreceptor.
- Tight junction between the cells form outer blood-retinal barrier.

2. Layer of Rods and Cones. It consists of the outer segments of the photoreceptors (rods and cones). Photoreceptors are the end organs of vision.

3. External Limiting Membrane. It is not a separate membrane. In fact, the numerous connections made between Muller cells and inner segments of photoreceptors give the appearance of a continuous membrane under light microscopy.

4. Outer Nuclear Layer. This layer contains the nuclei of rods and cones.

5. Outer Plexiform Layer. This layer contains presynaptic and postsynaptic elements of synapses that exist between the photoreceptors, bipolar cells and horizontal cells.

6. Inner Nuclear Layer. It contains the cell bodies and nuclei of bipolar cells, amacrine cells and horizontal cells.

7. Inner Plexiform Layer. It is the layer of synapse between bipolar cells, ganglion cells and amacrine cells.

8. Ganglion Cell Layer. It consists of ganglion cells, which are the output cells of the retina. They transmit visual information to the brain.

9. Nerve Fibre Layer. It consists of the axons of ganglion cells which pass through lamina cribrosa to form the optic nerve. These fibres remain unmyelinated in the retina, but become myelinated in the optic nerve.

10. Inner Limiting Membrane. It is formed by projections of the Muller's cells and separates the retina from vitreous.

Structural Characteristics of Fovea Centralis. Foveal region has the highest visual resolution because of following structural characterstics:

- Rods are absent and cone density is maximum.
- Foveal cones have unusually long and thin outer segments. This shape allows a high packing density.

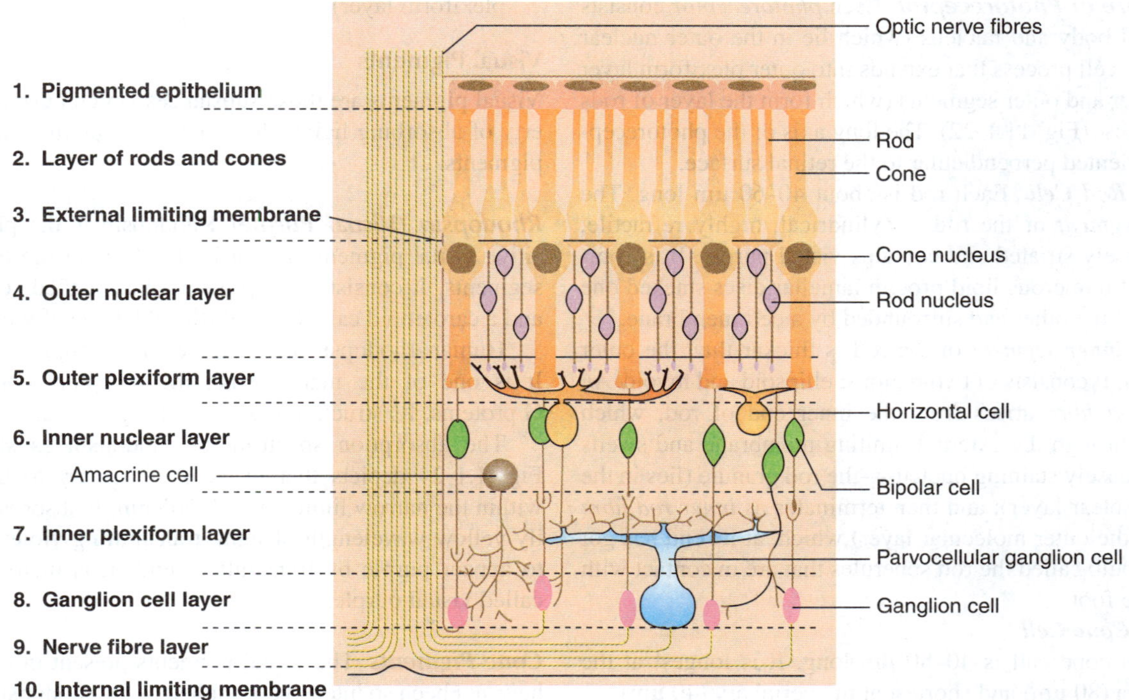

FIGURE 11.1-21 Microscopic structure of retina.

- All other inner layers of retina are pushed aside in this area. This arrangement allows light to reach the cones without having to pass through the inner layers of retina, and thereby reduces distortion of the image.
- The most central part of fovea (foveola) is devoid of even capillaries, while the rest of fovea contains fine capillaries but no large vessels which encircle this area.
- There is no convergence of efferents of the foveal cones. Each foveal cone relays to single ganglion cell. Hence, there is disproportionate large representation of the fovea in the visual cortex.

Photoreceptors

Density and Distribution of Photoreceptors

- Rods and cones *(photoreceptors)* are the end organs of vision which transform light energy into visual (nerve) impluse.
- Rods contain a photosensitive substance visual purple *(rhodopsin)* and subserve the peripheral vision and vision of low illumination (scotopic vision).
- Cones also contain a photosensitive substance and are primarily responsible for highly discriminatory central vision (photopic vision) and colour vision.
- There are about 120 million rods and 6.5 million cones.
- The highest density of cones is at fovea with an average of 199,000 cones/mm^2. The number of cones falls off rapidly outside the fovea.
- Rods are absent at the fovea in an area of 0.35 mm (rod-free zone) which corresponds to 1.25o of the visual field; but are present in a large number (160,000/ mm^2) in a ring-shaped zone 5-6 mm from the fovea.

Structure of Photoreceptor Each *photoreceptor* consists of a cell body and nucleus (which lie in the outer nuclear layer), a cell process that extends into outer plexiform layer and inner and outer segments (which form the layer of rods and cones) (Fig. 11.1-22). The long axis of the photoreceptor is oriented perpendicular to the retinal surface.

The Rod Cell. Each rod is about 40–60 **μ**m long. The *outer segment* of the rod is cylindrical, highly refractile, transversely striated and contains visual purple. It is composed of numerous lipid protein lamellar discs stacked one on top of the other and surrounded by a cell membrane.

The *inner segment* of the rod is thicker than the outer segment. It consists of two regions: ellipsoid and myoid. *An outer rod fibre* arises from the inner end of rod, which passes through the external limiting membrane and swells into a densely staining nucleus—the rod granule (lies in the outer nuclear layer); and then terminates as *inner rod fibre* (lies in the outer molecular layer) which, at its end has got an end bulb called the rod spherules that are in contact with the cone foot.

The Cone Cell

- Each cone cell is 40–80 **μ**m long. It is longest at the fovea (80 **μ**m) and shortest at the periphery (40 **μ**m)

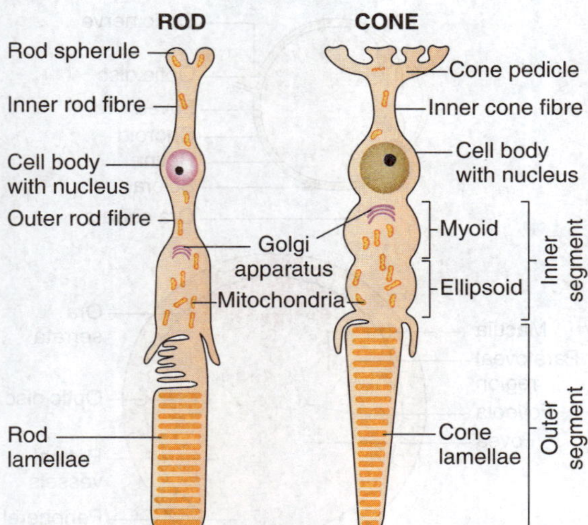

FIGURE 11.1-22 Microscopic structure of rod and cone cells.

- The *cone outer segment* is conical in shape, much shorter than that of rod and contains the iodopsin. The lamellar discs, which are narrower than those of the rods are, in fact, infoldings of plasma membrane. There are about 1000—1200 discs/cone.
- The *cone inner segment* and cilium are similar to the rod structures; however the cone ellipsoid is very plump and contains a large number of mitochondria.
- Unlike rod the inner segment of the cone becomes directly continuous with its nucleus and lies in outer nuclear layer. A stout cone inner fibre runs from the nucleus which at the end is provided with lateral processes called *cone foot* or *cone pedicle* (lies in the outer plexiform layer).

Visual Pigments

Visual pigments are those substances which have the property of absorbing light. These include *rhodopsin* and cone pigments.

Rhodopsin (Visual Purple) Rhodopsin is the photosensitive visual pigment present in the discs of the rod outer segments. It consists of a protein opsin (called scotopsin) and a carotenoid called retinal (the aldehyde of vitamin A).

Human rhodopsin has a molecular weight of 40,000. It is one of the many serpentine receptors coupled to G proteins. Its structure is shown in Fig.11.1-23.

The absorption spectrum of rhodopsin as shown in Fig.11.1-24 depicts that its peak sensitivity to light lies within the narrow limits of 493–505 nm. It absorbs primarily yellow wavelength of light, transmitting violet and red to appear purple by transmitted light; it is therefore also called visual purple.

Cone Pigments The visual pigments present in the cones have not been so intensively studied as the rhodopsin. There

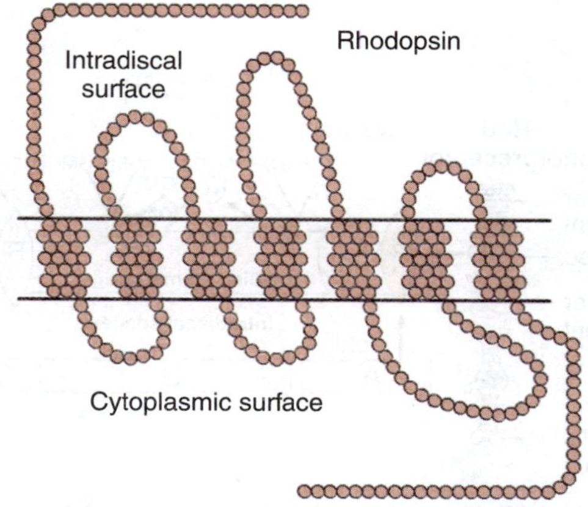

FIGURE 11.1-23 Structure of rhodopsin molecule.

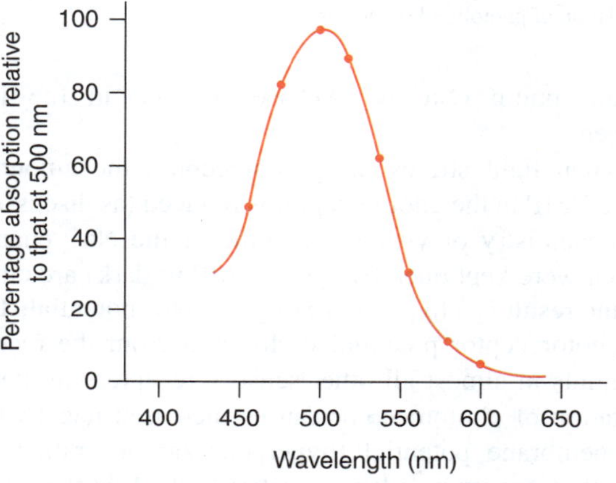

FIGURE 11.1-24 Absorption spectrum of rhodopsin.

are three kinds of cones in primates. Cone pigments are somewhat different from the rhodopsin, in that they respond to specific wavelength of light, giving rise to colour vision. These differences are present in the opsin portion of the molecule, whereas the chromophore 11-cis-retinal remains the same. The peak absorbance wavelength of the 'blue', 'green' and 'red' sensitive cones lie at about 435, 535 and 580 nm, respectively.

Light-induced Changes Light falling upon the retina is absorbed by the visual pigments and initiate *photochemical changes* which in turn trigger a sequence of events that cause phototransduction. The photochemical changes occurring in the rods and cones are similar, but they have been studied in detail in the rods and can be described under three headings:

- Rhodopsin bleaching,
- Rhodopsin regeneration and
- Visual cycle.

Rhodopsin Bleaching. As mentioned earlier the rhodopsin consists of a protein called *opsin* and a carotenoid called retinene (vitamin A aldehyde or 11-cis-retinal). The light absorbed by the rhodopsin converts its *11-cis-retinal* into *all-trans-retinal.* This light-induced isomerization of 11-cis-retinal into all-trans-retinal occurs through formation of many intermediates which exist for a transient period (Fig. 11.1-25). One of the intermediate compounds *(metarhodopsin II,* also called as activated rhodopsin) of the above isomerization chain reaction acts as an enzyme to activate many molecules of transducin. The activated transducin triggers the phototransduction (see page 1148)

The all-trans-retinal (produced from light-induced isomerization of 11-cis-retinal) can no longer remain in combination with the opsin and thus there occurs separation of opsin and all-trans-retinal. This process of separation is called *photodecomposition* and the rhodopsin is said to be bleached by the action of light.

Rhodopsin Regeneration. The all-trans-retinal separated from the opsin (as above), subsequently enters into the chromophore pool existing in the photoreceptor outer segment and the pigment epithelial cells (for this, close approximation of RPE and photoreceptor is must). The all-trans-retinal may be further reduced to retinol by alcohol dehydrogenase, then esterified to re-enter the systemic circulation.

The first stage in the reformation of rhodopsin, as shown in Fig. 11.1-25, is isomerization of all-trans-retinal back to 11-cis-retinal. The process is catalyzed by the enzyme *retinal isomerase*. Energy for the regeneration process is supplied by the overall metabolic pool of the photoreceptor outer segment. The 11-cis-retinal in the outer segments of photoreceptors reunite with the opsin to form

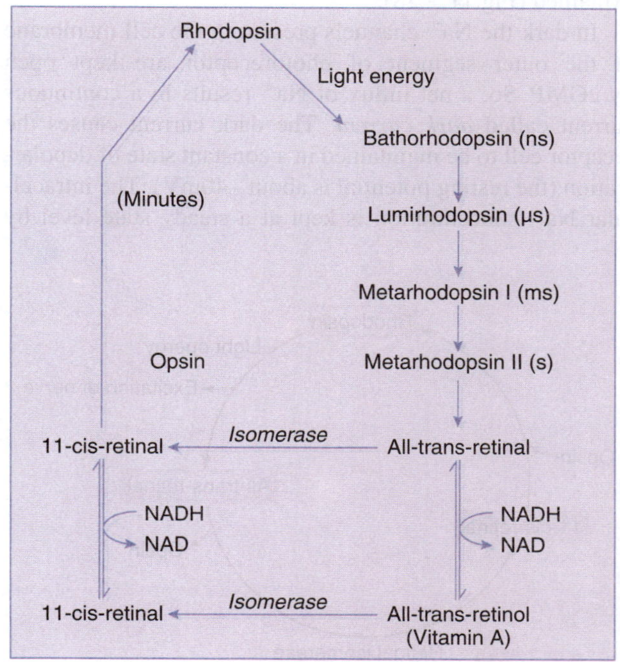

FIGURE 11.1-25 Light induced changes in rhodopsin.

rhodopsin. This whole process is called regeneration of the rhodopsin. Thus, the bleaching of the retinal photopigments occurs under the influence of light, whereas the regeneration process is independent of light, proceeding equally well in light or darkness. The amount of rhodopsin in the rods, therefore, varies inversely with the incident light.

Visual Cycle. In the retina of living animals, under constant light stimulation, a steady state must exist under which the rate at which the photochemicals are bleached is equal to the rate at which they are regenerated. This equilibrium between the photodecomposition and regeneration of visual pigments is referred to as *visual cycle* (Fig. 11.1-26).

Phototransduction

Phototransduction refers to conversion of light energy into nerve impulse. It involves a cascade of biochemical reactions in following steps (Fig. 11.1-27):

Activation of Rhodopsin. As described above, following exposure to light the rhodopsin undergoes a series of spontaneous transformation, leading to formation of an active form of rhodopsin the *metarhodopsin II.*

Activation of Transducin. The activated rhodopsin acts as an enzyme to activate many molecules of transducin (G-protein). When transducin gets replaced by GTP and the αsubunit separates.

Conversion of cGMP to GMP. The α subunit activates the many molecules of the enzyme phosphodiesterase (PDE) which catalyzes conversion of cGMP to GMP leading reduction in the concentration of cGMP within the photoreceptor.

Production of Receptor Potential. Reduction in the cGMP is responsible for producing receptor potential as explained (Fig.11.1-28):

In dark the Na^+ channels present in the cell membrane of the outer segment of photoreceptor are kept open by cGMP. So, a net influx of Na^+ results in a continuous current called *dark current.* The dark current causes the receptor cell to be maintained in a constant state of depolarization (the resting potential is about –40mV). The intracellular Na^+ concentration is kept at a steady state level by

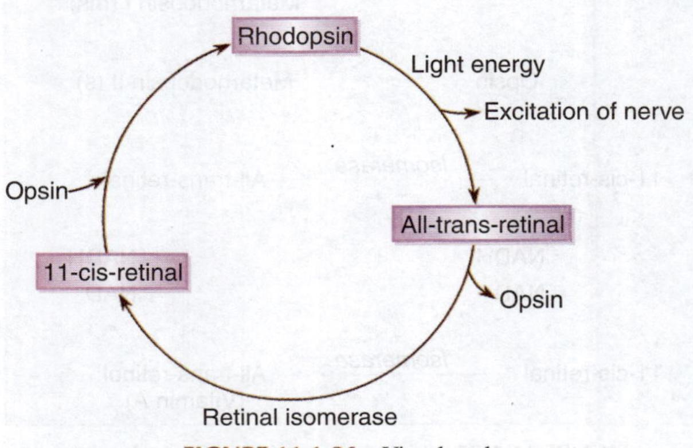

FIGURE 11.1-26 Visual cycle.

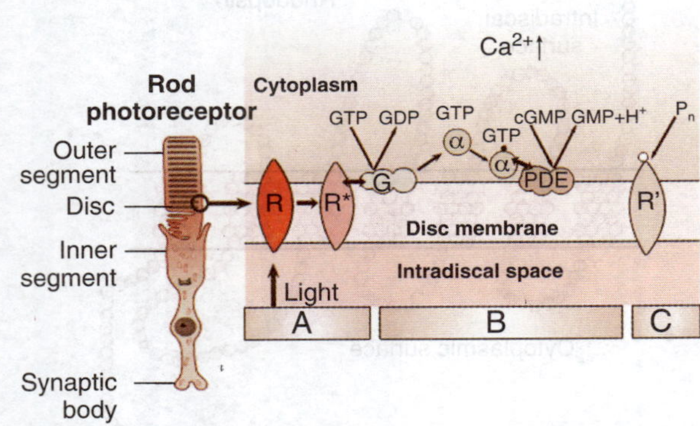

FIGURE 11.1-27 The scheme for reaction triggered by rhodopsin bleaching which affect cyclic GMP in the photoreceptors: **(A)** light induced conversion of rhodopsin to its active form; **(B)** activation of G-protein (G) and activation of cGMP phosphodiesterase (PDE) protein and **(C)** phosphorylation of photolysed rhodopsin.

sodium pump (Na^+-K^+-ATPase) located in the inner segment.

When light strikes the photoreceptor, the amount of cyclic GMP in the photoreceptor is reduced (as discussed in photochemistry of vision), so some of the Na^+ channels (which were kept open by cyclic GMP in dark) are closed, and the result is a hyperpolarizing receptor potential. Thus, the photoreceptor potential is different from the receptor potentials in almost all other sensory receptors in that the excitation of photoreceptor causes increased negativity of the membrane potential (hyperpolarization), rather than decreased negativity (depolarization) which is the characteristic of all other receptors. Normally, in dark, the electronegativity inside the rod membrane is about 40 millivolts and after excitation it approaches about 70 to 80 millivolts. Further, the eye is unique in that the receptor potential of the photoreceptors is local graded potential, i.e. it does not propagate and does not follow the 'all or none law'.

The sequence of events in photoreceptors by which incident light leads to production of a nerve impulse (*phototransduction*) are summarized in Fig.11.1-29.

Cone versus Rod Receptor Potential

The cone receptor potential has a sharp onset and offset, whereas the rod receptor potential has a sharp onset and slow offset. The curve relating the amplitude of receptor potentials to stimulus intensity have similar shapes in rods and cones, but the rods are much more sensitive. Therefore, rod responses are proportionate to stimulus intensity at levels of illumination that are below the threshold for cones. On the other hand, cone responses are proportionate to stimulus intensity at high levels of illumination when the rod responses are maximal and cannot change. That is why cones generate good response to change in light intensity above background but do not represent absolute illumination well, whereas rods detect absolute illumination.

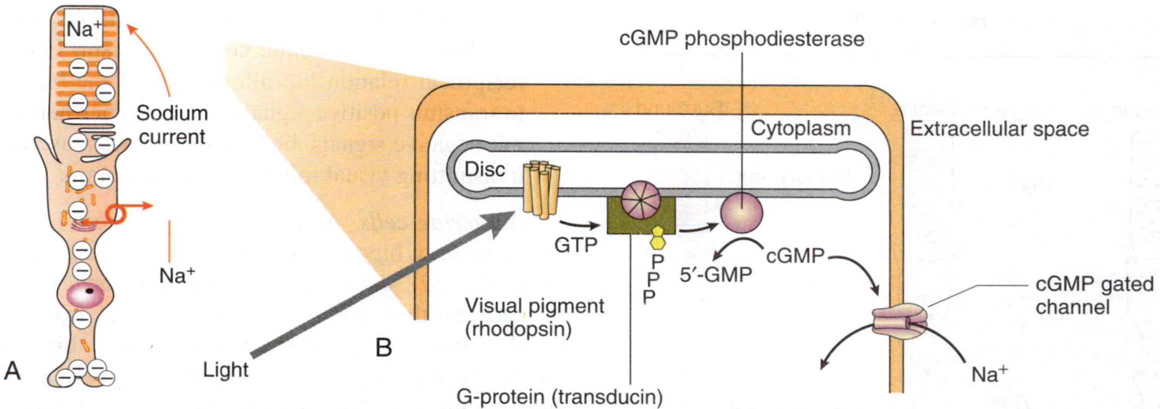

FIGURE 11.1-28 Potential changes in a photoreceptor: **(A)** in dark Na^+ channels are opened by the cGMP and due to Na^+ influx (dark current) results and membrane is kept depolarized (at resting membrane potential of –40 mV) and **(B)** when light falls on the retina the activated rhodopsin reduces intracellular levels of cGMP and consequently the Na^+channels are blocked. This results in hyperpolarization (photoreceptor potential).

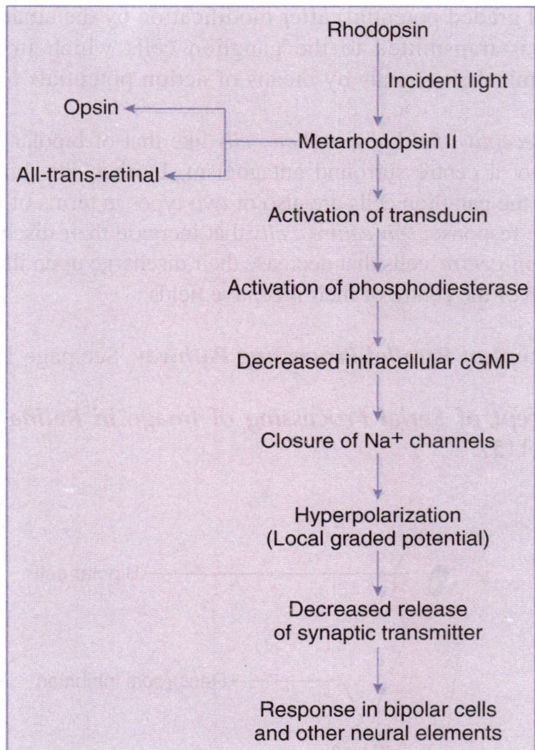

FIGURE 11.1-29 Sequence of events involved in phototransduction process in the photoreceptors.

Processing and Transmission of the Visual Impulse in Retina

The receptor potential generated in the photoreceptors is transmitted by *electrotonic conduction* (i.e. direct flow of electric current, not action potential to other cells of the retina, viz., horizontal cells, amacrine cells and ganglion cells). However, the ganglion cells transmit the visual signals by means of action potential to the neurons of lateral geniculate body and the later to the primary visual cortex.

Role of different cells in the processing of retinal image can be discussed in terms of following concepts which have been evolved in physiology of vision:

- Concept of receptive field,
- Concept of serial processing of the image (see page 1157) and
- Concept of parallel processing pathway (see page 1156).

Concept of Receptive Field The concept of receptive field has been evolved to explain the processing of visual signal. In general sense, the receptive field is defined as the influence area of a sensory neuron. It is circular in configuration.

Receptive field of individual photoreceptor is small and circular. Light falling in the receptive field hyperpolarizes the cell (as described above). In the dark, i.e. when the photoreceptor is depolarized, a neurotransmitter (glutamate) is released from its terminal. When hyperpolarized, the photoreceptor will therefore release less neurotransmitter.

Horizontal cells have a very large receptive field in comparison to the photoreceptor cell. A horizontal cell transmits signals horizontally in the outer plexiform layer from rods and cones to the bipolar cells. Their main function is to *enhance the visual contrast by causing lateral inhibition, i.e.* they play role in processing of *spatial information* (Fig.11.1-30).

Bipolar cells. There are two types of bipolar cells, one type of cells (which are inhibited by glutamate) are depolarized while the other (which are excited by glutamate) are hyperpolarized when the photoreceptors are excited (Figs. 11.1-30, 11.1-31). Thus, the two different types of bipolar cells provide opposing excitatory and inhibitory signals in the visual pathway.

- *Receptive field* of the bipolar cell is also circular in configuration *but* has *got centre-surround antagonism.* As shown in Fig. 11.1-31 in case of centre depolarizing cells (also called 'on cell'), the light striking the centre

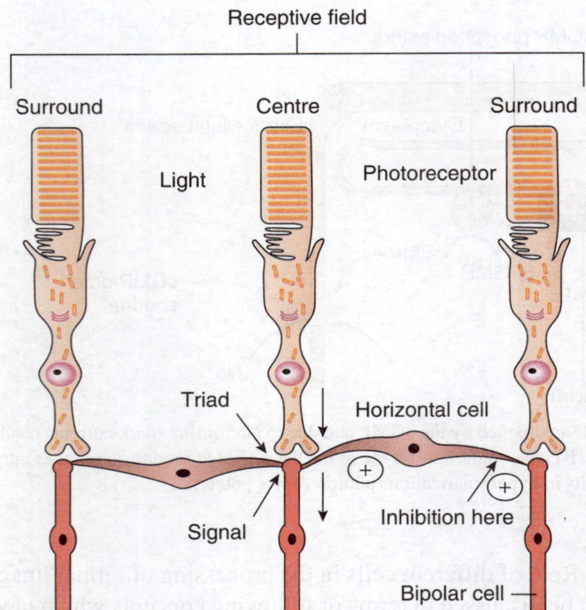

FIGURE 11.1-30 Horizontal cells showing phenomenon of lateral inhibition in the surround receptive plexiform layer. The central photoreceptor has been stimulated with light and inner portion of the cell membrane becomes more negative. The signal is transmitted upward to bipolar cell and horizontally to horizontal cells. This horizontal transmission results in inhibition of receptor bipolar synapse of neighbouring photoreceptor element. The stimulated bipolar cell may be hyperpolarized or depolarized.

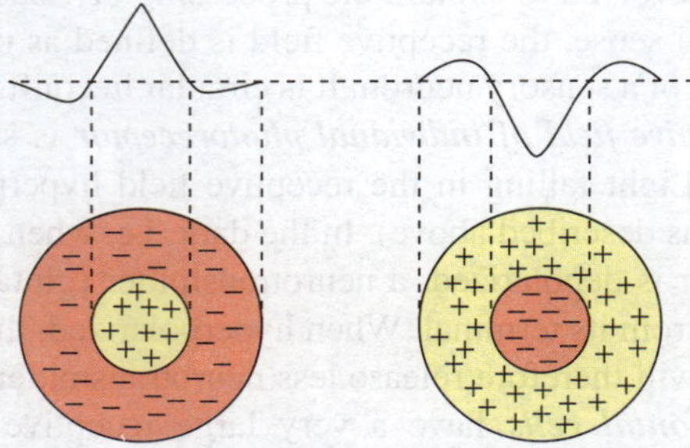

FIGURE 11.1-31 Showing the centre surround response to light in 'on' or centre depolarizing bipolar cell (left) and 'off' or centre hyperpolarizing bipolar cell (right). Plus (+) signs indicate region giving depolarizing response and minus (-) signs, a hyperpolarizing one.

of receptive field activates and the light striking the 'surround' inhibits bipolar cell output. The reverse occurs in the centre hyperpolarizing cell (also called as 'off cell') i.e. the light striking the 'centre' is inhibitory and the light striking the 'surround' is excitatory to bipolarcell output. The size of the centre of the bipolar cell receptive field is determined by the reach of its dendrites and that of the much larger 'surround' is determined by the spread of interconnected horizontal cells.

- The importance of the above-described reciprocal relationship between the depolarizing and hyperpolarizing bipolar cells is that it provides a second mechanism for lateral inhibition *(spatial information processing)* in addition to horizontal cell mechanism. Further, this reciprocal relationship allows half of the bipolar cells to transmit positive signals and the other half to transmit negative signals, both of these have a useful role in transmitting visual information to the brain.

Amacrine cells. Amacrine cells receive information at the synapse of bipolar cell axon with ganglion cell dendrite (Fig. 11.1-32) and use this information for *temporal processing.* Further, these cells receive input from different combinations of on-centre and off-centre bipolar cells. Therefore, the *receptive fields of amacrine cells* are mixture of on-centre and off-centre regions. Many different types of amacrine cells utilize at least eight different neurotransmitters. Thus, the contributions of amacrine cells to visual processing are complex.

Ganglion cells. The electrical response of bipolar cells (local graded potential) after modification by the amacrine cells is transmitted to the ganglion cells which in turn transmit their signals by means of action potentials to the brain.

Receptive field of ganglion cells like that of bipolar cells has got a centre surround antagonism. Further, like bipolar cells, the ganglion cells are also of two types in terms of their centre response: *'on-centre' cells* that increase their discharge and *'off-centre'* cells that decrease their discharge upon illumination of the centre of their receptive fields.

Concept of Parallel Processing Pathway See page 1156.

Concept of Serial Processing of Image in Retina See page 1157.

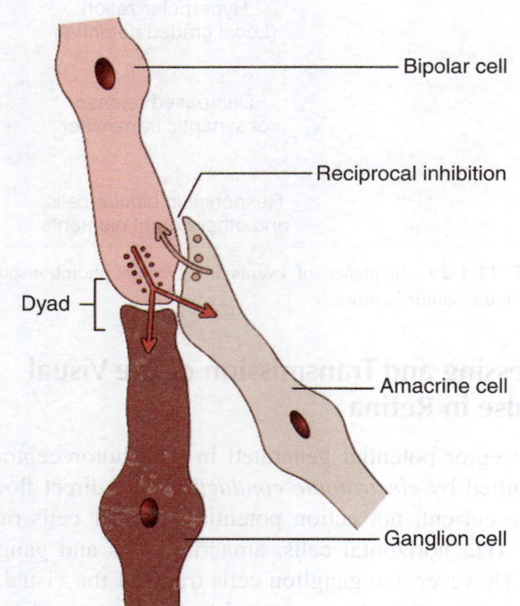

FIGURE 11.1-32 Showing bipolar-amacrine ganglion cell interaction.

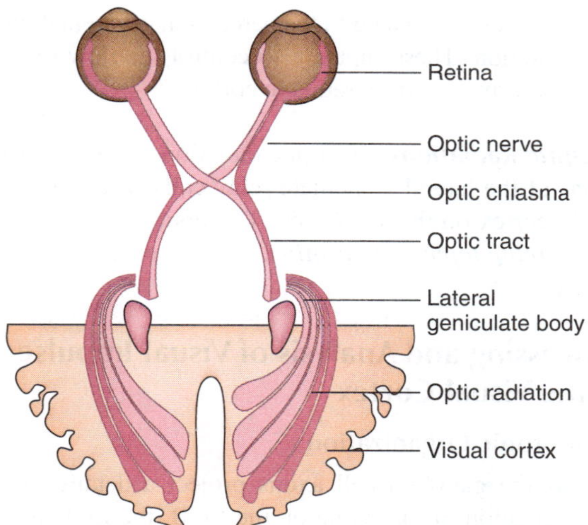

FIGURE 11.1-33 Components of visual pathway.

Synaptic Mediators in the Retina Various types of synaptic transmitters found in retina are: acetylcholine (secreted only by amacrine cells of retina), glutamate, GABA, serotonin, dopamine, glycine, substance P, TRH, GnRH, somatostatin, enkephlins, β endorphin, CCK, VIP, glucagon and neurotensin.

Processing and Transmission of Visual Impulse in Visual Pathway

The retina relays the visual information to the brain (occipital cortex) via visual pathway which comprises the optic nerve, optic chiasma, optic tract, geniculate body and optic radiations (Fig.11.1-33).

1. Optic Nerve Optic nerve fibres are axons of the retinal ganglion cells and carry the total output of retina. Arrangement of nerve fibres in the optic nerve head and distal region of the optic nerve (behind the eyeball) is exactly same as in the retina (Fig.11.1-34), i.e.

- ***Macular fibres*** which form papillomacular bundle pass straight in the temporal part of optic disc.
- ***Temporal fibres*** of retina arch above and below the papillomacular bundle as superior and inferior *arcuate fibres* and occupy upper temporal and lower temporal quadrants of the optic disc.
- ***Nasal fibres*** of retina come directly to the nasal half of the disc as superior and inferior radiating fibres.

2. Optic Chiasma It is a flattened structure lying above the pituitary fossa. Fibres originating from the nasal halves of the retinae decussate at the chiasma while the fibres from temporal halve of retinae remain uncrossed. It is to be noted that the nasal and temporal halves of retina are demarcated by a vertical line passing through the fovea and not through the optic disc). This implies that visual impulse from the temporal half of visual field goes to the opposite side while the input from the nasal half of the visual field remains in the same side (Fig. 11.1-33).

3. Optic Tracts These are cylindrical bundles of nerve fibres which originate from the posterolateral angle of chiasma and run outwards and backwards to end in the lateral geniculate body (LGB). They consist of temporal fibres of the same side and nasal fibres of the opposite side.

4. Lateral Geniculate Bodies These are oval structures situated at the posterior termination of the optic tracts.

Retinotopic Projection. The optic tract fibres, which are axons of retinal ganglion cells project a detailed spatial representation of the retina on the lateral geniculate body, with precise point-to-point localization.

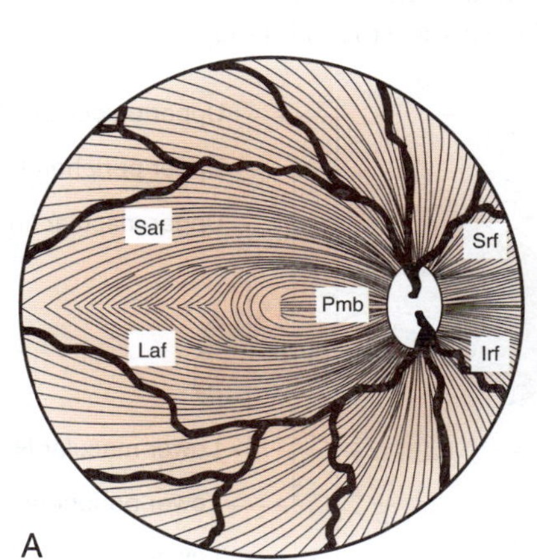

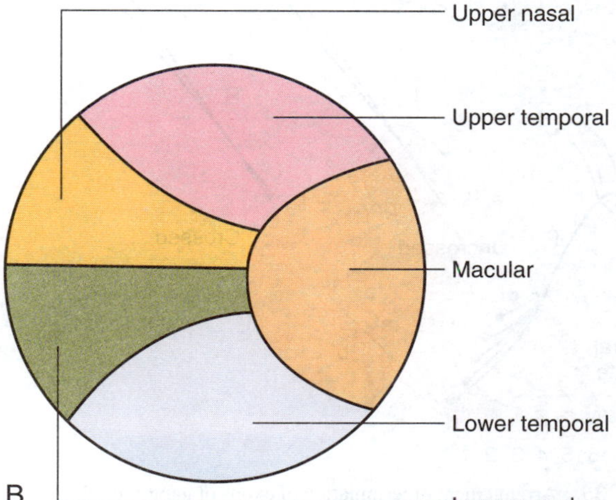

FIGURE 11.1-34 Arrangement of nerve fibres: **(A)** in the retina, optic disc and distal part of optic nerve and **(B)** in proximal region of optic nerve.

Lamellar Structure of Lateral Geniculate Body. Each LGB contains six well-defined layers. On each side layers 1,4 and 6 receive input from the nasal half of the contralateral eye, while layers 2, 3 and 5 receive input from the temporal half of the ipsilateral eye (Fig. 11-1-35). In each layer there is precise point-to-point representation of the retina, and all six layers are in register so that along a line perpendicular to the layers, the receptive fields of the cells in each layer are almost identical.

Magnocellular and Parvocellular Layers. The layers 1 and 2 of LGB have large cells and are called magnocellular layers, whereas layers 3 to 6 have small cells and are called parvocellular layers. The inputs to magnocellular layer come from the M ganglion cells of retinae while inputs to parvocellular layer come from the P ganglion cells of retinae.

Functions of LGB. Two principal functions served by LGB are:

1. ***Relay station.*** LGB serves as a relay station to relay the visual information from the ganglion cells to the visual cortex via parvocellular and magnocellular pathways, which travel through optic radiations to the visual cortex. The relay function is very accurate, so much so that there is exact point-to-point transmission with a high degree of spatial fidelity all the way from the retina to visual cortex. The signals from the two eyes are kept apart in LGB.
2. ***Visual perception and to 'gate' the transmission of signals,*** i.e. to control how much of the signals be allowed to pass to the cortex. It is worth noting that only 10–20% of the input to the LGB comes from the retina. The major inputs (80–90%) come as corticofugal fibres from the primary visual cortex and other brain regions. The feedback pathway from the visual cortex has been shown to be involved in the visual processing related to the perception of orientation and motion. These inputs also control the flow of visual information from retina to cortex

5. Optic Radiations The optic radiations are composed of axons of the lateral geniculate relay cells which project to visual cortex on the same side. The optic radiations maintain a *retinotopic organization* in their passage to visual cortex.

Processing and Analysis of Visual Impulse in the Visual Cortex

Retinotopic Organization

Just as the ganglion cell axons project a detailed spatial representation of the retina on the LGB, the LGB projects a similar point-to-point representation on the visual cortex. The visual cortex is, therefore, also called the *cortical retina,* since a true copy of the retinal image is formed here. It is only in the visual cortex that impulses originating from corresponding points of two retinae meet. Thus, the right visual cortex is concerned with the perception of objects situated to the left of the vertical median line in the visual fields, and the left visual cortex with the objects situated to the right.

Functional Anatomy and Organization of the Visual Cortex

Visual Areas

Classical Nomenclature. Classically, the visual cortex has been divided into:

- Primary visual cortex or striate cortex (area 17),
- Peristriate cortex or visual association area (area 18) and
- Parastriate cortex or visual association area (area 19).

1. ***Primary visual cortex,*** also called striate cortex or area 17 lies in the medial surface of the occipital lobe in and near the calcarine sulcus occupying parts of the lingual sulcus and coneum. Retina is represented in primary visual cortex as (Fig. 11.1-36):

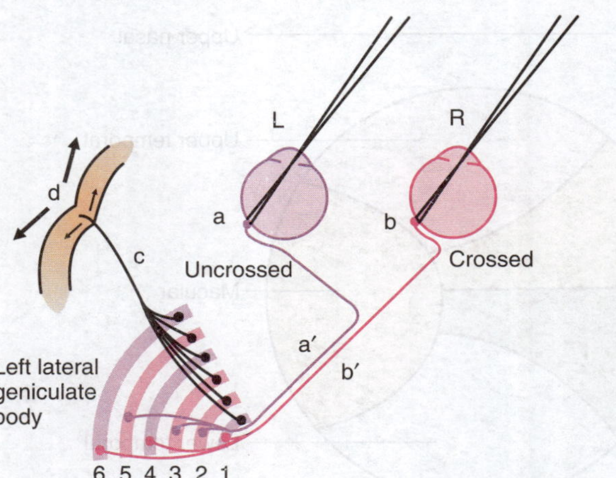

FIGURE 11.1-35 Arrangement of termination of axons of ganglion cells (second order neurons) of two eyes in the lateral geniculate body (LGB) (for explanation see text).

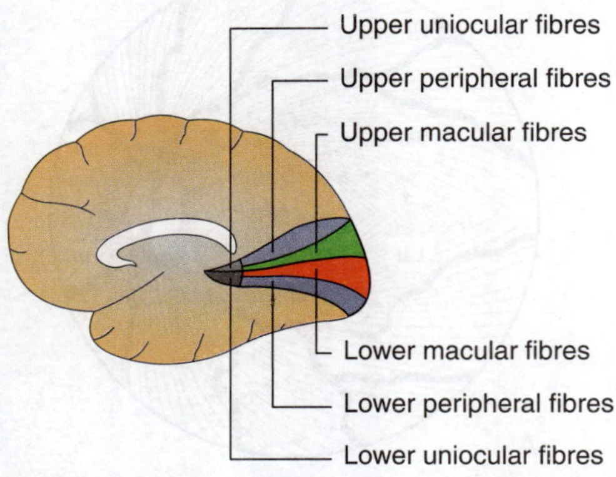

FIGURE 11.1-36 Arrangement of termination of retinal fibres in visual cortex.

  - Peripheral *part* in the anterior part of area 17, upper quadrants projects on the upper wall of the calcarine sulcus and lower quadrants on the lower walls of sulcus.
  - *Macular part* projects mainly to the posterior part of area 17 and anteriorly, to a thin strip along the calcarine sulcus. The macular area occupies nearly one-third of area 17.
2. ***Peristriate cortex*** or visual association area 18 lies in the walls of lunate sulcus.
3. ***Parastriate cortex*** or visual association area 19 lies in the cortex in front of the lunate sukus.

Modified Nomenclature of Visual Areas. It is now believed that some other parts of the brain are also involved in visual processing and so a modified nomenclature recognizing five visual areas has been described as:

- ***V1 (Visual area 1).*** It mainly includes primary visual cortex or Brodmann area 17.
- ***V2 (Visual area 2).*** It occupies the greater part of Brodmann area 18, but not the whole of it.
- ***V (Visual area 3).*** It occupies a narrow strip over the anterior part of area 18.
- ***V_4 (Visual area 4).*** It occupies the area 19.
- ***V5 (Visual area 5)*** or middle temporal (MT) area. It is located at the posterior end of superior temporal gyrus.

Histological Layers of Primary Visual Cortex Primary visual cortex, like other portions of cerebral cortex, has six distinct layers (Fig. 11.1-37). Layers I, II and III are thin and contain pyramidal cells. Layer IV is thickest and contains stellate cells. Layer IV may be further subdivided into layers, a, b, ca and c»; layers IV a + b contain the white stripe of Gennari. Layers V and VI are again relatively thin.

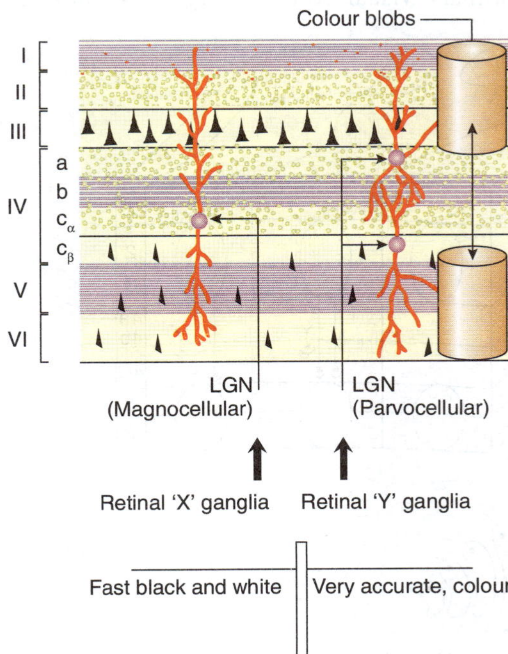

FIGURE 11.1-37 Layers of visual cortex.

Physiological Considerations of Visual Cortex

The present information available on physiology of the visual cortex is just a tip of iceberg. The much credit goes to Hubel and Wiessel for the present day knowledge. Some of the aspects of physiology of visual cortex which have been delineated, though incompletely, can be discussed under following headings:

- Concept of receptive field of striate cortex.
- Columnar organization of striate cortex.
- Serial versus parallel analysis of visual image.
- Role of extra-striate cortex in visual functions.
- Psychophysiological aspects of visual functions.

Concept of Receptive Field of Striate Cortex Unlike retinal ganglion cells and lateral geniculate neurons (which respond to both diffuse retinal stimulation and spot stimulus), the cortical neurons prefer stimuli in the form of straight line, bar or edge presented in the proper spatial orientation. Thus, in visual cortex the orientation and configuration of receptive field differ from those earlier points in the visual pathway. Depending upon the peculiarities of receptive fields, the cortical cells have been classified into three types:

- Simple cells,
- Complex cells and
- Hypercomplex cells.

Simple Cells. Simple cells are found mainly in layer IV of the primary visual cortex (area17) and form the first relay station within the visual cortex. These respond to bars of light, lines or edges, but only when they have a particular orientation. The orientation of a stimulus that is most effective in evoking a response is called the *receptive field axis orientation.* The receptive field of simple cells can be mapped with small spots of light into *on-areas* and *off-areas,* which like those of cells in the lateral geniculate body, are mutually antagonistic. However, unlike lateral geniculate neurons, the receptive fields of simple cells are arranged in parallel bands of 'on' and 'off regions, rather than concentric centre-surround arrangement of geniculate body (Fig. 11.1-38 A and B). Receptive fields of simple cells often have a central band that is either an 'on-region' or an 'off-region', with parallel flanking region on two sides that are opposite (Fig.11.1-38 C to G).

Thus, the simple cell receptive fields play an important role not only in the detection of lines and borders in the different areas of retinal image, but also detects the orientation of each line or border—that is whether it is vertical, or horizontal or lies at some degree of inclination. It is

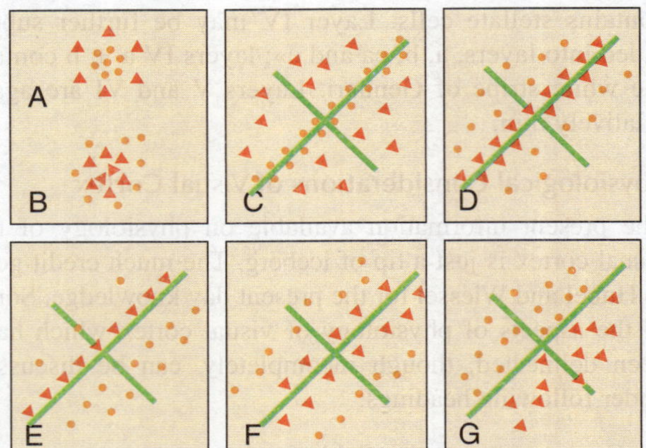

FIGURE 11.1-38 Showing arrangement of receptive fields of lateral geniculate body and primary visual cortex: **(A)** 'on centre' geniculate receptive field; **(B)** 'off centre' geniculate receptive field and **(C** to **G)**, arrangement of receptive field of simple cell. Dots represent areas that give excitatory responses (on response) and triangles represent areas that give inhibitory responses (offresponse). Receptive field axes are shown by continuous lines through field centres.

assumed that for each such orientation of a line a specific neuronal simple cell is stimulated.

Complex Cells. These cells are found in the cortical layers above and below layer IV of areas 17, 18 and 19 of visual cortex, and only rarely in layer IV itself. They resemble simple cells in requiring a preferred orientation of a linear stimulus but are less dependent upon the location of a stimulus in the visual field than the simple cells. They often respond maximally when a linear stimulus is moved laterally without a change in its orientation. Unlike simple cells it is not possible to map out distinct antagonistic 'on' and 'off' region in the receptive fields of complex cells. Complex cells often receive input from both eyes and are thus called binocular. The receptive fields of a given binocular complex cell are on corresponding parts of the two retinae and have identical receptive field properties.

Four types of complex cell receptive fields are described according to their preferred stimulus:

- Activated by a slit-non-uniform field,
- Activated by a slit-uniform field,
- Activated by an edge and
- Activated by a dark bar.

Thus, the complex cell receptive fields play an important role in the detection of lines, bars and edges, but especially so, when they are moving. In other words, by means of simple and complex cells, the person perceives the features, orientation, and movements of the objects. Therefore, simple and complex cells together are known as 'feature detectors'.

Hypercomplex Cells. These are found in cortical layers II and III of the areas 17, 18 and 19. These cells retain all the properties of complex cells but also have the added feature of requiring the line stimulus to be of a specific length. The stimuli to which they respond vary greatly, as does their complexity.

Four types of 'lower' hypercomplex cells and two categories of 'higher' hypercomplex cells were described by Hubel and Wiesel. Dreher has classified hypercomplex cells into two types: I and II.

Thus, the hypercomplex cells play a role in the detection of lines of specific length, angles or other shapes.

Columnar Organization of the Striate Cortex (Fig. 11.1-39)

The primary visual cortex is organized into vertically

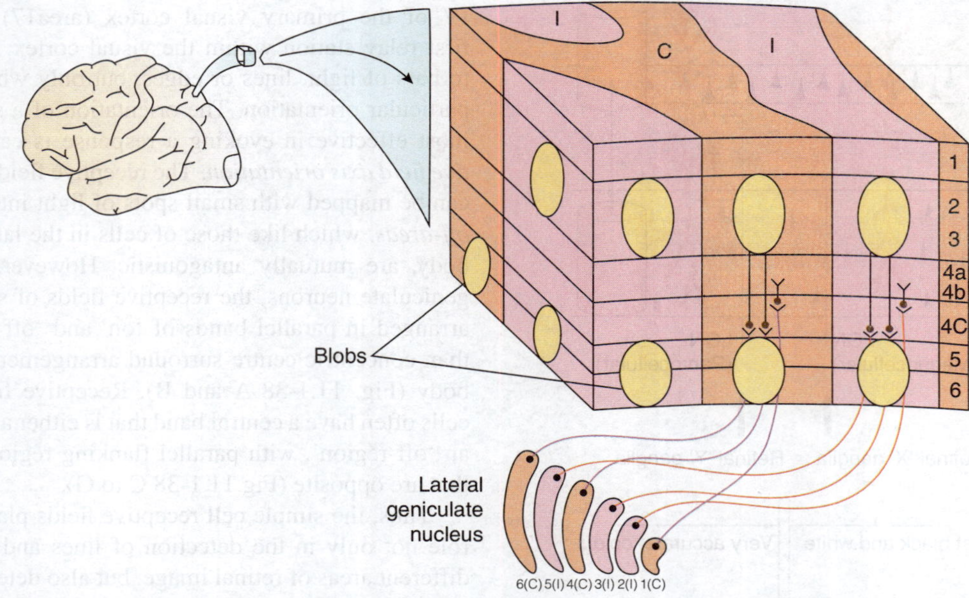

FIGURE 11.1-39 Organization of the orientation columns, ocular dominance columns and blobs in the primary visual cortex. I: Ipsilateral inputs; and C: contralateral inputs.

oriented functional modules called the *hypercolumns,* each of which processes visual information from a specific region of the visual field. The term hypercolumn refers to a set of columns responsive to lines of all orientation from a particular region in space. These vertically oriented columnar units are linked with one another by means of horizontal connections that link cells within a layer. Each hypercolumn includes sets of three types of vertical columns, which are (Fig. 11.1- 39):

- Orientation columns,
- Ocular dominance columns and
- Colour blobs.

Orientation Columns. Like the somatic sensory cortex, the primary visual cortex is organized into narrow columns of cells, running from the pial surface to the white matter. Thus, the orientation column is the unit of organization in the visual cortex which can be defined as *vertical grouping of cells with identical orientation specificity.* The visual cortex is thus organized into several million vertical columns of neuronal cells, each being about 30 to 100 jum wide and 2 mm deep.

It has been observed that the orientation preferences of neighbouring column differ in a systematic way; as one moves from column to column across the cortex, there are sequential changes in orientation preference of 5–10 degrees (Fig. 11.1-40). Thus, it is possible to speculate that for each ganglion cell receptive field in the visual field, there is collection of column in a small area of visual cortex representing the possible preferred orientation at small intervals throughout the full 360 degrees.

Ocular Dominance Columns. Ocular dominance columns refer to an independent system of columns which exist in the visual cortex with respect to the binocular input to cortical cells. As discussed earlier the simple cells in layer IV of striate cortex receive input from one eye only, whereas most complex and hypercomplex cells in layers above and below the layer IV receive input from both eyes. Although most cortical neurons are binocularly activated, there remains a strong monocular dominance. Neurons with receptive fields dominated by one eye are grouped alternately into left eye and right eye columns that are 0.25–0.5 mm in width (Fig. 11.1-41).

Thus, a group of binocular complex and hypercomplex cells in layers II, III, V and VI that receive a stronger input from one of the two eyes, along with the cells in layer IV that receive input from the same eye, is called an ocular dominance column.

The reason for the existence of rigorously ordered, complex binocular input to some complex cells is unknown but may have something to do with *binocular stereoscopic vision.*

The Colour Blobs. Interspersed among the primary visual columns are special column-like areas called *colour*

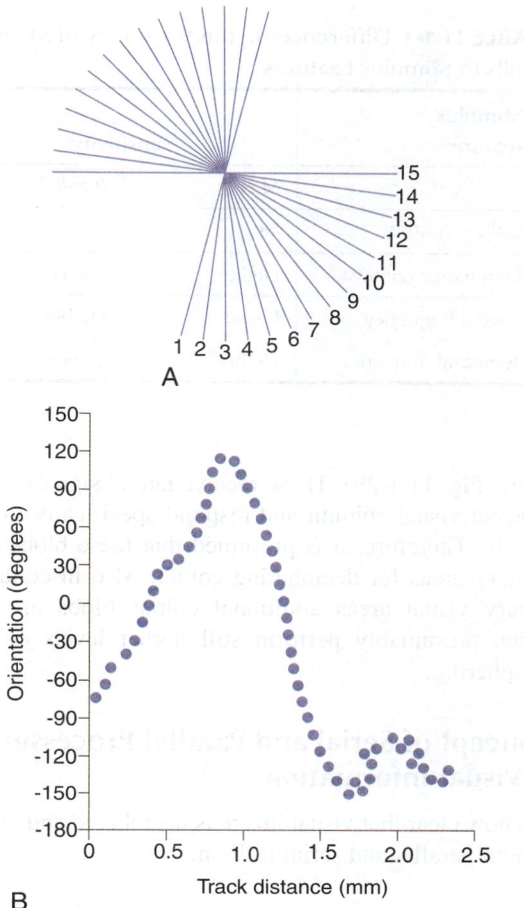

FIGURE 11.1-40 (A) Orientation preferences of 15 neurons encountered as a microelectrode penetrated the visual cortex obliquely. The preferred orientation changed steadily in a counterclockwise direction. **(B)** Results of a similar experiment plotted against distance the electrode travelled. In this case, there were a number of reversals in direction of rotation.

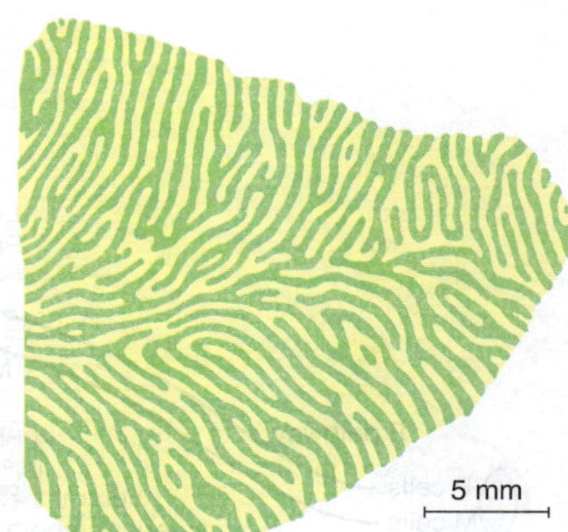

FIGURE 11.1-41 Representation of ocular dominance columns in a relatively large segment of monkey striate cortex of right occipital lobe. View is of layer IVc seen from above; ocular dominance column for one eye are in dark and those for the other eye in light. The foveal representation is to the right.

TABLE 11.1-1 Differences in the Sensitivity of M and P Cells to Stimulus Features

Stimulus feature	Sensitivity	
	M cell	*P cell*
Colour contrast	No	**Yes**
Luminance contrast	Higher	Lower
Spatial frequency	Lower	Higher
Temporal frequency	Higher	Lower

blobs (Fig. 11.1-39). These receive lateral signals from the adjacent visual column and respond specifically to colour signals. Therefore, it is presumed that these blobs are the primary areas for deciphering colour. Also in certain secondary visual areas additional colour blobs are found, which presumably perform still higher levels of colour deciphering.

Concept of Serial and Parallel Processing of Visual Information

It is now clear that visual image is deciphered and analyzed in both parallel and serial fashion.

Parallel Processing Pathways Two kinds of cells can be distinguished in the visual pathway starting from the ganglion cells of retina including neurons of the lateral geniculate body, striate cortex and extrastriate cortex. These are large cells (magno or M cells) and small cells (parvo or P cells). There are striking differences between the sensitivity of M and P cells to stimulus features (Table 11.1-1).

The visual pathway is now being considered to be made of two lanes: one made of the large cells is called magnocellular pathway, and the other of small cells is called parvocellular pathway. These can be compared to two lanes of a road. The M pathway and P pathway are involved in the *parallel processing* of the image, i.e. analysis of different features of the image.

Magnocellular Pathway. It is formed by the M cells and their processes (Fig. 11.1-42). M ganglion cells of the retina project to the magnocellular layers of the lateral geniculate nucleus (layer 1 and 2). The magnocellular projections from the LG nucleus project to the striate cortex first to layer IV c and then to layer IV. Cells in layer IV_B project directly to the middle temporal area (MT) and also the thick stripes in area V, from which cells also project to MT. From MT the M pathway extends to the posterior parietal cortex as dorsal cortical pathway.

Functions. Magnocellular pathway is concerned with the processing and detection of movement, depth and flicker feature of visual information. Thus, the parietal pathway appears to be dominated by the M input (e.g. the

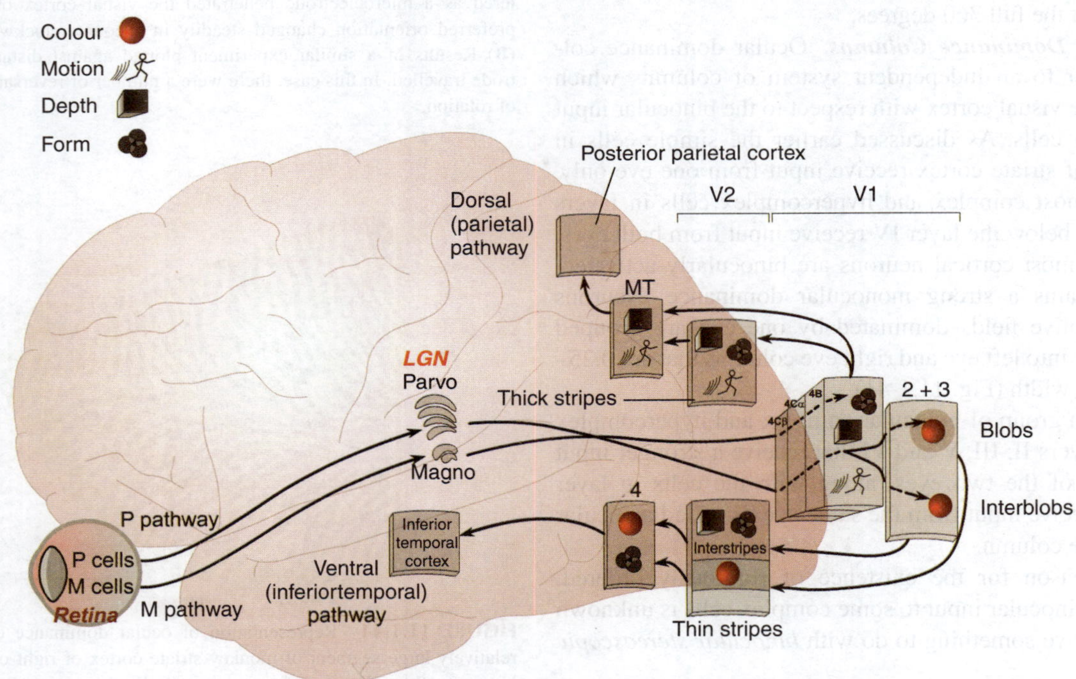

FIGURE 11.1-42 The magnocellular (M) and parvocellular pathway (P) from retina project through lateral geniculate body (LGB) to V_I. Separate pathways to temporal and parietal cortices course through the extrastriate cortex beginning in V_2.

inferior temporal pathway which depends upon both P and M inputs).

Parvocellular Pathway. It consists of P cells of visual system and their processes (Fig. 11.1-42):

- P ganglion cells of the retina project to the parvocellular layers of lateral geniculate nucleus (layers 3-6).
- Parvocellular projections from the LG nucleus project to the layer IV cR of striate cortex, from which cells project to the blobs and interblobs of V1.
- The blobs send a strong projection to the thin stripesin V, whereas interblobs send strong projection to the interstripes in V_2
- The thin stripe and interstripe area of V project to discrete subregions of V_4, from which the cells project to inferior temporal cortex as *ventral cortical pathway.*

Function. The parvocellular pathway is concerned with colour vision, texture, shape and fine details.

Concept of Serial Processing of Visual Information

The successive cells in the visual pathway starting from the photoreceptors to the cells of lateral geniculate body are involved in increasingly complex analysis of image. This is called sequential or serial processing of visual information.

Serial Processing in the Retina. In a sense, the processing of visual information in the retina involves the formation of three images:

- ***First image*** is formed by the action of light on the photoreceptor. Photoreceptors break up the image into small spots of light or darkness (much like a scanner that breaks down a picture into small pixels).
- ***Second image*** First image is converted into second image by bipolar cells. In the formation of second image, the signal is altered by horizontal cells which cause *spatial summation* by lateral inhibition.
- ***Third image.*** The second image is converted into third image by the ganglion cells. In the formation of third image, the signal is altered by amacrine cells which cause *temporal summation.* Thus, image processing in ganglion cells result in the sharpening of the image contrast. The image is thus analyzed mostly in terms of contours of the light-darkness boundaries and areas of uniform light or darkness elicit very little neural response. Thus, the image processing system in ganglion cells yields a high-contrast line diagram of the original image. There is a little change in the impulse pattern in the LGBs, so the third image reaches the occipital cortex.

Serial Analysis of Visual Image in the Visual Cortex. A hierarchical model for cell interconnections has been suggested in the visual cortex. The sequence from simple to complex and to hypercomplex forms a system of serial analysis with more and more details being deciphered. A complex cell is thought of as receiving input from several simple cells of the same orientation whose receptive fields are overlapping to produce the complex cell receptive field (Fig. 11.1-43). Since the complex cells are binocular and simple cells are mainly monocular, this adds support to the idea that complex cells are at a more advanced stage of processing.

Visual Perception

It is a complex integration of light sense, form sense, sense of contrast and colour sense. The receptive field organization of the retina and cortex are used to encode this information about a visual image.

The Light Sense

It is awareness of the light. The minimum brightness required to evoke a sensation of light is called the *light minimum.* It should be measured when the eye is dark adapted for at least 20–30 minutes.

The human eye in its ordinary use throughout the day is capable of functioning normally over an exceedingly wide range of illumination by a highly complex phenomenon termed as the *visual adaptation.* The process of visual adaptation primarily involves:

- *Dark adaptation* (adjustment in dim illumination) and
- Light adaptation (adjustment to bright illumination).

Dark Adaptation It is the ability of the eye to adapt itself to decreasing illumination. When one goes from bright sunshine into a dimly lit room, one cannot perceive the objects in the room until some time has elapsed. During this period eye is adapting to low illumination. The time taken to see in dim illumination is called *dark adaptation time.* The rods are much more sensitive to low illumination than cones. Therefore, rods are used more in dim light *(scotopic vision)* and cones in bright light *(photopic vision).*

Dark Adaptation Curve. Dark adaptation curve plotted with illumination of test object in vertical axis and

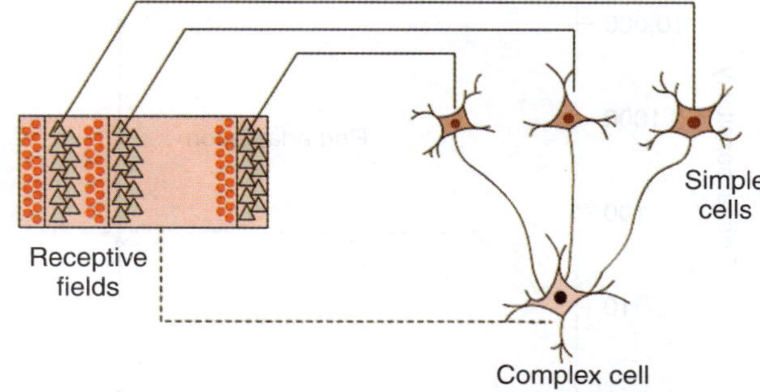

FIGURE 11.1-43 Hubel and Wesel's model of serial pathway explaining the organization of complex receptive fields. A number of cells with simple fields, of which three are shown schematically, are imagined to project to a single cortical cell of higher order. Areas marked with • represent the excitatory regions and those marked with △ represent the inhibitory region.

duration of dark adaptation along the horizontal axis shows that visual threshold falls progressively in the darkened room for about half an hour until a relative constant value is reached (Fig. 11.1-44). The dark adaptation curve plotted with retinal sensitivity along the vertical axis and duration of dark adaptation along the horizontal axis (Fig. 11-1-45) shows that the sensitivity of retina is very low on first entering the darkness, but within 1 minute the sensitivity has increased tenfold, that is, the retina can respond to light of one-tenth the previously required intensity. At the end of 20 minutes the sensitivity has increased about 6000-fold, and at the end of 40 minutes it has increased about 25,000-fold.

It can be seen that the decrease in threshold of the retina (Fig. 11.1-44), i.e. increase in sensitivity of retina (Fig. 11.1-45), proceeds in two steps: (i) the first is rapid, of short duration, and small in extent, and (ii) the second is slow, more prolonged, and larger. This indicates that two processes are at work, each having different characteristics, and that the break in the curve is the point at which one process is about to finish and the second one is just commencing. The analyses have revealed that the first plateau of the curve represents cone threshold (reached in about 5 minutes) and the second plateau represents rod threshold (reached after about 30 minutes). The inflection of the dark adaptation curve where the rod limb begins is called the cone-rod break or alpha point, and it usually occurs after 7 to 10 minutes of adaptation. The final rod phase of adaptation does not begin until 93% of rhodopsin has already regenerated.

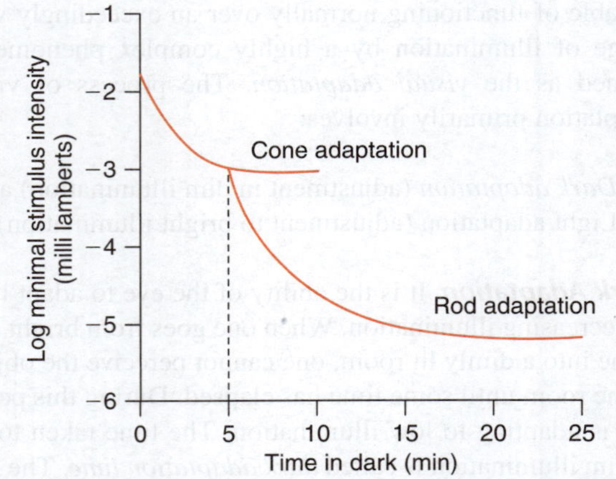

FIGURE 11.1-44 Dark adaptation curve plotted with illumination of test object in vertical axis and duration of dark adaptation along the horizontal axis.

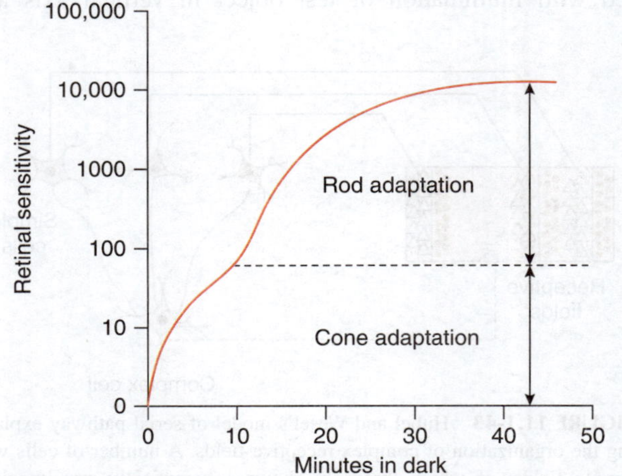

FIGURE 11.1-45 Dark adaptation curve plotted with retinal sensitivity along the vertical axis and duration of dark adaptation along the horizontal axis.

Mechanism of Dark Adaptation. Mechanism of dark adaptation involves:

1. ***Visual pigment mechanism.*** Dark adaptation primarily involves a reversal of the mechanism of light adaptation, i.e. regeneration of visual pigments (rhodopsin and cone pigments (see page 1146).
2. ***Change in pupillary size.*** Pupil dilates and can cause adaptation of approximately 30-fold because of changes in the amount of light allowed through the pupil.
   Neural mechanism. The mechanism of neural adaptation involves neurons of the visual chain in the retina itself. The neurobiological adaptation is based on feedback inhibition and the mechanism of adaptation that lies within the neuron itself.

Dark Adaptation and Vitamin A Deficiency. Severe deficiency of vitamin A elevates the threshold for dark adaptation curve due to depletion of photosensitive pigment. *Nyctalopia,* i.e. night blindness is an other important feature of vitamin A deficiency. Other causes of nyctalopia are retinitis pigmentosa and congenital night blindness.

Light Adaptation When one passes suddenly from a dim to a brightly lighted environment, the light seems intensely and even uncomfortably bright until the eyes adapt to the increased illumination and the visual threshold rises. The process by means of which retina adapts itself to bright light is called *light adaptation.* Unlike dark adaptation, the process of light adaptation is very quick and occurs over a period of 5 minutes. Strictly speaking, light adaptation is merely the disappearance of dark adaptation

Mechanism of Light Adaptation. It involves following processes:

1. ***Neural adjustment*** of sensitivity which takes place rapidly is more important and is responsible for the *transient effect* seen in light adaptation curve (Fig. 11.1-46 B to C).
2. ***Visual pigment mechanism*** involves reduction of quantity of rhodopsin and cone pigment because of their bleeching in light (see page 1147) and is responsible for the *photochemical effect* in the light adaptation curve (Fig. 11.1-46 D).
3. ***Pupillary mechanism.*** Pupil constricts in bright light and decreases the amount of light entering the eye.

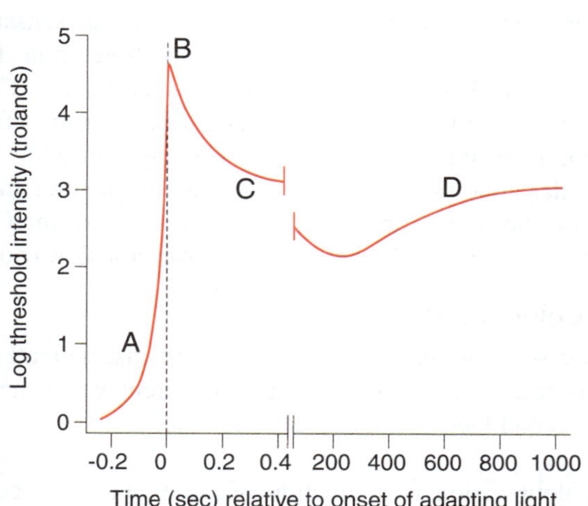

FIGURE 11.1-46 Time course of light adaptation measured by an increment threshold technique. **(A)** Anticipitory effect; **(B to C)** transient effect and **(D)** photochemical effect.

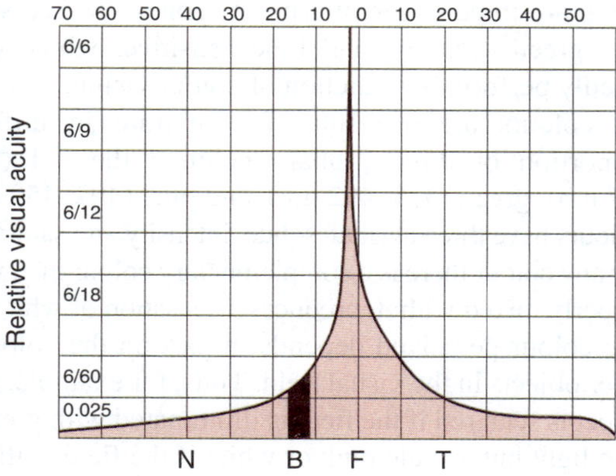

FIGURE 11.1-47 Visual acuity (form sense) in relation to the regions of the retina: N, nasal retina; B, blind spot; F, foveal region; and T, temporal retina.

The Form Sense

It is the ability to discriminate between the shapes of the objects. Cones play a major role in this faculty. Therefore, form sense is most acute at the fovea, where there are maximum number of cones and decreases very rapidly towards the periphery (Fig. 11.1-47). Visual acuity recorded by Snellen's test chart is a measure of the form sense.

Components of Visual Acuity In clinical practice, measurement of the threshold of discrimination of two spatially separated targets (a function of the fovea centralis) is termed visual acuity. However, in theory, visual acuity is a highly complex function that consists of the following components:

Minimum Visible. The ability to determine whether or not an object is present in an otherwise empty visual field is termed *visibility* or *detection.* This kind of task is referred to as the *minimum visible* or *minimum detectable function.* The limit of visibility reflects the absolute threshold of vision. The minimum visible spatial threshold level will depend upon the specification of stimulus such as size, shape, illumination and so on.

Resolution (Ordinary Visual Acuity). Discrimination of two spatially separated targets is termed resolution. The minimum separation between the two points, which can be discriminated as two, is known as *minimum resolvable.* Measurement of the threshold of discrimination is essentially an assessment of the function of the fovea centralis and is termed *ordinary visual acuity.* The distance between the two targets is specified by the angle subtended at the nodal point of the eye. The normal angular threshold of discrimination for resolution measures approximately 30 to 60 second arc; it is usually called the minimum angle of resolution (MAR).

The clinical tests determining visual acuity measure the form sense or reading ability of the eye. Thus, broadly, resolution refers to the ability to identify the spatial characteristics of a test figure. The test targets in these tests may either consist of letters (Snellen's chart) or broken circle (Landolt ring). More complex targets include gratings and checker board patterns.

Recognition. It is that faculty by virtue of which an individual not only discriminates the spatial characteristics of the test pattern but also identifies the patterns with which he has had some experience. Recognition is thus a task involving cognitive components in addition to spatial resolution. For recognition, the individual should be familiar with the set of test figures employed in addition to being able to resolve them. The most common example of recognition phenomenon is identification of faces. The average adult can recognize thousands of faces.

Minimum Discriminable or Hyperacuity. Minimum discriminable refers to spatial distinction by an observer when the threshold is much lower than the ordinary acuity. The best example of minimum discriminable is *vernier acuity*, which refers to the ability to determine whether or not two parallel and straight lines are aligned in the frontal plane.

Snellen's Test Types As mentioned earlier, in clinical practice, the measurement of visual acuity is considered synonymous with measurement of *minimal resolvable*, which in theory is just one component of the visual acuity. To measure the minimal resolvable, Snellen constructed certain test types, which are now routinely used to test the distant central visual acuity.

The fact that two distant points can be visible as separate only when they subtend an angle of 1 min at the nodal point of the eye, forms the basis of Snellen's test types. It consists of a series of black capital letters on a white board, arranged in lines, each progressively diminishing in size. The lines comprising the letter have such a breadth that

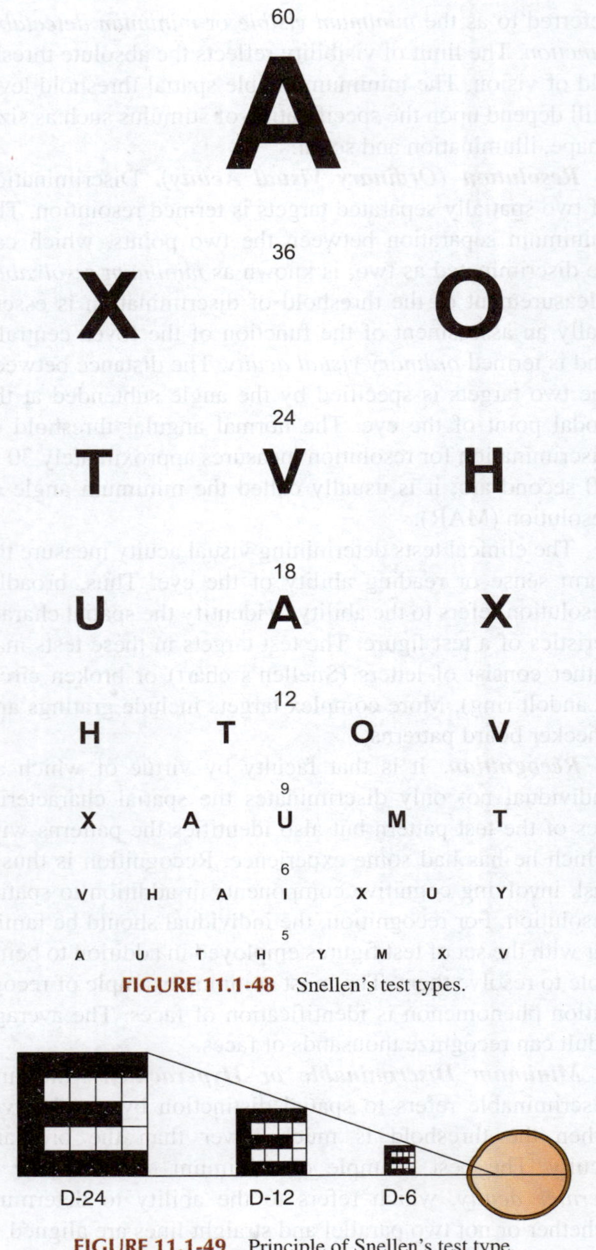

FIGURE 11.1-48 Snellen's test types.

FIGURE 11.1-49 Principle of Snellen's test type.

they will subtend an angle of 1 min at the nodal point. Each letter of the chart is so designed that it fits in a square, the sides of which are five times the breadth of the constituent lines. Thus at the given distance, each letter subtends an angle of 5 min at the nodal point of the eye (Fig. 11.1-48). The letter of the top line of Snellen's chart (Fig. 11.1-49) should be read clearly at a distance of 60 metres. Similarly, the letters in the subsequent lines should be read from a distance of 36, 24, 18, 12, 9, 6, 5 and 4 metres.

Critical Flicker Fusion Frequency When intermittent light stimuli are presented to the eye, a sensation of 'flicker' is evoked. As the frequency of presentation of the stimuli is increased a point is reached at which flicker sensation fuses to form the sensation of continuous stimulation. This frequency is known as the critical flicker fusion (CFF) frequency. The CFF frequency serves as a measure of the temporal resolving power of the visual system under the particular condition of stimulation. Motion pictures move because the frames are presented at a rate above the CFF, and movies began to flicker when the projector slows down.

The Colour Sense

Colour sense is the ability of the eye to discriminate between colours excited by light of different wavelengths. Some broad facts about colour vision are:

- Colour vision is a function of cones and thus better appreciated in photopic vision.
- The sensation of colour is subjective. Individuals are taught names for their colour sensations and subsequently use these names whenever the same sensation is obtained.
- There are three different types of cones viz. red sensitive, green sensitive and blue sensitive, which combinedly perform the function of colour vision.
- All colours are a result of admixture in different proportion of three primary colours: the red (723–647 nm), green (575–492 nm), and blue (492–450 nm)
- Colours have three attributes: hue, intensity and saturation.
- For any colour there is a complementary colour that, when properly mixed with it, produces a sensation of white.
- The colour perceived depends in part on the colour of other objects in the visual field. Thus, for example, a red object is seen red if the field is illuminated with green or blue light but as pale pink or white if the field is illuminated with red light.
- A normal person can see all wavelengths between violet and red. If the wavelength is shorter than that of violet, the light becomes ultraviolet (UV) and is beyond visibility. If the wavelength is greater than 750 nm, the light is infrared and is again beyond visibility. Human beings could have seen even UV light as blue cones retain some sensitivity at around 10 nm, but crystalline lens blocks all UV rays. Consequently after cataract operation, one can see the UV rays to some extent.
- In dim light all the colours are seen as grey; this is called Purkinje shift phenomenon.

Mechanism (Neurophysiology) of Colour Vision

Theories of Colour Vision. The process of colour analysis begins in the retina and is not entirely a function of brain. Many theories have been put forward to explain the colour perception, but two have been particularly influential:

1. Trichromatic Theory. The trichromacy of colour vision was originally suggested by Young and subsequently modified by Helmholtz. Hence, it is called Young-Helmholtz

theory. It postulates the existence of three kinds of cones, each containing a different photopigment and maximally sensitive to one of three primary colours viz. red, green and blue. The sensation of any given colour is determined by the relative frequency of the impulse from each of the three cone systems. In other words, a given colour consists of admixture of the three primary colours in different proportions. The correctness of the Young-Helmholtz's trichromacy theory of colour vision has now been demonstrated by the identification and chemical characterization of each of the three pigments by recombinant DNA technique, each having different absorption spectrum as (Fig. 11.1-50):

- ***Red sensitive cone pigment*** also known as *erythrolabe or* long wavelength sensitive (LWS) cone pigment absorbs maximally in a yellow portion with a peak at 565 nm. But its spectrum extends far enough into the long wavelength to sense red.
- ***Green sensitive cone pigment,*** also known as *chlorolabe*or medium wavelength sensitive (MWS) cone pigment absorbs maximally in the green portion with a peak at 535 nm.
- ***Blue sensitive cone pigment,*** also known as *cyanolabe or* short wavelength sensitive (SWS) cone pigment absorbs maximally in the blue-violet portion of the spectrum with a peak at 440 nm.

Thus, the Young-Helmholtz theory concludes that blue, green and red are primary colours, but the cones with their maximal sensitivity in the yellow portion of the spectrum are light at a lower threshold than green.

It has been studied that the gene for human rhodopsin is located on chromosome 3, and the gene for the blue-sensitive cone is located on chromosome 7. The genes for the red and green sensitive cones are arranged in tandem array on the q arm of the X chromosomes.

2. Opponent Colour Theory. The opponent colour theory of Herring points out that some colours appear to be 'mutually exclusive'. There is no such colour as 'reddish

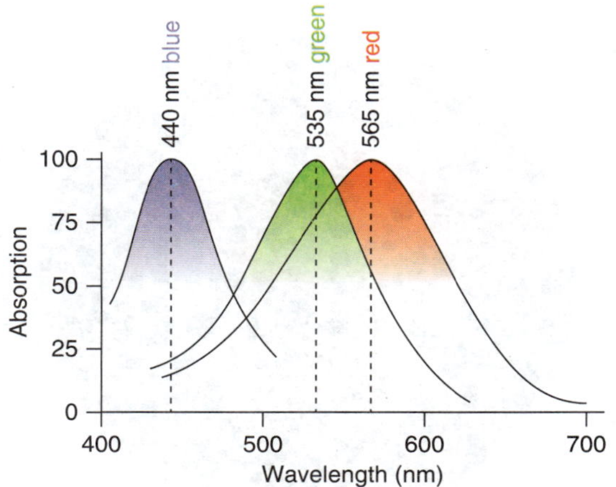

FIGURE 11.1-50 Absorption spectrum of three cone pigments.

green', and such phenomenon can be difficult to explain on the basis of trichromatic theory alone. In fact, it seems that both theories are useful in that:

- The colour vision is trichromatic at the level of photoreceptors, and
- Colouropponency at ganglion cell onward.

According to opponent colour theory, there are two main types of colour opponent ganglion cells:

a. ***Red-green opponent colour cells*** use signals from red and green cones to detect red/green contrast within their receptive field.
b. ***Blue-yellow opponent colour cells obtain a yellow signal*** from the summed output of red and green cones, which is contrasted with the output from blue cones within the receptive field.

Analysis of Colour Signals in the Visual Cortex. Colour information from the parvocellular portion of the LGB is relayed to the layer IVc of the *striate cortex* (area 17). From there, the information passes to the blobs in layers II and III. The neurons in the *blobs* lack orientation-specificity but respond to colours. Like the ganglion cells and LGB cells they are *centre-surround cells.* Many are *double-opponent cells,* which for example are stimulated by green centre and inhibited by green surround and are inhibited by red centre and stimulated by red surround. From the blobs colour information is relayed to thin strips in the visual association area and from there to a *specialized area concerned* with colour, which in human is in the lingual and fusiform gyri of occipital lobe.

Hierarchy of Colour Coded Cells The phenomenon of hierarchy of colour coded cells suggests a system of *serial analysis* of colour sense. The colour coded cells have been reported to be arranged in a hierarchical manner as: the *opponent colour cells* being located in ganglion cells and lateral geniculate neurons and the *double opponent cells* with either 'centre-surround' or bar-flank receptive fields in the layer IV of striate cortex. *Complex and hypercomplex colour coded cells* have been described in the layers II, III, V and VI of the striate cortex in the form of 'blobs'. This sequential arrangement suggests that perhaps the cells at one level of the hierarchy converge to form the receptive field of the cells at the next higher level.

Colour Blindness An individual with normal colour vision is known as *'trichromate'*. In colour blindness, faculty to appreciate one or more primary colours is either defective (anomalous) or absent (anopia). It may be congenital or acquired.

1. Congenital Colour Blindness. It is an inherited condition affecting males more (3–4%) than females (0.4%). It may be of the following types:

- Dyschromatopsia and
- Achromatopsia

i. Dyschromatopsia. Dyschromatopsia, literally means colour confusion due to deficiency of mechanism to perceive colours. It can be classified into:

- Anomalous trichromatism and
- Dichromatism.

a. *Anomalous trichromatism.* Here the mechanism to appreciate all the three primary colours is present but is defective for one or two of them. It may be of following types:

- *Protanomalous,* i.e. defective red colour appreciation,
- *Deuteranomalous,* i.e. defective green colour appreciation.
- *Tritanomalous,*i.e. implies defective blue colour appreciation.

b. *Dichromatism.* In this condition faculty to perceive one of the three primary colours is completely absent. Such individuals are called dichromates and may have one of the following types of defects:

- *Protanopia,* i.e. complete red colour defect.
- *Deuteranopia,* i.e. complete defect for green colour.
- *Tritanopia,* i.e. absence of blue colour appreciation.

Red green deficiency (protanomalous, protanopia, deuteranomalous and deuteranopia) is more common. Such a defect is source of danger in certain occupations such as drivers; sailors and traffic police. *Blue deficiency* (tritanomalous and tritanopia) is comparatively rare.

ii. Achromatopsia. It is an extremely rare condition presenting as cone monochromatism or rod monochromatism.

- ***Cone monochromatism*** is characterized by presence of only one primary colour and thus the persons are truly colour blind. Such patients usually have a visual acuity of 6/12 or better.
- ***Rod monochromatism*** may be complete or incomplete. It is inherited as an autosomal recessive trait. It is characterized by:
    - Total colour blindness and
    - Day blindness (visual acuity is about 6/60).

It may follow damage to macula or optic nerve. Usually, it is associated with a central scotoma or decreased visual acuity. It may manifest as:

- *Blue-yellow impairment,*
- *Red-green deficiency and*
- *Acquired blue colour defect* (blue blindness). It may occur in old age due to increased sclerosis of the crystalline lens. It is owing to the physical absorption of the blue rays by increased amber-coloured pigment in the nucleus.

Tests for Colour Vision. Commonly employed colour vision tests are:

1. Pseudo-isochromatic Chart Test. It is the most commonly employed test using Ishihara's plates. In this there are patterns of coloured and grey dots which reveal one pattern to the normal individuals and another to the colour deficients. It is a quick method of screening colour blinds from the normal (Fig. 11.1-51).

Another test based on the same principle is *Hardy-Rand-Rittler plate test.*

2. The Lantern Test. In this test, the subject has to name the various colours shown to him by a lantern and the judgement is made by the mistake he makes. *Eldridge-Green lantern* is most popular.

3. Farnsworth-Munsell 100 Hue Test. It is a spectroscopic test in which subject has to arrange the coloured chips in ascending order. The colour vision is judged by the error score, i.e. greater the score poorer the colour vision.

4. City University Colour Vision Test. It is also a spectroscopic test where a central coloured plate is to be matched to its closest hue from four surrounding colour plates.

5. Nagel Anomaloscope Test. In this test, the observer is asked to mix red and green colours in such a proportion that the mixture should match the given yellow coloured disc. The judgement about the defect is made from the relative amounts of red and green colours and the brightness setting used by the observer.

6. Holmgren Wool Test. In this the subject is asked to make a series of colour matches from a selection of skeins of coloured wools.

Contrast Sensitivity

Contrast sensitivity is the ability to perceive slight changes in luminance between regions which are not separated by definite borders and is just as important as the ability to perceive sharp outlines of relatively small objects. It is only the latter ability which is tested by means of the Snellen's test types. In many diseases loss of contrast sensitivity is more important and disturbing to the patient than the loss of visual acuity.

Encoding of Contrast Contrast is encoded when one ganglion cell is stimulated and its neighbour is inhibited.

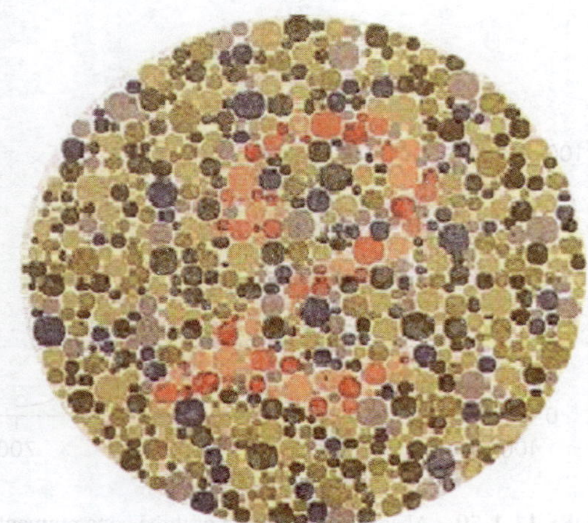

FIGURE 11.1-51 Ishihara chart.

At the border between light and dark areas of image, the neighbouring cells respond in opposite way, i.e.

- *In the lighted portion* of the border between light and dark the centre of the receptive field is illuminated, while its surround is not. Therefore, the on-centre ganglion cell activity is increased.
- *In the darkened portion,* the surround of the receptive field is illuminated, while its centre is not. Therefore, the on-centre ganglion cell activity is decreased.

When both the centre and surround of the receptive field are totally in the illuminated or darkened portion, of the image, no change in ganglion cell activity occurs.

Electrophysiological Tests

The electrophysiological tests allow objective evaluation of the retinal functions. These include: electroretinography (ERG), electro-oculography (EOG), and visually evoked response (VER).

Electroretinography ERG is the record of changes in the resting potential of the eye induced by a flash of light. It is measured in dark adapted eye with the active electrode (fitted on contact lens) placed on the cornea and the reference electrode attached on the forehead.

Normal record of ERG consists of the following waves (Fig.11.1-52):

- ***a-wave.*** It is a negative wave possibly arising from the rods and cones.
- ***b-wave.*** It is a large positive wave which is generated by Muller cells, but represents the activity of the bipolar cells.
- ***c-wave.*** It is also a positive wave representing metabolic activity of pigment epithelium.

Both scotopic and photopic responses can be elicited in ERG. Foveal ERG can provide information about the macula.

Uses. ERG is very useful in detecting functional abnormalities of the outer retina (up to bipolar cell layer), much before the ophthalmoscopic signs appear. However, ERG is normal in diseases involving ganglion cells and the higher visual pathway, such as optic atrophy.

Electro-oculography EOG is based on the measurement of resting potential of the eye which exists between the cornea (+ve) and back of the eye (-ve).

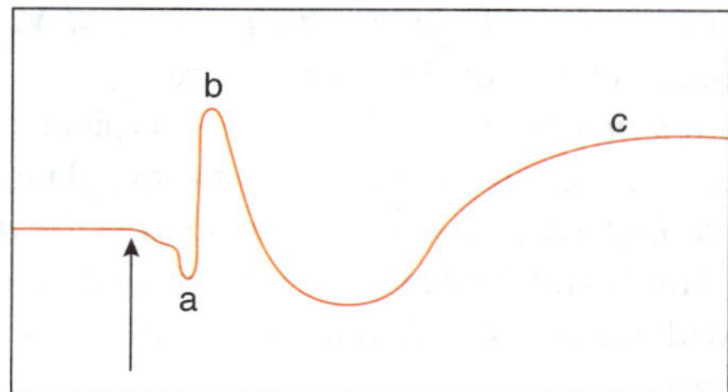

FIGURE 11.1-52 Components of normal electroretinogram (ERG).

Normally, the resting potential of the eye decreases during dark adaptation and reaches its peak in light adaptation.

Interpretation of results. Results of EOG are interpreted by finding out the Arden ratio as:

$$\text{Arden ratio} = \frac{\text{Maximum height of light peak}}{\text{Minimum height of dark peak}} \times 100$$

- *Normal curve* values are 185 or above.
- *Subnormal curve* values are less than 150
- *Flat curve* values are less than 125.

Uses. Since the EOG reflects the presynaptic function of the retina, any disease that interferes with the functional interplay between the retinal pigment epithelium and the photoreceptors will produce an abnormal or absent light rise in the EOG. Thus, EOG is affected in diseases such as retinitis pigmentosa, vitamin A deficiency, retinal detachment and toxic retinopathies. Hence, EOG serves as a test that is supplementary and complementary to ERG and in certain states is more sensitive than the ERG.

Visually Evoked Response As we know when light falls on the retina, a series of nerve impulses are generated and passed on to the visual cortex via the visual pathway. The changes produced in the visual cortex by these impulses can be recorded by electroencephalography (EEG). Thus visually evoked response (VER) is nothing but the EEG recorded at the *occipital lobe. VER* is the *only clinically objective technique available to assess the functional state of the visual system beyond the retinal ganglion cells.* Since there is disproportionately large projection of the macular area in the occipital cortex, the VER represents the macula-dominated response. VER is of two types depending upon the techniques used:

1. ***Flash VER.*** It is recorded by using an intense flash stimulation. It merely indicates that light has been perceived by the visual cortex. It is not affected by the opacities in the lens and cornea.
2. ***Pattern reversal VER.*** It is recorded using some patterned stimulus, as in the checker board. In it the pattern of the stimulus is changed (e.g. black squares go white and white become black) but the overall illumination remains same. The pattern reversal VER depends on form sense and thus may give a rough estimate of the visual acuity.

FIELD OF VISION AND BINOCULAR VISION

Field of Vision

The visual field is a three-dimensional area that can be seen around an object of fixation. The extent of normal visual field with a 5-mm white colour object is superiorly 60°, inferiorly 70°, nasally 60° and temporally 90° (Fig. 11.1-53). The field for blue and yellow is roughly 10° less and that for red and green colour is about 20° less than that for white. Perimetry

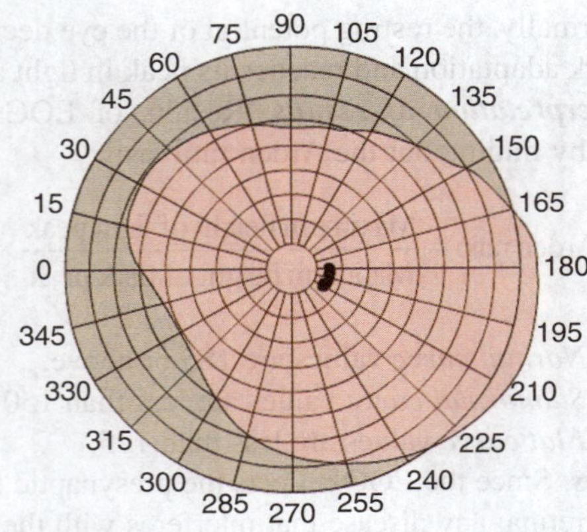

FIGURE 11.1-53 Extent of normal visual field.

with a red colour object is particularly useful in the diagnosis of bitemporal hemianopia due to chiasmal compression and in the central scotoma of retrobulbar neuritis.

Perimetry It is the procedure for estimating extent of the visual fields. It is of following two types:

1. ***Kinetic perimetry.*** In this the stimulus of known luminance is moved from periphery towards the centre to establish isoptres.
2. ***Static perimetry.*** This involves presenting a stimulus at a predetermined position for a preset duration with varying luminance.

Methods of Estimating the Visual Fields

A. Peripheral Field Charting

- Confrontation method
- Perimetry: Lister's, Goldmann's and automated.

B. Central Field Charting

- Campimetry or scotometry
- Goldmann's perimetry
- Automated field analysis.

1. ***Confrontation method.*** This is a rough but rapid and extremely simple method of estimating the peripheral visual field. Assuming the examiner's fields to be within the normal range, they are compared with patient's visual fields.
2. ***Lister's perimeter***. It has a metallic semicircular arc, graded in degrees, with a white dot for fixation in the centre. The arc can be rotated in different meridia. With the help of this perimeter extent of peripheral field is charted (Fig. 11.1-54).
3. ***Campimetry*** (scotometry) is done to evaluate the central and paracentral area (30°) of the visual field. The Bjerrum's screen is used and can be of size 1 metre or 2 metre square (Fig. 11.1-55). Initially the *blind spot* physiological scotoma is charted, which is normally located about 15° temporal to the fixation point. Dimensions of blind spots are horizontally 7–8° and vertically 10–11°. *Central/paracentralscotomas* can be found in optic neuritis and open angle glaucoma.
4. ***Goldmann's perimeter***. It consists of a hemispherical dome. Its main advantage over the tangent screen is that the test conditions and the intensity of the target are always the same. It permits greater reproducibility.
5. ***Automated perimeters*** are computer assisted and test visual fields by a static method. They automatically test suprathreshold and threshold stimuli and quantify depth of field defect.

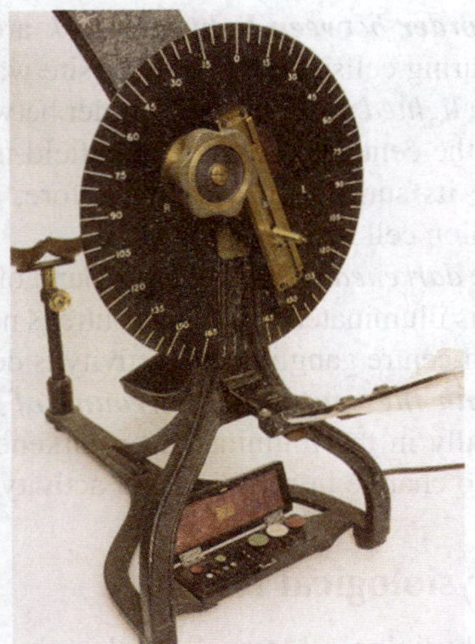

FIGURE 11.1-54 Perimeter.

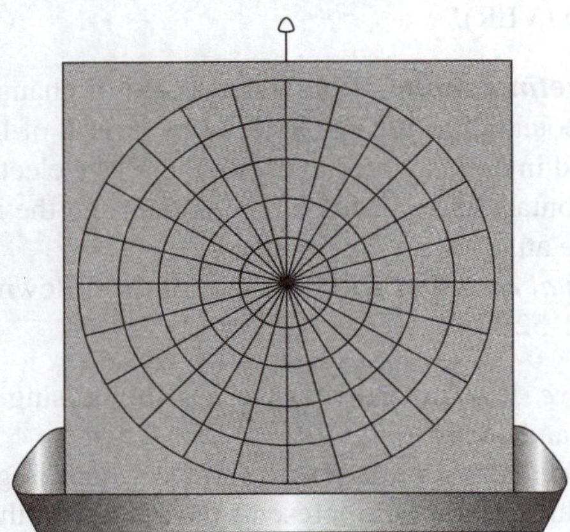

FIGURE 11.1-55 Bjerrum's screen.

Common Causes of Defects in the Field of Vision The most common causes of field defects are:

I. Glaucomatous Field Defects. A typical pattern of field defects is seen in patients with chronic glaucomas.

II. Field Defects in Lesions of the Optic Disc and Optic Nerve. Central and paracentral scotomas can be found in patients with papillitis (inflammation of the optic disc) and optic neuritis.

III. Fields Defects in Lesions of Visual Pathway. Salient features and important causes of lesions of the visual pathway at different levels (Fig. 11.1-56) are as follows:

1. Lesions of the Optic Nerve. These are characterized by marked loss of vision or complete blindness on the affected side associated with abolition of the direct light reflex on the ipsilateral side and consensual light reflex on the contralateral side. Near (accommodation) reflex is present. *Common causes* of optic nerve lesions are: optic atrophy and acute optic neuritis.

2. Lesions through Proximal Part of the Optic Nerve. Salient features of such lesions are: ipsilateral blindness, contralateral hemianopia and abolition of direct light reflex on the affected side and consensual on the contralateral side. Near reflex is intact.

3. Sagittal (Central) Lesions of the Chiasma. These are characterized by bitemporal hemianopia and bitemporalhemianopic paralysis of pupillary reflexes. These usually lead to partial descending optic atrophy. *Common causes* of central chiasmal lesion are: suprasellar aneurysms and tumours of pituitary gland.

4. Lateral Chiasmal Lesions. Salient features of such lesions are binasal hemianopia associated with binasalhemianopic paralysis of the pupillary reflexes. These usually lead to partial descending optic atrophy. *Common causes* of such lesions are distension of third ventricle causing pressure on each side of the chiasma.

5. Lesions of Optic Tract. These are characterized by incongruous homonymous hemianopia associated with contralateral hemianopic pupillary reaction (Wernicke's reaction).

6. Lesions of Lateral Geniculate Body. These produce homonymous hemianopia with sparing of pupillary reflexes, and may end in partial optic atrophy.

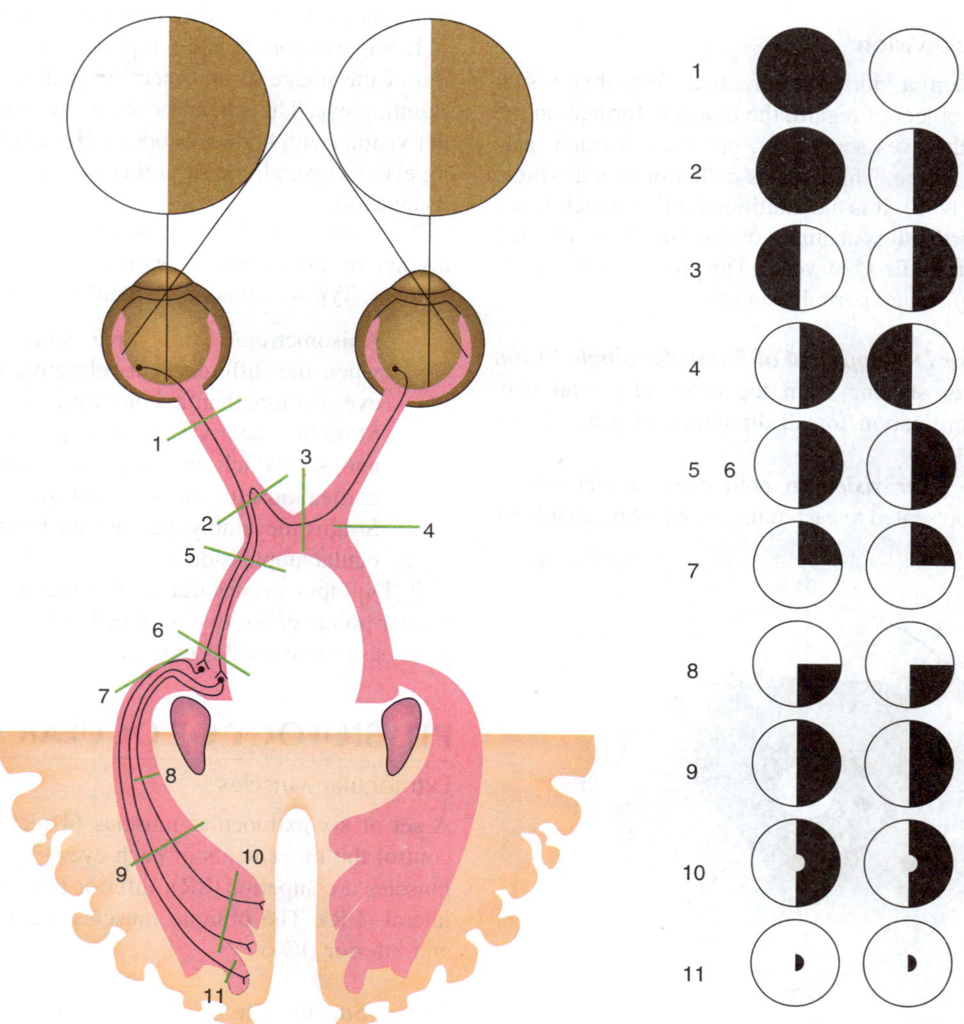

FIGURE 11.1-56 Lesions of the visual pathways at the level of: 1, optic nerve; 2, proximal part of optic nerve; 3, central chiasma; 4, lateral chiasma (both sides); 5, optic tract; 6, geniculate body; 7, part of optic radiations in temporal lobe; 8, part of optic radiations in parietal lobe; 9, optic radiations; 10, visual cortex sparing the macula; and 11, visual cortex, only macula.

7. Lesions of Optic Radiations. Their features vary depending upon the site of lesion. Involvement of total optic radiations produce complete homonymous hemianopia (sometimes sparing the macula). Inferior quadrantic hemianopia (*pie on the floor*) occurs in lesions of parietal lobe (containing superior fibres of optic radiations). Superior quadrantic hemianopia (*pie in the sky*) may occur following lesions of the temporal lobe (containing inferior fibres of optic radiations). Pupillary reactions are normal as the fibres of the light reflex leave the optic tracts to synapse in the superior colliculi. *Common lesions* of the optic radiations include vascular occlusions.

8. Lesions of the Visual Cortex. Congruous homonymous hemianopia (usually sparing the macula, is a feature of occlusion of posterior cerebral artery supplying the anterior part of occipital cortex. Congruous homonymous macular defect occurs in lesions of the tip of the occipital cortex following head injury or gun shot injuries. Pupillary light reflexes are normal and optic atrophy does not occur following visual cortex lesions.

Binocular Single Vision

Definition When a normal individual fixes his visual attention on an object of regard, the image is formed on the fovea of both the eyes separately; but the individual perceives a single image. This state is called binocular single vision (Fig. 11.1-57). It is a conditioned reflex which is not present since birth but is acquired during first 6 months and is completed during first few years. The process of its development is complex and partially understood.

Prerequisites for Development of Binocular Single Vision

1. ***Straight eyes*** starting from the neonatal period with precise co-ordination for all directions of gaze (motor mechanism).
2. ***Reasonably clear vision*** in both eyes so that similar images are presented to each retina (sensory mechanism).

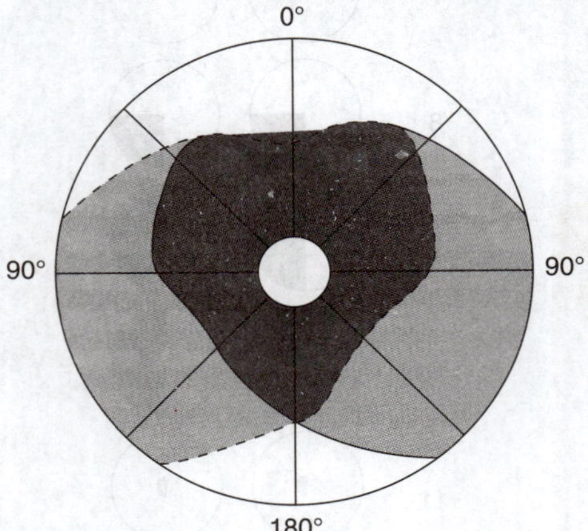

FIGURE 11.1-57 Monocular and binocular visual fields. The dashed outline depicts visual field of left eye and solid line, that of right eye. The common area (clear zone) is viewed by binocular vision and coloured areas are viewed by monocular vision.

3. ***Ability of visual cortex*** to promote binocular single vision (mental process).

Therefore, pathologic states disturbing any of the above mechanisms during the first few years of life will hinder the development of binocular single vision and may cause squint.

Grades of Binocular Single Vision There are three grades of binocular single vision, which are best tested with the help of a synoptophore.

- ***Grade I*** *Simultaneous perception.* It is the power to see two dissimilar objects simultaneously.
- ***Grade II****-Fusion.* It consists of the power to superimpose two incomplete but similar images to form one complete image.
- ***Grade III*** *Stereopsis.* It consists of the ability to perceive the third dimension (depth perception).

Anomalies of Binocular Vision Anomalies of binocular vision include suppression amblyopia and diplopia.

1. Suppression. It is a temporary active cortical inhibition of the image of an object formed on the retina of the squinting eye. This phenomenon occurs only during binocular vision (with both eyes open). However, when the fixating eye is covered, the squinting eye fixes (i.e. suppression disappears).

2. Amblyopia. It is an impairment of vision in the absence of any organic disease of ocular media and visual pathway. Types of functional amblyopia are:

- Anisometropic amblyopia which usually occurs when the difference in refractive error of the two eyes is more than 2.5 dioptres.
- Stimulus deprivation amblyopia (amblyopia ex anopsia) which may occur in children with cataract, corneal opacity and severe ptosis.
- Strabismic amblyopia results from prolonged uniocularsuppression.

3. Diplopia *occurs* due to formation of image on dissimilar points of the two retinae. It is the main symptom of paralysis of extraocular muscles.

PHYSIOLOGY OF OCULAR MOTILITY

Extraocular Muscles

A set of six extraocular muscles (4 recti and 2 obliques) control the movements of each eye (Fig. 11.1-58). Rectus muscles are superior (SR), inferior (IR), medial (MR) and lateral (LR). The oblique muscles include superior (SO) and inferior (IO).

Nerve Supply The extraocular muscles are supplied by third, fourth and sixth cranial nerves. The third cranial nerve (oculomotor) supplies the superior, medial and inferior recti and inferior oblique muscles. The fourth cranial

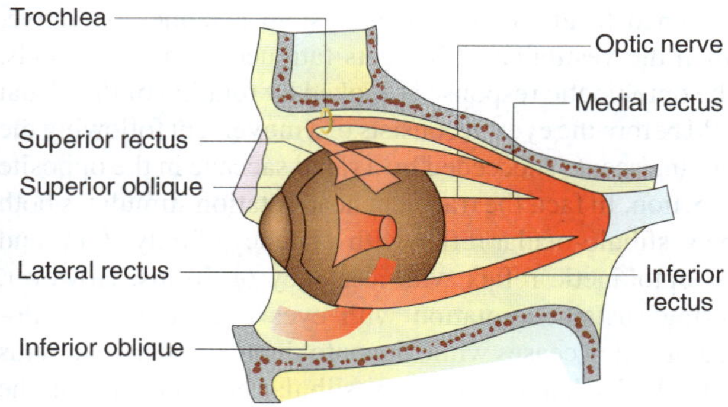

FIGURE 11.1-58 Extraocular muscles.

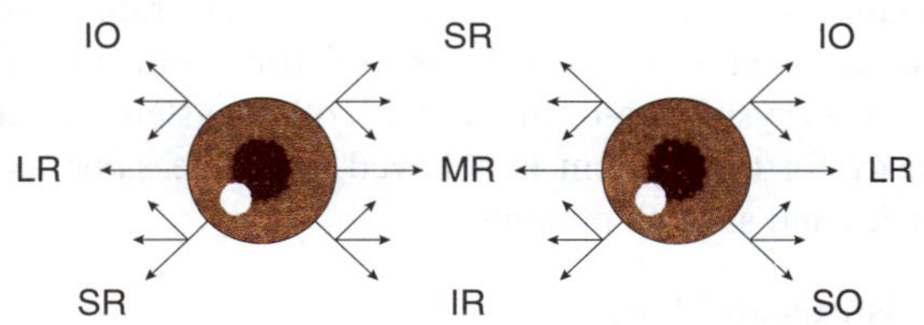

FIGURE 11.1-59 Action of extraocular muscles: SR (superior oblique); LR (lateral rectus); IO (inferior oblique); MR (medial rectus); IR (inferior rectus); and SO (superior oblique).

TABLE 11.1-2 Actions of Extraocular Muscles

Muscle	Primary action	Secondary action	Tertiary action
MR	Adduction	—	—
LR	Abduction	—	—
SR	Elevation	Intorsion	Adduction
IR	Depression	Extorsion	Adduction
SO	Intorsion	Depression	Abduction
IO	Extorsion	Elevation	Abduction

nerve (trochlear) supplies the superior oblique and the sixth nerve (abducent) supplies the lateral rectus muscle.

Actions The extraocular muscles rotate the eyeball around vertical, horizontal and anteroposterior axes. Medial and lateral rectus muscles are almost parallel to the optic axis of the eyeball; so they have got only the main action. While superior and inferior rectus muscles make an angle of 23° and reflected tendons of the superior and inferior oblique muscles of 51° with the optical axis in the primary position; so they have subsidiary actions in addition to the main action. Actions of each muscle (Fig. 11.1-59) are shown in Table 11.1-2.

Ocular Movements

Types of Ocular Movements

A. ***Uniocular movements*** are called 'ductions' and include:

1. *Adduction.* It is inward movement (medial rotation) along the vertical axis.
2. *Abduction.* It is outward movement (lateral rotation) along the vertical axis.
3. *Supraduction.* It is upward movement (elevation) along the horizontal axis.
4. *Infraduction.* It is downward movement (depression) along the horizontal axis.
5. *Incycloduction*(intorsion). It is a rotatory movement along the anteroposterior axis in which superior pole of the cornea (12 O'clock point) moves medially.
6. *Excycloduction* (extorsion). It is a rotatory movement along the anteroposterior axis in which superior pole of the cornea (12 O'clock point) moves laterally.

B. ***Binocular movements***. These are of two types: versions and vergences.

a. ***Versions,*** also known as conjugate movements, are synchronous (simultaneous) symmetric movements of both eyes in the same direction. These include:

1. *Dextroversion.* It is the movement of both eyes to the right. It results due to simultaneous contraction of right lateral rectus and left medial rectus.
2. *Levoversion.* It refers to movement of both eyes to the left. It is produced by simultaneous contraction of left lateral rectus and right medial rectus.
3. *Supraversion.* It is upward movement of both eyes in primary position. It results due to simultaneous contraction of bilateral superior recti and inferior obliques.
4. *Infraversion.* It is downward movement of both eyes in primary position. It results due to simultaneous contraction of bilateral inferior recti and superior obliques.
5. *Dextrocycloversion.* It is rotational movement around the anteroposterior axis, in which superior pole of cornea of both the eyes tilts towards the right.
6. *Levocycloversion.* It is just the reverse of dextrocycloversion. In it superior pole of cornea of both the eyes tilts towards the left.

b. ***Vergences,*** also called disjugate movements, are synchronous and symmetric movements of both eyes in opposite directions, e.g.

1. *Convergence.* It is simultaneous inward movement of both eyes which results from contraction of the medial recti.
2. *Divergence.* It is simultaneous outward movement of both eyes produced by contraction of the lateral recti.

Supranuclear Control of Eye Movements

There exists a highly accurate, still not fully elucidated, supranuclear control of eye movements which keeps the two eyes yoked together so that the image of the object of interest is simultaneously held on both fovea despite movement of the perceived object or the observer's head and/or body.

Following supranuclear eye movement systems have been recognized:

1. Saccadic system,
2. Smooth pursuit system,
3. Vergence system,
4. Vestibular system,
5. Optokinetic system and
6. Position maintenance system.

All these systems perform specific functions and each one is controlled by a different neural system but share the same final common path—the motor neurons that supply the extraocular muscles.

1. Saccadic System Saccades are sudden, jerky conjugate eye movements, that occur as the gaze shifts from one object to another. Thus, they are performed to bring the image of an object quickly on the fovea. Though normally voluntary, saccades may be involuntary aroused by peripheral, visual or auditory stimuli.

2. Smooth Pursuit Eye Movement System Smooth pursuit movements are tracking movements of the eye as they follow moving objects. These occur voluntarily when the eyes track moving objects but take place involuntarily if a repetitive visual pattern is displayed continuously. When velocity of the moving object is more, the smooth pursuit movement is replaced by *small saccades (catch-up saccades)*.

3. Vergence Movement System Vergence movements allow focusing of an object which moves away from or towards the observer or when visual fixation shifts from one object to another at a different distance. Vergence movements are very slow (about 20°/sec) disjugate movements. They have a latency of about 160 msec.

4. Vestibular Eye Movement System Vestibular movements are usually effective in compensating for the effects of head movements in disturbing visual fixation. These movements operate through the vestibular system (see page 1078).

Most rotations of the head do not involve angular rotations as fast as 300°/sec and the vestibular system can compensate for these. However, when the body is rotated at great speeds around a vertical axis (e.g. a skater performing a spin) eye movements show the so-called oculovestibular nystagmus, with a slow motion of the eyes in the opposite direction to that of rotation—this is initiated by the vestibular mechanism—followed by a quick jerky binocular 'return' movement in the direction of rotation. This sequence is repeated as long as the angular acceleration lasts. It is likely that the fast component of nystagmus is mediated by mechanisms similar to those responsible for saccades.

5. Optokinetic System This system helps to hold the images of the seen world steady on the retinae during sustained head rotation. This system becomes operative, when the vestibular reflex gets fatigued after 30 seconds. The optokinetic response is evoked by rotation of the visual field before the eyes. It consists of a movement following the moving scene, succeeded by a rapid saccade in the opposite direction. In fact, the transient head rotation stimulates both the vestibulo-ocular reflex with a latency of only 10 ms and the optokinetic reflex with a latency of 70 ms. However, during sustained rotation with eyes open the vestibulo-ocular reflex ceases while the optokinetic system maintains a steady discharge from the vestibular nuclei to sustain the compensatory optokinetic nystagmus.

6. Position Maintenance System This system helps to maintain a specific gaze position by means of rapid micromovements called *flicks* and slow micromovements called *drifts.* This system co-ordinates with other systems. ***Neural pathway*** for this system is believed to be the same as for saccades and smooth pursuits.

Strabismus and Nystagmus

Strabismus

Definition. Normally visual axes of the two eyes are parallel to each other in the 'primary position of gaze' and this alignment is maintained in all positions.

A *misalignment of the visual axes of the two eyes is called squint or strabismus.*

Manifest Squint (Heterotopia) It is of two types

- Concomitant strabismus and
- Incomitant strabismus.

1. ***Concomitant strabismus***. It is a type of manifest squint in which the amount of deviation in the squinting eye remains constant (unaltered) in all the directions of gaze; and there is no associated limitation of ocular movements.
   - ***Aetiology*** of concomitant strabismus is not clearly defined. The causative factors differ in individual cases. As we know, the binocular vision and co-ordination of ocular movements are not present since birth but are acquired in the early childhood. The process starts by the age of 3–6 months and is completed up to 5–6 years. Therefore, any obstacle to the development of these processes may result in concomitant squint. These obstacles can be arranged into three groups, namely sensory, motor and central.
2. ***Paralytic strabismus***. It refers to ocular deviation resulting from complete or incomplete paralysis of one or more extraocular muscles. The causative lesions may be neurogenic, myogenic or at the level of neuromuscular junction.

Nystagmus It is defined as regular and rhythmic to and fro involuntary oscillatory movements of the eyes.

Aetiology. It occurs due to disturbance of the factors responsible for maintaining normal ocular posture. These include disorders of sensory visual pathway, vestibular apparatus, semicircular canals, mid brain and cerebellum.

Features of Nystagmus. It may be characterized by any of the following features:

1. It may be *pendular or jerk nystagmus.* In pendular nystagmus movements are of equal velocity in each direction. It may be horizontal, vertical or rotatory. In jerk nystagmus, the movements have a slow component in one direction and a fast component in the other direction. The direction of jerk nystagmus is defined by direction of the fast component (phase). It may be right, left, up, down or rotatory.
2. Nystagmus movements may be *rapid or slow*.
3. The movements may be *fine or coarse*.
4. Nystagmus may be *latent or manifest*.

AQUEOUS HUMOUR AND INTRAOCULAR PRESSURE

Aqueous Production

The aqueous humour is a clear watery fluid filling the anterior chamber (0.25 ml) and posterior chamber (0.06 ml) of the eyeball. In addition to its role in maintaining a proper IOP it also plays an important metabolic role by providing substrates and removing metabolites from the avascular cornea and the lens. Constituents of normal aqueous humour are: water (99.9%), proteins (0.04%) and others in millimoles/kg are Na^+ (144), K^+ (4.5), Cl^-(110), glucose (6.0), lactic acid (7.4), amino acids (5), and inositol (0.1).

Aqueous humour is derived from plasma within the capillary network of ciliary processes. The normal aqueous production rate is 2.3 ml/min. The three mechanisms: *diffusion, ultrafiltration and secretion* (active transport) play a part in its production at different levels. The steps involved in the process of production are:

1. First of all, by *ultrafiltration,* most of the plasma substances pass out from the capillary wall, loose connective tissue and pigment epithelium of the ciliary processes. Thus, the plasma filtrate accumulates behind the non-pigment epithelium of ciliary processes.
2. The tight junctions between the cells of the non-pigment epithelium creates part of blood-aqueous barrier. Certain substances are actively transported *(secreted)* across this barrier into the posterior chamber. The active transport is brought about by Na^+-K^+ activated ATPase pump and carbonic anhydrase enzyme system. Substances that are actively transported include: sodium, chlorine, potassium, ascorbic acid, amino acids and bicarbonates.

Active transport of these substances across the non-pigmented ciliary epithelium results in an osmotic gradient leading to the movement of other plasma constituents into the posterior chamber by ultrafiltration and *diffusion.* Sodium is primarily responsible for movement of water into the posterior chamber

Control of aqueous formation. The diurnal variation in IOP certainly indicates that some endogenous factors do influence the aqueous formation. The exact role of such factors is yet to be clearly understood. Vasopressin and adenylyl cyclase have been described to affect aqueous formation by influencing active transport of sodium.

Ultrafiltration and diffusion, the passive mechanisms of aqueous formation, are dependent on the level of blood pressure in the ciliary capillaries, the plasma osmotic pressure and the level of IOP.

Drainage of Aqueous Humour

Aqueous humour flows from the posterior chamber into the anterior chamber through the pupil against slight physiologic resistance. From the anterior chamber the aqueous is drained out by two routes:

- Trabecular (conventional outflow) and
- Uveoscleral (unconventional) outflow.

A. Trabecular (Conventional) Outflow It is the main outlet for aqueous from the anterior chamber. Approximately, 90% of the total aqueous is drained out via this route. The aqueous outflow system includes the trabecular meshwork, Schlemm's canal, collector channels, aqueous veins and the episcleral veins (Fig. 11.1-60).

1. Trabecular Meshwork. It is a sieve-like structure through which aqueous humour leaves the eye. It consists of three portions:

- *Uveal meshwork,*
- *Corneoscleral meshwork and*
- *Juxtacanalicular (endothelial) meshwork.*

2. Schlemm's Canal. This is an endothelial lined oval channel present circumferentially in the scleral sulcus. The endothelial cells of its inner wall are irregular spindle-shaped and contain giant vacuoles. The outer wall of the canal is lined by smooth flat cells and contains the openings of collector channels.

Free flow of aqueous occurs from trabecular meshwork up to inner wall of Schlemm's canal which appears to provide some resistance to outflow.

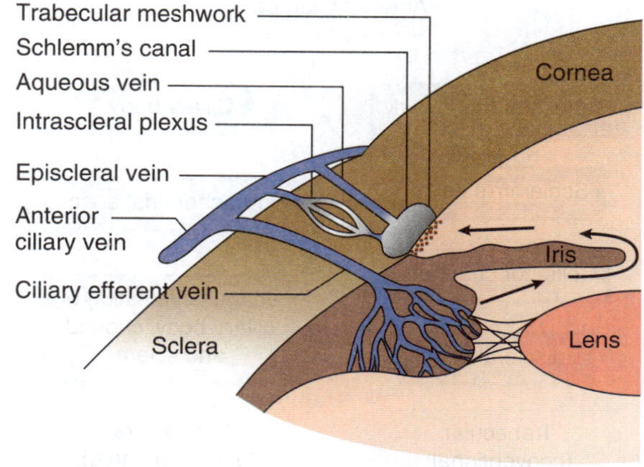

FIGURE 11.1-60 The aqueous outflow system.

Mechanism of aqueous transport across inner wall of Schlemm's canal. It is partially understood. *Vacuolation theory* is the most accepted view. According to it transcellular spaces exist in the endothelial cells forming inner wall of Schlemm's canal. These open as a system of vacuoles and pores, primarily in response to pressure, and transport the aqueous from juxtacanalicular connective tissue to Schlemm's canal.

4. Collector Channels. These, also called intrascleral aqueous vessels, are about 25–35 in number and leave the Schlemm's canal at oblique angles to terminate into episcleral veins in a laminated fashion. These intrascleral aqueous vessels can be divided into two systems (Fig. 11.1-60). The larger vessels *(aqueous veins)* run a short intrascleral course and terminate directly into episcleral veins (*direct system*). Many smaller collector channels form an intrascleral plexus before eventually going into episcleral veins (*indirect system*).

From Schlemm's canal the aqueous is transported via external collector channels into the episcleral veins by direct and indirect systems. A pressure gradient between IOP and intrascleral venous pressure (about 10 mm of Hg) is responsible for unidirectional flow of aqueous.

B. Uveoscleral (Unconventional) Outlow It is responsible for about 10% of the total aqueous outflow. Aqueous passes across the ciliary body into the suprachoroidal space and is drained by the venous circulation in the ciliary body, choroid and sclera.

The drainage of aqueous humour is summarized in the flowchart:

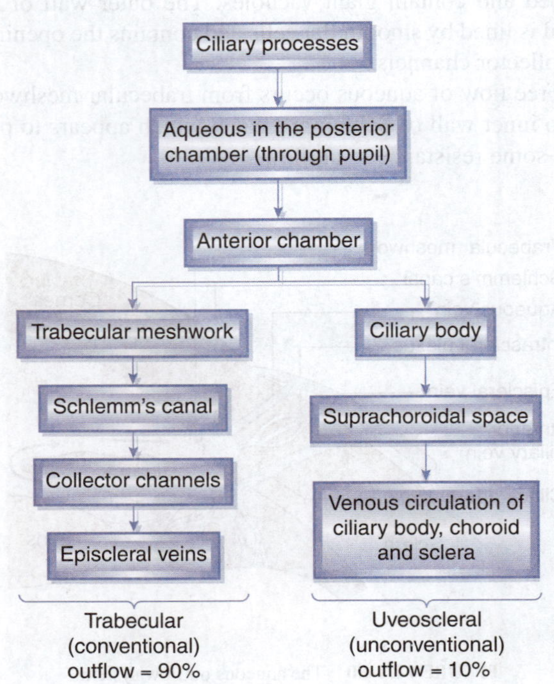

Maintenance of Intraocular Pressure

The IOP refers to the pressure exerted by intraocular fluids on the coats of the eyeball. The normal IOP varies between 10 and 21 mm of Hg (mean 16 ± 2.5 mm of Hg). The normal level of IOP is essentially maintained by a dynamic equilibrium between the formation and outflow of the aqueous humour. Various factors influencing IOP can be grouped as:

A. Local Factors

1. ***Rate of aqueous formation*** influences IOP levels. The aqueous formation in turn depends upon many factors such as permeability of ciliary capillaries and osmotic pressure of the blood.
2. ***Resistance to aqueous outflow (drainage).*** From the clinical point of view, this is the most important factor. Most of the resistance to aqueous outflow is at the level of trabecular meshwork.
3. ***Increased episcleral venous pressure*** may result in rise of IOP. The Valsalva manoeuvre causes temporary increase in episcleral venous pressure and rise in IOP.
4. ***Dilatation of pupil*** in patients with narrow anterior chamber angle may cause rise of IOP owing to a relative obstruction of the aqeuous drainage by the iris.

B. General Factors

1. ***Heredity.*** It influences IOP, possibly by multifactorial modes.
2. ***Age.*** The mean IOP increases after the age of 40 years, possibly due to reduced facility of aqueous outflow.
3. ***Sex.*** IOP is equal between the sexes in ages 20–40 years. In older age groups increase in mean IOP with age is greater in females.
4. ***Diurnal variation of IOP.*** Usually, there is a tendency of higher IOP in the morning and lower in the evening. This has been related to diurnal variation in the levels of plasma cortisol. Normal eyes have a smaller fluctuation (< 5 mm of Hg) than glaucomatous eyes (> 8 mm of Hg).
5. ***Postural variations.*** IOP increases when changing from sitting to the supine position.
6. ***Blood pressure.*** As such it does not have long-term effect on IOP. However, prevalence of glaucoma is marginally more in hypertensives than the normotensives.
7. ***Osmotic pressure of blood.*** An increase in plasma osmolarity (as occurs after intravenous mannitol, oral glycerol or in patients with uraemia) is associated with a fall in IOP, while a reduction in plasma osmolarity (as occurs with water drinking provocative tests) is associated with a rise in IOP.
8. ***General anaesthetics*** and many other drugs also influence IOP, e.g. alcohol lowers IOP, tobacco smoking, caffeine and steroids may cause rise in IOP. In addition there are many antiglaucoma drugs which lower IOP.

Glaucoma

Glaucoma is not a single disease process but a group of disorders in which IOP is raised above the tolerance limit of the affected eye, resulting in a damage to the optic nerve head and irreversible visual field defects.

This definition is not so simple as it apparently looks; since it is impossible to know the tolerance limit of the individual eye. Consequently the term *ocular hypertension* is used for cases having constantly raised IOP without any associated glaucomatous damage. Conversely, the term *normal* or *low tension glaucoma (NTG/LTG)* is suggested for the typical cupping of the disc and/or visual field defects associated with a normal or low IOP.

Types of Glaucomas

1. ***Congenital and developmental glaucomas*** occur due to developmental anomalies of the angle of anterior chamber.
2. ***Primary glaucomas*** occur without any obvious systemic or ocular cause, usually after the age of 40 years. These are of two types:
   - *Primary open angle glaucoma*, which occurs due to sclerosis of trabecular meshwork, and
   - *Primary angle closure glaucoma*, which occurs due to closure of the angle of anterior chamber
3. ***Secondary glaucomas*** are characterized by rise in IOP, secondary to some other ocular disease, e.g. phacomorphicglaucoma associated with swollen cataractous lens.

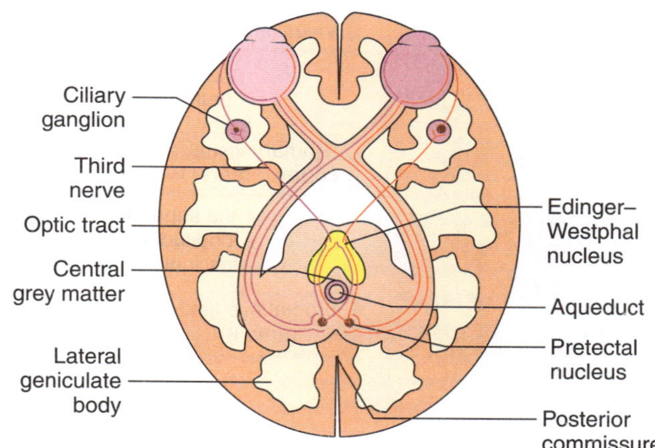

FIGURE 11.1-61 Pathway of the light reflex.

PHYSIOLOGY OF PUPIL

Pupillary Reflexes

Light Reflex When light is shone in one eye, both the pupils constrict. Constriction of the pupil to which light is shone is called *direct light reflex* and that of the other pupil is called *consensual (indirect) light reflex.* Light reflex is initiated by rods and cones.

Pathway of Light Reflex (Fig. 11.1-61). The *afferent fibres* extend from retina to the pretectal nucleus in the mid brain. These travel along the optic nerve to the optic chiasma where fibres from the nasal retina decussate and travel along the opposite optic tract to terminate in the contralateral pretectal nucleus. While the fibres from the temporal retina remain uncrossed and travel along the optic tract of the same side to terminate in the ipsilateral pretectal nucleus.

Internuncial fibres connect each pretectal nucleus with Edinger-Westphal nuclei of both sides. This connection forms the basis of consensual light reflex.

Efferent pathway consists of the parasympathetic fibres which arise from the Edinger-Westphal nucleus in the mid brain and travel along the third (oculomotor) cranial nerve. The preganglionic fibres enter the inferior division of the third nerve and via the nerve to the inferior oblique reach the ciliary ganglion to relay. Post-ganglionic fibres travel along the short ciliary nerves to innervate the sphincter pupillae.

Accommodation Reflex

During accommodation, when eyes are focused from distant to near object to achieve clear vision, three reactions occur; wiz.

- Changes in the radius of curvature of the lens (more convex) by contraction of ciliary muscles.
- Pupillary constriction (meiosis) by contraction of sphincter pupillae and
- Convergence of eyes due to contraction of medial recti of eye balls.

Near Reflex Near reflex occurs on looking at a near object. It consists of two components: (a) convergence reflex, i.e. contraction of pupil on convergence; and (b) accommodation reflex, i.e. contraction of pupil associated with accommodation.

Pathway of Convergence Reflex (Fig. 11.1-62). Its afferent pathway is still not elucidated. It is assumed that the afferents from the medial recti travel centrally via the third nerve to the mesencephalic nucleus of the fifth nerve, to a presumptive convergence centre in the tectal or pretectal region. From this the impulse is relayed to the Edinger-Westphal nucleus and the subsequent efferent pathway of near reflex is along the 3rd nerve. The efferent fibres relay in the accessory ganglion before reaching the sphincter pupillae.

Pathway of Accommodation Reflex (Fig. 11.1-62). The afferent impulses extend from the retina to the parastriate cortex via the optic nerve, chiasma, optic tract, lateral geniculate body, optic radiations and striate cortex. From the parastriate cortex, the impulses are relayed to the Edinger-Westphal nucleus of both sides via the occipitomesencephalic tract and the pontinecentre. From the Edinger-Westphal nucleus the efferent impulses travel along the third nerve and reach the sphincter pupillae and ciliary muscle after relaying in the accessory and ciliary ganglia.

For convergence reaction impulses from visual cortex reach the frontal eye field (area 8) through association fasciculus (superior longitudinal fasciculus). From frontal eye field the corticonuclear fibres project to the third nerve nuclei of both sides and through oculomotor nerves supply the medial recti of the eye balls.

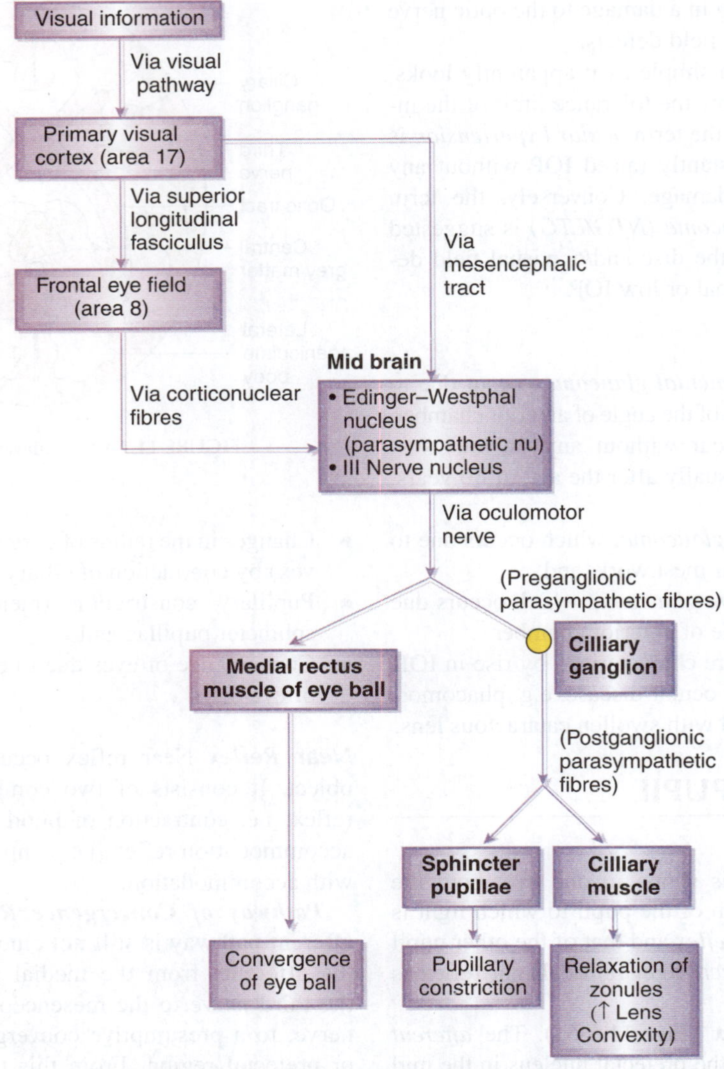

FIGURE 11.1-62 Pathway of the accommodation reflex.

Psychosensory Reflex It refers to dilatation of the pupil in response to sensory and psychic stimuli. It is very complex and its mechanism is still not elucidated.

Abnormalities of Pupillary Reactions

1. Efferent Pathway Defect. Absence of both direct and consensual light reflex on the affected side (say right eye) and presence of both direct and consensual light reflex on the normal side (i.e. left eye) indicates efferent pathway defect (sphincter paralysis). Near reflex is also absent on the affected side. Its causes include: effect of parasympatholytic drugs (e.g. atropine, homatropine), internal ophthalmoplegia and third nerve paralysis.

2. Wernicke's Hemianopic Pupil. It indicates lesion of the optic tract. In this condition, light reflex (ipsilateral direct and contralateral consensual) is absent when light is thrown on the temporal half of the retina of the affected side and nasal half of the opposite side; while it is present when the light is thrown on the nasal half of the affected side and temporal half of the opposite side.

3. Marcus-Gunn Pupil. It is the paradoxical response of a pupil of light in the presence of a relative afferent pathway defect (RAPD). It is tested by swinging flash light test.

4. Argyll Robertson Pupil (ARP). Here, the pupil is slightly small in size and reaction to near reflex is present but light reflex is absent, i.e. there is light near dissociation (to remember, the acronym ARP may stand for 'accommodation reflex present'). Both pupils are involved and dilate poorly with mydriatics. It is caused by a lesion (usually neurosyphilis) in the region of tectum.

5. The Adie's Tonic Pupil. In this condition reaction to light is absent and to near reflex is very slow and tonic. The affected pupil is larger (anisocoria). Its exact cause is not known. It is usually unilateral, associated with absent knee jerk and occurs more often in young women. Adie's pupil constricts with weak pilocarpine (0.125%) drops, while normal pupil does not.

Chapter 11.2

Sense of Hearing

FUNCTIONAL ANATOMY

The Ear

The mechanism of hearing is closely associated with the mechanism of equilibrium; therefore, the inner ear acts as an organ of hearing and equilibrium. For hearing, the sound waves have to pass through the three subdivisions of the ear, which are (Fig. 11.2-1):

- External ear,
- Middle ear and
- Internal ear.

External Ear

The external ear consists of the pinna (auricle) and the external auditory meatus.

- ***Pinna*** or auricle consists of a single convoluted plate of elastic cartilage covered by skin which is tightly attached to the underlying perichondrium.
  Functions. The pinna collects and reflects the sound waves into the external auditory canal.
  - In lower animals, pinna is more important, in whom it can be moved by muscular action in the direction of sound source.
  - In humans, the pinna is not moveable, but its peculiar shape aids in *discerning* the source of sound (e.g. in front of versus behind the head).
- ***External auditory meatus*** extends from the pinna to the tympanic membrane. It consists of two distinct portions: external one-third, cartilaginous portion and internal two-third, bony portions. It is lined with skin, which in the cartilaginous part secretes wax (from the ceruminous glands) and oil (from the sebaceous glands).

Middle Ear

Walls of Middle Ear The middle ear or the tympanic cavity is a six sided air-filled rectangular space in the petrous part of temporal bone with a roof, a floor, and an anterior, a posterior, a medial and a lateral wall (Fig. 11.2-2).

- ***Lateral wall*** is formed by tympanic membrane which shuts the medial end of external auditory meatus. The tympanic membrane is a cave-shaped structure with concavity directed towards the external auditory meatus. Point of maximum convexity is called umbo. It consists of connective tissue covered with skin on the outside and mucous membrane on the inside.

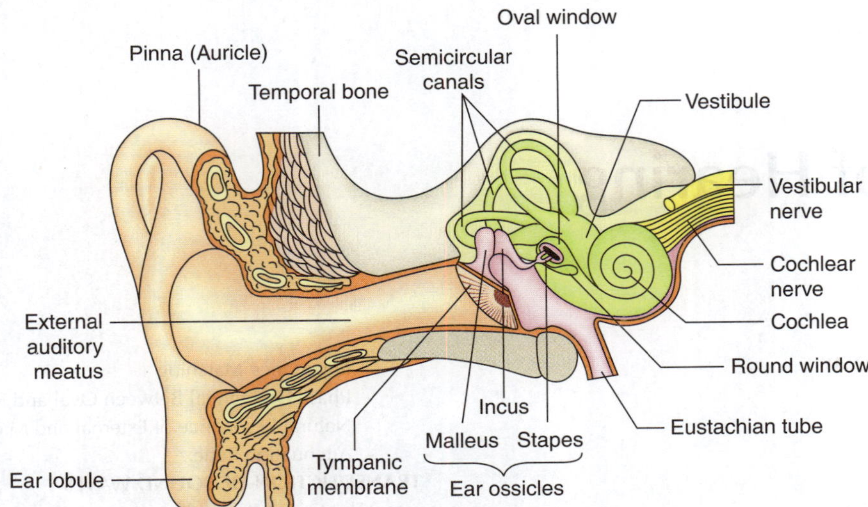

FIGURE 11.2-1 Structure of three subdivisions of the ear.

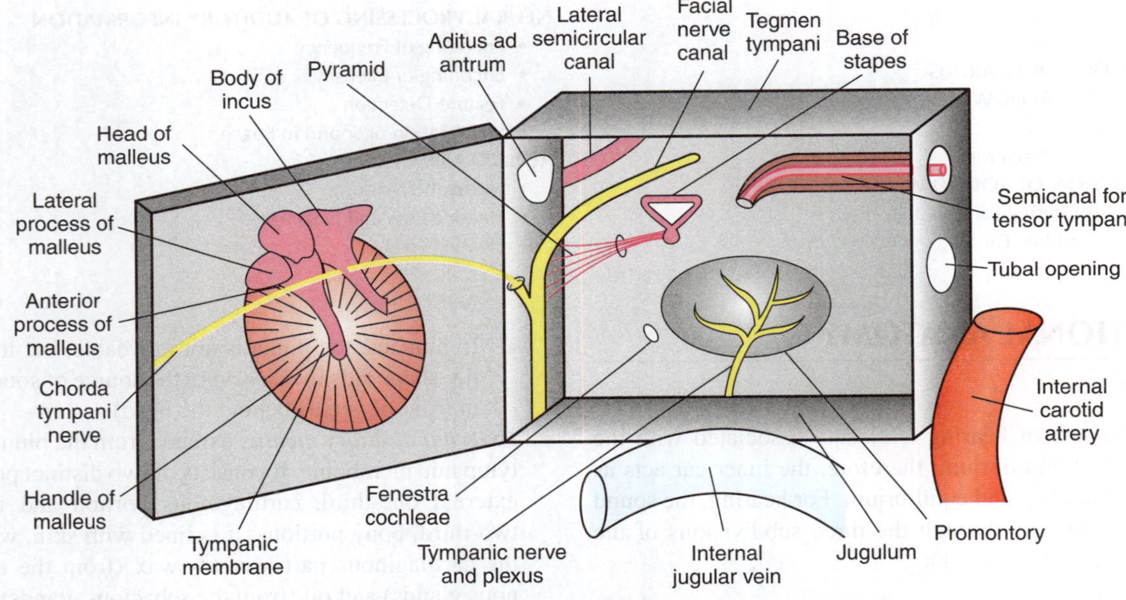

FIGURE 11.2-2 Schematic diagram of the six sided tympanic cavity (middle ear) with the lateral wall open to depict the features on various boundaries.

- ***Anterior wall*** contains two canals: upper one lodges tensor tympani muscle and lower one lodges the eustachian tube (Fig. 11.2-2).

  Eustachian tube or the pharyngotympanic tube connects the middle ear cavity with pharynx. Air can pass through this tube into the middle ear. Therefore, it serves the function of equalization of pressure on two sides of tympanic membrane. When its pharyngeal opening is blocked, e.g. in common cold, the air cannot pass into the tympanic cavity. The air present in the middle ear gets absorbed by the mucous membrane and the tympanic membrane is retracted inwards. As a result the vibrations of tympanic membrane get decreased or abolished, causing discomfort and loss of hearing.
- ***Posterior wall*** of the middle ear communicates with air cavities in the mastoid process.
- ***Medial wall*** (labyrinthine wall). It contains two windows (Fig. 11.2-2.):
  - ***Oval window*** (fenestra vestibuli) is present above, in which foot plate (face plate or stapes) is attached. It leads to the vestibule of the internal ear and

transmits the sound vibrations of the ossicles to the perilymph of scalavestibuli.
   - ***Round window*** (fenestra cochlea) is present, in the lower part, and is closed by a thin membrane called *secondary tympanic membrane*. It accommodates the pressure waves transmitted to the perilymph of the scala tympani.
- ***Roof.*** It is formed by a thin bone called the tegmen tympani of the petrous temporal bone and separates the middle ear from the middle cranial fossa.
- ***Floor.*** It is formed by a convex plate of bone which separates the middle ear from jugular fossa which lodges the superior bulb of the internal jugular vein.

Ear Ossicles The three ear ossicles (auditory ossicles) include malleus, incus and stapes. They are attached to each other by ligaments and form a chain (Fig. 11.2-3).

- ***Malleus.*** It resembles a mallet (hammer) and consists of a head, neck and three processes: the handle or manubrium, the lateral and anterior processes.
   - *Manubrium* (handle) of the malleus is connected to inner surface of the tympanic membrane.
   - *Head* articulates with incus posteriorly.
- ***Incus*** is the middle ossicle that resembles an anvil in shape. It consists of a body and two processes. The body of incus articulates with the head of malleus.
- ***Stapes.*** It resembles a stirrup. Its head articulates with the incus and the oval footplate contacts the membrane of the oval window of the cochlea.

Muscles of the Middle Ear The middle ear contains two muscles: the tensor tympani and stapedius.

Tensor Tympani. It arises from the wall of the semicanal for tensor tympani (Fig. 11.2-2) and is inserted into the handle of malleus. It is innervated by a branch of mandibular division of the fifth cranial nerve. It constantly pulls the handle of malleus inwards and thus keeps the tympanic membrane tensed. Due to this, vibrations on any portion of the tympanic membrane are transmitted to the malleus.

Stapedius. It arises from the posterior wall of the middle ear and is inserted on the neck of stapes. It is innervated by a branch from facial nerve and on contraction it pulls the footplate of stapes out from the oval window.

Function. Both muscles of the middle ear act simultaneously and reflexly in response to loud sound and attenuate the sound (see also page 1181).

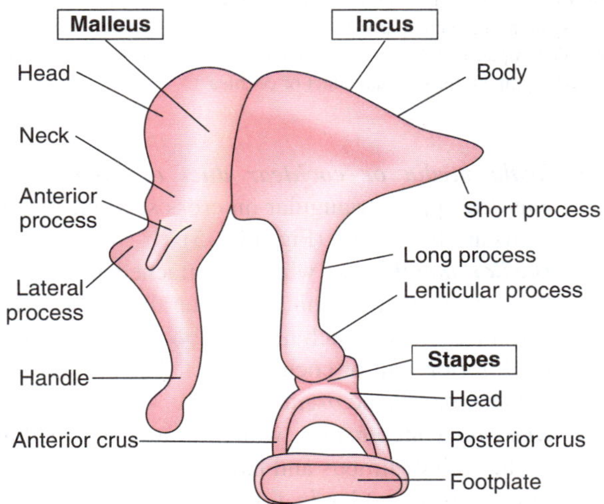

FIGURE 11.2-3 Ear ossicles and their parts.

Internal Ear

The internal ear or labyrinth is situated in the petrous part of the temporal bone. It consists of bony labyrinth and membranous labyrinth (Fig. 11.2-4).

- ***Bony labyrinth*** consists of three parts: vestibule, semicircular canals and the cochlea.
- ***Membranous labyrinth*** is lodged within the bony labyrinth. It is filled with endolymph (which resembles intracellular fluid) and is surrounded by perilymph (which resembles extracellular fluid in its composition). The inner ear can be divided into two main parts:
   1. *Vestibular receptor apparatus.* It consists of (Fig. 11.2- 4):
      - *Utricle and saccule*, which are lodged in the bony vestibule, and are collectively called *otolith organs*.
      - *Semicircular ducts*, which lie within the body of semicircular canals.

      Vestibular apparatus is concerned with equilibrium and is described on page 1074.
   2. *Auditory receptor apparatus* is formed by the *duct of cochlea* which lies within the bony cochlea.

Auditory Apparatus The bony cochlea containing membranous cochlear duct (which houses the organ of Corti) forms the so-called auditory apparatus (Fig. 11.2-4).

Bony cochlea is a spiral tube which in humans has a two and three fourth turns around a central bone called the *modiolus*.

The base of the modiolus is directed towards internal acoustic meatus and transmits vessels and nerves to the cochlea. Around the modiolus and winding spirally like the thread of a screw is a thin plate of bone called *osseous spiral lamina*. It divides the bony cochlea incompletely and gives attachment to the basilar membrane. Two membranes (basilar membrane and Reissner's membrane) divide the bony cochlea into three compartments (Fig. 11.2-5):

- Scala vestibuli,
- Scala media (membranous chochlear duct) and
- Scala tympani.

  Scala vestibuli and scala tympani are filled with perilymph and communicate with each other at the apex of cochlea through an opening called *helicotrema*.

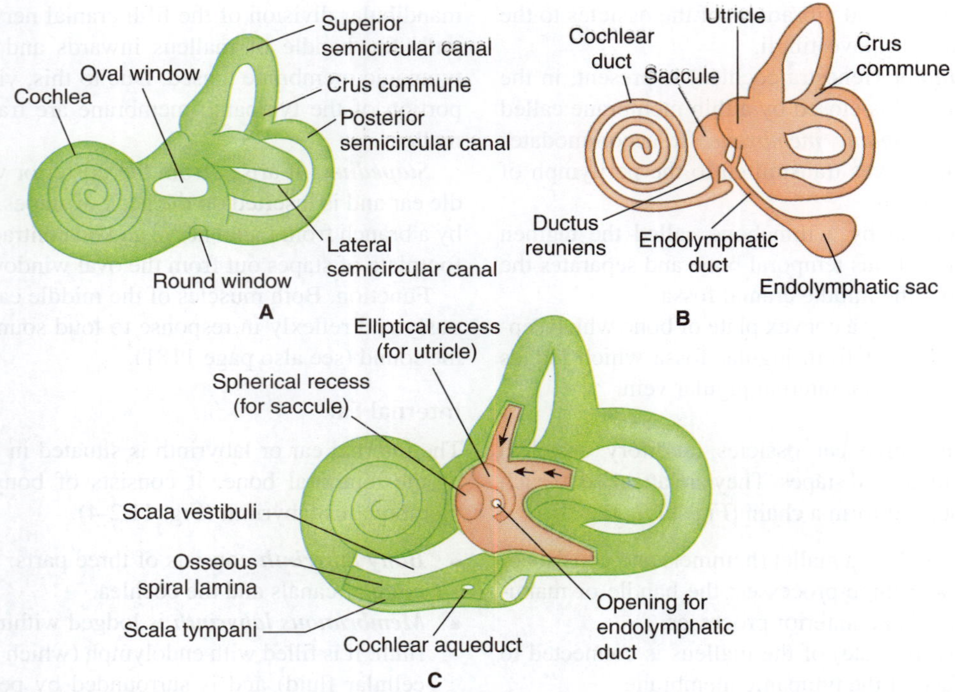

FIGURE 11.2-4 Structure of inner ear: (A) left bony labyrinth; (B) left membranous labyrinth and (C) cut section of bony labyrinth.

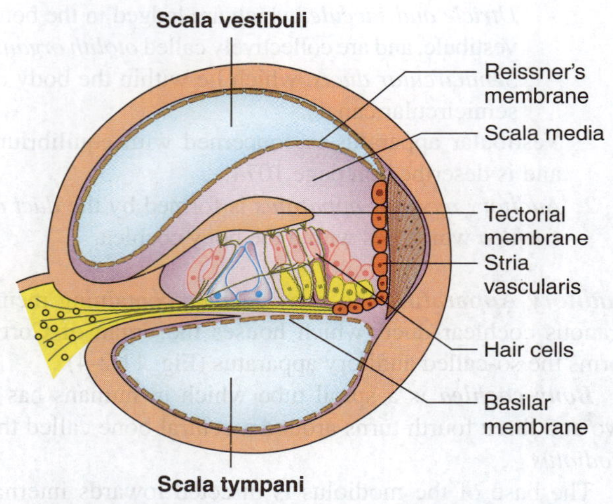

FIGURE 11.2-5 Vertical section through cochlea showing scalavestibuli, scala media (cochlear duct) and scala tympani. Note the location of organ of Corti over the basilar membrane in the cavity of cochlear duct.

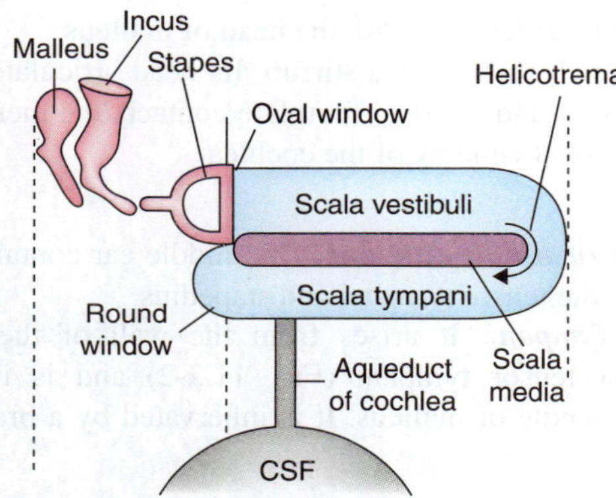

FIGURE 11.2-6 Diagrammatic depiction of arrangement of perilymphatic system, three compartments of cochlea (scalavestibuli, scala media and scala tympani), and ear ossicles of the middle ear. Note the CSF passes into scala tympani through aqueduct of cochlea

- ***Scala vestibuli*** is separated from the scala media by *Reissner's membrane* and is closed by the footplate of stapes which separates it from the air-filled middle ear (Figs 11.2-5 and 11.2-6).
- ***Scala tympani*** is separated from the scala media by the *basilar membrane* and is closed by *secondary tympanic membrane*. It is also connected with subarachnoid space through the aqueduct of cochlea (Figs 11.2-5 and 11.2-6).
- ***Scala media or cochlear duct or membranous cochlea*** appear triangular on cross section. Its three walls are formed by (Fig. 11.2-5):
- ***Basilar membrane,*** which is attached medially to the osseous spiral lamina and laterally to the fibrous spiral ligament (which lines the bony cochlea) forms the inferior wall of cochlear duct. The basilar membrane supports the *organ of Corti*.
- ***Reissner's membrane,*** which is attached medially to the wall of limbus and laterally to the upper margin of striavascular is forms the superior wall of cochlear duct.

- ***Striavascularis*** forms the lateral wall of cochlear duct. It consists of vascular epithelium and is concerned with secretion of *endolymph.*

Perilymph and Endolymph

- ***Perilymph*** is the fluid present in the scala tympani and scala vestibuli compartments of the cochlea. Its composition is similar to extracellular fluid (ECF) in that it is high in Na^+ and low in K^+.
- ***Endolymph*** is the fluid present within the scala media or the membranous cochlea. Its composition is similar to intracellular fluid (ICF) in that it is high in K^+ and low in Na^+. It is secreted by the stria vascularis which forms the lateral wall of scala media.

Organ of Corti. The organ of Corti, the sense organ of hearing, is situated on the top of the basilar membrane in the scala media (Fig. 11.2-5). It contains the auditory receptors or the peripheral receptors of sense of hearing. Important components of the organ of Corti are (Fig. 11.2-7):

1. Rods of Corti. These are two projections (inner and outer rods) from the basilar membrane into the scala media. In between the two rods is the *tunnel of Corti* which contains a fluid called cortilymph. The exact function of the rods and cortilymph is not known.

2. Hair Cells. Hair cells are receptor cells that transduce sound energy into electrical energy. Two groups of hair cells lie on the basilar membrane (Fig. 11.2-7).

- ***Inner hair cells.*** These form a single row of cells internal (i.e. medial) to the inner rod. These are about 3500 in number. These cells are probably more important in the transmission of auditory impulses. These are responsible for fine auditory transmission.
- ***Outer hair cells.*** These are about 20,000 in number and are arranged in three or four layers external (i.e. lateral) to the outer rod. These are responsible for *detecting the presence of sound.* They mainly receive efferent innervation from the olivary complex and are concerned with modulating the function of inner hair cells.

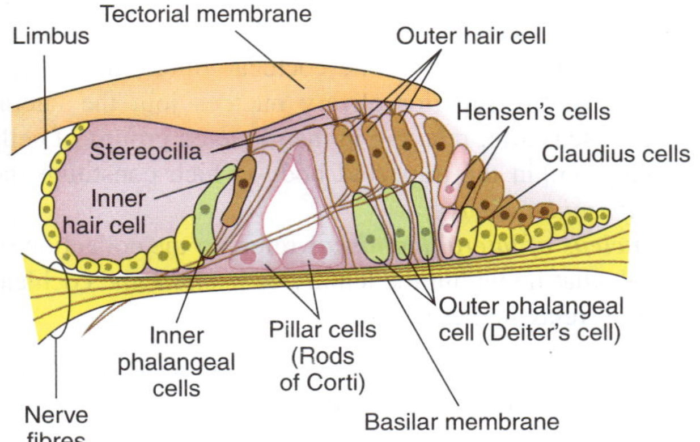

FIGURE 11.2-7 Structure of organ of Corti. Note the connections between tectorial membrane and cilia of hair cells.

Structure of a hair cell. The inner hair cells are flask-shaped while outer hair cells are cylindrical. On the upper surface of the hair cells are present tiny cilia (*stereo-cilia*) which protrude into the overlying tectorial membrane.

3. Supporting Cells of following type are known (Fig. 11.2-7):

- Inner phalangeal cells support the inner hair cells.
- Deiter's cells (outer phalangeal cells) are situated between the outer hair cells and provide support to the latter.
- Hensen's cells lie outside the Deiter's cells.
- Claudius cells lie outside the Hensen's cells.

4. Tectorial Membrane. It consists of gelatinous matrix with delicate fibres. It is a thin but stiff membrane made of glycoprotein material. This membrane is attached to the upper surface of spiral lamina, and its free edge extends just beyond the outermost neuroepithelial cells.

The shearing force between the hair cells and tectorial membrane produces the stimulus to hair cells.

Nerve Supply of Hair Cells Afferent fibres supplying the hair cells constitute the cochlear division of the eighth cranial nerve. Cell bodies of these fibres are located in the spiral ganglion

- ***Inner hair cells*** receive 90–95% of the afferent fibres and so are more important in the transmission of auditory impulses.
- ***Outer hair cells*** receive only 5–10% of the afferent fibres.

Note. There are about 30,000 fibres in each auditory nerve, so there is no net convergence of receptors on the first order neurons. Most of the afferent fibres, however, supply more than one hair cell and conversely, most of hair cells are supplied by more than one fibre.

Efferent fibres to the hair cells come from both the ipsilateral and contralateral sides via the olivocochlear bundle. Their cell bodies are situated in superior olivary complex. These fibres descend to join the eighth nerve. Outer hair cells receive most of the efferent fibres, while inner hair cells receive only a few efferent fibres. The efferent fibres are cholinergic and cause inhibition of afferent fibres by liberating a hyperpolarizing mediator which is probably acetylcholine (Ach). Thus, the outer hair cells are mainly concerned with modulation of the function of inner hair cells.

Auditory Pathways

Auditory pathways comprise following relay stations (Fig. 11.2-8):

- Spiral ganglion,
- Superior olivary nucleus complex, trapezoid nucleus and nucleus of lateral lemniscus.

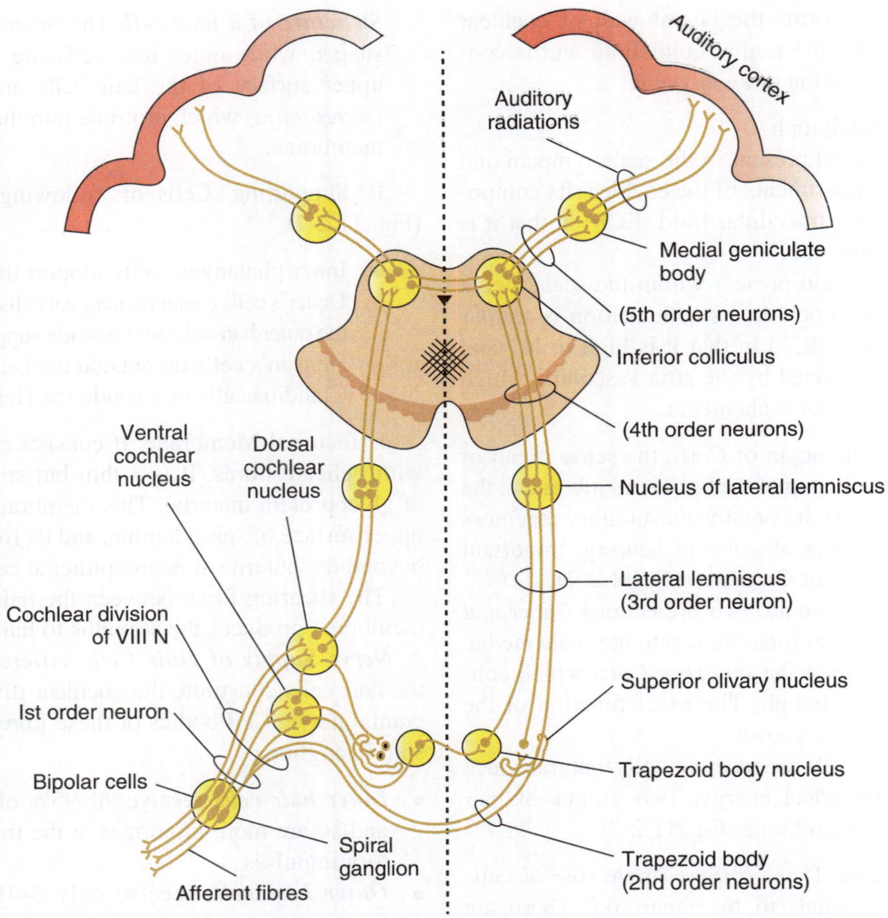

FIGURE 11.2-8 Central auditory pathways.

- Inferior colliculus,
- Medial geniculate body and
- Auditory cortex.

Spiral Ganglion ***First order neurons*** are the bipolar cells of the *spiral ganglion* which is situated in Rosenthal's canal (canal running along osseous spiral lamina).

- ***Dendrites*** of these bipolar cells constitute the afferent fibres innervating the hair cells.
- ***Axons*** of these bipolar cells form the cochlear division of the eighth cranial nerve. The cochlear nerve ends in the cochlear nuclei in medulla.

Cochlear Nuclei ***Second-order neurons*** have their cell bodies in the cochlear nuclei which are situated in the rostral part of medulla. There are two cochlear nuclei: dorsal and ventral.

The axons of second-order neurons from cochlear nuclei pass medially in the dorsal part of pons. Most of them cross to the opposite side, but some remain uncrossed.

- The crossing fibres of two sides form a conspicuous mass of fibres called the *trapezoid body*.
- Some crossing fibres run separately in the dorsal part of pons and do not form part of the trapezoid body.

Superior Olivary Nucleus Complex, Trapezoid Nucleus and Nucleus of Lateral Lemniscus ***Third-order neurons*** have their cell bodies mainly in the *superior olivary complex* (made up of a number of nuclei) and also in trapezoid nucleus and nucleus of lateral lemniscus.

- ***Superior olivary nuclear complex*** receive the large majority of lateral lemniscus fibres from the cochlear nuclei. Axons arising from the superior olivary complex form an important ascending bundle called the *lateral lemniscus*.
- ***Trapezoid nucleus.*** Some cochlear fibres that do not relay in the superior olivary nucleus join the lateral lemniscus after relaying in the scattered groups of cells lying within the trapezoid body (which constitute the *trapezoid nucleus*).
- ***Nucleus of lateral lemniscus*** refers to the collection of cells that lie within the lemniscus itself. Some cochlear fibres relay in these cells.

The fibres of *lateral lemniscus* ascend to the mid brain and terminate in the inferior colliculus.

Inferior Colliculus ***Fourth-order neurons*** have their cell bodies in *inferior colliculus* where the fibres of lateral lemniscus terminate. Fibres arising in the inferior colliculus enter the inferior brachium to reach the medial geniculate body.

Medial Geniculate Body ***Fifth-order neurons*** have their cell bodies in the medial geniculate body where most of the fibres arising in inferior colliculus terminate. Some fibres from the lateral lemniscus reach this body without relay in the inferior colliculus. Fibres arising in the medial geniculate body form the *acoustic radiation* which ends in the acoustic area of the cerebral cortex.

Auditory Cortex Major areas constituting auditory cortex present in the temporal lobe are:

- Primary auditory cortex (areas 41 and 42), and
- Auditory association areas (areas 22, 21 and 20), for details see page 973.

PHYSIOLOGY OF HEARING

Hearing, i.e. detection of sound waves may serve to warn of impending danger or localize friends. But most importantly, audition allows social communication. Physiology of audition can be discussed under following headings:

- Stimuli or sound waves,
- Conduction of sound waves,
- Transduction of sound waves,
- Neural transmission of signals and
- Encoding of signals.

Stimuli or Sound Waves

Definition Stimuli for the receptors of hearing are sound waves. Sound is a form of energy produced by a vibrating object. A sound wave consists of alternating phases of compression and rarefaction of molecules of the medium (air, liquid, or solid) in which it travels.

Physical Properties of Sound Physical properties of sound and certain terms which are frequently used in audiology and acoustics are (Fig. 11.2-9):

1. Speed of Sound. Speed or velocity of the sound waves is different in different media:

- *In the air*, at 0° C, at sea level, sound travels at a rate of approximately 330 m/sec (1100 ft/sec), while at 20° C it travels at a rate of 349 m/sec (1150 ft/sec).
- *In the water*, at 20° C, sound travels at much faster speed of 1450 to 1500 m/sec. The speed is faster in salt water as compared to fresh water. Further, the speed of sound in water slightly increases with temperature and altitude.

2. Frequency of Sound refers to number of waves per second.

- The *unit* of frequency is hertz (Hz).
- Range of human hearing is approximately 20–20,000 Hz.

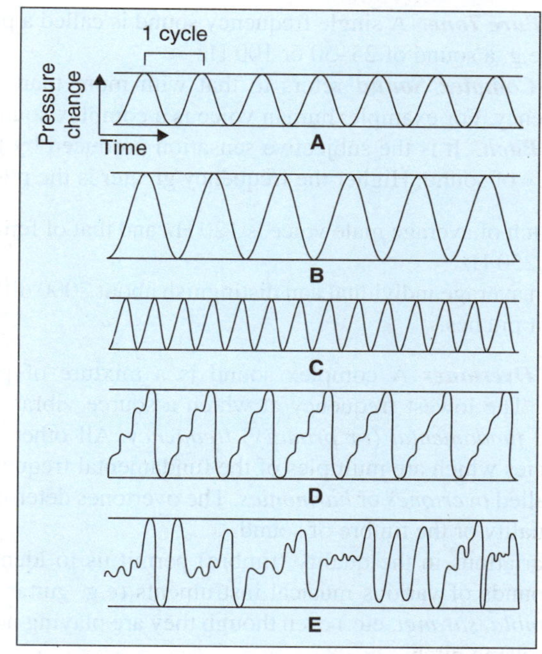

FIGURE 11.2-9 Characteristics of sound wave: **(A)** pure tones; **(B)** increase in amplitude (intensity) of sound wave thus the sound is louder; **(C)** increase in frequency (pitch); **(D)** complex waveform due to mixture of pure tones and overtones; determines the quality of sound (timbre) and **(E)** aperiodic irregular waveform (noise).

- Range of average speaking voice is approximately 2000–5000 Hz.

3. Amplitude (intensity) of Sound is the strength which determines its loudness. The intensity of sound is measured in terms of maximum pressure change at the tympanic membrane which is more commonly expressed as *sound pressure level* (SPL). The unit of SPL is decibel (dB), which is expressed as:

$$\text{dB} = 20.\log\frac{P_s\,(\text{Pressure of the stimulus sound})}{P_R\,(\text{Pressure of the reference sound})}$$

Reference (standard) pressure is 0.0002 dynes/cm^2. It is defined as a sound pressure that is just detectable, i.e. auditory *threshold.*

Thus, sound intensities are measured on a ratio scale using a subjective intensity (i.e. the threshold), rather than an arbitrary intensity, as a base.

At a distance of one metre, intensity of some common sounds is:

- Whisper : 30 dB
- Normal conversation : 60 dB
- Rock music : 90 dB
- Discomfort of the ear is produced by sounds of : 120 dB
- Pain in the ear is produced by sound of above (10^7 times threshold) : 140 dB

4. Pure Tone. A single frequency sound is called a pure tone, e.g. a sound of 25–50 or 100 Hz

5. Complex Sound refers to that with more than one frequency. For example, human voice is a complex sound.

6. Pitch. It is the subjective sensation produced by frequency of sound. Higher the frequency greater is the pitch.

- Pitch of average male voice is 120 Hz and that of female is 250 Hz.
- An average individual can distinguish about 2000 different pitches.

7. Overtones A complex sound is a mixture of pure tones. The lowest frequency at which a source vibrates is called *fundamental (or primary) frequency*. All other frequencies which are multiples of the fundamental frequency are called *overtones* or *harmonics*. The overtones determine the quality or the timbre of sound.

Variations in the quality (timbre) permit us to identify the sounds of various musical instruments (e.g. guitar, piano, *tabla, sarangi,* etc.) even though they are playing notes of the same pitch.

Conduction of Sound Waves

Role of External Ear External ear captures the sound waves.

Pinna collects and reflects the sound waves into the external auditory meatus. Its peculiar shape, in humans, aids in discerning the source of sound (e.g. in front versus behind the head).

External auditory meatus conducts the sound waves to tympanic membrane. Its S-shaped course:

- Helps in amplifying the sound waves.
- Prevents mechanical injury to the tympanic membrane and
- Helps in maintaining favourable temperature and humidity for normal functioning of the tympanic membrane.

Role of Middle Ear

Conduction of Sound Stimulus by Tympanic Membrane to Ear Ossicles. The sound waves that pass through the pinna and external auditory meatus strike the tympanic membrane. The presence of air at atmospheric pressure on both sides of the membrane enable it to vibrate. Eustachian tube does the function of equalization of pressure on two sides of tympanic membrane. The vibrating tympanic membrane causes the ear ossicles to vibrate. Thus, tympanic membrane acts as:

- ***Pressure receiver,*** i.e. it is extremely sensitive to pressure changes produced by sound waves.
- ***Resonator,*** i.e. starts vibrating with pressure changes produced by sound waves.
- ***Critically dampens,*** i.e. the vibrations of tympanic membrane cease immediately after the end of sound.

Conduction of Sound Waves Mechanically from Middle Ear to Inner Ear. Various mechanisms which play role during conduction of sound waves mechanically from the middle ear to inner ear are:

- Impedance matching mechanism,
- Phase differential between oval and round window,
- Natural resonance of external ear and middle ear and
- Attenuation reflex.

Impedance Matching Mechanism The air-filled middle ear conducts sound waves mechanically to the fluid-filled internal ear through the ossicular system. Effective transfer of sound energy from an air to a fluid medium is difficult because most of the sound is reflected as a result of the different mechanical properties of the two media, i.e. *impedance mismatching*. This fact can be appreciated by the observation that a person under water cannot hear any sound made in the air. This happens because 99.9% of the sound energy is reflected away from the surface of water because of the impedance offered by it. Exactly a similar situation exists in the ear when the air-filled middle ear has to conduct the sound to the fluid-filled inner ear. Nature has compensated for it by providing impedance matching mechanism to middle ear.

- The middle ear functions as impedance matching device, primarily by amplifying the sound pressure. It is accomplished by following three mechanisms (Fig. 11.2-10):
  1. ***Lever action of ossicles.*** Handle of malleus is 1.3 times longer than long process of incus, this provides a mechanical leverage advantage, due to which the middle ear ossicles increase the force of movement by 1.3 times.
  2. ***Hydraulic action of tympanic membrane*** is exerted because the effective vibratory area of the tympanic membrane (about 55 mm^2) is much greater than the stapes oval window surface area (about 3.2 mm^2). This size difference means the force produced by the sound is concentrated over a smaller area, thus amplifying the pressure exerted on the oval window (17 folds).

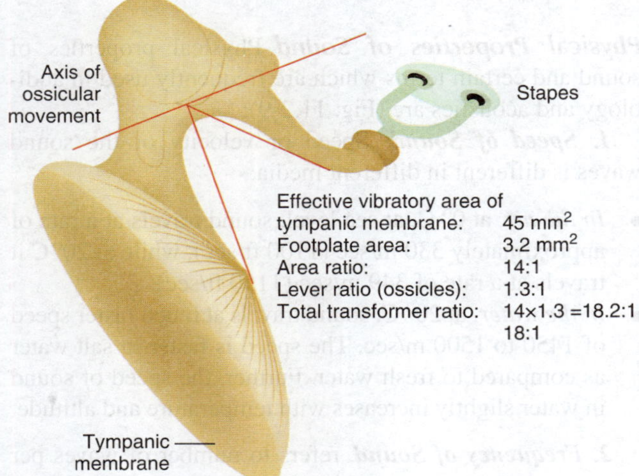

FIGURE 11.2-10 Amplification of sound pressure by the combined hydraulic effect of tympanic membrane and leverage effect of ear ossicles.

3. ***Curved membrane effect.*** Movements of the tympanic membrane are more at the periphery than at the centre where malleus handle is attached. This too provides some leverage.

Thus, the above three mechanisms together increase the sound pressure 22 fold (i.e. 17 × 1.3). In this way the impedance mismatching between the air-filled middle ear and fluid-filled inner ear is mostly compensated. Therefore, when the tympanic membrane and the ossicles are removed, and the sound waves strike the oval window directly, even very loud sounds are heard as whispers.

Minimum audibility curve. It is important to note that:

- Amplification of sound intensity is greatest between 1000-3000 Hz.
- Sounds below 16 Hz or above 20,000 Hz are not amplified at all.
- Because of the above, the human ear can perceive pitch of sound between 16-20000 Hz, but maximum sensitivity is between 1000–3000 Hz. This effect is the basis of so-called minimum audibility curve (Fig. 11.2-11).

Phase Differential between Oval and Round Window. Sound waves striking the tympanic membrane do not reach the oval and round windows simultaneously. There is a preferential pathway to the oval window because of the ossicular chain. Thus, when oval window is receiving wave of compression, the round window is at the phase rarefaction. If the sound waves were to strike both the windows simultaneously, they would cancel each other's effect with no movement of perilymph and no hearing. This acoustic separation of windows is achieved by the presence of intact tympanic membrane and a cushion of air in the middle ear around the round window.

Natural Resonance of External and Middle Ear. The external ear and middle ear due to the inherent anatomic and physiologic properties, allow certain frequencies of sound to pass more easily to the inner ear. The natural resonance of different structures is:

- External auditory canal 3000 Hz
- Tympanic membrane 800-1600 Hz
- Middle ear 800 Hz:
- Ossicular chain 500-2000 Hz

Thus (from the above) the greatest sensitivity of the sound transmission is between 500 and 3000 Hz, and these are the frequencies most important to human in day to day conversation.

Attenuation Reflex Attenuation reflex also called tympanic reflex or acoustic reflex is a preventive reflex which reduces sound pressure amplitude by affecting the mobility and transmission properties of the auditory ossicles.

- *Stimulus* for this reflex is loud sound.
- *Latent period* is 40–80 ms.
- *Reflex activity*. The two muscles of the middle ear (tensor tympani and stapedius) contract reflexively in response to intense sound.

Contraction of tensor tympani muscle pulls the malleus inwards whereas contraction of stapedius muscle pulls stapes outward. These two opposing forces make the ossicular system very rigid and therefore it fails to vibrate with the sound waves. Thus, sound is not allowed to enter inner ear (i.e. is attenuated or intensity is reduced by 30-40 decibel).

Advantages of attenuation reflex are:

- It prevents occurrence of damage to cochlea from the intense sounds like that of loud music, of jet aircraft etc.
- It attenuates and masks all the low frequency environmental sounds and allows the person to concentrate on the sound above 1000 Hz, where most of the prominent information in voice communication is transmitted.
- It occurs just prior to vocalization and chewing, which suggests that the middle ear muscles may act to reduce the intensity of the sounds produced by these activities.

Note. Because the latent period of attenuation reflex is 40–80 ms, sudden, brief, extremely loud sound such as due to bomb explosion or gun shot is likely to cause deafness due to damage to the cochlea.

Transduction of Sound Waves

Transduction of mechanical sound wave into electrical signal occurs in the organ of Corti of inner ear (revise structure of inner ear and organ of Corti given at page 1177). Steps involved in the process of transduction are:

Vibration of Basilar Membrane Sound waves from the middle ear are passed on to the inner ear through the oval window by in-and-out motion of the stapes (Fig. 11.2-12):

- Sound waves entering the inner ear from the oval window spread along the scala vestibuli as a travelling wave.

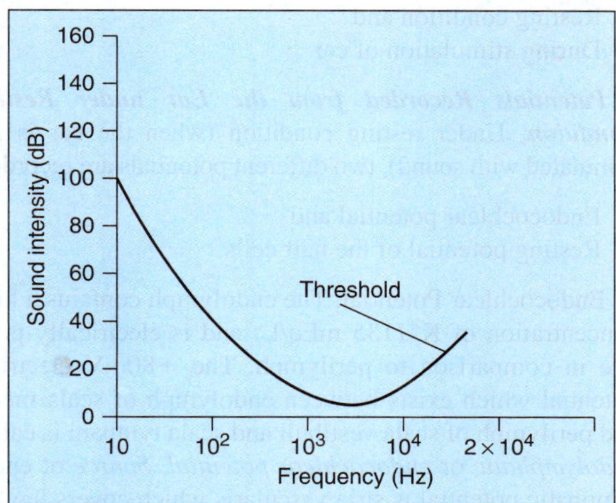

FIGURE 11.2-11 Minimum audibility curve.

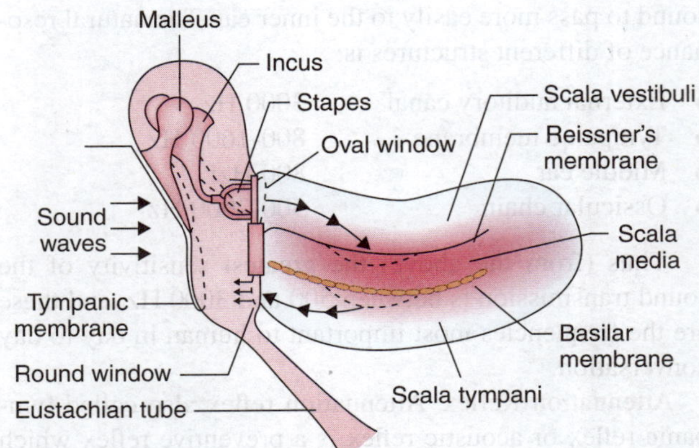

FIGURE 11.2-12 Diagrammatic depiction of the mechanism of vibrations of basilar membrane produced by in and out motion of stapes (for details see text).

- Most of the sound energy is transferred directly from the scala vestibuli to the scala tympani. Very little of the sound wave ever reaches the helicotrema at the apex of cochlea.
- As the sound energy passes from scala vestibuli to scala tympani, it causes the basilar membrane to vibrate. It is important to note that the part of the cochlea where height of pressure wave reaches its maximum varies with the frequency of sound (travelling wave theory of Von Bekesy (see page 1185).

Stimulation of the Hair Cells The up-and-down movements of the basilar membrane in turn cause the organ of Corti to vibrate up and down. The tops of the hair cells in organ of Corti are held rigid by the reticular lamina and the hair of the outer hair cells are embedded in the tectorial membrane (Fig. 11.2-13). Because the tectorial and basilar membranes are attached at different points on the limbus (Fig. 11.2-13A) they slide past each other as they vibrate up and down.

Owing to the shear forces set up by the relative displacement of basilar membrane and the tectorial membrane the stereocilia of hair cells bend back and forth as:

- When the organ of Corti moves up, the tectorial membrane slides forward relative to the basilar membrane, bending the stereocilia away from the limbus (Fig. 11.2-13B).
- When the organ of Corti moves down, the tectorial membrane slides backwards relative to basilar membrane and bends the stereocilia towards the limbus (Fig. 11.2-13C)

The bending of stereocilia stimulates (excites) the hair cells.

- *Depolarization occurs* when the stereocilia bend away from the limbus and
- *Hyperpolarization* occurs when the stereocilia bend towards the limbus.

Membrane Potential Changes in the Hair Cells The bending of the stereocilia produces a change in the membrane

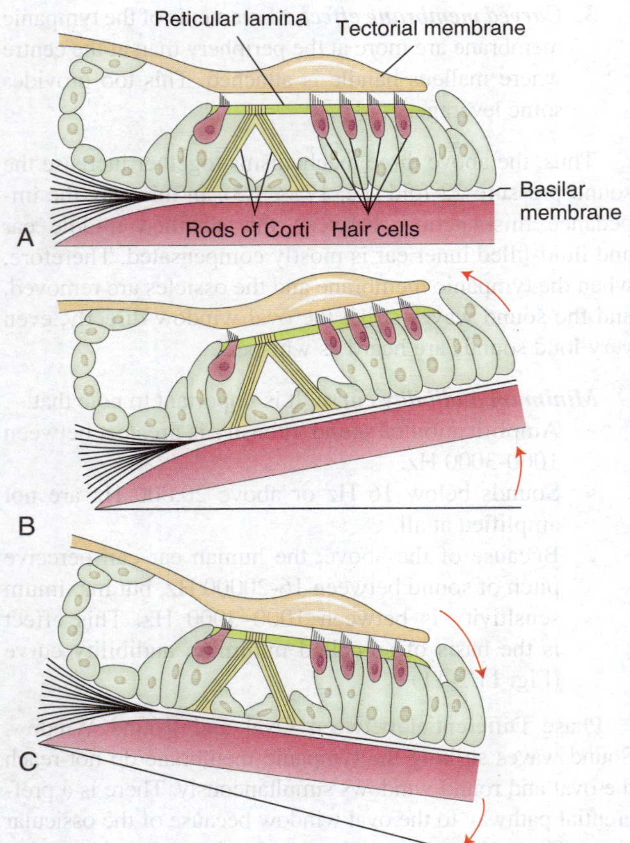

FIGURE 11.2-13 Demonstration of bending of stereocilia with movement of organ of Corti: **(A)** the tectorial membrane and basilar membrane are attached to limbus at different points; **(B)** upward movement of organ of Corti causes bending of cilia away from limbus and **(C)** downward movement of organ of Corti causes cilia to bend towards limbus.

potential of the hair cells proportionate to the degree of displacement (generator potential). The electrical activity of the inner ear can be considered as under:

- Resting condition and
- During stimulation of ear.

Potentials Recorded from the Ear under Resting Condition. Under resting condition (when the ear is not stimulated with sound), two different potentials are recorded:

- Endocochlear potential and
- Resting potential of the hair cells.

Endocochlear Potential. The endolymph contains a high concentration of K^+(135 mEq/L) and is electrically positive in comparison to perilymph. The +80mV electrical potential which exists between endolymph of scala media and perilymph of scala vestibuli and scala tympani is called *endolymphatic* or *endocochlear potential. Source* of endolymphatic potential is stria vascularis which covers the lateral wall of the scala media. The characteristic features of the cells of striavascularis which contribute to high K^+ concentration of endolymph are:

- High concentration of Na^+-K^+-ATPase and
- Presence of a unique electrogenic K^+ pump.

Resting Potential of the Hair Cells. Each hair cell has a negative resting membrane potential. Therefore, ICF is at a potential of –70 mV with respect to perilymph of scala tympani. At the upper end of hair cell the potential difference between ICF and endolymph is, therefore, –150 mV [–70–(+80)]. However, there is not much difference between K^+ concentration of endolymph and ICF. The large negative potential and lack of a K^+ concentration difference between the inside and outside of the hair cells make these cells very sensitive. Therefore, slightest movement of the hair stimulates the cells.

Potentials Recorded from the Ear on Stimulation. When the ear is stimulated by sound, two types of potentials can be recorded:

- Cochlear microphonic potential and
- Action potential in the auditory nerve.

Cochlear Microphonic Potential. When stimulated by the sound wave, the changes in membrane potential of the hair cells result from changes in cation conductance at their apical ends. The gating of K^+ channels is controlled by bending of stereocilia as:

- When the stereocilia bend away from the limbus, they cause K^+ channels to open; K^+ then flows into the cell and the *hair cell depolarizes*.
- When the stereocilia bend toward the limbus, they cause K^+ channels to close and the *hair cell hyperpolarizes*.

The sum of receptor potentials of a number of hair cells when recorded extracellularly is called *cochlear microphonic potential*. It is oscillatory event that can be recorded by placing one electrode in scala media and other electrode in scala tympani.

Cochlear microphonic potentials are similar to generator potential, because:

- These have no latency or refractory period,
- These do not obey all or none law and
- These are resistant to ischaemia and anaesthesia.

Relationship between intensity of sound and cochlear microphonic potential. The cochlear microphonic potentials recorded have the same form and polarity as that of the acoustic stimulus. The excitatory phase of cochlear microphonic potential (i.e. increasing negativity in scala media) is associated with a current flow outwards across the membrane of the nerve fibres (Fig. 11.2-14). As shown in Fig. 11.2-14, the base of cochlea responds to all frequencies of sound while the apex responds to only low frequencies of sound.

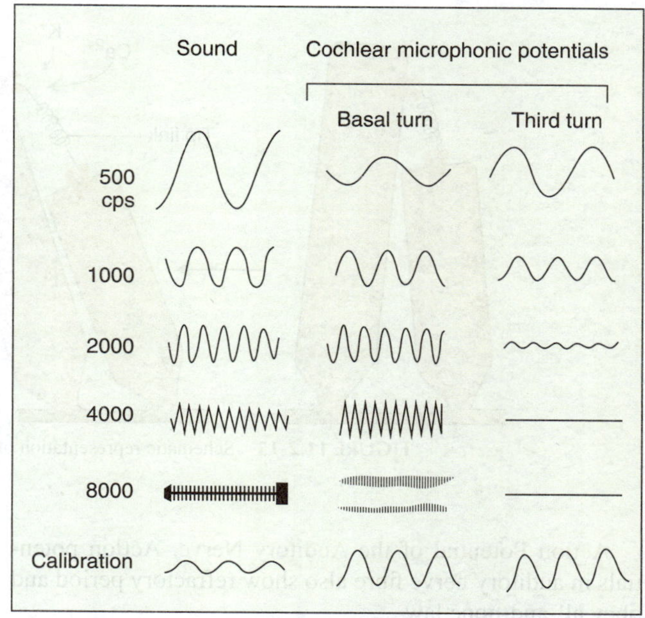

FIGURE 11.2-14 Relationship between the intensity (loudness) of sound and cochlear microphonic potentials recorded through basal turn and third turn of cochlea

Note. When organ of Corti is damaged by prolonged exposure to a loud tone, the cochlear microphonic potential produced by this particular band of frequency is abolished.

Genesis of action potential in afferent nerve fibres. The stereocilium of hair cells of organ of Corti are linked to the site of neighbouring hair cell by a very fine process called tip link. The arrangement is such that tip link tie the tip of stereocilium to the side of its higher neighbouring one stereocilium (Fig. 11.2-15). At the junction, mechanosensitive cation channels are present at the higher process. The events of genesis of action potential are as follows:

- When shorter stereocilia are pushed towards the higher neighbouring ones, the channels get open up and $K^+$and Ca^{2+} influx causes depolarization.
- The molecular motors (myosin based) present in the higher neighbouring process next moves the channel towards the base and thereby releasing tension in the tip link. This causes closure of the mechanosensitive cation channel and permits restoration of the resting state.
- The depolarization of hair cells causes release of neurotransmitter (glutamate), which initiates depolarization of neighbouring afferent neurons and causes generation of action potential.
- The K^+ that enters into the hair cells through mechanosensitive channels is recycled (Fig. 11.2-15). It enters through tight junctions into the neighbouring supporting cells and reaches into the striavascularis and secreted back into the endolymph, completing the cycle.

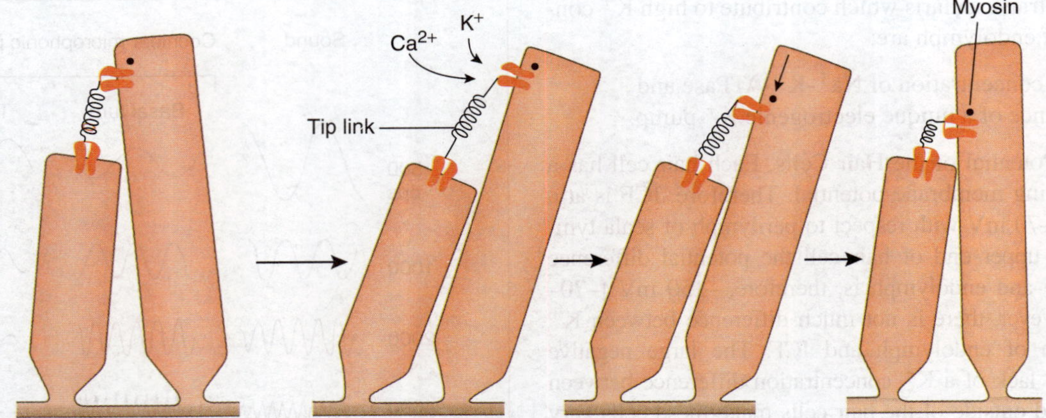

FIGURE 11.2-15 Schematic representation of the role of tip links in the responses of hair cells.

Action Potential of the Auditory Nerve. Action potentials in auditory nerve fibre also show refractory period and obey all-and-none law.

Loudness of the sound stimuli determine the frequency of action potentials in a single auditory nerve fibre (Fig. 11.2-16):

- *At low sound intensities,* each axon discharges to sounds of only one frequency called the characteristic frequency, which varies from axon to axon depending upon the part of cochlea from where the fibre originates.
- *At higher sound intensities* the individual axon responds to an increasingly wide range of sound frequencies.

Refractory period of auditory nerve fibre is 1 ms. Therefore, maximum rate of discharge through fibre can be only 1000 impulses/second. At a very low frequency (20–200 cycles/second) there is a synchronization between the sound frequency and the rate of discharge.

Neural Transmission of Signals

The electrical signals which emanate from transduction of the sound waves in the hair cells are transmitted through a complex auditory pathway which consists of following relay stations (Fig. 11.2-8)

- Spiral ganglion,
- Cochlear nuclei,
- Superior olivary nuclear complex, trapezoid nucleus and nucleus of lateral lemniscus,
- Inferior colliculus,
- Medial geniculate body and
- Auditory cortex.

Revise anatomical details of auditory pathway before proceeding further (see page 1177).

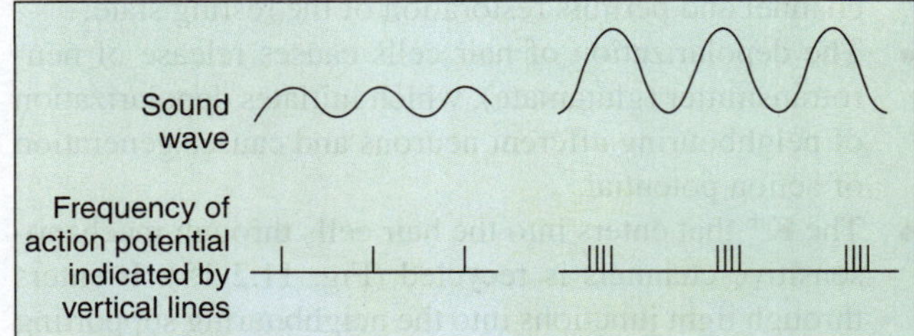

FIGURE 11.2-16 Effect of intensity of sound wave on action potential recorded from cochlear nerve fibres.

Salient Features of Auditory Pathway Some salient features of auditory pathway which need special emphasis are:

1. Bilateral Representation. From medulla onwards each ear is bilaterally represented in the auditory pathway with only slight proponderance in the contralateral pathway. Because of the bilateral representation lesion beyond medulla has slight effect on the auditory acuity.

2. Descending Pathway. There is not only an ascending auditory pathway but also a significant descending pathway forming feed-forward and feed-backward loops.

3. Role in Brain Stem and Spiral Acoustic Reflexes. Auditory pathway is also involved in the brain stem and spiral acoustic reflexes and brain stem mechanism for auditory visual reflexes. The integration of visual and auditory in-formation occurs due to interconnection of the superior and inferior colliculi.

4. Role in General Arousal. The auditory pathways in the brain stem give collaterals to the reticular formation and the cerebellum and thus play a role in general arousal.

5. Spatial Organization. The different parts of organ of Corti respond to tones of different frequencies from basilar to apical part of cochlea. Neurons receiving fibres from different parts of the spiral ganglion are arranged in a definite sequence in the cochlear nuclei. The tonotopicorganization which is prominent in cochlear nuclei is maintained in the superior olivary nucleus, inferior colliculus, medial geniculate body and auditory cortex. This *tonotopic organization* resembles the retinotopic organization of the visual pathway and somatotopic organization of the somatosensory system.

6. Features of Auditory Cortex. The auditory cortex exhibits following characteristic features:

i. *Tonotopic organization*, as described above and
ii. *Column organization*.

In addition to the tonotopic organization, the auditory cortex also exhibits feature extractions. For example, some neurons are selected for the direction of frequency modulation. Neurons in the primary auditory cortex form the so-called isofrequency, summation and suppression columns.

- ***Isofrequency columns.*** Neurons arranged in these columns have the same characteristic frequency.
- ***Summation columns.*** Neurons in these columns are more responsive to binaural than to monaural input.
- ***Suppression columns.*** Neurons in these columns are less responsive to binaural than to monaural stimulation and accordingly the response to one ear is dominant.

7. Features of Other Cortical Areas Concerned with Audition are:

i. ***Hemispheric specialization.*** Although the auditory area look very much the same on the two sides of the brain, there is marked hemispherical specialization. For example, Brodmann's area 22 is concerned with the processing of auditory signals related to speech. During language processing, it is much more active on the left side than on the right side. Area 22 on the right side is more concerned with melody, pitch and sound intensities.
ii. ***Plasticity of auditory pathways.*** There exists a great plasticity in the auditory pathways, i.e. they are modified by experience. Examples of auditory plasticity in humans include the following observations:
   - Individuals who become deaf before language skills are fully developed, viewing sign language activates auditory association areas.
   - Conversely, individuals who become blind early in life are demonstrably better at localizing sound than individuals with normal eyesight.
   - In right handed individual Planum temporal i.e. a portion of the posterior superior temporal gyrus involved in language related auditory process is larger in left cerebral hemisphere than in right .
   - Musicians have an increase in the size of auditory area activated by musical tones. They also have larger cerebellum than non-musicians, presumably because of learned precise finger movements.

Neural Processing of Auditory Information

Neural processing of auditory information involves:

- Encoding of frequency (pitch determination),
- Encoding of intensity (determination of loudness),
- Feature detection and
- Localization of sound in space.

Encoding of Sound Frequency The human auditory mechanism has a remarkable power to discriminate between the sounds in the 60–20,000 Hz range. Cochlear nerve fibres encode frequency of sound stimulus. *Duplex theory*, which includes both, place theory and frequency theory, is required to explain the frequency coding of sound.

Place Theory or Bekesy Travelling Wave Theory. This theory can explain the discrimination between sound frequencies above 2000 Hz and upto 20,000 Hz. Salient features of this theory are:

Basilar membrane is a mechanical analyser of source frequency. The basic pattern of movement of the basilar membrane is that of a travelling wave (Fig. 11.2-17). The high frequency sound waves produce waves of maximum height near the oval window, whereas low frequency sounds produce waves of maximum height near the helicotrema (Fig. 11.2-17). Correspondingly, the basilar membrane near the oval window vibrates in response to high frequency sounds. As the distance of the basilar membrane from the oval window increases there is gradual decrease in the frequency of sounds to which the membrane responds. Near the helicotrema the basilar membrane responds to very low frequency sound (Fig. 11.2-18). This differential response to different frequencies of sound is possible because of a systematic variation in the mechanical properties and along the basilar membrane. The basilar membrane is narrowest and stiffest at the base of cochlea (near the oval and round windows) and widest and most compliant at the apex of the cochlea (near the helicotrema).

Thus, as per the travelling wave theory of Von Bekesy, the higher frequencies are represented in the basal turn of cochlea and the progressively lower ones towards the apex (Fig. 11.2-19).

Different hair cells respond to different frequencies of sound depending upon their location on the basilar membrane. The auditory nerve fibre activated by a particular sound frequency is similarly dependent upon the location

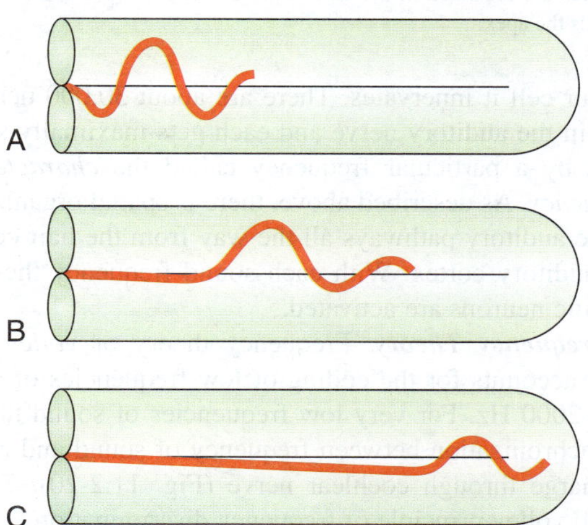

FIGURE 11.2-17 Travelling wave along the basilar membrane for **(A)** high, **(B)** medium and **(C)** low frequency sounds.

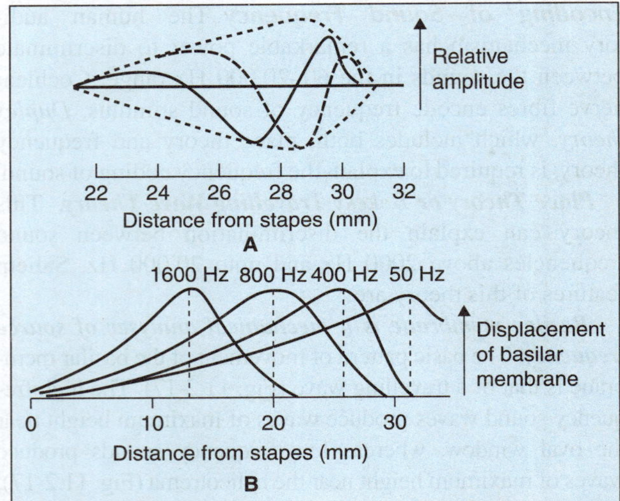

FIGURE 11.2-18 (A) Amplitude pattern of vibration of basilar membrane for a medium frequency sound wave and (B) displacement of the basilar membrane by the waves generated by stapes vibrations of frequencies shown at the top of each curve.

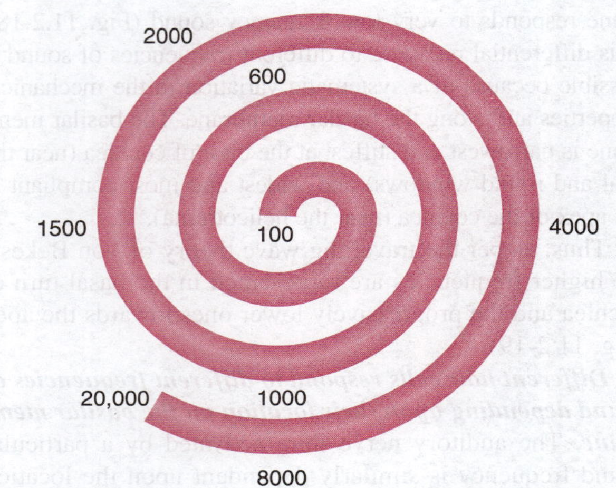

FIGURE 11.2-19 Frequency localization in the cochlea. Higher frequencies are localized in the basal turn and then progressively decrease towards the apex.

of hair cell it innervates. There are about 30,000 nerve fibres in the auditory nerve and each gets maximally stimulated by a particular frequency called the *characteristic frequency*. As described above, there is spatial organization of the auditory pathways all the way from the hair cells to the auditory cortex. With each sound frequency therefore specific neurons are activated.

Frequency Theory. Frequency theory or *volley principle* accounts for the coding of low frequencies of sound upto 2000 Hz. For very low frequencies of sound there is a synchronization between frequency of sound and rate of discharge through cochlear nerve (Fig. 11.2-20). This is called volley principle of frequency discrimination.

The importance of the volley principle is limited. The frequency of action potentials in a given auditory nerve

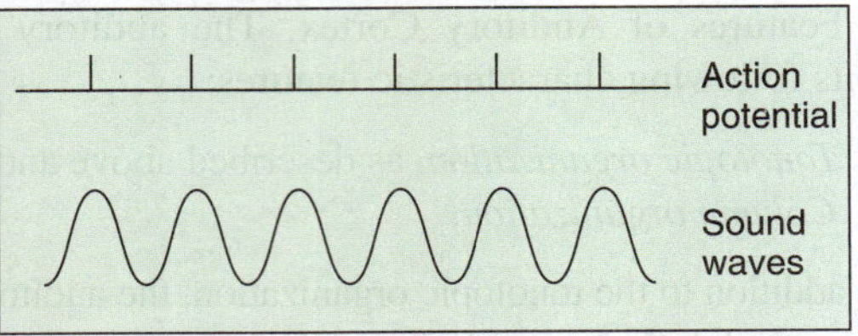

FIGURE 11.2-20 The volley effect, i.e. the auditory neuron fires an action potential to each sound wave.

fibre determines principally the loudness rather than the pitch of a sound.

Other Factors Affecting Pitch of Sound Pitch is the subjective sensation produced by *frequency of sound*. Therefore, higher the frequency greater is the pitch. However, discrimination of pitch also depends on some other factors which are:

- ***Loudness*** of sound also plays a part, low tones (below 500 Hz) seem lower and high tones (above 4000 Hz) seem higher as their loudness increases.
- ***Duration*** of sound also affects pitch to a minor degree. The pitch of a tone cannot be perceived unless it lasts for more than 0.01 sec and with durations between 0.01 and 0.1 s, pitch rises as duration increases.

Encoding of Intensity Encoding of sound intensity (loudness) occurs at the level of cochlear nerve fibres by following mechanisms:

- ***Increase in frequency of firing of an auditory nerve fibre.*** With the increase in intensity (loudness) of sound wave, the amplitude of vibration of the basilar membrane increases, which in turn increases the frequency of firing in an auditory nerve fibre.
- ***Increase in number of nerve fibres stimulation.*** As amplitude of vibration increases, a larger portion of the basilar membrane is vibrated and thus more and more hair cells are stimulated. This increases the number of auditory nerve fibres which are activated.
- ***Stimulation of inner hair cells.*** Certain hair cells (inner hair cells) are not stimulated unless the sound is very loud. Stimulation of these cells, therefore, apprise the nervous system that intensity of sound is high.

Feature Detection Higher auditory centres respond to particular features of sound stimuli. For example, cortical neurons may respond specifically to a shift from high-to low-frequency notes, which is why lesions of the auditory cortex may not impair the ability to discriminate frequency. Instead, lesions of auditory cortex cause a loss of ability to recognize a patterned sequence of sounds.

Location of Sound in Space A human can distinguish sounds originating from sources separated by as little as 1 degree. Binaural receptive fields (which is a feature of most auditory neurons above the level of cochlear nuclei) contribute to sound localization. In other words, relay nuclei in the brain stem (especially the superior olivary nuclei complex) mediate localization of sound sources. The auditory system uses following clues to judge the origin of sound:

- ***Time lag between the entry of sound in two ears.*** For example, if the sound originates from the right side of a person, it reaches the right ear earlier than the left ear. The interaural time differences is more important clue. The detectable time difference of 20μs, especially for relatively low-frequency sounds (below 3000 Hz). The medial superior olivary nuclei include many neurons responsive to low-frequency inputs.
- ***Differences in the intensity that reaches the two ears.*** Interaural intensity clues are most important for high-frequency stimuli (above 3000 Hz), because the head absorbs shorter wavelength sounds better than long wavelength sounds. The *lateral superior olivary*nu clei are most sensitive to high-frequency stimuli and thus differences in the sound intensity that reaches the two ears to provide information about the source of sound.
- ***Quality of sound.*** The sound coming directly infront of an individual differ in quality than coming from behind, because pinna is directed slightly forward. Therefore, quality of sound waves changes after reflection from pinnal surface, it moves up and down. Change in quality of the sound wave is an important factor in localizing the sound in vertical plane.

Neurons in the auditory cortex that receive input from both ears respond maximally or minimally when the time of arrival of a stimulus at one ear is delayed by a fixed period relative to the time of arrival at the other ear. This fixed period varies from neuron to neuron.

Sound localization is markedly disrupted by lesions of the auditory cortex.

APPLIED ASPECTS

- Noise and masking
- Hearing loss and deafness
- Hearing tests.

Noise and Masking

Noise Noise is defined as an aperiodic complex sound. There are three types of noise:

White Noise. It is a broad-band noise which contains all frequencies in audible spectrum. It is analogous to the white light which contains all the colours of the visible spectrum. It is used for masking.

Narrow-band Noise. It is a white noise, out of which certain frequencies above and below the given noise have been filtered out. Thus, its frequency range is smaller than the broad-band white noise. It is used to mask the tested frequency in pure tone audiometry.

Speech Noise. It is a noise having all frequencies in the speech range (300–3000 Hz). All other frequencies are filtered out.

Masking Masking refers to a phenomenon in which the presence of one type of sound decreases the ability of the ear to hear another type of sound. In other words, masking represents the inability of the auditory mechanism to separate the simultaneous stimulation into separate components. Masking is more effective for sounds with similar frequencies than with sounds for widely different frequencies. Low-frequency tones mask high frequency tones more easily than the reverse. Example of masking observed is the difficulty in conversation in noisy surroundings.

Clinical Applications. In clinical audiometry, one ear is kept busy by a sound while the other is being tested. Masking of non-test ear is essential in all bone conduction tests.

Hearing Loss, Deafness and Tinnitus

Hearing loss refers to impairment of hearing and its severity may vary from mild to profound.

Deafness is labelled when there is little or no hearing at all.

Degree of hearing loss. WHO 1980 recommended the following classification (Table 11.2-1) on the basis of pure tone audiogram taking the average of the thresholds of hearing for frequencies of 500,1000, and 2000 Hz.

Types of hearing loss. Hearing loss can be of three types:

- Conductive hearing loss,
- Sensorineural hearing loss and
- Mixed hearing loss.

1. Conductive Hearing Loss Any disease process which interferes with the conduction of sound from external ear to cochlea causes conductive hearing loss.

Causes. The causes of conduction hearing loss may lie in the:

- External ear: any obstruction in the ear canal, e.g. by wax (cerumen), tumours, atresia otitis externai.e inflammation of external ear (swimmer ear) etc.

TABLE 11.2-1 WHO Classification of Hearing Loss

Degree of hearing loss	Hearing threshold in better ear (average of 500, 1000, and 2000 Hz)
0 Not significant	0–25 dB
1 Mild	26–40 dB
2 Moderate	41–55 dB
3 Moderately severe	56–70 dB
4 Severe	71–91 dB
5 Profound	Above 91 dB
6 Total	

- Tympanic membrane, e.g. perforation.
- Middle ear cavity, e.g. fluid in the middle ear (as in otitis media).
- Ear ossicles, e.g. disruption of ear ossicles and fixation of ear ossicles (otosclerosis).
- Eustachian tube obstruction as in retracted tympanic membrane.

Characteristic Features

- Characteristically, hearing loss is partial and never complete because skull bones themselves conduct sound to the cochlea (bone conduction) and the basilar membrane can be set into vibrations.
- Hearing loss is fairly uniform throughout the frequency wave.
- Speech discrimination is good.

Hearing tests, see Table 11.2-2.

Management. Treatment of cause.

2. Sensorineural Hearing Loss Sensorineural (SN) hearing loss results from lesions of cochlea (*sensory type*) or eighth cranial nerve and its central connections (neural type).

Causes. SN hearing loss can be congenital or acquired.

- ***Congenital*** SN hearing loss is present at birth. It may be due to anomalies of the inner ear or damage to the hearing apparatus by prenatal or perinatal factors.
- ***Acquired*** SN hearing loss appears later in life. Cause may be genetic (delayed onset) or non-genetic.

Genetic causes of hearing loss include:

- Mutation of gene for connexin-26 protein. This defect prevents K^+ recycling through the sustantacular cells.
- Mutations in myosin like myosin VIIa, (associated with actin in hair cell processes); myosin -1b, (part of molecular motor that adjust tension on tip links); and myosine –VI (involved in formation of cilia).
- Mutation of α tectin – α tectin is one of the major proteins present in tectorial membrane.
- Pendered syndrome- associated with deafness and goiter is caused by mutation of multifactorial anion exchanger.
- Long QT syndrome in which a type of K^+ channel protein ($KVLQT_1$) is mutated. In normal individual K^+ channel is responsible for maintaining high K^+ concentration in endolymph and normal QT interval (see page 271).
- Bartter syndrome—Mutation of bartin, a membrane protein causes deafness and renal manifestations (see page 500.)

Causes of nongenetic acquired SN deafness are:

- *Infection* of labyrinth (viral, bacterial or spirochaetal).
- *Acoustic trauma*, i.e. injury to labyrinth or the eighth nerve.
- *Noise trauma or noise* induced hearing loss occurs due to prolonged exposure to industrial noise or at leisure activity causes high frequency hearing loss. The hair cells are damaged by excessive noise, the outer hair cells are more vulnerable than the inner cells.
- *Ototoxicity*. Certain drugs cause damage to inner ear, e.g. streptomycin, neomycin, quinine, chloroquine etc. These drugs specially cause damage to the outer hair cells or striavascularis.
- *Neoplasms*, e.g. acoustic neuroma.
- *Systemic disorders*, e.g. diabetes mellitus, hypertension etc.
- *Presbycusis* refers to gradual hearing loss associated with aging, occurs due to gradual loss of hair cells and neurons.

Characteristic Features

- Usually loss of hearing is complete.
- Speech discrimination is poor.
- Hearing loss may exceed 60 dB.

Hearing tests. See Table 11.2-2.

Management includes:

- Treatment of the cause when possible.
- Hearing aids for rehabilitation.

Cochlear implants are the devices which consist of-

- Microphone that picks up environmental sound.
- Speech processor that select and arrange these sounds
- Transmitter, receiver/stimulator that converts those sounds into electrical impulses.
- Electron array that sends impulses to auditory nerve.

Advantage. In a deaf person, though cochlear implants cannot restore normal hearing, but it can promote useful representation of environment sound. In adult onset deafness the person can learn to associate signals with sound that they remember.

With the help of cochlear implant with intensive therapy a deaf child can acquire language and speech skill.

Stem cell with the help of stem cells hair cells can be developed.

TABLE 11.2-2 Tuning Fork Tests and Their interpretation

Test	Normal	Conductive hearing loss	Sensorineural hearing loss
Rinne test	AC > BC Rinne +ve	BC > AC Rinne–ve	AC > BC in partial deafness
Weber test	Not lateralized	Lateralized towards affected ear	Lateralized towards healthy ear
Absolute boneconduction test	Same as examiners'	Same as examiners'	Reduced
Schwabach test	Equal	Better conduction in patient	Better conduction in examiner

3. Mixed Hearing Loss Both conductive and sensorineural hearing loss is present in the same ear and is *characterized* by:

- Air-bone gap indicating conductive hearing loss and
- Impairment of bone conduction indicating sensorineural hearing loss.

Tinnitus Tinnitus refers to ringing sensation in the ear. It is caused by irritative stimulation of either the inner ear or the vestibulocochlear nerve.

Hearing Tests

A. Clinical Tests of Hearing

1. Finger friction test. It is a rough and quick method for screening. In it thumb and index finger are rubbed near the ear and patient is asked to appreciate with eyes closed.

2. Watch Test. A clicking watch is brought close to the ear and the distance at which it is heard is noted.

3. Human Speech Voice Test. Normally, a conversational voice (60 dB) and whisper should be heard at 6 m with eyes closed (to avoid lip reading) in a quiet room. The commonly used *spondee* (phonetically balanced words) are: black-night, football, daydream or numbers with letters such as X3B, 2AZ, MOD etc. The distance at which the conversational voice is heard is measured.

4. Tuning Fork Tests. These tests are performed with tuning forks of different frequencies (commonly used are 256 and 512 Hz). These are quite useful in distinguishing conductive deafness from sensorineural deafness. Commonly used tests are:

i. ***Rinne test***. In this test air conduction (AC) of the ear is compared with bone conduction (BC). Base of a vibrating tuning fork is placed on the mastoid bone (Fig. 11.2-21A), and when he stops hearing, it is brought beside the meatus (Fig. 11.2-21B). If he still hears, AC is more than BC and Rinne test is positive.
- In normal subjects, Rinne test is positive.
- In conductive deafness, Rinne test is negative.
- In partial nerve deafness, Rinne test is positive.
- In complete nerve deafness, both bone conducted and air conducted sounds are not perceived.

ii. ***Weber's test***. In this test, base of the vibrating tuning fork is placed in the middle of the forehead (Fig. 11.2-21C) or vertex and patient is asked in which ear the sound is heard better.
- *Normally* the sound is heard equally in both ears.
- In *conductive hearing loss,* the sound is lateralized (better heard) towards affected ear. This is because the masking effect of environmental noise is absent in the affected ear.
- In *sensorineural hearing loss,* the sound is lateralized towards better ear, because the sound is reaching the normal cochlea through bone.

iii. ***Absolute bone conduction (ABC) test.*** In this test, patients' bone conduction is compared with that of the examiner (persuming that the examiner has normal hearing). External auditory meatus of both the examiner and the patient should be occluded (by pressing the tragus inwards), to prevent the ambience noise entering through air-conduction route.
- Normally, and in conduction deafness, both the examiner and the patient hear the fork for same duration of time.
- In sensorineural deafness, the patient hears the fork for shorter duration.

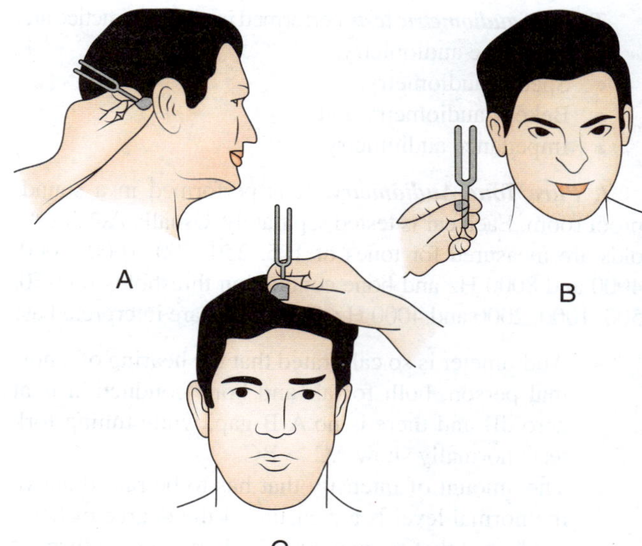

FIGURE 11.2-21 Tuning fork test: **(A)** test for bone conduction; **(B)** test for air conduction and **(C)** Weber's test.

iv. ***Schwabach's test.*** It is similar to the ABC test except that the external auditory meatus is not occluded in this test.
- *Normally*, both the examiner and the subject hear the sound equally well.
- In *conductive deafness* the patient hears the fork for longer period than the examiner (because there is no masking effect of environmental noise).
- In *sensorineural deafness*, the examiner hears the fork for a longer duration than the patient.

Table 11.2-2 summarizes the interpretation of tuning fork tests.

B. Audiometric Tests Audiometer is the device used to perform audiometry. Audiometry refers to measurement of auditory acuity (sharpness of hearing) using the audiometer. An audiometer consists of following main parts:

- Electronic oscillator. It can generate pure tones of frequencies ranging from low to high.
- Intensity dial. It helps to adjust the threshold intensity of hearing for each tone.
- Headphone. It helps to deliver the pure tones of various frequencies to each ear separately.

Types of audiometric tests performed in clinical practice are:

- Pure tone audiometry,
- Speech audiometry,
- Bekesy audiometry and
- Impedance audiometry.

1. Pure Tone Audiometry. It is performed in a soundproof room. Each ear is tested separately. Usually AC thresholds are measured for tones of 125, 250, 500, 1000, 2000, 4000 and 8000 Hz and bone conduction thresholds for 250, 500, 1000, 2000 and 4000 Hz. The results are interpreted as:

- Audiometer is so calibrated that the hearing of a normal person, both for air and bone conduction is at zero dB and there is no A-B gap, while tuning fork tests normally show AC > BC.
- The amount of intensity that has to be raised above the normal level is a measure of the degree of hearing loss at that frequency. It is charted in the form of a graph called *audiogram* (Fig. 11.2-22).
- Threshold of BC is a measure of cochlear function.
- Difference in the thresholds of air and bone conduction (A-B gap) is a measure of degree of conductive deafness.

2. Speech Audiometry. In this test, the patient's ability to hear and understand speech is measured. In it, a set of spondee words (two syllable words with equal stress on each, e.g. baseball, sunlight, daydream etc.) with variable intensity is delivered to each ear. Following two parameters are measured:

- Speech reception threshold (SRT), and
- Discrimination score (DS).

4. Bekesy Audiometry. It is a self-recording audiometry where various pure tone frequencies automatically move from low to high.

5. Impedance Audiometry. It is an objective test, which is particularly useful in children. It consists of two tests:

- Tympanometry and
- Acoustic reflex measurements.

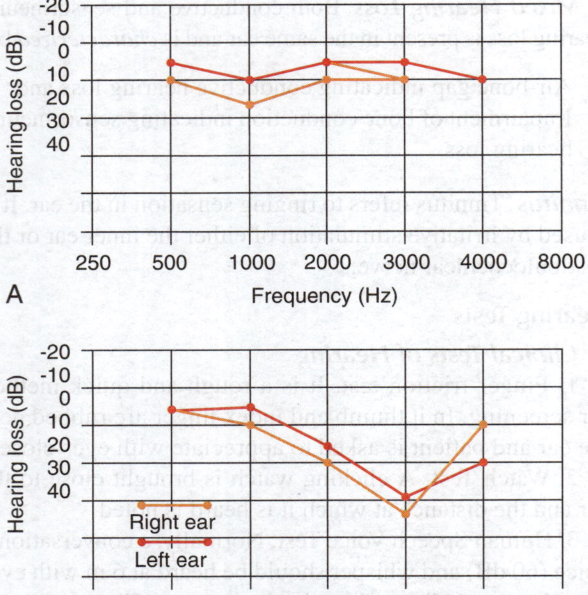

FIGURE 11.2-22 Audiogram showing: (A) normal hearing; (B) loss of 20 dB hearing for 3000 Hz frequency in both ears.

C. Special Tests for Hearing Certain special tests have been devised to illucidate different aspects of hearing loss. Some of these tests include:

- Recruitment,
- Short increment sensitivity index (SISI),
- Threshold tone decay test,
- Evoked response audiometry which includes:
  - Electro-cochleography (E CoG) and
  - Auditory brainstem responses (see page 1095).
- Otoacoustic emissions and
- Central auditory tests.

Chapter 11.3

Chemical Senses: Smell and Taste

THE SENSE OF SMELL

The sense of smell or olfaction is well developed in animals like dog and rabbit to give warning of the environmental dangers. Such animals are called *macrosomatics*. In humans, apes and monkeys (primates), the sense of smell is comparatively less developed, but still it is important for pleasure and for enjoying the taste of food. Therefore, the humans and primates are called *microsomatics*.

Site of Olfaction

The olfactory stimuli are detected by specialized receptors located on the free nerve endings of the olfactory nerves which are located in the:

- Olfactory mucosa of nose in human beings and
- Vomeronasal organ in reptiles and certain mammals.

Olfactory Mucosa In humans, the olfactory mucosa is confined to upper one-third of nasal cavity. It includes the roof of nasal cavity and the adjoining areas on the medial wall (septum) and superior nasal concha on the lateral wall (Fig. 11.3-1). The olfactory neuroepithelium is a patch of thin and dull yellow mucosa about 2.5 cm^2 in area. A mucous layer covers the entire epithelium.

Histological Structure. Histologically, the olfactory mucosa consists of three types of cells (Fig. 11.3-2):

1. ***Receptor cells.*** About 10–20 million receptor cells are present in the olfactory mucosa. These cells are bipolar neurons which lie between the supporting (sustentacular) cells. The dendrites of the receptor cells terminate in a knob from which 6–12 fine cilia project and form a dense mat into the mucous layer of the olfactory mucosa. Their axons are fine unmyelinated fibres which form the olfactory nerves.

   Characteristic features of olfactory receptor cells which differentiate it from other sensory neurons are:

   - These are the only sensory neurons whose cell bodies are closest to the external environment.
   - These cells have a short life span of about 60 days and get replaced by proliferation of basal cells. This

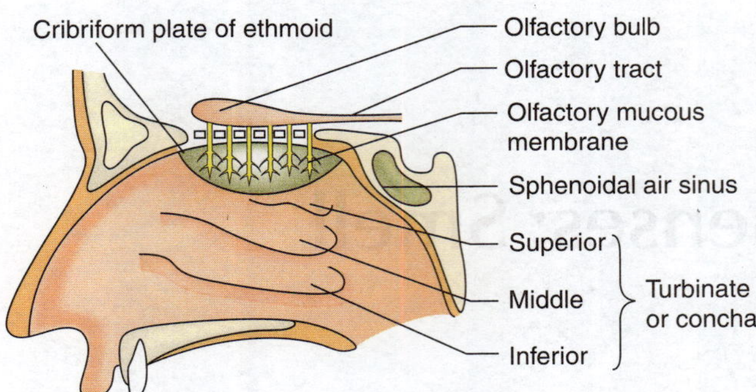

FIGURE 11.3-1 Location of olfactory mucosa.

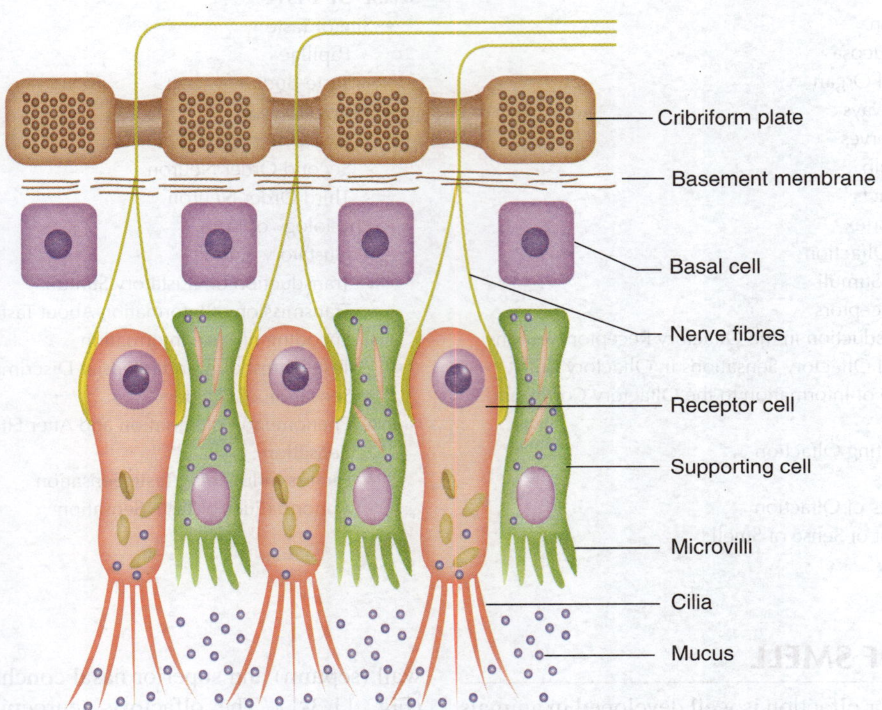

FIGURE 11.3-2 Histological features of olfactory mucosa.

natural turnover is a unique feature of these sensory neurons.

2. ***Supporting cells*** also known as sustentacular cells are columnar in shape. Microvilli extend from the surface of these cells into the mucous layer covering the olfactory mucosa. These cells secrete mucus.

   The *Bowman's glands* lying just under the basement membrane also secrete mucus.

3. ***Basal cells*** are stem cells from which new receptor cells are formed. As mentioned above, there is a continuous re placement of receptor cells by mitosis of basal cells.

Distinguishing features of olfactory mucosa from the surrounding respiratory mucosa of nasal cavity are:

- Presence of receptor cells,
- Presence of Bowman's glands,
- Absence of rhythmic ciliary beating (which is a characteristic feature of respiratory mucosa) and
- Presence of a distinctive yellow-brown pigment.

Nerve Supply of Olfactory Mucosa

- ***Special sensory nerves*** innervating the olfactory mucosa are 15–20 bundles of olfactory nerve fibres (first cranial nerve) which convey sense of smell.
- ***General sensory nerves*** supplying the olfactory mucosa are branches of trigeminal nerve (fifth cranial nerve). The irritative character of some odorants results from stimulation of free nerve endings of the trigeminal nerve. Therefore, vapours of ammonia are never used to test the sense of smell as they stimulate fibres of trigeminal nerve and cause irritation in the nose rather than stimulating the olfactory receptors.

Vomeronasal Organ It is a pouch-like structure found along the nasal septum in the nose of some animals (rodents and various other animals). Receptors present in vomeronasal organ are concerned with perception of odour that emanates from the *pheromones* and foodstuffs and are thus related to food and sex behaviour of the animals. Nerve fibres emerging from vomeronasal organ project to the *accessory olfactory bulb* and from those primarily to areas in the amygdala and hypothalamus that are concerned with reproduction and eating behaviour.

Vomeronasal organ is not well developed in humans, but there is anatomically separate and biochemically unique area of olfactory mucous membrane in a pit in the anterior third of the nasal septum which appears to be homologous structure.

Pheromones. These are hormone-like substances which emit specific odour and produce hormonal, behavioural, or other physiological changes in another animal of the same species. Usually a pheromone is secreted by an animal during mating season only. The smell of pheromones often is the cause of sex, which an animal follows to find out its mating partner which may be waiting at a distance. It is being assumed that pheromone also exists in humans and that there is close relationship between smell and sexual function.

Olfactory Pathways

Olfactory pathways comprise:

1. Olfactory Nerves. About 15–20 olfactory nerve filaments which consist of the axons of the bipolar olfactory neurons which pierce the cribriform plate on either side to reach olfactory bulb.

2. Olfactory Bulb. (Fig. 11.3-3). It is an oval flattened strip of gray matter lying on the cribriform plate which receives the olfactory nerve filaments. There is a point-to-point representation of olfactory mucosa in the olfactory bulb. The upper part of the mucosa is represented in the anterior part of bulb while the lower part is represented posteriorly. The olfactory bulb contains three types of cells: mitral cells, tufted cells and interneurons (granule cells and peri-glomerular cells). The mitral and tufted cells constitute second-order neurons.

- ***Dendrites of mitral and tufted*** cells branch and form synapses with the axon terminals of olfactory neurons (first-order neurons) to constitute globular masses called olfactory glomeruli. Olfactory axons converge extensively onto mitral cell dendrites, as many as axons from 1000 olfactory neurons synapse on the dendrites of a single mitral cell.
- ***Granule and periglomerular cells*** are inhibitory neurons. They form dendrodendritic reciprocal synapses with the dendrites of the mitral cells. The periglomerular cells also participate in the formation of olfactory glomeruli.
- ***Axons of the mitral and tufted cells*** leave the olfactory bulb and run in the olfactory tract.

3. Olfactory Tract. It lies in the olfactory sulcus on the orbital surface of the frontal lobe and proceeds backwards from each olfactory bulb to the region of anterior perforated

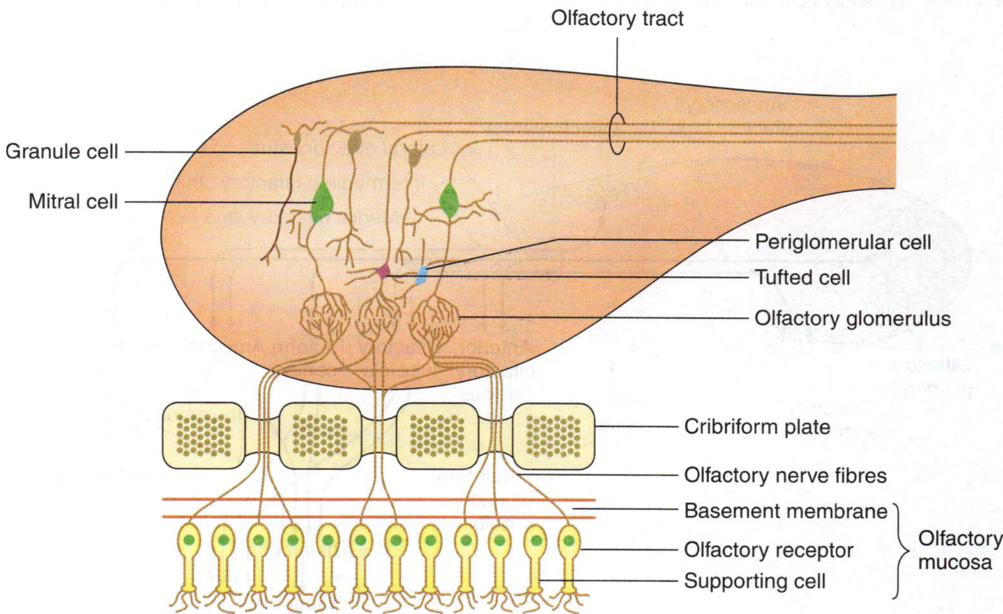

FIGURE 11.3-3 Diagrammatic depiction of the synapses between axons of olfactory neurons (first-order neurons) with the dendrites of mitral and tufted cells (second-order neurons) to form the olfactory glomeruli which lie in the olfactory bulb. The inhibitory neurons present in the olfactory bulb are granule cells and periglomerular cells.

substance on the base of brain where it divides into lateral, intermediate and medial olfactory striae (Fig. 11.3-4). *Olfactory trigone* refers to the flattened part of the olfactory tract, near the anterior perforated substance before it divides into the striae.

- ***Anterior olfactory nucleus***. It is made up of scattered neurons within the olfactory tract. Neurons in this structure receive synaptic connections from neurons of the olfactory bulb and send axons through the anterior commissure to excite inhibitory neurons on the contralateral olfactory bulb (Fig. 11.3-5).
- ***Olfactory striae***. Three striae are derived from each olfactory tract (Fig. 11.3-5):
  - ***Lateral olfactory stria.*** Axons of the lateral olfactory stria synapse in the primary olfactory receiving area which includes the *prepiriform cortex* (and in many animals the piriform lobe).
  - ***Medial olfactory stria*** includes projections to the *amygdaloid nucleus*, as well as to part of the cortex of the basal forebrain.
  - ***Intermediate olfactory stria*** terminates in the *olfactory tubercle*, an area of the cortex rostral to the anterior perforated substance.

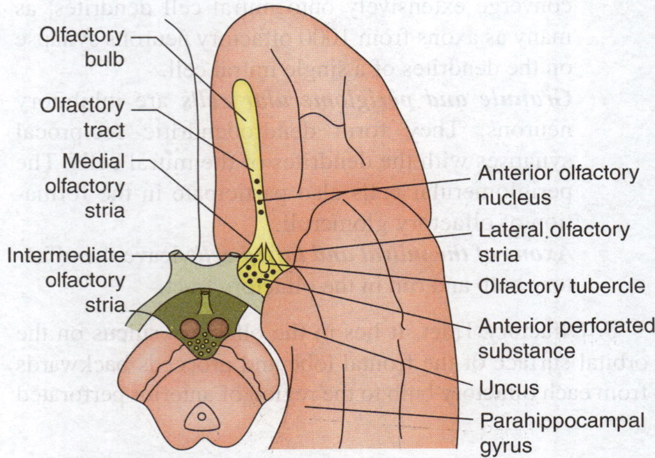

FIGURE 11.3-4 Olfactory bulb and olfactory tract.

4. Olfactory Cortex. It includes the anterior olfactory nucleus, prepiriform cortex, olfactory tubercle and amygdala. All these are parts of the limbic system.

Physiology of Olfaction

Odoriferous Stimuli The odoriferous (smell producing molecules) stimuli enter the nasal cavity while breathing. During quiet breathing, the air passes through the lower parts of the nasal cavity. Through eddy currents, however, some air does reach the olfactory epithelium. The amount of air reaching the olfactory mucosa can be increased by sniffing which causes turbulence in the airflow in the nasal cavity. Sniffing is an act of deep breathing (semi-reflex response) which occurs when a new odour is encountered. The odorant molecules must dissolve in the mucous layer (lining the olfactory mucosa) before they can come in contact with olfactory receptors.

Characteristic Features of Odorant Molecules. To be effective an odorant molecule must be:

- ***Volatile,*** because the olfactory receptors, respond to chemicals transported by the air into the nose.
- ***Water soluble*** (to some extent) to penetrate the watery mucous layer (lining the nasal epithelium) to reach receptor cell membrane.

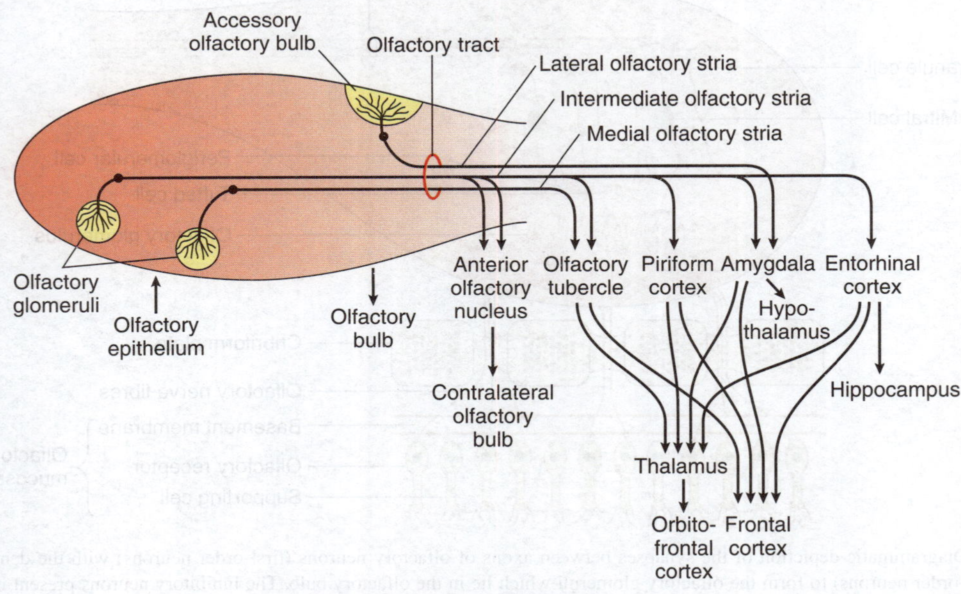

FIGURE 11.3-5 Olfactory pathways.

- ***Lipid soluble*** (to some degree), to penetrate the cell membranes of the olfactory receptor cells to stimulate those cells.

Types of Odorant Stimuli. There seems to be over 50 *primary smell sensations* (in contrast to three primary sensations of colour and four primary sensations of taste). Although the olfactory capability of humans is somewhat limited, compared with that of macrosomatic animals, nevertheless humans are able to perceive more than 10,000 different odorous molecules.

Common odours encountered are named as:

- *Aromatic or resinous odours*, e.g. camphor, lavender and cloves.
- *Fragrant odours*, e.g. perfumes and flowers.
- *Ethereal odours*, e.g. ether, chloroform.
- *Garlic odours*, e.g. garlic, onion and sulphur compounds.
- *Burning odours*, tobacco, burning of feathers, meat and bones.
- *Nauseating odours*, e.g. excreta, decomposed meat and vegetables.
- *Goat odours*, e.g. sweat, ripe cheese.
- *Repulsive odours*, e.g. odour of the bed bug.
- *Musky odours*, e.g. musk.

Olfactory Receptors The cilia of the olfactory neurons are specialized for odour detection. They have specific receptors for odorants as well as the transduction machinery needed to amplify sensory signals and generate action potentials in the neuron's axon. Some important points about olfactory receptors are:

- A large family of odorant receptors permits discrimination of a wide variety of odorants.
- A large multigene family (approximately 500) appears to code for as many as 1000 different types of odorant receptors.
- The odorant receptors belong to a large superfamily of structurally related receptor proteins that transduce signals by interactions with G-proteins.

Steps in Transduction in the Olfactory Receptor Neurons

1. Binding of Odorant Molecule to Receptors. As mentioned earlier the odorant molecules entering the nasal cavity dissolved in the mucous layer covering the olfactory mucosa. The cilia of olfactory neurons are projected into this mucous layer.

Role of odorant binding proteins (OBP). It has been suggested that the mucous layer covering the olfactory mucosa contains one or more OBP that concentrate and transfer the odorant molecules to the receptors present on the cilia of olfactory neurons. The OBPs are produced by the supporting cells. A unique OBP has been isolated in the nasal cavity is 18kDa. The OBPs serve following functions:

- They concentrate the odorant molecules on to the odorant receptors.
- They separate the hydrophobic (lipophilic ligands) from the air and transfer them to an aqueous phase.
- They may help in odour clearance by sequestering odorous molecules from the sites of recognition.

2. Activation of Receptor. The interaction of an odorant with its receptor induces an interaction between the receptor and a heterotrimetric G-protein. This interaction causes dissociation of α, β&γ subunits of G protein. The α subunit, which then stimulates adenylyl cyclase to produce cAMP.

3. Depolarization Receptor Potential. The increased intracellular cAMP opens cyclic nucleotide-gated (CNG) cation channels, leading to cation influx(Ca^{2+} and Na^{+}) and a change in membrane potential in the cilium membrane, i.e. produces a depolarizing receptor potential (Fig. 11.3-6).

4. Action Potentials. The receptor potential depolarizes the initial segment of the axon to threshold leading to the generation of action potentials in the sensory axon and the *transmission of signal to olfactory bulb.*

Note. A specific olfactory receptor does not respond to a particular compound or category of compounds. Instead, an individual receptor responds to many odours. Furthermore, no two receptor cells have identical responses to a series of stimuli. Sensory perception, therefore, is based on the pattern of receptors activated by the stimulus.

Processing of Olfactory Sensation in the Olfactory Bulb Odorant information is encoded spatially in the olfactory bulb. In the olfactory glomeruli, there is lateral inhibition mediated by periglomerular cells and granule cells (Fig. 11.3-3). Another potential source of signal refinement, or adjustment, is the multiple inputs to the olfactory bulb from the olfactory areas of the cortex as well as the basal forebrain and mid brain. Thus, sensory information is extensively processed, and perhaps refined in the olfactory bulb before it is sent to the olfactory cortex.

Transmission of Odorant Information to the Olfactory Cortex and Neocortex

- From the olfactory bulb the odorant information is first transmitted to *olfactory cortex* which includes piriform cortex, parts of amygdala, the olfactory tubercle and parts of entorhinal cortex.
- From the olfactory cortex, information is relayed to the frontal cortex (directly) and orbitofrontal cortex (via thalamus) (Fig. 11.3-5).

Note that the olfactory pathway is the only sensory system that does not have an obligatory synaptic relay in the thalamus. The olfactory tracts project directly to the olfactory cortex, while all other sensations are first processed

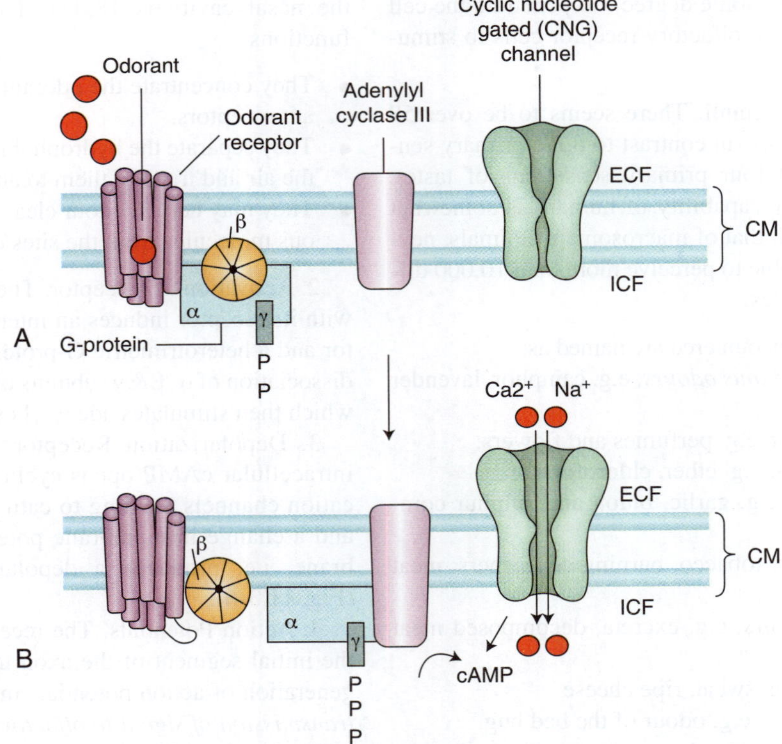

FIGURE 11.3-6 Transduction of olfactory signals. **A**; Receptor activation and **B**; depolarization.

in the thalamus before projection to cerebral cortex. This may reflect the phylogenetic primitiveness of the olfactory system. Further, because of this, olfactory stimuli have an unusually direct and widespread effect on emotions, motivation and certain kind of memory.

However, olfactory information does reach the mediodorsal nucleus of the thalamus, and olfactory information is then transmitted to the prefrontal and orbitofrontal cortex (neocortex).

Role played by different regions of cerebral cortex involved in processing of olfactory information is summarized as:

- ***Piriform cortex*** is activated by sniffing in humans.
- ***Amygdala*** and hypothalamus are probably involved with the emotional and motivational responses to olfactory stimuli as well as many of the behavioural and physiological effects of odour. In animals, effects of pheromones are also thought to be mediated by signals from the main and accessory olfactory bulbs to the amygdala and hypothalamus.
- ***Entorhinal cortex*** is concerned with olfactory memories.
- ***Neocortex (orbitofrontal and frontal cortex)*** is thought to be concerned with conscious discrimination of odours. People with lesions of orbitofrontal cortex are unable to discriminate odours.

Factors Influencing Olfactory Function

1. Threshold of Olfactory Receptors. The threshold of olfactory receptors varies from substance to substance. For example, methyl mercaptan, a substance which gives garlic its characteristic odour, has extremely low threshold. It can be smelled at a concentration of less than 500 mg/L of air (Table 11.3-1).

2. Intensity/Concentration of the Odour. Like taste receptors, the intensity discrimination of any odour by olfactory receptors is poor. The concentration of an odoriferous substance must be changed by about 30% before a difference can be detected.

- Solubility of the odorant. Relatively high water and lipid solubility are the characteristic of substances with strong odours.

3. Structural Configuration of Odorant. Odoriferous molecules are generally small and contain 3 to 20 carbon atoms. It is important to note that molecules with the same number of carbon atoms but different structural configurations have different odours.

4. Adaptation. Olfactory sensation adapts very rapidly with continued exposure to an odour. When one is continuously exposed to even the most disagreeable odour, perception of the odour decreases and eventually ceases. However, a brief exposure to fresh air allows one to smell the unpleasant odour again. Unlike adaptation of touch receptors, the

TABLE 11.3-1 Threshold Concentration of Some Odoriferous Substances

Substance	Concentration mg/L of air
Ethyl ether	5.83
Chloroform	3.30
Pyridine	0.03
Oil of peppermint	0.02
Iodoform	0.02
Butyric acid	0.009
Propyl mercaptan	0.006
Artificial musk	0.00004
Methyl mercaptan	0.0000004

adaptation of olfactory receptors may not be always functionally useful.

Physiological mechanisms responsible for olfactory adaptation are:

- ***Inactivation or desensitization*** of the receptor due to phosphorylation of the receptor by a protein kinase may occur following interaction of an odorant receptor with its ligand.
- ***Adjustment in the sensitivity of CNG ion channels to cAMP*** with different concentrations of odorant seems to be another physiological mechanism responsible for adaptation of olfactory neurons (when CNG A4 is knocked out, adaptation is slowed). This effect is conceptually analogous to light adaptation in the visual system, where light sensitivity is adjusted to match the intensity of light in the environment.

Applied Aspects

Abnormalities of Olfaction

1. Anosmia and Hyposmia. Anosmia is total loss of sense of smell while hyposmia refers to diminished olfactory sensitivity.

Causes of anosmia or hyposmia are:

- ***Injuries*** to olfactory nerves or olfactory bulb in fractures of anterior cranial fossa.
- ***Intracranial lesions*** like abscess, tumour or meningitis which may cause pressure on the olfactory tracts.
- ***Nasal obstruction*** due to nasal polyp, enlarged turbinates or marked oedema of nasal mucosa in allergic or vasomotor stimuli.
- ***Atrophic rhinitis,*** a degenerative disease of nasal mucosa also causes anosmia.
- ***Old age.*** Olfactory thresholds increase with advancing age, and more than 25% of humans over the age of 80 have an impaired ability to identify smells.
- ***Kallmann's syndrome.*** In this condition anosmia is associated with hypogonadism (see page 687).
- *Absence or disrupted function of receptors* is responsible for several dozen of different types of anosmias seen in humans.

2. Paraosmia or Dysosmia. It refers to distortion or perversion of smell. In it, person interprets the odours incorrectly. Often these persons complain of disgusting odours. ***Causes of paraosmia*** include:

- Recovery phase of post influenzal anosmia. The probable explanation for this is misdirected regeneration of nerves.
- Intracranial tumour should always be excluded in all cases of paraosmia.

Measurement of Sense of Smell

1. Qualitative Testing. Qualitatively, sense of smell can be tested by asking the patient to smell common odours such as onion, peppermint, rose, garlic or cloves from each side of the nose separately, with eyes closed.

2. Olfactometry is the method of quantitative estimation of sense of smell with the help of an instrument called olfactometer. *Olfactometer* consists of two glass tubes: outer and inner sliding one over the other. The inner tube is graduated. The inner surface of the outer tube contains the smelling substance. The curved end of the inner tube is introduced into the nostril and the subject is asked to breathe quietly. The distal end of the outer tube is closed and withdrawn gradually. The highest figure is noted as soon as the odour is perceived first of all. This reading gives the subject's threshold for smell in terms ofolfactories.

SENSE OF TASTE

Sense of taste (gustation) is a chemical sense that is stimulated by food and drink. It contributes considerably to the quality of life and is important stimulant for digestion. Taste must be distinguished from flavour, which includes the olfactory, tactile, and thermal attributes of food in addition to taste.

Site of Taste

The taste (gustatory) stimuli are detected by specialized chemoreceptors called taste receptors or taste cells. The taste receptors are clustered in the tastebuds located on the tongue, palate, pharynx, epiglottis and upper third of oesophagus.

Tongue, the main site of taste detection, contains numerous tastebuds on its dorsal surface. The mucous membrane of the dorsal surface of tongue exhibits numerous papillae, which increase the surface area of the mucosa available for taste receptors. The tastebuds are located in the walls of these papillae.

Papillae Papillae, present on the tongue, are of four types (Fig. 11.3-7):

1. Circumvallate Papillae. These are large (2–4 mm in diameter) papillae, about 10 to 12 in numbers, forming a

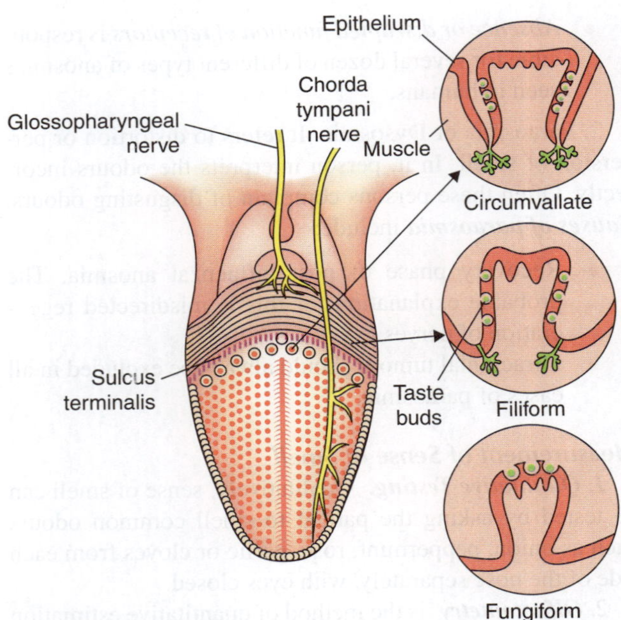

FIGURE 11.3-7 Structure and distribution of papillae on the tongue and arrangement of tastebuds in the three types of papillae. Innervation by the cranial nerves is also indicated.

single row in front of the sulcus terminalis. Sulcus terminalis is a V-shaped groove (with apex posteriorly), which separates the anterior two-thirds of the dorsum of tongue from the posterior one-third. Each circumvallate papilla is surrounded by a groove. About 200 tastebuds are located along the sides of each circumvallate papilla.

2. Fungiform Papillae. These are bright red, flat dot-like structures (each of about 1 mm in diameter) located in the anterior two-thirds of tongue along the edges, dorsum and tip. There are 8–10 tastebuds on each papilla.

3. Foliate Papillae. These are transverse mucosal folds, found on the posterolateral surfaces of the tongue anterior to the circumvallate papillae. Each foliate papilla has numerous tastebuds.

4. Filliform Papillae. These are small conical projections, covering the entire remaining surface of the dorsum of the anterior two-thirds of tongue, giving it a velvety appearance. They are arranged in rows parallel to the sulcus terminalis. They are not gustatory structures, i.e. *do not contain tastebuds*. However, they may play a role in breaking up food particles and also called *mechanical papillae* in contrast to the other three forms which are called gustatory papillae.

Taste Buds

Distribution. The tastebuds are concerned with the sensation of taste. As mentioned above, tastebuds are located on the tongue papillae, hard and soft palate, epiglottis, pharynx, and upper third of oesophagus.

Structure. Each tastebud is barrel shaped. Cluster of cells with a small opening (taste pore) in the surface that allows substances to reach the interior of the tastebud. Each tastebud measures about 50–70 μm in diameter and consists of following cells (Fig. 11.3-8):

1. ***Receptor cells.*** Each tastebud has about one hundred receptor cells (modified epithelial cells which have following characteristics:
   - The receptor cells are elongate, bipolar shaped and extend from the epithelial opening of the tastebud to its base.
   - The taste cells have a short life (about 10 days) and are continuously replaced by new taste cells differentiating from the basal cells.
   - Through the taste pore, microvilli (cilia) of all the taste cells protrude into the oral cavity and come in contact with the saliva.
   - The taste cells are innervated by sensory neurons (primary gustatory afferent fibres) at its basal pole. Although taste cells are nonneuronal epithelial cells, the contacts between these cells and sensory cells have morphological characteristics of chemical synapses.

   Each taste nerve fibre innervates taste cells in several taste buds and conversely, each taste bud is innervated by approximately 50 nerve fibres.
2. ***Basal replacement cells.*** These are small round cells present at the bottom of the taste bud (Fig. 11.3-8). They are thought to be stem cells which are continuously being differentiated into taste cells.
3. ***Supporting cells.*** In addition to taste cells and basal cells, the taste buds contain supporting or sustentacular cells.

Innervation. The special sensory nerve fibres innervating the taste cells come from the branches of the facial, glossopharyngeal and vagus nerve (7th, 9th and 10th cranial nerve, respectively). Further details of taste nerve fibres are described in the taste pathways. The tactile and temperature

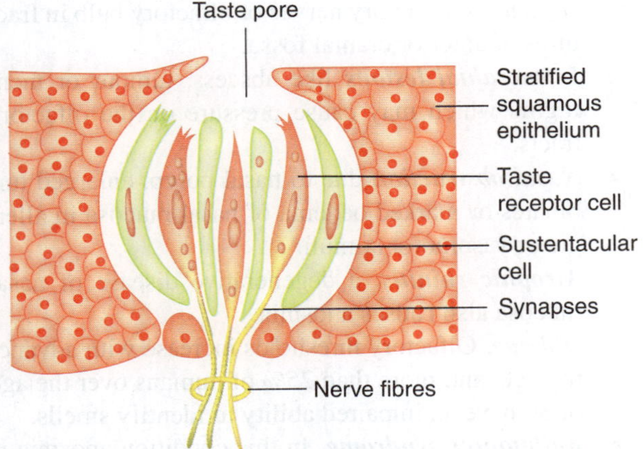

FIGURE 11.3-8 Structure of a taste bud.

receptors of the mouth, tongue and pharynx are innervated by the trigeminal nerve (fifth cranial nerve).

Taste Pathways

The taste pathways consist of three orders of neurons (Fig. 11.3-9):

First-order Neurons. The cell bodies of the first-order neurons innervating the taste cells in tastebuds are located indifferent ganglia of the 7th, 9th and 10th cranial nerves as:

- ***From the tastebuds located on anterior two-thirds of tongue,*** the taste fibres run in lingual nerve which branches from the chorda tympani nerve which is a branch of facial nerve. The cell bodies are located in the geniculate ganglion.
- ***From the tastebuds located on the posterior one-third of tongue,*** the taste fibres run in glossopharyngeal nerve. The cell bodies lie in the *superior and inferior ganglia* of this nerve.
- ***From the tastebuds located on pharyngeal aspect of tongue, epiglottis, hard and soft palate,*** the taste fibres run in the vagus nerve. The cell bodies are located in the superior and inferior ganglia of the vagus nerve.
- ***Termination of first-order neurons.*** Ultimately all the taste fibres, travelling in different cranial nerves join the tractus solitarius to terminate in the nucleus of tractus solitarius (Fig. 11.3-9).

Second-order Neurons. The cell bodies of second-order neurons of taste pathways are located in the *nucleus of tractus solitarius (NTS)* in the medulla. Axons of the second-order neurons cross the midline to join the medial lemniscus and terminate with the fifth cranial nerve fibres (carrying pain, touch and temperature fibres) in the ventral posterior medial nucleus of thalamus.

Third-order Neurons. The cell bodies of third-order neurons are located in the *ventral posterior medial nucleus of thalamus*. Axons of third-order neurons proceed to terminate in the inferior part of the postcentral gyrus, i.e. the part of sensory cortex called taste cortex (Fig. 11.3-9).

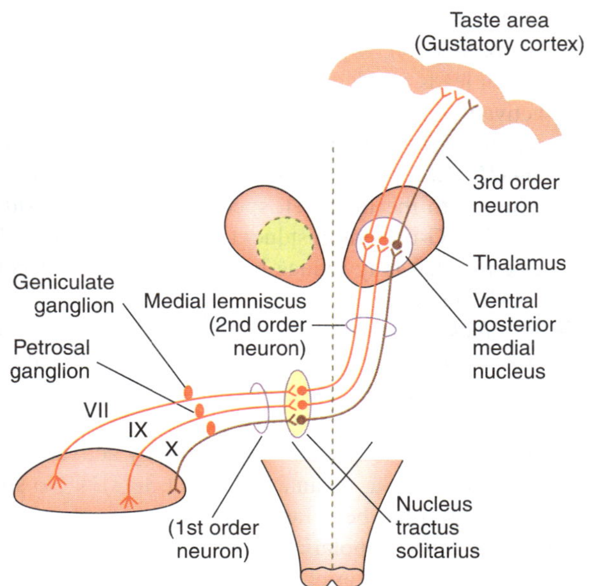

FIGURE 11.3-9 The taste pathways.

Physiology of Taste

Gustatory Stimuli

Types of Stimuli and Most Sensitive Areas of Tongue. As mentioned earlier, the tastebuds containing taste receptors are concerned with perception of sensation of taste. In humans, the tastebuds are located in the three types of gustatory papillae (Fig. 11.3-7). There are about 10,000 tastebuds, which after the age of 45 years start decreasing in number, resulting in blunting of taste sensations in old age.

Conventionally four basic types of taste sensations have been described: *sweet*, *salt*, *sour* and *bitter*. Recently, a fifth stimulus type called *umami* has also been considered in the list of basic tastes. All other taste sensations (hundreds in humans) are assumed to result from various combinations of these five primary (basic) taste sensations. In addition to the above, associated sensations of olfaction, heat, cold and texture contribute for different flavours. Earlier it was believed that there are special areas on the surface of tongue for each of the four conventional basic types of tastes; i.e. the sweet tastes are detected best at the tip of tongue, salty and sour tastes originate from the sides and bitter tastes are sensed best at the base (Fig. 11.3-10). However, it is now clear that all tastes are sensed from all parts of the tongue and adjacent structures containing tastebuds.

Substances Producing Primary (Basic) Taste Sensations
Primary (basic) taste sensations are produced by following (rapid taste producing) substances:

1. ***Sweet sensation*** is produced by a number of organic molecules including sugars, glycols, alcohols, aldehydes,

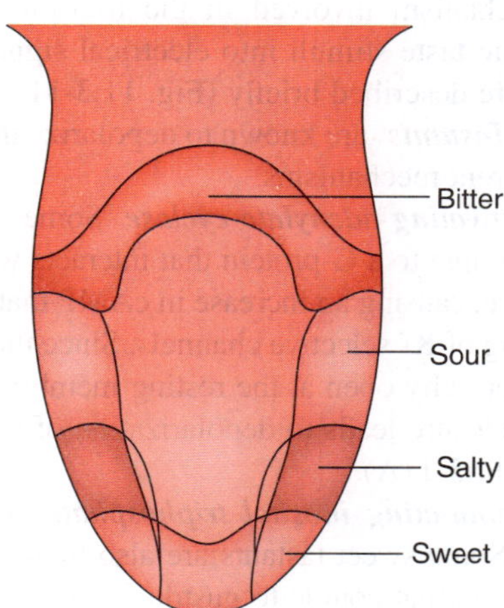

FIGURE 11.3-10 Distribution of four primary taste sensations (according to old view).

esters etc. Saccharin is a chemical 600 times as sweet as sucrose. Being noncalorigenic, it is often used as a sweetening agent for diabetic patients. Tip of the tongue was considered the area most sensitive to sweet stimuli.

2. ***Salty sensation*** is produced by the anions of ionizable salts especially the sodium chloride. The front half of each side of the tongue was thought to be the area most sensitive to salty stimuli (Fig. 11.3-10).
3. ***Sour sensation***. It is produced by acids; and the intensity of this sensation relates, to some degree, to the pH of stimulus solutions. As described above, the posterior half of each side of the tongue was the area considered most sensitive to sour stimuli (Fig.11.3-10).
4. ***Bitter sensation*** is produced by alkaloids such as quinine, caffeine, nicotine and strychnine. Many alkaloids are harmful when swallowed. Perhaps, the highly bitter taste has been given by the nature to these substances to prevent their ingestion by humans and animals.
5. ***Umami sensation***. It has been recently added to the four basic taste sensations. It is produced by glutamate particularly by monosodium glutamate used extensively in Asian cooking. This taste is pleasant and sweet but differs from the standard sweet taste.

Transduction of Gustatory Stimuli Transduction of gustatory stimuli into electrical signals is initiated at the level of receptors. The taste receptors are chemoreceptors which are stimulated by substances dissolved in the mouth by saliva. The dissolved substances act on the microvilli of taste receptors exposed in the taste pore of tastebuds. This interaction typically depolarizes the cell either directly or via the action of second messengers. This causes the development of *receptor potential* in the receptor cell which in turn generates action potential in the sensory nerves. The receptors for different taste modalities have been divided into two major types: Ligand gated channels (Ionotropic) and G protein coupled receptors (metabotropic)

The mechanism involved in the transduction of five types of basic taste stimuli into electrical signals is different. These are described briefly (Fig. 11.3-11):

1. Sweet Tastants are known to depolarize the taste cells by two different mechanisms:

i. ***By activating adenylate cyclase.*** Some sweet receptors couple to a G-protein that interacts with adenylyl cyclase, causing an increase in cAMP that leads to the closing of K^+selective channels. Since these channels are normally open at the resting membrane potential, their closure leads to depolarization of the taste cells (Fig. 11.3-11A).

ii. ***By stimulating inositol triphosphate (IP_3) production.*** Some sweet tastants are also thought to bind to receptors that couple to gustducin or a G-protein that stimulates IP_3 production. The increase in IP_3 is likely to cause the release of Ca^{2+} from intracellular stores.

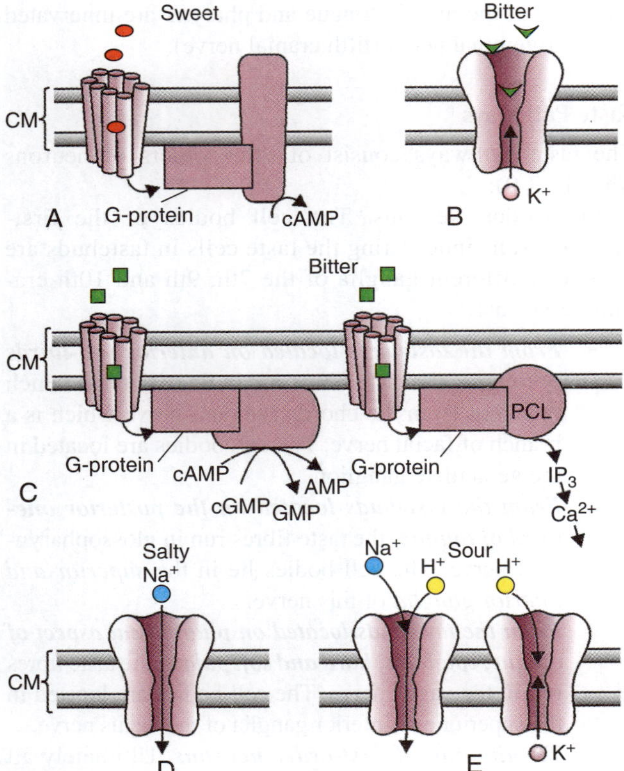

FIGURE 11.3-11 Transduction of basic taste stimuli (tastants) into electrical signals by different mechanisms: **(A)** sweet tastants; **(B** and **C)** bitter tastants; **(D)** salty tastants and **(E)** sour tastants (for details see text).

2. Bitter tastants are known to depolarize the taste cells by three different mechanisms (Fig. 11.3-11 B and C).

i. ***By stimulating inositol triphosphate (IP_3) production***. Some bitter tastants are thought to bind to receptors that couple to G-protein which stimulates IP_3 production. IP_3increases intracellular Ca^{2+} level, which leads to release of synaptic transmitter and the activation of the gustatory nerve fibre.

ii. ***By lowering intracellular levels of cAMP and cGMP.*** Receptors for some bitter tastants may be coupled to the taste cell-specific G-protein gustducin. The G-protein gustducin activates a phosphodiesterase that may reduce intracellular levels of both cAMP and cGMP.

iii. ***By blocking apical K^+ channel.*** At least one bitter stimuli, the quinine may depolarize the taste cells by blocking apical K^+ channels.

3. Salty Tastants depolarize taste cells by activating an amiloride-sensitive Na^+ channel. (Fig. 11.3-11D). No specific Na^+ receptor has been identified.

4. Sour Tastants depolarize the taste cells by permiation or blockade of apical ion channels by proteins. As shown in Figure 11.3-11E, sour taste can result from either the passage of H^+ through amiloride-sensitive Na^+ channels or from the blockade of K^+ channels, which are normally open at resting membrane potential.

5. Umami Taste is transduced by a specific type of truncated metabotopic glutamate receptor (mGluR4), and the agonists are purine 5-ribonucleotides such as AMP and GMP in the food. The way this produces depolarization is unsettled.

Transmission of Information about Taste to the Cortex

The detection of tastants is transduced into a receptor potential that induces action potentials in the taste cell and the release of neurotransmitter at synapses formed between the taste cell and sensory fibres. Each sensory fibre contacts a number of taste cells and each taste cell synapses with numerous sensory fibres. Thus the electrical activity recorded from a single sensory fibre represents the input of many taste cells. As described in the taste pathway (page 1199 Fig. 11.3-9), the signals carried by sensory fibres that innervate the tastebuds travel through several different nerves to the gustatory area of the nucleus of the solitary tract, which relay information to the thalamus. The thalamus transmits taste information to the gustatory cortex.

Encoding of Taste Information As described above, each sensory fibre carries information derived from a variety of taste stimuli. However, each fibre responds best to one of the five primary taste qualities. Thus, the encoding of a gustatory sensation is not a simple, labelled-line, chemical sensory system, instead, the identity of a taste stimulus appears to be encoded by a unique pattern of inputs from many separate fibres that provide components of the patterns for different stimuli. In this respect, taste coding may resemble sensory information coding in other systems, including the visual and auditory systems, where late steps in the processing of information involve a comparison of the activity of different cells that respond preferentially, but not exclusively, to certain features of sensory stimuli.

Taste Thresholds and Intensity Discriminations

Taste Threshold refers to minimum concentration at which a substance can be perceived . To be recognized as salty a substance need only be 0.01 M, whereas for quinine to be perceived as bitter, its concentration need only be 0.000008 M. This correlates with the notion that bitter serves a protective function against dangerous alkaloids, thus its intensity is high. The threshold concentration of some substances to which the tastebuds respond is shown in Table 11.3-2.

Intensity Discrimination. The ability of humans to discriminate differences in the intensity of tastes, like intensity discrimination in olfaction, is crude. A 50% change in the concentration of the substances being tasted is necessary before an intensity difference can be detected. Women are more sensitive to sweet and salt and less sensitive to sour.

TABLE 11.3-2 Threshold Concentration of Some Taste-Producing Substances

Substance	Taste	Threshold concentration (μmol/L)
Hydrochloric acid	Sour	100
Sodium chloride	Salt	2000
Strychnine hydrochloride	Bitter	1.6
Quinine	Bitter	8
Glucose	Sweet	80,000
Sucrose	Sweet	10,000
Saccharine	Sweet	23

Sensation of Flavours The multitude of different sensation of flavours that one experiences results from a combination of gustatory, olfactory and somatosensory inputs.

- ***Gustatory inputs***. The almost infinite variety of tastes are synthesized from the five basic taste components described earlier.
- ***Olfactory inputs*** are responsible for much of what we think as the flavour of foods. Volatile molecules released from foods or beverages in the mouth are pumped into the back of nasal cavity (retronasally) by the tongue, cheek and throat movements that accompany chewing and swallowing. Although the olfactory epithelium of the nose clearly makes a major contribution to sensations of taste, we experience taste as being in the mouth, not in the nose. It is thought that the somatosensory system is involved in this localization and that the coincidence between somatosensory stimulation of the tongue and retronasal passage of odorants into the nose causes the odorants to be perceived as flavours in the mouth.
- ***Somatosensory input*** frequently contributes to the sensation of flavour. This component includes the texture (consistency) and temperature of foods as well as pain sensations evoked by spicy and minty foods and by carbonation.

Phenomenon of Variation and After Effects in Taste Sensations It has been reported that taste sensations exhibit after reactions and contrast phenomena. These are similar in some way to visual after images and contrasts. Some of these occur due to chemical tricks, while others are considered to be the result of a true *central phenomenon.*

Factors Influencing Taste Sensation

1. Area of Stimulation. The perception of sense of taste is directly proportional to the area of tastebuds stimulated. Therefore, stimulation of a small area of the tongue by one drop of solution produces weaker sensation than the same solution by the whole mouth.

2. Temperature of the Tastant. An optimal response to taste producing substances is obtained when their temperature is between 30 and 40°C.

3. Age of the Person. After the age of 45 years, the number of tastebuds start decreasing resulting in the blunting of sensation of taste.

4. Sex. In general, women are more sensitive to sweet and salt and less sensitive to sour.

5. Adaptation. Taste sensation adapts rapidly when taste producing substance is kept for a long time in one place in the mouth. The adaptation is peripheral. Further adaptation to one acid produces adaptation to other acids, because H^+ is the stimulus in all cases.

6. Interaction between Taste Producing Substances also affects taste sensation. For example, the reduction of sour taste of fruits by sucrose is a well-known phenomenon.

7. Effect of Taste Modifying Proteins. A taste modifier protein, *miraculin*, has been discovered in a West African plant. When applied to tongue, this protein makes acids taste sweet.

8. Abnormalities of Taste Sensations obviously affect the various taste sensations.

Abnormalities of Taste Sensations

1. Ageusia. Ageusia refers to absence of taste sensation. ***Causes*** of ageusia are:

- *Lesions of mandibular* division of trigeminal nerve (through lingual branch of which the chorda tympani nerve reaches the tongue) cause loss of taste sensations in the anterior two-thirds of tongue.
- *Lesions of facial nerve* also leads to loss of taste sensations in the anterior two-thirds of tongue.
- *Lesions of glossopharyngeal nerve* are associated with absence of taste sensations from the posterior one-third of the tongue.
- *Drugs* likecisplatin, captopril and penicillamine, which contain sulphydryl groups, cause temporary loss of taste sensation. The reason for this effect of sulphydryl compounds is not known.
- *Familial dysautonomia*. It is a congenital widespread sensory disorder characterized by absence of taste sensations associated with other abnormalities such as postural hypotension, lacrimation, hyporeflexia and insensitivity to temperature and noxious stimuli.

2. Hypogeusia. Hypogeusia refers to diminished taste sensitivity. In it, the taste sensations are not completely lost but there occurs an increase in the threshold for different taste sensations. Many different conditions can produce hypogeusia are deficiency of vitamin B_{12} or zinc, tobacco chewing and aging.

3. Dysgeusia. Dysgeusia refers to disturbed sense of taste. It is a feature of temporal lobe syndrome, particularly when the anterior region of the temporal lobe is affected. Patient usually experiences paroxysmal hallucinations of taste and smell, which are usually unpleasant.

4. Selective Taste Blindness. Selective taste blindness is an inherited autosomal recessive trait characterized by markedly elevated threshold for phenyl thiocarbamide, i.e. PTC, (a chemical substance with very bitter taste). Such individuals are called *non-taster for PTC*. The defect is highly selective since there is no taste blindness to other substances producing bitter taste and to the substances producing salty, sour or sweet tastes. Probably, there is a particular receptor protein, which is not synthesized in these individuals.

5. Hypersensitivity to Taste particularly to bitter taste is called supertasters.

6. Taste Disturbances also occur in conditions in which levels of norepinephrine and serotonin are altered (e.g. during anxiety and depression) because these substances act as neuromodulators, thus contribute towards altered taste threshold.

Part III

Specialized Integrative Physiology

Section

Section 12

Specialized Integrative Physiology

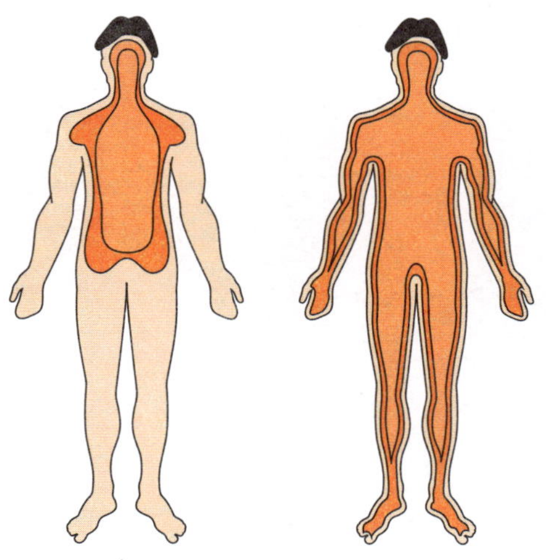

This section includes chapters on miscellaneous topics and not on different physiological aspects related to each other as is in the case of systemic physiology. In systemic physiology, each section, say for example the section on '*Respiratory System*', includes various chapters dealing with the different aspects of respiration. The only similarity between the various physiological aspects discussed in different chapters of this section is that each involves an integrated role of two or more than two systems to perform a highly specialized physiological activity. For instance, '*Physiology of Exercise*' includes integrated role of physiological activities related to skeletal muscle system, respiratory system, cardiovascular system, endocrinal and nervous system. Similarly, the chapter on '*Physiology of Body Temperature Regulation*' highlights the nicely integrated role of cardiovascular system, respiratory system, skin and the nervous system to perform the highly specialized task of regulating the body temperature. In other words, this section is perfect demonstration of unity in diversity. Various diverse aspects of physiology discussed in this section are enumerated above.

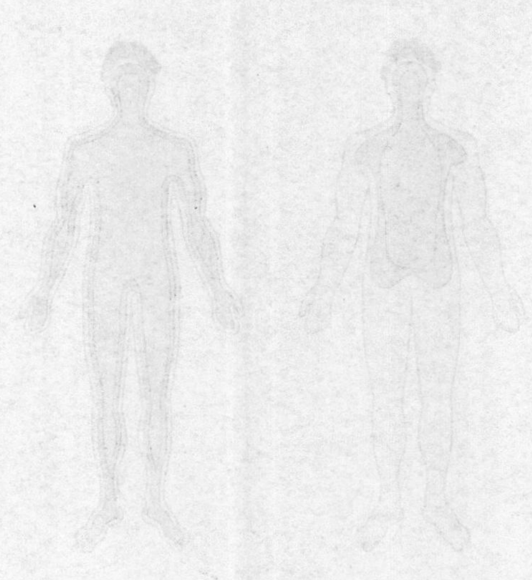

Chapter 12.1

Physiology of Exercise and Sports

INTRODUCTION

Physiology of exercise has generated significant interest and has gained importance because of:

- The current concern with physical conditioning and improvement in performance of athletes, sports persons, military and paramilitary personnel all over the world,
- Role of exercise in prevention of cardiovascular diseases and physical fitness of population groups,
- Role of exercise (stress tests) in evaluation of the cardiovascular and respiratory systems and
- Role of exercise in rehabilitation of the cardiac invalids.

Exercise: Types and Grading

Exercise, to be more precise, muscular exercise, is a period of enhanced energy expenditure by skeletal muscles, which is met by many complex adjustments of metabolism, respiration, circulation and temperature regulation.

Types of Exercise Exercise may be dynamic or isotonic and static or isometric.

Dynamic exercise involves isotonic muscle contractions. External work is involved in this type of exercise.

Static exercise involves isometric muscle contractions.

Quite a few changes in exercise depend on whether the exercise is predominantly isotonic or isometric. The differences in the two forms of exercise originate because isotonic exercise is associated with a fall in peripheral resistance, while isometric exercise is associated with a rise in peripheral resistance. The differences in the responses to two types of exercise will be summarized later.

Grading of Exercise WHO (1978) has classified muscular exercise into four grades depending upon the heart rate and oxygen consumption. Oxygen consumption can be expressed as litres per minute or as relative load index (RLI), i.e. percentage of maximum O_2 utilization. The oxygen utilization can also be expressed as MET (metabolic energy expenditure) test. One MET is equivalent to resting O_2 uptake of 250 ml/min for an average adult man and 200 ml/min for an average woman. Thus, exercise of two METs requires twice the resting metabolism and twice the amount of O_2 per minute and so on. The four grades of exercise are shown in Table 12.1-1.

Note. The figures shown in Table 12.1-1 are true for cold climates. In tropical countries like India, the environmental heat further increases the stress and even in moderate exercise heart rate increases like heavy exercise.

Muscles in Exercise

Muscle strength, power and endurance

For details see page 106.

Muscle metabolic systems in exercise

For details see page 111.

Adjustments to Exercise

Adjustments to physical (muscular) exercise depend upon the type of exercise, grade of exercise, cardiac reserve (i.e. efficiency of the heart), muscle power, training, motivation and the state of nutrition.

Response to exercise. The term 'response to exercise' is used to describe short-term adjustments to a bout of acute

TABLE 12.1-1 Grades of Exercise

	Grade level	Heart rate Beats/min	O_2 consumption L/min	Relative load index (RLI) (% of max. O_2 consumption)	METs
I	Light (mild)	<100	0.4–0.8	<25	<3
II	Moderate	100–125	0.8–1.6	25–50	3.1–4.5
III	Heavy	125–150	1.6–2.4>	51–75	4.6–7
IV	Severe	>150	2.4	>75	>7

exercise, which differ both in quantity and quality in trained and untrained individuals.

Effects of training. The term 'effect of training' is used to describe long-term adjustments (adaptations) to chronic exercise.

RESPONSES TO EXERCISE

Exercise, basically, is a period of enhanced energy expenditure. The energy for muscular exercise is provided by the increased fuel consumption, which is reflected as *greater O_2 consumption and CO_2 production.* The increased O_2 delivery to the tissues and removal of CO_2 from the tissues is achieved by:

- Cardiovascular responses to exercise,
- Respiratory responses to exercise and
- Changes at tissue levels during exercise.

In addition, endocrine responses to exercise occur and play a regulatory role by regulating the water loss and availability of fuel during exercise.

Oxygen Consumption during Exercise

Oxygen Consumption

Oxygen consumption during exercise. The energy for muscular work during exercise is provided by increased fuel consumption, which is reflected in greater O_2 consumption and CO_2 production.

Oxygen consumption (VO_2) during rest is about 250 ml/min, which increases linearly with severity of exercise up to a certain limit, beyond which a plateau is reached (Fig. 12.1-1).

Maximal oxygen consumption (VO_2 max) is the term used to define the level of oxygen consumption beyond which no further increase in O_2 consumption occurs with further increase in the severity of exercise.

- Thus VO_2 max refers to the maximum amount of oxygen that can be consumed by a person while performing severe exercise (irrespective of the demand).

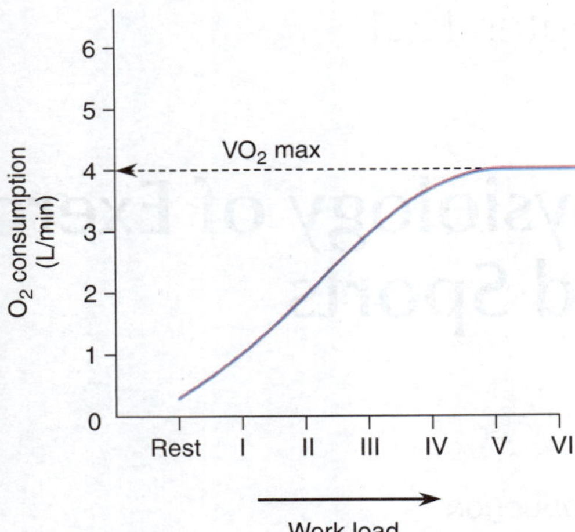

FIGURE 12.1-1 Oxygen consumption during exercise.

- Average VO_2 max in an adult is 3 L/min and in a trained athlete it may be as high as 5 L/min.
- VO_2 max is probably the best physiological indicator of a person's capacity to continue severe work, i.e. it determines the maximum *aerobic work capacity.*
- VO_2 max represents the highest attainable rate of aerobic metabolism during performance of rhythmic muscular work that exhausts the subject within 5–10 min.
- VO_2 max increases during childhood and reaches a peak during early adulthood, after that a gradual and steady decline takes place with the increasing age.
- VO_2 max of a normal individual is limited by the degree to which cardiac output can increase and not by the ventilatory capacity or oxygen diffusion capacity of the lungs. The ability of the active tissues to extract O_2 delivered by circulation or peripheral factors (muscle mass) may be the other possible limiting factors for VO_2 max.

Oxygen Deficit and O_2 Debt

The period of muscular exercise can be divided into three phases (Fig. 12.1-2):

1. Adaptation Phase refers to the beginning of muscular exercise (first 2–4 min) during which oxygen consumption increases linearly and reaches the maximal O_2 consumption (VO_2 max). The VO_2 max at this stage is much less than the oxygen demand; thus an *oxygen deficit* is established at the beginning of exercise which continues throughout the period of exercise. So, the energy requirement over and above the limits of O_2 consumption is met with by the anaerobic pathway.

2. Steady Phase of exercise is characterized by a maximum O_2 consumption (VO_2 max) throughout, i.e. a plateau phase of O_2 consumption and work done relationship. During this phase also, as mentioned above, the excess

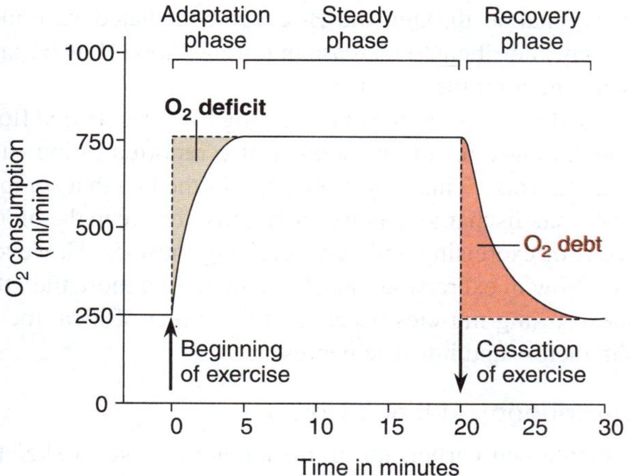

FIGURE 12.1-2 Oxygen deficit and oxygen debt.

energy requirement is met with by the anaerobic pathway, i.e. by breakdown of creatine phosphate and muscle glycogen. As a result of anaerobic release of energy in the muscles, the blood levels of lactic acid begin to rise steeply when the oxygen consumption exceeds 2 L/min (Fig. 12.1-3). In the blood, lactic acid is buffered by the bicarbonate buffer as:

$$H^+ + HCO_3^- \Leftrightarrow H_2CO_3 \Leftrightarrow CO_2 + H_2O$$

The extra CO_2 so evolved is removed by hyperventilation. Since CO_2 evolved is more than O_2 consumed, the respiratory quotient (CO_2 evolved/O_2 consumed) may reach 1.5–2 during severe exercise.

The anaerobic mechanism of energy release permits an individual to utilize energy far in excess of the capacity for oxidative metabolism. The amount of energy that a person may draw from the anaerobic metabolism in the muscle is limited by his tolerance for metabolic acidosis produced by the lactic acid. Trained athletes have greater tolerance for lactoacidosis than untrained individuals. Further, trained athletes produce smaller amounts of lactic acid for a given amount of submaximal work than an untrained individual.

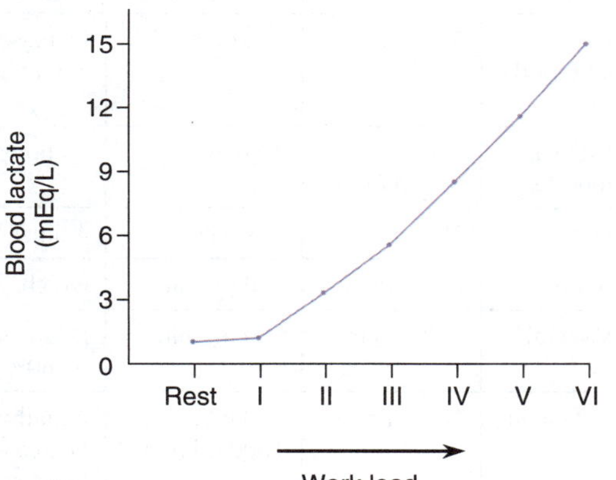

FIGURE 12.1-3 The relationship between blood lactate and severity of exercise.

3. Recovery Phase refers to the period after cessation of exercise during which extra amount of O_2 is consumed. The amount of extra O_2 consumed during recovery phase is called O_2 debt and is proportionate to the extent to which energy demands during exercise exceeded the capacity of aerobic synthesis of energy store, i.e. the extent to which *oxygen deficit* occurred during exercise. In other words, the O_2 deficit that occurs during exercise is repaid during the recovery phase, in the form of O_2 debt. The extra amount of O_2 consumed during recovery phase (O_2 debt) is used:

- To remove the excess lactate collected due to anaerobic glucose breakdown,
- To replenish the ATP and phosphoryl creatine store,
- To replace the small amounts of O_2 that has come from myoglobin and
- To resupply dissolved O_2 in tissue fluids and blood.

During recovery phase the respiratory quotient falls to low values since CO_2 is retained to form $HCO^-{}_3$ and lactate is mobilized by the Cori's cycle.

Cardiovascular Responses to Exercise

To meet the increased energy demand of muscles during exercise, the primary cardiovascular response is in the form of:

- Increase in the skeletal muscle blood flow,
- Redistribution of blood flow in the body,
- Increase in the cardiac output,
- Blood pressure changes and
- Changes in blood volume.

Skeletal Muscle Blood Flow

At rest the blood flow to the skeletal muscle is about 2–4 ml/100 g/min of muscle tissue. Since the whole body skeletal muscles weigh about 30 kg in adults, the total blood flow to the body muscles is about 750–800 ml/min which is about one-sixth of the cardiac output at rest. At rest about 20–25% of muscle capillaries have flowing blood.

During exercise. During strenuous exercise muscle blood flow can increase up to 20 times, i.e. about 50–80 ml/100 g/min muscle tissue or over 20 L/min to the whole body skeletal muscle mass. This is called *exercise hyperaemia.* This tremendous increase in muscle blood flow during exercise is made possible by:

- Arteriolar dilatation, and
- Opening up of closed capillaries which greatly increase the surface area and the rate of blood flow. During exercise, the blood flow to the muscle is intermittent (Fig. 4.6-9), because during each contraction, muscle fibres squeeze the blood vessels passing through them and thus the blood flow decreases or even stops. During relaxation period, muscle blood flow increases and

myoglobin acts as an O_2 acceptor and it yields its O_2 to the myofibres during subsequent muscle contraction.

Mechanisms of Increased Blood Flow during Exercise

1. Local Metabolic Control Mechanism is chiefly responsible for the tremendous increase in skeletal muscle blood flow during exercise (exercise hyperaemia) (see page 369). The muscle contraction increases the metabolic rate of tissue, which in turn reduces oxygen concentration in the muscle. The *decreased tissue pO_2* leads on to vasodilation. In addition, in the exercising skeletal muscles, there occurs accumulation of carbon dioxide, lactic acid, potassium ions, and hydrogen ions, and a rise in temperature. Each of these factor acts as a vasodilator. All these factors lead on to dilatation of arterioles and precapillary sphincters, and a 10- to 100-fold increase in the number of open capillaries in the skeletal muscle. The accumulated metabolites also maintain some increase in blood flow during recovery from the exercise.

The regulation of blood flow by local metabolic factors is a self-adjusting mechanism as explained. Vasodilatation increases blood flow, which brings in more oxygen and nutrients, and wash away the accumulated metabolites. When the demand is no longer heavy, the enhanced blood flow tends to reverse the changes which initiated vasodilatation.

2. Neural Control Mechanism. Vessels of the skeletal muscles are supplied by both sympathetic vasoconstrictor and sympathetic vasodilator fibres.

- ***Sympathetic vasoconstrictor control.*** Most of the basal tone of the resistance vessels of skeletal muscle is myogenic with very little contribution by noradrenergic sympathetic nerve fibres. Thus, it is obvious that exercise hyperaemia is independent of sympathetic discharge and is mainly due to metabolic factors as described above.
- ***Sympathetic vasodilator (cholinergic) fibres*** are unique to skeletal muscles. Previously, it was thought that these fibres are stimulated due to sympathetic overactivity in exercise and increase the blood flow to the muscles. However, now it has been established that the sympathetic vasodilator fibres dilate only the arterioles and not the precapillary sphincters and so do not increase the blood flow to muscles either during or before exercise (see page 338).

3. Humoral Control Mechanism. The skeletal blood vessels contain both α-adrenergic and β-adrenergic receptors. During strenuous exercise, norepinephrine and epinephrine are released into the systemic circulation from adrenal medulla which tend to produce vasoconstriction and vasodilatation by acting on α- and β-receptors, respectively. These two factors counter each other and hence may not contribute significantly to the increased skeletal blood flow during exercise. However, some authors do believe that adrenaline through the β-receptor-mediated vasodilation may contribute to increase in muscle blood flow before, during and after the exercise.

Blood Flow through Nonexercising Muscles Blood flow through nonexercising muscles is also reported to increase during exercise. This may be because of the fact that sympathoadrenal discharge may not distinguish between the blood vessels of exercising and nonexercising muscles. However, blood flow in exercising muscles is increased more than the nonexercising muscles because of the effect of local metabolic factors and intrinsic nerves.

Redistribution of Blood Flow

As mentioned earlier, the tremendous increase in skeletal muscle blood flow is possible due to increased cardiac output (discussed later in detail) and redistribution of cardiac output in the following manner (Table 12.1-2):

Coronary Blood Flow at rest is about 250 ml/min (about 70 ml/100 g tissue/min) with 70–80% coefficient of O_2 utilization. During exercise, coronary blood flow is increased by four to five times with 100% O_2 utilization. This occurs due to:

- ***Increased coronary blood flow*** due to sympathetic stimulation by the following mechanisms:
  - Increased activity of heart,
  - Increased cardiac output (≥5-fold) and
  - Increase in mean arterial pressure.
- ***Coronary vasodilatation*** produced by:
  - Catecholamine,
  - Hypoxia,
  - Fall in blood pH and
  - ATP and ADP

TABLE 12.1-2 Redistribution of Cardiac Output in Standing Posture during Exercise

	At rest	During heavy exercise	Change
Cardiac output Blood flow to	5 L/min	24 L/min	Increased by 5–6 times
• Skeletal muscles	750–800 ml/min	20 L/min	25 times
• Heart	250 ml/min	1 L/min	4 times
• Brain	750 ml/min	750 ml/min	No change
• Visceral	2600 ml/min	500 ml/min	Decreased by 80%
• Cutaneous	500 ml/min	400 ml/min 1000 ml/min	Initially decreased Later increased

Visceral Blood Flow is temporarily curtailed in coordination with increase in muscle blood flow. It is brought about by the increased sympathoadrenal discharge. Renal and splanchnic vessels have only sympathetic noradrenergic vasoconstrictor fibres and they respond to adrenaline with vasoconstriction because they are furnished with α-adrenergic receptors.

Splanchnic Blood Flow is decreased by 80% in severe exercise.

Renal Blood Flow is also decreased by 50–80% in severe exercise. Prolonged, heavy exercise may produce a condition known as *athletic pseudonephritis,* which is characterized by increase in proteins, cells and other abnormal substances in urine. It occurs because:

- Decreased renal blood flow produces glomerular capillary hypoxia and increases permeability to large molecules, and
- Increase in urine proteins in exercise

Cutaneous Blood Flow at rest is about 500 ml/min.

- *Decrease* in cutaneous blood flow occurs initially in the beginning of exercise due to reflex vasoconstriction.
- *Increase* in cutaneous blood flow is noted in sustained exercise when body temperature rises to dissipate the heat generated during exercise, as the blood flow through the skin is controlled predominantly by the requirements of temperature regulation.

Cerebral Blood Flow at rest is about 750 ml/min and remains unchanged during any grade of muscular exercise. This is because the blood flow through brain is governed primarily by local metabolites.

Adipose Tissue Blood Flow is increased by four times during exercise. This helps to deliver fatty acids mobilized from triglyceride stores to the working muscles.

Increase in Cardiac Output

Normal cardiac output is about 5–6 L/min. During exercise, the cardiac output is increased depending upon the severity of exercise. In maximum exercise it may increase by five to six times. Maximal cardiac output is greater in conditioned athletes than in unconditioned individuals (e.g. 30–35 L/min in Olympic-class runners compared with 15 L/min in unconditioned adults). Since cardiac output is the product of heart rate and stroke volume, an increase in both contributes to the increase in cardiac output during exercise (Fig. 12.1-4).

Increase in Heart Rate Heart rate increases linearly with the severity of exercise (Fig. 12.1-4) up to a maximum, which is determined by the subject's age. The *maximum heart rate* (HR max) is approximately equal to 210 − (0.65 × age in years), and is *unaffected by conditioning.* Increase in the heart rate causes palpitation that everyone has personally experienced during exercise. The increase in heart rate occurs as soon as exercise begins or may be seen even before the exercise begins (anticipatory tachycardia).

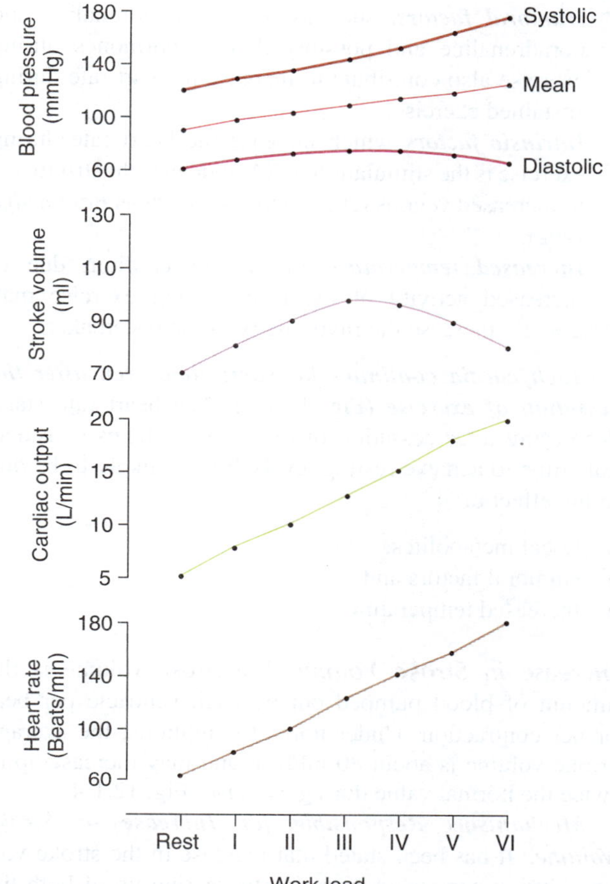

FIGURE 12.1-4 Effect of severity of muscular exercise on cardiovascular functions.

Factors Contributing to Tachycardia during exercise are:

- ***Increased sympathetic discharge*** which originates centrally, probably from the subthalamic movement centre whenever there is an increase in motor activity is responsible for tachycardia. Even the thought of exercise stimulates the hypothalamic defence area, bringing about intense sympathetic discharge and causing anticipatory tachycardia.
- ***Peripheral reflexes*** originating from the exercising muscles (muscle spindles, muscle-tendon receptors and organ of Corti) and joints are responsible for the increase in heart rate which occurs as soon as exercise begins.
- ***Local metabolic factors*** possibly contribute to the sustained increase in heart rate during prolonged exercise. Muscle tissue has free nerve endings that are stimulated by lactic acid, potassium ions and other metabolites, which collect in exercising muscles.

- ***Humoral factors,*** such as release of adrenaline and noradrenaline and possibly thyroid hormones during exercise also contribute to increase in heart rate during sustained exercise.
- ***Intrinsic factors*** which increase the heart rate during exercise is the stimulation of SA node in right atrium due to increased venous return. This is known as *Bainbridge reflex.*
- ***Increased temperature*** in the myocardium due to increased activity of the heart during exercise may directly increase the rhythmicity of the pacemaker.

Tachycardia continues for some time even after the cessation of exercise **(**Fig. 12.1-5**).** The heart rate starts decreasing after cessation of exercise but takes considerable time to achieve resting levels. This is likely to be due to the effect of:

- Local metabolites,
- Humoral factors and
- Increased temperature.

Increase in Stroke Volume The stroke volume is the amount of blood pumped out by each ventricle per beat or per contraction. Under normal conditions, the average stroke volume is about 80 ml/beat and may increase up to twice the normal value during exercise (Fig. 12.1-4).

Mechanisms Responsible for Increase in Stroke Volume. It has been stated that increase in the stroke volume during exercise occurs due to gearing up of both the control mechanisms, i.e.

- Intrinsic autoregulation or Frank–Starling mechanism (for details see page 288).
- Extrinsic regulation or autonomic and neural mechanism (for details see page 291) as explained:
  - ***In mild to moderate exercise,*** actual measurements of end-diastolic volume (EDV) and end-systolic volume (ESV) have revealed no change or even a decrease in EDV. At the same time, there is evidence of increased sympathetic discharge to the heart in the form of increased heart rate. It has been explained that *increased venous return* produced by skeletal vasodilatation, muscle pump action and increased respiration (thoracic pump) is tackled by *improved pumping of the heart* due to sympathetic activity and so the Frank–Starling mechanism does not operate. Therefore, it can be concluded that during mild to moderate exercise, the pumping ability of the heart is enhanced mainly by greater sympathetic discharge.
  - ***In severe exercise,*** when venous return is large enough to raise the end-diastolic volume, Frank–Starling mechanism also comes into play over and above the increased sympathetic discharge and thus results in very high cardiac output.
  - ***Important points to note*** are:
    - *Starling's law of heart* does not allow further increase in stroke volume once the heart rate increases to 120/min.
    - *Endurance training increases stroke volume* of the heart by increasing the ventricular end-diastolic volume. Thus, conditioned athletes can maintain any level of cardiac output at a lower heart rate than nonconditioned individuals.

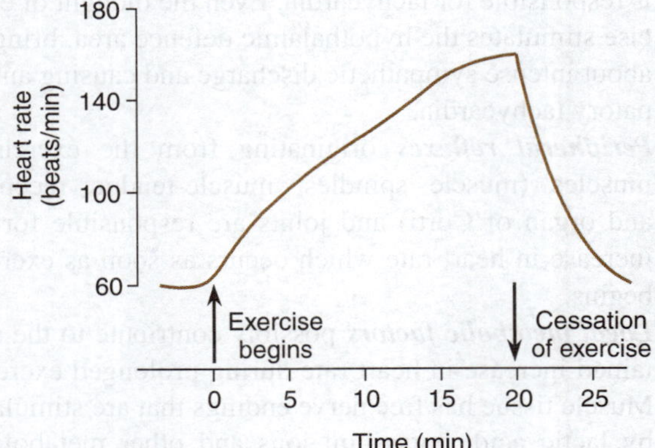

FIGURE 12.1-5 Heart rate response to moderate exercise.

Blood Pressure Changes during Exercise (Figs 12.1-4, 12.1-6)

In Systemic Circulation ***Systolic blood pressure*** is always raised by exercise, since it depends upon the cardiac output which is increased in exercise. The blood pressure remains elevated during exercise and is not reflexly corrected by baroreceptor reflex. This has been explained by the fact that the neurons descending from the hypothalamic defence centre inhibit the baroreceptor afferents.

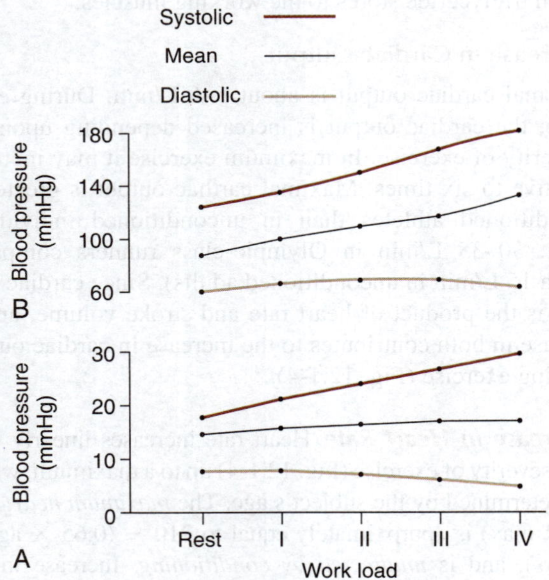

FIGURE 12.1-6 Blood pressure response to exercise: **A,** pulmonary; and **B,** systemic.

Diastolic blood pressure which primarily depends upon the peripheral resistance may mildly increase or decrease or remain unchanged depending upon the change in total peripheral resistance. Mostly the vasodilatation in the skeletal muscles balances the vasoconstriction in other tissues, so the diastolic blood pressure is usually not changed much.

Mean blood pressure is usually increased. It helps to increase the skeletal muscle blood flow by providing greater pressure head in the face of dilated resistance vessels.

In Pulmonary Circulation Pressure in the pulmonary artery does not rise much during exercise due to intrathoracic location of blood vessels which provide low resistance to blood flow, and due to marked increase in the number of open capillaries in lungs during exercise.

Systolic blood pressure in pulmonary artery may rise during heavy exercise to 25–30 mmHg from 15–20 mmHg at rest,

Diastolic blood pressure may rise from 5–8 mmHg at rest to 8–10 mmHg and

Mean blood pressure may reach to 15 mmHg from 8–12 mmHg at rest.

Changes in Blood Volume during Exercise

Blood volume during exercise is decreased by 15% resulting in haemoconcentration. Blood volume is decreased due to more plasma loss at the capillary level due to the following reasons:

- Increased hydrostatic pressure in capillaries, and
- Increased tissue fluid osmotic pressure due to accumulation of osmotically active metabolites in tissue spaces such as potassium, phosphate and lactic acid.

Advantages

- *Oxygen-carrying capacity of blood* is increased because of increased concentration of red blood cells.
- *Buffering capacity of blood* is increased due to increased concentration of plasma proteins.

Disadvantages

- *Blood flow decreases* due to increased viscosity of blood, and
- *WBC count increases* due to washing out of WBCs from storage places and bone marrow.

Summary of Cardiovascular Responses to Exercise

The cardiovascular responses to exercise are summarized in Fig. 12.1-7.

Respiratory Responses to Exercise

Exercise is the most frequently faced stress by the respiratory system in day-to-day life. During heavy exercise, up to 25-fold increase in O_2 consumption and CO_2 production may occur. The O_2 consumption does not decrease with training at any work load (i.e. training does not improve the body's efficiency unless muscle co-ordination is improved by practice). The respiratory system meets this metabolic demand so well that alveolar and arterial pO_2 and pCO_2 are practically maintained normal even during the most strenuous exercise. This is made possible by following respiratory responses to exercise:

I. Increase in Pulmonary Ventilation

The pulmonary ventilation increases linearly with the increase in intensity of exercise (O_2 consumption) until the anaerobic threshold is reached (Fig. 12.1-8). Anaerobic threshold is defined as the level of activity (exercise) that produces an elevation of blood lactate levels, which results from a shift from aerobic to anaerobic metabolism. The anaerobic threshold occurs at higher level of activity in conditioned athletes than in unconditioned individuals. The anaerobic threshold occurs at approximately 60% of the maximal exercise level, regardless of the level of physical fitness (Fig. 12.1-8). Above the anaerobic threshold, the pulmonary ventilation increases out of proportion to the increase in O_2 consumption because lactic acid that is generated imposes an additional respiratory drive. During this period the arterial pCO_2 may drop significantly, because excretion of CO_2 exceeds production (Fig. 12.1-8).

Pulmonary ventilation increases because of increase in depth as well as rate of respiration. As the severity of exercise is gradually increased, the depth of breathing (tidal volume) rapidly increases to an optimum value, beyond which ventilation is chiefly increased by increase in the rate of respiration. During quiet breathing at rest, the respiratory rate is about 12–14/min and the tidal volume is about 0.5 L and hence the pulmonary ventilation is about 12 to $14 \times 0.5 = 6$ to 7 L/min. During heavy exercise, the rate of respiration may increase to 40/min and the tidal volume to 2.5 L, increasing pulmonary ventilation to $40 \times 2.5 = 100$ L/min. Even during most strenuous exercise, pulmonary ventilation is seldom more than 100–120 L/min, i.e. it remains far below the maximum breathing capacity of the individual

Mechanism of Increased Pulmonary Ventilation Mechanism of increased pulmonary ventilation is still not fully understood. There are several factors which can explain a part of it, but not even all the known factors can account for the marked increase in pulmonary ventilation occurring in severe exercise. The probable factors are:

1. Neural Control Mechanisms have been suggested to play the main role than chemical mechanisms in increasing pulmonary ventilation during exercise. It has been supported by the observation that pulmonary ventilation increases abruptly just at the beginning of the exercise, followed by a further gradual increase as the exercise is continued. At the end of exercise, there occurs an abrupt moderate decrease followed by further decline during recovery period

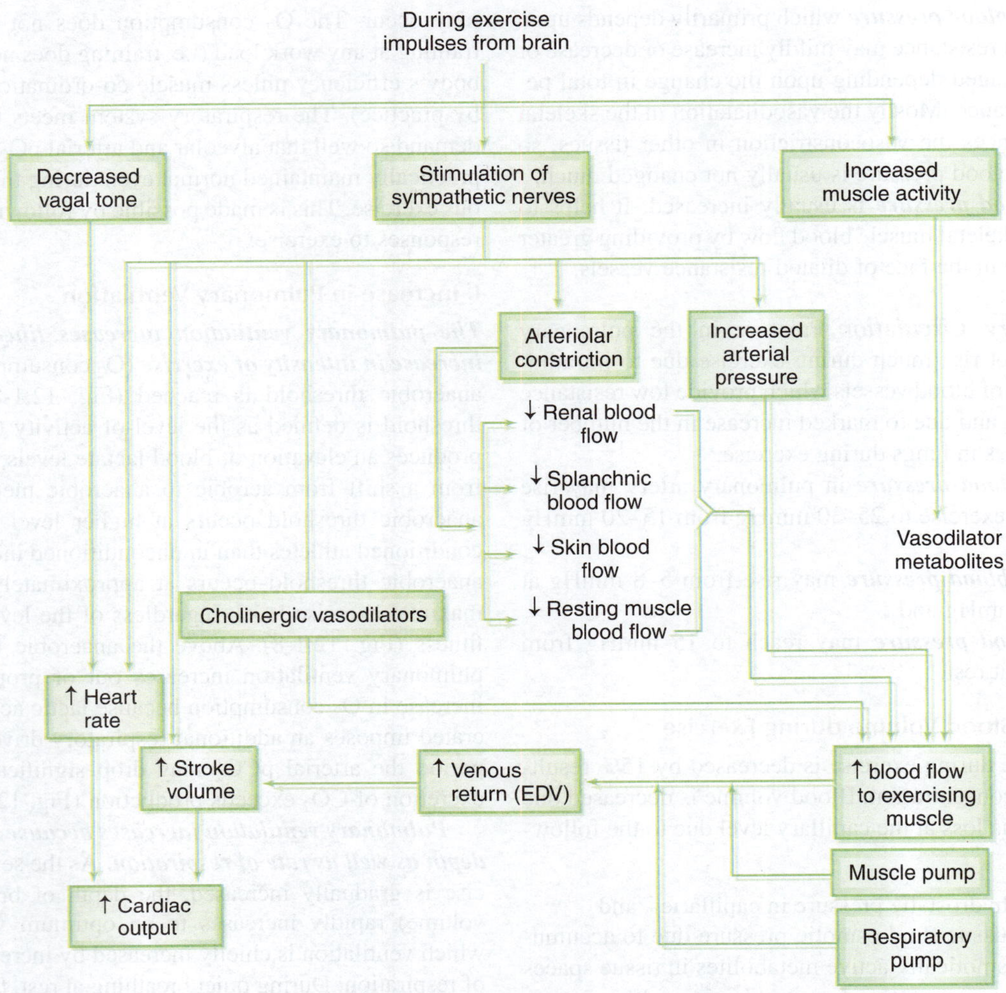

FIGURE 12.1-7 Summary of cardiovascular responses to exercise.

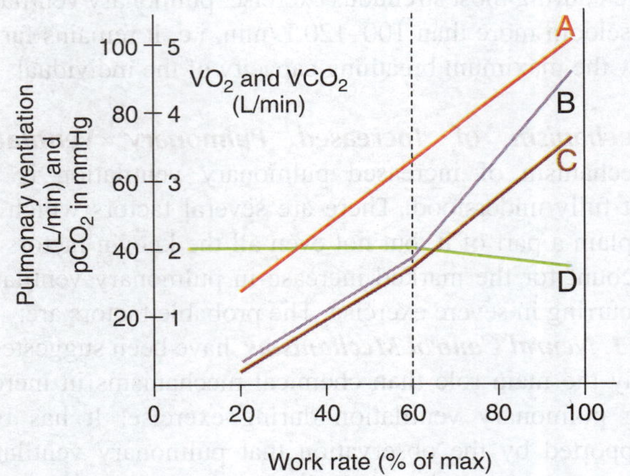

FIGURE 12.1-8 The effect of exercise on respiratory parameters of gas exchange: **A,** pulmonary ventilation; **B,** CO_2 excretion in expired air (VCO_2); **C,** oxygen consumption (VO_2); and **D,** arterial pCO_2. The dashed line indicates onset of anaerobic threshold.

(Fig. 12.1-9). The abrupt beginning and decline in pulmonary ventilation supports that some neuronal rather than chemical mechanism is responsible for it.

Neural control mechanisms which have been suggested to make contribution to exercise hyperpnoea are:

- ***Cerebral cortex,*** the seat of conscious thought and voluntary activity may be responsible for the anticipatory hyperpnoea, which may occur due to psychic stimuli just before the beginning of exercise.
- ***Afferent impulses from proprioceptors*** in the muscles and joints are at least partly responsible for exercise hyperpnoea.
- ***Increase in body temperature*** during sustained exercise may also make some contribution to exercise hyperpnoea through neural mechanism.

2. Chemical Mechanism does not play the main role in exercise hyperpnoea, as the alveolar and arterial pO_2 and

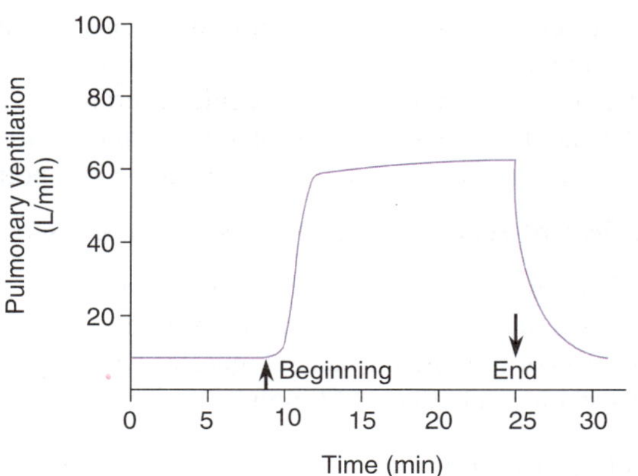

FIGURE 12.1-9 Ventilatory response to mild exercise showing abrupt change at beginning and at the end of exercise.

pCO_2 are well maintained during exercise. The following roles have been suggested, however:

- ***Accentuations of the normal oscillations*** in pO_2 and pCO_2 synchronous with respiration might stimulate the carotid body chemoreceptors and explain part of exercise hyperpnoea.
- ***Acidosis produced due to accumulation of lactic acid*** during severe exercise (above the aerobic threshold level) is responsible for increase in pulmonary ventilation which is out of proportion to the O_2 consumption. During this period, arterial pCO_2 may drop significantly.

3. Humoral Mechanisms are not reported to play any role in exercise hyperpnoea.

II. Increase in Oxygen Uptake in the Lungs

The oxygen uptake by blood in the lungs increases from 250 ml/min at rest to about 4 L/min during heavy exercise. This is made possible by the following changes:

1. Increased Pulmonary Perfusion. This happens due to increase in cardiac output from 5 L/min at rest to about 30 L/min during heavy exercise. This applies as much to the right ventricle as the left. Thus, during exercise about six times more blood passes through the lungs per minute and so more O_2 per minute is carried by the blood from the lungs.

2. Increased Alveolar Capillary pO_2 Gradient. During exercise, because of greater extraction of O_2 by the muscles, the O_2 content of the mixed venous blood reaching the lungs may be as low as 3 ml/100 ml of blood (compared with 14–15 ml% at rest). Thus the alveolar capillary pO_2 gradient is increased due to marked desaturation of the venous blood and so more O_2 is taken up by the blood in the lungs.

3. Increased Pulmonary Diffusion Capacity. About sixfold increase in pulmonary blood flow due to increased cardiac output during exercise is not accompanied by rise in the pressure in the pulmonary capillaries. This is made possible by the opening of several pulmonary capillaries which are closed at rest. As a result, the alveoli are better perfused with blood. The larger number of open up capillaries increases the surface area available for diffusion. In this way, there occurs threefold increase in the diffusion capacity of the lungs from 21 ml/min/mmHg at rest to about 65 ml/min/mmHg during exercise.

Changes at the Tissue Level

The cardiovascular and respiratory changes described above supply large amounts of O_2 from the alveolar air to the blood and remove equally huge amounts of CO_2 from the blood to the alveoli and ultimately to the atmosphere. The changes at the tissue level which facilitate transfer of large amount of O_2 from the blood to the exercising muscles and that of CO_2 from the tissues to the blood are:

- ***Blood Flow*** to the skeletal muscles is increased from 2–4 ml/min/100 g of muscles during strenuous exercise. Increased blood flow brings more O_2 to the tissue per minute. *Capillary bed* of the contracting muscles is dilated and many previously closed capillaries are open. Because of these changes, the mean distance from the blood to the tissue cells is greatly decreased; this facilitates movement of O_2 from the blood to the cells.
- ***Gradient of pO_2*** between capillary blood and tissue fluid is increased. This happens because during exercise contracting muscles extract more O_2 from tissue fluid. Due to increased gradient of pO_2 between capillaries and tissue fluid, more O_2 is removed from the capillary blood into the tissue fluid.
- ***O_2-Hb Dissociation Curve*** shifts to the right due to accumulation of CO_2, rise in temperature and rise in red blood cell 2,3-DPG. This results in a threefold increase in O_2 extraction from each unit of blood. Since there is associated (about 30-fold) increase in muscle blood flow (as mentioned above), so a net increase of about 100-fold in metabolic rate of muscle is possible during exercise.

Endocrinal Responses to Exercise

Endocrines play an important role in adjustment to exercise. However, it has still not been fully elucidated. The hormones that are increased during exercise along with the role played by them are given.

1. Antidiuretic Hormone (ADH) secretion is markedly increased during exercise. It helps to maintain fluid balance by reducing urine flow so that enough fluid is available for excessive sweating required to dissipate heat.

2. Adrenocorticotrophic Hormone (ACTH) is released during endurance events and probably helps by mobilizing fats for providing energy directly as well as by stimulating glucocorticoid secretion.

3. Endorphin secretion is significantly increased during exercise. They improve tolerance to discomfort associated with exercise by relieving pain. They also relieve mental stress and induce a feeling of well-being.

4. Cortisol secreted during exercise is helpful in reducing exercising stress. It also mobilizes proteins and fats. Fatty acids are particularly useful as fuel during exercise. Consequently, carbohydrates are spared to be used by the brain.

5. Aldosterone secreted during exercise reduces urinary loss of water and sodium like ADH. This helps to maintain fluid balance in the presence of excessive sweating during exercise.

6. Adrenaline and Noradrenaline secretion is increased significantly in intense exercise. These hormones mobilize fatty acids and glucose and thus improve the availability of fuel.

7. Insulin secretion is decreased during exercise. However, due to training tissue, sensitivity to insulin improves at rest and decreases during exercise. The improved sensitivity at rest accounts for the improvement in glucose tolerance test seen as a result of regular exercise. Because of this effect, exercise is considered one of the most useful components for the treatment of diabetes.

8. Glucagon. Prolonged exercise stimulates secretion of glucagon. It mobilizes glucose from glycogen and fatty acids from the adipose tissue, and thereby improves fuel availability during prolonged exercise.

EFFECTS OF TRAINING

Training to the body tissues is provided by different sets of exercise regimes. Endurance training (aerobic) produces different effects in the skeletal muscles than weight training. Training effects are specific for the particular muscle groups involved. Only aerobic exercises produce cardiovascular conditioning.

Usefulness of training to the body systems is highlighted:

- Training is most essential for the performance by athletes and sports persons, and it forms the main aspect of sports physiology.
- Training by regular physical exercise is likely to slow the ageing process, helps to prevent several degenerative and metabolic diseases and thereby makes life healthier and longer.
- One of the clear-cut benefits of exercise regime is psychological; patients who exercise regularly 'feel better'. Such effects may also be attributed to release of endorphins during exercise. Endorphins are reported to relieve mental stress and induce a sense of well-being, and even euphoria.
- Regular exercise is one of the most useful components of treatment of diabetes because it reduces insulin requirement by virtue of improvement in glucose tolerance.
- There is some evidence that regular exercise decreases the incidence and severity of myocardial infarctions, although there continues to be debate on this point.

Effects of training on the body tissues can be described as:

- Effects of training on cardiovascular system,
- Effects of training on respiratory system,
- Effects of training on skeletal muscles and
- Psychological effects of training.

Effects of Training on Cardiovascular System

Athletic training by regular exercise has a favourable influence on cardiovascular functions. Only aerobic exercises produce cardiovascular conditioning. *Optimal cardiovascular conditioning* requires attaining a heart rate of 60–70% of the maximum for 20–30 min, three to four times a week for at least 3 months. Athletic training produces following effects on the cardiovascular system:

1. Low Resting Heart Rate. Athletic training by some unknown mechanism increases the vagal tone. Consequently, trained athletes have low resting heart (50–60/min). This is useful during exercise because it increases the range through which the heart rate can increase without any change in the maximal heart rate. The maximal heart rate (HR max) is approximately equal to 210 − [0.65 × age in years], and is unaffected by conditioning.

2. Higher Resting Stroke Volume. The aerobic athletic training leads to cardiac hypertrophy and increase in end-diastolic volume which increase the resting stroke volume to about 105 ml compared with about 75 ml in an untrained individual.

3. Much larger Cardiac Output During Exercise. Because of the low resting heart rate and higher resting stroke volume, a trained athlete can achieve much larger cardiac output during exercise than an untrained individual as illustrated in Table 12.1-3 by arbitrary but plausible figures. An Olympic-class runner can achieve a maximal cardiac output of about 30–35 L/min compared with only 15 L/min in unconditioned adults.

Effects of Training on Respiratory System

1. Increase in Maximal Oxygen Consumption The O_2 consumption does not decrease with training at any work load, i.e. training does not improve the body's efficiency unless muscle co-ordination is improved by practice.

Maximal O_2 consumption (VO_2 max) increases by 5–20% by conditioning (athletic training) because of:

- Increase in cardiac output, and
- Increase in arteriovenous O_2 difference. *Values of VO_2* max (arbitrary but plausible) are:
- Average untrained male: 3600 ml/min,

TABLE 12.1-3 Effect of Aerobic Training on Cardiovascular Functions

	At rest		During maximal exercise	
	Untrained individual	*Trained athlete*	*Untrained individual*	*Trained athlete*
Heart rate (beats/min)	72	50	180	180
Stroke volume (ml/beat)	75	100	100	160
Cardiac output (L/min)	5	5	18	29

- Average trained male: 4000 ml/min and
- Male marathon runner = 5100 ml/min.

Of course, the maximum oxygen consumption increases during training, but high values in marathon runners may be partly genetically determined by factors such as large lung capacity in relation to body size and strength of respiratory muscles.

2. Increase in Maximal Minute Ventilation

- Endurance (aerobic) training increases maximal minute ventilation that is achieved during exercise but does not improve the maximum voluntary ventilation.
- Specific respiratory muscle training allows one to increase the duration and intensity of exercise.

3. Increase in Pulmonary Oxygen-Diffusing Capacity The oxygen-diffusing capacity is the rate at which O_2 diffuses from the alveoli into the blood per mmHg oxygen pressure. During exercise, diffusing capacity increases in a nonathlete from a resting value of 23 ml/min/mmHg to 48 ml/min/mmHg. Athletic training allows more increase in diffusion capacity of lungs for oxygen because by training the pulmonary capillary density increases.

4. No effect on Vital Capacity There is no consistent effect of training on vital capacity or other measures of pulmonary function. It implies that, in a healthy individual pulmonary function is usually not a limiting factor in determining the maximum intensity of exercise that one can undertake.

Effects of Training on Skeletal Muscles

Regular muscular exercise may lead on to following changes in the muscles:

Increased Muscle Strength due to training results from:

- *Increase in muscle mass,* which is entirely the result of an increase in the size of muscle fibres (*hypertrophy*) and not due to increase in the number of muscle fibres (hyperplasia). Further, it is observed that increase in muscle strength is out of proportion to the increase in muscle mass. Other factors which contribute to increase in muscle strength are:
- *More effective and efficient deployment of motor units* and
- *Increase in the production of contractile proteins* such as actin and myosin which is mediated by somatomedins. The increased amount of contractile proteins increases the cross-bridges available for generating force during muscle contraction.

Changes in the Muscle Fibres that enhance the capacity of the muscles to extract more O_2 and improve the ability of the muscle fibres to provide energy during prolonged exercise are:

- Increase in the capillary network which is demonstrated as significant increase in the capillary to muscle fibre ratio on muscle biopsy,
- Increase in the number of mitochondria in muscle fibres,
- Increase in the mitochondrial enzymes involved during oxidative metabolism,
- Increase in the muscle glycogen stores and
- Increase in the stored triglycerides.

Fast- and Slow-Twitch Muscle Fibres and Different Types of Exercise ***Fast-twitch muscle fibres*** generate a great amount of power in a short period of time, such as during a sprint. In other words, the fast-twitch fibres give a person the ability to rapidly and forcefully contract their muscles. Fast-twitch fibres are able to generate more power because:

- They are about twice as large in diameter as slow-twitch fibres, and
- The enzymes that release energy from the phosphogen and glycogen lactic acid energy systems are two- to threefold as active in the fast-twitch fibres.

Slow-twitch fibres are used in endurance exercise, i.e. prolonged lower leg muscle activity, such as marathons. The difference in the activities of fast-twitch and slow-twitch muscle fibres is because of following differences between the two types of muscle fibres. Slow-twitch fibres use more for endurance exercise while employing the anaerobic system of energy because in comparison to fast-twitch fibres they contain:

- Higher number of mitochondria,
- More myoglobin, which is a haemoglobin-like substance that combines with oxygen in muscle and
- More capillary density.

Training results in metabolic drift of both fast- and slow-twitch fibres towards the mitochondrial characteristics of slow muscle fibres, which are better suited for endurance events.

Psychological Effects of Training

Regular training improves the psychology of the individual and thus the psychic stimuli to vasomotor centre and respiratory centres are reduced. Consequently, during exercise there occurs:

- Less increase in sympathetic activity and
- Less decrease in parasympathatic activity.

Metabolic Effects of Training

Metabolic adjustments during exercise are the result of increase in energy stores and mitochondrial changes in the muscles described above. Due to these changes, the ability of the muscle to extract oxygen improves and there is shift towards aerobic metabolism, which is more efficient than anaerobic metabolism. Consequently, there is less accumulation of lactic acid and smaller fall in the pH of the body fluids. These changes facilitate mobilization of fatty acids from tissue stores into the blood. Shift in metabolism towards more utilization of fats is a very useful adaptation because fat stores are virtually unlimited compared with the extremely meagre glycogen store. So, fat utilization spares glycogen. As physical performance is a direct function of glycogen stores, endurance of the individual increases.

Summary of Effects of Training

In nutshell physical training decreases the O_2 deficit and thus increases the physical performance or fitness, which is inversely related to O_2 deficit. In summary, the physical training decreases O_2 deficit by the following effects:

1. Increasing maximal O_2 consumption (VO_2 max) because of:
   - Greater increase in cardiac output due to:
     - Low resting heart rate and
     - High resting stroke volume
   - Increase in arteriovenous O_2 difference.
2. Increasing oxygen availability by:
   - Increasing pulmonary diffusion.
3. Enhancing the capacity of the muscles to extract more O_2 due to:
   - Increase in capillary network in the muscle,
   - Increase in number of mitochondria in muscle fibres and
   - Increase in the mitochondrial enzymes.
4. Increasing the strength of muscles by hypertrophy.
5. Increasing the endurance of muscles by:
   - Metabolic changes leading to more utilization of fats as energy store and
   - Sparing of glycogen (physical performance is direct function of glycogen stores).
6. Psychological improvement makes it possible to perform better during exercise with:
   - Less increase in sympathetic activity and
   - Less decrease in parasympathetic activity.

All the aforementioned factors help in decreasing the dependence on anaerobic mechanism.

Chapter 12.2

Environmental Physiology

HIGH-ALTITUDE PHYSIOLOGY

Introduction

Atmosphere refers to the medium in which aerospace physiology occurs. This is divided into the following major zones:

- *Troposphere* extends from sea level to about 18 km (58,000 ft)
- *Stratosphere* extends from 18 to 50 km. The so-called *ozone layer* is found between 12 and 44 km.
- *Mesosphere* extends from 50 to 85 km.
- *Thermosphere* extends from 85 to 700 km.
- *Exosphere* extends beyond 700 km and is called true outer space.

Critical altitudes which are important from the physiological point of view are:

- *At 10,000 ft altitude,* usually no symptoms or some degree of hypoxia may be present, but the body can easily acclimatize to the lack of oxygen. Therefore, *high altitude* is classically defined as an altitude in excess of 10,000 ft (3 km).
- *An altitude of 18,000 ft* is the highest altitude at which permanent inhabitation is possible.
- *Above, 20,000 ft altitude,* hypoxia can endanger life, unless O_2 is added to the inhaled air.
- *At an altitude of about 35,000 ft,* modern aircraft commonly fly. The use of pressurized cabins in these aircraft helps to provide an environment similar to that at sea level.
- *Above 40,000 ft altitude,* the ozone layer starts.

Composition of air and effect of altitude on it. Composition of air (Table 12.2-1) does not change with altitude, i.e. composition of atmosphere (% of gases) remains constant from sea level to about 30,000 ft.

Barometric pressure and partial pressure of gases. Barometric pressure at sea level is 760 mmHg and it falls progressively with the increasing height (Table 12.2-2). With decrease in total pressure of air at increasing altitude, partial pressure of gases will change as:

- *According* to Dalton's law the total pressure of air (*P*) is equal to the sum of partial pressures of the gases contained, i.e. $P = pO_2 + pCO_2 + pN_2 + pH_2O$.
- *pH_2O in alveolar air* at sea level is 47 mmHg (Table 12.2-2). It is entirely determined by the body temperature and does not change with altitude. As the body can regulate and maintain the temperature at 37°C, so pH_2O remains constant at 47 mmHg.
- *pCO_2 in alveolar air* at sea level is 40 mmHg (Table 12.2-2) and depends upon the metabolic production of the body. As the metabolic production of CO_2 does not alter with increasing altitude, so the alveolar pCO_2 does not change with altitude until the breathing is affected by the effect of hypoxia.
- *pO_2 and pN_2 in alveolar air* at sea level are 104 and 569 mmHg, respectively. With increasing altitude there is decrease in total pressure of air. So, the pO_2 and pN_2

TABLE 12.2-1 Concentration and Partial Pressure of Gases in Atmospheric Air and Alveolar Air

	Atmospheric air		Alveolar air	
Gas	*Concentration (%)*	*Partial pressure (mmHg)*	*Concentration (%)*	*Partial pressure (mmHg)*
Nitrogen	78.62	597.0	74.9.	569
Oxygen	20.84	159.0	13.6.	104
Carbon dioxide	0.04	0.3	5.3.	40
Water vapour	0.50	3.7	6.2	47
Total	**100**	**760.0**	**100**	**760**

levels will decrease proportionately (as the pH_2O and pCO_2 remain unchanged).

- *Values of pO_2 in alveolar air and atmospheric* air at different altitudes are shown in Table 12.2-2.
- *Changes in the body at high altitude* are produced mainly by hypoxic *hypoxia* produced by falling pO_2. *Other factors* which produce changes in the body at high altitude are effects of expansion of gases, fall in atmospheric temperature, light rays and gravity.

Hypoxia at High Altitude

The effects of hypoxic hypoxia produced by decreasing pO_2 at high altitude depend upon:

- The level of altitude,
- Rate at which hypoxia develops, i.e. hypoxia occurs due to rapid ascent (acute hypoxia), or slow ascent (subacute hypoxia) and
- Duration of exposure to hypoxia, i.e. whether short-term stay or long-term stay (chronic hypoxia).

Barometric Pressure and pO_2 at Different Altitudes and Its Effect on the Body

The barometric pressure, partial pressure of oxygen (pO_2) and common effects at different altitudes are given in Table 12.2-2.

Stages of Hypoxic Hypoxia. In a classical mould, four stages of hypoxic hypoxia depending upon the value of pO_2 are described (Table 12.2-2):

1. ***Stage of indifference*** is usually characterized by no symptoms of hypoxia as pO_2 remains above 60 mmHg. This occurs up to an altitude of 10,000 ft.
2. ***Stage of reaction*** starts above 10,000 ft altitude and is characterized by development of moderate hypoxia up to 15,000 ft altitude at pO_2 levels of 40–60 mmHg. Hypoxic symptoms include:
   - *Cardiovascular involvement* in the form of tachycardia and hypertension,
   - *Respiratory symptoms* in the form of increased pulmonary ventilation and
   - *Early CNS involvement* in the form of impaired judgement, feeling of overconfidence, talkativeness, reduction in visual acuity and emotional outburst of laughing or crying, etc.
3. ***Stage of disturbance*** occurs when pO_2 values fall between 30 and 40 mmHg, usually between 15,000 and 20,000 ft altitude. It is characterized by development of severe hypoxia. In addition to the symptoms described above, the CNS involvement is aggravated.

Clinical Types of Hypoxic Hypoxia at High Altitude

Clinically, three types of hypoxia occurring at high altitude are described:

1. Fulminating hypoxia,
2. Acute hypoxia and
3. Chronic hypoxia (for details see page 461).

Clinical Syndromes Caused by High Altitude

The three specific entities (clinical syndromes) which need to be discussed in relation to the effects of low pO_2 at high altitude are:

- High-altitude pulmonary oedema (HAPO),
- Acute mountain sickness and
- Chronic mountain sickness.

High-Altitude Pulmonary Oedema High-altitude pulmonary oedema (HAPO) usually occurs as an effect of rapid ascent at high altitude (above 10,000 ft)

Individuals who develop HAPO. It is seen in the following individuals:

- About 75–80% individuals who engage in heavy physical work during the first 3–4 days after rapid ascent to high altitude develop HAPO.
- Individuals who are acclimatized to high altitude, stay for more than 2 weeks at sea level and then rapidly re-ascend at high altitude.

Mechanism of Development of HAPO. Since HAPO does not develop in individuals who ascend slowly at high altitude and avoid physical exertion for the first few days,

TABLE 12.2-2 Barometric Pressure, pO_2 and Common Effects at Different Altitudes

I Level of altitude [ft (km)]	II Barometric pressure (mmHg)	III Atmospheric air pO_2 (mmHg)	IV Alveolar air pO_2 (mmHg)	V Alveolar air pCO_2 (mmHg)	VI % oxygen saturation of haemoglobin	VII Common effects	VIII Stage of hypoxia
0 (sea level)	760	159	104	40	100	NIL	–
5000 (1.5)	630	130	80	40	95	No effects	
10,000 (3)	520	110	60	40	90	Usually no symptoms except at night there may be some reduction in visual capacity	**Stage of indifference** • The rapid ascent up to *10,000 ft is* safe zone of ascent • Classically high altitude is in excess of 10,000 ft • No hypoxia up to pO_2 60 mmHg
15,000 (4.5)	480	90	50	36	80	Effects of hypoxia in the form of CVS and respiratory system symptoms	**Stage of reaction** • At altitude 10,000–15,000 ft • Moderate hypoxic symptoms due to pO_2 40–60 mmHg
18,000 (5.5)	400	80	40	30	70	Above effects of hypoxia plus hypoxic symptoms due to involvement of CNS	**Stage of disturbance** • At altitude 15,000–20,000 ft • Severe hypoxia due to pO_2 30–40 mmHg • Needs to be treated with O_2 therapy
20,000 (6)	350	70	<40	<30	<70	Hypoxic symptoms due to CNS involvement aggravate. Unconsciousness occurs when Hb saturation falls below 60%	
30,000 (9)	226	47	21	24	20	Severe hypoxic symptoms even with oxygen therapy	**Critical stage** • Survival is not possible without O_2 therapy above 20,000 ft altitude called *critical* survival altitude
40,000 (12)	140	30	12	24	15		

so the mechanism of development of HAPO may probably be the following:

Sympathetic activity increased by physical work is over and above the sympathetic stimulation caused by hypoxia (due to low pO_2) and cold (as the temperature falls by 2°C for every 1000 ft increase in altitude).The resultant marked increase in sympathetic activity produces vasoconstriction leading to increase in pulmonary capillary hydrostatic pressure. Normally, pulmonary capillary hydrostatic pressure, which is less than 10 mmHg, and osmotic pressure of 25 mmHg, keeps the alveoli dry. Thus, increased pulmonary capillary hydrostatic pressure drives the fluid out of the pulmonary capillaries producing pulmonary oedema. When the hypoxia is very severe, even generalized oedema may develop by a similar mechanism.

Characteristics of HAPO include:

- It responds to rest and O_2 therapy because it occurs due to aggravation of hypoxia and not due to cardiovascular or lung disease.
- It is associated with increased pulmonary artery pressure, it also responds to calcium channel blockers such as nifedipine, which lowers the pulmonary artery pressure.

Acute Mountain Sickness Individuals who ascend to high altitudes gradually do not develop severe effects of hypoxia because the body gets some time to adjust to it.

Acute mountain sickness refers to the symptom complex which occurs in an individual residing at sea level, who ascends to a high altitude over a period of 1–2 days for the first time. The symptoms develop between 8 and 24 h after arrival at high altitude, and last for 4–8 days.

Characteristic Features of acute mountain sickness are headache, nausea, vomiting, irritability, insomnia, and breathlessness.

Cause of Acute Mountain Sickness is not definitely known, but it appears to be associated with cerebral oedema or alkalosis.

Mechanism of cerebral oedema. The low pO_2 at high altitude causes arteriolar dilation which is normally compensated by cerebral autoregulation. However, once the limit of the cerebral circulation autoregulatory mechanism is reached, there occurs an increase in capillary pressure that favours increased transudation of fluid into brain tissue.

Treatment. The symptoms of acute mountain sickness can be reduced by:

- ***Decreasing cerebral oedema*** by administration of large doses of glucocorticoids, and by
- ***Decreasing alkalosis*** by administration of acetazolamide. Acetazolamide decreases H^+ excretion through kidneys by inhibiting the enzyme carbonic anhydrase.

Chronic Mountain Sickness Chronic mountain sickness *(Monge's disease)* occurs in some long-term residents of high altitude who develop extreme polycythaemia, cyanosis, malaise, fatigue and exercise intolerance. These individuals must be removed to a lower altitude to prevent rapid development of fatal pulmonary oedema.

Physiological Compensatory Responses to High-Altitude Hypoxia

Two types of physiological compensatory responses known to occur in individuals exposed to high-altitude hypoxia are accommodation and acclimatization.

Accommodation refers to immediate reflex adjustments of the respiratory and cardiovascular system to hypoxia (for details see page 462).

Acclimatization refers to changes in the body tissues in response to long-term exposure to hypoxia, such as when a person living at sea level goes and stays at high altitude for a long time (for details see page 462).

Other Effects of High Altitude

Factors other than hypoxia which produce changes in the body at high altitude are:

- Effects of expansion of gases,
- Effects of fall in atmospheric temperature and
- Effects of light rays.

Effects of Expansion of Gases

According to Boyle's law of gases, the pressure (*P*) of a given mass of gas is inversely proportional to its volume (*V*), i.e. $p \propto \frac{1}{V}$.

Therefore at high altitude, barometric pressure and partial pressure of a gas is decreased, and its volume is increased. For example, if at sea level, with atmospheric pressure of 760 mmHg, the volume of a given gas is 1 L,

- *At an altitude of 18,000 ft* where atmospheric pressure is about 400 mmHg, the volume of gas increases to about *2 L* and
- *At an altitude of 30,000 ft* where atmospheric pressure is about 225 mmHg, the volume of the gas increases to about *3 L.*

Rapid Decompression refers to a situation when the body is suddenly exposed to low atmospheric pressure. Such a situation may be encountered when the cabin pressure failure accidentally occurs in an aircraft flying at high altitude. Immediately, all the body gases expand as expected as per Boyle's law of gases.

Effects of expansion of gases in the body are:

- *In gastrointestinal tract,* the expansion of gases may cause painful distension of stomach and intestines. This effect can be reduced by supporting the abdomen by a belt or by evacuation of gases while ascending rapidly.

- *In the lungs,* the expansion of gases may sometimes destroy the alveoli.
- *In the paranasal sinuses,* the expansion of gases may cause tissue damage.
- *Decompression sickness* may occur in an aviator if he is exposed to an ambient altitude in excess of about 22,000 ft (below this altitude, decompression sickness is almost nonexistent). This may happen as a corollary to rapid decompression.

Effects of Fall in Atmospheric Temperature

The atmospheric temperature falls by 2°C for every 1000 ft increase in altitude above sea level. Therefore, at different altitudes the atmospheric temperature changes as follows:

- At an altitude of 10,000 ft it is about 0°C,
- At an altitude of 20,000 ft it is about −22°C and
- At an altitude of 40,000 ft it is about –44°C.

Effects of low temperature on the human body depend not only on the atmospheric temperature, but also on wind velocity and humidity. The high wind velocity, as well as high humidity makes the cold more severe. For example, an atmospheric temperature of O°C, if accompanied by a wind velocity of 70 kmph, is equivalent to a temperature of –20°C when the air is still. Due to this, one feels colder while riding a motor cycle as compared to walking, or standing still.

In general, the effects of low temperature on the body can be described as:

- Effects of acute cold exposure (see page 1246), and
- Effects of long-term cold exposure (see page 368).

Effects of Light Rays

Ultraviolet (UV) rays at high altitude also cause many hazardous effects such as skin irritation.

PHYSIOLOGY OF HIGH ATMOSPHERIC PRESSURE

Introduction

Atmospheric pressure of 760 mmHg at sea level is considered one atmospheric pressure.

Pressure increases by 1 atmosphere for a depth of every 10 m (33ft) as one descends under water. Thus, a person under sea at a depth of 10 m (33 ft) is exposed to a pressure of 2 atmospheres, 1 atmosphere due to the air above the sea level and another 1 atmosphere due to 10 m column of water. As the depth under water increases, the pressure also increases proportionately (Table 12.2-3).

Decrease in volume of gases occurs due to compression as the pressure increases under water. According to Boyle's law, the volume to which a given quantity of gas is compressed is inversely proportional to the pressure. Therefore, 1 litre of volume of air at sea level with 1 atmospheric pressure compresses to ½ litre volume at a depth of 10 m under water, where pressure is 2 atmospheres. With further increase in the pressure, the volume decreases proportionately (Table 12.2-3).

TABLE 12.2-3 Effect of Sea Depth on Pressure and Volume of Gas

Depth [m (ft)]	Pressure (atmospheres)	Volume (L)
Sea level	1	1
10 (33)	2	1/2 (0.5)
20 (66)	3	1/3 (0.33)
30 (100)	4	1/4 (0.25)
40 (133)	5	1/5 (0.2)
50 (166)	6	1/6 (0.167)
60 (200)	7	1/7 (0.143)
90 (300)	10	1/10 (0.1)
120 (400)	13	1/13 (0.077)
150 (500)	16	1/16 (0.062)

High atmospheric pressure is met under following conditions:

- Deep sea diving,
- Going under the sea in submarines and
- Caisson's workers, i.e. the men who dig underwater tunnels, work in a chamber (Caisson's chamber) in which atmospheric pressure is high to prevent entry of water.

Physiological problems associated with life under high pressure may be classified as:

- Physiological problems at depth (due to compression effect of high atmospheric pressure), and
- Physiological problems of ascent (due to decompression phenomenon).

Physiological Problems under Depth

If appropriate preventive measures are not taken, then the individuals working at depth under water will face the following physiological problems:

Physiological Problems Due to Mechanical Effects of High Atmospheric Pressure

At a depth of more than 30 m (100 ft), due to the mechanical effects of increased atmospheric pressure, there may occur:

- Caving in of the chest,
- Damage to the face and
- Squeezing of air in the paranasal sinuses and middle ear.

Physiological Problems Due to Effect of High Pressure on Respiratory Gases

Air under high atmospheric pressure is breathed under water. At high atmospheric pressure, the partial pressure of oxygen (pO_2), nitrogen (pN_2) and carbon dioxide (pCO_2) also increases, producing the following physiological problems.

1. Effects of Increased pO_2 (Oxygen Toxicity) Oxygen toxicity may be acute or chronic.

Acute Oxygen Toxicity occurs on exposure to 4 atmospheric pressure of oxygen (pO_2 in lungs is approx. 3000 mmHg).

- Acute oxygen poisoning is typically characterized by nervous system complications as the *brain tissue is especially susceptible to acute oxygen poisoning.*
- *Mechanism of damage to nervous system* is as described. At 4 atmospheric pressure, the amount of oxygen dissolved is markedly increased to 9 ml/100 ml compared with about 2 ml at 1 atmosphere. This raises the tissues pO_2 level. At high tissue pO_2, the molecular oxygen is converted into active oxygen, i.e. superoxide anion (O_2^-) which is a free radical. The oxygen free radicals oxidize the polyunsaturated fatty acids of the cell membranes as well as the cellular enzymes, thus damaging the cellular metabolic system severely. Nervous tissues, because of their high lipid content, are especially susceptible to damage by oxygen free radicals producing nervous complications.
- *Nervous complications of acute oxygen poisoning* include disorientation, dizziness, convulsions and even coma.

Chronic Oxygen Toxicity occurs due to prolonged exposure (8–24 h) to oxygen at 1 or 1.5 atmospheric pressure. Chronic oxygen poisoning causes the following bronchopulmonary problems.

- *Irritation of airways* in the form of nasal congestion, sore throat, substernal discomfort, sneezing, coughing, and bronchoconstriction may occur after 8 h of exposure.
- *Pulmonary oedema and atelectasis* begin to develop after 12 h of exposure.
- *Bronchopneumonia* may be initiated when exposure is continued for more than 24 h. Bronchopneumonia is initiated because of inhibition of ability of lung macrophages to kill bacteria, and decreased production of surfactant.

2. Effects of Increased pN_2 (Nitrogen Narcosis) The partial pressure of nitrogen (pN_2) rises in the blood when an individual is made to breathe compressed air for an hour or more at high atmospheric pressure, deep underwater. Due to increased pN_2, the nitrogen dissolves *gradually* into the body fluids and more easily into fats. The cell membrane of neurons contains high lipid content, so more nitrogen is dissolved in the neurons of the brain. The nitrogen dissolved in the cell membranes of neurons alters the ionic conductance through the membrane, and finally decreases the neuronal excitability, producing nitrogen toxicity known as nitrogen narcosis.

Nitrogen narcosis is characterized by:

- *At a depth of about 120 ft* (4–5 atmospheric pressure), there occurs euphoric symptoms. The individual becomes jovial and carefree. These are followed by impairment of mental functions and intelligence.
- *At a depth of 150–200 ft* (about 6–7 atmospheric pressure), the individual becomes drowsy and has poor muscular co-ordination.
- *At a depth of 200–250 ft* (7–8 atmospheric pressure), the individual becomes extremely fatigued, weak and in stupor.
- *Beyond a depth of 250 ft* (above 8 atmospheric pressure), there occurs deep narcosis and the individual becomes unconscious and insensitive to stimuli (anaesthetized) and ultimately may even die.

Note. It is important to note that very short-lasting dives do not result in nitrogen narcosis, no matter how deep. This is because the nitrogen takes time to get dissolved.

3. Effects of Carbon Dioxide Build-Up Carbon dioxide build-up occurs when the individual rebreathes the CO_2 which he/she produces. This happens in the absence of an apparatus which absorbs CO_2 or releases expired CO_2 into the atmosphere. With the passage of time, pCO_2 in the body fluids may build up to reach toxic levels. The maximum tolerated CO_2 build-up is up to an alveolar pCO_2 of 80 mmHg, beyond which respiratory acidosis and carbon dioxide narcosis may occur.

Physiological Problems of Ascent

The two physiological problems which occur when an individual ascends back to sea level after sufficient exposure to high atmospheric pressure in the deep sea are:

- Decompression sickness, and
- Air embolism.

Decompression Sickness

Decompression sickness is also known as Caisson's disease, dysbarism, compressed air sickness, the bends and diver's palsy.

Cause of Decompression Sickness. As discussed earlier under high atmospheric pressure (deep in the sea), the nitrogen present in the breathed air is dissolved in the body fluids and fats in considerably increased amounts. When the individual ascends rapidly to sea level after sufficient exposure to high atmospheric pressure deep underwater, nitrogen is decompressed and escapes from the tissues at a faster rate. Being gas, it forms bubbles while escaping rapidly from the tissues. The gas bubbles block the blood vessels producing tissue ischaemia, and sometimes, result in tissue death. The symptoms produced by escaping gas bubbles constitute *decompression sickness.*

Symptoms of Decompression Sickness caused by the escape of nitrogen bubbles from the various tissues are:

- ***Pain in joints and muscles*** of legs or arms is the most frequently occurring symptom. The joint pain accounts for the term '*bends*' that is often used to describe decompression sickness. Pain is produced due to the escape of nitrogen bubbles from the myelin sheath of sensory nerves supplying the joints and muscles.
- ***Sensation of numbness,*** tingling or pricking (paraesthesia) and itching, may also be produced due to the escape of bubbles from the myelin sheath of sensory nerves.
- ***The chokes*** may also occur in patients with decompression sickness. The chokes refer to serious shortness of breath, which is often followed by severe pulmonary oedema, and occasionally, even death. This is caused by a massive number of microbubbles plugging the capillaries of the lungs.
- ***Paralysis*** of muscles may occur temporarily due to escaping nitrogen bubbles from the myelin sheath of motor nerves. This is called *diver's palsy* (one of the names of this disease).
- ***Coronary ischaemia*** or myocardial infarction may occur due to blockage of coronary capillaries by the nitrogen bubbles.
- ***Neurological symptoms*** like dizziness, paralysis of muscles, or collapse and unconsciousness, may occur due to blockage of blood vessels of brain and spinal cord.

Treatment of Decompression Disease. Tank decompression is used for treatment of decompression disease. The diver, i.e. the affected individual is placed in a pressurized tank and recompression is done, first to dissolve the N_2 bubbles, and then the pressure is lowered gradually back to normal atmospheric pressure. In this way, a slow decompression is performed so that body can get rid of N_2 without producing any harmful effects.

Air Embolism

Air embolism is another physiological problem which may occur during rapid ascent from a depth below the sea level.

Cause of Air Embolism. Air embolism, i.e. entry of air into the blood circulation occurs following a rupture of pulmonary capillaries, arteries and veins caused by sudden expansion of gases in the lungs due to a sudden fall in the atmospheric pressure (*explosive decompression*). Such a situation may typically occur in deep sea divers or Caisson's workers who breathe oxygen–helium mixture at high pressure. A similar situation may also occur in rockets (i.e. spacecraft where high pressure is maintained according to height of ascent). Due to accidental leakage in a pressurized cabin, sudden reduction in pressure occurs, causing expansion of gases in the lungs.

Manifestations of air embolism include chest pain, tachypnoea, systemic hypotension and hypoxaemia. In severe cases, air emboli may travel to the systemic circulation, block the blood flow to some vital organs and may even result in death.

Prevention of Physiological Problems Occurring at Depth and on Ascent

We have studied that without appropriate preventive measures, physiological problems occur at depth (oxygen toxicity and nitrogen narcosis) and on ascent (decompression disease and air embolism). So, professional sea divers and Caisson's workers must adopt some preventive measures to avoid occurrence of these problems.

Measures for Short-Duration Dive up to 20 m A short duration dive up to 20 m is made safe by adopting a simple and safe strategy in which the divers take a few rapid and deep breaths before diving which washes off carbon dioxide, nitrogen does not get enough time to dissolve and oxygen toxicity cannot occur as the diver holds the breath. Traditionally, pearls and sponge divers have been adopting this strategy.

Measures for Deeper and Longer Dives Deeper and longer dives can be made safer by adopting the following preventive measures.

1. Use of Breathing Apparatus. Use of breathing apparatus which delivers gas to breathe and either absorbs carbon dioxide (closed-circuit apparatus) or releases carbon dioxide as bubbles into the surroundings (open-circuit apparatus). An example of such an apparatus is SCUBA diving gear.

SCUBA diving. SCUBA (self-contained underwater breathing apparatus) is a compact arrangement for breathing which the diver can carry with him under water. In this apparatus, the air is compressed so that more air is carried in less volume and also the gas amounts to a substantial quantity even when the ambient pressure is high. The cylinder of compressed air is connected via a mask and tube for breathing through a valve. The valve ensures that whenever the diver makes an inspiratory effort, an appropriate quantity of compressed air is delivered and the expired air is released into the water (outside the apparatus). The amount of gas in SCUBA required for a deeper dive is more than that for a less-deep dive.

2. Use of Breathing Mixture Containing Helium and Low Oxygen Concentration. Use of breathing a mixture containing helium and low oxygen concentration is less harmful than natural air because:

- ***Low oxygen concentration*** prevents occurrence of oxygen toxicity.
- ***Helium when replaced with nitrogen*** provides following advantages:
  - Because of its smaller molecules and lower density than nitrogen it is easier to breathe, it diffuses faster and it is easier to eliminate its bubbles from the body.
  - The amount of helium trapped in the body under high atmospheric pressure is much less than that of nitrogen because its solubility in the body fluids is less than half that of nitrogen.
  - Being less toxic than nitrogen, its narcotic effect is only one-fifth that of nitrogen.

3. Slow Ascent or Use of Decompression Tank. Slow ascent with short stay at regular intervals, i.e. slow and stepwise ascent ensures that only a small amount of bubbles are formed at a time. They are eliminated before further ascent. In this way, decompression sickness can be prevented effectively.

Decompression tank is based on the principle of slow ascent. After a rapid ascent, the individual is placed in a pressurized tank whose pressure is lowered gradually to normal atmospheric pressure. Usually, no decompression is required after a 30 m dive for less than 30 min. Decompression for a period of 3 h is required for a 60-min dive at a depth of 60 m, and for a 20-min dive at a depth of 100 m.

Chapter 12.3

Physiology of Acid–Base Balance

GENERAL CONSIDERATIONS

Acids and Bases

Acids and bases. Acid refers to a substance that acts as proton (H^+) donor while base refers to a substance that accepts proton (H^+). Examples of a few acids and their corresponding base are:

Acid	*Base*
HCl	$H^+ + Cl^-$
H_2CO_3	$H^+ + HCO_3^-$

Alkalies refer to metallic hydroxides, e.g. NaOH and KOH. These compounds do not directly satisfy the criteria of bases. However, they dissociate to form metallic ion and OH^- which being the base accepts H^+ ions. Therefore, for all practical purposes, alkalies are considered bases.

Strong acid and bases. Acid or base having a strong tendency to dissociate into ions is called strong acid or strong base; and the acid or base having a weak tendency to dissociate into ions is called weak acid or weak base. In general, a strong acid has a weak base, while a weak acid has a strong base. For example, strong acid HCl has weak base Cl^-, and weak acid HCN has a strong base CN^-.

Ampholytes refer to the substances that can act both as acids and bases. Water is the best example of an ampholyte.

Concept of pH and H^+ Concentration

H^+ ion concentration. The acidic or basic nature of a solution is measured by H^+ ion concentration. Since the concentration of H^+ ions in biological fluids is exceedingly low, the conventional units such as mEq/L or moles/L, etc. are not commonly used to express H^+ ion concentration. For example, the normal Na^+ concentration of arterial plasma is about 140 mEq/L, whereas H^+ ion concentration is 0.00004 mEq/L.

pH is the term suggested to express H^+ ion concentration. pH is defined as the negative logarithm of H^+ concentration.

$$pH = -\log [H^+]$$

It is important to note that pH and (H^+) are inversely related. For example, pH of plasma with an H^+ ion concentration of 0.00004 mEq/L is 7.4, while pH of HCl with H^+ ion concentration of 150 mEq/L is 0.8.

Neutral pH, acidic pH and alkaline pH. Pure water has an equal concentration of H^+ and OH^- ions, i.e. 10^{-7} M each. Thus, pure water has pH of 7 which is neutral. Therefore, solutions with pH less than 7 are considered acidic and those with more than 7 are considered alkaline.

H^+ Concentration and pH of Biologic Fluids

The H^+ concentration and pH of some biologic fluids is depicted in Table 12.3-1.

TABLE 12.3-1 H^+ Concentration and pH of Biologic Fluids

Fluid	H^+ concentration		pH
	nEq/L	*mol/L*	
1. Pure water	100	1×10^{-7}	7.0
2. Blood			
Normal mean	40	3.98×10^{-8}	7.4
Normal range	44–36	4.36×10^{-8} to 3.6×10^{-7}	7.36–7.44
Acidosis (severe)	126	1.26×10^{-7}	6.9
Alkalosis (severe)	20	2.00×10^{-8}	7.7
3. Cerebrospinal fluid CSF (normal range)	44–36	4.36×10^{-8} to 3.6×10^{-7}	7.36–7.44
4. Gastric juice (pure)	100,000,000	1×10^{-1}	1.0
5. Pancreatic juice	10	1×10^{-8}	8.0
6. Urine			
Normal average	1000	1×10^{-6}	6.0
Maximum acidity	31,600	3.16×10^{-5}	4.5
Maximum alkalinity	10	1×10^{-8}	6.0
7. Intracellular fluid (ICF)	158	1.58×10^{-7}	6.8

MAINTENANCE OF BLOOD pH

General Considerations

Blood and Plasma pH

- The term blood pH always refers to plasma pH.
- Normal plasma pH is 7.4 (H^+ concentration ~40 nEq/L), which is higher than the intracellular pH of the erythrocyte (7.2).
- Plasma pH compatible with life varies from 7.7 to 6.9 (H^+ concentration is 20–120 nEq/L).
- At rest, normal pH of mixed venous blood is 7.38 compared with 7.41 of arterial blood, because of uptake of CO_2 by blood as it perfuses the tissues.
- Normally, the pH of ECF is maintained between a narrow range of 7.35 and 7.45.

Dietary and Metabolic Production of Acid and Bases

The daily consumed diet contains many acids and alkalies. The diet rich in animal proteins results in acid production while the vegetarian diet has an alkalizing effect on the body. In addition, cellular metabolism produces a number of acidic and alkaline substances that have an impact on the body pH. Finally, alkalies are normally lost in the faeces. As a net result, the dietary and metabolic products, add some acid to the body fluids; which need to be excreted daily at an equivalent rate so that acid–base balance can be maintained. If acid addition exceeds excretion, acidosis results, and conversely, if acid excretion exceeds addition, alkalosis results.

Acid Production by the Body The metabolic activities of the body are accompanied by production of two types of acids:

1. Volatile Acids. CO_2 is the volatile acid produced from the aerobic metabolism of cells. It is also a major end product in oxidation of carbohydrates, fats and amino acids. CO_2 accounts for over 12,000 mEq/L of H^+ per day. It is considered acid, because CO_2 combines with H_2O (by a reaction catalysed by carbonic anhydrase, i.e. (CA) to form weak acid H_2CO_3, which dissociates into H^+ and HCO_3 by the following reaction:

$$CO_2 + H_2O \overset{CA}{\rightleftharpoons} H_2CO_3 \rightleftharpoons H^+ + HCO_3^-$$

It is called volatile, because it is a gas, and under normal circumstances almost all the CO_2 is excreted by lungs.

2. Nonvolatile Acids, also called fixed acids contribute about 50–100 mEq H^+ per day, depending upon the diet. *These include:*

- *Sulphuric acid,* a product of sulphur containing amino acids such as cysteine, and methionine.
- *Phosphoric acid,* a product of phospholipid metabolism.
- *Hydrochloric acid,* a product of amino acids such as lysine, arginine and histidine.
- *Organic acids* are other fixed acids, that may be overproduced in disease:
  - *Lactic acid* produced in conditions of severe exercise, hypovolemia and circulatory shock,
  - *Acetic acid* and *β-hydroxybutyric acid* produced in conditions of starvation and uncontrolled diabetes mellitus, and
  - *Uric acid* produced in metabolism of nucleoproteins.

Production of Bases by the Body In normal circumstance, a negligible amount of bases is formed in the body.

- *HCO^-* produced by the metabolism of organic anions (e.g. citrate) offsets nonvolatile acid production to some degree.
- *Ammonia* produced in the amino acid metabolism is converted to urea; hence, its contribution as a base in the body is insignificant.

Defences against Changes in H^+ Concentration

There are three lines of defence to regulate the body's acid–base balance and maintain the blood pH (around 7.4):

I. ***Buffer systems of body fluid***. These:
- Form first line of defence,
- Act instantaneously in ECF and
- Immediately combine with H^+ to prevent changes in H^+ concentration and form a temporary measure to control changes in H^+ concentration.

II. *Respiratory mechanism* to regulate acid–base balance:
- Forms second line of defence,
- Acts within a few minutes,
- Acts via respiratory centre to regulate removal of CO_2 (and therefore H_2CO_3), and
- Forms a short-term measure to regulate changes in H^+ concentration.

III. *Renal mechanism* to regulate acid–base balance:
- Forms third line of defence,
- Takes days or weeks,
- Slow, but most powerful and effective in regulating pH,
- Acts by reabsorbing filtered HCO_3, generating new HCO_3^- and excreting H^+ as titrable acid and ammonium ion, and thus
- Provides a permanent solution to acid–base balance.

I. Buffer System: Primary Defence

Buffers. A buffer is a solution, consisting of a weak acid and its salt with strong base, which prevents a change in pH when H^+ ions are added to or removed from a solution. Buffers are most effective within 1.0 pH unit of the p*K* of the buffer (i.e. in the linear portion of the titration curve). Buffering capacity is dependent on the absolute concentration of salt and acid. It must be born in mind that a buffer cannot remove H^+ ions from the body. It temporarily acts as a shock absorbent to reduce the free H^+ ions. The H^+ have to be ultimately eliminated by the renal mechanism.

When acid is added to a buffer solution, its H^+ ion concentration is increased and the reaction is forced towards right leading to increase in undissociated molecules, therefore, increase in H^+ concentration is less.

When base is added to buffer, reaction shifts towards left; more H^+ ions are released from the buffer to combine with base, thereby limiting the decrease in H^+ concentration. ***Henderson–Hasselbalch equation*** which is used to calculate the pH in a buffer system can be derived as: The general equation for a buffer is

$$\mathrm{HA} \rightleftharpoons \mathrm{H^+} + \mathrm{A^-}$$

A^- represents any anion from a buffer (i.e. H^+ acceptor) and HA the undissociated acid from a buffer (i.e. H^+ do not). By the law of mass action, at equilibrium

$$K = \frac{[\mathrm{H^+}][\mathrm{A^-}]}{[\mathrm{HA}]} \quad (1)$$

where K = dissociation constant of the acid HA.

The equation, to represent free H^+ ion in a solution can be rewritten as:

$$[\mathrm{H^+}] = K = \frac{[\mathrm{HA}]}{[\mathrm{H^-}]} \quad (2)$$

We know that $\mathrm{pH} = \log \dfrac{1}{[\mathrm{H^+}]}$

By taking the reciprocals and logarithms (for log, multiplication becomes addition).

$$\log \frac{1}{[\mathrm{H^+}]} = \log\frac{1}{K} + \log\frac{[\mathrm{A^-}]}{[\mathrm{HA}]} \quad (3)$$

As $\log \dfrac{1}{K} = \mathrm{p}K$,

Equation (3) may be rewritten as:

$$\mathrm{pH} = \mathrm{p}K + \log\frac{[\mathrm{A^-}]}{[\mathrm{HA}]}$$

From this equation, it is evident that buffering capacity of a buffer system is greatest when amount of anions [A] and undissociated acid [HA] is same, i.e.

$$\frac{[\mathrm{A^-}]}{[\mathrm{HA}]} = 1, \text{ or } \log\frac{[\mathrm{A^-}]}{[\mathrm{HA}]}$$

Thus, pH = p*K*. Therefore, most effective buffers in the body are those with p*K* close to the pH in which they operate.

Isohydric principle states that when there is a change in H^+ concentration in the ECF, balance of all the buffer systems changes at the same time. According to this principle, all buffers in a common solution are in equilibrium with the same H^+ concentration, i.e.

$$[\mathrm{H^+}] = K_1 \times \frac{\mathrm{HA_1}}{\mathrm{A_1}} = K_2 \times \frac{\mathrm{HA_2}}{\mathrm{A_2}} = K_3 \times \frac{\mathrm{HA_3}}{\mathrm{A_3}}$$

where:

- K_1, K_2 and K_3 are dissociation constants of the three acids,
- HA_1, HA_2 and HA_3 are undissociated acids and
- A_1, A_2 and A_3 are the concentrations of free negative anions.

Classification of the Buffer Systems

Buffer systems in the body can be classified by different methods:

A. Bicarbonate Versus Nonbicarbonate Buffers

1. *Bicarbonate buffer* forms 53% of the buffering in the whole body. Out of it:
   - Plasma HCO_3^- contributes 35%, and
   - Erythrocyte HCO^- contributes 18%
2. *Nonbicarbonate buffers* form remaining 47% of the buffering in the whole body. With a contribution from:
   - Haemoglobin and oxyhaemoglobin 35%
   - Plasma proteins 7%
   - Organic phosphate 3%
   - Inorganic phosphate 2%

B. Extracellular Versus Intracellular Buffers

1. *Bicarbonate* (HCO_3) is the major extracellular buffer, which is produced from CO_2 and H_2O.
   - The p*K* of the CO_2/HCO_3 buffer pair is 6%.

2. *Phosphate* is a minor extracellular buffer.
   - The pK of H_2PO-/HPO^{-2} buffer pair is 68%.
   - Phosphate is most important as urinary buffer, excretion of H^+ as H_2PO_4- is called titrable acid.
3. *Plasma proteins* form the nonbicarbonate buffer in the blood and are responsible for 7% of the total buffering of blood.
4. *Haemoglobin,* though found intracellularly, is more conventionally regarded as part of the extracellular system (as described later).

C. Intracellular Buffers

1. *Organic phosphate,* e.g. AMP, ADP, ATP and 2,3-diphosphoglycerate (DPG).
2. *Proteins* of the skeletal muscle form 6 mEq/L.
3. *HCO^-* present in intracellular fluid of skeletal and cardiac muscles constitutes 12 mEq/L.
4. *Haemoglobin* is intracellular buffer but is considered an extracellular buffer as mentioned above.

Major Buffer Systems of the Body

The major buffer systems involved in the maintenance of body pH are:

- Bicarbonate buffer,
- Phosphate buffer and
- Protein buffer.

1. Bicarbonate Buffer System The carbonic acid–sodium bicarbonate (H_2CO_3–$NaHCO_3$) is the most predominant buffer system of the extracellular fluid and particularly the plasma H_2CO_3 in the body is formed by CO_2 and H_2O:

$$CO_2 + H_2O \xrightarrow[\text{anhydrase}]{\text{carbonic}} H_2CO_3$$

This reaction is catalysed by the enzyme carbonic anhydrase, which is present in the RBCs, walls of the lungs, alveoli and epithelial cells of renal tubules.

Dynamics of Bicarbonate Buffer System Carbonic acid dissociates into hydrogen and bicarbonate ions:

$$H_2CO_3 \rightleftharpoons H^+ + HCO_3^-$$

According to Henderson–Hasselbalch equation for this system:

$$pH = pK + \log\frac{[HCO_3^-]}{[H_2CO_3]} \quad (1)$$

The pK for the system in an ideal solution is low (about 3), and the amount of H_2CO_3 is small and hard to measure accurately. However, in the body, H_2CO_3 is in equilibrium with CO_2, i.e.

$$H_2CO_3 \rightleftharpoons CO_2 + H_2O$$

If the pK is changed to pK_1 and CO_2 is substituted for H_2CO_3, the pK_1 is 6.1

$$pH = 6.10 + \log\frac{[HCO_3^-]}{[CO_2]} \quad (2)$$

Since, the amount of dissolved CO_2 is proportionate to the partial pressure of CO_2 and the solubility co-efficient of CO_2 in mmol/L/mmHg is 0.0301, the clinically relevant form of this equation is as follows:

$$pH = 6.10 + \log\frac{[HCO_3^-]}{[.0301\ PCO_2]} \quad (3)$$

$[HCO_3^-]$ cannot be measured directly but can be calculated from the values of pH and pCO_2 which can be measured with suitable accuracy using pH and pCO_2 glass electrodes.

Blood pH and the ratio of HCO^- to H_2CO_3. The pH of arterial plasma with normal CO_2 tension (pCO_2) of 40 mmHg, and normal HCO^- concentration of 24 mmol/L can be calculated from the above equation (3) as below:

$$\begin{aligned} pH &= 6.10 + \log\frac{24\ \text{mmol/L}}{0.301 \times 40\ \text{mmHg}} \\ &= 6.10 + \log\frac{24}{1.2} \\ &= 6.1 + \log 20 \\ &= 6.1 + 1.3 \\ &= 7.4 \end{aligned}$$

The pK_1 of this system (6.1) is still low, relative to the pH of the blood (7.4), but the system is one of the most effective buffer systems in the body because the amount of dissolved CO_2 is controlled by respiration, and plasma concentration of HCO_3 is regulated by the kidney. Therefore, pH of ECF can be precisely controlled.

Actions of Bicarbonate Buffer System

1. ***Effective buffering of H^+.*** It is evident that at a blood pH 7.4, the ratio of bicarbonate to carbonic acid is 20%. Thus, the bicarbonate concentration is much higher (20 times) than carbonic acid in the blood. This is referred to as alkali reserve and is responsible for effective buffering of H^+.

   Addition of strong acid, e.g. HCl is followed by buffering of H^+ by following reaction:

$$\uparrow H^+ + HCO_3^- \rightarrow \text{More } H_2CO_3 \rightarrow CO_2 + H_2O$$

$$\downarrow$$

$$\text{Elimination of } CO_2 \leftarrow \uparrow \text{ Respiration}$$

2. ***Effective buffering of base,*** on addition the strong base (e.g. NaOH), is converted into a weak base ($NaHCO_3$), as shown:

$$NaOH + H_2CO_3 \rightarrow NaHCO_3 + H_2O \rightarrow Na^+ + HCO_3^-$$

- As a consequence, the concentration of H_2CO_3 decreases and that of HCO_3 increases. Therefore, more CO_2 combines with H_2O to form new carbonic acid.

$$H_2O + CO_2 \rightleftharpoons H_2CO_3$$

- Decrease in CO_2 (as above), inhibits the respiration, leading to correction of CO_2 deficiency.
- Increase in HCO_3^- is corrected by increased renal excretion of HCO_3^-.

2. Phosphate Buffer System

Inorganic Orthophosphate Buffer System. Inorganic orthophosphate buffer system is formed by sodium dihydrogen phosphate and disodium hydrogen phosphate ($NaH_2PO_4 \sim Na_2HPO_4$), which exist in at a plasma pH of 7.4 in a concentration ratio of 1:4.

Sites of Operation of NaH_2PO_4–Na_2HPO_4 Buffer

1. ***In ECF (plasma and interstitial fluid),*** the $HPO_4^{2-}/H_2PO_4^-$ buffer exists in small concentration (0.66 mmol/L) and thus contributes little to the buffering capacity of plasma. However, it is important to note that this buffer pair with a p*K* of 6.8 would be a more effective buffer than HCO_3^-/CO_2 system (p*K* = 6.1) if it were present in an appreciable concentration.
2. ***In intracellular fluid (ICF),*** the $HPO_4^{2-}/H_2PO_4^-$ forms an important buffer pair because:
   - Its concentration in ICF is high (6 mmol/L), and
   - Its p*K* (6.8) is much closer to pH of ICF (6.9).
3. ***In renal tubules,*** the $HPO_4^{2-}/H_2PO_4^-$ forms an effective extracellular buffer because:
   - Phosphate becomes greatly concentrated in the tubular fluid due to reabsorption of H_2O, and
   - pH of tubular fluid and urine is more acidic than the pH of ECF, i.e. is close to p*K* of phosphate buffer. The $HPO_4^{2-}/H_2PO_4^-$ system is a major elimination route for H^+ via the urine (see page 524).

Mechanism of Action of $HPO_4^{2-}/H_2PO_4^-$

- This nonbicarbonate buffer system can buffer both noncarbonic and carbonic acid.
- It equilibrates as:

$$H_2PO_4^- \rightleftharpoons H^+ + HPO_4^{2-}$$

- *On addition of strong acid,* e.g. HCl, it forms a weak acid:

$$HCl + Na_2HPO_4 \rightleftharpoons \underset{\text{(Weak acid)}}{Na\ H_2PO_4} + NaCl$$

- *On addition of strong base,* e.g. NaOH, it forms a weak base:

$$NaOH + NaH_2PO_4 \rightleftharpoons \underset{\text{(weak base)}}{Na_2HPO_4} + H_2O$$

Organic Phosphate Buffer System. Organic phosphates (such as AMP, ADP, ATP and 2,3-diphosphoglycerate, i.e. (2,3-DPG) exist in quantitatively significant amount in ICF (8.4 mmol/L), giving this compartment the capacity to effectively buffer both noncarbonic and carbonic acid, as well as alkali.

3. Protein Buffer System The protein buffer system of the blood is constituted by the plasma proteins and haemoglobin combinedly. The buffering capacity of proteins is dependent on the pK of ionizable groups of amino acids. The *imidazole group of histidine* (p*K* 6.7) is the most effective contributor of protein buffers:

Plasma Proteins Buffer System. Plasma proteins buffer system accounts for 15% of the buffering capacity of the whole blood. Plasma proteins are effective buffers because both their free carboxyl and free amino groups dissociate:

$$RCOOH \rightleftharpoons RCOO^- + H^+;$$

$$pH = pK^1\ RCOOH + \log\frac{[RCOO^-]}{[RCOOH]}$$

$$RNH_3^+ \rightleftharpoons RNH_2^+ + H^+;$$

$$pH = pK^1\ RNH_3 + \log\ (RNH_2)/(RNH_3)$$

Because of their amphoteric nature, plasma proteins can combine with acids and bases as:

- *In acidic pH,* the NH_2 group of the proteins acts as a base and accepts protons and is converted to NH_3.
- *In alkaline pH,* the -COOH group of the proteins acts as an acid and can donate a proton and thus becomes COO^-.
- *At normal pH* of blood, proteins act as acids and combine with cations (mainly sodium).

Haemoglobin Buffer System. Haemoglobin buffer system (Hb/HHb and $HbO_2^-/HHbO_2$) accounts for 35% of the total buffering capacity of the whole blood. It mainly buffers the fixed acids, besides being involved in the transport of gases (O_2 and CO_2).

Haemoglobin: intracellular versus extracellular buffer concept. Haemoglobin, though found intracellularly, is more conventionally regarded as part of the extracellular buffer system because:

- Haemoglobin is confined to the erythrocytes which are a cellular component of ECF,
- Haemoglobin is readily available for the buffering of extracellular acids and
- Haemoglobin is the primary noncarbonated buffer of the body.

Buffering system in haemoglobin is provided by dissociation of imidazole group of histidine residues:

```
        H                       H
       /C\                     /C\
    HN     NH+      ⇌      HN     N   + H+
    |       |              |      |
    HC  =  C – R           HC  =  C\
                                   R
```

Hb is a major buffer in blood, although between pH 7 and 7.7, it contributes relatively less to buffering capacity. This is because:

- Haemoglobin molecules are present in large amounts. One litre of whole blood contains about 150 g (2.3 mmol) of haemoglobin.
- Haemoglobin molecule contains 38 histidine residues.

Deoxyhaemoglobin (Hb) is a better buffer than oxyhaemoglobin (HbO_2), because the imidazole groups of Hb dissociate less than those of HbO_2, making Hb a weaker acid.

Titration curves for Hb and HbO_2 (Fig. 12.3-1) illustrating the importance of haemoglobin as a buffer indicates that:

- The complete deoxygenation of 1 mmol of HbO_2 to liberate 1 mmol of O_2 results in the neutralization of 0.7 mmol of H^+ without a change in pH (arrow AC in Fig. 12.3-1). Such a reaction is called *isohydric buffering*.
- When the oxyhaemoglobin (HbO_2) at pH 7.4 is completely reduced to deoxyhaemoglobin (Hb), there occurs an increase in pH (arrow AB, in Fig. 12.3-1).

II. Respiratory Mechanism for pH Regulation

Second line of defence against acid–base disorders is formed by the respiratory mechanism, which provides a short-term but rapid control. It acts via the respiratory centre, located in the medulla to regulate removal of CO_2 and therefore, carbonic acid (H_2CO_3) concentration in the blood.

Role of Respiratory Centres Respiratory centres are influenced by both CO_2 as well as H^+ concentration: through central and peripheral chemoreceptors.

1. Effect of CO_2. CO_2 influences the respiratory centre through peripheral as well as central chemoreceptors. The CO_2 is highly diffusible gas and can easily cross the blood–brain–CSF barriers and influence the medullary central chemoreceptors. In contrast, H^+ cannot cross these barriers easily. Therefore, central chemoreceptors are most sensitive to changes in arterial pCO_2 and less so to changes in H^+ concentration.

Under most circumstances, CO_2 production and excretion are matched and the usual steady state pCO_2 is maintained at 40 mmHg. Therefore, increases or decreases in pCO_2 do not occur due to change in production of CO_2, but either represents derangements of neural respiratory control or is due to compensatory changes in response to or primary alteration in plasma HCO_3^-.

2. Effect of pH. Changes in arterial blood pH (H^+ concentration) also influences pulmonary ventilation, chiefly through the peripheral (sino-aortic) chemoreceptors and helps in regulation of acid–base balance of the body even when the increase in H^+ concentration is not due to CO_2 but due to nonvolatile acids like sulphuric acid, phosphoric acid and/or lactic acid.

Respiratory response, as described later, does not occur in response to respiratory acid–base disorders but occurs in response to metabolic acid–base disorders only, and consists of:

1. *Hyperventilation*. It occurs in response to metabolic acidosis and results in lowering of pCO_2 to match the decreased (HCO_3^-).
2. *Hypoventilation* occurs in response to metabolic alkalosis and results in raising the pCO_2 to match the increased (HCO_3^-).

III. Renal Mechanism for pH Regulation

The kidneys regulate pH through three main processes:

- 'Reabsorption' of filtered HCO_3^-,
- 'Generation' of new HCO_3^- and
- H^+ excretion in the form of titrable acid and NH_4^+. For details see description of acidification of urine (page 524).

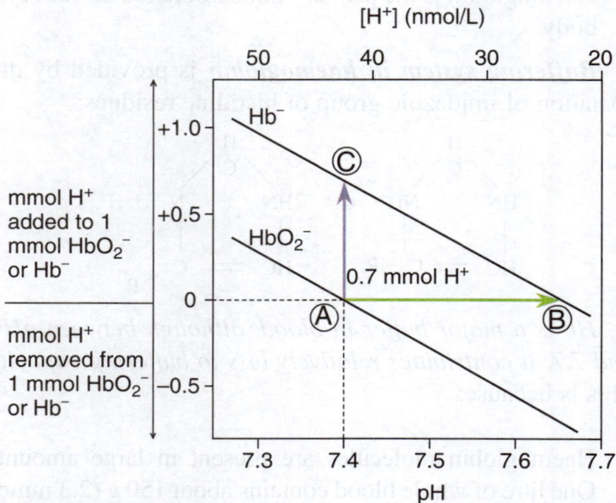

FIGURE 12.3-1 Titration curves for oxyhaemoglobin and deoxyhaemoglobin (for explanation see text).

ACID–BASE DISORDERS

Acidosis refers to decline in blood pH, while *alkalosis* refers to rise in blood pH. As described above, our body has been provided with an efficient system for the maintenance of acid–base equilibrium with a result that the pH of blood is almost constant (7.4). The blood pH compatible to life is 6.8–7.8, beyond which life cannot exist.

Acid–base disorders can be classified into two groups:

I. *The simple acid–base disorders* include:

- Metabolic acidosis,
- Metabolic alkalosis,
- Respiratory acidosis and
- Respiratory alkalosis.

II. *Mixed acid–base disorders* include:

- Metabolic acidosis and respiratory acidosis,
- Metabolic acidosis and respiratory alkalosis,
- Metabolic alkalosis and respiratory alkalosis and
- Metabolic alkalosis and respiratory acidosis.

Simple Acid–Base Disorders

The physiological aspects of single acid–base disorders are summarized in Table 12.3-2 and described:

Metabolic Acidosis

Physiological Disturbance that produces metabolic acidosis is either increased net nonvolatile acid load or loss of base (HCO_3^-).

TABLE 12.3-2 Summary of Characteristics of Simple Acid–Base Disorders

		Arterial plasma (approximate values)			Defence mechanism		
Disorder	Primary disturbance	*pH (normal 7.4)*	*HCO_3^- (mEq/L) (normal 24)*	*pCO_2 mmHg) (normal 40)*	*Buffering*	*Respiratory compensation*	*Renal compensation*
Metabolic acidosis	↓ Plasma HCO_3^-	↓ (7.28)	↓ (18)	→ (40)	ECF and ICF	Hyperventilation (↓pCO_2)	↑ H^+ excretion ↑ New HCO_3^- reabsorption
Metabolic alkalosis	↑ Plasma HCO_3^-	↑ (7.5)	↑ (30)	→ (40)	ECF and ICF	Hypoventilation (↑pCO_2)	↓ H^+ excretion ↓ New HCO_3^- reabsorption
Respiratory acidosis	↑ pCO_2	↓ (7.34)	↑ (25)	↑ (48)	ICF	None	↑ H^+ excretion ↑ New HCO_3^- reabsorption
Respiratory alkalosis	↓ pCO_2	↑ (7.53)	↓ (22)	↓ (27)	ICF	None	↓ H^+ excretion ↓ New HCO_3^- reabsorption

ICF: Intracellular fluid; ECF: Extracellular fluid; ↑ : increased; ↓ : decreased; → : normal.

Primary Disturbance in metabolic acidosis is *decreased plasma [HCO_3^-]* (which has either been used to buffer the extra fixed acid or lost from the body) producing a *low plasma pH*.

Causes of metabolic acidosis include:

1. ***Addition of nonvolatile acids*** to the body can occur in:
   - Diabetic ketoacidosis causing accumulation of acetoacetic acid and β-OH-butyric acid.
   - Lactic acidosis in hypoxia.
   - Methanol/formaldehyde intoxication which produces formic acid.
2. ***Loss of nonvolatile alkali*** from the body occurs in:
   - Diarrhoea (G1 loss of HCO_3^-),
   - Type 2 renal tubular acidosis (renal loss of HCO_3).
3. ***Failure of the kidney to excrete sufficient net acid to replenish HCO_3^- used to titrate the net daily acid load,*** as may occur in:
   - Chronic renal failure (failure to excrete H^+ as titrable acid and NH_4).
   - Type I distal renal tubular acidosis (failure to excrete titrable acid and NH_4).

Uncompensated Metabolic Acidosis characterized by a low plasma pH and low plasma HCO_3^- is expressed as:

$$\downarrow pH = pK + \log \frac{HCO_3^-}{pCO_2} \downarrow$$

Compensatory Mechanisms. When metabolic acidosis is produced by nonrenal factors, the respiratory and renal compensatory mechanisms tend to minimize the change in pH of blood. In renal failure, only respiratory compensation is possible.

1. ***Respiratory compensation.*** Increased (H^+) stimulates the respiratory centre through peripheral chemoreceptors and produces *hyperventilation* (Kussmaul *breathing*) which in turn decreases the arterial pCO_2 value and minimizes the degree of acidosis. Respiratory compensatory mechanism is prompt but short term.

   Compensated metabolic acidosis characterized by near normal pH with ↓pCO_2 to compensate the ↓HCO^-_3 is expressed as:

$$pH = pK + \log \frac{HCO_3^- \downarrow}{pCO_2 \downarrow}$$

2. ***Renal compensation*** is slow, but an effective mechanism to control metabolic acidosis. It consists of:
   - *Increased excretion of fixed H^+* as titrable acid and NH_4.
   - *Increased reabsorption of 'new HCO_3^-'*, which replenishes the HCO_3^- used in buffering the added fixed H^+.
   - *In chronic metabolic acidosis*, an adaptive increase in NH_3 synthesis helps in the excretion of excess H^+.

Hyperchloraemic versus Normochloraemic Metabolic Acidosis. ***Normochloraemic metabolic acidosis*** is characterized by decreased plasma (HCO_3^-) and low plasma pH with normal serum Cl^- levels. As described above, the metabolic acidosis caused by conditions adding nonvolatile acid to the body or due to renal failure to excrete H^+ is normochloraemic type of metabolic acidosis.

Hyperchloraemic metabolic acidosis is characterized by decreased plasma (HCO_3) and low plasma pH with an increase in plasma (Cl^-)

This type of metabolic acidosis occurs in:

- *Diarrhoea,* in which HCO_3^- is lost from the gut in exchange of Cl^-, and
- *Type 2 renal tubular acidosis*, in which failure to reabsorb HCO_3^- by kidneys is accompanied by excessive reabsorption of Cl^-.

Anion Gap Concept. Anion gap helps to differentiate the hyperchloraemic metabolic acidosis from normochloraemic metabolic acidosis.

According to law of electroneutrality, the total concentration of cations and anions in serum are equal. Routine serum electrolyte determinations measure essentially all cations but only a fraction of the anions. This apparent disparity between the total cation concentration and the total anion concentration is termed the anion gap (Fig. 12.3-2). It is a virtual measurement and does not represent any specific ionic constituent as shown (Fig. 12.3-2A):

$$[Na^+ + K^+ + Ca^+ + Mg^+] = [HCO_3^- + Cl^-$$
$$+ \text{Unmeasured anions}] \text{ (Anion gap)}$$
$$\therefore \text{Anion gap [AG]} = [Na^+ + K^+ + Ca^+ + Mg^+]$$
$$-[HCO_3^- + Cl^-]$$

Often the anion gap is calculated with Na^+ as the major cation, as K^+, Ca^{2+} and Mg^{2+} have a relatively minor quantitative contribution. The equation then becomes (Fig. 12.3-2B):

$$AG = [Na^+] - [HCO_3^- + Cl^-]$$
$$= [142 \text{ mEq/L}] - [25 \text{ mEq/L} + 105 \text{ mEq/L}]$$
$$= 142 \text{ mEq/L} - 130 \text{ mEq/L}$$
$$= 12 \text{ mEq/L}$$

The anion gap, which has a normal value of 12 ± 4 mEq/L, reflects the concentration of those anions which are actually present but are not determined routinely (i.e. other than HCO_3^- and Cl^-) and include polyanionic plasma proteins (primarily albumin), inorganic phosphates, sulphate and ions of organic acids.

Anion gap in metabolic acidosis. As mentioned above, in metabolic acidosis, the serum (HCO_3^-) decreases, since it is utilized in buffering the fixed acid. For electroneutrality, the concentration of another anion must increase to replace HCO_3^-. That anion can be Cl^- or the unmeasured anions (which constitute anion gap).

- *In normochloraemic metabolic acidosis,* the concentration of unmeasured anions is increased to replace HCO_3^- and hence the serum anion gap is increased (Fig. 12.3-2C).
- *In hyperchloraemic metabolic acidosis,* the concentration of Cl^- is increased to replace the HCO_3^-, so the serum anion gap is normal (Fig. 12.3-2D).

Metabolic Alkalosis

Physiological Disturbance that produces metabolic alkalosis is either addition of nonvolatile alkali or loss of H^+ from the body.

Primary Disturbance in metabolic alkalosis is *increased plasma* HCO_3^- producing a high plasma pH

Causes of metabolic alkalosis include:

1. ***Addition of nonvolatile alkali*** to the body, e.g. in:
   - Ingestion of antacids.
2. ***Volume contraction alkalosis*** may occur with:
   - Haemorrhage, and
   - Loop or thiazide diuretics.
3. ***Loss of H^+ from the body*** (a common cause) may occur in:
   - Vomiting (H^+ is lost from the stomach), and
   - Hyperaldosteronism (increased H^+ secretion by distal tubule).

Uncompensated Metabolic Alkalosis characterized by a high plasma pH and high plasma HCO_3^- is expressed as:

$$\uparrow pH = pK + \log \frac{HCO_3^- \uparrow}{pCO_2}$$

Compensatory Mechanisms

1. ***Respiratory compensation.*** Increased pH (or decreased H^+) inhibits the respiratory centre through peripheral chemoreceptors and produces *hypoventilation* which in turn elevates pCO_2 and thus normalizes plasma pH.

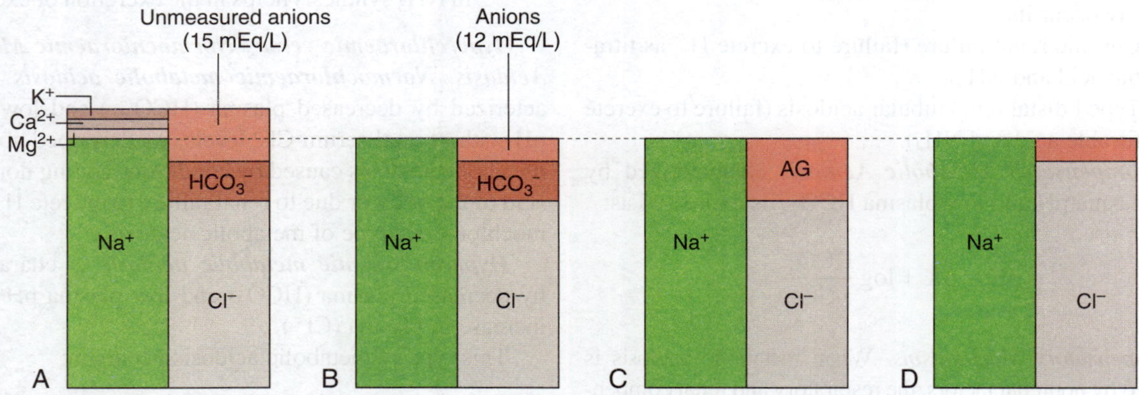

FIGURE 12.3-2 Concept of anion gap: **A,** normal ionogram showing the major cations (Na^+) and the minor cations (K^+, Ca^{2+} and Mg^{2+}). The major anions are HCO_3^- and Cl^- and the unmeasured anion constitute the anion gap; **B,** simplified ionogram showing Na^+ as the only cation and making the anion column fall as the Na^+ column; **C,** ionogram depicting increased anion gap in normochloraemic metabolic acidosis; and **D,** ionogram depicting normal anion gap but increased [Cl^-] in hyperchloraemic metabolic acidosis.

2. ***Compensated metabolic alkalosis*** characterized by near normal pH with ↑pCO_2 to compensate the ↑HCO_3^- is expressed as:

$$pH = pK + \log\frac{HCO_3^- \uparrow}{pCO_2 \uparrow}$$

Note. It is important to note that the magnitude of respiratory compensation is limited by the fact that hypoventilation results in decreased arterial pO_2 which stimulates the respiratory centres via peripheral chemoreceptors.

3. ***Renal compensation*** for metabolic alkalosis consists of:
   - *Decreased* H^+ *secretion* by the renal tubules, and
   - *Increased* HCO^- *excretion,* as the filtered load of HCO_3 exceeds the ability of renal tubule to reabsorb it. The urinary loss of HCO_3^- decreases the plasma level of HCO^- thereby restoring the pH of blood to near normal.

Note. It is important to note that if metabolic alkalosis is accompanied by ECF volume contraction (e.g. following persistent vomiting), the resultant hypovolemia becomes a strong stimulus for Na^+ reabsorption by increased H^+ secretion (because of Na^+/H^+ antiport system) and thus HCO_3^- reabsorption increases, worsening the metabolic alkalosis.

Respiratory Acidosis

Primary Disturbance in respiratory acidosis is *increased* pCO_2, which by mass action causes an increase in H^+ and thus lowers the blood pH.

Causes. The pCO_2 is increased due to decreased gas exchange across the alveoli because of following causes:

1. ***Inadequate ventilation,*** which may occur due to:
   - Drug-induced (opiates, sedatives, anaesthetics) depression of respiratory centres,
   - Weakening of respiratory muscles as in Guillain–Barré syndrome, polio, amyotrophic lateral sclerosis and multiple sclerosis and
   - Airway obstruction.
2. ***Impaired gas diffusion,*** may occur in cardiovascular diseases or lung diseases (e.g. adult respiratory distress syndrome, chronic obstructive pulmonary disease).

Uncompensated Respiratory Acidosis, characterized by low plasma pH and high pCO_2 is expressed as:

$$\downarrow pH = pK + \log\frac{HCO_3^-}{pCO_2 \uparrow}$$

Compensatory Mechanism. Note. There is no respiratory compensation for respiratory acidosis.

Buffering in respiratory acidosis, in contrast to metabolic acidosis, occurs almost entirely in the intracellular compartment.

Renal compensation. Increased pCO_2 supplies more H^+ to renal tubule cells for secretion which leads to:

- Increased excretion of H^+ as titrable acid and NH_3, and
- Increased reabsorption of new HCO_3^-
- The resulting increase in serum HCO_3^- helps to normalize the pH. Thus, acidosis is mostly but not completely compensated by the renal mechanism.

Acute versus Chronic Respiratory Acidosis As the renal compensatory response takes several days to develop; consequently, the respiratory acidosis can be divided into acute and chronic phases.

1. ***Acute respiratory acidosis*** is labelled, when not enough time has elapsed and the renal compensation has not yet occurred. During this phase, the body relies on intracellular buffering to minimize the change in pH. Because of intracellular buffering, plasma (HCO_3^-) increases 1 mEq/L for every 10 mm rise in pCO_2 during this period.
2. ***Chronic respiratory acidosis*** is labelled when renal compensation occurs. During this phase, plasma (HCO_3^-) increases 3.5 mEq/L for every 10 mm rise in pCO_2.
3. ***Compensated respiratory acidosis*** characterized by near normal pH with increased plasma HCO_3^- to compensate the increased pCO_2, is expressed as:

$$pH = pK + \log\frac{HCO_3^- \uparrow}{pCO_2 \uparrow}$$

Respiratory Alkalosis

Primary Disturbance in respiratory alkalosis is decreased pCO_2 associated with low (H^+) and thus, an elevated plasma pH.

Causes. The pCO_2 is decreased due to increased gas exchange in the lungs because of increased ventilation as seen in following conditions:

- Pneumonia and pulmonary embolus (ventilation rate is increased secondary to hypoxaemia),
- High altitude (ventilation rate is increased secondary to hypoxaemia),
- Psychogenic hyperventilation may occur as a response to anxiety or fear and
- Salicylate intoxication (hyperventilation occurs due to direct stimulation of medullary respiratory centres).

Uncompensated Respiratory Alkalosis, characterized by high plasma pH and low pCO_2, is expressed as:

$$\uparrow pH = pK + \log\frac{HCO_3^-}{pCO_2 \downarrow}$$

Compensatory Mechanisms. Note. There is no respiratory compensation for respiratory alkalosis.

Buffering in respiratory alkalosis, in contrast to metabolic alkalosis, occurs almost entirely in the intracellular compartment.

Renal compensation. Decreased pCO_2 causes a deficit of H^+ in the renal cells for secretion which leads to:

- Decreased excretion of H^+ as titrable acid and NH_4^+,
- Decreased reabsorption of new HCO_3^- and
- Decreased reabsorption of the filtered HCO_3^-.

The resulting decrease in serum (HCO_3^-) helps to normalize the pH. In this way, alkalosis is mostly but not completely compensated by the renal mechanism.

Acute versus Chronic Respiratory Alkalosis As the renal compensatory response takes several days to develop; consequently, the respiratory alkalosis can be divided into acute and chronic phases:

1. ***Acute respiratory alkalosis*** is labelled when not enough time has elapsed and renal compensation has not yet occurred. During this phase, the body relies on intracellular buffering to minimize the change in pH. Because of intracellular buffering plasma (HCO_3^-) decreases 2 mEq/ L for every 10 mmHg fall in pCO_2.
2. ***Chronic respiratory alkalosis*** is labelled when renal compensation occurs. During this phase, plasma (HCO_3^-) decreases by 5 mEq/L for every 10 mmHg reduction in pCO_2 by the renal compensatory mechanism as described above.

Compensated Respiratory Alkalosis, characterized by near normal pH with decreased plasma HCO_3^- to compensate the decreased pCO_2, is expressed as:

$$pH = pK + \log \frac{HCO_3^- \downarrow}{pCO_2 \downarrow}$$

Summary of Characteristics of Simple Acid–base Disorders. Various characteristics of simple acid–base disorders are summarized in Table 12.3-2.

Predicted Physiological Responses to Simple Acid–Base Disorders As described above, the primary respiratory disturbances (primary change in pCO_2) involve secondary metabolic responses (secondary change in HCO_3^-) and primary metabolic disturbances elicit predictable respiratory responses. Predicted physiological compensation in various acid–base disturbances is summarized in Table 12.3-3.

TABLE 12.3-3 Predicted Physiological Responses in Simple Acid–Base Disorders

Acid–base disorder	Primary disturbance	Predicted compensatory response
Metabolic acidosis	$\downarrow[HCO_3^-$	$\downarrow pCO_2$ by 1.30 mmHg/ mEq/L decrease in HCO_3^-
Metabolic alkalosis	$\uparrow[HCO_3^-]$	$\uparrow pCO_2$ by 0.7 mmHg/ mEq/L increase in HCO_3
Respiratory acidosis		
• Acute	$\uparrow pCO_2$	$\uparrow[HCO_3^-]$ by 0.1 mEq/L/ mmHg increase in pCO_2
• Chronic	$\uparrow pCO_2$	$\uparrow[HCO_3^-]$ by 0.4 mEq/L/ mmHg increase in pCO_2
Respiratory alkalosis		
• Acute	$\downarrow pCO_2$	$\downarrow[HCO_3^-]$ by 0.2 mEq/L/ mmHg decrease in pCO_2
• Chronic	$\downarrow pCO_2$	$\downarrow[HCO_3^-]$ by 0.4 mEq/L/ mmHg decrease in pCO_2

ANALYSIS AND CLINICAL EVALUATION OF ACID–BASE DISORDERS

Three-Step Approach for Analysis of Acid–Base Disorders

Three-step approach for analysis of acid–base disorders is summarized in Fig. 12.3-3. It consists of the following three steps:

- ***Step I.*** Estimate pH to know acidosis ($pH < 7.4$) or alkalosis ($pH > 7.4$).
- ***Step II.*** Detect primary disturbance to know whether the disorder is metabolic (primary disturbance of HCO_3^-) or respiratory (primary disturbance of pCO_2).
- ***Step III.*** Analysis of compensatory response can be done from the values of plasma HCO_3^- and pCO_2.

Determination of Anion Gap

As described above (page 1234), the determination of anion gaps is useful in differential diagnosis of metabolic acidosis. The anion gap is increased in metabolic acidosis due to ketoacidosis, lactic acidosis and other forms of acidosis in which organic anions are increased. It is not increased in hyperchloraemic acidosis.

Graphic Analysis of Changes in pH, pCO_2 and HCO_3^-

Acid–Base Nomogram Acid–base nomogram (Fig. 12.3-4) is the graphical display of changes in pCO_2 (curved lines in Fig. 12.3-4), plasma HCO_3^- and pH of arterial blood in respiratory and metabolic acid–base disorders. This nomogram is useful in predicting compensatory responses to simple acid–base disorder. While the shaded areas of nomogram show the 95% confidence limits for normal compensation in simple disturbances, finding acid–base values within the shaded area does not necessarily rule out a mixed disturbance. Note the shifts in HCO_3^- and pH as acute respiratory acidosis and alkalosis are compensated producing their chronic counterparts.

Davenport Diagram: Graphic Display of True Plasma pH, HCO_3^- and pCO_2 in Metabolic Acidosis and Alkalosis Fig. 12.3-5 is the typical graphical display of true plasma pH, HCO_3^- and pCO_2 in uncompensated and compensated

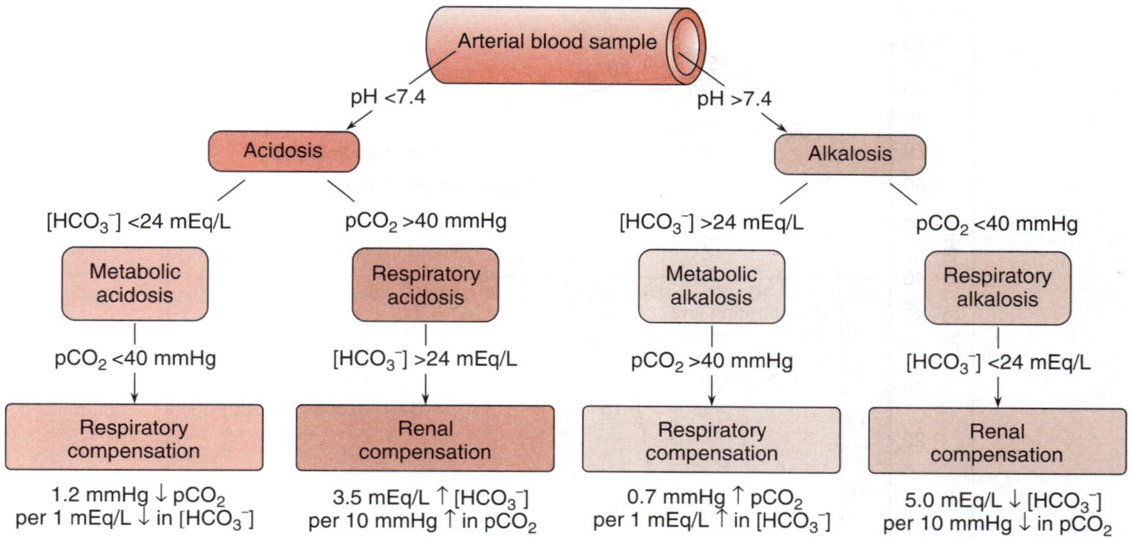

FIGURE 12.3-3 Algorithm of three-step approach for analysis of acid–base disorder.

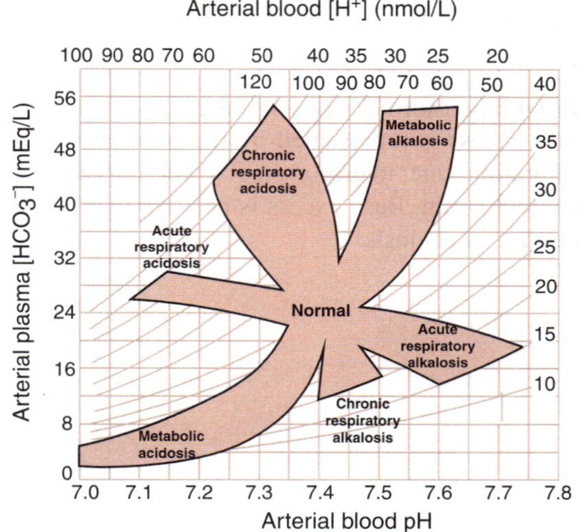

FIGURE 12.3-4 Acid–base nomogram (for explanation see text).

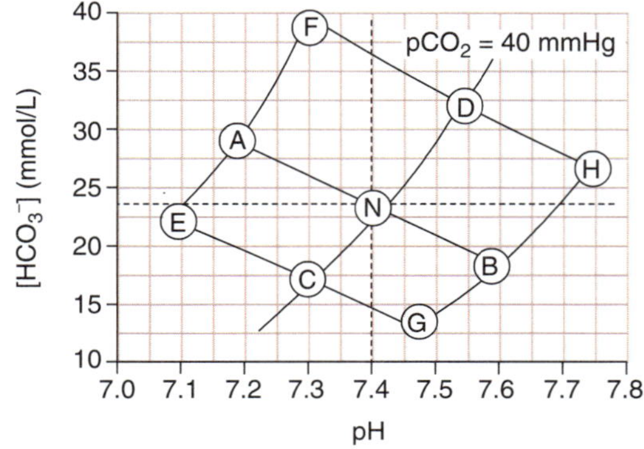

FIGURE 12.3-5 Interpretation of acid–base abnormalities using the pH–[HCO_3^-] diagram (Davenport diagram; for explanation see text). Acid–base nomogram (for explanation see text).

metabolic acidosis and metabolic alkalosis. It shows the relationship between pH and HCO_3^- at a constant pCO_2, and hence also called *pCO_2 isobar*. Thus, acid–base imbalances are determined graphically, with reference to the intercept of pCO_2 isobar of 40 mmHg (line CND, Fig. 12.3-5) and the normal buffer line (Line ANB, Fig. 12.3-5). The intercept of these two curves marks the point of normality (N) which is associated with a pH of 7.4 (the abscissa) and a [HCO_3^-] of 24 mmol/L (the ordinate). Thus, the point N is the triple intercept that defines the pH, [HCO_3^-] and pCO_2 of true arterial plasma of a normal individual.

Interpretation of acid–base abnormalities using pH, HCO_3^- diagram is made as:

- *Point A,* represents uncompensated respiratory acidosis,
- *Point B,* represents uncompensated respiratory alkalosis,
- *Point C,* represents uncompensated metabolic acidosis,
- *Point D,* represents uncompensated metabolic alkalosis,
- *Point E,* represents respiratory acidosis + metabolic acidosis,
- *Point F,* represents respiratory acidosis + metabolic alkalosis,
- *Point G,* represents respiratory alkalosis + metabolic acidosis and
- *Point H,* represents respiratory alkalosis + metabolic alkalosis.

Siggaard-Andersen Curve Nomogram Siggaard-Andersen (SA) curve nomogram (Fig. 12.3-6) has pCO_2 plotted on a log scale on the vertical axis and pH on the horizontal. This nomogram is helpful in clinical situations to plot the acid–base, a characteristic of arterial blood.

Protocol for Using SA Nomogram

- Arterial capillary blood is drawn anaerobically and pH is measured. pH of the same blood after equilibration

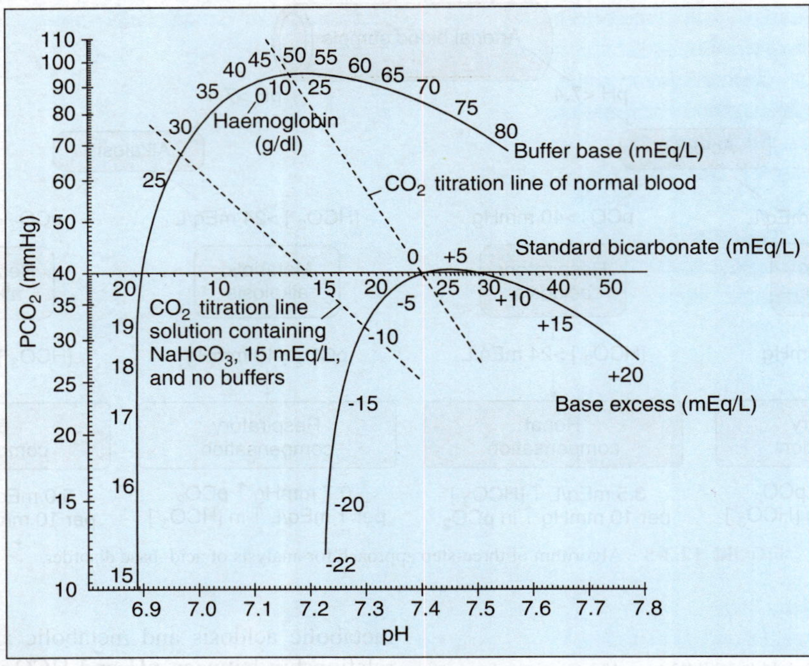

FIGURE 12.3-6 Siggaard-Andersen curve nomogram to plot the acid–base characteristics of arterial blood.

with each of 2 gas mixtures containing known amounts of CO_2 are determined.

- pH value at known pCO_2 levels are plotted and connected to provide CO_2 titration line from blood sample.
- pH of the blood sample before equilibration is plotted on this line and actual pCO_2 of sample read off the vertical line.

Following values can be determined:

- Standard HCO_3^- content of sample, i.e. measure of the alkali reserve of the blood.
- Buffer base (normal value 48 mEq/L).
- Base excess is represented by the point at which CO_2 calibration line intersects the lower curved scale on the nomogram. Base excess is positive in alkalosis and negative in acidosis.

Chapter 12.4

Physiology of Body Temperature Regulation

BODY TEMPERATURE

Homeothermic versus Poikilothermic Animals

Homeothermic animals, also called warm-blooded animals, are able to maintain their body temperature within a normal narrow range in spite of wide variations in the environmental temperature. Birds and mammals, including humans, belong to this category.

Poikilothermic animals, also called cold-blooded animals, do not have an efficient temperature-regulating system; therefore, their body temperature fluctuates with the fluctuations in the environmental temperature. The reptiles, amphibians and fishes belong to this category.

Normal Body Temperature

There is a slight variation in normal temperature at different parts of the body:

- ***Oral temperature,*** when measured with the help of a clinical thermometer, varies from 36.0 to 37.5°C (97.5–99°F) with an average of 37°C (98.6°F). Oral temperature is affected by hot and cold drinks and food, smoking, chewing gums and mouth breathing.
- ***Axillary temperature*** is slightly lower (about 0.5°C) than the oral temperature.
- ***Rectal and oesophageal temperatures*** are slightly higher (about 0.5°C) than the oral temperature.
- ***Superficial skin or surface temperature*** varies to some extent with the environmental temperature (see 'shell temperature').
- ***Extremities*** are generally cooler than the rest of the body.
- ***Scrotal temperature*** is carefully regulated at 32°C (89.6°F).

Concept of Core versus Shell Temperature. The body is hypothetically divided into core and shell (Fig. 12.4-1).

- ***Shell temperature,*** i.e. temperature of the limbs and the surface layer of trunk, i.e. skin and underlying structure exhibits variations of the temperature with the change in external temperature.

In cold weather, the temperature of the shell may be several degrees lower than the core temperature (Fig. 12.4-1A). This decreases the loss of body heat to the environment by conductional radiation. In hot environment, the shell

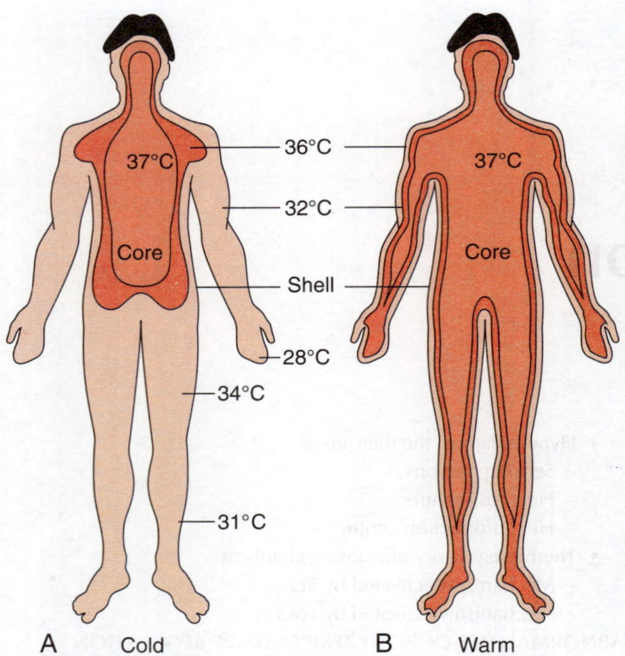

FIGURE 12.4-1 Concept of body core and shell temperature. Dark areas represent body core and superficial light areas represent body shell.

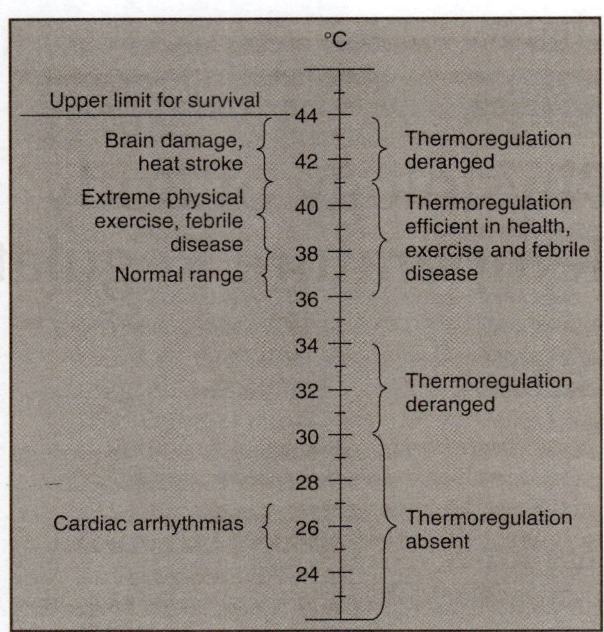

FIGURE 12.4-2 Effects of alteration of body temperature.

temperature approaches the core temperature (Fig. 12.4-1B), and this helps in heat loss by conduction and radiation.

- ***Core temperature,*** i.e. temperature of deeper body structures (e.g. temperature of intra-abdominal, intrathoracic and intracranial structures) is maintained strictly constant. It has been widely assumed to be an accurate index of the temperature of blood to which hypothalamic thermoregulatory receptors are exposed. The core temperature is always slightly more than the oral temperature (about 37.8°C or 100° F). Rectal, vaginal and oesophageal temperatures represent the core temperature. Oesophageal temperature taken at the heart level is a good index of rapid changes of cardiac and aortic blood temperature. Whereas, rectal temperature gives a poor reflection of rapid changes of blood temperature and may be misleading.

Lower versus Upper Lethal Core Temperature. As shown in Fig. 12.4-2, the *lower lethal core temperature* is about 26°C, at which cardiac arrhythmias occur and lead to death due to cardiac failure. *Upper lethal core temperature* is 43.5°C, which leads to death due to heat stroke. A core temperature of 41°C for prolonged periods produces irreversible brain damage.

Factors Affecting Body Temperature

I. Physiological Variations

1. Diurnal Variation. Body temperature is *highest* in the evening (after day's labour—between 5 and 7 p.m.) and *lowest* in early hour of morning (after night's rest between 2 and 4 a.m.). Difference between the two values may be 1°C. In the night workers, the rhythm is reversed. This diurnal variation is related to exercise and specific dynamic action of food. Fasting and absolute bed rest abolish this variation.

2. Age. *Infants* have imperfect regulation of temperature. Hence, range of variation is wider. A fit of crying may raise and a cold bath may lower the body temperature.

In old age, the body temperature tends to be subnormal due to decreased activity and decreased basal metabolic rate (BMR). In addition, due to compromised circulatory system, older individuals cannot tolerate extremes of environmental temperature.

3. Sex. *Females* have slightly low body temperature due to relatively low BMR and thick layer of subcutaneous fat (nonconductor). Further, due to thermogenic effect of progesterone, the body temperature is higher in *postovulatory phase* of menstrual cycle than in the preovulatory phase.

4. Size. Heat production and heat loss depend upon the ratio of mass to body surface area. In a mouse, heat production is 450 kcal/kg body weight/24 h, whereas in a horse it is only 14.5 kcal/kg body weight/24 h.

5. Food. Protein food, due to high specific dynamic action (SDA), may raise body temperature. The act of ingestion of food may also raise body temperature.

6. Exercise Increases Temperature. Only 25% of muscular energy is converted into mechanical work, the rest comes out as heat. Inability of heat-dissipating mechanisms to handle the greatly increased amount of heat produced increases body temperature. Further, there occurs resetting of the thermostat at a higher body temperature.

7. Atmospheric Conditions. Temperature, humidity and movement of air are directly concerned with the amount of heat loss from the surface and thus affect body temperature.

8. Sleep. Because of muscular inactivity, sleep results in a slight fall of body temperature.

9. Emotions. Body temperature may rise due to emotional disturbances. The rise of temperature may be as high as 2°C.

10. Posture, Piloerection and Clothing are also important factors that affect the body temperature. All animals and even humans may conserve heat or may prevent heat loss by curling up during exposure to cold.

II Pathological Variations

1. Hyperthermia or Fever refers to the pathologically raised body temperature. Common causes of fever are:

- *Pyrogens* are the toxic substances which raise the body temperature by affecting the hypothalamus. Pyrogens are released during infections (bacterial, viral, parasitic, etc.).
- *In hyperthyroidism*, body temperature is raised due to increased BMR.
- *Lesions of brain* and diabetes insipidus may be associated with raised temperature.

2. Hypothermia refers to lowered body temperature (below normal) due to some pathological causes, such as:

- Hypothyroidism,
- Hypopituitarism,
- Lesions in hypothalamus and
- Haemorrhage in certain parts of the brain particularly pons.

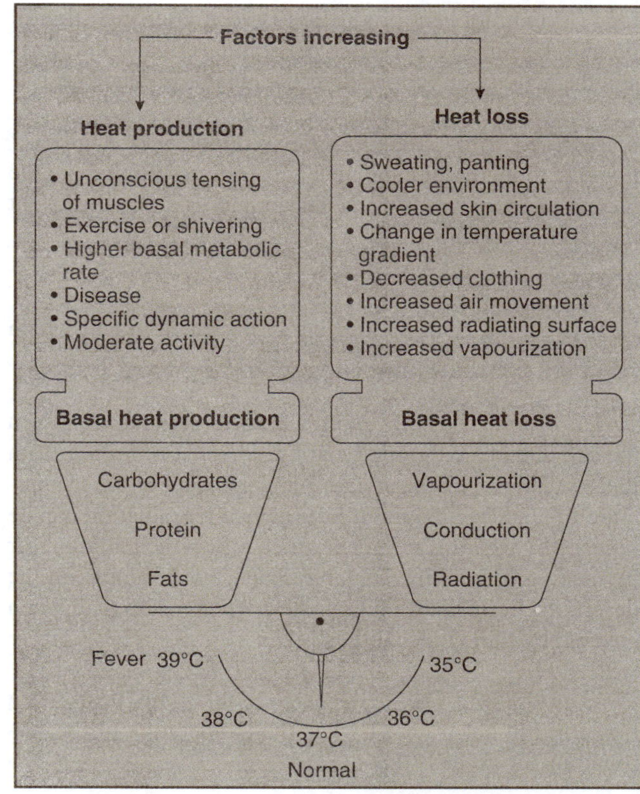

FIGURE 12.4-3 Balance between factors contributing to heat gain and heat loss from the body.

HEAT BALANCE

Heat balance refers to the balance between the mechanisms of net heat gains by the body and mechanisms of heat losses from the body (Fig. 12.4-3). The heat balance in the body is maintained by adjusting the heat production in accordance to heat loss and vice versa. In turn, the heat balance maintains the body temperature at a constant level.

Mechanisms of Heat Gain

The main mechanisms responsible for heat gain by the body are:

- Heat production in the body, and
- Heat gain from the environment.

Heat Production or Thermogenesis

Thermogenesis refers to heat production in the body by various physiological/metabolic processes which include:

1. Basal Metabolic Activity. The main mechanism responsible for heat production in the body is physiological oxidation of food materials, i.e. combustion of carbohydrates, proteins and fats; 1 g of each yields about 4, 4 and 9 calories, respectively. This is called *heat of metabolism*. Of all the organs, the liver contributes the highest amount of heat of metabolism. Heat produced by liver and heart is relatively constant.

2. Muscular Activity. Though heat produced by skeletal muscles is variable and depends upon the physiological activity, yet skeletal muscles are a major source of heat. The heat produced during muscular activity is called *heat of activity*. Muscular activities contributing to heat production are:

i. ***Muscle tone*** and unconscious tensing of muscles produce heat even when the individual is resting.
ii. ***During exercise,*** a great deal of heat is produced by the skeletal muscles.
iii. ***Respiratory muscle activity*** produces about 38% of activity heat.
iv. ***Shivering*** refers to muscle response to cold. It is characterized by oscillating rhythmic muscle tremors occurring at a rate of 10–20/s. During shivering, efferent impulses to skeletal muscles are controlled by descending pathways, primarily by hypothalamus, and heat production may increase several folds within seconds to minutes. As no work is performed during shivering, all the energy liberated by muscles appears as internal heat (*shivering thermogenesis*).

3. Specific Dynamic Action (SDA) of Food is the obligatory energy expenditure that occurs during assimilation of food. Maximum heat production is seen after ingestion of protein. During digestion, the peristaltic action of intestines and the activity of various digestive glands produce heat.

4. Nonshivering Thermogenesis refers to heat production due to increase in the metabolic rate resulting from the increased secretion of epinephrine and to a certain extent thyroid hormone.

Heat Gain from the Environment

Heat is gained from the objects in the environment which are hotter than the body by the following mechanisms:

1. Radiation. The body gains heat by *direct radiation* from the sun and heated ground and by *reflected radiation* from the sky. This type of heat gain is independent of the temperature of air. The amount of heat gained by radiation can be reduced by wearing garments which reflect the radiations or by making use of any available shade. For example, in the desert, the body takes up more heat when naked than when covered by thin white clothes.

2. Conduction. The body surface takes up heat when immersed in hot water or when the temperature of the surrounding air exceeds that of skin.

3. Ingestion of hot fluids and food can add a small amount of heat to the body.

4. Ventilation also adds to body heat in hot climates when air is heated.

Mechanisms of Heat Loss

Heat is lost from the body by the following routes:

- Heat loss from the skin,
- Heat loss from the lungs and
- Heat loss in the excreta.

I. Heat Loss from the Skin

Mechanisms of heat loss from the skin surface include (Table 12.4-1):

1. Radiation refers to transfer of heat from an object to another object with which it is not in contact. The magnitude of heat loss by radiation depends on the size of the body surface and the average temperature difference between the skin and the surrounding objects. About 50% of the total heat loss from the body occurs by radiation. The colour of clothing may play a part but the colour of human skin has no effect on the radiation.

2. Conduction refers to heat exchange between objects at different temperatures that are in contact with one another. The amount of heat transferred by conduction is proportionate to the temperature difference between the two objects.

TABLE 12.4-1 Mechanisms of Heat Loss from the Body

Mechanism	Amount of heat loss in calories		Percentage (%)	
Radiation	1500		50	70
Conduction and convection	600		20	
Evaporation of water from:				
• Skin	690	1000	20	27
• Lungs	210		7	
Warming inspired air	60		2	
Excreta (urine and faeces)	30		1	
Total	3000		100	

3. Convection refers to the movement of molecules of a gas or liquid at one temperature to another location that is at a different temperature. Thus, the heat loss through this process depends upon the temperature of the surrounding atmosphere. When the temperature of the surrounding atmosphere is low, heat is lost from the skin to the surrounding air. The molecules of air gradually get warmed and move away from the skin. Another layer of the cooler air takes its place. Thus, heat loss through convection depends upon the relative density and temperature of air and wind velocity.

Note. About 20% of heat is lost from the body by conduction and convection.

4. Evaporation. About 27% of the heat is lost by evaporation from the skin, mucous membranes and respiratory passages. Vaporization of 1 g (approximately 1 ml) of water resumes about 0.6 kcal of heat. Evaporation from skin only accounts for loss of 600 cal (20%) per day which occurs in two forms:

i. ***Insensible water loss (perspiration).*** Perspiration occurs due to continuous diffusion of fluid through the epidermis (in absence of sweating). It occurs over the entire body surface at a uniform rate and is largely independent of environmental conditions. Perspiration amounts to about 60 ml/day and is equivalent to heat loss by evaporation of approximately 400 kcal/day. But this heat loss is not under control and, therefore, cannot be changed as required.

ii. ***Evaporation of sweat.*** The eccrine sweat glands play a very important role in thermoregulation of the body. *Thermal sweating* from eccrine sweat glands increases when the external or internal body temperature rises (details are given). Sweat is vaporized from the skin, which decreases its temperature. Evaporation decreases to a great extent if the humidity of the atmosphere is high, and thus body temperature regulation becomes seriously affected.

Factors Affecting Cutaneous Heat Loss

1. ***Gradient between the temperature of the skin and the environmental temperature*** is the most important factor determining the cutaneous heat loss, especially by the radiation, conduction and convection mechanisms. The temperature of skin that depends upon the amount of heat reaching the surface from the deeper tissues can be varied by changing the blood flow to the skin depending upon the requirement. This is accomplished by the radiator system of the body.

   Radiator system of the body is formed by the cutaneous circulation. Blood vessels penetrate fatty subcutaneous insulator tissue and are distributed profusely beneath the skin. There is a venous plexus underneath the skin, which is supplied by inflow of blood from the skin capillaries. In exposed areas of the body, such as hands, feet and ears, there is arteriovenous anastomoses (blood is supplied to the plexus directly from the small arteries). The rate of blood flow through venous plexus can be varied as:

   - *When the cutaneous blood vessels are dilated,* the blood flow to the venous plexus can be increased up to 30% of the total cardiac output. As the warm blood fills the subcutaneous venous plexus, the skin temperature approaches the deep tissue temperature. It promotes heat loss.
   - *When the cutaneous blood vessels are constricted,* e.g. on exposure to extreme cold, the rate of blood flow to the venous plexus can be reduced to as low as 2–3% of cardiac output. Consequently, the skin temperature, especially of the hands and feet, becomes much lower than the deep tissue temperature (Fig. 12.4-4). In this way, heat loss is minimized by decrease in the temperature gradient between skin and environment.

   Changing flow of blood through skin is thus the effective mechanism of controlling heat loss. The skin therefore forms an effective radiator system.

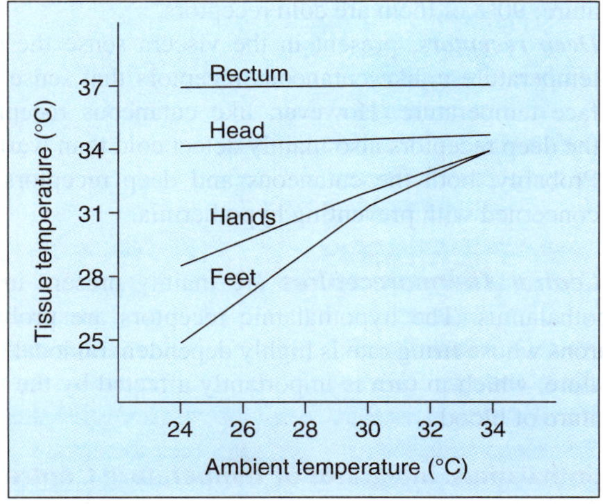

FIGURE 12.4-4 Effect of exposure of naked individuals to low ambient temperature on different parts of the body.

2. ***Insulator system***. The subcutaneous fat acts as the heat insulator for the body. Fat conducts heat only one-third as readily as other tissues. This insulation is important in maintaining the core temperature even though the skin temperature varies with that of the surroundings. Women have a thicker layer of subcutaneous fat than men; this is partly the reason why in winter, males feel more cold than the females. This is in spite of the fact that males produce more heat because of higher basal metabolic rate (BMR).
3. ***Piloerector muscle*** contracts in response to cold and causes erection of the hair. The layer of air entrapped between the hair acts as an insulator and thus reduces the cutaneous heat loss.
4. ***Clothing***. Woollen clothes offer better protection against cold than cotton clothes, because of larger amount of air entrapped in the former. In animals, the fur and feathers serve the same purpose more effectively.

II. Heat Loss from the Lungs

Heat loss from the lungs occurs by three processes:

1. ***Evaporation of Water*** in expired air causes heat loss. On an average, the water loss from the lungs is approximately 300 ml/day equivalent to heat loss of 200 kcal. It is the main mechanism through which heat is lost in dogs and sheep.

2. ***Warming Inspired Air*** to the body temperature accounts for 2% of heat loss in man.

3. ***Panting.*** Some mammals lose heat by panting. Panting refers to rapid shallow breathing which greatly increases the amount of water to be evaporated in the mouth and respiratory passages and thereby results in the heat loss.

III. Heat Loss in the Excreta

About 1% of the total body heat loss occurs in the excreta (urine and faeces).

REGULATION OF BODY TEMPERATURE

Like other homeothermic animals, humans have been provided with a *temperature control system* which maintains the internal (core) body temperature constant within the range of ±1°F of the normal temperature. Normal body temperature is the 'set point' in the system of temperature regulation. In humans, the set point of the temperature control system is approximately 98.6°F (37°C), although it normally varies somewhat diurnally, decreasing to a minimum during sleep. The set point can be altered by pathological status, for example, by the action of pyrogens, which induce fever (see page 1247).

Thermoneutral Zone Before discussing the temperature control system, it will be appropriate to know about the thermoneutral zone (TNZ). The thermoneutral zone refers to the range of ambient temperature within which the metabolic rate is at a minimum, i.e. at which the O_2 consumption at rest or when asleep is minimal and temperature regulation is achieved by nonevaporative physical processes alone (Fig. 12.4-5). The values of thermoneutral zone in naked humans are (Fig. 12.4-6):

- Adults: 26–28°C,
- Newborn infants: 32–34°C and
- Premature infants: 35°C.

Certain other terms which need mention are:

Critical Temperature. It is the lower limit of thermoneutral zone. Below it the metabolic heat production of a resting thermoregulating animal increases to maintain thermal balance (Fig. 12.4-5).

Preferred Ambient Temperature (PAT). It is the range of ambient temperature associated with thermal comfort. It is not the same as thermoneutral zone (TNZ). It is important to note that:

- When humidity is high the PAT would be lower than the TNZ, and
- When air movement is brisk the PAT would be higher than the TNZ.

Thermal Comfort is maximum when the skin temperature is about 33°C and also depends upon:

- Level of humidity,
- Amount of air movement,
- Level of body activity and
- Amount of clothing.

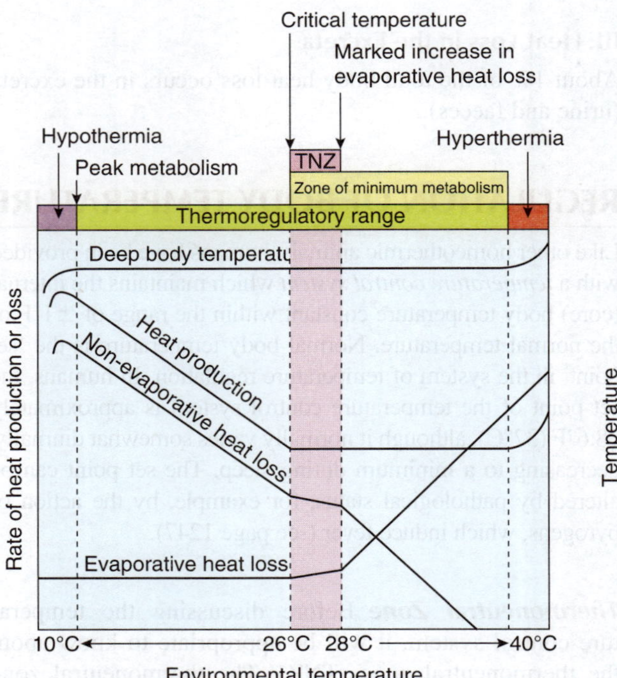

FIGURE 12.4-5 Thermoneutral zone and rate of heat production and heat loss in relation to environmental temperature.

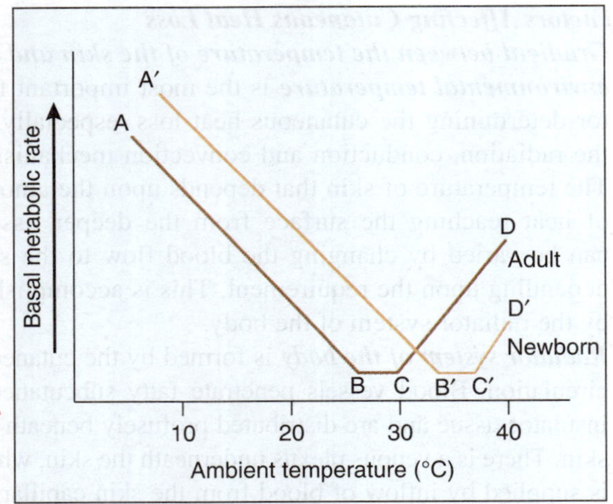

FIGURE 12.4-6 Thermoneutral zone of the newborn (B'-C') compared with that of an adult human (B-C).

Temperature Control System The temperature control system comprises the hypothalamus integrated autonomic, endocrine and skeletomotor responses. The components of the temperature control system are:

- Thermoreceptors,
- Hypothalamus, the thermostat and integrator of temperature control system and
- The thermoregulatory effector mechanisms.

Thermoreceptors

Thermoreceptors or temperature receptors which give information about the body temperature to the temperature control centre in the hypothalamus are of two types: peripheral thermoreceptors and central thermoreceptors.

1. Peripheral Thermoreceptors are present throughout the body in the skin and mucous membrane (and probably other organs such as muscle and viscera).

- ***Cutaneous thermoreceptors*** sense the ambient temperature; 90% of them are cold receptors.
- ***Deep receptors,*** present in the viscera sense the core temperature unlike cutaneous receptors that sense surface temperature. However, like cutaneous receptors, the deep receptors also mainly detect cold than warmth. Probably, both the cutaneous and deep receptors are concerned with preventing hypothermia.

2. Central Thermoreceptors are mainly present in the hypothalamus. The hypothalamic receptors are probably neurons whose firing rate is highly dependent on local temperature, which in turn is importantly affected by the temperature of blood.

Hypothalamus: Integrator of Temperature Control System

The integrator and many controlling elements for temperature regulation appear to be located in the hypothalamus.

The system acts as a *servo-mechanism* (a control system that uses negative feedback to operate another system) with a *set point* at normal body temperature (98.6°F or 37°C). The hypothalamic neurons involved in temperature regulation can be divided into three types, depending upon the function subserved by them:

- Sensing neurons or feedback detectors,
- Heat loss centre or antirise centre and
- Heat production and conservation centre or antidrop centre.

Sensing Neurons or Feedback Detectors. These neurons, located in the anterior hypothalamus, collect information about temperature from both the central as well as peripheral thermoreceptors.

Two types of neurons have been identified in this area, the *warm-sensitive neurons*, which respond to information from warmth receptors and *cold-sensitive neurons*, which respond to cold receptors.

The central and peripheral thermoreceptors rarely provide identical information about body temperature. In dealing with the body temperature, therefore, the hypothalamus calculates an integrated temperature from the feedback received.

Heat Loss Centre (antirise centre) along with the heat production and conservation centre form the two thermoregulatory systems. Each of this system has its own cut-off temperature at which the heating or cooling mechanisms are activated or deactivated.

Heat loss centre is composed of neurons in the preoptic region and anterior or rostral hypothalamus. It organizes the heat loss responses as illustrated:

- ***Electrical stimulation*** of this area produces heat loss by cutaneous vasodilatation, sweating, panting, and decreases heat production by inhibiting shivering.
- ***Lesions of heat loss centre,*** conversely, prevent sweating and cutaneous vasodilatation and they cause hyperthermia (neurogenic fever) when the individual is placed in a warm environment.

Heat Production and Conservation Centre (antidrop centre) is formed by the neurons in the area of *posterior or caudal hypothalamus* which is dorsolateral to the mammillary body. These neurons organize the heat production and conservation responses as illustrated:

- ***Stimulation*** of this area conserves heat by cutaneous vasoconstriction and activates heat production by evoking shivering and increasing the metabolic rate through the release of thyroid-stimulating hormone (TSH).
- ***Lesions*** in this area interfere with heat production and conservation, and they can cause *hypothermia* when the subject is in cold environment.

Thermoregulatory Effector Mechanisms

As described above, the effector mechanisms of thermoregulation are integrated by a thermostat located in the hypothalamus, and that the *hypothalamic thermostat* has a set point which is normally at 98.6°F (37°C). Error signals that represent a deviation from the set point, either due to raised or lowered body temperature, evoke responses that tend to restore body temperature towards the set point. These responses are mediated by autonomic, somatic and endocrine systems. The thermoregulatory effector mechanisms activated by hypothalamus can be grouped as:

A. ***Mechanisms activated by heat***
  I. *Mechanisms increasing heat loss:*
    1. Cutaneous vasodilatation,
    2. Sweating and
    3. Increased respiration/panting.
  II. *Mechanisms decreasing heat production:*
    1. Anorexia and
    2. Behavioural responses.

B. ***Mechanisms activated by cold***
  I. *Mechanisms conserving heat:*
    1. Cutaneous vasoconstriction,
    2. Piloerection and
    3. Behavioural mechanisms.
  II. *Mechanisms increasing heat production:*
    1. Shivering,
    2. Thermogenic chemical (nonshivering) thermogenesis and
    3. Behavioural responses.

A. Mechanisms Activated by Heat

I. Mechanisms Increasing Heat Loss

1. Cutaneous Vasodilatation As described on page 1243, the cutaneous vessels form the radiator system of the body. Cutaneous vasodilatation occurring on exposure to heat stresses increases cutaneous blood flow from 4–5 ml/100 g skin weight/min to as high as 150 ml/100 g of skin weight/min. By this, warm blood from the deeper tissues is brought to the surface, and heat loss by conduction, radiation and convection is facilitated as described above.

Mechanisms of cutaneous vasodilatation. Cutaneous vasodilatation is produced through a local effect, spinal reflex as well as through the hypothalamus.

i. ***Local effect.*** Body kinins released from the secretory activity of sweat glands cause local vasodilatation.
ii. ***Spinal reflex*** evoked by peripheral thermoreceptors produce localized vasodilatation.
iii. ***Hypothalamus controlled vasodilatation.*** Impulses from the heat loss centre of hypothalamus produce inhibition of the sympathetic discharge to cutaneous vessels causing vasodilatation and accumulation of blood in subpapillary venous plexus. The effect of sympathetic inhibition is particularly prominent in the hands, feet and ear lobules, where A-V anastomoses present in the skin are normally kept closed by the strong sympathetic discharge.

2. Sweating As mentioned earlier, the evaporation of sweat is the most important mechanism of heat loss, especially when a person is exposed to the environmental temperature greater than the body temperature.

Sweat glands. There are two types of sweat glands: eccrine and apocrine.

Eccrine sweat glands are distributed all over the body. Their ducts open on the surface of skin independent of hair follicles. These glands play the main role in thermoregulation of the body.

Apocrine glands are found in the skin of the axilla, pubic, circumareolar and circumanal areas. Their ducts open into a hair follicle above the opening of sebaceous glands. These glands do not have any thermoregulatory function.

Mechanism of heat-induced sweating. When the environmental temperature rises above the *thermal comfort level* (about 33°C), sweating is induced by three mechanisms: a local response, spinal reflex as well as through hypothalamus influence. The impulses from the heat loss centre of the anterior hypothalamus increase the impulse discharge in the sympathetic cholinergic fibres to the sweat glands. As a result, sweating starts suddenly, and the rate of sweating progressively increases with the increase in environmental temperature.

Rate of sweating, which is practically zero in cold weather, may reach to a maximum of 700 ml/h in bad weather. In very hot climate, sweat secretion may be over 10 L/day. Such a heavy sweating causes marked loss of body water and NaCl. This happens because body homeostasis mechanisms give priority to temperature regulation over water and electrolyte regulation. Therefore, in acute heat stress, death may occur due to severe dehydration and salt loss leading to circulatory failure.

Acclimatization of sweating mechanism is an adaptation which occurs following prolonged exposure to high environmental temperature. Acclimatization is very useful in conserving body NaCl as explained:

The composition of sweat produced by glandular epithelial cells is modified by the ductal cells when sweat passes through the ducts. The NaCl concentration in primary secretion from the glandular cells is about 60 mEq/L. When the rate of sweat formation is low, the primary secretion passes slowly through the ducts, and during this time most of the NaCl is reabsorbed by the ductal cells and the Na^+ concentration in the sweat may be as low as 5 mEq/L. On exposure to high temperature environment, the sympathetic stimulation of the gland is very strong and so the rate of secretion becomes high. The primary secretion quickly passes through the ducts, and so the time available for Na^+ reabsorption is decreased. As a consequence, more NaCl is lost in the sweat, to the extent of 15–30 g/day. However, a prolonged exposure to high environmental temperature leads to acclimatization which leads to gradual decrease in NaCl concentration in the sweat, so that even at high rate of sweat secretion its Na^+ concentration remains low.

Mechanism of acclimatization. Acclimatization occurs due to increased secretion of aldosterone (stimulated due to slight decrease in NaCl levels of body fluids because of excessive sweating before acclimatization). Aldosterone increases absorption of Na^+ and Cl^- from the duct. This reduces excretion of salt to 3–5 g/day compared with 15–30 g/day before acclimatization.

3. Panting Panting refers to rapid shallow breathing which increases heat loss by increasing water vaporization in the mouth and respiratory passages. In some animals, like dogs, panting is an effective means of heat loss. Because the breathing is shallow, it produces little disturbance in the arterial pCO_2 or pH.

II. Mechanisms Decreasing Heat Production and Heat Gain from Environment

1. Anorexia and Lethargy. A rise in ambient temperature produces anorexia and lethargy. Anorexia results in decreased food intake which decreases heat production because of decrease in specific dynamic action of food. Lethargy decreases muscular activity which decreases heat of activity.

2. Behavioural Responses include shelter in shade or a cooler place and preference for cold food and drinks. These acts decrease heat gain from the environment.

B. Mechanisms Activated by Cold

I. Mechanisms Conserving Heat

1. Cutaneous Vasoconstriction. As mentioned earlier (see page 1243), the immediate reflex response to cold is cutaneous vasoconstriction, which reduces the heat loss from the body core to the surface and thus conserves heat.

Mechanism. Like vasodilatation, cutaneous vasoconstriction is produced through:

- Direct local effect of cold,
- Local spinal reflex, evoked through peripheral thermoreceptors and
- Hypothalamus controlled cutaneous vasoconstriction. Impulses from 'heat production and conservation centre' (which is located in the posterior hypothalamus) increase the sympathetic discharge to the cutaneous vessels causing extreme vasoconstriction. The effect of increased sympathetic discharge is particularly prominent in the hands, feet and ear lobules where closure of A-V anastomoses (present in the skin) reduces the cutaneous blood flow to as low as 1 ml/100 g skin weight/min. As a result, the practically blood less skin prevents heat loss by becoming an insulating barrier between the warm core of the body and the cold environment.

2. Piloerection, i.e. cold-induced erection of the body hair, as mentioned earlier, entraps a layer of air in the hair,

which acts as an insulator and thus reduces the cutaneous heat loss.

3. Behavioural Responses which help heat conservation are:

- *Curling up while sleeping*. It reduces the body surface area in contact with the environment.
- *To put warmer clothes* also prevent heat loss.

II. Mechanisms Increasing Heat Production

1. Shivering Thermogenesis. When the heat loss prevented by cutaneous vasoconstriction is not sufficient to cope up with the environmental cold, heat production is increased by shivering (for details see page 1241). Shivering is evoked in response to impulses from the 'heat production and conservation centre' located in the posterior or caudal hypothalamus.

2. Chemical (Nonshivering) Thermogenesis refers to increased heat production due to increased cellular metabolism. It is associated with uncoupling of oxidative phosphorylation, i.e. the oxidation of foodstuffs is associated with release of heat rather than generation of ATPs. Chemical thermogenesis occurs because of the following effects:

i. ***Increased sympathetic stimulation and increased secretion of catecholamines*** (epinephrine and norepinephrine), which occurs as a part of response to cold. *Role of brown fat.* The amount of chemical thermogenesis occurring in response to increased catecholamine secretion is proportional to the amount of brown fat in the tissues, because the brown fat contains large number of special mitochondria where the uncoupled oxidation occurs. Adults do not have brown fat; therefore, heat production by this mechanism is increased by only 10–15%. However, in infants (who have brown fat in interscapular region, around the neck, behind the sternum and around the kidneys), increased secretion of catecholamines may increase heat production by 100%.

ii. ***Increased secretion of thyroxine*** also promotes chemical thermogenesis. After several weeks of exposure to severe cold, hyperplasia of thyroid gland and increased secretion of thyroxine can be demonstrated. This occurs because the cold temperature stimulates hypothalamic release of TRH, which in turn stimulates the secretion of TSH and thyroxine. Consequently, thyroxine secretion in winters is somewhat greater than in summers. In infants, even short exposure to cold increases thyroxine secretion.

3. Behavioural Responses associated with increased heat production are:

i. ***Hyperphagia*** helps in increased heat production because of specific dynamic action of food.

ii. ***Hyperactivity,*** e.g. in the form of rubbing of palms also increases heat production.

iii. ***Seeking out sources of heat,*** e.g. standing out in the sun, or heat fire and also consumption of hot food and hot drinks, help in gaining heat.

ABNORMALITIES OF BODY TEMPERATURE REGULATION

Fever

Fever, also known as *pyrexia,* refers to an increase in the body temperature above the normal range. It is the most common symptom/sign of the ill health.

Causes. Common causes of fever are:

1. ***Infections*** caused by bacteria, viruses, protozoa (e.g. malaria) and other infecting agents are usually associated with fever.
2. ***Tissue destruction,*** as in myocardial infarction, uninfected neoplasms, serum sickness and rheumatism, etc. is also associated with fever.
3. ***Pyrexia of unknown origin (PUO).*** This term is used when cause of fever cannot be ascertained.

Pathogenesis. Fever develops when the hypothalamic set point is reset at a higher temperature by the pyrogens as explained (Fig. 12.4-7):

Role of pyrogens. Toxins liberated from the infecting organism and tissue destruction act on the phagocytic cells (monocytes, macrophages and Kupffer cells) to produce cytokines that act as *endogenous pyrogens*. The pyrogens are polypeptides and include interleukin-I (IL-I) and other cytokines, which act on the anterior hypothalamus to increase the production of prostaglandin E_2. Prostaglandin E_2 acts on the hypothalamus to increase the thermostat 'set point'. This explains how drugs like aspirin, which prevent the formation of prostaglandin E_2 from arachidonic acid, act as antipyretics (which lower the temperature).

Production of fever. Once the thermostat set point is raised by the pyrogens, the heat-producing mechanisms and heat-conserving mechanisms of the body are activated till the body temperature equals the elevated hypothalamic thermostat set point, i.e. till fever is produced. Because of these mechanisms, during production of fever there occurs:

- Shivering (which produces heat),
- Skin vessels are constricted to minimize heat loss,
- Rate of metabolism is increased which increases further heat production and
- Chills are felt in fever when the heat-generating and heat-conserving mechanisms are active.

Termination of fever. When the causes producing pyrogens are removed, the set point of hypothalamic thermostat is reset back to normal. At this juncture, since the body temperature is higher than the set point of thermostat, the heat production is decreased and mechanisms of heat loss

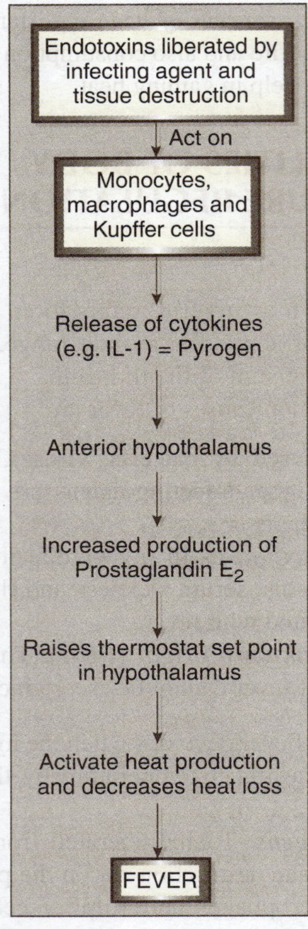

FIGURE 12.4-7 Pathogenesis of fever.

are activated. Because of these mechanisms, during termination of fever, there occurs:

- Cutaneous vasodilatation and
- Profuse sweating.

This sudden change in febrile condition associated with profuse sweating and red and hot skin is called *crisis* or *flush*. ***Beneficial effects of fever*** include:

- *Inhibition of growth of bacteria, viruses* and other infecting organisms occurs at high body temperature. Because of this effect, artificial flue therapy was used to treat infections before the advent of antibiotics.
- *Antibody production* is increased when body temperature is raised.
- *Growth of some tumours* is slowed down by the increased body temperature.

Harmful effects of fever include:

- Dehydration, negative nitrogen balance, loss of NaCl and alkalosis (because of hyperventilation).
- Permanent damage to brain, kidney and liver may occur when the core temperature is more than 41°C (hyperpyrexia) for prolonged period.
- Death may occur due to heat stroke when temperature rises above 43°C.

Heat Exhaustion and Heat Stroke

Heat Exhaustion refers to a condition of circulatory failure caused by excessive sweating following prolonged exposure to heat. It is characterized by dehydration, salt loss, decreased blood volume and decreased arterial pressure and syncope (fainting).

Heat stroke usually occurs when heavy physical work is performed in hot and humid environment. In this condition, normal response to increased ambient temperature (sweating) is impaired, and core temperature increases to the point of tissue damage. Convulsion, loss of consciousness and even death may occur when body temperature exceeds 41°C.

Hypothermia

Hypothermia results when the ambient temperature is so low that the body's heat generating mechanisms (e.g. shivering and metabolism) cannot adequately maintain core temperature near the set point. Infants and old people develop hypothermia more easily than the adults.

It has been observed that:

- At a rectal temperature of 28°C, the body's ability to spontaneously return the temperature is lost.
- Humans can tolerate body temperature of 21–24°C without permanent ill effects, i.e. if rewarmed with external heat, returns to a normal state. *Effects of hypothermia* on body include:
- Slowing of metabolic and physiologic processes,
- Retardation of glucose metabolism,
- Slowing of respiration and heart rate,
- Lowering of blood pressure,
- Slowing of reflexes and occurrence of muscular rigidity,
- Loss of consciousness and
- Death may occur when temperature remains below 25°C for some time.

Accidental Hypothermia occurs due to prolonged exposure to cold air or cold water, e.g. after ship wreck or accidents in high mountain. It is a serious condition and requires careful monitoring and prompt rewarming.

Induced Hypothermia. The fact that the human body can tolerate hypothermia (of 21–24° C) for quite some time without ill effects has been explained for use in heart and brain surgery. The induction of hypothermia during surgery is made easier with the use of anaesthesia and muscle relaxants, both of which abolish shivering.

Poikilothermia

Poikilothermia refers to a condition in which the individual is not able to maintain core body temperature during fluctuations in the environmental temperature. That is, with increase in the environmental temperature, the body temperature increases and with the decrease in environmental temperature, the body temperature decreases. Such a condition of impaired thermoregulation occurs in hypothalamic lesions and brain stem lesions that interrupt descending hypothalamic fibres to the spinal cord.

Malignant Hyperthermia

Malignant hyperthermia is caused in susceptible individuals by inhalation anaesthesia. It is characterized by a massive increase in oxygen consumption and heat production by skeletal muscle, which causes a rapid rise in body temperature. In susceptive individuals, a defective ryanodine receptor leads to excess Ca^{2+} release during muscle contraction triggered by stress (See page 109).

Chapter 12.5

Physiology of Growth and Behavioural Development

GROWTH AND DEVELOPMENT

The terms growth and development are intimately interdependent and interacting with each other. Growth per se refers to the increase in the physical size, as the child grows to adulthood, while development refers to maturity, i.e. improvement in the capability of the tissue. They are, therefore, termed together to signify a process of maturation, both in quality and quantity.

Growth Curves

Growth of different parts of the body does not follow a uniform pattern. The patterns of growth of different parts are described in the form of different growth curves (Fig. 12.5-1):

1. General Growth Curve shows two growth spurts: one in infancy, and another around puberty (Fig.12.5-1A).

General growth refers to increase in height, weight and growth of the skeletal muscle, blood volume, respiratory system, cardiovascular system, GIT and excretory system.

Infancy Growth Spurt. Weight and height are generally considered a good index of the child's growth potential and a delicate measure of the individual's health.

The first spurt of growth occurring in infancy is characterized by increase in birth weight to two times by 6 months of age, three times at 1 year of age, four times at 2 years of age. After this, the weight increases by about 2 kg per year till about 12 years of age.

Height increases in increments of 2–2.5 cm per month in the first year of postnatal life. Thereafter, it slows down (Table 12.5-1).

Adolescent Growth Spurt is characterized by rapid increase in weight gain, about 3.5 kg per year between 12 and 18 years of age (Table 12.5-1). During this period, rapid growth of bones is brought about by the various endocrinal influences. After this, the rate of growth again slows down. *Height* increase during adolescent growth of spurt varies between 4 and 7 cm per year depending on the genetic potential and endocrinal factors (Table 12.5-1).

2. Neural Growth Curve shows that brain, spinal cord and visual apparatus grow very rapidly after birth (Fig. 12.5-1B). At the end of the first year of postnatal life, the brain has already achieved 2/3rd and by the end of second year 4/5th of adult size. By 5 years of age, the brain is almost fully developed and the child is ready for education and training. The measurement of head circumference (which also increases with the growth of brain) is thus very important up to 3–5 years of age to get information of the developing brain inside.

3. Lymphoid Growth Curve The growth of lymphoid organs such as tonsils, adenoids, thymus, spleen, lymph nodes and lymphoid tissue of the intestine is very rapid in infancy and childhood and is followed by a partial involution at puberty (Fig. 12.5-1C). Because of this reason, the size of tonsils and adenoids at the age of 8–10 years is larger than in the adults. This is important to recognize that more enlargement of tonsils is not an indication for removing them surgically.

4. Gonadal Growth Curve The gonads and accessory organs of reproduction remain in dormancy in childhood and grow at a remarkable rate around puberty. Thus, gonadal growth pattern is essentially opposite to the neural growth pattern (Fig. 12.5-1D).

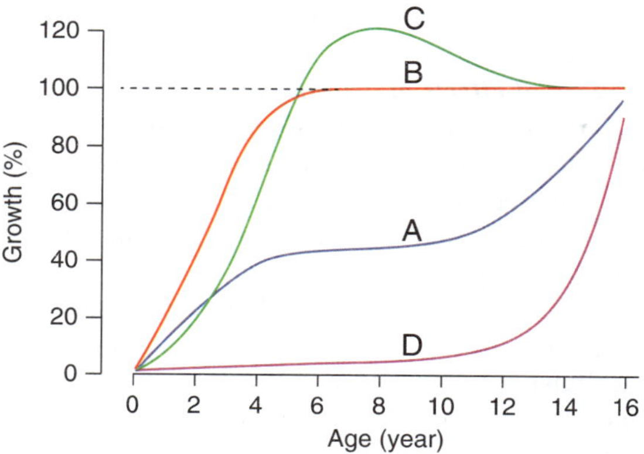

FIGURE 12.5-1 Different growth curves: **A,** general growth curve; **B,** neural growth curve; **C,** lymphoid growth curve; and **D,** gonadal growth curve.

TABLE 12.5-1 Mean Weight and Height at Different Ages in Indian Children

	Weight (kg)		Height (cm)	
Age	*Male*	*Female*	*Male*	*Female*
Birth	2.8	2.7	48.5	47.7
3 months	4.5	4.5	60.2	58.5
6 months	6.2	6.0	65	63.6
9 months	7.9	7.5	68.7	67.6
1 years	8.9	8.4	73.9	72.8
3 years	12.6	12	88.8	87.2
6 years	16.3	16	108.5	107.4
9 years	21.5	21.3	123.7	122.9
12 years	28.5	29.8	138.3	139.2
15 years	39.6	36.8	155.5	149.6
18 years	47.4	42.4	163.1	151.7

Source: Indian Council of Medical Research (ICMR).

Factors Affecting Growth

Marked differences existing between the growth and development patterns of various races and communities and different individuals in the same race and community are determined by various factors, which affect the growth:

1. Genetic Factors. The ultimate growth pattern of an individual is largely determined by the genetic inheritance, either maternal or paternal.

2. Hormonal Factors. The important hormones which affect the growth and development are:

i. *Growth hormone (GH)* secreted by anterior pituitary plays an important role in the growth and thus determines the height of an individual during childhood (see page 685). Therefore, deficiency of GH produces growth retardation known as *pituitary dwarfism*.

ii. *Insulin-like growth factor-1 (IGF-1),* as the name indicates chemically resembles insulin. It is one of the poly-peptides which are collectively known as somatomedins. IGF-1, like GH, promotes protein synthesis and epiphyseal growth. Some of its actions are opposite to GH.

iii. *Thyroxine* plays an important role in the growth and development by its direct action, and also indirectly by potentiating the release of GH and somatomedins (see page 704). Congenital deficiency of thyroxine results in a clinical condition called 'cretinism', which is characterized by retardation of physical as well as mental growth.

iv. *Sex hormones*. The oestrogens and androgens cause maturation and are important in the adolescent age. The anabolic actions of sex hormones, adrenal androgens, growth hormone and IGF-1 seem to potentiate each other, producing a marked growth spurt during puberty.

v. *Insulin* is an anabolic hormone and thus its role in growth and development cannot be overemphasized. Congenital deficiency of insulin results in juvenile diabetes mellitus. Retardation of growth is one of the characteristic features of juvenile diabetes mellitus.

Relative importance of different hormones at various stages of growth is (Fig. 12.5-2):

- *Thyroxine* is essential for growth in late fetal life and first few years of postnatal life (Fig. 12.5-2A).
- *Growth hormone* in contrast to thyroxine does not seem to be of critical importance during fetal and early postnatal life. Infants with congenital deficiency of GH have normal height and weight up to about 2 years of age, after which a decrease in the velocity of growth becomes apparent (Fig. 12.5-2B).
- *Insulin*, being an anabolic hormone, remains important during fetal as well as postnatal growth (Fig. 12.5-2C).
- *Sex hormones* are most essential around puberty and play an important role in the development of gonads as well as general growth (Fig. 12.5-2D).

3. Nutritional Factors. The major ingredients of diet, viz. proteins, fats, carbohydrates, minerals and vitamins are important for optimal growth, both pre- and postnatally. Protein and its various amino acids are essential for laying down the new tissues, for wear and tear and for specific metabolic functions. Their requirements are increased during active periods of growth.

Lack of nutritional factors affects normal growth even when the genetic and hormonal factors are normal. Undernutrition and malnutrition in childhood is responsible for smaller status, poor muscular development and generalized apathy in underdeveloped countries.

4. Illnesses. Congenital anomalies compatible with life are likely to retard the growth of the child. Acute illnesses

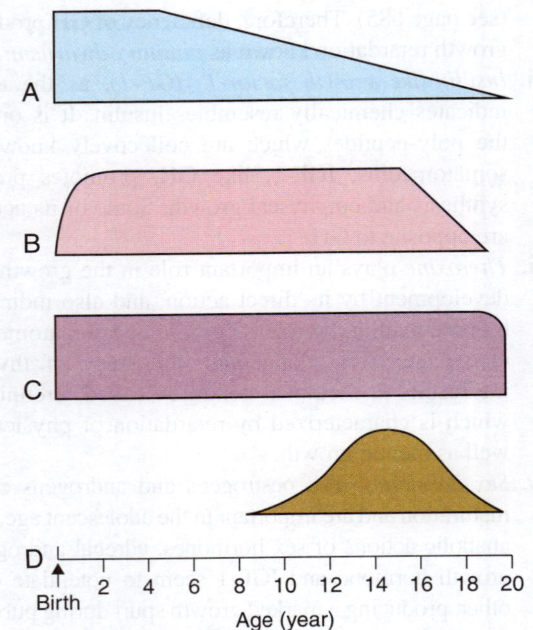

FIGURE 12.5-2 Relative importance of different hormones at various stages of growth: **A,** thyroxine; **B,** growth hormone; **C,** insulin; and **D,** sex hormones.

temporarily depress growth. Chronic long-standing illnesses, including long-standing infections, can markedly interfere with normal pattern of physical and mental growth and can produce permanent growth retardation.

5. Emotional Factors. Lack of love and security and a disturbed child–parent relationship result in various psychological and behavioural problems during childhood and adolescence, which result in distortion of normal development and achievement of maturity.

6. Internal Milieu. Normal metabolism and co-ordinate functioning of all the organs result in optimum growth. Disturbed internal metabolism in various liver and kidney diseases precludes normal growth.

7. Environmental Factors. The environment influences the growth pattern right from the intrauterine life. Faulty position of the fetus, faulty implantation of the ovum, rubella syndrome, etc. are amongst the earliest environmental factors influencing growth. Birth injuries during a difficult labour and other factors during natal period interfere with the normal development. Exposure to various seasonal variations has a similar effect. The countries in temperate zone have a small average height because of suboptimal environment. Lack of sunshine and poor personal hygiene also affect the normal growth.

8. Socioeconomic Factors also play an important role in growth and development of a child.

Growth Factors

Growth factors refer to a number of polypeptides which regulate the proliferation of cells in the embryonic and postnatal life and thus ultimately affect the growth of various tissues.

Pattern of effects of growth factors are:

1. Endocrine Effect. This pattern of effect is shown by some of the growth factors, which are released into the circulation and act at a distant site. Examples of the growth factors acting through the endocrine effect include growth hormone and erythropoietin.

2. Paracrine Effect. A growth factor is said to exert its paracrine effect when it is released by a cell into the extracellular environment, and it acts on the nearby cells. Platelet-derived growth factor or fibroblast growth factor acts in this fashion.

3. Autocrine Effect of a growth factor means that the growth factor acts on the cells which produce them.

Actions of Growth Factors. Actions of some of the important growth factors are summarized in Table 12.5-2.

BEHAVIOURAL DEVELOPMENT

Behavioural development of a child is studied through various responses which the child exhibits, following a natural or experimental stimulus. The developmental status depends not only on the age but also on the

TABLE 12.5-2 Actions of Commonly Known Growth Factors

Name of growth factors	Action
Growth hormone	General tissue growth
Insulin-like growth factor (IGF-1)	General tissue growth
Erythropoietin	Proliferation of red cell precursors
Thrombotin	Proliferation of platelet precursors
Colony-stimulating factors Granulocyte stimulating factor	Proliferation of granulocyte and monocyte
Lymphokines	Proliferation of lymphocytes
Epidermal growth factor (EGF)	Proliferation of epithelial cells, fibroblasts and glial cells
Platelet-derived growth factor	Growth of vascular smooth muscle
Fibroblast growth factor	Proliferation of fibroblast, endothelial cells and vascular smooth muscle
Nerve growth factor	Growth and maintenance of neurons

environment. The age determines the proper physical and biochemical growth of various constituent organs, and the environment determines the experiences during the process of learning. Hence, both the factors are essential to determine a particular behaviour which in other words could be called a milestone in the developmental process.

Behaviour Pattern Behaviour pattern can be divided into four groups, for the sake of convenience, to observe the development in different age groups (Gessel):

1. Motor Behaviour. *Gross motor behaviour* is the behavioural response in ventral suspension, supine, prone, sitting, standing and walking postures. *Fine motor behaviour* is seen in the form of grasp and manipulation of the objects, e.g. cube, pellet and string.
2. Adaptive Behaviour. This includes sensory and motor adjustments to objects and co-ordination of eyes and hands to adjust with the simple problem situations which are set before the infant.
3. Language Behaviour. This includes all visible and audible forms of communication whether by facial expression, gestures, postural movements, vocalisation of words, phrases or sentences and mimicry. Articulate speech depends upon social milieu and readiness of sensory, motor and cortical structures.
4. Personal–social Behaviour. A child's individual reaction depends primarily upon the neuromotor maturity and the social culture in which the child lives. These include bladder and bowel control, feeding abilities, sense of priority, self-dependence in play, co-operativeness and emotional responsiveness to various stimuli.

Developmental and Intelligent Quotient ***Developmental quotient (DQ)*** represents the proportion of normal development that is present at any given age. The measurement of the former depends upon the achievement of the adaptive behaviour, e.g. prehension, locomotion and manipulation.

$$DQ = \frac{\text{Maturity age}}{\text{Chronological age}} \times 100$$

Intelligent quotient (IQ). The child can make use of his intellectual capabilities at the age of 5–6 years, because mental development is almost complete by this age. Therefore, intelligent quotient can only be applied at this age, unlike that of developmental quotient which can be tested at any age after birth.

$$IQ = \frac{\text{Mental age}}{\text{Chronological age}} \times 100$$

Milestones Some of the important developmental milestones at different ages are depicted in Table 12.5-3.

TABLE 12.5-3 Developmental Milestones at Different Ages

Milestone (motor)	Age (weeks)
Holding of head with bobbing	12
Head control	16
Sitting with support	20
Sitting without support	26
Standing with support	32
Standing without support	36–40
Crawling on belly	30
Crawling on knees	32
Walking with support	45
Walking without support	52

Chapter 12.6

Physiology of Fetus, Neonate and Childhood

INTRODUCTION

An infant or a child is not a miniature or small adult, rather the difference between a child and adult is more than that of the size. The physiological responses to environmental stresses, diseases and drugs are a lot different in a child and an adult. It is because of the fact that some of the organs develop during different stages of infancy or childhood, and in other organs, the function is not as well developed as in an adult. The difference is maximum between a newborn and an adult, and this gap gradually narrows down with the growth of a newborn into an adult. There exist both quantitative as well as qualitative differences between physiological responses of a child and adult in each organ system. Therefore, this section discusses some basic differences and specific details of systemic physiology of the fetus, neonate and childhood and how it changes during progress towards adulthood.

ROLE OF PLACENTA IN FETAL PHYSIOLOGY

Uterine and Placental Circulation during Pregnancy

Uterine Circulation As described on page 838, the blood supply to the uterus comes through uterine arteries and fluctuates cyclically along with the menstrual cycle to fulfil the metabolic demands of myometrium and endometrium. During pregnancy, the uterine blood flow increases parallel to the increase in fetal weight and uterine size (Fig. 12.6-1A). During early pregnancy, a rise in the levels of oestrogen and progesterone leads to an increase in uterine blood flow which meets the increased O_2 demand. Eventually, the placenta develops and becomes the circulatory link between the mother and fetus. Owing to increasing demand of O_2 with the progression of pregnancy, more and more O_2 is extracted from the uterine blood and consequently in later part of pregnancy, the O_2 saturation of uterine blood falls (Fig.12.6-1B). As shown in Fig. 12.6-1A, the uterine blood flow increases tremendously (200–300 ml/min/kg of uterine mass including the fetus) during late pregnancy. To provide for it, the maternal cardiac output increases by 2–2.5 L/min near full term. Eighty per cent of the uterine blood flow enters the placenta. Just before parturition there occurs a sharp decline in uterine blood flow, but the significance of this is not yet known.

Placental Circulation Placenta, which forms the circulatory link between the mother and the fetus, also works as *fetal lung, fetal gut* and *fetal kidney*. It consists of two major portions (Fig. 12.6-2):

- ***Maternal portion of the placenta*** is in fact a large blood sinus. The maternal blood flows through the uterine

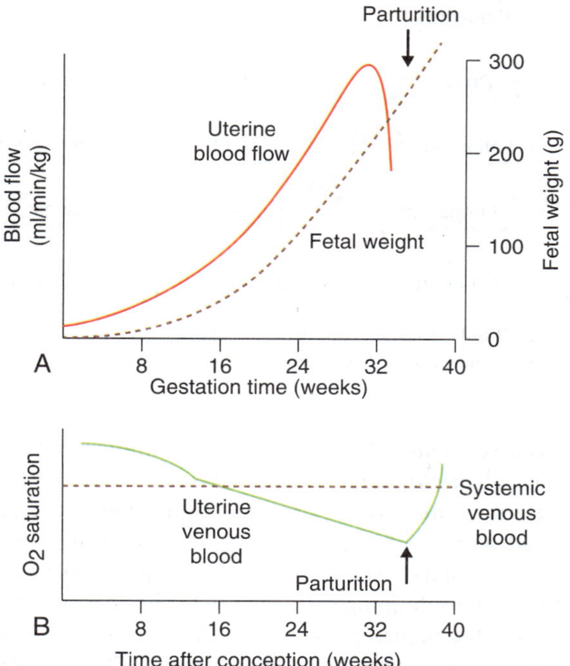

FIGURE 12.6-1 Uterine circulation during pregnancy: **A,** changes in uterine blood flow; and **B,** changes in the amount of O_2 in the venous blood.

arteries into the maternal sinuses and back through the uterine veins of the mother.

- ***Fetal portion of the placenta*** consists of placental villi. The fetal blood flows through umbilical arteries into the capillaries of placental villi and back through an umbilical vein into the fetus.

Exchange between Maternal and Fetal Blood Across Placental Membrane

As shown in Fig. 12.6-2, the placental villi containing fetal blood in capillaries project into and are then bathed by the blood in the maternal sinuses. Hence, in the placenta, the maternal and fetal blood does not mix with each other but are separated by the so-called placental membrane which consists (from fetal side) of following layers (Fig. 9.4-6, page 864):

- Endothelium and basement membrane,
- Surrounding mesenchymal tissue (connective tissue),
- Cytotrophoblast and its basement membrane and
- Syncytiotrophoblast.

All exchange of O_2, nutrients, and waste products between the maternal and fetal blood takes place through the placental membrane barrier.

1. Gaseous Exchange at Placenta: Placenta as Lung As shown in Fig. 12.6-2A, O_2 is taken up by the fetal blood and CO_2 is discharged into the maternal circulation across the placental membrane in a fashion analogous to O_2 and

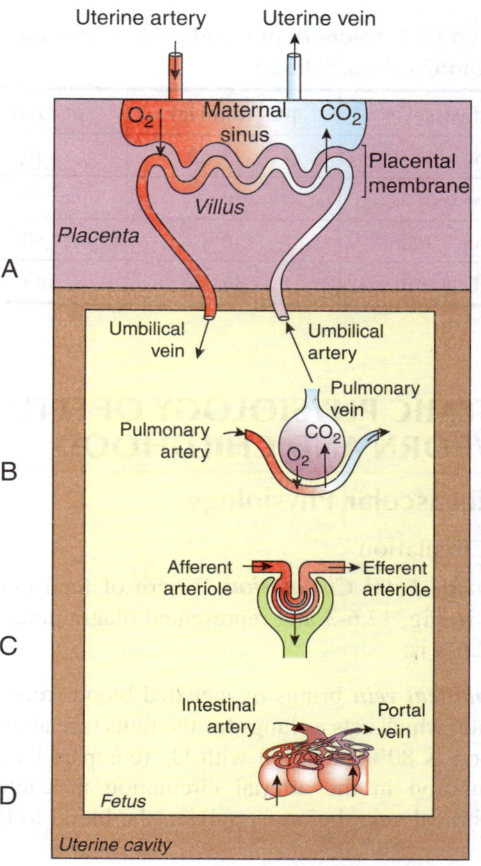

FIGURE 12.6-2 Placental circulation: **A,** diagrammatic depiction of exchange across placental membrane between mother and fetal blood; **B,** diagrammatic depiction of gas exchange across pulmonary alveolus during extrauterine life. Observe the similarity with the process in placenta. For practical purposes the umbilical artery can be compared to pulmonary artery and umbilical vein to pulmonary vein; **C,** diagrammatic depiction of nutrient absorption from the gut during extrauterine life. The similar process occurs in placenta where umbilical artery can be compared to intestinal artery and umbilical vein to portal vein; and **D,** diagrammatic depiction of glomerular filtration during extrauterine life. In the fetus similar process takes place at placenta where the umbilical artery can be compared to afferent arteriole and umbilical vein to efferent arteriole.

CO_2 exchange in the lungs across the alveolocapillary membrane (Fig. 12.6-2B). However, it is important to note that placental membrane (Fig. 9.4-6) is much thicker and less permeable than the alveolar membrane (Fig. 5.4-6), and, therefore, the exchange is much less efficient. Table 12.6-1 shows the values of gaseous interchange in the placenta.

2. Placental Transfer of Nutrients: Placenta as Gut
See page 868.

3. Excretion of Waste Products through Placenta: Placenta as Kidney
See page 868.

TABLE 12.6-1 Values of pO_2 and pCO_2 in the Maternal and Umbilical Cord Blood

Blood vessel	pO_2 (mmHg)	pCO_2 (mmHg)
Uterine artery	95	36
Uterine vein	50	40
Umbilical artery	20	50
Umbilical vein	35	43

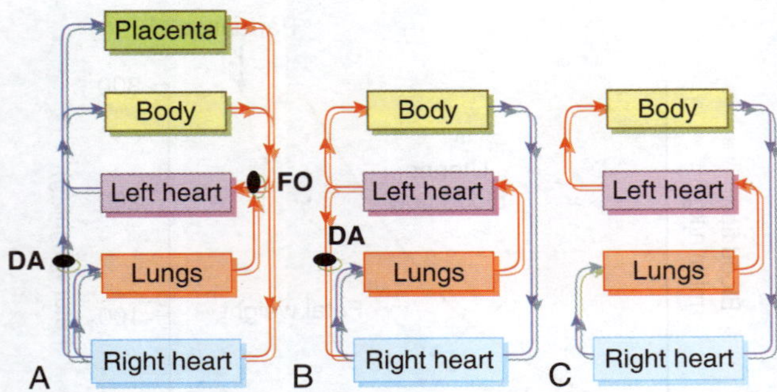

FIGURE 12.6-4 Diagrammatic depiction of circulatory pattern: **A,** fetus; **B,** newborn; and **C,** adult. DA; ductus arteriosus, FO; foramen ovale.

SYSTEMIC PHYSIOLOGY OF FETUS, NEWBORN AND CHILDHOOD

Cardiovascular Physiology

Fetal Circulation

Pattern of Fetal Circulation Pattern of fetal circulation shown in Fig. 12.6-3 and represented diagrammatically in Fig. 12.6-4 is:

- ***Umbilical vein*** brings oxygenated blood from the placenta, which acts as lungs for the fetus (see above). This blood is 80% saturated with O_2 (compared with 98% saturation in the arterial circulation in adults). The umbilical vein, before supplying the blood to the liver, bypasses some of the blood to the inferior vena cava through ***ductus venosus*** (Fig. 12.6-3).
- ***Inferior vena cava*** thus receives some blood (80% saturated with O_2) from the umbilical vein through ductus venosus, and other blood from the hepatic veins and systemic veins draining from the trunk and inferior extremities (26% saturated with O_2). The mixed blood from inferior vena cava (with approximate 67% saturation) then enters the right atrium.
- ***Right atrium*** receives blood from the inferior vena cava (saturation 67%) as well as superior vena cava (saturation 26%). The fate of blood entering the right atrium is very different from that in adults:
  - From the right atrium, majority of the blood coming from the inferior vena cava (saturation 67%) passes to the left atrium directly through the *foramen ovale* (an opening in the interatrial septum), and joins the blood coming from the pulmonary vein (saturation 42%). The mixed blood from left atrium (saturation 62%) passes on to the left ventricle.
  - From the right atrium, most of the blood coming from the superior vena cava (26% saturation) and small amount of that coming from the inferior vena cava (saturation 67%), passes into the right ventricle. This mixed blood from the right ventricle (saturation 52%) is pumped into the pulmonary artery. But, since the fetal lungs are collapsed, their vascular resistance is very high. Hence, only a small fraction of blood passes through the lungs to reach the left atrium via the pulmonary veins. Bulk of the pulmonary artery blood enters the descending aorta directly by a vascular connection called the *ductus arteriosus*.
- ***Left ventricle*** pumps the blood (with saturation 62%) into the ascending aorta, from where most of the blood goes into the vessels of the head and neck and forelimbs and only a small amount of blood goes to the descending aorta.
- ***Descending aorta*** thus receives blood mainly from the pulmonary artery through ductus arteriosus (with saturation 52%) and only a small amount from the left ventricle

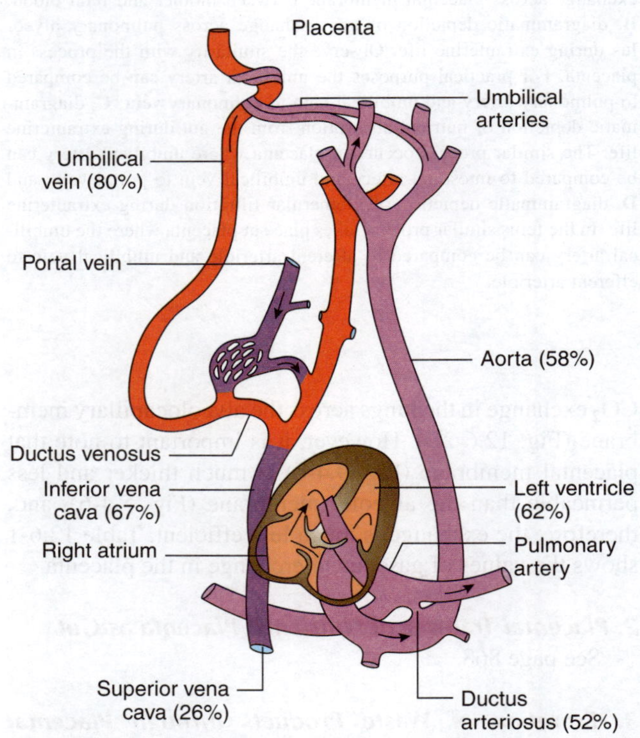

FIGURE 12.6-3 Pattern of fetal circulation with pO_2 in different components.

(with saturation 62%). The descending aorta then supplies the blood (with saturation 58%) to the whole of body (minus head and neck and forelimbs) and also to the placenta via *umbilical arteries* for oxygenation.

Special Features of Fetal Circulation

1. ***The two ventricles work in parallel*** (of in series in adults), because of the presence of foramen ovale (FO) and ductus arteriosus (DA), to drive the blood from the great veins into the arteries.
2. ***The two ventricles have equal thickness***. This is due to the fact that the right ventricle has to pump blood against considerable resistance. Firstly, because of high resistance of pulmonary vasculature, and secondly because of the reason that the major part of the right ventricular output is pumped into the aorta via the ductus arteriosus. The latter is possible only if the pulmonary artery pressure is higher than the aortic pressure. In fact, the fetal right ventricular systolic pressure is a few millimetres higher than the left ventricular pressure.
3. ***The two ventricles do not have similar cardiac output***. The left ventricular output is approximately 20% greater than the right ventricular output. The disparity between the outputs of two ventricles does not produce any haemodynamic complications because, unlike in adults, the ventricles work in parallel, as mentioned above.
4. ***Fetal heart pumps only 40% of the output to the systemic circulation and 60% to the placenta***. This is firstly because of the fact that fetal lungs are mainly nonfunctional, liver is partially functional and peripheral resistance of fetal vessels is high because of low level of activity. Secondly, the resistance of the placenta is low because of the large cross-sectional area of chorionic villi.
5. ***Oxygen saturation of the fetal arterial blood supplying the tissues is much lower (~60%) than that of adults (~98%)***. However, fetus shows remarkable adaptation to low pO_2, because of following compensatory mechanisms:
   - i. Greater affinity of fetal haemoglobin (HbF) for O_2 (see page 433),
   - ii. Greater concentration of haemoglobin in fetus (18–20 g%),
   - iii. Double Bohr's effect allows increased uptake of O_2 by the fetal blood (see page 868) and
   - iv. Fetal tissues, as well as blood vessels are highly resistant to the effects of hypoxia.

Neonatal Circulation

Changes in Circulation after Birth

1. Arrest of Umbilical Blood Flow and Placental Transfusion. Factors responsible for arrest of umbilical blood flow and placental transfusion are:

i. Vasoconstriction of Umbilical Vessels. Immediately after birth, there occurs sudden and marked reduction in blood flow through the umbilical vessels. It results from vasoconstriction of the umbilical vessels in response to:

- Mechanical stimulation,
- Exposure to cold air and
- Secretion of catecholamines from the infant's adrenal medulla due to stress.

ii. Tying and Cutting of the Umbilical Cord. The process which is initiated by nature by producing vasoconstriction is completed by the doctor by tying and cutting the umbilical cord.

Precautions to be taken while tying the umbilical cord

- Milking of the umbilical cord should not be done, because it can send so much blood to the infant that its circulation may get overloaded.
- Infant should be held at or slightly below the level of vagina; as it leads to transfer of an additional 60–80 ml of blood to the infant, which is very useful.
- Optimum time to tie the umbilical cord is 40–60 s after birth. Tying earlier than this will prevent the transfer of additional blood from placenta for the infant, and delay in tying may be associated with risk of blood flow from the infant to the placenta producing haemorrhagic anaemia.

2. Closure of Foramen Ovale. Factors leading to closure to foramen ovale are:

i. Reduction in Inferior Vena Cava–left Atrial Pressure Gradient. The valve of foramen ovale is held open before the birth by the pressure and momentum of blood flowing up to the inferior vena cava. After birth, closure of the umbilical circulation immediately decreases the volume of blood flowing up the inferior vena cava and causes contraction of ductus venosus within 1–3 h after birth. Consequently, there occurs a reduction in the inferior vena cava–left atrial pressure gradient favouring functional closure of the valve of foramen ovale.

ii. Decrease in Right Atrial and Right Ventricular Pressure. Following arrest of umbilical flow, after birth, the infant develops asphyxia (i.e. pO_2 is lowered and pCO_2 is raised). Fetal asphyxia leads to an intense peripheral chemoreceptor discharge resulting in initiation of breathing. The infant gasps several times and the lungs expand. The inflation of lungs after birth causes a 10% decrease in pulmonary vascular resistance. The decreased resistance causes a large drop in the after load of the right ventricle and lowers the right atrial and right ventricular pressure. The drop in the right-sided pressure causes pressure in the left atrium to exceed the pressure in the right atrium. This pressure reversal causes the flap-like valve to close over the foramen ovale.

The valve then normally fuses to the interatrial septum over the next few days.

Closure of the foramen ovale prevents the right-to-left flow of venous blood and thus improves the oxygenation of systemic arterial blood.

3. Changes in Pulmonary Circulation. Rapid fall in pulmonary artery pressure, which occurs following inflation of previously collapsed lungs (as described above), is accompanied with a six- to tenfold increase in pulmonary blood flow. In the fetus the pulmonary arterial pressure is slightly higher than that in the aorta and most of the output from the right heart passes through the ductus arteriosus to the aorta. After birth the position is reversed, for the aortic pressure rises and pulmonary artery pressure falls so that blood flow through the ductus arteriosus, which remains partially open for many hours after birth, occurs from the aorta to the pulmonary trunk, i.e. in the reverse direction to that which takes place in the fetus (Figs 12.6-4 A and B).

4. Closure of Ductus Arteriosus. The ductus arteriosus is almost as large as ascending aorta of the mature fetus and has a thick, smooth muscle wall. The closure of ductus occurs in three steps:

- Vasoconstriction with partial patency,
- Complete functional closure and
- Permanent sealing with fibrous tissue.

i. ***Vasoconstriction of ductus arteriosus occurs*** rapidly during the first few hours after birth but final functional closure takes place gradually over the next 1–3 days.

Factors responsible for constriction of ductus are:

- Rise in pO_2 of neonatal blood which occurs following inflation of the lungs after birth causes constriction of ductus. This is consistent with the higher incidence of persistent patency of the ductus associated with fetal distress at birth and with delivery at high altitude.
- Vasoconstrictor effect of catecholamines released due to stress of birth.
- Fall in levels of prostaglandins PGE and PGF_2, which help in keeping the ductus arteriosus patent during fetal life because of their vasodilator effect (therefore, inhibitors of prostaglandin synthesis like aspirin and indomethacin have been used clinically to promote closure of patent ductus arteriosus in premature babies).

Blood flow through constricted ductus after birth. For the first hour after birth, flow continues through the ductus in the fetal direction (i.e. right-to-left shunt from the pulmonary artery to the aorta), but subsequently the flow reverses due to reduction in pulmonary pressure and rise in aortic pressure (as described above).

Flow of blood through this constricted but slightly patent ductus is responsible for the murmur which may be heard by careful auscultation in the immediate neonatal period. The murmur though continuous, reaches a crescendo with each second heart sound.

ii. ***Functional closure of the ductus*** with complete muscular contraction occurs gradually over the next 1–8 days.

iii. ***Permanent sealing of the ductus lumen*** occurs 2–3 weeks after birth by replacement of musculature with fibrous tissue.

5. Changes in Cardiac Muscle. During fetal life, the two ventricles have almost similar thickness, because the pressure in the pulmonary artery is slightly greater than the aortic pressure. However, after birth, the left ventricular wall rapidly grows thicker as systemic arterial pressure rises, and the right ventricular wall becomes thinner than the left, as the pulmonary artery pressure falls after birth. It is important to note that the number of muscle fibres in the two ventricles is approximately the same and does not change from birth to adult life. The increase in left ventricular size after birth occurs due to increase in length and thickness of the individual fibres in response to increased left ventricular pressure. The redistribution of the myocardial blood flow with major portion getting directed towards left ventricular myocardium helps in this endeavour.

Status of Cardiovascular System after Birth

1. ***Heart rate***. Immediately after birth, the heart rate of an infant is approximately 140 beats/min. During infancy and childhood, heart rate decreases gradually and the adult values are reached only at puberty (Table 12.6-2).
   Sinus arrhythmia, i.e. variation in heart rate during two phases of respiration, can be observed in infants and children even during normal quiet breathing. In adults it is observed only during deep breathing.
2. ***Blood pressure***. At birth, the mean arterial blood pressure is approximately 80 mmHg. During the next few hours, it declines to about 65 mmHg. Thereafter, the blood pressure gradually increases throughout infancy and childhood to reach the adult values by the end of pubertal growth (Table 12.6-3).
3. ***Blood volume*** at birth is 300 ml or (90 ml/kg).
4. ***Cardiac output*** at birth is about 550 ml/min (which is two times as much in relation to body weight as in the adult).

TABLE 12.6-2 Heart Rate Values in Relation to Age

Age	Heart rate (beats/min)
Birth	140–150
1 month	130–140
1 year	110–115
5 years	105–110
10 years	95–100
15 years	80–85
Adults	70–80
Old age	Up to 100

TABLE 12.6-3 Blood Pressure Values in Relation to Age

Age	Blood pressure (mmHg)	
	Systolic	*Diastolic*
Birth	70–90	30–45
15 days	70	45
1 month	75	85
1 year	85	55
5 years	100	60
12 years	105	62
17 years	115	68
Adult	120	80
Old age	140	90

5. ***Electrocardiography (ECG)***. At birth, the ECG record shows all the normal waves; however, the right ventricular preponderance is indicated by mild right axis deviation. After a few months of postnatal life, the right axis deviation is no more evident. Left ventricular preponderance, indicated by mild left axis deviation is established between the ages of 6 and 8 years.

Congenital Heart Diseases

Congenital heart diseases occur either due to defective development of the embryonic heart or due to defect in the closure of three channels of communication (ductus venosus, ductus arteriosus and foramen ovale) after birth. A few common congenital heart diseases are described briefly.

1. ***Atrial septal defect (ASD)*** results from failure of foramen ovale to close. A very small symptomless defect is not uncommon. A large defect causes problem due to shunting of a large volume of blood from left atrium to right atrium, then to right ventricle and pulmonary arteries. Thus, initially the right ventricle is overburdened; and later on pulmonary hypertension may develop.
2. ***Ventricular septal defect (VSD)*** occurs due to defective development of interventricular septum. It is the most common congenital cardiac defect occurring in 1:500 live births. It is an acyanotic heart defect with left to right (L → R) shunt. The VSD may be small and isolated or may be a part of a complex congenital heart disease.
3. ***Patent ductus arteriosus (PDA)***. It is also an acyanotic congenital defect with left to right (L → R) shunt, as the blood flows from a high pressure vessel (aorta) to a low pressure vessel (pulmonary artery).
4. ***Tetralogy of Fallat***. It occurs due to defective development of an embryonic heart, and as the name indicates, consists of four components:
   - Ventricular septal defect (VSD),
   - Overriding of the aorta at the level of VSD,
   - Pulmonary stenosis (subvalvular) and
   - Right ventricular hypertrophy.

   Due to pulmonary stenosis and large VSD, the right ventricular pressure is elevated and leads to right to left (R → L) shunt resulting in mixing of unoxygenated and oxygenated blood that is pushed through the overridden aorta. Thus, there occurs tissue hypoxia which produces cyanosis (bluish discolouration of skin) and clubbing of the fingers in infancy or after first year of life. Capacity for physical exercise is limited.

Respiratory Physiology

Fetal Respiration

Placenta as Lung As described earlier (see page 1255 and 868), the placenta acts as the site of gas exchange for the fetus before birth.

Oxygen and Carbon Dioxide Transport in the Fetus
See page 868.

Fetal Breathing Movements Though gaseous exchange does not occur in fetal lung, the breathing movements do occur during fetal life. Since the lungs are filled with fluid with a viscosity and density many times that of air, the breathing movements lead to only small alterations in pulmonary volume. Thus, there is little mixing of amniotic fluid and lung fluids. It has been suggested that the purpose of these breathing movements in utero is to exercise and train the respiratory muscles for their function after birth. Ultrasound scanning technique reveals fetal breathing movements as early as 11 weeks gestation. Initially, irregular, they gradually become more regular.

Fetal Pulmonary Blood Flow and Peripheral Chemoreceptors

Pulmonary blood flow, during fetal life, is just a fraction of the right ventricular outflow because, due to high pulmonary vascular resistance, most of the right ventricular output is diverted to the aorta through the ductus arteriosus.

Peripheral chemoreceptors are fully developed in a fetus before birth. However, due to some unexplained mechanisms, there is no chemoreceptor discharge in spite of very low pO_2 in the fetal blood.

Pulmonary Surfactant

See page 405.

Respiratory Adjustments at Birth

Birth is the most traumatic event that the respiratory system must withstand during the entire life span of an individual. It involves sudden transfer from a situation in which no breathing effort is necessary to one in which continual breathing effort is indispensable.

Initiation of Breathing The essential changes which occur while shifting from perinatal respiration to postnatal respiration are summarized:

- ***Pulmonary fluid*** which fills the airway in the fetus, keeps the respiratory system at approximately functional residual capacity (FRC). Hence, a major requirement after birth is speedy replacement of fluid by the air so that the respiratory movements can be easier and more useful in terms of gas exchange. From the lungs, fluid is removed by following forces:
  - Part of this vital task is accomplished when the thorax is squeezed while passing through birth passages during delivery, and
  - Part of the fluid is absorbed into the pulmonary capillaries and lymphatics after birth, and some fluid is removed by evaporation.
- ***Alveolar epithelium,*** which has got a fluid secretory function in prenatal period, changes its function to fluid reabsorption after birth.
- ***Factors which stimulate first breath*** after the birth have been an interesting area of research and speculation, and probably are:
  - Squeezing of thorax during birth,
  - Lower temperature outside as compared to inside the uterus,
  - Sound, light, gravity and tactile and painful stimuli and
  - Fall in arterial pO_2 and rise in pCO_2 (asphyxia) due to suspension of fetal respiration for a small period during birth and mainly following arrest of umbilical flow (see page 465) is the main stimulant for initiation of breathing.

All the above factors are mediated through nerves, so these may be depressed if the mother receives general anaesthesia during labour, as the fetus is also anaesthetized.

- ***Intraplural pressure generated during first few breaths is very high,*** about 60 mmHg, since the lungs are partly fluid filled. The intense efforts required to expand the lungs slowly decrease and normalize in 2 weeks. During this period, *surfactant* is also produced lowering the surface tension which stabilizes the alveoli and allows the lung volume to increase steadily during first few weeks of life.
- ***Effects of initial breathing.*** After the first gasping breath, normal breathing pattern is gradually established within hours of the breathing. The neonate recovers from hypoxia, hypercapnia and acidosis present throughout fetal life and aggravated markedly by the process of birth and subsequent ligation of the umbilical cord.
- ***Neonatal resistance to hypoxia.*** It may be mentioned that even when the breathing is not initiated up to 10 minutes after birth, the neonate shows normal postnatal growth and development. Resistance to such a prolonged and severe hypoxia is a peculiar feature of neonatal physiology and does not occur in later life.
- ***Neonatal respiration and haematological changes.*** Haematological changes also take place after birth, because the adaptations in the form of high haemoglobin level and fetal type of haemoglobin which is necessary to cope with the hypoxic environment in uterus (pO_2 of oxygenated fetal blood is 30 mmHg and that of mother's blood in placenta is 50 mmHg) are no more required after birth. The haemoglobin level falls by haemolysis outplacing erythropoiesis, and the haemoglobin type changes to the adult variety soon after birth (see page 146).
- ***To conclude,*** it can be said that one set of mechanisms make it possible for the fetus to respire and survive in the uterus; and another set of mechanisms make the sudden transmission from the hypoxic but sheltered uterine environment to the normoxic but harsh extrauterine environment, a smooth journey. One can only marvel at the gently co-ordinated events involved in the process.

Status of Respiratory System after Birth

1. Number of Alveoli in the Lungs. About 20 million alveoli are present in the lungs at birth, and their number increases to the adult value of 300 million alveoli by the age of 8–10 years. After this age till the end of pubertal growth, the lungs increase in size because of increase in the size of alveoli rather than increase in their number.

2. Respiratory Rate of a newborn is very high (30–60/min) and gradually decreases during infancy and childhood. The adult values of respiratory rate are reached at about 10 years of age (Table 12.6-4).

3. Tidal air Volume at birth in a premature infant is 10–12 ml, while in a full-term newborn it is 16–18 ml and keeps on increasing throughout childhood, till the pubertal growth is completed (Table 12.6-4).

TABLE 12.6-4 Respiratory Rate and Tidal Air in Relation to Age

Age	Respiratory rate/min	Tidal air volume (ml)
Premature	40–80	10–12
Full term/newborn	30–60	16–18
1 year	20–40	48
2 years	20–30	90
5 years	20–25	175
10 years	15–20	400
15 years	15–20	400

4. Vital Capacity also continues to increase throughout childhood. It reaches to about 3.3 L at the age of 15 years.

5. Minute Ventilation at birth is about 140 ml/min. This is two times as great as in relation to body weight of an adult.

6. Functional Residual Capacity in a newborn is only half that of an adult in relation to body weight.

Applied Aspects

Respiratory Distress Syndrome
See page 406.

Blood and Immune Mechanisms

Erythropoiesis, Leucopoiesis and Thrombopoiesis

At 2 weeks of gestation, erythropoiesis begins in the mesenchymal tissue of yolk sac. Large RBCs with low haemoglobin concentration are produced at this stage.

At 2nd and 3rd month of gestation, the chief sites of erythropoiesis, leucopoiesis and thrombopoiesis are liver and spleen.

After 4 months of gestation, the chief site for erythropoiesis is bone marrow.

In postnatal life, bone marrow remains the only site of erythropoiesis. However, the extramedullary regions (liver and spleen) remain the potential sites of erythropoiesis when the entire bone marrow has been damaged (myelosclerosis).

Fetal Haemoglobin (HbF) and Adult Haemoglobin (HbA)

Characteristic features of HbF and HbA are described on page 146. The salient point to be noted is that HbF has higher affinity than the HbA. Up to 32 weeks of gestation, fetus RBCs contain only HbF; after which, HbA begins to be synthesized in low concentration. Consequently, by 36 weeks of gestation, the fetal RBCs contain 90% HbF and 10% HbA. After birth, synthesis of HbF practically ceases; consequently, its concentration in the newborn's blood declines linearly. At about 3–4 months of age almost all the RBCs contain HbA, and HbF is completely absent from the blood.

Characteristics of Blood in Newborn

1. Haemoglobin concentration is high (16–18 g%). It is related to low pO_2 of the fetal blood. Changes in Hb seen with age are depicted in Table 12.6-5.

2. RBC Count at birth is about 5.5–6.5 million/mm^3, which gradually decreases to 3–4 million/mm^3 by approximately 10–12 weeks of age due to absence of hypoxic stimulus of fetal life, and returns to normal within another 2–3 months (Table 12.6-5).

3. WBC Count at Birth, is nearly 20,000/mm^3 with preponderance of neutrophils (70%). It decreases to about 12,000/mm^3 with marked decrease in neutrophils (30%) by the end of 1 month. From the first month to 1 year of life, lymphocytes predominate. Normal adult values of WBC count are reached at 5–10 years of age (Table 12.6-5).

4. Coagulation Factors. *At birth,* though all the clotting factors and fibrinolysins are present in plasma, but the levels of prothrombin, factor V, VII and X are subnormal. *In the first week* of postnatal life, the levels of these clotting factors may decrease to a level to produce the so-called *haemorrhagic diseases of newborn,* which is characterized by bleeding from umbilicus, GIT and other internal organs. Premature infants are more prone to it. This occurs primarily because of deficiency of vitamin K and consequently decreased synthesis of vitamin K-dependent clotting factors by immature hepatocytes. That is why to prevent this disease, injection of vitamin K is given immediately after birth as prophylaxis.

At about 2–12 months of age, the adult values of all the clotting factors are reached.

5. Immunologic Functions. The newborn is competent to produce both T lymphocyte as well as B lymphocyte-mediated response.

- ***IgG levels.*** During intrauterine life, IgG levels are actively transferred from the maternal blood to the fetus. Consequently, at birth the newborn's plasma level of IgG is

TABLE 12.6-5 Hb Concentration, RBC Count and WBC Count in Relation to Age

Age	Hb concentration (g%)	RBC count (million/mm^3)	TLC per mm^3	DLC	
				Poly (%)	*Lymphocyte (%)*
1 day	18	6.0	20,000	70	20
1 month	16	4.7	12,000	30	60
3 months	10	4.0	11,000	35	55
1 year	12.5	4.5	10,000	45	50
5 years	13.0	4.7	8000	55	40
10 years	13.0	4.7	8000	60	35

TABLE 12.6-6 Levels of IgG, IgA and IgM (mg%) in Maternal and Fetal Blood (at Birth)

Immunoglobulin	Maternal blood (mg/100 ml)	Fetal blood (mg/100 ml)
IgG	1000	1230
IgA	350	07
IgM	125	15

even higher than the maternal plasma level (Table 12.6-6). However, soon the IgG levels decline rapidly to reach a level of 400–500 mg% within 1 week compared with over 1200 mg% at birth. At about 4 months of age, the infant's immunological apparatus starts manufacturing IgG and adult levels are reached by the age of 8 months.

- **IgA and IgM** are not transferred to the fetus; consequently, their levels are much lower at birth as compared to mother's level (Table 12.6-6). After birth, IgM begins to rise rapidly, reaching 30 mg% by the end of one week and 45 mg% at 6 months of age. IgA levels also begin to rise in infancy, but adult levels are reached by the age of 12–16 years.

Physiological Anaemia

At birth, the cord blood shows high concentration of erythropoietins, high Hb concentration (18 g%), and high RBC count (5.5–6.5 million/mm^3). It is related to low pO_2

After birth, the hypoxic stimulus present throughout intrauterine life disappears and the pO_2 is raised. Consequently, after one week of life there occurs complete cessation of RBC production in the bone marrow. As a result, by 10–12 weeks of life the Hb concentration may fall to as low as 9–10 g% and RBC count may be as low as 3–4 million/mm^3. This produces the so-called *physiological anaemia* of the newborn, which cannot be prevented even by administration of haematinics. The disappearance of erythropoietin and reticulocytes from the infant's blood support the explanation that physiological anaemia of newborn is related to disappearance of hypoxic stimulus after birth.

Nervous System

Neural growth is completed by 4–5 years of age (see page 1250):

- At the end of 1 year, 50%,
- At the end of 3 years, 75% and
- At the end of 5 years, 90% of postnatal growth is completed.

CNS weight:body weight relation is:

- At birth = 1:10,
- At 5 years = 1:20 and
- In an adult = 1:50.

Myelination begins during fetal life, but continues for several years postnatally.

Blood–brain barrier is not well developed at birth. This accounts for higher levels of protein, sugar and high white cell count in CSF of newborn compared with that in later childhood. This also explains the occurrence of kernicterus in an infant at that level of serum bilirubin which is harmless in an adult.

Visual apparatus becomes fully developed by 5 years of age. Salient points to be noted are:

- *Macula and fovea* of the retina are structurally and functionally differentiated by 4–6 months of age.
- *Colour perception* is fully developed by the age of 4–6 months.
- *Size of eyeball* at birth is small, so the infant is hypermetropic. Adult size is obtained by 5 years, when the child becomes emmetropic.
- *Visual acuity* becomes 6/6 by the age of 5–6 years.

Auditory apparatus is almost fully developed at term. Therefore, response to loud noise can be elicited just after birth.

Taste sensation is present at birth, but becomes sharp by the age of 2–3 months.

Visceral reflexes involved in swallowing, micturition, defaecation, sneezing and coughing are fully developed at birth.

Deep reflexes. Most of the tendon jerks can be elicited at birth except the ankle jerk. The Babinski's sign appears only a few weeks after birth and can be elicited during the next 1–2 years.

Gastrointestinal Physiology

GIT: During Fetal Life

Placental Transfer of Nutrients: Placenta as Gut As mentioned earlier, the transfer of nutrients to the fetus occurs from the maternal blood through placenta (see Fig. 12.6-2D and page 1255).

During fetal life, constant and plentiful supply of glucose reaches from the mother. Due to deficiency of enzymes like glucokinase and those for glycogenolysis and gluconeogenesis, the fetus is incapable of regulating blood sugar on its own. Thus, fetal glucose is regulated by maternal blood glucose level. Further, large amounts of free fatty acids and amino acids are transported to the fetus across the placenta, but they are used for tissue formation rather than for energy production.

Fetal Gastrointestinal Tract ***After 20 weeks,*** fetus ingests and absorbs large quantities of amniotic fluid.

At 24 weeks, fetal GIT functions approach that of normal newborn infant. Small quantities of *meconium* are continuously formed in the GIT and excreted from the bowels into the amniotic fluid. The meconium consists of unabsorbed residue of amniotic fluid and secretions from GIT mucosa and glands.

GIT: After Birth

The fetus gets the nutrients supply from the maternal blood through the placenta, which is suddenly cut-off after ligation of the cord. Since the newborn has to produce its own nutrient's supply, so the gastrointestinal function is fairly well developed at birth. Some of the salient features of GIT physiology of newborn are:

Digestive and Absorptive Functions

Salivary secretion, though present since birth, its rate of secretion increases over the next 6 months, due to maturation of the salivary glands.

Gastric HCl concentration is very high on the first postnatal day but within the next 10–15 days, the gastric acid secretion almost ceases. After a gap of 3–4 months, gastric acid secretion starts once again. The physiological significance of increased acidity of the stomach at birth, followed by a phase of achlorhydria for the next about 3 months, is not yet clear.

Pancreatic juice contains adequate concentration of lipase and proteolytic enzymes at birth. But the concentration of α-amylase is very low at birth and begins to increase a few months later. Therefore, a newborn is not able to utilize starch in the early postnatal life, rather may get severe diarrhoea.

Intestinal absorption of fats is less, thus milk with high fat content is inadequately utilized. However, due to presence of disaccharidases, the absorption of disaccharides is very efficient. Similarly, monosaccharides are also well absorbed right from birth.

Liver Functions The newborn has to fulfil the caloric requirements from carbohydrate-poor, fat-rich milk diet and a number of adaptive changes in the hepatic enzymes help in this transition.

Liver Functions are Quite Deficient During First Few Days, as the liver of newborn:

- Poorly conjugates bilirubin causing its less excretion,
- Poorly performs gluconeogenic function, decreasing blood glucose level to 30–40 mg%,
- Inadequately synthesizes plasma proteins producing hypoproteinaemia, and
- Inadequately synthesizes clotting factors producing even haemorrhagic disease of newborn, sometimes, especially in premature babies.

Fetal Liver Glycogen and Blood Glucose. During late fetal life, the activity of glycogen synthetase in the fetal liver increases. As a result, fetal liver is very rich in glycogen at birth. After ligation of the cord, the blood sugar level of the infant begins to fall and may reach 60 mg% within 1 h. Hypoglycaemia induces the secretion of glucagon, catecholamines and glucocorticoids. Presence of hepatic glucose-6-phosphatase in high concentration in the full-term infant helps to convert glycogen into glucose and, therefore, blood glucose recovers soon. However, the enzyme, involved in gluconeogenesis takes a few days to develop fully and thus account for occurrence of hypoglycaemia during first few days of life (as mentioned above). The problem of neonatal hypoglycaemia is more pronounced in premature babies.

Hepatic Bilirubin Excretion. *During fetal life,* the RBCs have a life span of approximately 70 days, and thus about 1.4% of circulating red cell mass is destroyed every day producing a large amount of bilirubin. However, the plasma bilirubin level usually remains below 1 mg%. Further, even during pathological state like Rh incompatibility when the production of bilirubin is markedly increased, the plasma bilirubin level does not exceed 5 mg%. This happens because of the fact that the lipid-soluble unconjugated bilirubin can cross the placental barrier. *After birth,* in the early postnatal life the hepatic conjugation enzyme UDP-glucuronyl transferase is not fully active, so conjugation with glucuronic acid is poor and so is the bilirubin excretion (as also mentioned earlier).

This explains the occurrence of physiological jaundice in first week of postnatal life. However, soon the enzyme activity begins to rise rapidly, and by the age of 15 days it even exceeds the adult level (Fig. 12.6-5). There seems to be some variation in the rate of increase of the hepatic conjugation enzyme activity. That is why some babies develop more severe physiological jaundice (with plasma bilirubin as high as 18 mg%) than others. Further, the risk of neonatal jaundice is more in premature neonates and those suffering from Rh incompatibility. Such infants are under the risk of developing kernicterus, since the blood–brain barrier is not well developed at birth (see above in nervous system).

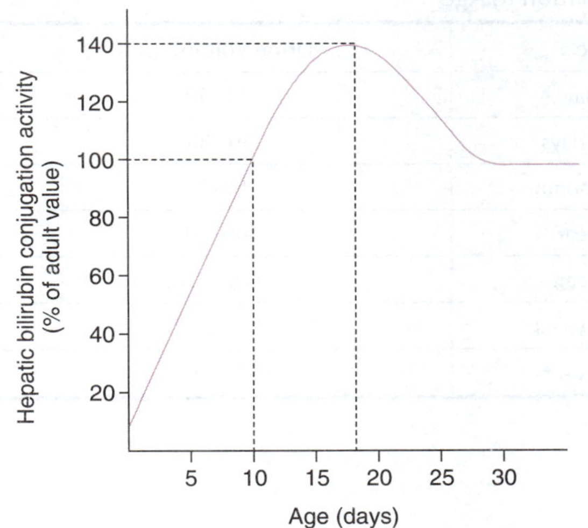

FIGURE 12.6-5 Changes in rate of hepatic conjugation of bilirubin during neonatal period.

Renal Physiology, and Fluid and Acid–base Balance

Anatomically the development of nephrons is fairly complete at birth, and no new nephrons are formed in the postnatal life. However, functionally the kidneys in infancy are immature and can manage to maintain normal blood chemistry as long as there is no homeostatic disturbance. In other words, there is very little margin of safety, hence important problems of infancy are dehydration, overhydration and acidosis as explained:

1. ***The fluid intake and fluid excretion*** in an infant is about 500 ml per day representing nearly 50% of the ECF volume. While an average adult takes and excretes about 2000 ml fluid per day, which represents only 15% of ECF volume (the daily average urinary volume at different age groups is shown in Table 12.6-7). Further, the ECF volume of the newborn infant per kg body weight is nearly double than the adult. Therefore, even a slight alteration of fluid balance due to diarrhoea, infection or solute overload may lead to rapidly developing fluid balance abnormalities.
2. ***Power of urinary concentration in an infant is poor.*** This is because of two main reasons:
   - At birth, 20% of the loops of Henle fail to reach the medulla in contrast to 1–2% in adults, and
   - Rate of urea secretion is low and so the osmolar gradient in medullary pyramids is slight. In turn, the low urea secretion of the neonate is because of the fact that the rate of deamination is low as more amino acids are utilized for tissue formation.

   Because of poor power of urinary concentration, the infant up to 1 year of age continues to pass iso-osmolar urine or even dilute urine in the face of severe dehydration. During infancy, the maximum urinary specific gravity may be only 1.008. Normal adult values of urinary concentration are reached by the age of 5–6 years.
3. ***Power of H^+ excretion is also poor in infancy.*** This is because of the fact that there is lesser glomerular filtration of phosphates, as well as, inadequate synthesis of ammonia by the tubular cells. Further, the rate of metabolism in infants is two times more in relation to body mass as in adults, i.e. two times as much acid is normally formed which produces tendency towards acidosis in infants.

TABLE 12.6-7 Average Daily Excretion of Urine in Relation to Age

Age	Urine volume (ml)
1 day	15–50
10 days	50–300
1 month	250–400
1 year	400–500
5 years	600–750
10 years	700–1500
15 years	1500–2000

It is once again repeated that all the above facts underline the risk of dehydration, overhydration and acidosis during infancy and the need for urgent treatment.

Temperature Regulation in Newborn and Infants

The temperature regulation mechanisms, as described in Chapter 12.4 on Physiology of Body Temperature Regulation, are operative in newborns and even in premature babies. The salient points which need special mention for temperature regulation in newborns and infants are:

1. ***Maintenance of body temperature presents greater problems in newborns and infants*** because of following reasons:
   - *Surface area* in relation to the body weight is greater than adults.
   - *Basal metabolic rate (BMR),* throughout the childhood, is relatively higher than the adult values and
   - *Sweating mechanism* is not fully developed during infancy.
2. ***Thermoneutral zone*** (see page 1243), for naked newborn infants (32–34°C in term infants and 35°C in premature infants), is higher than the naked adult (26–28°C) (see Fig. 12.4-6). The fact underlines two important implications:
   - Infants have poor tolerance to cold, and
   - While adjusting the temperature of the incubator for premature babies and of the labour room in general, the thermoneutral zone of the infant should be kept in mind.
3. ***Nonshivering or chemical thermogenesis*** is the most effective mechanism against cold in infants. Presence of brown adipose tissue in infants accounts for this fact (for details see page 1242).

Sexual Growth and Development

See page 805.

Chapter 12.7

Geriatric Physiology

INTRODUCTION

Ageing Ageing is a natural process. No one knows when old age begins. The biological age of the person is not identical with his chronological age. While ageing merely stands for growing old, senescence is an expression used for the deterioration in the vitality or the lowering of the biological efficiency that accompanies ageing. From a physiological standpoint, human ageing is characterized by a progressive constriction of the homeostatic reserve of every organ system. This decline, often referred to as homeostenosis, is gradual and progressive, although the rate and extent of decline vary.

The decline of each organ system appears to occur independently of changes in other organ systems and is influenced by diet, environment and personal habits as well as by genetic factors.

In other words, ageing can be defined as the time-related deterioration of the physiological functions necessary for survival and fertility. The science of ageing is often referred to as *gerontology*. The scientists studying the science of ageing are known as *gerontologists,* and the branch of medicine dealing with the problems of ageing is called *geriatric medicine*.

AGE-RELATED CHANGES IN DIFFERENT ORGAN SYSTEMS

I. Cardiovascular Changes

Changes in Heart

1. ***Myocardium*** may show the following changes:
   - Deposition of yellow–brown lipofuscin pigment.
   - Degenerative changes in the myofibrils and mitochondria.
   - Fibrotic lesions and sometimes amyloid deposits.
   - Capillary density may be decreased.
2. ***Valves*** show thickening and structural changes making the:
   - Aortic valve somewhat stenotic and
   - Mitral valve slightly incompetent.
3. Functional changes in the heart of elderly include:
   - *Heart rate* in resting conditions is unchanged, but the maximum heart rate during exercise declines.
   - *Maximum cardiac output* in response to exercise is decreased at the rate of 1% per year after the age of 40 years.
4. ***SA node automaticity*** and baroreceptor sensitivity is decreased with age. This leads to impaired blood pressure response to standing and volume depletion.
5. ***Electrocardiogram*** does not show any significant change with age. Therefore, any significant change in ECG of an elderly individual should be considered pathological.

Changes in Blood Vessels and Blood Pressure ***Blood vessels*** show gradual decrease in the number of elastic fibres and a progressive change in the characteristics of elastic tissue. There occurs deposition of calcium salts in the elastic and muscular type of arteries, as well as deposition of more collagen fibres resulting in decrease in the distensibility of the blood vessels.

Blood pressure. Systolic blood pressure is raised because of loss of elasticity in the aorta and its major branches, but there is little change in the diastolic blood pressure, resulting in widening of pulse pressure.

Blood flow to the various organs such as heart, brain and especially kidney is decreased.

II. Changes in Respiratory System

Structural changes in lungs. Alveoli become flatter and shallow, while alveolar ducts enlarge. The number of alveoli declines gradually due to progressive loss of interalveolar septa.

Pulmonary compliance is increased due to decrease in elasticity of the lungs.

Compliance of thoracic cage and mobility of the ribs are decreased due to calcification of costal cartilages.

Pulmonary blood vessels show age-related increase in wall thickness.

Functional changes occurring as a result of aforementioned changes in the lungs and thoracic cage are:

- *Functional residual capacity* of the lungs is increased by 50%.
- *Residual volume* is increased by 100%.
- *Vital capacity,* FEV_1, MBC and diffusion capacity for oxygen are significantly decreased.
- *Respiratory response to hypoxia and hypercapnia* is sluggish in the elderly.
- *Airways become more susceptible to collapse,* especially during expiration, because of reduced elastic recoil of thoracic cage. The collapse is more likely during exercise because of the high expiratory flow rate.
- *Arterial pCO_2 and pO_2.* The arterial pCO_2 is not changed, but arterial pO_2 is decreased by 10–15% due to an increase in physiological dead space. But it has no serious detrimental effect on the body.
- *Impairment of bronchiolar escalator function,* which occurs in old age, causes more serious problem, especially in smokers.

To summarize, the respiratory functions of the elderly show an overall impairment of ventilation, diffusion, ventilation/perfusion mismatch as well as regulation.

III. Gastrointestinal Tract Changes

Age-related changes noted in relation to GIT include:

1. ***Diminution of masticatory efficiency*** occurs due to teeth problems. With advancing age, teeth show *attrition* due to loss of first enamel and then even dentine and cement. In addition, several teeth are lost as a result of caries or periodontal diseases.
2. ***Difficulty in swallowing (dysphagia)*** may occur in extreme old age, because of frequent weakness of pharyngeal musculature and abnormal relaxation of cricopharyngeal muscle. Disordered oesophageal motility, especially at the lower end of oesophagus, may further compound this problem.
3. ***Reduction in gastric secretion*** leading to *achlorhydria* is seen in 25% of the individuals above 60 years of age. It results from age-related mucosal atrophy. Decreased gastric acidity causes decreased Ca^{2+} absorption from empty stomach. Achlorhydria also results in deficiency of iron and vitamin B_{12}.

   The secretion of pancreatic amylase is not affected in old age. Thus, as a whole, digestion and absorption of foodstuffs do not seem to be affected in old age, except for the deficiency of iron and vitamin B_{12}.
4. ***Age-related changes in small intestine*** include reduction in villus height and reduction in lactase activity in the brush border. These changes decrease absorptive capacity in the elderly. However, there is no marked decrease in the digestive or absorptive processes. Therefore, nutritional deficiency in an elderly individual cannot be attributed to malabsorption and actually reflects deficient intake of the nutrients.
5. ***Changes in liver*** include decrease in the number but increase in the size of hepatocytes, and an increase in fibrous tissue. But, because of large reserves the hepatic function is maintained at normal level even after 70 years of age. However, synthetic functions of liver such as protein synthesis, microsomal mixed function and oxidase activity required for hepatic metabolism of drugs and steroids are reduced in old age. Consequently, all the liver function tests show normal results except for a decrease in albumin/globulin ratio. Pigment excretion also remains normal.
6. ***Colon motility*** may be decreased in extreme old age resulting in constipation.

IV. Renal and Genitourinary Changes

1. ***Kidneys*** show progressive reduction in weight. Functional renal changes include:
   - *Decreased GFR* occurs in the elderly because of 30–40% decrease in the number of renal glomeruli by the age of 80 years. It leads to impaired excretion of certain drugs, which may produce toxicity at doses well tolerated in younger individuals.
   - *Decrease in tubular function,* both secretory and absorptive activity, leads to decreased urinary concentration and dilution abilities. This leads to delayed response to salt or fluid restriction/overload. There occurs nocturia. Maximum urinary osmolality is about 750 mOsm/kg (specific gravity 1.0) at the age of 80 years.
   - *Renal function* becomes borderline. Because of the large renal reserves, plasma concentration of creatinine and other nitrogenous waste products is not elevated. However, any type of circulatory stress may precipitate renal failure.
2. ***Prostate enlargement*** in elderly males is a frequent cause of increased residual urine volume. It may take the form of a disease (urinary incontinence or urinary retention).
3. ***Vaginal/urethral mucosal atrophy*** occurring in elderly females leads to dyspareunia and bacteriuria.

V. Changes in Endocrinal System

Endocrinal changes have even been implicated as the underlying mechanism of ageing. Age-related decrease in endocrinal function may occur due to any of the following changes:

- Decrease in plasma concentration of hormone due to decreased production or due to decrease in the concentration of binding proteins involved in the transport of hormone,
- Decreased responsiveness of the target cells,
- Alteration in the number or sensitivity of the hormone receptors or
- Diminished response to physiological stimuli for secretion of the hormone.

Age-related Changes Occurring in the Endocrinal System

1. ***Thyroid hormone*** secretion is definitely decreased. Up to a 50% decrease in the production is noted by the age of 80 years.
2. ***Impaired glucose homeostasis*** is frequently seen in old age. This seems to be due to diminished sensitivity of tissues to insulin, as the plasma levels of insulin are unaffected. It has been observed that, 2 h after the administration of glucose load, plasma glucose is about 30 mg% higher at the age of 70 years than in young adults.
3. ***Reproductive hormones*** show most consistent age-related changes. In females, plasma levels of oestrogen and progesterone are decreased after menopause. In males testosterone levels are decreased around the age of 70 years.
4. ***Anterior pituitary hormones*** secretion is not decreased.
   - FSH and LH levels in females are rather increased due to negative feedback effect exerted by the decreased plasma levels of oestrogen and progesterone.
   - Gonadotropin levels in males are raised because of negative feedback effect of lowered testosterone levels. The raised gonadotropin level induces an increase in testicular Leydig cell volume. But, because of the age-related changes, even the higher Leydig cell volume is not able to achieve the normal testosterone output.
5. ***ADH, renin and aldosterone*** levels are decreased in the old age. Changes in these hormones affect the renal functions, especially urinary concentration and dilution mechanism.
6. ***Vitamin D*** absorption and activation is decreased with age, and contributes to *osteoporosis* occurring in old age.

VI. Changes in Blood and Immune Mechanisms

1. ***Blood volume and blood cells.*** The blood cells (red blood cells, white blood cells and platelets) of elderly individuals are not significantly different from those of young individuals.
2. ***Haemopoietic marrow reserve*** is gradually decreased because of its replacement with fatty marrow as age advances. Long bones are first affected, followed by flat bones and lastly, the vertebrae.
3. ***Anaemia*** in elderly usually occurs due to deficiency of iron and vitamin B_{12}.
4. ***Senile purpura*** occurs due to defect in the capillary endothelium. Platelet count and function of blood coagulation usually remain normal in old age.
5. ***Raised ESR*** (up to 40 mm in first hour), seen in elderly, is related to increased plasma fibrinogen levels.
6. ***Immunological function*** is markedly depressed in old age. Both cell-mediated immunity and humoral immunity decline.
   - *Reduced immune surveillance* by T lymphocytes, at least in part, explains the greater incidence of malignancy in old age.
   - *Involution of thymus* is a well-known age-related change.
   - *T-cell autoreactivity and autoantibody titre* are, however, increased, probably due to diminished tolerance to antigens normally recognized as self.

VII. Changes in Musculoskeletal System

1. ***Muscular power***, characteristically, reduces progressively with ageing due to loss of muscle fibres (decreased lean body mass). The loss of muscle fibres is much greater than the number explained by loss of motor neurons in the CNS. Muscle fibres show deposition of lipofuscin and many other degenerative changes with age.
2. ***Muscle twitch*** reveals a prolongation of latency, contraction period and relaxation period. The maximum tension developed in a muscle in elderly is much less than in young adults.
3. ***Osteoarthritis,*** i.e. age-related degenerative changes in the joints start at the age of 40 years and become well marked by the age of 60–70 years.
4. ***Osteoporosis,*** i.e. age-related decrease in bone density is a characteristic feature of ageing. It is more marked in postmenopausal women than men of the same age group. Osteoporosis predisposes the elderly to fractures.
5. ***Changes in stature and posture*** occur mainly due to changes in the vertebral column, as long bones of the limbs do not show any significant change. Initially, there occurs thinning of the intervertebral disc only; osteoporotic changes cause a decrease in the height of individual vertebra after the age of 50–60 years. As a result of these changes, the height decreases progressively from 50 years onwards, with a prominent change at 70–80 years. Further, kyphosis and slight flexion at the hip and knee make an aged person look still smaller. A decrease of about 5 cm in height is reported to occur from 20 to 80 years of age, which increases to 10 cm by the age of 90 years.

VIII. Changes in Skin and Hair

1. ***Wrinkling of skin*** due to decreased elasticity, increased thinning of epidermis and dermis, and decreased subcutaneous fat is the hallmark of ageing.

2. ***Greying of hair,*** due to loss of melanin pigment, is universal in ageing.
3. ***Baldness*** in males is quite common, though growth of beard is not effected.
4. ***Loss of axillary and pubic hair*** in females occurs due to decreased levels of adrenal androgens.
5. ***Increase in facial hair growth*** may occur in females due to unopposed action of the residual adrenal androgens in the absence of oestrogens.
6. ***Sweat glands*** decrease in size and number; therefore, secretion of sweat as well as sebaceous glands is decreased.

IX. Changes in Central Nervous System

Both structural and functional changes in CNS are quite common with ageing.

1. ***Brain atrophy and neuronal loss*** is the most obvious change. By the age of 70 years, there may be 45% cell loss in cerebral cortex, and 25% loss in cerebellum. Atrophy of frontal lobes leading to shrinkage of gyri and enlargement of sulci is quite common.
2. ***Degenerative changes*** may occur in substantia nigra and lentiform nucleus. Degeneration in spinal cord occurs to a lesser extent than in the brain.
3. ***Other histological changes*** include accumulation of lipofuscin granules in almost all the neurons and glial cells, loss of synapses and gradual loss of dendrites.
4. ***Cerebral blood flow*** is decreased by 40% at the age of 70 years, and oxygen utilization is reduced by 25%.
5. ***Functions of neurotransmitters are impaired.*** Specifically, cholinergic deficit has been demonstrated in *Alzheimer's disease* (see also page 1127) and dopaminergic deficit in Parkinson's disease (see also page 944). Milder forms of cholinergic deficit may be responsible for *senile dementia,* and some degree of dopaminergic deficit may be responsible for *hypokinesia* of old age. Decrease in catecholamine synthesis may be responsible for depression in old age.
6. ***Reflexes*** tend to be sluggish or even absent. The ankle jerk is lost in most of the elderly individuals. Decreased righting reflexes result in increased body sway in old age.
7. ***Sleep changes*** occur in the form of decrease in stage 3 and 4 of non-REM sleep, while the total duration of sleep may not be decreased much. Very old people may not go into stage 4 of sleep at all and have early awakening. Numerous brief arousals occur and account for a feeling of no sleep or insomnia.

X. Changes in Autonomic Nervous System

There is also an age-related impairment of ANS function associated with the increased sensitivity to humoral factors. Common manifestations of decreased ANS function are:

1. ***Impaired temperature regulation*** in elderly individuals occurs because of the fact that exposure to moderate cold or hot environment does not produce expected vasoconstriction and shivering, or vasodilatation and sweating, respectively. Consequently, elderly are more prone to get hypothermia on exposure to cold and hyperthermia on exposure to heat.
2. ***Postural hypotension*** is of frequent occurrence in elderly. It is known to occur because of partial failure of baroreceptor mechanism.

XI. Changes in Special Senses

i. Age-related Ocular Changes

1. ***Presbyopia*** refers to age-related physiological insufficiency of accommodation, leading to failing vision for near or progressive increase in near point. It is as consistent an ageing effect as menopause in females. It usually starts at the age of 40, and by the age of 50, most of the normal individuals need glasses for near work. Decrease in the accommodating power of the crystalline lens with increasing age leads to presbyopia. It occurs due to:
   - Decrease in the elasticity and plasticity of the crystalline lens, and
   - Age-related decrease in the power of ciliary muscles.
2. ***Age-related cataract*** or the senile cataract refers to opacification of the crystalline lens, leading to progressively decreasing vision. Its age of onset and maturation is influenced by the hereditary and environmental factors.
3. ***Age-related corneal degeneration*** manifests as a ring-shaped, whitish opacity near the limbus, which is called *arcus senilis*.
4. ***Age-related macular degeneration (ARMD)*** is a cause of irreversible blindness in many elderly individuals after the age of 70 years.
5. ***Dry eye*** may occur in elderly individuals, more so in postmenopausal females because of age-related decrease in tear secretion.

ii. Age-related Changes in Ears

1. ***Presbyacusia,*** i.e. age-related impairment of hearing, especially for higher frequencies occurring due to degenerative changes in the organ of Corti (hair cells), ganglion cells as well as of temporal cortex, is not uncommon. Other factors contributing to prebyacusia are loss of elasticity of the tympanic membrane and basilar membrane, loss of neurons in the cochlea and atrophy of stria vascularis. The impaired sensitivity often leads to difficulty in understanding speech and the disturbances of localization of sounds.
2. ***Otosclerosis,*** characterized by age-related decrease in motility of middle ear ossicles, is another cause of deafness in old age.
3. ***Impairment of postural reflexes*** may occur due to age-related degenerative changes in hair cells of the crista ampullaris, and decreased endolymph production because of atrophy of the stria vascularis.

iii. Age-related Changes in Taste and Smell

1. ***Impairment in taste sensation*** in elderly is attributed to decrease in the number of tastebuds, from an average of 250 buds per papilla in childhood to about 90 buds per papilla by the age of 80 years.
2. ***Impairment in sensation of smell*** in the elderly is attributed to the decrease in smell receptors and partly to the loss of neurons in cerebral cortical centres.

THEORIES OF AGEING

Many theories have been put forward to explain the process of ageing, but none is able to explain all the queries. Most of the theories fall in one of the two main groups:

- Genetic theories of ageing, and
- Random damage theories.

I. Genetic Theories of Ageing These theories consider ageing to be the inevitable result of the genetic programme. The enthusiasm for genetic theories is fuelled by the following observations:

- The dramatic species-specific differences in maximal life span. For example, every dog grows old in about 10 years, while a human being takes about 60 years to reach the same level of senescence. Obviously, the difference lies in the genetic programme of two species.
- The strong correlation with the survival among the monozygotic compared with the dizygotic twins,
- Ageing cannot be prevented altogether, suggesting thereby that the gradual impairment of function is genetically programmed and
- The fact that a single mutation can prolong life span by more than 50% in some nematodes and mice is a very strong pointer to the role of genetics in ageing.

However, all genetic theories must account for the fact that evolutionary selection pressure is minimal following completion of reproduction.

Of the many genetic theories, some important are:

1. Programmed Senescence Theory. Programmed senescence theory of ageing holds that ageing follows a biological timetable, perhaps a continuation of one that regulates childhood growth and development. According to *programmed senescence theory,* ageing is the result of the segmental switching on and off of certain genes, with senescence being defined as the time when age-associated deficits are manifested.

2. Mutation Theory. This theory suggests that, since animals usually succumb to natural forces long before reaching their maximal life span, ageing might reflect mutations that impair long-term survival. These mutations would accumulate in the genome because there is no selection pressure to delete them.

3. Theory of Pleiotropic Antagonism. This theory proposes that ageing may be caused by the late and deleterious effects of the genes that are conserved because of the survival advantages they confer prior to reproduction.

4. Theory of Ecological Niches. This theory applies to ecological niches, where extrinsic hazards are relatively low. In such an environment, evolution might select the mutations that retard the ageing process, since these might allow an animal to produce and protect many more litters. In support of this theory, the rate of ageing in an isolated class of *Virginia opossums* was calculated to be roughly half of that seen in their less-fortunate cousins.

Many genetic theories previously postulated to mediate ageing which have not been borne out include:

- ***Isomatic mutation theory***. This theory postulated that ageing would result from cumulative spontaneous mutations.
- ***The error catastrophe theory***. This theory postulated that ageing would result from errors in the synthesis of proteins critical to the synthesis of genetic material or protein-synthesizing machinery.
- ***Intrinsic mutagenesis theory***. According to this theory, ageing is the result of ongoing intrinsic DNA rearrangements.

II. The 'Random Damage' Theories of Ageing All the 'random damage' theories are based on the possibility that the balance between ongoing damage and repair is disrupted. These theories differ in the emphasis placed on the increased damage (e.g. by free radicals, oxidation or glycation) versus deficient repair, as well as in the mechanisms that might mediate each. However, all share the observation that cell and organ repair capacity declines with age.

The 'random damage' theories include:

1. Free Radical Theory. Oxidation reactions in the cells are associated with the formation of free radicals, such as superoxide and hydroxyl radicals. For free radical scavenging, *antioxidant mechanisms* exist in the body in the form of glutathione, vitamin E, vitamin A and vitamin C. When these antioxidant mechanisms are overwhelmed, there occurs damage by the free radicals. The free radicals can possibly damage vital macromolecules such as DNA and proteins, and cause peroxidation of lipids in the membranes around cells and organelles. Although free radical theory is very popular, and antioxidants are being prescribed over enthusiastically by the physicians, neither has lipid peroxidation been demonstrated at the cellular level, nor has the beneficial effect of antioxidants been proven.

2. Cell Replication Theory. Depending upon the replicating capabilities, the cells in the body can be divided into three categories:

- *Cells which continuously replicate* include blood cells, epidermis cells and gastrointestinal cells.
- *Cells which replicate only under stress* (e.g. injury) include endothelial cells, hepatocytes and fibroblasts and
- *Cells which do not replicate at all* include neurons, myocardial and skeletal muscle cells,

It has been stated that replicating cells have a definite replicating limit. The cell replication theory suggests that ageing may represent a stage of life when replication of cell ceases, i.e. when repair is not capable to cope up with the damage.

Subsequent researches revealed that this replicative senescence was due to arrest of the cell cycles at the G_1/S phase, the point at which DNA synthesis begins. Recently, cell replication has also been linked to the length of *telomeric DNA*. With each cell division, roughly 50 of the total 2000 base pairs of the telomere are lost. Telomeric shortening might thus result in loss of gene accessibility, which is caused by metabolism. Together with cytoplasmic factors mediating arrest of DNA synthesis, telomeric shortening could also limit the cell's ability to divide and thereby replace cells loss to apoptosis.

3. Cross-linking Theory. This theory highlights that an accumulation of cross-linked proteins damages cells and tissues, slowing down bodily processes and results in ageing. In a process called *nonenzymatic glycosylation or glycation*, glucose molecules attach themselves to proteins, setting in motion a chain of chemical reactions that ends in the proteins binding together or cross-linking, thus altering their biological and structural roles. The process is slow but increases with time.

Cross-links, which have been termed as *advanced glycosylation end products* (AGEs), seem to toughen tissues and may cause some of the deterioration associated with ageing. AGEs have been linked to stiffening of the connective tissue (collagen), hardened arteries, clouded eyes, loss of nerve function and less efficient kidneys. These are deficiencies that often accompany ageing. They also appear at younger ages in people with diabetes, who have high glucose levels. Diabetes, in fact, is sometimes considered an accelerated model of ageing. Not only do its complications mimic the physiologic changes that can accompany old age, but also expectances. As a result, much research on cross-linking has focussed on its relationship to diabetes, as well as ageing.

MODULATING THE PROCESS OF AGEING

The quest for staying youthful and preventing ageing has led to many trials on modulating the process of ageing. However, ageing has proved to be an almost inevitable process. The only measures that have shown some progress in this regard are: caloric restriction and exercise.

Caloric Restriction. To date, the only intervention known to delay ageing and prolong the life span is caloric restriction, which has been proved in experimental animals. Although the underlying mechanism is still not determined, it is specific to caloric restriction rather than to the reduction of any dietary compound (e.g. fat intake) or supplementation with vitamins or antioxidants. Further, the effects of caloric restriction in humans are still unknown.

Exercise. There is still no conclusive evidence to document that exercise prevents ageing or not. However, definitely, exercise improves work capacity as assessed from maximum oxygen uptake. Physical exercise also improves cardiac performance and reduces musculoskeletal disability. Physical exercise is also reported to prevent age-related decline in resting metabolic rate.

Index

D

E

H

I

O

P

T

U

V

W

X

Y

Z